Textbook of
Family Medicine

Textbook of Family Medicine

NINTH EDITION

Robert E. Rakel, MD

Professor
Department of Family and Community Medicine
Baylor College of Medicine
Houston, Texas

David P. Rakel, MD

Associate Professor
Department of Family Medicine
University of Wisconsin School of Medicine and Public Health
Madison, Wisconsin

ELSEVIER
SAUNDERS

1600 John F. Kennedy Blvd.
Ste 1800
Philadelphia, PA 19103-2899

TEXTBOOK OF FAMILY MEDICINE, NINTH EDITION ISBN: 978-0-323-23990-5

Notices

Knowledge and best practice in this field are constantly changing. As new research and experience broaden our understanding, changes in research methods, professional practices, or medical treatment may become necessary.

Practitioners and researchers must always rely on their own experience and knowledge in evaluating and using any information, methods, compounds, or experiments described herein. In using such information or methods they should be mindful of their own safety and the safety of others, including parties for whom they have a professional responsibility.

With respect to any drug or pharmaceutical products identified, readers are advised to check the most current information provided (i) on procedures featured or (ii) by the manufacturer of each product to be administered, to verify the recommended dose or formula, the method and duration of administration, and contraindications. It is the responsibility of practitioners, relying on their own experience and knowledge of their patients, to make diagnoses, to determine dosages and the best treatment for each individual patient, and to take all appropriate safety precautions.

To the fullest extent of the law, neither the Publisher nor the authors, contributors, or editors, assume any liability for any injury and/or damage to persons or property as a matter of products liability, negligence or otherwise, or from any use or operation of any methods, products, instructions, or ideas contained in the material herein.

Library of Congress Cataloging-in-Publication Data
Textbook of family practice.
Textbook of family medicine / [edited by] Robert E. Rakel, David P. Rakel.—Ninth edition.
      p. ; cm.
Includes bibliographical references and index.
ISBN 978-0-323-23990-5 (hardcover : alk. paper)
I. Rakel, Robert E., editor.   II. Rakel, David, editor.   III. Title.
[DNLM: 1. Family Practice.   2. Evidence-Based Medicine.   3. Patient Education as Topic. WB 110]
RC46
610–dc23
                                                                                2014043849

Senior Content Strategist: Suzanne Toppy
Content Development Manager: Marybeth Thiel
Publishing Services Manager: Patricia Tannian
Project Manager: Kate Mannix
Design Direction: Julia Dummit

Printed in Canada

Last digit is the print number: 9   8   7   6   5   4   3   2   1

Although he is the founder and main editor of this text, I would like to dedicate my contribution as co-editor to my father, mentor, and friend, Robert Rakel. He started this text in 1971 when he perceived a need to give the generalist guidance on how to specialize in the whole person and family. Now in its 9th edition, his legacy continues within these pages and within more than 50 other texts he has authored and edited. The science has evolved, but the mission remains, which is to facilitate health with the patients and communities we are privileged to serve. I am grateful to have had the opportunity to learn from his artistry as a clinician, teacher, and father. We are truly lucky souls to be able to do this work together.

David P. Rakel

Contributors

Syed M. Ahmed, MD, MPH, DrPH
Senior Associate Dean for Community Engagement, Professor, Family & Community Medicine, Medical College of Wisconsin, Milwaukee, Wisconsin
Psychosocial Influences on Health

Erin Allen, MD
Assistant Professor, Department of Pediatrics, Baylor College of Medicine, Houston, Texas
Care of the Newborn

Heather Bartsch, MD
Assistant Professor, Family and Community Medicine, Baylor College of Medicine, Houston, Texas
Care of the Newborn

J. Mark Beard, MD
Associate Professor and Residency Program Director, Department of Family Medicine, University of Washington, Seattle, Washington
Common Office Procedures

Wendy S. Biggs, MD
Residency Program Director, Department of Family Medicine, University of Kansas, Kansas City, Kansas
Human Sexuality

Christopher F. Blanner, MD
Family Physician, Mercy Clinic Family Medicine, O'Fallon, Missouri
Contraception

Elizabeth Boham, MD, RD
Physician, The UltraWellness Center, Lenox, Massachusetts; Faculty, Institute of Functional Medicine, Federal Way, Washington
Obesity

Robert D. Brook, MD
Professor of Medicine, Division of Cardiovascular Medicine, University of Michigan, Ann Arbor, Michigan
Cardiovascular Disease

Charles S. Bryan, MD
Heyward Gibbes Distinguished Professor of Internal Medicine Emeritus, The University of South Carolina, Columbia, South Carolina
Infectious Diseases

J. Brian Byrd, MD
Clinical Lecturer of Internal Medicine, Division of Cardiovascular Medicine, University of Michigan, Ann Arbor, Michigan
Cardiovascular Disease

Kara Cadwallader, MD
Associate Clinical Professor of Family Medicine, Department of Family Medicine, Family Medicine Residency of Idaho, Boise, Idaho; Senior Medical Director, Family Planning, Planned Parenthood of the Great Northwest, Seattle, Washington
Gynecology

Doug Campos-Outcalt, MD, MPA
Chair, Department of Family, Community, and Preventive Medicine, University of Arizona College of Medicine, Phoenix, Arizona
Preventive Health Care

William E. Carroll, MD
Medical Director, Grant Medical Center Neurology and OhioHealth Stroke Network, Adjunct Assistant Professor of Neurology, Wexner Medical Center, The Ohio State University, Columbus, Ohio
Neurology

Chuck Carter, MD
Residency Director, Palmetto Health Family Medicine Residency; Associate Professor, Family and Preventive Medicine, University of South Carolina School of Medicine, Columbia, South Carolina
Urinary Tract Infections

Sulabha Chaganaboyana, MBBS
Family Medicine Resident, University of Kansas Medical Center, Kansas City, Kansas
Human Sexuality

Frederick Chen, MD, MPH
Chief of Family Medicine, Harborview Medical Center; Associate Professor, Department of Family Medicine, University of Washington, Seattle, Washington
Clinical Genomics

Carol L. Chervenak, MD
Medical Director, ABC House; Child Abuse Intervention Center serving Benton and Linn Counties, Albany, Oregon
Child Abuse

Isabelle Chughtai-Harvey, MD
Clinical Assistant Professor, Weill Cornell Medical College;
Family Medicine Residency Program, Department of
Family Medicine, Houston Methodist Hospital, Houston,
Texas
Hematology

Emily Collins, MD
Staff Psychiatrist, Atlanta VA Medical Center, Atlanta,
Georgia
Crisis Intervention, Trauma, and Disasters

Douglas Comeau, DO
Medical Director, Sports Medicine, Ryan Center for Sports
Medicine at Boston University, Boston Medical Center,
Boston, Massachusetts
Rheumatology and Musculoskeletal Problems

Joseph Connelly, MD
Residency Director, Department of Family Medicine,
Stamford Hospital/Columbia University, Stamford,
Connecticut
*Patients with Personality Disorders; Difficult
Encounters*

Deanna Corey, MD
Primary Care Sports Medicine, Department of Family
Medicine, Boston University School of Medicine, Boston
Medical Center, East Boston Neighborhood Health
Center, Boston, Massachusetts
Rheumatology and Musculoskeletal Problems

Earl R. Crouch, Jr., MD
Associate Professor of Pediatrics, Department of
Ophthalmology, Eastern Virginia Medical School,
Norfolk, Virginia
Ophthalmology

Eric R. Crouch, MD
Associate Professor of Ophthalmology, Assistant Professor
of Pediatrics, Eastern Virginia Medical School, Norfolk,
Virginia
Ophthalmology

Ruth DeBusk, PhD, RD
Clinical Dietitian and Geneticist, Family Medicine
Residency Program, Tallahassee Memorial HealthCare,
Tallahassee, Florida; Faculty, Institute for Functional
Medicine, Federal Way, Washington
Obesity

Philip M. Diller, MD, PhD
Fred Lazarus Jr Professor and Chair, Department of Family
and Community Medicine, University of Cincinnati
College of Medicine, Cincinnati, Ohio
Clinical Problem Solving

Rina Eisenstein, MD
Assistant Professor of Medicine, Division of General
Medicine and Geriatrics, Emory University School of
Medicine, Atlanta Veterans Affairs Medical Center,
Bronze Geriatric Clinic, Atlanta, Georgia
Delirium and Dementia

Robert Ellis, MD
Associate Professor, University of Cincinnati, Department
of Family and Community Medicine, Cincinnati, Ohio
Clinical Problem Solving

Karen Farst, MD, MPH
Associate Professor, Pediatrics, University of Arkansas for
Medical Sciences, Little Rock, Arkansas
Child Abuse

W. Gregory Feero, MD, PhD
Residency, Maine Dartmouth Family Medicine Residency,
Augusta, Maine
Clinical Genomics

Robert E. Feinstein, MD
Professor of Psychiatry, Vice Chairman for Clinical
Education Quality & Safety, Department of Psychiatry,
Colorado School of Medicine, Aurora, Colorado
*Crisis Intervention, Trauma and Disasters; Patients
with Personality Disorders; Difficult Encounters*

Blair Foreman, MD
Cardiovascular Medicine, P.C., Genesis Heart Institute,
Davenport, Iowa
Cardiovascular Disease

Luke W. Fortney, MD
Family Medicine, Meriter Medical Group, Madison,
Wisconsin
Care of the Self

Thomas R. Grant, Jr., MD
Professor, Clinical Community and Family Medicine,
Eastern Virginia Medical School, Norfolk, Virginia
Ophthalmology

Mary P. Guerrera, MD
Professor of Family Medicine & Director of Integrative
Medicine, Department of Family Medicine, University
of Connecticut School of Medicine, Farmington,
Connecticut
Integrative Medicine

Steven Hale, MD
Senior Physician, Orange County Health Department,
Florida Department of Health-Orange, Orlando, Florida
Alcohol Use Disorders

Kimberly G. Harmon, MD
Professor, Departments of Family Medicine and
Orthopaedics and Sports Medicine, Team Physician,
University of Washington, Seattle, Washington
Sports Medicine

Diane M. Harper, MD
Rowntree Professor and Chair of Family and Geriatric
  Medicine, Department of Obstetrics and Gynecology,
  School of Medicine, Department of Bioengineering,
  Speed School of Engineering, Departments of
  Epidemiology and Population Health and Health
  Promotion and Behavioral Health, School of Public
  Health and Information Sciences, University of
  Louisville, Louisville, Kentucky
Contraception

Joel J. Heidelbaugh, MD
Clinical Professor, Departments of Family Medicine and
  Urology, University of Michigan Medical School,
  Ann Arbor, Michigan
Gastroenterology

Vivian Hernandez-Trujillo, MD
Director, Division of Allergy and Immunology, Miami
  Children's Hospital, Miami, Florida
Allergy

Arthur H. Herold, MD
Associate Professor of Family Medicine, Department of
  Family Medicine, College of Medicine, University of
  South Florida, Tampa, Florida
Interpreting Laboratory Tests

Paul J. Hershberger, PhD
Professor, Department of Family Medicine, Wright State
  University Boonshoft School of Medicine, Dayton, Ohio
Psychosocial Influences on Health

N. Wilson Holland, MD
Associate Professor of Medicine, Division of General
  Medicine and Geriatrics, Emory University School of
  Medicine, Acting Designated Education Officer, Atlanta
  Veterans Affairs Medical Center, Atlanta, Georgia
Delirium and Dementia

Thomas Houston, MD
McConnell Heart Health Center, Columbus, Ohio
Nicotine

Mark R. Hutchinson MD
Professor of Orthopaedics and Sports Medicine, Adjunct
  Professor of Orthopaedics and Sports Medicine in
  Family Medicine, Head Team Physician, University
  of Illinois at Chicago, Chicago, Illinois
Common Issues in Orthopedics

Wayne Boice Jonas, MD
President & CEO, Samueli Institute, Alexandria, Virginia
The Patient-Centered Medical Home

Scott Kelley, MD
Clinical Lecturer, Department of Family Medicine,
  University of Michigan, Ann Arbor, Michigan
Gastroenterology

Sanford R. Kimmel, MD
Professor and Vice Chair, Family Medicine, University of
  Toledo College of Medicine and Life Sciences, Toledo,
  Ohio
Growth and Development

Alicia Kowalchuk, DO
Assistant Professor, Department of Family and
  Community Medicine, Baylor College of Medicine;
  Medical Director, InSight Program, Harris Health
  System; Medical Director, CARE Clinic, Santa Maria
  Hostel; Medical Director, Sobering Center, Houston
  Recovery Center, Houston, Texas
Substance Use Disorders

Jennifer Krejci-Manwaring MD
Assistant Professor, Department of Dermatology,
  University of Texas Health Science Center; Chief of
  Teledermatology, Audie Murphy Veteran's Hospital;
  Medical Director, Limmer Hair Transplant Center,
  San Antonio, Texas
Dermatology

David Kunstman, MD
Assistant Clinical Professor, Family Medicine, University
  of Wisconsin School of Medicine and Public Health;
  Associate Medical Director, Information Services,
  University of Wisconsin Health, Madison, Wisconsin
Information Technology

Jeanne Parr Lemkau, PhD
Professor Emerita, Departments of Family Medicine and
  Community Health, Wright State University, Dayton,
  North Carolina
Psychosocial Influences on Health

Russell Lemmon, DO
Assistant Professor, Department of Family Medicine,
  University of Wisconsin, School of Medicine and Public
  Health, Madison, Wisconsin
Neck and Back Pain

Jim Leonard, DO
Associate Professor, Department of Orthopedics and
  Rehabilitation, University of Wisconsin School of
  Medicine and Public Health, Madison, Wisconsin
Neck and Back Pain

David R. Marques, MD
Associate Director with OB, Department of Family
  Medicine, Grant Medical Center; Clinical Assistant
  Professor, Department of Family Medicine, The Ohio
  State University College of Medicine, Columbus, Ohio;
  Clinical Assistant Professor, Department of Family
  Medicine, Ohio University Heritage College of
  Osteopathic Medicine, Athens, Ohio
Neurology

James L. Moeller, MD
Sports Medicine Associates, PLC, Bloomfield Hills, Michigan; Associate Professor, Family Medicine and Community Health, Oakland University William Beaumont School of Medicine, Rochester, Michigan
Common Issues in Orthopedics

Scott E. Moser, MD
Professor, Department of Family and Community Medicine, University of Kansas School of Medicine–Wichita, Wichita, Kansas
Behavioral Problems in Children and Adolescents

Ethan A. Natelson, MD
Professor of Clinical Medicine, Weill-Cornell Medical College; Department of Medicine, Division of Hematology, Houston Methodist Hospital, Houston, Texas
Hematology

Kelli L. Netson, PhD
Assistant Professor & Pediatric Neuropsychologist, Rockhill Clinic Director, Department of Psychiatry & Behavioral Sciences, University of Kansas School of Medicine–Wichita, Wichita, Kansas
Behavioral Problems in Children and Adolescents

Mary Barth Noel, MPH, PhD
Professor, Department of Family Medicine, College of Human Medicine, Michigan State University, East Lansing, Michigan
Nutrition

John G. O'Handley, MD
Clinical Associate Professor, Department of Family Medicine, The Ohio State College of Medicine, Columbus, Ohio
Otorhinolaryngology

John W. O'Kane Jr., MD
Associate Professor, Departments of Family Medicine and Orthopedics and Sports Medicine, Head Team Physician, University of Washington, Seattle, Washington
Sports Medicine

Justin Osborn, MD
Assistant Professor, Department of Family Medicine, University of Washington, Seattle, Washington
Common Office Procedures

Heather L. Paladine, MD
Assistant Professor of Medicine at Columbia University Medical Center, Center for Family and Community Medicine, Columbia College of Physicians and Surgeons, New York, New York
Gynecology

Birju B. Patel, MD
VISN 7 Co-Consultant for Outpatient Geriatrics; Director, Bronze Geriatric Primary Care Clinic; Director, Mild Cognitive Impairment (MCI) Clinic; Chair, Atlanta VA Dementia Committee, Atlanta Veterans Affairs Medical Center; Assistant Professor of Medicine, Division of General Medicine and Geriatrics, Emory University School of Medicine, Atlanta, Georgia
Delirium and Dementia

Gabriella Pridjian, MD, MBA
Professor and Chairman, The C. Jeff Miller Chair in Obstetrics & Gynecology, Department of Obstetrics & Gynecology, Tulane University School of Medicine, New Orleans, Louisiana
Obstetrics

Sana Rabbi, MD
Family Medicine Resident, Department of Family Medicine, Houston Methodist Hospital, Houston, Texas
Hematology

David P. Rakel, MD
Associate Professor, Department of Family Medicine, University of Wisconsin School of Medicine and Public Health, Madison, Wisconsin

Robert E. Rakel, MD
Professor, Department of Family Medicine and Community Medicine, Baylor College of Medicine, Houston, Texas

Karen Ratliff-Schaub, MD
Associate Clinical Professor, Department of Pediatrics, The Ohio State University; Medical Director, Child Development Center, Developmental-Behavioral Pediatrics, Nationwide Children's Hospital, Columbus, Ohio
Growth and Development

Brian Christopher Reed, MD
Associate Professor, Department of Family & Community Medicine, Baylor College of Medicine, Houston, Texas
Substance Use Disorders

Elly Riley, DO
Assistant Professor, Department of Family Medicine, University of Tennessee Health Science Center, Jackson, Tennessee
Allergy

Brian Rothberg, MD
Associate Professor, Department of Psychiatry, University of Colorado School of Medicine, Aurora, Colorado
Anxiety and Depression

Justin Rothmier, MD
Physician, The Sports Medicine Clinic; Clinical Assistant Professor, Department of Family Medicine, University of Washington, Seattle, Washington
Sports Medicine

Chad Rudnick, MD
Physician, Miami Children's Hospital, Miami, Florida
Allergy

J. Chris Rule, MSW, LCSW
Instructor, Departments of Psychiatry and Family and
  Preventive Medicine, University of Arkansas for Medical
  Sciences, Little Rock, Arizona
Behavioral Change and Patient Empowerment

George Rust, MD, MPH
Professor, Department of Family Medicine, Morehouse
  School of Medicine; Co-Director, National Center for
  Primary Care, Morehouse School of Medicine, Atlanta,
  Georgia
Pulmonary Medicine

Christopher D. Schneck, MD
Associate Professor of Psychiatry, Department of
  Psychiatry, University of Colorado School of Medicine,
  Aurora, Colorado
Anxiety and Depression

Sarina B. Schrager, MD
Professor, Department of Family Medicine, University
  of Wisconsin, Madison, Wisconsin
Gynecology

Stacy Seikel, MD
Chief Medical Officer, Advanced Recovery Systems,
  Umatilla, Florida
Alcohol Use Disorders

Ashish R. Shah, MD
Otolaryngologist, OhioENT, Columbus, Ohio
Otorhinolaryngology

Nicolas W. Shammas, MD, MSc
Cardiovascular Medicine, P.C., Midwest Cardiovascular
  Research Foundation, Davenport, Iowa; Associate
  Professor of Clinical Medicine, University of Iowa
  School of Medicine, Iowa City, Iowa
Cardiovascular Disease

Robert Shapiro, MD
Professor, Department of Pediatrics, Cincinnati Children's
  Hospital Medical Center, Cincinnati, Ohio
Child Abuse

Mae Sheikh-Ali, MD
Associate Professor of Medicine, Associate Program
  Director, Endocrinology Fellowship Program, Division
  of Endocrinology, Diabetes, and Metabolism, University
  of Florida College of Medicine, Jacksonville, Florida
Endocrinology

Kevin Sherin, MD, MPH, MBA
Clinical Professor, Department of Family Medicine, Florida
  State University College of Medicine; Health Officer and
  Director, Florida Department of Health in Orange
  County, Florida Department of Health; Clinical
  Associate Professor, Department of Family Medicine,
  University of Central Florida College of Medicine,
  Orlando, Florida
Alcohol Use Disorders

Jeffrey A. Silverstein, MD
Orthopedic Surgeon, Sarasota Orthopedic Associates,
  Sarasota, Florida
Common Issues in Orthopedics

Charles W. Smith, MD
Executive Associate Dean for Clinical Affairs, Professor,
  Department of Family and Community Medicine,
  University of Arkansas for Medical Sciences, Little Rock,
  Arkansas
Behavioral Change and Patient Empowerment

Douglas R. Smucker, MD, MPH
Adjunct Professor, Department of Family and Community
  Medicine, University of Cincinnati; Program Director,
  Hospice and Palliative Medicine Fellowship Program,
  The Christ Hospital, Cincinnati, Ohio
*Interpreting the Medical Literature: Applying
  Evidence-Based Medicine in Practice*

Melissa Stiles, MD
Professor, Department of Family Medicine, University
  of Wisconsin, Madison, Wisconsin
Care of the Elderly Patient

P. Michael Stone, MD, MS Nutrition
Physician, Stone Medical, Ashland, Oregon; Faculty,
  Institute of Functional Medicine, Federal Way,
  Washington
Obesity

Margaret Thompson, MD
Associate Professor, Department of Family Medicine,
  Michigan State University College of Human Medicine,
  Grand Rapids, Michigan
Nutrition

Evan J. Tobin, MD
Clinical Assistant Professor, Otolaryngology–Head and
  Neck Surgery, The Ohio State University, Columbus,
  Ohio
Otorhinolaryngology

Peter P. Toth, MD, PhD
CGH Medical Center, Sterling, Illinois; Professor of Clinical
    Family and Community Medicine, University of Illinois
    School of Medicine, Peoria, Illinois; Professor of Clinical
    Medicine, Michigan State University College of
    Osteopathic Medicine, East Lansing, Michigan; Adjunct
    Associate Professor of Medicine (Cardiology), Johns
    Hopkins University School of Medicine, Baltimore,
    Maryland
    Cardiovascular Disease

Thuy Hanh Trinh, MD, MBA
Associate Medical Director, Houston Hospice; Adjust
    Assistant Professor, Family Medicine Department,
    Baylor College of Medicine, Houston, Texas
    Care of the Dying Patient

Jeff Unger, MD
President, Unger Primary Care, Rancho Cucamonga,
    California; Director of Metabolic Studies, Catalina
    Research Institute, Chino, California
    Diabetes Mellitus

Richard P. Usatine, MD
Professor of Family and Community Medicine, Professor
    of Dermatology and Cutaneous Surgery, University of
    Texas Health Science Center San Antonio; Medical
    Director, Skin Clinic, University Health System, San
    Antonio, Texas
    Dermatology

Kathleen Walsh, DO
Assistant Professor, Department of Medicine, University
    of Wisconsin School of Medicine and Public Health,
    Madison, Wisconsin
    Care of the Elderly Patient

Elizabeth A. Warner, MD
Associate Professor, Department of Internal Medicine,
    University of South Florida, Tampa, Florida
    Interpreting Laboratory Tests

Sherin E. Wesley, MD
Assistant Professor, Pediatrics, Family and Community
    Medicine, Baylor College of Medicine, Houston, Texas
    Care of the Newborn

Gloria E. Westney, MD
Associate Professor of Clinical Medicine, Department
    of Medicine, Pulmonary and Critical Care Medicine
    Section, Morehouse School of Medicine, Atlanta,
    Georgia
    Pulmonary Medicine

Russell White, MD
Clinical Professor of Medicine, Department of Community
    and Family Medicine, University of Medicine-Kansas
    City School of Medicine; Diplomate, American Board
    of Family Medicine; Fellow of the American College
    of Sports Medicine, Kansas City, Missouri
    Diabetes Mellitus

Lauren E. Wilfling, DO, MBA
Family Medicine Faculty Physician, Mercy Family
    Medicine Residency Program, Mercy Hospital, St. Louis,
    Missouri
    Contraception

Dave Elton Williams, MD
Daughters of Charity, New Orleans, Louisiana
    Obstetrics

George A. Wilson, MD
Senior Associate Dean for Clinical Affairs, Department of
    Community Health/Family Medicine, University of
    Florida College of Medicine, Jacksonville, Florida
    Endocrinology

Philip Zazove, MD
Professor and George A. Dean, MD, Chair, Department of
    Family Medicine, University of Michigan, Ann Arbor,
    Michigan
    Clinical Genomics

Contents

Video Contents

The first edition of *Textbook of Family Medicine* was published in 1973, just after the specialty of family practice, now family medicine, was approved by the American Board of Medical Specialties.

Although the practice of medicine has changed considerably since that first edition, the content of the specialty remains essentially the same. Our goal is to provide in one text the information essential to our discipline. While some family physicians, especially those in urban areas, no longer deliver babies, the breadth of knowledge required to practice comprehensive primary care remains unchanged. Because of the great deficit of primary care physicians in the United States, those trained in other specialties are often called upon to provide primary care. They may benefit significantly from the breadth of material presented here.

The entire content of this edition is available electronically and can be accessed by iPad, iPhone, PC, and Mac. In order to limit the size (and weight) of the book, some material (such as references) is available only online. Also available online are 38 videos from Elsevier's Procedures Consult. Videos range from how to repair a wound with tissue glue to performing a vasectomy. See the *Video Contents* for the full list.

This text is designed to be a resource for family physicians to help them remain current with advances in medicine.

It is especially valuable to those preparing for certification or recertification by the American Board of Family Medicine.

Following the policy we established in the first edition, most of the authors of this text are family physicians. The clinical chapters combine a family physician with an authority in the field to ensure that the material is current and relevant to the needs of the family physician.

This edition continues an evidence-based approach, giving the Strength of Recommendation (SOR) taxonomy in the Key Treatment boxes, focusing on Grade A recommendations. More than 1000 tables and color illustrations facilitate the rapid retrieval of essential information and are used to present in-depth data conveniently.

Although this text focuses on problems most frequently encountered in the primary care setting, significant attention is also given to potentially serious problems that would be dangerous if missed. Diagnosing a problem in its early, undifferentiated stage is much more difficult than after symptoms have progressed to the point that the diagnosis is evident.

Our thanks to the staff at Elsevier for their high publishing standards and insistence on quality.

Robert E. Rakel
David P. Rakel

PRINCIPLES OF FAMILY MEDICINE

1 *Family Physician*

ROBERT E. RAKEL

Key Points

- The rewards in family medicine come from knowing patients intimately over time and from sharing their trust, respect, and friendship, as well as from the variety of problems encountered in practice that keep the family physician professionally stimulated and challenged.
- The American Board of Family Practice was established in 1969 and changed its name to the American Board of Family Medicine in 2004. It was the first specialty board to require recertification every 7 years to ensure ongoing competence of its diplomates.
- The American Academy of Family Physicians (AAFP) began as the American Academy of General Practice in 1947 and was renamed in 1971.
- Primary care is the provision of continuing, comprehensive care to a population undifferentiated by age, gender, disease, or organ system.

- The most challenging diagnoses are those for diseases or disorders in their early, undifferentiated stage, when there are often only subtle differences between serious disease and minor ailments.
- The family physician is the conductor, orchestrating the skills of a variety of health professionals who may be involved in the care of a seriously ill patient.
- The most cost-effective health care systems depend on a strong primary care base. The United States has the most expensive health care system in the world but ranks among the worst in overall quality of care because of its weak primary care base.
- The greater the number of primary care physicians in a country, the lower the mortality rate and the lower the cost.

The family physician provides continuing, comprehensive care in a personalized manner to patients of all ages, regardless of the presence of disease or the nature of the presenting complaint. Family physicians accept responsibility for managing an individual's total health needs while maintaining an intimate, confidential relationship with the patient.

Family medicine emphasizes continuing responsibility for total health care—from the first contact and initial assessment through the ongoing care of chronic problems. Prevention and early recognition of disease are essential features of the discipline. Coordination and integration of all necessary health services (minimizing fragmentation) and the skills to manage most medical problems allow family physicians to provide cost-effective health care.

Family medicine is a specialty that shares many areas of content with other clinical disciplines, incorporating this shared knowledge and using it uniquely to deliver primary medical care. In addition to sharing content with other medical specialties, family medicine's foundation remains

clinical, with the primary focus on the medical care of people who are ill.

The curriculum for training family physicians is designed to represent realistically the skills and body of knowledge that the physicians will require in practice. This curriculum is based on an analysis of the problems seen and the skills used by family physicians in their practice. The randomly educated primary physician has been replaced by one specifically prepared to address the types of problems likely to be encountered in practice. For this reason, the "model office" is an essential component of all family medicine residency programs.

The Joy of Family Practice

If you cannot work with love but only with distaste, it is better that you should leave your work and sit at the

3

gate of the temple and take alms from those who work with joy.

KAHLIL GIBRAN (1883-1931)

The rewards in family medicine come largely from knowing patients intimately over time and from sharing their trust, respect, and friendship. The thrill is the close bond (friendship) that develops with patients. This bond is strengthened with each physical or emotional crisis in a person's life, when he or she turns to the family physician for help. It is a pleasure going to the office every day and a privilege to work closely with people who value and respect our efforts.

The practice of family medicine involves the joy of greeting old friends in every examining room, and the variety of problems encountered keeps the physician professionally stimulated and perpetually challenged. In contrast, physicians practicing in narrow specialties often lose their enthusiasm for medicine after seeing the same problems every day. The variety in family medicine sustains the excitement and precludes boredom. Our greatest days in practice are when we are fully focused on our patients, enjoying to the fullest the experience of working with others.

PATIENT SATISFACTION

Attributes considered most important for patient satisfaction are listed in Table 1-1 (Stock Keister et al., 2004a). Overall, people want their primary care doctor to meet five basic criteria: "to be in their insurance plan, to be in a location that is convenient, to be able to schedule an appointment within a reasonable period of time, to have good communication skills, and to have a reasonable amount of experience in practice." They especially want "a physician who listens to them, who takes the time to explain things to them, and who is able to effectively integrate their care" (Stock Keister et al., 2004b, p. 2312).

PHYSICIAN SATISFACTION

Physician satisfaction is associated with quality of care, particularly as measured by patient satisfaction. The strongest factors associated with physician satisfaction are not personal income but rather the ability to provide high-quality care to patients. Physicians are most satisfied with their practices when they can have an ongoing relationship with their patients, the freedom to make clinical decisions without financial conflicts of interest, adequate time with patients, and sufficient communication with specialists (DeVoe et al., 2002). Landon and colleagues (2003) found that rather than declining income, the strongest predictor of decreasing satisfaction in practice is loss of clinical autonomy. This includes the inability to obtain services for their patients, the inability to control their time with patients, and the freedom to provide high-quality care.

In an analysis of 33 specialties, Leigh and associates (2002) found that physicians in high-income "procedural" specialties, such as obstetrics-gynecology, otolaryngology, ophthalmology, and orthopedics, were the most dissatisfied. Physicians in these specialties and those in internal medicine were more likely than family physicians to be dissatisfied with their careers. Among the specialty areas most satisfying was geriatrics. Because the population older than 65 years in the United States has doubled since 1960 and will double again by 2030, it is important that we have sufficient primary care physicians to care for them. The need for and the rewards of this type of practice must be communicated to students before they decide how to spend the rest of their professional lives.

A study of medical students (Clinite et al., 2013) showed that most of them say that enjoying their work is the most important factor in selecting a specialty. Students who ranked primary care as their first choice ranked time with family, work/life balance, and personal time outside work high, and salary and prestige low. In comparison, students who were least interested in primary care ranked salary and prestige highest. It is clear what changes must be made if we are to increase the number of students entering primary care.

Development of the Specialty

As long ago as 1923, Francis Peabody commented that the swing of the pendulum toward specialization had reached its apex and that modern medicine had fragmented the health care delivery system too greatly. He called for a rapid return of the generalist physician who would give comprehensive, personalized care.

Dr. Peabody's declaration proved to be premature; neither the medical establishment nor society was ready for such a proclamation. The trend toward specialization gained momentum through the 1950s, and fewer physicians entered general practice. In the early 1960s, leaders in the field of general practice began advocating a seemingly paradoxical solution to reverse the trend and correct the scarcity of general practitioners—the creation of still another specialty. These physicians envisioned a specialty that embodied the knowledge, skills, and ideals they knew as primary care. In 1966, the concept of a new specialty in primary care received official recognition in two separate reports published 1 month apart. The first was the report of the Citizens' Commission on Medical Education of the American Medical Association, also known as the Millis Commission Report. The second report came from the Ad Hoc Committee on Education for Family Practice of the Council of Medical

---

Table 1-1   What Patients Want in a Physician

Does not judge.
Understands and supports me.
Is always honest and direct.
Acts as a partner in maintaining my health.
Treats serious and nonserious conditions.
Attends to my emotional as well as physical health.
Truly listens to me.
Encourages me to lead a healthier lifestyle.
Tries to get to know me.
Can help with any problem.
Is someone I can stay with as I grow older.

Modified from Stock Keister MC, Green LA, Kahn NB, et al. What people want from their family physician. *Am Fam Physician.* 2004a;69:2310.

Education of the American Medical Association, also called the Willard Committee (1966). Three years later, in 1969, the American Board of Family Practice (ABFP) became the 20th medical specialty board. The name of the specialty board was changed in 2004 to the *American Board of Family Medicine* (ABFM).

Much of the impetus for the Millis and Willard reports came from the American Academy of General Practice, which was renamed the *American Academy of Family Physicians* (AAFP) in 1971. The name change reflected a desire to increase emphasis on family-oriented health care and to gain academic acceptance for the new specialty of family practice.

SPECIALTY CERTIFICATION

The ABFM has distinguished itself by being the first specialty board to require recertification (now called *maintenance of certification*) every 7 years to ensure the ongoing competence of its members. Certification was achieved initially only by examination, with no "grandfathering" as had been the practice when other specialties were established. Recertification required the attainment of a specified amount of continuing medical education; a full, valid, and unrestricted license; the completion of an audit of office records; and successful performance on a recertification examination. These "firsts" raised the bar for specialty certification in the United States and established the ABFM as a leader and innovator among specialty boards. The logic of the ABFM's emphasis on continuing education to maintain required knowledge and skills has been adopted by other specialties and state medical societies. All specialty boards are now committed to the concept of recertification to ensure that their diplomates remain current with advances in medicine.

The maintenance of certification now requires that all diplomates comply with the ABFM policy on professionalism, licensure, and personal conduct; complete a combination of self-assessment modules and performance in practice activities every 3 years; accumulate at least 50 continuing medical education credits per year; and successfully pass the maintenance of certification examination every 10 years.

In 2003, the ABFM began transitioning diplomates from its old recertification paradigm into its new process, termed Maintenance of Certification for Family Physicians. By the end of 2009, this transition was complete, and the ABFM became the first specialty board to have all of its diplomates enrolled and participating in maintenance of certification.

The ABFM also offers subspecialty *certificates of added qualifications* in five areas: adolescent medicine, geriatric medicine, hospice and palliative medicine, sleep medicine, and sports medicine. In additional, a special pathway within the maintenance of certification pathway, Recognition of Focused Practice in Hospital Medicine, is offered to family physicians who primarily practice in the hospital setting. Combined residency programs are available and are offered conjointly by ABFM and the appropriate specialty board. These provide training in family medicine and preventive medicine (six programs), family medicine and psychiatry (five programs), family medicine and emergency medicine (two programs), and family medicine and internal medicine (two programs). These combined residencies make candidates eligible for certification by both specialty boards with 1 year less training than that required for two separate residencies through appropriate overlap of training requirements.

Definitions

FAMILY MEDICINE

Family medicine is the medical specialty that provides continuing and comprehensive health care for the individual and the family. It is the specialty in breadth that integrates the biologic, clinical, and behavioral sciences. The scope of family medicine encompasses all ages, both genders, each organ system, and every disease entity.

In many countries, the term *general practice* is synonymous with *family medicine*. The Royal New Zealand College of General Practitioners emphasizes that a general practitioner provides care that is "anticipatory as well as responsive and is not limited by the age, sex, race, religion, or social circumstances of patients, nor by their physical or mental states." The general practitioner must be the patient's advocate; must be competent, caring, and compassionate; must be able to live with uncertainty; and must be willing to recognize limitations and refer when necessary (Richards, 1997).

FAMILY PHYSICIAN

The family physician is a physician who is educated and trained in the discipline of family medicine. Family physicians possess distinct attitudes, skills, and knowledge that qualify them to provide continuing and comprehensive medical care, health maintenance, and preventive services to each member of a family regardless of gender, age, or type of problem (i.e., biologic, behavioral, or social). These specialists, because of their background and interactions with the family, are best qualified to serve as each patient's advocate in all health-related matters, including the appropriate use of consultants, health services, and community resources.

The World Organization of Family Doctors (World Organization of National Colleges, Academies and Academic Associations of General Practitioners/Family Physicians [WONCA]) defines the "family doctor" in part as the physician who is primarily responsible for providing comprehensive health care to every individual seeking medical care and arranging for other health personnel to provide services when necessary. Whereas the family physician functions as a generalist who accepts everyone seeking care, other health providers limit access to their services on the basis of age, gender, or diagnosis (WONCA, 1991, p. 2).

PRIMARY CARE

Primary care is health care that is accessible, comprehensive, coordinated, and continuing. It is provided by physicians specifically trained for and skilled in comprehensive first-contact and continuing care for ill persons or those with an undiagnosed sign, symptom, or health concern (i.e., the "undifferentiated" patient) and is not limited by problem origin (i.e., biologic, behavioral, or social), organ system, or gender.

It is "the provision of integrated, accessible health care services by clinicians who are accountable for addressing a large majority of personal health care needs, developing a sustained partnership with patients, and practicing in the context of family and community" (WONCA, 2013).

In addition to diagnosis and treatment of acute and chronic illnesses, primary care includes health promotion, disease prevention, health maintenance, counseling, and patient education in a variety of health care settings (e.g., office, inpatient, critical care, long-term care, home care). Primary care is performed and managed by a personal physician using other health professionals for consultation or referral as appropriate.

Primary care is the backbone of the health care system and encompasses the following functions:

1. It is *first-contact care*, serving as a point of entry for the patient into the health care system.
2. It includes *continuity* by virtue of caring for patients in sickness and in health over some period.
3. It is *comprehensive care*, drawing from all the traditional major disciplines for its functional content.
4. It serves a *coordinative function* for all the health care needs of the patient.
5. It assumes *continuing responsibility* for individual patient follow-up and community health problems.
6. It is a highly *personalized* type of care.

In a 2008 report, *Primary Health Care—Now More Than Ever*, the World Health Organization (WHO) emphasizes that primary care is the best way of coping with the illnesses of the 21st century and that better use of existing preventive measures could reduce the global burden of disease by as much as 70%. Rather than drifting from one short-term priority to another, countries should make prevention equally important as cure and focus on the rise in chronic diseases that require long-term care and strong community support. Furthermore, at the 62nd World Health Assembly in 2009, the WHO strongly reaffirmed the values and principles of primary health care as the basis for strengthening health care systems worldwide (WONCA, 2013).

PRIMARY CARE PHYSICIAN

A primary care physician is a generalist physician who provides definitive care to the undifferentiated patient at the point of first contact and takes continuing responsibility for providing the patient's care. Primary care physicians devote most of their practice to providing primary care services to a defined population of patients. The style of primary care practice is such that the personal primary care physician serves as the entry point for substantially all the patient's medical and health care needs. Primary care physicians are advocates for the patient in coordinating the use of the entire health care system to benefit the patient.

Patients want a physician who is attentive to their needs and skilled at addressing them and with whom they can establish a lifelong relationship. They want a physician who can guide them through the evolving, complex U.S. health care system.

The ABFM and the American Board of Internal Medicine have agreed on a definition of the generalist physician, and they believe that "providing optimal generalist care requires broad and comprehensive training that cannot be gained in brief and uncoordinated educational experiences" (Kimball and Young, 1994, p. 316).

The Council on Graduate Medical Education (COGME) and the Association of American Medical Colleges (AAMC) define generalist physicians as those who have completed 3-year training programs in family medicine, internal medicine, or pediatrics and who do not subspecialize. COGME emphasizes that this definition should be "based on an objective analysis of training requirements in disciplines that provide graduates with broad capabilities for primary care practice."

Although the number of medical students entering family medicine is far below the number needed in the United States for an effective health care system, things appear to be improving. The percentage of medical school graduates choosing family medicine residencies jumped nearly 10% between 2008 and 2013.

For the seventh consecutive year, the demand for family physicians outpaced the demand for other specialists. A 2013 survey noted more searches for family physicians (624) than for other specialists such as internal medicine (194) and psychiatrists (198). As a result, salaries for family physicians increased 6% from 2011 to 2012 (www.aafp.org/news-now/practice-professional-issues/20130916recruitingstudy.html).

Physicians who provide primary care should be trained specifically to manage the problems encountered in a primary care practice. Rivo and associates (1994) identified the common conditions and diagnoses that generalist physicians should be competent to manage in a primary care practice and compared these with the training of the various "generalist" specialties. They recommended that the training of generalist physicians include at least 90% of the key diagnoses they identified. By comparing the content of residency programs, they found that this goal was met by family medicine (95% of the time), internal medicine (91% of the time), and pediatrics (91% of the time) but that obstetrics-gynecology (47% of the time) and emergency medicine (42% of the time) fell far short of this goal.

Personalized Care

It is much more important to know what sort of patient has a disease than what sort of disease a patient has.

SIR WILLIAM OSLER (1904)

In the 12th century, Maimonides said, "May I never see in the patient anything but a fellow creature in pain. May I never consider him merely a vessel of disease" (Friedenwald, 1917). If an intimate relationship with patients remains the primary concern of physicians, high-quality medical care will persist, regardless of the way it is organized and financed. For this reason, family medicine emphasizes consideration of the individual patient in the full context of her or his life rather than the episodic care of a presenting complaint.

Family physicians assess the illnesses and complaints presented to them, dealing personally with most and arranging special assistance for a few. The family physician serves as the patients' advocate, explaining the causes and implications of illness to patients and families, and serves as an advisor and confidant to the family. The family physician receives great intellectual satisfaction from this practice, but the greatest reward arises from the depth of human understanding and personal satisfaction inherent in family medicine.

Patients have adjusted somewhat to a more impersonal form of health care delivery and frequently look to institutions rather than to individuals for their health care; however, their need for personalized concern and compassion remains. Tumulty (1970) found that patients believe a good physician is one who shows genuine interest in them; who thoroughly evaluates their problem; who demonstrates compassion, understanding, and warmth; and who provides clear insight into what is wrong and what must be done to correct it.

Ludmerer (1999a) focused on the problems facing medical education in this environment:

Some managed care organizations have even urged that physicians be taught to act in part as advocates of the insurance payer rather than the patients for whom they care. ... Medical educators would do well to ponder the potential long-term consequences of educating the nation's physicians in today's commercial atmosphere in which the good visit is a short visit, patients are "consumers," and institutional officials speak more often of the financial balance sheet than of service and the relief of patients' suffering (pp. 881–882).

Cranshaw and colleagues (1995) discussed the ethics of the medical profession:

Our first obligation must be to serve the good of those persons who seek our help and trust us to provide it. Physicians, as physicians, are not, and must never be, commercial entrepreneurs, gate closers, or agents of fiscal policy that runs counter to our trust. Any defection from primacy of the patient's well-being places the patient at risk by treatment that may compromise quality of or access to medical care. ... Only by caring and advocating for the patient can the integrity of our profession be affirmed (p. 1553).

CARING

Caring without science is well-intentioned kindness, but not medicine. On the other hand, science without caring

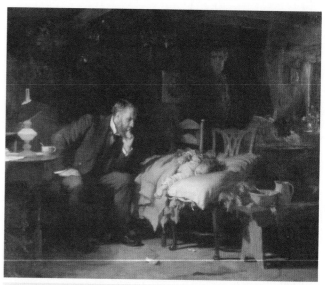

Figure 1-1 *The Doctor* by Sir Luke Fildes, 1891. (© Tate, London, 2005.)

empties medicine of healing and negates the great potential of an ancient profession. The two complement and are essential to the art of doctoring.

B. LOWN (1996, p. 223)

Family physicians do not just treat patients; they also care for people. This caring function of family medicine emphasizes the personalized approach to understanding the patient as a person, respecting the person as an individual, and showing compassion for his or her discomfort. The best illustration of a caring and compassionate physician is *The Doctor* by Sir Luke Fildes (Figure 1-1). The painting shows a physician at the bedside of an ill child in the preantibiotic era. The physician in the painting is Dr. Murray, who cared for Sir Luke Fildes's son, who died Christmas morning, 1877. The painting has become the symbol for medicine as a caring profession.

COMPASSION

The treatment of a disease may be entirely impersonal; the care of a patient must be completely personal.

FRANCIS PEABODY (1930)

Compassion means co-suffering and reflects the physician's willingness somehow to share the patient's anguish and understand what the sickness means to that person. Compassion is an attempt to feel along with the patient. Pellegrino (1979) said, "We can never feel with another person when we pass judgment as a superior, only when we see our own frailties as well as his" (p. 161). A compassionate authority figure is effective only when others can receive the "orders" without being humiliated. The physician must not "put down" the patients but must be ever ready, in Galileo's words, "to pronounce that wise, ingenuous, and modest statement—'I don't know.'" Compassion, practiced in these terms in each patient encounter, obtunds the inherent dehumanizing tendencies of the current highly institutionalized and technologically oriented patterns of patient care.

The family physician's relationship with each patient should reflect compassion, understanding, and patience combined with a high degree of intellectual honesty. The physician must be thorough in approaching problems but also possess a sense of humor. He or she must be capable of encouraging in each patient the optimism, courage, insight, and self-discipline necessary for recovery.

Bulger (1998, p. 106) addressed the threats to scientific compassionate care in the managed-care environment:

With health care time inordinately rationed today in the interest of economy, Americans could organize themselves right out of compassion. ... It would be a tragedy, just when we have so many scientific therapies at hand, for scientists to negotiate away the element of compassion, leaving this crucial dimension of healing to nonscientific healers.

Time for patient care is becoming increasingly threatened. Bulger (1998, p. 106) described a study involving a "good Samaritan" principle, showing that the decision of whether or not to stop and care for a person in distress is predominantly a function of having the time to do so. Even those with the best intentions require time to be of help to a suffering person.

Characteristics and Functions of the Family Physician

The ideal family physician is an explorer, driven by a persistent curiosity and the desire to know more (Table 1-2).

CONTINUING RESPONSIBILITY

One of the essential functions of the family physician is the willingness to accept ongoing responsibility for managing a patient's medical care. After a patient or a family has been accepted into the physician's practice, the responsibility for care is total and continuing. The Millis Commission chose the term "primary physician" to emphasize the concept of primary responsibility for the patient's welfare; however, the term *primary care physician* is more popular and refers to any physician who provides first-contact care and is essentially that person's personal physician.

The family physician's commitment to patients does not cease at the end of illness but is a continuing responsibility, regardless of the patient's state of health or the disease process. There is no need to identify the beginning or end point of treatment because care of a problem can be reopened at any time—even though a later visit may be primarily for another problem. This prevents the family physician from focusing too narrowly on one problem and helps maintain a perspective on the total patient in her or

Table 1-2 Attributes of a Family Physician*

A strong sense of responsibility for the total, ongoing care of the individual and the family during health, illness, and rehabilitation

Compassion and empathy with a sincere interest in the patient and the family

A curious and constantly inquisitive attitude

Enthusiasm for the undifferentiated medical problem and its resolution

Interest in the broad spectrum of clinical medicine

The ability to deal comfortably with multiple problems occurring simultaneously in a patient

Desire for frequent and varied intellectual and technical challenges

The ability to support children during growth and development and in their adjustment to family and society

The ability to assist patients in coping with everyday problems and in maintaining stability in the family and community

The capacity to act as coordinator of all health resources needed in the care of a patient

Enthusiasm for learning and for the satisfaction that comes from maintaining current medical knowledge through continuing medical education

The ability to maintain composure in times of stress and to respond quickly with logic, effectiveness, and compassion

A desire to identify problems at the earliest possible stage or to prevent disease entirely

A strong wish to maintain maximum patient satisfaction, recognizing the need for continuing patient rapport

The skills necessary to manage chronic illness and to ensure maximal rehabilitation after acute illness

Appreciation for the complex mix of physical, emotional, and social elements in personalized patient care

A feeling of personal satisfaction derived from intimate relationships with patients that naturally develop over long periods of continuous care, as opposed to the short-term pleasures gained from treating episodic illnesses

Skills for and a commitment to educating patients and families about disease processes and the principles of good health

A commitment to place the interests of the patient above those of self

* These characteristics are desirable for all physicians but are of greatest importance for family physicians.

his environment. Peabody (1930) believed that much patient dissatisfaction resulted from the physician's neglecting to assume personal responsibility for supervision of the patient's care: "For some reason or other, no one physician has seen the case through from beginning to end, and the patient may be suffering from the very multitude of his counselors" (p. 8).

Continuity of care is a core attribute of family medicine, transcending multiple illness episodes, and it includes responsibility for preventive care and care coordination. "This longitudinal relationship evolves into a strong bond between physician and patient characterized by trust, loyalty, and a sense of responsibility" (Saultz, 2003, p. 134). Trust grows stronger as the physician–patient relationship continues and provides the patient a sense of confidence that care will always be in his or her best interest. It also facilitates improved quality of care the longer the relationship continues.

The greater the degree of continuing involvement with a patient, the more capable the physician is in detecting early signs and symptoms of organic disease and differentiating it from a functional problem. Patients with problems arising from emotional and social conflicts can be managed most effectively by a physician who has intimate knowledge of the individual and his or her family and community background. This knowledge comes only from insight gained by observing the patient's long-term patterns of behavior and responses to changing stressful situations. This longitudinal view is particularly useful in the care of children and allows the physician to be more effective in assisting children to reach their full potential. The closeness that develops between physicians and young patients increases a physician's ability to aid the patients with problems later in life, such as adjustment to puberty, problems with employment, or marriage and changing social pressures. As the family physician maintains this continuing involvement with successive generations within a family, the ability to manage intercurrent problems increases with knowledge of the total family background.

By virtue of this ongoing involvement and intimate association with the family, the family physician develops a perceptive awareness of a family's nature and style of operation. This ability to observe families over time allows valuable insight that improves the quality of medical care provided to an individual patient. A major challenge in family medicine is the need to be alert to the changing stresses, transitions, and expectations of family members over time, as well as the effect that these and other family interactions have on the health of individual patients.

Although the family is the family physician's primary concern, his or her skills are equally applicable to the individual living alone or to people in other varieties of family living. Individuals with alternative forms of family living interact with others who have a significant effect on their lives. The principles of group dynamics and interpersonal relationships that affect health are equally applicable to everyone.

The family physician must assess an individual's personality so that presenting symptoms can be appropriately evaluated and given the proper degree of attention and emphasis. A complaint of abdominal pain may be treated lightly in one patient who frequently presents with minor problems, but the same complaint would be investigated immediately and in depth in another patient who has a more stoic personality. The decision regarding which studies to perform and when is influenced by knowledge of the patient's lifestyle, personality, and previous response pattern. The greater the degree of knowledge and insight into the patient's background, as gained through years of ongoing contact, the more capable is the physician in making an appropriate early and rapid assessment of the presenting complaint. The less background information the physician has to rely on, the greater the need to depend on costly laboratory studies, and overreaction to the presenting symptom is more likely.

Families receiving continuing comprehensive care have a decreased incidence of hospitalization, fewer operations, and fewer physician visits for illnesses compared with those having no regular physician. This results from the physician's knowledge of the patients, seeing them earlier for acute problems and therefore preventing complications that would require hospitalization, being available by telephone or by e-mail, and seeing them more frequently in the office for health supervision. Care is also less expensive because there is less need to rely on radiographic and laboratory procedures and visits to emergency departments.

Continuity of care improves quality of care, especially for those with chronic conditions such as asthma and diabetes (Cabana and Jee, 2004). Because about 90% of patients with diabetes in the United States receive care from a primary care physician, continuity of care can be especially important. Parchman and associates (2002) found that for adults with type 2 diabetes, continuing care from the same primary care provider was associated with lower Hb$_{A1c}$ values, regardless of how long the patient had diabetes. Having a regular source of primary care helped these adults manage their diet and improve glucose control.

Collusion of Anonymity

The need for a primary physician who accepts continuing responsibility for patient care was emphasized by Michael Balint (1965) in his concept of *collusion of anonymity*. In this situation, the patient is seen by a variety of physicians, not one of whom is willing to accept total management of the problem. Important decisions are made—some good, some poor—but without anyone feeling fully responsible for them. Both the patient and family often wonder who is in charge.

Francis Peabody (1930) examined the futility of a patient's making the rounds from one specialist to another without finding relief because the patient:

… lacked the guidance of a sound general practitioner who understood his physical condition, his nervous temperament and knew the details of his daily life. And many a patient who on his own initiative has sought out specialists, has had minor defects accentuated so that they assume a needless importance, and has even undergone operations that might well have been avoided. Those who are particularly blessed with this world's goods, who want the best regardless of the cost and imagine that they are getting it because they can afford to consult as many renowned specialists as they wish, are often pathetically tragic figures as they veer from one course of treatment to another. Like ships that lack a guiding hand upon the helm, they swing from tack to tack with each new gust of wind but get no nearer to the Port of Health because there is no pilot to set the general direction of their course (pp. 21-22).

Chronic Illness

The family physician must also be committed to managing the common chronic illnesses that have no known cure but for which continuing management by a personal physician is all the more necessary to maintain an optimal state of health for the patient. It is a difficult and often trying job to manage these unresolvable and progressively disabling problems, control of which requires a remodeling of the lifestyle of the entire family.

About 45% of Americans have a chronic condition. The costs to individuals and to the health care system are enormous. In 2000, care of chronic illness consumed 75 cents of every health care dollar spent in the United States (Robert Wood Johnson Foundation Annual Report, 2002).

Comorbidity, the coincident occurrence of coexisting and apparently unrelated disorders, is increasing as the population ages. Those age 60 years or older have an average of 2.2 chronic conditions, and physicians in primary care provide most of this care (Bayliss et al., 2003).

Diabetes is one of the most rapidly increasing chronic conditions. Quality of life is enhanced when care of patients with diabetes is provided in a primary care setting without compromising quality of care (Collins et al., 2009).

Quality of Care

Primary care provided by physicians specifically trained to care for the problems presenting to personal physicians, who know their patients over time, is of higher quality than care provided by other physicians. This has been confirmed by a variety of studies comparing the care given by physicians in different specialties. When hospitalized patients with pneumonia are cared for by family physicians or full-time specialist hospitalists, the quality of care is comparable, but the hospitalists incur higher hospital charges and longer lengths of stay and use more resources (Smith et al., 2002).

In the United States, a 20% increase in the number of primary care physicians is associated with a 5% decrease in mortality (40 fewer deaths per 100,000 population), but the benefit is even greater if the primary care physician is a family physician. Adding one more family physician per 10,000 people is associated with 70 fewer deaths per 100,000 population, which is a 9% reduction in mortality rate. Specialists practicing outside their area have increased mortality rates for patients with acquired pneumonia, acute myocardial infarction, congestive heart failure, and upper gastrointestinal hemorrhage. A study of the major determinants of health outcomes in all 50 U.S. states found that when the number of specialty physicians increases, outcomes are worse, but mortality rates are lower where there are more primary care physicians (Starfield et al., 2005).

Veerappa and colleagues (2011) found that increasing the number of family physicians practicing in the community is associated with reduced hospital readmissions and substantial cost savings. Thirty-day hospital readmission rates for pneumonia, heart attack, and heart failure decrease as the number of family physicians in the community increases. Conversely, increased numbers of physicians in all other major specialties (including general internal medicine) are associated with increased risk of readmission (Figure 1-2).

A comparison of family physicians and obstetrician-gynecologists in the management of low-risk pregnancies showed no difference with respect to neonatal outcomes. However, women cared for by family physicians had fewer cesarean sections and episiotomies and were less likely to receive epidural anesthesia (Hueston et al., 1995).

Patients of subspecialists practicing outside their specialty have longer lengths of hospital stay and higher mortality rates than patients of subspecialists practicing within their specialty (Weingarten et al., 2002). The quality of the U.S. health care system is being eroded by physicians being

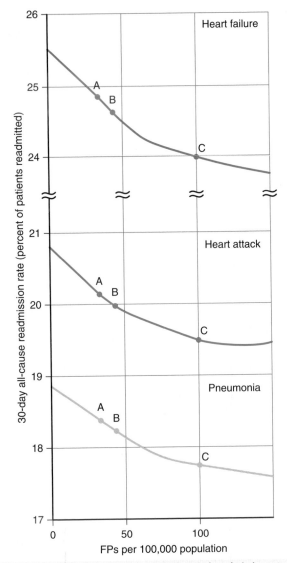

Figure 1-2 Actual and estimated 30-day hospital readmission rates in 2005 per county density of family physicians (FPs). **A,** Actual readmissions in 2005. **B,** Estimated readmissions with 46 FPs per 100,000 population. **C,** Estimated readmissions with 100 FPs per 100,000 population. (From Veerappa K, Culpepper L, Phillips RL, et al. FPs lower hospital readmission rates and costs. *Am Fam Physician.* 2011;83(9):1054.)

extensively trained, at great expense, to practice in one area and instead practicing in another area, such as surgeons practicing as generalists. Primary care, to be done well, requires extensive training specifically tailored to problems frequently seen in primary care.

As much-needed changes in the U.S. medical system are implemented, it would be wise to keep some perspective on the situation regarding physician distribution. Beeson (1974) commented:

I have no doubt at all that a good family doctor can deal with the great majority of medical episodes quickly and competently. A specialist, on the other hand, feels that he must be thorough, not only because of his training but also because he has a reputation to protect. He, therefore, spends more time with each patient and orders more laboratory work. The result is a waste of doctors' time and patients' money. This not only inflates the national health bill, but also creates an illusion of doctor shortage when the only real need is to have the existing doctors doing the right things (p. 48).

Cost-Effective Care

A physician who is well acquainted with a patient provides more personal and humane medical care and does so more economically than a physician involved in only episodic care. A physician who knows his or her patients well can assess the nature of their problems more rapidly and accurately.

The United States has the most expensive health care system in the world. In 1965, the cost of health care in the United States was just under 6% of the gross domestic product (GDP). It shot up to 16% of GDP in 2008 and continues to increase, with predictions it will reach 20% by 2015. Despite the most expensive health care, however, among industrialized nations, the United States ranks 29th in infant mortality, 48th in life expectancy, and 19th (of 19) in preventable deaths.

Although the rhetoric suggests it is worth this cost to have the best health care system in the world, the truth is that we are far from that goal. The WHO ranks the quality of health care in the United States at 37th in the world, well behind Morocco and Colombia. (For the standing of all countries, see the World Health Organization's ranking of the world's health systems under http://geographic.org/countries/countries.html). In a comparison of the quality of health care in 13 developed countries using 16 different health indicators, the United States ranked 12th, second from the bottom. Evidence indicates that quality of health care is associated with primary care performance. Of the seven countries at the top of the average health ranking, five have strong primary care infrastructures. As Starfield (2000) states, "The higher the primary care physician-to-population ratio, the better most health outcomes are" (p. 485).

Similarly, the greater the number of primary care physicians practicing in a country, the lower is the cost of health care. Figure 1-3 shows that in the United Kingdom, Canada,

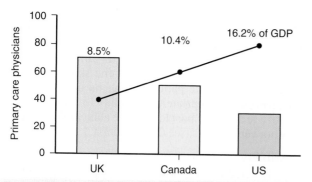

Figure 1-3 Inverse relationship between number of generalists and cost of health care in the United Kingdom, Canada, and the United States. *GDP,* Gross domestic product. (From Henry J. Kaiser Family Foundation. *Snapshots: Health Care Spending in the United States & Selected OECD Countries,* April 12, 2011. Available at kff.org/health-costs/issue-brief/snapshots-health-care-spending-in-the-united-states-selected-oecd-countries/)

and the United States, the cost of health care is almost inversely proportional to the percentage of generalists practicing in that country. Great Britain has twice the percentage of family physicians but about half the cost. Administration and profit (31%) of U.S. health care account for a major part of the high overhead cost (Woolhandler et al., 2003). For the same number of physicians, Canada has one "billing clerk" for every 17 in the United States (Lundberg, 2002).

Countries with strong primary care have lower overall health care costs, improved health outcomes, and healthier populations (Phillips and Starfield, 2004; Starfield, 2001). In comparing 11 features of primary care in 11 Western countries, the United States ranked lowest in terms of primary care ranking and highest in per-capita health care expenditures. The United States also performed poorly on public satisfaction, health indicators, and the use of medication (Starfield, 1994).

In the United States, the greater the number of primary care physicians, the lower the mortality rate, and conversely, the higher the specialist/population ratio, the greater the mortality rate. Adding one family physician per 10,000 people would result in 35 fewer deaths. Increasing the number of specialists, a process that continues in the United States, is associated with higher mortality rates and increasing cost. One third of the excessive cost is attributed to performance of unnecessary procedures (Starfield et al., 2005).

Uninsured Persons

Before the Affordable Care Act, the number of Americans without health insurance had been increasing by 1 million per year. In 2008, the number of uninsured persons was 16% of the U.S. population. The number of people who were *underinsured* was growing even more rapidly. Contrary to widespread belief, the problem is not confined simply to unemployed or poor persons. More than half of uninsured persons had annual incomes greater than $75,000, and 8 of 10 were in working families. In 2013, medical expenses were responsible for 62% of bankruptcies in the United States. This will certainly change with the Affordable Care Act, but the amount of change remains to be seen because many of those filing for bankruptcy already had medical insurance but were still overwhelmed by medical bills.

The United States is the only developed country that does not have universal health care coverage for all its citizens. According to Geyman (2002), "Today's nonsystem is in chaos. A large part of health care has been taken over by for-profit corporations whose interests are motivated more by return on investment to shareholders than by quality of care for patients" (p. 407).

The United Nations passed a resolution encouraging all governments to move toward providing universal access to affordable and quality health care. In 2013, the WHO published a World Health Report, "Research for Universal Health Coverage," that focused on the need for more research to assist countries in establishing universal health care.

The Institute of Medicine (IOM) report on the uninsured population, *Insuring America's Health: Principles and Recommendations,* called for "health care coverage by 2010 that is universal, continuous, affordable, sustainable, and enhancing of high-quality care that is effective, efficient, safe, timely, patient centered, and equitable. ... While stopping short of advocating a specific approach, the IOM's Committee on the Consequences of Uninsurance acknowledges that the single payer model is the most effective in ensuring continuous universal coverage that would remain affordable for individuals and for society" (Geyman, 2004, p. 635).

Family physicians account for a larger proportion of office visits to U.S. physicians than any other specialty. However, Geyman (2004, p. 631) observed problems:

The country's health care (non) system has undergone a major transformation to a market-based system largely dominated by corporate interests and a business ethic. The goal envisioned in the 1960s of rebuilding the U.S. health care system on a generalist base, with all Americans having ready access to comprehensive health care through a personal physician, has not been achieved. Overspecialization was a problem as long as 4000 years ago, when Herodotus in 2000 BC noted that "The art of medicine is thus divided: each physician applies himself to one disease only and not more."

Comprehensive Care

The term *comprehensive medical care* spans the entire spectrum of medicine. The effectiveness with which a physician delivers primary care depends on the degree of involvement attained during training and practice. The family physician must be trained comprehensively to acquire all the medical skills necessary to care for most problems. The greater the number of skills omitted from the family physician's training and practice, the more frequent is the need to refer minor problems to another physician. A truly comprehensive primary care physician adequately manages acute infections, biopsies skin and other lesions, repairs lacerations, treats musculoskeletal sprains and minor fractures, removes foreign bodies, treats vaginitis, provides obstetric care and care for newborn infants, gives supportive psychotherapy, and supervises diagnostic procedures. The needs of a family physician's patient range from a routine physical examination, when the patient feels well and wants to identify potential risk factors, to a problem that calls for referral to one or more narrowly specialized physicians with highly developed technical skills. The family physician must be aware of the variety and complexity of skills and facilities available to help manage patients and must match these to the individual's specific needs, giving full consideration to the patient's personality and expectations.

Comprehensive care includes complementary and alternative techniques that are of value in managing problems encountered in primary care (see Chapter 12). The book *Integrative Medicine* (Rakel, 2012) focuses on techniques that can be of value to the family physician but also identifies those than can be harmful or ineffective.

Management of an illness involves much more than a diagnosis and an outline for treatment. It also requires an awareness of all the factors that may aid or hinder an individual's recovery from illness. This approach requires consideration of religious beliefs; social, economic, or cultural problems; personal expectations; and heredity. An outstanding clinician recognizes the effects that spiritual, intellectual, emotional, social, and economic factors have on a patient's illness.

A family physician's ability to confront relatively large numbers of unselected patients with undifferentiated conditions and carry on a therapeutic relationship over time is a unique primary care skill. A skilled family physician has a higher level of tolerance for the uncertain than her or his consultant colleagues.

Society benefits more from a surgeon who has a sufficient volume of surgery to maintain proficiency through frequent use of well-honed skills than from one who has a low volume of surgery and serves also as a primary care physician. The early identification of disease while it is in its undifferentiated stage requires specific training; it is not a skill that can be automatically assumed by someone whose training has been mostly in hospital intensive care units.

Interpersonal Skills

One of the foremost skills of family physicians is the ability to use effectively the knowledge of interpersonal relations in the management of patients. This powerful element of clinical medicine may be the specialty's most useful tool. Physicians too often are seen as lacking personal concern and as being unskilled in understanding personal anxiety and feelings. There is a need to nourish the seed of compassion and concern for sick people that motivates students as they enter medical school.

Family medicine emphasizes the integration of compassion, empathy, and personalized concern. Some of the earnest solicitude of the "old country doctor" and his or her untiring compassion for people must be incorporated as effective but impersonal modern medical procedures are applied. The patient should be viewed compassionately as a person in distress who needs to be treated with concern, dignity, and personal consideration. The patient has a right to be given some insight into his or her problems; a reasonable appraisal of the potential outcome; and a realistic picture of the emotional, financial, and occupational expenses involved in his or her care. The greatest deterrents to filing malpractice claims are patient satisfaction, good patient rapport, and active patient participation in the health care process.

To relate well to patients, a physician must develop compassion and courtesy, the ability to establish rapport and to communicate effectively, the ability to gather information rapidly and to organize it logically, the skills required to identify all significant patient problems and to manage these problems appropriately, the ability to listen, the skills necessary to motivate people, and the ability to observe and detect nonverbal clues (see Chapter 13).

Accessibility

The mere availability of the physician is therapeutic. The feeling of security that the patient gains just by knowing he or she can "touch" the physician, in person or by phone, is therapeutic and has a comforting and calming influence. Accessibility is an essential feature of primary care. Services must be available when needed and should be within geographic proximity. When primary care is not available, many individuals turn to hospital emergency departments. Emergency department care is fine for emergencies, but it is no substitute for the personalized, long-term, comprehensive care a family physician can provide.

Many practices are instituting open-access scheduling, in which patients can be seen the day they call. This tells patients that they are the highest priority and that their problems will be handled immediately. It also is more efficient for the physician who cares for a problem early, before it progresses in severity and becomes complicated, requiring more physician time and greater patient disability.

Some physicians have turned to concierge medicine (also called boutique medicine, retainer-based medicine, and enhanced medical care for an annual fee) in which, for a monthly or annual fee, the physician promises to be available 24/7.

DIAGNOSTIC SKILLS: UNDIFFERENTIATED PROBLEMS

The family physician must be an outstanding diagnostician. Skills in this area must be honed to perfection because problems are usually seen in their early, undifferentiated state and without the degree of resolution that is usually present by the time patients are referred to consulting specialists. This is a unique feature of family medicine because symptoms seen at this stage are often vague and nondescript, with signs being minimal or absent. Unlike the consulting specialist, the family physician does not evaluate the case after it has been preselected by another physician, and the diagnostic procedures used by the family physician must be selected from the entire spectrum of medicine.

At this stage of disease, there are often only subtle differences between the early symptoms of serious disease and those of self-limiting, minor ailments. To an inexperienced person, the clinical pictures may appear identical, but to an astute and experienced family physician, one symptom is more suspicious than another because of the greater probability that it signals a potentially serious illness. Diagnoses are frequently made on the basis of probability, and the likelihood that a specific disease is present frequently depends on the incidence of the disease relative to the symptom seen in the physician's community during a given time of year. Many patients will never be assigned a final, definitive diagnosis because a presenting symptom or a complaint will resolve before a specific diagnosis can be made. Pragmatically, this is an efficient method that is less costly and achieves high patient satisfaction even though it may be disquieting to the purist physician who believes a thorough workup and specific diagnosis always should be obtained. Similarly, family physicians are more likely to use a therapeutic trial to confirm the diagnosis.

The family physician is an expert in the rapid assessment of a problem presented for the first time. He or she evaluates its potential significance, often making a diagnosis by exclusion rather than by inclusion, after making certain the symptoms are not those of a serious problem. Once assured, some time is allowed to elapse. Time is used as an efficient diagnostic aid. Follow-up visits are scheduled at appropriate intervals to watch for subtle changes in the presenting symptoms. The physician usually identifies the symptom that has the greatest discriminatory value and watches it more closely than the others. The most significant clue to the true nature of the illness may depend on subtle changes in this key symptom. The family physician's effectiveness is often determined by his or her knack for perceiving the hidden or subtle dimensions of illness and following them closely.

The maxim that "an accurate history is the most important factor in arriving at an accurate diagnosis" is especially appropriate to family medicine because symptoms may be the only obvious feature of an illness at the time it is presented. Further inquiry into the nature of the symptoms, time of onset, extenuating factors, and other unique subjective features may provide the only diagnostic clues available at such an early stage.

The family physician must be a perceptive humanist, alert to early identification of new problems. Arriving at an early diagnosis may be of less importance than determining the real reason the patient came to the physician. The symptoms may be the result of a self-limiting or acute problem, but anxiety or fear may be the true precipitating factor. Although the symptom may be hoarseness that has resulted from postnasal drainage accompanying an upper respiratory tract infection, the patient may fear it is caused by a laryngeal carcinoma similar to that recently found in a friend. Clinical evaluation must rule out the possibility of laryngeal carcinoma, but the patient's fears and apprehension regarding this possibility must also be allayed.

Every physical problem has an emotional component, and although this factor is usually minimal, it can be significant. A patient's personality, fears, and anxieties play a role in every illness and are important factors in primary care.

THE FAMILY PHYSICIAN AS COORDINATOR

Francis Peabody (1930), a professor of medicine at Harvard Medical School from 1921 to 1927, was ahead of his time. His comments remain appropriate today:

Never was the public in need of wise, broadly trained advisors so much as it needs them today to guide them through the complicated maze of modern medicine. The extraordinary development of medical science, with its consequent diversity of medical specialism and the increasing limitations in the extent of special fields—the very factors that are creating specialists—in themselves create a new demand, not for men who are experts along narrow lines, but for men who are in touch with many lines (p. 20).

The family physician, by virtue of his or her breadth of training in a wide variety of medical disciplines, has unique insights into the skills possessed by physicians in the more limited specialties. The family physician is best prepared to select specialists whose skills can be applied most appropriately to a given case, as well as to coordinate the activities of each, so that they are not counterproductive.

As medicine becomes more specialized and complex, the family physician's role as the integrator of health services becomes increasingly important. The family physician facilitates the patient's access to the whole health care system and interprets the activities of this system to the patient, explaining the nature of the illness, the implication of the treatment, and the effect of both on the patient's way of life. The following statement from the Millis Commission Report (Citizens' Commission, 1966) concerning expectations of the patient is especially appropriate:

The patient wants, and should have, someone of high competence and good judgment to take charge of the total situation, someone who can serve as coordinator of all the medical resources that can help solve his problem. He wants a company president who will make proper use of his skills and knowledge of more specialized members of the firm. He wants a quarterback who will diagnose the constantly changing situation, coordinate the whole team, and call on each member for the particular contributions that he is best able to make to the team effort (p. 39).

Such breadth of vision is important for a coordinating physician. She or he must have a realistic overview of the problem and an awareness of the many alternative routes to select the one that is most appropriate. As Pellegrino (1966) stated:

It should be clear, too, that no simple addition of specialties can equal the generalist function. To build a wall, one needs more than the aimless piling up of bricks, one needs an architect. Every operation which analyzes some part of the human mechanism requires it to be balanced by another which synthesizes and coordinates (p. 542).

The complexity of modern medicine frequently involves a variety of health professionals, each with highly developed skills in a particular area. In planning the patient's care, the family physician, having established rapport with a patient and family and having knowledge of the patient's background, personality, fears, and expectations, is best able to select and coordinate the activities of appropriate individuals from the large variety of medical disciplines. He or she can maintain effective communication among those involved, as well as function as the patient's advocate and interpret to the patient and family the many unfamiliar and complicated procedures being used. This prevents any one consulting physician, unfamiliar with the concepts or actions of all others involved, from ordering a test or medication that would conflict with other treatment. Dunphy (1964) described the value of the surgeon and the family physician working closely as a team:

It is impossible to provide high quality surgical care without that knowledge of the whole patient, which only a family physician can supply. When their mutual decisions ... bring hope, comfort and ultimately, health to a gravely ill human being, the total experience is the essence and the joy of medicine (p. 12).

The ability to orchestrate the knowledge and skills of diverse professionals is a skill to be learned during training and cultivated in practice. It is not an automatic attribute of all physicians or merely the result of exposure to a large number of professionals. These coordinator skills extend beyond the traditional medical disciplines into the many community agencies and allied health professions as well. Because of his or her close involvement with the community, the family physician is ideally suited to be the integrator of the patient's care, coordinating the skills of consultants when appropriate and involving community nurses, social agencies, the clergy, or other family members when needed. Knowledge of community health resources and a personal involvement with the community can be used to maximum benefit for diagnostic and therapeutic purposes and to achieve the best possible level of rehabilitation.

Only 5% of visits to family physicians lead to a referral, and more than 50% are for consultation rather than direct intervention. Surgical specialists are sent the largest share of referrals at 45.4% followed by medical specialists at 31% and obstetrician-gynecologists at 4.6%. Physicians consulted most frequently are orthopedic surgeons followed by general surgeons, otolaryngologists, and gastroenterologists. Psychiatrists are consulted the least (Forrest et al., 2002; Starfield et al., 2002).

The Family Physician in Practice

The advent of family medicine has led to a renaissance in medical education involving a reassessment of the traditional medical education environment in a teaching hospital. It is now considered more realistic to train a physician in a community atmosphere, providing exposure to the diseases and problems most closely approximating those she or he will encounter during practice. The ambulatory care skills and knowledge that most medical graduates will need cannot be taught totally within a tertiary medical center. The specialty of family medicine emphasizes training in ambulatory care skills in an appropriately realistic environment using patients representing a cross-section of a community and incorporating those problems most frequently encountered by physicians practicing primary care. For this reason, the model office is integral to training in family medicine because it imitates realistically the environment and kind of problems the student and resident will encounter in practice.

The lack of relevance in the referral medical center also applies to the hospitalized patient. Figure 1-4 places the health problems of an average community in perspective. In any given month, 800 people experience at least one symptom. Most of these people are managed by self-treatment, but 217 consult a physician. Of these, eight are hospitalized, but only one goes to an academic medical center. Patients seen in the medical center (with most cases used for teaching) represent atypical samples of illness occurring within the community. Students exposed to

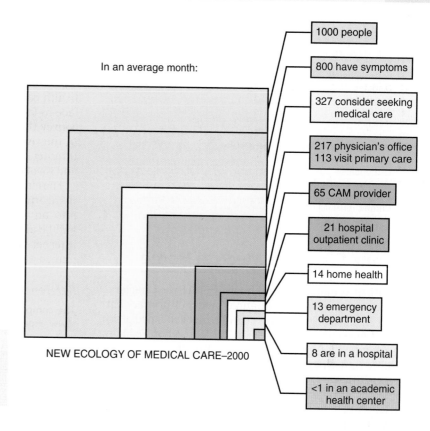

In an average month:

1000 people

800 have symptoms

327 consider seeking medical care

217 physician's office
113 visit primary care

65 CAM provider

21 hospital outpatient clinic

14 home health

13 emergency department

8 are in a hospital

<1 in an academic health center

NEW ECOLOGY OF MEDICAL CARE–2000

Figure 1-4 Number of persons experiencing an illness during an average month per 1000 people. *CAM,* Complementary and alternative medicine. (From Green LA, Fryer GE Jr, Yawn BP, et al. The ecology of medical care revisited. *N Engl J Med.* 2001;344:2021-2025.)

patients in only this manner develop an unrealistic concept of the types of medical problems prevalent in society and particularly those composing primary care. It focuses their training on knowledge and skills of limited usefulness in later practice.

PRACTICE CONTENT

Since 1975, the National Ambulatory Medical Care Survey conducted by the National Center for Health Statistics (NCHS) of the U.S. Department of Health and Human Services has annually reported the problems seen by office-based physicians (in all specialties) in the United States. The 20 most common diagnoses seen by physicians in their offices are shown in Table 1-3. Note that arthritis is fourth and diabetes mellitus sixth, reflecting the prominence of chronic diseases in practice. For those who think primary care is little more than caring for acute pharyngitis, note that it is ranked 19th. When only chronic conditions are listed (Table 1-4), arthritis is second and diabetes fourth.

Although hypertension is the most common problem encountered in offices (see Table 1-3), primary care physicians checked the blood pressure at 60% of the visits compared with only 20% of surgical specialists and 40% of visits to medical specialists (Woodwell and Cherry, 2002).

Available data concerning primary care indicate that more people use this type of medical service than any other and that, contrary to popular opinion, sophisticated medical technology is not normally either required or overused in basic primary care encounters. Most primary care visits arise from patients requesting care for relatively

Table 1-3 Rank Order of Office Visits by Diagnosis

1. Essential hypertension
2. Routine infant or child health check
3. Acute upper respiratory infections, excluding pharyngitis
4. Arthropathies and related disorders
5. Malignant neoplasms
6. Diabetes mellitus
7. Spinal disorders
8. Rheumatism, excluding back
9. General medical examination
10. Follow-up examination
11. Specific procedures and aftercare
12. Normal pregnancy
13. Gynecologic examination
14. Otitis media and eustachian tube disorders
15. Asthma
16. Disorder of lipoid metabolism
17. Chronic sinusitis
18. Heart disease, excluding ischemic
19. Acute pharyngitis
20. Allergic rhinitis

From Cherry DK, Woodwell DA, Rechtsteiner EA. 2005 *Summary: National Ambulatory Medical Care Survey.* National Center for Health Statistics, Advance Data Vital Health Statistics. No 387. Washington, DC, US Government Printing Office; 2007.

uncomplicated problems, many of which are self-limiting but which cause the patients concern or discomfort. Treatment is often symptomatic, consisting of pain relief or anxiety reduction rather than a "cure." The greatest cost-efficiency results when these patients' needs are satisfied while the self-limiting course of the disease is recognized, without incurring unnecessary costs for additional tests.

Table 1-4   Rank Order of Chronic Conditions, All Ages

1. Hypertension
2. Arthritis
3. Hyperlipidemia
4. Diabetes
5. Depression
6. Obesity
7. Cancer
8. Asthma
9. Chronic obstructive pulmonary disease
10. Ischemic heart disease
11. Osteoporosis
12. Cerebrovascular disease
13. Congestive heart failure
14. Chronic renal failure

Patient-Centered Medical Home

The patient-centered medical home (PCMH; see Chapter 2) has been proposed as an enhanced model of primary care by four medical organizations (family medicine, pediatrics, internal medicine, osteopathy) and is focused on reducing fragmentation of care and overcoming the reliance on specialty rather than primary care (Berenson et al., 2008; Rogers, 2008).

Primary care was encouraged to expand beyond its restrictive role as a provider of care to one that analyzes the needs of a community and focuses on those at risk of disease. This process was first described in the 1950s by Sydney Karf, who looked at the needs of his community in South Africa, whether or not they were his patients (Kark and Cassel, 1952; WONCA, 2013). The process involves identifying the health problems of a community, such as diabetes or obesity, developing a program to prevent the disease and care for people in the early stage, and then evaluating the effectiveness of the program (Longlett et al., 2001).

Looking toward the Future

The pace of medical progress may result in tomorrow's innovations exceeding today's fantasies. Family medicine in the future will be different as a result of technology. Every patient and physician is computer literate, with patients having access to the same sources of information as physicians. Patients are likely to have their own home page that contains their medical information and gives them access to whatever services they need (Scherger, 2005). Although the Internet is an excellent tool for consumers to access information about their health and for disseminating health care information, it will never be a substitute for a face-to-face discussion and physical examination. It cannot convey the worry in a voice or the subtle, nonverbal clues to the real reason for the patient's distress. However, the Internet does allow the individual patient to be more active and involved in his or her own care.

The electronic medical record allows the family physician to incorporate the latest evidence-based recommendations into an individual's care, write electronic prescriptions, and be alerted to drug interactions while seeing a patient. Internet-based textbooks such as this one will provide immediate access to information during patient visits.

References

The complete reference list is available online at www.expertconsult.com

Web Resources

www.aafp.org: The American Academy of Family Physicians' site with information for members, residents, students, and patients. Publishes the *American Family Physician, Family Practice Management Journal, Annals of Family Medicine,* and *AAFP News Now.* Sponsors the Family Medicine Interest Group (FMIG) for medical students.

www.adfammed.org: The Association of Departments of Family Medicine represents departments of family medicine in U.S. medical schools.

www.familydoctor.org: Family Doctor provides consumer health information, including tips for healthy living, search by symptom, immunization schedules, and drug information.

www.globalfamilydoctor.com: The World Organization of National Colleges, Academies and Academic Associations of General Practitioners/ Family Physicians (WONCA). The World Organization of Family Doctors is made up of 126 organizations in 102 countries.

www.napcrg.org: The North American Primary Care Research Group (NAPCRG) is committed to fostering research in primary care.

www.photius.com/rankings/healthranks.html: The World Health Organization's ranking of the quality of health care in 190 countries. Also available are life expectancy, preventable deaths, and total health expenditure (as percentage of gross domestic product).

www.stfm.org: The Society of Teachers of Family Medicine, representing 5000 teachers, publishes *Family Medicine, Annals of Family Medicine,* and the *STFM Messenger.*

www.theabfm.org: The American Board of Family Medicine, the second largest medical specialty in the United States. The site includes a link to *The Journal of the American Board of Family Medicine,* certification requirements, and reciprocity agreements with other countries.

2 Patient-Centered Medical Home

DAVID P. RAKEL and WAYNE BOICE JONAS

Key Points

- Continuous, healing-oriented relationships are the foundation on which the medical home, or "health home," is built. This is the interpersonal environment.
- The patient-centered medical home brings together health professionals to work collectively toward the health needs of the community through the creation of health teams.
- A continuous self-reflective process is required for the physician-leader to prevent burnout, maintain joy in her or his work, and create an optimal healing environment (OHE). This is the inner environment.

- The health home can have the greatest impact on community health by proactive incorporation of positive lifestyle behaviors. This is the behavioral environment.
- Patient empowerment involves providing accurate information in a manner that is understandable to the individual and creating a context that supports the patient's ability to make decisions.
- Infusing the elements of an OHE (including inner, interpersonal, behavioral, and external) within the medical home will encourage patient and team empowerment and enhance change toward positive health.

The intuitive mind is a sacred gift, and the rational mind is a faithful servant. We have created a society in which we honor the servant and have forgotten the gift.

ALBERT EINSTEIN

History

The concept of the "medical home" was first described in *Standards of Child Care* by the American Academy of Pediatrics (AAP) Council on Pediatrics Practice in 1967. It defined "ideal care" for children with disabilities as a practice that provided care that was accessible, coordinated, family-centered, and culturally effective.

The American Academy of Family Physicians (AAFP) used this concept to expand the characteristics based on discussions defining the future of family medicine. These characteristics described the "personal" medical home, which focused on bringing attention to the importance of continuous, relationship-centered, whole-system, comprehensive care for communities (Martin et al., 2004). In 2007, the AAP, AAFP, American College of Physicians (ACP), and American Osteopathic Association (AOA)

collaborated to define further the foundational principles of the patient-centered medical home (PCMH; Table 2-1). The goal of the medical home is to emphasize the importance of primary care in maximizing quality of care, health outcomes, and the patient experience, with improved cost efficiency, called "the "triple aim" by the Institute for Healthcare Improvement (IHI, 2014).

However, the ingredients of the medical home (or "health home") continue to be defined and modified based on the needs of the clinicians and communities that implement them. These ingredients and how they are delivered are key to the achievement of the lofty goals of the medical home and family medicine in general. This chapter discusses the most important ingredients for the medical home and the actions that the family physician can take to create one.

Healing, Curing, and the Goals of the Medical Home

Medicine in general and primary care in particular involve constant tension between the diagnosis and elimination of disease (cure) on one hand and the alleviation of suffering (healing) on the other. In this context, *healing* means

Table 2-1   Principles of a Patient-Centered Medical Home

1. Access to care based on an ongoing relationship with a personal physician who is able to provide first-contact, continuous, and comprehensive care
2. Care provided by a physician-led team of individuals within the practice who collectively take responsibility for the ongoing needs of patients
3. Care based on a whole-person (holistic) orientation in which the practice team takes responsibility for either providing care that encompasses all patient needs or arranges for the care to be done by other qualified professionals
4. Care coordinated and integrated across all elements of the complex health care system and the patient's community
5. Care facilitated by the use of office practice systems (e.g., registries, information technology, health information exchange) to ensure that patients receive the indicated care when and where they need and want it in a culturally and linguistically appropriate manner
6. Reimbursement structure that supports and encourages this model of care

Modified from American College of Physicians. *Joint Principles of the Patient-Centered Medical Home,* March 2007. http://www.acponline.org/advocacy/where_we_stand/medical_home/approve_jp.pdf.

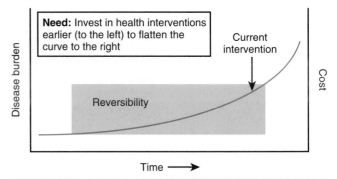

Figure 2-1 Profit in the current U.S. health care system is obtained focusing on the right of the curve. Investment toward the left of the curve will reduce disease burden and cost over time.

optimizing patients' responses to treatments and helping them cope emotionally and practically with whatever condition they face, even when cure is not possible.

In *The Nature of Suffering and the Goals of Medicine,* Cassell (2004) elegantly describes this tension and the continual erosion of healing practices under the pressure to apply more specific, technologic cures. In *A Time to Heal,* Ludmerer (1999) documents how, despite decades of efforts in curriculum change, these core values of healing in medical education have failed to gain significant traction under the forces driving the payment for cure-seeking behaviors.

Thus, physicians seeking to create a medical home that balances cure and healing face considerable challenges, especially in the delivery of healing. What are the essential components of such a health care home? How can they be delivered in the current medical context? What actions must a family physician take to create not only a practice that treats disease but an optimal healing environment (OHE) as well?

BALANCING TREATMENT OF DISEASE AND PROMOTION OF HEALTH AND HEALING

Health is largely a result of positive lifestyle behaviors that are often challenging to implement. Addressing issues such as smoking, obesity, substance abuse, and inactivity can reduce premature death by 40% (McGinnis et al., 2002; Schroeder, 2007). Positive lifestyle behaviors not only prevent premature death but also extend the average life expectancy by 14 years (Khaw et al., 2008). Currently, approximately 4 cents of every dollar spent for health care goes toward prevention and public health, with 96% spent on treating established disease (Lambrew, 2007). Two thirds of chronic disease is behavior-related and could be eliminated or mitigated by working interprofessionally to help guide patients toward healthy choices (McGinnis et al., 2002).

Behaviors that have the greatest impact on preventing chronic disease and its progression are (1) reducing exposure to toxic substances (tobacco, alcohol, drugs, pollution),

(2) movement and exercise, (3) healthy diet, (4) psychosocial integration and stress management, and (5) early disease detection and intervention (Jonas, 2009; McGinnis, 2003). For these behaviors to have an impact, the health home needs to be both designed and financially supported with the goal of health as its primary focus. This requires new models for funding that go beyond the disease-focused, payment-by-episode, high-throughput model of payment that currently dominates medicine. A primary care clinic that only works from this model will encourage shorter office visits while promoting reliance on expensive technologies that modify symptoms without addressing the cause of disease. The PCMH needs to push the curve in Figure 2-1 to the left by involving professionals who specialize in health promotion and flatten the disease progression curve and reduce the need for emergency and tertiary care.

ESTABLISHING AN OPTIMAL HEALING ENVIRONMENT

An OHE involves changes in the delivery and context of medical treatment rather than a specific treatment itself. Its goal is to infuse healing processes (salutogenesis) into any disease treatment. This means optimizing the effects of "meaning and context" in care process rather than ignoring or dismissing them as "placebo" effects (Jonas 2011). An OHE involves attending to three primary domains of care delivery: (1) the "inner" personal environment of the team and patient; (2) the "inter" personal or relationship environment of care delivery; and (3) the "external" behavioral and physical environment of the medical home (Chez and Jonas, 2005; Jonas et al., 2014).

The "treatment" itself is given the most credit in medicine when often it should not be so. A prescribed medication is valued for its "specific" medical influence, as deemed beneficial by randomized (placebo-) controlled trials (RCTs). This research focuses on the effects of the drug and attempts to control the context to reduce "nonspecific" (placebo) effects that may compromise the results. This helps physicians understand the specific effects of the drugs they prescribe, but it does not value those nonspecific effects that surround the prescribing of a medication. It is impossible, even undesirable, to remove all nonspecific effects from the patient encounter (Moerman and Jonas, 2002). "Meaning" and "context" effects are rooted in relationship-centered care, including empathy, trust, empowerment, and hope (Walach

Table 2-2 Optimal Healing Environments

Inner Environment to the Outer Environment

Healing Intention	Personal Wholeness	Healing Relationships	Healing Organizations	Healthy Lifestyles	Integrative Collaborative Medicine	Healing Spaces
Expectation	Mind	Compassion	Leadership	Diet	Person oriented	Nature
Hope	Body	Empathy	Mission	Movement	Conventional	Light
Understanding	Spirit	Social support	Culture	Relaxation	Complementary	Color
Belief	Family	Communication	Teamwork	Addictions	Culturally appropriate	Architecture
	Community					
Enhance awareness expectancy.	Enhance personal integration.	Enhance caring communication.	Enhance delivery process.	Enhance healthy habits.	Enhance medical care.	Enhance healing structure.

Modified from Jonas WB, Chez RA. Toward optimal healing environments in health care. *J Altern Complement Med.* 2004;10(suppl 1):S1-S6.

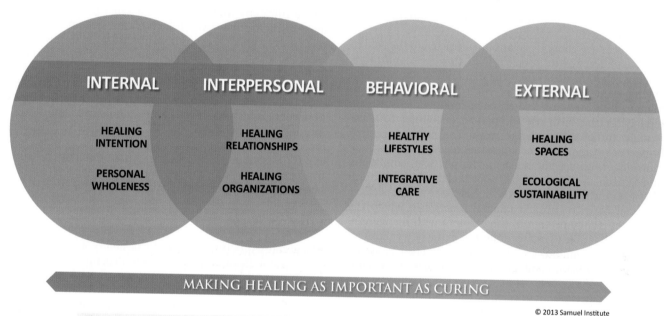

Figure 2-2 Optimal healing environments. (Used with permission from Samueli Institute, **www.SamueliInstitute.org**.)

and Jonas, 2004) Research on one of the most frequently prescribed drugs in primary care, selective serotonin reuptake inhibitors (SSRIs), shows that these work only about 6% to 9% better than placebos for mild to moderate depression (Kirsch et al., 2002; Turner et al., 2008). Both placebos and drugs work well and are often almost 60% effective. Therefore, if the drug only accounts for 9% of this effect, which factor accounts for the majority of the healing influence? Maybe researchers are not giving enough credit to the clinician and the nonspecific variables that surround the prescribing of the pill. Maybe it is simply the act of listening to people who are suffering and giving them a sense of understanding that there is something they can do to overcome the suffering. Maybe it is the interaction between two people before the medicine is prescribed that has the greatest healing effect. Psychiatrists gifted at developing a trusting relationship were found to have better effects with placebo in treating depression than their colleagues less talented at developing relationships who used active drugs (McKay et al., 2006). Acupuncture delivered with an enhanced clinical human encounter produces better effects than the same points treated by clinicians who do not form a therapeutic relationship (Kaptchuk et al., 2008; Kelley et al., 2009).

Family physicians do not need to wait for further research to create an OHE for patient care. Physicians already know that the factors summarized in Table 2-2 and Figure 2-2 help encourage the healthy unfolding of complex systems no matter what the disease or treatment. The most important part in influencing healing in others is focused on the left side of the table and starts with a self-reflective, internal process. Family physicians first need to understand the importance of continuously exploring their own awareness and health so they are prepared to do the same for their patients.

THE IMPORTANCE OF SELF-CARE

To care deeply for others, we must know how to care for ourselves. As Cassell (2004) says, "... virtually all the doctor's healing power flows from the doctor's self-mastery." True primary care, therefore, also includes what we do for ourselves. Up to 60% of practicing physicians report symptoms of "burnout" (Shanafelt et al., 2003; Spickard et al., 2002) with a higher incidence in primary care (Shanafelt, et al., 2012). This is associated with emotional exhaustion, depersonalization (seeing patients as objects), reduced empathy, and the loss of meaning in work. (See Chapter 6, Care of the Self.)

The characteristics lost in burnout are important ingredients in facilitating health and healing in others. If the health team physician leader is "burning out," the health home will not be healthy. When physicians practice healthy lifestyle behaviors, they are more likely to educate patients on the importance of these behaviors (Lewis et al., 1991) and to become more motivating to their patients toward positive change (Frank et al., 2000; Lobelo et al., 2009). Family physicians benefit from a self-reflective inquiry about personal balance toward health. This behavior will constantly be challenged and will require attention and "mastery."

Most primary care physicians are attracted to the field to make a difference in people's lives through continuous healing relationships. When the demands of the working environment tax the sense of control to maintain these relationships, stress and potential burnout can ensue. One remedy for this is to use the patient encounter to allow *meaning* to flow through the work. The healing-oriented primary care approach recognizes each patient as a unique individual with specific needs in the physical, emotional, and spiritual domains and sets aside both mental space and physical time to deal with those needs. To be aware of these personal needs requires a mindful practice in which the physician is fully present in the moment with the patient, where each is able to reduce suffering in the other (Epstein, 1999). This "mindfulness" approach has been found to enhance well-being and physician attitudes in patient-centered care (Krasner et al., 2009) and reduce stress, anxiety, and depression in primary care clinicians (Fortney, et al., 2013). It requires that physicians create physical time in the health home to sit and listen to patient stories (Rakel, 2008).

INVESTING IN RELATIONSHIP

The medical home is just that, a "home" where someone feels welcome, known, and part of a community. The ongoing relationship with patients provides insight into the complexity of their health care needs and honors the interactions among multiple health perspectives. It allows the clinician to use evidence-based guidelines while realizing that variability is the norm. The best care for one individual may not be best for another. Patient-centered care recognizes that care should be focused on the needs of the individual patient, not simply on a disease state. Ideally, the goal should be "relationship centered," encouraging attention to the unique needs of the patient to be well. Thus, creating healing relationships is a core goal of an effective medical home (Chez and Jonas, 2005).

The evidence for the benefits of continuous, relationship-centered primary care is solid and growing (Neumann et al., 2010). It has been found to improve quality of care (Starfield, 1991), reduce expenditures on diagnostic testing (Epstein et al., 2005), reduce hospital admissions (Gill and Mainous,

1998), and lower total health care costs (De Maeseneer et al., 2003). Having continuous, ongoing relationships with patients is often cited as the most rewarding aspect of being a family physician (Fairhurst and May, 2006). A systematic review of controlled trials on effective "team care," in which relationship-centered factors are formalized in the care process, has demonstrated reduced mortality and morbidity, improved morale of health care workers, and reduced costs of health care (Safran et al., 2006). Patients with diabetes who are cared for by physicians who rate high in empathy have lower Hgb A1C and low-density lipoprotein cholesterol levels (Hojat et al., 2011).

One health care system that restructured its whole organization around establishing long-term, trusting, accountable relationships in the community is the Southcentral Foundation Alaska Native Health Care model (Eby, 2007). This was the main request of the leaders of native Alaskans when they were asked what they wanted most in their public-owned health care system. Above all else, they valued the relationship with their physician, someone who "listens to them and takes time to explain things and who is able to coordinate effectively their overall care" (Gottlieb, 2007). The system made this its primary objective. This focus not only delivered a better patient experience, but it also improved clinical outcomes. After transforming their health model in 1999, urgent care and emergency department utilization decreased by 40%, specialist utilization by 50%, and hospitalization days by 30%. Customer satisfaction surveys showed that 91% rated their overall care as "favorable" (Gottlieb et al., 2008).

EMPOWERMENT

The greatest amount of suffering, disability, and cost occurs when the individual becomes more dependent on tertiary health care. The goal of the primary health team is to reduce this need. This requires that physicians empower individuals, families, and communities to understand what they can do to reduce the risk of disease and move the acuity curve in Figure 2-3 to the left. This will increase control of health by the individual, family, and community, with less dependence on the health care industry. To understand how best to work toward this goal, it is important to understand the process of empowerment.

Empowerment does not mean that patients do what is asked of them; this is *compliance*. Noncompliance is two people working toward different goals. Empowerment is a way of interacting in which accurate information is provided in a manner understandable to the individual that both respects and promotes patients' ability to make decisions for themselves. A patient's decision making occurs in the "inner," personal environment, influenced by external issues such as culture, family, peer group, work, and payment for care. Anderson and Funnell (2009) describe this well in their research on empowerment and diabetes care, reporting that 98% of diabetes care is "patient directed." When a patient is told to act a certain way, it is successful less than 5% of the time.

Empowerment is both a process and an outcome. The *process* requires that a health care partner recognizes individuals' unique needs and helps them think critically to make informed decisions on which they choose to act. This results in an *outcome* that individuals decide is best for them and their current situations. Health care practitioners cannot control their patients' decisions and thus cannot own the outcome. The clinician can recognize the psychosocial and emotional underpinnings that allow positive change to take place and then gradually and supportively work with the patient toward positive behaviors. As the

health guide of the community, the relationship-centered health home requires the development of health teams to facilitate this change.

Health Teams

Patient-centered, healing-focused care requires that primary care physicians evolve beyond "physician-centered care" that is restricted by the dwindling access of the one-on-one physician visit. The family physician of the future can be a leader in the creation of a team of health professionals who provide multiple paths to access care (Figure 2-4) (Grumbach and Bodenheimer, 2004). This may involve group visits, phone contact, e-mail, Facebook, Twitter, photo and video access, and other use of information technology. The goal should be a proactive, collaborative team effort that is not restricted to the in-office encounter and continuously moving toward meeting patient goals, not just expecting adherence to treatment guidelines (Nutting et al., 2009). Healing-oriented teams include the most appropriate clinicians for the health needs of the community. This process may be physician-led but not necessarily physician-dominant and may include nurses and nurse practitioners, physician assistants, psychologists and counselors, allied health practitioners, complementary and alternative practitioners, health coaches, and others to provide more effective care while reducing the threat of a physician shortage (Bodenheimer and Smith, 2013). Administrative office

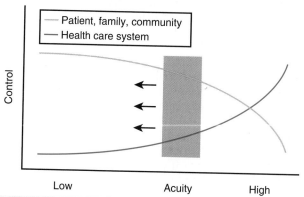

Figure 2-3 The Alaska Native Health Care model moved the slashed lines to the left, reducing dependence on the health care system and increasing control of the family. The goal is to flatten the curves to the right. The health care system should empower the family and community to maintain control of their health and make people less dependent on the "health rescue." (Modified from Gottlieb K, Sylvester I, Eby D. Transforming your practice: what matters most. *Fam Pract Manag.* 2008;15:32-38.)

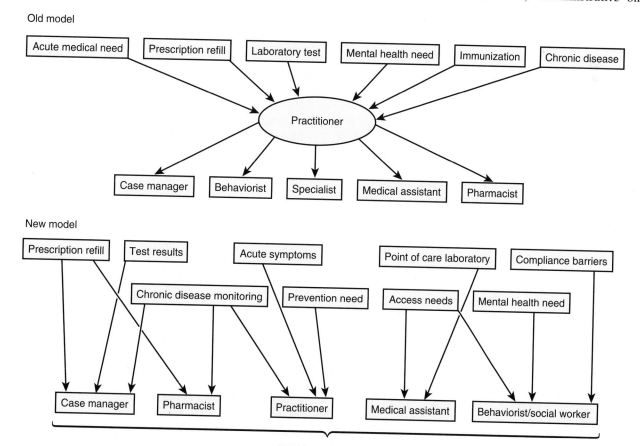

Figure 2-4 Traditional model versus new model of care showing multiple ways to access the health home (medical home).

Table 2-3 Defining Disciplinary Teams

Term	Definition
Multidisciplinary team	**Additive.** Composed of "more than two professionals from different health care disciplines who work with the same patient, set of patients, or clinical condition, but provide care independently of each other" (Choi and Pak, 2006) (interdisciplinary team building). For example, a patient may have visits with both a primary care practitioner (PCP) and physical therapist (PT). Although the PCP may view clinical notes or a report from the PT, the practitioners from the two disciplines usually do not interact.
Interdisciplinary team	**Interactive.** An ongoing and integrated care team of one patient, set of patients, or clinical condition. Team members develop collegial relationships with shared goals and joint decision making. They interact, supporting as well as questioning each other's opinions, and negotiate to develop health strategies based on the needs of the individual.
Transdisciplinary team	**Holistic.** Professionals learn from each other and in the process transcend traditional disciplinary boundaries, which may result in new knowledge. Often, the greater the difference between professions (epistemologic distance; e.g., engineering and humanities), the more likely insight will develop toward the creation of a new way to solve a problem.

Data from Choi BC, Pak AW. Multidisciplinarity, interdisciplinarity and transdisciplinarity in health research, services, education and policy. 1. Definitions, objectives, and evidence of effectiveness. *Clin Invest Med.* 2006;29:351-364 and Choi BC, Pak AW. Multidisciplinarity, interdisciplinarity and transdisciplinarity in health research, services, education and policy. 3. Discipline, inter-discipline distance, and selection of discipline. *Clin Invest Med.* 2008;31:E41-E48.

staff, with their frequent patient interactions, are also key members of the healing team, and, of course, the patient and his or her family, friends, caregivers, and community members frequently participate in important ways.

In 2003, the Robert Wood Johnson Foundation supported research to bring behavior change initiatives into primary care to address inactivity, unhealthy eating, smoking, and risky drinking (Cifuentes et al., 2005). Lessons learned from 17 practice-based research networks showed that health behavior change resources are enthusiastically received by practices and patients (Cohen et al., 2005; Woolf et al., 2005), and that practices that use multifaceted team-based interventions are more effective in promoting healthy behaviors than those providing isolated therapy (Goldstein et al., 2004; Prada, 2006; Solberg et al., 2000; Woolf et al., 2005).

When working within teams, it is important to understand the difference among multidisciplinary, interdisciplinary, and transdisciplinary team models (Table 2-3). Traditional *multidisciplinary* teams are often focused on disease states and are limited to specific organ systems. In multidisciplinary teams, clinicians work in isolation, with limited communication and collaboration. These models tend to focus on body parts or systems in isolation, not recognizing their interdependency. Developing a common

goal of health facilitation allows professionals to come together to develop *interdisciplinary* teams that encourage insight toward new ways of problem solving not previously in the group's consciousness. When a new insight develops, the interdisciplinary team becomes a *transdisciplinary* team as its members develop novel ways to create (or promote) health that transcend the "siloed" model of care (Choi and Pak, 2006; Soklaridis et al., 2007).

Accountable care organizations (ACOs) are an example of *interdisciplinary* communication and coordination of care to eliminate waste while improving care for specific disease-based conditions such as congestive heart failure (Berwick and Hackbarth, 2012). Although ACOs will benefit from patient-centered medical homes, they continue to focus within a disease-care paradigm and thus are not an example of *transdisciplinary* care. *Transdisciplinary* care will require teams that partner with patients and help them achieve their health goals. This transcendence asks the patient, "What do you want your health for?" The answer will direct the energy of the team, and the disease will often improve as a consequence.

WHO SHOULD COMPRISE THE HEALTH TEAM?

The family physician knows the population of the community served and their specific health care needs. This insight will define the professionals who will be of most benefit for health creation (promotion). For example, obesity is a significant health threat in many locales. A team of professionals working together toward sustained optimal weight for patients might include a registered dietician, an exercise physiologist, and a psychologist or mind–body practitioner to understand the interplay between stress and eating. The process to develop a health-oriented team for musculoskeletal health (back pain) is summarized in Table 2-4.

The health team may look different from a disease team, but there will be obvious overlap. For example, a health home may include a nutritionist or health coach who works with patients who have diabetes. This team member can also provide counseling for prediabetic persons and overweight youths to prevent the expression of a disease that is influenced by lifestyle choices.

HEALTH TEAM MODELS

There are many ways to develop health-oriented teams. The approach will depend on the needs of patients, the population served, the availability of team members, the size of the clinic, strategic needs, and the support of administration and clinic staff. Teams can be initiated in all sizes of clinics, from large, complex institutions to small, rural settings, and may take many forms. For example, a team may include only the family physician and two health coaches or medical assistants. This "teamlet" model extends the office visit to include communication before, during, and after the visit (Bodenheimer and Laing, 2007). The teamlet uses these opportunities to address patient needs and develops appropriate strategies. The health team's common mission is working toward the greatest improvement in the patient's quality of life.

The team members do not need to share the same space as long as they maintain communication and build

Table 2-4 Health-Oriented Team Creation Worksheet (Example: Achieving Optimal Back Health)

Task	Action
Health need of my community	Achieving optimal back health
Identify professionals to address health need.	1. Manual practitioner 2. Physical therapist 3. Psychologist or "mindfulness" instructor 4. Health coach
Delineate the team-focused goal/mission.	To empower patients to learn how to achieve their ideal back function and health
Name the health-oriented program.	"Back to Health" program
Create relationships among team members.	Team members to meet initially to develop program goal or mission and methods of interacting; periodic meetings as needed for team building and interactions around patient issues
Agree on team communication method.	Fax or e-mail will be sent to the team for referrals, findings, and discussion.
Follow up and promote sustainability.	Patient will meet periodically with health coach or nurse at the medical home to sustain lifestyle behaviors.

intermember relationships. This helps clinicians learn of each other's interests and talents in relation to common goals, fostering mutual understanding, trust, and respect. Without the team concept, there will simply be separate therapies and professionals working in isolation, causing fragmentation of care.

The most important ingredient in effective teams is trust—trust that each team member will play his or her particular part in care delivery and process improvement (Sargeant et al., 2008). Changing to an effective team approach takes humility and time and requires constant fine tuning and quality improvement. Miller and Crabtree (2005) have developed a comprehensive model of team care operations and describe effective techniques to build effective team processes. However, the physician can begin in any domain that fits the readiness of the practice (see Table 2-4), and the effects will often spread to other domains. The following checklist provides some places to start in a practice assessment format.

The Health Home Checklist

- Create a "home" where those who enter feel known and welcome. Patients will remember how they *felt* in a health home longer than what they are told. This starts with how they are greeted when then come in.
- Create a common mission supported by all health home members; for example, "To invest in a continuous healing relationship for the well-being of the community we serve."
- Provide multiple ways to access care from the most appropriate health professional, including using technology to provide interaction outside the office encounter (see Figure 2-4).

- Provide a variety of encounter visits that complement the one-on-one office visit. These may include group visits, e-mail, video access, support groups, and health promotion or disease-focused programs.
- Create relationships through open communication with a team of health professionals who are configured specifically for each patient to positively influence lifestyle behaviors or address specific disease states and management needs.
- Provide a way for the consumers (patients) to have input into what health-related programs or services are implemented based on their perceived needs and explicit goals.
- Provide an opportunity to understand the most important areas that patients believe need to be addressed for their long-term health. (See eBox 2-1, health agreement document online.)
- Learn to provide rapid and evidence-based information on lifestyle and conventional and complementary medicine in each team encounter.
- Review the space of the practice and develop a plan to make it less stress-inducing and more comfortable and conducive to communication and operations for the patient and team members.
- Make sure the health home resonates with that which gives family physicians meaning and purpose in their work. This will translate across the medical home, encouraging team acceptance while reducing the risk of burnout.

Lessons from Early Adaptors

A national demonstration project was launched in 2006 to implement and study the patient-centered medical home model. The findings of this project confirmed that this can be done, but change is slow and should recognize the unique aspects of each individual health team and the needs of its community. A strategy that may be successful for one health home will be different for another (Crabtree et al., 2010). In fact, many of the challenges that were encountered in shifting a culture from a throughput disease model to one of patient empowerment and population management are similar to the challenges seen in facilitating health in complex systems (Bitton et al., 2012). The characteristics of effective PCMH were found to include:

Interpersonal autonomy. Physicians needed to learn to work with teams, and the teams needed to understand and identify with their new roles (Cronholm et al., 2013).
Uniqueness. Every site had its own underlying story that influenced the projects they would work on. The talents and expertise of the team often directed projects that resulted in the most success (Alexander et al., 2013).
Leadership engagement. Success requires commitment from system leaders to provide resources needed for sustainability (True et al., 2013).
Communication. Invest in a communication plan that may include regular meetings and access to patients and team members through electronic health records for ongoing coordination of care and interprofessional collaboration.

Payment. It is difficult to sustain new payment models if there is no support for non–face-to-face work that is required to improve access and value. Be an advocate for policy change that pays for coordinated team-based care and the health outcomes the team has as their priority.

Patience. Creating patient-centered medical homes cannot be done in isolation because they are a foundational ingredient of a larger health care system that takes time to change. Celebrate each small step toward this cultural transformation.

Payment Models for the Health Home

In the past several years, it has become clear that a simple, office visit only, episode-based, disease treatment model alone will not allow for the optimal delivery of the patient-centered medical home. Although several elements of the Affordable Care Act favor the PCMH, transition to an effective payment model will be essential of those elements to work. Recently, the AAFP has embarked on a rethinking of how to align payment models for the "health home" (Family Medicine 2.0), examining everything from bundled capitated, per patient, per month models to blended models that still optimize preventive and postvisit care. Primary care is at the center of our health care delivery system and affects the functioning of both downstream care (tertiary, hospital, and emergency department care) and upstream care (prevention and population health). Family physicians can be the leaders in these efforts by pushing for the widespread adoption of global payment models as soon as possible even if they currently do not rely on those models for payment. The time for adequate investment in primary care has come.

Conclusion

Creating OHEs with health-oriented teams honors the concepts of the medical home as primary care physicians transition from medical care to health creation as a critical focus (see Table 2-2 and Figure 2-2). This is an exciting opportunity for professionals from varied disciplines to come together to work toward a common goal. The family physician's expertise in understanding the interplay of biopsychosocial systems makes this profession uniquely qualified to lead the implementation of these models of care.

The gift of primary care is the human connection that occurs within continuous healing relationships. Family physicians will succeed in providing efficient, cost-effective quality care if they invest in ingredients that are the most valuable yet most difficult to measure, the most important one being that nonquantifiable bond of intention, trust, and communication between the practitioner and patient in which both are transformed (Scott et al., 2008).

EVIDENCE-BASED SUMMARY

- Positive lifestyle behaviors have the largest effect on reducing morbidity and mortality for chronic disease (Khaw et al., 2008; McGinnis et al., 2002; Schroeder, 2007) (SOR: A).
- Team-based interventions are more effective in promoting healthy behaviors than are those that provide isolated therapy (Safran et al., 2006; Woolf et al., 2005) (SOR: B).
- Relationship-centered care improves quality of care and clinical outcomes (Starfield, 1991) (SOR: B).
- Relationship-centered care reduces health care costs (De Maeseneer et al., 2003; Epstein et al., 2005) (SOR: B).

Summary of Additional Online Content

The following content is available at www.expertconsult.com:
eBox 2-1 Health Agreement

References

The complete reference list is available online at www.expertconsult.com.

Web Resources

www.aafp.org/pcmh: Resources on the patient-centered medical home (PCMH) from the American Academy of Family Physicians.

http://www.pcpcc.org/about/medical-home: Patient-Centered Primary Care Collaborative site that includes a video to educate staff and colleagues about the PCMH.

samueliinstitute.org/our-research/optimal-healing-environments/ohe-framework: A graphic illustrating the components of an OHE.

samueliinstitute.org/our-services/assessment: A 360-degree assessment tool for making your clinic or health care setting an optimal healing environment.

www.transformed.com/Delta-Exchange: A community of clinicians, tools, and resources to help clinics transform to a PCMH (requires a monthly fee). Guides for creating an OHE in health care from the Samueli Institute.

www.transformed.com/mhiq/welcome.cfm: Module to calculate your medical home IQ. Gives a baseline practice assessment toward the creation of a medical home.

www.transformed.com/resources.cfm: Resources from TransforMED on transforming a medical practice to a medical home.

3 Psychosocial Influences on Health

SYED M. AHMED, PAUL J. HERSHBERGER, and JEANNE PARR LEMKAU

Key Points

- Factors that influence health include age, gender, and sexual orientation.
- Religious, ethnic, and cultural groups affect individual functioning.
- Individuals are affected by family composition, structure, and functioning.
- The health of an individual is influenced by work and school status.
- Individuals are affected by their social support network and significant others.
- Financial resources, including health insurance status, affect health status.
- Personal and family history of major loss, trauma, or illness should be integrated into the assessment of a patient's health status.

- Psychological functioning, including personality, defensive style, and current mental status, warrants evaluation.
- Self-control is a limited resource that can be replenished with healthy food, sleep, and practice.
- Data about the patient's physical environment, including home, neighborhood, and environmental hazards, are essential.
- The physician should elicit an account of recent stressors and changes in the patient's life.
- A collaborative physician–patient relationship that emphasizes physician listening is the foundation for sensitive psychosocial care.

- An overweight 11-year-old boy with abnormal lipids tells his family physician that his favorite activity is playing online video games.
- A middle-aged woman emphatically asserts that her blood pressure is elevated only when she has it taken in a medical setting.
- A single mother with a part-time job but no health insurance tells her doctor that she can only take medications that have low co-pays.

Psychosocial factors influence health. Assessing and treating patients in a manner that integrates psychosocial and biologic aspects of care is the essence of excellent family medicine and its greatest challenge. The following example is illustrative.

Mr. Ramirez is a 52-year-old man who lost his well-paying job as a software engineer several years ago. After 8 months of unemployment, he took a less satisfying job for less money. Mr. Ramirez has type II diabetes, diagnosed when he was 45 years old and well-controlled before he lost his job. He has taken diabetes education classes and can accurately describe what he must do to maintain good glucose control. Reluctantly, Mr. Ramirez acknowledges to his physician that he does not follow his diet as closely as he

once did and more frequently eats fast food. He also misses the exercise facility at his former workplace and struggles with motivation to exercise. His marriage "isn't as good as it used to be," and he reports decreased interest in sex. When the physician asks him about feelings of depression, Mr. Ramirez says that he never thought he was a weak person, but he just does not enjoy things as he once did. His physician summarizes the changes Mr. Ramirez has experienced in the past few years and acknowledges the emotional toll of such stress. She briefly describes how stress and depression make diabetes more difficult to control and how she and Mr. Ramirez can collaboratively work on strategies to improve his health and quality of life.

This case highlights the following three imperatives for providing care that is appropriately responsive to psychosocial issues:

1. The physician sees the person first, conceptualizing symptoms and behaviors in his social and psychological context and responding with sensitivity to the patient's experience and priorities.
2. The physician understands the interactive nature of multiple biopsychosocial variables and communicates this effectively to the patient.

Table 3-1   Psychosocial Influences: Conceptual Models

Biopsychosocial model
Systems approach
Stress and coping model
Life span perspective
Ethnomedical cultural model

Table 3-2   Five-Factor Model of Personality

1. Openness to experience: tendency to be curious and appreciative of a variety of experiences
2. Conscientiousness: proclivity to be self-disciplined, to plan, and to direct behavior toward achieving goals
3. Extraversion: preference for being around other people and to be enthusiastic and socially energetic
4. Agreeableness: inclination to be cooperative with others; strongly preferring harmony over disagreement
5. Neuroticism: propensity to experience negative emotions on an ongoing and regular basis

3. The physician fosters a supportive and empathic physician–patient relationship to provide the foundation for gathering information and intervening effectively.

As the case illustrates, biomedical factors may be only a small part of what patients bring to their physicians. The biomedical model, based on the assumptions of mind–body dualism, biologic reductionism, and linear causality, has resulted in miraculous achievements of high-technology medicine, but primary care physicians who restrict their attention to purely medical considerations are of limited use to their patients. Nevertheless, the shift from a biomedical to a biopsychosocial paradigm has been a major challenge to modern medicine.

In 1977, psychiatrist George Engel proposed a biopsychosocial model that included social and psychological variables as crucial determinants of disease and illness. According to his new framework, the subsystems of the body interact to produce successively more complex biologic systems, which are simultaneously affected by social and psychological factors. The organism is thus conceptualized in terms of complex interacting systems of biologic, psychological, and social forces, and neither disease nor illness is seen as understandable only in terms of smaller and smaller biologic components. Engel (1980) believed that systemic interactions of biopsychosocial factors were relevant to all disease processes and to the individual's experience of illness. Accordingly, understanding a person's response to a disease requires consideration of such interacting factors as the social and cultural environment, the individual's psychological resources, and the biochemistry and genetics of the disorder in the population (Brody, 1999).

In the following section, we present a number of conceptual models and perspectives that emphasize different but overlapping psychosocial dimensions that influence health (Table 3-1). These models can aid practicing physicians in thinking about their patients in psychosocial context and conceptualizing potentially helpful interventions. Subsequently, we elaborate on practical strategies for gathering and using psychosocial information in clinical practice and discuss a pragmatic approach to addressing psychosocial considerations in primary care. We conclude with brief discussions of evidence-based practice and how current challenges and trends in the health care system may affect the practice of family medicine.

Conceptual Models

THE BIOPSYCHOSOCIAL MODEL

As previously noted, the biopsychosocial model was proposed as a scientific paradigm by Engel (1977), who encouraged the clinician to observe biochemical and morphologic changes in relation to a patient's emotional patterns, life goals, attitudes toward illness, and social environment. Engel proposed that the brain and peripheral organs were linked in complex, mutually adjusting relationships, affected by changes in social as well as physical stimuli. Within this model, environmental and psychological stress is seen as potentially pathogenic for the individual. Emotions may serve as the organism's bridge between the meaning (or significance) of stressful events and the changes in physiologic function (Zegans, 1983). Engel urged physicians to evaluate the patient on biologic, psychological, and social factors to understand and manage clinical problems effectively (Wise, 1997). For example, a workplace accident could be seen as resulting from poorly designed equipment (social) and inattentiveness (psychological) brought about by low blood sugar (biologic). Similarly, the accident could result in damage to internal organs (biologic), distress (psychological), and lost income (social), any or all of which may become the focus of physician intervention.

Comprehensive evaluation of biopsychosocial dimensions would assess the following:

- Biologic factors, including genetics, medical history, and environmental factors that affect physiologic functioning (e.g., those causing cancer)
- Psychological factors, including affective, cognitive, and behavioral components, such as feelings, beliefs, expectations, personality, coping style, and health behaviors (e.g., exercise, diet, smoking) that contribute to patients' experience of health and illness
- Social factors, including access to health care, quality of available health care, social systems (e.g., family, school, work, church, government), social values, customs, and social support

Further discussion of biologic influences on health is beyond the scope of this chapter. Psychological and social factors known to affect health are discussed next.

Psychological Factors

Numerous psychological factors affect health. We discuss here a common approach to personality, the five-factor model, and an essential psychological resource for healthy behavior, self-control. We also review key findings from the literature on the relationship between emotions and health.

The most prominent approach to personality at present is the five-factor model (Goldberg, 1993). The five broad personality domains of this model, for which OCEAN is an acronym, are openness to experience, conscientiousness, extraversion, agreeableness, and neuroticism (Table 3-2). Research on the relationship of these factors to health

Table 3-3   Self-Control

Self-control is a limited resource, like a muscle. It can be replenished.
Self-control is used to:

- Regulate emotions
- Control thoughts
- Manage impulses
- Direct performance
- Make decisions

Self-control is replenished or strengthened through:

- Fuel (healthy food at regular intervals)
- Sleep
- Practice

People high in self-control tend to plan and adjust their schedules or environments to reduce demands on willpower (desired behaviors are more automatic, and temptations are minimized).

variables has generated several findings. Whereas conscientiousness has been associated with longevity among healthy individuals and better functional status in those with physical illnesses or impairments, neuroticism is consistently found to be negatively correlated with health (Bogg and Roberts, 2013; Goodwin and Friedman, 2006; Smith and Mackenzie, 2006). Agreeableness, extraversion, and openness to experience generally tend to have weaker associations with health.

Because personality style tends to be quite stable across the life span, physician focus on changing personality for health reasons is not a sensible pursuit. However, an understanding of a particular patient's personality can help guide the physician toward interventions that are more likely to be effective.

Because health behaviors are a major factor in the development of, management of, and morbidity from chronic illnesses, self-control or willpower is a critical psychological resource. Children with more self-control have been found to have better health as adults. Adults with more self-control have healthier behaviors. Research indicates that willpower operates like a muscle; it is a resource that people have in limited supply, and it can be exhausted (Baumeister and Tierney, 2011). Fortunately, it can also be replenished. Importantly, various demands for willpower draw from the same common resource. Willpower is used to control thoughts, regulate emotions, manage impulses (the task most commonly associated with willpower), and direct performance. Making decisions uses willpower. Numerous studies have demonstrated that tasks requiring willpower deplete the self-control resource, so that performance declines on subsequent tasks requiring willpower. Interestingly, when there are competing demands for the self-control resource, managing negative emotions predictably takes precedence over other demands. Given the multiple emotional and behavioral challenges associated with the management of chronic illness, a patient with excessive demands on the limited self-control resource is particularly vulnerable to worsening health. See Table 3-3 for a summary of key factors about self-control, including how it can be replenished.

The ongoing experience of chronic negative emotions (depression, anxiety, and anger) tends to be associated with poorer health. There is an extensive research literature linking negative affectivity and pessimism to adverse health outcomes (Peterson et al., 1988; Salovey et al., 2000). Although the experience of negative emotions is a natural part of the human experience, effective management of such emotions through cognitive strategies, active coping, and social support can be learned, and medications can be a helpful adjunct when negative emotional states are prolonged or severe.

Likewise, a large body of research indicates that positive emotional states are associated with better health and longevity. Happiness, optimism, and positive attitudes toward aging have been associated with 7 more years of life (Danner et al., 2001; Levy et al., 2002). Almost three decades of research have shown that an optimistic outlook has a positive effect on coping and on mental and physical health outcomes (Peterson and Steen, 2002). Family physicians have long recognized the importance of mobilizing and maintaining patient hopefulness through encouraging words that foster positive expectations of medical treatment. The demonstrated efficacy of placebos affirms the importance of this approach (Sobel, 1991).

Social Factors

A gradient between socioeconomic status (SES) and health is consistently found in epidemiologic studies (Marmot, 2004). Persons with less education and income tend to have poorer health than their better educated and richer counterparts. A recent analysis indicates that in the year 2000 in the United States, 245,000 deaths could be attributed to low education, 176,000 to racial segregation, 162,000 to low social support, and 133,000 to poverty (Galea et al., 2011). Interestingly, subjective SES (i.e., individuals' perceptions of where they view themselves on the social ladder) has an even stronger relationship to health than objective SES (Singh-Manoux et al., 2005). Negative affect, stress, pessimism, and a decreased sense of control are among the factors thought to contribute to the relationship between lower subjective SES and poorer health (Operario et al., 2004).

In general, social support reduces stress and contributes to more positive health outcomes. Social support refers to the process by which a social network provides psychological and material resources to enhance an individual's ability to cope with stress (Cohen, 2004). Both quantity and quality of support are important, and sources of support include spouses, lovers, friends, family, coworkers, and health care professionals. A person who has many friends but no confidant may have inadequate social support in a time of need. Some people report high levels of satisfaction with just a few close friends, but others require larger social networks.

There are several varieties of social support (Cohen, 2004). Emotional support involves the expression of caring, concern, and empathy toward the person and typically involves opportunities for the recipient to express emotions. Instrumental support involves providing some type of direct assistance, which might include financial resources, transportation, or help with daily tasks. Informational support involves giving advice or information relevant to an individual's situation.

Social support appears to undergird health by buffering the person against negative effects of stress, perhaps by affecting the cognitive appraisal of stress. When people encounter a strong stressor, such as a major financial crisis, individuals with high levels of social support may appraise the situation as less stressful than will those with low levels of support. Social support may further buffer the stress by modifying people's response to a stressor as they turn to friends for advice, reassurance, or material aid. Social integration, or participating in a broad range of social relationships, benefits health and well-being by enhancing self-esteem and fostering positive health behaviors in people who believe that others count on them. Social integration is beneficial, whether or not an individual is experiencing stress (Cohen, 2004).

Relationships also can involve significant negative social exchange and be harmful to health; negative interactions in troubled marriages have adverse effects on cardiovascular, endocrine, and immune system function (Robles and Kiecolt-Glaser, 2003). Recent research has found specific links between negativity in relationships and cellular aging, such as shortening telomere length (Uchino et al., 2012).

Misconceptions

Polan (1993) identified and addressed two common misconceptions about the biopsychosocial model. First, contrary to popular belief, a physician who is "humanistic" is not necessarily practicing biopsychosocial medicine. A physician can be ethical and caring but still neglect scientific knowledge from the social and behavioral sciences and relevant data from the patient's life. For example, compassion by itself is of limited usefulness to a physician who needs an effective treatment plan for a patient with asthma who smokes. Interventions should be informed by knowledge of the social environment and the individual psychology of the patient.

The second misconception is that people can be reduced to distinct biologic, psychological, and social categories or that their problems can then be expressed as a set of scientific principles from which diagnosis and treatment can be neatly derived. In fact, use of the biopsychosocial model increases rather than decreases the level of complexity required to understand patient status, introducing multiple avenues for intervention. Interpreting the biopsychosocial model as a new opportunity for reductionist thinking diminishes its power to inform more holistic treatment. Borrell-Carrio and colleagues (2004) proposed a biopsychosocially oriented clinical practice based on self-awareness, active cultivation of trust, an emotional style characterized by empathic curiosity, self-calibration to reduce bias, cultivation of emotional sensitivity to assist with diagnosis and therapeutic relationships, use of informed intuition, and communication of clinical evidence to foster dialogue.

Another important misconception is that educating patients about important biologic, psychological, social, or environmental factors will necessarily change behavior. Much of human behavior is automatic, cued by environmental or situational factors. Health behaviors are frequently less a product of thoughtful choices than of nonconscious factors (Sheeran et al., 2013). Although intention and motivation affect adherence to treatment regimens and health behavior recommendations, multiple other factors (e.g., depletion of self-control, media and peer influences, physical environment) play important roles.

THE SYSTEMS APPROACH

Humans are infinitely complex. Adequately conceptualizing a person in health or illness requires a systems approach that encompasses this complexity. The concept of systems was first developed by von Bertalanffy (1968) to refer to the dynamic interrelationships of various components. A systems approach rejects the notion of linear causality in favor of multidimensional and multidirectional models.

The systems approach has strongly influenced conceptualizations of family functioning. Smilkstein (1978) developed one of the first applications of "family systems" thinking for family medicine. Physician attention is important in the systemic interactions of family members and the impact of crisis, coping styles, and resources on family functioning. He incorporated these components into the "family APGAR" (adaptation, partnership, growth, affection, and resolve), a simple instrument and mnemonic device for assessing the functioning of a family system in health and illness (not to be confused with the newborn Apgar score).

THE STRESS AND COPING MODEL

General relationships among life stresses, coping resources, and health outcomes are presented schematically in Figure 3-1. This approach represents another example of the application of a systems model. In this model, health outcomes are impacted by how life stresses affect the individual. The effect of stress is moderated by the individual's appraisal and coping responses, personality, and the person's available social resources. Although the complex synergistic interactions that characterize these relationships are beyond the scope of this chapter, the major variables provide a basis for considering physician interventions.

Definitions of Stress

Stress has been variously defined as an environmental event, a response to an event or circumstance, and a process. One approach defines stress in terms of life events—as a stimulus—circumstances or events that require the person to adapt produce feelings of tension. These stressors may be major catastrophic events (e.g., natural disaster), major life events (e.g., death of a loved one), or recurrent daily hassles (e.g., need to manage a chronic medical condition).

Stress can also be seen as a response. For example, a person with a social phobia feels stressed at a party, experiencing a psychological state of nervousness with associated physical symptoms of dry mouth, palpitations, and sweating. This physiologic and psychological response to a stressor is often called *strain*.

A third approach emphasizes stress as a process in which "environmental demands tax or exceed the adaptive capacity of an organism, resulting in psychological and biologic changes that may place persons at risk for disease" (Cohen et al., 1995). Within this approach, stress includes stressors and strains along with the relationship between the person and the environment. The process involves transactions between the person and the environment, with each affecting and being affected by the other (Sarafino, 1990). "Adaptive capacity" is operationalized in terms of resilience and vulnerability; within this model, the physician considers aspects of a person's psychological makeup

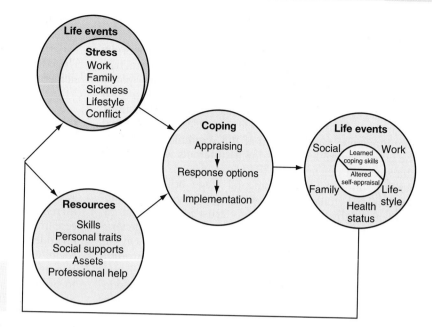

Figure 3-1 Stress, life events, and coping. (From Tunks E, Bellissimo A. *Behavioral Medicine: Concepts and Procedures*. Boston, Pergamon Press. Copyright 1991 Permagon Press.)

and social world that may render the patient more susceptible or more resilient (Steptoe, 1998).

Stress Appraisal and Coping

Every family physician sees patients under stress who present with a wide spectrum of stress-related symptoms and coping responses. How the individual interprets and copes with stress are as significant as the stressor itself. Cognitive appraisal of a stressor, rather than severity or duration alone, determines physiologic and behavioral responses (Epel et al., 1998).

Coping refers to how individuals manage the real or imagined discrepancy between environmental demands and their resources for addressing the stressful situation. According to Lazarus and Folkman (1984), adaptation to stress is mediated by appraisal (i.e., personal meaning of a stressor and one's sense of resources for dealing with it) and coping (i.e., thoughts and behaviors used to manage stress). Whereas with emotion-focused coping, a person directs energy to regulating internal feeling states, with problem-focused coping, a person directs attention to reducing the stressor or expanding resources for dealing with it (Sarafino, 1990). The effect of stressful life events on health is determined by many factors related to coping, including cognitive style, personality characteristics, and social and behavioral tendencies.

Personal Control

An individual's perception of the extent of his or her control in a stressful circumstance is a critical component of the appraisal process in coping. This includes control over the stressor as well as control over one's responses, whether problem-focused or emotion-focused. How a person deals with the loss of control precipitated by stressful life events can affect health outcomes.

Personal control can be defined as the feeling that one can make decisions and take effective action to produce desirable outcomes and avoid undesirable ones (Rodin,

1986). Mobilizing a strong sense of personal control can significantly reduce the impact of stressors on the individual, particularly when the response is appropriate to the circumstance. Sarafino (1990) classified personal control into the following five types:

1. Behavioral control involves the ability to take concrete action to reduce the impact of a stressor. For example, using a special breathing technique may help reduce pain.
2. Cognitive control involves the ability to use thought processes or strategies to modify the impact of a stressor. For example, focusing on a pleasant thought during suturing of a laceration may decrease the pain sensation.
3. Decisional control involves the opportunity to choose among alternative procedures or courses of action. For example, a victim of domestic violence may benefit from considering various options for when and how she will leave her abuser.
4. Informational control involves the opportunity to obtain knowledge about a stressful event, what will happen, why, and what consequences are likely. For example, a patient may feel less anxious about upcoming surgery upon learning more about managing discomfort from the procedure.
5. Retrospective control involves beliefs about causation of a stressful event after it has occurred. The attribution that the person makes about the adversity can affect future perspective and behavior. For example, attributing misfortune to factors that are temporary and specific leaves an individual feeling more optimistic than when misfortune is attributed to stable and global factors (Seligman, 1990).

Life stresses affect health outcomes. These effects are moderated not only by individual differences in genetics and pathophysiology but also by psychosocial factors. Psychosocial influences include appraisal and coping, personality traits, cognitive style, and such resources as social support.

THE LIFE SPAN PERSPECTIVE

The life span perspective emphasizes the importance of an individual's place on his or her personal developmental trajectory. Past development, current status, and anticipated developmental changes and challenges are taken into account. On the biologic level, changes in cellular functions occur from infancy through old age; decline in physical stamina is one manifestation of this dynamic change. On the psychological level, personality interacts with ongoing changes that occur across the life span (e.g., becoming a parent), and each developmental stage brings its own psychosocial challenges. Erikson's eight stages of development highlight the importance of trust issues in infancy, autonomy issues in early childhood, and issues of generativity and meaning in old age (Erickson, 1959). On the social level, family and peer relationships change throughout life, with significant implications for health, which may be either positive or negative. For example, the typical adolescent's shift toward greater reliance on peer relationships may lead to behaviors that endanger health, such as smoking or substance abuse. The death of a husband who has been physically abusive may lead to improved well-being for the surviving wife. The primary care physician needs to keep the life span model in mind and assist patients in addressing psychosocial factors that facilitate or block health and development.

THE ETHNOMEDICAL CULTURAL MODEL

Every encounter between a patient and a physician is a cross-cultural transaction. Each person brings to the physician–patient relationship a unique mix of culturally embedded attitudes, knowledge, and beliefs. Ethnicity, gender, religion, language, education, and personal history shape expectations and behavior on both sides of the relationship. A physician's cultural proficiency is instrumental in establishing rapport and gathering information for accurate and comprehensive diagnosis and treatment (Carrillo et al., 1999). The patient's acculturation status and cultural background are important to understand, and physicians should become familiar with the dominant cultural groups they serve.

The ethnomedical cultural model emphasizes cultural concepts relevant to health and illness (Kleinman et al., 1978), including patient beliefs and expectations about the body, illness, and treatment. Berlin and Fowkes (1983) operationalize this model in clinical encounters with their LEARN acronym, exhorting physicians to do the following:

- Listen with empathy a nd understanding to the patient's perception of the problem by eliciting the patient's explanatory model for the illness.
- Explain your perceptions or explanatory model in language the patient can understand.
- Acknowledge the differences and similarities between your explanatory model and that of the patient and discuss any significant discrepancies.
- Recommend treatment that you decide is optimal within your explanatory model.
- Negotiate treatment with the patient, seeking a compromise that is acceptable to the patient, is consistent with

your ethical standards, and uses the patient's social network when necessary.

The ethnomedical cultural model highlights cross-cultural elements in all physician–patient interactions.

Integration of Psychosocial Issues in Clinical Practice

Wynne (2003) states, "In the 'real' world of health care, systems thinking is more needed than ever before, but its increased complexity challenges both clinicians and researchers to the depths of their resources." Knowledge, attitudes, beliefs, emotions, behaviors, relationships, and social/environmental factors interact to affect the experience of illness or well-being. Accordingly, physicians' ability to promote health and relieve suffering depends on their ability to engage effectively in this complex web of interrelationships. This is a daunting task that depends on fostering a quality relationship over time, gathering sufficient biopsychosocial data about each patient, and integrating data with theoretic understanding to inform interventions.

The challenge for even the most astute physician is to assess and address psychosocially important issues within the limited time available for each patient. In a 10- to 15-minute period, a detailed evaluation of all relevant psychosocial factors is an impractical goal. Using a pragmatic approach that balances this goal with time constraints, a physician can maintain awareness of psychosocial cues and information in all patient encounters while restricting direct inquiry, depending on the specific situation. A physician may not need to elicit a detailed psychosocial assessment with every patient who presents with an upper respiratory infection, but knowing if the patient smokes would be useful, leading to further inquiry and potential smoking intervention.

Following pragmatic considerations, a physician should work collaboratively with patients to identify problems of highest priority and to address less pressing issues in subsequent encounters. For example, in the case of domestic violence, immediate needs for patient safety must be addressed. Addressing long-standing issues, such as dysfunctional means of coping with stress, must be a secondary concern in the face of the primary need to achieve safety. Similarly, every physician learns to place high priority on patient complaints of chest pain, adjusting questioning depending on the patient's age, gender, family history of coronary heart disease, and patient medical history. Nevertheless, the physician must look for psychosocial clues, evaluate stressors, and be aware of factors that suggest an anxiety or somatization disorder. These secondary factors can be addressed in more depth when the physician is assured that a cardiac crisis is not imminent.

COLLECTION OF PSYCHOSOCIAL DATA

In family practice settings, the most common and natural approach to gathering psychosocial data is interviewing the patient over time. Freud suggested that the major achievements of healthy development were the abilities "to work and to love," and this is often a good place to start. Where does this patient work, and how does he or she feel about the job, school, or household responsibilities? Who is "family" for this patient, and what is the nature of the support system? Detailed inquiries about work and love made in the context of the ongoing physician–patient relationship result in significant accretion of knowledge over time and make it easy to flag stressful changes in these important arenas.

Other important areas of inquiry include the patient's physical and social environment. Factors such as the quality of housing, neighborhood, food, and financial resources all affect patient safety, health care use, family stress, and physical health. Understanding the ethnic, religious, and political culture of a patient and family is important for guiding culturally appropriate care. Personal and family history, usually gathered gradually over time, can alert the physician to important family coping patterns, strengths, and liabilities. Of special importance is information on major personal family "dislocations," including losses, illness, and trauma. Knowledge of any traumatic encounters with previous health professionals or with previous medical procedures may help the physician anticipate and manage potential crisis situations.

Information from patient dialogue can be supplemented by standard measures such as health questionnaires (e.g., Short Form 36); screening inventories (e.g., Beck Depression Inventory); and stress, coping, and social support tools. Other means of gathering relevant data include informal interviews with family members, structured assessments (e.g., family APGAR), review of existing records (e.g., school records), consultation with nonmedical colleagues (e.g., psychologist, occupational therapist), observation of the patient's environment through home visits, and consultation with cultural informants and translators. Perhaps most important is the ongoing use of open-ended questions, so that important psychosocial data are elicited from the patient in the patient's own words.

INTERVENTIONS USING PSYCHOSOCIAL DATA

A comprehensive review of interventions addressing psychosocial influences in health is beyond the scope of this chapter and would require discussions of clinical psychology, social work, nursing, occupational therapy, and public health. Even in optimal circumstances, competency can be achieved only within a limited range. Realistically, family physicians should pursue basic proficiency in selected interventional strategies and additional training in areas of interest relevant to their specific practice needs and the population they serve. Here we discuss pragmatic interventions for practicing physicians based on the general model of stress, life events, coping, and health discussed earlier.

Because health outcomes are affected by stressful life events, coping (e.g., stress appraisal), and resources (e.g., personality, social support), addressing any of these dimensions can have a positive effect on functioning. As stress increases relative to available support and coping capacities, disequilibrium results. Put simply, interventions that decrease stress or enhance support tend to improve well-being. Physician attention to factors that exacerbate or

mitigate is always valuable. For example, because a new medical diagnosis is stressful but a loving partnership is a source of support, assuring the presence of a loving family member when bad news is to be shared with a patient may lessen its negative impact. Some life events, such as the death of a supportive partner, affect several elements in the model, as the bereaved partner confronts a major loss (stress) without the person who had previously offered comfort in such times (decreased support). Not surprisingly, persons who are grieving are at higher risk for experiencing health problems (Rogers and Reich, 1988), and a focus on their support systems and coping strategies is almost always warranted.

Interventions that should be part of the standard repertoire for family physicians are those that do no harm, usually help, and use traditional skills. Specifically, physicians can work with patients directly to reduce stress, to enhance or mobilize social support resources, and to reinforce or model positive stress appraisal and coping. Direct approaches to stress reduction may include intervening in the patient's environment (e.g., arranging respite care for an older patient to relieve stress on his middle-aged daughter) and allaying a patient's unrealistic fears about an illness. Social support can be enhanced directly through the provision of more contact with the physician or indirectly through mobilizing the patient to increase contact with family or friends. Physicians can support positive coping through instilling hope, modeling optimism, and encouraging patients who adapt. Reminding patients of personal strengths previously used to confront crises is also helpful. The physician often can implement these strategies by asking questions that allow the patient to respond in a broader perspective (e.g., "What do you remember doing to help you cope with the death of your good friend several years ago?"). Especially when behavior change is indicated, collaborating in discussing options rather than giving advice is more likely to be effective. One collaborative approach that has demonstrated efficacy is motivational interviewing (Rollnick et al., 2008; Rubac et al., 2005).

In the provision of care within a biopsychosocial model, interdisciplinary teams, rather than solo practitioners, have the advantage, and physicians can have more positive impact on their patients' lives when they harness the wisdom of colleagues from other fields through referral or consultation. Depending on physician training, interest, and time, these basic categories of intervention can be supplemented by a wide range of psychosocial interventions, from family therapy to behavior modification.

IMPORTANT TIMES FOR PSYCHOSOCIAL INTERVENTIONS

Interventions that attend to psychosocial issues are especially important at specific times in the provision of family medical care. Natural transitions in the family life cycle, such as the birth of a child or the death of a spouse, call on the physician to provide empathic support, assess the patient's support system, normalize emotional reactions, and provide anticipatory guidance as patients confront changing family roles and functioning.

When adherence or lifestyle issues impinge on health, interventions that focus on biologic mechanisms alone are likely to be ineffective. The health effects of substance abuse, domestic violence, poverty, or inactivity are often best addressed through attention to social environment and psychological concerns.

A dramatic change in patient symptoms also indicates consideration of psychosocial factors. A psychosocial crisis can provoke an exacerbation of a chronic condition (e.g., rheumatoid arthritis), a new manifestation of illness (e.g., myocardial infarction), or emotional-psychiatric symptoms (e.g., anxiety, trouble sleeping) best treated through stress reduction and symptomatic care.

A significant medical diagnosis may precipitate emotional distress or psychosocial upheaval and requires physician attention to the context of the patient's life. Effective physician intervention may involve anticipating the nature of the potential family crisis, including family members in discussions with the patient, and addressing family needs for support. Timely provision of accurate information can enhance a patient's sense of control. Direct support by the physician during the initial adjustment phase can minimize more serious emotional disruption.

Patients living with chronic illness require sensitive psychosocial care. Managing a chronic health problem challenges a person's ability to adhere to medical recommendations and to cope with other life stressors. Patients often cope in highly idiosyncratic ways. Pollin (1995) identified eight emotionally charged issues that patients with chronic illnesses inevitably confront: control, self-image, dependency, stigma, abandonment, anger, isolation, and death. These issues can often be effectively addressed within the physician–patient relationship and through judicious referral to support groups for chronically ill patients. As elaborated by Pollin, each issue can be met by an appropriate and helpful professional stance. In response to control issues, for example, professionals should help patients express their feelings of loss of control and identify areas where they may feel powerless. Normalizing the patient's feelings and fears is the first step in helping address control issues. The goal of intervening in regard to the issue of loss of control is to reinforce the patient's confidence in being able to cope with the demands of the medical condition.

Evidence-Based Practice

Increasingly, high-quality data are available that support the therapeutic efficiency of a variety of general and specific behavioral interventions relevant to primary care practice (Trask et al., 2002). A systematic review by Di Blasi and colleagues (2002) on the consequences of nonspecific effects of the physician–patient relationship found that providing information and emotional support contributed to recovery or improvement from physical illness. Because coping with stress and managing chronic illness often involve behavior change, physicians may use "motivational interviewing" approaches to assist these patients (Rollnick et al., 2008).

Much research demonstrates the efficacy of psychosocial interventions in diseases that have been historically viewed as purely medical, including cancer (Anderson et al., 2007; Edwards et al., 2008; Rehse and Pukrop, 2003; Spiegel et al., 1989) and diabetes (Bogner et al., 2007), and the efficacy of behavioral interventions such as exercise for cardiovascular disease (Taylor et al., 2004). Online resources are available to search for study results (see Web Resources at end of chapter).

Given the time constraints primary care physicians face and the expertise required to use behavioral interventions effectively, the physician should know behavioral health providers in the community and refer to them promptly and often. The evidence base for effective behavioral interventions in numerous psychiatric and psychosocial problems, as well as medical problems, continues to expand (e.g., mood and anxiety disorders, trauma victims). Highly effective treatments are underused when physicians underrefer to mental health professionals with specialized training and overrely on the use of psychotropic medicines alone. Unfortunately, even when guidelines are available that physicians could follow themselves, resistance to change impedes their implementation (Torrey et al., 2001).

KEY TREATMENT

- Providing information and emotional support contributes to the improvement and recovery from physical illness (SOR: A; Di Blasi et al., 2002).
- Negative emotions such as anger, anxiety, and depression are associated with poor health (SOR: B; Salovey et al., 2000).
- Positive emotions such as happiness, optimism, and a positive attitude have been shown to add 7 years to life (SOR: B; Danner et al., 2001; Levy et al., 2002).
- "Motivational interviewing" outperforms advice-giving in addressing a broad range of behavioral problems (SOR: A; Rubac et al., 2005).
- Exercise-based rehabilitation for patients with cardiovascular disease is associated with reduced cardiovascular- and all-cause mortality (SOR: A; Taylor et al., 2004).
- Treating depression in older patients with diabetes reduces mortality (SOR: A; Bogner et al., 2007).

The Patient-Centered Medical Home

Health care spending currently represents approximately 18% of the U.S. gross domestic product and is projected to surpass 20% within a decade (Sisko et al., 2009). There is ongoing concern about the number of uninsured and underinsured persons, although new legislation to expand insurance coverage took effect in 2014.

Numerous perspectives exist on how the health care system needs to change, but a consensus is emerging that focuses on the importance of primary care medicine and on managing chronic disease in the context of a high-quality physician–patient relationship (Bein, 2009). This consensus reflects the accumulating evidence that higher quality health care at lower cost is achieved when primary care is emphasized (Starfield et al., 2005).

The concept of the patient-centered medical home (PCMH) embodies this emerging emphasis. As discussed in Chapter 2, the numerous components of a PCMH (or "health home") include the use of an electronic health record, better access and scheduling processes, use of evidence-based medicine, more point-of-care services (e.g., multidisciplinary teams, group visits), and ongoing emphasis on quality improvement. Some argue that incremental change in this regard is insufficient and that transformation of practices is necessary (Nutting et al., 2009). Such transformation would include a broad, population-based approach to preventive services and chronic care beyond a "single patient at a time" approach. However, even within such a model, services would need to be individualized based on the patient's goals and unique situation, including attention to the psychosocial factors that affect chronic disease prevention and management.

These trends represent an opportunity for family medicine to take a leadership role in health care reform, with an emphasis on psychosocial aspects. The PCMH philosophy is consistent with family medicine's long-standing emphasis on whole-person care in the context of a high-quality physician–patient relationship. Ideally, the family physician in a PCMH will address the psychosocial needs of patients in collaboration with ancillary providers as needed.

Conclusion

To practice in a way that sensitively integrates psychosocial concerns, a physician needs to have a solid knowledge base in the social and behavioral sciences (Cuff and Vanselow, 2004). This general knowledge base complements specific knowledge of self, patients, practice, and community. Self-knowledge entails an honest assessment of the physician's knowledge base, skills, and attitudes relevant to comprehensive care. Acknowledging limitations in dealing with psychosocial issues in primary care is vital and can serve as an impetus for further training and the development of collaborative relationships with other professionals. A responsible physician feigns neither knowledge nor empathy but relies on an interdisciplinary network of professional and community resources to complement personal limitations.

As Osler (1904) emphasized, knowing what kind of person has a disease is as important as knowing the disease. Knowledge of each patient is requisite to the provision of sensitive psychosocial care, with attention to life stresses, coping, personality, and social resources. Furthermore, the physician needs to know details about the population he or she serves, including demographic, socioeconomic, cultural, and epidemiologic dimensions. Addressing psychosocial issues in a practice that serves an ethnically diverse, indigent population presents different challenges than addressing the needs of an affluent population from a familiar ethnic and cultural background. Understanding the practice also entails knowing the health care economics and current systems of care, which inevitably introduce challenges to comprehensive care.

References

The complete reference list is available online at www.expertconsult.com.

Web Resources

www.aafp.org/pcmh This resource from the American Academy of Family Physicians provides ready access to information about the patient-centered medical home movement.

www.cdc.gov Centers for Disease Control and Prevention. Information related to the protection of health and enhancement of quality of life.

www.cfah.org/hbns Health Behavior News Service. Disseminates the results of peer-reviewed research in the broad area of behavior and health.

www.motivationalinterview.org This website offers extensive resources on the topic of motivational interviewing.

4 Care of the Elderly Patient

MELISSA STILES and KATHLEEN WALSH

Family physicians are responsible for the care of increasing numbers of elderly patients and their unique and complex primary care needs. Older patients often have comorbidities; "polypharmacy"; and psychological, social, and functional impairments. These can lead to variability in presentation of health problems and make diagnosis and treatment challenging for the family physician.

This chapter discusses common geriatric syndromes and outlines a process by which family physicians can effectively and efficiently care for elderly patients. The main goal is to assist elderly persons to maintain function and quality of life with self-respect, preserving their lifestyle as much as possible. The chapter addresses functional assessment, falls, elder abuse, pressure ulcers, rational drug prescribing, and incontinence; geriatric conditions such as dementia, delirium, and depression are discussed in other chapters.

Geriatric Assessment

Key Points

- A comprehensive geriatric assessment includes a systematic approach assessing medical, functional, psychological, and social domains.
- A medication review is an essential component of a geriatric assessment.
- A multidisciplinary approach is used to identify intervention and management strategies.
- A questionnaire targeted to the geriatric assessment domains will expedite the patient visit.
- The goals of the geriatric assessment are to maintain function and preserve quality of life.

Longer life spans and aging "baby boomers" will double the population of Americans age 65 years and older over the next 25 years. The dramatic increase in life expectancy in the United States is the result of improved medical care and prevention efforts. In 2006, persons 65 years or older numbered 37.3 million and represented 12.4% of the U.S. population, about one in every eight Americans. The population 65 years of age and older increased from 35 million in 2000 to about 40 million in 2010, a 15% increase, and will increase to 55 million in 2020, a 36% increase for that decade. According to the Centers for Disease Control and Prevention (CDC, 2007), by 2030 there will be about 71.5 million older persons, more than twice their number in 2000 and about 20% of the U.S. population (Table 4-1).

There has been a significant shift in the leading causes of death for all groups from infectious disease and acute illnesses to chronic diseases and degenerative illnesses. Of the elderly population, approximately 8% experience severe cognitive impairment, 20% have chronic disabilities and vision problems, and 33% have restrictions in mobility and hearing loss (Freedman et al., 2002). There are also the predictable age-related structural and physiologic changes that occur with aging. External factors such as diet, occupation, social support, and access to health care can significantly influence the extent and speed of the physiologic decline (Sarma and Peddigrew, 2008; Tourlouki et al., 2009).

America's aging population is also marked by a more racially and ethnically diverse group of individuals. Simultaneously, the health status of racial and ethnic minorities lags far behind that of nonminority populations. The burden of many chronic diseases and conditions, such as hypertension, diabetes, and cancer, varies widely by race and ethnicity. Data from the 1997 to 2009 National Health Interview Survey (NHIS) indicated that 70.2% of non-Hispanic white adults aged 65 years or older reported very good or excellent health compared with 57% of non-Hispanic blacks and 58.8% of Hispanics (CDC, 2009).

There is a strong economic incentive for action. The cost of providing health care for an older American is three to five times greater than the cost for someone younger than 65 years of age. As a result, by 2030, the nation's health care spending is projected to increase by 25% because of these demographic shifts (CDC, 2009).

A comprehensive geriatric assessment is a systematic approach to the collection of patient data. The approach varies greatly, from single-physician evaluation with referral as needed to full teams of professionals evaluating all patients. The geriatric assessment can assist in developing an individualized approach to each patient (Table 4-2). It is imperative to recognize the unique "blueprint" of what characterizes each elderly patient, including age, ethnicity, education, religious or spiritual beliefs, traditions, diet, interests and hobbies, daily routines, medical illness and

Table 4-1   Population by Age and Gender, 2010*

	Both Sexes		Male	Female
Age	Number	Percent	Number	Number
All ages	310, 233	100.0	152,753	157,459
55-59 years	19,517	6.3	9,450	10,067
60-64 years	16,758	5.4	8,024	8,733
65-69 years	12,261	4.0	5,747	6,514
70-74 years	9,202	3.0	4,191	5,011
75-79 years	7,282	2.5	3,159	4,123
80-84 years	5,733	1.8	2,302	3,431
85 years and older	5,751	1.9	1,893	3,859

*Numbers in thousands.
Data from U.S. Census Bureau. *2010 Statistics*. http://www.census.gov/
compendia/statab/2012/tables/12s0009.pdf.

Table 4-2   Goals of Geriatric Assessment

1. Focus on preventive medicine rather than acute medicine.
2. Focus on improving or maintaining functional ability and not necessarily a "cure."
3. Provide a long-term solution for "difficult to manage" patients with multiple physicians, recurrent emergency department visits, and hospital admissions with poor follow-up.
4. Aid in the diagnosis of health-related problems.
5. Develop plans for treatment and follow-up care.
6. Establish plans for coordination of care.
7. Determine the need and site of long-term care as appropriate.
8. Determine optimal use of health care resources.
9. Prevent readmission into the hospital.

disabilities, language barriers, functional status, marital status, sexual orientation, family and social support, occupation, life experiences, and socioeconomic position.

The geriatric assessment can be divided into four categories: medical, functional, psychological, and social. Within each of these categories are a number of approaches, including use of office-based instruments that can aid in the collection of information and streamline the plan of care.

MEDICAL ASSESSMENT

The medical assessment includes a review of the patient's medical record, medication history (past and present), and a nutritional evaluation. On average, elderly patients have four to six diagnosable disorders, which may require the use of several medications. One disorder can affect another, and in turn a collective deterioration of both can lead to overall poor outcomes. Review of the patient's medical record should focus on conditions that are more common in elderly adults (geriatric syndromes) and in particular their risk factors.

Four shared risk factors—older age, baseline cognitive impairment, baseline functional impairment, and impaired mobility—have been identified within the five most common geriatric syndromes: pressure ulcers, incontinence, falls, functional decline, and delirium (Inouye et al., 2007). It is important that health care providers familiarize themselves with the common geriatric body area or system disorders that can directly influence these risk factors. Understanding the basic mechanisms involved in geriatric syndromes is essential to targeting therapeutic options.

During the medical assessment, the review of systems should be completed with special emphasis on sensory impairment, dentition, mood, memory, urinary symptoms, falls, nutrition, and pain. However, the U.S. Preventive Services Task Force (2013) recommends routine screening for visual and hearing impairment in older adults.

Hearing loss is the third most prevalent chronic condition in elderly people, after hypertension and arthritis, and its prevalence and severity increase with age. In persons age 65 to 75 years, the prevalence of hearing loss ranges from 20% to 40% (Cruikshanks et al., 1998; Rahko et al., 1985; Reuben et al., 1998), but in those older than age 75, it ranges from 40% to 66% (Ciurlia-Guy et al., 1993; Parving et al., 1997).

Screening for hearing loss can be accomplished using two office-based methods: the audioscope (objective) and a validated short questionnaire (subjective) (Ventry, 1982). The audioscope is a handheld instrument that functions as an otoscope and audiometer and can be used to visualize the ear canal and eardrum and remove cerumen if necessary. The audioscope is easy to use, with 87% to 96% sensitivity and 70% to 90% specificity (Abyad, 1997; Mulrow and Lichtenstein, 1991). The Hearing Handicap Inventory for the Elderly—Short Version (HHIE-S) is a subjective, 10-item, 5-minute questionnaire with an overall accuracy of 75% in identifying hearing loss (Mulrow et al., 1990).

A formal audiologic evaluation should be offered to any patient who fails a hearing screening. The evaluation can assist in determining the need for further testing or management, including hearing aid, medical treatment, or surgical intervention.

Review of the patient's current medication list, including over-the-counter (OTC) medications, as well as any drug allergies or previous adverse drug reactions (ADRs), is a necessary component of the geriatric assessment. ADRs (also called adverse drug events [ADEs]) are a significant public health issue, especially in the elderly population (Thomsen et al., 2007). Polypharmacy is defined as taking more than four medications and is an independent risk factor for both delirium and falls (Inouye, 2000; Moylan and Binder, 2007).

Patients or family members should be asked to bring in all the patient's prescription medications and supplements at the initial visit and periodically thereafter. Clinicians can make sure patients have the prescribed drugs, but possession of these drugs does not guarantee adherence. Patients should be asked to demonstrate their ability to read labels (often printed in small type), open containers (especially the child-resistant type), and recognize their medications. Pill boxes may be helpful in organizing the patient's medications by the week or month.

Nutritional evaluation is an integral part of the geriatric assessment. The type, quantity, and frequency of food eaten should be determined. Malnutrition and undernutrition can lead to health problems, including delayed healing and longer hospital stays. A reliable marker of nutritional problems is weight loss, specifically, more than 5% in the past month and 10% or greater in the last 6 months (Huffman, 2002). Clinicians should ask about any special diets (e.g., low carbohydrate, vegetarian, low salt) or self-prescribed "fad" diets. A nutritional screen can aid in further assessment of the patient's nutritional health and help guide

Directions: Read the statements below. Circle the number in the YES column if it applies to you or the person you are completing the questionnaire for. Add the circled numbers for the total.

	YES
I have an illness or condition that made me change the kind or amount of food I eat.	2
I eat fewer than two meals per day.	3
I eat few fruits or vegetables or milk products.	2
I have three or more drinks of beer, liquor, or wine almost every day.	2
I have tooth or mouth problems that make it hard for me to eat.	2
I don't always have enough money to buy the food I need.	4
I eat alone most of the time.	1
I take three or more different prescribed or over-the-counter drugs a day.	1
Without wanting to, I have lost or gained 10 lb in the last 6 months.	2
I am not always physically able to shop, cook, or feed myself.	2
TOTAL	

Total

0–2	Good! Recheck your nutritional score in 6 months.
3–5	You are at moderate nutritional risk. See what can be done to improve your eating habits and lifestyle. Your office on aging, senior nutrition program, senior citizens center, or health department can help. Recheck your nutritional score in three months.
6 or more	You are at high nutritional risk. Bring this checklist next time you see your doctor, dietitian, or other qualified health or service professional. Talk with them about any problems you may have. Ask for help to improve your nutritional health.

Figure 4-1 Nutrition questionnaires such as this (Determine Your Nutritional Health) can help in the assessment of the elderly patient's nutritional health. (Courtesy Nutrition Screening Initiative, Washington, DC, 2007. The Nutrition Screening Initiative is funded in part by a grant from Ross Products Division of Abbott Laboratories, Inc.)

interventions (Figure 4-1). Additional questioning should include weight loss and change of fit in clothing, amount of money spent on food, and accessibility of grocers with a variety of fresh foods.

The ability to chew and swallow should also be evaluated. It may be impaired by xerostomia (dryness of mouth), which is common in elderly persons. Decreased taste or smell may reduce the pleasure of eating, so patients may eat less. Patients with decreased vision, arthritis, immobility, or tremors may have difficulty preparing meals and may injure or burn themselves when cooking. Patients worried about urinary incontinence may reduce their fluid intake and thus may eat less food.

FUNCTIONAL ASSESSMENT

A primary goal of the geriatric assessment is to identify interventions to help patients maintain function and stay at home in independent living situations. The functional assessment focuses on activities of daily living (ADLs) and risk screening for falls. The basic ADLs include eating, dressing, bathing, transferring, and toileting. The instrumental ADLs (IADLs) consist of shopping, managing money, driving, using the telephone, housekeeping, laundry, meal preparation, and managing medications (Katz, 1983). Home health and social services referral should be considered for patients who have difficulty with the ADLs. A simple method of screening patients for gait and mobility problems

is to ask, "Have you fallen all the way to the ground in the past 12 months?" A positive screen should lead to a more thorough evaluation and consideration of a physical therapy referral (Ganz et al., 2007) (see "Falls Assessment" later in this chapter).

PSYCHOLOGICAL ASSESSMENT

The psychological assessment screens for cognitive impairment and depression, two conditions that significantly impact both the patient and the family. The most studied test to screen for cognition is the Mini-Mental State Examination, which is best for identifying patients with moderate or severe dementia. Depression can be readily screened with shorter versions of the original 30-item Yesavage Geriatric Depression Scale (GDS) (Yesavage et al., 1983). The five-item version of the GDS asks the following:

1. Are you basically satisfied with your life?
2. Do you often feel bored?
3. Do you often feel helpless?
4. Do you prefer to stay home rather than going out and doing new things?
5. Do you feel pretty worthless the way you are now?

A score of greater than two positive answers is positive (97% sensitivity, 85% specificity) (Rinalde et al., 2003). The Yale Depression Screen ("Do you often feel sad or depressed?") is a validated one-item GDS screening tool (Mahoney et al., 1994).

SOCIAL ASSESSMENT

It is important to assess the patient's living situation and social support when performing a geriatric assessment. The living situation should be evaluated for potential hazards, especially if the patient is identified as being at risk of falling. The social assessment also includes questions about financial stressors and caregiver concerns. Advance planning is a key component of the assessment and includes clarifying the patient's values and setting goals for care in case of future incapacity, including identifying the patient's "power of attorney" for health care.

SUMMARY

A geriatric assessment can identify frequent problems, thus leading to earlier interventions for the common medical and social concerns of the elderly population. It is important to remember, however, that patients may underreport medical problems because they worry about losing their independence. Patients may also be reluctant to repeat their health concerns to their primary care physician because they fear being perceived as having an emotional or psychiatric illness. Often, older patients rationalize their symptoms as being a "normal" component of aging.

The key to a successful geriatric assessment is to establish trust and effective communication between the patient and the physician. Allotting for adequate time during appointments and, if needed, scheduling frequent office visits are essential to the gathering of information. Inquiring about recent socioeconomic changes, functional losses, or life transitions is also important. The physician should obtain the patient's medical records before the first visit. A questionnaire targeted to the geriatric assessment domains should be completed by the patient, with family assistance if needed (Figure 4-2). Language, education, social support, economic status, and cultural and ethnic factors play a vital role in the patient's health care outcome. A multidisciplinary approach is used in interventions and management. Preserving function and maintaining quality of life are the primary goals of the geriatric assessment (Miller et al., 2000).

Falls

Key Points

- Falls result in significant morbidity, mortality, and functional decline.
- Patients should be asked about their history of falls and balance issues.
- Medication review is a key component of falls assessment.
- Multifactorial interventions can reduce the rate of falls.
- Exercise programs that focus on strength and balance training are most effective in preventing falls.

EPIDEMIOLOGY

Falls result in significant morbidity and mortality as well as an increased rate of nursing home placement. Each year, approximately 30% of persons older than age 65 years fall at least once, and the incidence increases with age. Up to 10% of falls result in serious injury. Falls are the leading cause of injury-related deaths in people older than 65 years (CDC, 2013). In the United States, hip fractures currently account for more than 300,000 hospitalizations, with a 1-year mortality rate of up to 33% (Sattin, 1992; Tinetti et al., 1988). By 2050, it is estimated that the worldwide number of hip fractures will rise to 6.26 million. Direct medical costs related to falls in adults age 65 years of age or older exceeded $19 billion in 2000 (Stevens et al., 2006).

Falls also cause functional limitations by both direct injury and indirect psychological consequences. Postfall anxiety leads to loss of self-confidence in ambulation and self-imposed limitations in activity. Postfall anxiety syndrome can also result in depression, social isolation, and increased risk of falls from deconditioning. Because the cause of falls is often multifactorial, the assessment and interventions target several areas (Nevitt et al., 1989).

RISK FACTORS

The multiple risk factors for falling can be categorized as intrinsic or extrinsic. Intrinsic risk factors include age-related physiologic changes and diseases that affect the risk of falling (Table 4-3). Extrinsic risk factors include medications and environmental obstacles. The risk of falling increases significantly in people with multiple risk factors. A prospective study found that 19% of older patients with one risk factor have a fall in a given year compared with 60% of older patients with three risk factors (Tinetti et al., 1988).

Taking four or more prescription drugs is itself a risk factor for falling. Also, several medication classes have a higher potential to cause falls, including tricyclic antidepressants, neuroleptic agents, serotonin reuptake inhibitors, benzodiazepines, and class 1A antiarrhythmic medications. Narcotic analgesics, antihistamines, and anticonvulsants are also associated with increased risk for falls (Ensrud et al., 2002; Rubenstein and Josephson, 2002).

Physical restraints have been used in an attempt to reduce falling. Although the focus here is on community-dwelling elderly persons, it is worth noting that use of physical restraints in nursing home and hospital settings does not reduce the risk of falling and is instead associated with an increased risk of injury (Neufeld et al., 1999). Since the 1980s, the use of physical restraints has been appropriately and dramatically reduced.

SCREENING

At present, no one screening test can be recommended to identify potential fallers (Gates et al., 2008). The two best predictors of falls are a history of falls and a reported abnormality in gait or balance (Ganz et al., 2007). "Have you had any falls in the past year?" is a simple screening question that can be answered by the patient or caregiver in a previsit

GERIATRIC HEALTH QUESTIONNAIRE

Date: _____ Birthdate: _____ Hosp #: _____

Name: _____ Address: _____

INSTRUCTIONS: PLEASE CIRCLE ANSWERS.

1. **General health:**   In general, would you say your health is:
                               Excellent / Very good / Good / Fair / Poor

                               How much bodily pain have you had during the past 4 weeks?
                               None / Very mild / Mild / Moderate / Severe / Very severe

2. **Activities of daily living:** Are you (I) independent (can do by myself); (A) require assistance (need help from another person); or (D) dependent (cannot do at all) with each of the following tasks?

Walking	I	A	D	Using telephone	I	A	D
Dressing	I	A	D	Shopping	I	A	D
Bathing	I	A	D	Preparing meals	I	A	D
Eating	I	A	D	Housework	I	A	D
Toileting	I	A	D	Taking medications	I	A	D
Driving	I	A	D	Managing finances	I	A	D

3. **Geriatric review of systems:**
    a. Do you have difficulty driving, watching TV, or reading because of poor eyesight?   Yes / No
    b. Can you hear normal conversational voice?   Yes / No
        Do you use hearing aids?   Yes / No
    c. Do you have problems with your memory?   Yes / No
    d. Do you often feel sad or depressed?   Yes / No
    e. Have you unintentionally lost weight in the past 6 months?   Yes / No
    f. Do you have trouble with control of your bladder?   Yes / No
        Do you have trouble with control of your bowels?   Yes / No
    g. How many falls have you had in the past year? _____
    h. Do you drink alcohol?   Yes / No
        If yes, how many drinks per week? _____

4. Do you live with anyone?   Yes / No
    If yes, who? Spouse / Child / Other / Relative / Friend
    Who would help you in an emergency? _____
    Who would help you with health care decisions if you were not able to communicate your wishes?
    _____

5. How many medicines do you take, including prescribed, over the counter, and vitamins? _____
    What is your system for taking your medications? Pill box / Family help / List or chart / None

6. Are you sexually active?   Yes / No

7. Has anyone intentionally tried to harm you?   Yes / No

8. Have you had a shot to prevent pneumonia?   Yes / No

9. Please draw the face of a clock with all the numbers and the hands set to indicate 10 minutes after 11 o'clock.

Memory: 3 item recall after 1 minute   (pen, dog, watch)   # recalled _____
Patient signature_____ Date _____
Reviewing physician _____ Date _____

Figure 4-2 Geriatric health questionnaires assist in gathering pertinent information regarding the functioning of the elderly patient. (From Jogerst GJ, Wilbur JK. Care of the elderly. In Rakel RE, ed. *Principles of Family Practice*, 7th ed. Philadelphia: WB Saunders; 2007:67-105.)

Table 4-3 Intrinsic Risk Factors for Falls

Age-related changes in vision, hearing, or proprioception
Decreased blood pressure response to postural changes
Delayed compensatory muscle response to postural changes
Age older than 80 years
Cognitive impairment
Depression
Functional impairment
History of falls
Visual impairment
Gait or balance impairment
Use of assistive device
Arthritis
Leg weakness

Table 4-4 Initial Evaluation of Falls

History	Circumstances of fall
	Presence of risk factors
	Medical conditions
	Medication review
	Functional abilities
Physical examination	Postural blood pressure
	CV examination focusing on rhythm and murmurs
	Visual acuity
	Neurological examination: strength, proprioception, cognition
	Musculoskeletal examination: ROM, joint abnormalities
	Gait and balance assessment
Diagnostic studies	None required routinely

CV, Cardiovascular; *ROM*, range of motion.

questionnaire. For patients who have not fallen, the pretest probability of a fall in the upcoming year ranges from 19% to 36%. Also, asking the patient, "Have you noticed any problems with gait, balance, or mobility?" is another simple screening question. Answering "yes" to either screening question warrants further assessment (Tinetti, 2003).

FALLS ASSESSMENT

Falls assessment should include a multifactorial evaluation beginning with the circumstances surrounding the fall(s), associated symptoms, risk factor assessment, and medication history (Table 4-4). The physician should ask about the environment (e.g., indoors or outdoors, dark or well lighted, time of day), environmental obstacles (e.g., throw rugs, door thresholds, stairs), and footwear worn at the time. The history should also include questions about prodromal symptoms (e.g., lightheadedness, dizziness) if there was a loss of consciousness or other symptoms of arrhythmias (i.e., palpitations). If available, information should be obtained from a witness. The evaluation should also include questions about risk factors, functional abilities, and medication history (American Geriatrics Society [AGS] et al., 2010).

Postural blood pressure and pulse are important assessments in the examination. Up to 30% of older persons have orthostatic hypotension, and although some may be asymptomatic, others become lightheaded and dizzy (Luukinen et al., 1999). The musculoskeletal examination should focus on range of motion in the legs, inflammatory or degenerative conditions of the leg joints, kyphosis, and abnormalities of the feet. The neurologic examination should include proprioception, coordination, muscle strength, and cognition. The cardiovascular examination should focus on detecting potential causes of falls (e.g., arrhythmias, aortic stenosis). Visual acuity and hearing should be assessed. Disturbances in gait and balance can be identified through the patient or caregiver's direct report or a simple office-based assessment, such as the "get up and go" test (Podsiadlo and Richardson, 1991). This test may be scored, timed, or used as an overall assessment of the patient's gait, stability, balance, and strength. The patient is asked to stand from a seated position, walk about 10 feet (3 m), turn around, walk back, and sit down again. If the patient needs to push off the chair or rock back-and-forth several times to arise, leg strength is diminished. The task should be completed within 10 seconds. Gait abnormalities, such as poor step height, decreased stride length, and shuffling, may be observed. A wide-based stance and slow, multiple-point turning may reveal poor balance.

Laboratory evaluation and imaging are based on the history and clinical findings. If an underlying metabolic abnormality is suspected (e.g., diabetes, anemia, dehydration), appropriate blood tests may assist in the diagnosis. If a patient is suspected of having syncope, cardiac rhythm monitoring (e.g., Holter or event monitor) is appropriate. An echocardiogram may be necessary for evaluation of a murmur. Neuroimaging with magnetic resonance imaging (MRI) or computed tomography (CT) is indicated for the evaluation of focal findings on neurologic examination.

MANAGEMENT

Evidence has demonstrated that a multifactorial approach and intervention strategy is needed to reduce the rate of falling in older patients (Figure 4-3). Because one of the most modifiable risk factors is medication use, medication review is a key component of management (Hanlon et al., 1997). The review should focus on decreasing the dose or discontinuing sedating medications. If orthostasis is present, adjustment of diuretics and antihypertensive medications should be considered. The role of vitamin D in fall prevention is questionable. Although it probably does not decrease the risk of falls, except in patients with low levels of vitamin D, supplementation should be started in patients with osteopenia or osteoporosis (Gillespie et al., 2012).

Supervised exercise programs should be considered for patients at high risk for falls; exercise can reduce the physical risk factors (Rose, 2008). Specifically, programs that focus on two of three exercise components (strengthening, balance training, and aerobic or endurance training) for a minimum of 12 weeks have shown the most benefit (Costello and Edelstein, 2008). Finally, home hazard evaluation and intervention is an essential component in the assessment of falls in elderly (AGS, 2010; Gillespie et al., 2012).

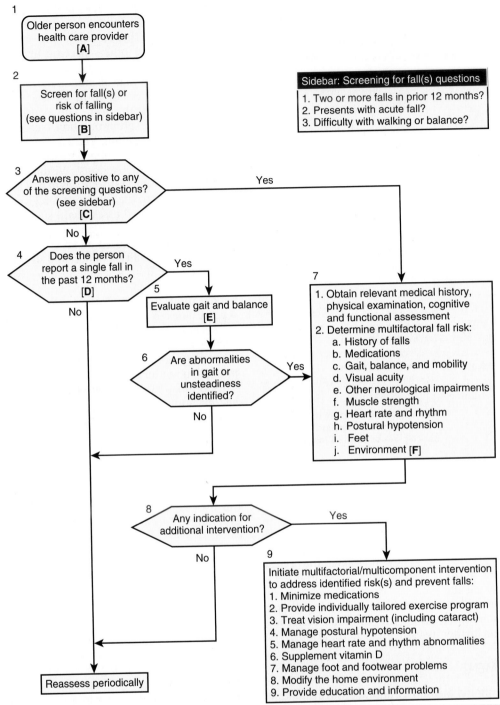

Figure 4-3 Practice guideline for the prevention of falls in older persons. (From American Geriatrics Society, British Geriatrics Society, and American Academy of Orthopedic Surgeons Panel on Falls Prevention: Guideline for the prevention of falls in older persons. *J Am Geriatr Soc.* 2001;49:664-672.)

KEY TREATMENT

- Risk factor assessment and multifactorial intervention reduce the rate of falls (SOR: A; Gillespie et al., 2012).
- Exercise programs that target more than two components reduce the rate of falls (SOR: A; Gillespie et al., 2012).

- Community-living elderly patients who have fallen or who have risk factors for falling should have their homes assessed for safety by occupational therapists (SOR: A; Gillespie et al., 2012).
- All older individuals should be asked at least once yearly about falls (SOR: C; AGS et al., 2010; Tinetti, 2003).

Elder Abuse

Key Points

- Elder abuse is underreported.
- Direct questioning for elder abuse is recommended.
- Physicians should recognize the physical and behavioral signs of abuse.
- A positive screening result for elder abuse should be followed by a safety assessment.
- Physician reporting requirements regarding elder abuse vary by state.

Elder abuse is a significant public health issue that physicians need to identify and address in both outpatient and inpatient settings. The prevalence of elder abuse is difficult to determine because its definition varies across U.S. states and other countries, and research is still limited in this area (Erlingsson, 2007). In a systematic review of international literature, estimates ranged from 3.2% to 27.5% based on population studies. More than 6% of the general population had reported abuse in the prior month (Cooper et al., 2008).

In the United States, the number of people age 65 years and older who have been victims of elder abuse ranges between 1 and 2 million. In 2000, adult protective services (APS) departments received approximately 470,000 reports. Of the types of abuse, elder "self-neglect" is most often reported. A prospective, population-based cohort study found that elder self-neglect was associated with a 5.82 times increased risk for mortality in the year after a report of self-neglect (Dong et al., 2009). From incidence studies, it is estimated that for every case reported, about five go underreported (National Elder Abuse Incidence Study, 1998). Underreporting stems from both patient issues (familial secrecy, denial, fear, shame) and provider issues (lack of awareness) (Kahan and Paris, 2003). Primary care physicians have the opportunity to detect early signs of elder abuse in patients with whom they have well-established relationships (Stiles et al., 2002).

DEFINITION

The National Center on Elder Abuse (2013) defines elder abuse as "a term referring to any knowing, intentional, or negligent act by a caregiver or any other person that causes harm or a serious risk of harm to a vulnerable adult." Although terms vary across states, elder abuse can be generally categorized into several types: physical abuse, emotional abuse, sexual abuse, exploitation, neglect, self-neglect, and abandonment (Table 4-5). Elder abuse is also classified by its setting. Domestic abuse occurs in the home of the victim. Institutional abuse occurs in a nursing home, hospital, assisted living center, or group home.

RISK FACTORS

Awareness of risk factors for abuse can increase the chance of identification and early intervention. Although research is ongoing, several characteristics of both the victim and

Table 4-5 National Center on Elder Abuse Definitions

Physical abuse	Inflicting or threatening to inflict physical pain or injury on a vulnerable elder or depriving him or her of a basic need
Emotional abuse	Inflicting mental pain, anguish, or distress on an elder person through verbal or nonverbal acts
Sexual abuse	Nonconsensual sexual contact of any kind
Exploitation	Illegal taking, misuse, or concealment of funds, property, or assets of a vulnerable elder
Neglect	Refusal or failure by those responsible to provide food, shelter, health care, or protection for a vulnerable elder
Abandonment	Desertion of a vulnerable elder by anyone who has assumed the responsibility for care or custody of that person
Self-neglect	Characterized as the behavior of an elderly person that threatens his or her own health or safety

From National Center on Elder Abuse. http://www.ncea.aoa.gov/faq/index.aspx.

Table 4-6 Screening Questions for Elder Abuse

Are you afraid of anyone at home?
Are you alone a lot?
Has anyone at home ever hurt you?
Has anyone taken anything that was yours without asking?
Does anyone at home make you uncomfortable or afraid?
Has anyone ever forced you to sign a document that you did not understand?
Are you kept isolated from friends or relatives?

the abuser should trigger further screening questions. Risk factors associated with the victim include shared living situations, history of dementia, and social isolation. Perpetrator risk factors include a history of mental illness (specifically depression), alcohol abuse, and financial dependency (Lachs and Pillemer, 2004).

SCREENING

There is no consensus that asymptomatic patients should be screened for elder abuse. The American Medical Association (AMA, 1992) suggests that all outpatients be screened for family violence, but the U.S. Preventive Services Task Force (2013) concluded that there was insufficient evidence for or against screening for older adults or their caregivers for elder abuse. Patients should be screened if there is a suspicion of elder abuse. The questions should be open ended, nonthreatening, and asked in a variety of ways to assess for the different forms of elder abuse (Table 4-6). A positive response should be followed by more direct questions as to the nature of the abuse. Direct questioning by physicians has been shown to increase reporting (Oswald et al., 2004).

CLINICAL MANIFESTATIONS

Certain behavioral and physical signs should raise suspicion for elder abuse. Behavioral signs in the caregiver

Table 4-7 Physical Signs of Elder Abuse

General	Weight loss, dehydration, and poor hygiene
HEENT	Traumatic alopecia; poor oral hygiene; absent hearing aids, dentures, or eyeglasses; subconjunctival or vitreous hemorrhage
Skin	Hematomas, welts, burns, bites, bruises, pressure sores
Genitorectal	Inguinal rash, fecal impaction
Musculoskeletal	Fractures, contractures

HEENT, Head, ears, eyes, nose, throat.

include answering for the patient, insisting on being present for the entire visit, failing to offer assistance, and displaying indifference or anger. Behavioral signs in an elderly patient include poor eye contact, hesitation to talk openly, or fearfulness toward the caregiver. Other indicators of possible abuse include confusion, paranoia, anxiety, anger, and low self-esteem. Physical signs that may signal neglect include poor hygiene, malnutrition, dehydration, pressure ulcers, and injuries (Table 4-7). Medication nonadherence may also be a warning sign of abuse.

ASSESSMENT

In suspected cases of abuse, the assessment includes a thorough history; physical examination; and functional, cognitive, and mental health assessments. The patient and the caregiver should be interviewed alone and separately (Abbey, 2009). Documentation begins with the description of the abusive or neglectful event, using the patient's words whenever possible. The duration, frequency, and severity of the abuse should be recorded. If injuries are present, a detailed description of the injuries and photographs, if available, should be documented. Whereas assessment of functional dependence can be helpful in recommending resources, evaluation of cognitive impairment is important in assessing both risk and capacity. The assessment should also include a mental health screening, with particular attention to depression, anxiety, insomnia, and alcohol abuse.

The elderly patient's caregiver should be assessed for caregiver stress and for risk factors for elder abuse, including alcohol abuse, depression, and financial dependency.

MANAGEMENT

Because the cause of elder abuse is often multifactorial, management involves a multidisciplinary approach with social workers and legal, financial, and APS representatives. The immediate management is determined by the safety and capacity assessments. Is the patient in any immediate danger? If so, acute hospitalization, safe home placement, and a protective court order may be indicated. If the patient lacks capacity, the physician should work with APS on options, including guardianship, financial management resources, and order of protection if indicated. In other cases, management should focus on using community resources to maintain the patient in the least restrictive environment. The emphasis is to decrease social isolation and caregiver stress. Interventions can include respite care, home health or custodial services, counseling, and drug or alcohol rehabilitation.

REPORTING REQUIREMENT

All 50 states have laws authorizing APS departments to intervene in cases of elder abuse. It is important for primary care physicians to know their state's requirements on mandatory reporting for elder abuse and which type of abuse (e.g., physical, emotional, sexual, financial) requires reporting. Higher rates of abuse have been documented in states that require public education regarding elder abuse and states that require mandatory reporting (Jogerst et al., 2003). Mandatory reporting laws in 42 states are controversial because they conflict with a competent elder's autonomy and with the physician–patient relationship. In such cases, physicians should explain their legal obligation to report and emphasize that the goal of reporting is to develop a care plan to assist the patient.

> **KEY TREATMENT**
>
> - Direct questioning by physicians for elder abuse increases the rate of reporting (Oswald et al., 2004) (SOR: B).
> - Older individuals should be screened for elder abuse (AMA, 1992) (SOR: C).

Pressure Ulcers

> ## Key Points
>
> ■ Preventive measures can reduce the incidence of pressure ulcers in elderly patients.
> ■ Classification is only one aspect of wound assessment.
> ■ Assessment of pressure ulcers includes identification of risk factors.
> ■ Pain assessment is an essential component of management.
> ■ Risk factor modification is the key to management of pressure ulcers.

Pressure ulcers are a common and serious public health issue, especially in the elderly population. The reported incidence is as high as 22% in the nursing home population and ranges from 4.7% to 9% up to 32% in the hospitalized population (Allman, 1997; Allman et al., 1995; Coleman et al., 2002; Kaltenthaler et al., 2001). The treatment costs related to pressure ulcers exceed an estimated $5 billion annually in the United States (Xakellis et al., 1995). Prevention is paramount and can reduce the incidence of pressure ulcers by 50%. A thorough assessment of the wound and potential risk factors is the key to management.

CLASSIFICATION

Wound assessment begins with classification, as initially proposed in 1989 by the National Pressure Ulcer Advisory Panel (NPUAP) and then adopted for the Agency for Health

Care Policy and Research (AHCPR) Pressure Ulcer Clinical Practice Guidelines (1992 and 1994). The NPUAP revised the stage I classification in 1998 and added two stages in 2007, suspected deep tissue injury and unstageable. The six classifications are as follows:

Suspected deep tissue injury: Purple or maroon, localized area of discolored skin or blood-filled blister caused by damage to underlying soft tissue from pressure and shear. The area may be preceded by tissue that is painful, firm, mushy, boggy, and warmer or cooler compared with adjacent tissue.

Stage I: Intact skin with nonblanchable redness of a localized area, usually over a bony prominence. Darkly pigmented skin may not have visible blanching; its color may differ from the surrounding area. The area may be painful, firm, soft, and warmer or cooler compared with adjacent tissue. Stage I may be difficult to detect in individuals with dark skin tones.

Stage II: Partial-thickness skin loss involving the epidermis, the dermis, or both. The ulcer is superficial and presents clinically as an abrasion, blister, or shallow crater, without slough.

Stage III: Full-thickness skin loss involving damage or necrosis of subcutaneous tissue that may extend down to, but not through, underlying fascia. The ulcer presents clinically as a deep crater with or without undermining of adjacent tissue.

Stage IV: Full-thickness skin loss with extensive destruction, tissue necrosis, or damage to muscle, bone, or supporting structures (e.g., tendons, joint capsules). Slough or eschar may be present on some parts of the wound bed, often with undermining and tunneling.

Unstageable: Full-thickness tissue loss in which the base of the ulcer is covered with slough (yellow, tan, gray, green, or brown) or eschar in the wound bed.

A wound cannot be accurately staged if eschar or slough is present. The staging system is useful only for initial classification because wounds do not heal predictably (Ferrell, 1997). Thus, it is important to include other factors when describing the wound to help assess treatment over time. These factors include size, type of exudate, and a description of the predominant tissue type. Size can be assessed by measuring the two largest diameters at right angles. The type and amount of exudate should be recorded. Exudate types include serous (clear or amber), sanguineous (bloody), or purulent (thick, yellow, or odiferous). The predominant tissue types are epithelial, granulation, necrotic, and eschar (AHCPR, 1992; Ferrell, 1997; Maklebust, 1997; NPUAP, 2007).

RISK FACTORS

An understanding of risk factors for pressure sore development is the key to prevention and management. Risk factors can be divided into extrinsic and intrinsic categories (Table 4-8).

Extrinsic Risk Factors

Extrinsic factors include direct pressure, shearing forces, friction, and moisture. Direct pressure results in hypoperfusion of the affected tissue, which can lead to hypoxia;

Table 4-8 Risk Factors for Pressure Sore Development

Extrinsic Factors	Intrinsic Factors
Pressure	Age
Shearing forces	Impaired mobility
Friction	Malnutrition
Moisture	Sensory impairment

acidosis; and, if prolonged, tissue death and necrosis. Pressure sores most frequently occur over bony prominences below the waist, including the sacrum, greater trochanter, malleolus, heel, ischial tuberosity, and fibular head. Of note, the heels are the second most common site for pressure ulcer development. As the prevalence of pressure ulcers at other sites has decreased or remained the same, the prevalence of heel pressure ulcers has increased.

Shearing forces result from traction on the skin, which causes a relative displacement of the underlying structures. This usually occurs when patients are positioned in bed more than 30 degrees or seated and then slide down. In these patients, the underlying sacrum is at risk for pressure sore development. Friction between the skin and a stationary source such as bedclothes or sheets is another factor. Care must be taken to avoid friction, especially during transfers in and out of bed. Excessive moisture can lead to skin maceration and subsequent skin breakdown. Common causes include incontinence, diarrhea, and excessive perspiration (AHCPR, 1994; Patterson and Bennett, 1995).

Intrinsic Risk Factors

Intrinsic risk factors for pressure ulcer development include age, conditions that impair mobility, malnutrition, and sensory impairment. Skin changes associated with aging (e.g., epidermal thinning, diminished vascularity) increase the susceptibility of older persons to shearing forces, pressure, and friction. Immobility can cause infrequent position changes, thus exposing an older person to prolonged pressure. Malnutrition, specifically an inadequate intake of calories or protein, has been associated with the development of pressure sores (Thomas, 2001). The AHCPR (1994) defines clinically significant malnutrition as a serum albumin level of less than 3.5 mg/dL, a total lymphocyte count of less than 1800 cells/mm^3, or body weight less than 80% of ideal weight. Supplementation of micronutrients involved in skin healing, such as ascorbic acid and zinc, has not been shown to prevent pressure sores or improve rates of healing. Sensory impairment, such as in diabetic neuropathy, can prevent an individual from responding appropriately to pressure-related discomfort (Patterson and Bennett, 1995; Reddy et al., 2006; Thomas, 1997, 2001).

Risk Factor Assessment Tools

The AHCPR's guidelines recommend that individuals with limited mobility be assessed on admission to hospitals, nursing homes, and home care programs for risk factors for pressure sore development. The most common assessment tool is the Braden scale (Pancorbo-Hidalgo et al., 2006). Risk factor identification and subsequent intervention are integral components of pressure sore prevention and management.

Table 4-9 Pressure Sore Risk Factor Modification

Implement	Avoid
Support devices to reduce pressure	Donut-type devices
Frequent repositioning	Massage over bony prominences
Positioning devices such as pillows	Raising head of bed above 30 degrees
Lifting devices such as a trapeze	Dragging the patient during transfers

MANAGEMENT

The principles of pressure sore management include modification of risk factors, nutritional support, maintaining a wound environment optimal for healing, and pain control.

Risk Factor Modification

The primary goal is to reduce pressure, shear, and friction over high-risk bony prominences (Table 4-9). This can be accomplished by frequent turning and repositioning while the patient is in bed (every 2 hours); frequent repositioning while sitting (every hour); and use of a support device to lower surface pressure, such as a foam, static air, alternating air, gel, or water mattress. Positioning devices such as pillows or foam wedges should be used to keep bony prominences (e.g., knees, ankles) from touching each other and high-risk areas from contacting the bed (e.g., heels). Donut-type devices should be avoided because the tissue within the ring can become necrotic from increased venous congestion.

Massage should be avoided over bony prominences because it can lead to deep tissue trauma. When positioning on the side, avoid pressure directly on the trochanter. To decrease the effect of shear forces, maintain the head of the bed at the lowest degree of elevation. To decrease the effect of friction lubricants, use protective films, dressings, or padding. Also, lifting devices such as a trapeze can be used to assist patients with limited mobility in transfers and repositioning (AHCPR, 1994; Bergstrom, 1997; Bluestein and Javaher, 2008; Reddy et al., 2006; Remsburg and Bennett, 1997).

Nutritional Support

Nutritional support emphasizing adequate protein and calorie intake is another key component of pressure sore management. Protein intake should be 1.0 to 1.5 g/kg/day. Caloric intake should be 30 to 35 kcal/kg/day. Some experts recommend supplementation with vitamin C and zinc, although evidence that either enhances wound healing is limited (AHCPR, 1994; Langer et al., 2003; Reddy et al., 2006; Thomas, 2001).

Debridement

Wound healing requires a moist environment, free of necrotic tissue and infection, which allows for granulation and reepithelialization. Debridement is often needed to remove necrotic tissue, slough, and eschar, which can be accomplished by sharp, mechanical, enzymatic, or autolytic techniques. The technique used depends on the patient's condition, location, clinical urgency, and overall goals for patient care. Debridement is not recommended for heel ulcers that have stable, dry eschar without edema or signs of infection (AHCPR, 1994; NPUAP, 2007).

Sharp debridement is appropriate for removing areas of thick eschar and necrotic tissue in extensive ulcers. Care must be taken to control pain when using this technique. Also, surgical debridement may cause transient bacteremia, and prophylactic antibiotics may be needed for high-risk patients.

Mechanical debridement includes wet-to-dry dressings; hydrotherapy; wound irrigation; and dextranomers, which are small beads of highly hydrophilic dextran polymers (e.g., Debrisan). Wet-to-dry dressings may be painful when changed and need be discontinued when the wound bed is clean to avoid desiccation (Ovington, 2001). Hydrotherapy is appropriate for pressure sores with thick exudate or necrotic tissue. Care must be taken not to place the wound too close to the jets. Irrigation pressures need to be high enough to adequately cleanse the wound but not too high to potentially cause tissue trauma. Safe and effective pressures are between 4 and 15 pounds per square inch (psi). Examples of safe irrigation devices include 35-mL syringe with 19-gauge needle or angiocatheter, water-jet device at the lowest setting, and saline squeeze bottle (250 mL) with irrigation cap.

Enzymatic debridement is accomplished by products that have proteolytic enzymes such as papain and urea (e.g., Accuzyme, Panafil) and collagenase. Typically used once daily, these products may damage healthy tissue and should not be used if infection is present. Thus, special care is needed in application, and use should be limited to short periods (<2 weeks).

Autolytic debridement involves the use of occlusive synthetic dressings that allow enzymes normally present within wounds to self-digest necrotic tissue. Occlusive dressings should not be used if the wound is infected or if there is a moderate amount of exudate (AHCPR, 1994; Cervo et al., 2000; Goode and Thomas, 1997).

Infection Control

In the majority of cases, infection can be prevented by adequate debridement and cleansing. Wounds should be cleansed daily and with dressing changes. Normal saline is the most appropriate solution for cleansing. Avoid skin cleansers and antiseptics that are cytotoxic, such as povidone–iodine, hydrogen peroxide, and acetic acid. Signs of a wound infection include delayed healing, increasing wound size, purulent exudate, pain, and foul odor. Initially, consider a trial of topical antibiotics, such as silver sulfadiazine cream (Silvadene), for 2 weeks. Superficial cultures of the wound are not helpful because they detect only the surface colonization. Ideally, bacterial tissue cultures should be performed to guide antibiotic coverage. Systemic antibiotics are reserved for patients with cellulitis, osteomyelitis, bacteremia, or sepsis (AHCPR, 1994).

Dressing Selection

Wound dressings provide a physiologically moist wound environment shown to enhance healing, reduce pain, debride necrotic tissue, and decrease infection rates in pressure sores. Dressing selection depends on the stage,

Table 4-10   Wound Dressing Properties

Wound Dressings	Absorbent Quality*	Debriding Action	Frequency of Dressing Change	Stage
Polyurethane films	None	None	Every 7 days or less	I, II
Amorphous hydrogels	Minimal to moderate	Autolysis	Every 7 days or less	II, III, IV
Hydrogel sheets	Minimal to moderate	Autolysis	Every 7 days or less	II, III
Hydrocolloids	Minimal to large	Autolysis	Every 7 days or less	II, III, IV
Polyurethane foams	Minimal to moderate	None	Every 7 days or less	II, III, IV
Foamed gels	Minimal to large	Autolysis	Every 7 days of less	II, III, IV
Alginates	Minimal to large	Autolysis	Daily to every 3 days	II, III, IV
Hydrocolloid–alginate	Minimal to large	Autolysis	Every 3 to 5 days	III, IV

*None, minimal, moderate, or large.

amount of exudate, size, site, and condition of surrounding skin. No moist-dressing type has proved superior to the others (Bouza et al., 2005). The main categories of modern dressings are polyurethane films, hydrocolloids, amorphous hydrogels, hydrogel sheets, polyurethane foams, foamed gels, alginates, and hydrocolloid–alginate combinations (Table 4-10).

For deep, stage III and stage IV pressure sores, packing is often needed to eliminate dead space. This can be accomplished with saline-moistened gauze, calcium alginates, gels, and dextranomers. After packing, the wound is covered with an occlusive or semiocclusive dressing. If excessive exudate is present, the dressing must have absorptive properties to control exudate without drying the wound bed. Examples include saline-moistened gauze, alginates, and combination hydrocolloid–alginate dressings.

Pressure sores should be evaluated weekly by a health care professional. Reevaluation of the treatment plan should be considered if there are not signs of healing within 2 weeks of treatment (Ferrell, 1997; Goode and Thomas, 1997).

Pain Control

The overall management of a patient with a pressure sore includes pain assessment and control. Patients should be assessed for pain related to the pressure sore. Management includes the appropriate use of analgesics and eliminating or modifying the source of the pain. This can be accomplished by repositioning, using support surfaces, and using wound dressings shown to reduce pain. Pain should be anticipated before dressing changes and debridement. Appropriate analgesia should be provided as needed.

Adjunctive Therapy

Numerous modalities have been attempted to expedite the wound healing process, but their role remains unclear. Examples include electrical stimulation, hyperbaric oxygen, ultrasonography, and hydrotherapy (Baba-Akbari et al., 2006; Kranke et al., 2004; Olyaee Manesh et al., 2006). Negative-pressure wound therapy has shown promise in the management of stage III and IV pressure ulcer (Banwell and Teot, 2003; Mendez-Eastman, 2004). Further research is needed to establish efficacy of adjunctive therapy for wound healing.

KEY TREATMENT

- Assess all support surfaces and patient factors for increased pressure and modify appropriately (AHCPR, 1994, Reddy et al., 2006) (SOR: A).
- Assess and manage the patient's nutritional status (AHCPR, 1994; Langer et al., 2003; Thomas, 2001) (SOR: B).
- Assess all patients for pain related to the pressure ulcer treatment or its treatment (AHCPR, 1994; NPUAP, 2007) (SOR: C).

Rational Drug Prescribing for Elderly Patients

Key Points

- Adverse drug events result in significant morbidity and a high rate of hospital admissions.
- Medications should be adjusted for the individual patient's renal function.
- Medication lists of elderly patients should be periodically reviewed, focusing on indications and side effects.
- One drug should not be used to treat the side effects of another medication.
- Pharmacists' recommendations should be incorporated in a rational drug-prescribing plan.
- The primary care physician plays an important role in addressing an array of pharmaceutical issues and concerns for elderly patients, including polypharmacy, adverse drug reactions, adherence, and undertreatment of certain conditions.

Medication use is common in the elderly population and increases with age. A population-based survey showed that 44% of men and 57% of women older than age 65 years used five or more medications weekly (Kaufmann et al., 2002). Although persons older than 65 years represent only 13% of the general population, they account for more than 30% of U.S. drug expenditures, totaling more than $73 billion in 2006 (Medical Expenditure Panel Survey, 2006). Polypharmacy is a major risk factor for ADEs. Up to 10% of emergency department visits and 10%

Table 4-11   Pharmacokinetic Changes in Older Persons

Absorption generally does not change
Longer half-life of lipophilic drugs
Increased amount of water soluble and free (active) drug
Decreased excretion

to 17% of hospital admissions are the result of ADEs (Hayes et al., 2007).

PHARMACOKINETICS AND PHARMACODYNAMICS

Knowledge of the physiologic changes that occur with aging is essential when prescribing medications to elderly patients. Changes in pharmacokinetics and pharmacodynamics can result in increased or decreased amounts of medication and drug-drug interactions (Table 4-11).

Pharmacokinetics refers to the body's response to the drug and includes absorption, distribution, metabolism, and elimination (excretion). Age-related gastrointestinal and skin changes have minimal effect on drug absorption, except for drugs that require active gastrointestinal transport (vitamins, minerals), which decreases with aging. The volume of distribution (Vd) is determined by degree of plasma protein binding and body composition. The changes in protein binding are not clinically significant, unless a condition (e.g., acute illness, malnutrition) is causing a marked decline in albumin. Water composition and lean body mass decrease with aging. Fat composition increases, resulting in a larger Vd of lipid-soluble drugs, such as benzodiazepines. Although liver function tests are unchanged, liver size and blood flow are somewhat reduced. The clinical significance is difficult to determine because there is such wide interindividual variation in hepatic metabolism. Drug elimination is mainly affected by a decrease in creatinine clearance. Also, decreased muscle mass causes a decrease in serum creatinine. Because serum creatinine may appear normal even when significant renal impairment exists, it is important to calculate clearance and adjust medication dosages accordingly (Cusak, 2004). The Cockcroft-Gault (1976) formula can be used to estimate creatinine clearance (eCcr).

$$Cr\ clearance = (140 - Age\,[yr]) \times (Actual\ body\ weight\,[kg])/(72 \times Serum\ Cr\,[mg/dL])$$

For women, multiply the result by 0.85. Of note, this formula is less accurate in extremely ill patients and those with moderate to severe renal insufficiency.

Pharmacodynamics refers to the end-organ response to a drug. Although not as well understood as pharmacokinetic changes, pharmacodynamic changes can lead to changes in receptor binding, a decrease in receptor number, and altered translation of response to a receptor. One clinical example involves β-adrenergic blockers and β-adrenergic agonists. With aging, there is a reduction in β-adrenergic activity in the cardiovascular and respiratory systems that can result in less responsiveness to β-blockers and β-agonists (Cooney and Pascuzzi, 2009).

COMMON PRESCRIBING ISSUES

Prescribing problems that can lead to ADEs include a failure to monitor medications appropriately, to prescribe clinically indicated medications, to educate patients, or to maintain continuity (Higashi et al., 2004). One well-researched problem is the use of inappropriate medications in elderly patients. In 1991, based on ADEs in the nursing home, an expert panel developed a list of drugs that should generally be avoided in the elderly population (Beers et al., 1991). The Beers criteria were updated in 2002 to include ambulatory and nursing facility populations (Fick et al., 2003/2004) and further updated in 2012 (AGS, 2012). Medications on the list are generally ineffective in elderly patients, have a higher risk for ADEs, or have safer alternatives (Table 4-12). The list also includes recommendations regarding medication dosages that generally should not be exceeded and medications to avoid in certain comorbid conditions. It is important to note that this list is only a guideline; if a patient has been taking one of the medications without adverse effects, it may not need to be discontinued.

On the other end of the spectrum is failure to prescribe clinically appropriate medications. Common oversights include a failure to prescribe a β-blocker for a patient with congestive heart failure or with a history of a myocardial infarction, aspirin in a patient with known coronary heart disease, or angiotensin-converting enzyme inhibitors for a patient with diabetes and proteinuria (Rosen et al., 2004; Sloane et al., 2004).

PRINCIPLES OF PRESCRIBING

With patients seeing multiple providers across different clinical settings, it is essential that the medication list remain updated. In one prospective observational study, 74% of patients were taking at least one medication of which their primary physician was unaware (Bikowski et al., 2001).

At least once yearly, ask your older patients to bring in all their medications, including over-the-counter medications. Use a checklist to review each medication (Table 4-13). With each medication, first and foremost, review the indication. Educating the patient about the indication can decrease ADEs and increase adherence (Garcia, 2006). Is the medication effective? Medications are often started for good clinical reasons but never revisited as to their efficacy. Are there side effects? Medications should be discontinued if there are intolerable side effects, and always consider an ADE as a cause of any new patient symptom. Avoid the "prescribing cascade," in which medications are started to treat an ADE. Does the medication require any laboratory monitoring? This may include direct drug levels (e.g., digoxin) or monitoring for side effects (e.g., electrolytes in patient taking hydrochlorothiazide).

Is the patient taking the medication? Medication nonadherence is a common and complex issue with both physician and patient factors. Depending on the definition, "nonadherence" ranges from 14% to 70% (DeSmet et al., 2007). Adherence is associated with the number of medications, cost, frequency of dosing, and patient's knowledge of the condition. It is important to obtain the patient's

Table 4-12 Drugs to Avoid or Limit in the General Elderly Population

Pharmacologic Agents	Comments
Drug Classes to Avoid	
Antihistamines	Nonsedating antihistamines (e.g., fexofenadine, loratadine) are considered safer
Antispasmodics	May result in anticholinergic side effects, sedation, and generalized weakness
Barbiturates	Highly addictive with many side effects; numerous other agents for sedation are preferred
GI antispasmodic drugs (e.g., dicyclomine, hyoscyamine)	Highly anticholinergic
Long-acting benzodiazepines (e.g., chlordiazepoxide, diazepam)	Short- or medium-acting agents are preferred; start with smaller doses
Muscle relaxants	May result in anticholinergic side effects, sedation, and generalized weakness
Specific Drugs to Avoid	
Amitriptyline	Highly anticholinergic; use newer antidepressants or less anticholinergic tricyclics
Chlorpropamide	Long half-life leads to increased risk of hypoglycemia; newer insulin secretagogues are preferred
Dipyridamole	May cause dizziness and hypotension
Disopyramide	Anticholinergic and negative inotropic properties
Doxepin	Highly anticholinergic; use newer antidepressants or less anticholinergic tricyclics
Indomethacin	Compared with other NSAIDs, risk of CNS, GI, and renal side effects is greater
Meperidine	Active metabolite normeperidine may accumulate and cause CNS stimulation and seizures
Meprobamate	Highly addictive; may worsen depression; other anxiolytics preferred
Methyldopa	Common side effects include depression, sedation, and edema; multiple antihypertensive options are available
Pentazocine	Mixed narcotic agonist–antagonist with potent CNS effects
Phenylbutazone	May cause severe bone marrow suppression; other NSAIDs are preferred
Propoxyphene	Weak narcotic pain reliever (probably no better than acetaminophen alone) but has same side profile as other narcotics
Reserpine	CNS side effects include sedation and depression; multiple antihypertensive options are available
Ticlopidine	More toxic effects than aspirin or clopidogrel
Trimethobenzamide	May cause extrapyramidal side effects; numerous alternative antiemetics are available
Drugs to Limit	
Digoxin	Limit to <0.125 mg/day in most elderly patients
Ferrous sulfate	Limit to <325 mg/day in most elderly patients
Spironolactone	>50 mg; avoid in patients with heart failure or creatinine clearance <30 mL/min

CNS, Central nervous system; *GI,* gastrointestinal; *NSAID,* nonsteroidal antiinflammatory drug.
Data from American Geriatrics Society 2012 Beers Criteria Update Expert Panel. American Geriatrics Society updated Beers criteria for potentially inappropriate medication use in older adults. *J Am Geriatr Soc.* 2012;60:616-631. http://www.americangeriatrics.org/files/documents/beers/2012BeersCriteria_JAGS.pdf.

Table 4-13 Medication Checklist

Is there a clear indication for this medication?
Is it working?
Are there side effects?
Is the patient taking the medication routinely?
Does the medication need laboratory monitoring?
Is it still needed?

perspective and concerns about medications in a nonjudgmental manner (Erice Medication Errors Research Group, 2009). Methods to increase adherence have focused on educational interventions and external cognitive aids. For short-term therapies, written information, counseling about the medication's indication and potential side effects, and personal phone calls increased adherence. The same effect was not seen for patients taking long-term medications (Haynes et al., 2008; McDonald et al., 2002).

Finally, the checklist should include asking if the medication is still needed. Has the patient's condition changed to where you can stop unnecessary drugs, such as preventive medications in a hospice patient?

Continuity of pharmacists is as important as continuity of physicians in decreasing medication errors. Encourage patients to use one pharmacy and inform the pharmacist of any medication changes. Seeking input from the pharmacist can reduce inappropriate prescribing (Garcia, 2006). With inpatient settings, pharmacists obtain more accurate medication histories from patients, reducing the rate and severity of ADEs (Carter et al., 2006; Reeder and Mutnick, 2008). Simplify the medication regimen by using once-daily dosing and generic drugs, if possible. Discontinue medications that have no indication or benefit (Carlson, 1996). When initiating medications, start one at a time at the lowest dose possible (Table 4-14).

The decision to prescribe a drug depends on many factors besides age, including the patient's functional status, comorbidities, other medications, and personal preferences and values. Physicians must be extremely vigilant in prescribing, especially for frail, elderly patients, carefully weighing the risks and benefits of any new medication. Periodic review of patients' medication list is essential for

Table 4-14 Principles of Prescribing

Periodically update and review the medication list.

Work with the community pharmacist.

Educate the patient about his or her medications.

Consider an adverse drug event as a cause of any new patient symptom.

Simplify the medication regimen.

Start one medication at a time.

monitoring adverse effects, potentially inappropriate drugs, drug–drug interactions, and drug–disease interactions.

KEY TREATMENT

- Current methods of improving medication adherence for chronic health problems are not predictably effective (Haynes et al., 2008; McDonald et al., 2002) (SOR: B).
- Certain drugs should be avoided or limited in the elderly patient (AGS, 2012) (SOR: C).
- Obtain local pharmacists' recommendations to reduce inappropriate prescribing and ADEs (Garcia, 2006) (SOR: B).
- Reviewing a medication list regularly can reduce polypharmacy and inappropriate prescribing (SOR: B).

Urinary Incontinence

Key Points

- Incontinence is a common medical problem in the elderly population, affecting up to 30% of women and 15% of men.
- Older women are more likely to have urge and stress incontinence, and older men are more likely to experience overflow and urge incontinence.
- Acute episodes of incontinence are more likely the result of underlying medical conditions (e.g., infection, hyperglycemia) or new medications (e.g., diuretics).
- Specific health risks, including depression and falls, have been linked to urinary incontinence in elderly patients.
- History, physical examination, urinalysis, and postvoid residual assessment are the key elements in categorization of incontinence.
- In the majority of patients, incontinence can be diagnosed and treated by the primary care provider.
- Treatment options for incontinence include behavior modification, pelvic floor exercises, pharmacologic agents, vaginal pessaries, urethral inserts, condom catheters, penile clamps, and surgical procedures.
- Systemic hormone replacement therapy may exacerbate incontinence.

Urinary incontinence, defined as involuntary leakage of urine, affects 25% to 30% of all adults in their lifetime. Although women report incontinence more often than men, both sexes are affected equally after the age of 80 years. The estimated prevalence of urinary incontinence in people older than 65 years of age ranges from 35% in community-dwelling individuals to more than 60% for those who reside in long-term care facilities (Goode et al., 2008; Song and Bae, 2007; Tennstedt et al., 2008). Incontinence not only increases in prevalence with age but also is considered part of a geriatric syndrome. Within the younger population, a specific condition of the lower urinary tract or its neurologic control is often the cause of urinary incontinence. In older persons, however, incontinence is often secondary to physiologic age-related changes, comorbidities, medications, and functional impairments.

Women spend almost $750 annually out of pocket for incontinence management, have significantly decreased quality of life, and are willing to pay almost $1400 per year for a cure. The annual costs of incontinence care are greater than annual direct costs for breast, ovarian, cervical, and uterine cancer treatments combined (Subak et al., 2006, 2008; Wilson et al., 2001).

Urinary incontinence is associated with increased morbidity and mortality. Studies have demonstrated an association between urinary incontinence and worsening in overall function. Health-related quality of life measurements have been found to decline in individuals with urinary incontinence (DuBeau et al., 2009; Ko et al., 2005; Teunissen et al., 2006). This decline has been seen in those living independently, in assisted living facilities, and in long-term care environments (DuBeau et al., 2006).

Specific health risks linked to urinary incontinence include depression, social isolation, urinary tract infections (UTIs), pressure ulcers, falls and fractures, decreased sexual activity, sleep deprivation, and increased caregiver stress (Brown et al., 2000; Griebling, 2006; Ory et al., 1986; Spector, 1994). Urinary incontinence is also found to be a common reason for institutionalization of elderly patients (Holroyd-Leduc et al., 2004).

AGE-RELATED CHANGES IN URINARY SYSTEM

Specific age-related changes in the urinary system can directly influence urinary continence. The pelvic floor muscles can lose tone and predispose women to uterine, bladder, and rectal prolapse, causing secondary urge incontinence. Overall bladder capacity also tends to decrease, limiting total volume and therefore increasing urge to urinate. Prostatic hypertrophy predisposes older men to increases in postvoid residual volumes. Older incontinent persons may also experience increased involuntary bladder contractions, exacerbating the problem.

PRESENTATION

Urinary incontinence presentations can be divided into acute ("transient") or chronic. Sudden onset of incontinence by potentially reversible and treatable conditions is referred to as acute urinary incontinence. Conditions contributing to acute incontinence include lower urinary tract conditions, stool impaction, delirium, fluid imbalance, impaired mobility, and medications (Table 4-15). These conditions not only precipitate acute urinary incontinence but can also contribute to chronic incontinence.

Chronic incontinence can be divided into five types: urge, stress, overflow, functional, and mixed (Table 4-16).

Table 4-15 Medications That Can Cause or Contribute to Geriatric Urinary Incontinence

Class	Mechanism of Action
Pain relievers	Urinary retention, fecal impaction,
Opioids	sedation, delirium, overflow
Antiinflammatories;	incontinence
COX-2 inhibitors	Increase fluid retention, nocturnal
Skeletal muscle	diuresis, functional incontinence
relaxants	Inhibit bladder contractions causing
	retention and overflow incontinence
Psychotherapeutics	Urinary retention, overflow incontinence
Antidepressants,	Sedation, delirium, immobility causing
antipsychotics	functional and overflow incontinence
sedatives and hypnotics	
Pain relievers	Increased fluid retention, nocturnal
NSAIDS, COX-2	diuresis and functional incontinence
inhibitors	Bladder relaxation, fecal impaction,
Opioids	sedation, retention, overflow
Skeletal muscle	incontinence
relaxants	Inhibit bladder contractions, overflow
	incontinence
Others	Inhibit bladder contractions, sedation,
Anticholinergics,	retention, and overflow incontinence
antihistamines	Lead to diuretic effect, depressed central
Alcohol, caffeine	inhibition, urge and overflow
	incontinence

COX, Cyclooxygenase; *NSAID,* nonsteroidal antiinflammatory drug.

Urge Incontinence

Urge incontinence is the most common type of incontinence identified in older ambulatory patients. It is defined as an abrupt, urgent sensation to urinate and results in loss of urine, with both large and small amounts. Urinary frequency and nocturia are often associated with urge incontinence. Detrusor overactivity is also associated, caused by age-related smooth muscle changes, central inhibitory pathway lesions, history of pelvic irradiation, and bladder sensory or motor innervation deficits. Urge incontinence with an elevated postvoid residual volume can occur when detrusor overactivity and impaired detrusor contractility occur simultaneously. Urinary frequency and retention are common in these patients, particularly those receiving anticholinergic medications.

Stress Incontinence

Stress incontinence is the unintentional loss of urine. It is most often associated with weakening of the pelvic floor muscles and subsequent hypermobility of the bladder outlet and urethra. Stress incontinence occurs with physical movement or activity, such as coughing, sneezing, laughing, or heavy lifting. Stress incontinence is often seen in older women with previous vaginal deliveries or pelvic surgery. It is also associated with lack of estrogen in the menopausal woman. Obesity can exacerbate the symptoms of stress incontinence.

Overflow Incontinence

Symptoms of overflow incontinence include a weak urine stream, dribbling, urinary hesitancy, frequency, and nocturia. These symptoms may overlap with other types of incontinence, influencing the diagnosis. The etiology of overflow incontinence includes detrusor muscle weakness, bladder outlet obstruction, or both. Medications such as narcotics, anticholinergics, and α-adrenergic blockers can contribute to overflow incontinence.

Functional Incontinence

Functional incontinence refers to leakage of urine caused by factors not directly associated with the bladder. Cognitive impairment (e.g., dementia), mobility disorders (e.g., Parkinson's disease), and inaccessible bathrooms are the most common contributing factors in functional incontinence. Factors may be temporary, as in a patient with a lower extremity fracture who is not able to transfer independently on and off the toilet.

Mixed Incontinence

Mixed urinary incontinence is the combination of two types of incontinence simultaneously, typically stress and urge incontinence. Mixed incontinence is the most common type in women, and the causes of the two forms may or may not be related. Detrusor hyperactivity with impaired contractility is a form of mixed incontinence specific to older adults. Symptoms include urinary frequency and urgency caused by uninhibited contractions of the detrusor smooth muscle. When patients try to void, the bladder does not contract sufficiently, and emptying is incomplete, leading to overflow incontinence.

EVALUATION

The initial step in the clinical evaluation is the identification of patients with urinary incontinence. Many older patients do not complain about incontinence to their health care providers because they are embarrassed or believe their symptoms are just part of normal aging. Direct questioning during the review of systems can help identify urinary incontinence: Do you have trouble with your bladder? Do you lose urine when you do not want to? Do you find that you have to wear pads or adult diapers for protection? (Fantl et al., 1996; Kane et al., 2004).

A thorough history and physical examination are important in the clinical evaluation of older patients with urinary incontinence. The main objectives of the workup are to diagnose and treat reversible causes, establish the principal type of urinary incontinence to help guide treatment, identify patients who may need subspecialty referral, and improve overall quality of life for the patient. After urinary incontinence has been identified, the evaluation should continue with a detailed incontinence history, including the type of leakage, frequency, duration, inciting factors, previous treatments, and overall treatment goals. The physical examination should include abdominal, genitopelvic, rectal, and neurologic evaluation. Health care providers need to be aware of the specific "red flags" to refer a patient for further urologic, gynecologic, or urodynamic evaluation (Table 4-17).

A urinalysis should be obtained in all patients to assess for UTIs, hematuria, or other medical conditions that may be associated with urinary incontinence. Persistent hematuria should prompt additional evaluation, including upper

Table 4-16   Basic Types, Causes, and Treatments of Persistent Urinary Incontinence

Types	Symptoms	History	Common Causes	Primary Treatment
Stress	Involuntary loss of urine with increases in intraabdominal pressure (e.g., cough laugh, exercise)	Patient can usually predict which activities cause leakage of urine	Urethral hypermobility Sphincteric dysfunction Radical prostatectomy	Scheduled voiding Pelvic muscle exercises (Kegel) Females: pessary, tampon during exercise; surgical bladder neck suspension or sling; urethral bulking agent Males: condom catheter, penile clamp; synthetic sling, artificial urinary sphincter
Urge	Leakage of urine because of inability to delay voiding after sensation of bladder fullness is perceived	Loss of urine may vary from minimal to complete emptying of bladder (if full) Urinary frequency and nocturia are common	Detrusor overactivity Neurologic disorders Spinal cord injury	Bladder training (including pelvic muscle exercises) Antimuscarinic therapy Topical estrogen (for severe vaginal atrophy or atrophic vaginitis)
Mixed	Combination of urge and stress symptoms	Variable; patient will usually identify which symptom is more bothersome	Combination of above causes	One or a combination of above, targeting most bothersome symptom(s) first
Overflow	Leakage of urine resulting from mechanical forces on an overdistended bladder, or from other effects of urinary retention on bladder and sphincter function	Usually does not occur unless bladder emptying is impaired Usually see postvoid residual volumes >200-300 mL	Detrusor failure Neurologic disorders Spinal cord injury Diabetes Anatomic obstruction	Bladder retraining; Surgical removal of obstruction Intermittent catheterization Indwelling catheterization
Functional	Urinary accidents associated with inability to toilet because of impairment of cognitive or physical functioning, psychological unwillingness, or environmental barriers	Physical or cognitive impairment May have lower urinary tract deficits	Mobility Impairment Cognitive Impairment	Behavioral interventions with toileting assistance Environmental adaptations Undergarments and pads

urinary tract imaging and cystoscopy. A postvoid residual volume (with ultrasound or catheterization) helps to exclude overflow incontinence. In clinical practice, a postvoid volume of less than 50 mL is regarded as normal, and in general, residual volumes greater than 200 mL are considered abnormal (Fantl et al., 1996).

Voiding (bladder) diaries can provide valuable information for the clinician and patient. The diary includes documentation of each urination episode and any associated symptoms of incontinence for three 24-hour periods. If possible, the patient can also record the amount of fluid intake and output (Abrams and Klevmark, 1996). Several patterns of abnormality can emerge from the voiding diary. For example, frequent small volumes can occur in patients with overactive bladder syndrome, detrusor overactivity, and some painful bladder conditions (e.g., cancer). Frequent large-volume voids are associated with polyuria, as seen in patients with excessive fluid intake and conditions causing polyuria (e.g., diabetes, hypercalcemia). Obstructive sleep apnea, physiologic aging, congestive heart failure, and medications can all cause nocturnal polyuria (Bryan and Chapple, 2004). A simple office tool that can help detect stress incontinence is the cough test. The patient is asked to produce a forceful cough with a comfortably full bladder to determine any urine leakage and potential stress incontinence.

TREATMENT

Several therapeutic options exist to help manage the different types of urinary incontinence. Many older adults prefer to start with conservative therapies such as behavioral modification techniques before considering medications or surgery. In many cases, several small behavioral changes together may lead to significant improvement in symptoms.

Behavioral Interventions

Particular beverages can aggravate the lower urinary tract symptoms in older adults. Alcohol, caffeine, and highly acidic citrus fruits and drinks are considered direct bladder irritants and may worsen incontinence symptoms. Alcohol has diuretic properties, causing increased urinary frequency. Weight loss may be beneficial for some patients, in particular women with stress incontinence. Nocturia is a common complaint for many elderly patients with multifactorial causes (Sugaya et al., 2008). Minimizing late-afternoon and evening fluid intake may decrease nocturnal episodes for some patients. Reduced production of antidiuretic hormone has been seen in patients with obstructive sleep apnea. Treatment of the sleep apnea may help reduce nocturia symptoms (Kujuba and Aboseif, 2008).

In older patients with symptoms of urinary urgency, timed voiding is often suggested. Many patients experience symptoms only when the bladder is full, so voiding more frequently will reduce the amount of bladder distention and the sense of urinary urgency. Older patients with cognitive or mobility impairments will often need assisted-toileting programs. Providing physical assistance in going to the toilet on a regular basis can reduce incontinence episodes (van Houten et al., 2007). Some patients benefit from bladder retraining, in which they are taught to delay voiding

Table 4-17 "Red Flag" Criteria to Refer an Older Patient with Incontinence to a Subspecialist

Significant uterine, bladder, or rectal prolapse

Surgery or radiation involving the lower urinary tract within the past 6 months

Two or more symptomatic urinary infections within the past 6 months

Greater than 5 red blood cells per high-power field on repeated urinalysis in the absence of infection

Postvoid residual volume >200 mL

Marked prostatic enlargement, prominent asymmetry, or induration of the lobes

Persistent symptoms after appropriate trials of behavioral or drug therapy

at progressively longer intervals (Wallace et al., 2004). Bladder retraining can take months and has the most benefit for patients with urge incontinence and those with mixed incontinence when combined with pelvic floor exercises (Teunissen et al., 2004). The patient is encouraged to focus on the sensations in the pelvis, complete pelvic floor contractions, and wait until the urgency sensation subsides before proceeding to the toilet.

Pelvic floor muscle (Kegel) exercises remain one of the mainstays of behavioral therapy in the treatment of urinary incontinence. The exercises involve repetitive contractions and relaxations of the pelvic floor muscles. They have been found effective in stress, urge, and mixed incontinence (Hay-Smith and Dumoulin, 2006). A simply way to teach women to identify and isolate the pelvic floor muscles is by having the patient squeeze the examiner's finger during vaginal examination. Squeezing the examiner's finger by contracting the anal sphincter during a rectal examination can help both men and women isolate the pelvic floor muscles.

Management with Devices

There are two main device options for women with primarily stress incontinence: pessaries and urethral inserts. Pessaries come in many different forms and sizes and have been used for hundreds of years for the treatment of pelvic organ prolapse and urinary incontinence in women. The support offered by the pessary helps in correcting the angles and contacts between adjacent organs, thus minimizing bladder irritation and spontaneous contractions that lead to incontinence. Women need to have pessaries fitted individually by a health care provider. Routine cleaning and care by either the patient or, in many cases, a health care provider is required. Urethral inserts are short silicone single-use tubes. The tube is placed in the urethra by the woman and held in place by a mineral oil–filled bulbous sheath that is located in the bladder neck. In a 2-year follow-up study of 150 women using the insert, mild urethral trauma (6.7%) and UTIs (31.3%) occurred (Sirls et al., 2002). The urethral insert has not seen as widespread use as the pessary.

Men with incontinence have a few device options, including condom catheters and body-worn urinal and penile clamps. A condom catheter is a well-known external collection device and is much safer than indwelling catheters, which have been associated with UTIs and patient discomfort (Saint et al., 2006). Several condom catheter brands and sizes are available, and most are latex free.

Another similar device is the body-worn urinal. Body-worn urinals consist of a rubber cone (into which the penis fits) and a flange (with a central hole through which the penis passes) that fits around the base of the penis. Body-worn urinals are secured in place by straps or specially designed support underwear as opposed to adhesive. The final male-specific option is the penile clamp. It is a device that is applied to the pendulous part of the penis, preventing urinary leakage, and is used primarily for stress incontinence. The clamps carry a risk of penile edema, urethral erosion, pain, and skin breakdown. Use over a short period of time and by cognitively intact men provides for an excellent discreet device option for male incontinence (Saint et al., 2006).

Absorbent Pads. Many older adults with urinary incontinence use some type of pad or undergarment to help with their urinary incontinence. Although these products play an important role in the management of incontinence symptoms, patients should be encouraged to seek other types of treatment if appropriate. The cost of these products can be significant and is not covered by Medicare or most other insurance plans. However, it is important to realize that these absorbent products can help older adults maintain their functional independence and participate in their preferred activities.

Pharmacologic Therapies

Various medications have been used to treat the different forms of urinary incontinence. However, most current medications are used for urge or mixed incontinence because there is little evidence that adrenergic agonists help stress incontinence (Alhasso et al., 2005) (Table 4-18). The anticholinergic, antimuscarinic medications prescribed for urge incontinence work by blocking cholinergic receptors in the bladder, which in turn diminishes bladder contractility. This class of medications is effective but has adverse side effects (e.g., dry mouth, constipation) related to the cross-reactivity with muscarinic receptors in the salivary glands and colon (Alhasso et al., 2006). Additional side effects include dry eyes, blurry vision, and risk of urinary retention. Anticholinergics can also worsen cognitive function in elderly patients or cause drug-induced delirium, mimicking dementia. Newer medications (e.g., Sanctura) that are theoretically more uroselective and preferentially bind to the muscarinic receptors in the bladder may be associated with fewer adverse side effects. Incontinence medications should not be prescribed to those patients with untreated closed-angle glaucoma and in memory-impaired patients already taking cholinesterase inhibitors to prevent further deterioration of memory function. The anticholinergic agents and cholinesterase inhibitors work in direct opposition and, if taken together, can lead to rapid loss of cognitive function (Sink et al., 2008).

α-Adrenergic antagonists are helpful in treating urge incontinence in men with benign prostatic hypertrophy (BPH). Hypotension is a common side effect with traditional α agents. The newer agents (e.g., Tamsulosin) have fewer adverse side effects and should be used in older men who have low blood pressure or episodes of dizziness. The

Table 4-18   Drug Treatment for Urinary Incontinence

Generic Drugs (Trade Name)	Dosages	Mechanisms of Action	Type of Incontinence
Antimuscarinic			
Darifenacin (Enablex)	7.5-15 mg QD	Lesson involuntary bladder contractions and increasing bladder capacity	Urge or mixed
Oxybutynin (Ditropan) (Ditropan XL) (Oxytrol) transdermal	2.5-5 mg TID 5-30 mg QD (extended-release XL) 3.9- mg patch Q4 days	Lesson involuntary bladder contractions and increasing bladder capacity	Urge or mixed
Solifenacin (Vesicare)	5-10 mg QD	Lesson involuntary bladder contractions and increasing bladder capacity	Urge or mixed
Tolterodine (Detrol) (Detrol XL)	1-2 mg BID 2-4 mg QD (extended-release XL)	Lesson involuntary bladder contractions and increasing bladder capacity	Urge or mixed
Trospium (Sanctura) (Santura XR)	20 mg BID 60 mg QD (extended-release XR)	Lesson involuntary bladder contractions and increasing bladder capacity	Urge or mixed
Estrogen			
Topical estrogen Topical cream Vaginal ring Vaginal tablets	0.5-1.0 g/day for 2 wk; then twice weekly One ring Q3 months One 25-μg tablet QD for 2 wk; then twice weekly	Strengthen periurethral tissues Increase periurethral blood flow	Urge associated with severe vaginal atrophy or atrophic vaginitis
Cholinergic Agonists			
Bethanechol (Urecholine)	10-30 mg TID	Stimulates bladder contraction	Overflow incontinence with atonic bladder
α-Adrenergic Antagonists			
Alfuzosin (UroXatral) Tamsulosin (Flomax) Terazosin (Hytrin)	10 mg QD 0.4 mg QD 1 to 10 mg QHS	Relax smooth muscle or urethra and prostate capsule	Urge and symptoms associated with BPH

BID, Twice daily; *BPH,* benign prostatic hypertrophy; *Q,* every; *QD,* every day, *QHS,* every night at bedtime; *TID,* three times daily.

addition of an antimuscarinic drug can be considered in men who are still symptomatic on α-antagonist therapy. For long-term treatment of overflow incontinence in men, 5α-reductase inhibitors alone or in combination have been shown to reduce the voiding symptoms from BPH as well as the incidence of urinary retention (McConnell et al., 2003).

Currently, no medications are approved by the Food and Drug Administration for the treatment of stress incontinence. Estrogen has been prescribed in the past for stress incontinence because it was thought to improve urethral thickness and vascularity and sensitize α-adrenergic receptors in the bladder neck musculature. However, a Cochrane review failed to demonstrate improvement in stress incontinence while patients were taking estrogen, and the incontinence may actually worsen with oral agents. Conversely, combination estrogen–progestin oral hormone therapy has been associated with increased frequency of incontinence. Topical estrogen in the same Cochrane review was mildly effective when prescribed for older women with urge incontinence related to atrophic vaginitis or severe vaginal atrophy (Cody et al., 2009; Grady et al., 2001; Rossouw et al., 2002).

Surgical Treatment

The sling procedure is the primary form of open surgical treatment in women with stress incontinence. Several variations of the procedure exist with relation to the exact location of the sling and the nature of the graft material used to make the sling. The principal function of the sling is to increase the outlet resistance and thus prevent urine leakage during periods of increased intraabdominal pressure. Initial success rates for the sling procedure range from 80% to 90% but decrease with time. Some women respond to other forms of therapy or elect to undergo another sling procedure (Anger et al., 2007).

Periurethral injection of bulking agents can be an effective treatment is some elderly women with stress incontinence. The procedure is minimally invasive and can be performed in the outpatient setting with rapid recovery and immediate results. To date, there is limited evidence that this can relieve stress incontinence in women (Keegan et al., 2007). One disadvantage is that treatment usually needs to be repeated with time. Injection therapy may be particularly useful in elderly women who are unable to undergo the more invasive sling procedure or who are symptomatic after a previous sling procedure. Older men with mild postprostatectomy stress incontinence may benefit from periurethral injection of bulking agents (Fantl et al., 1996).

KEY TREATMENT

- Pelvic floor exercises help with all types of urinary incontinence in women (Hay-Smith and Dumoulin, 2006) (SOR: A).
- Anticholinergic drugs are effective for overactive bladder syndrome but are associated with common side effects (Alhasso et al., 2006) (SOR: A).
- There is limited evidence that periurethral injection helps women with stress incontinence (Keegan et al., 2007) (SOR: A).

References

The complete reference list is available online at www.expertconsult.com.

Web Resources

www.aoa.gov The Administration on Aging offers comprehensive information about "seniors," including aging statistics and government programs.

www.ncbi.nlm.nih.gov/bookshelf/br.fcgi?book=hsahcpr&part=A5124 The Agency for Health Care Policy and Research's treatment of pressure ulcers guideline.

www.ncea.aoa.gov/NCEAroot/Main_Site/Index.aspx The National Center on Elder Abuse provides information on the prevention, diagnosis, and management of elder abuse, including available resources for physicians, patients, and families.

www.npuap.org The National Pressure Ulcer Advisory Panel provides up-to-date information on the prevention and management of pressure ulcers.

Podcasts

www.fammed.wisc.edu/our-department/media/615/geriatric-assessment An overview of geriatric assessment in the office.

www.youtube.com/user/WIFamilyMedicine#p/u/4%20%3/xIMJ1aVvch8 An overview of the assessment and management of elder abuse.

5   *Care of the Dying Patient*

ROBERT E. RAKEL and THUY HANH TRINH

Medical education and our professional attitude regarding patient care are oriented primarily toward sustaining life and curing disease. This is reasonable because not long ago, the major causes of death were infectious diseases, which usually attacked young people, who died before experiencing life. With the advent of antibiotics, it was possible to triumph over these diseases and prevent untimely death. Patients had a high probability of complete recovery. It is no surprise, therefore, that the medical profession emphasized preserving life at all costs and became preoccupied with the advancing technology that made such triumphs possible. Today, most people no longer die of acute illness but rather from chronic disease for which there is no cure. This calls for medicine to focus on improving the *quality* rather than the *quantity* of life and to recognize that the relief from suffering is superior to attempts to cure when there is limited likelihood of success. Patients with chronic diseases and those who are terminally ill benefit most from supportive therapy.

In previous centuries, it was assumed that life should be lived so that one would be able to "die well," but contemporary American culture has refused to accept death as a normal occurrence. Children and young adults have been conditioned to consider death from the viewpoint of the observer or disinterested third party. An individual's attitude toward his or her own death depends largely on experiences in dealing with the deaths of relatives or friends. Rather than a time of despair, sickness may be used as an opportunity for reflection. For some patients, it may be the first time they have faced their own mortality. Too often, however, this natural personal encounter has been depersonalized by removing the dying patient to an institutional setting.

Care of a terminally ill patient typically focuses on the disease, neglecting the patient as a whole person. The value of treatment must be interpreted on the basis of its net value to the individual. When additional treatments no longer provide benefits, the patient needs someone who provides personalized care with attention to the patient's emotional as well as physical comfort. The dying person often is isolated physically and emotionally from familiar surroundings and placed in a social setting that gives very low priority to an individual's personality, fears, and past experiences. Informed physicians, family, and friends can do much to help the terminal patient die with integrity and dignity. However, if dying is really to be accepted as a normal component of the life cycle, reintegration of the dying patient into the routine course of living is necessary.

The concept of quality care does not always demand that death be regarded as an enemy to be fought with every weapon at a physician's disposal. The technology of today makes it possible to keep people alive indefinitely, often without consideration for their quality of life. An obsession with quantity of life can adversely affect its quality; at times, a graceful death with dignity is preferable to lingering torment (LORAN Commission, 1989). Many people consider quality of life more important than quantity and want to leave while they still have something to say about it. The goal is to "respect the experience of living while supporting the process of dying" (Berlinger et al., 2013, p. 13).

The Physician's Attitude

Fewer than 10% of people die suddenly; more than 90% experience a protracted, life-threatening illness (Emanuel et al., 2003). Terminal illness is more taxing on the physician than sudden and unexpected death. Not surprisingly, an empathic family physician with a long patient relationship may be uncomfortable in dealing with the patient's impending death. Physicians are most uncomfortable when they feel helpless. Unfortunately, this leads to withdrawal from the patient who is terminally ill because the physician inappropriately feels helpless and impotent, when in fact a great deal of comfort and help can be provided. "Even the busiest doctor owes [the patient] courtesy and compassion" (Lieberman, 2013, p. 136).

While expressing concern and compassion for a terminal patient, the family physician still must maintain composure and objectivity to remain effective. Osler (1904) referred to this as "calm equanimity" and added, "Our equanimity is chiefly exercised in enabling us to bear with composure the misfortunes of our neighbors" (p. 8). Medicine long has emphasized the need for physicians to remain objective and deal with problems factually; if a physician is unable to do so effectively, attempts to hide emotion may lead the physician to adopt a facade that appears unsympathetic and insensitive to the patient's needs. A son reported that "with the worsening of my father's condition, the physician stopped being friendly and warm; his visits became rare and brief; his manner became quite detached, almost angry" (Seravalli, 1988, p. 1729).

Physicians sometimes lose enthusiasm for care when an illness has been recognized as incurable. If this occurs, interaction with the patient diminishes at the very time emotional support is needed most. Time-motion studies indicate that nurses and other ward personnel also spend less time with terminally ill patients when giving baths and providing routine care. Using videotape surveillance of terminally ill patients' rooms in a university hospital, Sulmasy and Rahn (2001) found that the average patient spent more than 10 hours alone while awake per day. Because abandonment is a major fear of terminally ill patients, we must remain aware of the need to reduce the time patients spend without human interaction by physicians, nurses, or family.

Compassion fatigue is a form of emotional exhaustion and diminished empathy more common in health professionals caring for dying patients. Symptoms parallel those of posttraumatic stress disorder—that is, hyperarousal in the form of disturbed sleep and irritability, avoidance of the patient, and intrusive thoughts or dreams relating to the provider's work with dying patients (Kearney et al., 2009).

During the terminal stages of a fatal illness, it is vital to the dying patient that the family physician maintain a warm and caring relationship and, through the strength of the doctor–patient bond, provide support for the patient.

A physician who is uncomfortable discussing impending death can discourage conversation in many subtle ways. Hospital rounds are made rapidly, perhaps in a superficial, lighthearted manner, never pausing long enough to give the patient an opportunity to express fears and concerns. Comments such as "everything will be all right" effectively close lines of communication with an intelligent patient who is fully aware of the seriousness of the situation. When the physician tells a patient, "Don't worry," the patient interprets this as, "Don't bother me." Patients are unlikely to initiate discussions regarding their fears of death or feelings of helplessness under such circumstances and remain silent or avoid these issues unless they think the physician is interested and will listen. The physician easily can squelch such conversation, but a slight indication of willingness to discuss the problems disturbing the patient often results in frank conversations, which relieve much of the patient's anxiety and reveal concerns that can be shared only with the physician.

THE "RIGHT TIME" TO DIE

Simpson (1976) described the "how dare you die on me" syndrome in which the patient has the "effrontery" to die before medical and nursing staff have used all the treatments in their repertoire. The patient is supposed to die "at the right time"—neither before all potential effective therapies have been tried nor too long after all palliative procedures have been used. Health professionals often need to believe that everything possible was done for the patient before death. These attitudes have developed because the health care process too often focuses more on professional expectations than patient needs.

We might consider what we have done to a patient who dies in the isolation of a laminar flow room without having been able to touch another person's hand during his last few weeks of life. Such treatment is a *false-positive,* a treatment inappropriate to the real needs of the patient (Saunders, 1976).

However, it is impossible for physicians to provide adequate support during this difficult time unless they have come to grips with their own mortality. Studies by the Group for the Advancement of Psychiatry have revealed that physicians are afraid of death in greater proportion than patient control participants (Aring, 1971). What better defense against death than to make one's full-time vocation fighting it?

Patients are often more willing to accept death than the physicians who treat them, and many fear that they will receive more aggressive treatment than they want. Based on interviews with seriously ill patients, 60% preferred that treatment focus on comfort even if it meant shortening their lives. The other 40% wanted life-extending care. Of those preferring comfort care, only 41% reported that treatment matched their wishes (Teno et al., 2002). In another study, more than half of physicians interviewed admitted they had provided overly aggressive care to patients (Solomon et al., 1993).

Many, if not most, patients will choose toxic chemotherapy even if there is only a slight chance of cure or even if it would prolong their life by only a few months. The concern is that they may choose this route on the advice of their physician even though they will be miserable for those remaining months. It is important to have a straightforward discussion with the patient about the quality and quantity of life with and without chemotherapy. More than 20% of Medicare patients with metastatic cancer had a new chemotherapy treatment regimen started in the 2 weeks before death (Earle et al., 2004).

Unfortunately, chemotherapy is better compensated than are discussions as to its need and potential side effects. It is no surprise that oncologists prefer third- or fourth-line chemotherapy to discussing hospice care. One patient received intrathecal chemotherapy 6 days before his death at a cost of $3400 (Harrington and Smith, 2008).

Communication

WHEN TO TELL THE PATIENT

The issue today is not so much whether to tell patients they have a terminal illness but rather how to share this information with them—because most patients know the nature of their disease process to some degree. Because they know their patients well, family physicians should be able to gauge patients' desire to be told and their capacity to withstand the shock of disclosure. When a terminal state of cancer is inevitable, most patients prefer to discuss such issues with their family physician rather than with their oncologist.

Key Points

- Abandonment is a major fear of dying patients, who spend an average of 10 awake hours alone per day.
- Listening and allowing patients to express their fears and concerns is of great therapeutic benefit.
- Touch and sitting with the patient convey support and compassion.
- Frequent assessment of the patient and family's desire for information must be accompanied by honest answers.
- Patients should be allowed as much control as possible to avoid fear of the unknown.
- When cure is not possible, much benefit can be derived from attention to daily symptom control.
- Avoid giving false hope but remember that hope and humor can be therapeutic.

Table 5-1   Useful Questions in Determining a Terminally Ill Patient's Needs and Wishes

What do you fear most?

What would you like to accomplish in the time left?

What is your highest priority?

How can I help you achieve this?

What has been most difficult about this illness for you?

How is your family (e.g., wife, husband, child) dealing with your illness?

Is religion important to you?

Patients who have end-of-life conversations with their family physician have lower health care costs during the final week of life. Better communication results in better quality of life and quality of death as well as lower cost (Zhang et al., 2009). End-of-life care is often fragmented among providers, leading to a lack of continuity of care and impeding the ability to provide high-quality, interdisciplinary care. A family conference to discuss a plan of care, which would include the patient if he or she were still capable of participating, is often initiated after the patient's functional decline (Berlinger et al., 2013). Enhanced communication among patients, families, and providers is crucial to high-quality end-of-life care (National Institutes of Health, 2004).

A frank discussion of death or how long the patient is expected to live may not be necessary or even indicated. A good understanding between the physician and patient may make open disclosure unnecessary. The physician's role may be primarily one of supporting patients during the progressive, terminal course of their illness. However, the physician who is uncomfortable with the subject of death should not use such a situation as an excuse to avoid discussing the issue. The family physician's primary responsibility is to take the time to evaluate the situation, make sure the patient's true desires have been assessed correctly, and provide whatever support is needed based on the patient's concepts and needs rather than those of the physician (Table 5-1). An institution's policies should recognize that, on occasion, a health care professional may choose to withdraw from a patient on religious or other moral grounds as a conscientious objection. The institutions should accommodate for this request without compromising standards of professional care and the rights of the patients. The physician should maintain the duty of care until the patient is transferred to another professional (Berlinger et al., 2013).

A physician who can deal with death honestly is able to focus more attention on the patient and can determine the patient's level of awareness by listening and observing nonverbal cues. Clues to the patient's wish to discuss the condition may simply be a deep sigh, a tear, or a shaky voice. The physician must be alert during busy hospital rounds for these or similar signs. The physician can pause to sit and encourage conversation if time permits or return later when more time is available. Whenever possible, however, the response should be at that moment because the patient is more likely to communicate freely in a spontaneous situation. Physicians who are uncomfortable in this situation may insulate themselves from the issue during hospital rounds by checking the bedside monitoring equipment or otherwise directing attention away from the patient, effectively ignoring overt as well as subtle clues to the patient's needs.

Talking with patients about their death can be difficult, but end-of-life discussions with patients do not result in greater emotional or psychological stress. On the contrary, worse outcomes are found in those who do not have these conversations. Such discussions result in less aggressive medical care near death and earlier hospice referrals. Wright and colleagues (2008) showed that quality of life deteriorates with a greater number of aggressive end-of-life interventions and improves with longer hospice care. Even if a patient has a short hospice stay of hours to days, the patient may still benefit from a higher quality of life because of better symptom management and spiritual support for both the patient and the family (Waldrop et al., 2009). A key benefit of hospice is bereavement support for the patient's family up to 13 months after the patient has died. When the patient is ready to discuss her or his impending death, the physician and patient are probably past the most difficult stage, and the physician needs merely to listen, accept the patient's feelings, and respond to questions honestly. Most patients raise questions that indicate how much they wish to know, provided the physician gives them the opportunity. The most supportive and facilitative act the physician can provide is to sit and ask the patient, "Do you have any questions?" When asked in a sincere manner, patients who are ready to talk about their death will take advantage of the opportunity, but they may be reluctant under other, more hurried circumstances.

Patients usually will indicate their desire to discuss their prognosis, as well as when they want to avoid the subject and focus on other topics. Even patients who fully accept their terminal process cannot remain constantly focused on that subject and must attend to more satisfying issues. Physicians should honor and respond to this need, just as they would respond to a desire to discuss pain or other problems.

What physicians say to dying patients is not nearly as important as their willingness to listen. One of the most comforting steps physicians can take in caring for the dying is to allow them to talk about their fears, frustrations, hopes, needs, and desires. *Talking about problems can be very therapeutic.* Patients who are permitted to examine and discuss their feelings about death and dying are grateful for the opportunity and usually become less anxious, experience less pain, and accept their situation more easily. If they are denied this opportunity, especially when the terminal process is obvious, they may be convinced that the time remaining is too terrible to be discussed, and their anxiety will be significantly increased. Often, terminally ill patients are more fearful of the manner in which death will occur (e.g., painful, alone and abandoned, weak and helpless) than they are of death itself.

Do all patients want to be told of their fatal illness, however? Surveys indicate that 80% to 90% of patients say they wish to be told, but many physicians prefer not to tell a patient that he or she is dying. Ward (1974) found that family physicians are more likely to discuss a fatal diagnosis with women than with men (22% vs. 7.5%) and more often with patients in the upper social class than the lower social class (24% vs. 5% for men; 30% vs. 26% for women). Physicians often wait until the patient is close to death before initiating end-of-life discussions with patients and their families. Patients with cancer often receive a more comprehensive discussion about end-of-life issues than patients with noncancer diagnoses (Abarshi et al., 2011). Promoting earlier discussion about end-of-life decisions helps patients and their families to better prepare for the changes to come. Medical students must be trained more adequately to assist their future patients with how to cope with the dying process. Allowing space to patients and family is beneficial for all participants in the discussion, combined with communication that includes active listening tailored to each patient's needs (Mazzi et al., 2013).

Most physicians tell a patient that he or she has terminal cancer if the patient asks a direct question but otherwise evade the issue and discuss it openly only with the family. In many cases, this is the most appropriate course of action; some patients clearly indicate that they cannot and do not wish to face the fact that they have an incurable disease. It is essential, however, that the physician evaluate the true nature of the patient's desire in the matter and neither avoid the issue when the patient wishes to discuss it nor force a discussion on an unwilling individual. "When the task of telling a patient about an onerous diagnosis is too easy, the doctor has become callous. When it is too difficult, he needs to examine his own guilt or anxiety" (Weisman and Brettell, 1978, p. 251).

Patients should be given adequate time to absorb the knowledge of the terminal nature of their illness and the opportunity to react appropriately before death intervenes. This is not possible if the physician procrastinates or rationalizes that it is better not to inform the patient. The process should not be allowed to advance to such a final a stage that inadequate time remains for individuals to react appropriately and put their affairs in order.

HOW TO TELL THE PATIENT

There is no need to answer questions the patient has not yet asked. One way to approach the subject is to ask patients what they think the problem is or how sick they think they really are. The response may be straightforward ("I think I have cancer"), or the patient may indicate a wish to avoid the issue by saying, "I hope it's nothing serious." The patient's condition can be revealed gradually or in stages, such as telling the patient after surgery that there is a suspicion of cancer but that further information will have to wait for the pathology report. The physician should observe the patient's response to this initial suspicion and, based on that reaction, choose a method for presenting subsequent information. Tumulty (1973) supported the concept of *gradualism* in informing a patient and the family of the terminal nature of the illness: "The total truth is revealed in small doses as the illness unfolds, affording the family the opportunity to get its feet under itself before another blow falls. ... The patient and the family need to be eased into the truth ... not slugged with it" (pp. 180-181).

Such a gradual disclosure is likely to lead to acceptance, but a harsh, sudden, or abrupt disclosure is likely to result in denial or severe depression. If the patient appears reluctant to accept the information, do not push the issue; merely make sure that openings for discussion are made available periodically and further information is provided when the patient is ready.

One statement is never appropriate: "There is nothing more that we can do." Such statements tell patients they are being abandoned and increase their feelings of isolation and vulnerability. There is *always* something the family physician can do to provide compassionate, comforting care to the patient and family even if it is only sitting at the bedside so the patient does not feel abandoned. *Distress* can take many forms: physical, emotional, and spiritual, as well as anticipating symptoms that may arise, such as pain, constipation, anxiety, depression, and nausea. Family physicians also can help by stopping or avoiding treatments and diagnostic procedures that hold little promise of improving the patient's quality of life, such as taking vital signs or turning patients in bed when they are trying to sleep. If a test will not lead to a change in treatment, the test is not indicated.

Delivering "Bad News"

When giving "bad news" to a patient, do so privately and without interruption (see eTable 5-1). Use language the patient can understand, allow the patient to be emotional, offer to help break the news to the patient's family and employer, and be sure that care providers know what the patient has been told (Field and Cassel, 1997).

Health care professionals caring for patients at the end of life should assess the patient's readiness to engage in the discussion and appreciate their level of understanding about the situation and how much they want to know. When physicians know the patient's preferences, they can tailor the discussion appropriately, checking periodically for the patient's level of comprehension and desire for more information. It is best to provide small amounts of information at a time, frequently assessing the patient's desire to continue. Also, besides comprehension, what are the patient's expectations?

When sharing information regarding a fatal diagnosis with a patient, eye contact, touch, and personal closeness are important. If possible, sit with the patient and hold his or her hand or touch the forearm. Such gestures convey a sense of support, closeness, and compassion, reinforcing

Table 5-2   Positive Language to Use with Dying Patients

I will keep you as comfortable as possible.

I will focus on maintaining your quality of life.

I want to help you live meaningfully in the time you have left.

I will do everything I can to help you maintain your independence.

Maintaining your independence and dignity will be my top priority.

I will do my best to fulfill your wish to remain at home.

Modified from Stone MJ. Goals of care at the end of life. *Proc (Bayl Univ Med Cent).* 2001;14;134-137.

verbal assurance that the patient will not be abandoned during the difficult time remaining. Be positive whenever possible (Table 5-2).

Sitting with the patient on the bed or at the bedside rather than standing puts the physician on the same level and conveys in a clear, nonverbal manner a willingness to talk and listen. In one study, physicians visited with hospitalized patients for exactly 3 minutes. Half the visits they sat down, and the other half they remained standing, a little removed from the bed. "Every one of the patients [with whom] the physician had sat down thought the physician had stayed at least 10 minutes. None of the ones [with whom] the physician remained standing estimated that it was as long" (Kübler-Ross, 1975, p. 20).

PROGNOSTICATING

One of the most difficult tasks in medicine is predicting how long someone with a terminal illness will live. People enjoy repeating stories of patients who survived long after the date their doctor predicted. In most cases, however, physicians tend to be overly optimistic, and short estimates are more accurate than longer ones (Evans and McCarthy, 1985).

In fact, physicians overestimate survival more than 60% of the time and underestimate it only 17% of the time (Christakis and Lamont, 2000). In addition to physicians overestimating prognosis, many patients believe their treatment at the end of their life (e.g., radiation) is intended to be curative, when in reality it is palliative. The better that physicians know their patients, the more they overestimate survival, probably hoping the best for patients they know well. The longer the physician has been in practice, the more accurate the prognosis. Most patients want optimistic physicians, but at some point, this optimism may delay palliative treatment.

Attempts have been made to develop indexes (e.g., Karnofsky score) to assist the physician in making objective estimates that correlate with actual survival. However, no accurate method is currently available, largely because of the multiple variables that influence when a patient dies. A good policy is to provide a conservative estimate. It is better to have the patient and family proud that they "beat the odds" or exceeded the physician's prediction than to have the patient die earlier than anticipated.

CONSPIRACY OF SILENCE

Honesty with the terminal patient will provide the greatest benefits. However, the physician frequently is torn between patient and family, with the patient saying, "Don't tell my wife because she can't handle it," while the wife is saying, "Don't tell my husband because he can't handle it." Although the wishes and desires of the family must be considered when deciding how to care for a dying patient, the physician's primary obligation is to the patient. The method of management must be based on the physician's knowledge of the patient and insight into the patient's desires, feelings, and approach to life. Despite all efforts at deception, the patient knows or will soon learn about his or her condition.

By cooperating with the family in a conspiracy of silence, information that really belongs to the patient is withheld. Only if the physician believes that the patient is not yet ready to cope with the information or sincerely wishes not to be told should the information be withheld; however, this is more often the exception than the rule. One patient said, "I knew it was cancer from the moment they started lying to me" (Lamerton, 1976, p. 28). Simpson (1976) described a 63-year-old woman whose family insisted she knew nothing of her inoperable gastric carcinoma. When visited by the physician, "She gave a dry chuckle: 'Only a little ulcer ... and my relatives down from Wales to see me for the first time in 15 years, and the priest here at 6 in the morning?'" (p. 193). When such a charade continues, terminally ill patients become increasingly more isolated because they are unable to communicate their concerns and fears honestly and openly with those closest to them. The elaborate schemes some families and physicians develop to "protect" the patient lead to great tension within the family, as everyone attempts to perpetuate the lie while continuing to interact with the patient.

Similarly, failure to provide the information to the patient's family can lead to a decrease in the quality of their relationship in the time remaining because the patient's tensions and fears are not understood by family members and friends. Dunphy (1976) described a patient with terminal cancer who asked that his wife not be told. He then quickly planned a world cruise, which they had wanted to take for some time. The wife, unaware of the reason for the hasty departure, was unhappy and complaining throughout the trip, while the husband saw himself as a silent martyr, trying to provide a final measure of happiness for his wife. Only after returning home and reminiscing on this miserable cruise did he tell his wife the truth and the reason for the precipitous departure. Had she been told earlier, their final days together could have been a pleasant and memorable experience. At a time when the terminally ill patient most needs closeness, a lie may serve to push them apart.

Denial

Most patients tend to deny the reality of their situation after being made aware of the terminal nature of their illness. Denial is one way of coping with or protecting oneself against overwhelming anxiety, which otherwise could be incapacitating. This reaction is more marked in a patient who is told abruptly without adequate preparation. Although denial is noted primarily when the patient first learns of impending death, it can appear in different degrees at different times. Even patients who have accepted the terminal nature of their illness will need to use denial periodically to avoid feelings of hopelessness. The mental burden of impending death is too heavy to carry all the time, and periodic relief is necessary to carry on customary activities and enjoy the limited time left. As Aring (1971) noted, La Rochefoucauld said, "Neither the sun nor death can be looked at steadily."

Patients who avoid asking about their illness or prognosis when the physician offers every opportunity usually are experiencing denial. Excessive denial usually means that the patient subconsciously knows the truth but wants to avoid facing it consciously. Even when repeatedly given the accurate diagnosis, some patients deny ever having been told. This denial provides constant emotional protection until the patient is ready to face the truth.

"Watch with Me"

The greatest fear of the dying patient is that of suffering alone and being deserted. There is less fear of a painful death than of the loneliness and alienation that may accompany it. A patient particularly dreads being abandoned by the physician in the face of death and may need increasing levels of professional support as the illness progresses. This is particularly true if family and friends are not able to cope with the deteriorating condition and begin to avoid contact, thus contributing further to the patient's feelings of loneliness and abandonment. If the patient believes that no one is available to discuss the situation openly and honestly, despair is likely to ensue. The patient's fear of the unknown is easier to cope with if his or her apprehension can be shared with a caring physician who provides comfort, support, encouragement, and even a modicum of hope.

Each new problem of the dying patient should be viewed as a nuisance requiring relief or removal and approached with the vigor that one would devote to an acute, short-term illness. When a fresh complaint arises, the patient should be reexamined and attempts made to relieve the symptom so the patient will not feel unworthy of further attention. If everyday nuisances can be controlled or lessened, the patient will believe that there is sincere concern for making her or his remaining life pleasant. The physician should give attention to details such as improving the taste of food by fixing or replacing dentures or stimulating the patient's appetite, eliminating foul odors, and suggesting occupational therapy to avoid boredom.

The physician should take advantage of every opportunity to touch and examine the patient rather than standing apart. Gentle palpation of areas of pain or merely taking a pulse can convey a sense of concern and warmth and provide comfort for an apprehensive and lonely patient. The physician and other health professionals can provide much support merely through conversation. The tendency to withdraw and reduce conversation contributes to the patient's sense of loneliness. Silence is an enemy of dying patients and increases their separation from society. Conversation is a social bond that affirms life and reduces anxiety by providing a means of catharsis. Saunders (1976) summed up the needs of a dying patient with the words of one patient: "Watch with me," asking that he not be abandoned in his final days. The readiness to listen and personal, caring contact are comforts that cannot be matched by modern "wonder drugs" and procedures.

When dying patients notice that people are avoiding them, they may interpret it as rejection because their condition has not improved or as the loss of love from family and friends, which is particularly traumatic because it tends to negate long-cherished relationships; the joys of a rewarding life can suddenly lose their value. The dying patient's contentment depends on maintaining warm relationships with loved ones as well as continuing other satisfying interpersonal relationships, including with the physician. If physicians and others withdraw from interaction with the terminally ill patient, much of the motivation for living disappears and is replaced by despair or terminal depression. The following plea to fellow health professionals is from a young student nurse who was terminally ill (Kübler-Ross, 1975):

I know you feel insecure, don't know what to say, don't know what to do. But please believe me, if you care, you can't go wrong. Just admit that you care. ... All I want to know is that there will be someone to hold my hand when I need it. I am afraid. Death may get to be a routine to you, but it is new to me. You may not see me as unique! .. If only we could be honest, both admit of our fears, touch one another. If you really care, would you lose so much of your valuable professionalism if you even cried with me? Just person to person? Then, it might not be so hard to die—in a hospital—with friends close by (p. 26).

Patient Control

We need to provide options to patients so they can actively participate in their care and feel a sense of control.

Terminally ill patients have a need to believe that they are still in control of their affairs as much as possible even though they have lost control of their bodies. They should be given the freedom to make choices and assume responsibility over as many aspects of their existence as possible. For many individuals, this is an essential part of living, and its loss may destroy their motivation to live. A terminally ill patient should be helped to focus on and cope with the realities of daily living because these problems remain very real and can serve as a diversion from constant preoccupation with the prospect of death. When patients have understanding and insight into the treatment and believe they still have some control over the decision-making process regarding their lives, they are more likely to cooperate with prescribed treatment regimens.

It is often fear of the unknown that makes a patient suspicious and resistant to therapy. Patients also should be given the opportunity to settle their affairs. Studies have shown that 40% of terminally ill patients are most concerned about being a burden to their family and friends and that 40% of the families of cancer patients become impoverished as a result of providing care for a family member (Emanuel et al., 2003). Concentration on financial business and putting the house in order is a pragmatic approach to active participation in the decision-making process. Some patients may have a burning desire to complete a cherished project, reconcile an estranged relationship, or visit particular places before they die. Positive motivation can be maintained by assisting them to focus on and deal with these issues.

A sense of control is more possible for the patient if pain is controlled and the patient is made comfortable. Sleep should not be forced with medication because some patients resist going to sleep, fearing they may never awaken, and others frequently have terrifying dreams.

The Importance of Hope

Hope is one of the essential ingredients of human existence, without which life is dark, cold, and frustrating. It maintains strength and gives substance to courage. In the presence of hope, suffering of all sorts still has some positive qualities. In its absence, suffering is a completely negative experience (Tumulty, 1973).

Hope allows patients to face the shortness of their lives constructively. Twycross (1986) defined hope as having "an expectation greater than zero of achieving a desired goal." Hope can also be defined as the patient believing in what is still possible. Anything that contributes to a sense of meaning or purpose in life fosters hope. Thus, belief in God or a higher being provides hope and may give a sense of meaning to suffering for some patients.

The physician should not raise false hopes or be overaggressive in treating a terminal illness to help the patient maintain hope. Some patients find it best to plan for a little time and hope for more. A false sense of hope may deflect the patient and family from finding final meaning and value in their remaining lives together.

Even patients with advanced cancer can maintain a positive outlook on life. The physician can help direct a patient toward an achievable goal, such as pain relief, support for the family from a hospice service, or making a trip to visit relatives.

Even laughter can contribute to hope. One patient said, "I may not have much control over the nearness of death, but I do have the power to joke about it." Also, recalling uplifting moments such as vacations or looking at old photograph albums can support hope. Memories of the past can serve to enrich the present (Herth, 1990).

Whereas having one's individuality accepted, honored, and acknowledged fosters hope, devaluation of personhood and a feeling of abandonment and isolation interfere with hope. Hope is also hindered by uncontrollable pain and discomfort. The continuation of pain after attempts to control it have failed contributes to the loss of hope (Herth, 1990).

Even when death is near, the patient can hope for a measure of happiness during the amount of time he or she has remaining. The physician can support the patient's hope for a good quality of life in the remaining time, for spiritual healing, and for a final phase of life that has integrity and dignity.

Hope is a potent force for patients to deal with their illness and to have a confiding relationship with a physician, spouse, or close friend, which can also help prevent depression. Every physician–patient encounter should leave the dying patient emotionally more able to deal with end-of-life issues. Always promote the patient's sense of hope (Ngo-Metzger et al., 2008).

DISCUSSING RELIGIOUS AND SPIRITUAL ISSUES

As patients approach the end of life and grapple with their mortality, their spiritual and religious concerns may be awakened or intensified. Although some physicians may be uncomfortable discussing a patient's spiritual and religious concerns, they can listen respectfully without judgment or discussion of religious views. Patients who believe that the physician really understands their concerns no longer feel isolated or alone in their final days (Low et al., 2002).

One way to approach this issue is to ask the patient, "Is faith or religion important to you in this illness?" In a study of patients with advanced cancer, 88% reported that religion and spirituality were important factors in adjusting to their illness (Balboni et al., 2007). Although religious coping can offer patients a sense of meaning and comfort when facing a life-threatening illness, it is somewhat surprising that a high level of religiousness is associated with preference for aggressive end-of-life care such as mechanical ventilation. These patients may have a greater trust that God will heal them through the treatment even when near death (Phelps et al., 2009).

Prolonging Living or Prolonging Dying?

It has been a long time since pneumonia was accepted as "the old man's friend." As one organic system after another slowed to a halt, the aged person was released from nausea, pain, delirium, and the degradation of lingering deterioration by finally developing pneumonia and dying. The family doctor merely showed concern and support; before antibiotics, there was not much to do but stand by and "let nature take its course." With improved medical care, however, a dying process that might have taken only a few days in previous years now may drag out for months (Veatch, 1972). Modern technology allows improved medical care to be taken to unrealistic extremes; one person was kept alive in a vegetative state for more than 37 years (LORAN Commission, 1989).

Protraction of the dying process is a modern epidemic. Some physicians seem to forget that their primary responsibility is to relieve suffering, not prolong it. Greater clinical skill often is required to provide daily supportive care than to cure acute illness. Tenderness and caring must be included in the protocols of terminally ill patients so that the ravaged patient is allowed to die peacefully, without tubing and respirators. Patients should be allowed "to experience those waning moments unencumbered by high-tech devices that serve only to impede their capacity for human interaction. Here it is the patient's comfort, not the caregiver's need 'to do something,' that should prevail" (LORAN Commission, 1989, p. 29).

In some situations, therapeutic restraint is necessary to permit a patient to die with dignity. When a cure is no longer possible, care should focus on the comfort of patient and family. At St. Christopher's Hospice in London, feeding is provided by human hands instead of nasogastric or intravenous tubes; "even if the patient does not get enough physical nourishment, he or she gets what is more important—the personal nourishment of someone who cares enough to sit by the bed several hours each day" (Nelson and Rohricht, 1984, p. 174).

Management of Symptoms

When fewer therapeutic options are available, the physician's involvement should increase. Even when no cure is possible, much can still be done to relieve pain and suffering. The family physician can help alleviate the fear, symptoms, and family stress that often make this a distressing time, keeping the patient as comfortable as possible and avoiding any impression of abandonment. A good death means being free of pain and unpleasant symptoms yet having the ability to make clear decisions and prepare for death.

Care of a dying patient can be one of the most rewarding aspects of the family physician's practice. Too often, however, the physician's discomfort with this stage of life contributes to the isolation and discouragement of the terminally ill patient. Unwarranted fears of respiratory depression, addiction, or tolerance prevent the prescribing of adequate amounts of analgesics. The resulting uncontrolled pain makes those final weeks a nightmare for all. Families may disintegrate as a result of the sleepless nights, fears, and guilt that come from trying to cope with uncontrolled symptoms.

Table 5-3 shows symptoms most often encountered in seriously ill hospitalized patients; some are predictable, and all are manageable to some extent. Rarely is a single symptom present, and most patients have two or more. Symptom severity can be decreased if anticipated and treated early. Eliciting and addressing the patient's concerns about anticipated suffering can often be as important as managing the symptoms. Good control of pain, nausea, and dyspnea can enable patients to die in the place of their

Table 5-3 Common Symptoms in Seriously Ill Hospitalized Patients

Symptom	Percentage of Total Patients	
	At Any Time	**Severe and Frequent**
Pain	51	23
Dyspnea	49	23
Anxiety	47	16
Depression	45	14
Nausea	34	6

From Expert Consult—Cecil Medicine, after Desbiens NA, Mueller-Rizner N, Connors AF Jr, et al., for the SUPPORT Investigators. The symptom burden of seriously ill hospitalized patients. *J Pain Symptom Manage.* 1999;17:248-255.

choosing with comfort and dignity. A study of patients in inpatient palliative care units showed that the quality of dying was associated with adequate symptom management and communication of the expected outcome to the family members (Choi et al., 2013).

The keys to symptom control, as in all areas of medicine, are a careful history and physical examination to determine the various causes of discomfort, as well as a broad knowledge of the therapeutic agents available.

PAIN CONTROL

Key Points

- Analgesics should be given regularly and in adequate doses. When titrated appropriately, analgesics do not cause addiction or respiratory depression.
- Oral morphine is the drug of choice for severe pain.
- Nonsteroidal antiinflammatory drugs (NSAIDs) are recommended for bone or joint pain, antidepressants or anticonvulsants for neuropathic pain, anticholinergics for cramping abdominal pain or bladder spasms, and antipsychotics for restlessness and confusion.
- Prevention and treatment of constipation is required for all patients receiving opioids.

Pain can be physical, psychological, emotional, or spiritual. It can also be a combination of chronic, somatic, visceral, and neuropathic pain. *Somatic* and *visceral* pain account for about two thirds of patients with pain and respond to conventional opioids. About 35% of patients have some degree of *neuropathic* pain, a shooting or stabbing, electric shock–like pain. *Chronic* pain is influenced by memories of past pain and the anticipation of future pain. The fear of worsening pain may distort the patient's perception of current discomfort. Frustration and anxiety may accentuate the pain. All these factors can lower the patient's pain threshold and greatly magnify even minor disturbances (Twycross, 1993).

Failure to treat the whole person often results in inadequate pain control for patients with terminal cancer. Fatigue, insomnia, anxiety, boredom, and anger all contribute to a lower threshold for pain. Rest, sleep, diversion, and companionship all help to increase the patient's tolerance for pain.

Analgesics should be given in adequate amounts to provide comfort. Giving analgesic doses both regularly and on an as-needed basis is ideal for pain management. Using only as-needed doses for moderate to severe pain is suboptimal because it contributes to a lower pain threshold and a need for increasing doses to relieve the pain. When medication is given regularly in adequate doses, the anxiety and fear that accentuate pain are avoided, and lower doses of the drug are effective because the patient no longer fears recurrent or "breakthrough" pain.

Nonpharmacologic Techniques

Nonpharmacologic pain management techniques include transcutaneous electrical nerve stimulation (TENS), exercise, heat, cold, acupuncture, cognitive therapies (relaxation, imagery, hypnosis, biofeedback), behavioral therapy,

Table 5-4   Guidelines for Dosing Data for Opioid Analgesics (see Table 5-5)

1	Evaluate pain for all patients using a 0-10 scale: A. Mild pain: 1-3 B. Moderate pain: 4-7 C. Severe pain: 8-10
2	For chronic moderate or severe pain, do the following: A. Give baseline medication around the clock. B. Order 10% of the total daily dose for PRN administration given every 1 to 2 hours for the PO route or every 30 to 60 minutes for the SC or IV route. C. For continuous infusion, PRN administration can be the hourly rate every 15 minutes or 10% of the total daily dose every 30 to 60 minutes. D. Adjust the baseline upward daily in an amount roughly equivalent to the total amount used for PRN. E. Negotiate with the patient the target level of relief, usually achieving a level at least <4.
3	In general, the PO route is preferable, then the transcutaneous, SC, and IV routes.
4	When converting from one opioid to another, some experts recommend reducing the equianalgesic dose by one third to half and then titrating as in guideline 2.
5	Elderly patients or those with severe renal or liver disease should start on half of the usual initial dose.
6	If parenteral medication is needed for mild to moderate pain, use half of the usual starting dose of morphine or an equivalent.
7	Refer to the *Physicians' Desk Reference* for additional fentanyl guidelines.
8	Naloxone (Narcan) should be used only in emergencies: Dilute 0.4 mg of naloxone with 9 mL of normal saline; give 0.1 mg (2.5 mL) by slow IVP until effect; and monitor patient every 15 minutes. It may be necessary to repeat naloxone again in 30 to 60 minutes.
9	Short-acting preparations should be used in the initial period and postoperatively. Switch to long-acting preparations when the pain is chronic and after the total daily dose is determined.

IV, Intravenous; *IVP,* intravenous push; *PO,* oral; *PRN,* as needed; *SC,* subcutaneous.
Adapted from Quill T, Holloway R, Shah M, et al. *Primer of Palliative Care.* 5th ed. Glenview, IL: American Academy of Hospice and Palliative Medicine; 2010.

psychotherapy, music therapy, and massage. Cold works especially well for neuropathic pain; heat works well for muscle spasm.

Opioids

A symptom-oriented history and careful examination may reveal a number of different sources of pain. Oral candidiasis, decubitus ulcers, constipation, and infected wounds all have specific remedies. Most patients with pain from cancer (and many with pain from non-neoplastic illnesses) require an opioid analgesic. Opioids are often the safest analgesics available, usually causing only temporary sedation and an increased need for laxatives. Opioid toxicity may manifest as myoclonus or nightmares; the patient may exhibit spontaneous jerking or pull the hand away when touched, which can be misinterpreted by others, making them reluctant to touch the patient. Morphine taken orally gives good relief for cancer pain but has some unwanted side effects, mainly constipation and nausea.

High doses of opioids may be necessary to obtain initial pain control in a patient with severe pain. Psychological dependence is rarely a problem in patients who receive appropriate opioid doses for chronic, severe cancer pain. When medication is given before the recurrence of pain, craving for medication does not occur. Physical dependence does occur with routine use, but withdrawal symptoms can be avoided by reducing a dose no more than 20% in any 2-day period.

In the past, physicians feared scrutiny by the U.S. Drug Enforcement Administration for using high doses of morphine to control pain. However, failure to use adequate doses of morphine may be a greater concern now because a physician was successfully sued for undertreatment of pain in a terminally ill patient. The proper combination of pain medications can relieve pain without clouding the mind or suppressing the spirit.

Concerns about addiction, respiratory depression, and tolerance usually are unwarranted in patients with severe pain (Twycross, 1993). If the dose is titrated carefully, the patient's pain (or dyspnea) usually can be controlled completely. Patients can still be alert and mentally clear even when they receive hundreds of milligrams of oral morphine every 4 hours (Bruera et al., 1990).

A number of effective oral opioid preparations are available (Tables 5-4 and 5-5). Start with oral morphine solution 2 mg every hour as needed for pain. If four or more doses are given in 24 hours, divide the total milligrams into every-4-hour doses the following day. Use breakthrough doses every hour as needed between scheduled doses. Do the same for each subsequent day. Titrate the morphine dose upward until analgesia lasts the full 4 hours even if large doses are required. Hydromorphone is a good alternative.

The particular drug used is less important than the method of administration. To *prevent* pain and end the cycle of uncontrolled pain followed by oversedation, an oral narcotic should be administered on a regular schedule around the clock. "Breakthrough" doses equal to about half the regular 4-hour dose can be used as needed for breakthrough pain.

Long-acting drugs such as methadone (half-life 48 to 72 hours) can be prescribed every 8 to 12 hours but are often unsuitable for booster doses. They accumulate over several days and are difficult to titrate, especially in patients who have fluctuating levels of pain or deteriorating renal or hepatic function. Methadone is a synthetic that has no cross-allergenicity with morphine. It is available in oral and injectable forms and has been successfully used via other

Table 5-5 Dosing Data for Opioid Analgesics

Medication	Equianalgesic Dose (for chronic dosing)		Usual Starting Doses Adult > 50 kg; for opioid-naive patients (♦ ½ dose for elderly or severe renal or liver disease)		Comments	Half-Life (hours)	Duration (hours)
	IM/IV	PO	Parenteral	PO			
Morphine	10 mg	30 mg	2.5-5 mg SC/IV q3-4h (♦ 1.23-2.5 mg)	5-15 mg q3-4h (IR or oral solution) (♦ 2.5-7.5 mg)	IR tablets (15, 30 mg) oral sol. (2 mg/ml, 4 mg/ml). Conc. (20 mg/ml) can give buccally. Morphine ER tablets (15, 30, 60, 100, 200 mg) q8-12h. Kadian ER pellets (10, 20, 30, 50, 60, 80, 100, 200 mg) q12-24h. Avinza ER pellets (30, 60, 90, 120 mg) q24h. Rectal suppositories (5, 10, 20, 30 mg). Not recommended in renal failure.	1.5-2	3-7
Oxycodone	Not available	20 mg	Not available	5-10 mg q3-4h (♦ 2.5 mg)	OxyIR capsule (5 mg); IR tablet (5, 10, 15, 0, 30 mg); Conc. sol (20 mg/ml). Oxycontin (10, 15, 20, 30, 40, 60, 80 mg)—due to high cost and potential for abuse, use only if failure or contraindication to morphine ER. Combos available with APAP or ibuprofen (generally not recommended). Not enough literature regarding dosing in renal failure. Use caution.	3-4	4-6
Hydromorphone	1.5 mg	7.5 mg	0.2-0.6 mg SC/IV q2-3h (♦ 0.2 mg)	1-2 mg q3-4h (♦ 0.5-1 mg)	Tablet (2, 4, 8 mg); oral liquid (1 mg/ml); Suppository (3 mg). Use carefully in renal failure.	2-3	4-5
Methadone (see text for dosing conversions)	½ oral dose 2 mg PO methadone = 1 mg parenteral methadone	Oral morphine: methadone ratio — 24 hour oral morphine / methadone ratio: <30 mg 2:1; 31-99 mg 4:1; 100-299 mg 8:1; 200-499 mg 12:1; 500-999 mg 15:1; 1000-1200 mg 20:1; >1200 mg Consider consult	1.25-2.5 mg q8h (♦ 1.25 mg)	2.5-5 mg q8h (♦ 1.25-2.5 mg)	Tablet (5, 10 mg): solution (1 mg/ml, 2 mg/ml, and concentrated 10 mg/ml). Usually q12h or q8h; long variable T1/2. Acceptable with renal disease; small dose change makes big difference. Tends to accumulate with higher doses; always advise "hold for sedation." Because of long half-life, do not use methadone prn unless experienced. When converting from oral to parenteral, cut dose in half for safety. When converting from parenteral to oral, keep dose the same.	15-190 (N.B. Huge variation)	6-12

Continued on following page

Table 5-5 Dosing Data for Opioid Analgesics (Continued)

Medication	Equianalgesic Dose (for chronic dosing)		Usual Starting Doses Adult > 50 kg; for opioid-naive patients (♦ ½ dose for elderly or severe renal or liver disease)		Comments	Half-Life (hours)	Duration (hours)
	IM/IV	PO	Parenteral	PO			
Fentanyl (see text for dosing conversions)	100 mcg single dose (T1/2 and duration of parenteral doses variable)	24 hr oral MS dose / Initial patch dose 30-59 mg / 12.5 mcg/h 60-134 mg / 25 mcg/h 135-224 mg / 50 mcg/h 225-314 mg / 75 mcg/h 315-404 mg / 100 mcg/h	25-50 mcg IM/IV q1-3h (♦ 12.5-25 mcg)	Transdermal path 12.5mcg/h q72h (Use with caution in opioid-naive and unstable patients because of 12-hour delay in onset and offset)	Transdermal patch (12.5, 25, 50, 75, 100 mcg) N.B.: Incomplete cross-tolerance already accounted for in conversion to fentanyl; when converting to other opioid from fentanyl, generally reduce the equianalgesic amount by 50% (see text, PDR). Acceptable with renal disease; monitor carefully if using long term. IV: very short acting; associated with chest wall rigidity. Oral lozenge (200 mcg start) and buccal tablet (100 mcg start) indicated for breakthrough cancer pain only (see PDR and package insert).	7 (Lozenge) 12-22 (Buccal) 13-22 (Transdermal)	60+ min (Lozenge) 120+ min (Buccal) (Both not well studied) 48-72 (Transdermal)
Meperidine	75-100 mg	300 mg	75 mg SC/IM q2-3h (♦ 25-50 mg) Generally not recommended	Not recommended	Not recommended for standard analgesia. May be useful for shivering and procedural analgesia/sedation. Toxic metabolites accumulate with repeated doses and with renal or hepatic disease. Contraindicated with MAOIs.	3-4	2-4
Codeine	130 mg	200 mg	15-30 mg IM/SC q4h (♦ 7.5-15 mg) IV contraindicated	30-60 mg q3-4h (♦ 15-30mg)	Tablet (15, 30, 60 mg); elixir 12 mg and 120 mg APAP/5 ml Tylenol #3 (30 mg with 300 mg APAP); Tylenol #4 (60 mg with 300 mg APAP) Monitor total APAP dose.	3	4-6
Hydrocodone	Not available	30 mg	Not available	5 mg q3-4h (♦ 2.5 mg)	Tablet—multiple brand and generic strengths ranging from 2.5-10 mg combined with 300-750 mg APAP Table (hydrocodone/ibuprofen: 7.5/200mg) Elixir 2.5 mg and 167 mg APAP/5ml Monitor total acetaminophen or ibuprofen dose.	3.3-4.5	4-6
Propoxyphene	Not available	130 ng (HCl) 200 mg (Napsylate)	Not available	Not recommended	Not recommended: relatively ineffective Capsule (propoxyphene HCl 65 mg) Tablet (propoxyphene N with APAP 50/325 or 100/650 mg) Monitor total acetaminophen dose.	6-12	4-6

*See Table 5-4 for Guidelines.

†New York State currently requires triplicate reporting.

‡Adults weighing more than 50 kg.

§Half dose for elderly patients or those with severe renal or liver disease.

IR, Immediate release; IVP, intravenous push; MAOI, monoamine oxidase inhibitor; meth, methadone; mod, moderate; morph, morphine; MS, morphine sulfate; PDR, Physicians' Desk Reference; sev, severe; sol, solution; SR, sustained release; TD, transdermal.

From Primer of Palliative Care (6th ed, Table 2.1), by TE Quill, KA Bower, RG Holloway, et al, 2014, Chicago, IL, American Academy of Hospice and Palliative Medicine, p. 15. ©2014 University of Rochester Medical Center. All rights reserved. Reprinted with permission.

Table 5-6 Dosing Data for Coanalgesics

Pain Source	Pain Character	Drug Class	Examples	Comments
Bones or soft tissue	Tenderness over bone or joint pain on movement	NSAIDs	Ibuprofen, 400 mg q4hr	Inexpensive; large pills
			Sulindac (Clinoril), 200 mg q12hr	Well tolerated; preferred in renal impairment
			Naproxen (Naprosyn susp, 125 mg/5 mL), 15 mL q8hr	Liquid preparation
			Indomethacin (Indocin, 50-mg caps or susp), q8hr	Suppository; more gastritis?
			Piroxicam (Feldene, 20-mg caps), qD	Easiest to swallow; more gastritis?
			Choline magnesium trisalicylate (Trilisate susp, 500 mg/5 mL), 15 mL q12hr	No platelet dysfunction; less problem with gastritis; less effective
			Celecoxib (Celebrex), 100 mg q12hr	Less GI toxicity; high cost
		Steroid	Dexamethasone 4-8 mg at 8 AM and 2 PM daily	Liquid available. Insomnia, vivid dreams possible
Nerve damage or dysesthesia	Burning or shooting pain radiating from plexus or spinal root	Tricyclic antidepressant	Amitriptyline (Elavil), 10-50 mg HS	Best studied; sedating; start with low dose
			Doxepin (Sinequan), 10-50 mg HS	10 mg/mL susp available
			Trazodone (Desyrel), 25-150 mg HS	Less anticholinergic effect; one third as potent as amitriptyline
		Anticonvulsant	Carbamazepine (Tegretol), 200 mg q6-12hr	Absorbed from rectum, unlike phenytoin
			Valproic acid (Depakene), 250 mg q8-12hr	Liquid available; can be absorbed rectally
			Gabapentin (Neurontin), 100-400 mg qd to qid	Often effective but expensive
		Steroid	Dexamethasone 4-8 mg at 8 AM and 2 PM daily	Liquid available. Insomnia, vivid dreams possible
Smooth muscle spasms	Colic: cramping, abdominal pain, bladder spasms	Anticholinergic	Glycopyrrolate 0.4 mg q 1hr PRN	Oral or parenteral
			Dicyclomine (Bentyl), 10 mg q4-8hr	Capsules
			Oxybutynin (Ditropan), 5-10 mg q8hr	Tablets
			Hyoscyamine (Levsin), 0.125 mg q4-8hr	Sublingual available
			Glycopyrrolate (Robinul), 2 mg q8hr 0.2 mg/mL IV or IM q4h PRN	

Cap, capsule; *GI,* gastrointestinal; *HS,* at bedtime; *IM,* intramuscular; *IV,* intravenous; *NSAID,* nonsteroidal antiinflammatory drug; *PRN,* as needed; *q,* every; *qd,* every day; *qid,* four times a day; *susp,* suspension.

routes. It is metabolized in the liver and has no active metabolites, making it especially useful in patients with renal insufficiency (Toombs and Kral, 2005). The cost of methadone, especially in the parenteral form, has recently skyrocketed, making it cost prohibitive in many settings. The availability of parenteral methadone is limited.

Slow-release morphine preparations such as MS Contin and Oramorph SR can provide excellent analgesia for 8 to 12 hours, and Kadian and Avinza last 12 to 24 hours. The shorter-acting, slow-release tablets may be given rectally when the patient cannot swallow (Wilkinson et al., 1992). Small, soluble tablets or concentrated solutions of morphine or hydromorphone can be given sublingually when the patient is too weak to swallow and can be used for both 4-hour and booster doses.

Fentanyl, a synthetic opioid, is available for use as a transdermal patch (Duragesic) in 12.5-, 25-, 50-, 75-, and 100-μg/hr strengths or a transmucosal lozenge on a stick (Actiq) in 200- to 1600-μg strengths. Because these products are expensive and deliver a wide variation of plasma levels (25-μg patch = 4 to 11 mg of oral morphine every 4 hours), they should be reserved for patients who cannot receive drugs by the oral or subcutaneous routes. However, the patches may not work in thin, malnourished elderly patients because they need a subcutaneous fat reservoir to work. There is no need to use injections when an adequate dose by mouth will work effectively.

Two opioid agents that are available orally are not recommended for cancer pain. Meperidine (Demerol) has a very low oral potency, a short duration of action, and a toxic metabolite that can cause tremors or even seizures (Kaiko

et al., 1983). Pentazocine (Talwin, Talacen) is an agonist–antagonist agent that is no more potent than aspirin with codeine and has a high incidence of psychotomimetic effects (hallucinations, confusion) in cancer patients.

Co-analgesics

Co-analgesics are drugs that potentiate the analgesic effects of opioids for particular types of pain (Table 5-6).

Bone Pain

Nonsteroidal antiinflammatory drugs are quite helpful in the alleviation of pain from lesions in bones or skeletal muscles. The nonacetylated salicylates (e.g., salsalate [Disalcid], choline magnesium trisalicylate [Trilisate]) are less toxic to the gastric mucosa and do not inhibit platelet function (Zucker and Rothwell, 1978) but are less potent analgesics. The newer nonsalicylate NSAIDs are more potent, more convenient, more expensive, and less toxic than aspirin. Although no single agent has been shown to be consistently more efficacious, particular patients do seem to favor one drug over another. If swallowing large tablets becomes a problem, piroxicam (Feldene) capsules, naproxen (Naprosyn) suspension, or indomethacin (Indocin) rectal suppositories may be used. The cyclooxygenase-2 (COX-2) inhibitor celecoxib (Celebrex) offers comparable analgesia and less gastrointestinal toxicity but at a higher risk of stroke or heart attack (which may not be an issue in the final weeks of life) and a higher cost. Steroids may also be a helpful adjuvant for bone pain. The steroid side effect of insomnia or vivid dreams may arise. Administering the doses of steroids earlier in the day, such as dexamethasone 4 mg at 8 AM and 2 PM daily, can prevent negative side effects.

Neuropathic Pain

For the burning, stabbing, or shooting pain caused by nerve damage, an anticonvulsant such as gabapentin (Neurontin), 100 to 400 mg orally one to four times a day, or pregabalin (Lyrica), 50 to 100 mg orally three times a day, may be a useful addition (Rosenberg et al., 1997). Amitriptyline or nortriptyline, in doses smaller than those used to treat depression (10-50 mg at bedtime), are often effective, but newer agents such as venlafaxine (Effexor) or duloxetine (Cymbalta) may be effective for neuropathic pain and have fewer side effects. If swallowing problems arise and a tricyclic drug is needed, doxepin (Sinequan) solution may be used. The addition of carbamazepine (200 mg three times daily) or valproate (Depakene, 250 mg three times daily) should be considered if the tricyclic agent alone is not adequate. Both doxepin and carbamazepine can be administered rectally in gelatin capsules (Storey and Trumble, 1992). Steroids are helpful in treating neuropathic pain.

Visceral Pain and Smooth Muscle Spasm

If smooth muscle spasms are not caused by a treatable condition, such as urinary tract infection from a nonessential Foley catheter, these are best treated with an anticholinergic agent such as dicyclomine (Bentyl) or oxybutynin (Ditropan). For severe cases, 0.6 to 1.6 mg of glycopyrrolate (Robinul) subcutaneously may be used (Storey et al., 1990). The physician must be alert for side effects such as dry mouth, constipation, and delirium.

ANXIETY AND DEPRESSION

If anxiety is severe enough to require drug therapy, a benzodiazepine such as lorazepam (Ativan), 0.5 to 1 mg two or three times a day, may be effective. Antidepressants such as nortriptyline (Pamelor), desipramine (Norpramin), and doxepin in low doses (25-75 mg at bedtime) have analgesic properties and can help with insomnia and agitation. Selective serotonin reuptake inhibitors (SSRIs) and serotonin–norepinephrine reuptake inhibitors (SNRIs) may also be effective. Mirtazapine may provide the advantage of improved sleep and appetite. Psychostimulants such as methylphenidate (Ritalin), 2.5 to 10 mg orally at 9 AM and 12 noon, take effect quickly and can relieve depression and pain in some terminally ill patients, especially when the prognosis is limited (Block, 2000). Quetiapine (Seroquel), an atypical antipsychotic beneficial for addressing bipolar disorder and schizophrenia, can also be used as an adjuvant antidepressant.

Grief and depression may appear similarly. The key to their differentiation is whether the patient is able to function. For example, a grieving patient will still function by taking his or her children to school or going to work and will temporarily improve on seeing his or her grandchildren, but depressed patients will not function appropriately.

In family members, *complicated grief,* also called "unresolved grief," is grief persisting more than 6 months and occurring at least 6 months after death. Normally, grief symptoms fade over time, but those of complicated grief linger or worsen, resulting in a chronic state of mourning. Although complicated grief can lead to depression, it may be distinct and associated with long-term functional impairment (Prigerson et al., 1995). Parents who have not successfully worked through their grief are at increased risk of mental and physical problems 4 to 9 years later (Lannen et al., 2008).

DELIRIUM OR AGITATION

Delirium or agitation is often seen in dying patients. It may result from the disinhibition of the nervous system that takes place. It is often concerning for family members because personality changes are associated with the delirium. This can result in the patient's attempting to get out of bed, when he or she is significantly weaker, increasing the risk of falling or harming caregivers. Haloperidol (Haldol) is an antipsychotic that is beneficial for restlessness or confusion. It can be administered orally, rectally, intravenously, or subcutaneously. It is reasonable to start with 0.5 or 1 mg every hour as needed for breakthrough restlessness and monitor over an initial 24 hours. If the patient requires three or more doses in a day, adding the total haloperidol, dividing evenly and scheduling the haloperidol regularly may be beneficial. Chlorpromazine (Thorazine) is an antipsychotic that is more sedating than haloperidol; the patient's family members may desire this sedating effect at a certain point in the patient's disease progression. Escalating the dose of the chlorpromazine may be necessary to treat progressively worsening agitated delirium (Bascom et al., 2013). Chlorpromazine, given subcutaneously, may cause more irritation to the injection site than haloperidol. Atypical antipsychotics may be used when there is a longer prognosis of weeks to months to decrease the side effects of extrapyramidal symptoms and tardive dyskinesia. Quetiapine (Seroquel) is favored over other atypical antipsychotics for patients with Parkinson disease or parkinsonian features because it improves delirium without worsening motor function (Friedman, 2011). When symptoms of anxiety and restlessness are both present, benzodiazepines are effective in treating these symptoms, as listed in the previous section on anxiety.

DYSPNEA

As with pain, dyspnea can have many causes. When anemia, bronchospasm, and heart failure have been excluded or treated, the focus should be on symptom control. Oxygen has been shown to be helpful for controlling dyspnea in patients with hypoxia but may be less convenient and more expensive than opioids. When the dose of opioid is titrated carefully to control the pain and is administered on a regular schedule, with additional doses available for breakthrough dyspnea, the patient can obtain excellent relief without significant respiratory depression (Bruera et al., 1990).

Evidence from 13 studies shows a valuable effect of morphine for dyspnea in advanced lung disease and terminal cancer. However, using nebulized versus oral opioids showed no additional benefit. Good-quality evidence shows that long-acting β-agonists are beneficial in the treatment of dyspnea in patients with chronic obstructive pulmonary disease (Qaseem et al., 2008).

Albuterol nebulizer treatments every 4 hours while the patient is awake may help relax the bronchospasms that often result in dyspnea and loosen the secretions that become more cumbersome as the respiratory muscles become weaker.

It may also be helpful to provide cool, moving air (open window, fan) and keep an unobstructed line of sight between the patient and the outside. Careful consideration should be given to the use of antibiotics for pneumonia in terminally ill patients. Because dyspnea can be controlled well without antibiotics, the physician must decide whether the antibiotics will improve the quality of life or just prolong the dying.

CONSTIPATION

Constipation can be more easily prevented than treated. When mobility and oral intake decrease and opioid analgesics are required, virtually every patient will require regular doses of laxatives to avoid distressing constipation. The laxative should be given once or twice *every* day and the amount increased to get a soft bowel movement every 1 to 2 days. Bulk laxatives are tolerated poorly and rarely are adequate for these patients. If docusate (Colace), 100 to 200 mg twice daily, is not effective, senna (Senokot), 1 to 4 tablets twice daily, should be added. Sorbitol 70% may be added in doses of 15 to 45 mL two or three times per day if the tablets are inadequate or if dysphagia causes aspiration risk when taking tablets. If a patient has gone several days without a bowel movement or is having small, frequent, liquid stools, an impaction may require manual removal. Bisacodyl (Dulcolax) 10-mg suppositories or sodium phosphate (Fleet) enemas may be needed occasionally until an effective oral regimen is found. Impaction may cause delirium, which can mimic pain. In these patients, the delirium may be improved with a simple enema.

NAUSEA AND VOMITING

In patients with nausea and vomiting, the physician should first look for a reversible cause such as constipation or gastritis from NSAIDs. If increased intracranial pressure is the cause, the patient may require steroids. Overfeeding may be the problem if a nasogastric or gastrostomy tube is in place. Metoclopramide (Reglan) is the agent of choice when an enormous liver limits gastric emptying or slow motility is causing early satiety. Many patients whose nausea and vomiting have not responded to prochlorperazine (Compazine) or promethazine (Phenergan) will be relieved by haloperidol (Haldol), 0.5 to 2 mg orally or subcutaneously every 4 to 8 hours. Effective and expensive preparations (usually unnecessary for hospice patients) that are approved for the treatment of nausea associated with chemotherapy include ondansetron (Zofran), granisetron (Kytril), dolasetron (Anzemet), and palonosetron (Aloxi). Parenteral fluids administered subcutaneously may provide some relief from the nausea. Either D5 ½ normal saline or normal saline is often effective, given about 1 L/day or 40 cc/hr. It can be administered as a rapid drip, if time is limited, so that the patient does not have to have a cumbersome fluid bag

all day. If the patient develops worsening respiratory secretions, increasing abdominal girth, or worsening extremity edema, it would be necessary to decrease or stop the parenteral fluids because it demonstrates that the patient's body is not able to process the fluid.

As with persistent pain, persistent nausea should be treated with regularly scheduled antiemetics. Combinations of antiemetics that have different modes of action may be needed. A combination of haloperidol with metoclopramide or dexamethasone may be effective. When oral antiemetics cannot be tolerated, rectal suppositories can be tried but rarely provide adequate control for persistent nausea and vomiting unless they are compounded from the potent agents just mentioned. Continuous subcutaneous infusions of metoclopramide, haloperidol, and the required opioid are more effective (Baines, 1988). Discontinuation of metoclopramide is recommended for complete bowel obstruction because this can worsen abdominal pain, nausea, and vomiting (Doyle et al., 2004). Even vomiting associated with complete bowel obstruction can be controlled *without* a nasogastric tube or gastrostomy with a continuous subcutaneous infusion of opioids, antiemetics, and anticholinergic agents (Baines et al., 1985). Octreotide (Sandostatin) has also been extremely effective.

HICCUPS

Persistent hiccups can be caused by any lesion affecting the phrenic nerve and by gastric distention or systemic problems, such as uremia. Oral treatment may include baclofen (Lioresal), 10 mg every 8 hours as needed; chlorpromazine (Thorazine), 25 to 50 mg every 4 to 6 hours as needed; metoclopramide, 10 to 20 mg every 6 to 8 hours as needed; or haloperidol, 1 to 2 mg every 4 to 6 hours as needed.

SUBCUTANEOUS ROUTE

When oral opioids or antiemetics cannot be tolerated because of nausea, vomiting, stupor, or extreme weakness, parenteral medications may be needed. Frequent intramuscular injections or frequent restarting of intravenous infusions can be painful and difficult to manage at home. In these cases, medications can be administered subcutaneously, either by intermittent bolus or by continuous infusion. At least 50 mL of medication per day can be infused through a small-gauge butterfly needle under the skin of the upper chest, arms, abdomen, or thighs using a portable pump. Morphine and hydromorphone have been shown to be safe and effective when administered by this route (Bruera et al., 1988). Methadone, metoclopramide, haloperidol, lorazepam, dexamethasone, glycopyrrolate, and parenteral fluids can also be administered subcutaneously (Destro et al., 2012).

Nutrition

Although uncontrolled pain is the principal complaint of many patients, the family's primary concern is often the patient not eating well. The causes of cancer cachexia are still poorly understood. Because patients seem to stop eating, lose weight, and eventually die, the natural assumption has been that even if physicians cannot effectively treat the cancer, they can at least treat malnutrition and thereby delay death.

The problem is that more harm than good can come from tube feedings or pushing multiple cans of supplement each day. The family may feel responsible if the patient loses weight and may feel guilty when the person dies. Unfortunately, the patient's final weeks become a struggle with the family over how much the person has eaten. One patient said, "Tell her to stop pushing that spoon into my face; I don't want any more!" This can be carried to extremes, such as inserting nasogastric tubes in patients who "do not cooperate." If they tug on the tube, their hands may be tied to the bed rails. A study of tube feedings in elderly patients revealed that within 2 weeks, 67% of patients with nasogastric tubes had attempted self-extubation, and 43% had aspiration pneumonia. Gastric or jejunal tubes had a lower self-extubation rate (44%), but 56% of the patients had aspiration pneumonia, 31% had a leak or infection at the insertion site, and 50% had a clogged or kinked tube (Ciocon et al., 1988). Another comprehensive analysis found evidence of many risks and no benefits from tube feeding in patients with advanced dementia (Finucane et al., 1999). Large volumes of supplemental feeding can cause painful gastric distention, nausea, diarrhea, and copious pulmonary secretions. Routinely checking residuals of gastric content before each tube feeding is beneficial. This can be done by gently pulling back on the syringe attached to the tube used for feeding to measure any fluid left in the stomach. If residuals are more than approximately 60 cc, then the patient may not be processing the tube feeding, so that the patient or family can see why decreasing or stopping the tube feeding would be in the patient's best interest.

There is no evidence that forced feeding of cancer or dementia patients prolongs life. Careful metabolic studies on force-fed cancer patients at the National Institutes of Health showed irreversibly increased metabolic rates from forced feeding. It was speculated that tumor growth was accelerated (Terepka and Waterhouse, 1956). Animal experiments have shown that growth rates of a variety of different cancers are nutrient dependent; the growth rate slows down with fasting or protein-free diets and speeds up with total parenteral nutrition (TPN) (Buzby et al., 1980; Stragand et al., 1979). In several trials, patients who received TPN plus chemotherapy were compared with those receiving chemotherapy alone. The TPN group died faster, especially patients with lung adenocarcinoma (Jordan et al., 1981), colorectal cancer (Nixon et al., 1981), and small-cell lung cancer (Shike et al., 1984). Pooling data on TPN and cancer through 1985, Klein and associates (1986) found that infections were more common in patients receiving TPN and that these patients were less responsive to chemotherapy and had shortened survival times. After reviewing all the clinical trials of parenteral nutrition in patients receiving cancer chemotherapy, the American College of Physicians (1989) concluded, "The evidence suggests that parenteral nutritional support was associated with net harm, and no conditions could be defined in which such treatment appeared to be of benefit. Thus, the routine use of parenteral nutrition for patients undergoing chemotherapy should be strongly discouraged."

What should be done to relieve the anorexia of patients with advanced cancer? eTable 5-2 lists a number of treatable causes of anorexia. Uncontrolled pain blunts any person's appetite and can be alleviated. Low-level nausea, oral candidiasis, and constipation can interfere with eating and can be treated effectively. Families can be taught to relieve xerostomia (dry mouth) using a small syringe filled with water or juice and to prepare soft foods. Corticosteroids and megestrol have been beneficial to some but can cause side effects. The most important service the family physician can provide is to allay guilt. An appropriate statement would be: "I do *not* believe that how much time your husband has or how comfortable he is depends on how much he eats." Family members can be counseled about offering pleasure feedings, not for nutrition but to bring back the pleasant memories of food that was enjoyable. Offering small amounts, about a handful at a time, can keep the portions from being overwhelming. Allowing the patient to take as much or as little as desired is best.

Where to Die

Death with dignity is easiest to accomplish when the patient dies amid the surroundings that gave meaning to his or her life and in the company of those whose companionship provided most of the rewards of living. Physicians too often deny this, however, in the medically conditioned struggle to prolong life. Medical technology has advanced to the point that too few patients are permitted to die at home even though improved diagnostic techniques identify the irreversible nature of a terminal process at an earlier stage. A sorry commentary, reflecting the abuse of technology, is the case of a man who had built his house with his own hands and wanted to die there but was prevented from doing so while physicians exhausted their therapeutic armamentarium in an attempt to prolong his life a few days or weeks. The family physician must remain in charge as the patient's advocate when the consultants want to continue aggressive therapy yet all the patient wants to do is be comfortable. The family physician must have the courage to discontinue aggressive therapy when the evidence points to its futility.

Charles Lindbergh is an excellent example of an individual who insisted on designing his final days in a manner that would preserve dignity and allow him to die as comfortably as possible. When dying of lymphoma, he refused to remain in a medical center on the East Coast and returned to his home in Hawaii, where he made final arrangements regarding his estate and discussed with friends and family the details of his memorial service and burial site. His death was as he preferred—quiet, dignified, private, and in the company of family and friends—a striking contrast to what it would have been had he not insisted on leaving the medical center.

Although 70% of Americans still die in institutions (39% in hospitals and 31% in nursing homes), polls show that 80% of them say they would rather die at home (Farber et al., 2002). Jacqueline Onassis is an example of a prominent person whose wish to die at home was respected. Similarly, Richard Nixon's wishes were respected when his physicians and family knew that he wanted no extraordinary means taken to keep him alive if he developed an illness that left him seriously debilitated, particularly intellectually.

Some patients do not want to be a burden to their families and pride themselves on being able to afford hospitalization or nursing home care. For some of these patients, the gradual withdrawal from family may be an emotional "letting go" that is necessary for all concerned in their particular family and circumstances. In other cases, the spouse simply may not be equipped physically or psychologically to deal with the loved one dying in the house over time. The important aspect is a network of support for all concerned, with no arbitrary judgment about the best approach. The family physician will be sensitive to the style of living and the style of dying that seem most appropriate in a given case after the options have been explained to the patient and family.

Hospice Care

Key Points

- Hospice care is intended for patients with a prognosis of 6 months or less.
- Most patients are referred too late, with a reported median survival time of only 3 weeks.
- A primary goal of a hospice is to support the patient's wish to die at home.
- The hospice team gives around-the-clock support to the family, relieves them at times to prevent burnout, and provides follow-up bereavement care for up to 1 year.

"Hospice" originally meant a way station for pilgrims and travelers, where they could be replenished, refreshed, and cared for if needed. The Irish Sisters of Charity viewed death as one stage of a journey. They opened hospices for dying patients in Dublin in 1879 and in London in 1905. These were places where dying people could be cared for when such care could not be managed at home.

Cicely Saunders was trained as a nurse and social worker in London in the 1940s. She cared for a dying cancer patient who made a £500 donation to "be a window" in the special home for the dying they both knew was needed. Saunders went to medical school and then worked in St. Joseph's Hospice in London from 1958 to 1965. She discovered the effectiveness of interdisciplinary team support, scheduled doses of oral opioids, and other methods to relieve the symptoms and stresses of her patients and their families. She opened St. Christopher's Hospice in south London in 1967, and the modern hospice movement was born. In 2008, there were almost 5000 hospices in the United States alone.

The hospice concept can benefit patients and families wherever death takes place. A hospice program consists of palliative and supportive services that provide physical, psychological, social, and spiritual care for dying persons and their families. Services are provided by a medically supervised interdisciplinary team of professionals and volunteers and are available both in the home and in an inpatient setting. Home care is provided as necessary: on a part-time, intermittent, regularly scheduled, or around-the-clock on-call basis. The hospice concept is directed toward providing compassionate care for people facing life-limiting illnesses or injuries. Hospice and palliative care involve a team-oriented approach to expert medical care, pain management, and emotional and spiritual support expressly tailored to the patient's needs and wishes. Support is provided to the patient's loved ones as well. At the center of hospice and palliative care is the belief that everyone has the right to die pain free and with dignity and that patients' families will receive the necessary support to allow them to do so (www.nhpco.org, 2009).

The principal requirement for hospice admission is a life-limiting illness with a prognosis of 6 months or less, if the disease runs its normal course, as certified by the patient's physician and the hospice physician. eTable 5-3 lists the standards of a hospice program as developed by the National Hospice and Palliative Care Organization (NHPCO).

The interdisciplinary hospice team consists of a patient care coordinator, a nurse, a physician, a counselor, a volunteer coordinator, and spiritual support. Medical services are on call 24 hours a day, 7 days a week. Continuity of care by the same group of team members provides a familiarity that is comforting to the patient. Volunteers are an integral part of the program and provide many helpful services. Hospice services are covered by Medicare, Medicaid, and most insurance companies to some extent. Some hospices are able to provide charity care.

To qualify for hospice under the Medicare Hospice Benefit, a patient should have a life expectancy of less than 6 months. Again, however, referrals are usually made much too late. A study of five hospice programs in Chicago showed that the median survival time after referral was only 24 days (Stone, 2001). In fact, 7% of patients referred to hospice die within hours of admission. This may be because survival estimates by physicians at admission are accurate only 20% of the time, 63% being optimistic and 17% pessimistic. The longer the physician had cared for the patient, the more optimistic the prediction. In 2011, the median (50th percentile) length of stay in a hospice was only about 19.1 days, and the average length of service was 69.1 days, with 35.8% enrolling in the last week of life (NHPCO, 2013). Family physicians should discuss hospice care when options are still available, not at the end of life.

SUPPORT FOR THE FAMILY

Families and close friends of the dying patient also suffer and should be supported. A good policy is for the physician not only to be sensitive to the needs of family members before death but to also follow up with the family after the patient dies with a phone call, letter, or home visit.

Hospice care is not focused only on the patient; the unit of care is the patient and family. The physical, psychological, and interpersonal needs of both the patient and the family are addressed. After a patient's death, family members may experience increased morbidity and mortality, emphasizing the need for greater family support from the physician. Unfortunately, most physicians do not routinely contact the family after a patient's death, so this need often goes unrecognized.

The "widower effect" is the likelihood that the surviving spouse will die shortly after the death of the partner. However, spouses of partners who received hospice care live longer than those whose spouses died without the benefit of hospice care, probably because hospice patients impose less stress on the family (Christakis and Iwashyna, 2003).

The hospice team provides follow-up bereavement care to the family up to 1 year after the patient's death. Family members who experience grief after the death of a loved one are more vulnerable to physical and other emotional disturbances than at any other time in their lives. They need help dealing with the grief, guilt, and symptoms associated with this emotional turmoil. The bereavement services of a hospice team can minimize these problems and can help family members cope with the pain of memories that arise from time to time, especially at holidays, birthdays, and other stressful occasions.

A man dying of cancer did not tell his family or friends in order to spare them. After his death, some admired his ability to suffer in silence, but many were angry and hurt, believing he did not think they were strong enough to suffer with him. The survivors not only were angry because he did not appear to need them but also were hurt because he did not even say good-bye (*New Age Hospice Horizons*, 1989).

The most remarkable contribution of the hospice movement is not that it provides a special and compassionate setting in which terminally ill persons can die without heroic measures but that the family becomes involved and comfortable in caring for the ill member. With the rapid increase of scientific and technologic competence in the field of medicine, families feel increasingly incompetent about the dying process. The hospice movement has reversed this trend and helps family members work with community support services to provide home care for many of these patients. When symptoms cannot be controlled at home, the hospice inpatient unit can provide medical and nursing expertise in a homelike setting.

SELECTING A HOSPICE

Most cities now have more than one hospice. Some organizations consist of volunteers with little or no medical expertise. Others have freestanding inpatient units and their own medical staffs. The questions in eTable 5-4 will help in the selection of a hospice.

Some patients and their families resist entering hospice for fear that their care will be taken over by a stranger and their personal physician will no longer be involved. That fear should be addressed directly by the family physician (Jemal et al., 2009). Many hospices employ a physician board certified in hospice and palliative medicine who can help with particularly difficult symptom problems. (See www.abhpm.org for a list of certified physicians in each area.)

SOCIAL SUPPORT AND RESOURCES IN THE COMMUNITY

See eAppendix 5-1 at www.expertconsult.com.

Advance Directives

An advance directive is a legal document that allows competent adults to express their intentions regarding medical

> ### Key Points
>
> - An advance directive is a legal document expressing a person's preferences regarding care in the event the person becomes unable to make decisions regarding care.
> - The most important item is the appointment of a health care surrogate as the patient's proxy.
> - Advance directives vary from simple to complex but still cannot cover every possibility.
> - A variety of state-specific advance care-planning documents are available on the Internet.

treatment in the event that they lose decision-making capacity because of a terminal illness. Types of advance directives are as follows:

- **Living will:** A form regarding the limitation of life-sustaining medical treatment in the face of a life-threatening illness.
- **Health care surrogate:** The appointment of a person to serve as the health care proxy (or medical power of attorney) to make medical decisions for an incapacitated patient. Ideally, these medical decisions would be based on the patient's preferences expressed in earlier discussions with the health care proxy.
- **Durable power of attorney:** Designates a person to make health, financial, and legal decisions if the patient is unable to do so.
- **"Do not resuscitate" (DNR) order, also known as Allow Natural Death (AND):** Determined by the physician and patient or the patient's health care surrogate or power of attorney.
- **Physician Orders for Life-Sustaining Treatment (POLST):** A set of medical orders based on the patient's wishes, as discussed with the patient's physician. This assures that health care professionals provide only the medical treatment that the patient desires to receive. This is currently endorsed with legislative support in 14 states, and it is in development in several other states.

If a person has only one action to take, it should be to appoint a health care surrogate as the person's proxy. Family physicians should encourage every patient to name a substitute decision maker, proxy, or surrogate who can represent the patient's wishes when needed. One problem is that often the surrogates named in the advance directive are not present to make decisions or are too emotionally overwrought to offer guidance.

Each state has its own laws governing advance directives, available at www.caringinfo.org.

Another site for useful advance directive information is:

www.familycaregiversonline.net/legal-resources

The Patient Self-Determination Act of 1991 requires hospitals and other health care institutions that receive Medicare or Medicaid funds to inform patients of their right to formulate advance directives. The purpose is to encourage greater awareness and use of advance directives so that situations of ambiguity can be avoided (Field and Cassel, 1997). The act requires hospitals to provide written information to all patients concerning their rights under state

---

Example of Medical Power of Attorney

I, _____, appoint _____ as my agent to make any and all health care decisions for me, except to the extent I state otherwise in this document. This Medical Power of Attorney takes effect if I become unable to make my own health care decisions and my physician certifies this fact in writing.

I sign my name to this Medical Power of Attorney on _____ (date).

Signature _____

Printed Name _____

Witnesses

Signature _____   Signature _____

Printed Name _____   Printed Name _____

Figure 5-1 Example of a living will.

law to refuse or accept treatment and to complete advance directives.

Almost 90% of Americans say that they would not want extraordinary steps taken to prolong their lives if they were dying, but only 20% have put that wish in writing in the form of a "living will." The version of the living will shown in Figure 5-1 has several advantages over others. It clarifies the person's preferences, and instead of locking elements arbitrarily in place, it leaves two witnesses as guardians of the individual's wishes and intentions, with discretion to use their judgment in the specific circumstances. This statement presumes goodwill on all sides and should be helpful to all concerned.

There is no one-size-fits-all approach to advance care planning. Some people prefer a simple approach, and others choose a more comprehensive, step-by-step process. The simple approach prevents support measures from being undertaken that should never have been initiated. It is best to have a patient both complete a living will and designate a health care surrogate to ensure that the person receives the desired medical care.

Although advance directives are not guarantees that the patient's wishes will be followed, without them, these wishes probably will not be followed. Since the case of Terri Schiavo, a 41-year-old woman whose feeding tube was removed in 2005 after a legal battle and political storm, patients are much more aware of the need to declare their feelings about life-sustaining treatment. The Schiavo case illustrates the importance of advance care planning to save both families and physicians considerable anguish.

Unfortunately, the legal restrictions arising out of the Schiavo case may be counterproductive. Courts in several states have now ruled that life-sustaining interventions must be continued in the absence of *clear and convincing evidence* that the patient would not want them. Despite efforts to make advance directives address a greater variety of terminal situations, it is almost impossible to state accurately the patient's wishes in every scenario. Advance directives are poorly equipped to cope with the complex clinical situations that often arise, emphasizing the need to appoint a health care surrogate.

In the past, end-of-life decisions were usually limited to deciding whether or not to use cardiopulmonary resuscitation (CPR). Now the range includes feeding tubes, hydration, hospitalization, antibiotic use, and terminal sedation. The more the family can focus on what the patient would want instead of what makes the family members feel most comfortable, the better will be the final decision (Lang and Quill, 2004). CPR can be lifesaving in some cases, but in most terminally ill patients, it is extremely unlikely to result in return of satisfactory cardiopulmonary function, survival to discharge from the hospital, or ability to live outside an institution. In a large multi-institutional study, physicians did no better than chance in identifying their seriously ill hospitalized patients' wishes to forgo CPR, and such wishes, even when known, rarely were respected when the physician believed that another course was more appropriate (Connors et al., 1995).

A relatively simple Advance Care Plan Document is available from Project GRACE (Guidelines for Resuscitation and Care at End-of-life) at www.projectgrace.org. A document that attempts to address a variety of clinical situations that may arise is the Medical Directive site at www.medicaldirective.org. This permits patients and physicians to download a scenario-based living will that includes six different scenarios to cover a variety of situations, plus a personal statement and a health care proxy. See Web Resources for additional sites and more information.

CARDIOVASCULAR IMPLANTABLE ELECTRONIC DEVICES

Many patients with end-stage cardiac disease have implantable electronic devices, such as pacemakers and implantable cardioverter-defibrillators (ICDs). To better prepare patients and their families, the family physician can discuss the risks and benefits of having or discontinuing these devices before an event in which the patient has a significant decline or hospitalization. Pacemakers are considered to neither prolong nor shorten the end of life. Discontinuing a pacemaker may result in angina or dyspnea, so continuing a pacemaker at the end of life is recommended. On the other hand, ICDs cause pain with shocks and are considered to be comparable to resuscitation efforts. At the end of life, when the goal is comfort only, discontinuing the ICD is indicated (Manaouil et al., 2012). The company that manufactures the device can assist with discontinuing the ICD. Also, placing a magnet the size of the ICD on the chest over the device can deactivate the ICD temporarily while the magnet is in place. ICD deactivation should be explicitly addressed in advanced care planning and at the end of life (Hastings, 2013, p. 167).

EUTHANASIA AND ASSISTED SUICIDE

See eAppendix 5-2 at www.expertconsult.com.

Summary of Additional Online Content

▶ **The following content is available at www.expertconsult.com:**

eAppendix 5-1 Social Support and Resources in the Community

eAppendix 5-2 Euthanasia and Assisted Suicide

eTable 5-1 Delivering "Bad News" to Patients

eTable 5-2 Management of Anorexia

eTable 5-3 Principles of Hospice Care

eTable 5-4 Questions to Ask When Selecting a Hospice

References

▶ **The complete reference list is available online at expertconsult.inkling.com.**

Suggested Readings

▶ **Available online at www.expertconsult.com.**

Web Resources

www.aarp.org American Association of Retired Persons. Consumer information regarding living wills, life after loss, and end-of-life issues.

www.aahpm.org The American Academy of Hospice and Palliative Medicine, a professional organization providing educational resources, jobmart, news, and challenges in symptom management.

www.adec.org Association for Death Education and Counseling. Educational resources on coping with loss, bereavement rituals, grief counseling, and other end-of-life issues.

www.americangeriatrics.org American Geriatrics Society. A variety of clinical practice guidelines and educational materials for those caring for older adults, including inappropriate medication use.

www.ampainsoc.org American Pain Society. Professional education regarding pain management and research.

www.asbh.org American Society for Bioethics and Humanities. Educational materials for health care professionals engaged in academic bioethics and the health-related humanities.

cancer.net American Society of Clinical Oncology. Patient information regarding symptom and disease management.

cancer.org American Cancer Society. Includes a complete listing of support programs and services in your area.

getpalliativecare.org Center to Advance Palliative Care. Tells patients where to find palliative care. Provides links to important websites, videos, and specific resources for clinicians, caregivers, the media, and policy makers.

www.abanet.org/aging Commission on Law and Aging of the American Bar Association. Consumer information on elder abuse, guardianship law, Medicare advocacy, and cognitive impairment.

www.agingwithdignity.org Develops a living will by answering five questions: medical care when incapacitated, medical treatment I want or do not want, how comfortable I want to be, how I want people to treat me, and what I want my loved ones to know.

www.cancer.gov National Cancer Institute. Complete listing of cancer treatment and ongoing clinical trials for the public and health care professionals.

www.caringinfo.org National Hospice and Palliative Care Organization. A layperson's guide to advance care planning. Provides free advance directives for each state, financial considerations, choosing a hospice, and grieving a loss.

www.compassionandchoices.org Compassion & Choices. Nonprofit organization to improve care and expand choice at the end of life, including links to Facing a Terminal Illness, Planning for the Future, and Help for a Loved One.

www.dyingwell.org Dying Well. Dr. Ira Byock's website. Includes resources on end-of-life care, grief and healing, and frequently asked questions about end-of-life experience and care.

www.epec.net The EPEC Project. Education of health care professionals in the essential clinical competencies of palliative and end-of-life care.

www.hospicefoundation.org Hospice Foundation of America. How to locate and choose a hospice, paying for hospice care, tools for caregivers, and so on.

www.nahc.org National Association for Home Care & Hospice. Trade association representing interests and concerns of home care agencies and hospices, including regulatory, legislative, and educational resources.

www.caregiveraction.org Caregiver Action Network. Tips and tools for family caregivers and information on agencies that provide caregiver support.

www.nhpco.org National Hospice and Palliative Care Organization, formerly National Hospice Organization. A professional organization that provides a large variety of educational programs and helps find a hospice or palliative care program.

www.nih.gov/nia National Institute on Aging. Publications and clinical trials on aging and disease and an online searchable database of health topics and contact information that provide help to elderly patients.

www.polst.org Physician orders for life-sustaining treatment. A form that complements but does not replace the advance directive. YouTube videos demonstrate its use in practice.

www.prepareforyourcare.org Prepare for Your Care. An easy-to-use online advance care planning tool. Includes easy-to-understand videos.

www.projectgrace.org Project GRACE. Includes an advance care plan document, examples of a living will in English and Spanish, and which states require it to be notarized.

www.uslivingwillregistry.com U.S. Living Will Registry. National registry that stores advance directives for access by medical professionals (membership required). Provides advance directive forms for all 50 states.

www.ycollaborative.com A consulting service that assists with advance directives, do not resuscitate orders, and medical powers of attorney.

6 *Care of the Self*

LUKE W. FORTNEY

Key Points

- Professional burnout is common among physicians and is considered an occupational hazard that significantly impacts patient care.
- Burnout is dynamic and changes along a spectrum depending on both the duration and degree of work-related stress.
- For many physicians, burnout starts as early as medical school but appears to be most significant mid-career, with primary care specialties being at greatest risk.
- Treatment and prevention of professional burnout involves a general, well-balanced approach to physical and mental health.
- Simple but persistent efforts using "The Formula for Good Health" and other tools are an effective evidenced-based approach to achieving wellness.
- Mindfulness is one form of mind-body medicine that is helpful for both burnout prevention and health promotion.
- A regular mind-body practice such as mindfulness can help physicians work through hard times and avoid being overwhelmed by stress.

The Burnout Trap

THE PHYSICIAN PREDICAMENT

Societies of the world have long recognized the fragile and challenging role that healers have played. Although highly regarded in most cultures, healers have also been charged by their communities to oversee and manage the inevitable afflictions of old age, sickness, and death. A culture's medicine-person is and has always been committed to a life of addressing suffering in an endless pursuit to restore and preserve health and balance in the body and mind. Prior to relatively recent advances in science and medical technologies, this endeavor has historically often been unsuccessful (Rakel and Weil, 2012).

Although the landscape, culture, technologies, and beliefs surrounding healing continue to evolve, the predicament has not. Every clinical encounter includes five general patient expectations: trust, compassion, accuracy, safety, and relief. No matter the location or situation, every patient seeks a physician who will establish a trusting therapeutic and compassionate partnership to accurately diagnose the problem and offer safe and effective treatment options that empower the patient. Unfortunately, mistakes, neglect, and bad luck will always be a part of medical practice. It can be very challenging dealing with the blame, guilt, remorse, grief, fear, and anger that come with the loss and injury that occasionally occur in medical practice.

The practice of modern medicine can be called a high-pressure, high-expectation, high-stakes profession that involves the persistent stress of navigating life-threatening issues on a regular basis, but often in a random and unanticipated way. Early psychology research showed that inescapable electric shocks administered to dogs leads to strong emotional stress, learned helplessness, and depression. Just like this classical conditioning experiment where repeated inescapable stress results in depression-like symptoms and learned helplessness (Seligman, 1972), similar effects are also observed among physicians who are subject to the continued, unrelenting, and unpredictable stresses of medical emergencies, overwhelming patient care duties, and beeping pager alerts in on-call situations (Arora et al., 2013). Over time these and other factors can have negative effects on health and quality of life for physicians (Sonneck and Wagner, 1996).

The modern physician predicament incorporates a wide range of stressors and influencing factors. Patient satisfaction scores are now commonly used in part to determine a physician's success and reimbursement, which can pose considerable strain, especially in treating conditions such as addiction, working with demanding patients with unrealistic demands, and managing U.S. Drug Enforcement Administration (DEA) schedule II and III medications, among many others. Furthermore, many physician roles involve not only patient care in clinic and hospital settings, but also teaching, oversight of advanced practitioners, and managerial responsibilities with increasing expectations for excellence (Nedrow et al., 2013).

The advent of electronic health records (EHRs) along with changes in billing, coding, documentation, and electronic patient communication pose new opportunities and challenges in a rapidly changing landscape of insurance coverage and prior authorization processes (Howard et al., 2013). What's more, physicians are independently accountable and licensed professionals who are finding themselves more and more as employees in large health care corporations. Nonetheless, physicians continue to be individually responsible for staying current with advances in medical research as it applies to patient care. In large corporate hospital environments, physicians must also skillfully navigate personal and professional boundaries with staff, administration, patients, and home life (Chen et al., 2013).

At times the conflicting interests of altruistic expectations from patients and the personal need for rest and limits on work-hour responsibilities can be overwhelming and exacerbate the underlying strain that comes from working with sick patients in an endless stream of crises (Sonneck and Wagner, 1996). In short, physicians are being asked more and more to be everything to everyone in every way all the time (Merton, 1966). It is important to also realize that all of these factors are stressors that come *in addition to* remaining proficient with medical skills in various areas of expertise. Add strain from one's personal life—family, home, and financial disruption—and it is easy to understand why today's physician will at times experience significant professional burnout.

To allow oneself to be carried away by a multitude of conflicting concerns, to surrender to too many demands, to commit oneself to too many projects, to want to help everyone in everything, is to succumb to violence. The frenzy neutralizes our work for peace. It destroys our own inner capacity for peace because it kills the root of inner wisdom which makes work fruitful.

—THOMAS MERTON

BURNOUT AMONG PHYSICIANS

Professional burnout is characterized as a loss of emotional, mental, and physical energy caused by continued job-related stress. It results from ongoing, unrelenting work stress without adequate time away from professional work duties for rest and recreation. The Maslach Burnout Inventory (MBI) is used worldwide and has been validated in samples of various professions, including health care workers (Maslach and Jackson, 1996). It is used to investigate job satisfaction using self-report measures that score three aspects of professional burnout syndrome: emotional exhaustion, depersonalization, and lack of personal accomplishment. A high degree of burnout is one in which a respondent has high scores on the Emotional Exhaustion and Depersonalization subscales and a low score on the Personal Accomplishment subscale (Maslach and Jackson, 1996). Among these, research suggests that emotional exhaustion represents the core burnout dimension among physicians (Lee et al., 2013), which is caused in large part by working long hours with significant off-duty personal-time intrusion (Chen et al., 2013).

Burnout appears to be more common among physicians than other professional groups, with primary care and emergency medicine specialties being at greatest risk (Fortney et al., 2013; Shanafelt et al., 2012; Sonneck and Wagner, 1996) (Figure 6-1). However, research comparing inpatient- to outpatient-based care does not support the belief that burnout is more frequent among hospitalists compared to clinic-based physicians (Roberts et al., 2013). Furthermore, compared with physicians in the early and late stages of their careers, middle career physicians appear to be particularly at risk (Dyrbye et al., 2013).

In general, there are three risk factors recognized as being independently associated with burnout for physicians: hours worked per week, experience of recent work or home conflict, and how that conflict was addressed or resolved (Dyrbye et al., 2011). Overall, up to 60% of all physicians report having experienced burnout at some point in their careers (McCray et al., 2008), with more than 40% experiencing burnout at any single point in time (Wallace et al., 2009). Perhaps the most concerning aspect of physician burnout is that it starts early, with up to 45% of medical students and 80% of medical residents reporting significant work-related burnout (McCray et al., 2008). A cross-sectional survey administered to senior medical students in New York found that 71% met criteria for burnout (Mazurkiewicz et al., 2012).

BURNOUT CAUSES

There are several factors that contribute to burnout (Table 6-1). Increasing workload is significant in primary care. In the United States, implementation of the Affordable Care Act is estimated to enroll 32 million previously uninsured citizens, which will increase demand for primary care services (Mann, 2011). In addition, an expanding elderly population, insufficient supply of new primary care physicians, increased physician attrition, low medical student interest in primary care specialties, and lower primary care services reimbursements compared with other medical specialties add further strain (Baron, 2010; Bell et al., 2002; Dyrbye et al., 2008; Dyrbye and Shanafelt, 2011).

There is a saying that the cobbler always wears the worst shoes. It has been observed that physicians, while striving to deliver high quality care to their patients, tend to give themselves suboptimal care and are less attentive to their own wellness (Wallace et al., 2009). An increasingly bureaucratic health care system also creates the higher likelihood of feeling alienated and depersonalized (Bell et al., 2002; McKinlay and Marceau, 2011). Furthermore, certain personality traits—for example, being highly driven, a strong sense of perfectionism, being strongly empathetic, feeling inadequate, having low self-esteem, and being the classic "type A" workaholic—may add greater risk to burnout syndrome (Table 6-1) (Vicentic et al., 2013).

Other personal factors that correlate with professional burnout (see Table 6-1) include the lack of coping skills for stress (Epstein, 1999; Nedrow et al., 2013), unhealthy habits such as smoking and alcohol abuse, and poor relationships with colleagues. Lack of time for self-care and feeling that there is not enough time in the day to complete necessary work tasks are other common physician concerns—while for some, regret of specialty choice can be a significant cause of burnout (Eckleberry-Hunt et al., 2009). From a medical practice perspective, increasing clinical demands, caring for a difficult or sociomedically complex patient panel, mounting productivity pressures, business or insurance concerns, keeping up with rapidly advancing technology and EHRs, lack of control over office

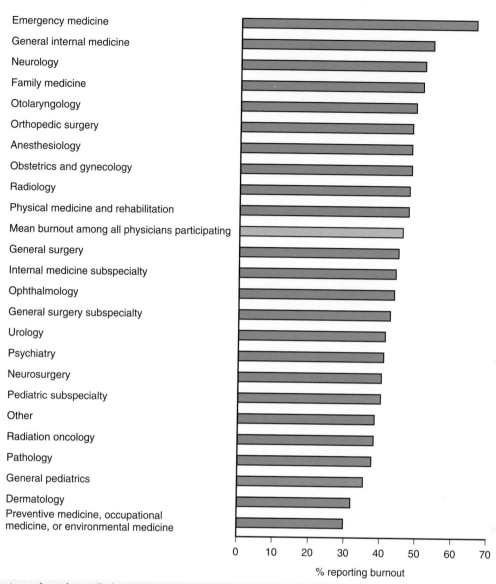

Figure 6-1 Burnout prevalence by medical specialty. (From Shanafelt TD, Bradley KA, Wipf JE, et al. Burnout and self-reported patient care in an internal medicine residency program. *Ann Intern Med.* 2002;136(5):358-367.)

Table 6-1 Risk Factors for Burnout

1. Highly driven, "workaholic," perfectionistic personality
2. Low self-esteem, feeling inadequate
3. Continued unabated work stress and long work hours
4. Poor relationships with colleagues
5. Difficulty resolving home and work relationship conflicts
6. Poor coping skills for stress (smoking, alcohol abuse, drug use, avoidance, confrontational)
7. Lack of time for self-care
8. Feeling there is not enough time in the day to complete work tasks
9. Regret of specialty choice
10. Lack of control over clinic schedule or office processes
11. Rapidly advancing electronic health records, changing insurance landscape
12. Increasing bureaucratization of health care
13. Complex and challenging patient panels

processes and one's schedule are additional physician concerns (Shanafelt et al., 2002). Finally, studies have also identified difficulty in resolving home and work conflicts as a major contributor to physician burnout (McCray et al., 2008; Dyrbye et al., 2014).

BURNOUT EFFECTS

Considerable evidence suggests that burnout negatively affects quality of patient care (Durning et al., 2013), with profound personal implications for physicians, including depression and suicidal ideation (Center et al., 2003; Devi, 2011; Dyrbye et al., 2008; Sonneck and Wagner, 1996). Furthermore, physician attrition because of burnout is both disruptive to continuity of patient care and costly to health care organizations (Scott, 1998). Once burnout is present, absenteeism increases, physician turnover increases, and overall job satisfaction decreases; but perhaps

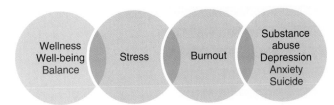

Figure 6-2 Burnout spectrum. (Adapted from West CP, Shanafelt TD. Physician well-being and professionalism. *Minn Med.* 2007;90(8):44-46.)

Table 6-2 Attributes That Protect Against Burnout
1. Having a healthy temperament and sense of humor
2. Being self-aware, reflective, and attuned to personal needs
3. Having meaningful core values
4. Having an optimistic philosophy of life and work
5. Having a nonjudgmental and forgiving attitude
6. Being compassionate and accepting of self and others
7. Feeling that one is making a difference in one's work
8. Having healthy boundaries and knowing when to say no or step away
9. Maintaining work and life balance with regular restorative time away from work
10. Having supportive and caring friends, family, and colleagues
11. Maintaining a balanced lifestyle of healthy diet, regular exercise, and attention to mind-body needs

most concerning is that physicians self-report increased suboptimal patient care and medical errors (McCray et al., 2008). Physician surveys also suggest that 50% of all physicians with professional burnout are also depressed and at risk for alcohol abuse (Brown et al., 2009; Shanafelt et al., 2002). This is especially concerning given that many aspects of patient care—physician self-reported medical error, lower empathy, early retirement, and lower patient satisfaction—are directly affected by physician burnout (Dyrbye and Shanafelt, 2011).

BURNOUT SPECTRUM

On one end of the burnout spectrum is wellness, well-being, and balance in one's personal and professional life (West and Shanafelt, 2007). However as stress increases and persists over time, scores of depersonalization and emotional exhaustion increase, while personal accomplishment measures decrease. The extreme end of the burnout spectrum includes substance abuse, depression, anxiety, and suicidal ideation (Figure 6-2). Death by suicide is considered a major occupational hazard for physicians (Center et al., 2003; Devi, 2011; Sonneck and Wagner, 1996). Among medical students, suicidal ideation is nearly double that of the general population (Dyrbye et al., 2008).

BURNOUT PROTECTION

Certain personal attitudes and perspectives appear to be protective against burnout (Table 6-2). Having a healthy temperament and sense of humor, along with being self-aware, reflective, and attuned to personal needs appears to be helpful. Additionally, having meaningful core values with an optimistic philosophy of life have also been identified as important protective traits (Jensen et al., 2008). Healthy, happy, and well-adjusted physicians also display nonjudgmental and forgiving attitudes, as well as a compassionate acceptance of self and others. Perhaps most importantly, feeling that one is making a difference in one's profession carries significant protection from burnout (Jensen et al., 2008). Fortunately, these skills can be learned and supported.

Finally, as the mind goes, so follows the body and vice versa. This fundamental truth of health was recognized long ago when Plato wrote, "The great error of our day is that physicians separate treatment of psyche from treatment of the body." Even today, this is more commonly recognized. For example, there have been more than 1000 trials that have examined the link between exercise and depression and anxiety (Kirby, 2005), with more than 80 meta-analyses showing significant benefit (North et al.,

1990). One study concluded that moderate regular exercise should be included as a viable means of treating depression, anxiety, and improving mental well-being (Fox, 1999). As the saying goes, "we have yet to find a disease that exercise does not help." When it comes to burnout, the importance of regular physical activity as it pertains to wellness cannot be overstated.

A Roadmap to Health and Wellness

The true healer knows that health can only be achieved by promoting a balance of body, emotions, mind, and spirit...first in oneself and then in one's patients.

—HOWARD SILVERMAN, MD

The effects of professional burnout go beyond depersonalization, emotional exhaustion, and low sense of accomplishment. In a ripple effect of consequences, continued unabated work stress can quickly move from health, well-being, and balance on one end of the spectrum and eventually lead to depression, anxiety, substance abuse, and various chronic diseases on the other end. Just as the burnout spectrum is dynamic and shifting from time to time, so is health and well-being, which must be cultivated and supported.

In general, health can be defined as decreased morbidity and mortality. The first rule of health, therefore, is to remove the obstacles to healing. From this perspective, unnecessary early death and suffering are overwhelmingly caused by tobacco use, poor diet, and lack of physical activity alone (Katz, 2013). Just these three adverse health behaviors are directly responsible for 8 out of every 10 deaths in the United States every year (McGinnis and Foege, 1993; Mokdad et al., 2004). Expanding on this, the Centers for Disease Control and Prevention (CDC) has identified four modifiable health risk behaviors—tobacco use, lack of physical activity, poor nutrition, and obesity—that are overwhelmingly responsible for most of the unnecessary illness, suffering, and early death in the United States every year (CDC, 2014; Katz, 2013).

At the same time, positive change in these four main modifiable health risk behaviors is at the root of preventing unnecessary suffering, while empowering patients and physicians alike to take direct personal action toward wellness in their own lives using straightforward and simple strategies that have dramatic effects on improving longevity and happiness (Kopes-Kerr, 2010; Formula for Good Health). One representative study from the large corpus of literature showing the profound benefits of healthy lifestyle behaviors found that by getting 3.5 hours of exercise per week, eating a healthy diet, not smoking, and having a body mass index (BMI) of less than 30 kg/m² reduced the risk of myocardial infarction (MI) by 81%, stroke by 50%, type 2 diabetes by 93%, and cancer by 36% over nearly 8 years. Adhering to all four of these health factors reduced overall risk of death and serious disease by 78% (Ford et al., 2009).

AVOID UNNECESSARY SUFFERING

A basic evidence-based strategy to reduce the risk of developing chronic disease and early death is comprised of the followed five elements (www.meriter.com/wellness; Kopes-Kerr, 2010):

1. Increase physical activity.
2. Eat healthier foods.
3. Avoid tobacco.
4. Consume moderate or no alcohol.
5. Acknowledge and address stress and the mind-body connection.

THE BASIC TENANTS OF WELLNESS: MIND-BODY CONNECTION

There are three main pillars to prevention and health: (1) what we put into the body (e.g., nutrition, medications, supplements, vitamins), (2) how we move the body (e.g., exercise, manual therapies, procedures), and (3) how we perceive the world (e.g., mind-body connection) (Figure 6-3). Mind-body awareness and practice, which are those things that address subjective areas such as emotions, the heart, meaning and purpose, and connection with others, may be the least recognized but most essential aspect of good health. For example, the INTERHEART study, which was a study of risk factors for first MI in more than 24,000 adults from 52 countries, found that psychosocial stress

was the second most significant risk factor for acute MI, behind smoking, but above hypertension and obesity (Rosengren et al., 2004). Another study found that severe emotional stress was the cause of 19 cases of reversible cardiomyopathy as demonstrated by objective measures such as decreased ejection fraction, prolonged QT interval electrocardiogram (ECG) findings, increased inflammatory monocyte infiltration, and elevated serum troponin and catecholamine levels, despite the fact that 95% of cases had normal cardiac arteries when visualized on catheterization (Wittstein et al., 2005). Yet another study found an inverse association between sense of humor and coronary heart disease. Of 150 participants who were given humorous manuscripts to read, those with existing heart disease were 45% less likely to laugh. Those who did laugh were less likely to have heart disease and hostility overall (Clark et al., 2001). Specific to professional burnout, research shows that there is an increased risk of cardiovascular disease, including metabolic syndrome, hypertension, overall poor health, and increased meta-inflammation, among chronically stressed mid-career physicians (Melamed et al., 2006; Spickard et al., 2002).

MINDFULNESS IN A MEDICAL CONTEXT

From these three main generalized areas of health (see Figure 6-3) are derived more specific aspects of healing that help guide decisions about what therapies and approaches are best suited from person to person for both illness and wellness (Figure 6-4). But before any therapeutic action can happen, it is essential to start with pausing, being present, and taking an objective inventory of one's current work and life situation before proceeding (Figure 6-5) (Rakel and Fortney, 2012).

The practice of mindfulness is a fundamental dimension of the mind-body connection that addresses every aspect of health. Mindfulness in a medical setting is considered a form of awareness training (Figure 6-6) that enables one to attend to aspects of experience in a nonjudgmental, nonreactive way, which in turn helps cultivate clear thinking, equanimity, compassion, and open-heartedness (Ludwig and Kabat-Zinn, 2008). The goal of mindfulness is compassionate informed action in the world, using a wide array of data, making correct decisions, better understanding the patient and oneself, and ultimately relieving suffering (Epstein, 1999). In this sense, mindfulness aims to maintain open awareness in one's experience in a way that generates a greater sense of emotional balance and well-being. Through the practice of mindfulness, unhelpful habitual thoughts and behaviors can be recognized, allowing for new and creative ways of responding.

MINDFULNESS AND BURNOUT

Growing research shows that the practice of mindfulness can have significant health benefits (Fortney and Taylor, 2010). Among physicians, mindfulness is helpful in both preventing and treating professional burnout. In practical terms, mindfulness operationalizes the notion that increased awareness leads to insight, which in turn leads to increased clarity in making healthy personal choices in any given moment (Epstein, 1999). A study published in *The Journal*

STATE OF HEALTH, BALANCE, AND WELLBEING

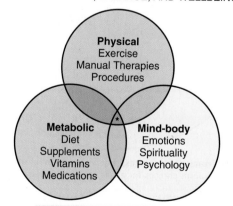

Figure 6-3 Three pillars of health.

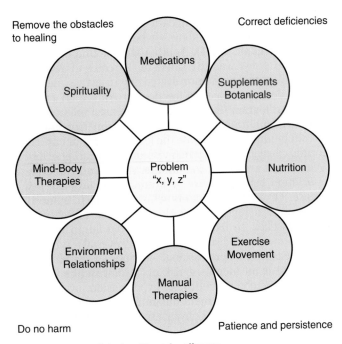

Remove the obstacles to healing

Correct deficiencies

Do no harm

Patience and persistence

General approach to health and wellness:
1. Awareness of the factors influencing burnout
2. Action steps toward wellness

Peripheral lifestyle factors: (1) Remove obstacles to health, such as smoking, overeating, sleep deprivation, and those lifestyle factors that are in direct competition to well-being. (2) Identify and correct obvious deficiencies (hypothyroidism, anemia, malnutrition, etc.). (3) Choose strategies that are not harmful and have low risk for harm. (4) Encourage patience and persistence with lifestyle changes.

Eight integrated approaches to addressing burnout and any health concern: (1) medications (non-habit-forming options for sleep, mood support, etc.); (2) OTC nutriceuticals that have evidence for safety and efficacy; (3) improving nutrition to include transition to a general healthy, antiinflammatory, whole-foods-based diet; (4) encouragement to increase movement, activity, exercise in any capacity; (5) manual therapies such as massage, acupuncture, etc.; (6) environment and relationships are those external factors that influence health such as air pollution, abusive relationships, toxic work/home settings, etc.; (7) mind-body therapies address internal factors such as emotions, beliefs, thoughts, and memory; (8) spirituality defined as that which gives meaning and purpose and/or is valuable, which may or may not be religious.

Figure 6-4 Integrated eight-wheel approach to health and wellness. OTC, over-the-counter. (Used with permission from Fortney L, Rakel D, Rindfleisch A, et al. Introduction to the integrative primary care: the health-oriented clinic. *Prim Care.* 2010;37(1):1-12.)

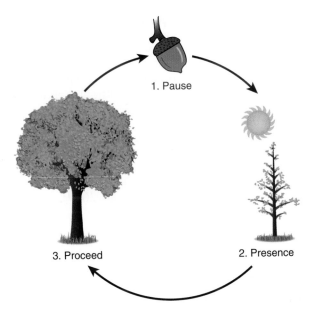

A 3-step exploration of health: practice in your practice
1. Pause: stop, take a breath, drop in, notice this moment
2. Presence: noticing thoughts, body sensations, and emotions without reactivity
3. Proceed: mindfully responding to whatever needs attention in this moment

Figure 6-5 Mindfulness in medicine: practice in your practice. (Used with permission from University of Wisconsin Integrative Medicine (http://www.fammed.wisc.edu/MINDFULNESS)

Practice:
1. In this moment, what is happening?
2. How does the experience change from moment to moment?

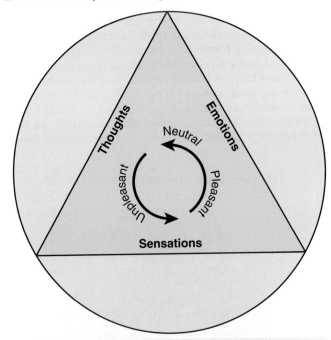

Figure 6-6 Triangle of awareness: becoming aware of things as they are, so as to inform choices for change. (From Fortney L. Chapter 98: Recommending meditation. In: Rakel D, ed. *Integrative Medicine.* 3rd ed. Philadelphia: Elsevier; 2012.)

of the American Medical Association demonstrated that mindfulness education for primary care physicians over 12 months was helpful in addressing burnout by improving mood and emotional stability. Another study then went on to demonstrate that even an abbreviated course in mindfulness adapted to the professional needs of primary care physicians significantly improved burnout, depression, anxiety, and stress. These positive effects were maintained and generally trended toward further improvements over the length of the 9-month study despite there being no booster sessions or formal follow-up trainings (Fortney et al., 2013).

This study helped show that mindfulness—even relatively brief training—for busy primary care physicians was sufficient in teaching meaningful mindfulness skills that led to significant improvements in burnout that persisted over a relatively long period of time. Similar to exercise, it appears that any amount of mindfulness training and practice is better than none at all when it comes to burnout, stress, health, and well-being (Podein, 2013). These and other findings further support growing evidence that suggests increased emotional awareness among physicians is associated with less burnout, higher work satisfaction, and higher patient satisfaction overall (Jensen et al., 2008; Weng et al., 2011).

MINDFULNESS IN MEDICINE:

Increased research and familiarization with mindfulness in the fields of neuroscience, psychology, and medicine have led to an increased understanding of consciousness and improved treatment for many health conditions, including burnout and stress. Practicing mindfulness (see Figures 6-5 and 6-6) can elicit physical ease and mental stability, which can provide a foundation for health and wellness as they directly influence one's ability to meet the challenges resulting from stress, burnout, and illness for patients and practitioners alike (Rakel et al., 2011). According to experienced meditation teacher Charlotte Joko Beck, the practice of mindfulness "provides a skill that affords a greater sense of self-determination—the ability to cultivate and draw upon inner resources to help meet all circumstances with equanimity and clarity."

Basic mindfulness practice addresses burnout by offering a simple yet effective tool to help ease many of the challenges, both personal and academic, encountered throughout medical training and practice. Medical students who participated in an 8-week mindfulness course showed reduced anxiety, reduced distress and depression, and increased levels of empathy (Shapiro et al., 1998). There is growing evidence that heightened present-moment awareness gained through mindfulness training improves attention and memory as well (Jha et al., 2007). Furthermore, research suggests that mindfulness meditation can help foster present-moment awareness that may reduce medical error and improve patient care by addressing faulty thinking such as snap judgments, distracted attention, inadvertent stereotyping, and other cognitive traps that lead to critical mistakes in patient care (Groopman, 2007). This line of thinking is contrary to previous conventional thinking that medical errors are derived from lack of knowledge. These cognitive processing errors can be avoided by paying attention to the process of thinking by the metacognitive practice of mindfulness (Epstein, 1999).

Research also shows that practitioners who themselves exhibit healthy habits are more effective in motivating patients to make significant positive change for health (Fortney et al., 2010; Frank et al., 2000). In a randomized controlled trial of 124 psychiatric inpatients managed by 18 psychology residents, patients of interns who received mindfulness training did significantly better than those patients treated by interns who did not receive mindfulness training (Grepmair et al., 2007).

CREATE YOUR OWN HEALTH PLAN

Preventive research widely shows the benefits of healthy behaviors, for both avoiding chronic disease and promoting good health. Within the three main areas of wellness (see Figure 6-3), it is clear that even very basic minimal efforts in exercise, nutrition, and mind-body care can have profound health benefits that can lead to reduced mortality and morbidity in the long run (Kopes-Kerr, 2010; Mokdad et al., 2004). In approaching both disease and wellness, the process starts with awareness of those factors that either directly contribute to poor health or create obstacles that interfere with healing and well-being (Fortney, 2010). Heavy alcohol use, smoking, and overindulgence of unhealthy foods are the most common things that inhibit the body's ability to heal and recover. Having a plan to guide the process of wellness can be helpful, and there are simple tools that can facilitate this (Table 6-3; see Figure 6-4) (see the Web Resources).

For busy primary care physicians, knowing when to step away, turn off the pager, and intentionally limit work responsibilities can be very challenging. The practice of "letting go," being more mindful, and living a balanced lifestyle may even seem impossible. However, the effect of burnout on patient care can have negative consequences, as well as negatively affect home life and relationships if a balance of rest, physical health, and work is not

Table 6-3 Strategies That Help Reduce Burnout

Cultivating balance, the "In's and Out's" of personal needs. In any given moment, ask, "What do I need?" Different things are needed in different situations from the perspective of physical, psychological, emotional, and spiritual aspects of life.

Physical	**Energy out**: Unburdening—to release tension and overstimulation in the body. Examples: Movement, exercise, physical activity. **Energy in**: Restorative—to increase energy when physically depleted. Examples: Rest, sleep, food, water.
Psychological	**Energy out**: Unburdening—actively seeking answers and resolving confusion. Examples: Analysis, insight, problem-solving, research, learning. **Energy in**: Restorative—taking in peace and equanimity, letting go of mental clutter and chatter. Examples: Meditation, silence, stillness, mental rest.
Emotional	**Energy out**: Unburdening—cathartic, get it out. Examples: Emotional expression such as journaling, singing, talking with a counselor, "shouting" technique. **Energy in**: Restorative—receiving emotional support and care. Examples: Love, laughter, kindness, positive touch.
Spiritual	Being aware and acknowledging what is personally meaningful in life, what provides a sense of wonder and awe, being connected to something and someone(s) beyond oneself—this may or may not be religious for each person. Examples: Cultivating connection with loved ones, being in nature, recognizing and expressing love, offering service and kindness to others, practicing prayer or meditation, experiencing joy, and pursuing an experience of being alive.

maintained. One study found that doctors who were more mindful with their patients were more upbeat, better listeners, and showed more empathy while remaining efficient in their daily work tasks (Beach et al., 2013). Another study from the University of Warwick found that happier people are more motivated to work harder and overall are more productive (Oswald et al., 2014). As the saying goes, "you can't give what you don't have." Resilience, however, is a dynamic, evolving process of healthy attitudes, mindful awareness, and constructive action steps toward good health (Fortney, 2012; Jensen et al., 2008) (see Figures 6-3 and 6-4).

Summary

It is important to remember that burnout is not static, but rather a dynamic process that changes over time along the burnout spectrum depending on various degrees and duration of work-life stressors (West and Shanafelt, 2007). Nonetheless, the absence of disease—in this case anxiety, depression, and stress—does not automatically imply the presence of health and well-being (WHO, n.d.). The full importance of the impact of happy, healthy clinicians on patient care cannot be overstated (Dyrbye, 2008; Wallace et al., 2009). The path to health and wellness among physicians and for patients starts with self-reflection, personal awareness, and small action steps that incorporate regular physical activity, a reasonably healthy diet, avoidance of substance abuse, and other work-life changes that may be appropriate from person to person (Ford et al., 2009) (see Table 6-3).

KEY TREATMENT

- Professional burnout is a significant occupational hazard for physicians, which has a negative effect on patient care and quality of personal and professional life (SOR: B) (Arora et al., 2013; Brown et al., 2009; Center et al., 2003; Chen et al., 2013; Devi 2011; Durning et al., 2013; Dyrbye et al, 2008; Dyrbye and Shanafelt, 2011; Eckleberry-Hunt et al., 2009; Fortney et al., 2013; Lee et al., 2013; McCray et al., 2008; Melamed et al., 2006; Scott, 1998; Shanafelt et al., 2002; Shanafelt et al.,

2012; Sonneck and Wagner, 1996; Spickard et al., 2002; Wallace et al., 2009).
- Emotional exhaustion and emotional awareness are the two most important aspects in recognizing and addressing burnout (SOR: B) (Dyrbye et al., 2013; Epstein, 1999; Jensen et al., 2008; Lee et al., 2013; McCray et al., 2008; Nedrow et al., 2013; Shapiro et al., 1998; Weng et al., 2011).
- Mindfulness training has been shown to reduce stress and burnout among medical professionals (SOR: B) (Beach et al., 2013; Epstein, 1999; Fortney et al., 2013; Krasner et al., 2009).
- Stress, poor diet, lack of exercise, and substance abuse are four modifiable risk factors that contribute to early mortality and morbidity (SOR: A) (CDC, 2014; Kopes-Kerr, 2010; McGinnis and Foege, 1993; Mokdad et al., 2004; Rosengren et al., 2004).
- Stress reduction, eating a healthy diet, getting a minimum of 2.5 hours of exercise a week, avoiding tobacco products, and drinking no to moderate alcohol significantly reduces the risk of chronic lifestyle-related disease and early death (SOR: A) (Ford et al., 2009; Fox, 1999; Katz, 2013; Kopes-Kerr, 2010; Mokdad et al., 2004).

Acknowledgment

Lisa Rambaldo, PsyD, for her help developing Table 6-3.

References

The complete reference list is available at www.expertconsult.com.

Web Resources

www.fammed.wisc.edu/mindfulness Comprehensive website for mindfulness in medicine, for personal use and for patient care.
www.fammed.wisc.edu/integrative/modules Evidence-based "Mind/Body Awareness Writing Exercises" that help address stress, trauma, and pain for physicians and patients.
www.fammed.wisc.edu/aware-medicine/self "Writing Your Personal Health Plan" and other self-awareness and self-care tools for physicians.
www.meriter.com/wellness An evidence-based roadmap and plan for improving general health, "The Formula for Good Health."
www.meriter.com/wellness General user-friendly exercise and nutrition prescriptions.

7 *Preventive Health Care*

DOUG CAMPOS-OUTCALT

Key Points

- Preventive interventions should be supported by high-level evidence of effectiveness and safety.
- Of all organizations and committees that make prevention recommendations, the U.S. Preventive Services Task Force (USPSTF) uses the most robust, evidence-based methodology.
- Other groups that make recommendations pertinent to prevention in the primary care and community setting are the Advisory Committee on Immunization Practices (ACIP) and the Community Preventive Services Task Force, both supported by the Centers for Disease Control and Prevention (CDC).
- Screening tests should be assessed for accuracy, safety, and effectiveness. Effectiveness means that screening results in an outcome that is better than occurs when the condition presents naturally and that the benefit gained exceeds harms caused.
- Screening tests can appear effective when they are not because of lead time and length biases.
- In low-prevalence conditions, even with accurate tests, the positive predictive value of the test will be low.
- One of the harms that can arise from screening is overdiagnosis, finding and treating disease, with the associated harms from diagnosis and treatment, when the condition would have resolved on its own or never progressed.
- Some behaviors that lead to bad health can be modified by brief interventions in a clinical encounter, others need more intensive interventions.
- A four-step approach of considering risk assessment, risk reduction, screening, and immunizations can assist family physicians in remembering to address prevention with each patient.
- Reducing "risks" for specific diseases found in observational studies should be tested in controlled clinical trials to see if risk reduction lowers the incidence of the disease.
- Tools available for risk reduction include behavior modification and chemoprevention.

- Physicians should offer to patients screening tests that have an A or B recommendation from the USPSTF.
- Physicians should offer and encourage patients to accept immunizations recommended by the ACIP.
- Preventive services offering the most benefit and those most acceptable to the patient should be prioritized.
- Smoking is the leading cause of preventable mortality and morbidity. Any patient who smokes should be encouraged to cease smoking and be offered nicotine replacement, medications, and support group referral.
- Accurately diagnosing and treating diseases of public health importance, such as sexually transmitted infections, influenza, and tuberculosis, helps control these diseases and prevent drug resistance.
- Family physicians can minimize the effects of communicable diseases in the community by providing recommended treatment for family members and other contacts of those with infectious diseases either with expedited partner therapy or by referring them to the public health department.
- Infection control practices should be enforced in the clinical setting.
- Physicians should report infectious diseases, cancers, and other reportable conditions as required by state and local reporting requirements.
- Clinic staff should be vaccinated as recommended by the CDC.
- Avoiding unnecessary or harmful testing and treatments and their associated harms should be considered part of the preventive practices of family physicians.
- Genomic and genetic testing holds promise for enhancing clinical prevention, but only a few tests have been proven effective at this time, and genetic risk profiling for chronic disease risk has not proven to be beneficial.
- Making prevention interventions routine, as part of the clinical system, helps to ensure a high level of performance.

Family Medicine and Prevention

Prevention is a large part of family medicine. Family physicians provide preventive health care on a daily basis and are frequently consulted by patients on how to stay healthy and avoid disease. Family physicians are also a part of the foundation of the nation's public health system, being the first contact for patients with illnesses of public health importance, a source of surveillance for disease prevalence, and a resource for dissemination of information that can protect the health of the public. This chapter will discuss all these roles and describe how to maximize the effectiveness of preventive services delivered.

Definitions of Prevention

Prevention can be divided into three categories: primary, secondary, and tertiary. Family physicians should consider how all three categories may benefit each patient.

Primary prevention results in the prevention of a disease or condition from occurring. Examples include vaccinations, which prevent an array of infectious diseases, and smoking cessation, which prevents myriad illnesses that result from sustained tobacco use. Primary prevention can be, but is not always, cost saving for society (more money is saved than spent). It often involves community-wide intervention (clean water and sanitation), and the benefits are often unseen and unappreciated by the public.

Secondary prevention involves screening asymptomatic individuals for a disease to detect it early, and with early intervention achieve a better outcome than with later detection and treatment. When testing is performed in those who are symptomatic, to diagnose or rule out a suspected condition, this is not screening, it is diagnostic testing. Screening applies only to those who are asymptomatic. Many disagreements over the value of screening result from not understanding this fundamental difference between screening and diagnostic testing.

Contrary to common belief, secondary prevention does not save money. It can lower morbidity and mortality and usually compares favorably in cost-benefit analyses to medical interventions such as cardiac bypass surgery, but it does not result in more money saved than spent. It can be, however, money well spent.

Tertiary prevention involves interventions that occur after a disease or condition is evident, in an attempt to make the affected person healthier and improve quality of life. An example is cardiac rehabilitation after myocardial infarction. Tertiary prevention also is not cost saving. Because tertiary prevention can prevent a repeat event, such as a second heart attack, it is frequently, although incorrectly, referred to as secondary prevention.

Evidence as the Foundation of Prevention

Solid evidence supporting the effectiveness and safety of an intervention is important. Family physicians are busy and need to use their time effectively, concentrating on providing services that actually result in improvements for their patients. In addition, with primary and secondary prevention, the interventions involve healthy, asymptomatic people. The physician does well to remember that it is hard to improve on the healthy, asymptomatic patient. It can be done, but in attempting to make someone healthier we should ensure that not only are we being effective, we are also being safe and not causing harm in the process.

For this reason the evidence threshold for action should be higher for prevention than for therapy. If a patient has a serious illness, the therapeutic imperative provides a rationale for using treatments that might be supported only by moderate quality studies and intermediate outcomes, if that is the best evidence that exists. For prevention, if the safety and effectiveness of the intervention is not based on high-quality evidence, it is better to wait for better evidence and concentrate on the many interventions available that are backed by strong evidence. It is difficult enough to fit all the proven interventions into a tight clinical schedule without spending time on those we are not sure make a difference.

Figure 7-1 illustrates the pyramid of evidence that is found in the medical literature. At the top of the pyramid, and providing the highest quality evidence, are high-quality systematic reviews and meta-analyses. Next come randomized controlled trials, followed by lesser quality-controlled trials. Below that are observational studies, which are much more subject to bias. Among observational studies, cohort and case-control studies provide more reliable information than cross-sectional studies. Correlational (ecological) studies and case reports are at the base, providing interesting information that should not be used as proof of effectiveness or causation but are useful for generating questions and providing direction for more in-depth research. A description of each type of study is provided in Chapter 9.

Accepted practice should not be altered based on a single observational study and rarely on a single randomized, controlled trial. Single studies are frequently cited to support one view or another, and this practice is called "cherry picking." The astute family physician will want to know that results are reproducible, will realize that more than one study on the topic probably exists, and will ask, "What does the totality of the evidence show?"

There are well-developed methods for assessing the quality of individual studies and for assessing the totality of the evidence. The individual family physician does not need to possess these skills and certainly does not possess the time necessary to properly research each possible prevention intervention; there are organizations and authoritative groups that perform these functions. However, the family physician should know what makes for a high-quality, truly evidence-based recommendation, and know which organizations can reliably be depended on to produce them.

The Institute of Medicine (IOM) has published guidance on how to conduct a high-quality systematic review (IOM, 2011c) and how to produce a high-quality, dependable guideline (IOM, 2011a). A high-quality guideline is based on a high-quality systematic review, preferably conducted by a noninterested, independent party. A high-quality systematic review should involve methods of finding all the

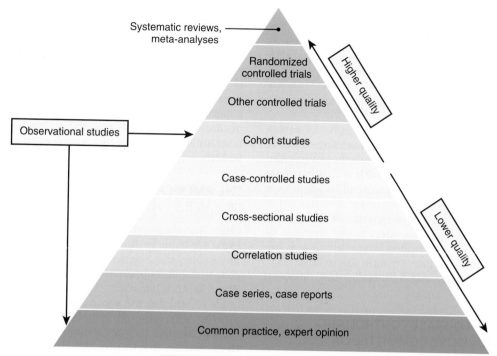

Figure 7-1 **The pyramid of evidence.**

existing evidence on the issue with clearly defined inclusion and exclusion criteria; a clear and accepted method of assessing each study and for summarizing and ranking all of the evidence; and several reviewers doing the assessment, using defined methods of resolving differences of opinion.

High-quality guidelines also involve a panel of experts with an array of skills, including how to assess the medical literature; conflict of interest policies that minimize and manage potential as well as real conflicts of interest; a methodology that assigns a strength of recommendation that reflects the best available evidence behind it; a limited number of clearly worded, unambiguous recommendations; an emphasis on patient-oriented outcomes, as well as options that allow for patient preferences; a consideration of potential harms as well as benefits; tools that assist with implementation, if they are available; and plans for periodic updating.

As described in the IOM report (2011a), many guidelines and recommendations currently do not meet these standards. This places family physicians in an awkward position, as poor-quality guidelines produced by specialty societies and special interest groups can be perceived as the gold standard because they come from the specialists who are seen as the experts in a particular topic. Some specialty societies produce high-quality guidelines, others do not. Specialist-dominated panels can be conflicted (setting out to defend current practices and justify payments), often do not consider potential harms, frequently are not prevention oriented, and may lack the members with the skills needed to assess the medical literature. This has resulted in the American Academy of Family Physicians (AAFP) developing its own prevention recommendations. These can be found on the AAFP website (www.aafp.org/patient-care/clinical-recommendations/cps.html).

THE UNITED STATES PREVENTIVE SERVICES TASK FORCE

The U.S. Preventive Services Task Force (USPSTF) was first created in 1984 as an independent panel of experts to provide guidance to physicians on the use of clinical preventive services. In 1998, it was placed under the sponsorship of the Agency for Healthcare Research and Quality (AHRQ), while maintaining its independent status, and provided with support to conduct scientific evidence reviews of a broad array of clinical preventive services and develop recommendations. The topics the task force addresses include screening tests, counseling, and preventive medications.

The USPSTF uses a rigorous and strict methodology of considering evidence and making recommendations after balancing documented benefits and harms (USPSTF, 2014). The task force does not consider the costs of the services being assessed or cost-benefit analyses. The interventions evaluated are often already in common use and frequently recommended by specialty and advocacy organizations before they have been thoroughly assessed for effectiveness and safety.

The USPSTF recommendations are separated into four categories: Level A recommendations are reserved for interventions with a clear predominance of benefits over harms backed by high-quality evidence. If evidence is not as robust, or the benefit/harm differential not as great but still in favor of benefits, a B recommendation is given. When benefits and harms are balanced, or overall benefit is minimal, it is assigned a C. Level D (a recommendation against) is assigned when no benefit exists or harms exceed benefits. If insufficient evidence exists to judge the balance of benefits and harms, the USPSTF is not compelled to make a practice recommendation and will assign it an I. Each recommendation made by the task force is accompanied by a description of the natural history of the condition, the types of interventions available, and the level of evidence that exists on their effectiveness and harms, as well as how the task force recommendation either agrees with or differs from those of other organizations. All USPSTF recommendations are found on their website (www.uspreventiveservicestaskforce.org/recommendations.htm).

The process used by the USPSTF is scientifically robust and is considered the gold standard for assessing evidence and making recommendations. The result, however, often leads to recommendations that are at odds with other organizations and advocacy groups, which tend to adopt new technologies before they are fully tested for effectiveness or safety. In addition, because of a reluctance to make a recommendation without strong evidence, the wording of USPSTF recommendations is often vague about the frequency of testing or screening, because the relative effectiveness of different screening frequencies has not been assessed.

THE CENTERS FOR DISEASE CONTROL AND PREVENTION ADVISORY COMMITTEE ON IMMUNIZATION PRACTICES

The Advisory Committee on Immunization Practices (ACIP) was created in 1964 to provide expert external advice and guidance to the director of the Centers for Disease Control and Prevention (CDC) and the Secretary of the U.S. Department of Health and Human Services (DHHS) on use of vaccines. The ACIP is an official federal advisory committee and is governed by the Federal Advisory Committee Act, which has strict requirements for public notification of meetings, allowing for public comment, and publication of minutes.

The ACIP recently adopted a new system for developing evidence-based recommendations that is based on a modification of the Grading of Recommendations, Assessment, Development and Evaluation (GRADE) approach (Guyatt et al., 2011). Key factors considered in the development of their recommendations include the balance of benefits and harms, type of evidence, values and preferences of the people affected, and health economic analyses. There are two categories of recommendations: category A (either for or against) applies to all persons in an age- or risk-factor-based group, while category B is a recommendation that is not meant to be universal but recognizes that a vaccination may be found to be appropriate for an individual within the context of a clinician-patient encounter. Evidence tables are used to summarize the benefits and harms and the strengths and limitations of the body of evidence. This new process brings the ACIP more in line with contemporary evidence-based processes (Ahmed et al., 2011).

THE NATIONAL HEART, LUNG, AND BLOOD INSTITUTE

The National Heart, Lung, and Blood Institute (NHLBI) in the National Institutes of Health produces guidelines on prevention and control of the major risks for cardiovascular diseases in adults, including two influential clinical guidelines; one on cholesterol and one on high blood pressure

(NHLBI, 2001, 2004). These and other guidelines regarding cardiovascular diseases can be found on their website (www.nhlbi.nih.gov/guidelines). The NHLBI, unfortunately, does not use methodology as strong as the USPSTF to produce their guidelines. Many of the recommendations are based on expert opinion, and the strength of the evidence supporting each recommendation is not readily apparent. They are, however, widely viewed as the standard of care. Both the cholesterol and high blood pressure guidelines are in the process of revision as this chapter is being written.

THE AMERICAN ACADEMY OF FAMILY PHYSICIANS

Clinical prevention recommendations to guide family physicians are made by the AAFP Commission on the Health of the Public and Science, and their recommendations are considered and approved by the AAFP Board of Directors. The AAFP has taken a strong evidence-based approach and tends to endorse the recommendations from the USPSTF and the ACIP, although not always. The AAFP approach to child preventive services is more conservative than that of the American Academy of Pediatrics (AAP), and it does not endorse AAP recommendations if they differ from those of the USPSTF or if they are not evidence based. The AAFP recommendations for clinical preventive services are listed at their website (www.aafp.org/patient-care/clinical-recommendations/cps.html).

THE AMERICAN ACADEMY OF PEDIATRICS AND BRIGHT FUTURES

The AAP endorses a set of periodic visits and clinical guidelines for children starting at birth and continuing to age 21 years. This set of recommendations is called *Bright Futures* and can be found on the AAP website http://www.aap.org/en-us/professional-resources/practice-support/Pages/PeriodicitySchedule.aspx. There is a set of recommended screening tests, developmental assessments, immunizations, and anticipatory guidance recommended for each visit. Due to a scarcity of research on the effectiveness of preventive services in infants and children, many of these recommendations are not based on high-quality evidence. The AAP acknowledges this by calling these recommendations "evidence informed." The AAFP has not endorsed the Bright Futures guidelines. They are, however, the basis for Medicaid preventive services for children and some quality-improvement programs use them as performance measures of quality in child preventive care.

THE COMMUNITY PREVENTIVE SERVICES TASK FORCE

The Community Preventive Services Task Force (CPSTF) was formed in 1996 and consists of 15 members appointed by the director of the CDC. They are tasked to make recommendations and develop guidance on which community-based health promotion and disease-prevention interventions work and which do not work, based on available scientific evidence. The CDC provides the CPSTF with technical and administrative support. This task force uses a strong evidence-based methodology that consists of systematic reviews of the evidence and tying recommendations to the strength of the evidence.

A challenge for the CPSTF is that community-wide recommendations are rarely subjected to controlled clinical trials so that methods of assessing and ranking other forms of evidence are required. The methods used by the CPSTF are described on their website (www.thecommunityguide.org/index.html). The recommendations made are contained in the Guide to Community Preventive Services, often called *The Community Guide*, which is also available on the website.

The Community Guide also provides evidence-based recommendations for increasing the use of preventive services in the clinical setting.

Paying for Preventive Services

The Patient Protection and Affordable Care Act (PPACA), Public Law 111-148, passed on March 23, 2010, established that a set of preventive health services shall be included without cost sharing by group health plans and health insurers offering group or individual health insurance. These services include:

- Those recommended with an A or B rating by the USPSTF.
- Immunizations that are recommended by the ACIP.
- Preventive services for infants, children, and adolescents that are included in guidelines supported by the Health Resources and Services Administration (HRSA), which in effect are those described in the Bright Futures initiative of the AAP.
- Additional services for women as provided for by guidelines supported by the HRSA. The HRSA contracted the task of developing this list to the IOM (2011b).

The intent of this provision in the PPACA is to provide an incentive to Americans to obtain evidence-based (or at least evidence-informed) preventive services to promote health and prevent disease. While on the surface it appears to provide an array of free preventive services, family physicians and patients need to appreciate that unanticipated expenses can occur from these services. As an example,

while colonoscopy screening for colorectal cancer every 10 years should be available without patient cost sharing (it is a level A recommendation by the USPSTF), a polypectomy performed during the procedure and follow-up testing are not covered by this PPACA provision and can result in significant out-of-pocket expenses.

Assessing Screening Tests

Many physicians and much of the public believe that screening and finding disease early is always beneficial. Many single-issue advocacy groups view screening as a key element in the control of their condition of concern. Family physicians simply do not have time to screen for every condition advocated, and should not screen for all of them, even if they did have time. Screening should only be conducted when the outcome of screening (finding the condition early and treating it) provides an outcome that is superior to waiting for the condition to become symptomatic. Additionally, the benefits provided by the screening test should outweigh any harms it causes.

Assessing the effectiveness of screening tests is not easy. Let us take an imaginary example. If screening for a cancer, labeled cancer of organ A, is detected by screening and then treated, life expectancy is 8 years. If the disease is detected by the presence of symptoms and then treated, life expectancy is 2 years. Does this prove that screening is effective? Many will answer that it does, including many practicing physicians (Wegwarth et al., 2012), but it does not. There are two biases in observational studies of this type that can affect the results: lead time bias and length bias (Figure 7-2). *Lead time bias* means that the disease is detected earlier, but the outcome is not changed. The point of death is not moved back; the disease was simply detected earlier making it seem that life expectancy is improved. *Length bias* comes from the fact that screening is more likely to find less aggressive disease. Cancers can have more aggressive and less aggressive forms. Aggressive forms leave little time from onset to symptoms to be detected by screening. Less aggressive forms exist in an asymptomatic state for an extended period and are more likely to be detected by screening, again leading to perceived increase in life expectancy.

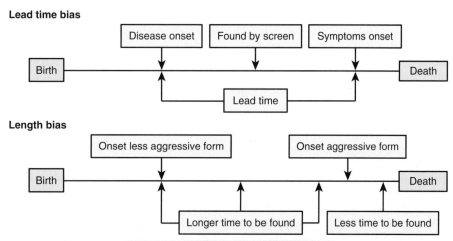

Figure 7-2 **Lead-time bias and length bias.**

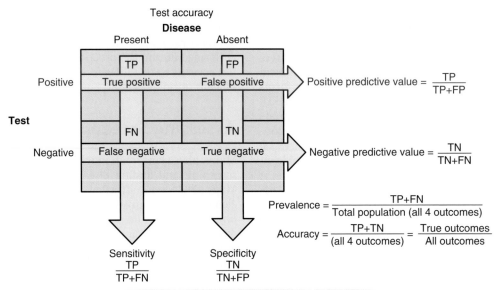

Figure 7-3 **Measures of accuracy in screening tests.**

Table 7-1 How Positive Predictive Value Changes with Prevalence*

Prevalence	1/100,000	1/10,000	1/1000	1/100 (10/1000)	1/10 (100/1000)
Number of true positives (TP)	1	1	1	10	99
Number of false-positives (FP)	100	10	1	1	1
Positive predictive value (TP/all positives)	1/101	1/11	1/2	10/11	99/100

*This example involves a test with a sensitivity of 99% and a specificity of 99.9% (false-positive rate of 1/1000) and the number tested equal to the denominator of the prevalence.

The only sure way to prove that screening is effective is to perform a controlled clinical trial in which a large number of people are randomly assigned to one of two groups: screening and no screening. They then need to be followed over time to determine the age-adjusted cancer A–specific death rates (using the previous example). If screening is effective in preventing death from cancer A, the death rate in the screened group should be lower than the unscreened group. In addition, the overall death rate should be lower. If both conditions are not met, the screening test is of questionable value. Very few screening tests have been evaluated with such rigor, and we are often left with making decisions about effectiveness on lower quality observational studies. However, a recommendation can still be made without a controlled clinical trial if the observational evidence is strong enough. This requires that there be a large difference between those screened and unscreened, and that the difference is found consistently in multiple studies in which potential biases have been controlled for.

Other factors that should be considered when assessing a screening test should include characteristics of the condition and the screening test. The condition should be serious (causing major mortality or morbidity) with a natural history that includes a lengthy asymptomatic period, and there should be an effective treatment for the condition or an intervention that prevents spread of the condition to others. The screening test should be readily available, relatively inexpensive, acceptable, and, above all, safe. This is because most of those being screened will not have the condition being screened for, and it is important not to cause them harm with screening.

In addition, the test should be accurate. Accuracy is measured by sensitivity, specificity, positive predictive value (PPV), and negative predictive value (NPV). These terms and how they are determined are illustrated in Figure 7-3. Sensitivity is the proportion of those with the condition who are detected by the test. Specificity is the proportion of those without the condition who are labeled as negative. Generally, as a test's sensitivity improves, specificity worsens and vice versa. PPV is the proportion of those with a positive test who actually have the condition, whereas NPV is the proportion of those who test negative who are condition free. While sensitivity and specificity are frequently reported as the most important statistic, from a physician and patient perspective, the predictive values are more critical.

It is possible to have a test with a very good sensitivity and specificity but a poor PPV. This occurs when the prevalence of the condition in the screened population (the pretest probability) is low. With rare conditions, even with very accurate tests, a positive test is more likely to be a false-positive than a true positive (i.e., it has a poor PPV). The effect of prevalence on PPV is illustrated in Table 7-1. This concept is very important for assessing screening tests because false-positives can cause harm.

Another statistical concept one must understand to assess screening tests is the difference between relative risk reduction and absolute risk reduction. Using another hypothetical example, if a screening test and early treatment result in a 50% reduction in mortality, this looks pretty impressive. But what if the reduction in mortality is from a rate of 2 per 100,000 to 1 per 100,000? That is a relative reduction of 50% but an absolute reduction of only 1 per

100,000. In this example, it is necessary to screen 100,000 people to save one life or, stated another way, the number needed to screen (NNS) is 100,000.

When assessing a screening test, it is important to ask about all these variables: sensitivity, specificity, PPV, NPV, NNS, and number needed to harm (NNH). It also is necessary to compare the benefits from testing to the harms caused by testing. Benefits can include improved outcomes resulting from early detection as well as, with infectious diseases, prevention of spread to others. Harm can result from both false-positive and false-negative results, complications that can result from further testing when the test is positive, and complications from the treatment for the condition.

It is increasingly appreciated that additional harm can occur from testing, called *overdiagnosis*. This occurs because not all disease detected by screening is destined to progress and cause morbidity and mortality. Sometimes the condition regresses or does not progress, or progresses so slowly that other conditions cause death first. An example of this is prostate cancer. Many prostate cancers detected by screening would never cause a man any problems. It would have gone unnoticed if the screening had not been performed. But almost all these men will undergo further diagnostic testing and then treatment, with significant resulting morbidity and even mortality caused by complications of these interventions. There is now an appreciation that overdiagnosis occurs as a result of cancer screening much more frequently than was previously known (Kalager et al., 2012).

Assessing Physician Counseling

Changing patients' behavior is difficult. An in-depth discussion on effective counseling and behavioral modification methods is in Chapter 8. While there are many behaviors that place a person at risk for current and future adverse health, not all of them are conducive to being modified by counseling in a clinical encounter. Since family physicians do not have time to counsel regarding all potential risky behaviors, it is important to focus on the ones that have the greatest effect on health and for which evidence of the effectiveness of counseling exists. The USPSTF provides guidance on this topic but frequently finds that evidence is insufficient to judge whether physician advice and counseling actually change behavior. This does not mean that a family physician should not provide counseling when insufficient evidence exists, but they should be aware that evidence is lacking about the effectiveness of counseling in that situation and that time might be better spent on interventions supported by stronger evidence.

Putting Prevention into Practice

There are many barriers to practicing preventive medicine in a family medicine clinical setting. These include time pressures, inadequate reimbursement, and lack of interest from the patient. These barriers can be overcome with a systematic and organized approach to prevention that is part of each patient encounter. A complete set of preventive

Table 7-2 Four-Step Approach to Prevention in a Clinical Encounter

Step 1: Risk assessment based on:	Age
	Gender
	Family history
	Medical history
	Occupation
	Socioeconomics
	Environment
	Behaviors:
	■ Diet
	■ Physical activity
	■ Sexual practices
	■ Alcohol, tobacco, and drug use
	■ Risk taking
Step 2: Risk reduction including:	Counseling and behavior modification Chemoprevention
Step 3: Screening	A and B recommendations from the USPSTF
Step 4: Immunizations	Immunizations recommended by the ACIP

ACIP, Advisory Committee on Immunization Practices; *USPSTF,* U.S. Preventive Services Task Force.

services can be provided as part of a periodic health assessment and wellness examination, which for most people does not need to be performed annually. They can also be approached incrementally, with the physician addressing a limited number of them at each visit. Neither approach has been proven superior to the other. Continuity of care is the family physician's ally in providing comprehensive preventive care, in that a little bit of prevention can be achieved at each visit and important prevention messages can be reinforced. With either approach, a four-step process (Table 7-2) can be used to consider

1. Risk assessment
2. Risk reduction
3. Screening
4. Immunizations

RISK ASSESSMENT

Each patient has a set of risks that can affect his or her health in the near or long term. These risks are based on age, gender, family history, medical history, current chronic diseases, occupation, socioeconomic factors, environment, and behaviors (diet; physical activity; sexual practices; alcohol, tobacco, and drug use; and risk taking). Some of these risks are modifiable; others are not. This information can be obtained at the first encounter or shortly thereafter, but it needs to be updated periodically. Knowing a patient's risks helps to focus risk reduction advice where it will have the greatest impact.

Table 7-3 lists the leading causes of death in the United States. The two leading causes of death are cardiovascular diseases and cancer. Figure 7-4 shows the time trends in these leading causes of mortality and demonstrates that age-adjusted death rates for cardiovascular diseases are declining while those for cancer and injuries are remaining relatively stable. Cancer will soon be the leading cause of death, and unintentional injuries has replaced cerebral vascular disease as the third leading cause. These data show that the largest improvements in population mortality can

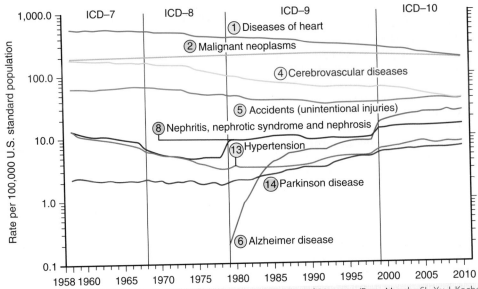

Figure 7-4 Time trends in the leading causes of death. *ICD,* International Classification of Diseases. (From Murphy SL, Xu J, Kochanek KD. Deaths: final data for 2010. *Natl Vital Stat Rep.* 2013;61:67.)

Table 7-3   Leading Causes of Death, United States, 2010

Cause	Number of Deaths	Percent of All Deaths	Rate per 100,000
Heart disease	307,384	24.9	202.5
Cancer	301,037	24.4	198.3
Unintentional injuries	75,921	6.2	50.0
Chronic lung disease	65,423	5.3	43.1
Stroke	52,367	4.2	34.5
Diabetes	35,490	2.9	23.4
Suicide	30,277	2.5	19.9
Alzheimer disease	25,364	2.1	16.7
Kidney disease	24,865	2.0	16.4
Influenza and pneumonia	23,615	1.9	15.6

From Heron M. Deaths: leading causes for 2010. *Natl Vital Stat Rep.* 2013;62(6):1-96. http://www.cdc.gov/nchs/data/nvsr/nvsr62/nvsr62_06.pdf.

Table 7-4   Actual Causes of Death, United States, 2000

Actual Cause	Number (%)
Tobacco	435,000 (18.1)
Poor diet and physical inactivity	400,000 (16.6)
Alcohol	85,000 (3.5)
Infectious diseases	75,000 (3.1)
Toxic agents	55,000 (2.3)
Motor vehicles	43,000 (1.8)
Guns	29,000 (1.2)
Sexual behavior	20,000 (0.8)
Illicit drug use	17,000 (0.7)

Data from Mokdad AH, Marks JS, Stroup DF, Gerberding JL. Actual causes of death in the United States 2000. *JAMA.* 2004;291:1238-1245.

Table 7-5   Deaths Attributable to Risk Factors, United States, 2009

Rank	Risk	Number of Deaths
1	Smoking	467,000
2	High blood pressure	395,000
3	Overweight and obesity	216,000
4	Physical inactivity	191,000
5	High blood glucose	190,000
6	High cholesterol	113,000
7	High dietary salt	102,000
8	Low omega-3 fatty acid intake	84,000
9	High trans fat intake	82,000
10	Alcohol intake	64,000

Data from Danaei G, Mozaffarian D, Taylor, et al. The preventable cause of death in the United States: comparative risk assessment of dietary, lifestyle and metabolic risk factors. PLoS Med. 2009;6(4):e1000058. doi:10.1371/journal.pmed.1000058. http://www.plosmedicine.org/article/info:doi/10.1371/journal.pmed.1000058.

be achieved by concentrating on the causes of cardiovascular diseases, cancer, and injuries.

The actual causes of death in the United States are listed in Table 7-4 and include unhealthy behaviors, most notably tobacco use, poor diets, lack of physical activity, and misuse of alcohol. Table 7-5 lists the risk factors for the leading causes of death and the number of deaths attributed to each. These behaviors and risk factors are prime targets for preventive interventions in the clinical setting.

Figure 7-5 demonstrates that the leading causes of death are quite different in younger age groups than older. In addition, race/ethnicity and socioeconomic factors change the magnitude of these causes. Family physicians knowing the epidemiology of disease and risks in their communities can focus in on the risks that have the greatest impact on their patients.

When assessing the risks linked to each of these leading causes of death and disability, it is important to remember that a "risk factor" identified in an observational study may not translate into reduced disease if that risk is eliminated.

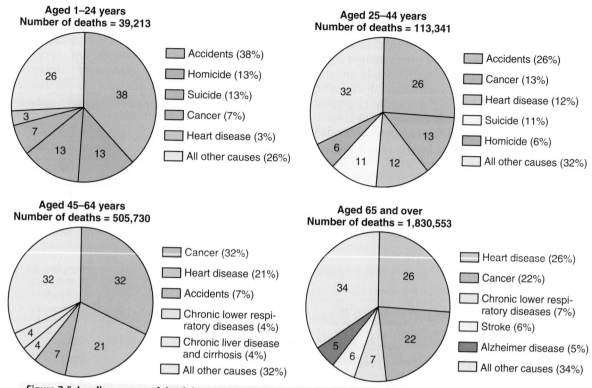

Aged 1–24 years
Number of deaths = 39,213

26   38   3   7   13   13

- Accidents (38%)
- Homicide (13%)
- Suicide (13%)
- Cancer (7%)
- Heart disease (3%)
- All other causes (26%)

Aged 25–44 years
Number of deaths = 113,341

32   26   13   6   11   12

- Accidents (26%)
- Cancer (13%)
- Heart disease (12%)
- Suicide (11%)
- Homicide (6%)
- All other causes (32%)

Aged 45–64 years
Number of deaths = 505,730

32   32   4   4   7   21

- Cancer (32%)
- Heart disease (21%)
- Accidents (7%)
- Chronic lower respiratory diseases (4%)
- Chronic liver disease and cirrhosis (4%)
- All other causes (32%)

Aged 65 and over
Number of deaths = 1,830,553

34   26   5   6   7   22

- Heart disease (26%)
- Cancer (22%)
- Chronic lower respiratory diseases (7%)
- Stroke (6%)
- Alzheimer disease (5%)
- All other causes (34%)

Figure 7-5 Leading causes of death by age. (From Minino AM. Death in the United States, 2011. *NCHS Data Brief.* 2013;115:1-8.)

Controlled clinical trials are needed to provide proof of improved outcomes from risk reduction. An example of a risk reduction intervention for which evidence exists is blood pressure control. It was shown in observational studies that hypertension is a risk for coronary heart disease and cerebral vascular disease. Following that discovery, controlled clinical trials showed that controlling blood pressure resulted in a reduction in these conditions. An example of a risk reduction effort that did not pan out is the use of antioxidants to prevent cancer. Observational studies indicated that lower intake of certain vitamins with antioxidant properties was associated with higher rates of certain cancers. However, controlled clinical trials of increased antioxidant intake failed to demonstrate reduced cancer rates (Boffetta et al., 2010; Gasiano et al., 2009; Zhang, 2008). Looking back at Table 7-5, there is good evidence that reducing risks 1 through 6 and 10 result in improved health outcomes. The evidence of benefit from reducing risks 7 through 9 is not as strong.

RISK REDUCTION

Once a patient's short and long-term health risks are known, the family physician can concentrate on reducing these risks. Time and effort is best spent on risk reduction that evidence demonstrates will result in improved outcomes. There are two major tools for reducing patients' risks for disease—behavioral change counseling and chemoprevention. Both can be applied as primary or tertiary prevention.

Information on how to provide effective behavioral change counseling is provided in Chapter 8. Because the leading causes of death are chronic diseases affected by behavior, with the harmful effects building up over a number of years, convincing younger adults to change unhealthy behaviors is challenging as is altering habits that have been practiced for long periods. We should keep in mind, however, that if behavior change is achieved in only a small percentage of patients, this can add up, on a population level, if all physicians applied the most effective counseling and behavior modification methods.

Some behaviors can be changed by brief counseling that can be provided in a clinical encounter. Table 7-6 lists those that are recommended by the USPSTF. Other behaviors are more difficult to change and require more intensive and multicomponent interventions. Table 7-7 lists behaviors in this category and the more intensive interventions needed to change them that are recommended by the USPSTF. In these instances the family physician can provide more intensive counseling themselves or defer to other health care professionals who have more time and training in this area.

Chemoprevention can be utilized as either a primary or tertiary prevention intervention. Those in Table 7-8 are primary interventions that are recommended by the USPSTF. Table 7-9 includes examples of other uses of medications for prevention in specific circumstances. These include those that are used commonly, such as medications to control high blood pressure and hypercholesterolemia, which can prevent cardiovascular disease, and medications to improve hyperglycemia in those with diabetes, which can prevent the microvascular complications of this chronic condition. Others are less common and need to be kept in mind when patients present after an event that places them at risk for a recurrence or have had an exposure to an infectious agent.

SCREENING

Secondary prevention, or screening for early detection of asymptomatic disease, is an important component of clinical prevention. As described previously, the USPSTF and the AAFP list screening tests that family physicians should offer to patients. The USPSTF offers a user-friendly electronic version of their recommendations called the Electronic Preventive Services Selector (ePSS). It can be downloaded to all types of electronic devices and used to search for recommended screening tests by age and gender (see http://epss.ahrq.gov/PDA/index.jsp). If the screening test is recommended only for certain risk groups, there is an attached tool to assist in measuring risk.

Family physicians should, over time, ensure that their patients have been offered screening tests with A or B recommendations. Table 7-10 lists screening tests recommended by the USPSTF for adults, and Table 7-11 lists screening tests and other preventive interventions the

Table 7-6 Conditions That Can Be Affected by Brief Counseling in a Clinical Encounter

Condition	Counseling	For Whom
Alcohol misuse	Brief behavioral counseling interventions to reduce alcohol misuse	Adults age 18 years and older engaged in risky or hazardous drinking
Skin cancer	Counseling about minimizing exposure to ultraviolet radiation to reduce risk for skin cancer	Children, adolescents, and young adults ages 10-24 years who have fair skin
Tobacco use	Tobacco cessation interventions	All those who use tobacco products
Tobacco use	Interventions, including education or brief counseling, to prevent initiation of tobacco use	School-aged children and adolescents

Data from U.S. Preventive Services Task Force. http://www.uspreventiveservicestaskforce.org/index.html.

Table 7-7 Behaviors That Require Intensive Counseling or Referral

Condition	Intensive Counseling or Referral	For Whom
Fall prevention	Counseling about exercise or physical therapy	Community-dwelling adults age 65 years and older who are at increased risk for falls
Cardiovascular disease risk reduction	Health diet counseling	Adult patients with hyperlipidemia and other known risk factors for cardiovascular and diet-related chronic disease
Intimate partner violence	Intervention services	Women of childbearing age who screen positive for intimate partner violence
Obesity, improvement in weight status	Intensive, multicomponent behavioral interventions	Obese adults and children
Sexually transmitted infections	High-intensity behavioral counseling to prevent sexually transmitted infections (STIs)	Sexually active adolescents and adults at increased risk for STIs

Data from U.S. Preventive Services Task Force. http://www.uspreventiveservicestaskforce.org/index.html.

Table 7-8 Chemoprevention Recommended by the U.S. Preventive Services Task Force

Chemoprevention	Condition to Prevent	When to Use	A or B Recommendation	Risk Group
Aspirin	Myocardial infarction	When the potential benefit due to a reduction in myocardial infarctions outweighs the potential harm due to an increase in gastrointestinal hemorrhage	A	Men ages 45-79 years
Aspirin	Ischemic stroke	When the potential benefit outweighs the potential harm of an increase in gastrointestinal hemorrhage	A	Women ages 55-79 years
Erythromycin ophthalmic ointment	Gonococcal ophthalmia neonatorum	All newborns	A	Newborns
Fluoride supplementation	Dental caries	When the primary water source is deficient in fluoride	B	Preschool children older than 6 months
Folic acid daily supplement containing 0.4-0.8 mg (400-800 µg)	Neural tube defects	All women	A	Women planning or capable of pregnancy
Iron supplementation	Iron deficiency	When at increased risk for iron deficiency	B	Children ages 6-12 months
Tamoxifen or Raloxifene	Breast cancer	Discuss chemoprevention and the potential benefits and harms of chemoprevention	B	Women at high risk for breast cancer and at low risk for adverse effects of chemoprevention
Vitamin D supplementation	Falls in the elderly	When at increased risk for falls	B	Community-dwelling adults age 65 years and older

Data from U.S. Preventive Services Task Force. http://www.uspreventiveservicestaskforce.org/index.html.

Table 7-9 Examples of Chemoprevention Not Addressed by the U.S. Preventive Services Task Force

- Isoniazid (INH) for treatment of latent tuberculosis (TB) and prevention of active TB
- Antivirals for influenza prevention in high-risk, exposed individuals
- Postexposure prophylaxis for human immunodeficiency virus (HIV) exposure from sexual contact or work-site exposure
- Antibiotics in contacts and household members of those with meningococcal and *Haemophilus influenza* type B meningitis
- Anticoagulants in those with atrial fibrillation and post deep vein thrombosis or pulmonary embolus
- Antibiotic prophylaxis in those with heart valves undergoing invasive procedures
- Postexposure prophylaxis after exposure to syphilis, gonorrhea, and chlamydia
- Treatment for high blood pressure, high cholesterol, diabetes control

Table 7-10 Screening Tests for Adults Recommended by the U.S. Preventive Services Task Force

Condition	Screening Test	A or B	For Whom
Abdominal aortic aneurysm	One-time screening for abdominal aortic aneurysm by ultrasonography	B	Men ages 65-75 who have ever smoked
Alcohol misuse	Screen for alcohol misuse	B	All age 18 years and older
High blood pressure	Screen for high blood pressure	A	All age 18 years and older
Breast cancer gene	Referral for genetic counseling and evaluation for *BRCA* testing	B	Women whose family history is associated with an increased risk for deleterious mutations in *BRCA1* or *BRCA2* genes
Breast cancer	Mammography every 2 years	B	Women 50-74 years
Cervical cancer	Screen with cytology (Pap smear) every 3 years or, for women ages 30-65 years who want to lengthen the screening interval, screening with a combination of cytology and human papillomavirus (HPV) testing every 5 years	A	Women 21-65 years
Chlamydia	Screen for chlamydia infection	A	Sexually active women age 24 and younger, older women at risk
Cholesterol abnormalities	Screen for lipid disorders	A	All men age 35 years and older and women age 45 and older if at increased risk of coronary heart disease
Cholesterol abnormalities	Screen for lipid disorders	B	All men ages 20-35 years and women ages 20-45 years if they are at increased risk for coronary heart disease
Colorectal cancer	Screen for colorectal cancer using fecal occult blood testing, sigmoidoscopy, or colonoscopy	A	All age 50-75 years
Depression	Screen for major depressive disorder when systems are in place to ensure accurate diagnosis, psychotherapy (cognitive-behavioral or interpersonal), and follow-up	B	All adults
Diabetes	Screen for type 2 diabetes	B	Asymptomatic adults with sustained blood pressure (either treated or untreated) greater than 135/80 mm Hg
Gonorrhea	Screen for gonorrhea infection	B	Sexually active women, if they are at increased risk for infection
Hepatitis C virus (HCV)	Screen for HCV	B	Adults at high risk for infection, including a one-time screening for adults born between 1945 and 1965
Human Immunodeficiency Virus (HIV)	Screen for HIV	A	All adults through age 65 years and older adults who are at increased risk
Intimate partner violence	Screen for intimate partner violence, such as domestic violence, and provide or refer women who screen positive to intervention services	B	Women of childbearing age
Obesity	Screen for obesity	B	All adults
Osteoporosis	Screen for osteoporosis	B	Women age 65 years and older and younger women whose fracture risk is equal to or greater than that of a 65-year-old white woman who has no additional risk factors
Syphilis	Screen for syphilis infection	A	Those at increased risk for syphilis infection
Tobacco use	Ask about tobacco use and provide tobacco cessation interventions for those who use tobacco products	A	All adults

Data from U.S. Preventive Services Task Force. http://www.uspreventiveservicestaskforce.org/index.html.

Table 7-11   Screening Tests and Other Interventions for Infants, Children, and Adolescents Recommended by the U.S. Preventive Services Task Force

Condition	Screening Test/Intervention	A or B Recommendation
Chlamydia infection	Screen for chlamydia infection in females if sexually active	A
Gonorrhea infection	Screen for gonorrhea infection if sexually active	B
Gonococcal ophthalmia neonatorum	Ocular topical medication for newborns	A
Hearing loss	Screen for hearing loss in newborns	B
Hemoglobinopathies	Screen for sickle cell disease in newborns	A
Human immunodeficiency virus (HIV) infection	Screen for HIV infection age 15 and older, younger if at risk*	A
Hypothyroidism	Screen for congenital hypothyroidism in newborns	A
Intimate partner violence	Screen for intimate partner violence, such as domestic violence, in women of childbearing age†	B
Iron deficiency	Iron supplementation for asymptomatic children ages 6-12 months who are at increased risk for iron deficiency anemia	B
Obesity	Screen children age 6 years and older for obesity	B
Phenylketonuria	Screen for phenylketonuria in newborns	A
Sexually transmitted infections	High-intensity behavioral counseling to prevent sexually transmitted infections (STIs) in all sexually active adolescents	B
Skin cancer	Counsel children, adolescents, and young adults ages 10-24 years who have fair skin about minimizing their exposure to ultraviolet radiation to reduce risk for skin cancer	B
Tobacco use	Provide interventions, including education or brief counseling, to prevent initiation of tobacco use in school-aged children and adolescents	B
Syphilis	Screen those at increased risk for syphilis infection	A
Vision	Vision screening for all children at least once between the ages of 3 and 5 years to detect the presence of amblyopia or its risk factors	B

*The American Academy of Family Physicians (AAFP) recommends routine screening starting at age 18 and screening at younger ages for those at risk.
†Reproductive age is considered to start at age 14. If an adolescent has an intimate partner relationship, screening is recommended.
Data from U.S. Preventive Services Task Force. http://www.uspreventiveservicestaskforce.org/index.html.

USPSTF recommends for infants, children, and adolescents. It is equally important not to provide screening tests that are not effective and/or are harmful, such as those given a D rating by the USPSTF (Table 7-12). These tables describing USPSTF recommendations were developed at the time of the writing of this chapter and reflect the USPSTF recommendations as of that time. Keeping up to date on screening recommendations is challenging. The USPSTF makes a new recommendation or updates an old recommendation about once a month. Physicians can sign up for periodic updates at the USPSTF website (www.uspreventiveservicestaskforce.org/announcements.htm).

IMMUNIZATIONS

One of the most effective forms of primary interventions available to family physicians is vaccines. The ACIP publishes updated immunization schedules annually. These include routinely recommended immunizations for infants, children, and adolescents (Figure 7-6), routinely recommended immunizations for adults starting at age 19 years (Figure 7-7), and catch-up recommendations for these two age groups (all can be found at www.cdc.gov/vaccines/schedules/index.html). The catch-up schedules are useful in determining what vaccines to provide to someone who is not completely vaccinated with recommended vaccines at the time of the clinical encounter.

Family physicians should take every opportunity and use systematic approaches to ensure that patients are completely protected from vaccine-preventable diseases. This can involve assigning a clinical team member to be a vaccine advocate, implementing standing orders for nurses and others to administer vaccines, sending electronic reminders when vaccines are due, and taking advantage of each clinical encounter to provide recommended vaccines unless a valid contraindication exits (Community Preventive Services Task Force, *Increasing Appropriate Immunizations*).

PRIORITIZING PREVENTIVE SERVICES

Given the large number of possible preventive interventions that can be implemented, it is often necessary to prioritize them and address the most important ones first and the others as time and continuity allow. Patient preferences are important to consider. Difficult choices are sometimes necessary when patients have multiple risks and comorbid conditions. Chronic diseases often occur concurrently, and the guidelines for each often are written from the assumption that only one disease is present. Research is being conducted on what preventive interventions will yield the greatest gains to patients with multiple chronic conditions and risks (Taksler et al., 2013). Family physicians and patients should prioritize together.

Table 7-12   U.S. Preventive Services Task Force D Recommendations (Screening Tests That Should Not Be Performed)

Infants, children, and adolescents	▪ Screening of asymptomatic adolescents for idiopathic scoliosis ▪ Screening for elevated blood lead levels in asymptomatic children age 1-5 years who are at average risk
Pregnant women	▪ Screening for bacterial vaginosis in asymptomatic pregnant women at low risk for preterm delivery ▪ Screening for elevated blood lead levels in asymptomatic pregnant women
Adults: chemoprevention	▪ Use of aspirin and nonsteroidal antiinflammatory drugs (NSAIDs) to prevent colorectal cancer in persons at average risk for colorectal cancer ▪ Routine use of medications, such as tamoxifen or raloxifene, for risk reduction of primary breast cancer in women who are not at increased risk for breast cancer ▪ Use of aspirin for stroke prevention in women younger than age 55 years and for myocardial infarction prevention in men younger than age 45 years ▪ Use of β-carotene supplements, either alone or in combination, for the prevention of cancer or cardiovascular disease ▪ Use of combined estrogen and progestin for the prevention of chronic conditions in postmenopausal women ▪ Use of estrogen for the prevention of chronic conditions in postmenopausal women who have had a hysterectomy ▪ Daily supplementation with 400 IU or less of vitamin D_3 and 1000 mg or less of calcium for the primary prevention of fractures in noninstitutionalized postmenopausal women
Adults: screening	**Cancer** ▪ Routine referral for genetic counseling or routine breast cancer susceptibility gene (*BRCA*) testing for women whose family history is not associated with an increased risk for deleterious mutations in breast cancer susceptibility gene 1 (*BRCA1*) or breast cancer susceptibility gene 2 (*BRCA2*) ▪ Teaching breast self-examination (BSE) ▪ Screening for cervical cancer in women younger than age 21 years ▪ Screening for cervical cancer in women older than age 65 years who have had adequate prior screening and are not otherwise at high risk for cervical cancer ▪ Screening for cervical cancer in women who have had a hysterectomy with removal of the cervix and who do not have a history of a high-grade precancerous lesion (i.e., cervical intraepithelial neoplasia [CIN] grade 2 or 3) or cervical cancer ▪ Screening for cervical cancer with human papillomavirus (HPV) testing, alone or in combination with cytology, in women younger than age 30 years ▪ Screening for testicular cancer in adolescent or adult males ▪ Screening for colorectal cancer in adults older than age 85 years ▪ Screening for ovarian cancer in women ▪ Screening for pancreatic cancer in asymptomatic adults using abdominal palpation, ultrasonography, or serologic ▪ Prostate-specific antigen (PSA)-based screening for prostate cancer **Cardiovascular and Lung Disease** ▪ Screening for abdominal aortic aneurism in women ▪ Screening for asymptomatic carotid artery stenosis in the general adult population ▪ Screening adults for chronic obstructive pulmonary disease (COPD) using spirometry ▪ Screening with resting or exercise electrocardiography (ECG) for the prediction of coronary heart disease (CHD) events in asymptomatic adults at low risk for CHD events ▪ Routine genetic screening for hereditary hemochromatosis in the asymptomatic general population **Infectious Disease** ▪ Screening for asymptomatic bacteriuria in men and nonpregnant women ▪ Screening for gonorrhea infection in men and women who are at low risk for infection ▪ Screening the general asymptomatic population for chronic hepatitis B virus infection ▪ Serological screening for herpes simplex virus (HSV) in asymptomatic pregnant women at any time during pregnancy to prevent neonatal HSV infection ▪ Serological screening for HSV in asymptomatic adolescents and adults ▪ Screening of asymptomatic persons who are not at increased risk for syphilis infection

Data from U.S. Preventive Services Task Force. http://www.uspreventiveservicestaskforce.org/index.html.

Examples of Putting the Four-Step Approach into Practice

EXAMPLE 1, YOUNG ADULT MALE

A 28-year-old male visits the clinic in October with a complaint of abdominal pain. The pain occurs after nights when he parties with friends, consuming 6 to 7 alcohol-containing drinks. He drinks some alcohol almost every day. He admits to occasionally driving home after these parties, but feels like he is not impaired, although he was cited for driving under the influence several months ago. He also admits to being in bar fights once or twice the past year. He smokes less than one pack of cigarettes per day and started at the age of 17 years and states he would like to quit. He denies any use of illicit drugs except occasionally smoking marijuana. He is an only child and both parents are alive with no health problems. There is no known history of cancer or early heart disease in his family. He currently takes no medications and has no chronic health problems. He has sex only with women, has had eight partners in the past year, and uses condoms irregularly. He works as an insurance adjuster in an office, exercises three to four times a week at the gym, lifting weights. He eats mostly fast food for convenience. He believes he has had all childhood vaccines but is not sure. His last tetanus shot was at age 22 years after a laceration. He is 5 ft 11 in tall and weighs 180 lb (body mass

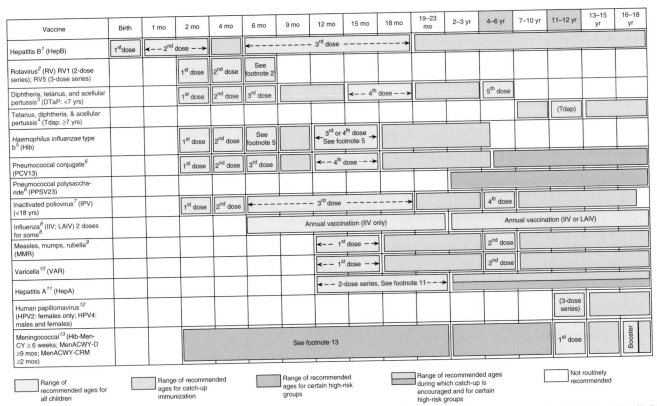

Vaccine	Birth	1 mo	2 mo	4 mo	6 mo	9 mo	12 mo	15 mo	18 mo	19–23 mo	2–3 yr	4–6 yr	7–10 yr	11–12 yr	13–15 yr	16–18 yr
Hepatitis B[1] (HepB)	1st dose	←– 2nd dose –→			←– – – – – – – 3rd dose – – – – – – →											
Rotavirus[2] (RV) RV1 (2-dose series); RV5 (3-dose series)			1st dose	2nd dose	See footnote 2											
Diphtheria, tetanus, and acellular pertussis[3] (DTaP: <7 yrs)			1st dose	2nd dose	3rd dose		←– 4th dose – –→					5th dose				
Tetanus, diphtheria, & acellular pertussis[4] (Tdap: ≥7 yrs)														(Tdap)		
Haemophilus influenzae type b[5] (Hib)			1st dose	2nd dose	See footnote 5		3rd or 4th dose See footnote 5									
Pneumococcal conjugate[6] (PCV13)			1st dose	2nd dose	3rd dose		←– 4th dose ·– –→									
Pneumococcal polysaccha-ride[6] (PPSV23)																
Inactivated poliovirus[7] (IPV) (<18 yrs)			1st dose	2nd dose	←– – – – – – 3rd dose – – – – – – →							4th dose				
Influenza[8] (IIV; LAIV) 2 doses for some[8]					Annual vaccination (IIV only)							Annual vaccination (IIV or LAIV)				
Measles, mumps, rubella[9] (MMR)							←– – 1st dose –→					2nd dose				
Varicella[10] (VAR)							←– – 1st dose –→					2nd dose				
Hepatitis A[11] (HepA)							←– – 2-dose series, See footnote 11 – –→									
Human papillomavirus[12] (HPV2: females only; HPV4: males and females)														(3-dose series)		
Meningococcal[13] (Hib-Men-CY ≥ 6 weeks; MenACWY-D ≥9 mos; MenACWY-CRM ≥2 mos)					See footnote 13									1st dose		Booster

Range of recommended ages for all children	Range of recommended ages for catch-up immunization	Range of recommended ages for certain high-risk groups	Range of recommended ages during which catch-up is encouraged and for certain high-risk groups	Not routinely recommended	

This schedule includes recommendations in effect as of January 1, 2014. Any dose not administered at the recommended age should be administered at a subsequent visit, when indicated and feasible. The use of a combination vaccine generally is preferred over separate injections of its equivalent component vaccines. Vaccination providers should consult the relevant Advisory Committee on Immunization Practices (ACIP) statement for detailed recommendations, available online at http://www.cdc.gov/vaccines/hcp/acip-recs/index.html. Clinically significant adverse events that follow vaccination should be reported to the Vaccine Adverse Event Reporting System (VAERS) online (http://www.vaers.hhs.gov) or by telephone (800-822-7967). Suspected cases of vaccine-preventable diseases should be reported to the state or local health department. Additional information, including precautions and contraindications for vaccination, is available from CDC online (http://www.cdc.gov/vaccines/recs/vac-admin/contraindications.htm) or by telephone (800-CDC-INFO [800-232-4636]).

This schedule is approved by the Advisory Committee on Immunization Practices (http://www.cdc.gov/vaccines/acip), the American Academy of Pediatrics (http://www.aap.org), the American Academy of Family Physicians (http://www.aafp.org), and the American Congress of Obstetricians and Gynecologists (http://www.acog.org).

Figure 7-6 Infant, child and adolescent immunization schedule. **These recommendations must be read with the footnotes shown on the Centers for Disease Control and Prevention (CDC) website.** For those patients who fall behind schedule or start late, see the Catch-Up Schedule from CDC website. (From CDC. *Recommended Immunization Schedule for Persons Aged 0 through 18 years—United States,* 2014. http://www.cdc.gov/vaccines/schedules/downloads/child/0-18yrs-schedule.pdf.)

index [BMI] 20.9 kg/m²). He is well developed and muscular. His blood pressure is 125/75 mm Hg.

Because he presents out of concern for his abdominal pain, this problem needs to be addressed first. However, doing a quick assessment (Step 1), it can be determined that his major health risks are smoking, alcohol misuse (which is likely contributing to his abdominal pain), unsafe sex, and risk-taking behavior. You can mention each of these to him quickly and focus on smoking, strongly advising him to quit, offering nicotine replacement, and providing information on smoking cessation support groups. You make a note to address the other two risks, which are related, at the follow-up visit. You advise a healthier diet and the addition of aerobic exercise to his weight lifting, even though the value of this advice in changing behavior is uncertain (Step 2).

Using the USPSTF ePSS you determine the recommended screening tests are human immunodeficiency virus (HIV), syphilis (although this may not be indicated if the rate of heterosexual syphilis in the community is low), lipid disorders (since he is at higher risk for cardiovascular disease due to his smoking), high blood pressure (done at this first visit and to be repeated at each follow-up visit), obesity (done with the initial height and weight measurement), and depression (which can be deferred to a future visit). HIV testing and a nonfasting cholesterol and high-density lipoprotein (HDL) cholesterol level can be performed on a blood sample taken in the office, in addition to any diagnostic blood tests needed (Step 3).

You can ask him to try to find his childhood vaccine record at his parent's house to bring to the next visit and offer him influenza vaccine and tetanus toxoid, reduced diphtheria toxoid, and acellular pertussis vaccine (Tdap) today (Step 4).

EXAMPLE 2, OLDER ADULT MALE

A 61-year-old male is in the clinic for a routine visit for several medical conditions including hypertension, hypercholesterolemia, obesity, and osteoarthritis of his right knee. His medications include lovastatin, hydrochlorothiazide, enalapril, and acetaminophen. He has had no recent hospitalizations or surgery. He smoked in the past but quit 15 years ago, currently drinks a glass of wine several times a week, uses no illicit drugs and denies past use, has been married to his wife for 35 years, and has no extramarital sexual partners. He has three children, all grown and out of the house, and three grandchildren, one of them

Recommended adult immunization schedule, by vaccine and age group¹

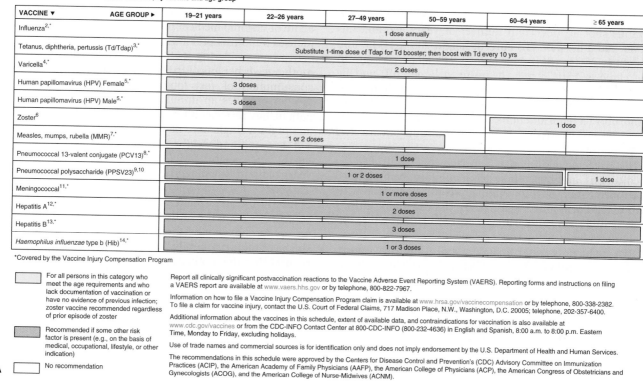

VACCINE ▼ AGE GROUP ►	19–21 years	22–26 years	27–49 years	50–59 years	60–64 years	≥ 65 years
Influenza[2,*]	1 dose annually					
Tetanus, diphtheria, pertussis (Td/Tdap)[3,*]	Substitute 1-time dose of Tdap for Td booster; then boost with Td every 10 yrs					
Varicella[4,*]	2 doses					
Human papillomavirus (HPV) Female[5,*]	3 doses					
Human papillomavirus (HPV) Male[5,*]	3 doses					
Zoster[6]					1 dose	
Measles, mumps, rubella (MMR)[7,*]	1 or 2 doses					
Pneumococcal 13-valent conjugate (PCV13)[8,*]	1 dose					
Pneumococcal polysaccharide (PPSV23)[9,10]	1 or 2 doses					1 dose
Meningococcal[11,*]	1 or more doses					
Hepatitis A[12,*]	2 doses					
Hepatitis B[13,*]	3 doses					
Haemophilus influenzae type b (Hib)[14,*]	1 or 3 doses					

*Covered by the Vaccine Injury Compensation Program

For all persons in this category who meet the age requirements and who lack documentation of vaccination or have no evidence of previous infection; zoster vaccine recommended regardless of prior episode of zoster

Recommended if some other risk factor is present (e.g., on the basis of medical, occupational, lifestyle, or other indication)

A   No recommendation

Report all clinically significant postvaccination reactions to the Vaccine Adverse Event Reporting System (VAERS). Reporting forms and instructions on filing a VAERS report are available at www.vaers.hhs.gov or by telephone, 800-822-7967.

Information on how to file a Vaccine Injury Compensation Program claim is available at www.hrsa.gov/vaccinecompensation or by telephone, 800-338-2382. To file a claim for vaccine injury, contact the U.S. Court of Federal Claims, 717 Madison Place, N.W., Washington, D.C. 20005; telephone, 202-357-6400.

Additional information about the vaccines in this schedule, extent of available data, and contraindications for vaccination is also available at www.cdc.gov/vaccines or from the CDC-INFO Contact Center at 800-CDC-INFO (800-232-4636) in English and Spanish, 8:00 a.m. to 8:00 p.m. Eastern Time, Monday to Friday, excluding holidays.

Use of trade names and commercial sources is for identification only and does not imply endorsement by the U.S. Department of Health and Human Services.

The recommendations in this schedule were approved by the Centers for Disease Control and Prevention's (CDC) Advisory Committee on Immunization Practices (ACIP), the American Academy of Family Physicians (AAFP), the American College of Physicians (ACP), the American Congress of Obstetricians and Gynecologists (ACOG), and the American College of Nurse-Midwives (ACNM).

Vaccines that might be indicated for adults based on medical and other indications¹

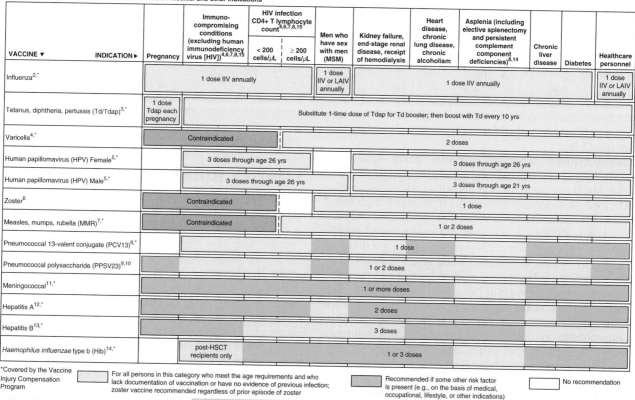

VACCINE ▼ INDICATION ►	Pregnancy	Immuno-compromising conditions (excluding human immunodeficiency virus [HIV])[4,6,7,8,15]	HIV infection CD4+ T lymphocyte count[4,6,7,8,15] < 200 cells/μL	HIV infection CD4+ T lymphocyte count[4,6,7,8,15] ≥ 200 cells/μL	Men who have sex with men (MSM)	Kidney failure, end-stage renal disease, receipt of hemodialysis	Heart disease, chronic lung disease, chronic alcoholism	Asplenia (including elective splenectomy and persistent complement component deficiencies)[8,14]	Chronic liver disease	Diabetes	Healthcare personnel
Influenza[2,*]	1 dose IIV annually	1 dose IIV annually	1 dose IIV annually	1 dose IIV annually	1 dose IIV or LAIV annually	1 dose IIV annually	1 dose IIV annually	1 dose IIV annually	1 dose IIV annually	1 dose IIV annually	1 dose IIV or LAIV annually
Tetanus, diphtheria, pertussis (Td/Tdap)[3,*]	1 dose Tdap each pregnancy	Substitute 1-time dose of Tdap for Td booster; then boost with Td every 10 yrs									
Varicella[4,*]	Contraindicated	Contraindicated		2 doses							
Human papillomavirus (HPV) Female[5,*]		3 doses through age 26 yrs				3 doses through age 26 yrs					
Human papillomavirus (HPV) Male[5,*]		3 doses through age 26 yrs				3 doses through age 21 yrs					
Zoster[6]	Contraindicated	Contraindicated		1 dose							
Measles, mumps, rubella (MMR)[7,*]	Contraindicated	Contraindicated		1 or 2 doses							
Pneumococcal 13-valent conjugate (PCV13)[8,*]		1 dose									
Pneumococcal polysaccharide (PPSV23)[9,10]		1 or 2 doses									
Meningococcal[11,*]		1 or more doses									
Hepatitis A[12,*]		2 doses									
Hepatitis B[13,*]		3 doses									
Haemophilus influenzae type b (Hib)[14,*]		post-HSCT recipients only		1 or 3 doses							

*Covered by the Vaccine Injury Compensation Program

For all persons in this category who meet the age requirements and who lack documentation of vaccination or have no evidence of previous infection; zoster vaccine recommended regardless of prior episode of zoster

Recommended if some other risk factor is present (e.g., on the basis of medical, occupational, lifestyle, or other indications)

No recommendation

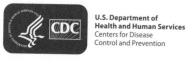

U.S. Department of Health and Human Services
Centers for Disease Control and Prevention

These schedules indicate the recommended age groups and medical indications for which administration of currently licensed vaccines is commonly indicated for adults ages 19 years and older, as of February 1, 2014. For all vaccines being recommended on the Adult Immunization Schedule: a vaccine series does not need to be restarted, regardless of the time that has elapsed between doses. Licensed combination vaccines may be used whenever any components of the combination are indicated and when the vaccine's other components are not contraindicated. For detailed recommendations on all vaccines, including those used primarily for travelers or that are issued during the year, consult the manufacturers' package inserts and the complete statements from the Advisory Committee on Immunization Practices (www.cdc.gov/vaccines/hcp/acip-recs/index.html). Use of trade names and commercial sources is for identification only and does not imply endorsement by the U.S. Department of Health and Human Services.

B

Figure 7-7 Adult immunization schedule. These recommendations must be read with the footnotes shown on Centers for Disease Control and Prevention (CDC) website. (From CDC. *Recommended Adult Immunization Schedule—United States,* 2014. http://www.cdc.gov/vaccines/schedules/downloads/adult/adult-schedule.pdf.)

born just 3 weeks ago. Both parents are still alive at ages 89 and 90 years. He does not exercise regularly. He had a tetanus shot an uncertain number of years ago and has never had a flu shot. His current height is 5 ft 10 in. and weight is 250 lb (BMI 35.9 kg/m^2). His blood pressure in the clinic is 130/75 mm Hg (using a large cuff) and he reports a similar reading when he checks it at home. His fasting labs, obtained a week before the clinic visit, demonstrate normal renal functions, a cholesterol level of 155 mg/dL, an HDL cholesterol level of 35 mg/dL, and glucose level of 95 mg/dL.

His risks include obesity, hypertension (controlled on medication), and hypercholesterolemia (also being treated with medication but not optimally controlled). Using the NHLBI cardiovascular disease (CVD) risk calculator (http://cvdrisk.nhlbi.nih.gov/calculator.asp), his risk of a myocardial infarction in the next 10 years is 12%.

Risk reduction could include obesity intensive educational interventions. To be effective in assisting him to lose weight, this will need to consist of setting weight loss goals, improving diet and increasing physical activity, addressing barriers to change, self-weight monitoring regularly, and setting strategies to maintain lifestyle changes. Today you can ask him to go online and assess his diet and obtain advice on how to improve his diet at the DHHS website (www.healthfinder.gov/HealthTopics/Category/health-conditions-and-diseases/diabetes/eat-healthy). A plan for regular follow-up and monitoring should be established.

Recommended chemoprevention includes continued treatment for hypertension and hypercholesterolemia to reduce risks of cardiovascular disease. If he has no history of bleeding disorders, he might benefit from daily low-dose aspirin, and this can be discussed. At age 61, with a 12% risk of a heart attack, daily aspirin will prevent about four heart attacks per 100 men over 10 years (see www.uspreventiveservicestaskforce.org/uspstf09/aspirincvd/aspcvdrsf2.htm).

Recommended screening includes being tested for colorectal cancer (with colonoscopy, sigmoidoscopy, or fecal occult blood testing), HIV and hepatitis C virus, hyperlipidemia (not applicable since he is on treatment), high blood pressure (not applicable since he is on treatment), obesity (done), depression using one of the scales linked on the USPSTF website (www.integration.samhsa.gov/images/res/PHQ%20-%20Questions.pdf), and type 2 diabetes (done with the preclinic laboratory work). He does not meet the criteria to screen for syphilis (men who have sex with men, commercial sex workers, persons who exchange sex for drugs, and those in adult correctional facilities).

Immunizations that are recommended include influenza vaccine annually, herpes zoster, and Tdap. Tdap and influenza vaccine are especially important if he is going to be in contact with his 3-week-old grandchild. You should mention that Tdap and influenza are also recommended for his wife for the same reason.

EXAMPLE 3, EARLY ADOLESCENT FEMALE

A 12-year-old African American female visits the clinic with her mother because the mother felt it was time for her daughter to have a checkup. The patient is seen at first with the mother and then alone. The patient is well, with no acute or chronic medical problems. She started having her menses 6 months previously and states she is not sexually active or considering it. She is active in sports, and her mother feeds her lots of fruits and vegetables and minimizes consumption of fast foods and sweetened drinks. The mother provides an immunization record that shows the patient has received all recommended childhood vaccines except for a single dose of varicella vaccine. The patient is 5 ft 4 in. tall and weighs 120 lb (75th percentile for both height and weight; BMI 20.6 kg/m^2). Her mother is 45 years old and was diagnosed with breast cancer earlier in the year.

Risk factor assessment shows that injuries from a motor vehicle crash are the most likely cause of death in this age group. A more detailed family history is important to see if she has a high-risk family history for breast cancer. You can request that the mother gather this information to present at a future visit.

Risk reduction should include counseling about tobacco avoidance. Skin cancer behavioral counseling is recommended only for those with fair skin color, not African Americans and others with dark skin.

Recommended screening includes tests for depression, which can be performed using one of the tools on the USPSTF website, and obesity (done).

Recommended immunizations include Tdap, meningococcal conjugate vaccine (MCV4), human papillomavirus (HPV) first dose of a three-dose schedule, varicella dose 2 (catch up), and annual influenza vaccine.

Bright Future recommendations for this age group include measuring blood pressure, checking vision, performing a psychosocial and behavioral assessment, and providing anticipatory guidance focused on substance abuse and safety. The USPSTF states that the evidence is insufficient to recommend for or against these interventions.

EXAMPLE 4, ELDERLY FEMALE

An 85-year-old female visits the clinic for her annual examination to have her migraine medication refilled. She has occasional migraine headaches that are relieved by sumatriptan. She lives alone, walks 2 miles daily, and reports no health problems. She has no problem getting out of a chair. Her height is 5 ft 10 in. and weight is 165 lb (BMI 23.7 kg/m^2). Her family history shows no cancer or cardiovascular risks. She is 30 years post menopause, and other than a multivitamin each day, takes no medicine. She received a pneumococcal shot at age 65, a Tdap 4 years ago, and a zoster vaccine 5 years ago. She receives a flu shot each year. All of her children (4) and grandchildren (8, the youngest being age 5 years) live in the local area. Her blood pressure has never been high and today is 125/75 mm Hg.

Influenza and pneumonia are risks for this patient since she is around her school-age grandchildren, and the influenza vaccine has low effectiveness in those age 85 years old.

Risk reduction can best be achieved in this woman through advising influenza and pneumococcal vaccines for her children and grandchildren and avoiding unnecessary screening tests. The only screening tests recommended for her are for osteoporosis, obesity (done), high blood pressure (done), and depression (which she refuses). She is current on all other recommended vaccines.

This woman is best left alone, other than the screening for osteoporosis to prevent iatrogenic illnesses.

The Family Physician as the Foundation of the Public Health System

Although applied prevention in the clinical setting is important for individualized health and wellness, family physicians should realize that the largest improvements in the health of the public at large come from community-wide, public health interventions. Table 7-13 lists just some of the important public health interventions of the last century that have led to significant decreases in morbidity and mortality.

Each state and local political jurisdiction has some kind of official public health presence. At the local level, these are referred to as *local health departments*, which are subunits of city, county, or other regional government jurisdictions. All states have state public health departments, and the major public health department at the national level is the CDC, although important public health functions are also carried out by other federal agencies. The major roles and functions of local, state, and national health departments include disease surveillance and reporting, infectious disease control, infectious disease outbreak response, emergency preparedness and response, and chronic disease prevention.

The public health infrastructure, however, provides minimal direct clinical care, and depends on family physicians and other primary care providers to fulfill vital public health functions that contribute to improved community health. These functions are listed in Table 7-14. Screening tests, immunizations, and risk reduction have already been discussed in this chapter. Other important functions include

accurately diagnosing and treating diseases of public health importance, such as sexually transmitted infections, influenza, and tuberculosis; providing recommended treatment for family members and other contacts to infectious diseases or referring them to the public health department; reporting of infectious diseases, cancers, and other reportable conditions as required by state and local reporting requirements; enforcing infection control practices in the clinical setting; and providing advice to infectious patients on how to avoid spreading disease. Avoiding unnecessary or harmful testing and treatments should also be considered part of the prevention package offered by family physicians.

Family physicians should be continually aware of the epidemiology of disease in their communities, which diseases are endemic, which ones are not, and which infectious diseases are occurring at increased rates as part of an epidemic or seasonal increase. Local and state health departments as well as the CDC provide routinely updated epidemiological information through a variety of communication outlets. This knowledge assists physicians in making more accurate clinical diagnoses and providing appropriate treatments. The CDC and state health departments provide recommendations on how to diagnose and treat infectious diseases such as sexually transmitted infections, influenza, tuberculosis, and many others. A list of the most commonly used recommendations and their location on the CDC website is contained in Table 7-15. Following these official guidelines assists in providing accurate surveillance data, helps control infectious disease outbreaks, and assists in preventing antibiotic resistance.

When an infectious disease is discovered in a patient, the family physician should think about the implications of this for the family and the community. Family members may benefit from immunizations and/or chemoprevention depending on the disease. Some states allow treatment of sexually transmitted infections and other infectious diseases for contacts of patients, without directly examining the contact. This is called expedited partner therapy (EPT), and it not only benefits the contact but can also prevent reinfection of the patient. Examples of when EPT can be

---

Table 7-13 Major Public Health Achievements of the Past Century

- Vaccination
- Motor-vehicle safety
- Safer workplaces
- Control of infectious diseases
- Prevention of deaths from coronary heart disease and stroke through risk factor reduction
- Safer and healthier foods
- Maternal and child health programs
- Family planning
- Fluoridation of drinking water
- Tobacco use prevention

Centers for Disease Control and Prevention (CDC). Ten great public health achievements—United States 1900-1999. *MMWR Morb Mortal Wkly Rep.* 1999;48(12):241-243.

Table 7-14 Important Public Health Functions of Family Physicians

- Provide and promote recommend immunizations
- Provide screening tests recommended by the U.S. Preventive Services Task Force (USPSTF)
- Avoid providing unproven and/or harmful screening tests
- Use effective methods to modify risky behaviors
- Accurately diagnose and treat diseases of public health importance, such as sexually transmitted infections, influenza, and tuberculosis
- Either provide treatment for exposed family members and other contacts of infectious diseases or refer to the public health department
- Adhere to reporting requirements for infectious diseases, cancers, and other reportable conditions
- Enforce infection control practices in the clinical setting
- Provide advice to infectious patients on how to avoid spreading disease
- Avoid unnecessary and harmful testing and treatments

Table 7-15 Commonly Referenced Guidelines on Diseases of Public Health Importance

Diseases	Guideline Location
Sexually Transmitted Diseases ■ Treatment guidelines and updates	http://www.cdc.gov/std/treatment/2010/default.htm
Tuberculosis ■ Diagnosis, treatment of active and latent tuberculosis	http://www.cdc.gov/tb/publications/guidelines/Treatment.htm#treatment
Influenza ■ Vaccinations ■ Diagnosis and treatment ■ Outbreak control ■ Pre- and postexposure chemoprevention	http://www.cdc.gov/flu/professionals/index.htm

Table 7-16 Policies for Respiratory Hygiene in Health Care Settings

- Signs at entrances asking patients to inform office staff if they have symptoms of a respiratory infection
- Signs describing expectations regarding respiratory hygiene and demonstrating the correct way to cover the mouth and nose with a tissue when coughing or sneezing; proper disposal of tissue and hand cleansing after contact with respiratory secretions
- Offering masks to those who are coughing and not practicing respiratory hygiene
- Providing readily available tissues and hand sanitizer and no-touch receptacles for tissue disposal

useful include chlamydia and trichomonas infections. Family physicians who live in states where EPT is not legal and those who are not comfortable providing EPT should either recommend the exposed contact see a physician for assessment and treatment or refer the patient to the local health department. A current catalogue of the legal status of EPT by state can be found at the CDC Expedited Partner Therapy web page (www.cdc.gov/std/ept/default.htm/).

Much of the public health surveillance system depends on reports that come from clinical settings. Hospitals, physicians, and other providers are required to report to the local health department occurrences of specific infectious diseases. In some locations, new diagnoses of cancers are also required. Family physicians should be aware of what the reporting requirements are in the locale of their practice. These requirements usually specify that individual cases should be reported; however, in some instances, the requirement applies only to suspected outbreaks or multiple cases. Anytime family physicians detect an infectious disease that is out of the ordinary, with potential to spread in the community, they should consult with a public health department, either local or state.

Most of the required reports request information about the patient that includes name, address of residence, and phone number. If this information is required, it is exempt from the requirements of the Health Insurance Portability and Accountability Act (HIPAA), and the patient's consent to report is not required. The public health department uses this information for a variety of purposes, including detailed surveillance, contact notification, and implementation of preventive measures.

A clinical setting can be the source of spread of infectious disease in the community. Sick, infectious patients visit physician offices and clinics, and measures need to be taken to insure that spread of disease does not occur in these settings, to other patients as well as to physicians and staff. Measures that can be taken fall into five categories: policies on respiratory hygiene, policies on hand hygiene, immunization of staff, triage policies, and use of personal protective equipment (PPE). Policies on all these areas should be in place and enforced. A checklist of what the CDC considers minimum expectations for the prevention of infections in the outpatient setting can be found at its

Healthcare-associated Infections web page (www.cdc.gov/HAI/settings/outpatient/checklist/outpatient-care-checklist.html).

Respiratory hygiene means covering the nose and mouth with a disposable tissue when coughing and sneezing. This should be an expectation for patients and staff. Measures that can be taken to encourage and enforce respiratory hygiene are listed in Table 7-16. Health care personnel should wash or sanitize their hands after every patient encounter. Patients should be instructed to use frequent hand washing when sick. Hand sanitizer should be readily available in clinical areas and waiting rooms.

Office design and triage policy can assist in physically and temporally separating sick, infectious patients from others. Potentially infectious patients can be placed in a separate waiting area and/or asked to come in during specified time periods. However, if respiratory and hand washing policies are adhered to, having those with common respiratory infections use common waiting areas and examination rooms is acceptable. Other infectious diseases require more stringent measures. Fever accompanied by rash is particularly problematic. Measles, rubella, and varicella can all present this way and are highly infectious. Those presenting with rash and fever can be placed into a designated "rash room" and kept confined there until the diagnosis is clarified. If a highly infectious disease is suspected or confirmed, the room should not be used for other patient encounters for a time period as determined by the public health department.

Physicians and other health care personnel are at increased risk of exposure to infectious diseases and should take measures to protect themselves and thereby also protect their patients and families. All health care personnel should be vaccinated according to CDC recommendations (Table 7-17). Having unvaccinated personnel in a clinical setting causes a risk to them, their families, and patients. They are also a liability risk to the practice. PPE should be used any time an exposure to a potentially infectious body fluid occurs. Details on the proper use of PPE are on the CDC web page, Healthcare-associated Infections (www.cdc.gov/HAI/prevent/ppe.html).

When a family physician detects an infectious disease in a patient, advice should be given on how to prevent the spread of the disease to the patient's family, friends, and the community. A list of advice that can be provided is in Table 7-18.

As noted earlier, the last important role for family physicians in practicing optimal preventive medicine is to avoid

Table 7-17 Vaccines for Health Care Personnel

Vaccines	Recommendations in Brief
Hepatitis B	If you do not have documented evidence of a complex hepatitis B vaccine series, or if you do not have an up-to-date blood test that shows you are immune to hepatitis B (i.e., no serologic evidence of immunity or prior vaccination), then you should: ■ Get the 3-dose series (dose #1 now, #2 in 1 month, #3 approximately 5 months after #2). ■ Get anti-hepatitis B surface antigen (HBs) serologic tested 1-2 months after dose #3.
Flu (Influenza)	Get 1 dose of influenza vaccine annually.
MMR (Measles, Mumps, and Rubella)	If you were born in 1957 or later and have not had the MMR vaccine, or if you do not have an up-to-date blood test that shows you are immune to measles, mumps, and rubella (i.e., no serologic evidence of immunity or prior vaccination), get 2 doses of MMR, 4 weeks apart. For health care workers (HCWs) born before 1957, see the Advisory Committee on Immunization Practices (ACIP) recommendations.
Varicella (Chickenpox)	If you have not had chickenpox (varicella), if you have not had varicella vaccine, or if you do not have an up-to-date blood test that shows you are immune to varicella (i.e., no serologic evidence of immunity or prior vaccination), get 2 doses of varicella vaccine, 4 weeks apart.
Tdap (Tetanus, Diphtheria, Pertussis)	Get a one-time dose of Tdap as soon as possible if you have not received Tdap previously (regardless of when previous dose of Td was received). Get Td boosters every 10 years thereafter. Pregnant HCWs need to get a dose of Tdap during each pregnancy.
Meningococcal	Those who are routinely exposed to isolates of *Neisseria meningitides* should get 1 dose.

From the Centers for Disease Control and Prevention (CDC). *Recommended Vaccines for Healthcare Workers.* http://www.cdc.gov/vaccines/adults/rec-vac/hcw.html.

Table 7-18 Advice to Patients to Prevent Spread of Infectious Disease

■ The patient should stay at home while most infectious to avoid infecting others. If patients have to leave the home, they should strictly follow respiratory hygiene.
■ At home, place patients in a separate room or separate them physically from other household members as much as possible.
■ Limit the number of household members having contact with the patient.
■ Follow hand hygiene after contact with the patient or the patient environment and waste products. This includes handwashing with soap and water or use of an alcohol-based hand rub.
■ Consider having the patient wear a surgical mask.
■ Immunize household members if appropriate.
■ Wash dishes, utensils, and laundry in warm water and soap.
■ Consider chemoprophylaxis for household members if it is available and recommended.
■ Household members should watch for symptoms and seek care at their first appearance.
■ Nonhousehold members should not enter the home. If nonhousehold members need to enter the home, they should avoid close contact with the patient.

unnecessary and harmful testing and treatments. This at first glance seems clear cut, but there is good evidence that in daily medical practice many tests and treatments provided are not necessary and result in harm (Kale et al., 2013; Korenstein et al., 2012) Antibiotics for upper respiratory infections is one example. The AAFP and other specialty organizations have joined forces in an initiative called "Choosing Wisely." Each organization has developed a list of testing or interventions that should not be performed, or done only in specific circumstances. The AAFP list of 15 such interventions is contained in Table 7-19. Unnecessary testing and treatments are costly and harmful, and avoiding them is good preventive medicine.

Intergenerational Aspects of Prevention in the Family

Family physicians have the opportunity to appreciate and achieve intergenerational benefits of preventive interventions within families and households. Influenza and pneumococcal vaccines in infants and children provide added protection to elderly family members—who are at the highest risk of morbidity and mortality from these respiratory infections—through herd immunity and reduced disease transmission. Pertussis immunization of adolescents and adults of all ages provides a cocoon of protection around infants who have high rates of serious complications from pertussis and are not fully protected by the vaccine until they have received a full primary series. Other infectious diseases can spread among family members, and ways to minimize this have already been discussed in this chapter.

In addition, chronic diseases tend to be common among family members because of common genes and common environments, and interventions to prevent these conditions can spread their effects through the household. For example, smoking cessation helps prevent disease not only in the smoker but also in the whole family by preventing exposure to secondhand smoke. Improved diets and increased physical activity can be family activities, which lead to improved health for those with obesity and diabetes and contribute to a reduced risk for everyone else in the household.

Genomics and Prevention

The human genome project has led to a better understanding of the genomic basis of responses to specific

Table 7-19 American Academy of Family Physicians "Choosing Wisely" List

1. Do not do imaging for low back pain within the first 6 weeks unless red flags are present.
2. Do not routinely prescribe antibiotics for acute mild-to-moderate sinusitis unless symptoms last for 7 or more days or symptoms worsen after initial clinical improvement.
3. Do not use dual-energy x-ray absorptiometry (DEXA) screening for osteoporosis in women younger than 65 or men younger than 70 with no risk factors.
4. Do not order annual electrocardiograms (ECGs) or any other cardiac screening for low-risk patients without symptoms.
5. Do not perform Pap smears on women younger than 21 years of age or who have had a hysterectomy for noncancer disease.
6. Do not schedule elective, nonmedically indicated induction of labor or cesarean deliveries before 39 weeks, 0 days gestational age.
7. Avoid elective, nonmedically indicated inductions of labor between 29 weeks, 0 days and 41 weeks, 0 days, unless the cervix is deemed favorable.
8. Do not screen for carotid artery stenosis in asymptomatic adult patients.
9. Do not screen women older than 65 years of age for cervical cancer who have had adequate prior screening and are not otherwise at high risk for cervical cancer.
10. Do not screen women younger than 30 years of age for cervical cancer with human papillomavirus (HPV) testing alone or in combination with cytology.
11. Do not prescribe antibiotics for otitis media in children ages 2 to 12 years of age with nonsevere symptoms when the observation option is reasonable.
12. Do not perform voiding cystourethrograms routinely in first febrile urinary tract infection in children ages 2 to 24 months.
13. Do not routinely screen for prostate cancer using a prostate-specific antigen (PSA) test or digital rectal examination.
14. Do not screen adolescents for scoliosis.
15. Do not require a pelvic examination or other physical examination to prescribe oral contraceptive medications.

From American Academy of Family Physicians. *Fifteen Things Physicians and Patients Should Question.* http://www.aafp.org/dam/AAFP/documents/about_us/initiatives/choosing-wisely-fifteen-questions.pdf.

medications, adverse drug reactions, and the underlying inheritability of many conditions. Rapidly evolving scientific advances in genomics, along with reduced costs of genomic tests, holds the promise of one day each person knowing their whole genome. While theoretically this will lead to more accurate targeting of drug therapy, fewer adverse drug reactions, and targeted risk reduction activities, the full translation of this new science into useful and effective clinical interventions is pending the demonstration of clinical utility and improved clinical outcomes.

Genomic tests should be evaluated for effectiveness just as should other screening tests. So far, evidence-based groups that have assessed genetic and genomic tests used for predicting risk for chronic diseases, such as diabetes, coronary heart disease, and obesity, have not endorsed their use because they have not proven to be clinically useful; they do not provide much information beyond that obtained from a family history and traditional risk factors (EGAPP Working Group, 2010, 2013). In addition, it is not clear

that people will take any action to improve their health or risks based on this information.

However, testing for two conditions that cause higher risks for cancer have been found to result in improved outcomes: breast cancer genes and Lynch syndrome. The USPSTF recommends that women with high-risk family histories for breast and uterine cancer be counseled about the *BRCA* gene test (USPSTF, n.d.). Patients who have a *BRCA* gene can reduce their chances of breast and ovarian cancer with bilateral mastectomy and oophorectomy. First-degree relatives of those with Lynch syndrome, discovered to be the cause of colon cancer, can be tested to see if they carry the same mutation, and if they do, they can benefit from earlier and more frequent colonoscopy. This has led to a recommendation to test all of those with newly diagnosed colon cancer for Lynch syndrome and counseling of first-degree relatives of those with this inherited disorder (EGAPP Working Group, 2009).

Family physicians will need to stay current with advances in genomics and use discretion when deciding when to use genomic tests and genomic-based interventions, adopt them when the evidence merits it, and avoid unnecessary and potentially harmful testing.

Office Systems as an Aid to Prevention

In a busy clinical setting, prevention can easily be relegated to the back bench. It takes effort to adhere to recommendations for counseling, chemoprevention, screening, and vaccines. Reporting of infectious diseases to the health department can be overlooked. Making prevention interventions routine, as part of the clinical system, helps ensure a high level of performance. Examples of systemization that can occur include electronic health record reminders to providers of recommended preventive services for each patient; flagging of infectious diseases that need to be reported; standing orders for immunizations; alerts when targets such as blood pressure and blood glucose levels are exceeded; and automatically generated reminders for patients that can be sent using electronic media. Other system-wide interventions with good evidence of effectiveness include group education sessions for diabetes self-management and increasing breast cancer screening; team-based approaches to assist patients in managing chronic conditions such as high blood pressure, diabetes, and high cholesterol; and periodic assessment and feedback to providers on performance on prevention measures (Community Preventive Services Task Force, *Cardiovascular Disease Prevention, Diabetes Prevention and Control,* and *Obesity Prevention and Control*). Individual team members can be charged with specific responsibilities such as assessing each patient's vaccine status or ensuring that hand sanitizers and tissues are readily available. Immunization schedule wall charts can be posted in waiting areas and examination rooms, and prevention-oriented patient education materials can be placed so they are easily seen and obtained. The key is making all aspects of prevention a priority and finding ways to make it happen.

References

The complete reference list is available at
www.expertconsult.com.

Web Resources

http://www.cdc.gov *Centers for Disease Control and Prevention*
http://www.thecommunityguide.org/index.html *Community Preventive Services Task Force*

http://www.thecommunityguide.org/vaccines/index.html *Community Preventive Services Task Force article, Increasing Appropriate Immunizations*
http://www.uspreventiveservicestaskforce.org/index.html *U.S. Preventive Services Task Force*

8 Behavioral Change and Patient Empowerment

CHARLES W. SMITH and J. CHRIS RULE

Key Points

- Patients are responsible for their own health.
- Patient engagement and shared decision-making is more likely to result in better patient outcomes.
- Motivational interviewing can help patients make important changes.

Although most people find it very difficult to change behavior, they often do so in the interest of achieving positive health outcomes. This chapter introduces you to the concept of "participatory medicine" and challenges you to think of patient relationships in a new way, as a partnership, and to facilitate the notion that patients are, in fact, responsible for their own health. Patients will never achieve meaningful, lasting behavior change unless the decision is their own. And, they will not feel empowered to make change unless they have access to enabling tools and methods. Motivational interviewing (MI) is one technique that can be used by providers to help patients initiate and implement important change processes. This approach is presented later in this chapter.

Traditional Physician Role

Physician training often involves techniques and advice about how to "lead" or "direct" the patient to change, whether the goal is adherence to treatment recommendations, smoking cessation, or dietary changes to achieve weight loss. As a result of taking on this provider-centric, directive role, physicians often mistakenly assume responsibility for patient outcomes. This can foster paternalistic interaction, cause frustration, and contribute to provider burnout. Embracing the notions of shared decision-making, patient engagement, and patient empowerment frees both patient and provider to form a more equal relationship and allows the patient to receive appropriate guidance and

advice. This type of relationship is more likely to result in the patient taking responsibility for making the necessary changes to achieve optimal health (Stewart et al., 2000). Examples that support this approach can be seen in the Kaiser Permanente HealthConnect Collaborative Cardiac Care Case Study, which reported that patient engagement resulted in prevention of 135 deaths and 260 costly emergencies and increased achievement of patient's cholesterol goals from 26% to 73%; and it resulted in the percent of patients screened for cholesterol levels increasing from 55% to 97% (Munro, 2013).

Evolution of the Care Model

The dominant care model in Western medicine has been the biomedical model. The traditional provider role places the physician in an illness/disease paradigm. This model has sustained the health care system for more than a century and has resulted in much success. Yet the system cries out for change, in part because of the perceived negative consequences on patient health outcomes. An alternative approach, the patient-centered, participatory, patient-engagement paradigm, focuses more on health promotion and maintenance of a healthy lifestyle. One of the early "disruptive" forces that led to the evolution of the traditional medical model was Michael Balint, who used his dual training in medicine and psychiatry to explore the way emotions affect symptoms. He also emphasized the importance of the role of the physician himself and the doctor-patient relationship (Balint, 1957). Engel (1977), building on the works of general systems theorists, first proposed the biopsychosocial model, which embraces the complexities of genetics, physiology, family history, family dynamics, environmental stress, and stress-related illness, as well as social and cultural factors. It also takes into account that many deeply personal factors affect the expression of symptoms and one's response to, and recovery from, illness.

The "medical model" focuses on making a diagnosis and providing treatment to eliminate the disease, and it has been largely successful. Yet the obdurate rate of change for certain chronic diseases illustrates that this model has significant limitations. Likewise, while the biopsychosocial model and Balint's blend of the medical/psychosocial approach to care are helpful in understanding patient behavior, they do not provide readily applicable practice approaches that help doctors and patients achieve optimum health outcomes. Nevertheless, these pioneers provided the background and basis for an exciting new approach by encouraging patients to be active participants in narrating their stories to their physicians (Engel, 1997). This may provide a more effective approach, namely, participatory medicine.

The Participatory Medical Model

The medical and biopsychosocial models describe how providers view their patients. But in the realm of interaction and the doctor-patient relationship, patients and providers alike are calling for a new model of care in which the provider assumes a new, less authoritative role that seeks to engage the patient more actively in the care process. This participatory model assumes that patients will actively learn about their condition, prepare questions for provider visits, collaborate with other patients with similar conditions, and take an active role in making lifestyle changes to improve health and manage their own conditions.

The participatory health model goes hand in hand with the introduction of the Internet and mobile technology. And it embraces the enormous impact the Internet is having on health care. (Reynolds, 2013). But these changes also complicate the doctor-patient relationship, bringing to light multiple, potentially conflicting sources of information from online journals, websites, and blogs that must be reconciled. So then, how can this reconciliation best take place and how will we, as providers, facilitate the role of patients within the participatory model of care?

In this new model of care, patients will receive guidance, tools, and information that foster active participation in their care and effective collaboration with providers. In addition to engaging in research about their health and their medical conditions, patients will network with online communities to discover which treatments, providers, and facilities work best. Through the network effect of communicating with other engaged patients, they will become more aware of their responsibilities for maintaining health. This approach will be even more effective as home monitoring devices become routinely available (Kruse et al., 2013).

As providers increasingly adopt electronic communication options, clinical care will shift to a "care anywhere" model. Office visits will become much less important and less frequent. Most routine follow-up, medication refills, review of blood pressure, adjustment of medications, and other former office-based interactions will be conducted online. Office visits will only take place when a hands-on examination, interaction, or procedure is needed. This new care model will be less costly, more patient-centered, more convenient, and will lower barriers to accessing care. These electronic methods of communication may include e-mail, web-based secure messaging, videoconferencing, mobile phone conversations, text messaging, and instant messaging (Epstein and Street, 2011).

But, as with most things, these sweeping changes are not without risk and potential negative outcomes. Increasing dependence on online communication removes the valuable role of face-to-face communication and nonverbal communication. Thus it will risk missing subtle clinical clues that may otherwise be detected within an office setting. Further, it is difficult to be certain that someone other than the assumed patient is communicating online, so there is also a risk of fraudulent activity occurring. And state medical regulations generally limit the extent to which a provider may give online advice or prescription medications without a previously established doctor-patient relationship or an in-office evaluation before communicating online. So this, appropriately in most cases, limits the breadth of online provider-patient communication.

The Birth of the "e-Patient Revolution"

"e-Patients: How They Can Help Us Heal Healthcare," a Robert Wood Johnson white paper, articulated this emerging change in health care and introduced the participatory model for U.S. health care (Ferguson et al., 2007). More recently, the Affordable Care Act, with its emphasis on patient-centered medical homes and accountable care organizations (ACOs), is in the early stages of implementation. The effectiveness of these health reforms will depend to a great extent on how successful we are in activating and engaging patients to become participatory partners. Ferguson also noted that people provide their own care 80% to 98% of the time and thus self-care is actually the predominant care mode (Figure 8-1). He also noted that, with the advent of the Internet and the accompanying massive access to information, the triangle is becoming "flipped"; that is, self-care is now more encouraged, more routine, and more accepted than previously (Figure 8-2). Ferguson believed that patients are now more knowledgeable about their health and in a better position to use health professionals in a coequal, consultative mode (participatory model) than to continue to function as passive patients.

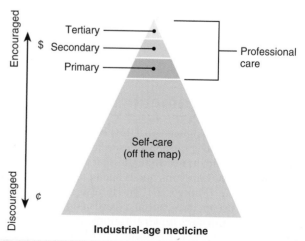

Figure 8-1 Importance of self-care. (From Ferguson T. Consumer health informatics. *Healthc Forum J.* 1995;38(1):28-33.)

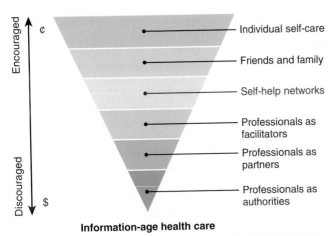

Figure 8-2 Emergence of individual self-care. (From Ferguson T. Consumer health informatics. *Healthc Forum J.* 1995;38(1):28-33.)

Patient- and Family-Centered Care

Medical teachers have emphasized the preeminent role of the provider in making the diagnosis, giving staff and patients "orders" to be carried out, and performing follow-up checks. The picture is one of the providers as "all knowing" and as "captains of the ship" who must remain in control within the medical setting. This focuses all of the pressure on the provider to perform well and places the patient in a passive role that often results in suboptimal outcomes.

In recent years, the patient-centered care movement has gained in popularity. Practicing patient-centered care embodies a number actions and strategies, including shared decision-making, open communication between physician and patient through patient portals, text messaging, e-mails and social media, MI, and being available and responsive during regular hours and after hours (Bergeson and Dean, 2006). Hospitals have encouraged and embraced this movement by building online portals that allow patients to review laboratory and radiography reports, request or make appointments, and communicate with clinical staff. Hospitals have also engaged individuals to serve in patient and family advocacy roles, including formation of patient advisory committees. Many institutions have also begun to add patients to hospital committees, boards, and work groups. This patient participation in the governance of health care organizations is a necessary addition if we are going to effectively bring the patient's voice and perspective into the way these entities function (Luxford et al., 2011).

Patient Engagement

The term "patient engagement" has become a "hot buzz" phrase recently and is variably interpreted and very difficult to measure. Munro notes that the search phrase returns more than 500,000 results and is a lead topic for speakers and conferences (Munro, 2013). He also notes that it is important to use metrics, not just words and platitudes, to measure how providers and institutions move into patient engagement programs. Kernisan (2013) defines patient engagement as fostering a fruitful collaboration in which patients and clinicians work together to help the patient progress toward mutually agreed-on health goals. It requires providers to work collaboratively with patients to determine which health outcomes are important, which ones to pursue, and how they should be pursued. This allows us to engage in meaningful partnerships with patients. Allowing patients to make these choices will be a very different mindset for many providers.

The Patient-Centered Medical Home

The patient-centered medical home (PCMH) concept has been embraced by many organizations and policy groups and is widely regarded as a key tool to reform health care. It involves a team approach to care and describes a wide variety of services to provide high-quality care to patients with chronic illnesses (Robert Graham Center, 2007). It also appeals to healthy patients who want to prevent illness and maintain optimum health.

Utilizing the principles of the PCMH is a practical way to shift physicians' attitudes and practices toward the participatory medicine model. It points to new roles for both patients and providers. It requires physicians to become more involved in and supportive of patient education. It involves a multidisciplinary team approach to care, with each member of the team practicing "at the top of their license." These teams often include mental health professionals, nutritionists, pharmacists, and other professional providers. And it will profoundly alter the provider business model, with widespread adoption and expansion of information technology (IT) capabilities, more accessible and more frequent modes of communication, and reconfigured incentives and rewards for all stakeholders. Many believe that it will ultimately bring an end to the fee-for-service reimbursement method of paying for medical services (NCQA, 2011).

This approach has profound implications for patient and provider interaction. No longer will the care system be based primarily on an "office visit" model. Physicians will be reimbursed for "monitoring" their overall practice population and will receive incentive payments for agreed-on, desired outcomes. Because payment to providers will not be based solely on office visit charges, there will be greater incentives to communicate in other ways, including phone, e-mail, text messages, and social media.

The National Committee for Quality Assurance (NCQA) created a certification standard for PCMH that was modified in 2011 (Peek and Oftedahl, 2010). This list comprises the six basic standards:

1. Enhance access and continuity.
2. Manage population.
3. Plan and manage care.
4. Provide self-care support using community resources.
5. Track and coordinate care.
6. Measure and improve performance.

Meeting these standards involves a significant redesign of the primary care physician office team, including utilization of nurse care managers, greatly expanding access to care, and involving patients in goal-setting and self-management. It also involves a commitment to evaluation of the patient experience and making appropriate modifications. And it involves significant additional investments in personnel, IT systems, and training. Thus if this model is to be sustainable, payers of health care services will need to take these additional costs into consideration in their reimbursement for this care.

Patient/Provider Collaboration

Adopting and following the principles outlined for the PCMH moves providers from traditional means of communication between doctor and patient. No longer does the provider supply "doctor's orders," but the paradigm has evolved toward the patient and provider conducting collaborative conversations and exchanging ideas. Providers will engage patients to participate in their care and will encourage them to be actively involved. Providers will also invite the patient to provide feedback about the care received. This feedback will include identification of, and reporting, medical errors (Allen, 2012; Pear, 2012).

Physicians and patients will find new ways to use social media to communicate with patient groups who have similar conditions (e.g., Association of Cancer Online Resources at www.acor.org). Physicians will commonly prescribe "information therapy" to give patients the material they need to manage their own health care. Similarly, patients will provide physicians with insights they have gleaned from their own experience and from their social network (Reinders et al., 2011). Most physicians will have interactive practice websites and an electronic portal through which patients can request an answer to a clinical question or renewal of a prescription.

Information Technology and Participatory Medicine

The use of electronic medical records (EMRs) and other technology tools will play a major role in this new model of health care. There will be easy mechanisms within the EMR for follow-up after every encounter (Smith and Graedon, 2012). Physicians will send communication to the patient electronically or give printed information, depending on patient preference and technical access, generated from the EMR. Laboratory and imaging results will be shared, along with interpretative comments and any necessary instructions. Physicians and patients will use e-mail or secure messaging to discuss changes in status, provide progress reports, or communicate other important information. Rather than establishing fixed intervals for when follow-up will occur, there will an ongoing dialogue made possible by these online tools.

Access to health applications (apps) currently available on smartphones and tablets will play a central role in the future of health care. Patients will use apps to help guide weight loss, promote exercise programs, and monitor chronic conditions (Lim, 2013). Patients with cardiac problems will be able to obtain and transmit an electrocardiogram to their providers (Seppala, 2013). Touch-sensitive devices will be used to monitor pulse, respiratory rate, and oxygen saturation (Bloom, 2013). Patients with diabetes will measure their glucose on a connected glucometer and transmit the results directly from their devices, allowing consultation and medication adjustments to be made without the necessity of an office visit.

Health Behavior Change and Motivational Interviewing

> **Key Points**
>
> - Health behavior change and MI are patient-centered approaches that promote change, empower patients to address ambivalence, and improve patient engagement in their health care.
> - Brief MI and health behavior change (HBC) interventions in clinical settings are more effective than no treatment and are generally equal to other viable treatments of longer duration and cost.

BACKGROUND AND KEY PRINCIPLES

Motivational interviewing is one good way to engage the patient in the process of positive change. Developed by Miller (1983) as a promising way to treat alcoholism, MI has most recently been defined as "a collaborative person-centered form of guiding to elicit and strengthen motivation for change" (Miller and Rollnick, 2009, p. 137). Often described by its creators as more than a series of techniques and skills, MI is a way of being with patients that empowers them to improve their own health, addresses resistance and barriers to change, and fortifies their ability to maintain these changes over time. Miller and Rollnick (1991) adapted and expanded MI to work with various patient populations in substance abuse treatment settings (see Miller and Rose, 2009, for an extensive background on the development of the method). In the past two decades, a strengthening evidence base has demonstrated that MI can be adapted to many different patient health problems in a wide variety of settings. Rollnick and colleagues (2008), in their book *Motivational Interviewing in Health Care*, identify four guiding principles of MI. These are captured in the mnemonic **RULE:**

1. **R**esist the "righting reflex"—recognize that correcting the patient can produce a paradoxical effect (i.e., "Don't try to fix it, and don't give advice").
2. **U**nderstand your patient's motivations—the desire for change and the goals to achieve must come from the patient not the provider.
3. **L**isten to your patient—use empathic, active listening; this changes the mindset that the provider has all the answers.
4. **E**mpower your patient—understand that the outcomes will be better when patients are active participants in their own care and take responsibility for the change process.

Prochaska and DiClemente (1984) developed their transtheoretical model, also known as the stages of change theory, to provide a structure that providers can use to track a patient's progress through health behavior change. This

Table 8-1 Stages of Change Theory
1. Precontemplation: not yet considering change
2. Contemplation: evaluating reasons for and against change
3. Preparation: planning for change
4. Action: making the identified change
5. Maintenance: working to sustain changes
6. Relapse: backsliding into old behavior patterns

Table 8-2 OARS for Brief Counseling
Open-ended questions, e.g., "How are you feeling about your health these days?"
Affirmation, e.g., "You may not be at your goal yet, but look at how far you've come."
Reflective listening, e.g., "It sounds as though you don't feel confident about making this change but you do want to change."
Summaries, e.g., "Let me summarize what we've just talked about."

From McAndrews JA, McMullen S, Wilson SL. Four strategies for promoting healthy lifestyles in your practice. *Fam Pract Manag* 18(2):16-20, 2011.

model has five key stages that are used to identify where a patient is in the process and tailor the appropriate intervention to this change. These can be used as a way to open the dialogue about change behaviors with the patient, and the provider can use the process to monitor treatment. The stages are listed in Table 8-1.

The sixth step or stage that is commonly seen in clinical settings is "backsliding" or relapse (see Table 8-1). This part of the transtheoretical process can occur at almost any level and is central to understanding how patients' health behavior is often cyclical as they move back and forth in their decision-making and maintenance of healthier behaviors. This model can serve as a complement to MI in clinical practice. There are several guiding philosophies that undergird MI, which make it an excellent approach within the PCMH model. MI specifically, and health behavior change (HBC) more broadly, are becoming essential tools in clinical practice and support providers' shift to the patient engagement movement and to practicing more patient-centered medicine. With a patient-centered approach, the patient works in collaboration with the provider to set the agenda for treatment; this contrasts with a provider-centered approach in which the physician or other health care team member determines the agenda for the patient and directs treatment. The collaboration between patient and team is seen as essential because the goals must start with what the patient is willing and able to do. This supports patient self-efficacy, autonomy, and expertise, and it creates belief in the patient's own capacity to change and implement these new healthier behaviors.

Key to the success of applying MI to patient care requires several provider behaviors, some of which fly in the face of the formal instruction that physicians receive. One of these is termed "rolling with resistance" or the denial that the patient may put forward. This keeps the encounter from becoming a confrontation or tug-of-war between patient and provider. Providers also need to be acutely aware of how to enhance a patient's readiness by helping the patient identify the real or perceived obstacle to change by resolving the patient's ambivalence. By enhancing patients' self-efficacy, providers become more active collaborators in their patients' health.

Empathy for the patient is a key component, as it allows the provider to really "start where the patient is" and promotes a deeper understanding of what it is like to be that patient as they face his or her health challenges. With this empathic stance, both the provider and the patient recognize that the motivation to change comes from the patient. The provider does not have to convince the patient to change or give sage advice about how this should be done. The mnemonic, OARS, is the basis for patient-centered interventions in brief counseling; it is a path that leads to empathic connection with the patient (Miller and Rollnick,

2002; Table 8-2). These basic microcounseling skills have been shown to work well with all types of patients considering a health behavior change. These interpersonal communication skills help a clinician capture what has been referred to as the "spirit" of MI, and this is often cited by the founders of the model as the most critical aspect of using this method properly (Miller and Rose, 2009).

EVIDENCE FOR HEALTH BEHAVIOR CHANGE AND MOTIVATIONAL INTERVIEWING

Recent meta-analyses and review articles across a variety of disciplines have further solidified the evidence for MI and other patient-empowering methods to bring about positive health outcomes (Britt et al., 2004; Burke et al., 2004; Martins and McNeil, 2009; Rubak et al., 2005). Numerous strategies for changing health behaviors have also received attention in recent years (Martins and McNeil, 2009; Rubak et al., 2005). MI has been shown in dozens of controlled trials to produce significant change in client health behaviors in general and in substance use in particular. Randomized trials showing benefit from MI have been completed with patients with alcohol, tobacco, and substance abuse problems, type 2 diabetes, hypertension, gambling addiction, and weight reduction (Miller et al., 2004). Given the wide breadth of articles and subjects covered, this section will focus on those studies that address a few of the problems commonly seen in family medicine practice.

HBC and MI complement the approaches being used in the management of a variety of chronic illnesses in health care settings. The "way of being with patients" that is the central aspect of MI and is a component of many chronic disease models being used to address these complex problems helps the provider address the problems in new ways. By dealing with a patient's feelings and thoughts and ambivalence using MI, there seems to be much less resistance and better adherence to treatments. As with all models, this one is not a panacea, but there are strong indications that MI and HBC approaches can have positive impacts on a wide range of illnesses and effect behavior change in many populations where other standard methods have come up short (Miller and Rose, 2009).

MOTIVATIONAL INTERVIEWING AS APPLIED TO COMMON PROBLEMS IN FAMILY MEDICINE

Diet Changes, Obesity, and Reducing Body Mass Index

More than three dozen studies have been conducted since 1999 that have investigated the effects of MI on changes in diet, for weight loss, to reduce body mass index (BMI), and to increase physical activity (see Martins and McNeil, 2009, for a review, and Armstrong et al., 2011). These studies, mostly randomized controlled clinical trials, have demonstrated moderate to strong support for MI and other HBC interventions. They used several MI methods to achieve their results, including empathic understanding; opened-ended questions to assess for readiness to change; scaling questions for importance and confidence to create discrepancy and to track progress; and multiple sessions of varying number and duration (10-40 minutes). In-person meetings by a variety of providers as well as telephone calls were used as the primary interventions and as follow-up or maintenance interventions. The most robust findings have been in the areas of maintaining dietary and weight loss changes and lowering BMI based on goals agreed on between patient and the provider. A recent review by Rose and colleagues (2013) summarized that provider advice, including some studies in which MI was used, produces a greater level of health behavior change and commitment to weight loss goals. The long-term value of MI in this area seems well established at this point. In the review by Rubak and colleagues (2005), the combined effect estimates of using MI to produce decreases in body mass index indicate that it can and should be used. The growing weight of the evidence supports using these techniques and this style of counseling with overweight and obese patients.

Case Example of a Participatory Encounter

See Box 8-1.

Hyperlipidemia

Several studies have investigated the effect of MI on lowering cholesterol level, and the results have been mixed. Brug and colleagues (2007) found that dietitians trained in using MI with patients with type 2 diabetes attained a significantly larger self-reported change in their saturated fat scores than dieticians who were not trained in MI in newly diagnosed patients. Other risk behaviors for type 2 diabetes such as glycemic control and body mass were no different than the controls. A study that compared two interventions, one of which was MI, for lowering lipid levels and dietary fat intake showed positive results for both interventions, which were sustained for 12 months (Mhurchu et al., 1998). Additionally, numerous other studies with a wide range of populations, age ranges, and from a broad diversity of cultures have demonstrated that using standard MI interventions to lower serum cholesterol has a strong enough positive effect to suggest its use over other methods (Martins and McNeil, 2009; Rubak et al., 2005).

Diabetes Care

There have been a large number of studies over the past 15 years investigating the impact of MI and other HBC approaches on patients with diabetes (see Rubak et al., 2005 for a review; DiLillo and West, 2011). Most of these studies have yielded positive or mixed (positive-neutral) results when comparing MI- or HBC-focused interventions to controls. The most salient changes have been where intervention groups who have received MI have experienced larger reductions in weight, significantly lower hemoglobin A1c values, improved dietary changes, increased activity

levels, an enhanced motivation to learn about their diabetes, and an improved outlook on maintaining behavior change (Channon et al., 2003, 2007; Rubak et al., 2009). West and colleagues (2007) studying a group of overweight women with type 2 diabetes found that MI enhances patient weight loss at 6 and 18 months, as well as leads to significantly reduced hemoglobin A1c levels. However, this study also found that the motivation to change for African American patients seemed to diminish over time. This observation calls into question the clinical durability of MI with some populations; however, there are promising studies being undertaken with adolescents that combine MI with other treatment strategies (Stanger et al., 2013). This will be an important area of future research as MI techniques are refined to discover how best to meet the needs of special populations. Team-based care for diabetes management has become the norm, involving physicians, nurses, care managers, social workers, psychologists, support groups, and lay volunteers. HBC and MI help to educate patients, facilitate change, and maintain patient adherence at all levels of care. Given all the available evidence, these techniques have been shown to empower patients to be more engaged with their diabetic care. They have the potential to make the provider's work more efficient and effective in reducing more costly levels of care. With further data, this may be where the greatest benefits of MI are realized.

TRAINING AND GROWTH OF MOTIVATIONAL INTERVIEWING

In the past 30 years since these approaches were conceived, the current widespread use of MI and HBC methods across a variety of disciplines illustrates that they have moved beyond emerging trends. Currently there is a need for expanded training and teaching of these methods and principles across the health care system. Having emerged from the discipline of psychology, these methods are being used in medical residency programs from family medicine to obstetrics/gynecology, and from internal medicine and pediatrics to psychiatry. They are also widely used in colleges of nursing, public health, schools of social work, and other health-related professions. The adoption of MI and HBC as part of standard curricula is in the beginning stages in medical school and other health care fields, so future professionals should have a stronger grounding in HBC and the basics of MI as essential tools. However, this has been helped along by recent reports from the Association of American Medical Colleges (AAMC, 2011) and the Accreditation Council for Graduate Medical Education (ACGME) that place strong emphasis on the physician-patient relationship, the psychosocial aspects of the human condition, the communication skills and advanced interpersonal competencies necessary to provide excellent care, and the importance of methods and techniques as found in MI and the HBC literature. Important support for these efforts could come from the accreditation bodies for PCMH as these methods are increasingly seen as cost-effective approaches that involve the entire health care team, especially the patient.

In the spirit of collaborative care, with provider and patient working together in MI, Triana and colleagues (2012) recently demonstrated how a standardized MI

Box 8-1 Case Example of a Participatory Encounter

Mrs. Smith is 59 years old, is 20 pounds overweight and has an average blood pressure of 145/98 mm Hg and a fasting glucose of 135 mg/dL. Her hemoglobin A1c is 7.2%, indicating that she has previously undiagnosed diabetes mellitus. She complains of bilateral knee pain, which makes it hard to exercise. Radiographs of the knees confirm the diagnosis of moderately severe osteoarthritis. She also has complained of hot flashes, insomnia, and depression.

When Ms. Smith calls the office to arrange for a new patient visit, she is enrolled in the office's patient portal, which allows her to submit her medical history and all of her insurance and demographic information online prior to her visit. When she arrives in the office, she checks in using a computerized kiosk and, because she has been preregistered, the process takes less than 2 minutes. She is brought back to the examination room a little ahead of her scheduled visit.

The doctor uses a questioning method informed by the spirit of motivational interviewing (MI). Open-ended questioning begins the visit, and the doctor actively listens to allow the patient to tell her story in her own way. This empowers the patient to inform the doctor of her concerns and what her most important issues are from her perspective. She expresses concerns about the diabetes diagnosis and her knee pain.

Using another key technique of MI and health behavior change, the doctor might use a scaling question or review with the patient a "confidence/readiness ruler" to assess the patient's confidence and the level of importance she places on making the necessary changes. This could be in a customized, tablet-based handout synched with the clinic electronic medical record (EMR), or it could be administered as a handout by a patient-centered medical home (PCMH) team member (nurse, medical assistant, or diabetes care manager) depending on the patient's health literacy level. The doctor (who has already reviewed her online history) reviews her laboratory results and discusses the medication choices for her to consider. Instead of making hasty decisions, the doctor then uses this information to

- Affirm how the patient is feeling about making these significant changes.
- Resolve any ambivalence she may be having to the recommended changes in her medication regimen, diet, and activity levels.
- Summarize the biomedical and psychosocial aspects of care into an integrated plan that is personalized and fits with the patient's level of readiness to change.

After reaching common ground the follow-up plans flow easily.

Because this MI approach blends client-initiated information with the doctor's medical knowledge and clinical judgment, the process is collaborative and the patient feels empowered to be more involved in the decision-making. The patient and doctor reach common ground on the patient's medications.

In addition to the core concerns, the doctor and patient discuss additional supports that the patient can receive through the PCMH. She is given an appointment with the nutritionist and with the diabetes educator for later that week. She is also given a web address for an online diabetes support group, and several diabetes care apps that the physician is familiar with are recommended for her to track her blood glucose levels and dietary changes.

To address the patient's second agenda item, the doctor and patient repeat the OARS process as detailed in Table 8-2. They reach mutual agreement to use ibuprofen for her knee pain and decide on a referral to a physical therapist who specializes in hydrotherapy for osteoarthritis. The patient also indicated that she is willing to try some alternative methods so she is provided with information about a certified acupuncturist to help treat her arthritis pain. She is referred to a well-respected website that specializes in home remedies and is encouraged to look over the options listed for treatment of arthritis and knee pain and select any that she is comfortable with. She is asked to log her results for later sharing with the care team.

She is encouraged to use the patient portal to provide blood glucose levels, ask questions, and provide feedback about the effectiveness of her medications. She uses a connected glucometer, along with a new mobile application on her smart phone, to upload her blood glucose data directly to her medical team. She is also given an opportunity to join the patient advisory group that the practice is forming, and she is invited to the first meeting 3 days from now. She is given a follow-up appointment with the physician in 3 months but is reminded that scheduling is "open" so she can come back sooner, or anytime she has a need. At the end of the visit, she receives a brief online feedback survey inviting her to give the doctor and his staff feedback about the visit and what suggestions she may have to improve her experience. She notes on this form that the office staff gave her incorrect information about her group diabetes visit and so the outdated information on the patient forms was promptly corrected for future patients.

She is referred to the psychologist who is integrated with the PCMH to help assess and treat her depression. The psychologist uses brief MI along with cognitive behavioral therapy (CBT) interventions to target the depressive symptoms. MI is used at each visit to affirm, support, and encourage the patient as she makes these changes that affect her overall health. In addition, she is given a web address for an online support group for depression, and is encouraged to log on to Psych Central (www.psychcentral.com) to review its array of resources and patient tools.

A couple of days later, she develops an annoying cough and is starting to have abdominal pain, so she logs onto the patient portal and asks the office team about these symptoms. The nurse who is monitoring the portal messages contacts the physician, who decides to switch her medication from the angiotensin-converting enzyme (ACE) inhibitor she is taking to a β-blocker. He also suggests that she stop taking the ibuprofen, try substituting acetaminophen (Tylenol), and take a proton pump inhibitor, omeprazole (Prilosec), for a 2-week trial. She is asked to log on and provide an online update in 48 to 72 hours.

Two days later, her abdominal pain and her cough have resolved. Her blood pressures are in normal range, but her blood glucose levels are still running from 120 to 150 mg/dL. She is urged to continue the current course and check back online after her nutrition visit, her group visit, and her diabetes education visit.

Two weeks later, on the same dose of diabetes medication, with the benefit of her classes and counseling, she logs back in and proudly reports that her glucose levels have come back into the normal range. She returns to the office 3 months later, feeling great, in good control of her health issues, and confident with the PCMH team's approach.

curriculum can be presented as part of an intensive block rotation for family medicine and psychiatry. This study reinforces the crucial need for continued one-on-one coaching and individual feedback as part of MI training, and it recognizes that increasing the self-efficacy of the learner is essential if clinical practice changes are the goal (Miller et al., 2006). Current research is helping establish a common core of MI that includes skills, training in the spirit of MI, eliciting change talk, and rolling with resistance (Söderlund et al., 2011); however, the authors caution that the results are not strong enough in all studies due to methodological issues. A recent study by Seale and colleagues (2013), in which MI-based training was shown to have relatively small effects in residents' behavior, underscores the difficulty of instilling these methods into their clinical communication skills during this stage of their careers. Despite mixed results so far, one of the benefits of MI's application across a variety of clinical settings and its implementation by providers with a variety of professional backgrounds suggests that this approach is well-suited for the PCMH model of care (VanBuskirk and Wetherell, 2013).

With its widespread adoption in primary care settings, MI has the potential to evolve into an essential clinical tool, much like taking a history and physical, with common practice guidelines and interventions that can be taught reliably. The Motivational Interviewing Network of Trainers (MINT) has established an international group of trainers and a set of criteria for certification for MI (http://www.motivationalinterviewing.org/motivational-interviewing-training). A series of assessment tools (such as the Motivational Interviewing Treatment Integrity [MITI] scale) are being used to validate the core elements of MI and the gains that are made after training in MI (Moyers et al., 2005).

CHALLENGES AND LIMITATIONS TO MOTIVATIONAL INTERVIEWING

As research progresses and MI continues its wide use in health care settings, there are limitations about which providers should be concerned. As several review articles point out, a number of studies fail to provide enough information on the details of each intervention. The measures and assessment tools for MI are still in initial stages of development and require larger validation studies. Additionally, while strong review studies and meta-analyses in the past 5 to 10 years have illustrated significant results, the efficacy of MI and HBC for producing the desired effects in every health problem being studied is not consistent across the board. As with many methods born out of clinical practice and based on experiential, interpersonal communication, the use and applications of MI and HBC techniques in practice has outpaced the research on their validity.

KEY TREATMENT

- Motivational interviewing (MI) has been shown to have moderate to significant and clinically relevant effects on

a range of health, mental health, and substance use conditions when compared to control groups in randomized trials in recent meta-analyses and reviews (SOR: A) (Lundahl et al., 2010; Martins and McNeil, 2009; Rubak et al., 2005; VanBuskirk and Wetherell, 2013).

- Training practitioners in MI can be cost-effective and seems to work best when accompanied by 1 : 1 coaching and individual feedback to enhance behavioral rehearsal of specific clinical skills (SOR: B) (Lundahl and Burke, 2009; Miller et al., 2006).
- MI lends itself to cross-disciplinary clinical settings such as patient-centered medical homes, which are common to family medicine. (SOR: B)

References

The complete reference list is available at www.expertconsult.com.

Web Resources

Participatory Medicine and Patient Empowerment Web Resources

http://acor.org This is one of the largest, most successful patient support groups for cancer patients, a major patient-empowerment resource for anyone with any type of cancer.

http://e-patients.net This is a participatory medicine "blog" where the leaders of the participatory medicine (PM) movement frequently post key issues from the provider and the patient sector.

http://e-patients.net/e-Patients_White_Paper.pdf This is the white paper that initially lays out the principles of participatory medicine and is regarded as the founding document of the e-patient movement.

http://www.jopm.org This is the online, peer reviewed *Journal of Participatory Medicine* where ideas, editorials, narratives, and research about PM and patient empowerment are published.

http://participatorymedicine.org This is the Society for Participatory Medicine website, where you can join the community of participatory medicine advocates.

http://patients.about.com/od/empowermentbasics/a/wisepatient.htm Patient advocate Trisha Torrey provides this practical guide to becoming an empowered patient.

Motivational Interviewing Resources

http://www.buildmotivation.com/online-training.php Provides a comprehensive series of training resources for MI by Great Lakes Training, Inc., The Center for Strength Based Strategies.

http://www.motivatehealthyhabits.com/html Helpful book and website with free resources for patients and training materials by Rick Botello, MD, of the University of Rochester.

http://www.motivationalinterviewing.org This is the motivational interviewing (MI) website. It provides resources for and information on MI and includes general information about the approach, as well as links, training resources, and information on reprints and recent research.

http://www.nova.edu/gsc/forms/mi_rationale_techniques.pdf Motivational Interviewing Strategies and Techniques: Rationales and Examples is an excellent brief overview with examples of change talk and MI language by Sobell and Sobell (copyright 2008).

http://www.psychologytools.org/motivational-interviewing.html PsychologyTools is a good source for free handouts that can be used for training and teaching or with clinical populations.

http://www.samhsa.gov/co-occurring/topics/training/change.aspx Substance Abuse and Mental Health Services Administration (SAMHSA). Co-Occuring Disorders.

http://www.youtube.com/watch?v=s3MCJZ7OGRk Introduction to MI video by Bill Matulich, PhD, Motivational Interviewing Network of Trainers.

9 Interpreting the Medical Literature: Applying Evidence-Based Medicine in Practice

DOUGLAS R. SMUCKER

Key Points

- Interpreting the medical literature is a task any physician can do, particularly when using common, evidence-based summaries that are available at low or no cost.
- The studies should report statistically significant results that are applicable to the physician's population of patients and that should evaluate important patient-oriented outcomes, including potential harms.
- When potentially changing practice behavior, the physician should assess whether the evidence is from high-quality studies replicated over time.
- The medical literature is an evolving body of evidence, and each physician should develop a personal plan to keep up with important changes in medicine and strategies to answer more immediately important clinical questions at the point of care.
- Summary measures, such as the number needed to treat, can help physicians interpret research findings in a way that better informs patient care decisions.

Building Clinical Evidence from Published Research

Evidence-based medicine (EBM)—asking clear, relevant clinical questions, finding appropriate studies, critically appraising the literature, and implementing changes in practice behavior—has become an essential part of medical care. Most busy physicians do not have the time nor the background to answer critically the questions that arise in practice. Primary care physicians identify 2.4 clinical questions for every 10 encounters (Barrie and Ward, 1997), but they spend less than 15 minutes on average with each patient. Evidence about common primary care problems is accumulating at an overwhelming pace, and the broad scope of family medicine presents important challenges. Other barriers to the use of EBM include lack of evidence that is pertinent to an individual patient, quick access to information at the point of care, and potentially negative impacts on the art of medicine (McAllister et al., 1999). How can diligent physicians narrow the gap between their current behaviors and best practices?

In this chapter, hormone replacement therapy (HRT) for postmenopausal women is used as a case example to understand the evolution of medical practice based on the changing landscape of published evidence over time and to review concepts important to interpreting the medical literature. These concepts form the basis for practical EBM tools that family physicians can use to answer important clinical questions.

Evidence that supports interventions such as HRT usually begins with observational studies, including unblinded case series, case-control studies, and cohort studies, and it culminates in randomized controlled trials (RCTs) (Figure 9-1). To better understand how we arrived at the current clinical understanding of HRT and its effects on heart disease, this chapter reviews the progression of research studies and evidence over the past 40 years. A series of observational studies in the 1970s and 1980s led to regular prescribing of HRT to prevent a number of significant health conditions in postmenopausal women. Common types of observational studies are case-control studies and cohort studies.

CASE-CONTROL STUDIES

Case-control studies are often the first step in a progression of building clinical evidence because they are relatively inexpensive and rapid studies to complete. Case-control studies always look backward in time (i.e., they are

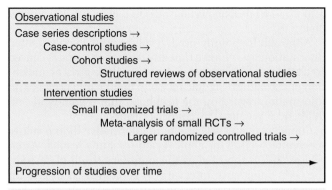

Observational studies
Case series descriptions →
    Case-control studies →
        Cohort studies →
            Structured reviews of observational studies

Intervention studies
    Small randomized trials →
        Meta-analysis of small RCTs →
            Larger randomized controlled trials →

Progression of studies over time

Figure 9-1 Common progression of research in building the strength of evidence. *RCTs*, Randomized controlled trials.

retrospective studies) to determine a statistical association between an exposure and an outcome. To complete a case-control study of the association of HRT and coronary heart disease (CHD), a researcher would identify a group of cases (i.e., women with CHD) and a group of controls (i.e., women without CHD) and look back in time to determine how many women in each group had taken HRT. The association between exposure (i.e., HRT) and outcome (i.e., CHD) in a case-control study is typically summarized by a statistical measure called an *odds ratio*. An odds ratio is an estimation of the true relative risk for the outcome in question. A common form of bias in a case-control study is recall bias: errors in accurately determining whether cases and controls had exposure to HRT in the past.

COHORT STUDIES

Cohort studies are often the next step in building the strength of evidence regarding an association between an exposure and an outcome. Cohort studies typically look forward in time (i.e., they are prospective studies) and are generally more expensive and take longer to complete than case-control studies. However, compared with case-control studies, they provide a more accurate estimate of the relative risk for women who take HRT and those who do not. A cohort study is also an observational study—one that observes outcomes in groups but does not assign participants to a particular exposure or treatment. In a cohort study of HRT and CHD, a researcher would identify a group of women taking HRT and a similar group of women who have chosen not to take HRT, and the researcher would then follow them over time and count the number of CHD events. Because outcome events may be uncommon in each group and may take many months to occur, cohort studies often require large numbers of participants and long follow-up periods to show significant differences between groups.

The primary statistical measure from a cohort study is relative risk. This is a ratio of the rate of CHD events among women who choose to take HRT divided by the rate among women who choose not to take HRT. A common form of bias in cohort studies related to prevention is the healthy user bias, when participants who choose one preventive measure (e.g., HRT) also tend to make healthier lifestyle decisions (e.g., diet, exercise) that may also prevent the measured outcome (i.e., CHD).

Beginning with case-control studies and then using larger cohort studies, early observational research showed that HRT might reduce the incidence of CHD, fractures, and colorectal cancer. These observational studies also suggested that the same therapy might cause harm, with a slightly increased risk of breast cancer, stroke, and venous thromboembolism. On balance, however, even a small positive impact of HRT on preventing CHD was thought to far outweigh the potential adverse effects of HRT.

STRUCTURED REVIEWS AND META-ANALYSIS

After a number of studies are completed, whether cohort studies or initial small RCTs, these are often reviewed and summarized in publications called *structured reviews*. Occasionally, data from a series of studies are combined using a statistical technique called *meta-analysis*, which allows increased statistical power to determine the weight of evidence from a series of studies. The use of HRT was greatly increased during the 1990s based on a number of case-control and cohort studies and on three meta-analysis studies that further suggested that HRT was protective against CHD (Pettiti, 1998).

In 1991, an editorial in the *New England Journal of Medicine* concluded that "a consensus of epidemiologic reports has demonstrated that women who are given postmenopausal estrogen therapy have a reduction of about 40% to 50% in the risk of ischemic heart disease as compared with women who do not receive such therapy" (Goldman and Tosteson, 1991). Prescribing HRT for disease prevention became a de facto standard for postmenopausal women through the 1990s.

THE POWER OF RANDOMIZED CONTROLLED TRIALS

In RCTs, study participants are randomly allocated to two or more groups and then assigned to receive an intervention such as HRT or to receive no active treatment (i.e., placebo or to continue with their usual care). RCTs greatly add to the confidence of measured results because the structure of an RCT helps to eliminate many of the inherent biases that are common in observational studies. Because participants in an RCT are randomly assigned to treatment and control groups, they are less likely to have differences in other factors that might also prevent or promote heart disease.

The decreased likelihood of systematic bias in an RCT may explain why HRT appeared to be protective in cohort studies but later proved to be harmful in large RCTs. Because RCTs have this inherent ability to decrease many important potential forms of bias (but are not immune to biases themselves), they are considered the strongest form of evidence for measuring the true association between the HRT treatment and CHD outcomes (Ebell et al., 2004). Despite decades of work, dozens of observational studies, and structured reviews that strongly suggested a protective effect of HRT for CHD, a single, large RCT trumped them all and caused a sudden reversal in physicians' prescribing behavior.

The results of the Women's Health Initiative (WHI) study, released in 2002, sent a shock wave through the medical community (WHI Writing Group, 2002). For the first time, a large, randomized trial showed that HRT—given to otherwise fairly healthy postmenopausal women—caused a statistically significant increase in CHD events. Within days of the release of the WHI primary results, many women called their physicians to decide whether they should continue with HRT. Many physicians drastically changed their prescription of HRT based on the WHI; within 9 months, prescriptions of the most popular formulation of HRT decreased by as much as 61% (Majumdar et al., 2004). Perhaps more than any other single study in modern medical history, the WHI report dramatically changed a widespread, common medical practice.

Understanding the Statistical Significance of Study Results

Reports from RCTs such as the WHI study frequently include relative risk as a summary measure of differences between the treatment and placebo groups (Table 9-1). To arrive at the relative risk, the researcher first measures the incidence rate of an outcome in each of the two study groups (i.e., treatment and placebo). The incidence rate for each group is a ratio of the number of new outcome events, such as CHD events, divided by the number of patients at risk for the outcome in that group over a specific period. In multiyear studies, the average annual incidence rate is often reported as a summary measure. In a placebo-controlled RCT, the relative risk is then calculated as a ratio of the incidence rate for the treatment group divided by the incidence rate for the placebo group (see Table 9-1).

How can a physician determine whether the reported relative risk from a study is significant enough to influence clinical decisions? Typically, the statistical significance of the summary measure is reported, which in this case is relative risk. Statistical significance is usually summarized in published studies by a p value for a given summary measure. The p value describes the statistical probability that the observed difference between the groups could have happened simply by chance alone. A p value of less than 0.05 is the arbitrary cutoff most often used for "statistical significance." A $p < 0.05$ means that there is less than a 1 in 20 (5%) probability that a difference as large as that observed would have occurred by chance alone; a $p = 0.04$ means a

1 in 25 (4%) probability; a $p = 0.06$ means a 1 in 16 probability (6%).

Although frequently used, p values provide only limited information: the chance that any difference found is caused by chance, or random error. A p value alone gives no indication of the clinical significance of a finding and provides no information regarding the likelihood that a finding of "no difference" is caused by chance or random error.

Confidence intervals are more informative than p values when interpreting the clinical value of study results. When relative risk is reported as the summary result of a study, the 95% confidence interval (CI) is often used to give an indication of the precision of the estimated relative risk. The 95% CI describes the range within which there is a 95% probability that the true relative risk (RR) is in that range. An RR of 1.0 indicates no difference. For example, if a study reported an RR of 2.5 with a 95% CI of 2.3 to 2.7, we could be reasonably certain (95% certain) that the true RR was no less than 2.3 and no greater than 2.7. Our conclusion would be that the estimated RR of 2.5 is fairly precise. However, if RR was reported as 2.5 with a 95% CI of 1.1 to 5.0, the true RR could be as low as 1.1 (almost no difference) or as high as 5.0 (a fivefold difference), a more imprecise estimate of the RR.

Confidence intervals also provide a better measure than p values of the precision for concluding that there is no difference in an RR. Any 95% CI that includes RR = 1.0 indicates that there may be no difference. However, an RR of 1.05 with a 95% CI of 0.99 to 1.11 is almost certainly a finding of no difference (i.e., a narrow CI), whereas an estimated RR = 1.4 with a 95% CI interval of 0.99 to 1.7 is much less precise (i.e., a wide CI). Even though the 95% CI contains 1.0 in the latter example, there may still be a true difference that was not able to be detected in this study.

Interpreting Study Results: Statistical and Clinical Significance

Although the WHI showed a statistically significant increase in the RR of CHD events among women who were randomly assigned to take HRT, it is important to consider the absolute difference in CHD events between the two groups to understand the strength of the association and to discuss the risk of HRT treatment with individual patients. Calculating absolute risk (in addition to RR) is a helpful way to understand the level of risk that HRT may add for a group of women who are at risk for CHD events (Table 9-2).

In the WHI study, the RR of CHD for participants who took HRT was 1.29, with a 95% CI that did not cross 1.0 (95% CI, 1.02-1.63). This figure (RR = 1.29) can generally be interpreted as HRT being associated with a 29% increase in CHD events. This summary measure was reported widely in medical journals and the mainstream press.

When reported in terms of RR, the weight of the association between HRT and CHD sounds ominous (i.e., a 29% increase). However, in terms of absolute risk attributable to HRT treatment, a less portentous picture emerges (see Table 9-2). In the WHI study, women taking HRT had an average rate of CHD events of 0.37% per year, or 37 events per 10,000 women each year, and those in the placebo

---

Table 9-1 Understanding Study Results

Typical summary rates from randomized, controlled trials:

$$\text{Incidence rate} = \frac{\text{Number of new cases of disease over a defined period}}{\text{Number of persons at risk during the period}}$$

$$\text{Relative risk (RR)} = \frac{\text{Incidence rate among the treated group}}{\text{Incidence rate among the placebo group}}$$

Summary measures that may be more meaningful for clinicians:

Attributable risk (AR), or risk difference = (Incidence rate among treated group) − (Incidence rate among placebo group)

Number needed to treat (NNT) or number needed to harm (NNH) = Reciprocal of AR, or 1/AR

Table 9-2   Examples of Summary Rates from the Women's Health Initiative Study

The following equations show how to take a summary rate commonly reported in published studies (i.e., relative risk) and calculate a summary measure (e.g., number needed to treat, number needed to harm) that may be more useful in describing the results to clinicians and patients. The example considers the average annual incidence rates and relative risk for coronary heart disease (CHD) events in the Women's Health Initiative (WHI) study on the effects of hormone replacement therapy (HRT):

Average annual incidence among HRT-treated women
= 37 CHD events/year/10,000 women

Average annual incidence among placebo-treated women
= 30 CHD events/year/10,000 women

$$\text{Relative risk of CHD} = \frac{37 \text{ CHD events}/10{,}000 \text{ women}}{30 \text{ CHD events}/10{,}000 \text{ women}} = 1.29 \text{ (adjusted)}$$

The relative risk describes a relative 29% increase in CHD events. It may be more useful to consider the absolute difference in incidence rates between the two groups to understand the magnitude of the potential risk for a given patient:

$$\text{Attributable risk (AR)} = \frac{37 \text{ CHD events}}{10{,}000 \text{ women}} - \frac{30 \text{ CHD events}}{10{,}000 \text{ women}}$$

$$= \frac{7 \text{ additional}}{10{,}000 \text{ women}} \text{ CHD events}$$

The number needed to harm (NNH) can be calculated to describe, on average, how many women must be treated for 1 year to cause one additional CHD event attributable to HRT:

$$\text{NNH} = \frac{1}{7 \text{ CHD events}/1000 \text{ women}} = \frac{10{,}000}{7} = 1430$$

Data from Women's Health Initiative (WHI) Writing Group: Risks and benefits of estrogen plus progestin in healthy postmenopausal women, *JAMA* 288:321-333, 2002.

group had an annual rate of 0.30%, or 30 events per 10,000 women each year. Although the adjusted RR of CHD is 1.29 (0.37 divided by 0.30), the attributable risk or risk difference between the two groups is 0.07% (0.37 minus 0.30). In other words, approximately seven additional cases of CHD occurred for 10,000 women using HRT during each year over the course of the study. The attributable risk of the treatment group can be summarized as the number needed to harm (NNH) or, if a study reports a beneficial effect, the number needed to treat (NNT). In this case the NNH was approximately 1430; on average, for every 1430 patients treated with HRT, one additional CHD event occurred each year (i.e., the inverse of the risk difference, 0.07, or 10,000 divided by 7) (see Table 9-2). The NNH or NNT is often a more understandable and useful summary of study outcomes when physicians and patients weigh the risks and benefits of a particular therapy (Bhandari and Haynes, 2005).

Other Keys to Interpreting Clinical Evidence

One of the major tasks in interpreting whether the results of a study should change practice is to determine whether all relevant patient-oriented outcomes were considered. For example, when considering evidence regarding the prevention of fractures, it is important to distinguish among studies that measure physiologic outcomes (e.g., serum calcium), intermediate outcomes (e.g., bone density), and patient-oriented outcomes (e.g., fractures). Whenever possible, practice decisions should be based on outcomes patients would deem important. For example, in a trial of HRT for osteoporosis, a decrease in fracture incidence would be a more convincing finding than a change in an intermediate outcome such as bone density. Likewise, all important harms (i.e., risks) and financial end points (i.e., costs and savings) should be reported and considered. In a trial of a new antiresorptive agent, the rate of esophagitis, gastritis, and esophageal perforation, along with such measures as patient satisfaction, costs, and global well-being, should all be considered in balance with any improvement in fracture incidence.

When assessing the benefits and harms of such a new treatment, appropriate competing alternatives (including no treatment at all) should be compared. Typically, such a comparison may take the form of a "balance sheet," a table comparing each intervention in terms of benefits, harms, and economic end points. Many studies are randomized, placebo-controlled trials in which some patients receive an active intervention and others receive a placebo or sham intervention. Alternatively, a study may use an active comparator, an intervention already known to be effective. Each of these approaches has pros and cons, but the most important point to remember is that just because a study shows statistical significance in a single measure, it does not mean that all appropriate patient-oriented outcomes were considered.

When a study shows no effect, the question of power is raised. Put in simple terms, power is the ability to detect the effect of an intervention; it depends on the number of patients in the study, the magnitude of effect of the intervention, and the variability of the effect from one subject to another. For some interventions, even a small effect may be important. For example, many nonpharmacologic treatments for hypertension (e.g., salt restriction) have relatively modest but important effects. Clinicians should generally be skeptical of small studies that show negative results. Examining the confidence intervals is the easiest way to assess whether the study sample was too small and therefore did not have the statistical power to detect a clinically important difference (as reflected by wide confidence intervals).

When a study is positive or shows statistically significant results, it is important to consider whether the findings are clinically significant and applicable to your practice. For example, if a study showed a drug reduces the risk of heart attack by one in a million patients, we would probably be skeptical about its clinical utility, even if the outcome was statistically significant. Likewise, a study showing that daily borscht reduces fractures in a group of Russian dockworkers may not be applicable to patient populations in the United States. Findings of a study done in a controlled research setting may differ from outcomes experienced in real-world practice. An intervention for osteoporosis requiring daily injections may be demonstrated to be efficacious among carefully selected participants in a clinical trial, but in the average practice setting its effectiveness may be more limited.

Table 9-3 Evidence-Based Medicine Skills and Techniques: Online Learning Resources

Online Learning Resource	Description
Evidence-Based Medicine Course; Michigan State University (MSU); http://omerad.msu.edu/ebm/index.html	Developed for the MSU Primary Care Faculty Development Fellowship Program, this free web-based course introduces the basic concepts of evidence-based medicine, information mastery, and critical appraisal of the medical literature.
Introduction to Evidence-Based Practice; Duke University Medical Center Library and the Health Sciences Library at the University of North Carolina at Chapel Hill; http://guides.mclibrary.duke.edu/ebmtutorial	This free online tutorial provides a basic introduction to the principles of evidence-based practice and covers skills in building good clinical questions, strategies for efficient PubMed literature searches, and critical appraisal of studies.
Centre for Evidence-Based Medicine; University of Oxford; www.cebm.net	The Oxford University CEBM offers conferences, workshops, online PowerPoint presentations, and other tools for effective practice and teaching of evidence-based medicine.
KT (Knowledge Translation) Clearinghouse; Funded by the Canadian Institute of Health Research; http://ktclearinghouse.ca	Website materials are provided by a collaborative effort between St. Michael's Hospital Toronto and the University of Toronto, Faculty of Medicine, and offer a wide range of training and tools for learning evidence-based medicine skills.
JAMAevidence; American Medical Association; http://jamaevidence.com	Free online access to content from the JAMA series *The User's Guides to the Medical Literature, The Rationale Clinical Examination,* and many other resources to learn skills in critical appraisal of the literature and evidence-based medicine techniques.

Clinicians frequently rely on the synthesis of many studies, rather than a single study, to change our practices. Such reviews can be systematic, in which rigorous attempts are made to uncover all studies, published and unpublished, in English and in other relevant languages, or they may be more limited reviews that consider only a portion of the published literature. Some use formal mathematical methods to combine the results of studies (i.e., meta-analysis), and others are qualitative and synthesize data according to an author's overall judgment. Common biases to consider related to published reviews include whether all sources of evidence were considered; how disparate results were combined; whether relevant patient-oriented outcomes were assessed; if there was adequate attention to the quality of the studies and their generalizability; and whether the authors analyzed why differences in outcomes may have occurred based on such factors as study design, population, and intervention. Published reviews, including systematic reviews and clinical guidelines, have become increasingly important tools for the busy clinician.

It is important to understand basic concepts for interpreting and applying research results (Bhandari and Haynes, 2005). Clinicians may move beyond the basic skills in searching the literature and critically appraising individual research studies by using online EBM tools and educational resources or by attending EBM training courses (Table 9-3). The ability to critique original research using a structured approach is facilitated by using widely available worksheets and tools. However, sifting through original research studies can be a tedious, impractical process for busy clinicians.

Using Evidence at the Point of Care

Finding evidence to inform clinical practice no longer requires clinicians to critically appraise individual research studies. Many practical EBM tools are available to help physicians quickly access comprehensive, expert reviews of published studies in the middle of a busy practice. Online searchable databases provide useful summaries of expert analysis of published clinical research for a wide variety of

clinical questions. Certain online resources require a paid subscription but may be available to clinicians through institutional subscriptions at a local hospital medical library or academic health center (Table 9-4). Others are free to access on the web or through applications on handheld digital devices and offer physicians a practical first step for rapidly accessing published evidence as part of daily patient care. Examples of freely available online resources include (see links and descriptions in Table 9-4):

- Systematic reviews and meta-analyses from the Cochrane Database of Systematic Reviews, or by searching PubMed using their Clinical Queries tool.
- Critically appraised topics and clinical guidelines from the National Guideline Clearinghouse.
- The *Trip* database, a clinical search engine that draws on multiple sources for systematic reviews and guidelines.

Once a clinician becomes familiar with searching online databases, identifying and reviewing published evidence can be accomplished quickly and at the point of care (Ebell, 1999). The following case describes examples of relevant information that a busy clinician can access using free online EBM resources described in Table 9-4.

CASE EXAMPLE

A 40-year-old woman sees you because she is experiencing severe vasomotor symptoms (i.e., hot flashes). These symptoms are keeping her awake at night. She had a total abdominal hysterectomy and oophorectomy 6 months ago because of enlarging uterine fibroids. She has a family history of heart disease and she is concerned about cardiovascular risks associated with HRT. What is the current evidence regarding cardiovascular risks of HRT for this patient? How should you counsel this patient?

A free search was performed using the Clinical Queries page in PubMed (www.ncbi.nlm.nih.gov/pubmed/clinical). When typing "HRT" into the Clinical Queries search box, a drop-down list of frequently entered queries automatically appears, and "menopause HRT" was chosen. The first

Table 9-4   Examples of Resources for Identifying Evidence-Based Medicine Information at the Point of Care

Information Source Access	Description	Paid Subscription Required?
DynaMed™; https://dynamed.ebscohost.com	Physician authored, clinically organized evidence summaries and expert opinion, organized in a searchable resource that can be used efficiently at the point of care to answer clinical questions.	Yes. Free trial available.
UpToDate®; www.uptodate.com/home/product	Synthesis of evidence and expert opinion on topics in multiple specialties, organized to provide practical answers to clinical questions at the point of care.	Yes
Cochrane Reviews; www.cochrane.org/cochrane-reviews	The Cochrane Collaboration is an international, nonprofit, independent organization that has produced and disseminated thousands of highly detailed systematic reviews of health care interventions. Seen by many as the gold standard of systemic evidence-based reviews.	Free searches and reviews of abstracts. Access to full reports requires subscription.
Family Physicians Inquiries Network (FPIN); www.fpin.org	Virtual learning community with point-of-care answers to clinical questions using structured, critical reviews of the literature, with a strong focus on topics relevant to family practice and other primary care specialties.	Yes
PubMed Clinical Queries; www.ncbi.nlm.nih.gov/pubmed/clinical	The Clinical Queries section of PubMed, a search engine for MEDLINE provided by the National Library of Medicine, conducts focused searches of published clinical studies and systematic reviews. A free Clinical Queries tutorial is available online.	Free
National Guideline Clearinghouse; www.guideline.gov	This public resource for evidence-based clinical practice guidelines is organized by the U.S. Federal Agency for Healthcare Research and Quality.	Free
Trip Database; www.tripdatabase.com	A meta-search engine that retrieves information from multiple evidence-based resources and databases.	Free

article listed from this simple search was a structured review of HRT and cardiovascular risk, including studies published since the 2002 WHI study (Hodis and Mack, 2014). The search and review of this article took approximately 5 minutes. The authors' conclusions include the following statement:

The totality of the data show that HRT decreases coronary heart disease and overall mortality when started in women who are less than 60 years old and/or less than 10 years post-menopausal, providing a "window-of-opportunity."

A second search using the free online database *Trip* (www.tripdatabase.com) with the keywords "hormone replacement therapy menopause" resulted in a list of clinical guidelines. Limiting the search to "Guidelines/USA" and scanning the first few listed titles showed a 2012 guideline and position statement of the North American Menopause Society and a link to a free online copy of the guideline through the National Guideline Clearinghouse (North American Menopause Society, 2012). This systemic review and guideline summarizes both the risks and benefits of HRT. Search of the *Trip* database and review of this guideline took approximately 4 minutes. Summary recommendations of the guideline include the following statement:

Women experiencing premature menopause are at increased risk of osteoporosis and, possibly, cardiovascular disease, and they often experience more intense symptoms than do women reaching menopause at the median age. Therefore, HRT generally is advised for

these young women until the median age of menopause when treatment should be reassessed.

This case outlines how a physician with access to searchable databases can quickly review an array of clinical evidence and published guidelines. Such resources are based on systematic evaluations of evidence and can provide clinicians with practical guidance at the point of care. EBM, information mastery, and the application of knowledge at the point of care remain works in progress. By developing a basic understanding of these resources and tools, physicians' care for patients can be more effective, safe, and efficient.

> ### Key Points
>
> - Do not assume that statistical significance is the same as clinical significance.
> - Do not rely on pharmaceutical representatives or experts who may be biased in their presentation of information.
> - Consider the potential harms and economic effects of an intervention.
> - Do not assume that results even from a well-done study are applicable to your population of patients.
> - Do not fail to use the many comprehensive sources of evidence-based information.

References

The complete reference list is available at www.expertconsult.com.

Web Resources

See Tables 9-3 and 9-4.

10 *Information Technology*

DAVID KUNSTMAN

Introduction

Information technology in medicine is a topic that has moved from concept and convenience to a critical operational and patient care need. The trend toward this received a big push in 2009 with the introduction of the Health Information Technology for Economic and Clinical Health (HITECH) Act. This act set aside $27 billion in incentives through Medicare and Medicaid for health care organizations to achieve "meaningful use" in the use of their electronic health records (EHRs).

Health care providers have been challenged to incorporate data entry skills into the patient care visit. They have also reaped benefits from the information and knowledge gained from the analysis of that data. Improvements in device technology, clinical work flows, and interface design are continually improving these efforts.

Patients are now witnessing the effects of this technology revolution from within our formal health care structure and from multiple other sources. The Internet remains a powerful tool for health information, but the introduction of the app store in 2008 and smartphone technology has pushed this into everyday life, including the examination room.

Electronic Health Records

EHRs were first discussed in the 1970s. Since then, there has been an evolution of the electronic storage of patient medical information, and at its heart is structured data. The entry and organization of this data is critical to the success of every process going forward. Each data element has a location, and data obtained from individuals or devices populate values to this location. A strong data governance structure is essential to maintain this order. Without governance, individuals will seek their own solutions, and the downstream benefits of structured data will be lost.

This governance group should look toward the needs of the organization and consumers of data when determining data architecture. Each request for a new data field should come with a discussion about where the data will ultimately be used. Examples of areas to include in this discussion are coding, compliance, business office, legal, clinic operations, clinical research, and, ultimately, patient needs.

The ability to enter values into the determined fields needs to be reasonable and practical so that individuals will choose to do the right thing. Tools to aid this may include graphical, tabular, or audible entry. Digital imaging and video are also becoming popular methods of entry.

One emerging technology that will aid entry is called *natural language processing*. This has the ability to analyze unstructured data similar to the original progress notes of years past. The notes are then parsed into specific data elements for inclusion in the electronic record.

ELECTRONIC HEALTH RECORD USABILITY

Adoption of the use of EHRs in a large part is affected by usability, or being "user friendly." Simply defined, this is the effectiveness, efficiency, and satisfaction with which specific users can achieve a specific set of tasks in a particular environment (Schoeffel, 2003). Usability was felt to be a major factor in the slow adoption of EHRs in the United States. In 2009, the Healthcare Information and Management Systems Society (HIMSS) defined a set of key principles behind EHR usability (HIMSS EHR Usability Task Force, 2009).

- Simplicity of design: Show the information minimally necessary to accomplish a task.
- Naturalness: Allow the ability for the user to be automatically familiar with the application.
- Consistency: Enable predictability of behaviors, layouts, and concepts between screens and work flows.
- Minimizing cognitive load: Present information needed to make the correct decision and desired outcome easy to perform.
- Efficient interactions: Minimize the number of steps it takes to complete the task.
- Forgiveness and feedback: Allow the user to explore without fear of bad outcomes through the use of feedback.
- Effective use of language: Provide language that is concise and unambiguous.
- Effective information presentation: Make good use of data density, color, and readability.

■ Preservation of context: Avoid distractions common with screen changes and dialog boxes.

OPTIMIZATION

The complexity of patient care and EHR software make it extremely difficult for all clinical operation processes to be taught effectively on day 1. In addition, software is constantly evolving, and new clinical needs arise on a frequent and sometimes emergent basis. Optimization of EHR use becomes essential maintenance. Users of the system will need regular reminders of software processes, especially those that are infrequently used. New processes will need to be introduced as well. Communication may take several forms. The training team becomes helpful for this, as does the use of advanced users in a train-the-trainer model. Written or electronic materials in a push or pull model may also be needed for those users requiring asynchronous learning.

MEANINGFUL USE

Meaningful Use is a Medicare and Medicaid EHR incentive program to provide financial incentives for "meaningful use" of a certified EHR. As of June 2014, 479,941 eligible professionals and 4741 hospitals (Medicaid and Medicare) have enrolled in the Meaningful Use program. The Meaningful Use program is comprised of three stages as summarized in Table 10-1 (HealthIT.gov, 2014). To receive incentives, attestation to specific criteria needs to begin by 2014, and the payments are made over a number of years (HealthIT.gov, 2014). The last year for incentives in the Medicare group is in 2015 and in 2021 for the Medicaid group.

COMPUTERIZED DECISION SUPPORT

Computerized decision support (CDS) is a key component of the Meaningful Use program. It relies on structured data within the EHR to output knowledge to the organization or consumer. The EHR software analyzes data and applies rules to identify patterns or critical values deserving of attention. A key concept here is that the correct data is presented to the correct audience in the correct format at the correct time.

An organization does need to be careful and balance the amount of clinical decision support with the operational work flows. Too many alerts, or "alert fatigue," may counteract the benefits of the intended support. A governance body tasked with monitoring the amount and perceived importance level of support is quite helpful here.

PATIENT PORTALS

Stage II of the Meaningful Use program calls for increased use of patient portals. These portals provide access to things such as messaging to providers, refill requests, appointment requests, notifications, and in some cases, full medical record access. As of 2013, it is estimated that 28% to 40% of patients have access to this technology. There has been concern by providers, but multiple organizations have now started providing patients direct viewing of their entire medical record with good results. The use of these patient portals not only gives patients more information about their health but allows them to participate in their health care. The use of questionnaires and direct entry of medical history is an area that is evolving. Not only may this be done manually, but device makers are starting to incorporate this technology into consumer products such as scales, blood pressure cuffs, and glucometers.

In a multinational study of 9100 patients by Accenture, 41% of U.S. patients said they would be willing to switch doctors to gain access to their records. Eighty-four percent of those patients felt they should have access to their records while only 36% of providers shared this view (Accenture, 2013).

TECHNOLOGY CONSIDERATIONS

With the advance of EHR, electronic means of obtaining data became essential. Equipment that was designed to provide a paper output now needs to also include a method to interface with EHRs. Examples of this technology include cardiac monitoring, radiologic and visible light imaging, audiometric screening, and diabetes monitoring.

Table 10-1 Stages of Meaningful Use Incentive Program

Stage 1: Data Capture and Sharing Meaningful Use Criteria Focus on:	Stage 2: Advance Clinical Processes Meaningful Use Criteria Focus on:	Stage 3: Improve Outcomes Meaningful Use Criteria Focus on:
Electronically capturing health information in a standardized format	More rigorous health information exchange (HIE)	Improving quality, safety, and efficiency, leading to improved health outcomes
Using that information to track key clinical conditions	Increased requirements for e-prescribing and incorporating laboratory results	Decision support for national high-priority conditions
Communicating that information for care coordination processes	Electronic transmission of patient care summaries across multiple settings	Patient access to self-management tools
Initiating the reporting of clinical quality measures and public health information	More patient-controlled data	Access to comprehensive patient data through patient-centered HIE
Using information to engage patients and their families in their care		Improving population health

Adapted from *EHR Incentives & Certification: How to Attain Meaningful Use.* HealthIT.gov; page modified April 10, 2014. http://www.healthit.gov/providers-professionals/how-attain-meaningful-use.

In evaluating this equipment, not only is it essential that the interface exists, but that interface must be compatible with EHRs. Cost considerations need to include the device itself, device maintenance fees, estimated years of service, initial interface fees, and maintenance of that interface. A good first step is to inquire with the EHR vendor about device compatibility. A centralized process for coordinating purchases of this equipment is also quite helpful.

Technical teams will also need to consider the storage of this digital information going forward. This consideration will include location, format, size requirements, and ability to review or recover the data. For that technology preceding electronic interfaces, a robust scanning solution must also be included.

Mobile Technology

By some measures, smartphone owners check their phones 150 times/day (Kvedar, 2013). A quarter of Americans in one survey say they would trust a symptom checker website or mobile application as much as they would their doctor (PMLive, 2013). Another study of 2000 patients and covering 20 disease states found that 90% of patients would accept the offer of a mobile app, while only 66% of respondents would accept prescription medicine from their doctor (Royal Philips Electronics, 2012).

Mobile technology applications are largely unregulated. Those applications that either control a regulated medical device or turn a smartphone into a regulated medical device may soon fall under the jurisdiction of the U.S. Food and Drug Administration (FDA). Several websites exist to give guidance to clinicians and patients about these applications (e.g., mobihealthnews at http://mobihealthnews.com and iMedicalApps at http://www.imedicalapps.com).

A survey conducted by the University of Pennsylvania found that the top eight mobile medical applications for 2012 were

1. Epocrates Essentials
2. MedCalc
3. Medscape Mobile
4. DynaMed
5. VisualDx
6. Micromedex
7. Skyscape
8. Diagnosaurus DDx

These applications are excellent references to clinicians and may also benefit patients. Physicians may consider "prescribing" applications to patients for uses of therapy, reference, or tracking. When considering applications to suggest to patients, consider the patient's likelihood to use, the developer of the application, and ratings that are often available on the developer or app store site (Table 10-2). It is best practice to try the application yourself when feasible.

Engaging Patients

Stage 2 of the Meaningful Use program will make more of the medical record available directly to the patient in the

Table 10-2 Medical Apps for Patients

Condition	App	Developer Website
Nutrition and diet	Lose It!	www.loseit.com
	SparkPeople	www.sparkpeople.com
	CalorieKing	www.calorieking.com
	MyFitnessPal	www.myfitnesspal.com
Stress management	Stress Check Pro	www.azumio.com
	Breathe2Relax	www.t2health.org
	Insight Timer	https://insighttimer.com
Exercise	MyFitnessPal	www.myfitnesspal.com
	Endomondo	www.endomondo.com
	Runtastic	www.runtastic.com
General knowledge	WebMD	www.webmd.com

form of the problem list. Although the introduction of the computer to the examination room was a recent phenomenon for many, the computer must now become an interactive learning tool. A few considerations for this include:

1. Position the computer between the health care provider and the patient so the patient may view information along with the provider. Pivot arms on monitors will greatly improve this interaction.
2. Keep patients first. Always greet patients before logging in. At the proper time, introduce the computer as a tool in their medical care.
3. Assure patients about the safety of their data and perhaps make specific mention about logging off to protect their data.
4. Position print devices convenient to the patient flow or alternatively encourage the patient to be involved in a patient portal.

Ultimately, patients may interact more directly with their charts and update information. Beginning to educate them about the problem list in the examination room may serve as a good primer for this.

Security

The Health Insurance Portability and Accountability Act (HIPAA) of 1996 ensured individual rights of patients and added specific privacy and security protections. The scope of this was expanded in 2013 along with the breech notification requirements under the HITECH Act of 2009. Providers play an important part in assuring the continued confidentiality of the patient record. Patient information may be shared for the purposes of treatment, but a few key points to be aware of follow:

- Understand what is protected health information (PHI) and what may be disclosed and authorization that may be needed.
- Provide safeguards such as individual passwords, private areas for viewing PHI, and policies and procedures for the release of PHI.
- Access only that information that is required to perform your job.
- Never discuss PHI in public areas or present PHI to individuals who are not involved in the care of the patient.

- Report any suspected breeches of PHI to your privacy officer immediately.

More information about privacy practices may be found at the U.S. Department of Health and Human Services website (www.hhs.gov/ocr/privacy/index.html). The Meaningful Use incentive program also has additional information about Privacy and Security at its website (www.healthit .gov/providers-professionals/ehr-privacy-security).

Conclusion

We are just beginning to see the impact of health information technology as we use the data stored now in EHRs and other databases. Beyond data acquisition, we derive knowledge and ultimately wisdom. The attention to structure and usability becomes essential to maintain integrity and trust.

Usability remains a top priority for health care providers and patients, and we should not forget the critical and personal interactions we have in the clinical setting. We should strive for seamless acquisition and understanding of data as we move this technology forward.

Finally, data security must guide our behavior and interactions. As health care providers, we are trusted with the most intimate details of our patient's lives and we must not breach that trust.

References

The complete reference list is available at www.expertconsult.com.

Web Resources

See Table 10-2.

Suggested Reading

Hoyt RE, Yoshihashi A, editors: *Medical Informatics: A Practical Guide for Healthcare and Information Technology Professionals*, ed 4, Raleigh, NC, 2010, Lulu.com.

11 Clinical Problem Solving

PHILIP M. DILLER and ROBERT T. ELLIS

Introduction

Practicing family medicine is a continual confrontation of problems besetting the human condition, and a goal for many family physicians is to become a master problem solver. Having a front row seat to the joys and tragedies, the drama and the misery that patients experience through the life cycle provides ample opportunity to gain mastery.

The purpose of this chapter is to outline a systematic approach to problem solving commonly used by family physicians. Before presenting the model for clinical problem solving, we review the context of family medicine practice that shapes problem solving by family physicians. By taking a systematic approach to solve problems and using point-of-care information resources, the physician can minimize or at least control some of the uncertainty common in practice.

There are four primary tasks to solve clinical problems: (1) begin to understand the problem in clinical terms, (2) define and select the problem or problems to address, (3) discuss and create treatment and solution options and eventually selecting an agreed-on management plan, and (4) monitoring response to treatment. The model for clinical problem solving can be used as a guide to improve the process and identify the challenges associated with the process to prevent errors. The intent of this chapter is to describe how to move toward mastery as a problem solver, and in turn, achieve desired patient outcomes of care.

The Principles of Family Medicine Define the Context for Solving Clinical Problems

The principles characterizing family medicine (Green et al., 2004) that shape the context for clinical problem solving include (1) deep understanding of whole person care, (2) provision of comprehensive care, (3) first contact care ensuring patient access, (4) continuity of care, and (5) commitment to team-based care.

WHOLE PERSON CARE

Patient problems presenting to family physicians are legion; anything having to do with the human condition can be encountered by family physicians. The family physician must first be a student of humanity and have a working knowledge of the five dimensions of being human: (1) physical, (2) psychological, (3) social, (4) spiritual, and (5) chronological (life cycle). Each dimension can be problem generating and require a treatment or solution. Some problems can be very simple, such as a sore throat that is easily diagnosed, and have a fairly standard course of treatment. At the other end of the spectrum a patient could come in with a congestive heart failure but then live on the street, have no insurance coverage, and have poorly controlled mental health problems. Thus patients can present with a multiplicity of problems, and these problems often are interactive, making it harder to control any one of them with singular solutions. As a result, family physicians need to have a fairly broad-based approach to solving problems, and this requires a very big search net in seeking to understand the nature of the problems.

COMPREHENSIVE CARE

Applying a taxonomy of visit types can also aid in understanding problems commonly seen in family medicine. Patients can be seen by family physicians for acute, self-limited illness, chronic disease, mental health problems, maternity care, prevention and wellness issues, and administrative needs such as disability evaluations or return-to-work notes. In addition, patients could have end-of-life concerns, including nursing home placement or a need for palliative care or hospice services. Thus the patient problems addressed by family doctors are many because of the multiple human dimensions, but also because of the breadth of comprehensive services offered by family physicians in the health system.

FIRST CONTACT CARE

Family physicians are on the frontlines and are often the entry point for patients who seek care, and as a result, problems present early in the course of an illness. Patients present with symptoms when the disease is not defined, is undifferentiated, and the illness is yet to be organized for the patient. This aspect of seeing patients in an undifferentiated state, when a physician only has a few facts or objective signs of disease, presents challenges and underscores how widespread uncertainty is when trying to define the problem. Family physicians need to be comfortable with uncertainty and to understand that time is an ally in sorting out patient problems. Family physicians also have to be versed in probabilities and consider likelihood ratios for what signs and symptoms mean. Such information can assist in deciding whether an intervention is needed or if a watch-and-wait approach is appropriate.

The family physician provides access to care in a multitude of settings, including home, office, hospital, nursing home, or even a factory. Each setting brings contextual data into play, and understanding the setting or the limitations of the setting can be helpful in solving patient problems. Resources available to the patient to be included in the solution or treatment plan may be setting-specific.

CONTINUITY OF CARE

Family physicians create longitudinal relationships with patients and as a consequence gain valuable prior knowledge of patients used to individualize problem solving. The accumulated knowledge of patients leads to efficiency in understanding patients' problems and then designing treatment solutions. For example, patients with chronic obstructive pulmonary disease (COPD) may have baseline respiratory distress but having adapted are reasonably comfortable with an oxygen saturation of 89%, and when they come in with a little additional distress, a decision needs to be made to hospitalize or closely watch them as outpatients. Having had prior episodes and knowing exactly how the patient responds and what is necessary, physicians are much more comfortable in that area of uncertainty about what the next steps should be in the care of the patient. Contrast this with an emergency department physician who has no prior knowledge of this patient, discovers an oxygen saturation of 88%, is concerned with how distressed the patient looks, and decides to admit the patient to the hospital. Understanding the problem as well as the context for that unique patient is fundamental to making patient-centered clinical decisions in practice.

TEAM-BASED CARE

Finally, an additional context factor for family physicians is the health system, a complex and evolving health environment in which different treatment options or innovative care models can be put into place. Increasingly, care managers are part of the emerging primary care delivery team included in the patient-centered medical home experience. The family physician also needs to be aware of what resources are in the health system, and the new and emerging innovations in care that can lead to potentially better patient outcomes.

Tasks and Steps Used by Family Physicians to Solve Clinical Problems

Figure 11-1 illustrates a systematic step-by-step approach to problem solving. There are four primary tasks, with each task having specific steps: (1) beginning to understand the problem in clinical terms, (2) defining the problem(s) to address, (3) formulating solutions and treatment, and (4) monitoring the response or testing the solution based on actual results. Family physicians perform these tasks in solving clinical problems. This problem-solving approach encompasses many of the fundamental steps of doctoring, including data gathering, clinical reasoning, defining the diagnosis, considering prognosis, generating a treatment plan, and monitoring the response to treatment.

BEGINNING TO UNDERSTAND PROBLEM(S) IN CLINICAL AND CONTEXTUAL TERMS

The first part of the *data-gathering step* is to take the traditional disease-focused approach: listening to the patient's chief concern or complaint, taking a medical history, doing a physical examination, and requesting needed laboratory or imaging data. This traditional approach is structured to elucidate physical diagnoses. Simultaneously, the family physician is also seeking focused data about the patient as a person, and these data include information of the five human dimensions. Patient-as-person data can be a source of nonphysical problems and influence possible solutions to the problems.

The chronological, or seasons-of-life, dimension is readily appreciated during the encounter and is valuable to note because the cause of the patient's symptoms may be age-related. For example, the causes of constipation in a 4-month-old infant are very different from a middle-age person who has constipation of recent onset. The same symptom is present, but there are very different diagnostic possibilities because of the patient's age.

The psychological dimension includes not just mental health diagnoses but also personality, intelligence, attention, ability to process information, mood, and emotional states such as fear and anxiety that are part of the conversation. Any of these can be source of problems for the patient or influence a solution.

A family physician actively scans the patient's social dimension for potential problems. Social dimension is often divided into five different areas (Berkman and Kawachi, 2000): (1) relationships at the individual level, such as a person's family unit or source of social support; (2) the work environment; (3) social status (e.g., educational level); (4) socioeconomic position (e.g., poverty); and (5) community relationships and norms. All can be a source of problems but can also set the stage for potential solutions. Such information is often critical in creating effective solutions to patient's problems.

The spiritual dimension can also be a source of problems and potential solutions for patients. Patients can attribute diseases as punishment from God or as a struggle with

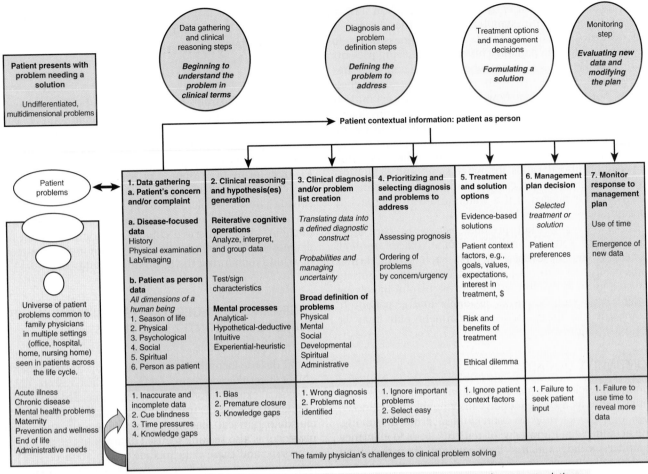

Figure 11-1 Steps family physicians take to define clinical problems and create patient-centered treatment solutions.

purpose and meaning in life. Alternatively, patients may draw on strong spiritual beliefs or a religious community for solace and support.

In addition to these five human dimensions, the role the person plays as patient can also be a source of problems. For example, the ideal patient is expected to follow through on treatment plans, but nonadherence to the plan is a common problem in practice. Trying to understand the factors causing noncompliance become part of the physician's search and demand a solution if patient adherence is to be achieved.

Family physicians elicit and search for "data" related to the physical diagnosis, the various human dimensions, the role of the patient to understand the multitude of problems, and also to generate an active problem list.

The second step after data gathering is *clinical reasoning*. In reality, this goes on simultaneously while gathering the data. The physician conducts specific mental operations that initially include sorting and sifting, analyzing, and interpreting the data. Signs and symptoms have different meanings diagnostically and prognostically (Wilson, 1926). The physician often uses two broad categories of mental operations on the gathered data (Croskerry, 2009). The first is an analytical or a systematic algorithmic approach to hypothesis generation. Questions are ordered sequentially, with the patient's answers directing the next line of questions. In a very systematic way, the physician is sifting and sorting information as it comes forth to get to a likely answer to the hypothesis. The second broad mental operation

category is intuitive processing. Here the physician is using prior experience and pattern recognition to sort information in a much more efficient, rapid manner. Intuitive processing is much quicker, but it also has a higher likelihood of error.

One aspect of sorting and sifting data and hypothesis generation is the value of that information in raising or lowering the likelihood of a specific diagnosis. In clinical practice, knowing likelihood ratios of specific signs (McGee, 2012), symptoms, and tests (or a combinations of these, for example, severity of illness scales) (Kellet, 2008) is valuable in defining the probability of a disease and its outcomes. In addition to the likelihood ratios, family physicians are assisted in defining clinical problems by knowing the prevalence and incidence of a specific disease in the community. Such information may not be readily available, but, for example, based on the season of year, monitoring the emergence of communicable disease (e.g., Centers for Disease Control and Prevention [CDC] flu map website) and hearing of patients with flu in the community, a physician's suspicions for flu are elevated when a patient comes in with runny nose, cough, fever, and diffuse body aches. Such information helps with generating probabilities in the same way Will Pickles' work on the incubation periods of certain infectious diseases (Pickles, 1939) allows a physician encountering a jaundiced patient to increase the likelihood of a diagnosis of infectious hepatitis by knowing when the patient was exposed to another person with that condition.

DEFINING THE PROBLEM(S) TO ADDRESS

The next step includes making a *clinical diagnosis, defining the problem(s)*, and *creating a problem list*. Diagnosis is a translation of symptoms and signs into a medical disease category or classification scheme. Diagnosis is the naming of the clinical problem based on the patient's signs and symptoms. Diagnosis is laden with meaning, assigning a pathobiological process responsible for the patient's signs and symptoms. The signs and symptoms understood in pathobiological terms begin to demystify and move the process to a specific prognosis and suggest treatment options.

For the family physician, patient problems do not end with a physical diagnosis. Glenn (1984) reminded us that diagnosis for family physicians is much broader and includes problems of the kind alluded to earlier of psychological, social, and spiritual dimensions of being human. Neglecting these problems in the treatment of disease often leads to poor outcomes because of the interaction of problems that permeate the patient's life. An important aspect of helping a patient is to classify these other problems as well and recognize how they are shaping the experience of disease (illness).

An important part of the discussion in generating an active problem list is to gain agreement with the patient on what the problems are and which ones are the most important. Getting to agreement on patient problems (and their treatment) influences the outcomes of care (Stewart, 1995).

The next step in clinical problem solving is *prioritizing and selecting the diagnosis and the problems to address*. This is really not as simple as it sounds, and it is an important part of the process because in practice, faced with multiple problems, the physicians must decide what to address first and in what order (Balint, 1964). Some solutions or treatments are easy, such as writing for a medication, whereas others require much effort by the patient and physician (e.g., behavior changes). A physician's expertise or comfort level influences what problem a physician or patient may choose.

Another factor is the level of concern or urgency to the problems. The patient with suicidal ideation in crisis needs immediate response to treatment, as opposed to somebody who has a nagging fatigue and back pain due to the repetitive stresses of life who may have depression; the sense of urgency is different. A patient may have strong feelings about what is most important and that influences what problem is addressed first. All are part of the conversation on deciding and prioritizing what problems need to be addressed.

The prognosis of the problem also shapes how the physician orders and prioritizes what problem should be addressed. A new diagnosis of cancer, for example, changes a person's life trajectory in the short term as well as the long term. With a new cancer diagnosis, the focus of attention for that patient carries heightened concern and anxiety about what the diagnosis portends for the future and how the cancer is going to impact his or her ability to function in his or her various work or family roles, and such considerations shape the nature of the treatment plan. Thus knowing the prognosis of specific conditions and what their natural history could be with or without treatment is included in formulating solutions and treatment options.

FORMULATING SOLUTIONS AND TREATMENT OPTIONS

Once the problem is understood, defined, and prioritized and agreement is achieved between the physician and patient, the physician and patient can then begin to explore treatment and solution options. Increasingly the physician takes an evidence-based approach to deciding treatment options (Sackett et al., 1991). Some treatments have a strong evidence base with clear likelihood of response to treatment. In practicing evidence-based medicine, the physician often uses point-of-care resources to help guide care decisions. In addition, there are also patient decision aids (O'Connor, 2001) available to help patients understand the risks and benefits of treatment. A selected set of electronic resources is shown in Table 11-1.

Table 11-1   Point of Care Resources Available to Assist with Clinical Problem Solving

Resource	Description	Type	Free
5-Minute Clinical Consult	Quick and concise clinical reference: not a lot of details but good for a quick overview of medical conditions	App, Web	No
AHRQ ePSS	Easy-to-use USPSTF guidelines: enter patient demographics and get patient-specific recommendations	App, Web	Yes
Epocrates	Popular drug reference	App	Yes
MedCalc	Free reference of more than 300 formulas, scoring, scale, and classification systems	App	Yes
MediMath Medical Calculator	More than 140 of the most important medical calculators and scoring tools	App	Yes
Mediquations Medical Calculator	More than 230 formulas and scoring systems	App	No
Medscape	Popular decision support tool that includes medical news, clinical information, drug information, procedure videos, and medical calculators	App, Web	Yes
Shots by STFM	Easy-to-use immunization program based on CDC guidelines; includes vaccine info and schedules if using combination shots	App	Yes
Skyscape	Decision-support tool that includes clinical information, drug information, and medical calculators	App	Yes
UpToDate	Comprehensive evidence-based resource; requires a subscription	App, Web	No

AHRQ, Agency for Healthcare Research and Quality; *CDC*, Centers for Disease Control and Prevention; *ePSS*, Electronic Preventive Services Selector; *STFM*, Society of Teachers of Family Medicine; *USPSTF*, U.S. Preventive Services Task Force.

In addition to knowing the evidence for specific treatments, patient context factors also impact the treatment plan options. Patient expectations, values, and willingness to pursue specific treatment plans come into play (Janz and Becker, 1984). Common to family medicine practice are patients who do not like to take medications and would prefer to use alternative approaches to treat physical problems. Thus, increasingly, family physicians should be knowledgeable of the integrative medicine approaches that can be used to complement some of the medical approaches to create a management plan that patients will accept.

Patient context factors also play into modifying the treatment plan in other ways. Specifically, concern for quality-of-life issues may want the physician to steer away from aggressive treatment plans that actually lead to lower quality of life. Patients have specific goals they want to accomplish in a certain period of time, and they will delay following through on some medical interventions before they have achieved these other goals. Even though there may be a very strong and compelling evidence base for a specific treatment plan, patients make choices based on other values and goals.

In addition, ethical issues arise in practice and shape and influence decisions. If a person is trying to weigh the benefits of treatment versus harm, and if one available treatment option will cause more harm than another, a patient may decide to avoid the harmful approach even if the patient knows there may be increased risk of premature mortality. Family physicians often handle ethical dilemmas that arise in practice as part of any management plan or decisions patients face.

All this information involving the treatment options is used to select the specific management plan on which the physician and patient agree to move forward. Including patient preferences is an important element in selecting that management plan.

MONITORING THE RESPONSE: TESTING THE RESPONSE BASED ON ACTUAL RESULTS

Monitoring the response to treatment is an important part of the problem-solving process because a plan ultimately must produce the desired results—a good outcome. When a patient presents early in the course of an illness, it is often not clear exactly what the problem is, but with the passage of time more data come forth and the physician can better understand the problem and adjust the treatment plan. In a similar way the response to treatment in time may help clarify what the problem actually might be. For example, a patient comes in with dyspepsia and the physician starts a medication for acid disease. In follow-up, the physician can monitor whether the patient responded to treatment and is able to confirm that the diagnosis is acid dyspepsia. That response may lead to evaluate for *Helicobacter pylori* infection and, in turn, offer treatment to eradicate the problem.

In monitoring the response to treatment, the physician and patient begin to gain further understanding of the problem, and the physician specifically gains practical experiential knowledge of what works and what does not. Time will tell if the problem was understood and defined correctly and if the treatment was effective. In this way, monitoring the response to treatment is a source of learning and helps with future problem solving.

Challenges to Clinical Problem Solving

The data-gathering step can be associated with potential errors that lead to poor problem solving. For example, having inaccurate or incomplete data leads to a limited understanding of the problem and, in turn, to ineffective solutions. Another factor related to data gathering is insufficient clinical knowledge to collect key data and ask important questions. The pressures of practice can limit the time allowed to gather information. As a result, the history may be a little bit briefer, the physical examination may be incomplete, and as a result, important data are not obtained.

Clinical reasoning errors using intuitive processing may lead a physician to prematurely close the search for a diagnosis; quick judgments of the problem based on prior pattern recognition may not be reliable. Knowledge gaps could also impact clinical reasoning abilities with analytical processing. If a physician's knowledge is incomplete, then a very limited algorithmic or analytical approach will be used compared with another physician who has a very detailed knowledge base and can go very deep in questioning to clarify the patient's story. Finally, clinical reasoning can be influenced by faulty assumptions (biases) and, as a consequence, lead to flawed diagnostic impressions and perception of problems.

In prioritizing and selecting problems, it is possible the physician can choose to ignore important problems because they are more difficult to manage than others. The physician may select easy problems rather than tackle those that are more frustrating and difficult to address. For example, changes in behavior to help people to lose weight for hypertension are much harder to accomplish than writing a prescription for hypertension medication. Depending on the degree of difficulty and resources available, patients may choose not to address certain problems.

In designing treatment options and solutions, physicians may ignore patient context factors, such as patient-driven goals or gaining agreement with the plan. Physicians may take a paternalistic approach and exclude patient input in the management plan. Sometimes paternalism is needed, but other times physicians create solutions not acceptable to patients. Patients may simply feign agreement and leave knowing they will not follow through.

Finally, in monitoring response to the management plan the physician may fail to pursue or seek new data and/or not try to understand the problem in a new way. The physician may not recognize how time can help in confirming whether the problems are correct or whether the treatment plan is working.

Conclusion

Effective clinical problem solving occurs when a family physician uses a systematic approach. This chapter offers a systematic approach to problem solving that outlines the specific tasks and describes specific steps to arrive at effective solutions. Patient involvement is critical throughout the whole process. Family physicians who debrief their problem solving skills and identify areas for improvement in time become master problem solvers, and in turn become trusted advisors to their patients. In the current environment of outcomes-based medicine, becoming a master clinical problem solver—creating care for the unique patient that leads to positive outcomes—cannot be overly emphasized.

References

The complete reference list is available at www.expertconsult.com.

12 Integrative Medicine

MARY P. GUERRERA

Key Points

- Terms and definitions that describe complementary and alternative medicine (CAM) are diverse and evolving.
- Integrative medicine combines CAM and conventional medicine.

The level of integration of conventional and CAM therapies is growing. That growth generates the need for tools or frameworks to make decisions about which therapies should be provided or recommended, about which CAM providers to whom conventional medical providers might refer patients, and the organizational structure to be used for the delivery of integrated care. The committee believes that the overarching rubric that should be used to guide the development of these tools should be the goal of providing comprehensive care that is safe and effective, that is collaborative and interdisciplinary, and that respects and joins interventions from all sources. (IOM, 2005)

Many countries now recognize the need to develop a cohesive and integrative approach to health care that allow governments, health care practitioners and, most importantly, those who use health care services, to access T&CM [Traditional & Complementary Medicine] in a safe, respectful, cost-efficient and effective manner. A global strategy to foster its appropriate integration, regulation and supervision will be useful to countries wishing to develop a proactive policy towards this important—and often vibrant and expanding—part of health care. (WHO, 2013)

In these tumultuous times of health care reform, family physicians find themselves on a threshold: a place of great professional promise as well as uncertainty. Will they step through this historic doorway with newfound meaning and professional identity? Will they create new practice models, new ways of delivering care, and new methods of collaborating across the spectrum of healing practices and health professionals? Work is already underway with initiatives such as patient-centered medical homes (PCMHs) and accountable care organizations (ACOs). In addition, the field of family medicine has taken the lead and is currently pioneering work bringing complementary and alternative medicine (CAM) and integrative medicine into residency training and clinical care (Benn et al., 2009; Lebensohn et al., 2012; Locke et al., 2013).

How will these relatively new and evolving areas of health care optimize and revitalize the practice of family medicine? This chapter describes these new fields, assesses proposals by U.S. medical organizations, and addresses the challenges for practitioners applying current research techniques to these diverse and complex healing approaches and systems. Core principles and specific examples of CAM encountered by the practicing family physician are presented with relevant evidence and helpful tips.

Complementary and alternative medicine is based on multiple healing traditions practiced long before conventional Western medicine. Emerging from diverse cultural traditions worldwide, these approaches to health and healing offer the wisdom of their unique perspective on the human condition. Many traditional practices, including those of conventional medicine, share common roots and philosophies and uphold the sacred call to relieve the suffering of others. Family physicians should keep an open mind as they explore these dimensions of CAM.

What Is Complementary and Alternative Medicine?

Various definitions have been used to describe the array of approaches and philosophies commonly referred to as CAM. As the field has evolved, so has the terminology. Unconventional, unproven, alternative, complementary, holistic, integrative, and integral are some of the most common examples of terms in current use.

Historically, medical pluralism has long existed in the United States (Kaptchuk and Eisenberg, 2001a). Over the past few decades, *alternative medicine* has become a more recognized entity within conventional medicine. Because of the public's growing use of CAM, the National Institutes of Health (NIH) created an Office of Alternative Medicine (OAM) in 1992, with the intention of bringing its scientific expertise "to more adequately explore unconventional medical practices" (NCCAM, 2000). Because of Americans' ongoing and increasing use of CAM, the OAM was expanded to the *National Center for Complementary and Alternative Medicine* (NCCAM) in 1998, guided by the following mission statement (2000, p 17): "We are dedicated to exploring complementary and alternative healing practices in the context of rigorous science, training researchers, and disseminating authoritative information to the public and professional communities." After a decade of work in the field, NCCAM has become a leading resource for helping the public and health professionals better understand this rapidly growing area of medicine. The center's name has led to the more widespread use and recognition of CAM as the defining term for this field. NCCAM's free website contains a wealth of information, including the following definitions (2014):

- **Complementary and alternative medicine** are terms often used to mean the array of health care approaches with a history of use or origins outside of mainstream medicine. NCCAM generally uses the term "complementary health approaches" when discussing the practices and products we study for various health conditions. Although some scientific evidence exists, the list of what is considered to be CAM changes continually as the therapies that are proved to be safe and effective become adopted into conventional health care and as new approaches to health care emerge.
- **Alternative medicine** refers to using a non-mainstream approach **in place** of conventional medicine.
- **Complementary medicine** generally refers to using a non-mainstream approach **together with** conventional medicine.
- *Integrative medicine* and *integrative health care* combine this array of non-mainstream health care approaches together with conventional medicine.

The NCCAM has classified CAM into five categories, or domains (Figure 12-1). Currently NCCAM finds it useful to consider these approaches as falling into one of two subgroups: natural products or mind and body practices. Examples of alternative or whole medical systems include homeopathy, naturopathy, and Ayurveda (**eAppendix 12-1** provides a glossary of CAM terms). Although there are a variety of approaches to the complex taxonomy of CAM (Kaptchuk and Eisenberg, 2001b), the NIH system is most often used.

Another term, *holistic medicine*, also describes these practices and philosophy. The American Holistic Medical Association (AHMA), founded in 1978, is a membership organization for physicians and other health professionals seeking to practice a broader form of medicine than that currently taught in allopathic medical schools (Table 12-1). "Holistic medicine is the art and science of healing that addresses care of the whole person—body, mind, and spirit.

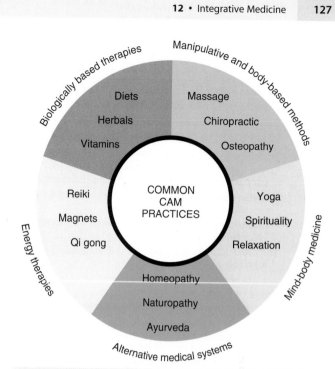

Figure 12-1 The National Center for Complementary and Alternative Medicine (NCCAM) groups' complementary and alternative medicine (CAM) practices into five domains, recognizing that there can be some overlap among them. *Biologically based therapies* use substances found in nature, such as herbs, special diets, or vitamins (in doses outside those used in conventional medicine). *Energy therapies* involve the use of energy fields, such as magnetic fields or biofields (i.e., energy fields that some believe surround and penetrate the human body). *Manipulative and body-based methods* are based on manipulation or movement of one or more body parts. *Mind-body medicine* uses a variety of techniques designed to enhance the mind's ability to affect bodily function and symptoms. *Alternative* or *whole medical systems* are built on complete systems of theory and practice. Often, these systems have evolved apart from and earlier than the conventional medical approach used in the United States.

The practice of holistic medicine integrates conventional and complementary therapies to promote optimal health and to prevent and treat disease by addressing contributing factors" (AHMA, 2014).

In 1981, the nursing profession, guided by a group of nurses dedicated to bringing the concepts of holism to every arena of nursing practice, founded the American Holistic Nursing Association (AHNA). "Holistic nursing is defined as 'all nursing practice that has healing the whole person as its goal' (AHNA, 1998). Holistic nursing is a specialty practice that draws on nursing knowledge, theories, expertise, and intuition to guide nurses in becoming therapeutic partners with people in their care. This practice recognizes the totality of the human being—the interconnectedness of body, mind, emotion, spirit, social/cultural, relationship, context, and environment" (AHNA, 2014).

Integrative medicine, a term brought into popular use by Andrew Weil, MD, founder and director of the innovative University of Arizona Center for Integrative Medicine, describes how CAM and conventional medicine is practiced together (Rakel and Weil, 2003, p 6):

Integrative medicine is healing oriented and emphasizes the centrality of the doctor-patient relationship. It

Table 12-1   Important Events in Complementary and Integrative Medicine

Year	Event
1978	American Holistic Medical Association is founded.
1981	American Holistic Nurses Association is founded.
1992	U.S. Office of Alternative Medicine (OAM) is established.
1996	U.S. Food and Drug Administration (FDA) approves acupuncture needles for use by licensed practitioners.
1998	National Center for Complementary and Alternative Medicine (NCCAM) is established, replacing OAM.
1999	Consortium of Academic Health Centers for Integrative Medicine (CAHCIM) is formed in response to increasing public interest in complementary and alternative medicine (CAM) and grows to 57 members by 2013.
2000	American Board of Medical Acupuncture is established, with a certifying examination for physicians to demonstrate proficiency in the specialty of medical acupuncture.
2000	President Clinton appoints James S. Gordon, MD, to chair the first White House Commission on Complementary and Alternative Medicine Policy (WHCCAMP).
2002	WHCCAMP submits final report with administrative and legislative recommendations for maximizing the benefits of CAM for all Americans.
2005	Institute of Medicine (IOM) releases report on CAM in the United States. NCCAM releases 5-year strategic plan.
2006	CAHCIM sponsors the first North American Research Conference on Complementary and Integrative Medicine.
2009	IOM Summit on Integrative Medicine and the Health of the Public. CAHCIM sponsors a second research conference. NCCAM prepares its third strategic plan.
2011	Veterans Heath Administration (VHA) launches a new Office of Patient-Centered Care and Cultural Transformation for "whole health."
2013	World Health Organization (WHO) Traditional Medicine Strategy 2014-2023 is published to set the course for global traditional and complementary medicine.
2014	American Board of Integrative Medicine offers its first certifying examination.

focuses on the least invasive, least toxic, and least costly methods to help facilitate health by integrating allopathic and complementary therapies. These are based on an understanding of the physical, emotional, psychologic, and spiritual aspects of the individual.

In general, the terms *holistic* and *integrative* seem to best convey the ideal blending of conventional and unconventional medicine "in that both imply a balanced, whole-person–centered approach and involve a synthesis of conventional medicine, CAM modalities, and other traditional medical systems, with the aim of prevention and healing as a basic foundation" (Lee et al., 2004, p 10).

The term *integral* has recently emerged in the literature. First noted several decades ago in the book *Mind, Body and Health: Toward an Integral Medicine* (Gordon et al., 1984), its original use may be traced to the work of Sri Aurobindo, an Indian mystic and political leader. The term has been popularized by contemporary philosopher and transpersonal psychologist Ken Wilber (2005), as applied in the context of his *integral theory*. Many thought leaders in the field of health and healing, including the Institute of Noetic Sciences (IONS), support these concepts and encourage further research into what may be considered the beginnings of a paradigm shift in medicine (Schiltz, 2005). The following excerpt captures the essence of the deep change and transformation that integral medicine calls for (Wilber, 2005, pp xxx-xxxi):

The crucial ingredient in any integral medical practice is not the integral medical bag itself—with all the conventional pills, and the orthodox surgery, and the subtle energy medicine, and the acupuncture needles—but the holder of that bag. Integrally informed health-care practitioners, the doctors, nurses, and therapists, have opened themselves to an entire spectrum of consciousness—matter to body to mind to soul to spirit—and who have thereby acknowledged what seems to be happening in any event. Body and mind and spirit are operating in self and culture and nature, and thus health and healing, sickness and wholeness, are all bound up in a multidimensional tapestry that cannot be cut into without loss.

Family physicians know this to be true. They practice with the intention to care for the whole patient within the context of a continuous healing relationship while honoring the rich complexity and interplay of family, community, and environment. They acknowledge the personal and interpersonal effects of health and illness and are trained to consider the behavioral and social aspects of a person's life as well as the biomedical factors.

Now is the time not only to reclaim its roots, but also to move primary care into expanded dimensions and possibilities of health and healing. Family medicine is the ideal discipline to champion this movement and to actualize changes that will begin to heal the failing U.S. health care system. Whether it is called holistic, integrative, or integral, family physicians are collectively evolving toward a more compassionate and sustainable system of care that may ultimately be called *good medicine.*

Complementary and Alternative Medicine Use in the 1990s

Key Points

- Almost 40% of U.S. adults and 12% of children use complementary and alternative medicine (CAM) therapies.
- The number of adult Americans using CAM rose by 38% between 1990 and 1997 and has remained stable between 2002 and 2007.
- CAM is used more by women, by those with higher levels of education and income, and by those who were recently hospitalized.
- Most patients do not disclose CAM use to their physicians.
- Most patients use CAM and conventional care together.

The first major study of CAM use in the United States was conducted in 1990 by David Eisenberg and colleagues (1993), who published a landmark paper in the *New England Journal of Medicine*. Serving as a wake-up call to conventional medicine, the data from this national telephone survey of 1539 English-speaking adults estimated that one of three Americans (34%) had used a CAM therapy in the prior year. The study estimated that those using CAM had made 425 million visits to complementary medicine practitioners—more than all office visits to primary care physicians in that same time frame! The out-of-pocket costs for these CAM services were approximately $14 billion a year. The striking statistics alerted mainstream medicine and prompted further inquiry into the growing phenomenon of the public's use of CAM.

In 1997, Eisenberg and colleagues conducted a follow-up to the 1990 study, again using a national telephone survey of English-speaking adults (2055). The findings, published in the *Journal of the American Medical Association* in 1998, showed that the number of Americans using CAM rose by 38% (60 to 83 million) and that visits to CAM practitioners increased from an estimated 427 million to 629 million. Overall, 42% of Americans were estimated to be using at least one CAM therapy in the prior 12 months. With regard to costs, conservative estimates put expenditures for CAM professional services at $21.2 billion, with approximately $12.2 billion paid as out-of-pocket expenses (Eisenberg et al., 1998).

Most concerning was the finding that although CAM use had increased over the 7-year period, the number of patients informing their doctors of such use had not changed—approximately 60% to 70% of CAM users in 1990 and 1997 did not discuss their use of CAM with their physicians. Lack of communication was noted again in a 2006 NCCAM/American Association of Retired Persons (AARP) survey of adults 50 or older revealing only one-third of CAM users had talked to their physicians about their CAM use (NCCAM/AARP, 2007). Given this fact and the potential for untoward side effects, it is essential that physicians and all other health professionals ask patients about their

Table 12-2 Guidelines for Advising Patients Who Seek Alternative Therapies

Ask; don't tell.
Be willing to listen and learn.
Communicate and **c**ollaborate.
Diagnose.
Explain and **e**xplore options and preferences.

use of CAM. In addition to NCCAM's "Time to Talk" campaign, several approaches have been suggested (Eisenberg, 1997); Table 12-2 lists an ABC format especially useful for the busy clinician (Sierpina, 2001).

Complementary and Alternative Medicine Use in the 21st Century

Data on the U.S. population's use of CAM was collected in 2002, 2007 (published), and 2012 (publication pending). Considered the most comprehensive and reliable findings on Americans' use of CAM, these studies were conducted by the NCCAM and the National Center for Health Statistics (NCHS), part of the Centers for Disease Control and Prevention (CDC). For the first time, detailed questions regarding CAM were added into the 2002 edition of the NCHS National Health Interview Survey (NHIS), an annual study interviewing tens of thousands of Americans about their health- and illness-related experiences. The 2002 and 2007 studies were completed by approximately 30,000 families through adults 18 years or older who spoke English or Spanish. The study reflected CAM use during the 12 months before the survey. The 2007 survey included expanded questions on 36 types of CAM therapies commonly used in the United States: 10 practitioner-based therapies, such as acupuncture, and 26 other, self-care therapies not requiring a practitioner. CAM therapies included in the surveys are listed in Table 12-3, and the terms are defined in eAppendix 12-1.

As shown in Figure 12-2, CAM use increased from 36% of U.S. adults in 2002 to 38% in 2007, or almost 4 of 10 adults (Barnes et al., 2004, 2008). For the first time, the 2007 survey collected data on CAM use in children (<18 years), showing 12% use, or 1 in 9 children. The top 10 CAM therapies for both adults and children are shown in Figure 12-3. Significant increases in adults' use of deep breathing, meditation, massage, and yoga occurred over the 5 years of the study. Another notable NCCAM/AARP study focused on CAM use in adults older than 50 years. Approximately two-thirds (63%) had used one or more CAM therapies (NCCAM/AARP, 2007). The most common reasons cited for not discussing CAM included: the physician never asked (42%), the patient did not know they should ask (30%), and there was not enough time during the office visit (19%). Of those using CAM, 66% did so to treat a specific condition and 65% for overall wellness. For details on CAM costs in the United States, see eFigures 12-1 to 12-3 online.

Table 12-3 Complementary and Alternative Medicine Therapies Included in 2002 and 2007 National Health Interview Surveys

Acupuncture*
Ayurveda*
Alternative practitioner*†
Biofeedback*
Chelation therapy*
Chiropractic care*
CAM†
Deep breathing exercises
Diet-based therapies
Vegetarian diet
Macrobiotic diet
Atkins diet
Pritikin diet
Ornish diet
Zone diet
Energy healing therapy*
Folk medicine
Guided imagery
Homeopathic treatment
Hypnosis
Massage*
Meditation
Megavitamin therapy
Movement therapy†
Alexander technique
Feldenkrais
Pilates
Trager psychophysical integration
Natural nonvitamin and nonmineral products (e.g., herbs, other
    products from plants, enzymes)
Naturopathy*
Osteopathic manipulation*†
Prayer for health reasons
Prayed for own health
Others ever prayed for your health
Participate in prayer group
Healing ritual for self
Progressive relaxation
Qi gong
Reiki*
Tai chi
Traditional healer*†
Botanica
Curandero
Espiritista
Hierbero (yerbera)
Native American healer
Shaman
Sobador
Yoga

CAM, Complementary and alternative medicine.
Definitions of these therapies are provided in the glossary of eAppendix
    12-1.
*Indicates a practitioner-based therapy.
†Indicates addition to 2007 survey.

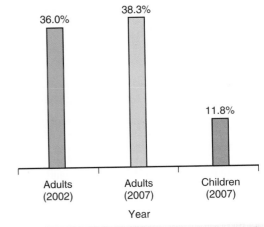

Figure 12-2 Complementary and alternative medicine (CAM) use by U.S. adults (2002, 2007) and children (2007). (From Barnes PM, Bloom B, Nahin R. Complementary and alternative medicine use among adults and children: United States, 2007. *Natl Health Stat Rep.* December 2008;(12):1-23.)

WHO IS MORE LIKELY TO USE COMPLEMENTARY AND ALTERNATIVE MEDICINE AND WHY?

Consistent with data from the 2002 NHIS study, CAM use by adults in 2007 was more prevalent among women; adults age 30 to 69; those with higher education level, not poor, or living in the West; former smokers; and those hospitalized in the prior year (Barnes et al., 2008). CAM use was positively associated with number of health conditions and number of physician visits in the previous year. When concerned about cost or unable to pay for conventional care, adults were more likely to use CAM. For children, the 2007 data show no gender difference. For all therapies combined, CAM use was highest among adolescents age 12 to 17 years (16%) versus children age 5 to 11 years (11%) or preschool children age 0 to 4 years (8%). Children's use of CAM increased as their parents' education or income level increased, and when families were unable to afford conventional medical care. Children with a parent or other relative who used CAM were about five times as likely (23%) to use CAM as children whose parent did not (5%).

Figure 12-4 shows the disease or condition for which adults and children are most likely to seek CAM. The 2002 survey also addressed the important question: Why do people use CAM? Previous studies revealed general issues of the overuse of technology and a reductionist approach to care, managed-care time constraints limiting visits and eroding the physician-patient relationship, and the explosion of Internet-based information on CAM. Astin (1998) found that along with being more educated and reporting poor health status, most alternative medicine users were not dissatisfied with conventional medicine but rather found these health care alternatives to be more congruent with their own values, beliefs, and philosophic orientations toward health and life. Only 4.4% reported relying primarily on CAM therapies for their health care. A subsequent study of patients using both CAM and conventional care also found that use of CAM did not primarily reflect dissatisfaction with conventional care (Eisenberg et al., 2001).

Reasons for CAM use reported in the 2002 NHIS study are shown in Figure 12-5, with slightly more than one-half of all respondents believing CAM *combined with* conventional medicine would be helpful.

TRENDS IN COMPLEMENTARY AND ALTERNATIVE MEDICINE USE

The 2002 and 2007 NHIS data show that although the overall prevalence of CAM use by adults had remained relatively stable (36% and 38%, respectively), there have

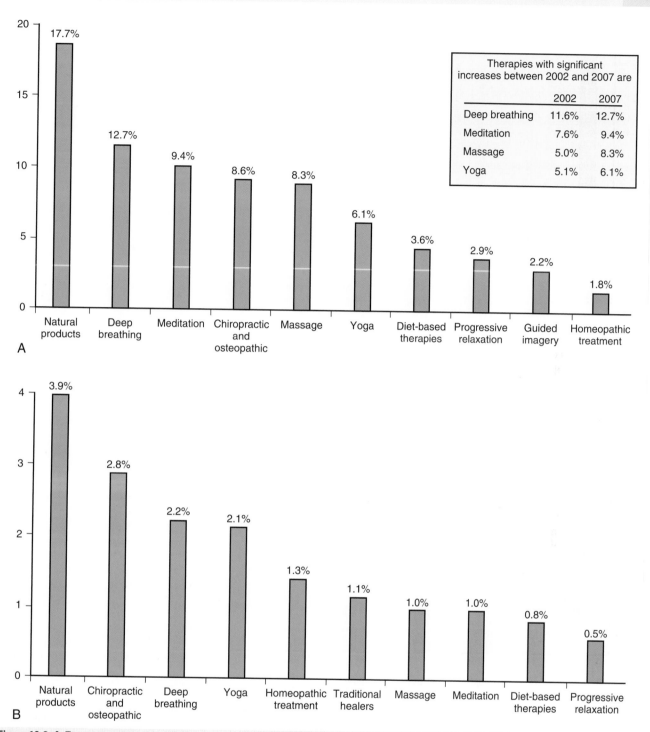

Figure 12-3 A, Ten most common complementary and alternative medicine (CAM) therapies among adults in 2007. **B,** Ten most common CAM therapies among children in 2007. (From Barnes PM, Bloom B, Nahin R. Complementary and alternative medicine use among adults and children: United States, 2007. *Natl Health Stat Rep.* December 2008;(12):1-23.)

been significant increases in some therapies, including acupuncture, deep-breathing exercises, massage therapy, meditation, naturopathy, and yoga (see Figure 12-3). Several factors may account for this growth, including increasing state licensure of some of the practices and greater public awareness of their use through the press and Internet resources. Characteristics of adult and pediatric CAM users are similar in that education, poverty status,

geographic region, number of health conditions, physician visits in the prior year, and delaying or not receiving conventional care because of cost are all associated with CAM use. Overall reasons for CAM use fall into two equal categories: (1) treating a variety of health problems, especially pain, and (2) promoting general health and wellness. Much of CAM use is "self-care" and is mostly used with conventional care.

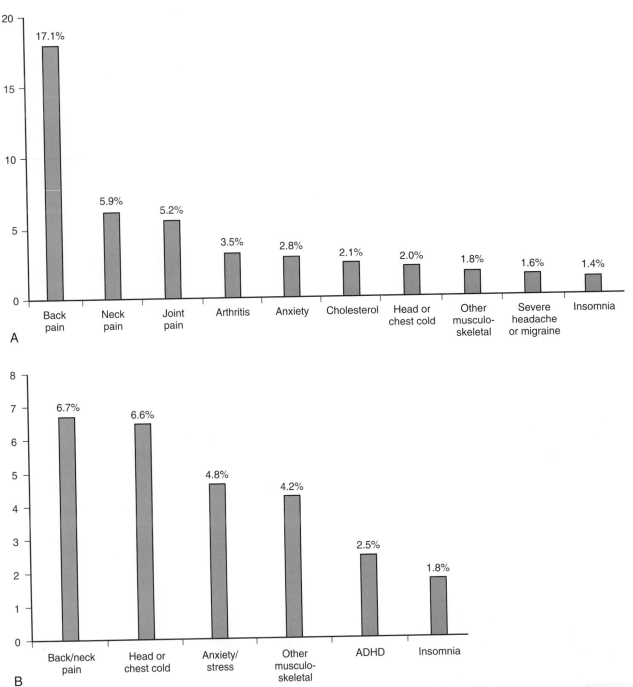

Figure 12-4 A, Disease or condition for which complementary and alternative medicine (CAM) therapies are most frequently used among adults in 2007. **B,** Disease or condition for which CAM therapies are most frequently used among children in 2007. *ADHD,* Attention-deficit/hyperactivity disorder. (From Barnes PM, Bloom B, Nahin R. Complementary and alternative medicine use among adults and children: United States, 2007. *Natl Health Stat Rep.* December 2008;(12):1-23.)

Important U.S. Reports

Key Points

- The White House Commission on complementary and alternative medicine (CAM) created a blueprint for public policy and health care transformation in 2002.

- The Institute of Medicine's 2005 CAM report and 2009 summit called for expanding research, education, and clinical application.
- CAM challenges conventional research methods.
- CAM creates opportunities for innovative studies.
- The National Institutes of Health (NIH) National Center for Complementary and Alternative Medicine 2010 Strategic Plan sets an agenda for more CAM research.

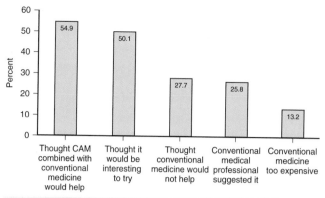

Figure 12-5 Reasons people use complementary and alternative medicine (CAM) therapies. (From Barnes PM, Powell-Griner E, McFann K, Nahin RL. Complementary and alternative medicine use among adults: United States, 2002. *Adv Data*. May 2004;(343):1-19.)

Table 12-4 Guiding Principles: 2002 White House Commission on Complementary and Alternative Medicine Policy

1. A wholeness orientation in health care delivery
2. Evidence of safety and efficacy
3. The healing capacity of the person
4. Respect for individuality
5. The right to choose treatment
6. An emphasis on health promotion and self-care
7. Partnerships are essential for integrated health care
8. Education as a fundamental health care service
9. Dissemination of comprehensive and timely information
10. Integral public involvement

Over the past two decades, several important reports have addressed CAM and integrative medicine in the United States. This section summarizes the major themes and recommendations.

WHITE HOUSE COMMISSION 2002 REPORT

The White House Commission on Complementary and Alternative Medicine Policy (WHCCAMP) 2002 report was the culmination of 18 months of in-depth work of a committee of 20 appointed commissioners. Their task was to provide the president, through the secretary of Health and Human Services, with a report containing legislative and administrative recommendations that would ensure a public policy that maximized the potential benefits of CAM to all. Specifically, the commission addressed the coordination of research to increase knowledge about CAM products; the education and training of health care practitioners in CAM; the provision of reliable and useful information about CAM practices and products to health care professionals; and guidance regarding appropriate access to and delivery of CAM. Table 12-4 lists the 10 guiding principles the commission endorsed for their process of making recommendations. The final report lists 29 recommendations and more than 100 action steps as a blueprint for shaping future CAM policy.

INSTITUTE OF MEDICINE 2005 REPORT AND 2009 SUMMIT

The Institute of Medicine (IOM) of the National Academy of Sciences acts as a private, nonprofit society of scholars engaged in research dedicated to the promotion of science and technology for the public good. Because of the American public's increasing use of CAM and the many concerns regarding safety, efficacy, and information access, a report was commissioned and a committee charged to explore the emerging scientific, policy, and practice questions. The 300-page report released in 2005 gave specific recommendations in the domains of research, education, and clinical care; new and innovative approaches to research were considered essential. The IOM Committee Chair placed a "call to action" to researchers (Bondurant and Sox, 2005, p 150):

Ignoring CAM is not an option. The widespread use of CAM by patients is a mandate to the scientific community to improve our relatively weak scientific understanding of CAM practices. Moreover, health professionals have a duty to their patients to bring these 2 worlds of contemporary medical practice together. The path to this outcome begins with adopting the same standards of evidence.

In 2009, IOM and the Bravewell Collaborative convened a 3-day summit, Integrative Medicine and the Health of the Public. More than 600 scientists, academic leaders, policy experts, health practitioners, advocates, and other participants from various disciplines examined the practice of integrative medicine, its scientific basis, and its potential for improving health. Note how the recurring themes and shared values listed in Table 12-5 resonate with the principles of family medicine and the foundations of the PCMH. Family physician Victor Sierpina shared a vision for integrative medicine and the physician of the future (Table 12-6).

NATIONAL CENTER FOR COMPLEMENTARY AND ALTERNATIVE MEDICINE STRATEGIC PLAN 2010

Now in its third cycle of 5-year strategic planning, NCCAM continues to explore CAM healing practices in the context of science, train CAM researchers, and disseminate authoritative information to public and professional communities. NCCAM's course for 2010-2014 is to create priority areas of CAM research to focus efforts that would best serve public need while meeting fiscal realities, as guided by four factors: (1) scientific promise, (2) extent and nature of practice and use, (3) amenability to rigorous scientific inquiry, and (4) potential to change health practices. A recent, new research priority is focused on symptom management, specifically the role of mind-body interventions in managing pain and common chronic disease symptoms. (Briggs and Killen, 2013)

Nahin and Strauss (2001) and Ahn and Kaptchuk (2005) discuss the unique challenges that CAM presents to conventional research approaches in evidence-based medicine.

Table 12-5   Recurring Perspectives from the Institute of Medicine Summit on Integrative Medicine and the Health of the Public

Vision of optimal health	Alignment of individuals and their health care for optimal health and healing across a full life span.
Conceptually inclusive	Seamless engagement of the full range of established health factors—physical, psychological, social, preventive, and therapeutic.
Life span horizon	Integration across the life span to include personal, predictive, preventive, and participatory care.
Person-centered	Integration around, and within, each person.
Prevention-oriented	Prevention and disease minimization as the foundation of integrative health care.
Team-based	Care as a team activity, with the patient as a central team member.
Care integration	Seamless integration of the care processes, across caregivers and institutions.
Caring integration	Person- and relationship-centered care.
Science integration	Integration across approaches to care (e.g., conventional, traditional, alternative, complementary), as the evidence supports.
Policy opportunities	Emphasis on outcomes, elevation of patient insights, consideration of family and social factors, inclusion of team care and supportive follow-up, and contributions to the learning process.

From Institute of Medicine (IOM). *Integrative medicine and the health of the public: summary of the February 2009 summit.* Washington, DC: National Academies Press; 2009, p 5.

Table 12-6   How the Physician of the Future Will Function

The Care Process Is ...	The Doctor's Role Will Be ...
Patient-centered	A navigator
Team based	Part of a multidisciplinary team
High touch, high tech	Grounded in the community
Genomic and personalized	Support of social and environmental policies promoting health
Preventive	
Integrative	
And Supports Patients Through ...	**And Will Follow ...**
Complementary and alternative practices	Evidence-based, outcome-focused practices
Belief that the body helps heal itself	Principles for creations of healing environments
	The lead of empowered patients

From Institute of Medicine (IOM). *Integrative medicine and the health of the public: summary of the February 2009 summit.* Washington, DC: National Academics Press; 2009, p. 43.

Many CAM study therapies are complex and heterogeneous compared with the more familiar single-drug trial of biomedicine. As such, innovative research strategies, such as those for sham acupuncture, will need to be continually developed. CAM may help the science of medicine to further evolve, as reflected on by Linde and Jonas (1999):

The continuing interface between orthodox and unorthodox medicine today provides the opportunity for new research strategies and methodologies to arise. By purposefully maintaining a creative tension between the established and frontier, we can advance scientific methods and more clearly define the boundaries and purpose of the scientific process for medicine.

Integrating Complementary and Alternative Medicine into Practice

Key Points

- Nutrition, mind-body medicine, and spirituality are core elements of integrative medicine practice.
- Strong evidence supports mind-body medicine for coronary artery disease, low back pain, and headache.
- Acupuncture is a safe and efficacious adjunctive treatment for several musculoskeletal conditions.
- Energy medicine researchers use current technologies to explore the frontiers of CAM.

Because the field of CAM and integrative medicine is so broad and includes so many different approaches and modalities, this section reviews core elements and then explores three common CAM modalities with evidence of efficacy: acupuncture, yoga, and homeopathy. Energy medicine, an important frontier of the CAM field, is also discussed.

CORE ELEMENTS OF INTEGRATIVE MEDICINE

Nutrition, mind-body medicine, and spirituality are considered core elements of an integrative medicine approach and often are applied during patient consultation. These elements also tend to be cost-effective and patient empowering. Considered the foundation of good health and enhanced healing, nutritional principles are key elements in most treatment plans.

The adage "food is medicine" is becoming ever more important as the United States, as well as other world populations, face impending epidemics of diabetes and obesity. Research has shown the health benefits and cost-effectiveness of the Mediterranean diet for primary and secondary prevention of metabolic syndrome (Kastorini et al., 2011). When the new food pyramid was released by the U.S. federal government (MyPyramid.gov), critics such as Walter Willett commented, "This is a huge lost

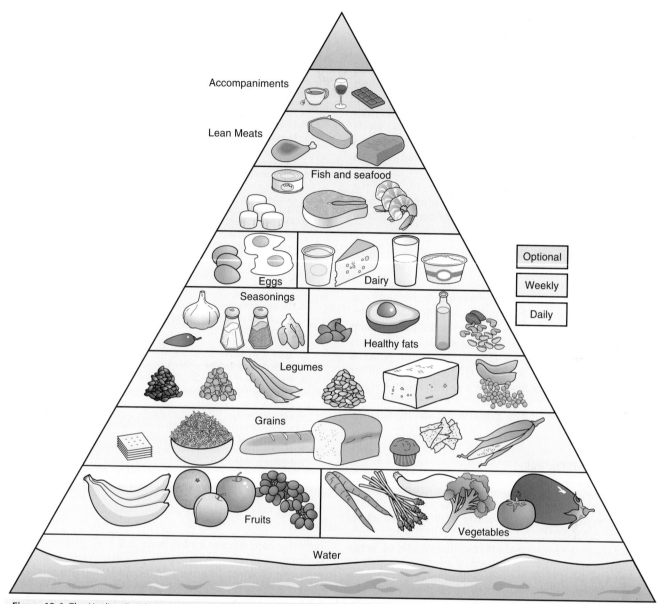

Figure 12-6 The Healing Foods Pyramid emphasizes "healing foods," which are known to have healing benefits or essential nutrients; plant-based choices, which create the base and may be accented by animal foods; variety and balance of color, nutrients, and portions sizes; a healthful environment; and "mindful eating" to savor and focus on the food being eaten. (Courtesy Monica Myklebust, MD, and Jenna Wunder, MPH, RD, University of Michigan Integrative Medicine Clinical Services, Regents of the University of Michigan. http://med.umich.edu/umim/food-pyramid/index.htm.)

opportunity to convey information about healthy food choices that could benefit Americans enormously. ... The pyramid tells nothing of healthy food choices" (Mitka, 2005, p 2581).

Other options are considered in the Healing Foods Pyramid (Figure 12-6). While developing the best nutrition advice for the diverse people seen at the University of Michigan's Integrative Medicine Clinic, family physician Monica Myklebust found various recommendations for the prevention and treatment of obesity, mood disorders, heart disease, diabetes, chronic pain, and inflammation. The result of her work is a user-friendly tool that brings all of these data together. Omega-3 fatty acids, antioxidants, medicinal seasonings, soy, chocolate, and tea are all considered. For example, green tea offers a variety of health benefits, with emerging evidence for prevention of cancer, stroke, and cardiovascular disease (Schneider and Segre,

2009). Health concerns regarding the sources of U.S. food and recommendations for organic and wild food are discussed. The Healing Foods Pyramid is available as a web-based interactive version (http://med.umich.edu/umim/food-pyramid/index.htm). The top is left open to be filled in by what individuals feel may complete and customize their pyramid.

A particular aspect of nutrition that has received increasing attention for its value in lessening inflammation is that of fish oil (i.e., omega-6 and omega-3 fatty acids). Omega-3 fatty acids consist of eicosapentaenoic acid (EPA) and docosahexaenoic acid (DHA) and are mostly found in fatty fish, such as herring and salmon. Because inflammation plays a role in several common conditions, such as cardiovascular disease, asthma, arthritis, psoriasis, and inflammatory bowel disease, research has explored the role of omega-3 fatty acids in reducing symptoms and improving outcomes.

Practical applications for recommending fish oil in the primary care setting included the following (Oh, 2005):

1. The American Heart Association recommends 1 gram (g) per day for all patients with documented coronary artery disease through diet or through supplementation.
2. For patients with mild or persistent hypertriglyceridemia, use of 2 to 4 g per day of fish oil may lower levels by 20% to 50% to reach NIH National Heart, Lung, and Blood Institute (NHLBI) Adult Treatment Panel (ATP) III goals.
3. For those with rheumatoid arthritis, doses of 2.6 to 6 g per day for at least 8 to 12 weeks are optimal and may reduce or eliminate nonsteroidal antiinflammatory drug (NSAID) use.

Monitoring for clinical bleeding and for low-density lipoprotein (LDL) cholesterol and glycemic response should be considered for patients taking doses higher than 3 g/day, especially if they are diabetic. Unfortunately, because our waters are polluted with heavy metals, avoiding fish known to have high methyl mercury levels (especially by women who are pregnant and of childbearing age) is an important precaution when discussing fish oil use with patients (Williams, 2005). Along with fish oil consumption, other dietary modifications are also known to help lessen inflammation; Table 12-7 shows guidelines for prescribing an antiinflammatory diet (Rakel, 2003; Rakel and Rindfleisch, 2006).

MIND-BODY MEDICINE

The area of CAM with perhaps the most extensive research base is mind-body medicine, which encompasses a diverse array of practices that overlap many traditions and whole systems of care. Astin and colleagues (2003, p 131) concluded, "There is now considerable evidence that an array of mind-body therapies can be used as effective adjuncts to conventional medical treatment for a number of common clinical conditions." They found strong evidence to support mind-body approaches in the treatment of low back pain, coronary artery disease, headache, insomnia, preparing for surgical procedures, and in the management of disease-related symptoms of cancer, arthritis, and urinary incontinence.

Given the relative ease of learning and employing such techniques, NCCAM has made research into mind-body medicine a priority. Mind-body medicine approaches may enhance healing and optimize health. They may be recommended to most patients for health maintenance and disease management and could easily be incorporated into a PCMH through group visits or health coaches. In addition, a study of 70 primary care physicians who participated in an intensive mindfulness education program over 1 year showed dramatic improvements in mindfulness skills, burnout, mood disturbance, and empathy (Krasner et al., 2009). An accompanying editorial noted that the study "demonstrates that training physicians in the art of mindful practice has the potential to promote physician health *through* work." Also, recognizing and enhancing the meaning derived from the practice of medicine using these skills may "protect against burnout and promote

Table 12-7 Guidelines in Prescribing an Antiinflammatory Diet

1. Omega-3 and omega-6 fatty acids are essential polyunsaturated fatty acids (i.e., they cannot be made by the human body).
2. The ratio of omega-6 to omega-3 fatty acids in the average Western diet has steadily increased in the past 100 years. The standard American diet has a ratio of omega-6 to omega-3 of more than 20:1, but the ideal range is less than 4:1.
3. To follow an antiinflammatory diet, take the following steps:
   a. Decrease red meat, poultry, and dairy intake.
   b. Increase the intake of omega-3 fatty acids, such as cold-water fish, flaxseed, walnuts, and green leafy vegetables.
   c. Even one meal of cold-water fish weekly reduces the risk of cardiac arrest. Consuming fish twice each week is ideal. If this is not possible, fish oil supplements can be taken at a dose of 500-2000 mg twice daily.
   d. An alternative is ground flax seeds or flaxseed oil. Flax should be freshly ground because it can spoil after exposure to light or heat. Supplementation can be provided with 500-2000 mg of flax oil twice daily.
   e. Reduce foods that contain omega-6 fatty acids, including the following:
      (1) Margarine.
      (2) Oils made from corn, cottonseed, grapeseed, peanut, safflower, sesame, soybean, or sunflower (avoid partially hydrogenated oils).
      (3) Foods with a long shelf life, such as crackers and chips.
   f. Cook with monounsaturated oils such as olive or canola oil.
4. Consider this dietary approach to treat the following:
   a. Heart disease or associated risk factors
   b. Inflammatory rheumatic disorders
   c. Autoimmune diseases
   d. Chronic pain
5. Low-carbohydrate, high-protein diets tend to have high omega-6 fat content and should be used with caution.
6. It may take up to 6 months to see the full clinical effects of an antiinflammatory diet.

From Rakel D, Rindfleisch A. Integrative medicine. In: Rakel RE, ed. *Essential family medicine: fundamentals and case studies.* Philadelphia: Saunders; 2006, pp. 132-141.

patient-centered care for the benefit of both physicians and their patients" (Shanafelt, 2009, p 1340). A recent abbreviated mindfulness intervention adapted for primary care clinicians was associated with reductions in indicators of job burnout, depression, anxiety, and stress (Fortney et al., 2013) and a multicenter study found that clinicians who rate themselves more mindful engage in more patient-centered communication and have more satisfied patients (Beach et al., 2013).

Online **eAppendix 12-2** highlights a well-known and well-studied mind-body technique called *mindfulness-based stress reduction* (MBSR) and includes a short audio sample of mindful breath work for the interested reader to try.

SPIRITUALITY

Another area thought to be integral to a whole-patient integrative medicine approach to care is spirituality. This broad and controversial subject is well reviewed (e.g., Sierpina and Sierpina, 2004); some key issues are considered here. Working definitions and terms from the Samueli Conference on Definitions and Standards in Healing Research (Dossey, 2003) include the following:

■ *Spirituality* encompasses the feelings, thoughts, experiences, and behaviors that arise from a search for that which is generally considered sacred or holy. Spirituality is usually considered to involve a sense of connection with an absolute, imminent, or transcendent spiritual force, however named, as well as the conviction that meaning, value, direction, and purpose are valid aspects of the universe.

- **Religion** is the codified and ritualized beliefs and behaviors of those involved in spirituality, usually taking place within a community of like-minded individuals.
- **Prayer** is communication with an absolute, imminent, or transcendent spiritual force, however named. Such communication may take a variety of forms and may be theistic or nontheistic in nature, as in some forms of Buddhism. *Intercessory prayer* is an appeal to such a force to influence another person or thing. *Healing prayer* is an appeal to such a force for the healing and recovery of self or others. *Directed prayer* is offered with a specific outcome in mind. *Nondirected prayer* is offered with no specific outcome in mind, such as, "Thy will be done," or "May the best outcome prevail."

Given recent statistics on prayer from the 2002 NHIS and Gallup Polls over the past six decades (showing that more than 90% of Americans believe in God or a universal spirit), it is not surprising that proponents and critics have agreed that taking a spiritual history is essential to a comprehensive and culturally sensitive medical consultation. Just as challenging as asking patients about substance abuse, domestic violence, and sexual practices, a spiritual history helps elucidate how spiritual beliefs or religious practices may impact health and health-related choices. Such discussions may be most relevant during times of a new diagnosis, loss of a loved one, onset of depression, or terminal illness. Continuity of care and sensitivity to the biopsychosocial aspects of a patient's life foster the rapport to facilitate such discussion. Such inquiry may also help engage support systems or identify deep conflicts. Although not all physicians may be comfortable addressing spirituality with their patients, referrals to colleagues in pastoral care and chaplaincy are options to consider.

Interviewing seven physicians recognized as leaders in the field of healing research, Egnew (2005, pp 258 and 255) found that "healing was defined in terms of developing a sense of personal wholeness that involves physical, mental, emotional, social and spiritual aspects of human experience." The central theme in the responses provided an operational definition of healing: "Healing is the personal experience of the transcendence of suffering."

Various models have been suggested as guides to taking the spiritual history (Table 12-8) (Anandarajah and Hight, 2001; Kinney, 1999; Puchalski and Romer, 2000).

ACUPUNCTURE, YOGA, AND HOMEOPATHIC REMEDIES

Three areas of CAM are most likely to be encountered in the family physician's office: acupuncture, yoga, and homeopathic remedies. As shown in Table 12-9, these three areas are components of whole systems or *nonallopathic* medical systems of care: *acupuncture* within traditional Chinese medicine (TCM), *yoga* as a part of Ayurveda, and *homeopathic remedies* as the mainstay of homeopathy. Many family

Table 12-8 Spiritual Assessment Tools

FICA MNEMONIC

F: Faith or belief—What is your faith or belief?
I: Importance and influence—Is it important in your life? How?
C: Community—Are you part of a religious community?
A: Awareness and addressing—What would you want me as your physician to be aware of? How would you like me to address these issues in your care?

HOPE MNEMONIC

H: Hope—What are your sources of hope, meaning, strength, peace, love, and connectedness?
O: Organized—Do you consider yourself part of an organized religion?
P: Personal spirituality and practices—What aspects of your spirituality or spiritual practices do you find most helpful?
E: Effects—How do your beliefs affect the kind of medical care you would like me to provide?

THREE QUESTIONS

1. What helps you get through tough times?
2. Who do you turn to when you need support?
3. What meaning does this experience have for you?

physicians have pursued professional training in these fields and are now integrating new skills and perspectives into their practice. The Society of Teachers of Family Medicine (STFM) *Group on Hospital Medicine and Procedural Training* has proposed that acupuncture become an advanced procedure within the scope of family medicine training (Kelly, 2009).

Although challenging to research, trials have shown acupuncture efficacious as an adjunctive therapy in osteoarthritis of the knee (Berman et al., 2004) and as a complement to standard therapy for the debilitating effect of pelvic girdle pain during pregnancy (Elden et al., 2005). Cochrane reviews have shown that acupuncture benefits patients with chronic low back pain, neck pain, and headache (migraine and tension) (Kelly, 2009). A meta-analysis evaluating 33 randomized controlled trials (RCTs) of acupuncture for acute and chronic low back pain concluded that acupuncture effectively relieves chronic low back pain, although no evidence suggests that it is more effective than other active therapies (Manheimer et al., 2005). A more recent review found acupuncture a reasonable referral option for chronic pain (Vickers et al., 2012).

Excellent reviews of acupuncture's theory, efficacy, and practice (Kaptchuk, 2002; Nielsen and Hammerschlag, 2004) cite the 1997 NIH Consensus Development Panel findings on acupuncture. After reviewing all available evidence from RCTs up to 1997, the panel concluded that clear evidence shows that acupuncture is efficacious for adult postoperative and chemotherapy nausea and vomiting and for postoperative dental pain. The panel also reported that acupuncture should be considered a useful adjunct for addiction, stroke rehabilitation, osteoarthritis, headache, low back pain, tennis elbow, menstrual cramps, carpal tunnel, and fibromyalgia (NIH, 1998).

Yoga, a widely popular and rapidly increasing CAM practice in the United States, has its roots in ancient India and is a Sanskrit word that means "yoke" or "union." The original goal of practicing these postures was to purify and

Table 12-9 Nonallopathic Medical Systems

TRADITIONAL CHINESE MEDICINE

Philosophy: Qi and other substances flow through the body through various channels, or meridians. Yin and yang (i.e., passive and active) and the five elements (i.e., wood, fire, earth, metal, and water) have competing influences on various body parts. Excesses or deficiencies of these cause illness. Pain is blocked qi.

Diagnostics: A specific diagnosis is not needed. Information is gathered by the four kanbing: looking (i.e., observation of posture, coloring, gait, demeanor, appearance of the tongue); asking about the status of the 11 basic areas, including body temperature, sleep, fluid metabolism, pain, and digestion; listening to the body's sounds, including breathing, voice, and peristalsis; and palpation of the affected site and the pulse. The pulse is thought to have three parts that correlate with the status of different parts of the body.

Therapeutics: Acupuncture is the insertion of needles into various points along the qi meridians. Moxibustion is the burning of moxa (*Artemisia vulgaris*) on or near meridian points. Gua sha is pressing the skin with a hard, round-edged instrument to create petechiae. Cupping is the creation of a vacuum in a cup and applying the vacuum pressure to the skin. Tui na is manipulation or massage with specific hand movements. Plum blossom is a cluster of needles that is moved along a meridian. Herbal therapies typically are combinations of multiple herbs mixed specifically for the individual patient.

AYURVEDA

Philosophy: The concept emerged in India 5000 years ago, and it incorporates five elements and three types of energy, or doshas. *Vata* is the dosha associated with movement, *pitta* governs metabolism, and *kapha* maintains structure. Diet, lifestyle, and relationships shape a person's energy and define health status. Ancient texts divide illnesses according to subspecialties, many of which are the same as for biomedicine.

Diagnostics: Factors that may have weakened the person's defenses are considered, such as genetics, trauma, diet, habits, seasonal affects, climate, age, balance of the doshas, emotions, metabolism, and acts of God. A full physical examination includes evaluation of pulses, speech and voice, eyes, tongue, and the appearance of the urine and feces.

Therapeutics: Approaches include prevention, detoxification, reestablishment of one's unique constitutional balance. Foods, emotions, and behaviors are used to adjust dosha levels. Panchakarma is used to remove aggravated doshas and toxins. Components of panchakarma include therapeutic vomiting, use of purgatives or laxatives, nasal administration of medications, blood purification (traditionally by blood-letting, now more often with teas), and therapeutic enemas.

NATUROPATHY

Philosophy: The body is able to heal itself by means of the healing power of nature. Healing occurs through a diet of natural, unrefined foods; adequate exercise; avoidance of environmental toxins; proper elimination of body wastes; and positive thoughts and emotions. Key principles in patient care include doing no harm, taking a preventive approach, and focusing on maintenance of health rather than just on the treatment of disease. The naturopath's goals are to educate, empower, and motivate.

Diagnostics: Methods may draw from any number of approaches, including laboratory testing not commonly performed in a biomedical setting.

Therapeutics: Approaches can include nutrition, botanicals, homeopathy, Chinese medicine, physical medicine (e.g., ultrasound, massage, manipulation), hydrotherapy (e.g., baths, steams, wraps, colonic irrigation), and various detoxification regimens.

HOMEOPATHY

Philosophy: Homeopathy is based on the law of similars, which holds that medicines can produce the same symptoms in healthy people that they cure in those who are ill. Remedies are used in the smallest quantity possible, which can often mean they are diluted to the point that not even a molecule of the original therapeutic substance remains in solution.

Diagnostics: A detailed history is taken relating to the specific nature of symptoms. For example, otitis media is treated differently based on the mood of the child, which ear is sore, the nature of the fever, and the nature of the pain.

Therapeutics: A remedy that has elicited a similar set of symptoms in a healthy patient is given in minute quantity to the ill person. The degree to which a remedy is diluted is given as a Roman numeral. For example, a 6X solution has been diluted to one-tenth of its strength six times (i.e., to 10^{-6} of the original strength), and a 200C solution has been diluted to 1/100 of its original strength 200 subsequent times (i.e., to 10^{-400} of its original strength).

From Rakel D, Rindfleisch A: Integrative medicine. In: Rakel RE, ed. *Essential family medicine: fundamentals and case studies.* Philadelphia: Saunders; 2006, pp 132-141.

prepare the body for higher states of consciousness. *Hatha yoga*, as described in Table 12-10 along with other types of movement therapies, has many different styles and is the most popular form taught and practiced in the United States today. Because most yoga instructors are not medical professionals, it is recommended to refer a patient to a teacher with several years' experience. A study of the efficacy of yoga on pregnancy outcome ($N = 335$) concluded that an integrated approach to yoga during pregnancy was safe and that it improved birth weight and decreased preterm labor and intrauterine growth retardation with no complications (Narendran et al., 2005). A recent study of 90 patients with chronic low back pain who participated in a 24-week trial of yoga twice a week showed those receiving the yoga intervention experienced decreased levels of pain, functional disability, and depression (Williams et al., 2009). The International Association of Yoga Therapists (IAYT) is a worldwide organization for yoga teachers, therapists,

and researchers (www.iayt.org). The Yoga Alliance (www.yogaalliance.org), formed in 1999, sets minimum training standards for yoga teachers. Both organizations provide sound resources for professionals and the public.

Perhaps the most controversial of CAM therapies, *homeopathy* seems to defy biomedicine's attempts to decipher its mechanism of action. Particularly perplexing is the concept that the more dilute the remedy, the more potent is its effect. Founded by the German physician Samuel Hahnemann (1755-1843), homeopathy is still widely accepted and practiced in Europe and is now experiencing a renaissance in the United States. A brilliant linguist and scholar, Dr. Hahnemann developed the Principle of Similars, in which "like cures like" based on his medical translation work and personal experience of malaria symptoms after taking *Cinchona* bark, which was then the treatment for the disease. A critical overview of homeopathy by Jonas and colleagues (2003) reviewed the research regarding specific conditions

Table 12-10 Commonly Used Movement Therapies

Therapy*	Description	Research
Hatha yoga	Focuses on the use of postures (asanas) and breathing exercises (pranayama); traditionally used in India to purify the body and maximize the impact of meditation practice; many different schools; must be used with caution by those with glaucoma, retinal detachment, or at high risk for muscle strain or fracture.	Most trials are quite small. Positive benefits likely for musculoskeletal and other types of pain; lowering autonomic nervous system sympathetic tone; decreasing histamine effects of FEV_1 in asthmatic patients; reducing blood pressure; improving headaches, diabetes, osteoarthritis, rheumatoid arthritis; overall improvement in balance, endurance, and vitality.
Tai chi	Developed more than 5000 years ago; movement and breathing, often associated with specific flowing movement patterns, are used to affect the flow of energy, or qi.	Useful adjunctive therapy for arthritis and cardiovascular disease. Helpful for improving postural stability and decreasing fall risk in older adults.
Qigong (Qi gong)	Part of traditional Chinese medicine; also used to cultivate qi; includes breathing exercises, meditation, and physical movement; used in the martial arts and to generate energy to be used in healing.	Most studies conducted in China. Potentially useful for hypertension, decreasing overall stroke and mortality rates compared with controls, decreasing peripheral vascular resistance, increasing bone density; improvement of blood flow to brain (e.g., adjunctive treatment for memory loss, dizziness, insomnia, vertigo); improvement of cardiac output, ejection fraction, and valve function.
Feldenkrais	Developed by Moshe Feldenkrais in the 1950s; gentle movements and manipulation enlisted to retrain the body with new movement patterns.	Limited randomized trial–based research. Used to promote flexibility and posture, decrease back pain, and improve vocal cord function.

From Rakel D, Rindfleisch A. Integrative medicine. In: Rakel RE, ed. *Essential Family Medicine: Fundamentals and Case Studies.* Philadelphia: Saunders; 2006, pp 132-141.

FEV_1, Forced expiratory volume in 1 second.

*Other therapies include *Alexander technique,* which uses minimal effort to maximize efficiency of muscle use and alleviate problems associated with poor posture, and *Pilates,* which also uses exercises and other techniques used to strengthen postural muscles.

and the placebo effect. After analyzing systematic reviews of clinical trials, the authors concluded, "Despite skepticism about the plausibility of homeopathy, some randomized, placebo-controlled trials and laboratory research report unexpected effects of homeopathic medicine. However, the evidence on the effectiveness of homeopathy for specific clinical conditions is scant, is of uneven quality, and is generally poorer quality than research done in allopathic medicine" (p 397).

Known for his groundbreaking research showing homeopathic treatment of allergic rhinitis more effective than placebo (Taylor et al., 2000), David Reilly of Glasgow, Scotland, commented on the increasing scientific validation for homeopathy over the past decade. Noting that studies reviewed show positive evidence for overall effect and citing the growing prospective, observational research that indicates beneficial outcomes, Reilly (2005) points out that homeopathy can offer therapeutic options when conventional care has failed or reached a plateau, no conventional treatments exist, conventional treatments are contraindicated, side effects of conventional treatments are not tolerated, and patients are reluctant to accept conventional care. An important distinction clouds other areas of medical research: "The two dimensions of care need to be considered: the direct effects of the remedy and the therapeutic impact of the method of approach on the patient" (p 30). Believing that the homeopathic approach is helping to reintroduce a holistic perspective in medical practice, Reilly concludes, "The evidence mosaic for homeopathy reinforces clinicians' and patients' experiential knowledge that this approach can make a valuable contribution to care, especially when applied with a whole person perspective and integrated with conventional knowledge" (p 31).

ENERGY MEDICINE: FRONTIER SCIENCE OF COMPLEMENTARY AND ALTERNATIVE MEDICINE

The practice of CAM presents many challenges to Western science. How does acupuncture work, and what is *qi*? How can dilute homeopathic remedies induce effects on biologic systems? What are the *chakras,* or energy centers, so integral to yoga and Ayurveda? These mysteries present us with opportunities for new discoveries and an expansion of our healing capacities **(eAppendix 12-3)**. Many scientists are showing how research in biophysics and biomagnetism is helping to elucidate the subtle energies of biologic systems, including those of humans. Advanced technologies such as functional magnetic resonance imaging and infrared thermography are demonstrating amazing images that seem to correlate with empiric knowledge **(eAppendix 12-4)**.

Open-minded scientists are helping to bridge the worlds of CAM and conventional medicine by linking research findings to those of clinical practice (Oschman, 2002). "Let us document each of these fascinating clues. We will connect the dots by describing an information system in the body that is the missing link for many phenomena that have seemed hopelessly inexplicable in the past. It is a system that is responsible for extraordinary feats of perception, movement, and healing" (Oschman, 2003, p. xiv).

Conclusion

Complementary and alternative medicine is an evolving area of health care used by approximately 4 in 10 adults and 1 in 9 children in the United States. As a diverse system

Table 12-11 Precautions in Complementary and Alternative Medicine

1. *Primum non nocere* (first, do no harm).
2. Patients may encounter complications if they abandon effective, conventional therapies in favor of complementary and alternative medicine (CAM).
3. Medicolegal issues and certification or qualification requirements of practitioners are important topics, not covered in this chapter.

of varied approaches and philosophies of healing, CAM is usually incorporated into conventional health care as integrative medicine. CAM presents opportunities to expand the current research paradigm to meet the challenges of studying its multidimensional approach to health and healing. Prominent organizations such as the IOM and World Health Organization (WHO) have placed a call to action to the medical community to advance knowledge and clinical applications in this field. Family physicians, specialists in caring for the whole person though a continuous, healing relationship, are in the ideal discipline to advance the integration of safe and effective CAM into their repertoire to optimize the health of their patients (Table 12-11). Ultimately, complex terminology will subside as the essence of integrative medicine becomes good family medicine.

KEY TREATMENT

- Fish oil supplementation can benefit heart health (Bucher et al., 2002; Wang et al., 2004), hypertriglyceridemia (Balk et al., 2004), and rheumatoid arthritis (Fortin et al., 1995; MacLean et al., 2004) (SOR: A).
- Acupuncture should be considered as a treatment option for common painful conditions such as chronic low back pain (Furlan et al., 2005; Yuan et al., 2008), neck pain (Fu et al., 2009, Trinh et al., 2006), and headache (migraine, tension) (Linde et al., 2009a, 2009b) (SOR: A).
- Green tea is associated with decreased risk of stroke and cardiovascular disease (Kuriyama et al., 2006) and may help prevent cancer of the breast (Sun et al., 2006a),

gastrointestinal tract (Sun et al., 2006b), and prostate (Kurahashi et al., 2008) (SOR: B).
- Yoga reduces functional disability, pain, and depression in people with chronic low back pain (Williams et al., 2009) (SOR: B).
- Mindful communication may improve physician well-being and attitudes associated with patient-centered care (Kearney et al., 2009; Krasner et al., 2009) (SOR: C).

Summary of Additional Online Content

The following content is available at www.expertconsult.com:

eFigures 12-1 to 12-10

E-APPENDIX 12-1 GLOSSARY OF COMPLEMENTARY AND ALTERNATIVE MEDICINE (CAM) TERMS

E-APPENDIX 12-2 MIND-BODY EXPERIENTIAL AND MINDFULNESS RESEARCH

E-APPENDIX 12-3 ENERGY HEALING MODALITIES

E-APPENDIX 12-4 HIGHLIGHTS OF ACUPUNCTURE RESEARCH AND FINDINGS

References

The complete reference list is available at www.expertconsult.com.

Web Resources

http://www.abpsus.org/integrative-medicine American Board of Integrative Medicine credentials physicians in the field of integrative medicine.

www.integrativemedicine.arizona.edu Arizona Center for Integrative Medicine. Offers innovative education in integrative medicine.

www.imconsortium.org Consortium of Academic Health Centers for Integrative Medicine. Includes 57 member institutions throughout North America who are advancing the field of integrative medicine in the domains of education, research, and clinical care.

www.nccam.nih.gov National Center for Complementary and Alternative Medicine, part of the National Institutes of Health (NIH). Offers excellent complementary and alternative medicine (CAM) resources for both patients and clinicians.

http://nccam.nih.gov/timetotalk/ "Time to Talk." NCCAM's educational campaign to encourage patients and clinicians to discuss their use of CAM. Download a toolkit for your office.

http://apps.who.int/iris/bitstream/10665/92455/1/9789241506090 _eng.pdf World Health Organization (WHO) 10-year plan for Traditional and Complementary Medicine (T&CM).

13 Establishing Rapport

ROBERT E. RAKEL

Rapport comes from the French *en rapport*, which means "in harmony with." Rapport is most easily established during the patient's first visit, and achieving rapport enhances the likelihood that the patient will comply with the treatment plan. When rapport has been established, patients are more likely to forgive a less than perfect experience or an unexpected poor clinical outcome.

Even the most knowledgeable and skilled physician will have limited effectiveness if he or she is unable to develop rapport with patients. Unfortunately, rapport is one of those intangibles that is more than the sum of its parts. Rapport is not analyzed easily within any one body of knowledge. The basis of rapport, however, is the development of communication skills that instill in patients a sense of confidence and trust by conveying sincerity and an interest in their care and well-being. The patient's satisfaction and compliance with the physician's instructions (both measures of rapport) depend on the ability of the physician to communicate understanding, compassion, and genuine interest in the patient and to display a thorough approach to solving the patient's problems. Patient satisfaction also is related to the physician's efforts in educating patients about the disease process and motivating them to participate in their treatment.

Failure of communication between physician and patient also can affect the outcome of treatment, often as seriously as an error in treatment. More complaints against physicians result from a breakdown of the caring aspect of the doctor-patient relationship than from the technical quality of treatment.

Most complaints against physicians—and those that too frequently lead to legal action—are the result of a lack of communication between physician and patient. The potential for a serious problem always exists when a patient is inadequately informed regarding a diagnostic procedure, treatment, prognosis, or anticipated cost. The misunderstandings that result cause unnecessary expense and grief for both parties.

Similarly, the worries that result from distorted information can jeopardize the physician-patient relationship. When a patient is discussed on hospital rounds or with a colleague in the office, take care that the discussion is not within the patient's hearing distance or within that of other patients. Patients overhearing the conversation may believe the comments apply to them, or they may know the patient involved and relay the information in a distorted manner. Fragments of such conversations, overheard by the patient

or others, are too easily taken out of context and can become the focus of fearful fantasies that only serve to increase uneasiness and apprehension.

Compassion, interest, and *thoroughness* are essential components of successful patient care. These features traditionally have been embodied in the term *bedside manner,* which also connotes qualities of concern, kindness, friendliness, wit, and cheerfulness, all of which result in an atmosphere of trust and confidence between physician and patient. The physician with the best bedside manner may be the one who makes no special effort to communicate these feelings but acts in a concerned, natural, and comfortable manner.

Oliver Wendell Holmes said that to be effective, the physician should "speak softly, be well-dressed, have quiet ways and have eyes that do not wander" (1883, p. 388). Lack of eye contact may be interpreted as a lack of concern. A good first impression is certainly great help in establishing rapport. It takes less than 7 seconds to form a first impression. You do not get a second chance to create a first impression. The physician should approach the patient in an assured, confident manner with a smile and a handshake if the occasion is appropriate.

Personal appearance is a significant part of nonverbal communication. Patients consider house staff who wear white coats with conventional street clothes as more competent than those who wear scrub suits. If white coats are worn, the patient sees only the collar, tie, and shoes, and it is therefore important to keep these items neat.

Posture is also important in conveying an image of confidence and competence. Standing erect, moving briskly with head up and stomach in, is better than slouching. Energetic people seldom slump; they sit upright and appear alert. A listless or lethargic appearance can be interpreted as lack of concern.

Before entering the examining room or hospital room to see a patient, review the record briefly and become familiar with the patient's name and its proper pronunciation. If the pronunciation is unusual or difficult, place phonetic markings on the chart as a reminder for future use. Repeat the patient's name when first given it to confirm the pronunciation, and then use the name twice in the first minute to help it register. Review the medical record for particular aspects of the previous visit that should be remembered and commented on, such as the illness treated at that time, family conditions, or other problems. Patients will believe that the well-informed physician is truly interested in them. Additional courtesy, such as opening the door and assisting patients with their coats (especially elderly patients), shows a consideration that aids in establishing and maintaining rapport.

Respect

Patients should believe that their comments are being listened to, carefully considered, and taken seriously. They must believe that the physician values their comments and opinions before trusting him or her with information of a more personal nature. As long as the physician's attitude toward the patient embodies respect, concern, and kindness and a sincere effort is made to understand the patient's difficulties, the patient will overlook or forgive myriad other problems.

Oliver Wendell Holmes advised patients to "Choose a man who is personally agreeable, for a daily visit from an intelligent, amiable, pleasant, sympathetic person will cost you no more than one from a sloven or a boor, and his presence will do more for you than any prescription the other will order" (1883, p. 391).

A lack of confidence, rather than an excess of it, may lead physicians to appear aloof and unconcerned. Too often, physicians think that a godlike image of omnipotence is necessary for the maintenance of the patient's respect and confidence. It is usually a lack of self-confidence that causes physicians to retreat behind this protective image, which limits their ability to help. Secure physicians are freer to establish close personal relationships with patients without fearing their position will be threatened. A physician with a positive self-image is also willing to recognize and admit the limits of personal competence and feels comfortable seeking help from a colleague when such consultation is of value to the patient's care.

The bond of mutual respect is enhanced if the physician makes positive statements about other people. Patients find it difficult to respect a physician who is regularly detractive, making negative statements about other people or other physicians. Any comments that can be interpreted as "building yourself up by tearing someone else down" merely accomplish the reverse.

The effectiveness of physicians depends on the degree of their insight into the limitations of their personalities and the psychological defenses that distort their perceptions of patients. Physicians must recognize patients or situations that make them unreasonably angry or provoked (e.g., a whining, complaining individual who shows no interest in being rehabilitated, preferring a role of social dependency). The physician's emotions, if they go unrecognized, can serve as a barrier to the development of mutual respect. If the physician is aware of negative feelings toward a patient, an effort can be made to avoid showing signs of irritation or anger. It has been said that clenching of the physician's fist is a clinical sign of a hysterical patient. The physician should attempt to remain objective and analyze the situation for its diagnostic value.

Patients with trivial complaints or somatic manifestations of emotional disease sometimes are given less attention than those with clear-cut organic abnormalities. The frequency with which a physician complains about the triviality and inappropriateness of patients' problems has been found to be related to the volume of patients seen and the degree to which the physician feels overburdened. The more patients that physicians see and the more overloaded their practices, the more likely they are to describe patients' complaints as trivial, inappropriate, or bothersome. Physicians who have more time or take more time per patient, and who investigate the patient's complaints more thoroughly, frequently uncover significant factors and less often tend to view the complaints as trivial. Respect for patients involves taking their fears and apprehensions seriously and withholding value judgments. Patients who frequently seek help for nonspecific somatic and functional complaints may be depressed (Widmer et al., 1980).

Patient Satisfaction

A close relationship exists between rapport and patient satisfaction, and this chapter deals with the many facets of that relationship. It is important that the physician make an effort to understand what patients are "going through" (not only their pain and discomfort, but also the effect these have on their lives) and communicate this understanding to them.

Most studies indicate that patient satisfaction depends on information and the degree to which the patient understands the illness. Joos and associates (1993) found that patients whose desires for information and attention to emotional and family problems went unmet were significantly less satisfied with their physicians than those whose desires were met. Even patients with chronic diseases who had lived with the problem for years had questions they wanted answered. Their satisfaction was related more strongly to the desire for information and affective support than to whether the physician conducted examinations and tests. The greater the patients' satisfaction, the more likely they are to comply with treatment recommendations.

Although patient satisfaction is strongly associated with the length of the visit, it can be further enhanced by spending some time talking about nonmedical topics. Even brief chatting about the weather or something nonmedical can give the impression that more time was taken with the patient, thereby reducing the feeling of being rushed through the visit (Gross et al., 1998).

PATIENT DISSATISFACTION

In a typical business, only 4% of customers voice their dissatisfaction. The other 96% say nothing, and 91% never return. This has led to many practices conducting regular patient satisfaction surveys so that problems can be identified.

Communication

The patient should be able to gain access to the clinician on the phone, by e-mail, or by an early appointment without having to run an obstacle course created by an overly protective staff. Delay in returning a phone call may result in a patient remaining home all day waiting; if the call is not returned at all, the negative effect on rapport is great.

Unwillingness to make communication convenient for the patient usually results in a spiral of increasingly frequent attempts to reach the physician and mounting frustration for everyone. In contrast, physicians who give a high priority to communicating discover that most patients are considerate and even protective of the physician's time. At the beginning of a practice, patients do a certain amount of testing to determine a physician's accessibility; physicians who pass the test find that they are rarely inconvenienced by unnecessary calls or patient visits.

VERBAL COMMUNICATION

Much of the communication process in the clinical interview centers on verbal interchange. Symptoms, past medical history, family medical history, and psychosocial data are transmitted primarily by verbal means. The chief complaint is extremely important because it explains why patients believe they need the physician's help.

Patients who do not mention a concern and who withhold requests are less satisfied with their care and experience less improvement in their symptoms. Bell and colleagues (2001) found that 9% of patients had one or more unvoiced desires and were most hesitant to ask their physician for referrals and for physical therapy. These patients were also less likely to trust their physician. This is an important reason to be sensitive to subtle clues that the patient may be suppressing something important to them. What the patient does *not* say may be as important as what the patient says.

"Slips of the tongue" or major areas of omission (e.g., a married person who never mentions a spouse) may signify problem areas that, when explored, help establish the interviewer as a perceptive person who understands the underlying issues. The interviewer constantly must consider, "Why is the patient telling me that?" Even simple, casual remarks may be the patient's way of broaching issues of great concern; the man who says, "Oh, by the way, a friend of mine has been having some chest pain when he walks a lot. Do you think that sounds serious?" may actually be talking about his own concern that he is unable to face directly. A child may be brought to the office with a trivial problem so that the mother has a chance to discuss with the physician something that is troubling her; the child is a calling card, signaling the need to open the communication channel. The physician who is sensitive to these subtle clues and encourages the patient to discuss what is actually troublesome will find that the rapport established allows future interviews to be much more open and direct.

HAND-ON-THE-DOORKNOB SYNDROME

The patient's parting phrase is sometimes a clue to the primary reason for the visit, or it may reflect another issue of great concern that is emotionally threatening and could not be voiced until adequate courage was summoned at the moment of departure. It sometimes surfaces as a last, desperate attempt to communicate because, with a hand on door, escape is readily accessible if the physician's reaction is unfavorable. Reasons for this hidden communication by the patient are important and must be recognized and addressed. Because of fear of rejection or humiliation, the patient may test the physician with minor complaints before mentioning the real reason for the visit (Quill, 1989). The physician must be alert to any unusual behavior during an interview (e.g., slips of the tongue, unexpected responses, overenthusiastic denials) and should search further for the underlying reason for the visit when a patient presents with a trivial complaint that appears inappropriate. It is a good practice to ask the patient routinely at the end of a visit, "Is there anything we have not covered, or anything else you would like to ask me?"

Patients with a fear of cancer, for example, often are unable to voice their concern to the physician. Instead, they present with somatic complaints or contrived reasons that necessitate a complete examination. They are hopeful that the examination will allay their fears without it being necessary to express them openly. A female patient presenting for a complete physical examination actually may be concerned over the possibility of a carcinoma of the breast, which her elder sister might have had at the same age or for which a friend recently had surgery. Such situations emphasize the need for a complete family history and a discussion of any patient concerns in an effort to allow these feelings to surface. Attention then should be paid to alleviating the anxiety. Apprehension regarding cancer is widespread, and the only cure for this fear often is a therapeutic conversation with the physician.

Physicians in private practice who have established rapport during an ongoing relationship with patients communicate more easily than do physicians seeing a patient for the first time in an emergency department (ED). Korsch and Negrete (1972) showed that ED physicians did more talking than the patients, although their perception was just the opposite. This was attributed to interaction with unfamiliar patients by house staff in a setting where the stress level is high and the orientation therapeutic. However, Arntson and Philipsborn (1982) found that physicians in private practice for 26 years who knew their patients and saw them in a low-stress situation for diagnosis or health maintenance also talked more than the patients (twice as long). One difference in the two settings was a strong, reciprocal affective relationship between physician and patient in the private office. If either made an affective statement, the other would respond similarly, whereas in the ED, patients expressed twice as many affective statements as did the physicians.

VOCABULARY

The use of appropriate vocabulary assists in establishing rapport by ensuring easy and accurate communication. Phrasing questions in simple language appropriate to the patient's level of understanding and avoidance of medical jargon help establish a sense of working together. The patient's cultural background and educational level should be considered, and the physician should avoid using slang or a contrived accent because the patient will detect the artificiality and consider this patronizing.

Patients prefer to be enlightened, and they demand maximum insight into their care. It is best to start all explanations at a basic level and proceed only as rapidly as the patient's understanding permits. An analysis of 1057 audiotaped patient interviews with 59 primary care physicians and 65 surgeons showed that in 9 of 10 cases, patients did not receive good explanations of proposed treatments or tests (Braddock et al., 1999).

Medical terminology should be avoided unless it is familiar to the patient. For example, some patients have interpreted "lumbar puncture" to mean "an operation to drain the lungs." No longer does the physician gain a therapeutic advantage by writing prescriptions in Latin or impressing the patient with medical terms.

Metaphors can be harmful and are often used without the physician being aware of the negative connotation, unknowingly raising the patient's anxiety level. Attempts to coerce a patient into having surgery with phrases such as "you are living on borrowed time" may cause anxiety and increase postoperative morbidity (Bedell et al., 2004).

Physicians should be sure of what patients mean to convey by their word selection and make certain they are operating at a common level of understanding. When the patient says he or she "drinks a little," inquire further to clarify "a little." If the patient "spits up blood," determine whether it is truly spitting or really vomiting. A major barrier to accurate interpersonal communication is the tendency of people to react to a statement from their own points of view, rather than attempting to interpret it from the speaker's vantage point. If a question exists regarding the clarity of the interpretation, it is best to repeat it to the speaker's satisfaction. Contract negotiators have found that when parties in a dispute realize that they are being understood and each party sees how the situation appears to the other, there is less need to exaggerate and act defensively. Korsch and Negrete (1972) found that some of the longest interviews between physician and patient were caused by failures in communication; they had to spend considerable time trying to "get on the same wavelength." An analysis of the conversations revealed that less than 5% of the physician's conversation was personal or friendly in nature, and that although most of the physicians believed that they had been friendly, fewer than half of patients had this impression.

NONVERBAL COMMUNICATION

Verbal communication occupies so much of daily social interaction that nonverbal communication often is ignored. However, much that is said is unspoken. Communications specialists have demonstrated convincingly that nonverbal messages play a major role in validating or contradicting verbal messages, with great influence as communication symbols in their own right. When there is conflict between the verbal and nonverbal, believe the latter.

Communication between two people is usually one-third nonverbal, although some say communication is 93% nonverbal and 7% verbal (Secrets of Body Language, 2008). What is said verbally often is emphasized nonverbally, and personal attitudes and emotions usually are communicated at the nonverbal level. Nonverbal communicative signals are under less censorship from conscious control than are verbal messages, so they are likely to be more genuine.

Charles Darwin held that there is a unique pattern of nonverbal actions for each emotion. In *Expressions of the Emotions in Man and Animals* (1872), Darwin suggested that emotional expressions are evolutionary remnants of previous adaptive behavior that persist even though currently useless. Snarling as a sign of aggression is one example. Although recent knowledge indicates that emotional expression is learned and genetically mediated, Darwin's idea of a unique pattern of actions has been shown for depression and anxiety and is likely in the future to be demonstrated for other emotional states.

PARALANGUAGE

Paralanguage is the voice effect that accompanies or modifies talking and often communicates meaning. It includes velocity of speech (e.g., fast, slow, hesitant), tone and volume of voice, sighs and grunts, pauses, and inflections. Urgency, sincerity, confidence, hesitation, thoughtfulness, gaiety, sadness, and apprehension all are conveyed by qualities of voice. McCaskey (1979) believes that the literal interpretation (i.e., definition) of words accounts for only 10% of communication between two people, whereas facial expression and tone of voice account for up to 90% of the communication.

There is a real difference between verbal and vocal information. The *verbal message* refers to the words literally transmitted. The *vocal message* includes the emotional quality, the tone of voice, and the frequency and length of pauses—information that is lost when the words are written. Tone of voice, for example, can reverse the meaning of words. Sarcasm is a common example of a contradiction between vocal and verbal messages. Comparative studies have shown that when the vocal and verbal messages transmit contradictory information, the vocal is more accurate.

Physicians should be alert to subtle changes of tone, such as when patients ask whether everything will be all right. Are they asking for reassurance, showing fear, or doubting the diagnosis? Rather than concentrating exclusively on *what* patients are saying, the astute physician will concentrate on *how* they are saying it.

In a study of recordings of surgeons who had been sued and those who had not, the sued group could be identified by their tone of voice. They sounded dominant, whereas the nonsued group sounded less dominant and more concerned. "In the end it comes down to a matter of respect, and the simplest way that respect is communicated is through tone of voice" (Gladwell, 2005, p. 43).

TOUCH

A close personal interest in the patient can be communicated by the appropriate use of touch. The most socially acceptable method in this country is a handshake, enabling the physician to establish early contact with the patient (Colgan, 2009). The handshake, properly used, can convey to the patient sincerity and interest as well as security and poise. It is an inoffensive intrusion into the other person's area of privacy and can be extended under certain circumstances to include the application of the left hand to the lower or upper arm. This technique is often used by politicians to emphasize sincerity and concern (Figure 13-1). A variation of the politician's handshake is the "double-hander," which some equate to a miniature hug.

Politicians also "gain the upper hand" by positioning themselves to the right of the other person so that when

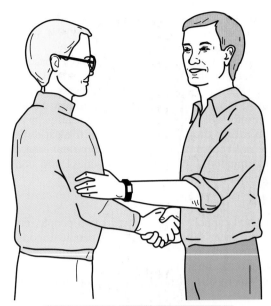

Figure 13-1 The politician's handshake.

shaking hands theirs is on top. Another way to show dominance is to make sure they go through a door last, often with a pat on the back. This shows that the one going through the door last is in charge. This was well illustrated when President Clinton welcomed the Israeli and Palestinian leaders into a building and each insisted the other go first. While this would be considered polite in the United States, in the Middle East it reflects a power struggle. The winner (the last one through the door) emphasizes this with a pat on the back as the other enters (Secrets of Body Language, 2008).

The handshake as a traditional greeting of friendship began by the raising of exposed hands by two approaching individuals to give evidence that they held no weapons. This proceeded to the grasping of hands or, in the Roman society, the forearms. In the United States, a firm handshake is most acceptable. Usually, the limp or "wet dishrag" handshake indicates lack of interest or insincerity, especially if it is rapidly withdrawn. A moist palm is a sign of nervousness or apprehension, and the "halfway there," fingers-only handshake indicates reluctance or indecision. However, the handshake continues to be modified culturally, and a person should be extremely wary of misinterpreting another person's handshake without understanding his or her cultural background.

In the past in China, the Confucian code of etiquette dictated that there should never be a touching of persons, and even today, Chinese officials may appear reluctant to grasp an extended hand; a Chinese man formerly shook his own hand (Butterfield, 1982). Some young people in the United States have modified the traditional palm-to-palm handshake to a grasping of the thumb and thenar eminence and continue to develop new variations reminiscent of the secret handshakes of fraternal groups.

Touching can be an effective method for communicating concern or compassion and can break down some of the defensive barriers to communication. Caution should be exercised, however, not to use it excessively or earlier than is socially permissible. If used without adequate preparation, touch can be interpreted as an invasion of privacy and a forward and inconsiderate act. During the physical examination, it is best to talk before touching by explaining to the patient what will be done next. Studies of primates have shown that touching gestures usually are considered nonaggressive and calming in nature. When used properly by the physician, touch can be facilitative and welcome.

The tremendous symbolic value of touch as a healing power was demonstrated during the Middle Ages, when people sought relief from scrofula (i.e., tuberculous lymphadenitis) through the king's touch, or royal touch, despite the notoriously low cure rates. This power has been transferred to physicians, and patients often feel better after a routine physical examination. Friedman (1979) stated that 85% of patients leaving a physician's office feel better even if they have not received medication or treatment, and 50% of patients in the waiting room feel better in anticipation of the help they will receive.

Touch, or "laying on of hands," may promote healing, especially if it is imbued by the patient with a special symbolic value. Franz Mesmer (1734-1815) was among the first to emphasize the medical importance of laying on of hands. Mesmer, however, believed that there was a magnetic power in his hands, which he called "animal magnetism" and which he applied to ailing individuals. His theory was unscientific, and although he became famous for successfully treating a number of hysterical patients, he finally was discredited by a committee that included Benjamin Franklin and Antoine Lavoisier. They found his treatments to be without magnetism and essentially useless. They did agree, however, that he had helped many people and had brought about many cures. They attributed these cures to unknown factors rather than to the animal magnetism he claimed. Mesmerism was the forerunner of hypnosis, initially called "artificial somnambulism," developed by Puységur, a disciple of Mesmer.

The magic of touch can be good medicine, especially when combined with concern, support, and reassurance. *Stroking*, a special kind of touching, describes a physical or symbolic recognition of a person's finer attributes. A stroke may be a kind word, a warm gesture, or a simple touch of the hand. Infants deprived of touch and stroking suffer mental and physical deterioration. Adults also require stroking to maintain a healthy emotional state. Stroking occurs when an interchange between two people leaves one or both with a good or fulfilled feeling.

Lightly touching someone's elbow for less than 3 seconds can give you up to three times the chance of getting what you want (Pease and Pease, 2004). Elbow touching works better in places where touching is not the cultural norm, such as Great Britain and Germany.

BODY LANGUAGE

It is said that body language is the unspoken truth. The astute physician will cultivate observational skills that enable the detection of hidden or subtle clues to diagnosis contained in the patient's nonverbal behavior. *Kinesics* is the study of nonverbal gestures, or body movements, and their meaning as a form of communication. However, specific gestures and their interpretation are of importance only when judged in the context of the circumstances surrounding them. Body language alone does not reveal the entire behavioral image any more than verbal language does alone. Just as one word does not make a sentence or even have much meaning without the sentence, a single gesture has clinical relevance only as part of a sequence of actions. Although they have significance, individual signs are not reliable when they stand alone; they are meaningful only when considered in the context of a person's total behavioral pattern.

When there is *congruence* between the verbal and nonverbal message—when the gesture conveys the same message as the spoken word—communication and its meaning are probably in agreement. When a person indicates something different from the other, however, the *nonverbal* message usually is more accurate. Unless body language, tone of voice, and words spoken all match, look more closely for the reason.

Attempts by the patient to mask feelings can be detected readily by observing body behavior. True feelings are more likely to leak through conscious efforts to conceal feelings. Likewise, a physician's attempt at deception will be detected by patients and can destroy confidence and damage rapport. Positive verbal communication (e.g., "You're looking better today") accompanied by negative nonverbal cues will be interpreted by the patient as insincere. For example, a patient who is not told the true nature of a terminal illness usually knows it anyway and may distrust family, friends, and physician if they persist in the charade.

In a medical school commencement address, Alan Alda (star of TV's *M*A*S*H*) challenged new physicians to be able to read a patient's involuntary muscles as well as their radiographic studies. He asked, "Can you see the fear and uncertainty in my face? If I tell you where it hurts, can you hear in my voice where I ache? I show you my body, but I bring you my person. Will you tell me what you are doing and in words I can understand? Will you tell me when you don't know what to do?" (*Time*, May 28, 1979, p. 68). The physician will see the fear and uncertainty in the patient's face only if she or he is looking at the patient rather than the medical record. Alda's statement reflects the concern and compassion that patients desire. By using appropriate body language, the physician can convey this attention and concern in the most effective manner possible.

Body Position

The body position when sitting can show various degrees of tension or relaxation. The tense person sits erect with a fairly rigid posture. A person who is moderately relaxed has a forward lean of approximately 20 degrees and a side lean of up to 10 degrees. A very relaxed position (usually too relaxed for physicians interacting with patients) is a backward lean (i.e., recline) of 20 degrees and a sideways lean of more than 10 degrees.

Higher patient satisfaction is associated with a physician's forward body lean and rotation of the torso toward the patient. Larsen and Smith (1981, p. 487) found that "the patient also responds more favorably to the physician who relaxes his chin in his hands and gazes directly at the patient, rather than a physician who elevates his chin (unsupported) as if to imply a more superior status." Physicians whose communication styles have been

considered patient oriented have been observed to change body position more frequently than physicians whose conversations were physician centered.

An attempt should be made, whenever possible, to sit rather than stand when interviewing a patient. Rapport is improved if the physician does not intimidate the patient by placing him or her in a submissive position. Patients feel more comfortable and less helpless speaking in a sitting position rather than prone. Sitting on the patient's bed is usually not recommended, but for some patients, it is an effective means of establishing closeness and conveying warmth in a relaxed yet attentive manner.

Mirroring

When good rapport exists between two people, each will mirror the other's movements. Some people unconsciously establish rapport with another by mirroring that person's movements or body posture (Key, 1980) (Figure 13-2). Disruptions in this mirroring may signal that one member

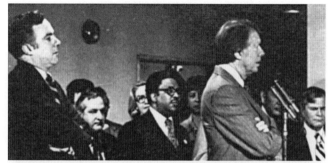
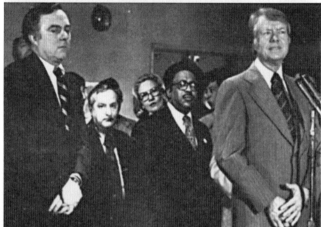
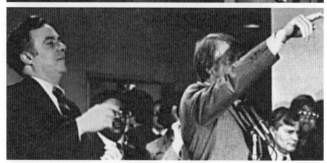

Figure 13-2 Joseph Califano *(left),* Secretary of Health, Education and Welfare, mirrors his boss, President Jimmy Carter, through his posture and gestures. (From Key MR, ed. *The relationship of verbal and nonverbal communication.* New York: Mouton; 1980, p. v.)

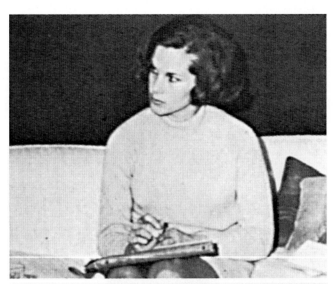

Figure 13-3 This woman signals attentiveness and seriousness by holding very still, cocking her head, and looking intently at the speaker. (From Scheflen AE. *Body language and the social order—Communication as behavioral control.* Englewood Cliffs, NJ: Prentice-Hall; 1972.)

disagrees with what the other has said or feels betrayed or insulted but cannot express this idea verbally. If the physician notices this sudden disruption of mirroring activity by the patient, more attention should be focused on the comment that led to the change of position. Renegotiation or further explanation may be indicated. A powerful way to establish rapport is to match intentionally the body language of another.

Head Position

Typically, the head is held forward in anger and back in defiance, anxiety, or fear. It is down or bowed in sadness, submissiveness, shame, or guilt. The head tilted to one side indicates interest and attention (Scheflen, 1972) (Figure 13-3); under certain circumstances, this can be a flirtation. The erect head indicates self-confidence and maturity. It is almost impossible to tilt the head in front of someone who is not trusted or of whom we are afraid.

When listening to a patient, the physician should show interest and concern by an attentive position, which is best illustrated by sitting forward in the chair with an interested, attentive facial expression and the head slightly tilted. Darwin was one of the first to notice that animals assume a head tilt when listening intently.

Face

The human face can create more than 7000 expressions using 44 muscles (Cleese, 2001); some say 10,000 expressions are possible (Ekman, 2003).

Darwin (1872) proposed that cultures throughout the world express similar emotions or states of mind with remarkably uniform body movements. His information was gathered from missionary friends working with aborigines, persons under hypnosis, infants, and patients with mental disease. He also studied blind and deaf persons who, without benefit of learning from others, were observed to raise eyebrows when surprised and shrug their shoulders to indicate helplessness.

Darwin held that the facial expression of emotion, when undisguised, is independent of culture and is identical throughout the world. The facial expressions of joy, sadness, and anger are the same in the Australian aborigine, the American farmer, and the Norwegian fisherman (Ekman, 2006). Various cultures, however, do disguise the facial expression in different ways. In American culture, the mouth is used most often to disguise feelings. A person in a social gathering may be smiling, although inwardly sad or angry. The eyebrows, eyes, and forehead are least affected by these cultural disguises and are the most consistently dependable indicators of emotion. The current popularity of Botox injections, however, may mask these expressions by showing no wrinkling of the forehead. "A 50-year-old person with no wrinkling has almost certainly had some kind of cosmetic procedure or treatment." (Hartley and Karinch, 2010, p. 88). As Shakespeare wrote, "I saw his heart in his face" (*The Winter's Tale*, Act I, Scene II).

Ekman and Friesen (1975) found that the facial expressions of fear, disgust, happiness, and anger were the same in countries with widely disparate languages and cultures. They used composite facial photographs to show how each part of the face contributes to the expressions of emotion, especially surprise, fear, disgust, anger, happiness, and sadness. In American culture, when people want to disguise their true feelings and convey a more socially acceptable impression, they do so by smiling. This may be especially true in patients who are sad or depressed. Figure 13-4 is a composite showing sadness in the eyes, brow, and forehead being masked by a smile.

Smile

A genuine smile can be helpful in quickly establishing a friendly atmosphere and developing a warm, interpersonal relationship. A grin can be the physician's most effective weapon for breaking down resistance or apprehension in patients, especially children or young adults. A number of studies have shown that patients are more positively disposed to physicians who smile. The smile must be genuine, however; patients can easily spot a phony smile.

Smiles are controlled by the zygomatic major muscles that connect to the corners of the mouth and the orbicularis oculi muscles. The latter are not under conscious control and reveal a true smile that involves characteristic creases around the eyes (crow's feet). A genuine smile lights up the whole face; one that does not is more likely a deception (Ekman et al., 2005). In Figure 13-5, *A*, the man on the left has a broad nonenjoyment smile whereas on the right there is true enjoyment shown by the eyes. Similarly, in Figure 13-5, *B*, the genuine smile on the right pulls back both the mouth and the eyes. An excellent overview of facial expressions can be viewed on the DVD *The Human Face* by John Cleese (2001).

Micro-Expressions

Ekman and Friesen (1975) describe micro-expressions as a valuable indication of masking or deception. "Micro-expressions are caused by the face's all too rapid efficiency in registering inner feelings" (Morris, 1977, p. 110). Most facial expressions last more than 1 second, but micro-expressions last only about one-fifth of a second (Ekman, 2003). This is approximately the time it takes to blink an

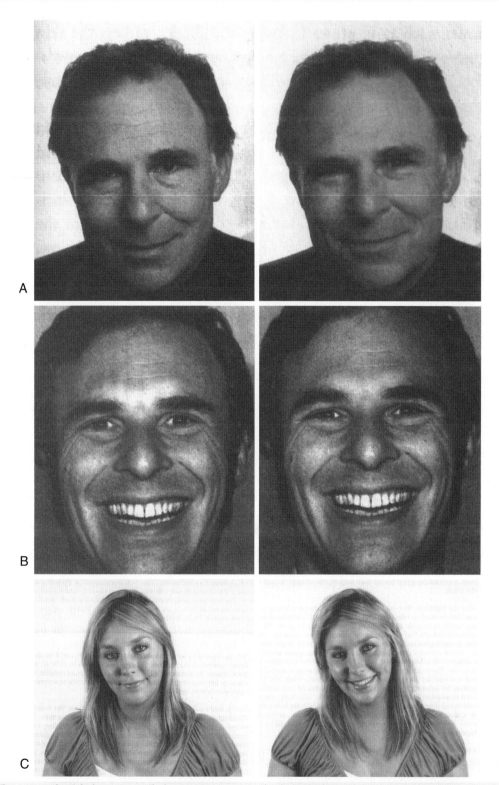

Figure 13-4 A, The man on the right has a true smile, his eyes are narrower, cheeks are higher and their contour has changed. **B,** Both have a broad smile but the one on the left has a broad, nonenjoyment smile while the one on the right shows true enjoyment. **C,** Compare the insincere smile on the left with a genuine smile on the right that pulls back both the mouth and the eyes. (A and B, From Ekman P. *Emotions revealed: recognizing faces and feelings to improve communication and emotional life.* New York: Henry Holt; 2003, pp. 207, 208; C, From Kuhnke E. *Body Language for Dummies.* Chichester, England: Wiley; 2007, pp. 66-67.)

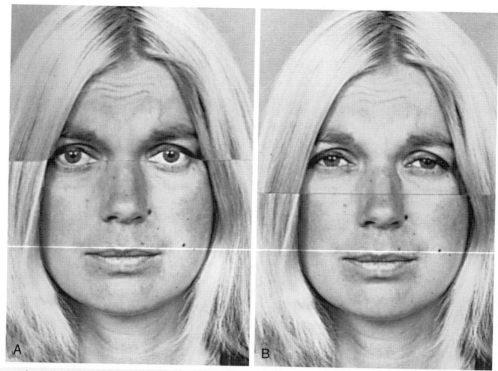

Figure 13-5 Sadness shown in the eyes and forehead (the mouth is neutral). The importance of the eyelids can be seen because the person on the right (**B**) is obviously sadder than the one on the left (**A**) but differs only in that a sad lower eyelid has been substituted for a neutral lower eyelid. (From Ekman P, Friesen WV. *Unmasking the face: a guide to recognizing emotions from facial clues.* Englewood Cliffs, NJ: Prentice-Hall; 1975.)

eye, and micro-expressions easily can be missed if the physician is not carefully observing the patient. Micro-expressions tend to occur when emotion is concealed unwittingly by repression or deliberately by suppression. They are seen when the patient begins to show a true facial expression, senses this, and immediately neutralizes or masks the expression. Some micro-expressions are complete enough to show the true emotion felt, but most often, they are squelched to such an extent that the physician has only a clue that the patient is concealing some emotion.

Most expressions last about 2 seconds (0.5 to 4 seconds). Surprise is the briefest expression (Ekman, 2003).

Eyes

The eyes are probably the principal organs of expression. They are so important to a person's appearance that when anonymity is desired, only the eyes need to be covered. The eyebrows have been shown to have 40 different positions of expression and the eyelids have 23. Consider the magnitude of possible combinations when all facial elements are involved as indicators of expression. The message conveyed by each position can be further modified by the length of a glance and its intensity.

In most cultures, good rapport is enhanced when one's gaze meets the other's 60% to 70% of the time. When we talk, we maintain eye contact about 40% of the time and 80% when listening. Ninety percent of the gaze will be in a triangular area between the eyes and the mouth (Pease and Pease, 2004). On meeting, two people will scan each other's face for about 3 seconds, then briefly gaze downward. An upward eye break may be disconcerting or convey a lack of interest (Lewis, 1989) (Figure 13-6).

The eyes can give more information for some emotions than others. Knapp (1978) found that the eyes were better than the brow, forehead, or lower face for the accurate portrayal of fear but were less accurate for anger and disgust. Even the lower eyelid alone can convey considerable information. In Figure 13-5, it is apparent that the person in *B* depicts more sadness than the one in *A*, but the pictures differ in only one respect: the lower eyelid.

It has long been known that *pupils* dilate when the person sees something pleasant and contract when something unpleasant is viewed. This involuntary signal can be a valuable indication of what is really going on. Asian jade dealers wore dark glasses so that no one could see their pupils dilate when they discovered an especially valuable piece of jade. Likewise, a magician doing card tricks can tell when a pre-selected card is seen by a subject because of the sudden pupil enlargement. In one experiment (Hess, 1975), the pupils of males dilated when the men were shown photographs of nude females and constricted for nude males. Homosexuals demonstrated the opposite. Dilated pupils also can indicate that listeners are interested, whereas constricted pupils suggest that they do not like what is being said (or viewed).

Sincerity is expressed with the eyes. The best method for conveying sincerity is frequent eye contact, a technique most appropriately used when listening to the other person. One trait of good listeners is that they constantly look at the speaker. A listener who does not maintain eye contact but continues to look down or away from the speaker may be shy, depressed, or indicating rejection of the speaker or the comments being made. One patient said, "I had one student doctor who looked at his toes instead of me. If he ever opens

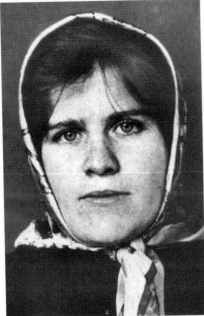

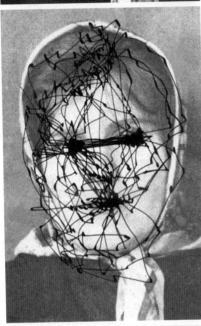

Figure 13-6 Record of eye movements made by a person looking at a photograph of a young girl's face.

a practice, I don't believe I would trust him." Conversely, speakers frequently may break eye contact when talking and are permitted a distant stare when formulating ideas and selecting phrases. However, they still should try to make frequent, although less prolonged and intense, eye contact.

A special form of human-to-human awareness is conveyed by eye contact. Prolonged eye contact, or staring, can be offensive. Monkeys can be provoked to combat by a person staring at them because it represents a threat of aggression. Under other circumstances, however, staring can be flirtatious, emphasizing that the meaning of eye behavior depends on other factors in the situation.

The acceptability of eye contact varies significantly among different cultures. In the United States, focusing the

eyes on the speaker indicates respect and attention, regardless of the age of the individuals involved. However, Mexican Americans tend not to maintain as much eye contact while listening as do other Americans and may look away from the speaker more often. This is not a sign of disrespect or inattention. In Latin American countries, a younger person may be thought disrespectful if his or her eyes meet those of the adult who is speaking. A physician could be considered seductive in that culture if he or she maintained steady eye contact while talking to a patient. In the United States, it is impolite to maintain eye contact with a stranger for more than 3 seconds, but Europeans believe that longer periods of eye contact are normal. The physician needs to consider the patient's cultural background when interpreting the meaning of eye contact behavior. Looking away from the speaker from time to time may be a sign of respect and sensitivity rather than the opposite. At the same time, the physician's failure to look a patient in the eye can be dehumanizing and can cause the patient to feel more like an object than a person. Patients are most comfortable when the physician looks at them approximately 50% of the time and are uncomfortable when eye contact is avoided. Some feel that rapport is improved if a person's gaze is met 60% to 70% of the time (Kuhnke, 2007).

The frequency of eye contact also can provide clues to whether the patient is anxious or depressed. The eyes of anxious patients blink frequently or dart back and forth. They look at the interviewer as frequently as low-anxiety patients but maintain eye contact for less time on each gaze. Similarly, the patient may interpret the physician's lack of eye contact as indicative of anxiety or discomfort, even rejection.

Frequent blinking of the eyes can be a sign of pressure or stress. In a political debate between Senator Bob Dole and President Bill Clinton in 1996, Dole blinked an average of 105 times per minute, showing more pressure than Clinton's 48 times per minute.

Depressed patients maintain eye contact only one-fourth as long as nondepressed patients. Downward contraction of the mouth and a downward angling of the head are also cues to depression. As with the anxious patient, there is no difference in frequency of eye contact in the depressed patient; the difference is only in the duration of contact.

Patients with abdominal pain caused by organic disease are more likely to keep their eyes open during palpation of the abdomen than those with nonspecific pain (Gray et al., 1988). The patient with genuine abdominal tenderness may apprehensively watch the physician's hand as it approaches the tender area.

Hands

The hands will be droopy and flaccid with sadness, fidgety or grasping in anxiety, and clenched in anger. When a speaker joins her or his hands, with fingers extended and fingertips touching, it is called *steepling* and indicates confidence and assurance in the comments being made (Figure 13-7). It can be taken to extremes if held too high and convey arrogance instead of self-assurance (Kuhnke, 2007).

Palms usually are held in the palm-in position. Turning the palms outward can be a subtle courting behavior (usually used by women), but it more likely indicates a warm and friendly greeting (Davis, 1975).

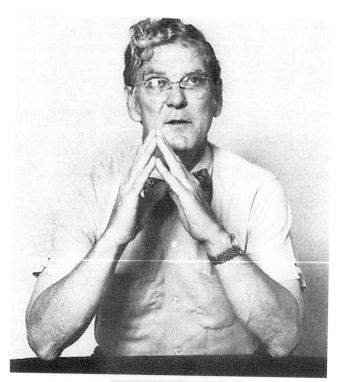

Figure 13-7 Steepling.

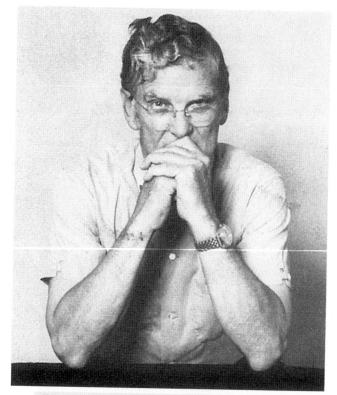

Figure 13-8 The defensive or "doubting Thomas" position.

The hands of an anxious patient can be observed to shake when holding a pen, to twitch, or to be braced unnaturally. The white-knuckle pose of tightly locked fingers can be an effort to mask anxiety.

Hands can be a subtle indicator of the urge to interrupt. Be alert for this sign in a patient so that important information will not be suppressed, and the patient can be given every opportunity to supply valuable information. Indications of this urge to interrupt are a slight raising of the hand or perhaps the index finger only, pulling at the earlobe, or raising the index finger to the lips. The latter gesture also may indicate an attempt to suppress a comment and should alert the physician to inquire further and elicit the hidden information. A patient listening in "The Thinker" position, with the index finger across the lips or extended along the cheek, or one sitting with elbows on the table and hands clenched in front of the mouth, although listening intently, may not believe or understand the physician's words (Figure 13-8). The physician should take additional time to amplify the issue or explain the diagnosis or treatment regimen further.

Arms

Although folded arms are found in all cultures, this is considered a discovered action rather than an inborn trait because it is a natural position of comfort that is as easily discovered by the African tribesman as the New York banker. It is the subtle ways in which the arms are held that can give clues to underlying emotions. Crossed arms can be a defensive posture, indicating disagreement with another's view, or it can be a sign of insecurity. It can also be nothing more than a position of comfort and should, as with all other signs, be considered in the context of the individual's total behavior.

Notice the manner in which the arms are crossed. Are they relaxed in the normal position of comfort, or are they in a self-hugging posture, reflecting insecurity or sadness and indicating a need for reassurance? Anger can be seen in clenched fists that are held tightly against the body in a holding-back manner, preventing them from hitting (Figure 13-9). If the patient has assumed a position of resistance or defensiveness, sitting with arms and legs crossed and perhaps with body turned away, search for the reason for this defensiveness and try to eliminate it. Perhaps a recommendation that the patient stop smoking is threatening and difficult to accept. In that case, it is important to make an additional effort to explain the rationale for the recommendation; do not hurry over it with a brief comment or admonition.

Men who are under stress will often cross their hands in front of them as if protecting their genitals, called the fig-leaf position or "protecting the precious." Women may cross arms over their abdomen referred to as "egg protecting" (Hartley and Karinch, 2010).

Legs

Although crossing the legs is a common position of comfort, it can also indicate a shutting out of or protection against the outside world. If crossed legs in a patient confirm the total kinesic picture of resistance, including crossed arms and other signals discussed earlier (Figure 13-10), make every effort to identify the reason for the resistance and correct it before proceeding further. Likewise, locked ankles can indicate defensiveness. Diagnostic information obtained from a resistant patient is likely to be incomplete, and instructions are unlikely to be followed.

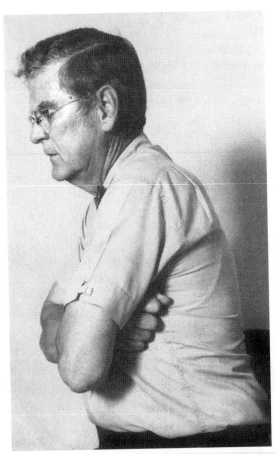

Figure 13-9 The resistant position, suggesting suppressed anger.

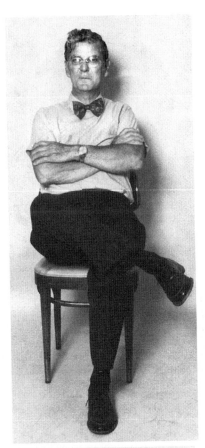

Figure 13-10 The defensive position.

When seated, a person's legs are pointed in the direction of interest and if disinterested will point away. Similarly, when legs are crossed, the upper knee dictates the direction of interest.

Notice the position of the feet and their movement. As with fidgety hand movements, anxiety is associated with the fidgety, constantly moving foot. An anxious or scared person may sit forward in the chair with feet placed in the ready-to-run position, with one foot in front of the other. The angry person is more likely to place the feet widely apart in a position of stability, whereas the feet of a sad person tend to move in a slow, circular pattern.

Gestures

The thumbs-up sign in the United States means "good going," but in some Islamic countries, it is the equivalent of an upraised middle finger. Similarly, the extended hand with palm forward means "stop" in the United States, but in West Africa, it is an insult greater than the upraised middle finger.

Joining the thumb and index finger in a circle to indicate "OK" is an insult in many Latin American countries and in France means zero or worthless. In Texas, raising the index and little finger with the middle two fingers folded down is the "Hook 'em Horns" gesture of the University of Texas Longhorns, but in parts of Africa this gesture is a curse and in Italy it means your spouse is unfaithful.

American television and the movies have dulled these differences worldwide, although some still exist. In the 1978 movie *Inglorious Bastards* (remade in 2009) the American posing as a German was detected because he displayed the number 2 using index and middle fingers, whereas Europeans would hold up the thumb and index finger with the thumb being number 1.

Preening

Preening gestures, such as the male pulling up socks, adjusting a tie, or combing hair and the female adjusting clothing or using a mirror to review makeup, may not necessarily be seductive in nature but can be an attempt to establish rapport and good interpersonal relations. If the preening is intended to be flirtatious, however, the woman may cross her legs, place a hand on her hip, caress her leg, or stroke the arm or thigh in some fashion. The flirtatious male typically uses gaze holding and head tilt to accentuate normal preening gestures or may stretch to make himself look larger. Both genders may use "accidental" touching as a flirting signal. When someone's attention is completely focused on the other, legs, knees, and feet are usually extended in the direction of the other. The physician should remain alert to the accentuation of normal preening gestures into courtship actions to identify the seductive patient and deal with the issue early, before unknowingly encouraging the patient to proceed further along this course.

Respiratory Avoidance Response

The respiratory avoidance response involves a frequent clearing of the throat when no phlegm or mucus is present. All animals exhibit a respiratory avoidance response as a

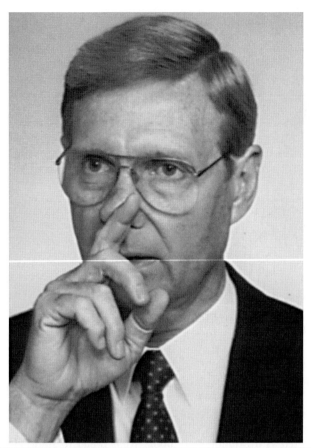

Figure 13-11 The nose rub, a variation of the respiratory avoidance response.

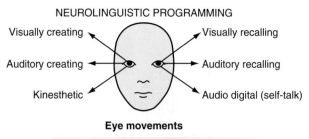

Figure 13-12 Neurolinguistic programming.

means of clearing something unpleasant or undesirable from the respiratory tract. This action also can be a nonverbal indication of disgust or rejection. When physicians find themselves doing this, they should observe the accompanying circumstances and notice whether posterior pharyngeal mucus is truly present.

Nose Rub

Another component of the respiratory avoidance response is the nose rub (Figure 13-11). This involves a light or subtle rub of the nose with the index finger and signals rejection of a statement being made by the subject or by another individual. The nose rub to relieve an itch is usually vigorous and involves a repeated series of rubs, whereas that of the respiratory avoidance response is soft and consists of one or two light strokes, often involving nothing more than a light flick of the nose. Morris (1977, p. 111) described the nose flick as "a reflection of the fact that a split is being forced between inner thoughts and outward action." It can be associated with lying or with the struggle to appear calm while suppressing anger or discomfort. During Bill Clinton's testimony to the grand jury regarding his affair with Monica Lewinsky, he rarely touched his nose when telling the truth, but when he lied he gave a split-second frown, then touched his nose. During the testimony he touched it 26 times (Pease and Pease, 2004). Variations of the nose rub include pulling at the earlobe, scratching the side of the neck or rubbing one eye. Someone aware of the nose rub will often notice it

in themselves and realize they are uncomfortable with what is being said by themselves or others. Watching for this during interviews on television may indicate the person being interviewed is uncomfortable with the question, or the person asking may realize it is a "testy" point.

This sign can be quite useful in patient interviewing. For example, the physician may ask a patient, "How are things at home?" The patient may answer, "Fine," but then clears his or her throat and lightly rubs the nose with the index finger. He or she is actually saying, "I don't like what you are asking me," or "I feel uncomfortable with my answer; things really aren't going very well at home." If there is a cause to pursue the issue further, a simple comment such as "Really?" or "You mean not even an occasional argument?" may lead to a flood of information masked by the previous response.

Verbal-Nonverbal Mismatch

Another indication that what a patient is saying may be in conflict with what is being felt is a verbal-nonverbal mismatch, such as when the patient answers "fine" to "how are things between you and your husband?" while looking sad and avoiding eye contact (Quill, 1989). If the patient answered negatively to the question, "Have you ever had a venereal disease?" and at the same time exhibited a nose rub, this topic should be followed up with a similar inquiry later, perhaps while doing the physical examination, when the patient may feel more comfortable after better rapport has been established.

Other clues that the patient may not be telling the truth or that there are repressed feelings are asymmetric facial expressions and a prolonged smile or expression of amazement. Almost all authentic facial expressions fade after 4 or 5 seconds (Ekman, 1985).

Neurolinguistic Programming

Neurolinguistic programming (NLP) involves the eye movements performed while thinking and depends on whether a person is thinking visually, aurally, or kinesthetically. A right-handed person who is visually oriented will look up and to his or her left when recalling something visually, but up and to the right if creating something visually or, in other words, making it up or lying. Similarly, a right-handed person will look sideways to his or her left when recalling sounds and sideways to the right when imagining sounds (Ritch, 2004). A person who is looking up and to his or her right (i.e., your left) probably is imagining things he or she has never seen before. This technique is used by police investigators when interviewing suspects. A left-handed person will respond in opposite directions (Brooks, 1989; Zellmann, 2004) (Figure 13-12).

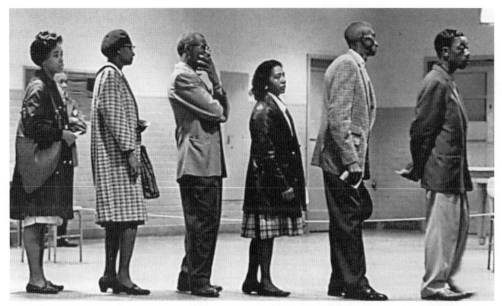

Figure 13-13 The "body bubble" surrounding strangers in a queue. (Courtesy Magnum Photos, New York.)

DETECTING LYING

In addition to looking up and to the right to create an image or a fact, a person who is lying is also likely to do the following:

- Cover the mouth with hand.
- Rub or flick the nose.
- Scratch the neck.
- Pull at the ear, or rub behind the ear.
- Rub one eye.
- Blink excessively (although absence of blinking is also possible).
- Have a micro-expression indicating something is different than what is said.
- Avoid making eye contact.
- Use arms and hands less.
- Be defensive rather than aggressive.
- Change manner or posture abruptly.

The liar will also rarely touch the other person or point a finger at them or others, and the story will not include negative details (Lieberman, 1998). The liar is not comfortable with silence and may speak more than normal to convince the other. Persons suspected of lying should be encouraged to talk because verbal and nonverbal clues will then be easier to detect (Vrij, 2005). Liars are also likely to slouch, unlike a confident person, who will sit upright. Remember that it takes a combination of verbal and nonverbal clues to detect lying, and no single action is likely to be dependable other than to raise doubt or suspicion.

PROXEMICS: SPATIAL FACTORS

Proxemics is the study of how people unconsciously structure the space around them. This structuring varies with every culture. North Americans, for example, maintain a protective "body bubble" of space about 2 feet in diameter around them when they interact with strangers or casual acquaintances. Violators of that space are considered intruders and cause the person to become defensive (Figure 13-13). In the Middle East, no such bubble exists, and it is proper to invade this area. In fact, not to do so may be interpreted as unfriendly and aloof. Arabs prefer to stand close enough to touch and smell the other person. Americans, however, if forced to stand close together, as on a crowded subway, will use their eyes (i.e., distant gaze) to maintain a more proper distance. An arm's length is a good measure of the appropriate personal distance for most people. A wife can stand inside her husband's bubble, but she will be unhappy if another woman invades this sphere of privacy, and vice versa.

Robert Frost said, "Good fences make good neighbors." In suburbs and small towns, people are more likely to talk to each other while in their backyards if a fence indicates the boundary than if there is a communal yard (McCaskey, 1979). Marking the boundary helps maintain territoriality and actually brings the neighbors closer together than when there is no fence.

Intimate space has been classified as that ranging from close physical contact to 18 inches, *personal space* from 18 inches to 4 feet, *social space* from 4 feet to 12 feet, and *public space* from 12 feet and beyond (Lambert, 2008). Placing a desk between two people shifts personal space to social space. The office desk also can be a barrier to communication when it is placed between the physician and patient, thereby emphasizing the illusion of the physician's importance and power. There may be occasions when this is desired, but it usually is not necessary in a family physician's office. Office furniture should be arranged so that a minimum number of obstacles lie between physician and patient.

Automobiles magnify the size of one's personal space up to 10 times. Compare the relationship of two people having a conversation with that of "road rage" when one invades the other's space by cutting in front of them.

HIDDEN OR MASKED COMMUNICATION AND PATIENTS' EXPECTATIONS

Although the average person has a symptom about every 6 days, he or she visits a physician only once every 4 months. Some people visit a physician much more frequently than others for the same symptom. The group who visits more frequently tends to have a higher level of anxiety, fear, grief, or frustration. It is the physician's responsibility to search for, identify, and treat organic disease if it is present, but in about one half of cases, none will be found. It is equally important to identify the reason for these visits—the basis for the heightened concern or increased anxiety. A person may see a minor symptom as a potential catastrophe if she or he thinks it may be a sign of cancer similar to that causing a parent's death. Is the patient really there "just for a blood pressure check," or because of concern about the condition of his or her coronary arteries since a friend recently had an acute myocardial infarction? If the physician deals only with the symptoms, the real concerns may go undetected, and the result will be a dissatisfied and noncompliant patient.

Barsky (1981, p. 492) cautioned, "Patients who express dissatisfaction with their medical care should be questioned about this, as they may be dissatisfied because their real motivation in seeking care has not been illuminated." He also advised the physician to investigate the patient's current life stresses when visits are made if there is no change in clinical status.

Patients may come to a physician because of what they imagine is causing their symptoms rather than because of the symptoms themselves. Identifying what patients hope can be done for them—focusing on their expectations for the visit—often reveals hidden reasons for the visit. The physician should be sure to address the patient's expectations and make certain that the interpretation is correct. Rapport and satisfaction will be enhanced if the physician identifies and satisfies the patient's expectations for the visit. Dissatisfaction results when these expectations go unmet.

LISTENING WELL

A good family physician must be a good listener. Of all the communication skills essential to rapport, the ability to listen well is probably the most important. All the information in the world about body language, vocal messages, and nonverbal cues is of limited value unless it helps the family physician be a better listener.

As Lown (1996) states, "In the brief time available to take a history, the aim is to obtain, in addition to essential facts, insight into the human being. This seems easy, but listening is the most complex and difficult of all the tools in a doctor's repertory. One must be an active listener to hear an unspoken problem" (p. 10). The appearance of readiness to listen is aided by bending forward and maintaining eye contact. The physician can discourage a patient from talking by looking away or writing in the medical record. Well-chosen questions can be rendered useless by inappropriate nonverbal behavior. Even great questions are of no value if you do not know how to listen.

For many people, the opposite of talking is not "listening" but rather "waiting to talk." It is impossible to listen attentively when you are planning what to say next. Besides, learning to listen is more difficult than learning to ask good questions (Dimitrius and Mazzarella, 1999).

The average listening efficiency of most people is only 25% because we do not concentrate on what is being said. Effective listening requires focus on what is being said and on voice tone, facial expression, and body movements. Hearing what someone says and truly listening to what they are saying is quite different (Zellmann, 2004).

Analyses of physician-patient interviews reveal that, on average, the physician rather than the patient does most of the talking, although when questioned, physicians usually imagine the reverse. In general, the less the physician says during an interview, the more the patient will say.

Boredom is one of the most difficult states to conceal. It is very difficult to appear attentive and interested if you are bored, and it takes considerable effort to appear interested (Dimitrius and Mazzarella, 1999).

SILENCE

Silence can be as effective a means of eliciting further information as direct questions. The timing is important, however, and silence should be used as a technique only when the physician is relatively certain that there is more information to follow the last statement. A shift of position or a nod and a smile, properly timed and coupled with silence, can be more effective than an encouraging comment. Nonverbal encouragement to continue is less distracting and may be more facilitative than the verbal form.

Attorneys use silence in the courtroom to get witnesses to say more than they had intended. They wait silently as if the witness has not given a complete answer, and usually they do receive additional information. Silence can be effective as long as the patient feels more inclined to fill the void than the physician. This is of value, however, only when there is more information to be obtained. It is said that Charles DeGaulle thought that silence was the ultimate power tool, and in his speeches, he gained control by looking at the audience, never breaking eye contact, and saying nothing.

INTERRUPTION

The patient may be following a line of thought and may be about to open up more but must stop and refocus if the physician captures the patient's attention with a question. The physician should interrupt a patient's statement only if it is necessary to change the conversation to a new topic, clarify an issue, elicit information not produced spontaneously, offer reassurance, or reduce patient anxiety.

Physicians usually use closed-ended questions to interrupt the patient and thereby inappropriately control the interview. Beckman and Frankel (1984) found that 69% of patients (52 of 74) had only 18 seconds to complete their initial complaint before being interrupted by their physician. This usually occurred after the patient stated only a single concern, and it effectively halted the further flow of information from the patient. This prematurely terminates opportunities for patients to present their primary concerns. Only one of the 52 patients subsequently returned to and completed the opening statement. In these recorded office interviews, only 23% of the patients were permitted to complete their list of problems uninterrupted; when they were, the complete statements usually took less than 60 seconds, and none required more than 2.5 minutes.

HUMOR

The art of medicine consists of amusing the patient while nature cures the disease.

　　　　　　　　　　　　　　　　　　—VOLTAIRE

Humor can be helpful in establishing rapport and can strengthen the physician-patient relationship. It can be used to "break the ice" and is most useful if it communicates the feeling that "we are all in this together." Humor is an effective way for physicians to appear human while supporting and empathizing with their patients. Physicians who score high in empathy also tend to have a good sense of humor (Hampes, 2001). Empathic humor can promote a stronger physician-patient relationship and enhance the effectiveness of other, more traditional as well as nontraditional forms of therapy (Berger et al., 2004).

Care must be taken, however, because humor can be a two-edged sword that can cut either way if used inappropriately. The least risk is when the humor is self-deprecating or focused on neutral topics such as the weather or parking. It can even alienate the patient if they feel the joking around is inappropriate at the very time they want serious attention paid to their problem.

More research is needed on the value of humor in medicine so that we will know when and how to use it effectively. Norman Cousins, former editor of the *Saturday Review*, had ankylosing spondylitis. He received 3 hours of pain relief after watching comedy videotapes of *The Three Stooges* and *Abbott and Costello* but obtained only one-half hour of pain relief from an oral analgesic. Some physicians write prescriptions for patients to laugh out loud three times each day. In India, more than 600 Laughter Clubs convene for 15 to 20 minutes at the beginning of each day to laugh out loud. Even a fake laugh makes one feel better throughout the day. Laughter boosts the immune system and even forced laughter leads to a good feeling and relieves stress and anger (Cleese, 2001).

Physicians who express interest in patient opinions and who use humor more often are sued less often. Tasteful humor can reduce anxiety and create a bond of friendship, but humor used inappropriately can magnify the distance between patient and physician, especially if it belittles the patient.

See eAppendix 13-1 online for interviewing effectively (including facilitating techniques) and eAppendix 13-2 for care with caring.

Summary of Additional Online Content

The following content is available at www.expertconsult.com:

eAppendix 13-1 Interviewing Effectively

eAppendix 13-2 Care with Caring

References

The complete reference list is available at www.expertconsult.com.

Web Resources

www.blifaloo.com/info/flirting-body-language.php Male and female flirting signals, eye contact, and mirroring. Also contains a link to "How to Detect Lies" plus tips on improving memory.

www.changingminds.org Covers a variety of body language message clusters, including aggressive, attentive, deceptive, romantic, and submissive.

www.wikihow.com/Read-Body-Language Good overview of the major components of body language; includes a video demonstration.

14 *Interpreting Laboratory Tests*

ELIZABETH A. WARNER and ARTHUR H. HEROLD

The use of the clinical laboratory to evaluate patients for the presence or absence of disease involves all medical and surgical specialties. Physicians in all areas of medical practice are dependent on laboratory testing to arrive at a correct diagnosis. Because many factors increase the uncertainty associated with a test result, physicians need to understand the limitations of interpreting test results.

Clinical decision making using diagnostic laboratory testing is based on the assumption that a given test is accurate and precise. Diagnostic test *accuracy* is the ability of a test to distinguish patients with a disease from those who are disease free (Leeflang et al., 2008). Test accuracy is not necessarily fixed; accuracy may vary among patient populations and with different clinical conditions. *Precision* is a measure of the reproducibility of a test measurement when the same specimen is rechecked under the same circumstances. Sources of imprecision include biologic variability and analytic variability. *Biologic variability* is the variation in a test result in the same person at different times because of physiologic processes, constitutional factors, and extrinsic factors (McClatchey, 2002) (Table 14-1). *Analytic variation* refers to the variation in repeated tests on the same specimen and relates to analytic technique and specimen processing. With current technology, biologic variation plays a larger role than analytic variation in most laboratory tests.

The Concept of "Normal"

The result of a laboratory test is compared with a reference standard, which traditionally has indicated values that are seen in healthy persons. Using the terms "normal results" or "normal range" implies that there is a clear distinction between healthy and diseased persons, when in reality there is considerable overlap.

The current standard of comparison for laboratory results is the *reference range*, which is frequently defined by results that are between chosen percentiles (typically the 2.5th to 97.5th percentiles) in a healthy reference population. Several problems are encountered when deriving a reference range. Often, the reference population is not representative of persons being tested. Differences in gender, age distribution, race, ethnicity, or the setting (hospitalized vs. ambulatory patients) between the reference population and the person receiving the test may be present. The person being tested should be tested under similar physiologic conditions (e.g., fasting, sitting, resting) as the reference population. The size of the reference population may be too small to include a representative range of the population.

Two statistical methods, parametric and nonparametric, are generally used to define the reference intervals. The *parametric* method applies when the results of the sample population fit a normal gaussian distribution, with a bell-shaped curve around the mean. In this case, the 2.5th and 97.5th percentiles can be calculated using statistical formulas. When the reference values do not follow a normal distribution, *nonparametric* methods are used, arranging the results from the reference subjects in ascending order, and identifying values between the 2.5th and 97.5th percentiles as within the reference range.

Reference ranges for a particular test can be the manufacturer's suggested reference range or may be modified because of differences in the population using the laboratory. The Clinical Laboratory Improvement Act (CLIA) of 1998 has defined three requirements for reference values: the normal or reference ranges must be made available to the ordering physician; the normal or reference ranges must be included in the laboratory procedure manual; and the laboratory must establish specifications for performance characteristics, including the reference range, for each test before reporting patient results. Using the manufacturer's reference range is valid when the analytic processing of the test is the same as that done by the manufacturer and when the population being tested is similar to the reference population used to define the reference range. When selecting a reference range that includes 95% of the test results, 5% of the population will fall outside the reference range for a single test. When more than one test is ordered, the probability increases that at least one result will be outside the reference range. Table 14-2 compares the number of independent tests ordered with the probability of an abnormal result being present in healthy persons.

Evaluating a Test's Performance Characteristics

Given that tests are not totally accurate or precise, one must have a way to quantify these shortcomings. A test's ability to discriminate diseased from nondiseased persons is defined by its sensitivity, specificity, and positive and negative predictive values. Table 14-3 shows how each is calculated. Sensitivity and specificity are inherent technical aspects of a test and are independent of the prevalence of disease in

Table 14-1   Biologic Variables That Affect Test Results

Biologic rhythms	Circadian
	Ultradian
	Infradian
Constitutional factors	Age
	Gender
	Genotype
Extrinsic factors	Posture
	Exercise
	Diet
	Caffeine use
	Medication
	Alcohol use
	Pregnancy
	Intercurrent illness

From Holmes EA: The interpretation of laboratory tests. In McClatchey KD, ed. *Clinical laboratory medicine.* 2nd ed. Philadelphia: Lippincott Williams & Wilkins; 2002, p 98.

Table 14-2   Probability That a Healthy Person Will Be Labeled as Abnormal with Multiple Test Ordering

Number of Independent Tests	Probability of an Abnormal Result (%)
1	5
2	10
5	23
10	40
20	64
50	92
90	99
Infinity	100

From Burke MD: Laboratory tests. Basic concepts and realistic expectations. *Postgrad Med*, 1978;63:55.

Table 14-3   Diagnostic Test Performance Characteristics

Finding	Disease Present	Disease Absent
Test positive	True positive (TP)	False positive (FP)
Test negative	False negative (FN)	True negative (TN)

Sensitivity = TP/(TP + FN); Specificity = TN/(TN + FP)
Positive predictive value = TP/(TP + FP); Negative predictive value = TN/(TN + FN).

the population tested. However, given that diseases have a spectrum of manifestations, sensitivity and specificity are improved if the population is heavily weighted with patients who have advanced (vs. early) illness.

Sensitivity is defined as the percentage of persons with the disease who are correctly identified by the test. *Specificity* is the percentage of persons who are disease-free and correctly excluded by the test. The *positive predictive value* is defined as the percentage of persons with a positive test who actually have the disease, whereas the *negative predictive value* is the percentage of persons with a negative test who do not have the disease. Predictive value is influenced by the sensitivity and specificity of the test and the *prevalence* (the percentage of people in a population who at a given time have the disease).

Separating Diseased from Disease-Free Persons

Under ideal circumstances, sensitivity and specificity approach 100%. In reality, they are lower. The best currently available test to decide who is diseased or disease-free could be imperfect and have sensitivities and specificities in the 80% range. Moreover, discrepancies between a test's efficacy and its effectiveness are common. *Efficacy* is a test's performance under ideal conditions, whereas *effectiveness* is its performance under usual circumstances. Tests under development are evaluated under highly rigorous criteria, but in clinical practice, inadvertent error can be introduced into the technical performance or interpretation of the test results. Also, test values for the diseased and disease-free populations overlap.

A cutoff value may be chosen to separate "normal" from abnormal (Figure 14-1). This decision is arbitrary and involves selecting a balance between sensitivity and specificity. The receiver operating characteristic (ROC) curve is a graphic analysis used to identify a cutoff that minimizes false-positive and false-negative results (Figure 14-2). The sensitivity and specificity are calculated for a number of cutoff values, with the variables *1-Specificity* plotted on the *x* axis and *Sensitivity* plotted on the *y* axis. Each point on the curve represents a cutoff for the test. A perfect test would have a cutoff that allowed both 100% sensitivity and 100% specificity. This would be a point at the upper-left corner of the graph. The most efficient cutoff for a single test is the one that gives the most correct results, represented by the value that plots nearest to the upper-left corner of the graph.

The optimal cutoff depends on the purpose of the test and essentially is a risk/benefit analysis. In situations where disease detection is most important, the cutoff may be chosen that maximizes sensitivity at the expense of decreasing specificity. If disease exclusion is the goal, sensitivity and negative predictive value need to be maximized. It is important that negative results be *true* negatives as opposed to false negatives, so that a negative test has correctly excluded the individual as having disease. Similarly, if disease confirmation is the goal, specificity and positive predictive value are critical. It is important that positive results are *true* positives and not false positives, so that healthy persons are not misidentified, especially when treatments (e.g., surgery) have serious risks.

The predictive value of a test is directly related to the pretest probability of disease. When the prevalence of disease is high in the population, a positive test result is expected and a negative result is not expected, because the disease is common. Similarly, when the prevalence is low, a negative test result is anticipated because few people have the disease. These characteristics of predictive value become clinically useful when one compares the outcome of a positive or negative test result with the pretest probability of disease (Figure 14-3). Prevalence (pretest probability of disease) is plotted against predictive value for a positive and negative test. Note that a test result loses its ability to discriminate those who have disease from those who do not at the extremes of prevalence. If disease probability is low, a positive or negative result does not change the posttest

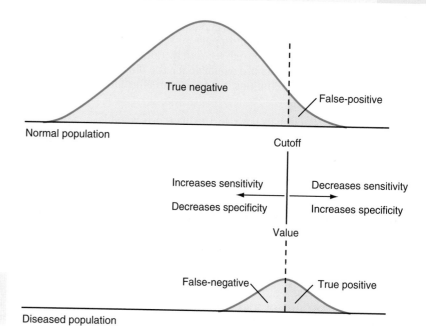

Figure 14-1 Effect of changing a test's cutoff value on disease classification. (Modified from Cebul RD, Beck LH. *Teaching clinical decision making.* Westport, CT: Praeger; 1985, p. 4.)

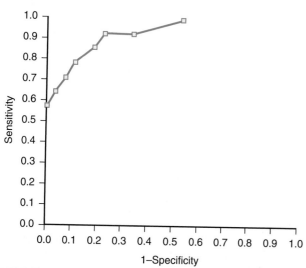

Figure 14-2 Receiver operating characteristic (ROC) curve showing the effect of changing the cutoff values for separating disease from no disease. (From Tetrault GA. Laboratory statistics. In Henry JB, ed. *Clinical diagnosis and management by laboratory methods.* 20th ed. Philadelphia: Saunders; 2001.)

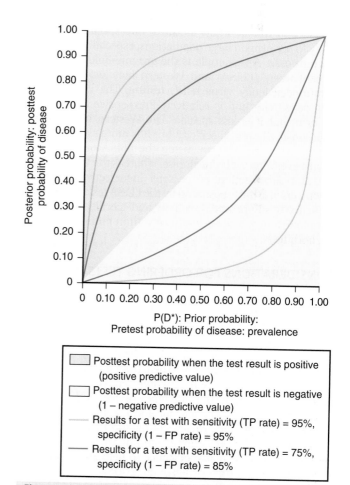

Figure 14-3 The relationship between pretest and posttest probability of disease based on a positive or negative test result. *FP,* False-positive; *TP,* true positive. (From Sackett DL, Haynes RB, Guynett GH, et al. *Clinical epidemiology.* 2nd ed. Boston: Little, Brown; 1991, p. 92.)

probability much—it is still low. Conversely, if disease probability is high, the posttest results, whether positive or negative, do not substantially alter an already high probability of disease being present. The predictive value has the greatest power to discriminate those with disease from those who are disease free in the mid-pretest probability range, near 50%. A positive test result suggests a higher posttest probability of disease than a negative result.

MULTIPLE TEST ORDERING

For many diseases, more than one test is available for diagnostic or screening purposes. The dilemma then becomes whether a positive result on several tests must be present before the diagnosis is confirmed, or whether a single positive test is sufficient to label the person as diseased. The various possibilities will have an impact on sensitivity and specificity if the tests are viewed separately. Consider the example in which two tests are available for the diagnosis of a disease. Three combinations can lead to an affirmative diagnosis:

1. If one of the two tests is positive, the diagnosis is made.
2. A positive result for both tests is required before the diagnosis is confirmed.
3. The second test is performed only if the first is positive, and the person is labeled as diseased only if the second is also positive.

The first combination will increase sensitivity and decrease specificity in comparison with each test alone, and the second combination will decrease sensitivity and increase specificity. These effects on sensitivity and specificity for multiple test ordering are similar to shifting the cutoff point for a single test.

The value of performing a second test only when the first is positive generally comes into play when the first test is significantly less expensive and easier to administer than the second test but is less specific, although highly sensitive. The second test is highly sensitive and specific but more costly to perform on large populations, especially for screening purposes. An example is the enzyme-linked immunosorbent assay (ELISA) and Western blot test for human immunodeficiency virus (HIV) testing. The ELISA has a high sensitivity and is relatively inexpensive and easy to perform, but it is less specific. The Western blot test has high sensitivity and specificity, but it is more expensive and more difficult to perform. Using the ELISA first identifies almost everyone with the disease, whereas the Western blot excludes the fraction of persons incorrectly labeled as having disease (false positives) by the ELISA test. This testing sequence has improved sensitivity and specificity over each test alone and is more cost-effective than initially performing both tests.

CONSIDERATIONS FOR ORDERING TESTS

In addition to diagnostic accuracy, the other important consideration in test ordering is the ultimate effect on the patient. What actions will be taken, based on the test results? What are the expected benefits or harms that might occur, based on a positive or a negative result? Will ordering a particular test be more likely to help than harm the patient? Unfortunately, at present, randomized controlled trials (RCTs) that examine the outcomes of test-and-treatment strategies are not available for most clinical situations. Thoughtful systematic reviews of diagnostic test accuracy, linked with clinical evidence examining treatment options, may be the best available evidence to help guide decisions on diagnostic testing (Cornell et al., 2008).

The following section presents an overview of 40 commonly ordered tests. Each section discusses the physiologic significance of the test, a typical range of reference values, and a listing of some common disease states that might explain an abnormal result. The reference ranges for each test are intended as guides and may differ from the reference ranges used by different laboratories, depending on the reference population and the test methodology.

Table 14-4   Causes of Decreased Albumin Levels

Reduced Absorption	Decreased Synthesis
Malabsorption	Chronic liver disease
Malnutrition	
Protein Catabolism	**Increased Losses**
Infection	Nephrotic syndrome
Hypothyroidism	Cirrhosis
Burns	Protein-losing
Malignancy	enteropathies
Chronic inflammation	Hemorrhage
Dilutional	
Syndrome of inappropriate antidiuretic hormone secretion (SIADH)	
Intravenous hydration	

ALBUMIN

Albumin is a transport protein that is produced mainly in the liver and maintains osmotic pressure. Albumin has a long half-life (20 days) and a small (approximately 5%) daily turnover. In humans, albumin levels increase from birth up to age 1 year, thereafter remaining stable at approximately 3.5 to 5.5 grams per deciliter (g/dL) throughout adult life. Albumin levels are reduced with advancing liver disease, nephrotic syndrome, protein-losing enteropathy, malnutrition, and some inflammatory diseases (Table 14-4). Elevations of serum albumin are unusual except in dehydration.

In severe acute infection, reduced albumin production combined with increased catabolism causes a reduction in serum albumin levels beginning in 12 to 36 hours and reaching a maximum nadir in about 5 days. As a marker for malnutrition, however, albumin levels decline relatively late. Albumin levels are most helpful in the evaluation of edema, liver disease, and proteinuria.

The difference between the serum albumin level and the albumin in ascites fluid, the serum-ascites albumin gradient (SAAG), can help differentiate portal hypertension from other causes of ascites. SAAG greater than 1.1 g/dL is seen with portal hypertension; SAAG less than 1.1 g/dL suggests another cause of the ascites, such as peritoneal inflammation or malignancy.

Most of the albumin filtered through the kidneys is reabsorbed, so significant urinary albumin is a sign of abnormal renal function. Large amounts (>300 mg/dL) of albumin can be detected on standard urine dipsticks. *Microalbuminuria* is defined as a persistent increase of urinary albumin that is below the detectable range of the standard dipstick test. Microalbuminuria is a marker for early diabetic nephropathy and also predicts macrovascular disease. Urinary albumin can be assayed from a spot urine specimen, which is corrected by the urine creatinine, or a 24-hour urine collection. A 24-hour urinary albumin excretion in mg/day equates to the same numeric value for the spot urine albumin (mg)/creatinine (g) ratio. Therefore the reference ranges for each test are normal less than 30, microalbuminuria 30 to 300, and clinical albuminuria greater than 300. Factors that may interfere with the test accuracy include strenuous or prolonged exercise, upright posture, hematuria, menses, genital or urinary infections, congestive heart

Table 14-5 Causes of Increased Alkaline Phosphatase Levels

Bone origin	Paget disease
	Osteomalacia
	Rickets
	Hyperparathyroidism
	Metastatic disease
Liver origin	Extrahepatic biliary obstruction
	Pancreatic cancer
	Biliary cancer
	Common bile duct stone
	Intrahepatic obstruction
	Metastatic liver disease
	Infiltrative diseases
	Hepatitis
	Primary biliary cirrhosis
	Sclerosing cholangitis
	Cirrhosis
	Passive hepatic congestion
Other causes	Drugs
	Phenobarbital
	Phenytoin
	Chlorpropamide
	Hyperthyroidism
	Temporal arteritis

failure, uncontrolled hypertension or uncontrolled hyperglycemia, and high protein or high salt intake.

ALKALINE PHOSPHATASE

Alkaline phosphatase (ALP) is found in a wide variety of tissues, including the liver, bone, intestine, and placenta. The reference value for ALP depends on age and gender, with higher levels in childhood, adolescence, and pregnancy. A typical reference range in an adult is 25 to 100 U/L. In adults, the source of an elevated ALP is the liver, bone, or medication (Table 14-5). Mild ALP elevations (one to two times above reference range) can occur with parenchymal liver disease, such as hepatitis or cirrhosis. Marked ALP elevations occur with infiltrative liver disease or intrahepatic or extrahepatic biliary obstruction. A persistently elevated ALP level can be an early sign of primary biliary cirrhosis. In cholestatic liver disease, bilirubin and *γ-glutamyltransferase* (GGT) levels are increased as well, with less prominent elevations in aminotransferase levels. To confirm a hepatic source of an elevated ALP level, one can simultaneously measure GGT, which is elevated in obstructive liver disease but not with bone disease. Imaging studies of the liver, by sonography or computed tomography (CT), can define an anatomic basis for obstruction in the setting of an elevated ALP level of hepatic origin.

AMINOTRANSFERASES

Liver chemistry tests are widely used to assess for liver disease. Common markers of hepatocellular damage are the aminotransferases, *aspartate aminotransferase* (AST) and *alanine aminotransferase* (ALT). While AST is also found in other tissues, such as the heart, skeletal muscle, and blood, ALT is more specific for liver. The aminotransferases are released by hepatocytes with cell injury or death. While the current reference range is approximately 10 to 40 U/L for AST and 15 to 40 U/L for ALT, some advocate that the current upper limit of normal for ALT should be lowered (Pacifico et al., 2013). Studies examining healthy people with normal body mass index (BMI), normal glucose and lipid values, and no hepatotoxic medication find that the 95th percentile for ALT is 30 IU/L in men and 19 IU/L in women. The magnitude of the elevation of aminotransferases and the ratio of AST to ALT can help suggest the cause of liver disease but does not necessarily correlate with the severity of underlying liver disease or the prognosis. In fact, normal or minimally elevated aminotransferases may be seen in patients with end-stage liver disease. Mild elevation (more than five times the upper limit of normal) of the ALT or AST, with ALT greater than AST, is frequently found with chronic liver disease, including chronic viral hepatitis, fatty liver, and medications. Probably the most common cause of persistently elevated unexplained aminotransferases is fatty infiltration of the liver. Less common causes of mildly elevated aminotransferases with ALT greater than AST include autoimmune hepatitis, hemochromatosis, α-1-antitrypsin disease, Wilson disease, metastatic disease, and cholestatic liver disease. Mild aminotransferase elevations with AST greater than ALT are more suggestive of alcohol-related liver disease but can also occur with cirrhosis and fatty liver. With alcoholic hepatitis, AST levels typically are approximately twice ALT levels, but the AST levels rarely are greater than 300 U/L. Marked elevations (greater than 15 times upper limit of normal) of AST and ALT suggest significant necrosis, such as seen in acute viral or drug-induced hepatitis, in ischemic hepatitis, or as can occur with acute biliary obstruction (Green and Flamm, 2002). When AST is elevated without elevation of ALT, one should consider extrahepatic causes, particularly myocardial or skeletal muscle sources. When AST and ALT are elevated approximately the same, a hepatic origin is most likely. eTable 14-1 compares the differences in liver function tests between hepatocellular and obstructive disorders.

Lactate dehydrogenase (LDH) is elevated in liver disease but is nonspecific; it is also found in skeletal muscle, cardiac muscle, blood, and some pulmonary disorders. Measurement of LDH rarely adds useful information to the evaluation of liver disease. GGT is a microsomal enzyme that is inducible by alcohol and certain drugs, including warfarin and some anticonvulsants. Although not specific for alcohol abuse, GGT is the most sensitive liver enzyme for alcohol abuse.

AMYLASE AND LIPASE

Pancreatic disease, particularly *acute pancreatitis,* is often associated with elevations in amylase and lipase. Table 14-6 lists common causes of elevated amylase and lipase. Lipase measurements are recommended over amylase measurements to diagnose acute pancreatitis because of their greater sensitivity and specificity. Reference ranges vary among assays. Amylase and lipase values increase 3 to 6 hours after the onset of acute pancreatitis, both peaking at approximately 24 hours. Amylase levels fall to normal in 3 to 5 days; lipase levels return to normal in 8 to 14 days. Because of exocrine insufficiency caused by recurrent pancreatitis, amylase levels tend to be lower when alcohol is the cause of pancreatitis, as opposed to gallstone or drug-induced pancreatitis. Pancreatitis is likely when the amylase

Table 14-6 Causes of Elevated Amylase and Lipase Levels

Amylase	Lipase
PANCREATIC DISEASES	
Acute pancreatitis	Acute pancreatitis
Chronic pancreatitis	Chronic pancreatitis
Pancreatic pseudocyst	
Pancreatic cancer	
Pancreatic trauma	
NONPANCREATIC DISEASES	
Salivary gland disorders	Diabetic ketoacidosis
Intestinal perforation, ischemia, or obstruction	Small bowel obstruction
Diabetic ketoacidosis	Acute cholecystitis
Perforated peptic ulcer	Renal failure
Ruptured ectopic pregnancy	
Renal failure	
Macroamylasemia	
Pregnancy	

is elevated to three times the upper limit of normal. When lipase levels are more than five times normal, pancreatitis is virtually always present. A normal amylase value, however, does not exclude pancreatitis, especially when induced by hypertriglyceridemia.

ANTINUCLEAR ANTIBODIES

Antinuclear antibodies (ANAs) are autoantibodies against parts of the cell's nucleus. When associated with symptoms of connective disease, such as arthritis, Raynaud phenomenon, or fever, ANA testing can help diagnose certain collagen vascular disorders (eTable 14-2). The likelihood that an ANA test will help with diagnosis depends on the pretest probability of disease. ANA tests are reported as negative (no staining) or positive at the highest cutoff of dilution of the serum that shows immunofluorescent nuclear staining. If positive, the description of the pattern is noted. When the ANA test is positive, testing for specific nuclear antigens should be guided by the clinical findings.

Although the ANA is 95% sensitive for *systemic lupus erythematosus* (SLE), it is not specific and is seen in other diseases. Higher titers are more specific for SLE but may be seen in the other autoimmune diseases. About 20% of normal people have an ANA titer of 1:40 or higher, and 5% have a titer of 1:160 or higher. In a series of referrals to a rheumatology clinic for a positive ANA, no patients with an ANA of less than 1:160 were diagnosed with ANA-associated rheumatic diseases. (Abeles and Abeles, 2013). Less than 5% of patients with definite SLE have a negative ANA titer. Because of the high prevalence of positive ANAs in normal people, physicians need to reserve the diagnosis of SLE for patients who have clinical findings compatible with SLE. ANA titers correlate poorly with relapses, remission, and severity of disease and are not helpful in monitoring the course or response to therapy. ANA testing should be ordered when a connective tissue disease is considered, but it is not generally helpful in the evaluation of nonspecific complaints, such as fatigue, widespread pain, or low back pain (Solomon et al., 2002).

For patients with a positive ANA titer, further testing for specific nuclear antibodies can be obtained, guided by the pattern and titer of ANA staining and the clinical findings. Patients with low titer ANA who do have additional clinical findings that suggest an ANA-associated disease should have no further testing. The interpretation of testing for specific nuclear antigens can also be difficult; most of the "specific" antigens are not 100% specific for a particular disease and need to be interpreted in the clinical context. The anti-DNA test is highly specific for SLE, with about 95% specificity but only 50% to 60% sensitivity.

BILIRUBIN

Bilirubin is produced by catabolism of heme in extrahepatic tissues. Hepatocytes conjugate the bilirubin, and it is then excreted into bile. Blood bilirubin levels are a function of production rate and biliary excretion. Total bilirubin is a combination of lipid-soluble *unconjugated* bilirubin and water-soluble *conjugated* bilirubin. Total bilirubin is less than 1.5 mg/dL and is normally primarily unconjugated bilirubin. The initial step in the evaluation of an elevated bilirubin level is to distinguish conjugated (direct) from unconjugated (indirect) hyperbilirubinemia.

Probably the most common cause of unconjugated hyperbilirubinemia is *Gilbert syndrome,* a benign condition that affects up to 5% of the population. In Gilbert syndrome, only the unconjugated bilirubin is elevated; the rest of the liver enzymes are normal. Other causes of unconjugated hyperbilirubinemia include hemolysis, ineffective erythropoiesis (as in megaloblastic anemias), or a recent hematoma. With normal hepatic function, hemolysis is not associated with bilirubin levels greater than 5 mg/dL. In an asymptomatic person with mildly elevated unconjugated hyperbilirubinemia (<4 mg/dL), a presumptive diagnosis of Gilbert syndrome can be made if there are no medications that cause elevated bilirubin, there is no evidence of hemolysis, and the liver enzymes are normal (Green and Flamm, 2002). Conjugated hyperbilirubinemia generally occurs with defects of hepatic excretion, including extrahepatic biliary obstruction, intrahepatic cholestasis, cirrhosis, hepatitis, and toxins.

BLOOD UREA NITROGEN AND CREATININE

Measurements of blood urea nitrogen (BUN) and creatinine have been used to estimate renal function. The reference range for BUN level is 7 to 18 mg/dL. Elevations in BUN, however, are not specific for intrinsic renal disease and can be seen with hypovolemia, increased protein intake, corticosteroid use, hypercatabolism, and gastrointestinal bleeding. With volume deletion, urea is reabsorbed by the tubules, and the BUN is elevated proportionately more than creatinine. The BUN-to-creatinine ratio can help differentiate prerenal and postrenal causes of renal insufficiency from intrinsic renal disease. Ratios of 10:1 suggest intrinsic renal pathology; ratios greater than 20:1 suggest prerenal or postrenal causes. BUN can also be reduced in severe liver disease, malnutrition, and with the syndrome of inappropriate antidiuretic hormone secretion (SIADH).

Currently creatinine is the most widely used laboratory test to estimate glomerular filtration rate (GFR). A product of muscle metabolism, serum levels of creatinine are related to muscle mass, age, gender, race, and dietary meat intake. At normal renal function, most of the urinary creatinine excretion is from glomerular filtration, with about 5% to 10% from tubular secretion. As GFR declines, a larger proportion of creatinine excretion is from tubular secretion. Some drugs, including cimetidine, trimethoprim, fenofibrate, and salicylates, can block the secretion of creatinine and falsely elevate creatinine levels, particularly in the setting of a low GFR. Creatinine levels increase as renal function is reduced in a parabolic fashion: At higher levels of renal function, large drops in GFR are reflected with small changes in creatinine; at lower levels of renal function, small changes in GFR are reflected in larger changes in creatinine. Although serum creatinine has long been used to estimate renal function, current guidelines from the National Kidney Foundation recommend using *estimated GFR* (eGFR) from serum creatinine to report kidney function. Many clinical laboratories now automatically report the eGFR using the Modification of Diet in Renal Disease (MDRD) equation. This equation uses age, serum creatinine, and gender to estimate the GFR, expressing GFR in $mL/min/1.73\ m^2$. The MDRD eGFR is reasonably accurate when estimating eGFRs less than 60 mL/min; however, it may underestimate eGFR at higher GFRs (Ferguson and Waikar, 2012). In addition, the equations were developed in persons with chronic kidney disease and may not accurately calculate GFR in elderly, nonwhite, or healthy persons.

CALCIUM

The total calcium level is a measurement of free (also called *ionized*) calcium, protein-bound calcium, and a chelated fraction. Approximately 50% of total calcium is ionized, 40% to 50% is bound to albumin, and 5% to 20% is bound to other ions. Only the free or ionized portion of calcium is physiologically active. Because of the binding of calcium with albumin, simultaneous measurements of calcium and albumin need to be performed to interpret calcium abnormalities. For every 1 g/dL that serum albumin is decreased below 4 g/dL, the estimated serum calcium is corrected by adding 0.8 mg/dL to the measured calcium level. An alternative is to measure ionized calcium levels in patients with abnormalities of serum albumin. The reference range for serum calcium is 8.5 to 10.5 mg/dL and for ionized calcium, 4.65 to 5.28 mg/dL. A single serum calcium measurement is not precise enough to reliably diagnose hypercalcemia; an initial abnormality of calcium should be repeated. Both dehydration and prolonged tourniquet use can cause elevated calcium levels.

The etiology of *hypercalcemia* is either hyperparathyroidism or malignancy in more than 90% of hypercalcemic patients. In the ambulatory setting, most patients with hypercalcemia have hyperparathyroidism. Thiazides can also cause mild hypercalcemia; the typical patient is an older woman. The intact *parathyroid hormone* (PTH, parathormone) levels can differentiate hyperparathyroidism from other causes of hypercalcemia. Nonhyperparathyroid causes of hypercalcemia will give low or "normal" intact PTH levels in a setting of hypercalcemia, whereas the PTH

Table 14-7 Causes of Calcium Abnormalities

Hypercalcemia

Hyperparathyroidism (primary and secondary)	Granulomatous diseases
Malignancies	Sarcoidosis
Breast, lung, prostate, renal, myeloma, T-cell leukemia, lymphoma	Tuberculosis
	Chronic renal failure
Drugs	Immobilization
Thiazide diuretics	Hyperthyroidism
Milk-alkali syndrome	
Vitamin D intoxication	

Hypocalcemia

Hypomagnesemia	Drugs
Hypoparathyroidism	*Loop diuretics*
Malabsorption of calcium or vitamin D	*Phenytoin*
Acute pancreatitis	*Phenobarbital*
Rhabdomyolysis	*Cisplatin*
Hyperphosphatemia	*Gentamicin*
Chronic renal failure	*Pentamidine*
Transfusion of multiple units of citrated blood	*Ketoconazole*
	Calcitonin
	Bisphosphonates

level will be increased in hyperparathyroidism. Typically the hypercalcemia of hyperparathyroidism is modest, with calcium levels less than 11 mg/dL and minimal symptoms. Hospitalized patients are more likely to have malignancy as a cause of hypercalcemia. Calcium levels greater than 13 mg/dL are usually associated with malignancy. Occasionally, patients with a family history of hypercalcemia show a reduction in calcium excretion and have familial hypocalciuric hypercalcemia. Other causes of hypercalcemia are related to increased gastrointestinal (GI) absorption, increased bone resorption, and decreased renal excretion (Table 14-7).

Perhaps the most common cause of a low total calcium level is a *low albumin level*. When hypocalcemia is found, one should establish that the serum albumin is normal. If serum albumin is also reduced, one should perform the above correction or obtain an ionized calcium level. Another important cause of hypocalcemia is *hypomagnesemia*, which can lead to PTH resistance or reduced PTH secretion. Correction of the magnesium deficiency usually results in correction of the hypocalcemia. Other causes of hypocalcemia are listed in Table 14-7.

CARCINOEMBRYONIC ANTIGEN

Carcinoembryonic antigen (CEA), an oncofetal glycoprotein antigen, is used in the evaluation of patients with adenocarcinomas of the GI tract, especially colorectal cancer. CEA may be elevated in benign as well as malignant diseases (eTable 14-3). CEA is not recommended as a screening test for occult cancer (including colorectal) because of its low sensitivity and specificity. Its main value is in monitoring for persistent, metastatic, or recurrent colon cancer after surgery. A preoperative elevation should return to normal in 6 to 12 weeks (CEA half-life, 2 weeks) if all disease has been resected (Duffy et al., 2013). CEA has an approximate 60% sensitivity for detecting recurrence in the patient whose postoperative CEA value has returned to normal. The adult reference range for CEA is 2.5 ng/mL or less for nonsmokers and 5.0 ng/mL or less for smokers. The degree of CEA elevation correlates with tumor bulk at diagnosis and therefore with prognosis. Values less than 5 ng/mL before therapy suggest localized disease and favorable prognosis, whereas levels greater than 10 ng/mL suggest extensive disease and a worse prognosis. About 30% of patients with metastatic colon cancer have normal CEA levels. Benign diseases do not usually produce CEA levels greater than 5 to 10 ng/mL. For an individual patient, repeat testing or longitudinal monitoring should be conducted at the same laboratory with the same methods because of variability among assays. A 20% to 25% increase in plasma concentration is considered a significant change. A rising CEA level may detect recurrent disease 2 to 6 months before it is clinically apparent.

COAGULATION STUDIES

The most common coagulation studies, *prothrombin time* (PT) and *partial thromboplastin time* (PTT), are used to evaluate patients with clotting disorders or to monitor patients taking heparin or oral anticoagulants. PT, a simple and inexpensive test for evaluating the extrinsic coagulation pathway, is the time in seconds for citrated plasma to clot after the addition of calcium and thromboplastin. Test accuracy depends on proper collection and instrument technique. Common uses include monitoring anticoagulant therapy with warfarin, evaluating liver function (because the liver synthesizes most of the clotting factors), and screening for coagulation disorders of the extrinsic system. PT is prolonged by defects in factors I (fibrinogen), II (prothrombin), V, VII, and X. Previously, PT measurements exhibited variability across laboratories because of differences in thromboplastin sensitivity. To correct for the type of thromboplastin used, the *international normalized ratio* (INR) is used to report PT results for patients taking oral anticoagulants. The INR is calculated as follows:

$$INR = (Patient\ PT/Control\ PT)ISI$$

The ISI is the international sensitivity index of the thromboplastin used at the local laboratory. Provided by the test's manufacturer, ISI reflects the responsiveness of the thromboplastin used in the PT test. The reference range for the PT and the INR in a non-anticoagulated patient is approximately 11 to 13 seconds and 0.9 to 1.1, respectively. The PT is prolonged with vitamin K deficiency, including those with fat malabsorption syndromes, recent broad-spectrum antibiotic use, and premature infants. In addition, severe liver disease, alcoholism, deficiencies of clotting factors, and circulating anticoagulants can prolong the PT. The PT is not affected by platelet disorders or platelet count. The target INR varies with specific indications. In general, an INR goal of 2.5 (range, 2.0-3.0) is generally accepted for the treatment of venous thromboembolic disease and atrial fibrillation, and 3.0 (range, 2.5-3.5) for patients at risk for arterial thromboembolism, including those with mechanical heart valves.

The *activated* PTT (aPTT, or simply PTT) is used to evaluate the intrinsic coagulation pathway, monitoring heparin therapy, screening for hemophilia A and B, and detecting clotting inhibitors. PTT is the time in seconds for citrated plasma to clot after a contact activator is added to plasma and incubated at 37° C for 5 minutes. Thromboplastin and calcium are added and the time to clot formation is recorded, which should be within 10 seconds of the control. PTT is abnormally prolonged in most patients with coagulation disorders (approximately 90%) and is therefore the best screening test in persons suspected of having a clotting disorder. PTT screens for all coagulation factors that lead to thrombin formation except VII and XIII. These factors include factors I, II, V, VIII (antihemophiliac), IX (Christmas), X, and XII (Hageman). PTT is useful to evaluate patients with a known, suspected, or active bleeding disorder; consumptive coagulopathy (e.g., disseminated intravascular coagulation); disorder of fibrin clot formation; or fibrinogen deficiency. In addition, PTT is prolonged with deficiency of the Fletcher (prekallikrein) and Fitzgerald factors, warfarin or heparin therapy, lupus anticoagulant, and vitamin K deficiency. PTT is significantly shortened by hemolysis, is affected by high or low hematocrit, but is not affected by platelet dysfunction or count. A prolonged PT or PTT can be caused by either a factor inhibitor or a deficiency of a clotting factor. To differentiate the two, a mixing study can be performed. When the abnormality is corrected after mixing with normal blood, a factor deficiency is likely. Failure to correct after mixing suggests the presence of a factor inhibitor.

When monitoring heparin therapy, the most widely used target for anticoagulation is a PTT 1.5 to 2.5 times the upper limit of normal. However, because of the great variation in thromboplastins used in different PTT assays, PTT results vary widely among laboratories. At present, there is no standardization similar to the INR for PTT results. Therapeutic heparin levels, as measured by antifactor Xa units, are approximately 0.3 to 0.7 antifactor Xa IU/mL. With plasma concentrations of heparin at 0.3 antifactor Xa IU/mL, investigators have found that mean PTT values ranged from 48 to 108 seconds, depending on the laboratory methods used. The American College of Chest Physicians recommends that each laboratory determine the PTT range that corresponds to a therapeutic heparin level (Garcia et al., 2012).

COBALAMIN (VITAMIN B$_{12}$) AND FOLATE ACID DEFICIENCY

Vitamin B$_{12}$ or folate deficiency may be suspected when a macrocytic anemia (mean corpuscular volume [MCV] >100 fL) or pancytopenia is present. Vitamin B$_{12}$ deficiency, but not folate deficiency, is also associated with neurologic symptoms, including paresthesias, numbness, ataxia, and cognitive decline. The megaloblastic anemia is identical for both folate and vitamin B$_{12}$ deficiency. *Megaloblasts* are enlarged blastic cells (precursors to the erythroid and myeloid cell lines) found in the bone marrow and caused by aberrant DNA synthesis. The peripheral blood smear typically shows the presence of oval macrocytes, hypersegmented neutrophils (>5% neutrophils with five lobes or any neutrophil with six lobes). The reticulocyte count is usually decreased.

The clinician must distinguish folate from vitamin B$_{12}$ deficiency, because supplementing one will not correct the symptoms from deficiency of the other—that is, folate replacement will not improve the neuropsychiatric

Table 14-8 Cobalamin (Vitamin B$_{12}$) and Folate Deficiency

Most Common Cause	Vitamin B$_{12}$ Deficiency	Folate Deficiency
Inadequate intake	Strict vegetarian diet (rare) Alcoholism, elderly patients	Malnutrition Alcoholism
Increased need	Pregnancy, lactation	Pregnancy, lactation, infancy Neoplasia, hyperthyroidism, hemolysis
Defective absorption or storage	Decreased intrinsic factor (e.g., pernicious anemia, congenital deficiency of intrinsic factor, gastrectomy) Zollinger-Ellison syndrome Pancreatitis Ileal mucosal disease (e.g., sprue, regional enteritis, surgery, lymphoma) Tapeworm infestation, other parasites Bacterial overgrowth in blind-loop syndrome Drugs (e.g., colchicine, aspirin, metformin)	Malabsorption caused by: Drugs (e.g., anticonvulsants, antituberculosis agents, oral contraceptives, folate antagonist) Jejunal mucosal disease (e.g., amyloidosis, sprue, lymphoma, surgery) Liver disease (cirrhosis, hepatoma)

abnormalities caused by vitamin B$_{12}$ deficiency. The neurologic signs and symptoms of vitamin B$_{12}$ deficiency may precede hematologic abnormalities. Vitamin B$_{12}$ and folate deficiency often coexist because some causes overlap (Table 14-8).

The reference range for vitamin B$_{12}$ is often listed as 200 to 900 pg/mL; however, it is now recognized that a significant portion of patients with vitamin B$_{12}$ levels of 200 to 400 pg/mL have symptoms of vitamin B$_{12}$ deficiency. Vitamin B$_{12}$ levels may be falsely elevated in patients with anti-intrinsic factor antibodies, folate deficiency, and pregnancy. Because vitamin B$_{12}$ is a cofactor in the conversion of methylmalonic acid to succinyl coenzyme A (CoA) and homocysteine to methionine, deficiencies of vitamin B$_{12}$ will lead to increased levels of methylmalonic acid and homocysteine. Folate is required in the conversion of homocysteine to methionine, but not in the conversion of methylmalonic acid to succinyl CoA. Folate deficiency is associated with elevated homocysteine, but not methylmalonic acid. Testing for methylmalonic acid and homocysteine is often recommended to confirm if patients with levels in the low-normal range actually have vitamin B$_{12}$ or folate deficiency. However, one study examining patients in the ambulatory care setting with symptoms compatible with vitamin B$_{12}$ deficiency found significant intraindividual variability in vitamin B$_{12}$, methylmalonic acid, and homocysteine levels. More importantly, they found that many patients with symptoms compatible with vitamin B$_{12}$ deficiency and normal vitamin B$_{12}$, methylmalonic acid, and homocysteine had a clinical response to pharmacologic doses of vitamin B$_{12}$ (Solomon, 2005). Because of the limitations of vitamin B$_{12}$ assays in diagnosing vitamin B$_{12}$ deficiency, some recommend a clinical trial of vitamin B$_{12}$ with predetermined clinical endpoints in patients with compatible clinical findings (Stabler, 2013).

Folate levels greater than 4 ng/mL are considered normal; levels of 2 to 4 ng/mL are indeterminate, and levels less than 2 ng/mL are diagnostic of folate deficiency in the absence of recent fasting. A person in negative folate balance will become serum deficient before tissue folate stores decrease; therefore, a low serum folate level indicates a negative folate balance, but not necessarily tissue folate deficiency. Intake of folate may normalize serum levels initially, so serum folate levels should be determined before a hospitalized or potentially deficient patient is fed, takes vitamins, or is given a transfusion. In a person with borderline folate levels, either measurement of homocysteine or red blood cell (RBC) folate levels may be helpful to confirm the diagnosis.

COMPLETE BLOOD COUNT

The complete blood count (CBC) measures circulating blood cells, including RBCs, white blood cells (WBCs), and platelets (eTable 14-4). Current technology uses electronic cell counters that can count and size the cells, providing an estimate of cell volume (MCV) and variation in cell size (red cell distribution width [RDW]), and give a five-part WBC differential, including neutrophils, lymphocytes, monocytes, eosinophils, and basophils (Tefferi et al., 2005). Typically, peripheral blood smears are prepared for manual review only when requested or when automated hematology analyzers flag abnormal results. By analyzing large numbers of cells, current instruments can generate more accurate data than by manual review for most parameters. Indications for manual review of a blood smear include the evaluation of hemolysis, RBC inclusions, myelodysplasia, megaloblastic changes, thrombocytosis, thrombocytopenia, leukocytosis, and immature or abnormal cells (Bain, 2005).

Red Blood Cells

A mild *anemia* is the most common abnormality found on a CBC. Factors that help determine whether further testing should be performed include the degree of anemia and the presence of other abnormalities in the CBC. The first step is to classify the anemia, based on MCV, as microcytic (<80 fL), normocytic (80-100 fL), or macrocytic (>100 fL). With a *microcytic* anemia, the most important test is the ferritin level, which suggests iron deficiency anemia when less than 30 ng/mL. With a *normocytic* anemia, potentially treatable causes should be excluded (e.g., recent bleeding, hemolysis, renal insufficiency, vitamin deficiency). Other causes of a normocytic anemia (e.g., anemia of chronic disease, primary bone marrow disorders) may need a bone marrow biopsy for definitive diagnosis. For a *macrocytic* anemia, important determinations are the medication history, alcohol use, and vitamin B$_{12}$ or folate deficiency.

Erythrocytosis refers to a hematocrit above the reference range. In *true* erythrocytosis, the total circulatory RBC mass is increased, whereas in *relative* erythrocytosis, the RBC mass is normal but the plasma volume is decreased, so the

Table 14-9 Classification of Erythrocytosis

RELATIVE ERYTHROCYTOSIS

Diminished plasma volume

ABSOLUTE ERYTHROCYTOSIS

Genetic disorders
Familiar polycythemia
High oxygen affinity hemoglobins
Primary marrow disorders
Polycythemia vera
Secondary conditions with appropriately increased erythropoietin, secondary to hypoxia
Chronic pulmonary disease
Right to left shunts
Sleep apnea syndrome
High altitude
Carbon monoxide poisoning
Secondary conditions with inappropriately increased erythropoietin production
Renal carcinoma
Hepatocellular carcinoma
Cerebellar hemangioma
Post-renal transplant
Polycystic kidney disease
Drugs
Androgens
Exogenous erythropoietin

Table 14-10 Common Causes of Leukocytosis or Leukopenia Stratified by White Blood Cell Type

Leukocytosis	
Neutrophilia	Infections, leukemia, rheumatic and autoimmune disorders, neoplastic disorders, chemicals, trauma, endocrine and metabolic disorders, hematologic disorders, drugs
Eosinophilia	Infectious diseases, parasitic infections, allergic diseases, myeloproliferative and neoplastic diseases, cutaneous diseases, gastrointestinal diseases
Basophilia	Allergic reactions, chronic myeloid leukemia, myeloid metaplasia, polycythemia vera, ionizing radiation, hypothyroidism, chronic hemolytic anemia, splenectomy
Monocytosis	Infections, neoplastic disorders, gastrointestinal disorders, sarcoidosis, drug reactions, recovering from marrow suppression
Lymphocytosis	Viral infections, lymphocytic leukemia, other infectious diseases, neoplastic disorders
Leukopenia	
Neutropenia	Overwhelming bacterial infection, viral infection, drug reaction, ionizing radiation, hematopoietic diseases, hypersplenism, anaphylactic shock, cachexia, autoimmune disease
Eosinopenia	Acute stress (usually physical), acute inflammatory states, Cushing's syndrome, corticosteroids
Basopenia	Sustained treatment with glucocorticoids, acute infection or stress, hyperthyroidism
Monocytopenia	Onset of steroid therapy; hairy cell leukemia
Lymphopenia	Immunodeficiency disorders, adrenocortical hormone excess, chemotherapeutic drugs, irradiation, impaired drainage of intestinal lymphatics, advanced lymphomas and carcinomas, anorexia

From Speicher CE. *The right test.* 3rd ed. Philadelphia: Saunders; 1998, pp. 281-283.

hematocrit is elevated. With true erythrocytosis, elevated erythropoietin levels suggest a secondary cause and can help distinguish secondary erythrocytosis from polycythemia vera (Table 14-9).

White Blood Cells

The WBC count is often requested to support a diagnosis of infection or an inflammatory process, or to monitor the course of a disease or response to treatment. The cell types that make up the WBC count include neutrophils (segmented and band forms), lymphocytes, monocytes, eosinophils, and basophils. *Bands* are immature neutrophils, and *segmented* forms are mature neutrophils. To diagnose neutropenia, the *absolute neutrophil count* (ANC) should be determined by multiplying the total WBC count by the percentage of bands plus mature neutrophils (segmented forms). With severe neutropenia, the ANC drops below 500 cells/mm^3, and the patient is at increased risk for infections. Causes of neutropenia include drug reactions, bacterial and viral infections, hematopoietic diseases, cachexia, hypersplenism, and autoimmune diseases. Lymphopenia is present when the lymphocyte count is less than 1500 cells/mm^3 in the adult or 3000 cells/mm^3 in children. Causes of lymphopenia include immunosuppressant drugs, corticosteroid therapy, viral infections (including HIV), and genetic immunodeficiencies.

Leukocytosis, or an elevated WBC count, occurs when the total WBC count is greater than 10,000 cells/mm^3. An elevated WBC count may be the result of a reactive process (leukemoid reaction) or leukemia. Leukemoid reactions can result from infections, toxic conditions, neoplasms, myeloproliferative diseases, and other hematologic disorders. The first step in the evaluation of leukocytosis is to determine what type of WBC is elevated. Leukocytosis may be caused by neutrophilia, eosinophilia, basophilia, monocytosis, or lymphocytosis (Table 14-10).

Platelets

Platelets, cellular fragments of the bone marrow precursor-cell megakaryocytes, are essential to clot formation and have a life span of about 10 days. Clinically, a disorder in platelets is usually suspected in a patient with excessive bleeding, typically from a mucocutaneous source or after trauma. Clinical evidence of bleeding does not occur until the platelet count drops below 50 to 70 × 10^3/μL. Platelet counts of less than 10 to 20 × 10^3/μL are associated with major spontaneous bleeding. *Thrombocytopenia* may be caused by disorders of production, distribution, or destruction (Table 14-11). In evaluating thrombocytopenia, one should first examine the peripheral smear for platelet clumping, or repeat the test using sodium citrate as the anticoagulant. *Thrombocytosis,* or an increased platelet count, may be caused by a reactive process or a myeloproliferative disorder. Reactive processes do not usually produce platelet counts greater than 1000 × 10^3/μL. Common causes of thrombocytosis include iron deficiency, acute blood loss, inflammatory disorders, malignancies, splenectomy, and myeloproliferative disorders.

Table 14-11 Causes of Thrombocytopenia

Decreased Production	Increased Destruction
Congenital disorders	Immune thrombocytopenia
Radiation or chemotherapy	Drugs
Vitamin B$_{12}$ or folate deficiency	Quinine
Drugs	Quinidine
Systemic lupus erythematosus	Heparin
Aplastic anemia	Sulfa drugs
Acute leukemia	Valproic acid
Lymphomas	Disseminated intravascular coagulation (DIC)
Alcohol abuse	Hemolytic-uremic syndrome
Viral infections, including human immunodeficiency virus (HIV)	HELLP (hemolysis, liver dysfunction, and low platelets) syndrome
Splenic sequestration	Sepsis
	Cardiopulmonary bypass
	Toxemia of pregnancy, eclampsia

CARBON DIOXIDE OR BICARBONATE

Acid-base disturbances are often recognized by abnormalities in the carbon dioxide (CO_2) content of blood, which is composed primarily of bicarbonate (HCO_3^-), with small amounts of carbonic acid and dissolved carbon dioxide. The reference range for CO_2 is 22 to 29 mmol/L. A reduced serum bicarbonate concentration frequently suggests *metabolic acidosis*, particularly when combined with a low pH. An elevated serum bicarbonate level frequently occurs with *metabolic alkalosis*. Bicarbonate is often used as a buffer for excess acid production, and levels are reduced in metabolic acidosis. In the evaluation of acidosis, calculation of the serum *anion gap* is helpful in determining the cause of the acidosis, as follows:

The normal anion gap is 10 to 12 mmol/L. An increased anion gap generally indicates the presence of metabolic acidosis with elevation of unmeasured ions, such as lactic acid, phosphates, sulfates, and ketoacids. A normal anion gap acidosis is seen with bicarbonate losses and increased chloride reabsorption and most frequently occurs with chronic diarrhea, but also with certain types of renal tubular acidosis. Low anion gaps can occur with hypoalbuminuria, congestive heart failure, and occasionally, multiple myeloma.

An elevated serum bicarbonate level frequently occurs in the setting of metabolic alkalosis. Metabolic alkalosis can be generated by loss of acid, such as in vomiting, but normally the kidney corrects the abnormality promptly by excreting excess bicarbonate. To maintain a metabolic alkalosis, the kidney must not be able to excrete excess bicarbonate. This abnormality usually occurs in the setting of volume depletion, when sodium reabsorption is enhanced and the sodium must be accompanied by an anion to maintain electroneutrality. In the absence of available chloride in the urine, bicarbonate is reabsorbed with sodium, thereby maintaining the alkalosis. Urine chloride levels less than 10 mmol/L are present with chloride-responsive metabolic alkalosis, such as vomiting with volume depletion. Elevated urine chloride (>20 mmol/L) are associated with mineralocorticoid excess, such as hyperaldosteronism and hypercortisolism.

C-REACTIVE PROTEIN

An acute-phase reactant glycoprotein, C-reactive protein (CRP), is associated with inflammation. CRP is one of the first proteins to become elevated after an inflammatory process has begun and disappears rapidly when inflammation subsides. In healthy persons, CRP levels are usually less than 0.8 mg/L and are often below the detection limit for standard assays. Serum levels may increase dramatically to exceed 100 mg/L in the presence of bacterial and viral infections, inflammation, severe trauma, surgery, neoplastic proliferation, tissue injury, necrosis, and transplant rejection. Moderate elevations may be seen with myocardial infarction, autoimmune diseases, rheumatic fever, pregnancy, obesity, and postoperatively. CRP is not affected by age, race, or food intake and does not have significant circadian variation. Drugs that may reduce or suppress CRP levels by controlling inflammation include statins, fibrates, niacin, nonsteroidal antiinflammatory drugs (NSAIDs), steroids, salicylates, angiotensin-converting enzyme (ACE) inhibitors, and β-adrenergic blockers. Compared with the ESR, the CRP rises earlier, returns to baseline sooner, and is less influenced by altered physiologic states.

The levels of CRP used to assess atherosclerotic risk are much lower than those associated with inflammation, and highly sensitive immunoassays CRP tests (hsCRP; cardiac-CRP) can accurately measure to a lower limit of 0.3 mg/L. Many studies have found that hsCRP levels predict the long-term risk of myocardial infarction, ischemic stroke, peripheral vascular disease, and all-cause mortality in healthy subjects (Greenland, 2010). The hsCRP can be used to further evaluate patients judged to be at intermediate risk for the development of coronary heart disease (those with 10-year coronary heart disease [CHD] risk of 10% to 20%). CRP levels are divided into tertiles: low risk (<1.0 mg/L), average risk (1.0-3.0 mg/L), and high risk (>3.0 mg/L). A CRP in the highest tertile is associated with a twofold risk of major coronary events compared with a CRP in the lowest tertile. Unexplained levels of hsCRP levels higher than 10 mg/L should be repeated and evaluated for noncardiovascular causes, such as infection or inflammation (Smith et al., 2004).

ERYTHROCYTE SEDIMENTATION RATE

The erythrocyte sedimentation rate (ESR) is one of the oldest laboratory tests still in clinical use. The test measures the distance that erythrocytes (RBCs) fall in a column of anticoagulated blood in 1 hour. Plasma proteins known as *acute-phase reactants* facilitate erythrocyte aggregation, which in turn affects the rate at which the solid component of blood will settle in a capillary tube. The plasma proteins most responsible for this aggregation (rouleaux formation), in decreasing order, are fibrinogen, beta (β-) globulins, alpha (α-) globulins, gamma (γ-) globulins, and albumin. Inflammatory, infectious, neoplastic, and collagen vascular diseases increase the ESR. The ESR is helpful in the diagnosis of *polymyalgia rheumatica* and *temporal arteritis*; otherwise, it is both nonsensitive and nonspecific. In studies of patients with biopsy-proven temporal arteritis, 90% of patients had an ESR greater than 30 mm/h with mean ESR of 90 mm/h. About 4% of patients with biopsy-proven

Table 14-12 Factors Affecting the Erythrocyte Sedimentation Rate

Increase	Decrease	No Effect
Anemia	Polycythemia	Body temperature
Macrocytosis	Microcytosis	Recent meal
Female gender	Spherocytosis	Aspirin
Advanced age	Extreme leukocytosis	NSAIDs
Second- and third-trimester pregnancy	Sickle cell disease	First-trimester pregnancy
Hypoalbuminemia	Excessive anticoagulant	
Tilted ESR tube	Short ESR tube	
High room temperature	Low room temperature Clotted blood sample	

ESR, Erythrocyte sedimentation rate; *NSAID*, nonsteroidal antiinflammatory drug.

temporal arteritis have a normal ESR (Smetana and Shmerling, 2002). When there is strong clinical evidence for temporal arteritis and a normal ESR, however, a temporal artery biopsy or a trial of corticosteroids should be considered. Although used to follow the response to corticosteroid therapy in polymyalgia rheumatica and temporal arteritis, ESR should be used in conjunction with clinical findings. Typically, ESR drops within a few days of corticosteroid therapy, falling to a level that is higher than normal. In addition, relapse can occur without ESR elevation.

Table 14-12 lists physiologic, pathologic, and technical factors that alter ESR, which is higher in women than men and higher in older persons. To determine ESR for healthy adult men, age in years is divided by 2, and for women, age in years plus 10 is divided by 2. Clinical considerations for using ESR have been defined (Brigden, 1998; Sox and Liang, 1986). It should not be used as a screening test for disease in asymptomatic persons. As a single test after a normal history and physical examination in asymptomatic persons, ESR contributes to disease detection of a serious illness in less than 6 of 10,000 persons. The underlying cause of an elevated ESR is usually apparent by the history and physical examination, especially for extreme elevations of about 100 mm/h. Many cases of unexplained elevated ESR are transient and not associated with serious disease. If no obvious cause is seen for elevated ESR, repeating the test in several months is recommended, rather than searching for occult disease.

FECAL OCCULT BLOOD TEST

The fecal occult blood test (FOBT) is used to detect blood loss in the stool that is not clinically apparent. Patients who report rectal bleeding or those with frank blood by rectal examination should undergo further diagnostic evaluation and do not need an FOBT. The two main FOBTs commercially available are the *guaiac-based tests*, which detect pseudoperoxidase in the heme portion of hemoglobin, and *immunochemical tests*, which detect the globulin portion of human hemoglobin.

The basis of the guaiac test is that the pseudoperoxidase of hemoglobin oxidizes guaiac to form a blue-colored quinone compound, after the addition of a hydrogen peroxide developer. The likelihood of a positive guaiac test is related to the amount of blood present in the stool. Several factors have an impact on FOBT performance characteristics. Bleeding from proximal GI lesions, including the right colon, may allow for degradation of the heme, which will then not catalyze the guaiac reaction. The myoglobin or hemoglobin in red meat can give a false-positive reaction, although ingesting 8 oz of cooked red meat daily has only a 5% probability of giving a positive test result. Peroxidase-rich raw vegetables and fruits (turnips, parsnips, horseradish, artichokes, mushrooms, radishes, broccoli, cauliflower, beets, apples, oranges, bananas, melons, grapes, pears, plums, cantaloupe) may give a false-positive result if fecal specimens are tested immediately after collection. However, plant peroxidases are unstable with time; therefore, if a specimen is developed several days after collection, the likelihood of a false-positive test result because of plant peroxidases is reduced.

Gastric irritants such as aspirin, NSAIDs, and excessive alcohol consumption may also produce positive results. Oral iron supplements and acetaminophen do not affect the guaiac test. Ascorbic acid (vitamin C) in excess of 250 mg/day or multivitamins with vitamin C may cause a false-negative result because ascorbic acid is a reducing agent and interferes with the oxidation of guaiac. Other antioxidants should also be avoided.

The processes of collecting and processing FOBTs are important in the evaluation of the results. Delaying the processing of the slides allows for dehydration of the specimen, which allows degradation of peroxidase activity and will decrease the sensitivity of testing. The delay between preparation and laboratory testing should not exceed 6 days. The issue of rehydration of dried slides with water is controversial. Rehydration of slides increases sensitivity and decreases specificity (false-positive rate increases) (Bresalier, 2010). Patients should not collect specimens until 3 days after menses have stopped or if obvious rectal bleeding or hematuria is noted. For 3 days before testing, patients should avoid ingesting red meat, vegetables with high amounts of peroxidase (broccoli, turnip, cantaloupe, cauliflower, radishes), aspirin, NSAIDs, and vitamin C. The detection of the blue color of a positive test may be affected by other factors, including a thick stool smear, exposure to high ambient temperatures, and black stools from iron ingestion.

About 2% to 6% of asymptomatic adults have a positive FOBT test, 10% of whom have cancer and 20% to 30%, adenomas. The rest have upper GI sources of bleeding, non-neoplastic lower GI sources of bleeding (e.g., hemorrhoids), or no identified source of bleeding. With home-based testing, FOBT has best been studied using a regimen of three stools. Because only one specimen is obtained during a digital rectal examination (DRE), a single digital FOBT has poor sensitivity and therefore cannot be recommended as the sole test for screening for colon cancer.

Newer fecal immunochemical tests (FITs) are based on an antigen-antibody reaction that is specific for human hemoglobin. They do not react with animal hemoglobin or peroxide-containing foods. Moreover, the FIT is not affected by ingestion of vitamin C, iron, or rehydration, so no dietary restrictions are required. However, globulin levels are reduced in high temperatures and with a delay in testing, which might reduce the sensitivity. Because globulin is broken down in the upper GI tract, the globulin tests do not detect bleeding from the upper GI tract as readily as guaiac-based tests. Current immunochemical tests use either one or two stool samples. The sensitive guaiac based tests (Hemoccult Sensa) and the FITs are more sensitive than Hemoccult II for colorectal cancer and advanced adenoma detection. Specificity for FIT testing is variable compared with sensitive guaiac-based tests, but probably similar. Several studies have shown participation rates are higher with the immunochemical tests than with guaiac-testing, likely because of the lower number of stool samples in the testing and the lack of dietary restrictions.

GLUCOSE

The reference range for a fasting plasma glucose level is between 70 and 99 mg/dL. *Hypoglycemia* is best documented by a plasma venous glucose level less than 50 mg/dL, although there is considerable variability in the level of hypoglycemia that causes symptoms. Asymptomatic hypoglycemia in a patient not taking insulin or oral hypoglycemic agents may be a laboratory artifact caused by ongoing metabolism of glucose in the specimen, especially if a delay has occurred in processing the specimen. The diagnosis of hypoglycemia is best made with typical symptoms associated with a laboratory confirmation of venous hypoglycemia, followed by relief of symptoms after ingesting glucose. The glucose tolerance test (GTT) can produce hypoglycemia in normal persons and should not be routinely ordered in the evaluation of hypoglycemia.

Hypoglycemia can be defined as iatrogenic, postprandial, or fasting. *Postprandial* hypoglycemia occurs after meals and is usually mild and self-limiting. *Alimentary* hypoglycemia occurs when patients have rapid gastric emptying. Insulin levels rise rapidly after a meal and fall more slowly than glucose levels, which results in hypoglycemia. *Fasting* hypoglycemia is seen much less often than reactive hypoglycemia and may be a harbinger of more severe disease, including insulin-producing pancreatic tumors and hepatic, adrenal, or renal insufficiency, or it may be the result of excess insulin or sulfonylurea administration. True fasting hypoglycemia needs to be confirmed by a prolonged fast, with simultaneous measurement of glucose and insulin. This technique can help determine whether the hypoglycemia is associated with excess insulin.

Diabetes mellitus is characterized by *hyperglycemia*. The American Diabetes Association has defined *normal* fasting plasma glucose as less than 100 mg/dL (5.6 mmol/L), *prediabetes* as 100 to 125 mg/dL (5.6-6.9 mmol/L), and diabetes mellitus as 126 mg/dL (7.0 mmol/L) or greater.

GLYCOSYLATED HEMOGLOBIN (HEMOGLOBIN A$_{1c}$)

The glycosylated hemoglobin (hemoglobin A$_{1c}$ [HbA$_{1c}$]) fraction measures nonenzymatic glycosylation of hemoglobin, which is related to level of glucose concentration over the life span of the erythrocyte. The HbA$_{1c}$ fraction can be used to estimate glucose control in the previous 2 to 3 months. In persons with normal erythrocyte survival, the glucose levels in the last 30 days contribute to 50% of the

HbA$_{1c}$, whereas the glucose levels in the preceding 90 to 120 days contribute only 10% to the HbA$_{1c}$ measurement. HbA$_{1c}$ can be reported in the familiar percentage combined with the HbA$_{1c}$-derived average glucose (ADAG) (Saudek et al., 2008). Using the National Health and Nutrition Examination Survey (NHANES) III data that the population average for HbA$_{1c}$ was 5.17 with standard deviation (SD) of 0.45, the International Expert Committee (2009) selected an HbA$_{1c}$ of 6.5% (approximately 3 SD above average) as the cutoff point to diagnose diabetes mellitus, with confirmation by a fasting glucose greater than 126 mg/dL or oral GTT greater than 200 mg/dL, or a repeat HbA$_{1c}$ greater than 6.5%. Screening with HbA$_{1c}$ identifies fewer individuals with diabetes than either plasma glucose or GTT. Goals for achieving optimal control of diabetes are controversial, but a reasonable goal in most persons is an HbA$_{1c}$ less than 7%. Conditions that shorten erythrocyte survival, such as hemolysis or recent bleeding, give a lower HbA$_{1c}$ level. Black patients tend to have a slightly higher HbA$_{1c}$ levels (by 0.2-0.3) than white patients (Inzucchi, 2012).

HELICOBACTER PYLORI

A spiral, urease-producing bacterium, *Helicobacter pylori*, is associated with almost 90% of duodenal ulcers. Testing is indicated in patients with either active or previously documented peptic ulcer disease, in the evaluation of dyspepsia who have no "alarm features," and for patients with a history of gastric mucosa-associated lymphoid tissue (MALT) lymphoma (MALToma) (Chey and Wong, 2007). Several tests can be performed during endoscopy. Rapid urease testing of a biopsy specimen has sensitivity over 90% and specificity over 95%, with results available within 1 to 24 hours. The sensitivity of rapid urease tests is reduced by drugs that treat *H. pylori*, including bismuth, antibiotics, and proton pump inhibitors (PPIs). Histologic examination of gastric biopsies can also detect *H. pylori*. Culturing *H. pylori* has a lower yield, is more expensive, and is not widely done.

There are three nonendoscopic methods to detect *H. pylori* infection. Serologic tests for immunoglobulin G (IgG) antibody to *H. pylori* can identify previous infection and have sensitivity of approximately 88% but specificity of only 70% to 80%. Serologic tests are inexpensive and have a good negative predictive value. The positive predictive value depends on the prevalence of *H. pylori*. Even though titers may decline slowly after eradication of the organism with antibiotics, these tests have limited use in evaluation of the effectiveness of antibiotic therapy and cannot reliably distinguish current from past infection.

The value of *H. pylori* antibody testing in the evaluation of uninvestigated dyspepsia depends on the prevalence of *H. pylori* infection. In areas of high prevalence (>20%), serologic testing may be cost-effective for a test-and-treat strategy. In areas of lower prevalence, the low positive predictive value of serology limits its usefulness; either stool antigen testing or urea-breath is more accurate. Antibody testing is inexpensive and has a very good negative predictive value.

Urea breath tests using carbon 13 (^{13}C)–urea or ^{14}C-urea can detect ongoing replication of *H. pylori*. These tests are most helpful in determining whether *H. pylori* has been successfully eradicated after a course of treatment, but they can also confirm active infection. After the ingestion of labeled urea, urease-producing *H. pylori* organisms break down the urea and produce labeled CO_2, which is absorbed into the circulation and exhaled, and can be measured by collecting an exhaled breath sample in a bag. False-negative breath tests may occur with the recent use of antibiotics, bismuth, or PPIs. Most studies find the sensitivity and specificity of the urease breath test to be greater than 95%.

Testing for *H. pylori* antigen in the stool by immunoassay has been found to have sensitivity over 90% and specificity approaching 100%, thereby making it an accurate noninvasive method to diagnose active *H. pylori* infection in untreated patients. As in urea breath testing, recent antibiotics, PPIs, and bismuth can cause false-negative results. Stool tests can also be used to confirm eradication, but no sooner than 4 weeks after completion of therapy. A rapid stool *H. pylori* antigen test is now available for on-site testing.

HEPATITIS SEROLOGY

Hepatitis A virus (HAV), hepatitis B virus (HBV), and less often hepatitis C virus (HCV) are the usual causes of acute viral hepatitis. A person with symptoms of acute hepatitis should have these four hepatitis serologies performed: immunoglobulin M (IgM) anti-HAV, hepatitis B surface antigen (HBsAg), IgM hepatitis core antigen (anti-HBc), and anti-HCV. At present, stool and blood assays for HAV antigen are not available. The diagnosis of hepatitis A is made by the detection of IgM anti-HAV during acute illness. A positive anti-HAV with only IgG anti-HAV indicates previous infection.

In hepatitis B, HBsAg is the earliest serologic marker of infection and is present before elevation of the aminotransferases. If HBsAg is present for more than 6 months, the patient should be considered chronically infected (carrier). Previous hepatitis B vaccination is indicated by the presence of anti-HBs only. After infection, antibodies to HBsAg (anti-HBs) typically indicate immunity to hepatitis B and appear several weeks to months after HBsAg disappears. The gap between the presence of HBsAg and anti-HBs is the "window period"; during this time anti-HBc can be detected in the blood. Anti-HBc can be differentiated into an IgM anti-HBc, which indicates recent infection, and an IgG anti-HBc, which indicates previous infection. HBeAg, a subparticle of core antigen, is present only when HBsAg is present and is a marker for infectiousness. Anti-HBe appears after HBeAg disappears, indicates decreasing infectivity and a good prognosis, and remains detectable for years. HBV DNA testing can be used to determine if the patient is a candidate for antiviral therapy. *Hepatitis delta virus* (HDV) infection coexists with hepatitis B in about 4% of hepatitis B infections and carries an increased mortality rate. HDV depends on the presence of HBV for expression and replication and can cause acute or chronic infection.

Hepatitis C occasionally presents as acute hepatitis, but more frequently is detected in the evaluation of patients with elevated aminotransferases or chronic liver disease. In 2012, the Centers for Disease Control and Prevention (CDC) recommended one-time screening for hepatitis C in persons in the United States born between 1945 and 1965, regardless of risk factors. The commonly available screening test is an enzyme immunoassay that detects antibodies to hepatitis C. The antibody test is usually detectable about 8 to 12 weeks after exposure. In a patient with a positive anti-HCV test, further testing for HCV RNA is recommended to confirm active HCV infection. A positive anti-HCV antibody and a negative HCV RNA suggest either a false-positive screening test or previous hepatitis C exposure with resolution of the infection. Quantitative HCV-RNA (viral load) and genotype testing should be performed prior to treatment.

HUMAN IMMUNODEFICIENCY VIRUS

The diagnosis of HIV infection usually depends on the detection of antibodies to the virus. The recommended screening test for HIV infection is an initial enzyme immunoassay, the ELISA test, which can detect the presence of antibody to HIV 2 to 8 weeks after infection. An initially positive ELISA should be repeated, and repeatedly positive ELISAs need to be confirmed by a more specific test, most often the Western blot. Sensitivity and specificity of this testing pattern are both greater than 99.5%. A positive ELISA combined with a negative Western blot should be considered a false-positive HIV test and indicates that HIV infection is not present. A positive ELISA and an indeterminate Western blot result can be a marker for early HIV infection or advanced acquired immunodeficiency syndrome (AIDS), or it can be a false-positive test result. The predictive value of a positive HIV test depends on the prevalence in the population being tested.

Rapid HIV tests are currently available that check saliva, whole blood, and plasma. The whole-blood tests measure capillary blood with a finger stick and do not require centrifugation. These tests are interpreted visually, do not require instrumentation, and provide test results in minutes. Rapid tests may be preferred for testing in patients who are not likely to return for results of standard testing, for pregnant women at delivery with no HIV testing during their pregnancy, and for testing during occupational exposure. Rapid tests for HIV have both similar sensitivity and specificity greater than 99.5%, and also require confirmation.

Tests to measure HIV directly include quantitative HIV RNA testing by polymerase chain reaction (PCR), which measures viral load or actual viral replication. Quantitative HIV RNA measurements are useful in evaluating indeterminate Western blot results and acute HIV infection, when the patient presents before seroconversion. Because neonates born to HIV-infected mothers often have maternal antibodies for months, early testing with HIV DNA PCR can identify infants with HIV infection. Newer combination fourth-generation p24 antigen-HIV antibody tests may shorten the window period between acute HIV infection and detection, and can be used in postexposure testing for health care professionals (Kuhar et al., 2013). In 2006, the CDC recommended routine, voluntary HIV screening for all patients age 13 to 64 in any health care setting.

IRON STUDIES

Iron deficiency is the most common type of anemia worldwide and therefore a significant cause of human morbidity. Other than menstrual blood losses, negligible iron is lost in a healthy person. Normally, regulation of iron absorption in the proximal small intestine controls iron balance. Iron deficiency results from increased need (growth of infancy or childhood, pregnancy), excessive loss (menstruation, hemorrhage, GI loss), inadequate intake (iron-deficient diet), or defective absorption (gastrectomy or sprue). In adult men or postmenopausal women with adequate iron stores, it takes 3 to 4 years for these stores to be depleted once negative iron balance starts.

During early *iron deficiency anemia*, the erythrocytes may be normochromic normocytic, and later the peripheral blood smear may show microcytosis, anisocytosis, poikilocytosis, and hypochromia. The reticulocyte count is low, and RDW is high (>16). Bone marrow stores of iron are decreased or absent. Serum iron has marked diurnal variation (higher in morning, lower later in day) and is increased transiently after meals. Because morning levels determine the reference range, iron levels should be performed on a fasting morning specimen. Obtaining a serum iron level without determining the level of transferrin (*total iron-binding capacity* [TIBC]) is of limited value. Serum iron is decreased with inflammation, infection, and ascorbate deficiency and increased with iron ingestion, transfusions, liver disease, aplastic anemia, and ineffective erythropoiesis. The total iron-binding capacity or transferrin is not subject to diurnal fluctuation, but it is reduced in chronic inflammation and malnutrition. The serum ferritin is the best indirect marker for the assessment of iron stores. The conventional cut off of a ferritin under 10 to 15 ng/mL is virtually diagnostic of iron deficiency anemia. However, using cutoffs of 30 ng/mL still results in a 92% sensitivity and 98% specificity for the deficiency of iron deficiency (Mast et al., 1998). Serum ferritin is an acute-phase reactant and can be elevated in some patients with liver disease, malignancy, or inflammatory or infectious diseases. In a patient with chronic inflammation, a rule of thumb is to divide the ferritin level by 3, and if lower than 20 ng/mL, suspect coexisting iron deficiency. Less than 10% of people with ferritin levels higher than 100 ng/mL have iron deficiency. Hemolysis may cause falsely high levels of serum iron (eTable 14-5).

Iron overload, typically related to hemochromatosis or to repeated transfusions, is associated with elevated iron, transferrin saturation, and ferritin levels. While a transferrin saturation more than 60% in men and more than 50% in woman has a 90% sensitivity in detecting symptomatic homozygous hemochromatosis, several guidelines recommend a cutoff of more than 45% in both men and women to allow greater detection of individuals at earlier stages of the disease. Ferritin levels of more than 300 ng/mL in men and 200 ng/mL in women are suggestive of iron overload, in the absence of chronic inflammation or liver disease.

LIPID PROFILE

Lipid levels are often obtained to evaluate cardiovascular risk. There are four major classes of lipoproteins: chylomicrons, very-low-density lipoprotein (VLDL) cholesterol (VLDL-C), low-density lipoprotein (LDL) cholesterol (LDL-C), and high-density lipoprotein (HDL) cholesterol (HDL-C). Approximately 60% to 70% of plasma cholesterol is carried as LDL-C. A direct association is seen between increased LDL-C and the risk of CHD. HDL-C functions in the reverse transport of cholesterol to the liver and carries apolipoprotein A-1. HDL-C accounts for about 20% to 30% of total cholesterol. HDL-C and CHD have a strong independent inverse relationship; for every 1-mg/dL decrease in HDL, the risk of coronary artery disease (CAD) increases 2% to 3%. The Adult Treatment Panel (ATP) III of theNational Cholesterol Education Program (NCEP Expert Panel, 2001) recommended lipid screening as a tool to promote cardiovascular disease risk reduction. The standard lipid profile, as recommended by the ATP III, consists of direct measurement of total cholesterol, HDL-C, and triglycerides, with a calculated LDL-C, obtained after a 9-hour fast. The Friedewald formula for calculating LDL is LDL = total cholesterol − HDL − triglycerides/5.

The Friedewald formula for estimating LDL is not valid in the following three conditions: when there are chylomicrons present, when the triglycerides are higher than 400 mg/dL, and when there is dysbetalipoproteinemia (type III hyperlipidemia). Hypertriglyceridemia and dysbetalipoproteinemia lead to underestimations of the LDL. Using the Friedewald formula, some non-LDL lipoproteins—intermediate-density lipoprotein (IDL) and lipoprotein (a)—are included in the LDL calculation. Measurements of direct LDL, although more costly, give more accurate values than calculations using this formula in patients with hypertriglyceridemia. Nonfasting total cholesterol and HDL measurements give reliable assessment of CHD risk without the need to measure triglycerides (Di Angelantonio et al., 2009). The American Heart Association (AHA) 2010 guidelines recommend against the use of measurements of lipoprotein subfraction, particle size, and density in asymptomatic adults for cardiovascular risk assessment, because there is no evidence that these measures improved predictive capacity over standard lipid panel (Ip et al., 2009). While an analysis showed a higher CHD risk in individuals with higher LDL particle numbers, the risk was similar to that of non-HDL cholesterol as a risk (El Harchaoui et al., 2007). Lipoprotein(a) levels have shown modest correlations with stroke and CHD risk, but because of concerns with standardization of measurement and lack of strong evidence of benefit of additional risk prediction beyond transitional risk factor assessment, the AHA recommended against testing in asymptomatic individuals.

There are a number of sources of physiologic and analytic variation in lipid measurements. Failure to fast before the test elevates the triglycerides and leads to an underestimation of the LDL. The total cholesterol and HDL are not significantly different in the fasting or postprandial state. Dietary changes begin to become apparent in lipid measurements in approximately 1 to 2 weeks; therefore, patients should have a stable diet for 3 weeks before testing. Morning specimens are preferred because triglycerides have diurnal variation—lowest in the morning, highest in the afternoon. Recent illness or surgery, including myocardial infarction, stroke, or cardiac catheterization, can lower lipid measurements for several weeks. For major illness or injury, it may be necessary to wait 2 to 3 months before measurement. Cholesterol levels decrease 24 hours after myocardial infarction and remain depressed for up to 12 weeks. Table 14-13 lists some drugs that can affect the lipid components. Major causes of secondary dyslipidemia also include

Table 14-13 Effects of Drugs on Lipid Values

Drug	Total Cholesterol	LDL Cholesterol	HDL Cholesterol	Triglycerides
Thiazide diuretics	↑	↑	–	↑
β-Blockers	–	–	↓	↑
α-Blockers	↓	↓	↑	↓
ACE-inhibitors	–	–	–	–
Calcium-channel blockers	–	–	↑	↑
Unopposed estrogens	↓	↓	↑	↑
Unopposed progestogens	–	↑	↓	↑
Tamoxifen	↓	↓	–	–
Raloxifene	↓	↓	–	–
Isotretinoin	↑	↑	–/↓	↑
Protease inhibitors	↑	–	–	↑

ACE, Angiotensin-converting enzyme; *HDL,* high-density lipoprotein; *LDL,* low-density.
Adapted from Mantel-Teeuwisse AK, Kloosterman JM, Maitland-van der Zee AH, et al. Drug-induced lipid changes: a review of the unintended effects of some commonly used drugs on serum lipid levels. *Drug Saf.* 2001;24(6): 443-456.

Table 14-14 Causes of Magnesium Abnormalities

Hypermagnesemia

Overingestion (usually in setting of renal insufficiency)	Renal insufficiency
	Addison disease
Antacids	Hypothyroidism
Cathartics	Lithium intoxication
Laxatives	

Hypomagnesemia

Gastrointestinal causes	Drugs
Low-magnesium diet	Diuretics (thiazide and loop)
Malabsorption	Digitalis
Diarrhea	Cyclosporine
Renal tubular disorders	Cisplatin
Ketoacidosis	Aminoglycosides
Alcohol abuse	Proton pump inhibitors
	Amphotericin B

diabetes mellitus, hypothyroidism, nephrotic syndrome, and obstructive liver disease.

MAGNESIUM

Magnesium levels are not routinely included in standard chemistry panels, so abnormalities of magnesium frequently go unrecognized. The reference range of serum magnesium concentration is 1.7 to 2.2 mg/dL (1.5-1.7 mEq/L, or 0.75-0.95 mmol/L). The most common cause of *hypermagnesemia* is excess magnesium intake in a patient with chronic kidney disease (Table 14-14). Symptoms of hypermagnesemia are seen with levels greater than 4 to 6 mg/dL.

Hypomagnesemia is more common than hypermagnesemia. The three mechanisms causing hypomagnesemia are reduced intestinal absorption from malnutrition or malabsorption, increased urinary losses, and intracellular shifts. Hypomagnesemia is typically associated with alcohol abuse, hypokalemia, hypocalcemia, chronic diarrhea, and ventricular arrhythmias. Symptoms occur with serum concentrations less than 1 mEq/L. Clinically, hypomagnesemia is associated with neuromuscular hyperirritability, including tremors, tetany, and rarely, seizures. In distinguishing renal wasting from extrarenal losses as the cause of hypomagnesemia, a 24-hour urine excretion of greater than 24 mg or a spot urine fractional excretion of magnesium greater than 2% suggests that the cause of hypomagnesemia is excessive renal losses.

MONONUCLEOSIS (EPSTEIN-BARR VIRUS INFECTION)

Mononucleosis is a common viral infection, particularly in adolescents and young adults. Typical symptoms include fever, pharyngitis, cervical lymphadenopathy, and fatigue. Typically, mononucleosis is associated with an infection by the Epstein-Barr virus (EBV). Laboratory findings include leukocytosis, with greater than 50% lymphocytes and more than 10% atypical lymphocytes. Almost 90% of patients with mononucleosis have abnormal liver enzymes. Mononucleosis is typically diagnosed by detecting a *heterophile antibody*, which is a nonspecific response to EBV infection. The heterophile antibody response is an IgM antibody that will agglutinate with the surface antigen of sheep and horse RBCs, but not with guinea pig kidney cells. Monospot tests are done with rapid slide agglutination procedures and horse RBCs to detect the heterophile antibody. Heterophile antibodies are negative in about 25% of patients in the first week of infection, and in 5% to 10% of patients in the second week or later (Luzuriaga and Sullivan, 2010). The heterophile antibody usually persists for 3 to 6 months after an acute infection, less frequently up to 1 year. The heterophile antibody has an overall false-negative rate of 10% to 15%, except in children younger than the age of 12, where the false-negative rate is higher. False-positive heterophile antibodies can occur with rubella, hepatitis, other viral infections, and lymphoma.

When the heterophile antibody is negative or the features of infectious mononucleosis are atypical, the disease can be confirmed with specific Epstein-Barr antibodies. Acute or recent infection is thought to be present if four serologic criteria are found: positive IgM to viral capsid antigen (VCA); high titers (>1:320) of IgG to VCA; positive early antigen antibody (anti-EA); and initial absence of antibody to Epstein-Barr nuclear antigens (EBNAs). The most useful

EBV-specific antibody to diagnose acute mononucleosis is the IgM VCA, which appears soon after the onset of symptoms and has sensitivity of 91% to 98% and specificity of 99%. Convalescent testing should document the appearance of IgG EBNA and disappearance of IgM VCA and anti-EA.

Syndromes mimicking infectious mononucleosis, but with negative heterophile antibodies, are considered *heterophile-negative* infectious mononucleosis. The most common syndromes are related to cytomegalovirus infection and toxoplasmosis. Occasionally, viral hepatitis, rubella, lymphoma, leukemia, and the drugs isoniazid and phenytoin can cause a mononucleosis-like syndrome. As acute HIV infection can present with similar symptoms, consideration should be given to testing for HIV nucleic acid in patients with risk factors for HIV infection. Because heterophile antibodies are not uniformly positive early in the disease, serial tests may often be needed weekly to confirm mononucleosis. Specific serologic tests for EBV and now PCR are relatively expensive and take longer to obtain results, so they are generally reserved for unclear cases and are not necessary in most patients with infectious mononucleosis. In an adolescent or young adult with appropriate clinical symptoms, heterophile antibodies are 95% sensitive and specific.

NATRIURETIC PEPTIDES (B-TYPE NATRIURETIC PEPTIDE AND N-TERMINAL PRO–B-TYPE NATRIURETIC PEPTIDE)

Blood levels of natriuretic peptides are used in the evaluation of *heart failure.* Cardiac cells release natriuretic peptides in response to stretch and wall tension. Ventricular myocytes release a pro–B-type natriuretic peptide (pro-BNP), which is cleaved into the active B-type natriuretic peptide (BNP) and the inactive N-terminal pro-BNP (NT–pro-BNP). Levels of both BNP and NT–pro-BNP increase with age, in renal insufficiency, and are higher in women; obesity is associated with lower BNP levels. Some medications, including spironolactone, ACE inhibitors, and angiotensin receptor blockers, lower BNP/NT–pro-BNP levels. Other conditions that increase natriuretic peptides include myocardial ischemia, atrial fibrillation, pulmonary embolus, pulmonary hypertension, chronic kidney disease, and sepsis.

The major established use of BNP testing is evaluating *acute dyspnea,* when the cause is uncertain, to differentiate whether the etiology is from heart failure versus another cause. In the setting of acute dyspnea, natriuretic levels are more accurate than clinical judgment in excluding or diagnosing acute decompensated heart failure. A normal level in a patient with acute dyspnea has a high negative predictive value and suggests that heart failure is unlikely the etiology. The optimal cutoffs for BNP/NT–pro-BNP vary with age. BNP less than 100 pg/mL or NT–pro-BNP less than 400 pg/mL makes the diagnosis of heart failure unlikely. Levels of BNP greater than 400 pg/mL or NT–pro-BNP greater than 2000 suggest heart failure (Dickstein et al., 2008). Elevated levels of BNP and NT–pro-BNP also are predictive of death or increased cardiovascular events. There is some evidence that the use of natriuretic peptid testing to guide heart failure therapy may improve clinical

outcomes, and clinical trials are ongoing to help determine optimal approaches (Januzzi, 2012).

PHOSPHORUS

Disorders of phosphorus metabolism are caused by variations in dietary intake, phosphorus excretion, and transcellular shifts. The reference range for serum phosphorus level is approximately 2.5 to 4.8 mg/dL in adults and 4.0 to 6.0 mg/dL in children. Because postprandial phosphorylation of glucose can decrease serum phosphorus levels, fasting specimens are more accurate. *Hyperphosphatemia* most often occurs in the setting of reduced renal excretion from renal insufficiency. Other causes of hyperphosphatemia include excess phosphate ingestion, either orally or with phosphate-containing enemas, hypoparathyroidism, and spurious causes such as thrombocytosis. Less common causes include acromegaly, hyperthyroidism, acidosis, and massive cell lysis from hemolysis, rhabdomyolysis, and tumor lysis after chemotherapy.

Hypophosphatemia is defined as a serum phosphorus level below 2.5 mg/dL. Clinically significant hypophosphatemia occurs at levels less than 1.5 mg/dL. The three major mechanisms associated with hypophosphatemia are decreased intestinal absorption, increased phosphate loss from the kidney, and increased phosphorus shift into the bones. Decreased absorption occurs most often with antacid use. Persistent hypophosphatemia most frequently results from disorders causing increased phosphate loss in the kidney, including hyperparathyroidism, vitamin D deficiency, renal tubular disease, chronic acidosis, and rickets. Intracellular shifts into cells and bones during acute respiratory alkalosis, refeeding after starvation, hyperalimentation, intravenous carbohydrate administration, rapid tumor growth, treatment of respiratory failure, or diabetic ketoacidosis can cause hypophosphatemia (Bacchetta and Salusky, 2012). If the cause of hypophosphatemia cannot be determined based on the history, a fractional excretion of phosphorus less than 5% suggests that the etiology is not from inappropriate renal loss; if the fractional excretion is more than 5%, it implies that the problem is renal; renal wasting of phosphorus. ($FE_{Pi(\%)} = [(P_{urine}/P_{plasma}) \times 100 \times (Cr_{plasma}/Cr_{urine})]$ where P_{urine} and P_{plasma} are urine and plasma concentrations of phosphorus and Cr_{plasma} and Cr_{urine} are plasma and urine concentrations of creatinine, respectively.)

POTASSIUM

Potassium is the most abundant *cation* in the body and has a much higher concentration in the intracellular space than in extracellular fluids. Normal potassium levels are maintained despite fluctuating potassium intake by adjustments in renal secretion of potassium. *Hyperkalemia* is defined as a serum potassium level greater than 5.1 mmol/L. Occasionally, hyperkalemia can be an artifact (pseudohyperkalemia) of phlebotomy, associated with thrombocytosis, leukocytosis, or hemolysis during phlebotomy. In a patient with hyperkalemia of no apparent cause, a plasma potassium level can eliminate these effects on the potassium measurement. Because the normal response to increased potassium intake is to increase excretion, hyperkalemia is not likely to be attributed to increased intake unless there is

Table 14-15   Causes of Abnormal Potassium Levels

Hyperkalemia	Hypokalemia
PSEUDOHYPERKALEMIA	**INADEQUATE DIET**
Thrombocytosis	Malnutrition
Leukocytosis	Alcoholism
Prolonged tourniquet use during venipuncture	
Hemolysis	
REDUCED EXCRETION	**RENAL LOSSES**
Oliguria	Diuresis
Renal failure	Renal tubular acidosis, proximal and distal types
Hyporeninemic hypoaldosteronism	
Adrenal insufficiency	Hypomagnesemia
Type IV renal tubular acidosis	Hyperaldosteronism
	Cushing syndrome
CELLULAR SHIFTS	**CELLULAR SHIFTS**
Acute acidosis	Alkalosis
Insulin deficiency	β-Adrenergic therapy
Rhabdomyolysis	Catecholamine excess
DRUGS	**DRUGS**
β-Blockers	Thiazide diuretics
Angiotensin-converting enzyme inhibitors	Loop diuretics
	Epinephrine
Angiotensin receptor blockers	Albuterol
Spironolactone	Licorice
Triamterene	Glucocorticoids
Amiloride	Mineralocorticoids
NSAIDS	
Heparin	
Cyclosporine	
Pentamidine	

NSAID, Nonsteroidal antiinflammatory drug.

a deficiency in potassium excretion. Shifts of potassium from intracellular to extracellular fluids, such as with acute metabolic acidosis, crush injury, burns, insulin deficiency, β-adrenergic blockade, and hemolysis, can be associated with a transient hyperkalemia. Persistent hyperkalemia is usually caused by decreased potassium excretion. Potassium excretion by the kidney is flow dependent; therefore, oliguria and anuria are important causes of hyperkalemia. Because aldosterone deficiency is an important cause of decreased potassium excretion, hyperkalemia is seen with hyperreninism, hypoaldosteronism, type 4 renal tubular acidosis, and drugs that inhibit aldosterone (Table 14-15).

Hypokalemia is associated with a serum potassium level of less than 3.5 mmol/L. Symptoms are nonspecific and include muscular weakness. Occasionally, hypokalemia is associated with sustained inadequate potassium intake, particularly in patients with alcohol abuse. Transient episodes of hypokalemia are associated with increased extracellular to intracellular potassium shifts and occur with catecholamine increase, hyperinsulinemia, and adrenergic drugs such as bronchodilators. More frequently, hypokalemia is a result of loop or thiazide diuretic therapy or GI losses of potassium, such as with protracted vomiting, diarrhea, and laxative abuse. Other causes of hypokalemia include hypomagnesemia, drugs, metabolic alkalosis, skin losses, and increased urinary losses. In cases when the cause of hypokalemia is not apparent, measuring urinary potassium is helpful. A random urine potassium-to-creatinine ratio greater than 15 mEq/gm creatinine suggests renal wasting (Groeneveld et al., 2005).

PREGNANCY TESTS

Current pregnancy tests use immunoassays to measure the beta subunit of human chorionic gonadotropin (hCG). Serum assays and sensitive urine assays can now detect pregnancy approximately 1 week after conception. Home pregnancy tests have variable sensitivity, ranging from about 50% to 97% sensitive when done on the first day of the missed period, and nearly 100% sensitive at 11 days after the missed period. The most common reason for a false-negative home pregnancy test is incorrect timing, such as performing the test too soon, so it is recommended to repeat a home test if the initial test is negative (Cole, 2012).

In the first 4 to 8 weeks of pregnancy, serum hCG levels double approximately every 2 days. Failure to double in 48 to 72 hours suggests an ectopic pregnancy or abnormal intrauterine pregnancy. For the first 2 weeks after conception, serum levels of hCG are higher than those in urine. However, beginning at approximately 3 weeks and for the remainder of the pregnancy, urine levels are higher than serum levels. Levels of hCG return to normal approximately 2 weeks after delivery. After an abortion, levels return to normal in approximately 3 to 8 weeks. Other conditions that can raise hCG levels include gestational trophoblastic neoplasms, such as hydatidiform mole and choriocarcinoma. False positive pregnancy tests are uncommon but may be seen in women who have heterophile antibodies and in perimenopausal women who produce pituitary hCG.

PROSTATE-SPECIFIC ANTIGEN

Prostate-specific antigen (PSA) is a glycoprotein produced by the epithelial cells of the prostate. This protein circulates in the serum and can become elevated because of benign and malignant conditions of the prostate. Fifty percent to ninety percent of PSA is protein bound and the remainder is free. PSA is used as a tumor marker for the screening, diagnosis, and management of prostate cancer. PSA lacks specificity for cancer, however, because it can be elevated in benign conditions such as benign prostatic hypertrophy (BPH) and prostatitis. Estimates suggest that a PSA higher than 4 ng/mL has sensitivity of 70% to 80% and specificity of 60% to 70% for prostate cancer. Factors other than prostate cancer can affect the PSA level (Table 14-16). Both prostate biopsy and transurethral resection of the prostate (TURP) can elevate the PSA, but DRE does not cause significant elevations in PSA.

Although elevations of the PSA are associated with increased risk of prostate cancer, the upper limit of normal of 4 ng/mL is arbitrary. PSA levels increase with age and recent sexual activity and are reduced with the use of 5-α-reductase inhibitors. During an initial screening examination, prostate cancer was found in 27% of men with PSA levels of 4.1 to 9.9 ng/mL and 59% with PSA higher than 10 ng/mL (Hernandez and Thompson, 2004) (eTable 14-6). However, prostate cancer is found in 23.9% of men with PSA of 2.1 to 3.0 ng/mL and 26.9% with PSA of 3.1 to 4.0 ng/mL (Thompson et al., 2004). The positive predictive value (PPV) of the PSA is doubled if the patient also has an abnormal DRE. A normal PSA does not exclude cancer; 20% to 40% of men with organ-confined prostate cancer

Table 14-16 Noncancer Factors That May Influence Prostate Specific Antigen

Factor	Change
Acute urinary retention	Increase
Androgens	Increase
Antiandrogens	Decrease
Bed rest	Decrease
Benign prostatic hypertrophy	Increase
Cirrhosis	Increase
Cystoscopy	Increase
Digital rectal examination	Not significant
Diurnal variation	No change
Ejaculation	Increase
Extensive exercise	Increase
Finasteride	Decrease
Physiologic variation	May fluctuate by 30%
Prostatic message	Increase
Prostate needle biopsy	Increase
Prostatitis	Increase
Radial prostatectomy	Decrease
Radiation therapy	Increase initially then decrease
Transurethral resection of the prostrate	Increase
Transurethral ultrasound of the prostrate	No change
Urethral instrumentation	Increase

will have PSA within the reference range. The use of PSA velocity, free PSA/total PSA, and urinary prostate cancer antigen 3 (PCA3) for screening is unproven.

The use of PSA for screening for prostate cancer remains controversial. Although it is clear that PSA testing can lead to earlier detection of prostate cancer, it is not clear that early diagnosis and treatment offer significant reduction in overall mortality. Estimates suggest that 1 prostate cancer death is prevented in 1000 men aged 55 to 69 screened every 1 to 4 years over a decade, although 110 cases will be diagnosed (Carter et al., 2013). A significant number of men diagnosed with prostate cancer by PSA screening have a tumor that would never have become symptomatic. In addition to screening, PSA is used to monitor the response to treatment for localized prostate cancer. After radical prostatectomy, PSA levels should become undetectable. Any detectable levels suggest residual or recurrent tumor and may occur months or years before becoming clinically apparent. PSA levels fall after radiation therapy, although they usually do not become undetectable. A PSA recurrence has been defined as three successive increases in the PSA level after radiation therapy.

TOTAL PROTEIN

Total protein includes albumin and globulin. The factors that affect the total protein level include changes in fluid status, the balance of protein synthesis and catabolism, and protein losses. While dehydration can cause a relative increase in serum protein concentration, volume expansion causes a relative decrease in protein concentration. Elevated protein levels in the absence of dehydration are usually related to increased globulin levels. As previously discussed,

acute-phase reactants are proteins that are increased in inflammatory conditions and include CRP, haptoglobin, fibrinogen, ceruloplasmin, and α_1-antitrypsin.

Serum protein *electrophoresis* separates proteins based on their mobility in an electric field and can provide a visual estimate of albumin and globulin levels. The five bands on the electrophoresis column include albumin, α_1-globulin, α_2-globulin, β-globulin, and γ-globulin. The immunoglobulins are found primarily in the γ region. Diffuse elevations in the γ region can occur with chronic infections, liver disease, autoimmune disorders, and granulomatous diseases. A monoclonal spike in the γ region indicates proliferation of a single immunoglobulin, as seen in myeloma or a monoclonal gammopathy of uncertain significance. Immunoglobulin abnormalities noted on protein electrophoresis can be further characterized by *immunofixation*, which can confirm a monoclonal immunoglobulin and can determine the heavy or light chain type of the immunoglobulin.

RHEUMATOID FACTOR AND ANTI–CYCLIC CITRULLINATED PEPTIDE ANTIBODIES

The diagnosis of rheumatoid arthritis (RA) is usually made based on clinical findings, supported by laboratory testing. In 2010, the American College of Rheumatology/European League against Rheumatism classification criteria included the laboratory tests of rheumatoid factor (RF) and anti–cyclic citrullinated peptide antibodies (ACPAs) in the criteria for the diagnosis of RA. The mainstay of testing has been the RF, which is an autoantibody directed against the Fc portion of the IgG molecule. The sensitivity of RF is approximately 54% to 88% and the specificity 48% to 92%, depending on the method used (Lee and Schur, 2003). RF is not specific for RA and may be detected in the serum of persons with other rheumatoid conditions, chronic infections, or inflammatory conditions, as well as in healthy older adults.

Results are usually reported as a titer determined by using a tube dilution method. A significant titer is 1:80 or greater. In RA, titers are often 1:640 to 1:520 but can even be found up to 1:320,000. Very high titers more likely indicate severe disease or systemic involvement. Increasing serial titer elevations can be used to monitor RA disease progression but not response to therapy. RF titers may decrease during remission, but only rarely do they become undetectable. The ESR is a better index of disease activity.

The ACPA test complements RF in the diagnosis of RA. ACPAs have been found to be present in RA early in the disease course and have a high predictive value for developing RA. The sensitivity and specificity of the ACPA is 60% to 80% and 85% to 98%, respectively. The advantage of ACPA over RF is that it is much more specific for RA. In patients with a moderate pretest probability of RA, positive ACPA significantly increases the likelihood of RA (Shmerling, 2009).

SODIUM

Disorders of body fluid balance are categorized as hypoosmolar, when there is excess water to solute balance, or hyperosmolar, when there is reduced water to solute balance. Given that sodium is the primary solute in the body, these disorders are manifested as either hyponatremia or hypernatremia. The reference range for serum sodium concentration is 135 to 145 mmol/L. In the evaluation of abnormal sodium levels, it is helpful to measure or calculate the plasma osmolality, which typically has a range of 280 to 295 mOsm/kg H$_2$O. The osmolality can also be calculated using the following formula:

$$Calculated\ osmolality = (2 \times Na) + (BUN/2.8) + glucose/18$$

This formula gives comparable results to measured osmolality, except in the presence of significant unmeasured solutes, such as mannitol or radiologic contrast dyes.

In most cases, *hyponatremia* is associated with hypoosmolality (eTable 14-7). Pseudohyponatremia can be seen with very elevated glucose or protein levels, causing artifactually low serum sodium levels; in these cases measured plasma osmolality is normal. Hyponatremia can be associated with normal or increased measured osmolality in the presence of other osmotically active substances, such as glucose and mannitol. In the setting of hyperglycemia, every 100 mg/dL rise in glucose lowers serum sodium by 1.6 mmol/L.

The diagnostic evaluation of hypoosmolar hyponatremia should begin with an assessment of the patient's volume status and urine electrolytes (Verbalis et al., 2013). Hyponatremia can occur in states of volume deficiency, euvolemic states, or hypervolemic conditions (Table 14-17). *Hypovolemic hyponatremia* can occur with GI, renal or third space losses, and patients typically demonstrate clinical findings of hypovolemia. With nonrenal causes, the urine Na$^+$ should be less than 30 mmol/L and the urine osmolality higher than 100 mOsm/kg H$_2$O. Hypovolemic hyponatremia responds readily to isotonic fluid replacement.

Hypervolemic hyponatremia can occur with advanced congestive heart failure, cirrhosis, nephrotic syndrome, and renal failure in the presence of total-body sodium overload and edema. In these disorders, effective renal blood flow is reduced, thus stimulating the release of arginine vasopressin (AVP), also known as antidiuretic hormone (ADH), which reduces renal excretion of water. Both sodium and water are increased, but water is increased proportionally more than sodium. In the absence of diuretic therapy, urine sodium is generally less than 30 mmol/L, and urine osmolality is over mOsm/kg H$_2$O.

Euvolemic hyponatremia is caused by an excess in body water. The most common cause of *euvolemic hyponatremia* is the syndrome of inappropriate ADH secretion (SIADH), which occurs when the stimulus for ADH secretion is not related to osmolarity or reduced renal blood flow. No edema is present, although mild volume expansion and a modest increase in weight are seen. Continued release of ADH occurs despite low plasma osmolarity. Criteria for diagnosis of SIADH include (1) the presence of hypoosmolality (P$_{osm}$ < 275 mOsm/kg H$_2$O); (2) urine sodium level greater than 30 mmol/L, assuming adequate sodium intake; (3) urine osmolality greater than 100 mOsm/kg H$_2$O; (4) clinical euvolemia; and (5) absence of diuretic therapy, hypothyroidism, and glucocorticoid deficiency. Other clinical findings that suggest SIADH includes a uric acid level less than 3 mEq/dL and BUN less than 10 mg/dL. Serum ADH (AVP) levels are not helpful because most causes of hyponatremia are associated with elevated AVP (ADH) levels. The major causes of SIADH are drugs and pulmonary and central nervous system diseases. SIADH can respond to fluid restriction or correction of the underlying disorder. Another cause of euvolemic hyponatremia is called *primary polydipsia*, which occurs in people who consume massive amounts of water and have very large volumes of urine. In general, plasma osmolarity is mildly decreased. These individuals have low urine sodium and dilute urine. The hyponatremia readily responds to a reduction in fluid intake.

Hypertonic disorders are associated with excess water losses compared with solute losses. Clinically manifested as hypernatremia, this serious electrolyte abnormality generally occurs in the setting of a significant underlying medical illness. The primary causes are deficient water intake or excessive water excretion. For example, when a patient has significant diarrhea, hypernatremia can develop when the patient cannot ingest enough water to compensate for the loss. When the clinical evaluation is not clear, measurement of urine osmolality is helpful. In the setting of hypernatremia and insufficient water intake, the urine should be maximally concentrated, higher than 800 mOsm/kg H$_2$O. In the setting of hypernatremia, if the urine osmolality is less than 800 mOsm/kg H$_2$O, a renal concentrating defect is present. This can be seen with hyperglycemia, an osmotic diuresis, or diabetes insipidus. A rise in urine osmolality after administering desmopressin (DDAVP) will distinguish central diabetes insipidus from nephrogenic diabetes insipidus.

Less frequently, hypernatremia can occur in a setting of increased total-body sodium from an excessive exogenous sodium load. Hypertonic intravenous fluids, saltwater near-drowning, and hypertonic dialysis can cause hypernatremia.

STREPTOCOCCAL TESTING

Acute pharyngitis is a frequent office diagnosis, but the only common form of pharyngitis that requires antibiotic

Table 14-17 Classification of Hyponatremia

Clinical Findings	Causes
VOLUME DEPLETION Tachycardia Hypotension Urine sodium <30 mmol/L (if nonrenal losses) Urine osmolality >100 mOsm/k H$_2$O Increased urine osmolarity	Gastrointestinal losses: vomiting, diarrhea Renal losses: diuretics, chronic renal failure, salt-wasting nephropathies Skin losses: burns Third-space losses: pancreatitis
VOLUME OVERLOAD Edema Urine sodium <10 mEq/L Urine osmolarity high	Congestive heart failure, nephrotic syndrome, cirrhosis
Euvolemic	**SIADH**
No edema or evidence of dehydration Urine sodium >30mmol/L (unless sodium-restricted diet) Urine osmolality >100 mOsm/kg H$_2$O Normal thyroid and adrenal function Psychogenic polydipsia	CNS disorders: infection, mass lesion, head trauma Pulmonary: lung cancer, infection Drugs: chlorpropamide, opiates, nicotine, phenothiazines, vincristine, SSRIs

CNS, Central nervous system; *SIADH,* syndrome of inappropriate diuretic hormone; *SSRI,* selective serotonin reuptake inhibitor.

treatment is that caused by *group A β-hemolytic streptococci* (GABHS). Approximately 20% to 30% of children and adolescents and 5% to 15% of adults with sore throat have streptococcal pharyngitis. Suggestive clinical features include fever, no cough or rhinorrhea, tonsillar exudates or beefy-red pharynx, and tender anterior cervical lymphadenopathy. Because of the overlap in symptoms between viral and strep pharyngitis, the 2012 American Society of Infectious Disease guidelines recommend testing, unless the patients has symptoms clearly suggestive of a viral etiology. For an acutely ill patient, the *rapid antigen detection test* (RADT) and traditional bacterial throat culture are available to identify GABHS. In the setting of pharyngitis and a typical syndrome, a positive culture or RADT is sufficient to begin treatment. The sensitivity of both is affected by throat swab technique. Testing should be done of both tonsils or tonsillar pillars and the posterior pharynx. Antigen or bacterial recovery from the throat is increased by rigorous swabbing. The RADT has the advantage of giving immediate results, which allows for early antibiotic therapy and thus decreases the duration of illness, complications, and contagiousness. Recent antibiotic use may give a false-negative result. The major limitation of rapid streptococcal tests is low sensitivity (70% to 90% on average), but specificity is approximately 95%. Therefore, a positive test can be accepted as evidence of disease and therapy begun without further testing. However, a negative result does not exclude the possibility of GABHS as the source of the pharyngitis. Children and adolescents with a negative RADT should have a throat culture for confirmation. Because of the low incidence of streptococcal pharyngitis and the extremely low risk of rheumatic fever in adults, the American Society of Infectious Diseases supports the use of RADT alone in adults, without confirmation by cultures (Shulman et al., 2012).

The throat culture is performed on sheep blood agar plate under aerobic conditions. If proper collection and plating technique are used, throat culture sensitivity is 95% and specificity 99.5%. With poor technique, sensitivity can be as low as 30%. Previous antibiotic use may diminish the colony count. If clinical conditions suggest the presence of other pharyngeal pathogens, such as *Neisseria gonorrhoeae*, the laboratory test should be altered because different collection and plating techniques are required. Throat culture results are generally reported 24 to 28 hours after plating. Antibiotic sensitivities are not routinely reported because GABHS is uniformly sensitive to penicillin.

SYPHILIS TESTING

The sexually transmitted disease (STD) syphilis is usually diagnosed with serologic testing. Although darkfield microscopy can identify spirochetes in fluid obtained from lesions of primary syphilis, the test has many false-negative readings, and most physicians are not trained to perform these tests. PCR for *Treponema pallidum* DNA is now commercially available for diagnosing primary syphilis using a swab from an ulcer, with early reports showing good sensitivity and specificity.

The major serologic tests for syphilis are the nonspecific nontreponemal Venereal Disease Research Laboratories (VDRL) and rapid plasma reagin (RPR) tests, which measure antibody production to a cardiolipin-cholesterol-lecithin antigen, and the specific treponemal antibody tests, which measure antibodies against the spirochete *T. pallidum.* Because of false-positive results in each of these tests, the use of both types of tests are required for a diagnosis. The usual screening for syphilis is a two-step process, beginning with the RPR or VDRL test, followed by specific treponemal antibody testing for confirmation. However, some laboratories are now performing treponemal enzyme immunoassay (EIA) tests first, followed by nontreponemal tests for confirmation of current infection.

The RPR or VDRL is reported as a titer of the highest dilution giving a positive test. The VDRL usually becomes positive approximately 1 to 4 weeks after the development of a chancre. The highest titers of nontreponemal tests are seen in secondary syphilis. The sensitivity of the RPR or VDRL is 78% to 86% in primary syphilis, 100% in secondary syphilis, and 95% to 98% in latent syphilis. Titers of VDRL or RPR parallel disease activity. After appropriate treatment of primary or secondary syphilis, titers decline and usually become negative within 1 year. A fourfold decline in titers 6 months after treatment suggests an adequate response to treatment of primary or secondary syphilis. A fourfold rise in titers after treatment suggests reinfection. Low titers may persist after treatment of late and latent syphilis. Approximately 20% of nontreponemal screening tests are false positive; false-positive tests usually have titers less than 1:8. Causes of false-positive nontreponemal tests include autoimmune disorders, HIV infection, infectious mononucleosis, endocarditis, and lymphoma.

The treponemal tests, such as the fluorescent treponemal antibody absorption (FTA-ABS) test or *T. pallidum* enzyme immunoassay (EIA), are used to confirm infection in a patient with a positive nontreponemal test. The treponemal tests are reported as positive or negative. The FTA has a sensitivity of 84% in primary syphilis and almost 100% in other stages of syphilis. The specificity is 96%; approximately 1% of the population has a false-positive treponemal antibody. Treponemal tests remain positive in 95% of patients, even after treatment, and are not used to monitor treatment response and cannot distinguish active from treated syphilis. If using treponemal EIA for screening, the CDC recommends performing a standard nontreponemal test after a positive treponemal EIA to guide treatment decisions. If the nontreponemal test is negative, then a different treponemal test should be performed to confirm infection. If the second treponemal test is positive, those without a history of treatment should be treated and those with a prior history of treatment should be offered treatment if there is a likelihood of reexposure (Workowski and Berman, 2010). Rapid testing using point-of-care testing for immunoassays against treponemal antigens is now available. The sensitivities appear to be from 84% to 97%, and the specificity is 92% to 98%.

In neurosyphilis, cerebrospinal fluid (CSF) abnormalities include elevated protein, a lymphocytic pleocytosis, and a positive VDRL. The CSF VDRL is the preferred test because it is more specific than the CSF FTA. However, the sensitivity is low enough that a negative CSF VDRL does not rule out neurosyphilis. In congenital syphilis, the diagnosis can be difficult because both FTA and VDRL antibodies can be transferred passively to newborns, and their identification at birth in the baby does not necessarily indicate infection. Passively transmitted antibodies generally decline in the first 2 months of life. If titers rise after birth, congenital syphilis is likely. Testing using specific *T. pallidum* EIA IgM may allow earlier diagnosis of congenital syphilis.

TESTOSTERONE

Evaluating men for low testosterone should be done only when there are clear signs and symptoms of androgen deficiency. Serum testosterone levels are highest in the morning, fluctuate by season, and are subject to episodic secretion and measurement variations. Therefore, the standard is to obtain more than one sample between 8:00 and 10:00 a.m. Other factors that affect testosterone levels include acute and chronic systemic illnesses, some medications including opioids and glucocorticoids, eating disorders, excessive exercise, and changes in the sex hormone–binding globulin (SHBG). The SHBG is affected by weight; diabetes mellitus; aging; thyroid, renal, and liver disease; acromegaly; HIV infection; and medications.

Most of the circulating testosterone is tightly bound to SHBG or loosely bound to albumin, while only about 0.5% to 3% is unbound, free testosterone. Bioavailable testosterone refers to the free plus albumin-bound fraction. Measuring the total serum testosterone is generally adequate. Checking the free or bioavailable testosterone concentration is usually necessary only when the total is low or conditions that affect the SHBG are present. The free and bioavailable testosterone tests cost significantly more than the total testosterone. The reference range for total, bioavailable, and free testosterone varies by laboratory and assay. In individuals with repeatedly low testosterone levels, measuring the luteinizing hormone (LH) and follicle-stimulating hormone (FSH) levels can help distinguish primary from secondary hypogonadism. These gonadotropins are high in primary (testicular) and low in secondary (pituitary) hypogonadism.

The serum testosterone level at which therapy should begin is unknown. Generally older men with low testosterone levels and men with borderline levels who are asymptomatic or have nonspecific symptoms should not be treated. The treatment goal is the minimal testosterone level that improves symptoms but no more than the mid normal reference range (Bhasin et al., 2010).

THYROID TESTING

Currently available tests for assessing thyroid function measure functional activity of the thyroid, the hypothalamic-pituitary-thyroid axis, or thyroid hormone levels. The third-generation thyroid-stimulating hormone (TSH) test is the best method to confirm or exclude primary thyroid disease in an ambulatory population. TSH is produced by the pituitary and is inhibited by circulating thyroxine (T_4) and triiodothyronine (T_3). In general, a normal TSH level is approximately 0.5 to 5 mIU/L and excludes hyperthyroidism or primary hypothyroidism. Supersensitive tests measure TSH at levels at least as low as 0.01 mIU/L. TSH levels less than 0.1vmIU/L suggest hyperthyroidism. Levels of 0.1 to 0.5 mIU/L may represent subclinical hyperthyroidism or excess thyroid hormone administration. Levels of 6 to 10 mIU/L are often considered subclinical hypothyroidism, are usually associated with normal free T_4 levels, and are not usually associated with symptoms. In patients with subclinical hypothyroidism, the presence of thyroid antibodies suggests a risk of conversion to frank hypothyroidism of about 5% per year. Symptomatic hypothyroidism occurs with TSH levels greater than 10 mIU/L. The TSH test is also the best way to monitor the results of replacement or suppressive therapy. Although the TSH level is an excellent screen for thyroid function in ambulatory patients, it must be interpreted with caution in acutely ill patients. TSH levels should be used to diagnose thyroid disorders in acutely ill hospitalized patients only when less than 0.1 mIU/L or greater than 20 mIU/L. TSH levels can be decreased by glucocorticoids, dopamine, and octreotide.

Measurements of circulating thyroid hormone should be obtained to confirm abnormal TSH levels. Measurement of free T_4 levels measure the total amount of hormone in blood, free and protein bound. Total T_4 or T_3 levels can be misleading in the setting of protein-binding abnormalities, such as estrogen therapy and liver disease. An approximate reference range in the adult for free T_4 is 0.7 to 2.5 ng/dL and for free T_3 0.2 to 0.5 ng/dL. Free T_3 testing is usually not necessary. One exception is in early hyperthyroidism, when the TSH is suppressed, free T_4 is normal, and free T_3 is elevated.

Primary hypothyroidism accounts for more than 95% of cases of hypothyroidism and is associated with an elevated TSH and reduced free T_4. *Central hypothyroidism* (secondary or tertiary) is associated with low free T_4 and normal to low TSH. Primary hyperthyroidism is associated with a suppressed TSH and elevated free T_4. Subclinical hyperthyroidism is associated with a reduced TSH but normal free T_4 and T_3 levels.

The radioactive iodine uptake scan measures 24-hour thyroid uptake of a labeled quantity of radioactive iodine. In normal persons, uptake is 8% to 30%. Lower limits of normal cannot be reliably differentiated from hypothyroidism in the radioactive iodine uptake scan. Its major value is to help identify causes of thyrotoxicosis associated with low levels of iodine uptake, such as thyroiditis and fictitious hyperthyroidism from overingestion of thyroid hormones. Other causes of reduced thyroid hormone uptake include recent iodine contrast administration and amiodarone.

URIC ACID

Uric acid is produced in the liver as a byproduct of purine metabolism. Measurement of uric acid is useful in the evaluation of *gout* and monitoring of certain types of chemotherapy. Uric acid levels are increased in situations with increased dietary purine intake, reduced excretion, or increased production. In addition, volume status affects uric acid secretion. With a decrease in extracellular volume, uric acid excretion declines, and serum uric acid levels increase. Conversely, volume expansion increases uric acid excretion and leads to *hypouricemia*. Several drugs inhibit the reabsorption of uric acid in the kidney and therefore lead to *uricosuria* (Table 14-18).

Table 14-18 Causes of Hyperuricemia

Overproduction

Myeloproliferative disorders	Psoriasis
Polycythemia vera	Toxemia of pregnancy
Hemolytic anemia	Ethanol
Malignancies	

Decreased Excretion

Renal failure	Hyperparathyroidism
Volume depletion	Diabetic ketoacidosis
Hypothyroidism	

Drugs

Thiazides	Pyrazinamide
Furosemide	Cyclosporine
Aspirin (low dose)	Niacin
Ethambutol	Vitamin B_{12} therapy

Table 14-19 Expected Results on Urine Opiate Screen and Gas Chromatography/Mass Spectometry

Prescribed Opioid	Opiate Immunoassay	GC/MS
Morphine	Positive	Morphine Codeine
Codeine	Positive	Codeine Morphine Hydrocodone
Hydrocodone	Positive/negative*	Hydrocodone hydromorphone
Hydromorphone	Positive/negative*	Hydromorphone
Oxycodone	Positive/negative*	Oxycodone Oxymorphone
Oxymorphone	Negative	Oxymorphone
Methadone	Negative	Methadone
Fentanyl	Negative	Fentanyl

GC/MS, gas chromatography/mass spectometry.
*Depends on the cross-reactivity of the opiate assay with the prescribed drug; varies among assays.

Progressively higher levels *of hyperuricemia* predict the likelihood of gout; however, most authorities believe that asymptomatic hyperuricemia should not be treated. At 37° C, saturation in plasma occurs when uric acid levels are greater than 6.8 mg/dL. Most patients with gout have uric acid levels greater than 7 mg/dL at some time, but they can have normal serum uric acid levels at the time of an acute gouty attack. Although a biologically significant uric acid level is greater than 6.8 mg/dL, the upper limits of "normal" based on population studies are 7.7 mg/dL for men and 6.8 mg/dL for women. The incidence of gout is approximately 5% per year in men with uric acid levels greater than 9 mg/dL, but only 0.5% per year in men with uric acid levels of 7.0 to 8.9 mg/dL.

A distinction between production of uric acid and reduced uric acid excretion as a cause of hyperuricemia may be helpful in evaluating patients with gout. Underexcretion is identified when the *fractional excretion* (excretion of uric acid/excretion of creatinine) is less than 6%. When a person is consuming a standard diet, excretion of uric acid greater than 800 mg/day is considered *hyperuricosuria*. Follow-up testing for patients with hyperuricosuria can be repeated on a low-purine diet, with 24-hour excretion of uric acid greater than 600 mg indicating uric acid overproduction. Of patients with gout, an estimated 90% have reduced uric acid excretion, and less than 10% have overproduction of uric acid as the cause. Drugs that lower serum uric acid include losartan, amlodipine, fenofibrate, and atorvastatin.

URINE DRUG SCREENS

The standard urine drug screen in a clinical setting is a panel of immunoassays designed to detect common drugs of abuse. The panel can include the five drugs required by federal workplace testing: amphetamines, cocaine, opiates, marijuana, and PCP. Panels can also include other classes of drugs, such as benzodiazepines, and more specific assays for synthetic opioids, such as oxycodone, methadone, and fentanyl. Point-of-care testing kits can be ordered for office use that are individualized to the need of the practice. These point-of-care tests provide results in minutes and have generally good sensitivity.

Urine drug screens use cutoff points to define a positive and negative test. These cutoffs are somewhat arbitrary, are chosen mainly to maximize sensitivity and specificity, and do not correlate with the degree of impairment or toxicity. Urine that contains a drug concentration below the cutoff will be reported as negative, even though the drug is present. With standard drug screens, the immunoassays can produce false-positive results. In clinical settings, confirmatory testing using more specific tests, such as gas chromatography/ mass spectometry (GC/MS) or liquid chromatography/mass spectrometry (LC/MS), may be ordered to confirm either the presence or absence of a drug.

Generally, drugs and their metabolites are detectable in urine tests for about 3 days after use. A notable exception is marijuana, which can be present in the urine for weeks after heavy use. Urine drug screens have significant limitations, which are not always recognized. For example, most immunoassays for "opiates" are designed to detect heroin and measure codeine, which is a byproduct of heroin and morphine metabolism. However, synthetic opioids such as fentanyl or methadone do not cross-react with "opiate" immunoassays and will produce a negative result. Oxycodone has variable cross-reactivity with standard opiate assays. See Table 14-19 for a chart listing "expected" results on urine opiate screens and GC/MS. Urine drug panels with specific assays for oxycodone, hydrocodone, methadone, and fentanyl are available for monitoring chronic opioid therapy.

VITAMIN D

Vitamin D is now recognized not only for its importance in preventing rickets, but also in preventing osteopenia, osteoporosis, muscle weakness, and falls. Testing levels of vitamin D can be considered in patients at increased risk of vitamin D deficiency, including elderly patients and those with osteoporosis, osteopenia, fat malabsorption, chronic kidney disease, and increased skin pigmentation. The term "vitamin D" includes vitamin D_2 and vitamin D_3. Vitamin

D$_2$ (calciferol) is manufactured from the plant sterols in yeast, and vitamin D$_3$ (cholecalciferol) is manufactured from lanolin. Vitamin D is hydroxylated by the liver into 25-hydroxyvitamin D [25(OH)D], the major circulating form of vitamin D in the body. The kidney converts 25(OH)D into 1,25-dihydroxyvitamin D [1,25(OH)$_2$D], which is the active form of vitamin D (Rosen, 2011).

The laboratory diagnosis of vitamin D deficiency relies on measuring the levels of 25(OH)D. Measuring 1,25(OH)$_2$D is not recommended in clinical practice because it is not a reliable indicator of vitamin D status. 1,25(OH)$_2$D has a half-life of only 4 hours, whereas 25(OH)D has a half-life of about 3 weeks. In addition, vitamin 1,25(OH)$_2$D levels can actually increase with vitamin D deficiency because increasing PTH levels stimulate the conversion of 25(OH)D to 1,25(OH)$_2$D.

The serum 25(OH)D is a measurement of vitamin D intake and that made in the body after sun exposure. Although some laboratories may report 25(OH)D$_2$ and 25(OH)D$_3$ levels, it is the total level that is used clinically to monitor vitamin D status. PTH rises when the 25(OH)D levels are less than 30 ng/mL. Although laboratories may list 20 to 100 ng/mL as the reference range for 25(OH)D, most experts define a preferred level of 25(OH)D as 30 to 60 ng/mL, with deficiency defined as less than 20 ng/mL and insufficiency as 20 to 30 ng/mL.

Summary of Additional Online Content

The following content is available at www.expertconsult.com:

eTable 14-1 Pattern of Liver Function Elevation

eTable 14-2 Conditions Associated with Positive Antinuclear Antibody Test

eTable 14-3 Conditions Associated with Elevated Carcinoembryonic Antigen Level

eTable 14-4 Complete Blood Count Components

eTable 14-5 Iron-Related Laboratory Measurements in Common Anemias

eTable 14-6 Positive Predictive Value of Total Prostate-Specific Antigen for Prostate Cancer

eTable 14-7 Classification of Hypernatremia

References

The complete reference list is available at www.expertconsult.com.

Web Resources

http://labtestsonline.org/understanding/analytes/ Developed by the American Association for Clinical Chemistry, this site allows patients to search for explanation of specific tests.

www.nlm.nih.gov/medlineplus/laboratorytests.html An overview for patients that explains basic laboratory principles, and gives links to other resources.

http://www.uspreventiveservicestaskforce.org/ Homepage of the U.S. Preventive Services Task Force (USPSTF), which lists recommendations for screening tests.

PART TWO

PRACTICE OF FAMILY MEDICINE

15 *Infectious Diseases*

CHARLES S. BRYAN

As a boon to humankind, the taming of yesteryear's infectious diseases ranks alongside anesthesia, aseptic surgery, and improved public health. Still, infections cause about one third of deaths worldwide, are a leading cause or contributor to deaths in developed nations, and present an array of challenges as new pathogens emerge and old pathogens become drug resistant. Factors contributing to the burden of infectious diseases in the United States include an aging population, medical progress (as in the treatment of cancer, cardiovascular diseases, and degenerative joint disease), immigration, HIV/AIDS, the emergence of new pathogens and of drug resistance in old pathogens, suburbanization, homelessness, incarceration, outdoor activities, and international travel.

Most family physicians will find that infectious diseases account for much of the joy and some of the sorrow of their careers. Self-limited infections comprise much of the throughput of daily office practice, but avoiding tragedy when nonspecific symptoms and signs portend life-threatening illness requires constant vigilance. This chapter focuses mainly on principles and diagnosis. Drug dosages are omitted; these are now universally available through electronically based resources, and no drug should be prescribed without thorough knowledge of routes of elimination; side effects; drug–drug interactions; status for use during pregnancy; and dose adjustments necessary for impaired kidney or liver function, unusually large body mass, and extremes of age.

Principles

This section reviews some principles fundamental to preventing, diagnosing, and managing infectious diseases in family medicine.

THE PATHOGENESIS OF INFECTIOUS DISEASES

The germ theory of disease as developed by Robert Koch, Louis Pasteur, and others during the 19th century held that a single virulent pathogen caused a specific disease. The germ theory has since become more nuanced, and Koch's postulates for establishing pathogenicity continue to evolve.

Several concepts are useful for understanding the pathogenesis of infection:

1. A *formula for infection* holds that the likelihood of clinical infection is proportionate to the product of the virulence (*V*) of an invading microorganism multiplied by the number (*N*) of microorganisms, divided by the resistance (*R*) of the host—that is, likelihood of infection = $(V \times N)/R$. Only highly virulent organisms, such as the agents of tuberculosis (TB), tularemia, and plague, require just a few microorganisms to make a healthy person sick. Less virulent organisms require large numbers or impaired host resistance.

2. The *epidemiologic triad* consists of a *reservoir* for a potential pathogen in the animate or inanimate environment; a *means of transmission* such as physical contact, droplets, contaminated food or water, or an insect vector; and a *susceptible host*, whose resistance to disease (as expressed in the "formula for infection") may have been reduced by disease, trauma, or drugs.

3. *Colonization*—the multiplication of a potential pathogen on an epithelial surface—is a common event that is occasionally (but not usually) followed by *invasion* of subepithelial tissues resulting in disease.

4. *Exogenous* microorganisms are those acquired from the animate or inanimate flora; *endogenous* microorganisms belong to the patient's microbial flora. *Endogenous* microorganisms can be permanent (e.g., *Escherichia coli*, enterococci, and anaerobic bacteria in the colon) or *transient colonizers* (e.g., *Streptococcus pneumoniae* and *Neisseria meningitidis* in the upper respiratory tract).

5. A *locus minoris resistentiae* (place of least resistance) occurs whenever the integrity of tissue is disrupted by trauma, a foreign body, or an implanted device. Such a locus creates a safe haven for microorganisms by depriving access by host defenses.

Let us illustrate these concepts with the case of a 17-year-old high school football player who, during a Friday night game, bruised his hip while going through the line. The next evening, as he prepared for a date, he squeezed a pimple. A week later he presented the emergency department with fever, chills, and pain, redness, and swelling over

Key Points

- Concepts useful for understanding the pathogenesis of infection include the formula for infection, the epidemiologic triad, endogenous versus exogenous flora, colonizing flora, and the *locus minoris resistentiae*.
- Protocols for managing common and usually self-limited infections such as upper respiratory infections (URIs) and urinary tract infections (UTIs) should include checklists for symptoms and signs that might portend more serious illness.
- A thorough history and physical examination, combined with simple laboratory tests such as the complete blood count and urinalysis, should precede request for expensive "send-out" studies.
- A system should be in place for reviewing laboratory results, especially critical results such as positive blood cultures and acid-fast bacillus (AFB) cultures. Failure to notice and act upon positive results can lead to tragedy.
- Evaluation for immunodeficiency in patients with frequent URIs or recurrent boils (furunculosis) is seldom worthwhile.
- Common misconceptions about contraindications for vaccines include mild illness, present antibiotic therapy, disease exposure or convalescence from an acute illness, pregnancy in the household, breastfeeding, premature birth, allergies to products that are not contained in the vaccine, the need for tuberculin skin testing, and the need for multiple vaccines.
- Before prescribing presumptive (empiric) antibiotics, one should clarify the syndrome, estimate its severity, ask whether it is treatable, consider the most likely pathogen(s), and assess the patient's comorbidities.
- For a returning traveler who presents with new medical complaints, the clinician should make two lists of diagnostic possibilities: one for destination-related illnesses and the other for diseases that might have occurred had the patient stayed home.
- An office practice should have in place an infection control plan and promote a "culture of cleanliness."

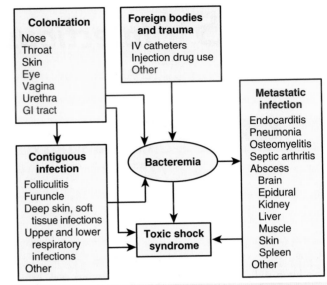

Figure 15-1. Dynamics of colonization and infection by *Staphylococcus aureus*. Nasal colonization often precedes contiguous infection, which can lead to bacteremia. Bacteremia carries the potential for serious infection in deep organs and tissues, especially when a *locus minoris resistentiae* is present. Toxin-producing strains can cause the staphylococcus toxic shock syndrome. *GI*, Gastrointestinal; *IV*, intravenous.

THE HISTORY AND PHYSICAL EXAMINATION

Symptoms suggestive of infectious disease prompt the clinician to search for a *syndrome*. Usually, the likely diagnosis is quickly apparent. For the more common syndromes seen in family medicine—for example, the common cold, otitis media, acute pharyngitis, and acute uncomplicated cystitis—it is helpful to design, maintain, and regularly update office protocols that can be implemented by physician extenders. Such protocols should ideally contain checklists to catch unusual symptoms and signs that might indicate something more serious.

The chief complaint should be recorded verbatim along with a statement as to its *duration*. Was the onset gradual or sudden? Was there an identifiable *prodrome*? It is useful to ask: "When was the *last time* you were in your usual state of health?" This question, which may have to be asked repeatedly, sometimes yields the first hint of a serious underlying problem.

The physical examination should include accurate vital signs, including a measurement (not an estimate) of the respiratory rate. Experienced clinicians often begin the physical examination by looking at the patient's hands. Splinter hemorrhages in the nail beds, Osler nodes, small pustules (Figure 15-2), or Janeway lesions (painless small red spots on the palms) suggest endocarditis, as do petechial lesions on the palpebral conjunctiva. A careful history and physical examination should always precede and can often eliminate the need for expensive laboratory tests.

USE OF LABORATORIES

The Clinical Laboratory Improvement Act (CLIA) and its amendments now preclude many and perhaps most primary care clinicians from performing in-office tests such as the complete blood count (CBC), differential blood count, and

the hip. Blood cultures revealed *Staphylococcus aureus*, and further studies confirmed *S. aureus* osteomyelitis of the upper femur.

This case illustrates the dynamics of colonization and invasive infection by *S. aureus* (Figure 15-1), an organism of intermediate virulence that requires large numbers of bacterial cells to cause disease unless host defenses are compromised. A locker room full of colonized teammates promoted the patient's *S. aureus* nasal colonization, which led to a tiny abscess in a hair follicle, which led to small numbers of *S. aureus* in his bloodstream after he squeezed the pimple. Disruption of capillaries in the metaphyseal end of his femur produced a small hematoma (a *locus minoris resistentiae*) in which a few *S. aureus* bacteria escaped host defenses; otherwise, he would never have known of their presence. Thinking in epidemiologic and pathophysiologic terms usually allows the inquisitive clinician to formulate a plausible story about why an infection occurred in a particular person at a particular time. Serious infection is usually an accidental event in a world in which each of us lives intimately with billions of microorganisms.

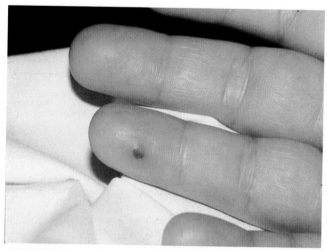

Figure 15-2. A small pustule ("purulent purpura") on the finger of a patient with *Staphylococcus aureus* endocarditis.

examination of specimens stained with Gram's method. These are considered to be of moderate complexity and require expense and inconvenience to assure compliance with CLIA regulations. Family physicians commonly rely on three types of laboratories:

1. An in-house laboratory, typically for CLIA-waived tests, provider-performed microscopy, and phlebotomy service for send-out specimens
2. A laboratory at a local hospital or other facility for most types of routine cultures, fungal cultures, mycobacterial (AFB) cultures and stains, and various serologic tests
3. One or more reference laboratories

Communication with laboratories can be time consuming but is of crucial importance, especially when results do not support a strong clinical impression. Here are some suggestions for effective use of laboratories:

1. Do not overlook the value of the total white blood cell (WBC) count, differential count, and platelet count and examination of the urine sediment. These often provide subtle clues to serious illness.
2. *C-reactive protein* (CRP), which is superseding erythrocyte sedimentation rate (ESR) as a marker of inflammation (because it is less influenced by noninflammatory factors), is useful for diagnosing infection and monitoring the efficacy of therapy (Ansar and Ghosh, 2013).
3. The *procalcitonin level* is increasingly used as a biomarker of sepsis but must be interpreted in the context of other findings (Wacker et al., 2013).
4. *Blood cultures* should be obtained before antibiotics are given to patients with predispositions to endocarditis.
5. *A system should be in place for reviewing laboratory results*, especially critical results such as positive blood cultures and AFB cultures. Failure to notice and act on positive results can lead to tragedy.
6. It is often useful to ask the laboratory to *hold a serum specimen* for the possibility that further testing may be needed, especially for situations requiring paired acute and convalescent samples.
7. It is usually inappropriate to obtain specimens for culture from predictably colonized drainage, body surfaces, or

fluids. Examples include swabs from ulcers or open wounds, sinus tract drainage, nasal swabs (except to look for *S. aureus* colonization), and nasopharyngeal swabs for patients with otitis media.
8. Do not send a swab specimen when a generous amount of purulent material is available, as from an incision and drainage procedure.

An array of new procedures, most of them nucleic acid based, are available in special situations, and exciting new tests loom on the horizon (Mitsuma et al., 2013).

IMPAIRMENTS OF HOST DEFENSES

Careful clinicians keep in mind their patients' predispositions to specific diseases (Table 15-1). Such host factors include age and common acquired diseases; immunosuppressive drugs; and, less often, primary (congenital) immunodeficiency disorders.

Common Acquired Conditions Predisposing to Infection

Poorly controlled diabetes mellitus impairs neutrophil function, predisposing to several unique syndromes (malignant otitis externa, rhinocerebral mucormycosis, and polymicrobial osteomyelitis of the small bones of the feet) and to gas-forming infections; soft tissue infections, including necrotizing fasciitis; and UTIs. Patients with diabetic sensory polyneuropathy should take scrupulous care of their feet, including daily inspection.

Acute alcohol intoxication predisposes to pneumonia. Habitual alcohol use impairs maturation of neutrophils in the bone marrow and depresses cell-mediated immunity. Patients with alcohol-related liver disease are vulnerable to overwhelming sepsis (the "ALPS syndrome" denotes alcoholic liver disease, leukopenia, and pneumococcal sepsis, but gram-negative bacilli can also be responsible) and spontaneous bacterial peritonitis. Spontaneous bacteremia—most often caused by infection with *E. coli*—also occurs. *Vibrio vulnificus* septicemia associated with severe cellulitis with formation of bullae is associated with alcoholism, cirrhosis, and the ingestion of raw oysters.

Anatomic or functional asplenia carries a lifetime risk—estimated to be as high as 5%—of overwhelming sepsis with high mortality rates. *S. pneumoniae* causes about 60% of cases; other causes include *Haemophilus influenzae*, *N. meningitidis*, various aerobic gram-positive and gram-negative bacteria, *Capnocytophaga canimorsus* (after dog bites), and babesiosis (in areas endemic for this tickborne parasite). The risk of overwhelming sepsis after splenectomy is greatest during the first 2 years. All patients with anatomic or functional asplenia should receive the pneumococcal, meningococcal, and *H. influenzae* vaccines.

Immunosuppressive Drugs

Corticosteroids promote infections mainly by impairing neutrophil, lymphocyte function, and wound healing. A general consensus holds that doses of 10 to 15 mg of prednisone equivalent, given for at least 2 months, impairs lymphocyte function. Common opportunistic pathogens

Table 15-1 Some Host Factors Predisposing to Infectious Diseases

Host Factor	Selected Infections
POPULATION-RELATED HOST FACTORS	
Refugees and international adoptees	Hepatitis B, hepatitis C, hepatitis D (delta agent), CMV, HIV, measles, TB, syphilis, intestinal pathogens, cysticercosis, malaria
Homeless persons	Pneumococcal pneumonia; meningococcal disease; TB; parasitic diseases; periodontal diseases; common skin infections, including cellulitis, arboviral encephalitis, and trench fever (*Bartonella henselae* and *Bartonella quintana*)
Incarcerated persons	Sexually transmitted diseases, HIV, TB, hepatitis B and C
UNDERLYING DISEASES OR CONDITIONS	
Diabetes mellitus	See text
Alcoholism and liver disease	Pneumonia, lung abscess, anaerobic pleuropulmonary infection, lung abscess, spontaneous bacterial peritonitis, TB
Injection drug use	Hepatitis A, B, C, and D (delta agent); skin and soft tissue infections, including *S. aureus* infections and necrotizing fasciitis; intravascular infections, including endocarditis and septic arthritis
Splenectomy	Overwhelming sepsis caused by *Streptococcus pneumoniae* or other pathogens (see text)
Spinal cord injury	UTIs, decubitus ulcers, pneumonia (the leading cause of death)
Organ transplant recipients	CMV infection (usually after the first month), EBV infection (which may cause posttransplantation lymphoproliferative disease), polyomavirus BK virus infection (which in kidney transplant recipients may cause nephropathy and organ rejection), *Pneumocystis jiroveci* pneumonia, invasive aspergillosis, strongyloidiasis
Granulocytopenia (absolute granulocyte count <1000/mL of blood)	Bacterial sepsis; fungal sepsis; invasive mold infections including aspergillosis, bowel ulcers (neutropenic enterocolitis or "typhlitis")

CMV, Cytomegalovirus; *EBV*, Epstein-Barr virus; *TB*, tuberculosis; *UTI*, urinary tract infection.

associated with impaired lymphocyte function include viruses (notably DNA viruses such as the herpesviruses but also RNA viruses, including human papillomavirus [HPV] and measles virus), intracellular bacteria (notably *Mycobacterium tuberculosis*; *Listeria monocytogenes*; and *Nocardia*, *Salmonella*, *Brucella*, and *Legionella* spp.), fungi (notably *Cryptococcus neoformans*, the regional mycoses, and *Pneumocystis jiroveci*), and parasites (e.g., *Toxoplasma gondii* and *Strongyloides stercoralis*). Patients receiving corticosteroids should know to watch for infection because signs and symptoms are rendered subtle by the blunted immune response.

Biologic agents commonly used for diseases such as rheumatoid arthritis, notably monoclonal antibodies directed against tumor necrosis factor, and other inflammation-inducing cytokines also predispose to opportunistic pathogens associated with impaired lymphocyte function. The infectious risk varies among the available biologic agents. Rituximab, a monoclonal antibody directed against CD20 B cells, has been associated with bacterial infections and, rarely, with progressive multifocal leukoencephalopathy (PML).

Primary Immunodeficiency Disorders

Rare primary immunodeficiency disorders presenting in childhood—for example, X-linked agammaglobulinemia, DiGeorge syndrome, severe combined immunodeficiency syndromes, chronic granulomatous disease, reticular dysgenesis, Chédiak-Higashi syndrome, and ataxia-telangiectasia—are beyond the scope of this chapter. Here, we review several immunodeficiency disorders that may present during adolescence or early adulthood:

1. *Selective IgA deficiency* occurs worldwide in one in every 300 to 700 persons but seldom predisposes to infection. A few patients have recurrent infections, especially URIs, atopic disorders, or autoimmune disorders. Anaphylaxis can result from the administration of blood products or intravenous immune globulin.

2. *Common variable immunodeficiency* occurs worldwide in about one in 25,000 persons and predisposes to frequent sinopulmonary infections, ear infections, conjunctivitis, chronic lung diseases, autoimmune disorders ($\approx$25% of patients), gastrointestinal disorders (including inflammatory bowel disease, malabsorption, and pernicious anemia), and lymphoma. Diagnosis is usually made by measuring serum levels of IgG, IgA, and IgM. If the levels are low but not extremely low (i.e., below 200 mg/dL), one can confirm the diagnosis by testing the antibody response to vaccines (e.g., the pneumococcal and tetanus vaccines). Immune globulin replacement therapy reduces the incidence of infections.

3. *Inherited deficiencies in the complement system*, which consist of about 30 known proteins, occur in about 0.03% of all persons and are usually inherited as autosomal recessive traits. Predisposition to disease varies according to which protein is deficient. Affected patients are predisposed to recurrent mild or serious bacterial infections. Deficiency of certain components (properdin, C3, factor H, and factor I) predisposes to infection by encapsulated organisms such as *S. pneumoniae*. Deficiency of late-acting components (C5, C6, C7, and C8) predisposes to disseminated meningococcal and, less commonly, gonococcal infection. Screening for complement deficiencies is accomplished by testing for total hemolytic complement (CH_{50}).

4. The recurrent infection hyperimmunoglobulin E syndrome (known as Job syndrome, after the biblical personage) usually becomes apparent during childhood but may present later in life. Features include recurrent skin

and soft tissue infections, especially staphylococcal; recurrent sinopulmonary infections; dry eyes; and phenotypic abnormalities in bone structure. Immunoglobulin E levels are dramatically elevated.

5. Immunoglobulin G subclass deficiency, diagnosed by low levels of one or more subclasses (IgG_1, IgG_2, IgG_3, and IgG_4), is controversial. Patients suspected of this and other subtle abnormalities of humoral immunity (e.g., "specific antibody deficiencies" in which immunoglobulin levels are normal but patients fail to respond to a specific antigen) should probably be referred to an immunologist.

Extensive immunologic evaluation for "frequent colds" or frequent "boils" (furunculosis) is seldom worthwhile unless there are other reasons to suspect immunodeficiency.

IMMUNIZATION

Active immunization consists of the administration of vaccines or toxoids, which induces an immune response. *Passive* immunization, which will not be considered further here, consists of the administration of an exogenously produced immunoglobulin. All family physicians should stay abreast of nationally recommended vaccines for the general population (Advisory Committee on Immunization Practices, 2014; also available at http://www.cdc.gov/vaccines) and should be aware of special recommendations for immunocompromised persons (Rubin et al., 2014). (See Figures 7-6 and 7-7 for current immunization recommendations.)

Vaccines are of two broad types. *Live attenuated vaccines* are produced by modifying the disease-causing "wild form" of a virus or bacterium into an innocuous form, which induces an immune response after multiplying in the recipient. With rare exception (mainly orally administered agents such as the live polio vaccine), such vaccines usually confer immunity with a single dose. Commonly used live attenuated vaccines include those for measles, mumps, rubella, polio, yellow fever, varicella, influenza (the live, intranasally administered vaccine), zoster, and (formerly) vaccinia for smallpox. Because they replicate in the recipient, live attenuated vaccines must be given cautiously if at all to immunocompromised persons.

Inactivated vaccines are derived from killed viruses or bacteria and, in the case of bacteria, may consist of either the whole organism or fractional components such as toxoids, subunits, or polysaccharide surface antigens. An effective immune response often requires multiple doses spaced over time. Periodic booster inoculations may be necessary to sustain protective antibody levels. Inactivated bacterial vaccines may consist of the entire organism or fractional components such as toxoids, subunits, and polysaccharide surface antigens. Inactivated vaccines include those for polio, influenza (the intramuscularly administered vaccine), hepatitis A, hepatitis B, acellular pertussis, diphtheria, tetanus, botulism, *S. pneumoniae, H. influenzae* type b, and *N. meningitidis*. Because they do not replicate in the recipient, inactivated vaccines can be given safely to immunocompromised persons.

A practice should have in place two reminder systems: one for its staff members and the other for its patient population. Many vaccines should be mandatory for staff members. All patients except children younger than 6 months of age should be urged to receive the annual vaccine against influenza. Teenage girls should be encouraged to receive the HPV vaccine to reduce the incidence of condyloma and risk of cervical cancer (Herweijer et al., 2014); persons older than 60 years of age should receive the varicella-zoster (shingles) vaccine to reduce the risk and severity of shingles and postherpetic neuralgia. Physicians and staff should hone arguments for those who refuse vaccines or, worse, refuse them for their children. Herd immunity is everyone's responsibility.

Contraindications to vaccines are relatively few. Valid contraindications include allergy, mainly type I allergy (anaphylaxis, angioedema, urticaria, and bronchospasm), and severe illness. As stated earlier, inactivated vaccines (but not live vaccines) may be given if indicated to immunosuppressed persons; the same holds for pregnant women. Anyone with a history of Guillain-Barré syndrome developing within 6 weeks of receiving the influenza vaccine should not receive the influenza vaccine. Recent administration of a blood product is a relative contraindication to a live attenuated vaccine because the blood product may have contained antibodies that will render the vaccine ineffective. Care should be taken administering the MMR (measles, mumps, and rubella) and MMRV (measles, mumps, rubella, and varicella) vaccine when there is a history of seizures because these vaccines carry a small risk of febrile seizures in children. The acellular pertussis, DTaP (diphtheria, tetanus, and acellular pertussis, and varicella vaccines do not carry a similar risk.

Many people erroneously think that vaccines are contraindicated during mild illness, present antibiotic therapy, disease exposure or convalescence from an acute illness, pregnancy in the household, breastfeeding, premature birth, allergies to products that are not contained in the vaccine, the need for tuberculin skin testing, and the need for multiple vaccines. Screening questionnaires for vaccine administration can be found at sources such as the Immunization Action Coalition (http://www.immunize.org).

Adverse reactions to vaccines most commonly consist of pain and erythema at an injection site or fever. Syncope sometimes occurs, especially among adolescents and young adults. Anaphylactic reactions—the symptoms of which include flushing, facial edema, swelling of the mouth or throat, dyspnea, and wheezing—are life threatening. Facilities administering vaccines should therefore have available supplies and procedures for managing anaphylaxis.

ANTIMICROBIAL AGENTS

Antimicrobial therapy is of three types: presumptive (empiric) therapy when the microbial etiology is unproven, precise (targeted) therapy after isolation of the infecting microorganism(s), and preventive (prophylactic) therapy in certain well-defined situations.

Presumptive (Empiric) Antimicrobial Therapy

The decisions about whether to prescribe presumptive therapy and what agents to describe depend on answers to structured questions (Figure 15-3). The *presumed infectious*

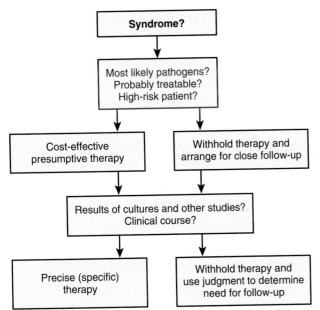

Figure 15-3. Decision making about antimicrobial therapy for infectious disease begins with accurate definition of the patient's syndrome.

syndrome should be defined as accurately as possible. The *severity* of the syndrome and the presence of *underlying conditions* such as serious diseases, use of immunosuppressive drugs, and advanced age affect (1) the decision to give antibiotics or "watch and wait" and (2) if presumptive therapy is given, the decision whether to cover most of the potential pathogens or just the more likely ones. What is the margin for error? One must also decide whether to admit the patient to the hospital and, if not, the frequency of follow-up.

Precise (Targeted) Antimicrobial Therapy

All aspects of a serious or potentially serious illness should be reviewed within 48 to 72 hours after the initial encounter. Within this time frame, (1) the causative pathogen will usually have been isolated if it is ever to be isolated (rare exceptions include mycobacteria, fungi, and certain fastidious bacteria) and (2) the patient will have shown improvement if the drug regimen covers the pathogen(s) and no complicating factor such as an undrained abscess is present. The choice of drugs should be revisited. *De-escalation* consists of narrowing the spectrum of antimicrobial coverage based on the specific microorganism(s) isolated and the clinical response. Overcoming the reluctance to "leave things as they are because the patient is getting better" usually works to the patient's advantage because unnecessarily broad coverage predisposes to colonization by drug-resistant organisms and risks collateral damage such as drug reactions and colitis caused by infection with *Clostridium difficile*.

Preventive (Prophylactic or Preemptive) Antimicrobial Therapy

Preventive antimicrobial therapy works best when given within 1 hour of a planned invasive procedure in which infection would be disastrous. Preventive therapy works less well when drugs are given over extended period or indefinitely, but there are nevertheless well-defined indications for such therapy. Examples include prophylaxis against *P. jiroveci* and *Mycobacterium avium* complex infections in patients with advanced HIV disease, prophylaxis against recurrent bacterial cystitis in sexually active women, and use of antiviral agents to protect solid organ transplant recipients from serious cytomegalovirus (CMV) infection.

Specific Antimicrobial Agents

Knowledge of antimicrobial spectrum of activity, pharmacokinetics, pharmacodynamics, and drug–drug interactions aids antibiotic selection, as does knowledge of local antibiotic susceptibility patterns. Table 15-2 lists commonly used antibiotics by class and mechanism of action, with selected comments on precautions. A general knowledge of the efficacy, safety, and cost of commonly used antibiotics is essential. The practice of "thinking generically" even if one prescribes by trade names promotes awareness of new developments (including adverse drug reactions) as these appear in the literature.

Outpatient Parenteral Antimicrobial Therapy

A few family physicians may become involved with programs for outpatient parenteral antimicrobial therapy; more commonly, clinicians will find themselves monitoring such therapy, often in patients who have been released from the hospital. Clinicians should be aware of various temptations (including financial incentives) to prescribe parenteral therapy when orally administered drugs would suffice. Examples of drugs that when given orally provide nearly 100% bioavailability include trimethoprim–sulfamethoxazole (TMP-SMX), the fluoroquinolones (e.g., levofloxacin), metronidazole, and chloramphenicol (seldom used today because of rare cases of aplastic anemia). Patients on outpatient parenteral antimicrobial therapy should be monitored not only for serum drug levels (as for vancomycin and the aminoglycosides) and renal function but also for the potential for sepsis related to vascular access lines.

TRAVEL AND GEOGRAPHIC MEDICINE

Travelers are well advised to review destination-specific recommendations, now widely available on the Internet. Perhaps the most useful website is that of the travel health section of the Centers for Disease Control and Prevention (CDC) (http://www.cdc.gov/travel). Other federally sponsored websites include the CDC's Health Information for International Travel (http://www.cdc.gov/mmwr) and the U.S. State Department's travel warnings (http://www.state.gov/travel).

Travelers to developing countries should know precautions against traveler's diarrhea. Most travelers are advised to use bismuth subsalicylate (Pepto-Bismol) for prevention; loperamide (Imodium) for symptomatic treatment; and a fluoroquinolone for severe (*not* mild or moderately severe) diarrhea, which is usually of bacterial etiology (notably, *E. coli* and *Campylobacter, Salmonella,* and *Shigella* spp.). Traveler's diarrhea can also be caused by viruses (especially rotaviruses and, on cruise ships, noroviruses) and protozoa (notably *Cryptosporidium* spp., microsporidia, and *Giardia*

Table 15-2 Common Antibiotics by Class

Antimicrobial Class (Action)	Selected Agents	Selected Comments
β-lactams (disrupt cell wall synthesis by inhibiting formation of peptidoglycan cross-links)	*Penicillins:* penicillin V, penicillin G *Aminopenicillins:* ampicillin, amoxicillin, bacampicillin *Antistaphylococcal penicillins:* methicillin, nafcillin, oxacillin, dicloxacillin *Extended-spectrum penicillins:* ticarcillin, piperacillin *β-lactam–β-lactamase inhibitor combinations:* ampicillin–sulbactam; amoxicillin–clavulanate; ticarcillin–clavulanate; piperacillin–tazobactam *Carbapenems:* imipenem, ertapenem, meropenem, doripenem *Monobactam:* aztreonam *First-generation cephalosporins:* cefazolin, cephalexin *Second-generation cephalosporin:* cefuroxime *Third-generation cephalosporins:* ceftriaxone, cefotaxime, ceftazidime, cefdinir *Fourth-generation cephalosporin:* cefepime *Fifth-generation cephalosporin:* ceftaroline *Cephamycins:* cefoxitin, cefotetan	When patients give a history of allergy to penicillin or other β-lactam antibiotics, the adverse reaction and the year of its occurrence should be recorded. Type 1 (IgE-mediated allergy) is defined by anaphylaxis, urticaria, angioedema, or bronchospasm. Type 1 cross-reactivity occurs among all β-lactam antibiotics with the singular exception of aztreonam. However, the risk of type 1 cross-reactivity between penicillins, carbapenems, and cephalosporins is low (< 3% to 5%). Neurotoxicity, manifested by somnolence, coma, and seizures, is potentially fatal and is dose related; carbapenems confer the highest risk. Carbapenems are active against most aerobic and anaerobic bacteria; holes in coverage include MRSA, *Stenotrophomonas maltophilia, Burkholderia cepacia, Legionella* spp., and *Corynebacterium jeikeium*. Aztreonam is active only against aerobic gram-negative bacilli; it can be used safely in patients with a history of type 1 allergy to other β-lactams. Cephalosporins lack coverage against enterococci, thus predisposing to enterococcal superinfection. All broad-spectrum antibiotics predispose to *C. difficile* colitis.
Glycopeptides (disrupt cell wall synthesis, apparently by steric hindrance of the formation of backbone glycan chains)	Vancomycin, telavancin	Penetrate poorly into CSF Complications include infusion-related "red man's syndrome," nephrotoxicity, and thrombocytopenia. Monitoring of trough serum levels is recommended for safety. Telavancin, compared with vancomycin, is more active on a weight basis against gram-positive bacteria, including MRSA (i.e., the minimum inhibitory levels are lower) and has a longer serum half-life but has greater nephrotoxicity.
Lipopeptide (disrupts cell membrane, creating holes that allow potassium efflux)	Daptomycin	Daptomycin is inactivated by pulmonary surfactant and is therefore not effective for pneumonia. Rhabdomyolysis can occur; the serum CPK level should be monitored weekly. Severe eosinophilic pneumonia can occur.
Oxazolidinones (disrupt protein synthesis at the 50S ribosomal subunit)	Linezolid, tedizolid	Prolonged courses can cause myelosuppression (≤10% of patients) and potentially irreversible peripheral and optic neuropathy. When used in combination with serotonergic agents (e.g., SSRIs), can cause a serotonin release syndrome. Useful for pneumonia caused by MRSA because of excellent penetration into lungs
Glycylglycine (disrupts protein synthesis at the 30S ribosomal subunit)	Tigecycline	Nausea and vomiting are prominent after initial doses. Approved for complicated skin and skin structure infections, intraabdominal infections, and community-acquired pneumonia. Use for nonapproved indications has been associated with *increased* mortality; hence, a "black box" warning.
Folate antagonist (inhibit nucleic acid synthesis)	Trimethoprim–sulfamethoxazole (TMP-SMX)	Active against numerous bacteria Near 100% bioavailability Trimethoprim component causes benign increases in serum creatinine. Sulfa component confers risks of serious allergic reactions, including Stevens-Johnson syndrome. Side effects include nephrotoxicity, hyperkalemia, bone marrow suppression, and photosensitivity.
Fluoroquinolones (inhibit various topoisomerase enzymes and DNA gyrase)	Ciprofloxacin, levofloxacin, gemifloxacin, moxifloxacin, norfloxacin, ofloxacin	Can cause QTc prolongation with risk of torsades de pointes Risk of tendonitis and tendon rupture is increased by concomitant corticosteroid use Avoid in pregnancy and in children because of cartilage malformation. Other side effects include photosensitivity and dysglycemia.
Nitroimidazole (appears to disrupt DNA and inhibit nucleic acid synthesis by poorly understood mechanisms)	Metronidazole	Active against most anaerobic bacteria and some parasites Near 100% oral bioavailability Causes disulfiram reactions; avoid concurrent alcohol use (even with the vaginal preparation). High doses cause nausea and vomiting. Prolonged use can cause neurotoxicity, including encephalopathy and sensory or motor peripheral neuropathy.

Continued on following page

Table 15-2   Common Antibiotics by Class (Continued)

Antimicrobial Class (Action)	Selected Agents	Selected Comments
Tetracyclines (inhibit protein synthesis at the 30S ribosomal subunit)	Tetracycline, doxycycline, minocycline	Avoid during pregnancy and in children younger than 8 years of age because of teeth discoloration* (see RMSF). Photosensitivity, skin discoloration (minocycline), esophagitis (doxycycline) Avoid coadministration of oral tetracyclines and multivalent cations (e.g., calcium and magnesium).
Macrolides (inhibit protein synthesis at the 50S ribosomal subunit)	Azithromycin, clarithromycin, erythromycin, fidaxomicin	Can cause QTc prolongation with risk of torsades de pointes Drug–drug interactions secondary to 3A4 inhibition (clarithromycin, erythromycin) Side effects include nausea, vomiting, diarrhea; dysgeusia (clarithromycin). Fidaxomicin, a "nonabsorbable" agent marketed to treat refractory *Clostridium difficile* infection, can cause hypersensitivity reactions.
Lincosamide (inhibits protein synthesis at the 50S ribosomal subunit)	Clindamycin	Classically associated with *Clostridium difficile* colitis Active against most anaerobic bacteria other than *C. difficile* and against many gram-positive aerobic bacteria Susceptibility testing against gram-positive bacteria includes a "D-test" to screen for drug-resistant subpopulations of bacteria. Side effects include nausea, vomiting, diarrhea, and abdominal cramping.
Rifamycins (inhibit DNA-dependent RNA synthesis)	Rifampin, rifapentine, rifabutin, rifamixin	These drugs should never be used alone because of the potential for emergence of resistance. Risk of hepatitis increases with concurrent use of isoniazid or pyrazinamide. Allergic reactions include interstitial nephritis.
Aminoglycosides	Streptomycin, gentamicin, tobramycin, amikacin	Nephrotoxicity, although usually reversible, is associated with increased mortality rates among hospitalized patients. Auditory and vestibular toxicity are irreversible. Can also cause neuromuscular blockade
Polymyxins	Polymyxin B, colistimethate	Use may possibly expand because of continued emergence of resistant gram-negative bacilli. Risk of nephrotoxicity and neuromuscular blockade may be less than previously reported. Nevertheless, consultation should probably be sought before use.
Nitrofuran (inhibits protein, DNA, RNA, and cell wall synthesis by unclear mechanisms)	Nitrofurantoin	Acute pulmonary reactions result from hypersensitivity. Chronic pulmonary toxicity, usually after >6 months of use, includes pulmonary fibrosis that can be misdiagnosed as heart failure. Nausea, vomiting, and headache are the most common side effects.
Streptogramins (inhibit protein synthesis at the 50S ribosomal subunit)	Quinupristin–dalfopristin	Separately, quinupristin and dalfopristin are bacteriostatic. In combination, these agents are synergistic against gram-positive bacteria. Indications are vancomycin-resistant *Enterococcus faecium* and MRSA. Toxicity includes phlebitis. Side effects include arthralgia, myalgia, nausea, vomiting, and diarrhea.
Phosphonic acid derivative (blocks cell wall synthesis by inactivating enolpyruvyl transferase)	Fosfomycin	Broadly active against many gram-negative and gram-positive bacteria Used to treat UTIs, usually as a single megadose

CSF, Cerebrospinal fluid; *CPK*, creatine phosphokinase; *MRSA*, methicillin-resistant *Staphylococcus aureus*; *SSRI*, selective serotonin reuptake inhibitor; *UTI*, urinary tract infection.
*See text regarding use of tetracyclines in children with suspected Rocky Mountain spotted fever (RMSF).

and *Isospora* spp.). Travelers should take full supplies of their maintenance medications (indeed, a slight excess to allow for delays). Parting advice might include reminders that accidents (notably, road accidents) are the most common cause of travel-related death and that risk of sexually transmitted disease, including HIV, runs high in some destinations.

For a returning traveler who presents with new medical complaints, the clinician should make two lists of diagnostic possibilities. One list contains destination-related illnesses; the other list contains diseases that might have occurred had the patient stayed home. It is important to include a travel history whenever one evaluates a patient for a possible infection of unclear etiology because some travel-related illnesses have long incubation periods; examples include TB, HIV/AIDS, brucellosis, and leishmaniasis.

Malaria is now the major infectious cause of death among returning U.S. travelers and is discussed below in the section on parasites. Other potentially fatal diseases include typhoid fever. Febrile illnesses in travelers returning from the Caribbean can be caused by dengue ("break bone fever") and, since 2013, chikungunya ("chik fever"), both caused by viruses transmitted by *Aedes* mosquitoes. Febrile illnesses in travelers can also be caused by rickettsial infection and, rarely, yellow fever.

INFECTION CONTROL

Everything should be done to minimize the risk that people entering a facility to improve their health will leave with newly acquired pathogens. An office infection control plan should include written procedures for cleaning and disinfection of instruments, management of infectious waste, proper storage of sterilized supplies, wiping down of examination tables and horizontal surfaces at the end of

each day, and an employee health policy that extends to all physicians and staff. The plan should be supervised by a designated person (often a nurse) empowered to implement corrective measures. The practice should promote a "culture of cleanliness" that starts with strong emphasis on hand hygiene.

Syndromes

INFECTIOUS DISEASE EMERGENCIES

The clinician should memorize the essential features of various life-threatening infections that may present with nonspecific symptoms and signs. Table 15-3 discusses some of these syndromes; others are discussed elsewhere in this chapter.

Key Points

- Patients with suspected infection should be evaluated for severity: sepsis, sepsis syndrome, severe sepsis, and septic shock.
- Differential diagnosis of the "flulike illness" includes sepsis caused by *S. aureus* or gram-negative bacilli, Rocky Mountain spotted fever (RMSF), septic abortion, and malaria.
- Infectious causes of the "worst headache ever" include meningitis, brain abscess, RMSF, sphenoid sinusitis, and falciparum malaria.
- Necrotizing infections of skin, fascia, and muscle constitute a diverse group of syndromes of which *necrotizing fasciitis* is the most common. Necrotizing fasciitis should be considered whenever tissue injury to the skin or subcutaneous tissue is accompanied by *and muscle* constitute a diverse group of syndromes that should be considered whenever tissue injury to the skin or subcutaneous tissue is accompanied by systemic toxicity, pain disproportionate to physical findings; marked swelling; or blebs, bullae, or crepitance.
- Fever with localized pain or tenderness over the spine suggests vertebral osteomyelitis or spinal epidural abscess.
- Blood cultures should be obtained before antibiotics are prescribed to patients with conditions predisposing to endocarditis, such as regurgitant murmurs, congenital heart disease, or prosthetic heart valves.
- Acute bacterial meningitis can be misdiagnosed as "gastroenteritis" at the first clinical encounter because of prominent nausea.
- When an adolescent or young adult presents with a flulike illness and does not seem acutely ill but *might* have meningococcal disease, prescribe a "buddy check" whereby someone checks on the patient several hours after bedtime.
- Patients with fever with lethargy, impaired speech, bizarre behavior, or hallucinations should be evaluated for herpes simplex virus (HSV) encephalitis.
- Unusual causes of cellulitis include infection with *Aeromonas hydrophila, H. influenzae, S. pneumoniae, Cryptococcus neoformans, Erysipelothrix rhusiopathiae,* and *Streptococcus iniae.*
- Malignant otitis externa usually occurs in patients with diabetes mellitus, is caused by *Pseudomonas aeruginosa,* involves the temporal bone, and can extend into the brain.

- When patients present with suspected pneumonia, one should ask whether the problem could be something else (e.g., pulmonary embolism), whether the severity warrants hospitalization, and whether an unusual microorganism could be responsible.
- Clinical judgment takes precedent over a negative "rapid flu test" result whenever someone presents with typical symptoms of influenza at a time when influenza is prevalent in a community.
- Routine stool cultures have a low yield except in patients with severe disease or patients with the dysentery syndrome (small, frequent stools with blood and mucus).
- Patients older than 50 years of age with *Salmonella* gastroenteritis should receive antibiotics because of the risk of mycotic aneurysm of the aorta.
- Amebiasis should be excluded before steroids are prescribed for presumed first-episode ulcerative colitis.
- About 2% to 3% of patients with *C. difficile* colitis develop severe complications such as toxic megacolon or perforation of the colon; marked leukocytosis (WBC count >30,000/mm^3) strongly suggests severe disease.
- Treatment of asymptomatic bacteriuria, even when accompanied by pyuria, should be discouraged in elderly patients and in patients with obstructive uropathy because such treatment encourages colonization by difficult-to-treat microorganisms.
- Gonococcal infection is underdiagnosed in women, who are prone to develop pelvic inflammatory disease (PID), infertility, and disseminated infection with the gonococcal arthritis–dermatitis syndrome.
- Up to half of patients with RMSF do not have rash during the first week of illness; diagnostic clues include thrombocytopenia, hyponatremia, and mild elevation of aminotransferases.
- Serologic testing for Lyme disease should be discouraged for patients with nonspecific symptoms, who have not had documented erythema chronicum, and who have not spent much time in a highly endemic geographic area.
- Primary care clinicians play essential roles in the diagnosis, management, and prevention of HIV disease, which is highly treatable for patients who are able to comply with all recommendations.

Table 15-3   Classic Presentations of Some Infectious Diseases

Presentation	Cause(s)
Acute flulike illness with fever, malaise, myalgias, or arthritis	Septicemia caused by *Staphylococcus aureus* or gram-negative bacilli, endocarditis, RMSF, septic abortion, malaria, primary HIV infection
"Worst headache ever"	Meningitis, brain abscess, encephalitis, RMSF, sphenoid sinusitis, falciparum malaria
Severe, progressive, unilateral retroorbital or frontal headache	Septic cavernous sinus thrombosis
Fever, headache, stiff neck, nausea, and vomiting in previously healthy college student (especially a freshman)	Meningitis caused by *Neisseria meningitidis*, meningococcemia
Fever, headache, and altered mental status in an older adult with paranasal sinus tenderness, an abnormal chest examination, or a red tympanic membrane	Meningitis caused by *Streptococcus pneumoniae*
Low-grade fever and altered mental status in a frail elderly nursing home resident	Meningitis caused by *S. pneumoniae*, *Listeria monocytogenes*, or an aerobic gram-negative bacillus
Fever, headache, and focal neurologic signs	Brain abscess, subdural empyema, intracranial epidural abscess
Fever and localized back pain progressing to weakness of the lower extremities, with impaired bowel or bladder function	Spinal epidural abscess (usually caused by *S. aureus*)
Fever with flulike illness in an older person with a history or physical findings of valvular heart disease and evidence of heart failure	Endocarditis caused by *S. aureus* on the aortic or mitral valve
Fever with flulike illness in an injecting drug user with patchy pulmonary infiltrates on chest radiographic examination	Endocarditis caused by *S. aureus* on the tricuspid or pulmonic valve
Fever with flulike illness in a patient with known cirrhosis and who has recently ingested raw oysters who may have skin lesions suggesting cellulitis with bullae	Sepsis caused by *Vibrio vulnificus*
Fever, sore throat, tenderness over the anterior aspect of the neck or along the sternocleidomastoid muscle	Lateral or retropharyngeal space infection, septic thrombosis of the internal jugular vein (Lemierre syndrome)
Sore throat with difficulty breathing; pharynx relatively normal on physical examination	Acute epiglottitis
Severe localized pain over a seemingly trivial skin or soft tissue lesion, with or without a systemic toxicity	Necrotizing fasciitis
Severe localized pain over a skin lesion that contains bullae, watery discharge, or crepitance	Clostridial myonecrosis (gas gangrene) or necrotizing fasciitis
Fever with toxicity and a painful lymph node, with history of outdoors activity in the southwestern United States	Bubonic plague
Flulike illness progressing to hypotension and pulmonary edema in a patient with history of outdoors activity in the southwestern United States	Hantavirus pulmonary syndrome
Rapid onset of dyspnea, fever, diaphoresis, and cyanosis in a patient recently treated for "viral upper respiratory infection"	Inhalational anthrax due to bioterrorism
Fever with lethargy and confusion, personality change, or impaired speech	Herpes simplex encephalitis
Severe sepsis syndrome (sepsis with evidence of impaired organ perfusion) in a patient with a scar over the left upper quadrant of the abdomen	Fulminant postsplenectomy infection syndrome, most commonly caused by *S. pneumoniae* or *Haemophilus influenzae*
Returning traveler with fever, headache, and systemic toxicity	Malaria caused by *Plasmodium falciparum*
Shock, multiorgan failure, and diffuse erythroderma suggesting a sunburn, usually in a younger person	Toxic shock syndrome caused by *S. aureus*
Shock, multiorgan failure, and localized skin lesion with severe pain in a middle-aged or older person	Toxic shock syndrome caused by *Streptococcus pyogenes* (group A streptococcus)
Fever with abdominal pain and back pain in an older person with atherosclerosis and a recent diarrheal illness	Mycotic aneurysm of the abdominal aorta caused by *Salmonella* spp.
Ascending flaccid paralysis in a young person who has been in a tick habitat	Tick paralysis
Descending paralysis, symmetric cranial nerve palsies, dilated pupils, dry mouth, and furrowed tongue	Botulism
Fever with relative bradycardia, bilateral patchy pulmonary infiltrates, mild elevation of the aminotransferases, and history of exposure to wild rabbits or other animals	Tularemia

RMSF, Rocky Mountain spotted fever.

The Sepsis Syndrome: Differential Diagnosis of the Flulike Illness

Primary care clinicians frequently see patients with fever, malaise, myalgia, and other constitutional symptoms. When localizing symptoms are few, when the patient does not appear ill or "toxic," and when physical examination is unrevealing, such patients are often presumed to have a "flulike illness" or "viral syndrome." Some of these patients, however, have life-threatening disease. Examples include septicemia caused by *S. aureus* or aerobic gram-negative bacilli, septic abortion, endocarditis, and RMSF. The clinician's task is to determine which patients require close observation, special laboratory studies, and empiric antimicrobial therapy.

The following definitions express the stages of sepsis in ascending order of severity:

1. *Sepsis* denotes clinical evidence of infection plus a host response: fever (temperature >38.0 °C [100.4 °F]) or hypothermia (temperature <96.8 °F [36.0 °C], tachycardia (heart rate >90 beats/min), tachypnea (respiratory rate >20 breaths/min or $PaCO_2$ <32 mm Hg), and both quantitative and qualitative changes in circulating WBCs (total WBC count >12,000 cells/mm^3 or <4,000 cells/mm^3 or >10% band neutrophils in the differential count).
2. *Sepsis syndrome* denotes sepsis plus evidence of impaired organ perfusion. Evidence of impaired organ infusion includes altered mental status, decreased urine output, and low oxygen saturation by pulse oximetry. Lactic acidosis may also be present.
3. *Severe sepsis* denotes sepsis associated with organ dysfunction, hypoperfusion, or hypotension. Hypoperfusion abnormalities include oliguria and altered mental status. Hypotension is defined as systolic blood pressure less than 90 mm Hg or a decrease of greater than 40 mm Hg from the patient's baseline in the absence of hypotension.
4. *Septic shock* is defined as sepsis with hypotension despite adequate fluid resuscitation along with perfusion abnormalities such as lactic acidosis, oliguria, or alteration in mental status.

The concept of a *systemic inflammatory response syndrome* expresses the idea that the body responds in a fixed number of ways to a wide variety of insults. Thus, shock with acute respiratory syndrome and renal failure can result not only from infectious disease but also, for example, from acute hemorrhagic pancreatitis.

It cannot be stressed too strongly that *S. aureus* sepsis often presents as an undifferentiated flulike illness. Patients with *S. aureus* sepsis can progress rapidly to sepsis syndrome, severe sepsis, septic shock, and refractory septic shock.

Faced with a patient with possible sepsis syndrome, the clinician has three tasks:

1. Look for clues of infection and its severity by careful history and physical examination (including pulse oximetry if available).
2. Determine whether the patient's general appearance, underlying condition, or findings on CBC (notably, leukocytosis, leukopenia, bandemia, or thrombocytopenia) warrant admission to the hospital.
3. Assure close follow-up if it is deemed that admission to the hospital is not warranted.

Necrotizing Fasciitis and Other Necrotizing Infections of Skin, Fascia, and Muscle

A survey of members of the Infectious Diseases Society of America (IDSA) conducted by the present author indicated that *necrotizing fasciitis* more than any other infectious disease emergency is likely to result in misdiagnosis with disastrous consequences. *Necrotizing infections of skin, fascia, and muscle* constitute a diverse group of syndromes that should be considered whenever tissue injury to the skin or subcutaneous tissue is accompanied by any combination of (1) blebs, bullae, or crepitance (all of which suggest gas formation); (2) marked swelling; (3) pain disproportionate to the physical findings; (4) bluish-gray skin discoloration; and (5) systemic toxicity.

Necrotizing fasciitis caused by group A streptococci has received lay attention as the "flesh-eating bacteria syndrome." Many affected patients have features of the streptococcal toxic shock syndrome. A second type of necrotizing fasciitis is caused by various aerobic and anaerobic bacteria, often in combination. The resulting syndromes include *nonclostridial anaerobic cellulitis, synergistic necrotizing cellulitis,* and *Fournier's gangrene* (which involves the perineum; lower abdominal wall; and, in males, the scrotum and penis; many patients have underlying diabetes mellitus). *Clostridial myonecrosis (gas gangrene)* is a fulminant, necrotizing infection of muscle with marked toxicity caused by toxin-producing clostridial strains, notably *C. perfringens.* Up to 3000 cases occur in the United States each year, most of which are related to trauma or penetrating injury. A spontaneous form occurs in patients with cancer and is frequently caused by *Clostridium septicum.* Pain is often the initial complaint. When the infection affects an extremity, patients often note that the limb feels "heavy." The skin becomes dark and often mottled, with edema and multiple bullae. Crepitus is usually less marked than in clostridial cellulitis.

Necrotizing skin and soft tissue infections require a high index of diagnostic suspicion. Leukocytosis (total WBC count >15,400/mm^3) and hyponatremia (serum sodium level <135 mmol/L) were shown in one study to help distinguish necrotizing fasciitis from less severe soft tissue infections. Imaging studies, especially magnetic resonance imaging (MRI), help clarify the diagnosis but surgical exploration is usually necessary to define the type and extent of the infection. Appropriate initial antimicrobial therapy should cover both aerobic and anaerobic pathogens. Removal of all involved tissue by wide debridement (and sometimes amputation) is necessary to prevent death.

KEY TREATMENT

- Non–penicillin-allergic patients with necrotizing fasciitis caused by *Streptococcus pyogenes* (group A streptococci) should be treated with penicillin G combined with clindamycin (to inhibit toxin production) (SOR: A).
- Non–penicillin-allergic patients with community-acquired necrotizing fasciitis of mixed microbial etiology should be treated with three drugs, such as ampicillin–sulbactam plus clindamycin plus ciprofloxacin (SOR: A).
- Penicillin G is the drug of choice for gas gangrene (anaerobic myonecrosis) caused by infection with *Clostridium perfringens* (SOR: A).

Spinal Epidural Abscess

Spinal epidural abscess was, in the author's survey of IDSA members, the second most likely serious infection to be misdiagnosed with unfortunate results. The full-blown triad consists of fever, localized pain, and tenderness over the spine and symptoms and signs of spinal cord compression (impaired bowel or bladder function and then weakness or paralysis of the lower extremities). A flulike prodrome often signifies bacteremia caused by *S. aureus*, the most common causative organism. Patients suspected of this diagnosis should have a prompt MRI and be hospitalized because prompt surgical drainage, combined with antimicrobial therapy, is nearly always necessary for successful outcome.

Staphylococcal and Streptococcal Toxic Shock Syndromes

The toxic shock syndromes are caused by strains of *S. pyogenes* (group A streptococci) and *S. aureus* that produce unique toxins that function as superantigens, causing lymphocytes to produce massive quantities of inflammatory cytokines. These syndromes present as acute illnesses with fever, hypotension, tachycardia, and tachypnea. Staphylococcal toxic shock syndrome is usually preceded by a short flulike prodrome with chills, malaise, and generalized aching. A flulike prodrome is less common in streptococcal toxic shock syndrome, in which patients typically have symptoms and signs of localized infection, most commonly on an extremity and with severe pain. Suspicion of either syndrome should prompt hospitalization.

KEY TREATMENT

- Empiric therapy of staphylococcal toxic shock syndrome in non–penicillin-allergic patients consists of high-dose antistaphylococcal antibiotics (SOR: A).
- Treatment of streptococcal toxic shock syndrome consists of high-dose penicillin G combined with clindamycin to suppress toxin synthesis (SOR: A).

Endocarditis

The term "infective endocarditis" usually refers to infection of the heart valves, but other surfaces can be affected, such as the endocardium adjacent to a ventricular septal defect. "Endarteritis" refers to an identical process affecting a large blood vessel, such as a patent ductus arteriosus. Endocarditis is uniformly fatal without treatment. The diagnosis can be masked by prior antibiotic therapy. The primary care clinician's task is to know when to suspect endocarditis, when to request blood cultures, when to obtain special studies such as echocardiography, and when to refer patients for hospitalization.

The manifestations of endocarditis are caused by (1) continuous presence of microorganisms in the bloodstream; (2) embolism from the vegetations; (3) circulating immune complexes; and (4) destruction of cardiac tissue, causing heart failure and arrhythmias. "Viridans" streptococci are historically the most common causes of endocarditis, but staphylococci were more common in some recent series. Enterococci cause up to 18% of cases. Coagulase-negative staphylococci and fungi are important causes in patients with prosthetic valves. The many uncommon microorganisms causing endocarditis sometimes have specific associations, such as the well-known association of *Streptococcus gallolyticus* (formerly known as *Streptococcus bovis*) endocarditis or bacteremia with colorectal neoplasia.

Blood cultures are the keys to diagnosis. The modified Duke criteria for "definite" or "possible" endocarditis also take into account findings on echocardiography, predisposing heart conditions or injection drug use, documented vascular phenomena (evidence of embolism, telltale skin lesions, and other events), and immunologic phenomena. Classic "subacute" endocarditis caused by viridians streptococci typically unfolds over weeks to even months, and patients often seek medical assistance for complaints that seem unrelated to the heart. Therefore, when patients with predisposing conditions (e.g., regurgitant murmurs, new murmurs, prosthetic valves, or congenital heart disease) have indications for antibiotics, it is prudent to obtain blood cultures even when an alternative diagnosis seems clear-cut.

Blood cultures are positive in most patients with endocarditis. When endocarditis is strongly suspected and blood cultures are sterile, one should discuss alternative culture methods with the microbiology laboratory. The most common cause of "culture-negative" endocarditis is prior antibiotic therapy. Exposures that suggest unusual causes include cats (*Bartonella* spp.), cattle (*Coxiella burnetii*), goats or wild pigs (*Brucella* species), and psittacine birds (*Chlamydia psittaci*). Serology (IgM and IgG) is useful for all of these possibilities and also for *Mycoplasma* spp.; urinary antigen may be helpful for endocarditis caused by *Legionella* spp. Fungal endocarditis can be caused by *Candida* spp., *Histoplasma capsulatum*, and *Aspergillus* spp.

Patients with strongly suspected endocarditis should be hospitalized.

Meningococcal Disease

Meningococcemia with or without meningitis is one of the few infectious diseases capable of killing a previously healthy person within hours. It mainly affects children, adolescents, and young adults (notably, college freshmen) but can occur at any age. Initial symptoms are often nonspecific. A prodromal URI may be followed by a flulike illness with fever, chills, malaise, generalized aching, headache, nausea, and vomiting. A petechial rash, found in up to 60% of patients, appears first on the ankles, wrists, axillary folds, and points of pressure (as from elastic) (Figure 15-4). The rash later becomes purpuric. When a patient is seen in the ambulatory setting, the patient does not seem especially sick, and yet *might* have meningococcemia—for example, a patient with low-grade fever, mild headache, and nausea—a "buddy check" is recommended: (1) ascertain that the patient has someone who can check on him or her during the night, (2) have the designated "buddy" awaken the patient about 4 hours after bedtime, check the patient's level of consciousness, and look for "little red spots" on the aforementioned sites, and (3) report to the emergency department if there is any deterioration.

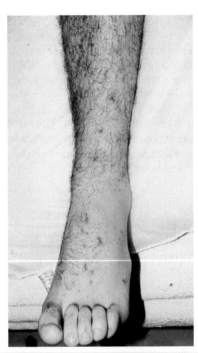

Figure 15-4. Petechial rash over the foot, ankle, and lower extremity in a college freshman with meningococcemia.

KEY TREATMENT

- Patients in whom meningococcemia is strongly suspected should be given ceftriaxone as soon as possible (ideally, after obtaining blood cultures) and then hospitalized (SOR: A).

Acute Bacterial Meningitis and Aseptic Meningitis

Acute bacterial meningitis is a medical emergency variably characterized by fever, headache, meningismus (stiff neck), nausea, vomiting, and altered mental status. None of these symptoms is sufficiently sensitive to exclude meningitis by its absence. The presentation is subtle in about 15% of patients, especially in young children and elderly adults. Nausea and vomiting may predominate during the early stages, leading to a misdiagnosis of gastroenteritis.

Meningitis caused by *H. influenzae* type b now affects only about two in every 100,000 children because of wide vaccination against this microorganism. *N. meningitidis* is the most common cause of meningitis in children, adolescents, and young adults. The quadrivalent meningococcal conjugate vaccine covers four of the five major meningococcal serotypes; the exception is serogroup B, which causes about one third of cases of invasive meningococcal disease in the United States.

S. pneumoniae causes meningitis in all age groups and is the most common cause in older adults. The majority of patients with pneumococcal meningitis, unlike most patients with meningococcal meningitis, have a predisposing condition such as otitis media, sinusitis, pneumonia, or basilar skull fracture. The diagnosis of pneumococcal meningitis is often delayed because another condition—for example, acute alcoholism, severe pneumonia, or

neurologic disease—might account for the patient's sluggishness. Less common causes of bacterial meningitis include *Streptococcus agalactiae* (the group B streptococcus), especially in children; *Listeria monocytogenes* in elderly adults and debilitated or immunosuppressed individuals; and aerobic gram-negative bacilli in neonates, elderly persons, and patients who have undergone neurosurgical procedures. A subacute or chronic onset of symptoms of meningitis raises the possibility of tuberculous or fungal meningitis.

When acute bacterial meningitis is suspected, lumbar puncture (LP) should be performed as soon as possible unless symptoms and signs (e.g., localizing neurologic findings) suggest an intracranial mass lesion. The cerebrospinal fluid (CSF) formula—that is, the combination of the WBC count and differential, glucose, and protein—often confirms the diagnosis or steers the clinician in the right direction. A high WBC count ($>1000/mm^3$) with a predominance of polymorphonuclear neutrophils, a low glucose level (<40 mg/dL or <40% of the simultaneous blood glucose), and a high protein content (>160 mg/dL) are nearly diagnostic of acute bacterial meningitis. Gram stain sometimes indicates the causative microorganism. In patients with aseptic meningitis (discussed later), the CSF WBC count is usually lower, the glucose level usually normal, and the protein content either normal or slightly elevated. When immediate LP is not feasible or when it is deemed best to exclude central nervous system (CNS) mass lesion by computed tomography (CT), it may be prudent to give an initial dose of an antibiotic (usually ceftriaxone) before the LP.

KEY TREATMENT

- Recommended empiric antimicrobial therapy for acute bacterial meningitis is age related (SOR: A).
- Vancomycin plus a third-generation cephalosporin are recommended between the ages of 1 month and 50 years (SOR: A).
- Adjunctive dexamethasone is recommended for infants and children with *H. influenzae* type b meningitis but not if they have already received antibiotics (SOR: A).
- Ampicillin is often added in older adults to cover *Listeria monocytogenes*, and when aerobic gram-negative bacilli are a possibility, patients should receive a drug active against *P. aeruginosa* until the diagnosis is clarified (SOR: B).
- Most adult patients—especially those with proven or suspected pneumococcal meningitis—should receive adjunctive dexamethasone therapy to blunt the intense inflammatory response that causes much of the disability (SOR: B).

Aseptic Meningitis

Aseptic meningitis is discussed here only because it needs to be distinguished from acute bacterial meningitis because the correct diagnosis of aseptic meningitis spares the patient expense and inconvenience. The term "aseptic meningitis," which in practice is basically synonymous with "viral meningitis," was coined in the 1930s to denote a clinical syndrome characterized by fever, headache, photophobia, unrevealing microbiologic studies on CSF, and a self-limited course without treatment. Enteroviruses are the most common proven cause and usually cause aseptic meningitis during the summer and fall months. Affected patients often complain of a severe headache—which is sometimes greatly relieved by LP—but mental status is normal, and they do not appear acutely ill. The CSF differential count may show a predominance of polymorphonuclear leukocytes when the patient is first seen. However, repeating the LP within the next 24 hours, even within 4 to 6 hours, reveals a predominantly lymphocytic pleocytosis despite withholding antibiotics. The prognosis for aseptic meningitis is, by definition, excellent, although occasional patients experience one or more recurrences.

Not infrequently, a patient who has received antibiotics presents with symptoms and signs suggesting aseptic meningitis. The differential diagnosis then includes aseptic meningitis versus *partially treated bacterial meningitis*. Partial treatment of bacterial meningitis may cause the CSF pleocytosis to become predominantly lymphocytic and the CSF glucose level to return toward normal. However, the CSF protein level usually remains elevated. Testing the CSF for bacterial antigens or bacterial DNA may be useful in this situation.

Encephalitis

Encephalitis is a life-threatening process characterized pathologically by inflammation of the brain parenchyma and clinically by neurologic abnormalities, including altered consciousness, localizing (focal) symptoms and signs, and seizures. Of the more than 100 microbial causes, *HSV* ranks first in importance for U.S. clinicians because of its potential severity and the availability of effective drug therapy.

Herpes simplex virus encephalitis usually begins with fever and lethargy and progresses rapidly to stupor and torpor. Impaired speech, bizarre behavior, or hallucinations suggest involvement of the temporal and frontal lobes, which can be confirmed by neuroimaging (for which MRI is more sensitive than CT). The CSF usually shows a lymphocytic pleocytosis, although the leukocyte count is normal in about 5% of patients. Red blood cells are usually present in the CSF, reflecting the necrotizing nature of the inflammatory process. Polymerase chain reaction (PCR) testing of CSF for herpes simplex viruses (HSV-1 and HSV-2) has a sensitivity of greater than 95% and a specificity of nearly 100%. Occasionally, the PCR test has a false-negative result early in the infection. Death and residual disability are common even with treatment.

Arboviruses causing encephalitis in the United States include the *St. Louis encephalitis virus* (which often strikes elderly adults and homeless individuals), the *Eastern equine encephalitis virus* (with a mortality rate in humans as high as 33%), the *California encephalitis virus* (which, similar to HSV, can cause a severe encephalitis with long-term sequelae and behavioral disorders in survivors), and *West Nile encephalitis virus*. West Nile virus, carried by migrating birds and transmitted to humans mainly by *Culex* mosquitoes; has since 1999 been recognized in most U.S. states; causes symptomatic disease (typically fever, often with rash and lymphadenopathy) in about 20% of infected persons; and results in serious CNS disease in fewer than 1% of persons, many of whom are elderly. The spectrum of CNS disease caused by West Nile virus includes encephalitis, meningoencephalitis, meningitis, and myelitis with flaccid paralysis. Diagnosis of arboviral encephalitis is usually made by serologic testing; virus-specific IgM antibodies can be detected in CSF and serum in nearly all cases by the 10th day of illness. There is no specific treatment. Uncommon and rare causes of encephalitis in the United States include rabies; dengue; yellow fever; and, in immunocompromised persons, HHV-6 and JC virus (the cause of progressive multifocal leukoencephalopathy [PML]).

Suppurative Intracranial Infections (Parameningeal Infections)

The term *parameningeal infection* encompasses syndromes that require prompt diagnosis and usually surgical drainage: brain abscess, subdural empyema, septic thrombosis of the dural veins, and epidural abscess. Neuroimaging (with MRI being superior to CT) simplifies the diagnosis.

Brain abscess often evolves slowly. The classic triad—headache (present in ≈70% of patients), fever, and focal neurologic signs—is present in fewer than half of adults. Streptococci, especially anaerobic streptococci (peptostreptococci) and *Streptococcus anginosus*, are the most common bacterial causes, but *S. aureus* and aerobic gram-negative bacilli can also be involved.

Subdural empyema usually results from sinusitis, especially frontal sinusitis, and should be suspected when a patient with sinusitis gradually develops severe headache with nausea or vomiting.

Cavernous sinus thrombosis usually results from contiguous spread of infection from a nasal furuncle (hence, the admonition not to "squeeze a pimple" in the so-called dangerous area of the face), ethmoid or sphenoid sinusitis (Figure 15-5), or dental infections. *S. aureus* is the most common pathogen (≈70% of cases) followed by streptococci, gram-negative bacilli, and anaerobic bacteria. The

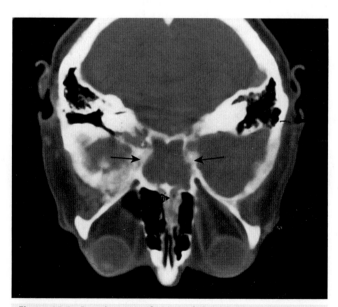

Figure 15-5. Complete opacification of the sphenoid sinusitis, presenting as the "worst headache ever" and leading to a fatal outcome because of misdiagnosis. *Arrows* indicate sphenoid sinuses.

classic presentation consists of headache, photophobia, unilateral periorbital edema, and bulging of the eye (proptosis). Examination of the eye may reveal ptosis; chemosis; and palsies involving the third, fourth, fifth, and sixth cranial nerves, with disturbance of lateral gaze (sixth nerve palsy) being the most common. The pupil may be dilated and sluggishly reactive. Suspicion of cavernous sinus thrombosis should prompt immediate hospitalization, imaging studies, and institution of antimicrobial therapy directed broadly against the aforementioned pathogens.

Botulism

Botulism, caused by an extremely potent neurotoxin produced by *Clostridium botulinum,* is uncommon in the United States but occasionally causes outbreaks and is a potential agent of bioterrorism. The disease typically presents with symmetric cranial nerve palsies and descending motor paralysis; other features include blurred vision, diplopia, dilated pupils, dry mouth, normal blood pressure, mental alertness despite the striking neurologic deficits, and intact sensation. Conditions that mimic botulism include stroke, Guillain-Barré syndrome, myasthenia gravis, diphtheria, and organophosphate poisoning. Infant botulism, now the most common form in the United States, often begins with weakness, including a weak cry, feeding problems, irritability, and hypotonia. Aggressive intensive care with mechanical ventilation enables patients to survive. An antitoxin is available from the CDC.

Tetanus

Tetanus (called "lockjaw" because of the characteristic rigidity of the masseter muscles) affects more than 100 persons in the United States each year, mainly older persons and especially older women. All of its manifestations are attributed to a toxin. The portal of entry is often trivial and overlooked. Dystonic reactions to neuroleptic drugs and other central dopamine antagonists can resemble tetanus; however, patients with dystonic reactions tend to show lateral neck turning and respond to diphenhydramine or benztropine. Strychnine poisoning resembles tetanus. Patients with suspected tetanus should be hospitalized.

Bioterrorism

Family physicians are crucial to the early recognition of bioterrorism because—unlike terrorism with chemical or physical agents—affected persons may be widely dispersed before disease manifestations appear. Potential agents of bioterrorism have been grouped into three categories designated A, B, and C. *Category A* organisms are easily disseminated from a central source or readily transmitted from person to person, cause high mortality, and may disrupt society. These include the agents of smallpox, anthrax, plague, tularemia, botulism, and certain viral hemorrhagic fevers. *Category B* organisms are moderately easy to disseminate, cause low mortality but considerable morbidity, and pose problems in recognition. These include the agents of salmonellosis, shigellosis, cryptosporidiosis, hemorrhagic colitis (*E. coli* 0157:H7), Q fever (*Coxiella burnetii*), and viral encephalitis. *Category C* includes organisms that could be bioengineered in the future with the potential to cause high morbidity and mortality with a major impact on public health. These include multi-drug-resistant *M.*

tuberculosis (TB), tickborne hemorrhagic fever viruses, tickborne encephalitis virus, Nipah virus, and various respiratory viruses. Bioterrorism should be suspected whenever clinicians encounter either a large number of cases of severe illness in previously healthy persons or a single case of a rare infectious disease. Other clues are higher morbidity and mortality than would be expected from a common disease; failure of a common disease to respond to the usual therapy; disease with an unusual geographic or seasonal distribution; outbreaks of unexplained disease in animals that precede or accompany severe illness in humans; and outbreaks associated with common exposures, including water sources and ventilation systems.

SKIN AND SOFT TISSUE INFECTIONS

Infections of skin and soft tissue are common in family medicine and must sometimes be distinguished from life-threatening conditions such as necrotizing fasciitis, discussed earlier. A rapid increase in ambulatory care visits for skin infections in the United States, estimated to now exceed 14 million visits per year, is attributed in part to the spread of methicillin-resistant *S. aureus* (MRSA). Issues for primary care clinicians include (1) when to suspect that skin lesions reflect a systemic illness, such as endocarditis; (2) when to treat empirically without special studies; (3) when to obtain Gram stains, cultures, or—if necrotizing soft tissue infection is a possibility—imaging studies such as MRI; (4) when to supplement incision and drainage of abscesses with antibiotics; and (5) when to hospitalize.

Impetigo and Ecthyma

Nonbullous impetigo is a superficial vesiculopustular infection of the stratum corneum, usually seen in children during the summer months. The vesicles quickly rupture to form thick, "stuck-on" golden-yellow to honey-colored crusts. *S. pyogenes* (group A streptococci) is the classic cause, but in some localities, *S. aureus* is now more common. Most cases are self-limited, although poststreptococcal glomerulonephritis can develop.

Ecthyma resembles nonbullous impetigo in that it usually caused by group A streptococci or staphylococci and begins with vesicles that become pustules and then rupture. Ecthyma differs from nonbullous impetigo in that (1) it occurs most commonly on the lower extremities; (2) occurs in other age groups besides young children, especially in elderly adults; (3) extends through the epidermis, leaving a "punched out" ulcer with raised violaceous margins; and (4) usually calls for systemic antibiotics. "Uncomplicated ecthyma" must be distinguished from *ecthyma gangrenosum* caused by systemic infection (notably, *P. aeruginosa*) and usually featuring a necrotic eschar in the center of the lesion.

Bullous impetigo usually occurs in infants and young children, is caused by *S. aureus* strains that produce an exfoliative toxin, and is characterized by vesicles that evolve into large flaccid bullae. Rupture of the bullae leaves exposed, moist, red skin before the formation of a thin, light brown, "varnish-like" crust. The mild form is self-limited, but a generalized form (the *staphylococcal scalded skin syndrome*, also called *pemphigus neonatorum* when it affects neonates) is life threatening.

- Topical mupirocin is recommended for localized nonbullous impetigo, although resistant bacterial strains occur (SOR: A).
- Oral antibiotic therapy with agents active against *S. pyogenes* and *S. aureus* may be required for nonbullous impetigo presenting with multiple lesions and for patients who fail topical therapy (SOR: A).

Folliculitis, Furuncles, Carbuncles, and Skin Abscesses

Folliculitis (pyoderma involving the hair follicles and apocrine glands) affects nearly everyone at one time or another and is usually self-limited. Occasionally, it progresses to larger lesions (furuncles and carbuncles). The characteristic "unit lesion" is a 2- to 5-mm erythematous papule that often contains a small pustule at its apex. The lesions are typically multiple and often pruritic. When over the bearded area of the face, the condition is known as *sycosis barbae*. Most cases in outpatients are caused by *S. aureus*. *P. aeruginosa* causes widespread folliculitis in patients exposed to contaminated hot tubs, whirlpools, swimming pools, or wet suits. Other gram-negative bacilli sometimes cause folliculitis in patients who have received prolonged courses of antibiotics for acne or rosacea. *Candida albicans* and *Malassezia furfur* cause folliculitis in patients who are immunocompromised, who have diabetes mellitus, or who have received antibiotic or steroid therapy.

Variants of folliculitis include (1) *eosinophilic folliculitis* ("itchy folliculitis"), which occurs mainly in HIV-infected patients, especially over the trunk but also over the face; (2) *pseudofolliculitis barbae* ("razor bumps" or "ingrown hairs"), a papular or pustular inflammatory reaction affecting persons with curly hair (especially African American men) who shave; (3) "*steroid acne*," a folliculitis resulting from systemic or topical corticosteroid therapy, sometimes caused by *Pityrosporum ovale*; (4) *viral folliculitis*, most commonly associated with herpesvirus infection in immunocompromised persons; and (5) *papular drug eruptions* ("acneiform dermatoses").

Furuncles ("boils") are thought to arise from folliculitis. "Furunculosis" refers to multiple or recurrent furuncles. These lesions are 1 to 2 cm in diameter (or about the size of a marble) and are nearly always caused by *S. aureus*. The time-honored treatment consists of warm, wet compresses to promote "coming to a head" with spontaneous drainage. Patients should be advised not to apply pressure or squeeze lesions because of the risk of bacteremia. Frequent recurrences (furunculosis) are usually frustrating to manage; many methods have been tried, but none is uniformly effective. Scrupulous hygiene and frequent bathing are often combined with an attempt to suppress *S. aureus* nasal carriage because many (perhaps most) patients are carriers. Limited experience suggests that a strategy of repeating a 5-day course of 2% mupirocin nasal ointment every month may be cost effective. Individualized treatment is recommended; a flowchart for patients might include separate columns for date; results of cultures, including nasal cultures; topical and systemic antibiotic therapy administered; and new furuncles with their locations and treatment.

Carbuncles are deeper, complex lesions, typically located over the nape of the neck, the back, or the thighs. Some patients with carbuncles meet the criteria for the sepsis syndrome.

Skin abscesses differ from furuncles and carbuncles in that they are deeper and do not necessarily arise in hair follicles. They are usually caused by *S. aureus*, and in recent years community-acquired MRSA (CA-MRSA) has become an extremely important etiology. Patients often give a spurious history of "spider bite" that evolved into an angry-looking furuncle or skin abscess with surrounding erythema. Incision and drainage may be necessary for large fluctuant lesions, and primary care physicians are well advised to learn newer approaches to drainage (Singer and Talan, 2014). IDSA guidelines published in 2011 suggest that adjunctive antibiotic therapy is unnecessary for patients without complicating factors (see later discussion). There is now broad consensus that antibiotics are overused for uncomplicated skin infections, including abscesses. Randomized placebo-controlled trials of TMP-SMX for skin abscesses in children and adults showed no significant benefit over drainage alone, although patients receiving antibiotic were slightly less likely to develop new lesions (Singer and Talan, 2014). However, many clinicians prefer to prescribe an adjunctive antibiotic, most commonly TMP-SMX, because alternatives such as linezolid are usually prohibitively expensive. Results of a recent study suggested that about half of antibiotic prescriptions for uncomplicated skin infections were avoidable—that is, complicating factors as listed were absent (Hurley et al., 2013).

- Most patients (≈90%) with fluctuant skin abscesses respond to drainage, and antibiotic therapy does not significantly improve the outcome (SOR: A).
- Indications for antibiotic therapy in patients with skin abscesses include involvement of an area that is difficult to drain (e.g., the face, the hands, or the genitalia), multiple foci of infection, rapid progression with associated cellulitis, diabetes mellitus, HIV infection, serious coexisting diseases or immunosuppressive therapy, temperature above 38.0 °C (100.4 °F), and extremes of age (younger than 3 years or older than 75 years).
- When antibiotics are indicated for patients with skin abscesses, drugs of choice include TMP-SMX, tetracycline, and clindamycin—with the caveat that up to 50% of CA-MRSA strains are resistant to clindamycin, and inducible resistance occurs.

Erysipelas and Cellulitis

"Cellulitis," a clinical diagnosis, denotes a spreading infection in the subcutaneous tissue. *Erysipelas* is a rapidly progressive superficial form of cellulitis usually caused by *S. pyogenes* (group A streptococci). The involved skin is usually a bright, fiery red and sharply demarcated from uninvolved skin (Figure 15-6). Erysipelas most commonly occurs on the lower extremities, often with bright red "lymphangitic

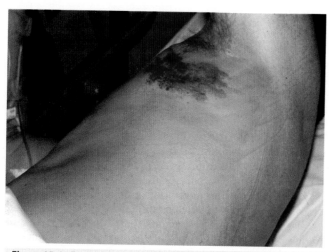

Figure 15-6. Erysipelas (superficial cellulitis) of the chest and abdominal walls caused by *Streptococcus pyogenes*. Note the primary lesion below the axilla and the sharp demarcation between normal and inflamed skin.

streaks" leading toward tender regional lymph nodes. *Cellulitis other than erysipelas* is commonly caused by *S. pyogenes*, *S. aureus*, or both. The line of demarcation between involved and uninvolved skin is blurred, in contrast to erysipelas, and lymphangitic streaks are seldom present. Abscess formation or extension into fat or fascial layers may occur. The history and the patient's demographics may suggest an alternative etiology, such as *Aeromonas hydrophila* when wounds have been exposed to fresh water; *V. vulnificus* when wounds have been exposed to saltwater or brackish water; *H. influenzae* in children; miscellaneous aerobic gram-negative bacilli in immunocompromised patients and patients with diabetes mellitus; non–group A β-hemolytic streptococci in frail elderly persons; *S. pneumoniae* in immunocompromised patients and persons with alcoholism; *Cryptococcus neoformans* in patients taking immunosuppressive medication; *Erysipelothrix rhusiopathiae* when abrasions have been exposed to freshwater fish, shellfish, meat, hides, or poultry; and *S. iniae* from similar exposure to raw fish, notably tilapia.

Imaging studies such as MRI may be advisable when clinical findings raise the possibility of necrotizing fasciitis, as discussed earlier. Blood cultures should be obtained when severe systemic toxicity is present; however, the yield is low. Aspiration of the lesion for culture may be helpful (up to 30% yield) in immunocompromised persons; the technique is to inject a small amount of sterile saline *without preservative* into unbroken skin and then pull back on the syringe and inoculate a blood culture bottle.

Recurrent Cellulitis

Approximately 17% of patients with lower extremity cellulitis develop recurrence within 2 years. Risk factors for recurrence include tibial lesions, dermatitis, large body size, chronic peripheral edema, malignancy, and dermatitis. Treatment of predisposing conditions such as dermatitis, support stockings, skin hygiene, and decolonization in patients with MRSA may be beneficial.

Diabetic Foot Ulcer Infections

Diabetic foot infections are distressingly common and often lead to amputation. Evaluation should be at three levels: the patient as a whole (including glucose control), the affected limb (whether sensory polyneuropathy and peripheral vascular disease are present), and the wound itself. Evaluation of the wound includes (1) determining whether the wound is infected, defined by purulence or by at least two of the classic signs of inflammation (erythema, warmth, tenderness, pain, and swelling or induration); (2) whether infection, if present, is superficial or deep; and (3) whether osteomyelitis is present. Recurrent or deepening foot ulcers suggest bone involvement, as does a positive "probe-to-bone test" (i.e., passing a sterile stainless-steel instrument to the depth of the wound produces a "click" on striking bone), but MRI is the most sensitive way to establish or exclude osteomyelitis short of bone biopsy. Patients with severe infections should be hospitalized, as should patients with moderately severe infections with complicating factors such as poor home support.

Bite Wound Infections

Animal bites prompt about 1% of emergency department visits in the United States, are most commonly inflicted by dogs (80%), and occur most often on the distal extremities, but may also be on the head or neck of children. *Pasteurella multocida* is the most frequent isolate, but cultures reveal on average about five species of aerobic and anaerobic bacteria. Dog bites necessitate evaluation for rabies transmission. Human bites, which include clenched-fist injuries ("fight bites"), are likely to involve not only anaerobic bacteria and streptococci but also *Eikenella corrodens*, a gram-negative bacillus usually resistant to first-generation cephalosporins and macrolides.

KEY TREATMENT

- For non–penicillin-allergic patients with animal bite wounds, treatment should consist of orally administered ampicillin–clavulanate or intravenously administered ampicillin–sulbactam, depending on the severity (SOR: B).
- Human bite wounds should be treated with intravenous ampicillin–sulbactam or cefoxitin (SOR: B).
- Prophylactic antibiotic therapy after human bites reduces the incidence of infection (SOR: C).
- Prophylactic antibiotic therapy after bites (of any kind) of the hand reduces the incidence of infection (SOR: B), and a hand surgeon should be consulted if the tendons or bones of the hands are likely to be involved (SOR: A).
- Patients should be given tetanus immunization if necessary (SOR: A) and postexposure prophylaxis against HIV if indicated (SOR: B).

UPPER RESPIRATORY INFECTIONS

Upper respiratory infections (URIs) comprise at least half of all symptomatic illness in a community and exact tolls measurable as morbidity, absenteeism from school and work, direct health care costs, and overuse of antibiotics. Most URIs are self-limited, but progression to life-threatening illness occurs, and progression to chronic disease is common.

The Common Cold (Acute Viral Rhinosinusitis)

The common cold is an acute-self-limited catarrhal syndrome limited to the mucosal membranes of the upper respiratory tract and responsible for about three fourths of all illnesses in young infants and up to half of illnesses in adults. About half of cases are caused by rhinoviruses; about 10% by coronaviruses; and the rest by other viruses, including respiratory syncytial virus (RSV), adenoviruses, and influenza and parainfluenza viruses. Rhinoviruses remain viable on skin or objects for at least 2 hours and are transmitted most efficiently by direct contact.

The common cold is a clinical diagnosis based largely on symptoms: a sore or scratchy throat at onset, nasal congestion or obstruction (CT scan shows abnormalities of the paranasal sinuses in up to 87% of cases, hence the alternative term "viral rhinosinusitis"), and cough ("chest cold") in about 30% of cases beginning the fourth and fifth days. In young children, alternative diagnoses include foreign body and *streptococcal nasopharyngitis. Allergic rhinitis* differs from the common cold by seasonal occurrence, itchy eyes, and more than 20% eosinophilia in nasal secretions. *Persistent, low-grade bacterial sinusitis* is recognized by long duration of symptoms. High fever, chills, myalgias, signs of meningeal irritation, or proptosis should prompt consideration of another diagnosis.

Well-controlled trials are lacking for most agents purported to help. The published literature provides mild support for ipratropium bromide and zinc lozenges but little support for antihistamines, decongestants, antiinflammatory drugs, and herbal regimens, including *Echinacea*. Nearly all authorities agree that antibiotics should be discouraged. Preventive measures include hand hygiene, use of disposable tissues by persons with colds, avoidance of hand contact with patients or fomites, and the vitamins supplied in a normal diet. Decontamination of surfaces with phenol-alcohol (Lysol) reduces transmission.

The *severe acute respiratory syndrome* (SARS), which begins with symptoms suggesting the common cold but progresses to full-blown acute respiratory distress syndrome (ARDS) and is therefore life threatening, appeared in Southeast Asia in 2002 and was shown to be caused by a newly recognized coronavirus designated SARS-CoV. More recently, in 2012, a similar illness appeared on the Arabian Peninsula, has been designated the *Middle East respiratory syndrome* (MERS), and has been shown to be caused by a coronavirus designated MERS-CoV. These syndromes raise the disturbing possibility that coronaviruses could become major causes of mortality or even an agent of bioterrorism.

Sinusitis

See Chapter 18, Otorhinolaryngology.

Otitis Externa

Otitis externa, a spectrum of conditions caused by infection, allergy, or primary skin disease, affects up to 10% of all persons during their lifetimes. The spectrum includes:

1. *Acute localized otitis externa* beginning as one or more pustules or furuncles in the ear, usually caused by *S. aureus*, presenting as itching, pain, swelling, redness, and sometimes decreased hearing and with one or more small pustules or furuncles in the ear canal on physical examination.
2. *Acute diffuse otitis externa (swimmer's ear)* presenting as severe and even intolerable earache (otalgia), itching, discharge, and hearing loss, most commonly caused by *P. aeruginosa*, and with diffuse erythema and edema in the ear canal on examination.
3. *Erysipelas* involving the concha and ear canal, caused by group A streptococci (*S. pyogenes*), presenting with a diffusely red and painful ear and with hemorrhagic bullae sometimes seen on the walls of the ear canal.
4. *Chronic otitis externa*, presenting with mild discomfort and flaking of the skin of long duration, often with a history of frequent use of antibiotic-containing otic preparations.
5. *Eczematous otitis externa*, presenting with severe itching and with physical findings of scaling of the skin surface with crusting, oozing, and erythema, reflects involvement of the ear by skin disease such as

contact dermatitis, seborrheic dermatitis, and atopic dermatitis.

6. *Malignant otitis externa*, also called *invasive otitis externa*, usually affecting patients with diabetes mellitus and caused by *P. aeruginosa*. The clinical course is often deceptively subacute or chronic: (1) initial symptoms and signs suggest uncomplicated otitis externa; (2) multiple courses of ear drops prove unhelpful; (3) the epithelium of the ear canal becomes macerated with cellulitis, formation of polypoid granulation tissue, persistent pain, continued drainage from the ear (otorrhea), and hearing loss; and (4) brain involvement becomes manifest by meningitis or cranial nerve palsies (VII, IX, X, and XII). It is thought that the causative bacteria, having burrowed below the epithelium of the ear canal, slip through gaps between the ear cartilages (fissures of Santorini), gain access to the temporal bone (causing osteomyelitis), and then extend into the base of the brain. Appropriate management includes imaging (MRI with gadolinium enhancement), aggressive debridement of the ear canal by an otolaryngologist, and systemic antimicrobial therapy directed against *P. aeruginosa*.

Except for the latter syndrome, patients with otitis externa can usually be managed conservatively with local care and topical otic preparations (containing appropriate antimicrobial agents when indicated), but patients with severe disease or complete occlusion of the ear canal should be referred to an otolaryngologist.

Otitis Media and Mastoiditis

Acute otitis media is mainly but not exclusively a disease of childhood, is caused by various virulent bacteria, and is optimally diagnosed by demonstrating reduced mobility of the tympanic membrane by pneumatic otoscopy. Tympanocentesis is required for accurate microbiologic diagnosis and should be considered in newborn infants, when the illness is unusually severe, when the patient fails to respond to antibiotics, or when a suppurative complication is confirmed or suspected. Acute otitis media must be distinguished from *otitis media with effusion* (*serous otitis media*), which consists of an asymptomatic or hyposymptomatic middle ear effusion without fever or otalgia.

Chronic suppurative otitis media is a complication of acute otitis media, usually occurring when a defect is present in the tympanic membrane, such as a perforation or the presence of a tympanostomy tube. It is accompanied by purulent drainage (otorrhea). Mastoiditis is invariably present. The associated bacteria vary depending on whether an infected *cholesteatoma* is present; cholesteatomas typically contain anaerobic bacteria and may therefore impart a foul odor. When cholesteatoma is not present, gram-negative bacilli, including *P. aeruginosa* and *E. coli*, are often found.

Mastoiditis, which before the advent of antibiotics was often a dramatic illness with a high incidence of intracranial complications, usually presents today as an indolent, low-grade, and often painless infection of the temporal bone. Spontaneous resolution is rare if it occurs at all.

Complications of chronic suppurative otitis media and mastoiditis include bone destruction, subperiosteal abscess, facial paralysis, labyrinthitis, petrositis, and—more dangerously—brain abscess, subdural abscess, epidural abscess, and septic thrombosis of one or more venous sinuses.

Acute Pharyngitis: Group A Streptococcal Pharyngitis versus Viral Pharyngitis

Acute pharyngitis (sore throat) is one of the most common problems in clinical practice and, more often than not, of viral etiology. The usual clinical problem consists of recognizing and treating pharyngitis caused by group A streptococci (*S. pyogenes*), which accounts for about 15% to 30% of cases in children between the ages of 5 and 15 years and about 5% to 15% of cases in adults. Accurate diagnosis of streptococcal pharyngitis is desirable to prevent overuse of antibiotics; reduce the duration and severity of symptoms; reduce disease transmission; and, in children, prevent suppurative complications and acute rheumatic fever (a nonsuppurative complication). Through the years, numerous clinical criteria have been proposed for identifying patients likely to have group A streptococcal pharyngitis rather than viral pharyngitis, which is more common in all populations. In general:

1. In children younger than 3 years of age, symptoms are atypical and may be protracted. The term "streptococcosis" has been applied to the triad of prolonged nasal congestion and discharge, low-grade fever, and tender cervical lymphadenopathy. Children younger than 1 year of age may present with fussiness, decreased appetite, and low-grade fever.
2. In children older than 5 years of age, the following clinical features increase the likelihood of streptococcal pharyngitis to greater than 50% but do not suffice for accurate diagnosis: the presence of pharyngeal exudates, palatal petechiae, or a scarlatiniform rash; vomiting; and tender cervical lymphadenopathy. Various scoring systems have been devised, but none obviates the need for diagnostic testing.
3. In adults, a checklist known as the Centor system uses four criteria: fever, tonsillar exudates, tender cervical lymphadenopathy, and absence of a cough. It has been suggested that patients with two or fewer of these four criteria do not need diagnostic testing or antibiotics unless they are at high risk for severe infections (e.g., patients with poorly controlled diabetes mellitus, immunocompromised persons, and those receiving long-term steroid therapy).

Protocols for managing acute pharyngitis in family medicine should take into account the numerous potential etiologies beyond streptococcal pharyngitis and viral pharyngitis.

KEY TREATMENT

- Rapid antigen detection tests or throat cultures should be obtained in patients with suspected streptococcal pharyngitis (SOR: A).
- Patients with proven streptococcal pharyngitis should be treated with penicillin or ampicillin or, in the case of penicillin allergy, a first-generation cephalosporin (if not allergic) or macrolide antibiotic (SOR: A).

- Postponing therapy for 24 to 48 hours while awaiting the results of throat culture does not reduce the efficacy of treatment. Indeed, therapy has been shown to effectively prevent nonsuppurative sequelae, such as acute rheumatic fever, even if begun 9 days after the onset of symptoms (SOR: A).

Acute Pharyngitis: Exclusion of Dangerous Syndromes

The differential diagnosis of acute pharyngitis includes at least five medical emergencies:

1. *Acute epiglottitis (supraglottitis)*: This is a life-threatening cellulitis of the epiglottis and adjacent structures occurring mainly in children and usually but not always caused by *H. influenzae* type b. Children usually present with a sudden onset of fever, dysphonia, dysphagia, and difficulty breathing. The child often leans forward and drools. Children with suspected acute epiglottis should undergo emergency endotracheal intubation because airway obstruction carries an 80% mortality rate. Most authorities agree that no attempt should be made to confirm the diagnosis (by laryngoscopy or imaging) before securing an airway. Adults are more likely to present with severe sore throat, odynophagia, and sensation of airway obstruction.
2. *Peritonsillar abscess (quinsy)*: This diagnosis is suggested by medial displacement of a tonsil or bulging of the ipsilateral soft palate. Patients usually present with severe sore throat on the side of involvement, fever, and a "hot potato" or muffled voice. Trismus (spasm of the muscles of mastication on opening the mouth) occurs in about two thirds of patients. Swelling of the neck and ipsilateral ear pain are also common, as is pooling of saliva or drooling.
3. *Submandibular space infection (Ludwig's angina)*: This diagnosis is suggested by a tender, symmetric, "woody" induration in the submandibular area in a patient whose symptoms may include fever, chills, malaise, stiff neck, mouth pain, drooling, and dysphagia, and who may—as in children with acute epiglottitis—lean forward in an effort to increase the diameter of their airway.
4. *Retropharyngeal space infection*: This diagnosis often presents with a bulge in the posterior wall of the pharynx or swelling of the lateral aspect of the neck and is usually caused by mixed aerobic and anaerobic bacteria.
5. *Septic thrombosis of the internal jugular vein (Lemierre syndrome)*: This diagnosis is usually caused by *Fusobacterium* spp. (an anaerobic bacterium in the normal flora) and accompanied by fever, septic pulmonary emboli, and pleural effusions.

Acute Pharyngitis: Other Microbial Etiologies

Uncommon but serious causes of sore throat include the following:

1. *Diphtheria*: Diphtheria, which is now rare in the United States, classically presents as a sore throat with a gray, adherent pseudomembrane that is easily mistaken for an exudate. Classically, diphtheria has a slow onset and marked systemic toxicity.

2. *Anaerobic pharyngitis (Vincent's angina)*: This uncommon infection is caused by a mixture of anaerobic bacteria and spirochetes, with group A streptococci and *S. aureus* sometimes having a role. Patients present with purulent exudates, and the breath often has a foul odor. Complications include peritonsillar abscess and septic thrombosis of the internal jugular vein.
3. *Kawasaki disease*: Sore throat in young child with conjunctivitis, erythema of the lips, strawberry tongue, edema of the hands and feet, and rash raises this diagnostic possibility, which can involve the coronary arteries.
4. *Yersinia enterocolitica*: Exudative pharyngitis and tender cervical lymphadenopathy can be part of a fulminant febrile illness with a high mortality rate; other features include abdominal pain with or without diarrhea. Outbreaks have resulted from contaminated food or beverages.
5. *Primary HIV infection (acute retroviral syndrome)*: The symptoms may include sore throat in addition to fever, weight loss, lymphadenopathy, rash, and splenomegaly.
6. *N. gonorrhoeae*: Although seen mainly in sexually active adolescents, gonococcal pharyngitis can occur at any age. The pharynx may appear erythematous with exudates or may appear normal despite positive cultures.
7. *Tularemia*: The typhoidal form of tularemia, which results from inhalation of the organism, typically begins with fever and sore throat suggesting streptococcal pharyngitis.

Less serious causes of sore throat include:

1. *Infectious mononucleosis*: Mononucleosis caused by Epstein-Barr virus (EBV) can present with sore throat and prominent pharyngeal exudates mimicking streptococcal pharyngitis. Pharyngitis is usually milder in mononucleosis caused by CMV.
2. *Arcanobacterium hemolyticum*: Pharyngitis caused by this bacterium occurs mainly in adolescents. A scarlatiniform rash on the extensor surfaces of the upper extremities—which does not peel, unlike the rash of scarlet fever—occurs in about half of patients and is highly suggestive. The organism grows slowly on sheep agar blood plates and is resistant to penicillin; erythromycin is the drug of choice.
3. *HSV*: Pharyngitis occurs mainly in adolescents and is usually caused by HSV-1. Nearly half of patients have exudates. Vesicles and shallow ulcers on the palate, sometimes confluent, are suggestive, but only a minority of patients have "fever blisters" on their lips.
4. *Influenza*: Sore throat is sometimes the chief complaint, but other symptoms such as myalgia, headache, cough, and severe fatigue soon predominate.
5. *Non–group-A β-hemolytic streptococci*: Groups C and G streptococci can cause pharyngitis clinically indistinguishable from that caused by *S. pyogenes*, sometimes in outbreaks from a common food source. Some researchers report frequent pharyngitis caused by group C streptococci among college-aged students.
6. Miscellaneous causes: These include *Mycoplasma pneumoniae*, *Chlamydophila pneumoniae* (previously known as *Chlamydia pneumoniae*), *Treponema pallidum* (syphilis), and numerous viruses.

LOWER RESPIRATORY INFECTIONS

Lower respiratory tract infections are common in family medicine; are responsible for much of the overuse of antibiotics; and remain common causes of death, especially among elderly individuals.

Acute Bronchitis ("Chest Cold") and Tracheobronchial Infections without Pneumonia

Acute bronchitis ("chest cold") is extremely common, usually of viral etiology, and results in overuse of antibiotics. The term "acute infectious bronchitis" is sometimes used to distinguish this entity from other causes of cough, and the term "tracheobronchitis" is sometimes used for accuracy because the trachea is also inflamed. The incidence of acute bronchitis is highest in children younger than 5 years of age, with another peak among elderly adults. The disease is seasonal and most common in midwinter.

Most cases (95% by some estimates) are caused by viruses. All of the common viruses affecting the upper respiratory tract have been implicated. *M. pneumoniae* and *C. pneumoniae* may cause protracted cases of bronchitis. *Bordetella pertussis*, the agent of whooping cough, has become an important cause of acute bronchitis in adults with cough lasting more than 3 weeks.

The onset is typically preceded by a prodrome of at least 24 hours with symptoms of common cold and pharyngitis. A dry cough signifying inflammation of the early airway evolves into a cough productive of moderate amounts of mucopurulent sputum. Fever, headache, myalgias, and retrosternal chest pain or discomfort may be present. Physical examination often reveals tracheal tenderness, and auscultation of the lung may reveal a few coarse crackles and occasional wheezes. The patient rarely appears toxic.

More than 90% of patients with cough lasting longer than 3 weeks have the postnasal drip syndrome, asthma, gastroesophageal reflux, or drug-induced cough (of which angiotensin-converting enzyme [ACE] inhibitors are now the most common cause). Isolation of *B. pertussis* requires special media and 5 to 7 days of incubation. The organism can be identified more rapidly by a direct fluorescein-labeled antibody method.

Acute bronchitis provides an excellent opportunity to counsel patients about smoking.

KEY TREATMENT

- Numerous trials indicate that antibiotics confer only modest benefit for acute bronchitis and should be reserved for patients at high risk of complications, including elderly adults, those with chronic lung disease, and those with compromised host defenses (SOR: A).
- Patients with prolonged bronchitis caused by *M. pneumoniae* and *C. pneumoniae* may respond to therapy with a tetracycline or macrolide antibiotic (SOR: B). More than one course of antimicrobial therapy may be required for bronchitis caused by *C. pneumonia*, which can cause a stubborn respiratory illness (SOR: B).

- Pertussis should be treated with macrolide antibiotics (erythromycin, azithromycin, or clarithromycin) (SOR: A).
- Adults should strongly consider making the acellular pertussis vaccine (contained in the TDaP vaccine) part of their routine immunizations.

Acute Exacerbations of Chronic Bronchitis

The American Thoracic Society (ATS) defines chronic bronchitis—which is caused mainly by cigarette smoking—as excessive sputum production with cough, present on most days for at least 3 months a year and for at least 2 successive years and without an underlying disorder such as TB or bronchiectasis. This common disorder affects up to 25% of the adult population and can progress to full-blown chronic obstructive pulmonary disease. The extent to which acute exacerbations of chronic bronchitis are caused by treatable infections remains controversial. Current opinion holds that most exacerbations of chronic bronchitis are caused by viruses or noninfectious agents, even though cultures of sputum often show nontypeable strains of *H. influenzae*, *S. pneumoniae*, *M. catarrhalis*, or other bacteria. Still, evidence suggests that recurrent bacterial infections in patients with chronic bronchitis contribute to deterioration of pulmonary function. Short (5 to 7 days) courses of antibiotics, although controversial and usually effecting only modest improvement in airflow, are usually given to patients with markedly impaired baseline pulmonary function because of the serious consequences of respiratory failure.

KEY TREATMENT

- Patients with acute exacerbations of chronic obstructive lung disease and who present with increasing shortness of breath and purulent sputum should be treated with antibiotics (SOR: A).
- Amoxicillin–clavulanate or fluoroquinolones (other than ciprofloxacin) are now preferred by some authorities over older drugs such as doxycycline, TMP-SMX, and amoxicillin for acute exacerbations of chronic obstructive lung disease (SOR: B)
- The practice of giving prophylactic antibiotics through the winter months is not supported by solid evidence and should be discouraged (SOR: B).
- Patients with chronic obstructive lung disease should receive the pneumococcal vaccine and yearly immunization against influenza (SOR: A).

Bronchiectasis

Bronchiectasis is an acquired disorder characterized anatomically by abnormal dilatation of bronchi and bronchioles and clinically by chronic productive cough and frequent lower respiratory infections. Its prevalence fell dramatically after the introduction of broad-spectrum antibiotics and vaccines against measles and pertussis. Specific causes include (1) *necrotizing pneumonia* in which treatment has been delayed; (2) *cystic fibrosis*, often as the presenting manifestation; (3) *allergic bronchopulmonary aspergillosis* in which the diagnosis has been delayed; (4) *immunodeficiency syndromes*; (5) the *dyskinetic cilia syndromes*; and (6) possibly

Helicobacter pylori infection. *M. avium–intracellulare* complex (MAC) infection is not infrequently associated with bronchiectasis in women (see later discussion under Mycobacterial Infections).

Patients with advanced bronchiectasis have daily cough productive of large amounts of thick, mucopurulent, tenacious sputum. However, most patients produce lesser amounts of sputum, at least during the early stages, and cough may be nonproductive ("dry bronchiectasis") or even absent. Dyspnea and hemoptysis are common.

Ultrasensitive, high-resolution CT scanning, now the imaging procedure of choice, demonstrates bronchial wall thickening and luminal dilatation. Workup includes a CBC and differential, quantitative immunoglobulin levels (IgA, IgG, and IgM), sputum Gram stain and culture for routine pathogens, and sputum culture for mycobacteria (AFB culture) and fungi. Screening tests for allergic bronchopulmonary aspergillosis include differential blood count (looking for eosinophilia), IgE level, and testing for precipitating antibodies to *Aspergillus* spp. Cystic fibrosis should be suspected when bronchiectasis begins in childhood, adolescence, or young adulthood.

There is no curative treatment other than resection of the involved portion of the lung. High-dose antibiotic therapy should be prescribed for episodes of fever associated with increased sputum production.

Bronchiolitis ("Wheezy Bronchitis" or "Asthmatic Bronchitis")

Bronchiolitis is a common disease of early childhood characterized by wheezing and nearly always caused by a virus, most typically RSV. The diagnosis is based on clinical findings and a self-limited course, with improvement beginning between the third and seventh days of the illness. Antibiotics are not indicated except for the rare patient with bacterial superinfection, but patients should be observed closely until improvement occurs. Some evidence suggests that the combined use of glucocorticoids and nebulized epinephrine may reduce the need for hospitalization, but the data should be interpreted cautiously (Fernandes and Hartling, 2014).

Acute Community-Acquired Pneumonia

Pneumonia remains a leading cause of death and the most common infectious cause of death in developed countries. Data suggesting a 28-fold increased cost for managing the disease on an inpatient basis prompted a renewed effort to identify patients who can be safely managed on an outpatient basis (Wunderink and Waterer, 2014). Unfortunately, it is difficult to make a precise etiologic diagnosis of pneumonia, especially at the first clinical encounter. In the past, many physicians placed much emphasis on examination of a carefully obtained Gram stain of sputum. In recent decades, more emphasis has been placed on grading the severity of the disease and treating accordingly.

Attack rates are highest at the extremes of life: younger than 4 years and older than 65 years of age. The incidence peaks during the winter months.

The distinction between "classical bacterial pneumonia" (lobar pneumonia typically caused by *S. pneumoniae*) and "atypical pneumonia" (classically caused by *M. pneumoniae*) has become blurred but remains conceptually useful. Classic bacterial pneumonia primarily involves inflammation of the alveoli, resulting in purulent sputum, elevated WBC count (or, in some patients, low or normal WBC count with excess band neutrophils on differential count), and peripherally located pleuritic chest pain. Atypical pneumonia primarily involves inflammation of the tracheobronchial mucosa and the interstitium of the lungs, resulting in nonpurulent (and scanty) sputum, normal WBC count, and centrally located, substernal chest pain. Classic pneumococcal pneumonia usually begins abruptly, but the onset is more likely to be gradual in atypical pneumonia (Table 15-4).

The diagnosis of acute pneumonia is usually based on the history, physical findings, and chest radiographic examination. Acute pneumonia is distinguished from chronic pneumonia (see later discussion) on the basis of the history. Three essential questions are:

1. Is the problem pneumonia or something else? The following should be considered: pulmonary thromboembolism (arguably the most common cause of "atypical pneumonia"), congestive heart failure with an associated viral URI or "viral syndrome," hypersensitivity pneumonitis caused by drugs or thermophilic actinomycetes, bronchiolitis obliterans organizing pneumonia (also known as cryptogenic organizing pneumonia), idiopathic acute eosinophilic pneumonia (characterized by a high fever, bilateral pulmonary infiltrates, and respiratory failure. Peripheral blood eosinophilia is usually absent, in contrast to chronic eosinophilic pneumonia [Carrington's syndrome]), foreign body aspiration, connective tissue diseases, pulmonary alveolar proteinosis, allergic bronchopulmonary aspergillosis, tumors (especially choriocarcinoma), pulmonary hemorrhage (as in Goodpasture's syndrome and mitral stenosis), and inhalation of freebase cocaine ("crack lung syndrome" characterized by fever, hypoxemia, hemoptysis, respiratory failure, and diffuse alveolar infiltrates).

2. How severe is the pneumonia and is hospitalization required? Guidelines for making these determinations continue to evolve. A Pneumonia Severity Index (PSI), which includes 20 variables and requires the use of a decision support tool, stratifies patients into five groups. The CURB-65 system offers a more practical way to grade severity of pneumonia, using five prognostic variables: confusion (based on a specific mental status test or disorientation to time, place, and person), urea (blood urea nitrogen >20 mg/dL), respiratory rate (>30 breaths/min), blood pressure (systolic pressure <90 mm Hg or diastolic pressure <60 mm Hg), and age >65 years. One point is given for each variable; patients with a score of 2 should be admitted to the hospital, and patients with a score of 3 or greater should be considered for admission to the intensive care unit. These criteria should not replace clinical judgment, which should take into account the patient's ability to maintain oral intake, knowledge of the patient's comorbidities, living situation, proclivity toward substance abuse, ability to comply with a drug regimen, and cognitive impairment. Pulse oximetry to assess the adequacy of oxygenation should ideally be performed in patients selected for outpatient management.

3. What is the most likely causative organism? Although the current style of practice in the United States places less emphasis on predicting the causative organism

than was formerly the case—with the admonition that blood cultures should be obtained before treatment for patients who require hospitalization (SOR: A) and a hospital quality indicator—clinicians should be familiar with the spectrum of etiologies (Tables 15-4 to 15-6).

Pneumococcal pneumonia continues to be the most common proven cause of severe community-acquired pneumonia, accounting for about two thirds of cases of pneumonia with positive blood cultures. Viral URI predisposes. Risk factors for invasive pneumococcal disease

Table 15-4   Clues to the Etiology of Pneumonia from the History

History	Suggested Etiologies
Sudden onset	Acute bacterial pneumonia, most often caused by *Streptococcus pneumonia*
Gradual onset	"Atypical" pneumonia, often caused by *Mycoplasma pneumoniae* or *Chlamydophila pneumoniae*
Respiratory illness in the family	*Mycoplasma pneumoniae*, RSV, influenza
Recent exposure to small children	*Mycoplasma pneumonia*, RSV
Chronic bronchitis or chronic obstructive lung disease	*S. pneumoniae. Haemophilus influenzae. Moraxella catarrhalis. Chlamydophila pneumoniae. Pseudomonas aeruginosa*
Nursing home resident or recent hospitalization	*S. pneumoniae, H. influenzae*, aerobic gram-negative bacilli, RSV
Alcoholism	*S. pneumoniae*, aerobic gram-negative bacilli (notably *Klebsiella pneumoniae*), mixed anaerobic and aerobic bacteria ("mouth flora"), *Mycobacterium tuberculosis*
Altered mental status, seizures, alcoholism, recent dental manipulation	"Mouth flora aspiration pneumonia" (mixed anaerobic and aerobic bacteria), *S. pneumoniae*
Homelessness or incarceration	*S. pneumoniae; M. tuberculosis*
Injection drug use	*Staphylococcus aureus* (consider septic pulmonary emboli from right-sided endocarditis), *S. pneumoniae*
Home use of small-volume nebulizers	*Pseudomonas aeruginosa*; other aerobic gram-negative bacilli
Recent influenza A or B	*S. pneumoniae, S. aureus*, group A streptococci (*S. pyogenes*)
Diabetic ketoacidosis	*S. pneumoniae, S. aureus*
Exposure to contaminated aerosols (showers, air coolers, water supplies), hotel or cruise ship stay in previous 2 weeks	*Legionella pneumophila* (legionnaire's disease)
Cystic fibrosis	*P. aeruginosa, S. aureus, Burkholderia cepacia*
B-lymphocyte disorder (agammaglobulinemia, multiple myeloma, chronic lymphocytic leukemia)	*S. pneumoniae*
Sickle cell anemia	*S. pneumoniae*
Exposure to birds (parakeets, cockatoos, budgerigars)	*Chlamydia psittaci* (psittacosis)
Exposure to cows, sheep, goats, or parturient cats	*Coxiella burnetii* (Q fever)
Exposure to tissues or body fluids of rabbits, foxes, or squirrels	*Francisella tularensis* (tularemia)
Exposure to raw wool, goat hair, animal hides, cattle, pigs, or horses	*Bacillus anthracis* (anthrax)
Exposure to ground squirrels, rats, chipmunks, or prairie dogs	*Yersinia pestis* (plague)
Exposure to rodent droppings, urine, or saliva; exploration in the "four corners" area of the southwestern United States	Hantavirus pulmonary syndrome
Exposure to water contaminated with animal urine or to wild rodents, dogs, cattle, pigs, or horses	*Leptospira* spp. (leptospirosis)
Military recruit	*Neisseria meningitidis*, adenovirus type 4 or 7
Travel to the southwestern United States or southern California, especially if exposed to a windstorm	*Coccidioides immitis* (coccidioidomycosis)
Travel to Ohio or Mississippi river valleys; exposure to bat droppings or to dust from soil enriched by bird droppings; exploration of a cave	*Histoplasma capsulatum* (histoplasmosis)
Travel to Southwest Asia, West Indies, Australia, Guam, or South or Central America	*Burkholderia pseudomallei* (melioidosis)
Weight loss	*M. tuberculosis*, postobstruction pneumonia behind endobronchial carcinoma
Pulmonary alveolar proteinosis	*Nocardia* spp. (nocardiosis)
HIV disease (early)	*S. pneumoniae, H. influenzae, M. tuberculosis*
HIV disease (late, with CD4 lymphocyte count <200/mm^3)	As above plus *Pneumocystis jiroveci, Cryptococcus neoformans, Histoplasma capsulatum, Aspergillus* spp., *Pseudomonas aeruginosa*, and nontuberculous mycobacteria (especially *Mycobacterium kansasii*)
Associated acute arthritis	Drug reaction or connective tissue disease
Suspicion of bioterrorism	*Bacillus anthracis* (anthrax), *Yersinia pestis* (plague), *Francisella tularensis* (tularemia)

RSV, Respiratory syncytial virus.

Table 15-5   Clues to the Etiology of Pneumonia from the Physical Examination

Finding	Suggested Etiologies
Relative bradycardia	Viral infection, tularemia, *Mycoplasma pneumoniae*, legionnaire's disease, psittacosis
Altered mental status	Associated meningitis, TB, fungal disease, legionnaire's disease, endocarditis
Prominence of symptoms "outside the chest," such as headache and diarrhea	Legionnaire's disease
Poor oral hygiene with foul odor to the breath	"Mouth flora" aspiration pneumonia (mixed aerobic and anaerobic bacteria)
Bullous myringitis	*M. pneumonia*
Skin lesions	Atypical measles, varicella-zoster, fungal pneumonia, nocardiosis, staphylococcal pneumonia with bacteremia
Erythema multiforme	*M. pneumoniae*
Erythema nodosum	Histoplasmosis, coccidioidomycosis, TB
Ecthyma gangrenosum	*Pseudomonas aeruginosa, S. aureus*
Relatively clear lung fields to auscultation despite impressive infiltrates by imaging	*M. pneumoniae, Chlamydophila pneumoniae*
Splenomegaly	Psittacosis, typhoid fever, brucellosis, endocarditis

TB, Tuberculosis.

Table 15-6   Clues to the Etiology of Pneumonia and Their Implications from Chest Radiography or Computed Tomography

Finding	Suggested Causes and Implications
Lobar consolidation	*Streptococcus pneumoniae*; less commonly, gram-negative bacilli
Multilobar consolidation	Hospitalization should be strongly considered
Bilateral lower lobe involvement	Consider thromboembolism, including septic embolism, chronic aspiration pneumonia, *Mycoplasma pneumoniae* pneumonia
Patchy bilateral infiltrates	Right-sided endocarditis, septic embolism, "atypical pneumonia" (especially tularemia)
Radiography or CT scan much more impressive than physical examination would suggest	Atypical pneumonia (especially *M. pneumoniae* pneumonia); pulmonary embolism
Volume loss	TB, carcinoma
Miliary pattern	TB, histoplasmosis, coccidioidomycosis, bacterial sepsis
Pulmonary nodules	Fungal infection (especially cryptococcosis), septic pulmonary embolism, *Legionella micdadei* pneumonia
Cavitary lesions	Aspiration pneumonia, gram-negative bacillary pneumonia, TB, cavitary carcinoma
Massive pleural effusion	*Streptococcus pyogenes* (group A streptococcus)
Hilar lymphadenopathy	TB, pertussis, tularemia, pneumonic plague, carcinoma
Clear chest radiograph despite strong suspicion of pneumonia	Experimental studies and anecdotal reports support the idea that occasional patients with pneumonia have normal chest radiographs because of dehydration; infiltrates "blossom" after administration of IV fluids

CT, Computed tomography; *IV*, intravenous; *TB*, tuberculosis.

include extremes of age, alcoholism, HIV disease, end-stage renal disease, sickle cell disease, diabetes mellitus, dementia, malnutrition, malignancy, diseases affecting B lymphocyte function, and immunosuppressive disorders. Risk factors for pneumococci with reduced susceptibility to penicillin G (defined by minimum inhibitory concentration >2 μg/mL for nonmeningeal isolates) include extremes of age (2 years or younger or 70 years or older), prolonged hospitalization, recent β-lactam antibiotic therapy, attendance at a day care center (either as a child or staff person), residence in a nursing home, or chronic disease (e.g., cirrhosis or chronic lung disease).

H. influenzae is a frequent cause of pneumonia in elderly patients and in patients with serious underlying diseases, including chronic obstructive lung disease. The pneumonia usually has a patchy or segmental distribution, which is characteristic of bronchopneumonia rather than lobar pneumonia.

S. aureus pneumonia, when community acquired, tends to be an acute, fulminant pneumonia. *S. aureus* is an uncommon cause of community-acquired pneumonia, explaining only about 1% of cases, except during influenza epidemics. Influenza virus markedly predisposes to staphylococcal colonization of the respiratory mucosa. Staphylococcal pneumonia tends to be a necrotizing process with abscess formation. In children, chest radiography may show air pockets known as pneumatoceles.

Group A streptococcal (*S. pyogenes*) pneumonia, which is rare except during influenza epidemics, often features the rapid development of a large empyema requiring chest tube drainage.

Klebsiella pneumoniae pneumonia is a relatively common cause of pneumonia in patients with alcoholism and often assumes a lobar pattern especially of the upper lobes. *E. coli* and other aerobic gram-negative bacilli are relatively common causes of pneumonia in the frail elderly.

P. aeruginosa, although a common cause of nosocomial pneumonia, is rarely associated with community-acquired pneumonia in patients without underlying lung disease or severe debility.

Pneumonia caused by "mouth flora" bacteria (mixtures of aerobic and anaerobic bacteria with anaerobes usually predominating) occurs most frequently in patients with alcoholism or poor oral hygiene. "Mouth flora" pneumonia in an edentulous patient should prompt suspicion of endobronchial obstruction caused by lung cancer. A foul odor of the breath is present in many but not all affected patients. Lung abscess or empyema is common.

M. pneumoniae is a cell wall–deficient organism with particular affinity for respiratory epithelium. Patients with *M. pneumoniae* pneumonia may have a second pulmonary pathogen. This disease mainly affects adolescents and younger adults and most commonly involves the lower lobes, sometimes with pleural effusions. Bullous myringitis (erythema of the tympanic membrane with a "bleb") occurs in fewer than 5% of patients but has a high positive predictive value for *M. pneumoniae* pneumonia. The chest radiography commonly shows infiltrates that are more extensive than physical examination would suggest. Extrapulmonary manifestations, which can dominate the clinical course, include hemolytic anemia, rashes (including the Stevens-Johnson syndrome), CNS complications (ranging in severity from aseptic meningitis to transverse myelitis), cardiac complications (including myocarditis), and polyarthralgia. Diagnosis is most commonly made by measuring IgM and IgG antibodies to *M. pneumoniae*.

Pneumonia caused by *C. pneumoniae*, in contrast to *M. pneumoniae* pneumonia, predominantly affects older persons. Younger persons infected with *C. pneumoniae* are more likely to manifest pharyngitis than pneumonia. Symptomatic *C. pneumoniae* pneumonia is usually, but not always, a relatively mild illness, but recovery is typically slow.

Legionnaire's disease is a relatively common cause of pneumonia in some geographic areas. Clinically severe cases tend to occur in persons with compromised host defenses, often in the setting of chronic obstructive lung diseases, immunosuppression, or advanced age. The urine antigen test for *L. pneumophila* serogroup 1 has a sensitivity of about 80% and a specificity approaching 100%; this serogroup accounts for about 80% of cases of legionnaire's disease.

Psittacosis (ornithosis) caused by *Chlamydia psittaci* is a rare cause of pneumonia (most commonly, with consolidation of a lower lobe) in the United States; other presentations of psittacosis include a typhoidal illness with fever, malaise, relative bradycardia, and hepatosplenomegaly; a mononucleosis-like syndrome with fever, sore throat, lymphadenopathy, and hepatosplenomegaly; fever of unknown origin (FUO); and a nonspecific flulike illness. Diagnosis is based on serology. Doxycycline is the drug of choice.

Macrolides are now recommended for previously healthy persons with community-acquired pneumonia who do not have risk factors for penicillin-resistant pneumococci and do not have indications for hospitalization except in regions with high rates (>25%) of macrolide-resistant *S. pneumoniae* (SOR: A). When patients have comorbidities or have received antimicrobials within the previous 3 months, alternatives include fluoroquinolones *other than ciprofloxacin* (SOR: A) or third-generation cephalosporins combined with either a macrolide or doxycycline (SOR: B).

For patients with comorbidities and who require hospitalization, reference should be made to protocols for antibiotic selection now in place at most, if not all, U.S. hospitals. For patients not requiring admission to an intensive care unit, combined therapy with a β-lactam agent (e.g., ceftriaxone) plus either a macrolide or doxycycline is often prescribed (SOR: A), with fluoroquinolones being recommended for penicillin-allergic patients.

Health Care–Associated Pneumonia

In 2005, the ATS and IDSA designated "health care–associated pneumonia" as a third category of pneumonia based on patient population—that is, a category in addition to the previous categories of "community-acquired pneumonia" and "hospital-acquired pneumonia." The definition of health care–associated pneumonia includes residing in an extended-care facility for 2 days or more during the preceding 90 days, receiving home infusion therapy or wound care as an outpatient, and attending a hemodialysis center during the preceding 30 days. This entity has become somewhat controversial. A recent analysis of 24 studies confirmed that patients with health care–associated pneumonia, compared with patients with "community-acquired pneumonia" without the listed risk factors, were more likely to have pneumonia caused by MRSA or aerobic gram-negative bacilli, including *P. aeruginosa* (Chalmers et al., 2014).

INFLUENZA

Influenza causes about 36,000 deaths in the United States each year, or about the same number as caused by traffic accidents. Influenza viruses infecting humans are classified as A, B, and C (rare), with influenza A viruses being classified further on the basis of changes in the antigenic characteristics of envelope glycoproteins known as hemagglutinin (H) and neuraminidase (N) antigens. The RNA genome of influenza A viruses is constantly undergoing rearrangement. *Antigenic shifts* denote major changes in the viral genome and often precede endemics and pandemics. *Antigenic drift* reflects minor changes associated with more localized outbreaks. The influenza B virus is less inclined to mutate; antigenic drifts in its H antigen occur, but antigenic shifts have not been reported.

The names assigned to influenza viruses disclose their identities. Consider, for example, the viruses represented in the 2013 to 2014 quadrivalent vaccine. The virus designated "A (H1N1)/California/7/2009" identifies an influenza A virus with hemagglutinin type 1 and neuraminidase type 1 (thus, H1N1) first isolated in California in 2009 as the seventh strain in a sequence. Antigenic shifts in the influenza virus—such as the recently recognized H5N1 and H3N7 influenza A viruses in birds—carry the potential for global pandemic influenza because few humans have naturally occurring protective antibodies. Influenza B vaccines have only one recognized type of the H antigen and one of the N antigen, and hence their designations are shorter. Thus, "B/Massachusetts/2/2012" identifies an influenza B virus isolated in Massachusetts during 2012 as the second strain in a sequence. Outbreaks of influenza A attack 10%

to 20% of the general population, with high rates especially in children attending day care centers and in institutions such as nursing homes. Pandemics of influenza A can attack more than 50% of the general population.

The clinical spectrum of influenza ranges from a self-limited illness resembling the common cold to death from overwhelming viral pneumonia within a few hours. Adults can often date to the hour the onset of symptoms, such as throbbing headache, photophobia, myalgia, sore throat, substernal soreness, nonproductive cough, and disabling fatigue. Preschool children tend to have fever, rhinitis, pharyngitis, vomiting, and diarrhea. In elderly patients, the course is often dominated by high fever, nasal obstruction, lassitude, and diarrhea. In all age groups, the constitutional symptoms may be more impressive than the respiratory symptoms (Memoli et al., 2014).

More than 10 "rapid flu tests," which provide results within 15 minutes, have been approved by the U.S. Food and Drug Administration (FDA). In general, their sensitivity is about 50% to 70% and their specificity about 90% to 95%. These tests are especially useful for making treatment decisions about patients with flulike symptoms in the absence of reported influenza in a community. However, a negative rapid flu test result should never be the basis for excluding influenza when a patient presents with compatible symptoms and signs of influenza and the disease is prevalent in a community. The symptoms of influenza overlap with other viral respiratory infections; recent data suggest that RSV commonly causes acute respiratory illness in older adults, although the onset is usually more gradual compared with influenza (Sundaram et al., 2014). And even when influenza seems obvious, the possibility of other life-threatening diseases should be kept in mind (Figure 15-7).

Pneumonia is the major life-threatening complication. *Primary influenza pneumonia*, which should be suspected when high fever and dyspnea persist for more than several days, is more common among elderly and immunocompromised individuals but can also affect previously health young adults. *Secondary bacterial pneumonia* should be

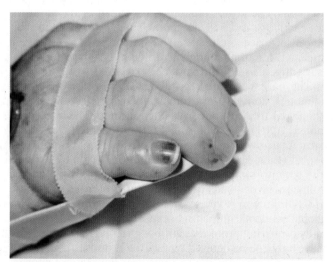

Figure 15-7. Keys to the diagnosis of *Staphylococcus aureus* endocarditis in a patient presenting with fever and heart failure at the peak of an influenza A epidemic included small embolic lesions in the skin and a large splinter hemorrhage beneath a nailbed.

suspected whenever a patient who seemed to be improving takes a dramatic turn for the worse. It is most often caused by *S. pneumoniae* (up to half of all cases), but *S. aureus* is also common in this setting.

We now know that influenza is mainly a disease of children, who spread the virus to their parents, grandparents, and others. Again, everyone older than 6 months of age should receive the annual flu vaccine barring a strict contraindication.

KEY TREATMENT

- Patients with severe, complicated, or progressive influenza if diagnosed within the first 2 days of illness should be treated with an antiviral agent, which may reduce the duration of illness and the risk of serious complications. Oseltamivir and zanamivir are currently recommended for this purpose (SOR: A).
- Oseltamivir (Tamiflu) is given in a dose of 75 mg twice daily. Higher doses do not seem to improve efficacy (SOR: B).
- Antiviral drug therapy is not recommended for patients with uncomplicated influenza with symptoms of more than 48 hours' duration (SOR-A).

GASTROINTESTINAL AND INTRAABDOMINAL INFECTIONS

Acute intraabdominal infection, mainly infectious diarrhea, is second only to cardiovascular disease as a cause of death worldwide. In the United States, acute gastroenteritis is second only to viral respiratory disease as a cause of acute illness. Most episodes are self-limited, but infectious diarrhea and various foodborne diseases annually account for more than 500 deaths. Other intraabdominal infections are relatively common and present dilemmas in diagnosis and management. Family medicine clinicians should know the following diagnostic pitfalls:

1. Acute bacterial meningitis is (to reiterate) sometimes misdiagnosed as "gastroenteritis" because of prominent nausea and vomiting.
2. Intrathoracic disorders such as pneumonia, pulmonary thromboembolism, and acute myocardial infarction sometimes present as pain in the upper abdomen. Conversely, pain in the lower chest can reflect intraabdominal pathology.
3. Unrecognized esophageal disease with reflux can cause asthma, persistent sore throat, and chronic aspiration pneumonia. The latter can lead to bronchiectasis and nontuberculous mycobacterial infection.
4. Fever with right lower abdominal pain suggesting acute appendicitis (pseudoappendicitis syndrome) can be caused by *Yersinia enterocolitica* (the usual cause), *Salmonella enteritidis* or *S. typhi*, or *Campylobacter jejuni*.
5. Abdominal pain in a person with diabetes mellitus can indicate a life-threatening syndrome such as emphysematous pyelonephritis or emphysematous cholecystitis.
6. Abdominal pain, fever, or evidence of sepsis in a person with cirrhosis and ascites should suggest the possibilities of spontaneous bacterial peritonitis or spontaneous bacteremia.

7. Abdominal pain and evidence of sepsis in an elderly person should raise the possibility of an "acute abdomen" caused by such disorders as acute cholecystitis, diverticulitis, perforation of the colon, acute appendicitis, or ruptured aortic aneurysm.

8. Abdominal pain and fever in a patient who has recently had diverticulitis, cholecystitis, or pancreatitis should raise the possibility of intraabdominal abscess.

Food Poisoning

Central food processing and distribution and the trend toward meals away from home make food poisoning an increasingly important problem in the United States, with about 5000 outbreaks being reported each year. A cause is determined in about two thirds of outbreaks, usually bacteria (75%) but also chemical agents (17%), viruses (6%), and parasites (2%). Symptoms range from mild facial flushing ("Chinese restaurant syndrome") or gastroenteritis to life-threatening paralysis or colitis. Onset of symptoms within an hour suggests a chemical agent. Onset between 1 and 6 hours suggests ingestion of a preformed toxin, usually in food contaminated with *S. aureus* or *Bacillus cereus*; vomiting and crampy abdominal pain are the usual symptoms, but diarrhea occurs in about one third of cases. Onset between 8 and 16 hours raises a number of possibilities, especially bacteria such as *C. perfringens* and enterotoxin-producing strains of *B. cereus*; characteristic symptoms are crampy abdominal pain and diarrhea—symptoms that can be caused by many enteric pathogens. Investigation is seldom indicated for an individual case, but the simultaneous occurrence of two or more cases should prompt notification of local health authorities.

Infectious Diarrhea

Acute diarrhea is extremely common in family medicine. The clinician's first task is to decide whether the problem is infectious or noninfectious (Figure 15-8). The focus here will be mainly on diarrhea as it presents in adolescent or adult patients. Noninfectious causes of diarrhea include food allergies, endocrine disorders, inflammatory bowel disease, and drugs (including cocaine), which should be considered in the differential diagnosis of ischemic colitis with abdominal pain and bloody diarrhea in a young or middle-aged adult. Findings suggesting medically important diarrhea warranting further investigation include high fever (≥38.5 °C [101.3 °F]), profuse watery diarrhea with severe volume depletion, severe abdominal pain (especially in a person older than 50 years of age), bloody diarrhea, diarrhea in a patient with hemolytic anemia or renal failure, the dysentery syndrome (small-volume stools with blood and mucus), duration longer than 3 days, advanced age (79 years or older), an immunocompromised state, or the occurrence of many similar cases suggesting a community outbreak. Acute bloody diarrhea is an urgent medical problem.

The distinction between "small bowel diarrhea" and "large bowel diarrhea" (Table 15-7) is conceptually useful and clinically relevant despite considerable overlap. About 90% of cases of acute, community-acquired infectious diarrhea in the United States represent "small bowel" diarrhea characterized by infrequent watery stools. About 5% to 10% of cases represent "large bowel" diarrhea or the *dysentery syndrome*, characterized by frequent small-volume

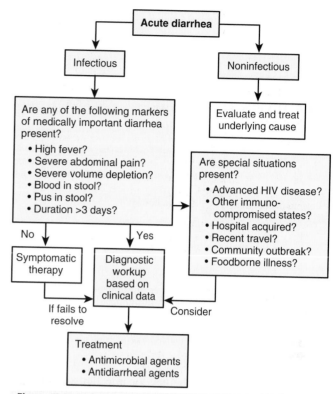

Figure 15-8. Evaluation of an adolescent or adult patient with acute diarrhea is based on the answers to a series of structured questions.

stools that often contain blood and mucus. Diagnostic workup has a higher yield in the dysentery syndrome than in "small bowel diarrhea," a situation in which routine stool cultures are discouraged.

Gross inspection of stool facilitates the distinction between noninflammatory and inflammatory diarrhea (see Table 15-7). Patients should bring a specimen to the office in a convenient container, such as a large, sealed glass jar. When the presence of blood and mucus suggests inflammatory diarrhea, the stool should be examined for WBCs. The traditional method is rapid and inexpensive: a drop of stool is placed on a glass slide, a drop of methylene blue is added, a coverslip is applied, and the preparation is examined using the high-dry or oil-immersion lens of the microscope. The commercially available Lactoferrin stool WBC test (Leuko-Test) may be more sensitive. Stool cultures, toxin assays, and microscopic examination for ova and parasites should be obtained on a selected basis based on the overall clinical picture, often taking into account the appearance of the tool and the presence or absence of fecal WBCs. Surveys indicate that only 0.6% to 6% of routine stool cultures yield pathogens, suggesting the need for greater selectivity.

KEY TREATMENT

- Most patients with diarrhea should be treated symptomatically, with attention to fluid and electrolyte replacement and judicious use of antimotility drugs (SOR: A).
- Antimotility agents should be avoided in patients with bloody diarrhea, who might have colitis caused by *C. difficile* or Shiga toxin–producing *E. coli* (SOR: A).

Table 15-7   Comparison of Small Bowel Diarrhea and Large Bowel Diarrhea

Parameter	Small Bowel Diarrhea	Large Bowel Diarrhea
Medical synonym	Noninflammatory diarrhea	Inflammatory diarrhea (dysentery)
Vernacular term	"The runs"	"The squirts"
Character of stools	Watery	Semiformed, typically with mucus and blood
Frequency of stools	Infrequent	Frequent
Pain on defecation	Usually absent	Often present
Pathophysiology	The small bowel secretes excessive fluid or fails to absorb fluids; the large bowel functions normally as a reservoir and therefore stores a large volume of fluid until overdistention prompts a bowel movement, typically on an urgent basis.	The colon is inflamed and therefore fails in its normal function as a reservoir, prompting frequent, small-volume bowel movements, which are often painful because of inflammation involving the rectum.
Polymorphonuclear leukocytes in the stool	Seldom present	Usually present
Fever	Usually absent	Often present
Associated symptoms	Abdominal cramping, bloating, and gas; symptoms of volume depletion (dehydration) if severe	Systemic toxicity; pain and tenderness in the lower quadrant of the abdomen
Classic prototype	Cholera	Shigellosis
Some important considerations	Viruses; enterotoxigenic *Escherichia coli* (traveler's diarrhea), protozoa (including giardiasis and cryptosporidiosis)	*Campylobacter jejuni*, Shiga toxin–producing strains of *E. coli* (especially *E. coli* O157:H7); amebiasis; also consider noninfectious causes such as ulcerative colitis and ischemic colitis

- Specific antimicrobial therapy for infectious diarrhea is recommended for at least six situations encountered in primary care in the United States: traveler's diarrhea, shigellosis, *C. difficile* colitis, *C. jejuni* infection, *Salmonella* gastroenteritis in persons older than 50 years of age, and proven infection by certain parasites.

Shiga-Toxin-Producing *Escherichia Coli* (*E. coli* O157:H7 and Other Serotypes). Strains of *E. coli* that produce Shiga toxin account for fewer than 1% of all cases of infectious diarrhea in primary care, but stool cultures are positive for these strains in up to 8% of patients with infectious diarrhea whose stools are visibly bloody. Most of these infections result from beef, notably undercooked hamburgers. Patients with hemorrhagic colitis caused by *E. coli* O157:H7 and other serotypes should be hospitalized because of the risk of severe complications, including *hemolytic-uremic syndrome*.

KEY TREATMENT

- Antimotility drugs should be avoided, especially in children, because they increase the duration and extent of exposure to the toxin (SOR: A).
- Antibiotics convey a 17-fold increased risk of hemolytic-uremic syndrome and should therefore not be used (SOR: A).

Salmonella Species. Typhoid fever has been eliminated as a major public health problem in the United States and other developed countries, although occasional cases still occur, mainly in returning travelers. Enteric infections from nontyphoidal *Salmonella* spp. are extremely common in the United States as elsewhere because of the wide presence of *Salmonella* in foodstuffs, especially poultry and eggs. *Salmonella* infections encompass at least five syndromes:

1. *Gastroenteritis caused by nontyphoidal species* is usually manifested as nausea, vomiting, and diarrhea 6 to 48 hours after ingestion of contaminated food or water. Stools are usually loose, of moderate volume, and without blood, and cultures are usually positive.
2. *Bacteremia with endovascular infection* can manifest as mycotic aneurysm (especially of the aorta, Figure 15-9); infection of vascular grafts; or, rarely, endocarditis. Blood cultures, if obtained, are positive in up to 4% of patients with *Salmonella* gastroenteritis, but the bacteremia is usually transient unless host factors present a *locus minoris resistentiae*. Advanced atherosclerosis of the aorta predisposes to colonization and then infection.
3. *Localized metastatic infections* can present as CNS infections; osteomyelitis or septic arthritis (especially in the context of sickle cell disease or immunosuppression); soft tissue infections; UTI (notably in the presence of stones; malignancy; renal transplant; or, in some parts of the world, schistosomiasis); and, rarely, other syndromes.
4. An *asymptomatic carrier state* occurs in 0.2% to 0.6% of persons with nontyphoidal salmonellosis, is more common in women and in persons with abnormalities of the biliary tract, and assumes importance in the food industry.
5. *Enteric fever* (typhoid fever caused by *S. typhi* and *paratyphoid* fever caused by other species) classically begins as a stepwise fever that becomes sustained (i.e., the temperature does not return to the baseline). Diarrhea is seldom the presenting complaint, and about 30% of patients, mainly adults, have constipation rather than diarrhea. Abdominal pain, sometimes with small "rose spots" on the trunk and abdomen, develops during the second week, and serious complications—including perforation of the bowel or hemorrhage—occur during the third week. Blood cultures are positive in 40% to 80% of

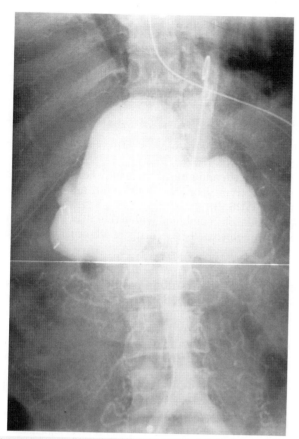

Figure 15-9. Mycotic aneurysm of the abdominal aorta demonstrated by aortography in a patient who had recently had *Salmonella* gastroenteritis.

cases, stool cultures in 30% to 40%, and bone marrow cultures in up to 98%.

KEY TREATMENT

- Antimicrobial therapy for gastroenteritis caused by non-typhoidal strains of *Salmonella* spp. is recommended for patients with more severe disease and for those predisposed to complications (namely, persons younger than 2 years of age or older than 50 years of age, those with malignancy or impaired T-lymphocyte function, those with disorders that cause "phagocyte blockade," and those with vascular grafts) (SOR: B).
- When antimicrobial therapy is indicated, current drugs of choice are TMP-SMX or a fluoroquinolone (SOR: B).

***Shigella* Species.** *Shigella* spp., the classic cause of dysentery (see Table 15-7) are highly communicable. *S. dysenteriae* serogroup 1 (the Shiga bacillus) is the most virulent *Shigella* species and an important cause of morbidity and mortality in young children worldwide. *S. sonnei*, which causes a relatively mild disease, accounts for 60% to 80% of shigellosis in the United States. The highest attack rates occur in children between 1 and 4 years of age. Although the inflammatory response is severe, it is relatively superficial, and bacteremia is therefore uncommon.

KEY TREATMENT

- Antimicrobial therapy for dysentery caused by *Shigella* spp. consists of TMP-SMX or a fluoroquinolone (SOR: A).

***Campylobacter* Species.** *C. jejuni*, now the most common bacterial pathogen isolated from stool cultures in the United States, mainly affects small children, adolescents, and young adults. Fever and abdominal pain are the usual presenting complaints. Atypical features include a severe flulike illness, a pseudoappendicitis syndrome (*C. jejuni* has been isolated in up to 3% of persons undergoing surgery for acute appendicitis), and acute colitis suggesting inflammatory bowel disease (ulcerative colitis or Crohn's disease). Other complications include cholecystitis, pancreatitis, hepatitis, peritonitis, the hemolytic-uremic syndrome, exacerbation of preexisting inflammatory bowel, and a Guillain-Barré variant known as the Miller-Fisher syndrome (in which cranial nerves are affected in addition to the ascending polyneuritis). *Campylobacter fetus* less commonly causes diarrhea, but, having a marked predilection for vascular sites, can also cause endocarditis, pericarditis, and thrombophlebitis.

KEY TREATMENT

- *C. jejuni* enteritis is usually treated with erythromycin (SOR: B).
- Most patients with severe gastroenteritis caused by *C. jejuni* and nearly all patients with *C. fetus* gastroenteritis should be hospitalized (SOR: A).

***Yersinia* Infection.** Two *Yersinia* species, *Yersinia enterocolitica* and *Yersinia pseudotuberculosis*, cause gastroenteritis indistinguishable from other types of inflammatory diarrhea and most commonly affect young children. Localization of the bacteria to the lymphoid tissue in the ileum (Peyer patches) and mesenteric lymph nodes causes a clinical syndrome closely mimicking acute appendicitis (the *pseudoappendicitis syndrome*). *Yersinia* spp. can also cause liver abscesses in patients with iron overload syndromes or diabetes mellitus. When yersiniosis is suspected, the laboratory should be notified to use special media for processing stool cultures.

KEY TREATMENT

- Antibiotics are not recommended for most enteric *Yersinia* infections (SOR: C).
- Regimens for severe infections or infections in immunocompromised persons caused by *Yersinia* spp. include TMP-SMX, fluoroquinolones, or combination therapy with doxycycline and an aminoglycoside (SOR: B).

***Vibrio* Infection.** Cholera, caused by *Vibrio cholerae*, is the classic cause of noninflammatory but life-threatening diarrhea. Stimulation of the adenyl cyclase system by the organism's toxin results in massive secretory diarrhea from a histologically normal small intestine, risking death from dehydration unless treated aggressively. *Vibrio parahemolyticus* is an important cause of gastroenteritis associated with ingestion of inadequately cooked or uncooked seafood (notably, raw oysters). Explosive watery diarrhea is usually the first symptom. Although usually mild, *V. parahemolyticus* infection can be fatal in young children, elderly adults, and severely debilitated individuals. *V. vulnificus*, previously discussed in this chapter, causes bloodstream and soft tissue infections but seldom causes diarrhea.

Viral Gastroenteritis. Viruses—notably rotaviruses and noroviruses—are the most common causes of diarrhea in the United States, but the disease is usually mild. *Rotaviruses* cause diarrhea mainly in children younger than 5 years of age but can also cause serious diarrhea in elderly adults, especially in long-term care facilities. Noroviruses are transmitted person to person; result in extensive fecal shedding; and cause large outbreaks of diarrhea in contained environments such as cruise ships, health care institutions, and schools. Diarrhea begins abruptly, often with nausea and vomiting (*winter vomiting disease*); stools are watery; and symptoms usually resolve after 3 days.

Parasitic Diarrheas. Parasitic causes should be considered in patients with diarrhea lasting more than 7 days. Of the numerous causes of parasitic diarrhea throughout the world (see later section on Parasites), the most important in the United States are three protozoa: *Giardia lamblia*, *Cryptosporidium parvum*, and *Entamoeba histolytica*. Molecular-based technologies are replacing traditional microscopy ("stool for ova and parasites") for diagnosis because the latter has low sensitivity. In a recent study, real-time PCR was 100% sensitive and specific for detecting these three protozoa, but traditional microscopy was only 38% sensitive (although nearly 100% specific) (Van Lint et al., 2013).

Giardiasis can be acquired from lake or stream water; contaminated food; or personal contact, especially in day care centers. *Giardia lamblia*, a flagellated protozoan, is found in many mammals, including beavers, dogs, and cats. *Giardia* cysts resist chlorination of water but are killed by boiling. Campers, who are at high risk, should therefore boil water obtained from streams or lakes. Diarrhea, when it is established, is usually protracted. Cysts can be hard to find in stools; a commercially available immunoassay is now recommended.

Cryptosporidiosis in immunocompetent persons is often asymptomatic or the cause of a mild and self-limited diarrhea. Treatment is not recommended. Large outbreaks of diarrhea caused by *Cryptosporidium parvum* have resulted from contamination of municipal water supplies. In persons with advanced HIV disease, cryptosporidiosis is a major cause of severe, intractable diarrhea. Diagnosis is usually made by partial acid-fast staining of stools or by newer antigen detection methods.

Amebiasis, caused by *E. histolytica*, is highly prevalent in many developing countries, in certain institutional settings in the United States, and among recent immigrants from Mexico. Up to 90% of persons with *E. histolytica* are asymptomatic cyst passers. Some infected persons have acute nonspecific diarrhea with bloody stools. The disease can present as fulminant colitis, mainly in children; this presentation can be misdiagnosed as ulcerative colitis; hence, amebic disease should be excluded if steroids are to be used for presumed first-episode ulcerative colitis.

Nonpathogenic amebae, notably *E. dispar*, can be confused with *E. histolytica* on microscopic examination. Antigen-detection methods are available for testing stool samples for *E. histolytica*, and serologic tests are usually positive in patients with liver abscess, the major systemic complication.

KEY TREATMENT

- Metronidazole is the drug of choice for giardiasis (SOR: A).
- Paromomycin and nitazoxanide have been used for treatment for cryptosporidiosis, but results are often unsatisfactory (SOR: B).
- Metronidazole, combined with either diiodohydroxyquin or paromomycin, is the drug of choice for amebiasis (SOR: A).

***Clostridium difficile* Infection.** Diarrhea is a relatively common complication of antimicrobial therapy and is associated with *C. difficile* in about 10% to 30% of cases. Pseudomembranous colitis caused by *C. difficile* occurs in about one in 10,000 courses of antibiotic therapy in ambulatory patients. Primary care clinicians are likely to encounter *C. difficile* in three groups of patients: (1) patients given broad-spectrum antibiotics—most commonly ampicillin, amoxicillin, newer cephalosporins, and clindamycin; (2) patients recently released from the hospital; and (3) patients in long-term care facilities. Asymptomatic *C. difficile* colonization is common, and the spores (which resist common disinfectants, including alcohol-based hand sanitizers) often contaminate the environment. The occurrence of person-to-person transmission mandates scrupulous hand hygiene with soap and water after direct contact with patients known or suspected to be colonized by this organism. *C. difficile* colitis typically presents as watery diarrhea with a low-grade fever and abdominal pain. About 2% to 3% of patients have serious complications, including ileus, toxic megacolon (maximum colonic diameter ≥ 7 cm), intestinal perforation, and protein-losing enteropathy. Marked leukocytosis (WBC count >30,000 mm^3) indicates severe disease, in which fecal polymorphonuclear leukocytes (PMNs) can usually be demonstrated.

The recent introduction of PCR-based molecular testing for *C. difficile* toxin A and B genes has simplified the diagnosis because the newer assays have near 100% sensitivity. However, these assays cannot distinguish infection from asymptomatic colonization. Endoscopic evaluation of the colon is generally reserved for cases in which the diagnosis is in doubt. Although optimum therapy of *C. difficile* remains controversial, all authorities agree on one point: broad-spectrum antimicrobial therapy should be stopped if at all possible.

KEY TREATMENT

- Drugs that alter normal intestinal motility should be avoided in patients with colitis caused by *C. difficile* (SOR: A).
- Orally administered metronidazole is recommended for mild to moderately severe cases of colitis caused by *C. difficile* (SOR: A).

- Orally administered vancomycin is recommended for severe cases of *C. difficile* colitis (SOR: B).
- The array of alternative agents now includes fidaxomicin, but no treatment is entirely satisfactory for patients with severe disease or frequent relapses (SOR: B).
- *C. difficile* colitis recurs in about 20% of patients, and numerous measures, including fecal transplantation, continue to be studied (SOR: C).

URINARY TRACT INFECTIONS

Urinary tract infections are the most common bacterial infections encountered in family medicine, affect perhaps half of all persons during their lifetimes, and are becoming increasingly problematic because of the emergence of drug-resistant strains of uropathogenic *E. coli*. UTI is mainly a disease of women except during early infancy and late adulthood (Barber et al., 2013).

The term "UTI" denotes a diverse group of conditions having in common the presence of microorganisms in bladder urine with or without symptoms and signs of disease. The term a*symptomatic bacteriuria* denotes the presence of greater than 10^5 colony-forming units (CFUs) of bacteria per milliliter of urine. Current opinion holds that lower counts (as little as 10^3 CFU/mL of urine) should be given credence in symptomatic patients (those suspected of having cystitis or pyelonephritis) and in patients whose specimens are obtained directly from an indwelling catheter. *Uncomplicated UTI*, in which infection is confined to the urinary bladders, is mainly a disease of women. About one in three women develop UTI requiring treatment by early adulthood. *Complicated UTI* implies the presence of predisposing anatomic, functional abnormalities; is more difficult to treat; and requires aggressive evaluation and patient follow-up. Some authorities maintain that *all* UTIs in patients other than young, healthy, nonpregnant women should be considered complicated.

Many authorities suggest abandoning the terms "lower" and "upper" UTI, but these terms are conceptually useful for indicating which patients need urologic intervention. The term "lower UTI" refers to infection at or below the level of the bladder and in clinical practice is synonymous with "cystitis," a syndrome characterized by dysuria (pain on voiding), frequency, urgency, and variable suprapubic tenderness. "Lower UTI" also encompasses prostatitis, urethritis, and infection of the periurethral glands. The term "upper UTI" refers to infection above the level of the bladder—that is, of the ureters, kidneys, and perirenal tissues. This term usually implies pyelonephritis .but can also denote intrarenal abscess ("renal carbuncle," usually caused by *S. aureus*) and perinephric abscess. *Obstructive uropathy* refers to obstruction of urine flow at any level.

Urine culture remains the gold standard for diagnosis but is unnecessary in most cases of uncomplicated UTI. Grossly clear urine has a negative predictive value of 91% or greater for significant bacteriuria. Combined use of the leukocyte esterase-nitrite test (by dipstick analysis of urine) has a sensitivity of 70% to 90% for UTI. Most patients with symptomatic UTI have pyuria. Urine culture should be obtained for patients with complicated UTI and for patients with recurrent uncomplicated UTI if the recurrences are not clearly related to sexual activity. Because the bacteria that usually cause UTI multiply rapidly at room temperature, false-positive cultures can result when specimens are not plated out or refrigerated promptly. The pretest probability of a positive urine culture is increased by a history of UTI symptoms, back pain, hematuria, or bacteriuria by dipstick analysis.

Asymptomatic Bacteriuria

Asymptomatic bacteriuria as defined above is relatively common in certain patient groups. Screening for asymptomatic bacteriuria is strongly recommended in the first trimester of pregnancy because pregnant women are at increased risk of acute pyelonephritis. Screening is discouraged in most patient populations. Eradication of the infecting microorganism commonly results in bladder colonization by a more difficult-to-treat pathogen.

> **KEY TREATMENT**
>
> - Antibiotic therapy for asymptomatic bacteriuria is indicated (1) during pregnancy, (2) in young children with vesicoureteral reflux, (3) in selected patients with urologic problems or ureteral obstruction (especially when such patients are scheduled for implant surgery of any kind, in which transient bacteremia might have disastrous consequences), (4) in renal transplant recipients during the early postoperative period, and (5) for patients with severe granulocytopenia (SOR: A).
> - In other patient groups, notably elderly patients and especially elderly women, treatment of asymptomatic bacteriuria can be distinctly harmful and is therefore not recommended (Mody and Juthani-Mehta, 2014) (SOR: A).
> - When a patient has asymptomatic bacteriuria caused by a microorganism resistant to the usual antibiotics or treatable only with a relatively toxic agent (e.g., an aminoglycoside antibiotic), it is often best to (1) record the presence of the microorganism in the patient's medical record and (2) prescribe antibiotics when and if the patient develops any combination of fever, flank tenderness, or documented bacteremia (SOR: B).
> - The presence of pyuria in a patient with asymptomatic bacteriuria does not constitute an indication for antibiotic therapy (SOR: C).

Uncomplicated Cystitis in Nonpregnant Adolescent and Adult Women

Uncomplicated acute cystitis in nonpregnant adolescent and adult women is typically caused by *E. coli* or, during the spring and summer months, *Staphylococcus saprophyticus* (Table 15-8). Diagnosis is usually based on symptoms: urinary urgency and frequency, dysuria, suprapubic discomfort, and cloudy urine. Vaginitis and genital herpes simplex infection should be excluded. The presence of fever or flank pain (i.e., pain experienced at the costovertebral angle, or "over the kidney") strongly suggests acute pyelonephritis. Patients with acute pyelonephritis often have "lower urinary tract" symptoms, but patients with infection confined to the lower urinary tract seldom, if ever, experience fever and chills. A wealth of experience supports the

Table 15-8   Some Microorganisms Causing Urinary Infection and their Clinical Correlates

Microorganism	Clinical Correlates
Escherichia coli	Causes >70% of uncomplicated UTIs and many complicated UTIs. Uropathogenic strains possess *P. fimbriae* (pyelonephritis-associated pili) to bind to urinary tract epithelial cells and thereby colonize the bladder. Certain strains known as ST131 strains exhibit high levels of resistance to antibiotics.
Staphylococcus saprophyticus	A coagulase-negative staphylococcus species causing up to 15% of uncomplicated UTIs in women and more common during the spring and summer months. It can be distinguished from other coagulase-negative staphylococci by its resistance to novobiocin.
Proteus mirabilis	A urea-splitting gram-negative bacillus that causes the urine to be alkaline (pH ≥7), thereby promoting the formation of struvite calculi capable of becoming large "staghorn" calculi that can completely obstruct the renal pelvis.
Aerobic gram-negative bacilli other than *E. coli* and *P. mirabilis*	*Klebsiella* spp. occasionally cause uncomplicated community-acquired UTI, but the presence of species of aerobic gram-negative bacilli usually signifies complicated UTI, typically in patients who have received multiple courses of antibiotics, have indwelling bladder catheters, or who have undergone urologic intervention.
Enterococci	The presence of enterococci in the urine usually correlates with some combination of prior antimicrobial therapy, urologic instrumentation, or obstructive uropathy. Enterococci seldom cause acute symptomatic UTI (Hooton et al., 2013). However, enterococcal UTI is a risk factor for enterococcal endocarditis.
Staphylococcus aureus	The presence of *S. aureus* in the urine can represent a "spillover" from bacteremia rather than infection of the urinary tract per se, although exceptions may occur, especially in older men with obstructive uropathy. *S. aureus* bacteriuria can also signify the presence of an intrarenal abscess (renal carbuncle).
Group B streptococci (*Streptococcus agalactiae*)	Group B streptococci rarely cause acute cystitis in healthy young women (Hooton et al., 2013). However, group B streptococci can cause symptomatic UTI in older patients with risk factors for complicated UTI.
Staphylococcus epidermidis	*S. epidermidis* is a frequent contaminant of urine cultures because of its heavy presence in normal skin flora. Symptomatic UTI occurs mainly in persons with indwelling urinary catheters.
Candida albicans and other yeasts	The tendency of yeast cells to clump together makes the "10^5 CFU/mL of urine" less accurate for defining "significant" growth of yeasts in urine culture compared with bacteria. Yeasts are usually encountered in catheterized patients who have received multiple courses of antibiotics. Patients are often asymptomatic, and treatment is often not required. However, yeasts can infect the kidneys and can give rise to "fungus balls" that obstruct the ureters.
Lactobacillus spp., *Gardnerella vaginalis*, and *Mycoplasma* spp.	These microorganisms have been implicated as causes of UTI, but their relative importance is unclear.
Adenoviruses	Adenoviruses occasionally cause acute hemorrhagic cystitis, mainly in children and young adults.

UTI, Urinary tract infection.

practice of managing first episodes of uncomplicated cystitis, and recurrent episodes clearly related to sexual activity, with short (3-day) courses of antimicrobial agents without a urine culture.

Of great current concern is the emergence throughout the world of uropathogenic *E. coli* strains of sequence type 131 (ST131 strains) (see Table 15-8), which often exhibit high-level resistance to multiple antibiotics.

KEY TREATMENT

- Fluoroquinolones and β-lactam antibiotics should no longer be used as empiric therapy for acute cystitis because of the emergence of resistance among uropathogenic *E. coli* (SOR: A).
- Common treatment options for uncomplicated cystitis include TMP-SMX, nitrofurantoin, and fosfomycin (SOR: A). Most patients improve rapidly; failure to improve should raise the possibility of a complicating factor (SOR: A).
- Forcing fluids has not been proven to be beneficial for acute cystitis (SOR: B).
- Cranberry juice is probably unhelpful unless taken in large quantities (SOR: B).
- Strategies for prevention and treatment of recurrent UTI in young, nonpregnant women include patient-initiated

self-treatment of symptomatic episodes, continuous low-dose prophylaxis, and postcoital prophylaxis. A recent analysis of the literature indicated daily low-dose nitrofurantoin to be the most effective of five alternatives for this purpose (Eells et al., 2014) (SOR: B).

Acute Pyelonephritis

Acute pyelonephritis usually arises from ascent of bacteria from the bladder to the renal medulla. Pyelonephritis in patients with structurally normal urinary tracts is usually caused by uropathogenic *E. coli* strains. Other aerobic gram-negative bacilli come into play in patients with complicated urologic histories. Fever, flank pain, nausea, and vomiting—with or without symptoms of lower UTI (dysuria, frequency, urgency)—suggest the diagnosis. PID is often misdiagnosed as acute pyelonephritis. Pelvic examination should therefore be undertaken when risk factors for sexually transmitted disease (STD) are present. Pyuria is nearly always present, and microscopic examination of the urine may reveal WBC casts (Figure 15-10). Urine culture should be performed because the nitrite test lacks sensitivity and will not provide the information about the causative organism that will be needed if initial therapy fails. Blood cultures should be performed in patients who require hospitalization. A pregnancy test should be obtained if the

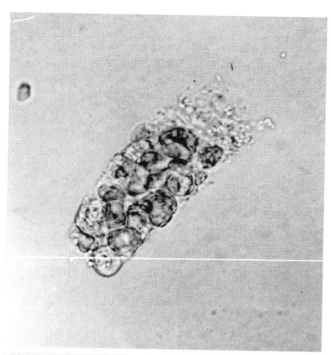

Figure 15-10. A white blood cell cast, in the setting of pyuria, fever, and flank pain, is essentially pathognomonic of acute pyelonephritis.

reliability of contraception is in doubt or menses are irregular.

KEY TREATMENT

- Patients with acute pyelonephritis and severe symptoms including nausea and vomiting should be started on parenteral antibiotic therapy, such as ceftriaxone (SOR: A).
- Indications for hospitalization include severe sepsis, uncertainty about the diagnosis, and inability to maintain hydration (SOR: A).
- Outpatient therapy often suffices for nonpregnant women with mild to moderately severe disease and who can be expected to be compliant with treatment (SOR: A).
- When the infecting microorganism is susceptible to the chosen drug, marked improvement usually occurs within 72 hours unless ureteral obstruction, renal or perinephric abscess, or other serious complication is present. Failure to respond within 72 hours should prompt evaluation of the urinary tract by CT scan or ultrasound examination. Imaging studies are also indicated in patients who have had two or more recurrences of acute pyelonephritis (SOR: A).

Complicated Urinary Tract Infection in Adults

Complicated UTI (as defined earlier) often begins more insidiously. Gradually worsening symptoms sometimes antedate the diagnosis by weeks or months, as opposed to less than 3 days in most cases of acute uncomplicated pyelonephritis. Complicated UTI should also be suspected when standard therapy of upper UTI fails to effect clinical

improvement (return of temperature and WBC to normal) within 5 days.

Perinephric abscess is typically associated with urinary calculi, diabetes mellitus, or both. *Renal cortical abscess* (renal carbuncle, often a result of *S. aureus* bacteremia) may present with symptoms suggesting acute pyelonephritis but responds poorly to therapy. Imaging studies (CT scan or ultrasonography) facilitate these diagnoses. *Xanthogranulomatous pyelonephritis* is an unusual variant of chronic pyelonephritis usually seen in middle-aged women with history of recurrent UTI. The lesion is usually unilateral, and imaging studies typically show a large, nonfunctioning kidney with several stones or a staghorn calculus. This entity can be confused with malignancy. *Emphysematous pyelonephritis* is a rare gas-forming infection of the renal parenchyma, usually seen in patients with diabetes mellitus, with a high risk of multiorgan failure and death. Diagnosis is now made by CT scan. Aggressive urologic intervention sometimes obviates the need for nephrectomy to save the patient's life.

Urinary Tract Infections in Adult Men

About half of adult men, and perhaps most men who survive well into their eighties, seek medical attention for UTI during their lifetimes. Men with UTI usually undergo imaging procedures to exclude obstructive uropathy. *Acute bacterial prostatitis* presents with some combination of fever, dysuria, pelvic or perineal pain, and pyuria. Rectal examination, which is painful and can cause bacteremia, should be avoided when the diagnosis seems straightforward. Initial antibiotic coverage, unless guided by Gram stain or spun urine sediment, should include drugs with broad-spectrum activity against aerobic gram-negative bacilli and gram-positive cocci. The diagnosis of *chronic bacterial prostatitis* is usually made in the course of investigating the cause of recurrent UTI or asymptomatic bacteriuria. Rectal examination often shows a tender and boggy prostate, but findings may be normal. Urinalyses and urine cultures taken before and after prostate massage (the four-cup test) can be useful but cannot exclude this diagnosis. Antimicrobial therapy must be prolonged, typically for 4 to 12 weeks, and is made difficult by the poor penetration of many antibiotics into the prostate. Occasional patients have granulomatous prostatitis caused by TB or fungi (notably, blastomycosis, coccidioidomycosis, and cryptococcosis; rarely histoplasmosis), which is suggested by failure to respond to antibiotics and by the finding of an indurated, firm, or nodular prostate. *Epididymitis* in young adults is most often the result of STD; epididymitis in older adults is usually caused by gram-negative or gram-positive bacteria and is associated with prostatic disease.

SEXUALLY TRANSMITTED DISEASES

The serious health consequences of STDs disproportionately affect women, children, and adolescents, especially among racial and ethnic minority groups. Barriers to effective STD prevention include lack of public awareness, inadequate training of health care professionals, and sociocultural misconceptions of the risks and consequences. Some studies suggest that fewer than 50% of family physicians obtain adequate histories of sexual practices in their new patients despite the obvious role of primary care in prevention. The focus here is mainly on recognition; family medicine physicians can stay current with evolving treatment recommendations through the CDC's website (http://www.cdc.gov/std/treatment).

Urethritis, Vaginitis, Cervicitis, and Pelvic Inflammatory Disease in Women

Consequences of STDs in women include infertility, fetal complications including death, and the end results of unrecognized syphilis and gonorrhea.

Urethritis (inflammation of the urethra, characterized by a burning sensation during urination or itching or discharge at the urethral meatus) in women, usually caused by *N. gonorrhoeae*, *Chlamydia trachomatis*, or HSV, presents with some combination of dysuria, urinary frequency, and lower abdominal pain. It must be differentiated from acute cystitis, which, similar to urethritis, is often preceded by sexual activity. When in doubt, patients should be tested for gonorrhea and *C. trachomatis* infection; nucleic-acid based tests on urine or on urethral specimens are highly sensitive and specific.

Vaginitis is discussed in the chapter on gynecology.

Cervicitis (inflammation of the cervix) is a common but poorly understood condition that has been found in 32% to 45% of women attending STD clinics and is often asymptomatic. Cervicitis can present with vaginal discharge, postcoital bleeding, or deep dyspareunia. *Mucopurulent cervicitis* is defined by the presence of a mucopurulent discharge from the endocervical os or by friability or easily induced bleeding when the endocervix is first touched by a swab. *Trichomonas vaginalis* is the most common cause, but other important causes include *N. gonorrhoeae* and *C. trachomatis*. In about 40% of cases, no pathogen is identified, and some cases are presumed to be of noninfectious etiology. Management of sexual partners should be based on the suspected or detected infection in the index patient if contact occurred within the preceding 60 days.

Pelvic inflammatory disease—inflammation of the upper female genital tract and related structures—can manifest as endometritis, salpingitis, adnexitis, tuboovarian abscess, pelvic peritonitis, perihepatitis, or chronic pelvic pain. Salpingitis predisposes to tubal pregnancy, tuboovarian abscess, and infertility. The risk for tubal-factor infertility is 7% after one episode of PID and increases to 28% after 3 or more episodes. Women with PID have a 7- to 10-fold increased risk of ectopic pregnancy, which accounts for 9% of all pregnancy-related deaths. Most cases of PID begin with *C. trachomatis* and/or *N. gonorrhoeae* infection. Damage to the fallopian tube mucosa allows invasion by opportunistic bacteria from the vaginal flora: gram-negative bacilli, various anaerobic bacteria, group B streptococci, and genital mycoplasmas. The clinical spectrum of PID ranges from asymptomatic infection to mild endometritis or salpingitis to generalized peritonitis. Women with gonococcal PID may present with abdominal pain of less than 3 days' duration; women with chlamydial PID tend to present with abdominal pain of longer than 1 weeks' duration. The minimum criterion for a clinical diagnosis of PID consists of one or more of the following: lower abdominal tenderness, adnexal tenderness, and cervical motion tenderness. Empiric therapy should be given when all three of these are present. Additional criteria that support the diagnosis are temperature of 38.3 °C (101 °F) or above, an abnormal cervical or vaginal discharge, an elevated ESR or CRP level, or documentation of cervicitis caused by *N. gonorrhoeae* or *C. trachomatis* by culture or nucleic acid–based tests.

The approach to treatment of PID includes the decision whether to hospitalize, patient education, follow-up, and treatment of sex partners. Antimicrobial therapy should include coverage against *N. gonorrhoeae*, *C. trachomatis*, anaerobic bacteria, streptococci, and gram-negative bacilli.

Urethritis in Men

Causes of urethritis in men include *N. gonorrhoeae*, *C. trachomatis*, *Ureaplasma urealyticum*, *Mycoplasma genitalium*, and occasionally *Trichomonas vaginalis*, HSV, syphilis, and various bacterial pathogens. Whereas gonococcal urethritis usually causes purulent discharge and dysuria, nongonococcal urethritis usually causes a scant, mucoid discharge and may be asymptomatic. Up to 30% of men with gonococcal urethritis, discussed in more detail later, have concomitant chlamydial infection. Some studies suggest that up to two thirds of cases of nongonococcal urethritis in men are undiagnosed. Treatment depends on the etiology.

Chlamydia trachomatis Infection

Chlamydia trachomatis is one of the most common sexually transmitted pathogens, especially between the ages of 15 and 24 years. In men, the spectrum includes urethritis, proctitis, epididymitis, and reactive arthritis. In women, the spectrum includes urethritis, bartholinitis, cervicitis, endometritis, salpingitis, tuboovarian abscess, ectopic pregnancy, pelvic peritonitis, and perihepatitis. Among women with gonorrhea, 30% to 50% have concomitant *Chlamydia* infection. Multiple exposures to different chlamydial serotypes may be a risk factor for carcinoma of the cervix. About 75% to 90% of cases of chlamydial cervicitis are asymptomatic. Infected men commonly have urethritis. Nucleic acid amplification tests are now widely used for diagnosis. Appropriate specimens in women include vaginal swabs, endocervical swab, self-collected vulvovaginal swabs, and urine; appropriate specimens in men include urethral swabs and urine.

Gonorrhea

N. gonorrhoeae, similar to many sexually transmitted pathogens, is usually (95%) symptomatic and easily diagnosed in men but is a more subtle and dangerous pathogen in women. About 10% to 20% of women develop acute salpingitis or PID. Underdiagnosis in women can lead to disseminated gonococcal infection, which most commonly presents as septic arthritis or tenosynovitis, sometimes with tender, necrotic skin nodules with an erythematous base on the distal extremities (the *gonococcal arthritis–dermatitis syndrome*). Rare complications include endocarditis and meningitis.

Gram stain of urethral exudates has a high sensitivity (90% to 95%) for men with symptomatic gonococcal urethritis but is much less reliable in women. Nucleic acid amplification tests (notably, PCR) have largely replaced Gram stain and culture for diagnosis of gonorrhea in the United States but do not provide information about drug susceptibility. Fluoroquinolones are no longer used for treatment of gonorrhea because of the high prevalence of resistance. Gonococci increasingly show resistance to other agents, and few new drugs are in the pipeline (Hook and Van der Pol, 2013).

Syphilis

Syphilis, caused by the spirochete *Treponema pallidum*, remains a public health concern in the United States with disproportionately high rates in various racial and ethnic groups and in HIV-infected persons, in whom the disease can be difficult to treat. *Primary syphilis* typically presents 2 to 6 weeks after exposure as a painless, indurated ulcer *(chancre)* with well-defined borders and a clean base, usually on the genital mucosa but sometimes on the oral or anorectal mucosa. *Secondary syphilis*, which develops in 60% to 90% of persons with untreated primary syphilis, is a systemic disease caused by dissemination of treponemes and is characterized by combinations of fever; generalized lymphadenopathy; headache; sore throat; arthralgias; rash; and, less often, involvement of the CNS, eyes, liver, and kidneys (as immune-complex glomerulonephritis). *Latent syphilis* is defined by reactive serologic tests without evidence of disease. *Tertiary (late) syphilis* presents as cardiovascular disease (aortic aneurysms, aortic regurgitation, and coronary stenosis), neurologic disease (as general paresis, tabes dorsalis, CNS gumma [inflammatory mass with necrotic center]), and other syndromes that earned syphilis the reputation of "great masquerader."

Definitive diagnosis of primary syphilis is based on demonstrating spirochetes by dark-field microscopy or direct immunofluorescence. Diagnosis of other states of the disease is based largely on serologic tests, which include both nontreponemal tests (notably, rapid plasma reagin [RPR] test and, for CSF, the Venereal Disease Research Laboratory [VDRL] test) and specific treponemal tests, notably the microhemagglutination–*Treponema pallidum* (MHA-TP) test. Secondary syphilis is the only stage of the disease in which serologic testing is reliable, the RPR being 99% sensitive and the MHA-TP 100% sensitive. Tertiary (late) syphilis is usually diagnosed by the combination of a reactive RPR and a confirmatory test (e.g., the MHA-TP) combined with clinical symptoms and signs consistent with the disease.

Benzathine penicillin G is used for non–penicillin-allergic patients with early syphilis and their recent (within 90 days) sex partners. Indications for CSF evaluation include neurologic, auditory, ophthalmic, or cardiovascular signs (e.g., aortic regurgitation); treatment failure (defined by failure of the nontreponemal titers to decrease fourfold, e.g. from 1 : 32 to 1 : 8, within 6 months of therapy for primary or secondary syphilis); and latent syphilis in the setting of HIV disease. High-dose penicillin G given intravenously remains the treatment of choice for non–penicillin-allergic patients with late syphilis. Latent syphilis (detected by nontreponemal serology, confirmed by specific treponemal serology, and—by definition—with exclusion of late syphilis by LP) is treated with several courses of benzathine penicillin G.

Other Causes of Genital Ulcers

Most genital, anal, and perianal ulcers in the United States are caused by HSVs (discussed later in the section on herpesviruses) or syphilis. *Chancroid*, caused by *Haemophilus ducreyi*, is endemic in some parts of the United States and causes a soft, painful ulcer *("soft chancre")* in contrast to the hard, painful ulcer of syphilis. The diagnosis is usually clinical because media for isolating *H. ducreyi* are not widely available. A painful ulcer combined with tender lymphadenopathy is highly suggestive, but syphilis and HSV infection must be excluded in every case. Various treatments are usually curative. The painless genital ulcer of *lymphogranuloma venereum* is typically inconspicuous; the early course is dominated by massive suppurative inguinal lymphadenopathy *(buboes)* and the late course by abscesses, fistulas, strictures, and sinus tracts. The diagnosis is usually confirmed by serology, and treatment consists of doxycycline combined with drainage of buboes and abscesses.

Human Papillomavirus Infection

Human papillomavirus infection is the most common viral STD worldwide. In the United States, the incidence of HPV has been especially high among college students (35% to 43%), minorities, and persons with multiple sex partners. Most genital HPV infections are subclinical and transmitted by sexual contact. Approximately 100 types of HPV have been identified. About 30 types have been shown to infect the anogenital area; these have been divided into "low-risk" and "high-risk" groups based on their associations with anogenital cancer. HPV types 6 and 11 are found in about 90% of cases of condylomata acuminata (genital warts) but are rarely associated with cancer. On the other hand, HPV types 16, 18, 31, and 35 have been associated with squamous cell cancer of the vulva, vagina, cervix (with about 95% of squamous cell carcinomas of the cervix being positive for HPV DNA), penis, and anus. None of the several treatment measures assure a cure.

MUSCLE, BONE, JOINT, AND ORTHOPEDIC HARDWARE INFECTIONS

These infections are nearly always serious, requiring hospitalization or consultation.

Pyomyositis

Pyomyositis, an acute infection most commonly affecting the large muscles of the lower extremities or trunk, is fairly common in parts of the tropics but uncommon in the United States; about 95% of cases in the tropics and about two thirds of cases in the United States are caused by *S. aureus*. There is often a history of blunt trauma, causing a *locus minoris resistentiae*. Pyomyositis is also associated with HIV disease, injection drug use, and defects in host defenses. Imaging studies, notably MRI, enable the diagnosis. Patients should be hospitalized and receive both intravenous antibiotics and surgical drainage because untreated pyomyositis often progresses to severe sepsis and death.

Osteomyelitis

Osteomyelitis—infection of bone—is of diverse etiologies and commonly presents diagnostic and therapeutic dilemmas. According to one of several classifications, osteomyelitis is of three broad types: (1) hematogenous, (2) related to trauma or contiguous infection, and (3) polymicrobial osteomyelitis of the small bones of the feet in patients with diabetes mellitus. Osteomyelitis commonly complicates compound fractures and contributes to nonunion.

Acute hematogenous osteomyelitis most often involves the metaphyses of long bones (notably, of the tibia and fibula) in children and adolescents and the spine in adults (Petola and Pääkkönen, 2014). *S. aureus* is the most common cause, but numerous bacteria and other organisms (notably, *M. tuberculosis* and fungi) sometimes cause acute hematogenous osteomyelitis. Some patients present with few, if any, symptoms of local infection, the illness being dominated by fever and systemic toxicity. However, careful palpation often reveals localized areas of tenderness. Vertebral osteomyelitis should be considered in all adults with unexplained fever; palpation or percussion of the entire spine may yield the first diagnostic clue. The WBC count is usually elevated, as are ESR and CRP, and blood culture results are often positive. MRI is more sensitive than plain radiographs for early diagnosis. Because therapy must be prolonged—at least 6 weeks—it is extremely important to secure a microbiologic diagnosis even if this requires bone biopsy for culture. Aggressive treatment of acute osteomyelitis reduces the risk of chronic osteomyelitis, which carries a lifelong risk of relapse.

SEPTIC ARTHRITIS

Acute septic arthritis in previously healthy persons is mainly caused by *S. aureus* and usually involves the large joints of the extremities. The affected joint is hot and swollen, and synovial fluid usually shows greater than 50,000 WBCs, predominantly neutrophils. *N. gonorrhoeae* should be considered in sexually active individuals; *P. aeruginosa* should be considered in injection drug users (in whom septic arthritis commonly affects unusual joints such as the sternoclavicular and sacroiliac joints), and gram-negative bacteria should be considered in patients with such risk factors as advanced age, rheumatoid arthritis, prosthetic joints, other joint surgeries, diabetes mellitus, skin infections, and immune suppression. TB and fungal infection should always be considered in subacute and chronic cases. Diagnosis depends largely on synovial fluid analysis and culture; when gonococcal septic arthritis is suspected, it is useful to inoculate culture media at the bedside after arthrocentesis. Treatment of septic arthritis consists of high-dose antimicrobial therapy; an orthopedic surgeon should be consulted for complicated cases requiring drainage.

Reactive Arthritis

Reactive arthritis, formerly known as "Reiter's syndrome" and now classified as a spondyloarthropathy, affects joints of the lower back, hand, feet, knees, and ankles. It occurs most often in men, has a strong association with the *HLA-B27* gene, and often follows (as a presumed immunologic reaction) urethritis caused by *C. trachomatis* or enteritis caused by *Campylobacter*, *Salmonella*, *Shigella*, or *Yersinia* spp. The onset can be acute, subacute, or chronic, and the diagnosis is made on clinical grounds.

Orthopedic Hardware Infections

Infections of prosthetic joints or of hardware used for stabilization of fractures can present with acute symptoms and signs or as pain, loosening of components, and subtle signs of inflammation months to years after implantation. Most infections result from wound contamination during surgery; clinical presentation is acute or subacute if caused by *S. aureus* but usually chronic if caused by coagulase-negative staphylococci. Rarely, infection is caused by wound dehiscence. Recent studies suggest that *S. aureus* bacteremia carries a substantial risk (18% to 60%) of infecting a preexisting prosthetic joint, which acts as a *locus minoris resistentiae*. Management of these infections is difficult and usually involves an orthopedic surgeon and an infectious diseases specialist working in concert with the primary care clinician.

Table 15-9 Some Ticks and Their Diseases in the United States

Tick	Appearance	Geographic Distribution	Characteristics	Diseases
American dog tick (*Dermacentor variabilis*)	Dark brown; rounded mouth parts	Widely distributed east of the Rocky Mountains and in limited areas on Pacific Coast	Favors trails and roadsides near clearings; commonly found on dogs	RMSF; human granulocytotropic ehrlichiosis; tularemia
Blacklegged tick (deer tick) (*Ixodes scapularis*)	Dark brown; long mouth parts	Northern form: eastern and central United States to Virginia; southern form: southern United States to Mexico	Favors edges of paths and roads; adults active in fall, winter, and spring; immature forms (nymphs) active in spring and summer	Northern form: Lyme disease, human granulocytotropic anaplasmosis; babesiosis (the feeding habits of the southern form make it an unlikely vector of human disease)
Lone star tick (*Amblyomma americanum*)	Red-brown; long mouth parts; white spot on the back of females	Southeastern and eastern United States	Bites aggressively in southern areas	Human monocytotropic ehrlichiosis; tularemia; STARI syndrome
Gulf Coast tick (*Amblyomma maculatum*)	Brown females with mouth parts and metallic markings on scutum*	Coastal areas along the Atlantic Coast and Gulf of Mexico	Bites aggressively	*Rickettsia parkeri* rickettsiosis (a form of spotted fever)
Rocky Mountain wood tick (*Dermacentor andersoni*)	Dark brown; white markings on scutum*	Rocky Mountains and adjacent areas	Favors bushy vegetation	RMSF; tularemia; tick paralysis
Western blacklegged tick (*Ixodes pacificus*)	Similar to *I. scapularis*	Canadian Pacific coast through California	Favors wild grasses and low vegetation in both urban and rural settings	Lyme disease; human granulocytotropic anaplasmosis; can also cause type I hypersensitivity reactions[†]
Relapsing fever ticks (*Ornithodoros turicata* and other species)	A gray soft tick up to 1 cm in diameter	Southwestern and south-central United States to northern Florida; Rocky Mountains	Found especially in rodent-infested rustic mountain cabins	Relapsing fever
Brown dog tick (*Rhipicephalus sanguineus*)	Red-brown; slightly longer than most other tick species	Probably the most widely distributed tick in the world	Dogs; prefers warm, dry, indoor conditions	RMSF
Amblyomma cajennense (Cayenne tick)	Mottled brown body; large black region on the abdomen of adult females	Southern United States, extending into Latin America and South America	Likes grassy areas with horses (a preferred host)	RMSF

*Scutum: a dorsal plate found on hard ticks.
[†]Type I hypersensitivity reactions: anaphylaxis, angioedema, urticaria, and bronchospasm.
RMSF, Rocky Mountain spotted fever; STARI, Southern tick-associated rash illness.

TICKBORNE DISEASES

As insect vectors for human disease, ticks rank first in North America and second to mosquitoes worldwide. A small number of the nearly 900 known species of ticks account for most tick-transmitted diseases of humans in North America (Table 15-9). Tick-related diseases occur mainly during the warmer parts of the year, peaking during the summer. Preventive measures include avoiding tick habitats during peak seasons; wearing light-colored clothing; covering most of the body (e.g., long-sleeved shirts, trousers, socks, and shoes); covering exposed areas with DEET-containing repellant; and checking the body (including the hair, neck, axilla, and genital areas) for ticks on a regular basis. The best way to remove a tick is to grasp the mouthparts (attachment point) with forceps and then pull gently until the tick releases. The use of chemicals or flames may cause the tick to break, potentially increasing the risk of transmission. The area should be cleaned thoroughly after ensuring removal of the entire tick, including the embedded mouth.

Rocky Mountain Spotted Fever

Rocky Mountain spotted fever, the most important life-threatening tickborne illness in the United States, is transmitted by several tick species (see Table 15-9). Five states (Arkansas, the Carolinas, Oklahoma, and Tennessee) account for 56% of cases. *Rickettsia rickettsii*, the causative organism, has a tropism for vascular endothelium, which explains at least in part the severe, generalized nature of the disease. After an incubation period of 2 days to 2 weeks, patients present with fever, chills, headache, malaise, myalgia, and other symptoms, often followed by multiorgan failure with seizures and coma. A maculopapular rash begins within 2 to 5 days on the extremities, classically involves the palms and soles, and evolves into a petechial rash. However, the rash may be absent in more than half of patients during the first week and never develops in up to 10% of patients (so-called "Rocky Mountain spotless fever"). The nonspecific presenting symptoms and signs present a diagnostic challenge. Common laboratory findings include thrombocytopenia, mild elevations in liver enzymes, and hyponatremia.

- Suspicion of RMSF should prompt strong consideration for empiric therapy with doxycycline because serum antibodies may not be detectable until 7 to 10 days after onset, and therapeutic delays increase the mortality rate. The remote risk of staining the teeth with a short course of doxycycline should not preclude its use in children (SOR: A).
- Chloramphenicol may be an alternative in severe disease but should be avoided in pregnancy (specifically the third trimester) given the risk of gray baby syndrome (SOR: A).

Ehrlichiosis and Anaplasmosis

Ehrlichiosis and anaplasmosis are caused by at least five species of obligate intracellular bacteria that infect and destroy WBCs (monocytes or neutrophils, depending on the species). The resulting tick-transmitted diseases in the United States include (1) *human monocytotropic ehrlichiosis* caused by *Ehrlichia chaffeensis*, (2) *human granulocytotropic ehrlichiosis* caused by *Ehrlichia ewingii*, and (3) *human granulocytotropic anaplasmosis* caused by *Anaplasma phagocytophilum* (see Table 15-9). After an incubation period of 1 to 2 weeks, patients present with some combination of fever, chills, headache, malaise, myalgia, gastrointestinal symptoms, cough, rash, and confusion. Common laboratory abnormalities are mild anemia, thrombocytopenia, leukopenia, and mild to moderate elevation of the aminotransferases. Characteristic morulae (clusters of bacteria) are sometimes seen in peripheral blood smears. Nucleic acid–based tests offer promise, but a retrospective diagnosis is usually based on serology, ideally on paired acute and chronic serum samples.

- Doxycycline is the drug of choice for both adults and children with ehrlichiosis or anaplasmosis.

Babesiosis

Babesiosis is a protozoan infection caused in the northeastern United States by *Babesia microti* and transmitted by two species of *Ixodes* tick or, rarely, by blood transfusion. Symptoms and signs of babesiosis include fever, chills, diaphoresis, malaise, fatigue, gastrointestinal symptoms, jaundice, mild splenomegaly, and rarely hepatomegaly. The disease is usually mild in immunocompetent persons but severe in asplenic or immunocompromised persons. Laboratory findings include hemolytic anemia, thrombocytopenia, mild elevations of the aminotransferases, and acute renal failure. The organisms can often be visualized within erythrocytes on peripheral smear, and *Babesia* DNA can be demonstrated in blood by PCR. Two-drug regimens are used for treatment; infectious diseases consultation should be considered.

Lyme Disease

Lyme disease is the most common tickborne infection in the United States, where it is caused by *Borrelia burgdorferi* and transmitted by two species of ticks (see Table 15-9). Symptoms and signs of the initial infection include malaise, headache, fever, myalgia, arthralgia, lymphadenopathy, and a rash known as erythema migrans (a "target" or "bull's eye" lesion with central clearing). Patients with disseminated disease may have cardiac conduction defects, myocarditis, transient oligoarthritis, seventh-nerve palsy (Bell palsy, which is sometimes bilateral), and meningitis or meningoencephalitis. Laboratory findings may include an elevated ESR and mild elevation of the aminotransferases. When meningitis is present, the CSF fluid typically shows a lymphocytic pleocytosis with mildly elevated protein and normal glucose. A single prophylactic dose of doxycycline (200 mg) may be given within 72 hours of confirmed tick exposure in highly endemic areas. Untreated patients are at risk of late complications, most commonly migratory arthritis commonly (85% of patients) involving the knee.

Most authorities agree that serologic testing for Lyme disease should be strongly discouraged for patients with nonspecific symptoms (e.g., fatigue and myalgia) who have not spent considerable time in a geographic area highly endemic for Lyme disease. Also, only the enzyme-linked immunosorbent assay (ELISA) test should be ordered. The result of the Western blot test (and, notably, the test for IgM antibodies by Western blot) is often false positive when the pretest probability of Lyme disease is low (as one would predict from Bayes' theorem).

- Drugs of choice for Lyme disease without CNS involvement are doxycycline, amoxicillin, and cefuroxime, given for 14 to 21 days (SOR: A).
- Ceftriaxone is the drug of choice for Lyme disease with CNS involvement (SOR: A).
- Controlled trials indicate that antibiotics are not useful for so-called "chronic Lyme disease," a controversial entity (SOR: A).

Tularemia

Tularemia can be transmitted by several tick species (see Table 15-9). The disease is classified on the basis of its portal of entry as ulceroglandular, glandular, oropharyngeal, oculoglandular, typhoidal, or pneumonic. Symptoms include fever, chills, headache, malaise, fatigue, anorexia, myalgia, chest discomfort, cough, sore throat, and gastrointestinal symptoms. Relative bradycardia is often present. Common laboratory findings are thrombocytopenia, hyponatremia, and elevations of the aminotransferases and creatine phosphokinase. The diagnosis is based on a fourfold change in antibody titer in paired sera or on the isolation of the organism, which, however, can be hazardous to laboratory personnel. A positive immunofluorescent antibody test result supports the diagnosis. Prophylaxis may be given with doxycycline after a confirmed exposure.

- Tularemia should be treated with streptomycin or gentamicin (SOR: A).

Emerging Tickborne Diseases

The *STARI* (Southern tick-associated rash illness) *syndrome* denotes a mild, flulike illness accompanied by a rash suggestive or typical of erythema migrans associated with a bite of the Lone Star tick and with negative serologic test results for Lyme disease. This syndrome was first described in Missouri and in the southeastern United States but now occurs in other regions such as the Midwest and the mid-Atlantic states. A spirochete, *Borrelia lonestari,* has been suspected but not proven to be the cause. Patients have been treated with doxycycline, but the efficacy of drug therapy is unknown because serious long-term consequences have not been established.

Powassan, so named after the town of Powassan, Ontario, where a young boy died from an apparently new disease, is caused by an RNA virus transmitted by various *Ixodes* ticks and by *Dermacentor* ticks. The disease presents as encephalitis, which is fatal in about 10% of cases and results in permanent neurologic deficits in about half of survivors. There have been about 50 known deaths in the United States at the time of this writing. Diagnostic tests have limited availability, and there is no known effective treatment.

American tick bite fever, also known as *Rickettsia parkeri* after the causative organism, features a maculopapular rash but can be differentiated from RMS by the presence of an eschar (a black wound) at the site of inoculation. The epidemiology and distribution of this disease in the United States remain to be elucidated. Doxycycline has been used for therapy.

364D rickettsiosis, a recently recognized disease, likewise features an eschar at the site of the tick bite. The distribution of the disease and the full spectrum of its manifestations remain to be determined.

FEVER OF UNCLEAR ORIGIN

Unexplained fevers are common in primary care, but most resolve within 1 or 2 weeks. The classic definition of FUO, known as the Petersdorf-Beeson criteria, consists of (1) an illness of at least 3 weeks' duration, (2) measured temperature greater than 38.3 °C (101 °F) on several occasions, and (3) no diagnosis after 1 week of intensive diagnostic efforts in the hospital. These criteria have been modified by today's emphasis on performing diagnostic procedures in ambulatory settings, and the spectrum of illnesses causing FUO continue to evolve as advances in imaging, microbiology, and serology enable earlier diagnosis. Various subsets of FUO (e.g., health care–associated FUO, immune-deficient FUO, and HIV-related FUO) are also recognized. There are more than 100 documented causes of "classic FUO," but even infectious diseases specialists see relatively few patients who fulfill the modified Petersdorf-Beeson criteria. Still, a general familiarity with the major causes of "true FUO" (Table 15-10) is useful because these disorders may be encountered in other ways. Patients whose FUO remains undiagnosed after intense evaluation often do well on long-term follow-up. Drugs should always be considered as causes of FUO in the ambulatory setting. The best approach is to discontinue all nonessential drugs; in most instances,

a definite downward trend in temperature occurs within 72 hours.

As a general rule, with the exception of elderly patients and patients receiving antiinflammatory drugs, it is useful to insist that "fever" be defined by a measured temperature of greater than 38.3 °C (101 °F). Extensive testing for lesser degrees of temperature elevation is usually unproductive unless patients have symptoms or signs strongly suggesting a disease of one or another category. A few patients present with prolonged (i.e., for more than several days) fever (temperature >38.3 °C [101 °F]) without localizing symptoms and signs, but a careful history and physical examination usually provide diagnostic clues.

Occasional patients exhibit *periodic fever,* defined by recurrent febrile illnesses usually lasting 1 to 3 days with fever-free intervals of at least 14 days. Some of these patients have hereditary periodic fever syndromes (e.g., familial Mediterranean fever, Muckle-Wells syndrome, hyperimmunoglobulin D syndrome, and TNF receptor-1–associated periodic syndrome); others are ultimately found to have a discernible cause, but in many cases, no cause is found, yet the patient remains well apart from the recurrent fevers.

Fever and Rash

Numerous diseases cause fever with rash or other lesions of the skin and mucous membranes (Table 15-11). *Adult Still disease* (see Table 15-10) and *acute rheumatic fever* (see Table 15-11) present with fever and arthritis or arthralgia, sometimes with a subtle rash. *Kawasaki disease,* a systemic vasculitis of unknown cause, mainly affects children but occasionally presents in adolescents and young adults. Patients should be hospitalized or referred to a consultant.

Leptospirosis, which in the United States occurs mainly in persons exposed to water or soil contaminated with animal urine, may cause a systemic disease with fever, chills, headache, nausea, vomiting, abdominal pain, and conjunctival suffusion. Patients who become jaundiced are at high risk of death from multiorgan failure. The diagnosis should be suspected in febrile patients potentially exposed to leptospirosis through such outdoor activities as farming, ranching, freshwater swimming, white-water rafting, or hunting.

Parvovirus B19 causes a characteristic "slapped cheek" rash in children (erythema infectiosum or fifth disease) but in adults is more likely to present with symmetric polyarthralgia or polyarthritis affecting mainly the small joints of the hands and feet and often accompanied by rashes that can be maculopapular, purpuric, or lacy and reticular. The diagnosis is made by demonstrating IgM antibodies. Parvovirus DNA can be demonstrated in blood by PCR, but positive results occur in otherwise healthy persons. The virus selectively infects red blood cell precursors, which can be disastrous in pregnant women, persons with high red blood cell turnover, and immunosuppressed persons.

Fever and Lymphadenopathy

Fever with lymphadenopathy has many potential causes, including malignancy (Table 15-12). Tender lymph nodes greater than 1.5 cm in diameter—especially if firm or fluctuant—usually signify a pathologic process. Lymph node biopsy is frequently appropriate when a diagnosis is not readily apparent by history; physical examination; and initial laboratory tests, including serologic tests. The more

Table 15-10 Some Causes of Classic Fever of Unknown Origin

Disease	Comments and Clues
INFECTIONS	
Tuberculosis	Mainly, disseminated (miliary) and extrapulmonary TB. Consider repeated physical examinations, bone marrow biopsy and culture, and liver biopsy and culture.
Intraabdominal abscess and other occult abscesses	Some cases remain elusive despite investigations with ultrasonography, CT, and MRI.
Hepatobiliary disease	Suggested by elevation of the serum alkaline phosphatase; consider recurrent bouts of ascending cholangitis (Charcot intermittent fever) caused by sepsis from gram-negative bacteria.
Endocarditis	Look for subtle clues in the skin and mucous membranes; apply protocols for evaluating suspected "culture-negative endocarditis" with various culture methods and serologic tests.
UTI	Atypical urinary tract infections include renal abscess (renal carbuncle) and perinephric abscess.
CMV infection	An important cause of FUO in younger persons who do not appear ill and have a paucity of physical findings; serology is helpful.
Miscellaneous infections	These include sinusitis, catheter-related infections, osteomyelitis, malaria, brucellosis, psittacosis, and disseminated fungal disease.
TUMORS	
Leukemias, lymphomas, and multiple myeloma	Look for the hectic "Pel-Ebstein" fever pattern of Hodgkin disease, although this is relatively uncommon; severe itching at night is a helpful clue.
Solid tumors	Carcinoma of the kidney may present as FUO without other manifestations. Many tumors cause fever when liver metastases are present.
CONNECTIVE TISSUE DISEASES	
Adult Still disease	Clues include a double-quotidian pattern (two fever spikes per day), sore throat, arthritis or arthralgia, lymphadenopathy, an evanescent salmon-pink rash, leukocytosis, and high serum ferritin level.
Temporal arteritis	A major cause of FUO, especially in older patients. Clues include diplopia or other visual symptoms, pain on chewing (intermittent masticatory claudication), and extremely high ESR (>100 mm/hr) or CRP.
Polyarteritis nodosa and other forms of vasculitis	Clues to polyarteritis include peripheral neuropathies (mononeuritis multiplex), renal involvement with active urine sediment, and occasionally eosinophilia. Other forms of vasculitis causing fever include hypersensitivity angiitis, Wegener granulomatosis, and vasculitis accompanying rheumatoid arthritis.
MISCELLANEOUS CAUSES	
Granulomatous diseases	Sarcoidosis, Crohn disease, and granulomatous hepatitis of unclear origin can cause FUO. Diagnosis requires biopsy and rigorous exclusion of infection.

CMV, Cytomegalovirus; *CRP*, C-reactive protein; *CT*, computed tomography; *ESR*, erythrocyte sedimentation rate; *FUO*, fever of unknown origin; *MRI*, magnetic resonance imaging; *TB*, tuberculosis; *UTI*, urinary tract infection.

Table 15-11 Some Diseases Associated with Fever and Rash

Disease	Morphology of Rash	Distribution of Rash
Acute rheumatic fever	Macules, erythema marginatum (erythematous, annular, or polycyclic macules that spread rapidly), subcutaneous nodules	Erythema marginatum on trunk or extremities; subcutaneous nodules on extensor surfaces near joints
Babesiosis	Petechiae, purpura, ecchymoses	Generalized
Coccidioidomycosis	Papules, nodules, plaques, ulcers, papulopustules	Head
Cryptococcosis	Papules, plaques, nodules, palpable purpura, cellulitis, pyoderma gangrenosum–like ulcers	Head and neck
Disseminated candidiasis	Erythematous papules and nodules	Trunk and extremities
Disseminated gonococcal infection	Macules, papules, vesicles, and petechiae initially, which may evolve into hemorrhagic vesiculopustules	Distal extremities, typically near an infected joint
Ecthyma gangrenosum and *Pseudomonas* sepsis	Erythematous to purpuric macules, hemorrhagic vesicles, bullae, nodules, or painless ulcers with a central necrotic, black eschar	Especially in axillary and anogenital regions
Ehrlichiosis	Usually, macules and papules; may be petechial; diffuse erythema is sometimes seen	Trunk
Epidemic typhus	Macules, papules, petechiae	Axillary folds, trunk, extremities (characteristically the face, palms, and soles are spared)
Herpes zoster and disseminated herpes zoster	Grouped vesicles on an erythematous base; hemorrhage bullae; in the disseminated form, large ulcers and plaques	Herpes zoster (shingles) has a dermatomal distribution; disseminated herpes zoster is generalized

Table 15-11 Some Diseases Associated with Fever and Rash (Continued)

Disease	Morphology of Rash	Distribution of Rash
Histoplasmosis	Ulcers, papules, plaques, purpura, abscesses, nodules, mucosal ulcerations	Generalized
Infective endocarditis	Petechiae, purpura, Osler nodes, Janeway lesions, splinter hemorrhages	Petechiae and purpura on heels, shoulders, legs, oral mucosa, conjunctivae; Osler nodes on digits (especially pulps of fingers and toes); Janeway lesions on palms and soles; splinter hemorrhages on nail plates
Kawasaki disease	Erythema (most often raised, deep red, plaquelike eruption); swelling of hands and feet; involvement of mucous membranes (dry, fissured lips, strawberry tongue; oropharyngeal erythema; conjunctival suffusion; later, desquamation)	Generalized, especially on trunk and extremities; accentuation in perineal area
Leptospirosis	Macules, papules, urticaria (wheals), purpura	Trunk
Lyme disease	Macules, papules, erythema chronicum (target or bulls-eye lesion)	Trunk, lower extremities; classically a single lesion but multiple lesions can be present
Meningococcemia and purpura fulminans	Petechiae, macules, papules, purpura (may become ecchymotic)	Generalized, especially on the lower extremities; neck and face usually spared
Murine typhus	Macules, papules, morbilliform rash	Begins on inner surfaces of arms and axillae; quickly becomes generalized, involving especially the trunk (limited involvement of face, palms, and soles)
Mycoplasma pneumoniae infection	Maculopapular or morbilliform rash most common; a variety of rashes can be seen, including urticaria, erythema multiforme (including Stevens-Johnson syndrome), erythema nodosum, and papulovesicular lesions	Variable
North American blastomycosis	Inflammatory papules and nodules with crusts; hyperkeratotic plaques with central ulceration	Face and extremities
Parvovirus B19 infection in children	"Slapped cheeks" rash (erythema infectiosum)	Face
Parvovirus B19 infection in adults	Variable: maculopapular, purpuric, or lacy and reticular	Usually the extremities, especially distal ("gloves and socks")
Primary HIV infection	Macules, papules, mucocutaneous ulcers, palatal papules	Face, trunk
Rat-bite fever caused by *Spirillum minus*	Maculopapular, later becoming petechial	Begins on abdomen; progresses to extremities; may involve palms and soles
Rat-bite fever caused by *Streptobacillus moniliformis*	Maculopapular or petechial	Most extensive on extremities; typically around joints; may become generalized
Rocky Mountain spotted fever	Macules, papules; later becomes petechial	Wrists and ankles initially, then palms and soles; finally, centripetal spread to face, trunk, and more proximal aspects of extremities
Scarlet fever (usually *Streptococcus pyogenes*)	Diffuse erythema with punctuate elevations ("sandpaper skin"); linear striations (Pastia lines) or confluent petechiae (which can be demonstrated on arms by applying a tourniquet)	Generalized, with sparing of area around mouth ("circumoral pallor")
Secondary syphilis	Macules, papules, mucous patches, condylomata lata; rash is sometimes pustular	Usually generalized with involvement of palms and soles; sometimes confined to palms and soles or to face
Staphylococcal toxic shock syndrome	Scarlatiniform rash (diffuse erythema, which can resemble sunburn); strawberry tongue; desquamation late in the course	Generalized
Streptococcal toxic shock syndrome	Localized area of cellulitis or necrotizing fasciitis; sometimes general erythema as well	Localized or generalized
Stevens-Johnson syndrome and toxic epidermal necrolysis	Macules, plaques, target lesions (both typical and atypical), vesicles, bullae, erosions and blisters of mucous membranes	Generalized
Typhoid fever *(Salmonella typhi)*	Slightly raised pink macules that blanch on pressure (rose spots)	Trunk, anteriorly and posteriorly (typically in crops of about 10 to 20 lesions)
Vibrio vulnificus infection	Large, hemorrhagic bullae are characteristic; also, cellulitis, lymphangitis	Especially on lower extremities

Table 15-12   Localized and Generalized Lymphadenopathy of Infectious Etiology

Lymph Node Group	Some Principal Considerations
Cervical	Pharyngitis of diverse causes, mycobacterial lymphadenitis (both TB and nontuberculous mycobacteria), Kawasaki disease, localized infections of the scalp, rubella (occipital lymphadenopathy)
Supraclavicular	Granulomatous diseases, including TB (supraclavicular and scale lymph nodes often indicate malignancy)
Axillary	Localized infection of the upper extremities, cat scratch disease
Subpectoral	When cellulitis or subpectoral abscess develops presentation can suggest an intraabdominal infection
Epitrochlear	Localized infection of upper extremities, cat scratch disease, sporotrichosis, herpetic whitlow
Inguinal and femoral	STDs (notably, syphilis, lymphogranuloma venereum, herpes simplex, and chancroid), localized infection of lower extremities
Iliac	Suppurative lymphadenitis with abscess formation, usually caused by *Staphylococcus aureus*; can be difficult to diagnose
All lymph nodes (generalized lymphadenopathy)	Heterophile-positive mononucleosis (EBV), heterophile-negative mononucleosis (CMV), HIV infection, secondary syphilis, TB, histoplasmosis, brucellosis, tularemia, measles, dengue

CMV, Cytomegalovirus; *EBV,* Epstein-Barr virus; *STD,* sexually transmitted disease; *TB,* tuberculosis.

common diseases causing fever and lymphadenopathy tend to have a benign course.

Cat scratch disease is a relatively common, slowly progressive, usually self-limited regional lymphadenitis caused by *Bartonella henselae* and mainly affecting children who have had contact with a cat (typically a kitten or feral cat). Tender, occasionally suppurative lymphadenopathy occurs most often in the cervical or axillary regions. A single lymph node is involved in about half of cases. Complications include *Parinaud's ocular glandular syndrome* (granulomatous conjunctivitis with preauricular lymphadenitis), atypical pneumonia, granulomatous hepatitis, prolonged fever, encephalopathy, neuroretinitis (with star-shaped macular exudates), and osteomyelitis. Serologic testing for IgM and IgG antibodies has a 95% sensitivity and 98% specificity for diagnosis.

Toxoplasmosis in immunocompetent persons can present mainly as fever and lymphadenitis. Cats are the usual source of infection (mainly by cleaning litter boxes), but ingestion of undercooked meat (including lamb in many countries and venison in the United States) can also transmit the disease. Testing for IgM antibodies spares the patient the need for lymph node biopsy, which, if done, usually shows prominent clusters of epithelioid histiocytes surrounding the germinal centers.

HIV/AIDS

Since its recognition in 1981, HIV infection and its end-stage manifestation, AIDS, have become global concerns, affecting more than 34 million people worldwide and more than 1.1 million people in the United States, where about 50,000 new infections occur each year. About 50% of HIV-infected persons worldwide and about 15% of HIV-infected persons in the United States are unaware of their infection. HIV disease, which is spread mainly by sexual contact but also by blood exposure and mother-to-child transmission, disproportionately affects African Americans and Hispanics and Latinos.

Combination antiretroviral therapy (ART) has transformed HIV from a uniformly fatal disease to a chronic condition that is well tolerated provided the patient complies with therapy. Primary care clinicians are pivotal to early diagnosis, comprehensive care, and prevention.

Management in the primary care setting reduces the stigma of the disease and helps patients cope with attendant mood disorders, life adjustments, and social problems. Primary care clinicians who wish to assume responsibility for all aspects of the disease, including the selection of ART regimens, must invest time and effort to stay current with this rapidly evolving area of medicine. Most family medicine clinicians will find it advantageous to manage HIV-infected patients in partnership with a physician who makes this disease a substantial part of his or her practice (or, in many communities, an HIV treatment center).

HIV belongs to the viral group Retroviridae (retroviruses) and subgroup Lentiviridae (lentiviruses). Its RNA genome undergoes frequent mutations; although the average time for viral replication is about 2 days, about 10^7 mutations take place every minute leading to genetic variations. Such variations mandate strict adherence to a multidrug ART regimen to delay the emergence of drug-resistant strains. After initial infection, there is a burst of viral replication with a high level of viremia. Some, but not all, patients develop within 2 to 4 weeks (range, 1 to 6 weeks) the acute retroviral syndrome, which may present as a flulike illness, sometimes with a maculopapular rash; as a heterophile-negative mononucleosis syndrome (occasionally the Monospot test result is false positive); or as aseptic meningitis. The patient then remains asymptomatic for months to years but is fully capable of spreading the virus to others. The quantitative HIV RNA level (viral load) declines from its postinfectious peak and becomes relatively stable at a "set point" reflecting a balance between viral replication and the host response. The CD4 count gradually declines, and because CD4+ T lymphocytes are crucial to cell-mediated immunity, severe complications or death usually results after months to years (median, 2 to 3 years; range 1 to >15 years). AIDS is defined by a CD4 count less than $200/mm^3$ or by certain opportunistic infections or tumors that seldom occur in immunocompetent persons. Advances in therapy make the distinction between "HIV infection" and "AIDS" less relevant than was formerly the case.

Diagnosis of HIV Infection

HIV-infected persons come to medical attention either as a result of testing for infection or seeking help for symptoms and signs of illness. The United States Prevention Services

Task Force and the CDC now recommend voluntary testing in all health care settings after informing individuals and allowing them to opt out. Early diagnosis increases access to care and enables earlier treatment, delaying progression and reducing the risk of transmission. In the past, serologic diagnosis depended on an ELISA test followed by a confirmatory Western blot test. Newer fourth-generation HIV enzyme immunoassay (EIA) tests detect both HIV antibodies and the HIV p24 antigen, on average 6 to 7 days after infection. Rapid screening tests are inexpensive, quick, and easy to perform (<20 minutes' turnaround time), require no instrumentation, and are CLIA waived.

Testing for HIV is strongly recommended when patients between the ages of 13 and 64 years present with any of the following: (1) STDs; (2) constitutional symptoms such as fever, night sweats, anorexia, and weight loss; (3) thrush (oropharyngeal candidiasis); (4) herpes zoster in persons younger than 50 years of age; (5) asymptomatic generalized lymphadenopathy; and (5) oral hairy leukoplakia (white spike-like lesions on the lateral edges of the tongue, which represent crystals of EBV). HIV-infected persons are more likely to have severe or prolonged aphthous stomatitis and any of several skin conditions, including seborrheic dermatitis, psoriasis, molluscum contagiosum, recurrent herpes simplex, and folliculitis.

P. jiroveci pneumonia, the opportunistic infection that in June 1981 brought what is now called HIV/AIDS to world attention, remains a common presentation in persons who have not sought HIV testing or, if tested, were lost to follow-up. The onset is often insidious over weeks to even months with cough, shortness of breath, and low-grade fever. Chest radiography classically shows diffuse bilateral infiltrates, but findings may be normal in up to 30% of patients. The causative organism, now considered a fungus rather than a protozoan, can often be demonstrated in induced sputum or specimens obtained by bronchoalveolar lavage. Many, and perhaps most, patients are now treated empirically when the disease is suggested by symptoms, signs, hypoxemia, and elevation of the serum lactic dehydrogenase level. High-dose TMP-SMX is the treatment of choice in patients without a history of hypersensitivity to sulfa drugs and is supplemented with corticosteroids when hypoxemia is severe ($PaO_2 \leq 70$ mm Hg on room air). Other AIDS-defining infections include cryptococcosis, CNS toxoplasmosis (usually with multiple ring-enhancing mass lesions on CT or MRI), CMV retinitis, and disseminated *M. avium* complex disease, for which a single AFB blood culture has a 90% to 95% sensitivity. Other patients seek medical attention because of multiple firm, slightly raised or nodular, 0.5- to 2-cm violaceous or dark red skin lesions determined on biopsy to be Kaposi sarcoma.

Initial Management of HIV Disease

Diagnosis of HIV disease should prompt education about the nature of the disease, reassurance of the possibility of a near-normal life *contingent on* adherence to a drug regimen, and aggressive follow-up with peer and substance counselors and the local health department for contact investigation. All new patients should have the following tests: CD4 count, quantitative HIV RNA (viral load), HIV genotype test (to screen for drug resistance), CBC, serum creatinine (and calculated creatinine clearance), urinalysis, tuberculin skin test (or interferon-γ release assay), anti-*Toxoplasma* IgG serology, hepatitis B screening (HBsAg, anti-HBsAg, anti-HBc, with vaccination against HBV for those who are susceptible to infection), hepatitis C virus antibody (with quantitative HCV RNA if positive), serology for syphilis (RPR), screening for gonorrhea and chlamydia infection, and chest radiography. Patients other than men who have sex with men (who can be assumed to be CMV seropositive) should have serology for CMV (anti-CMV IgG), and all women should have a cervical Pap test screening for trichomoniasis (SOR: A) (Aberg et al., 2014).

It is now recommended that ART be prescribed to *all* HIV-infected patients. At the time of this writing (February 2014), three one-pill, once-daily regimens are available, Atripla (efavirenz plus tenofovir plus emtricitabine), Complera (rilpivirine plus tenofovir plus emtricitabine), and Stribild (elvitegravir plus cobicistat plus tenofovir plus emtricitabine) (Johnson and Saravolatz, 2014). Optimally, the family physician, the consultant, and the patient should share (and maintain individually) a flow sheet with four columns: the date, the patient's CD4 count (CD4+ T lymphocyte count/mm^3 of blood), the patient's viral load (copies of HIV viral RNA/mm^3 of blood), and the patient's ART drug regimens. Monitoring therapy includes not only CD4 counts and viral loads but also watching for drug side effects such as dyslipidemia, glucose intolerance, and renal abnormalities. Patients should receive routine vaccines, including annual flu shots; should receive the pneumococcal vaccine; and should be vaccinated against hepatitis B if they lack anti-HBsAg antibodies.

Patients who are stable on ART with suppressed viral loads and CD4 counts greater than 200 per mm^3 for more than 2 to 3 years can be seen as infrequently as every 6 months, with monitoring of their viral loads every 6 months (SOR: A) and CD4 counts every 6 to 12 months (SOR: B). Recently diagnosed patients, those with acute illnesses, and those who are failing ART or who have recently changed ART need to be seen more frequently. The viral load should be monitored more frequently after initiation or change in ART (preferably within 2 to 4 weeks and no longer than 8 weeks, with repeat testing every 4 to 8 weeks until the viral load becomes undetectable) (SOR: B). Because the CD4 count can fluctuate up to 30%, at least two CD4 counts 4 to 8 weeks apart are necessary to assess the immunologic stage of the patient's disease.

KEY TREATMENT

- All patients with confirmed HIV disease should be treated with highly active antiretroviral drugs (SOR: B).
- Patients with HIV disease must understand the extreme importance of compliance with their drug regimens (SOR: A).

Pregnancy and HIV

All HIV-infected women of childbearing age should be asked about their desires regarding pregnancy upon initiation of care and regularly thereafter. Pregnant women should receive ART, irrespective of their immunologic or virologic status, to prevent infection of the fetus (SOR: A). Infants exposed to HIV in utero should receive antiretroviral postexposure prophylaxis and undergo HIV diagnostic testing at 10 to 21 days of life, 1 to 2 months of age, and 4 to 6 months of age (SOR: B).

Postexposure Prophylaxis

Postexposure prophylaxis (PEP) should be considered for health care workers and others who may have been exposed to HIV-infected blood during work or line of duty and also for those who may have been exposed by sexual assault, unprotected casual sex, or sex with a partner considered at high risk for infection. PEP should be given as soon as possible; logic suggests "the sooner the better," and animal models suggest PEP is unlikely to work if initiated more than 72 hours after exposure. When persons seek PEP, two questions should be asked:

1. Was the exposure risky? All sexual exposures should be considered risky, but in other settings, risky exposures are defined as blood contact by percutaneous injury (especially if blood was present in hollow needle); blood contact by splash to mucous membranes (eyes, mouth, and nose); or contact of nonintact skin with blood, tissue, or potentially infected body fluids.
2. Was the source risky? The source patient should be identified and tested for HIV, preferably with a rapid test.

If the answer to both questions is yes, drugs should be given. Because anxiety runs high after potential exposure to HIV, it is often best to start PEP when the facts are unclear or the patient is in doubt, deferring for one to several days the decision whether to complete the 28-day course.

KEY TREATMENT

- Recommended PEP for HIV at the time of this writing is the combination of twice-daily raltegravir (Isentress) and once-daily tenofovir–emtricitabine (Truvada) (Kuhar et al., 2013) (SOR: B).

Preexposure Prophylaxis

In June 2012, based on studies in heterosexual and homosexual persons, the FDA approved the use of tenofovir plus emtricitabine (TDF–FTC) for the prevention of HIV transmission among sexually active individuals at high risk for HIV transmission.

Pathogens

The purpose of this section is to help family physicians round out their understanding of infectious diseases and to review briefly some pathogens not discussed elsewhere in this chapter.

DRUG-RESISTANT AND UNUSUAL BACTERIA

Drug-resistant bacteria are now commonplace (John and Steed, 2013). Some infections have become untreatable because of a lack of any effective antibiotic.

MRSA is perhaps the most problematic bacterial pathogen now seen in family medicine. The distinction between hospital-acquired and community-acquired MRSA strains

Key Points

- Problematic drug-resistant bacteria include MRSA, vancomycin-resistant *Enterococcus faecium*, uropathogenic T131 strains of *E. coli*, and gram-negative bacilli expressing extended-spectrum β-lactamases and carbapenemases.
- Eight human herpesviruses are now recognized; HHV-6 causes roseola infantum (sixth disease), a major cause of febrile seizures in young children, and HHV-8 causes Kaposi sarcoma in patients with advanced HIV disease.
- *Candida albicans* remains susceptible to fluconazole, but *Candida krusei* is intrinsically resistant to fluconazole, and up to 25% of *Candida glabrata* strains are now resistant.
- Cryptococcal meningitis and tuberculous meningitis should be considered in patients with chronic or persistent headache and neurologic signs, including slow deterioration of mental function.
- Primary care clinicians who live in regions endemic for histoplasmosis, blastomycosis, or coccidioidomycosis should be thoroughly familiar with these diseases and their protean manifestations.
- Although TB remains problematic in certain populations in the United States, a positive acid-fast bacillus stain or culture is now more likely to indicate a nontuberculous mycobacterium.
- Malaria caused by *Plasmodium falciparum* is the most common cause of infection-related death in returning U.S. travelers and constitutes a medical emergency.

is becoming blurred, but the latter are often susceptible to broad-spectrum antibiotics such as TMP-SMX, doxycycline, and clindamycin. MRSA strains are often less susceptible to vancomycin (minimum inhibitory concentration [MIC] ≥2 μg/mL) than was formerly the case. Serious infections caused by such strains are often treated with high-dose vancomycin (aiming for trough serum levels of 20 μg/mL or higher), daptomycin (for nonpulmonary infections), or linezolid. Recent studies demonstrate that infectious diseases consultation and use of an evidence-based bundle reduce the mortality rate from *S. aureus* bacteremia (López-Cortés et al., 2013; Schmidt et al., 2014).

Coagulase-negative staphylococci are the most problematic bacteria for implant surgeons because of their ability to promote formation of biofilms ("slime") around devices of all types, including prosthetic joints, prosthetic heart valves, cardiac pacemakers and defibrillators, vascular access catheters, CSF shunts, and others. Device removal is usually necessary. Coagulase-negative staphylococci are often multiresistant and, similar to MRSA, often show reduced susceptibility to vancomycin. Of more than 16 species of CNS, *S. epidermidis* is the most common and *S. lugdunesis* the most aggressive.

Enterococci have always posed therapeutic problems (especially when causing endocarditis), but the emergence of vancomycin-resistant enterococci (VRE, which are usually *E. faecium* rather than the more common *E. faecalis*) presents therapeutic dilemmas.

The α-hemolytic and nonhemolytic "viridians" streptococci, similar to enterococci, are commensal organisms that assume clinical importance mainly as causes of endocarditis or infections in patients with deficient host defenses. These organisms are often less susceptible to penicillin G and ampicillin than was formerly the case. A subgroup of viridans streptococci variably known as the *Streptococcus anginosus* or *Streptococcus milleri* group is capable of causing severe infections, including brain abscess and pneumonia.

S. pneumoniae (the pneumococcus) often shows low-level (and occasionally high-level) resistance to penicillin and the third-generation cephalosporins, prompting the recommendation for combined therapy with ceftriaxone and vancomycin for life-threatening pneumococcal pneumonia and for pneumococcal meningitis.

Aerobic gram-negative bacilli now commonly resist many antibiotics, and occasionally all antibiotics. In many U.S. communities, *E. coli* resistance to ampicillin exceeds 50%, resistance to the fluoroquinolones exceeds 30%, and many isolates are resistant to TMP-SMX and other agents. Uropathogenic T131 strains (see Table 15-8) have previously been discussed. Gram-negative bacilli become resistant to the β-lactam antibiotics (see Table 15-2) by producing β-lactamase enzymes, of which there are several families: penicillinases, cephalosporinases, broad-spectrum β-lactamases, extended-spectrum β-lactamases, and carbapenemases. Carbapenemases are of concern because the carbapenems (see Table 15-2) are often the last resort for gram-negative bacillary infection. Isolates of *P. aeruginosa*, *Acinetobacter* spp., and other gram-negative bacilli are frequently resistant to aminoglycoside antibiotics.

Anaerobic bacteria are usually treated empirically because most hospital laboratories do not offer routine susceptibility testing. Historically, chloramphenicol, then clindamycin, and now metronidazole have been the drugs of choice especially for infections likely to involve the *Bacteroides fragilis* group of anaerobic bacteria. *B. fragilis* has now demonstrated its ability to be metronidazole resistant. Other anaerobes that may exhibit unique susceptibility patterns include *Prevotella*, *Fusobacterium*, and *Clostridium* spp., *Bilophila wadsworthia*, and *Sutterella wadsworthensis* (Brook et al., 2013).

Family physicians should have passing familiarity with certain infrequently isolated bacteria. Helpful acronyms include HACEK for certain fastidious gram-negative bacteria that sometimes cause endocarditis (*Haemophilus parainfluenzae*, *Haemophilus aphrophilus*, *Haemophilus paraphrophilus*, *Actinobacillus actinomycemcomitans*, *Aggregatibacter aphrophilus*, *Corynebacterium hominis*, *Eikenella corrodens*, and *Kingella kingae*) and MYSPACE for aerobic gram-negative bacilli that often pose problems because of drug resistance (*Morganella morganii*, *Yersinia enterocolitica*, *Serratia marcescens*, *Providencia* species, *Proteus vulgaris*, *P. aeruginosa*, *Acinetobacter* spp., *Citrobacter* spp., and *Enterobacter* spp.).

Higher bacteria of clinical importance—called "higher" because they produce branching, filamentous forms resembling fungi—are the *Actinomycetes* (anaerobic bacteria that cause actinomycosis) and *Nocardia* spp. (obligate aerobic bacteria that cause nocardiosis). *Actinomyces* species produce characteristic "sulfur granules," and *Nocardia* spp. are often recognized microscopically by their weakly acid-fast branching filaments. The classical clinical presentations of actinomycosis are cervicofacial, pulmonary, and intraabdominal disease, typically with draining sinus tracts. Nocardiosis causes pneumonia and brain abscess and opportunistic infection in immunocompromised persons.

HERPESVIRUSES

The herpesviruses are large DNA viruses that establish lifelong latent infection by poorly understood processes. Nearly 100 herpesviruses have been isolated from various animal species, eight of which are currently recognized as human pathogens (Table 15-13). Transmission usually involves person-to-person contact with transfer of an infected body fluid onto a susceptible tissue such as the eye, mouth, respiratory tract, or urogenital mucosa. Several classes of antiviral drugs are available, all of which should be used with

---

Table 15-13 Human Herpesviruses

Herpesvirus	Virus	Major Diseases	Route of Transmission
1	Herpes simplex type 1	Herpes labialis, herpes stomatitis, keratitis, skin lesions (herpes gladiatorum; herpes whitlow), genital ulcers, encephalitis, multiple congenital abnormalities	Close contact for both types; sexual contact especially for type 2; skin-to-skin contact in other forms, including herpes gladiatorum
2	Herpes simplex type 2		
3	Varicella-zoster virus	Varicella; herpes zoster (localized and disseminated); pneumonia, encephalitis, myelitis, cerebellar ataxia	Contact or respiratory
4	Epstein-Barr virus	Heterophile-positive mononucleosis, lymphomas, nasopharyngeal carcinoma, meningoencephalitis, lymphoproliferative syndrome (transplant recipients)	Saliva
5	Cytomegalovirus	Heterophile-negative mononucleosis; fever of unknown origin; in immunocompromised patients, retinitis, colitis, radiculopathy; multiple congenital abnormalities	Contact; bloodborne; transplantation; congenital
6	Herpes lymphotropic virus	Roseola infantum (exanthema subitum) in children (HHV-6B); numerous possible associations with various diseases including multiple sclerosis	Contact or respiratory
7	HHV-7	Fever, rash, and febrile seizures in children	Unknown
8	HHV-8	Kaposi sarcoma (common) and primary effusion lymphoma (uncommon) in persons with HIV disease; may also cause multicentric Castleman disease	Possible exchange of body fluids

HHV, Human herpesvirus.

careful attention to routes of elimination, side effects, and drug–drug interactions,

In family medicine, antiviral drug therapy for herpesvirus infections consists almost entirely of nucleotide analogues: acyclovir, valacyclovir, famciclovir, ganciclovir, and valganciclovir. The oral bioavailability of acyclovir is only about 10% to 20% and decreases as the dose is increased. Valacyclovir is a prodrug of acyclovir that is almost completely converted to acyclovir after oral administration. Similarly, the oral bioavailability of ganciclovir is only about 5%; valganciclovir is a prodrug with superior oral bioavailability. Other drugs active against herpesviruses include cidofovir and foscarnet; these are used in special situations (Evans et al., 2013; Field and Vere Hodge, 2013).

Human Herpesviruses 1 and 2 (HSV-1 and HSV-2)

Human herpesviruses 1 and 2 are commonly known as HSV-1 and HSV-2. These viruses cause ulcers of the lips (herpes labialis) and buccal mucosa (herpes stomatitis), keratitis, skin lesions (e.g., herpetic whitlow involving the fingers, or herpes gladiatorum involving any part of the body), encephalitis (especially HSV-1), aseptic meningitis (especially HSV-2), congenital disease of the newborn, pneumonia (rare), and—of greatest concern to family physicians—lesions of the genital tract. The characteristic lesion is a vesicle on an erythematous base. Vesicular lesions are typically grouped and may be confluent. A survey of men and women age 14 to 49 years between 2005 and 2010 revealed a 54% seroprevalence of HSV-1 and a 16% seroprevalence of HSV-2.

Genital lesions are predominantly caused by HSV-2, but HSV-1 causes a significant percentage of cases. Genital herpes simplex affects about one in six persons in the United States between the ages of 14 and 49 years and is usually acquired by sexual contact, although oral-to-genital transmission occurs. Primary genital herpes often begins with fever, chills, headache, malaise, and localized pain or paresthesia before the appearance of the highly characteristic grouped vesicles. Involvement of the vulva can be especially painful. Extragenital manifestations include disturbances of bowel and bladder function; extensive ulcerations of the buttock, groin, and thighs; aseptic meningitis; transverse myelitis; and sacral radiculopathy.

Serologic testing is generally unhelpful. Viral culture is highly sensitive if done during the vesicle stage of the disease. However, PCR has become the diagnostic procedure of choice. Determining whether genital herpes is caused by HSV-1 or HSV-2 has prognostic implications because HSV-2 is associated with more frequent recurrences. All patients should receive counseling, as should asymptomatic sex partners.

KEY TREATMENT

- Antiviral drugs (acyclovir and valacyclovir) reduce the severity and duration of symptoms during the first episode of genital herpes but do not reduce the frequency of recurrence or the risk of transmission to others (SOR: A).
- Recurrent episodes of genital herpes, for which famciclovir is also approved, can be treated episodically or with continuous suppressive therapy (SOR: B).
- Strains of HSV-1 and HSV-2 resistant to the above agents are uncommon in primary care; foscarnet is usually effective but has significant nephrotoxicity (SOR: B).

Varicella-Zoster Virus

Varicella-zoster virus causes chickenpox (varicella) and shingles (herpes zoster), the latter usually resulting from reactivation of latent virus in a dorsal root ganglion. Varicella is highly contagious. Before the advent of routine vaccination in 1995, varicella typically occurred in preschool and school-aged children. A prodrome with fever, headache, and sore throat is followed by the widespread appearance of vesiculopustules on an erythematous base. The hallmark of varicella is the presence of lesions in all stages of development—in contrast to smallpox, in which the lesions are at the same stage of development at a given time. Patients are contagious 1 to 2 days before the onset of the rash and remain contagious until all of the lesions are crusted, typically 4 to 7 days after appearance. Most cases in immunocompetent persons are self-limited. Complications include secondary bacterial infections (including necrotizing fasciitis caused by group A streptococci), pneumonia, cerebellar ataxia, and encephalitis. The virus is dangerous during pregnancy; it can cause severe pneumonia in the mother, loss of the fetus, and—in cases of severe material varicella during the first half of pregnancy—a fetal varicella syndrome with irreversible abnormalities.

Herpes zoster (shingles) occurs mainly in older and immunocompromised persons, with an annual incidence in the United States of about four cases per 1000 persons. The dermatomal distribution of the vesiculopustular rash is virtually diagnostic. Complications include postherpetic neuralgia (the incidence of which sharply increases with age), ocular involvement (herpes zoster ophthalmicus, which should prompt urgent referral to an ophthalmologist), ear involvement with facial paralysis (the Ramsay Hunt syndrome), skin and soft tissue infections (including, again, necrotizing fasciitis), meningoencephalitis, pneumonia, hepatitis, acute retinal necrosis, and death—especially when the disease appears in disseminated form in immunocompromised persons.

KEY TREATMENT

- Acyclovir, if started within the first 24 hours, can reduce the severity and duration of varicella (SOR: A).
- Antiviral drug therapy reduces the incidence of postherpetic neuralgia (SOR: B).
- Administration of varicella vaccine to a susceptible child within 3 days of exposure may modify or prevent disease (SOR: A).
- Older (>60 years) immunocompetent persons should be urged to receive the varicella-zoster (shingles) vaccine even if they previously had herpes zoster (SOR: A).

Epstein-Barr Virus and Cytomegalovirus

These clinically important viruses, the respective causes of heterophile-positive and heterophile-negative mononucleosis, have been previously discussed in this chapter; some additional manifestations are shown in Table 15-13. Deep

Table 15-14 Selected Antifungal Drugs

Antimicrobial Class (Action)	Selected Agents	Selected Comments
Polyenes (bind to ergosterol in fungal cell membranes, disrupting the steric integrity of the membrane)	**Amphotericin preparations:** Amphotericin B deoxycholate, amphotericin B lipid complex, amphotericin B cholesteryl sulfate, amphotericin B liposomal **Agents for oral or topical use:** Nystatin, candicidin, others	Amphotericin B deoxycholate revolutionized the treatment of deep fungal infections but is nephrotoxic. Other toxicities include infusion-related fever, nausea, vomiting, and hypotension; hypokalemia and hypomagnesemia; metabolic acidosis; and nephrogenic diabetes insipidus. The newer "lipid formulations" are less toxic but much more expensive.
Antimetabolite pyrimidine analogue (disturbs binding of essential proteins; inhibits fungal DNA synthesis)	Flucytosine	Initially developed as an antimetabolite, flucytosine has significant myelotoxicity, including fatal bone marrow failure. Serum levels should ideally be monitored when therapy is prolonged, especially in patients with impaired renal function.
Azole compounds (inhibit lanosterol demethylase, a cytochrome enzyme of the P450 group, blocking synthesis of ergosterol)	**Imidazoles:** Ketoconazole, others **Triazoles:** Fluconazole, itraconazole, voriconazole, others	Toxicity in humans derives largely from effect on P450 enzymes. Use should take into account all drugs the patient is taking because of the potential for serious drug interactions.
Echinocandins (inhibit glucan synthesis in the cell wall by the enzyme 1,3-β glucan synthase)	Anidulafungin, caspofungin, micafungin	More reliable coverage against *all* Candida spp. than fluconazole No clinically useful activity against *Cryptococcus* spp. Potential for drug–drug interactions Generally well tolerated
Allylamines (inhibit squalene epoxidase, an enzyme required for ergosterol synthesis)	Terbinafine, amorolfine, butenafine, naftifine	Mainly used for topical therapy for dermatologic conditions such as ringworm, athlete's foot, and tinea cruris (jock itch) Rare indications for systemic use
Griseofulvin (small molecule unrelated to other antifungals; binds to keratin precursor cells; on entering fungi, interferes with microtubules, thus inhibiting mitosis)	Griseofulvin	Mainly used for oral therapy of dermatophytosis with severe involvement of nails, hair, or large body surface areas Contraindicated in pregnancy, severe liver disease, systemic lupus erythematosus, and porphyria Antagonizes oral anticoagulants and contraceptives Decreases absorption of phenobarbital

infections caused by CMV, which occur mainly in immunocompromised patients, require referral; drugs include ganciclovir, valganciclovir, cidofovir, and foscarnet.

Other Human Herpesviruses

HHV-6 B, discovered in 1986, causes the childhood illness *roseola infantum* (also known as *exanthema subitum* or "sixth disease"), which is perhaps the most common cause of febrile seizures in children between the ages of 6 and 24 months. About 95% of adults are seropositive for HHV-7, but its role in disease is unclear. HHV-8 has emerged as the apparent cause of *Kaposi sarcoma* in HIV-infected persons, in whom it also causes *primary effusion lymphoma*. HHV-8 may also cause *multicentric Castleman disease*.

FUNGI

Only about 150 of the nearly 250,000 identified species of fungi are known to cause disease. Noninvasive, superficial fungal infections of the skin and related structures (dermatophytosis) are discussed in the chapter on dermatology. Here we will mainly discuss candidiasis; sporotrichosis; and the "deep" mycoses, including the three major "regional" mycoses in the United States: histoplasmosis, coccidioidomycosis, and blastomycosis. The major antifungal drugs are shown in Table 15-14.

Candidiasis

Candidiasis, commonly known among the laity as "yeast infection," encompasses a wide range of mucosal, skin, and nail infections. Oral candidiasis (thrush) takes several forms: pseudomembranous, erythematous, and hyperplastic candidiasis; denture-related stomatitis (involving Candida spp. in about 90% of cases), angular stomatitis (involving *Candida* spp., often as a mixed infection with *S. aureus*, in about 80% of cases), and median rhomboid glossitis. Candida vulvovaginitis is discussed in the chapter on gynecology; its male counterpart is candidal balanitis—infection of the glans penis, usually in persons who are uncircumcised. The multiple forms of cutaneous candidiasis and nail infection (onychomycosis) are covered in the chapter on dermatology. Esophageal candidiasis is a major problem in advanced HIV/AIDS infection and is usually treated with azole compounds (fluconazole or others, see Table 15-14).

Candida bloodstream infection (candidemia) is most likely to present in primary care practices as sepsis related to vascular access devices, especially in patients receiving hyperalimentation. Removal of the access device must be supplemented with antifungal drugs. *Candida albicans*, which is nearly always susceptible to fluconazole, is the most common isolate, but other *Candida* species may come into play. *Candida krusei* is intrinsically resistant to fluconazole and should be considered a distinct possibility whenever a patient who has recently taken fluconazole has a positive blood culture for *Candida* spp. Up to 25% of *Candida glabrata* isolates are now resistant to fluconazole. Complications of invasive candidiasis include endophthalmitis with the potential for permanent vision loss, osteomyelitis, and septic arthritis. *Candida* peritonitis results from infection of a peritoneal dialysis catheter but also occurs in patients with intraabdominal infection or necrotizing pancreatitis. *Candida* endocarditis usually occurs in patients with prosthetic heart valves; blood cultures may be sterile despite large vegetations with potential to cause embolism to major arteries.

- The isolation of *Candida* spp. from a blood culture should prompt a request to the laboratory for speciation, and empiric therapy either with fluconazole (if the patient is not severely ill and the likelihood of *C. krusei* or *C. glabrata* is low) or an echinocandin compound (SOR: A).
- Amphotericin B remains an alternative, with the caveat that 2 *Candida* spp.—*Candida lusitaniae* and *Candida guilliermondi*—are often resistant to amphotericin B (or will develop resistance during therapy) (SOR: A).

Cryptococcosis

There are more than 30 known species of *Cryptococcus*, of which two, *Cryptococcus neoformans* and *Cryptococcus gattii*, are recognized human pathogens. The former has a worldwide distribution and is the usual cause of disease; the latter has a more local distribution, including the Pacific Northwest in the United States and British Columbia in Canada. Similar to most deep fungal infections, cryptococcosis is usually acquired by inhalation. Pulmonary disease, which can resemble pneumonia or even metastatic cancer, is sometimes discovered accidentally on a chest radiograph taken for another reason. Meningitis is the most common clinical manifestation of cryptococcosis in both immunocompetent and immunocompromised persons. Between 80% and 90% of recognized cases of cryptococcal meningitis now occur in persons with HIV/AIDS, and other cases are associated with corticosteroid therapy, lymphomas, or other conditions that suppress T-cell immunity. Immunologically intact persons with cryptococcal meningitis sometimes give a history of exposure to accumulations of aged bird droppings, such as roosting sites, attics, or vacant old buildings.

- Initial therapy for cryptococcal meningitis should be started in the hospital and usually consists of amphotericin B plus flucytosine whether for immunocompromised persons (SOR: A) or immunocompetent persons (SOR: B), for whom high-dose fluconazole is an alternative.

Sporotrichosis

Sporotrichosis, caused by *Sporothrix schenckii*, is encountered in primary care mainly as the syndrome of nodular lymphangitis—nodular swellings along the path of lymphatic vessels, often with recognizable linear streaks (Figure 15-11). Less commonly, this syndrome is caused by *Nocardia brasiliensis*, *Mycobacterium marinum*, *Leishmania* spp., *Francisella tularensis*, *Mycobacterium kansasii*, and various other fungi and pyogenic bacteria, including staphylococci and streptococci. Biopsy or aspiration of tissue for culture is usually required for determining the causative organism.

- Itraconazole is the drug of choice for sporotrichosis (SOR: A).

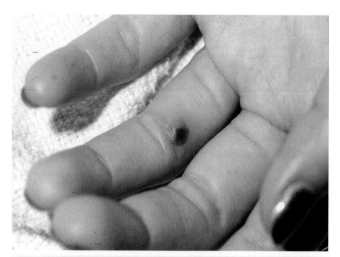

Figure 15-11. Hemorrhagic vesicular lesion on an erythematous base in a patient with the gonococcal arthritis–dermatitis syndrome. The lesion will rupture, leaving a tender, necrotic nodule.

Histoplasmosis

Histoplasma capsulatum is a dimorphic fungus (i.e., it assumes a yeast form in tissues but is a mold in the environment and in cultures) endemic to the soil of the Ohio and Mississippi river valleys but found occasionally throughout much of the world. Most persons residing in endemic areas become infected, but fewer than 10% come to medical attention. The disease assumes several forms. Acute pulmonary histoplasmosis is usually a mild disease but can cause high fever; chest radiographs show patchy infiltrates. Mediastinal lymphadenopathy often develops and usually remains asymptomatic; considering the possibility of histoplasmosis can spare the patient an unnecessary surgical exploration. Healed pulmonary histoplasmosis typically leaves pulmonary calcifications similar to those of healed TB. Inhalation of massive numbers of spores, especially if previous infection has conferred some degree of immunity, can cause miliary granulomatosis of the lungs that heals, leaving a "buckshot" pattern of calcification. Acute progressive disseminated histoplasmosis, which carries a mortality rate of 83% to 100% if untreated, should be considered in immunocompromised patients, especially those with HIV disease. The diagnosis can sometimes be made on peripheral blood smear. Subacute progressive disseminated histoplasmosis should be suspected in patients with combinations of fever, weight loss, localizing symptoms (especially of the gastrointestinal tract or CNS), hepatomegaly, punched-out mouth ulcers, and cytopenias. Other forms include isolated chronic cavitary lung disease, pulmonary nodules (which can enlarge over time, suggesting lung cancer), mediastinal fibrosis (which can obstruct major blood vessels and cause heart failure), broncholithiasis, and adrenal insufficiency. Urine and serum antigen tests are especially useful in persons with HIV disease, but definitive diagnosis of histoplasmosis is based on culture.

- Amphotericin B is the drug of choice for disseminated and severe pulmonary infection (SOR: A).
- Itraconazole is useful in other situations (SOR: A).

North American Blastomycosis

North American blastomycosis, caused by the dimorphic fungus *Blastomyces dermatitidis*, resembles histoplasmosis in many respects: endemicity in the Mississippi and Ohio river basins; acquisition by inhalation; pulmonary disease as the usual manifestation; disseminated disease, especially in severely immunocompromised persons; and use of amphotericin B for severe disease (SOR: A) but with a definite role for itraconazole. Blastomycosis differs from histoplasmosis in that it is more likely to be symptomatic (50%, vs. <10% for histoplasmosis) and more likely to secondarily involve the skin, bone, and genitourinary tract. As with histoplasmosis, serum and urine antigen tests are available, but diagnosis is optimally made by culture. However, the diagnosis is strongly suggested by a potassium hydroxide (KOH) preparation of pus, skin scrapings, or sputum, which reveals budding yeasts with a distinctive appearance: a highly refractile cell wall and a single, broad-based daughter yeast (in contrast to other budding yeasts).

Coccidioidomycosis

Coccidioidomycosis, caused by the dimorphic fungus *Coccidioides immitis*, is endemic in the southwestern United States (notably, southern Arizona, central California, southern New Mexico, and western Texas) and parts of Central and South America. The disease should be suspected in tourists and travelers returning from these areas. As with histoplasmosis and blastomycosis, the disease is acquired by inhalation, usually takes the form of pulmonary disease, but occasionally disseminates especially in persons with HIV/AIDS. Pulmonary manifestations include patchy pneumonia, pleural effusion, nodules, thin-walled cavities (≈8% of patients), and chronic fibrocavitary pneumonia. Most acute pulmonary infections are self-limited and do not require treatment. Dissemination may involve the skin (with papules, nodules, plaques, or ulcers), bones, joints, and CNS. Coccidioidal meningitis carries the potential for CNS vasculitis with ischemic stroke or hemorrhage. IgM and IgG antibody tests are useful but culture is required for definitive diagnosis. Management of coccidioidomycosis involves many subtleties; the IDSA guidelines should be consulted.

Aspergillosis

Aspergillus spp. are saprophytic molds found worldwide, frequently colonizing mucosal surfaces, commonly contaminating laboratory culture specimens, and causing a spectrum of clinical syndromes:

1. *Allergic bronchopulmonary aspergillosis*, a hypersensitivity disease of the respiratory tract occurring especially in patients with asthma or cystic fibrosis, discussed earlier under the discussion of bronchiectasis
2. *Aspergilloma (fungus ball)*, developing within a preexisting lung cavity or in a paranasal sinus, is often asymptomatic but may cause life-threatening hemoptysis or, when involving a paranasal sinus, recurrent bacterial infection and locally invasive disease
3. *Superficial aspergillosis*, typically occurring as chronic otitis externa caused by *Aspergillus niger*
4. *Asymptomatic colonization of mucosal surfaces*
5. *Invasive aspergillosis*, usually in the lungs (80% to 90% of cases) of immunocompromised persons (most commonly in the setting of severe granulocytopenia) as a fulminant, rapidly progressive disease. Definitive diagnosis requires tissue biopsy because positive cultures, even if obtained by bronchoscopy, can reflect contamination. A characteristic CT appearance includes the "halo sign" and the "air-crescent sign."

Mucormycosis

The term "mucormycosis" denotes invasive tissue infection by one or another of a diverse group of molds belonging to the order Mucorales. Most affected patients have a predisposing factor such as diabetes mellitus (poorly controlled or with a recent history of ketoacidosis), extensive trauma, burns, or an immunocompromised state. *Mucoraceae* species, such as *Aspergillus* spp., invade the walls of blood vessels, causing infarction and gangrene of tissues. Patients with rhinocerebral mucormycosis sometimes have on physical examination localized black (infarcted) areas on the nasal or palatal mucosa. Extension to the brain is life threatening. Pulmonary mucormycosis, similar to invasive pulmonary aspergillosis, occurs mainly in patients with severe prolonged granulocytopenia.

Less Common Deep Fungal Infections

Fungi belonging to the genus *Fusarium*, which cause infection in immunocompetent persons after traumatic inoculation, cause three major syndromes: fungal keratitis; onychomycosis; and chronic infections of skin, muscle, bone, or joints. The latter include *mycetoma (Madura foot)*, a slowly progressive and often painful destruction caused by various saprophytic foil fungi, including *Fusarium* spp.

Pseudallescheria boydii (the sexual or perfect stage of the organism) and *Scedosporium apiospermum* (the asexual or imperfect stage of the same organism) can cause a localized, recalcitrant infection in immunocompetent hosts. *P. boydii* occasionally causes invasive fungal sinusitis, meningitis, or disseminated infection.

The *dematiaceous fungi* are characterized by a melanin-like pigment in their cell walls that confers a dark-brown or black appearance to their hyphae or spores in tissue specimens and cultures. They cause a disease known as phaeo-hyphomycosis. The most severe form consists of invasive fungal sinusitis, which may spread to the brain.

MYCOBACTERIA

Tuberculosis remains the most important mycobacterial disease worldwide, but its incidence has been steadily declining in the United States, coincident with better control of HIV/AIDS. However, TB remains prevalent among disadvantaged populations, such as frail elderly adults, immigrants, injection drug users, homeless persons, the inner city poor, and persons infected with HIV. Today's family medicine clinicians are more likely to encounter nontuberculous mycobacteria, especially *M. avium–intracellulare*.

Tuberculosis

Tuberculosis usually presents as a pulmonary disease but is extrapulmonary in 10% to 25% of patients worldwide. Extrapulmonary TB takes one of three forms: disseminated (miliary) TB, which is more common in children and in immunosuppressed persons; "serosal" TB (tuberculous pleurisy, meningitis, pericarditis, peritonitis, and arthritis); and TB of solid organs (including tuberculous osteomyelitis and TB of the adrenal glands, formerly the usual cause of Addison disease).

Pulmonary TB typically manifests as some combination of fever, night sweats, productive cough, hemoptysis, anorexia, and weight loss. Imaging typically reveals upper lobe cavitary lesions (reactivation TB) but can also disclose consolidation in the apex of a lower lobe or base of an upper lobe (primary TB) or nodular lesions, with or without lymphadenopathy. In HIV-infected persons, TB may be more severe, the clinical findings atypical, and the chest radiographic findings are occasionally normal.

Latent TB is defined by a positive tuberculin skin test result or a positive interferon-γ release assay (the QuantiFERON-TB Gold test and the T-SPOT TB Test) without evidence of disease. The latter tests offer the convenience of a one-time blood sample, greater specificity for *M. tuberculosis*, and lack of an anamnestic response on repeat testing. A positive test result by either method should prompt consultation with guidelines for preventive therapy against TB with isoniazid.

Patients with AFB-positive sputum smears confirmed by molecular methods—and also those with positive AFB smears and a high index of suspicion for TB—should be started on a multidrug regimen. The standard therapy in the United States consists of isoniazid (INH), rifampin (RIF), pyrazinamide (PZA), and ethambutol (EMB). Patients at low risk of having a multidrug-resistant strain of *M. tuberculosis* are generally considered no longer contagious after 2 weeks of therapy even though it may take longer (≤8 weeks) for the sputum to become AFB smear negative. Pulmonary TB is treated for 6 months irrespective of host status, including HIV status, and should be supervised by the local or state health department.

Disseminated TB results from lymphohematogenous spread. The term "miliary" derives from the resemblance of the small granulomatous lesions to millet seeds, but granuloma formation may be absent in immunocompromised persons (notably, HIV-infected persons), children, pregnant women, or persons with alcoholism and liver disease. The presentation is often subtle. The diagnosis may require tissue biopsy.

Unexplained pleurisy, pericarditis, peritonitis, or chronic arthritis with effusion should prompt consideration of TB, but the most treacherous syndrome of "serosal TB" is TB meningitis because diagnosis is difficult, and permanent brain damage can result. Use of PCR on CSF represents a distinct advance; in a small series, a multiplex PCR had 94% sensitivity and 100% specificity for culture-confirmed TB meningitis.

See Chapter 16 on pulmonary medicine for more information.

Nontuberculous Mycobacteria

Nontuberculous mycobacteria—also known as atypical mycobacteria or as mycobacteria other than tuberculosis (MOTT)—are typically environmental organisms, are not transmitted from one person to another, and are often of little or no significance when isolated from clinical specimens. However, their clinical importance is increasing. Most hospital laboratories lack the supplies necessary to identify these organisms, and thus the clinician should know when to request referral of the isolate to a reference laboratory.

Pulmonary disease associated with NTM includes at least four syndromes:

1. Chronic cavitary pulmonary disease in patients with underlying chronic obstructive pulmonary disease, typically in white male cigarette smokers and resembling upper lobe cavitary TB but usually milder. The responsible microorganism is usually MAC or *M. kansasii*.
2. Nodular or reticulonodular pulmonary disease, often with bronchiectasis and typically in a thin white woman older than 50 years of age (the so-called Lady Windermere syndrome). These patients sometimes have a pectus excavatum deformity or mitral valve prolapse. MAC is the usual pathogen, but *M. kansasii* and *M. abscessus* also cause this syndrome.
3. Bronchiectasis in patients with cystic fibrosis. The usual isolates are MAC or *M. abscessus*, and it can be difficult to determine whether these isolates represent colonization or infection.

Chronic lower lobe pneumonia often presents as a hazy infiltrate in a patient predisposed to aspiration, usually as a result of disease of the lower esophagus. Opportunistic mycobacteria isolated in this setting include *M. fortuitum*, *M. abscessus*, *M. smegmatis*, and MAC. Because colonization by the ubiquitous organisms is commonplace, a single positive culture does not suffice for diagnosis of disease. Guidelines for diagnosis and treatment issued by the American Thoracic Society (the website is referenced in the following) should be consulted, but in general, diagnosis of nontuberculous mycobacterial disease requires (1) a compatible clinical syndrome; (2) appropriate exclusion of other diagnoses; and (3) multiple positive culture results. Transbronchial biopsy may also be required.

Distinctive syndromes of extrapulmonary disease caused by nontuberculous mycobacteria include:

1. *Cervical lymphadenitis* (scrofula), typically painless and unilateral and sometimes associated with fistula formation, occur most often in young children. MAC causes about 80% of cases in the United States; *M. scrofulaceum* also causes this syndrome, as does *M. tuberculosis* (TB). Surgical excision rather than drainage should be performed to avoid the formation of a sinus tract.
2. A lymphocutaneous syndrome resembling sporotrichosis, which constitutes an occupational hazard for those who keep aquariums and can also result from puncture wounds inflicted by fish or crabs, is caused by *M. marinum*. Outbreaks have been related to swimming pools.
3. Postoperative infections, typically occurring in incision sites or after cosmetic surgery (e.g., after breast augmentation), can result from rapidly growing mycobacteria: *M. fortuitum*, *M. chelonei*, and *M. abscessus*. When suspected, AFB cultures should be requested and the laboratory alerted to look for nontuberculous mycobacteria.

4. Unusual rheumatologic infections in tendon sheaths, bone, or bursa can be caused by MAC and *M. marinum*.
5. A painless, mobile, nodular swelling of the skin that evolves into extensive skin and soft tissue destruction with larger ulcers on an extremity occurs in tropical and subtropical climates, is known as "Buruli ulcer," and is caused by *M. ulcerans*.
6. Positive blood cultures in patients with vascular access catheters occur occasionally in patients being treated for cancer and are associated with high fever that responds to catheter removal and antibiotic therapy. The most common isolate (86% of cases) in one series was *M. mucogenicum*.

Leprosy

Leprosy, caused by *M. leprae*, affects between 100 and 200 persons in the United States each year, occurs mainly (85% of cases) in immigrants, and is endemic in several southern states (Louisiana, Arkansas, Texas, and Mississippi). Lepromatous leprosy, manifested by symmetric skin nodules, plaques, and dermal thickening and causing facial disfiguration ("leonine" facies), occurs in persons with essentially no immunity to *M. leprae*. Tuberculoid leprosy, a less severe form, features asymmetrically distributed skin plaques and involves the peripheral nerves. The *anesthetic plaque*—a focally hypopigmented skin lesion with loss of touch and pain sensation—is the hallmark of tuberculoid leprosy. In lepromatous leprosy, but not in tuberculoid leprosy, dermal macrophages are stuffed with *M. leprae*, an organism that still defies culture in artificial media.

PARASITES

With a few exceptions, most physicians in the United States seldom encounter or even think about parasitic diseases. The epidemiologic history is crucially important to diagnosis and management. Recent and remote travel, occupation, socioeconomic status, recreation, animal exposures, and living arrangements provide valuable clues. Immunocompromised persons, including those with HIV disease, are subject to reactivation of parasitic infections that would otherwise lie dormant; these include toxoplasmosis, cryptosporidiosis, and disseminated strongyloidiasis.

Malaria

Malaria, the most important parasitic disease in terms of mortality, is caused by five species of *Plasmodium*: *P. falciparum*, *P. vivax*, *P. ovale*, *P. malariae*, and *P. knowlesi*. The clinical hallmark is fever manifested by a three-phase paroxysm: a "cold stage" with chills or shaking lasting 15 minutes to several hours, a "hot stage" of high fever lasting several hours, and drenching sweats. Fever occurring with clockwise regularity typifies malaria caused by *P. vivax*, *P. ovale*, and *P. malariae*. *P. falciparum* is life threatening, as is *P. knowlesi*, which since its recent description in macaque monkeys in Southeast Asia has been shown to infect humans. *P. falciparum* infects red blood cells of all ages, giving rise to massive parasitemia; it also adheres to endothelial cells, resulting in microvascular disease. Complications include obstruction of brain capillaries with delirium, seizures, and coma (cerebral malaria); renal failure with hemoglobinuria ("blackwater fever"); pulmonary edema; and hypoglycemia. Malaria must be considered in any returning traveler with fever. Diagnosis is made by examining thick and thin blood films. The CDC maintains a Malaria Hotline (855-856-4713), which is available to the public during normal working hours and can be contacted at all times at (770-488-7100).

Other Parasitic Diseases

Family physicians should be prepared to encounter a few parasitic diseases (e.g., lice, pinworms, scabies, and toxoplasmosis), should recognize several others that may occasionally present in their practices depending on the geographic region (e.g., cutaneous larva migrans, echinococcosis, swimmer's itch, and—for practices with Hispanic immigrants—cysticercosis), should be aware that dirofilariasis can lead to an unnecessary thoracotomy, and should warn their young patients who enjoy warm freshwater ponds and lakes against activities such as diving that risk primary amebic meningoencephalitis (Table 15-15). Family physicians may occasionally encounter patients with

Table 15-15 Selected Parasites

Disease	Parasite (Usual Transmission)	Comments
Amebiasis*	*Entamoeba histolytica*	See text
Amebic meningoencephalitis*	*Naegleria fowleri* (enters CSF through cribriform plate; associated with warm freshwater lakes and ponds)	Rapidly progressive with mortality rate of about 95% Diagnosis can be made by demonstrating trophozoites on a wet mount of CSF
Angiostrongyliasis	*Angiostrongylus cantonensis* (ingestion of raw or undercooked snails or other vectors)	Eosinophilic meningitis or meningoencephalitis
Ascariasis*	*Ascaris lumbricoides* (food or beverages contaminated with *Ascaris* eggs)	Pulmonary symptoms with eosinophilia (PIE syndrome) Intestinal obstruction, mainly in children Pancreatic and biliary obstruction, mainly in adults
Babesiosis*	*Babesia microti* (in United States)	See text
Chagas disease (American trypanosomiasis)†	*Trypanosoma cruzi* Reduviid bugs (Triatominae)	Acute: febrile illness sometimes with lymphadenopathy, local swelling at site of bite (chagoma), and edema of eyelids Late: dilated cardiomyopathy, megaesophagus, megacolon, neuropathy

Continued on following page

Table 15-15 Selected Parasites (Continued)

Disease	Parasite (Usual Transmission)	Comments
Clonorchiasis	*Clonorchis sinensis* (ingestion of undercooked, smoked, or pickled freshwater fish)	Acute: fever and right upper quadrant pain caused by gallbladder obstruction Chronic: cholangiohepatitis; recurrent cholangitis; cholangiocarcinoma
Cryptosporidiosis*	*Cryptosporidium parvum* and others	See text
Cutaneous larva migrans ("creeping eruption," "ground itch," "sandworms")*	*Ancylostoma braziliense* (skin contact with contaminated soil, as by walking barefoot on beaches frequented by dogs)	Intensely pruritic, serpiginous, erythematous eruption often complicated by secondary bacterial infection induced by scratching
Cyclosporiasis*	*Cyclospora cayetanensis* (ingestion of contaminated fruits and vegetables)	Watery diarrhea, usually self-limited Outbreaks in United States traced to contaminated lettuce or raspberries
Cysticercosis†	*Taenia solium* (ingestion of undercooked pork or of raw vegetables grown in fields irrigated with untreated sewage water)	Cystic lesions in brain (neurocysticercosis) with seizures and hydrocephalus Subcutaneous nodules Eye involvement
Diphyllobothriasis*	*Diphyllobothriasis* (ingestion of raw or undercooked fish)	Nausea, vomiting, diarrhea, abdominal pain, weight loss Megaloblastic anemia (tapeworm competes for vitamin B_{12})
Dirofilariasis*	*Dirofilaria* spp. (mosquito bites; principle hosts are dogs, wolves, foxes, and raccoons)	Inflammatory nodules under skin or conjunctiva Pulmonary lesions that appear as coin lesions
Fasciolopsiasis	*Fasciolopsis buski* (ingestion of raw aquatic plants)	Diarrhea, abdominal pain, anemia Obstruction of biliary or pancreatic ducts Allergic reactions
Giardiasis*	*Giardia lamblia*	See text
Hookworm*	*Necator americanus* (United States); *Ancylostoma duodenale* (skin contact with egg-contaminated soil)	Pruritic lesions at site of penetration ("ground itch") Iron-deficiency anemia Intellectual impairment and growth retardation in children
Echinococcosis (hydatid disease)*	*Echinococcus granulosus, E. multilocularis, E. vogeli, E. oligarthrus* (ingestion of eggs)	Slow-growing masses in liver or other organs: "alveolar cysts" (*E. granulosus*, the most common form); "multilocular cysts" (*E. multilocularis*); "polycystic disease" (rare; *E. vogeli* and *E. oligarthrus*) Anaphylaxis from cyst rupture (whether spontaneous, traumatic, or during surgical extraction)
Hymenolepiasis	*Hymenolepis nana; H. diminuta* (ingestion of eggs)	Usually asymptomatic May cause anorexia, abdominal pain, diarrhea, perirectal itching, and irritability
Lice*	*Pediculus humanus capitis, Pediculus humanus corporis, Phthirus pubis* (person-to-person contact [*Pediculus humanus capitis* and *Phthirus pubis*], also clothing or bed sheets [*Pediculus humanus corporis*])	Intense pruritus (from allergic reaction) often with excoriation and secondary bacterial infection from scratching in all forms Body lice (*P. humanus corporis*) can transmit epidemic typhus, trench fever, and epidemic relapsing fever Pubic lice (*Phthirus pubis*) should prompt investigation for other sexually transmitted diseases
Loa loa filariasis (subcutaneous filariasis)	*Loa loa* microfilaria (tabanid flies, mainly deerflies and mango [mangrove] flies)	Usually asymptomatic Local swellings (calabar swellings) in extremities caused by allergic reactions Subconjunctival involvement ("African eye worm")
Lymphatic filariasis (Bancroftian filariasis; elephantiasis)	*Wuchereria bancrofti, Brugia malayi, Brugia timori* (mosquitoes)	Elephantiasis: edema, often massive, secondary to lymphatic obstruction
Malaria†	*Plasmodium vivax, P. ovale, P. malariae, P. falciparum, P. knowlesi*	See text
Ocular larva migrans*	*Toxocara canis* (ingestion of eggs)	Visual defects secondary to endophthalmitis, uveitis, or chorioretinitis Retinal lesion can mimic retinoblastoma, leading to enucleation
Onchocerciasis (river blindness)	*Onchocerca volvulus* (black flies)	Skin: itching and inflammation Eyes: visual defects caused by involvement of nearly any part of the eye (second only to trachoma as leading cause of blindness worldwide)
Paragonimiasis	*Paragonimus westermani* (ingestion of inadequately cooked or pickled crab ["drunken crabs'] or crayfish)	Acute: diarrhea, fever, urticaria, hepatosplenomegaly, eosinophilia Lungs: nodules or cavities with hemoptysis ("endemic hemoptysis") Can involve other organs, including the brain
Pinworm (enterobiasis)*	*Enterobius vermicularis* (usually, ingestion of eggs)	Perianal itching

Table 15-15 Selected Parasites (Continued)

Disease	Parasite (Usual Transmission)	Comments
Scabies* ("7-year itch")	*Sarcoptes scabiei* (usually, skin-to-skin contact)	Rash with intense itching and superficial borrows, often in a row Crusted scabies (formerly known as "Norwegian scabies"): severe form mainly in elderly and immunocompromised persons
Schistosomiasis	*Schistosoma mansoni, S. haematobium, S. japonicum;* occasionally other schistosomes (contact with water inhabited by freshwater snails)	Numerous symptoms depending on the species—organ damage is mainly caused by an immune reaction to eggs Portal hypertension (with varices) and pulmonary hypertension *(S. mansoni, S. japonicum)* Cystitis with risk of bladder cancer *(S. haematobium)*
Sleeping sickness (African trypanosomiasis)	*Trypanosoma brucei gambiense, T. brucei rhodesiense* (tsetse flies)	Acute: fever, headache, pruritus, arthralgia Late: confusion, insomnia, loss of coordination, numbness
Strongyloidiasis*	*Strongyloides stercoralis;* occasionally, *S. fülleborni*	Skin symptoms, including *larva currens,* a rapidly progressive migratory dermatitis with a wide band of urticaria and perianal involvement Diarrhea, abdominal pain, weight loss *Hyperinfection syndrome* occurs in immunosuppressed patients
Swimmer's itch (cercarial dermatitis)*	Various species of *Schistosoma* (skin penetration by larvae)	Itchy papules (inflammatory immune reaction)
Toxoplasmosis*	*Toxoplasma gondii*	See text
Trichinosis*	*Trichinella spiralis,* others (ingestion of undercooked pork or wild game)	Usually asymptomatic Acute: muscle pain, fever, weakness, periorbital edema, splinter hemorrhages in nails Rarely, myocarditis, encephalitis, pneumonia
Visceral larva migrans*	*Toxocara canis, T. cati,* other nematodes (ingestion of eggs in contaminated soil [often from pica in young children] or unwashed meat and vegetables)	Usually mild and self-limited. Abdominal pain, cough, fever, wheezing, irritability Rarely, cardiac or CNS in involvement

CNS, Central nervous system; *CSF,* cerebrospinal fluid; *PIE,* pulmonary infiltrates with eosinophilia.
*Endemic in all or parts of the United States (in some instances, in restricted populations or geographic areas).
†Seldom acquired in the United States but may be encountered in returning travelers and in Hispanic immigrants.

delusions of parasitosis, a heterogeneous disorder that can be surprisingly difficult to manage.

PRIONS

Prions are transmissible proteins that, although lacking genetic material, cause disease in humans characterized by progressive neurologic deterioration, leading to death and pathologically by spongiform changes in the brain parenchyma. Of the five known syndromes in humans, the most important in the United States is Creutzfeldt-Jakob disease. Useful for diagnosis are MRI (which can be suggestive but diagnostic) and measurement of 14-3-3 protein in CSF (which has low sensitivity and specificity). Surgical procedures should be avoided because of the risk of contaminating instruments and exposing health care workers to this untreatable disease.

Acknowledgments

The author acknowledges the assistance of Divya Ahuja, Helmut Albrecht, Majdi N. Al-Hasan, P. Brandon Bookstaver, Babatunde Edun, Jeffrey W.W. Hall, Joseph Horvath, Sangita Dash, Elizabeth Nimmich, Kamla Sanasi-Bhola, and Sharon Weissman.

References

The complete reference list is available at www.expertconsult.com.

Web Resources

aidsinfo.nih.gov This website includes federally approved guidelines for treatment of HIV disease, a database on drugs, information about clinical trials, and patient education materials.

www.cdc.gov Information from the Centers for Disease Control and Prevention is alphabetized on this website. Especially valuable are the guidelines for vaccine use and the destination-specific recommendations for travelers.

www.idsociety.org/idsa_practice_guidelines The clinical practice guidelines of the Infectious Disease Society of America are alphabetized on this website and provide up-to-date consensus recommendations.

www.thoracic.org/statements Statements from the American Thoracic Society include essential recommendations pertaining to TB and pneumonia.

16 Pulmonary Medicine

GEORGE RUST and GLORIA E. WESTNEY

Lung Disease in Primary Care

Breathing and the heartbeat draw the line between life and death. Pulmonary disease, respiratory symptoms, and respiratory failure are common high-impact conditions. For example, asthma is the most common chronic disease of childhood. Lung cancer is now the leading cause of cancer death for both men and women in the United States. Lung cancer accounts for 28% of cancer deaths in men and 26% of cancer deaths in women (American Cancer Society, 2013). In part because of the global spread of tobacco, the World Health Organization (WHO) now lists chronic obstructive pulmonary disease (COPD) as the fifth leading cause of death, with an expected 30% increase over the coming decade (World Health Organization, 2013).

SMOKING AND OTHER RISK FACTORS FOR LUNG DISEASE

The Centers for Disease Control and Prevention (CDC) describe smoking as the single most preventable cause of premature death in the United States, contributing to more than 440,000 deaths per year, or one in every five deaths (CDC, 2013a). People who smoke have more than a 20-fold increase in risk of death from lung cancer and a 10-fold increase in risk of death resulting from bronchitis or emphysema. For women in the United States, almost twice as many deaths are caused by lung cancer than by breast cancer. Worldwide, there were 5 million deaths attributable to smoking in 2000, almost 2 million of which were related to lung cancer and other lung diseases. The WHO projects a doubling of smoking-related deaths by 2020 (Ezzati, 2003).

Smoking cessation is the most important factor in preventing lung and cardiovascular disease and all-cause mortality. Avoidance of secondary exposure to smoke, especially in the household, is also important in preventing childhood infections and asthma, as well as adult cancers (US Department of Health and Human Services, 2006). Secondhand smoke is linked to nearly 50,000 deaths per year, most caused by heart disease.

Even simple physician advice to quit smoking provides a marginal benefit of 2.5% of patients quitting successfully (Lancaster and Stead, 2004). Interventions that combine counseling plus education or group strategies plus pharmacologic treatment with nicotine replacement or specific medications can achieve sustained quit rates of 25% to 30% (Hughes et al., 2004; Solomon et al., 2005; Stead and Lancaster, 2005). The Agency for Healthcare Research and Quality (AHRQ, 2008) has provided a comprehensive update to previous clinical guidelines for smoking cessation and treating tobacco dependence. Counseling is most effective when it includes both practical problem solving and social support. Pharmacologic treatment, such as nicotine replacement, bupropion, and varenicline, has proved effective but is most effective when combined with counseling or group programs. The Legacy Foundation reports that ex-smokers have an average of eight quit attempts before ultimately sustaining a tobacco-free lifestyle. Table 16-1 defines a strategy for helping patients to quit smoking by a simple mnemonic of "five A's" (ask, advise, assess, assist, arrange). Motivational interviewing is an effective and nonjudgmental behavioral technique that helps the patient discover their own motivations for quitting. Physicians can also play a key role in community-oriented primary care, helping to establish effective quit smoking groups and other smoking cessation programs, as well as influencing clean indoor air policies and enforcement of laws regarding sale of tobacco to minors.

DIAGNOSTIC TOOLS IN PULMONARY MEDICINE

History and Physical Examination

Diagnosis starts with the patient history and physical examination. Pulmonary symptoms may be evaluated by traditional history-of-present-illness questions, such as the character and quality of the symptoms, duration, onset, timing, exacerbating and alleviating factors, efforts at self-treatment, and the patient's own understanding of what is causing the symptoms. For example, the symptoms of asthma may be variously described by patients as shortness of breath, wheezing, whistling, "wheezling,"

Table 16-1   The Five A's: Strategies to Help Patients Quit Smoking

Ask	**Systematically identify all tobacco users at every visit.**
	Implement an office-wide system that ensures that, for *every* patient at *every* clinic visit, tobacco use status is queried and documented.
Advise	**Strongly urge all tobacco users to quit.**
	In a clear, strong, and personalized manner, urge every tobacco user to quit.
Assess	**Determine willingness to make a quit attempt.**
	Ask every tobacco user if he or she is willing to make a quit attempt at this time (e.g., within the next 30 days).
Assist	**Aid the patient in quitting.**
	Help the patient with a quit plan; provide practical counseling; provide intratreatment social support; help the patient obtain extratreatment social support; recommend use of approved pharmacotherapy except in special circumstances; provide supplementary materials.
Arrange	**Schedule follow-up contact.**
	Schedule follow-up contact, either in person or via telephone.

From Global Initiative for Chronic Obstructive Lung Disease (GOLD); Global Strategies for the Diagnosis, Management, and Prevention of COPD, Updated 2014. Table 3.2, Brief Strategies to Help the Patient Quit; p. 20; http://www.goldcopd.org/uploads/users/files/GOLD_Report_2014_Jun11.pdf.

chest tightness, tight breathing, or poor exercise tolerance. In addition, patients often self-medicate with nonprescription and prescription medications, as well as using herbal and nonmedicinal alternative therapies, which they typically do not report to their personal physician unless specifically asked (Braganza et al., 2003).

In addition to general history taking, a detailed history of respiratory exposures and risk factors is essential. Smoking is perhaps the most important pulmonary risk factor. A detailed smoking history includes age of first smoking, quantity smoked, number of years as a smoker, other tobacco use, previous attempts to quit, and an assessment of the level of nicotine addiction. Family history can reveal relatives with immunoglobulin E (IgE)–mediated allergy or *atopy* (allergic rhinitis, asthma, eczema, nasal polyps, or aspirin hypersensitivity) or even more serious genetic risk factors, such as cystic fibrosis (CF) or α_1-antitrypsin deficiency. Perinatal history of premature birth, neonatal respiratory failure, and ventilator care can lead to bronchopulmonary dysplasia and chronic lung disease in children who survive neonatal intensive care.

Taking a good occupational history is also essential, asking about the specific type of work the patient performs, as well as past jobs. In addition, the clinician should ask two key questions:

1. Have you ever been exposed to fumes, gases, or dusts?
2. Do your symptoms get better when you are away from work, during weekends and vacations?

Physical examination begins with vital signs. For example, tachypnea out of proportion to fever may be the first presenting sign of childhood pneumonia. The degree of respiratory difficulty may also be observed in the form of obvious shortness of breath, the work of breathing, the use of accessory respiratory muscles, and the patient's need to take a breath in midsentence (described as *three-to-four-word dyspnea*). General examination can also reveal either peripheral or central cyanosis. Clubbing of the nails can indicate chronic lung disease. Morbid obesity may be associated with obstructive sleep apnea, right-sided heart failure *(cor pulmonale)*, or both.

Examination of the chest begins with inspection and progresses to percussion, palpation, and auscultation (Fitzgerald & Murray, 2005). Inspection can reveal chest deformities (pectus excavatum or flail chest) or spinal deformities (kyphosis or scoliosis) that interfere with breathing, or an enlarged anteroposterior (AP) diameter in adults with chronically hyperexpanded lungs. Adults with morbid obesity or prior chest trauma that restricts chest wall motion can have pulmonary function tests (PFTs) consistent with restrictive lung disease of extrapulmonary origin. Infants and children in respiratory distress may have intercostal retractions.

Palpation can identify thoracic wall abnormalities, mass lesions, or tenderness and show asymmetry of chest wall expansion. Percussion of lung fields should normally be resonant. Dullness to percussion can indicate fluid in the pleural space or consolidation of the lung itself, with fluid filling the normally air-filled alveolar spaces. Both of these conditions also produce decreased breath sounds over the affected area. Hyperresonant lung fields on percussion can indicate the hyperexpansion of obstructive lung disease or even pneumothorax.

Auscultation should include listening over the upper, middle, and lower lung fields of each lung posteriorly, as well as over the apices and mid-lung fields anteriorly. The right middle lobe of the lung and the lingula of the left lung can only be heard anteriorly. In addition to identifying areas of decreased breath sounds, the quality of lung sounds on auscultation can further differentiate underlying lung pathology. Normal (vesicular) lung sounds are continuous. Other continuous breath sounds include wheezing (sibilant or musical rhonchi) and bronchial (tubular) breath sounds (sounds like "Darth Vader" or breathing through a snorkel), which occur normally over the trachea or upper anterior chest wall but indicate pathology when heard in the peripheral lung fields. Discontinuous breath sounds include the sound of small alveolar sacs popping open in fluid-based lung consolidation, which are heard as adventitial lung sounds, such as fine rales or crackles. This can occur in both bases, as in congestive heart failure, or in a more localized area, as in a lobar pneumonia. The sound has been described as similar to tufts of hair being rubbed together close to the ear.

Because decreased breath sounds and dullness to percussion can represent either fluid in the pleural space or consolidation of the lungs themselves, additional physical findings can help differentiate the two conditions. Vocal

Table 16-2 Physical Findings in Common Pulmonary Disorders

Disorder	Inspection	Palpation	Percussion	Auscultation
Bronchial asthma (acute attack)	Hyperinflation; use of accessory muscles	Impaired expansion; decreased fremitus	Hyperresonance; low diaphragm	Prolonged expiration; inspiratory and expiratory wheezes
Pneumothorax (complete)	Lag on affected side	Absent fremitus	Hyperresonant or tympanitic	Absent breath sounds
Pleural effusion (large)	Lag on affected side	Decreased fremitus; trachea and heart shifted away from affected side	Dullness or flatness	Absent breath sounds
Atelectasis (lobar obstruction)	Lag on affected side	Decreased fremitus; trachea and heart shifted toward affected side	Dullness or flatness	Absent breath sounds
Consolidation (pneumonia)	Possible lag or splinting on affected side	Increased fremitus	Dullness	Bronchial breath sounds; bronchophony; pectoriloquy; crackles

Modified from Hinshaw HC, Murray JF. *Diseases of the chest.* 4th ed. Philadelphia: Saunders; 1980:23.

fremitus and tactile fremitus are increased in lung consolidation but decreased in pleural effusion. Localized *egophony* ("e-to-a" changes) indicates consolidation of that segment or lobe of the lung; it is not present in pleural effusion except in a small band just above the upper edge of the effusion.

Signs of bronchial inflammation, mucus, and obstruction in the bronchial tree include coarse crackles and wheezes (sonorous or musical rhonchi). Additionally, in normal vesicular breathing, the duration of the inspiratory phase is longer than the expiratory phase, typically 90% of the expired air is exhaled in the first second. Prolongation of the expiratory phase is an early sign of obstruction even before wheezing develops. The diagnostic implications of these physical examination findings are summarized in Table 16-2.

PULMONARY FUNCTION TESTING

Key Points

- Obstructive lung disease is diagnosed by demonstrating a ratio of forced expiratory volume in 1 second (FEV_1) to forced vital capacity (FVC) (or FEV_1/FEV_6 ratio) of less than 70%.
- Improvement in FEV_1 of at least 12% and at least 200 mL from prebronchodilator to postbronchodilator measurement is considered evidence of reversibility of airway obstruction.
- Restrictive lung disease can be diagnosed using office spirometry if the FVC is reduced to less than 80% of predicted while maintaining a normal FEV_1/FVC ratio (i.e., no obstruction).

Pulmonary function testing is essential for detecting lung disease and for differentiating obstructive from restrictive lung disease. PFTs may be done in a hospital-based pulmonary function laboratory or, more often, in the outpatient setting using office spirometry. The simplest PFT is the *peak expiratory flow rate* (PEFR), measured by handheld mechanical peak-flow meters given to patients for self-management and used in office settings and emergency departments (EDs) for quick assessment during acute exacerbations of asthma. PEFR is the maximum flow generated during

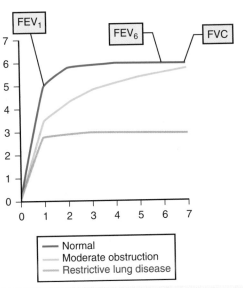

Figure 16-1 Time-volume spirometry curve showing measurement of forced expiratory volume in 1 second (FEV_1), forced vital capacity (FVC), and forced expiratory volume in 6 seconds (FEV_6) and curves for obstructive versus restrictive lung disease.

expiration performed with maximal force ("Take a deep breath and blow out as hard and as fast as you can").

Previous office spirometry units were bulky and required frequent recalibration, but modern units are small, computerized, and often self-calibrating. The quality of testing is important. The patient should be seated comfortably and instructed appropriately. An adequate PFT must include three valid measures (quick start, good effort, maintenance of forced expiration for at least 6 seconds with no cough) and three relatively similar results (FVC varying by <200 mL).

Results of office spirometry are presented both graphically and numerically, with actual values compared with values predicted by the patient's age, height, and gender. Figure 16-1 shows the points at which two critical values, FEV_1 and FVC, are measured on the time-volume curve. Figure 16-2 shows a typical flow-volume loop for patients that compares normal PFTs with obstructive lung disease and restrictive lung disease (Zoorob et al., 2002). Increasingly, the 6-second end point, or FEV_6, is being used as a

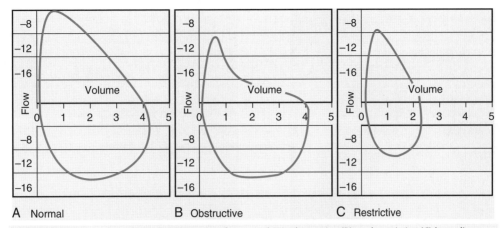

Figure 16-2 Flow-volume loop showing curves for normal (**A**), obstructive (**B**), and restrictive (**C**) lung disease.

reliable and reproducible surrogate measure that can replace FVC for patients who are unable to complete forced expiration beyond 6 seconds.

The key parameters of office spirometry are the FEV_1, the FVC, and the FEV_1/FVC ratio (percentage of exhaled volume blown out in first second of exhalation). The diagnosis of obstructive lung disease is made by demonstrating an FEV_1/FVC ratio (or FEV_1/FEV_6) of less than 70%. This means that the patient has exhaled less than 70% of FVC (full volume of air exhaled) in the first second of exhalation. Other tests of airway obstruction are the *midmaximal expiratory flow rate* (MMEF, or FEF_{25-75}), which is the average expiratory flow over the middle half of expiration, that is, flow rate during the time when 25% to 75% of the FVC is exhaled. This measure has been described as representing small airway obstruction, but it is less reproducible and has not been included in clinical guidelines for managing patients with obstructive lung disease. However, MMEF can be an early indicator of lung damage caused by smoking or occupational pneumoconioses. The FEF_{25} and FEF_{75} are moment-in-time measures of expiratory airflow and are therefore subject to significant patient-to-patient variability unrelated to clinical factors.

One other dimension of office spirometry in diagnosing and managing obstructive lung disease is to measure these parameters before and after a dose of inhaled β_2-adrenergic agonist is given. Improvement in FEV_1 of at least 12% and at least 200 mL from prebronchodilator to postbronchodilator measurement is considered evidence of reversibility of airway obstruction. Complete reversibility helps establish the diagnosis of asthma, and it is also useful in guiding therapy by establishing the potential efficacy of medications. For example, some patients with COPD are more responsive to anticholinergic medications such as inhaled ipratropium, but others are more responsive to inhaled β_2-agonists such as albuterol.

For restrictive lung disease, the "gold-standard" test is the *total lung capacity* (TLC), which is a measure of maximal exhaled air (FVC) plus residual capacity (RC). However, this can only be tested in pulmonary function laboratories that can test the patient in a sealed chamber. For practical purposes in the primary care setting, restrictive lung disease can be diagnosed using office spirometry if the FVC is reduced to less than 80% of predicted in the presence of a normal FEV_1/FVC ratio (i.e., no obstruction). One other test

that is available in pulmonary function laboratories but not in office spirometry is the *diffusion capacity* (DLCO), which is a measure of the diffusion of carbon monoxide across the alveolar-capillary membrane. Clinical reductions in DLCO can occur with thickening of the alveolocapillary membrane, which can be a sign of interstitial fibrosis.

CHEST RADIOGRAPHY AND OTHER DIAGNOSTIC IMAGING

Despite major advances in imaging technology, the chest radiography is still an important diagnostic modality that can clearly reveal signs of pneumonia, COPD, heart failure, tuberculosis (TB), lung masses, and pleural effusion. Figure 16-3 shows a chest radiograph with right middle lobe pneumonia. Although the posteroanterior (PA) radiograph shows some consolidation, it is attenuated by the overlying projection of a normal lower lobe. The lateral radiograph, however, shows the classic wedge-shaped profile of a consolidated right middle lobe.

Chest radiography is also widely used in evaluating patients with suspected exposure to TB because of symptoms, personal contact, or a positive intradermal purified protein derivative (PPD) test result. Figure 16-4 shows the patchy infiltrates and hilar adenopathy typical of pulmonary TB, although TB can have a variety of presentations on chest radiography, including adenopathy, pleural scarring, infiltrates, cavitary lesions, and miliary TB.

Chest radiography can also be helpful in diagnosing nonpulmonary causes of shortness of breath, as in the case of congestive heart failure, with enlarged heart, bibasilar consolidation, small pleural effusions, and prominent pulmonary vasculature. In other conditions such as asthma, chest radiography findings can be quite normal despite significant respiratory compromise.

Chest computed tomography (CT) scan plays an important role in diagnosing lung disease. High-resolution CT (HRCT) can identify pulmonary nodules and hilar lymph nodes at much smaller sizes than can chest radiography, and it is therefore important in diagnosing and staging lung cancers. CT can also detect lung abscess, vascular lesions, and pleural scarring or masses. Whereas early COPD or emphysematous changes can be difficult to detect with even HRCT, additional techniques such as minimum-intensity projection can aggregate data from adjacent slices and, by

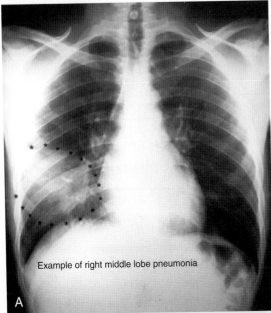

Example of right middle lobe pneumonia

A

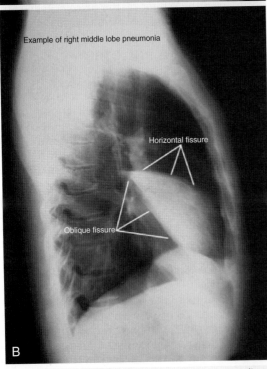

Example of right middle lobe pneumonia

Horizontal fissure

Oblique fissure

B

Figure 16-3 Posteroanterior (**A**) and lateral (**B**) chest radiographs showing right middle lobe pneumonia. (From Department of Neurobiology and Developmental Sciences, University of Arkansas for Medical Sciences, Little Rock. http://anatomy.uams.edu/anatomyhtml/xrays/xra_atlas39.html and http://anatomy.uams.edu/anatomyhtml/xrays/xra_atlas5.html.)

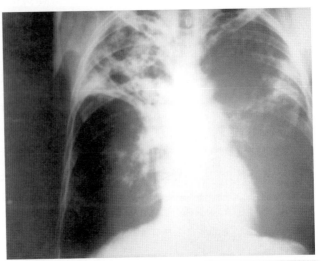

Figure 16-4 Chest radiograph showing tuberculosis with upper lobe fibrotic patchy infiltrates and hilar adenopathy. (From Centers for Disease Control and Prevention, Public Health Image Library, Image 2543. http://phil.cdc.gov/phil/home.asp.)

history and currently smoke or have quit within the past 15 years (US Preventive Services Task Force, 2013). When small, noncalcified pulmonary nodules are detected by CT, the likelihood of malignancy is influenced by nodule size, density, number of nodules, and growth over time, combined with patient factors such as age, smoking history, gender, spirometry, occupational history, and endemic granulomatous disease (Libby et al., 2004).

Positron emission tomography scans using ^{18}F-fluorodeoxyglucose (FDG-PET) are becoming increasingly useful in evaluating lung cancers and lymphomas. The ability to define anatomy and metabolism—that is, glucose uptake within the tumor—makes the PET scan useful for staging; detecting node involvement; and defining resectability, tumor response to therapy, and tumor recurrence (Avril and Weber, 2005). Diagnosing solitary pulmonary nodules is a common challenge in primary care. A meta-analysis of studies comparing dynamic CT, magnetic resonance imaging (MRI), FDG-PET, and single-photon emission computed tomography (SPECT) scans based on positive and negative likelihood ratios for identifying malignant versus nonmalignant solitary nodules found that all four were similarly accurate (Cronin et al., 2008). Nuclear medicine studies such as gallium scans are also used extensively in evaluating pulmonary symptoms in patients with human immunodeficiency virus (HIV) infection or acquired immunodeficiency syndrome (AIDS) and are discussed in more detail in the section on HIV-related pulmonary infections.

Other imaging studies have more specific indications. One nuclear medicine study long used in primary care is the ventilation/perfusion (V/Q) scan. This is specifically performed to rule out pulmonary embolism (PE), revealed by focal perfusion defects in adequately ventilated areas. This V/Q mismatch, in the absence of underlying lung pathology, is consistent with a high probability of PE. Unfortunately, patients can also demonstrate matching V/Q defects, which can occur when blood flow is shunted away from an underventilated area of the lung. Scans with no perfusion defect reflect a low probability for significant PE. Other tests

subtracting vascular and other tissue densities not consistent with lung parenchyma and air, demonstrate small air pockets consistent with early emphysema.

Imaging modalities such as spiral CT have been demonstrated to be effective in detecting early lung cancer in patients with high-risk smoking histories. The United States Prevention Services Task Force (USPSTF) now recommends yearly low-dose CT-scan screening for lung cancer in adults aged 55 to 80 years who have a 30 pack-year smoking are increasingly taking the place of V/Q scans (see later discussion).

BRONCHOSCOPY

Fiberoptic bronchoscopy allows direct visualization of the bronchial tree. It is useful for diagnosing conditions that require culture of a lower respiratory tract infection by bronchoalveolar lavage (BAL) or conditions such as bronchogenic carcinoma that require tissue diagnosis by transbronchial biopsy. Sometimes these techniques are combined, as in the diagnosis of *Pneumocystis jiroveci (carinii)* pneumonia (PCP), for which the sensitivity of bronchoscopy with BAL is approximately 86% and with transbronchial biopsy is 87% (Broaddus et al., 1985). A comparative assessment of different bronchoscopic techniques in obtaining culture specimens in cases of ventilator-associated pneumonia found no significant difference between blind bronchial brushings and bronchoscope-assisted lavage, bronchoscope-directed brushings, or even blind endotracheal aspirates (Wood et al., 2003). Rates of complications (including hemoptysis and pneumothorax) with traditional bronchoscopy are in the range of 0.5% to 1.0% without biopsy and up to 6.8% with transbronchial biopsy (Pue and Pacht, 1995). In a pulmonary fellowship program, the rate of complications for all bronchoscopies performed (with and without biopsy) was 2.06% (Ouellette, 2006). Therapeutic interventions using bronchoscopy are also increasing, and lesions are treated through the bronchoscope with laser, cryotherapy, electrocautery, and stents (Rafanan and Mehta, 2000).

Newer diagnostic techniques include fluorescent bronchoscopy, which can be more sensitive for detecting early endobronchial tumors (Gilbert et al., 2004; Moghissi et al., 2008), and virtual bronchoscopy, which uses sophisticated software to reconstruct images from HRCT scans to create three-dimensional imagery without invasive testing. This technique has been found useful in planning partial lung resection surgery, for example, but it cannot provide bronchoscopy's direct visualization of color, texture, or friability of the bronchial mucosa (Finkelstein et al., 2004).

MEASUREMENT OF BLOOD GASES

Measurement and monitoring of blood gases can be invasive or noninvasive. Transcutaneous pulse oximetry is the most widely used noninvasive test. It provides a fairly accurate measure of oxygen saturation (So_2) of hemoglobin at values ranging from 70% to 100% by measuring the difference between oxyhemoglobin and reduced hemoglobin in the absorption of light of specific wavelengths. So_2 of 98% corresponds to an arterial oxygen partial pressure (Pao_2) of 100 mm Hg and 95% to a Pao_2 of 80 mm Hg, demonstrating the challenge of interpreting a test with a 95% confidence interval of ±5%. An oxygen saturation of less than 89% corresponds to a Pao_2 of less than 60 mm Hg. Decreased tissue perfusion or color changes caused by jaundice or intravascular dyes can degrade accuracy. Arterial oxygen levels can also be measured transcutaneously ($tcPo_2$) with a skin surface oxygen electrode, but its accuracy is also affected by tissue perfusion, skin temperature, and other factors.

Exhaled carbon dioxide can also be measured noninvasively, most often in the intensive care unit (ICU) for patients on mechanical ventilation or in operating rooms during general anesthesia. Capnography, colorimetric techniques, and CO_2 sensors can detect failure of mechanical ventilation or improper endotracheal tube placement, which generate hypercapnia secondary to hypoventilation.

The invasive technique most often used for measuring oxygen, CO_2, and acid–base blood chemistries is the arterial blood gas (ABG) measurement. Although it requires an arterial needle puncture and several milliliters of blood, it is highly accurate and reproducible. ABG measurement is indicated in any patient with acute respiratory distress or in managing patients with respiratory failure. In addition to Pao_2 and arterial carbon dioxide partial pressure ($Paco_2$) measurements, ABG testing also provides a measure of pH, bicarbonate (HCO_3^-), and the anion gap, which can be used to detect respiratory (rather than metabolic) causes of acidosis and alkalosis. Patients with moderate to severe COPD can have chronic hypoxia plus chronic hypercapnia (decreased Pao_2 and increased $Paco_2$). They can also show signs of primary respiratory acidosis (reduced pH with elevated CO_2) and a compensatory metabolic alkalosis (partial normalization of the pH despite elevated $Paco_2$) mediated by renal HCO_3^- retention. Nomograms or software used in personal digital assistants allow simultaneous plotting of pH, CO_2, and HCO_3^- to facilitate interpretation of mixed respiratory and metabolic acid–base disturbances.

COMMON PULMONARY SYMPTOMS

Shortness of Breath

A common presenting symptom in pulmonary disease is shortness of breath. The fundamental question in patients presenting with recent-onset or episodic shortness of breath is this: Is it a lung problem, a heart problem, or something else? The most common pulmonary causes of chronic or repeated episodes of shortness of breath include asthma, smoking-related COPD, chronic lung infections (TB and HIV-related infections), and occupational pneumoconiosis. Acute-onset shortness of breath can be caused by acute exacerbations of any of these chronic conditions, by acute infections such as pneumonia or acute bronchitis, or by spontaneous pneumothorax. Among otherwise healthy children, shortness of breath can be related to asthma, bronchiolitis, pneumonia, or upper airway problems such as croup or epiglottitis. Chronic shortness of breath in children can be related to poorly controlled asthma, bronchopulmonary dysplasia from infancy, or chronic diseases (e.g., CF).

The cardiovascular system is the other organ system most often linked to shortness of breath. In adults, congestive heart failure (CHF) is a leading cause of recent-onset shortness of breath among middle-aged and older adults. In addition to shortness of breath, patients might report symptoms of wheezing from the pulmonary congestion, often referred to as *cardiac asthma*. Differentiating early CHF from pulmonary causes of dyspnea can be a challenge in middle-aged or older patients who smoke or have other chronic medical conditions. Other cardiac conditions associated with shortness of breath include pericarditis and cardiomyopathy, as well as congenital heart defects in infants presenting with respiratory distress. Vascular conditions include chronic pulmonary hypertension and PE in the setting of acute-onset shortness of breath.

Along with the history and physical examination, testing can help in ruling out pulmonary versus cardiac causes of dyspnea. Physicians often begin diagnostic testing with electrocardiography (ECG) and even echocardiography to rule out cardiac causes of shortness of breath, but simple history, auscultation of the heart and lungs, chest radiography, and office spirometry can also help diagnose or rule out common pulmonary causes of shortness of breath. Improvement on weekends or nonworkdays can suggest an occupational exposure, and a prolonged expiratory phase with expiratory wheezing suggests obstructive lung disease. Orthopnea and pedal edema suggest a cardiac cause. Bibasilar rales suggest fluid in the lower lung fields from CHF. ECG can approximate chamber enlargement and identify arrhythmias that might decrease ventricular filling time. Echocardiography can measure ejection fraction and systolic or diastolic dysfunction indicating heart failure, local wall motion abnormalities suggesting ischemic disease, and valvular abnormalities. Levels of B-natriuretic protein have a 90% sensitivity and 76% specificity for CHF; levels less than 100 pg/mL make CHF unlikely as the principal cause of shortness of breath or wheezing (Mueller et al., 2005). Chest radiography can help rule out pulmonary or other thoracic mass lesions, lung infections, granulomatous or interstitial lung disease (ILD), pleural disease, pneumothorax, and cardiomegaly, supplemented with CT as needed. Although young patients with normal physical examination findings have a low yield on chest radiography, up to 86% of patients older than 40 years with dyspnea have an abnormal chest radiograph (Benacerraf et al., 1981). Spirometry showing an FEV_1/FVC ratio less than 70% is diagnostic of obstructive lung disease, and an FVC less than 80% of predicted value in the presence of a normal FEV_1/FVC ratio suggests restrictive lung disease.

Many patients present primarily with dyspnea on exertion. The 6-minute walking exercise test is a valid measure of exercise tolerance (compared with maximal exercise testing) in patients with COPD and other pulmonary conditions, as well as in various stages of CHF. It can be performed in primary care settings to assess functional disability and response to therapy (American Thoracic Society [ATS], 2002; Lipkin et al., 1986). In patients with pulmonary hypertension, the distance walked with encouragement in 6 minutes in a controlled environment is also a strong independent predictor of mortality (Miyamoto et al., 2000).

Formal cardiac ECG stress testing by exercise treadmill can quantify the level of exercise tolerance and diagnose cardiac ischemia or angina-equivalent conditions, in which a person has ischemia-induced shortness of breath but no chest pain. However, the test has a sensitivity of only 63% and specificity of 74% (86% specificity in the setting of three-vessel or left main coronary artery disease) (Gibbons et al., 1997). Other types of cardiac stress testing, such as exercise echocardiography or the nuclear medicine thallium treadmill test, can be more specific (see Chapter 27) (Mayo Clinic, 1996). The American College of Cardiology and American Society of Echocardiography published a consensus guideline on the appropriate use of stress echocardiography for specific clinical scenarios (Douglas et al.,

2008). For patients unable to exercise, increased cardiac work may be induced pharmacologically, but dipyridamole and adenosine can each cause bronchospasm and should be avoided in patients with asthma or any other obstructive lung disease or undiagnosed pulmonary conditions (Tak and Gutierrez, 2004).

The presentation of patients with acute-onset shortness of breath requires more urgent evaluation. In addition to history and physical examination, a peak-flow test, chest radiography, ECG, complete blood count, and pulse oximetry or ABG testing may be done in short order. Further testing or treatment is guided by the differential diagnosis generated by this initial evaluation. Cardiac isoenzymes and troponin levels can help rule myocardial infarction in or out. If asthma is suspected, responsiveness to a trial of inhaled bronchodilator is both diagnostic and therapeutic. Antibiotics are initiated in cases of pneumonia or other pulmonary infection, and HIV testing can help in cases of suspected opportunistic infections (e.g., PCP).

Any suspicion of PE as a cause of acute shortness of breath requires specific diagnostic evaluation to allow quick intervention in this potentially life-threatening condition. Acute-onset shortness of breath coupled with pleuritic chest pain, hemoptysis, wedge-shaped pulmonary infarct lesions on chest radiographs, and an S1Q3 pattern on ECG can all point specifically to a diagnosis of PE, but most patients have a more nonspecific presentation. All patients with acute-onset shortness of breath with no apparent cause should be evaluated for PE. Physical examination for signs of deep vein thrombosis (DVT) (e.g., asymmetry in calf or thigh diameter, calf tenderness, Homans sign) are relatively insensitive and nonspecific, but other tests (e.g., D-dimer, CT angiography) can more accurately confirm the presence of significant underlying DVT. Clinical decision rules using objective scoring algorithms help establish pretest probability, which in turn enhances the predictive value of other tests for PE (Wells et al., 2000) (see later discussion).

Cough

Cough is also a common presenting symptom in primary care. Although cough can be part of a constellation of symptoms that leads to a specific diagnosis, it can also be the primary symptom in an undifferentiated patient. In these cases, the diagnosis must be obtained through a combination of careful history, physical examination, limited diagnostic testing, and often a trial of empiric therapy. Several elements of the history guide the initial differential diagnosis, especially a history of smoking, immunocompromise (HIV/AIDS or cancer chemotherapy), chronic pulmonary disease, medication use (angiotensin-converting enzyme [ACE] inhibitors), specific occupational exposures, or exposure to TB patients or TB-endemic areas.

Acute episodes of cough, defined as less than 3 weeks, are almost always caused by an acute infection (usually viral) or an acute exacerbation of chronic disease such as asthma or COPD, and the first rule should be to "do no harm" (primum non nocere) by treating conservatively and using time as a diagnostic test. Most episodes of acute cough caused by infection are viral in origin, mainly viral upper respiratory tract infections or acute bronchitis. Acute bacterial infections include sinusitis as well as bacterial overgrowth in exacerbations of chronic bronchitis or COPD. Fever, hemoptysis, or significant shortness of breath in association with cough indicates a chest radiograph or other immediate diagnostic evaluation. Frank hemoptysis can require urgent bronchoscopy for diagnosis and potentially for treatment (electrocoagulation of bleeding site). Without evidence of bacterial infection (clear evidence of sinusitis or pneumonia), previously healthy patients should generally be treated symptomatically without antibiotics unless symptoms persist for more than 3 weeks.

Foreign body aspiration is a diagnostic consideration in children with either acute or chronic cough. Exacerbations of asthma, as well as infections by *Bordetella pertussis* (whooping cough) or *Bordetella parapertussis*, can lead to a persistent cough for as long as 3 to 8 weeks. Cough might indeed be the only symptom experienced by some patients with asthma (cough-variant asthma). In patients with underlying chronic bronchitis or COPD, antibiotics may be indicated during episodes of increased shortness of breath, wheezing, hypoxia, or limitations of activity if accompanied by a sudden change in sputum from thin and clear to thick or copious or yellow-green. Other subacute or chronic infections include bronchiectasis, which can manifest with a cough productive of mucopurulent, blood-tinged, or foul-smelling sputum. In children with chronic productive cough or recurrent pulmonary infections, CF must be considered. Survivors of premature birth with mechanical ventilation in neonatal intensive care may have chronic lung disease with acute exacerbations.

In adults, the most common causes of chronic cough in nonsmokers are postnasal drip, asthma, gastroesophageal reflux disease (GERD), and ACE inhibitors (Holmes and Fadden, 2004). Among smokers, chronic bronchitis, bronchiectasis, and bronchogenic carcinoma (lung cancer) must also be considered. Additional elements of the history can suggest other diagnoses. For example, occupational exposures can suggest specific diagnoses such as coal miner's lung or farmer's lung. Immigration from or travel to TB-endemic areas could suggest TB.

After the history and physical examination, chest radiography is the most valuable diagnostic test in evaluating the patient with chronic cough. Chest radiography can reveal infections (atypical pneumonia or TB), mass lesions (carcinoma), granulomatous disease (sarcoidosis), or evidence of occupational lung disease. Radiography can also reveal nonpulmonary causes of chronic cough, such as early CHF or pleural lesions. Office spirometry may also be performed to rule out obstructive lung disease.

In an otherwise healthy nonsmoker with chronic cough and normal chest radiography findings, a trial of simple measures may be indicated. Persons being treated with an ACE inhibitor should be switched to alternative medication. Patients with occupational exposures should avoid the exposure or use protective equipment and should begin keeping a log to document the association of symptoms with days spent in workplace areas of exposure. Patients with signs of allergic rhinitis or postnasal drip may begin a simple trial of antihistamines. Patients with symptomatic GERD may begin taking a protein pump inhibitor (e.g., omeprazole) or H_2 antagonist. In some cases, chronic cough is the only symptom of GERD, and a successful trial of these agents is diagnostic.

Follow-up is essential, and the primary care practitioner must document instructions to patients that those who do not respond to empiric therapy in 2 to 3 weeks need further diagnostic evaluation. If asthma is suspected and initial office spirometry revealed normal pulmonary function, a simple approach is to ask the patient to keep a log of symptoms and morning peak-flow meter readings. In patients with an abnormal chest radiography findings or in smokers with chronic cough that does not respond to empiric therapy, HRCT scan or even bronchoscopy may be indicated to rule out malignancy. Less common conditions may also present as chronic cough. These include sarcoidosis, TB, and other granulomatous or ILDs, as well as pulmonary manifestations of autoimmune disease, such as rheumatoid arthritis (RA) or systemic lupus erythematosus (SLE).

Patients with HIV/AIDS or other compromise of the immune system deserve specific evaluation (Chapter 15). HIV testing may be indicated in patients with any risk factors because pulmonary symptoms can be the first manifestation of symptomatic HIV disease. In patients known to be HIV positive, tests in addition to chest radiography and HRCT could include gallium scan, PET, bronchoscopy with BAL for stains and cultures, PPD, and sputum testing for PCP.

Obstructive Lung Disease

The most common chronic lung diseases that have a major global impact on disability and health care costs are three obstructive lung diseases: asthma, COPD, and chronic bronchitis. Some patients have features of more than one of these conditions, such as a patient with asthma (acute episodes of reversible obstruction) who also has chronic bronchitis (cough productive of phlegm at least 3 months of the year for at least 2 years in a row) or an adult patient with asthma who is developing some level of irreversible decline in pulmonary function. COPD alone can ultimately result in pathologic signs of emphysema, a diagnosis previously made only with tissue pathology or large blebs on radiography but increasingly visible with high-resolution imaging.

ASTHMA

Key Points

- Asthma is defined as an inflammatory, episodic, obstructive lung disease that is completely reversible.
- Self-management is focused on improving symptom-free function and decreasing risk of adverse outcomes through control of environmental triggers, regular peak-flow monitoring, action plans, and long-term controller medications, a combined strategy that can prevent or abort most flare-ups of asthma.
- All patients with persistent asthma (daytime symptoms more than twice a week or nocturnal symptoms more than twice a month) should be treated with daily long-term control medication, preferably an inhaled corticosteroid (ICS).
- Eliminating passive exposure to smokers is the most important intervention in eliminating environmental triggers.

Asthma is a chronic inflammatory airway disease characterized by recurring acute episodes of reversible airway obstruction, with return to normal lung function between episodes. Although bronchospasm is a component of the reversible airway obstruction, recent clinical guidelines have emphasized the inflammatory pathophysiology of asthma (National Heart, Lung and Blood Institute, 2007). Therefore, the clinician must treat and prevent the inflammation that leads to mucosal edema, secretions, histologic remodeling of the airways, and bronchospasm of smooth muscle origin.

Epidemiology and Risk Factors

Asthma is the most common chronic disease of childhood and affects many adult patients as well. The prevalence of asthma is increasing rapidly worldwide. It now affects more than 300 million people and causes the loss of more than 15 million disability-adjusted life-years (DALY) each year (Global Initiative for Asthma, 2006). Asthma prevalence is increasing in many countries and is not decreasing globally, despite some indications of decreased emergency care use linked to improved care (Anandan et al., 2010). In the United States, National Health Interview Survey (NHIS) data (National Center for Health Statistics, 2011) suggest that 20 million Americans would report currently having asthma (72 per 1000 people). Asthma affects an estimated 6.1 million children nationally (83 per 1000). There were 384,588 hospital admissions with a principal diagnosis of asthma in the United States in 2011, with an average charge per hospitalization of more than $20,000. That same year, total hospital charges for asthma admissions in the United States added up to $8 billion (Agency for Healthcare Research & Quality [AHRQ], 2011a). Focusing on children, asthma was the primary diagnosis for more than 700,000 childhood ED visits in 2011, and one in 10 of these children seen in the ED were hospitalized (AHRQ, 2011b).

Asthma is also a high-disparity condition. Low-income, uninsured, and minority patients with asthma consistently receive worse care and have worse outcomes compared with patients with asthma in the general population (Lang and Polansky, 1994). Hospitalization rates in the United States are 3.3 times higher for black than for white patients (National Center for Health Statistics, 2011). Publicly insured and uninsured patients are significantly more likely to be hospitalized and to seek ED care during acute exacerbations (Targonski et al., 1995).

The strongest risk factors for developing asthma are exposure to household smokers and a family history of asthma or atopy (asthma, atopic dermatitis, or allergic rhinitis). A family history of nasal polyps or aspirin hypersensitivity can also suggest a risk for IgE-mediated atopic disease. Data are mixed on the impact of breastfeeding and early exposure to pets as protective factors in the development of asthma (Adler et al., 2005), although the benefits of puppies and breastfeeding should be self-evident.

Clinical Presentation and Diagnosis

A complete history in patients suspected of having asthma should include the frequency and severity of recent symptoms and should distinguish between daytime and nocturnal symptom frequency, a factor that is also important in staging asthma. A history of past or present smoking (tobacco or other drugs) is essential, as is an inquiry about current passive exposure to smokers in the household or occupational secondary exposure to tobacco smoke (e.g., bartenders, restaurant staff). The clinician should also inquire about activities, acute illnesses, or environmental exposures that trigger episodes; a family history of asthma or atopic disease; and a detailed occupational history. Some patients are also exposed to bronchial irritants through hobbies such as woodworking or oil painting.

Symptomatically, patients can present with complaints of chronic or acute episodic shortness of breath, wheezing, chest tightness, or a chronic cough (often at night). If they already have a diagnosis of asthma, they may report relief with rescue inhalers such as albuterol. Some patients, especially children, only have nocturnal cough, a syndrome known as *cough-variant asthma*, but others have symptoms precipitated mostly by exercise or by breathing in cold air.

On physical examination, the patient might have obvious difficulty breathing or audible wheezing during an acute episode. Patients with significant shortness of breath can have difficulty completing a full sentence without taking a breath. Inspection can reveal nasal flaring, breathing through pursed lips, central or acral cyanosis, hyperexpansion of the chest, or use of accessory respiratory muscles. In more extreme cases, patients appear to have respiratory exhaustion, central or distal cyanosis, or even a blunting of mental status.

On auscultation, the earliest sign of airway obstruction is a prolonged expiratory phase (expiratory phase longer than inspiratory phase). A more obvious sign of asthma is expiratory wheezing. Wheezing can sometimes be brought out by forced expiration, performed by asking the patient to blow out forcefully while the examiner listens over the second intercostal space at the right sternal border. More severe cases of obstruction can result in both inspiratory and expiratory wheezing. In the most severe cases, wheezing might not be audible at all because airflow is minimal. In these cases, wheezing becomes much more prominent as airflow improves. Another sign of severity of an acute episode is *pulsus paradoxus*, defined as a decrease in systolic blood pressure of more than 20 mm Hg during inspiration.

A more objective measure of pulmonary function during an acute exacerbation of asthma is to measure the peak flow of air during forced expiration using a simple, low-cost peak-flow meter. Airflow is measured in liters per second. The best of three attempts is recorded as the peak-flow measurement. Results can be measured against nomograms based on the patient's age, gender, and height, but a better measurement is to compare the patient's peak flow during the acute episode against his or her baseline or best performance during a period of complete remission from asthma signs or symptoms.

When patients present with a history of asthma-like symptoms in the primary care setting, the diagnosis can be confirmed with office spirometry, a form of pulmonary function testing. The essential criterion for a diagnosis of airway obstruction is an FEV_1/FVC ratio of less than 70%. To diagnose asthma, the clinician must also demonstrate reversibility with inhaled bronchodilators, either through the patient's history or improvement in the FEV_1 of greater than 200 mL or 12%. Because asthma is defined as an obstructive lung disease that is completely reversible between episodes, testing in the office during asymptomatic periods might not demonstrate airway obstruction. In this case, it is helpful for the patient to use a peak-flow meter at home, testing three times each morning and recording the best value, as well as testing during symptom episodes. The record of these values can be reviewed with the family physician to aid in diagnosis, as well as for coaching the patient in self-management and prevention of future episodes.

Chest radiography is not always indicated if the patient has a classic history of episodic airway obstruction, especially if it is reversible with β-agonist rescue inhalers. In infants and children, however, the physician must distinguish upper airway causes of obstruction from obstructive lung disease. Examples include croup or laryngotracheobronchitis, epiglottitis, and foreign bodies lodged in the upper airway. In infants and older adults, the clinician must also exclude so-called cardiac asthma, which manifests as wheezing or other signs of airway obstruction related to pulmonary edema or CHF. In these patients, chest radiography is clearly indicated.

Patients older than 40 years who have new-onset asthma should have a complete workup to rule out other causes of airway obstruction. Many clinicians order chest radiography in all patients with new asthma, although there is a low rate of finding pathology in otherwise healthy older children and young adults. Chest radiographs obtained during an acute episode of asthma can give false-positive findings of infiltrates or atelectasis.

Treatment

The National Asthma Education and Prevention Program (NAEPP) guidelines provide a comprehensive and evidence-based approach to the clinical care of asthma (National Heart Lung and Blood Institute, 1997; NAEPP Expert Panel Report 3, 2007). Unfortunately, there is a large gap between best practice guideline-based care and usual care, as measured by compliance with these national guidelines (Thier et al., 2008) and by the clinical outcomes achievable when these guidelines are followed.

Acute Exacerbations. The mainstay of treatment for acute exacerbations of asthma is an inhaled β-agonist medication such as albuterol. Although β-agonist medication is typically administered in the ED or physician's office with a nebulizer machine, a meta-analysis of controlled trials showed that a handheld metered-dose inhaler with a spacer device is at least as effective as a nebulizer in delivering albuterol and achieving a clinical response, as measured by pulmonary function and by clinical outcomes such as hospitalization (Castro-Rodriguez and Rodrigo, 2004). Adding ipratropium bromide to albuterol nebulizer treatments for patients with severe airflow obstruction in the acute ED setting produces additional bronchodilation, resulting in fewer hospital admissions (Plotnick and Ducharme, 2000; Rodrigo and Castro-Rodriguez, 2005).

Additional modalities of treatment include oxygen by nasal cannula or mask, and intravenous (IV) fluids for hydration. Short-term administration of systemic corticosteroids has also been demonstrated to be effective. Corticosteroids may be given intravenously (methylprednisolone), intramuscularly (dexamethasone or equivalent), or orally (prednisone or methylprednisolone). When given for 3 to 5 days as burst or pulse-dose therapy, steroids do

Table 16-3 MAP for Asthma Care

Management plan	What do I do every day to control my asthma?
Action plan	What do I do when I have acute symptoms or my peak-flow meter values are dropping?
Prevention plan	What can I do to control asthma triggers and prevent acute flare-ups?

not need to be tapered to prevent adrenal suppression. However, patients with chronic or severe exacerbations of asthma may require prolonged tapering to prevent rehospitalization for recurrence of airway obstruction.

Intravenous magnesium sulfate has also shown significant benefit in decreasing the rate of hospitalization of ED patients with acute asthma and in improving pulmonary function and clinical symptom scores (Cheuk et al., 2005). The most recent NAEPP Expert Panel Report (NAEPP Expert Panel Report 3, 2007) now recommends considering using IV magnesium sulfate or heliox-driven albuterol nebulizer treatments in patients who have failed to respond to 1 hour of conventional asthma therapy. Heliox alone (in place of oxygen) is not effective (Rodrigo et al., 2003). Children treated with theophylline during hospitalizations for acute asthma exacerbations required more albuterol treatments and had longer hospital stays than children not treated with theophylline (Goodman et al., 1996).

Chronic Care and Disease Management. To achieve optimal outcomes, each patient should have a personal asthma care plan, which can be summarized in the mnemonic MAP (Table 16-3). The *management* plan refers to daily medications or activities such as measuring peak flow; an *action* plan is needed for specific steps to take in the event of increased symptoms or deteriorating peak-flow values; and a *prevention* plan focuses on understanding personal and environmental triggers, such as avoiding passive exposure to cigarette smoke and eliminating dust mite and cockroach antigens. Treatment is focused on reducing symptoms, increasing functional capacity, and reducing the risk of adverse outcomes (missed school days, ED visits, hospital admissions, and death).

Appropriate chronic care requires appropriate staging of the clinical severity of asthma. Stage 1 is intermittent, and stages 2, 3, and 4 all represent persistent (mild, moderate, and severe) disease. Criteria for classification of patients into stages 1 to 4 are shown in Figure 19-1 and 19-2. This staging of asthma is done based on the level and frequency of symptoms or airflow obstruction before beginning treatment. The patient's step is determined by the *most severe* feature, and classification refers to symptoms *before* starting treatment. Pharmacologic treatment of asthma is linked to this classification, as shown in the treatment algorithm (see Figures 19-3 and 19-4).

A critical decision point is to decide if the patient has *persistent* disease as described by these criteria. Evidence suggests that primary care clinicians routinely underclassify the severity of asthma and thus undertreat with daily antiinflammatory, long-term control medications. NAEPP guidelines suggest that only patients with truly intermittent disease—that is, patients with normal peak flow readings, daytime symptoms no more than twice a week, and nighttime symptoms no more than twice a month—should be

Table 16-4 Estimated Comparative Daily Doses for Inhaled Corticosteroids for Adolescents (Age 12 Years) and Adults

Drug	Amount	Daily Dose (µg)		
		Low	**Medium**	**High**
Beclomethasone HFA	40 or 80 µg/puff	80-240	>240-480	>480
Budesonide DPI	90, 80, or 200 µg/inhalation	180-600	>600-1200	>1200
Flunisolide	250 µg/puff	500-1000	>1000-2000	>2000
Flunisolide HFA	80 µg/puff	320	>320-640	>640
Fluticasone				
HFA/MDI	44, 110, or 220 µg/puff	88-264	>264-440	>440
DPI	50, 100, or 250 µg/inhalation	100-300	>300-500	>500
Mometasone DPI	200 µg/inhalation	200	400	>400
Triamcinolone acetonide	75 µg/puff	300-750	>750-1500	>1500

DPI, Dry powder inhaler; *HFA,* hydrofluoroalkane; *MDI;* metered-dose inhaler.
From National Heart, Lung and Blood Institute, NHI, Expert Panel 3 (EPR3). Guidelines for the Diagnosis and Management of Asthma. National Asthma Education and Prevention Program (NAEPP) Coordinating Committee, 2007. http://www.nhlbi.nih.gov/guidelines/asthma/asthgdln.htm.

treated with intermittent medication alone. All other patients—those with mild, moderate, or severe persistent disease—should be treated with daily antiinflammatory, long-term control medication such as an inhaled corticosteroid (ICS). One study has been cited as providing evidence allowing intermittent therapy of patients with mild to moderate persistent asthma, but the study results actually found that daily budesonide therapy produced greater improvements in prebronchodilator FEV_1, bronchial reactivity, sputum eosinophils, exhaled nitric oxide levels, scores for asthma control, and the number of symptom-free days but not in postbronchodilator FEV_1 or in reported quality of life (Boushey et al., 2005).

A meta-analysis found that ICSs reduced asthma exacerbations by 55% compared with placebo or short-acting β-agonists, and long-acting β-agonists (LABAs) reduced flare-ups by only 26% (Sin et al., 2004). Similarly, a Cochrane Database review found that inhaled steroids at a dose equivalent to 400 µg/day of beclomethasone are more effective than leukotriene antagonists and that ICSs should be considered first-line monotherapy for persistent asthma. Patients with mild to moderate disease achieve similar levels of asthma control taking low doses (200 µg/day) as high doses (500 µg/day) of fluticasone, and side effects are greater with higher doses. A dose equivalency chart for inhaled steroids is shown in Table 16-4. Unfortunately, adherence to daily ICSs can be as low as 20% in real-world surveillance outside of clinical trials (Rust et al., 2013).

New approaches to monitoring therapy by measuring the fraction of exhaled nitric oxide (FE_{NO}) could theoretically allow better adjustment of inhaled-corticosteroid doses but have not been widely adopted (Smith et al., 2005). High-dose ICSs are useful primarily in weaning patients from oral steroids.

Other second-line long-term control agents include long-acting beta agonists (LABAs; salmeterol, formoterol), long-acting anticholinergics (tiotropium), leukotriene receptor antagonists (LTRAs), inhaled mast cell stabilizers (cromolyn, nedocromil), and theophylline. Although each has demonstrated efficacy, none is as effective as ICSs. When low-dose ICSs are not providing complete remission, the clinician may add a second medication or increase the inhaled steroid dose to moderate levels. In a controlled trial of an inhaled LABA (formoterol) versus theophylline versus a leukotriene antagonist (zafirlukast) as second-line agents added to ICS therapy, Yurdakul and colleagues (2002) found that the LABA was more effective in preventing exacerbations and had fewer side effects than the other options. A Cochrane review of 12 controlled trials also found that LABAs were more effective than leukotriene antagonists as add-on therapy to inhaled steroids (Ram et al., 2005). Concern persists, however, that LABAs can increase mortality rates when used as monotherapy in the absence of ICSs (Abramson et al., 2003b). Adding tiotropium bromide to low-dose ICS therapy is superior to doubling the dose of the ICS and equivalent to adding a LABA (SOR: A; Peters et al., 2010). The leukotriene synthesis inhibitor zileuton appears to improve pulmonary function and decrease need for β-agonist but causes significant elevations of liver transaminases in 2% to 3% of patients (Nelson et al., 2007).

Immunotherapy also appears to be effective. A Cochrane review found that allergen immunotherapy reduces asthma symptoms and use of asthma medications at a level similar to that of ICSs (Abramson et al., 2003a). A third-line therapy is the once- or twice-monthly injection of monoclonal anti-IgE antibodies (omalizumab), an expensive therapy that is associated with a 98% to 99% reduction in free IgE and significantly fewer exacerbations of asthma, even allowing some patients to be weaned from ICSs (Walker et al., 2003).

Prevention

Even though dust mites are usually mentioned as a controllable environmental trigger, a Cochrane review of 49 controlled trials found no evidence that either physical or chemical methods aimed at reducing exposure to house dust mite allergens had any benefit (Gotzsche et al., 2004). On the other hand, a controlled trial of an intervention to reduce cockroach and dust mite allergens *and* passive exposure to tobacco smoke among urban children with atopic asthma was effective in reducing both allergens in the home and asthma symptom days (Morgan et al., 2004). Teaching patients to self-monitor and self-manage their asthma using an action plan and ongoing review with their physician is effective in reducing exacerbations and symptoms (Gibson et al., 2002). For children, parents of other children with asthma can serve effectively as peer counselors and may be especially effective in reducing cultural and linguistic barriers (Flores et al., 2009). As with most pulmonary diseases, the most effective preventive strategy is to eliminate smoking as a risk factor from the patient, the household, and the workplace.

- Daily ICSs significantly reduce exacerbations and hospitalizations in patients with persistent asthma and are significantly more effective as first-line long-term control agents than any alternative agents (Sin et al., 2004) (SOR: A).
- LABAs are more effective than leukotriene antagonists as add-on-therapy to inhaled steroids. Because most benefits of ICS are achieved at lower doses, adding a LABA to a low or medium dose of ICS is preferred over using a higher dose of ICS. LABAs should not be used as monotherapy because of a higher risk of death (Food and Drug Administration black box warning) (NAEPP EPR-3; Ram et al., 2005) (SOR: A).
- Adding ipratropium bromide to albuterol nebulizer treatments for patients with severe airflow obstruction in the acute ED setting produces additional bronchodilation, resulting in fewer hospital admissions (Plotnick and Ducharme, 2000; Rodrigo and Castro-Rodriguez, 2005) (SOR: A).
- Theophylline is an acceptable (but not preferred) alternative to LABA for second-line long-term control treatment in combination with ICSs, but theophylline or aminophylline should not be used in the acute treatment of ED or in-hospital patients (SOR: A).
- Teaching patients to engage in effective self-management improves clinical outcomes (Gibson et al., 2002) (SOR: A).
- Nurse care managers, community health workers, and parents as peer counselors can improve asthma self-management and clinical outcomes (SOR: B).

CHRONIC OBSTRUCTIVE PULMONARY DISEASE AND CHRONIC BRONCHITIS

Consensus statements from the Global Initiative for Chronic Obstructive Lung Disease known as the GOLD guidelines (Global Initiative, Global Strategy, 2014) define COPD as a postbronchodilator FVC of less than 80% of predicted in a patient with evidence of airway obstruction (FEV_1/FVC ratio <70%) that is not completely reversible (Global Initiative Pocket Guide, 2014). Although some patients with asthma, especially those who smoke, can progress to varying degrees of irreversibility consistent with COPD, the underlying pathophysiology and inflammatory mechanisms in asthma are distinct from those found in patients with COPD.

Epidemiology and Risk Factors

In large part because of the global spread of tobacco addiction, WHO estimates that COPD is already the fifth leading cause of death and will soon be the fifth leading cause of disability as well. In the United States, there were 729,030 hospital admissions with a principal diagnosis of chronic obstructive lung disease in 2011, with an average length of stay of 4.4 days and in-hospital mortality rate of 1.4%. One third of these admissions were in relatively young 45- to 64-year-old adults (AHRQ, 2011c).

Smoking is the most important risk factor for COPD and causes ongoing damage in COPD patients, as measured by an accelerated decline in FEV_1 compared with nonsmokers or ex-smokers. Among COPD patients who have quit smoking, exposure to secondhand smoke can also be a trigger factor for acute exacerbations, as can variation in environmental air quality (ozone and small particulates). In many countries, indoor kitchen smoke can be a major source of damage to the respiratory tract in settings where daily cooking over indoor fires or charcoal is common. Other trigger factors for acute exacerbations include acute upper respiratory infections, sinusitis, exposure to dust or pet dander, and intercurrent illness. However, when patients reach a more severe stage of illness in which pulmonary reserves are minimal, almost any small change (e.g., fatigue, stress, change in weather) can trigger an exacerbation.

The other major risk factor for the development of COPD is the inherited disorder α_1-antitrypsin deficiency. The recognition of this disease and its cellular mechanisms of injury to the lung have led to a specific understanding of protease and antiprotease imbalance as one mechanism of disease progression of emphysematous COPD. Any patient who develops COPD without a significant smoking history, any patient with a strong family history of COPD, and any patient developing clinically significant COPD before age 45 years should be screened for α_1-antitrypsin deficiency. A detailed discussion of genetic counseling of patients with α_1-antitrypsin deficiency or carrier state can be found in the ATS and European Respiratory Society (2003) consensus standards.

Clinical Presentation

Chronic obstructive pulmonary disease includes the two overlapping clinical conditions of chronic *bronchitis* and *emphysema*, which can coexist in the same patient. A practical clinical approach is to diagnose COPD by documenting obstruction that is not completely reversible on pulmonary function testing and then assess whether the patient also has a component of chronic bronchitis—that is, cough productive of phlegm at least 3 months of each year for at least 2 years. Some patients meet this criterion for chronic bronchitis before developing clinical or spirometric evidence of obstructive lung disease. The international GOLD guidelines no longer categorize this as stage 0 COPD because of insufficient evidence that patients will inevitably progress to obstructive lung disease.

Often, patients who smoke have had a chronic smoker's cough for years and present for medical treatment only when symptoms such as shortness of breath on exertion or at rest begin to appear. The hallmark symptom of symptomatic COPD is progressive and persistent shortness of breath. Because of the built-in reserve of the pulmonary system, such functional disability often is not noticed until there is a substantial decline in pulmonary function and substantial damage to lung parenchyma. Still, the U.S. Preventive Services Task Force recommends not screening routinely with spirometry for obstructive lung disease or declining lung function.

Comorbidities are often present, and they must be co-managed with COPD if patients are to have optimal clinical outcomes and quality of life. For example, CHF can eventually occur after years of elevated right-sided pulmonary pressure (right-sided failure leading ultimately to biventricular failure), or patients might simply experience smoking-related myocardial infarctions and coronary ischemia in parallel with their COPD. Symptomatic COPD has a powerful adverse effect on quality of life, and a substantial proportion of patients with COPD develop comorbid depression. Chronic hypoxia and air hunger can also generate significant anxiety.

Diagnosis and Severity Assessment

By the time many patients present for treatment, the diagnosis of COPD is apparent. In addition to symptoms of dyspnea, chronic productive cough, and functional limitations, patients can show physical findings of lung hyperexpansion (increased lung span on percussion, increased thoracic AP diameter, and use of accessory muscles of respiration). Extrathoracic signs include peripheral or central cyanosis, nail clubbing, and signs of increased central venous pressure or even right-sided heart failure. Table 16-5 presents the differential diagnosis and distinguishing features of COPD suggested by the GOLD guidelines. Any patient who develops COPD without a significant smoking history, or any patient developing COPD before age 45 years, should be screened for α_1-antitrypsin deficiency. HRCT can help identify granulomatous or ILDs or provide evidence of bronchiectasis.

Spirometry is the key to making a formal diagnosis, as well as for grading the severity of illness. COPD may be diagnosed when obstructive lung disease is not fully reversible, defined as a postbronchodilator FVC of less than 80% of predicted in a patient with evidence of airway obstruction (FEV_1/FVC ratio <70%). A pattern of restrictive lung disease (FVC < 80% of predicted in the presence of a normal FEV_1/FVC ratio) would suggest alternative diagnoses, such as pulmonary fibrosis, sarcoidosis, autoimmune conditions, or primary CHF.

Although there are several classification systems for severity of COPD, the ATS guidelines and the international GOLD standards are similar. They are based on spirometric criteria—the presence of obstruction and the level of impairment in FEV_1—and correlate strongly with exacerbations and 3-year mortality but less so with perceived quality of life and functional limitations. According to the TOwards a Revolution in COPD Health (TORCH) study, moderate COPD (GOLD 2) has a 3-year mortality rate of 11% compared with 24% for very severe COPD (GOLD 4) (Calverly et al., 2007). One validated survey instrument recommended by the Global Initiative on COPD is the eight-item COPD Assessment Test (CAT), which assesses a broader range of symptoms than just breathlessness, which is the focus of the modified British Medical Research Council (mMRC) scale (GOLD, 2013b). A CAT score greater than or equal to 10 is considered a high score with regard to categorizing symptoms for treatment decisions. The 6-minute walk test is another way to assess COPD by its impact on daily activities. A distance of less than 149 meters walked in 6 minutes of encouraged walking indicates more severe functional limitation, and a distance

Table 16-5 Differential Diagnosis of Chronic Obstructive Pulmonary Disease* (GOLD Guidelines)

COPD	Onset in midlife Symptoms slowly progressive Long smoking history Dyspnea during exercise Largely irreversible airflow limitation
Asthma	Onset early in life (often childhood) Symptoms vary from day to day Symptoms at night and early morning Allergy, rhinitis, or eczema is also present Family history of asthma Largely reversible airflow limitation
Congestive heart failure	Fine basilar crackles on auscultation Chest radiograph shows dilated heart, pulmonary edema Pulmonary function tests indicate volume restriction, not airflow limitation
Bronchiectasis	Large volumes of purulent sputum Often associated with bacterial infection Coarse crackles or clubbing on auscultation Chest radiograph or CT shows bronchial dilation or bronchial wall thickening
Tuberculosis	Onset at all ages Chest radiograph shows lung infiltrate Microbiologic confirmation High local prevalence of tuberculosis
Obliterative bronchiolitis	Onset at a younger age and in nonsmokers May have history of RA or fume exposure CT on expiration shows hypodense areas
Diffuse panbronchiolitis	Most patients are male and nonsmokers Almost all have chronic sinusitis Chest radiography and HRCT show diffuse small centrilobular nodular opacities and hyperinflation

*These features tend to be characteristic of the respective diseases but do not occur in every case. For example, a person who has never smoked may develop chronic obstructive pulmonary disease (COPD), especially in the developing world where other risk factors may be more important than cigarette smoking, and asthma may develop in an adult and even elderly patients.

CT, Computed tomography; *HRCT*, high-resolution computed tomography; *RA*, rheumatoid arthritis.

From Global Initiative for Chronic Obstructive Lung Disease: Pocket Guide to COPD Diagnosis, Treatment, and Management: A Guide for Health Professionals; Updated 2014. Table 2, p.8. http://www.goldcopd.org/uploads/users/files/GOLD_Pocket_2014_Jun11.pdf.

farther than 350 meters indicates minimal limitation (Celli et al., 2004).

Treatment

Acute Exacerbations. The course of COPD is characterized by patients' daily coping with chronic obstruction, punctuated by episodic exacerbations that can be life threatening and only partially responsive to treatment. Initial evaluation includes the patient's assessment of the severity of symptoms, plus physical examination, chest radiography, and ABG tests. Predicting which patients can be safely discharged from the ED versus those who need to be hospitalized requires evaluation of both clinical and psychosocial indicators (Smith et al., 2000).

Chest radiography can reveal underlying causes of an acute exacerbation, such as pneumonia or CHF. ABGs are useful in assessing initial hypoxia and hypercapnia but also in monitoring the patient's response to judicious use of supplemental oxygen administered by nasal cannula or mask. Although relief of hypoxia reduces symptoms and improves cardiac function, it can also decrease the respiratory drive in a patient with chronic hypercapnia and partially compensated respiratory acidosis. For this reason, ABGs should be repeated within 30 minutes after starting oxygen, and ongoing hypoxia may be monitored with pulse oximetry (although oximetry becomes less accurate at SO_2 levels <70%).

An immediate response is expected from inhaled β_2-agonist therapy in asthma, but the response to bronchodilators in acute exacerbations of COPD can be modest. Some patients are more responsive to anticholinergic bronchodilators such as ipratropium, and others respond to β_2-agonist agents, so these therapies are often combined in the acute setting. At home, patients can increase the dose or frequency of current medications or add a short-term agent to their chronic therapy (e.g., adding albuterol doses to LABA or adding ipratropium to chronic tiotropium therapy). Either spacer devices or mechanical nebulizer delivery systems may be used. Treatment of acute exacerbations of COPD with systemic corticosteroids (administered orally or parenterally) can reduce treatment failures by more than 50% and improve short-term dyspnea and PFT results, but there is some increase in adverse effects (Wood-Baker et al., 2005). Continuing these systemic steroids beyond 2 weeks has not been shown to have a significant benefit.

Other acute treatments for COPD exacerbations include the nonspecific phosphodiesterase (PDE) inhibitors such as theophylline and aminophylline, which have some bronchodilating effect and may also have a positive effect on the central drive to breathe, on diaphragmatic contractility, and on some mechanisms of bronchial inflammation. More specific PDE-4 inhibitors such as roflumilast have anti-inflammatory effects and significantly improve FEV_1 while reducing exacerbations (McIvor, 2007) but have significant gastrointestinal (GI) side effects as well as mental health concerns (depression and suicidal thoughts). Their role in the treatment of COPD remains uncertain.

Antibiotics are indicated if there are signs of pneumonia, sepsis, or other bacterial infection. Recent changes in sputum production (copious, thick, multicolored, or blood tinged) just before the exacerbation can indicate bacterial overgrowth of chronically inflamed bronchial mucosa, another indication for antibiotics. Because of chronic bacterial colonization, second- and third-generation antibiotics may provide greater benefit.

Indications for hospitalization include the severity of underlying illness, significant worsening during this exacerbation, failure of home or outpatient treatment efforts, significant comorbidities (CHF, arrhythmias, or electrolyte imbalance), and underlying pneumonia or other acute causes. Indications for admission to the ICU or perhaps even intubation and mechanical ventilation include severe dyspnea unresponsive to initial therapy; change in mental status (e.g., confusion, lethargy); or severe or worsening hypoxia (PaO_2 < 40 mm Hg), hypercapnia ($PaCO_2$ > 60 mm Hg), or respiratory acidosis (pH < 7.25). In a meta-analysis of treatment strategies for patients hospitalized with an exacerbation of COPD, Quon and colleagues (2008) found that systemic corticosteroids decreased treatment failures by 46% and hospital stay by 1.4 days, although risk of hyperglycemia increased almost sixfold. Antibiotics also decreased treatment failures by 46% and the in-hospital mortality rate by 78%. Noninvasive positive-pressure ventilation (NPPV) reduced the risk of intubation by 65%, the in-hospital mortality rate by 55%, and hospital stay by 1.9 days. Noninvasive intermittent positive-pressure ventilation (NIPPV) is an option for treating moderate to severe respiratory failure in patients who have normal mental status, are stable hemodynamically, and do not have a high risk for aspiration. About 80% of patients improve symptomatically within 4 hours of initiating NIPPV (Putinati et al., 2000; Wijkstra, 2003). On the other hand, chronic nocturnal use of NIPPV has yet to show significant benefit (Wijkstra et al., 2003).

Perhaps just as important as managing the pulmonary disease is to make sure other conditions do not complicate the exacerbation. Unless there are specific contraindications, a patient hospitalized for COPD exacerbation should be started on subcutaneous heparin to prevent DVT. Cardiac monitoring is often indicated in the ED and beyond to assess and treat related arrhythmias or cardiac ischemia. Electrolyte abnormalities are quite common, especially in the setting of rapidly changing $PaCO_2$ and acid–base balance. The incidence of pneumonia in ICU patients ranges from 7% to 40%, and the mortality rate from ventilator-associated pneumonia can be as high as 50%. Prophylactic antibiotics can reduce the incidence of respiratory infections in ICU patients by up to 50%, but antibiotics do not reduce the mortality rate (Liberati et al., 2004). Comorbid anxiety and depression are both extremely common and can benefit from consultation and collaborative care with behavioral health specialists.

Chronic Care and Disease Management. Each patient with COPD also needs an ongoing care plan, which includes the MAP elements described for asthma patients (daily management plan, action plan for acute exacerbations, and prevention plan). The treatment of acute exacerbations is described earlier, but each patient should have an individual action plan for increasing symptoms to prevent hospitalization. Such action plans might include symptoms or signs that would trigger a call to the physician, as well as use of short-acting β_2-agonists (albuterol, terbutaline), short-acting anticholinergic (ipratropium), or oral steroids. Use of short-course antibiotics triggered by changes in phlegm (increased sputum or change in sputum from clear to yellow-green) is common but untested by controlled trials.

A meta-analysis of controlled trials assessed the impact of various modalities of treatment for COPD (Sin et al., 2003). Outcome measures included hospitalizations, exacerbation rates, and health-related quality of life. ICSs, long-acting β_2-agonists (salmeterol, formoterol), and the long-acting anticholinergic tiotropium each decreased exacerbation rates by 20% to 25% in patients with moderate to severe COPD. The greatest effect was in patients with a FEV_1 of 1 to 2 L. Combining ICSs with a long-acting β_2-agonist provided modest additional benefit (30% reduction

Table 16-6   Treatment Guidelines for COPD Symptoms and Risk

Category	Symptoms	Risk	First Choice Treatment	Alternative Treatments
A Low symptoms / low risk	Low (CAT score < 10)*	Low Low = GOLD grade 1-2 and 0-1 exacerbations per year	Short-acting inhaled β-agonist or anticholinergic prn*	Long-acting inhaled β-agonist or anticholinergic (or combine both short-acting classes)
B High symptoms / low risk	High (CAT score > 10)	Low Low = GOLD grade 1-2 and 0-1 exacerbations per year	Long-acting inhaled β-agonist *or* long-acting anticholinergic	Long-acting inhaled β-agonist *and* long-acting anticholinergic
C Low symptoms / high risk	Low (CAT score < 10)	High High = GOLD grade 3-4 or > 2 exacerbations per year	Inhaled corticosteroid *plus* long-acting inhaled β-agonist *or plus* long-acting anticholinergic	Long-acting inhaled β-agonist *and* long-acting anticholinergic or either of these plus a PDE-4 inhibitor
D High symptoms / high risk	High (CAT score > 10)	High High = GOLD grade 3-4 or > 2 exacerbations per year	Inhaled corticosteroid *plus* long-acting inhaled β-agonist *and plus* long-acting anticholinergic	Inhaled corticosteroid *plus* either long-acting inhaled β-agonist or long-acting anticholinergic *and plus* a PDE-4 inhibitor

*Short-acting inhaled β-agonist or anticholinergics (or both) may be considered for add-on as needed (prn) use at any level. Consider theophylline in special circumstances (cost, tolerance of or response to other therapies).
CAT, Chronic obstructive pulmonary disease assessment test; *PDE,* phosphodiesterase.
Table summarizing Global Initiative (GOLD) guidelines for treatment of COPD, see Tables 4 and 7 (pp. 10,19) of Global Initiative Pocket Guide, 2014.

in exacerbations). Tiotropium may be added to ICSs and LABAs as triple therapy (Decramer et al., 2009). Oral theophylline also appears to have some beneficial effects as an antiinflammatory nonspecific PDE-inhibiting bronchodilator but perhaps also in increasing the central drive to breathe. As a result, there are improvements in FEV_1, PaO_2, and $PaCO_2$, although these must be weighed against potentially significant side effects of theophylline, such as nausea, tremors, and palpitations.

Pharmacologic therapy of COPD is guided by focusing on the parallel goals of decreasing symptoms (to enhance functional capacity and quality of life) and reducing the risk of adverse outcomes (hospitalization and death). Based on high versus low symptoms (measured by CAT or mMRC scales) and high versus low risk (measured by spirometry and exacerbations), patients are placed in A, B, C, or D categories in the GOLD treatment guidelines. For example, some patients may have a high symptom burden but be categorized as low risk based on spirometric pulmonary function measures (GOLD grade 1 or 2) and a low frequency of hospitalization; they would be category B for treatment purposes. Other patients may have a relatively low daily symptom burden, but based on spirometry (GOLD 3 or 4) or frequency of hospitalization (two or more per year), they are categorized as high risk and therefore treatment category C. High-symptom, high-risk patients are category D in this schema. Treatment guidelines for each category of COPD symptoms and risk are summarized in Table 16-6.

Nonpharmacologic therapies have shown mixed results. Home oxygen therapy decreases dyspnea and increases survival time significantly in those with hypoxia at rest ($PaO_2 < 60$ mm Hg) but not in those with only exertional or nocturnal hypoxia (Crockett et al., 2000). NPPV has not been shown to improve COPD outcomes except in severely hypercapnic patients ($PaCO_2 > 55$ mm Hg, or 50-54 mm Hg in presence of nocturnal oxygen desaturation or multiple hospitalizations in past year). Pulmonary rehabilitation focuses on improving strength, cardiopulmonary fitness, and exercise tolerance, and nutrition improves health status, as measured by the St. George's Respiratory Questionnaire (SGRQ) and Chronic Respiratory Questionnaire (CRQ) but does not appear to decrease hospitalization or mortality rates (Lacasse et al., 2001). Pulmonary rehabilitation appears to be beneficial in COPD and other chronic pulmonary diseases and is recommended by joint guidelines published by the American College of Chest Physicians (ACCP) and the American Association of Cardiovascular and Pulmonary Rehabilitation (AACVPR) Evidence-Based Clinical Practice Guidelines (Ries et al., 2007).

One disease management program using self-management and telephone follow-up showed a 36% reduction in hospitalizations and a 45% reduction in mortality in COPD patients (Bourbeau et al., 2003), but other trials of disease management programs have not shown such benefit. Despite evidence of significant nutritional deficits in patients with moderate to severe COPD, neither nutritional supplements to increase antioxidants (vitamin E or beta-carotene) nor nutritional supports to increase caloric intake have been demonstrated to improve outcomes or functional status in patients with COPD.

Surgical therapy using lung volume reduction surgery can improve quality of life and exercise tolerance in selected patients with FEV_1 less than 30% to 40% of predicted values (Fishman et al., 2003; Geddes et al., 2000; Goldstein et al., 2003). However, surgery does not improve 5-year mortality rate and can actually worsen the short-term mortality rate (National Emphysema Treatment Trial Research Group, 2001).

Prevention

Smoking cessation is the most important factor in preventing COPD and is the cornerstone of COPD treatment to prevent exacerbations and progressive loss of pulmonary function (Man et al., 2003). The decline in pulmonary function as measured by FEV_1 can be halved (from 60 to 30 mL/year) if COPD patients quit smoking (Anthonisen et al., 1994). Physician advice to quit smoking alone has some impact, and combined interventions (counseling plus education or group strategies plus pharmacologic treatment with nicotine, bupropion) can achieve at least 25% long-term quit rates even in COPD patients. Use of spirometry for screening and early diagnosis of COPD to enhance smoking cessation interventions among smokers does not improve smoking cessation rates or other clinical outcomes. Avoidance of secondary exposure to smoke, especially in the household, is also important. In two thirds world settings, this can mean replacing indoor open fire cooking with kitchen stovepipes or chimneys.

Influenza vaccine should be administered every year; it can reduce hospitalizations and deaths from pneumonia, cardiovascular disease, and all causes by 30% to 40% (Govaert et al, 1994; Nichol et al, 2003). Because the influenza vaccine is now recommended for all persons older than 6 months of age, special attention should be paid to immunizing child and adult family members, caregivers, health professionals, and other contacts of the person with COPD. Pneumococcal vaccine is also indicated in all patients with COPD, and patients should be revaccinated after 10 years if the first pneumococcal vaccine was administered before age 65 years. Vaccination rates are increasing nationwide, but they are still significantly lower among uninsured people and among racial and ethnic minority populations (CDC, 2003b). Family physicians can improve vaccination rates in their own practice by establishing standing orders for influenza and pneumococcal vaccination (CDC, 2003c, 2009) and can play a key role in encouraging high vaccination rates in schools, senior health centers, and the community.

One critical role for family physicians in the chronic management of COPD is to facilitate open discussions with patients and family members about end-of-life issues such as therapy during acute exacerbations. Although this has become routine in the management of cancer patients, the 5-year survival rate of patients with severe stages of COPD (as well as heart failure and other chronic organ failure) is often worse than that of many cancers. Many patients have a strong desire to avoid mechanical ventilation, only to end up intubated, unconscious, and having difficulty being weaned from the ventilator. Often, family members are asked to assist in end-of-life decision making after complications occur in the course of COPD even though they have not previously discussed such issues with the patient. Facilitating such family discussions, providing templates for living wills and health care power of attorney forms, and referring for legal or psychological or pastoral counseling can dramatically ease a family's confusion and pain during these episodes and in the panoply of issues associated with death and dying.

KEY TREATMENT

- Smoking cessation is the best intervention to slow the long-term rate of decline in FEV_1 (Anthonisen et al., 1994) (SOR: A). All patients should be counseled on smoking cessation; combining effective behavioral therapies (behavioral group therapy, social support) with pharmacologic therapy (nicotine replacement therapy, antidepressants) (Hughes et al., 2004; Lancaster and Stead, 2004; Stead and Lancaster, 2005) (SOR: A).
- To increase efficacy and reduce side effects, inhaled bronchodilators are preferred over oral formulations, and long acting are preferred over short acting. (SOR: A).
- LABAs provide significant benefits in airflow limitation measures, health-related quality of life, and use of rescue medication but have no effect on mortality or decline of pulmonary function (GOLD, 2013; Rodrigo et al., 2008) (SOR: A).
- Long-acting anticholinergics such as tiotropium reduce exacerbations and hospitalizations while improving health status but do not slow the progressive decline in pulmonary function (SOR: A).
- Among patients with COPD, ICS use for at least 24 weeks is associated with a significantly increased risk of serious pneumonia but not death, especially among those using the highest dose of ICS and those with the lowest baseline FEV_1 (Drummond et al, 2008; Singh et al., 2009) (SOR: A).
- Triple therapy, adding tiotropium to a combined LABA and ICS inhaler, appears to add incremental benefit in improving lung function and quality of life and reducing exacerbations (SOR: B).
- Pulmonary rehabilitation, including patient education and cardiopulmonary exercise training, significantly improves clinical outcomes and health-related quality of life and decreases hospital admissions as well as COPD-related anxiety and depression (SOR: A), with some evidence for survival benefit (SOR: B).
- Home oxygen therapy decreases dyspnea and increases survival significantly in patients with resting PaO_2 less than 60 mm Hg but not in patients with normal oxygen levels or with hypoxemia only on exertion (Crockett et al., 2000) (SOR: A).

ACUTE RESPIRATORY FAILURE

Acute respiratory failure can be the result of acute pulmonary infections; exacerbations of chronic pulmonary disease; or other conditions, such as PE, tension pneumothorax, or sepsis.

Clinical Presentation and Diagnosis

The clinical presentation of acute respiratory failure is usually obvious, although some patients slip into respiratory failure while being treated for initially less serious conditions such as pneumonia or acute exacerbations of CHF, asthma, or COPD. Acute respiratory failure can have either or both of two components: inadequate oxygenation (hypoxia) and inadequate ventilation (resulting in hypercarbia and respiratory acidosis). Although patients might initially present with severe shortness of breath, the hypoxia and increased $PaCO_2$ can ultimately lead to suppression of respiratory centers in the brain, as well as lethargy, stupor, or coma.

An especially serious form of respiratory failure that can occur is acute respiratory distress syndrome (ARDS), which can occur in patients with severe trauma, especially those who have received massive blood transfusions, overwhelming pneumonia, septic shock, and the acute chest syndrome associated with sickle cell disease.

Indications for intubation and mechanical ventilation include hypoxia and hypoventilation unresponsive to pharmacologic intervention and supplemental oxygen delivery by mask or cannula. Patients unable to protect their own airway because of central nervous system (CNS) depression or inadequate gag reflex might also need intubation. The detailed management of mechanical ventilation is beyond the scope of this chapter, but ventilation can be thought of in terms of ventilator settings that increase or decrease *ventilation* (ventilator mode, respiratory rate, and tidal volume) and ventilator settings that improve *oxygenation:* forced inspiratory oxygen concentration (FIO_2) and continuous positive airway pressure (CPAP) or positive end-expiratory pressure (PEEP).

Weaning patients from the ventilator, especially those with chronic lung disease, can be challenging. Reintubation carries risks of trauma and of ventilator-associated pneumonia. Protocols based on objective criteria (vs. individual clinical judgment) significantly reduce time, costs, and complications related to weaning patients from mechanical ventilation.

OTHER CHRONIC BRONCHIAL DISEASES

Bronchiectasis

Bronchiectasis is both a chronic airway infection and a disease of chronic lung inflammation. Bronchiectasis might be more common outside the United States (Tsang and Tipoe, 2004). Clinical course can be progressive or indolent. Cough is the predominant symptom, and some patients have significant hemoptysis, shortness of breath, or both. Malodorous (fetid) breath is a characteristic symptom. Bronchiectasis not associated with a genetic disorder is designated non-CF bronchiectasis.

Antibiotics are given over the long term using antipseudomonal antibiotics either orally or as aminoglycosides nebulized for inhalation. Macrolide antibiotics such as azithromycin appear to have antibiotic and antiinflammatory effects in treating bronchiectasis. A Cochrane review found a small but significant benefit for prolonged antibiotic therapy in the treatment of patients with purulent bronchiectasis (Evans et al., 2003). Sputum cultures should be monitored for the presence of fungal (*Aspergillus*) and mycobacterial organisms as well because they can complicate the polymicrobial mix of organisms in these patients (Morrissey and Evans, 2003). Bronchodilators, oxygen, and even noninvasive pulmonary ventilation may be tried when bronchial obstruction becomes a major component of pulmonary impairment. Surgical resection of affected lung segments can be helpful in patients with localized disease (Greenstone, 2002).

Cystic Fibrosis

Cystic fibrosis is a genetic disease attributed to autosomal recessive defects on a single gene of chromosome 7. It affects membrane functions in mucus-secreting glands (e.g., sweat glands), the pancreas, and GI and respiratory tracts. Diagnosis of CF is suspected in the presence of pancreatitis and chronic or recurrent lung infections in infants or children. Definitive diagnosis may be made with a sweat chloride test. Treatment of CF has improved significantly over the past decades. Patients now routinely live into adulthood, and now more adults are living with CF than children. Family physicians and internists (in partnership with subspecialists) are increasingly involved in the care of patients with this complex condition.

Specific treatment modalities for CF include physical therapy; nutrition therapy; mucolytics; antibiotics; and increasingly, antiinflammatory therapies. Self-administered airway clearance techniques appear to be as effective as chest physiotherapy (Main et al., 2005). Antibiotics must be broad-spectrum and antipseudomonal agents and often are given in combination during exacerbations or acute infections. In recent years, inhaled tobramycin has become effective antibiotic therapy in bronchiectasis and CF. Antiinflammatory therapy includes oral corticosteroids and ibuprofen; azithromycin has both antibiotic and antiinflammatory properties. ICSs, methotrexate, and protease replacement do not appear to be effective (Prescott and Johnson, 2005). Delivery of gene therapy directly to the respiratory tract is the ultimate hope to achieve cure or long-term remission in CF patients.

Acute Infectious Diseases

BRONCHIOLITIS IN CHILDREN

Bronchiolitis is a viral infection associated with bronchial obstruction. It occurs most often in the fall and winter. About half of all children experience bronchiolitis during the first 2 years of life, with a median age of 6 months. *Respiratory syncytial virus* (RSV) is the most common causative organism, but other viruses (adenovirus, influenza, parainfluenza, and rhinovirus) can also cause bronchiolitis.

Clinical Presentation

Typically, an infant or toddler presents with routine signs and symptoms of upper respiratory infection, such as cough, sneezing, rhinitis, and low-grade fever. Dyspnea and irritability and perhaps audible wheezing soon follow. Tachypnea and nasal flaring are typical, along with signs of airway obstruction, such as a hyperexpanded chest and wheezing on auscultation, with a prolonged expiratory phase. Chest radiographs can show air trapping, peribronchial thickening, atelectasis, and patchy infiltrates. Premature infants and children with chronic disease are at special risk for respiratory failure or complications such as bacterial pneumonia, and up to 5% of patients require hospitalization for severe respiratory distress.

Treatment

Infants with mild bronchiolitis may be managed at home using fluids, antipyretics, and β_2-agonists if needed. Indications for hospitalization of children with bronchiolitis include age younger than 6 months, hypoxemia ($PaO_2 < 60$ mm Hg or $SO_2 < 92\%$), rapid deterioration, apnea, or poor oral intake.

Hospitalized infants should receive fluids (orally or intravenously) and supplemental humidified oxygen. Aerosolized bronchodilators, including aerosolized epinephrine, decrease airway obstruction. Aerosolized ribavirin may be used in infants or children with underlying risk factors, but a meta-analysis of eight randomized controlled trials (RCTs) found no benefit for antiviral agents in general use. A systematic review of glucocorticoid treatment found no benefit in any subgroup of patients with bronchiolitis (Patel et al., 2004), and glucocorticoids do not appear to prevent postbronchiolitic wheezing (Blom et al., 2007). Epinephrine treatment is better than placebo and might have a slight advantage over salbutamol in treating bronchiolitis in outpatient settings, but benefit has not been proved in hospitalized patients (Hartling et al., 2004). A Cochrane review concluded that nebulized hypertonic (3%) saline may significantly reduce the length of hospital stay and improve other clinical indicators in infants with acute viral bronchiolitis (Zhang et al., 2008).

Some patients ultimately have asthma, with the first episode diagnosed as bronchiolitis, but RSV has not been shown to be a causative agent of chronic asthma. A systematic review found treatment with RSV immune globulin to be effective in preventing hospitalizations and admission to the ICU but not in lowering mortality rates (Wang and Tang, 1999). Children with severe apnea or respiratory failure might require intubation and mechanical ventilation. Antibiotics are only indicated if secondary bacterial infection occurs.

Prevention

Smokers in the household predispose infants to bronchiolitis, and families should be counseled to make all homes with infants or children smoke free. In a small group of infants with underlying lung disease, heart disease, or low birth weight, monthly RSV hyperimmune gamma globulin has been proved to offer some protection from severe disease. Although influenza is a relatively infrequent cause of bronchiolitis, expanded recommendations for influenza vaccination include all children age 6 to 23 months as well as all close contacts of children from birth through 23 months of age.

ACUTE BRONCHITIS

A frequently diagnosed infection in children and adults, acute bronchitis is typically a viral respiratory infection with lower tract symptoms, such as cough, phlegm, hoarseness, or wheezing. This syndrome should be distinguished from acute exacerbations in patients with chronic bronchitis, who are more vulnerable, who might be colonized with different bacterial flora in the respiratory tract, and who might require more aggressive treatment. In acute bronchitis in otherwise healthy patients, viral causes predominate. RSV and rhinovirus are common causative organisms even during influenza season.

Treatment of acute bronchitis in otherwise healthy patients should be primarily supportive because the condition is largely self-limited. Patients with underlying pulmonary disease or even smokers may have a higher rate of pulmonary complications (e.g., secondary pneumonia) or exacerbation of COPD. Options for symptomatic treatment include air humidifiers, cough suppressants, and antipyretic analgesics. Although β-agonists are sometimes prescribed, there is no evidence for a treatment benefit in the absence of measurable airway obstruction.

Antibiotic use is controversial. Because the most frequent cause is viral, bronchitis has often been overtreated with antibiotics, which would be a preventable source of antibiotic resistance. However, in patients with a productive cough persisting beyond 10 to 14 days, treatment with antibiotics may be indicated to treat bacterial co-infection, especially in smokers or in patients with underlying pulmonary disease. In a study of community-acquired acute bronchitis in France, polymerase chain reaction (PCR) testing revealed that 4.1% of patients were infected with *Chlamydia pneumoniae* and 2.3% with *Mycoplasma pneumoniae* (Gaillat et al., 2005).

A systematic review of RCTs comparing antibiotic therapy with placebo in the treatment of acute bronchitis or acute productive cough without underlying cause found a significant benefit for the antibiotic therapy, as measured by days of illness, persistent cough, and abnormal lung findings on examination (Smucny et al., 2004). An increase in adverse effects in the antibiotic-treated group compared with the placebo group outweighed many of these benefits, however, and caution in using antibiotics unnecessarily to prevent the spread of antibiotic-resistant bacteria is still valid at the population level. The specific choice of antibiotic seems to have little impact, despite known patterns of bacterial resistance in most communities. A systematic review of controlled trials that compared azithromycin with amoxicillin or amoxicillin–clavulanic acid in patients with clinical evidence of acute bronchitis, pneumonia, and acute exacerbation of chronic bronchitis found no significant advantage for using the macrolide antibiotic (Panpanich et al., 2004).

PNEUMONIA

Key Points

- Pneumonia causes more than 1 million hospitalizations per year in the United States.
- Influenza vaccine should be administered every year to patients older than 50 years and to those with chronic lung disease, diabetes, immune dysfunction, or other chronic organ failure.
- Patients should be revaccinated with pneumococcal vaccine after 10 years if the first vaccine was administered before age 65 years.
- Although atypical pathogens commonly cause community-acquired pneumonia (CAP), controlled trials show that β-lactam antibiotics are as effective as macrolides and quinolones in most cases.

Pneumonia is an infection of the lungs that leads to consolidation of the usually air-filled alveoli. It occurs in all age groups and can be caused by various agents, including viruses, bacteria, mycobacteria, mycoplasma, and fungi. Systemic viral infections such as influenza A or B in adults and measles or varicella in children can also lead to bacterial pneumonia.

Epidemiology and Risk Factors

Pneumonia or influenza is the primary diagnosis in over a million hospital admissions per year in the United States, with an in-hospital death rate of 3.3%. Aggregate charges ("the national bill") for these hospitalizations add up to over $35 billion per year (AHRQ, 2011d).

Clinical Presentation

Patients with pneumonia can present with cough, fever, dyspnea, or malaise. Cough can be productive or nonproductive and blood tinged or with frank blood. The clinical presentation of pneumonia in otherwise healthy patients often follows one of two patterns that can indicate the cause. A rapid onset of cough and shortness of breath with a high fever can indicate classic bacterial lobar pneumonia such as that produced by a pneumococcus. Physical findings after consolidation occurs include decreased breath sounds, dullness to percussion, and egophony on the affected side. The white blood cell (WBC) count is often elevated ($>15,000 \times 10^3/mm^3$), with a predominance of neutrophils. A smoldering onset with low-grade fever and fewer constitutional symptoms can indicate an atypical pneumonia, which can be caused by organisms such as respiratory viruses or by *Mycoplasma, Chlamydia,* or *Legionella* spp.

Patients with new-onset pneumonia can be categorized by whether they are living at home in a community setting or living in a nursing home or other institutional setting. Patients who have had prolonged hospitalizations or who live in nursing homes may be colonized with gram-negative organisms (e.g., *Serratia, Pseudomonas* spp.), anaerobes, or multidrug-resistant (MDR) bacteria.

Patients with pneumonia can be further categorized by whether they are immunocompetent or immunocompromised. Patients with immunodeficiencies (including HIV/AIDS) can present with opportunistic organisms including *P. jiroveci (carinii)*, cryptococci, *Coccidioides immitis*, atypical mycobacteria, and fungi. Alcoholism can predispose patients to lung infections with *Haemophilus influenzae* or to aspirated anaerobic organisms such as *Peptostreptococcus* or *Bacteroides* spp.

In children, signs of pneumonia can include malaise, cough, chest pain, tachypnea, and intercostal retractions. Children with viral pneumonias have a less toxic appearance, with low-grade fever, wheezing, and cough. Children with bacterial pneumonia appear more acutely ill, with a high-grade fever, chills, cough, and dyspnea. The earliest diagnostic clue in children may be tachypnea disproportionate to degree of fever.

In infants, potential causes of pneumonia are tied to specific periods in the first few months of life. Pneumonia in the newborn is often linked to bacteria that colonize the mother's vaginal flora. Group B streptococcal infections can occur within the first 48 hours of life or appear at 7 to 10 days after birth. Other neonatal infections include gram-negative organisms such as *Escherichia coli*. Although *Chlamydia* infections of the eye can appear in newborns at 1 to 2 weeks of age, chlamydial pneumonia is typically diagnosed in infants age 6 to 8 weeks. Other causes of pneumonia in infants age 1 to 3 months include *Ureaplasma urealyticum* and cytomegalovirus (CMV).

Viral pneumonias are most common in preschool and older children. Viral upper respiratory infections or bronchiolitis can also predispose to a bacterial pneumonia. Bacterial pathogens are responsible for only 10% to 30% of all cases of infectious pediatric pneumonia. *Streptococcus pneumoniae* has been the most common bacterial cause of childhood pneumonia, but it is declining in the face of universal pneumococcal vaccination. *H. influenzae* type B pneumonia is associated with bacteremia and other deep tissue infections (e.g., meningitis, arthritis, cellulitis) but also has declined significantly with universal immunization. *Staphylococcus aureus* causes an aggressive pneumonia that can be complicated by acute respiratory failure, pneumatoceles, or empyema. Staphylococcal pneumonia typically occurs after a staphylococcal skin infection or a systemic viral illness such as varicella (chickenpox) or measles.

Diagnosis

Cases of pneumonia are often diagnosed presumptively based on the clinical presentation and perhaps a radiograph. Chest radiography findings in viral pneumonias include patchy or streaky, often bilateral, interstitial patterns and hyperinflation of the lungs. Bacterial pneumonias show classic lobar consolidation and alveolar infiltrates, although radiography findings typically lag behind the clinical course by 1 to 2 days and can be completely normal on day 1. Parapneumonic pleural effusions can also occur.

Sputum Gram stain and culture may be performed but have a low yield. Some bacterial agents such as *Legionella* may be identified by antigen detection from blood samples. *Mycoplasma pneumoniae* infection may be diagnosed with a positive cold agglutinin test of peripheral blood. Sputum smears and cultures for acid-fast bacilli (AFB) are appropriate when there has been possible contact with TB patients, in TB-endemic areas, or when clinical findings suggest TB. Invasive procedures (e.g., BAL, lung aspiration, bronchoscopy) are reserved for special circumstances, such as diagnosing pneumonia in the immunocompromised host or in ventilator-associated pneumonias.

Treatment

Although treatment of CAP is common in primary care, there are many controversies. Clearly, many patients may be managed on an outpatient basis (Segreti et al., 2005). Use of a formal instrument such as the pneumonia severity index (PSI) or CURB-65 can more accurately identify patients eligible for outpatient treatment (IDSA/ATS, 2007). The choice of oral antibiotic in the outpatient setting must cover common causes of bacterial pneumonia. Many treatment guidelines suggest using antibiotics that cover atypical organisms such as *Mycoplasma* and *Legionella* spp., but there is insufficient evidence to support any specific antibiotic strategy in the outpatient treatment of CAP (Bjerre et al., 2004). Treatment should be continued for a minimum of 5 days and at least 48 to 72 hours beyond the patient's last signs of fever or clinical instability.

In cases of pneumococcal pneumonia with bacteremia, there is limited evidence to suggest that dual therapy with a β-lactam antibiotic and an antibiotic with coverage of atypical organisms results in lower case-fatality rates than using a β-lactam alone. A meta-analysis of studies comparing the effectiveness of a β-lactam antibiotic with antibiotics active against atypical pathogens in nonsevere CAP found no advantage for the antibiotics that were active against atypical pathogens (Shefet et al., 2005). This was true even on subgroup analysis for patients infected with *M. pneumoniae* and *C. pneumoniae*, but there was a significantly lower treatment failure rate in the small number of patients with *Legionella* infections (relative risk [RR], 0.40) treated with a macrolide antibiotic (Mills et al., 2005). Patients with significant comorbidities or chronic organ failure and those at risk for drug-resistant *S. pneumoniae* should be treated with a respiratory fluoroquinolone or combination of β-lactam and macrolide antibiotic (IDSA/ATS, 2007).

Indications for hospitalization of any patient include failure to respond or tolerate oral antibiotics, moderate to severe respiratory distress, significant deficit in oxygenation (alveolar-arterial [A-a] O_2 gradient), more than one area of lobar consolidation, empyema, immunosuppression, abscess formation, pneumatocele, underlying cardiopulmonary disease, and high-risk PSI score. Two additional factors are the patient's age (e.g., infants younger than age 2 months, elderly patients) and comorbidities (underlying pulmonary or cardiovascular disease).

Even in the hospital, not all patients must be treated with IV antibiotics (Marras et al., 2004). The patient might require hospitalization for dehydration or oxygen therapy, but in select cases, oral antibiotics may be equally effective, cost less, and require fewer days in the hospital than IV antibiotic therapy. Other patients may start receiving IV antibiotics in the hospital, but an algorithm that provides for an early switch to oral antibiotics and early discharge can reduce hospital stay.

Treatment of neonatal pneumonia should target group B streptococci and gram-negative organisms such as *E. coli*. Older children with suspected bacterial pneumonia should be treated with antibiotics that provide appropriate coverage for *H. influenzae* and *S. pneumoniae*. Pneumonia in children older than 5 years should also include macrolide coverage for *M. pneumoniae*. When symptoms recur or persist for longer than 1 month, further evaluation for an underlying condition should be undertaken (TB skin test, serum immunoglobulin, bronchoscopy, barium swallow, sweat chloride test).

Prevention

Approximately half of all cases of adult pneumonia can be prevented by annual administration of influenza vaccine plus a one-time pneumococcal vaccine when indicated (Vu et al., 2002). Vaccination with inactivated influenza vaccine is appropriate for all age groups, but the live, attenuated influenza vaccine given by nasal spray is approved for use only in healthy patients ages 5 to 49 years. To prevent community spread of influenza, the CDC recommends that influenza vaccine be given to all persons older than 6 months of age.

Health care workers are an important source of transmission of influenza from infected patients to other medically vulnerable patients. Therefore, they also should be immunized, preferably with inactivated vaccine if they have close contact with severely immunocompromised persons. Health care workers or family members vaccinated with live, attenuated influenza vaccine should avoid contact with severely immunosuppressed patients for at least 7 days after vaccination.

A systematic review suggests that pneumococcal vaccination does not significantly reduce all-cause mortality or overall rates of pneumonia, but it is specifically effective in preventing invasive pneumococcal disease (Dear et al., 2003).

Two types of vaccine are available for immunizing against invasive pneumococcal disease. Pneumococcal conjugate vaccine (PCV13) is recommended for all children younger than 5 years old and for adults with specific risk factors. All adults age 65 years and older and younger adults and children with specific risk factors should receive pneumococcal polysaccharide vaccine (PPSV23) covering 23 serotypes of the disease. The Advisory Committee on Immunization Practices (ACIP) recommends that "those who received one or more doses of PPSV23 before age 65 years for any indication should receive another dose of the vaccine at age 65 years or older if at least 5 years have elapsed since their previous PPSV23 dose. If a dose of PPSV23 was received at age 65 years or later, no additional doses of PPSV23 are recommended." Elderly persons with unknown vaccination status should be administered one dose of vaccine. Specific indications for pneumococcal vaccines are listed in Table 16-7.

KEY TREATMENT

- Treating uncomplicated CAP with a macrolide or respiratory quinolone has no proven treatment advantage over cephalosporin or aminopenicillin therapy (Mills et al., 2005; Shefet et al., 2005), unless patients have significant comorbidities or other risk factors (IDSA/ATS, 2007) (SOR: A).
- Oral antibiotic therapy for uncomplicated CAP is safe and effective in outpatient or inpatient settings in patients younger than 65 years with no preexisting lung disease or other chronic disease with stable vital signs and no evidence of hypoxia or sepsis (Bjerre et al., 2004; Marras et al., 2004) (SOR: A).
- Influenza vaccination and pneumococcal vaccine are demonstrably effective among elderly patients and those with chronic disease (Vu et al., 2002) (SOR: A).

Chronic Infectious Diseases

TUBERCULOSIS

Tuberculosis is caused by infection with *Mycobacterium tuberculosis*, transmitted by airborne exposure from close contact with infected patients. Pulmonary infection is the most common form, although extrapulmonary TB from hematogenous spread (meningitis, peritonitis, renal or adrenal TB, spinal TB [Pott's disease], others) can occur in young children, elderly people, persons in high-endemic areas, and patients with impaired immunity or malnutrition.

Table 16-7   Medical Conditions or Other Indications for Administration of PCV13 and Indications for PPSV23 Administration and Revaccination for Adults 19 Years of Age or Older

Risk Group	Underlying Medical Condition	PCV13 Recommended	PPSV23* Recommended	Revaccination at 5 Years after First Dose
Immunocompetent persons	Chronic heart disease[†]		✓	
	Chronic lung disease[‡]		✓	
	Diabetes mellitus		✓	
	CSF leaks	✓	✓	
	Cochlear implants	✓	✓	
	Alcoholism		✓	
	Chronic liver disease		✓	
	Cigarette smoking		✓	
Persons with functional or anatomic asplenia	Sickle cell disease or other hemoglobinopathies	✓	✓	✓
	Congenital or acquired asplenia	✓	✓	✓
Immunocompromised persons	Congenital or acquired immunodeficiencies	✓	✓	✓
	HIV infection	✓	✓	✓
	Chronic renal failure	✓	✓	✓
	Nephrotic syndrome	✓	✓	✓
	Leukemia	✓	✓	✓
	Lymphoma	✓	✓	✓
	Hodgkin disease	✓	✓	✓
	Generalized malignancy	✓	✓	✓
	Iatrogenic immunosuppression[§]	✓	✓	✓
	Solid organ transplant	✓	✓	✓
	Multiple myeloma	✓	✓	✓

*All adults 65 years of age or older should receive a dose of PPSV23, regardless of previous history of vaccination with pneumococcal vaccine.
[†]Including congestive heart failure and cardiomyopathies.
[‡]Including chronic obstructive pulmonary disease, emphysema, and asthma.
[§]Diseases requiring treatment with immunosuppressive drugs, including long-term systemic corticosteroids and radiation therapy.
CSF, Cerebrospinal fluid; *PCV13,* pneumococcal conjugate vaccine; *PPSV23,* pneumococcal polysaccharide vaccine.
From Centers for Disease Control and Prevention. Pneumococcal conjugate vaccine (PCV-13) and pneumococcal polysaccharide vaccine (PPSV-23), Table 1. http://www.cdc.gov/vaccines/vpd-vac/pneumo/vac-PCV13-adults.htm#recommendations.#.

Key Points

- Eighty percent of TB cases come from 22 high-burden nations.
- Sputum cultures can confirm the diagnosis of TB, but they also are important for identifying patterns of drug resistance.
- PCR techniques looking for genetic polymorphisms can provide more rapid diagnosis of drug-resistant TB.
- Latent infection (positive skin test result in asymptomatic patient with normal chest radiograph) is treated with 6 to 9 months of isoniazid or 4 months of rifampin.
- Treatment of active pulmonary TB requires a multidrug regimen for 6 to 12 months; cultures should be negative in 80% of patients within 2 months.

Epidemiology and Risk Factors

In many parts of the world, TB is one of the most common causes of fatal respiratory infection; 80% of cases come from 22 high-burden nations. WHO (2005) estimated 8.8 million new TB cases worldwide in 2003, including 674,000 HIV-infected patients, with 1.7 million deaths attributed to TB. TB cases are falling or stable in most regions but increasing in Africa. In North America, TB rates rose during the 1980s, but since 1992, TB rates have been in decline. MDR TB is a rising problem. Worldwide, 3% of newly diagnosed TB cases are MDR TB, as are 15% of previously treated TB cases.

Children, elderly people, and immunocompromised patients are especially vulnerable. In the United States, 22% of TB cases occur in older adults, with the highest rates in elderly residents of long-term care facilities (Thrupp et al., 2004). The most important risk factor for developing TB is having household or other close contact with a patient who has active TB.

Clinical Presentation

Tuberculosis can be a life-threatening infection. For pulmonary TB, symptoms include cough, fever, dyspnea, night sweats, and weight loss or failure to gain weight. The few physical findings other than weight loss can include wheezes, rales, or signs of consolidation in the affected lung field. Hematogenous spread can lead to signs of extrapulmonary infection. Patients with an initial diagnosis of CAP might instead have TB. Patients with CAP who have symptoms suggesting TB or who do not respond to antibiotic treatment, who have upper lobe infiltrates or cavitary lesions, who come from endemic areas, or who have persistent cough or hemoptysis should be evaluated for TB (Kunimoto and Long, 2005).

For patients with symptoms or with a positive PPD result, chest radiograph and sputum cultures for AFB are required. Typical chest radiograph findings include hilar or mediastinal lymphadenopathy, patchy infiltrates, apical scarring, and pleural effusions, but a cavitary lesion or miliary pattern (typical millet-seed granulomas scattered diffusely throughout lung fields) more specifically suggests TB.

Diagnosis

Skin testing is still the best method of testing for latent infection by prior exposure to *M. tuberculosis.* Intradermal testing with 5 tuberculin units (0.1 mL) of PPD is more accurate than multiprong tine testing. Interpretation depends on the patient's risk of disease. Patients with a history of direct exposure to active cases of TB, or with impaired immunity such as HIV, should be considered to have a positive test if the area of induration is greater than 5 mm at 48 to 72 hours. Most other patients should be considered positive with induration greater than 10 mm. Very-low-risk patients (age > 5 years, no history of exposure, normal immune system, low rates of TB in population) may be considered positive only with induration greater than 15 mm. These criteria are summarized in Table 16-8 (Centers for Disease Control and Prevention, 2000). Persons vaccinated with bacille Calmette-Guérin (BCG) vaccine may still be accurately tested with PPD skin testing. For high-risk populations, a percentage tuberculin response higher than 15 on the QuantiFERON-TB test (QFT) performed on venous whole blood is moderately correlated with a positive skin test result. Neither PPD nor QFT is recommended as routine screening in low-risk populations (Centers for Disease Control and Prevention, 2003a).

Clinical diagnosis in endemic areas is often based on history of exposure, clinical signs, AFB smears, and chest radiography findings (see Fig. 16-4). Sputum cultures can confirm the diagnosis and also are important for identifying patterns of drug resistance. In infants and young children, sputum AFB smears and cultures plus gastric aspirates each morning for 3 days yield the diagnosis only 50% of the time. Other cases may need to be treated presumptively based on exposure, symptoms, and chest radiographs. In culture-negative cases of TB, it is essential to find the index case and to obtain sputum cultures and drug sensitivities from that patient to guide therapy for patients with negative cultures but active disease.

Laboratory diagnosis of TB historically has relied on the use of sputum smears for AFB and culturing of the *M. tuberculosis* organism. Culture results can require 2 to 8 weeks, but more rapid methods can detect early growth within 5 to 14 days (Katoch, 2004; Schluger, 2003). Gene amplification using PCR techniques can be performed on sputum samples for rapid results, as well as on cerebrospinal fluid (CSF), gastric or pleural aspirates, and urine. PCR is highly sensitive (95%-98%) for diagnosing TB from sputum in smear-positive and culture-positive cases, but it has lower sensitivity (57%-78%) for smear-negative and culture-positive cases (Rattan, 2000). PCR may also be used on organisms obtained from early growth on positive cultures to detect drug resistance more rapidly, taking advantage of the genetic polymorphisms in the *M. tuberculosis* organism, which are almost always associated with drug resistance. Although positive results are highly specific, failure to detect mutations does not entirely rule out drug resistance (Hazbon, 2004; Nachamkin et al., 1997).

Treatment

A positive PPD skin test result in an asymptomatic patient with a normal chest radiograph and negative HIV test result represents latent infection with no active disease. A 6- to 9-month course of isoniazid is effective in treating this latent infection and in preventing the development of active TB. Isoniazid therapy is associated with clinical hepatitis in approximately 0.6% of treated patients (Smieja et al., 1999). An effective alternative is rifampin for 4 months. The short course of two drugs, rifampin and pyrazinamide, for 2 months is no longer recommended because of evidence of increased liver toxicity with this combination (CDC, 2001). Treatment of positive PPD latent infection is indicated even in patients with a history of BCG vaccination and is also effective in patients co-infected with HIV (Wilkinson et al., 1998).

Table 16-8 Criteria for Tuberculin Positivity by Risk Group

Reaction > 2 mm of induration	■ HIV-positive patients ■ Recent contacts of TB patients ■ Fibrotic changes on chest radiograph consistent with prior TB ■ Patients with organ transplants and other immunocompromised patients (receiving equivalent of >15 mg/day of prednisone for >1 mo)*
Reaction > 10 mm of induration	■ Recent immigrants (i.e., within last 5 yr) from high-prevalence countries ■ Injection drug users ■ Residents and employees† of high-risk congregate settings 　■ Prisons and jails 　■ Nursing homes and other long-term care facilities for elderly persons 　■ Hospitals and other health care facilities 　■ Residential facilities for AIDS patients 　■ Homeless shelters ■ Mycobacteriology laboratory personnel ■ Persons with high-risk conditions 　■ Silicosis 　■ Diabetes mellitus 　■ Chronic renal failure 　■ Some hematologic disorders (e.g., leukemias, lymphomas) 　■ Other specific malignancies (e.g., head or neck or lung carcinoma) ■ Weight loss >10% of ideal body weight ■ Gastrectomy ■ Jejunoileal bypass ■ Children younger than 4 yr of age or infants, children, and adolescents exposed to high-risk adults
Reaction > 15 mm of induration	■ Persons with no risk factors for TB

*Risk of tuberculosis (TB) in patients treated with corticosteroids increases with higher dose and longer duration.
†For persons who are otherwise at low risk and are tested at the start of employment, a reaction of >15 mm of induration is considered positive.
Centers for Disease Control and Prevention, 2000. Table 7, Criteria for Tuberculin Positivity by Risk Group. Morbidity and Mortality Weekly Report (MMWR), Targeted Tuberculin Testing and Treatment of Latent Tuberculosis Infection; June 9, 2000. 49(RR06);1–54.

Treatment of active pulmonary TB requires a multidrug regimen for 6 to 12 months. For new drug-sensitive cases of uncomplicated pulmonary TB, the WHO recommends a 6-month protocol of four drugs (isoniazid, rifampin, pyrazinamide, and ethambutol) for the first 2 months, continuing with two drugs (isoniazid, rifampin) for the next 4 months (SOR: A) (WHO, 2009). Culture and drug susceptibility testing (DST) should be performed on all previously treated TB patients, with DST focusing at least on sensitivity to isoniazid and rifampin. In settings where rapid molecular-based DST is available, the results should guide the choice of drug treatment regimen. Rapid molecular-based DST or culture-based DST is strongly recommended in guiding treatment for HIV-positive patients.

In countries with high prevalence of isoniazid resistance and no routine DST, ethambutol may be continued throughout the 6-month course along with isoniazid and rifampin. Whenever possible, treatment should be taken daily unless dosing is directly observed. Treatment with intermittent therapy 2 days per week has been less effective than daily therapy in RCTs (Mwandumba and Squire, 2001). Repeat cultures should be obtained after 2 months of treatment, when 80% of patients have negative cultures. Cavitary lesions, or persistent positive cultures after 2 months of therapy, are indications for an extended 9-month course of treatment.

Directly observed therapy (DOT) is indicated for patients with specific risk factors for treatment failure caused by noncompliance, but RCTs in a variety of settings have not clearly demonstrated benefit over traditional public health strategies (Volmink and Garner, 2003). Enhanced DOT appears to be more effective. Table 16-9 lists strategies of social supports, barrier reduction, compliance monitoring, and incentives that can be blended in a broad-based strategy to ensure treatment compliance and cure (American Thoracic Society, CDC, IDSA, 2003). The WHO reports an 82% success rate for TB treatment worldwide, although the prevalence of MDR TB is increasing.

Treatment of patients who have positive PPD and radiography evidence of TB but negative sputum smears depends on the level of clinical suspicion for active TB. When suspicion is high, multidrug therapy should be initiated pending culture results. If cultures come back negative but the patient shows clinical or radiographic signs of improvement after 2 months of treatment, the patient is assumed to have culture-negative TB, and treatment should be completed using isoniazid and rifampin. If culture remains negative and there is no sign of clinical or radiographic improvement, treatment may be discontinued after 2 months. For patients at low suspicion of TB, no treatment is indicated pending culture results. If cultures remain negative and the patient is asymptomatic with no progression on chest radiography, a standard course of treatment for latent TB (isoniazid for 9 months or rifampin for 4 months) is indicated.

Prevention

The most important elements of prevention are screening for exposure, detection and follow-up of active cases, and prophylaxis of infected but clinically asymptomatic patients. PPD testing and treatment of latent infection is a more effective strategy than BCG vaccination in patient

Table 16-9 Broad-Based Strategy to Ensure Tuberculosis Treatment Adherence and Cure

Enablers	Incentives
Interventions to assist the patient in completing therapy	Interventions to motivate the patient, tailored to individual patient wishes and needs and thus meaningful to the patient
Transportation vouchers	
Child care	
Convenient clinic hours and locations	
Clinic personnel who speak the languages of the populations served	
Reminder systems and follow-up of missed appointments	Food stamps or snacks and meals
Social service assistance (referrals for substance abuse treatment and counseling, housing, and other services)	Restaurant coupons
	Assistance in finding or provision of housing
Outreach workers (bilingual or bicultural as needed; can provide many services related to maintaining patient adherence, including provision of DOT, follow-up on missed appointments, monthly monitoring, transportation, sputum collection, social service assistance, and educational reinforcement)	Clothing or other personal products
	Books
	Stipends
	Patient contract
Integration of TB care with care for other conditions	

DOT, Directly observed therapy; *TB,* tuberculosis.
American Thoracic Society, CDC, & IDSA Guidelines for treatment of tuberculosis, *Am J Respir Crit Care Med* 167:603–662, 2003.

Table 16-10 Latent Tuberculosis Infection Treatment Regimens

Drugs	Duration	Interval	Minimum no. of Doses
Isoniazid	9 mo	Daily	270
		Twice weekly with DOT	76
Isoniazid	6 mo	Daily	180
		Twice weekly with DOT	52
Isoniazid and rifapentine	3 mo	Twice weekly with DOT	12
Rifampin	4 mo	Daily	120

DOT, Directly observed therapy.
Centers for Disease Control and Prevention, 2014. Treatment of Latent TB Infection (updated Feb 7, 2014); http://www.cdc.gov/tb/topic/treatment/ltbi.htm.

populations with a relatively low incidence of pulmonary TB, but in highly endemic areas, infant BCG vaccination strategies can reduce childhood TB infection rates by as much as 50% (Colditz et al., 1995). Patients with a positive PPD result but no symptoms and negative chest radiography findings should be treated with an effective regimen such as isoniazid daily for 9 months or rifampin for 4 months or other regimens as listed in Table 16-10.

Maintaining an effective public health infrastructure, including TB surveillance, screening, and contact tracing, is essential. Sputum culture and sensitivity testing is an increasingly relevant component of an effective public health strategy to identify and contain the spread of MDR TB.

- A 9-month course of isoniazid or a 4-month course of rifampin is effective in preventing development of active TB in asymptomatic patients with a positive PPD test result and negative chest radiography findings (i.e., latent infection) even in patients with HIV co-infection (Smieja et al., 1999; Wilkinson et al., 1998) (SOR: A).
- Treatment with intermittent therapy 2 days per week has been less effective than daily therapy in RCTs (Mwandumba and Squire, 2001) (SOR: A).
- BCG vaccine effectively reduces infection rates by about 50% in highly endemic populations (Colditz et al., 1995) (SOR: B).
- Positive PPD test results require diagnostic evaluation even in patients with prior BCG vaccination.

AIDS-RELATED INFECTIONS

Key Points

- Specific opportunistic infections are associated with HIV, and bacterial CAPs are also common.
- More than half of HIV-infected patients with CD4+ counts less than 200 cells/μL experience an AIDS-related opportunistic infection within the next 2 years.
- TB is common in HIV patients. TB worsens the clinical course of HIV infection, and HIV infection complicates TB management.
- HRCT scan is the best imaging study for diagnosing HIV-related pulmonary infections.
- Inactivated influenza and pneumococcal vaccines are recommended for HIV-infected patients who are still able to mount a significant immune response.

HIV/AIDS by definition compromises our host defense capacity for fighting otherwise benign infections. Some of the most common opportunistic infections in patients with HIV/AIDS affect the lungs as their target organ.

Epidemiology and Risk Factors

Table 16-11 shows the relationship between opportunistic infections and specific levels of immunocompromise as measured by CD4$^+$ lymphocyte counts; 200 cells/μL is a critical threshold for prophylactic treatment (CDC, NIH, IDSA, 2013). More than half of HIV patients with CD4$^+$ counts below this level experience an AIDS-related opportunistic infection in 2 years.

Human cases of PCP are now understood to be caused by *P. jiroveci*. Most healthy children have been infected asymptomatically with *P. jiroveci* by age 4 years (Pifer et al., 1978), allowing cases in HIV patients to occur either by reactivation or by new exposure. Without antiretroviral therapy (ART) or PCP prophylaxis, more than 70% of HIV-infected patients could be expected to experience PCP, with a 20% to 40% mortality rate (Phair et al., 1990). With widespread use of effective antiretroviral therapy, the incidence of PCP among HIV-infected patients in Western nations is now less than one case per 100 person-years (Buchacz et al., 2010).

Table 16-11 Risk Factors Associated with Development of Major Opportunistic Infections in HIV-Infected Patients

Infection	CD4$^+$ Count Risk Threshold (cells/mm^3)	Other Risk Factors
Pneumocystis jiroveci (carinii) pneumonia (PCP)	≤200	Prior PCP
		Present CD4$^+$ cells <14%
		Fever of unexplained etiology
		Presence of oral candidiasis
Mycobacterium tuberculosis	Any	Tuberculin skin test (PPD) positive
		Exposure to infectious contact
Mycobacterium avium complex	≤50	Prior respiratory or GI colonization
		Prior opportunistic disease
		High viral load (>105 copies/mL)
CMV disease	≤50	Seropositive (IgG antibodies to CMV)
		CMV viremia
		Prior opportunistic disease
		High viral load (>105 copies/mL)
Cryptococcal meningitis	=50-100	Environmental exposure
Toxoplasmosis	=100-200	Seropositive (IgG antibody to Toxoplasma gondii)
Candida esophagitis	≤100	Prior Candida colonization
		High viral load (>105 copies/mL)
Cryptosporidiosis	≤100	Environmental exposure (contaminated water, soil, animal exposure)
Histoplasmosis	≤100	Exposure (endemic areas: Midwest, Southwest United States)
Coccidioidomycosis	≤100	Exposure (endemic areas: Southwest United States, Mexico)

CMV, Cytomegalovirus; *GI*, gastrointestinal; *PPD*, purified protein derivative. Guidelines for the Prevention and Treatment of Opportunistic Infections in HIV-Infected Adults and Adolescents, 2013

Clinical Presentation

A wide range of clinical presentations can occur with opportunistic infections in HIV/AIDS. PCP can manifest with cough, tachypnea, and fever. Chest radiographs may be relatively normal early in the course of disease but eventually may show diffuse, bilateral, symmetric interstitial infiltrates in a butterfly pattern or ground-glass appearance. Hypoxia, Pao$_2$ less than 70 mm Hg, and an increased A-a O$_2$ gradient are typical. Pneumothorax occurring in a patient infected with HIV suggests PCP, which typically produces pneumatoceles as lung tissue is destroyed.

Clinicians should also have a high index of suspicion for pulmonary TB in HIV-infected patients. Presentation of pulmonary TB is fairly typical (upper lobe patchy infiltrates with or without cavitation) in patients with normal CD4 counts, but patients with more severe immune suppression often have atypical lung presentations (lobar infiltrates or miliary pattern) or extrapulmonary forms of TB. In severely immunocompromised patients, sputum AFB cultures can be positive even in the presence of normal chest radiograph.

The attention to opportunistic infections should not diminish clinical suspicion for bacterial pneumonia as a cause of significant morbidity and mortality in HIV-infected patients. *S. pneumoniae, H. influenzae, Pseudomonas aeruginosa,* and *S. aureus* are the most frequently isolated organisms (Rimland et al., 2002). Patients present with typical symptoms such as fever, tachypnea, cough, and constitutional symptoms and a pattern of lobar pneumonia or other infiltrates on chest radiography.

Diagnosis

Diagnosis of PCP may be obtained from laboratory testing, histopathology, and imaging studies. Histochemical stains and direct immunofluorescent studies can confirm the organism's presence in induced sputum, but sensitivities are much greater (90%-99%) when specimens are obtained from BAL or transbronchial biopsy (Cruciani et al., 2002). Open lung biopsy is the gold standard and may be safer than bronchoscopic techniques for patients with bleeding disorders.

Nuclear medicine and CT studies are also used extensively in evaluating pulmonary symptoms in patients with HIV/AIDS. For example, HRCT scan can show a patchy, ground-glass appearance or characteristic pneumatoceles in PCP. Gallium-67 scintigraphy is also useful. In a study of 57 immunocompromised patients with pulmonary infections, the first-choice diagnosis suggested by CT was accurate in most fungal infections (95.0%) and PCP (87.5%) but was less accurate for bacterial (73.7%) and viral (75.0%) infections and missed both cases of mycobacterial infection (Demirkazik et al., 2008). A gallium scan showing diffuse increased uptake in the lungs of an HIV-infected patient can also suggest PCP. Sensitivity is high (>90%), but specificity can be as low as 51%. Features of an abnormal gallium scan that increase specificity and positive predictive value include increased uptake in the lungs in the presence of a normal chest radiograph, intensity of uptake in the lung (greater than liver uptake), and a diffuse heterogeneous pattern. In a comparative study of gallium scanning versus HRCT in HIV/AIDS patients with pulmonary symptoms but normal or near-normal chest radiographs, HRCT resulted in both higher positive predictive values (86%) and negative predictive values (88%) than gallium scintigraphy (62% and 73%) (Kirshenbaum et al., 1998).

Sequential thallium and gallium scanning may be performed when Kaposi sarcoma is suspected. The combination of a positive thallium and negative gallium scan is highly specific for Kaposi sarcoma, but sensitivity is decreased by the presence of opportunistic infections, which can make the gallium scan positive as well. Other nuclear imaging studies include cell-surface peptide receptor-binding molecules radiolabeled with indium or technetium (van de Wiele et al., 2002).

Prevention and Treatment

The treatment of HIV is covered in Chapter 15. However, there are specific opportunities for preventing pulmonary opportunistic infections in HIV-infected patients (Clumeck and Wit, 2003; Guidelines for Prevention & Treatment, 2013). ART has transformed HIV/AIDS into a chronic disease in which CD4$^+$ counts can often be maintained

above levels at which opportunistic infections are likely. However, PCP prophylaxis is still indicated for patients with CD4 counts below 200 cells/mm^3 or a history of oropharyngeal candidiasis.

When an opportunistic infection leads to the initial diagnosis of HIV/AIDS, treatment with ART and agents effective against the opportunistic infection may be begun simultaneously. Fever and worsening of clinical symptoms several weeks after ART initiation may be related to recovery of the patient's immune function, described as an "immune reconstitution or reactivation syndrome," and must be differentiated from treatment failure or progression of disease by measuring serial CD4$^+$ counts and RNA viral loads.

Trimethoprim–sulfamethoxazole (TMP-SMX) prophylaxis has been demonstrated to prevent episodes of *P. jiroveci* pneumonia and to enhance survival in patients with low CD4 counts (D'Egidio et al., 2007). Oral dapsone, inhaled pentamidine, or atovaquone are alternatives for patients unable to tolerate TMP-SMX. It is also used to treat PCP infections, although the side effects of TMP-SMX are significantly higher in HIV/AIDS patients. Corticosteroids are added for patients with significant respiratory distress or hypoxemia.

Tuberculosis worsens the clinical course of HIV infection, and HIV infection complicates the management of TB (Sharma et al., 2005). All HIV-infected patients should undergo PPD testing for latent infection with *M. tuberculosis.* A PPD reaction greater than 5 mm is considered positive in an HIV-infected patient. If the PPD result is negative but the CD4 count is below 200 cells/mm^3, then the patient should be retested after treatment reduces viral load and restores adequate CD4 levels to greater than 200 cells/mm^3. The interferon-γ release assay (IGRAs) for TB may be more sensitive than the TB skin test and less cross-reactive with BCG, but its role in routine practice (e.g., to replace or combine with the PPD) has not been fully established. If chest radiograph findings are negative and there are no other signs of active pulmonary or extrapulmonary TB, an appropriate treatment regimen for latent TB should be initiated. Treatment of latent TB reduces significantly the risk of developing active TB in HIV patients with a positive skin test result (Volmink and Woldehanna, 2004). Regimens are similar to those used in HIV-negative patients, but if isoniazid is chosen, the duration of treatment is 9 months rather than 6 months and given with pyridoxine supplements. Standard treatment regimens for active TB appear to be effective in HIV patients as well, but trials will determine the optimum duration, regimen, and dosing frequency in patients with TB and more severe HIV-related immunocompromise. Detailed guidelines for the combined treatment of TB and HIV to maximize outcomes while minimizing drug–drug interactions are available and frequently updated on the CDC's website (CDC, 2013b).

Mycobacterium avium complex (MAC) infections can be prevented with clarithromycin or azithromycin. Disseminated MAC infection often manifests with signs in multiple organ systems, and typically occurs in patients with severe immunocompromise (CD4 count <50 cells/mm^3). Localized pneumonia can occur in patients with more intact immune function receiving ART.

Although other prophylactic regimens are available to prevent systemic viral or fungal infections, a survival benefit has not been demonstrated. Inactivated influenza and

23-valent pneumococcal vaccines are recommended for HIV patients who are still able to mount a significant immune response and should be initiated early in the disease, with annual influenza vaccine each year thereafter. Live vaccines should not be used.

- Treatment of latent TB (positive skin test result) reduces risk of progression to active TB in HIV/AIDS patients (Volmink and Woldehanna, 2004) (SOR: A).
- Influenza vaccine is indicated for HIV/AIDS patients (SOR: A).
- Treatment of asymptomatic HIV-infected patients with TMP-SMX significantly reduces pulmonary infections with *Pneumocystis* pneumonia (Grimwade et al., 2003) (SOR: A).

Fungal Infections of the Lung

Endemic mycoses (histoplasmosis, coccidioidomycosis, and paracoccidioidomycosis) can cause primary pulmonary infections in exposed patients as well as reactivation syndromes in patients with HIV or other causes of immune suppression. The incidence of these infections has decreased with the widespread use of ART for HIV infection. Fungal infections related to *Aspergillus* spp. are more widespread geographically, but the incidence of aspergillosis has also decreased with increasing ART use.

EPIDEMIOLOGY AND RISK FACTORS

Histoplasmosis *(Histoplasma capsulatum)* is most common in basins of the Ohio and Mississippi rivers. Blastomycosis *(Blastomyces dermatitidis)* is found in this same area of the United States as well as in portions of Canada. Coccidioidomycosis *(Coccidioides immitis)* is prevalent in desert areas of the southwestern United States, and paracoccidioidomycosis *(Paracoccidioides brasiliensis)* is the most common endemic mycosis in Central and South America. Airborne exposure to local soil is a risk factor. In South Asia and Southeast Asia (especially India, China, Thailand, and Vietnam), *Penicilliosis marneffei* is another significant endemic mycosis affecting HIV/AIDS patients (Randhawa, 2000).

Aspergillosis occurs most often in the context of immune suppression, especially in HIV-infected patients with CD4[+] lymphocyte counts less than 50 cells/μL. Leukopenia, systemic corticosteroids, bone marrow transplantation, and broad-spectrum antibiotic therapy also increase risk for aspergillosis.

CLINICAL PRESENTATION

Presentation of any of the endemic mycoses depends on the patient's underlying immune status, as well as on the degree of exposure. For example, in patients with significant immune suppression (CD4[+] lymphocyte counts <150/μL), histoplasmosis can manifest with signs and symptoms of disseminated multiorgan infection, but patients with more intact immune symptoms can have more localized pulmonary symptoms and signs. Blastomycosis is often a self-limited infection, but it can lead to chronic pneumonia or skin, musculoskeletal, or CNS involvement (Pappas, 2004). Cough, dyspnea, and fever, with or without weight loss or night sweats, are the most common symptoms (Baumgardner et al., 2004). Coccidioidomycosis similarly can manifest as a self-limited pulmonary infection. In the case of intense exposure or in immunosuppressed patients, it can manifest as a severe fulminant pulmonary infection with ARDS or as a disseminated infection (peritonitis, lymphadenopathy, skin nodules, meningitis, musculoskeletal or liver involvement).

Respiratory disease caused by *Aspergillus* can take the form of pseudomembranous tracheitis or invasive pneumonia. Pseudomembranous tracheitis can lead to airway obstruction. Both respiratory syndromes are associated with cough, fever, dyspnea, and hemoptysis, and pneumonia also produces hypoxia. Chest radiography can show diffuse interstitial infiltrates or even signs of pulmonary infarction caused by fungal invasion of vascular tissue.

DIAGNOSIS

In disseminated histoplasmosis, *Histoplasma* antigen is detectable in blood or urine with 85% to 95% sensitivity. For isolated pulmonary histoplasmosis, BAL or transbronchial biopsy may be required. *Coccidioides* organisms may be cultured or seen on histopathologic tissue stains or detected by serologic tests of blood or CSF. *Aspergillus* spp. may be cultured from sputum samples, which is sufficient for diagnosis in the presence of a typical clinical syndrome and no alternative diagnosis. More definitive diagnosis may be made by BAL (50% sensitivity) or open-lung biopsy.

TREATMENT

Acute, uncomplicated pulmonary histoplasmosis may be treated with watchful waiting in patients with normal immune systems (Wheat et al., 2004). Severe disseminated histoplasmosis or severe diffuse pulmonary histoplasmosis is treated with the liposomal form of amphotericin B initially followed by 12 weeks of oral itraconazole therapy and then lifelong itraconazole prophylaxis. New antifungal agents such as voriconazole, posaconazole, caspofungin, and micafungin are potential alternatives (Herbrecht et al., 2005; Ruhnke, 2004). Detailed treatment guidelines for the management of histoplasmosis and blastomycosis infections are available from IDSA (Chapman et al., 2008; Wheat et al., 2007).

For coccidioidomycosis and blastomycosis, amphotericin B is usually chosen for initial therapy. Less serious infections might respond to fluconazole or itraconazole, and some treatment success has been demonstrated with voriconazole (Bakleh et al., 2005). Meningitis is treated with fluconazole or intrathecal amphotericin B. The CDC recommends treatment with voriconazole for invasive aspergillosis.

PREVENTION

The most important means of preventing fungal pulmonary infections is the ART of HIV/AIDS. HIV patients treated for histoplasmosis or coccidioidomycosis require chronic suppressive therapy with itraconazole or alternative antifungal therapy for life. TMP-SMX prophylaxis for PCP might also be protective against paracoccidioidomycosis. Education and protective gear (protective masks) during digging, excavation, and construction projects or cave exploration in endemic areas can help prevent acute pulmonary infections caused by high-level environmental exposures.

Vascular Disease

PULMONARY EMBOLISM

Key Points

- Clinical decision rules using objective scoring algorithms help establish pretest probability and enhance the predictive value of other tests for PE.
- A negative *quantitative* D-dimer test result by enzyme-linked immunosorbent assay (ELISA) less than 500 µg/L can effectively rule out PE in patients with low or intermediate pretest probability of disease.
- HRCT scan with contrast can be performed on the lungs and the deep veins of the legs at the same time in a PE protocol.
- Hemodynamically stable patients with submassive PE may be treated with dose-adjusted IV or fixed-dose subcutaneous heparin.
- Hemodynamically unstable patients with massive PE may be treated with thrombolytics or embolectomy.
- Prophylactic therapy is not effective if initiated after a clot has begun to form, so venous thromboembolism (VTE) prophylaxis with subcutaneous heparin should be part of standard hospital admitting orders unless specifically contraindicated.

In the 19th century, Rudolf Virchow defined the pathologic process of PE, in which blood clots, usually from DVTs in one or both legs, break off and are trapped in the pulmonary arterial system, leading to pulmonary infarct, decreased oxygenation of venous blood returning from the periphery, and elevated right-sided pressures in the heart (Dalen, 2002). Two thirds of emboli reach both lungs and lodge in large or intermediate pulmonary arteries, most often in the lower lobes.

Epidemiology and Risk Factors

In 2003, there were 98,921 hospitalizations in the United States during which PE was diagnosed, generating charges of nearly $2 billion. The in-hospital mortality rate was 3% (Health Care Utilization Project, 2003). The importance of rapid diagnosis and treatment was underscored by Dalen and Alpert in 1975, who estimated that only 6% of PE deaths at that point in medical history occurred in patients diagnosed and treated for PE (Dalen, 2002).

The most important cause of PE is DVT, and both conditions are included under the broader term *venous thromboembolism*. Virchow's triad of risk included hypercoagulability, stasis, and vascular injury. Patients can develop DVT after surgery (especially hip or pelvic surgery), major trauma, prolonged hospitalization or bed confinement, or even prolonged sitting in a confined space (air travel, bus or car trips,

medical school lectures). Patients at highest risk are those with a past history of DVT. Additional risk factors include smoking, cancer, obesity, pregnancy, heart disease, stroke, burns, and medications (e.g., estrogen therapy). Patients with inherited risk include those with antithrombin III deficiency, hyperhomocysteinemia, protein C or protein S deficiency, and factor V Leiden mutation, as well as those with acquired hypercoagulable states such as the antiphospholipid syndrome.

Clinical Presentation

Any suspicion of PE as a cause of acute shortness of breath requires specific diagnostic evaluation and quick intervention in this potentially life-threatening condition. Acute-onset shortness of breath coupled with pleuritic chest pain, hemoptysis, wedge-shaped pulmonary infarct lesions on chest radiograph, and S1Q3 pattern with tachycardia on ECG can all point specifically to a diagnosis of PE, but most patients have a nonspecific presentation. Collateral circulation from bronchial arteries makes pulmonary infarction relatively uncommon. Massive PE can lead to acute right ventricular failure and cardiovascular collapse. PaO_2 greater than 80 mm Hg in room air and a normal A-a O_2 gradient make the diagnosis less likely but do not completely exclude PE. All patients with acute-onset shortness of breath with no apparent cause should be evaluated for PE.

Diagnosis

Diagnosing PE includes an evaluation for DVT. Physical examination for signs of DVT (asymmetry in calf or thigh diameter, calf tenderness, Homans sign) are relatively insensitive and nonspecific, and other tests (venous Doppler ultrasonography or spiral CT with contrast) can more accurately confirm the presence of significant underlying DVT.

When suspected, PE must be confirmed or ruled out with a high degree of certainty. Failure to treat could be life threatening, but treatment carries significant risks as well. Clinical decision rules using objective scoring algorithms help establish pretest probability (high, intermediate, or low), which in turn enhances predictive value of other tests for PE (Ebell, 2004). One common decision tool uses only history and physical examination variables (Wells et al., 2001), and another scoring system adds variables from chest radiography and ABG measurements (Wicki et al., 2001).

Several qualitative, semiquantitative, and quantitative laboratory methods are available for measuring D-dimer. Any negative D-dimer test result can help exclude the diagnosis of PE in patients with low pretest probability of disease, but for patients with moderate pretest probability, only quantitative D-dimer test by ELISA less than 500 µg/L can effectively rule out PE. Spiral CT with contrast and magnetic resonance angiography (MRA), two alternative imaging studies widely replacing V/Q scan, are more accessible and accurate in patients with underlying heart or lung disease, and perhaps more accurate for centrally located than peripheral emboli. Spiral CT also offers the advantage of potentially diagnosing other conditions, and when ordered in a PE protocol may be combined with CT of the lower extremities to evaluate possible DVTs. Table 16-12 summarizes the results of strategies for excluding the diagnosis of PE (using criteria of posttest probability <5%) or for

Table 16-12 Diagnostic Tests to Exclude or Confirm Diagnosis of Pulmonary Embolism

Pretest Probability Based on Objective Clinical Decision Rules	Exclude Diagnosis (PE < 5%)	Confirm Diagnosis (PE > 85%)
Low clinical probability (10%)	Negative D-dimer (quantitative or semiquantitative) Negative spiral CT scan Negative MRA Low-probability V/Q scan	Positive pulmonary angiogram (no other test is adequate to confirm positive diagnosis of PE in a patient with low prior probability)
Moderate clinical probability (35%)	Quantitative D-dimer<500 μg/L (by ELISA method) Normal or near-normal lung scan Negative spiral CT scan *in combination with* negative venous Doppler ultrasonography of leg veins	Positive spiral CT scan High-probability V/Q scan Positive MRA Positive venous Doppler ultrasonography of leg veins
High clinical probability (70%)	Negative pulmonary angiogram (no other test is adequate to exclude or rule out diagnosis of PE in a patient with a high prior probability)	Positive spiral CT scan High-probability V/Q scan Positive MRA Positive echocardiogram ultrasound

CT, Computed tomography; *ELISA*, enzyme-linked immunosorbent assay; *MRA*, magnetic resonance angiography; *PE*, pulmonary embolism. *V/Q*, ventilation/perfusion ratio.

confirming the diagnosis (posttest probability >85%) (Roy et al., 2005).

Treatment

The options for treatment of PE include anticoagulation, thrombolysis, and (rarely) surgery. With controlled trials ongoing, no clear recommendation yet exists for thrombolysis in all cases of PE. One trial of alteplase plus heparin showed significantly decreased mortality in patients with submassive PE compared with patients treated only with heparin (Konstantinides et al., 2002). However, a meta-analysis of all RCTs comparing thrombolytic therapy with heparin in patients with PE showed a survival benefit only in studies that included hemodynamically unstable patients (patients with massive PE). In trials that excluded these patients, there was no benefit found for thrombolysis (mortality rate slightly worse for thrombolytic therapy) (Wan et al., 2004). Treatment of DVT with thrombolytics has also been studied, and although venous blood flow may be improved and post-DVT syndrome decreased, there is a significant risk of hemorrhagic complications such as stroke.

In massive PE with cardiovascular collapse, thrombolysis is often used, but emergency pulmonary embolectomy is an option in settings in which cardiothoracic surgery can be mobilized rapidly. Dauphine and Omari (2005) reported on 11 patients with massive PE treated with emergency embolectomy. Of the seven patients who did not have preoperative cardiac arrest, all survived to hospital discharge. One of the four patients who experienced cardiac arrest preoperatively also survived to discharge.

For patients who are hemodynamically stable and have less than massive pulmonary emboli, the initial treatment choice is dose-adjusted, IV unfractionated heparin or fixed-dose, subcutaneous low-molecular-weight heparin (LMWH). A meta-analysis comparing these two therapies in VTE treatment found odds ratios favoring LMWH in both the rate of recurrence and the rate of bleeding complications, but these differences were not statistically significant (Erkens and Prins, 2010). LMWH by fixed-dose subcutaneous injection is at least as safe and effective as traditional dose-adjusted, unfractionated heparin therapy. Anticoagulation with warfarin is indicated for at least 3 to 6 months after an initial PE episode, and lifetime therapy may be warranted for patients with hypercoagulability or

recurrent episodes. Patients with recurrent episodes unresponsive to anticoagulation might benefit from surgical placement of an inferior vena cava filter.

Prevention

Primary prevention of PE begins with prevention of DVT. Trauma, hip or pelvic surgery, general surgery, and hospitalization or prolonged bed rest put patients at significant short-term risk. Many cases of VTE can be prevented in these patients if prophylaxis is initiated promptly. Prophylactic therapy is not effective if it is initiated after a clot has begun to form, so it is crucial to include VTE prophylaxis (subcutaneous heparin as well as mechanical interventions) on admitting orders for most patients admitted to a hospital for surgery or for serious medical conditions. Clinicians currently underuse prophylactic therapies recommended in various clinical guidelines. They should order heparin prophylaxis on admission automatically unless there is a specific contraindication or the patient is clearly not at risk rather than ordering prophylaxis only when risk factors are obvious (Tooher et al., 2005). When DVT begins in the legs, prompt diagnosis and therapy can provide effective secondary prevention of the more life-threatening PE.

KEY TREATMENT

- DVT prophylaxis begun routinely on hospital admission, unless specifically contraindicated, can prevent many in-hospital PE episodes (Tooher et al., 2005) (SOR: A).
- An algorithm using clinical indicators, quantitative D-dimer test, and various imaging studies (spiral CT with contrast, MRA, venous Doppler ultrasonography) can effectively rule in (>85% probability) or rule out (<5% probability) PE (Roy et al., 2005) (SOR: A).

PULMONARY HYPERTENSION

Pulmonary hypertension is diagnosed when pulmonary artery pressures exceed normal levels, and symptoms ensue. The condition may be either primary or secondary to other causes, which can be pulmonary, cardiac, or systemic in origin.

Epidemiology and Risk Factors

Secondary causes of pulmonary hypertension include chronic lung disease (COPD and chronic bronchitis), cardiac disease (congenital defects, mitral stenosis, left atrial myxoma), autoimmune or inflammatory conditions such as scleroderma and SLE (Paolini et al., 2004), and granulomatous disease such as sarcoidosis. Certain drugs (fenfluramine) can also cause the condition, as can chronic liver disease with portal hypertension. Some patients experience pulmonary hypertension as a complication of arterial clotting or chronic damage from single or multiple episodes of PE.

Primary pulmonary hypertension is diagnosed when there is no obvious cause of the condition, and there is a familial form of the disease as well. Persistent pulmonary hypertension of the newborn occurs in 1.9 neonates per 1000 live births and results from shunting through a patent foramen ovale and ductus arteriosus, with or without pulmonary hypoplasia (Greenough and Khetriwal, 2005).

Clinical Presentation

Symptoms include easy fatigability, exertional dyspnea, chest pain, dizziness or lightheadedness, and syncope. Underlying pulmonary or cardiac disease can mask the diagnosis in early stages. Pulmonary hypertension is often diagnosed late with signs of right-sided heart failure. Patients with COPD, pulmonary fibrosis, sarcoidosis, or recurrent PE who have evidence of right-sided heart failure (cor pulmonale) should be evaluated for pulmonary hypertension as well.

Diagnosis

In the primary care office, patients can have signs of right-sided chamber enlargement on ECG. Echocardiography may also suggest increased right-sided pressures and decreased cardiac index and can be performed both at rest and during exercise. It may also reveal cardiac causes of secondary pulmonary hypertension (Bossone et al., 2005). Definitive diagnosis is made by recording of a pulmonary artery pressure greater than 25 mm Hg on catheterization.

Treatment

Nonspecific treatments of pulmonary hypertension include loop diuretics, digoxin, and anticoagulant therapy with warfarin when indicated. Traditional therapies include dihydropyridine calcium channel blockers such as nifedipine or amlodipine, which can modestly decrease pulmonary arterial pressures in vasoresponsive patients but can also cause sudden death in nonvasoresponsive patients (Humbert, 2004; Malik et al. 1997).

Other therapies include prostacyclins such as epoprostenol and treprostinil; both are pulmonary and systemic vasodilators but must be given by continuous IV infusion through an indwelling catheter or by subcutaneous injection (treprostinil) (Paramothayan et al., 2005b). Iloprost is an inhaled form of prostacyclin apparently with fewer side effects that can improve exercise capacity and symptom scores, but it requires frequent dosing (Baker and Hockman, 2005). Side effects and economic costs are significant obstacles to the use of all these agents. Bosentan is a nonselective endothelin receptor antagonist, and sitaxsentan is a

selective endothelin receptor antagonist. Both improve functional status and physiologic measures in pulmonary hypertension (Liu and Cheng, 2005).

Sildenafil, which inhibits PDE-5 in the pulmonary vasculature, has also been approved for this indication based on results of a controlled trial that showed it improved 6-minute walk distance, New York Hearth Association functional class, pulmonary artery pressure, cardiac index, and oxygenation. Sildenafil (2005) is also less expensive than the prostacyclins and endothelin receptor antagonists. Dipyridamole also has some PDE-5 activity.

Inhaled nitric oxide is a selective pulmonary vasodilator that is often used to treat persistent pulmonary hypertension of the newborn. In adults with pulmonary hypertension, a 2-year trial of inhaled nitric oxide therapy combined with dipyridamole demonstrated improvements in exercise capacity, symptoms, and hemodynamic measures (Perez-Penate et al., 2005). A European consensus panel has released guidelines for the use of nitric oxide in this condition (Germann et al., 2005).

Surgical therapies may be general (lung transplant) or specific, as in the repair of congenital shunting lesions, mitral stenosis, or atrial defects. Pulmonary thromboendarterectomy is effective in some patients with pulmonary hypertension associated with saddle pulmonary embolus (Olsson et al., 2005).

OTHER PULMONARY DISEASES OF THE PULMONARY VASCULATURE

Wegener granulomatosis is a small-vessel vasculitis that can manifest either with shortness of breath or hemoptysis or with progressive pulmonary fibrosis caused by repeated small hemorrhages at the alveolar level. It usually combines pulmonary features with glomerulonephritis. Tissue biopsy of either the lung or the kidney may be diagnostic. Clinical manifestations result from the combination of vasculitis, glomerulonephritis, and necrotizing granulomas of the respiratory tract. CT may be more sensitive than MRI for diagnosis of pulmonary lesions.

Diffuse alveolar hemorrhage may result from autoimmune collagen vascular disease or vasculitis, Goodpasture syndrome, and other vasculitides. *Goodpasture syndrome* results from the formation of anti–glomerular basement membrane antibodies, which can also attack the lung capillary membranes. Primary pulmonary vasculitides affect mostly small vessels, but systemic conditions can affect vessels of all sizes. *Churg-Strauss syndrome* is a small-vessel vasculitis that often manifests first as asthma. Most patients also have maxillary sinusitis, allergic rhinitis, or nasal polyposis. GI, neurologic, and cardiac involvement often follows. The condition responds well to systemic steroids, but patients can require long-term low-dose prednisone as maintenance therapy (Guillevin et al., 2004).

Pulmonary Complications of Sickle Cell Disease

Patients with sickle cell disease have complications that can manifest with pulmonary signs and symptoms. For example, patients with sickle cell disease are especially vulnerable to capsular bacteria such as *Streptococcus pneumoniae* (pneumococcus) and *Haemophilus influenzae*, and they can present with acute lobar pneumonia, sepsis, or even pneumonia-related ARDS. Pneumococcal and *H. influenzae* type b vaccines, in combination with penicillin prophylaxis, have significantly reduced (but not eliminated) rates of serious infections with these organisms (Hord et al., 2002).

Acute chest syndrome is an acute syndrome of varying origins in patients with sickle cell disease. One third of patients with this syndrome have an identified infectious cause. Fewer than one in 10 has a documented fat embolism. Postulated mechanisms in most patients with no identified cause include hypoxia-induced pulmonary vasoconstriction, with microclot formation and decreased levels of nitric oxide and other chemical mediators of vasodilatation, inflammatory response, and cellular protection (Stuart and Setty, 2001). Hydroxyurea therapy promotes production of hemoglobin F and appears to decrease the likelihood or severity of acute chest syndrome. Nitric oxide therapy might be of use acutely in acute chest syndrome or chronically in the treatment of pulmonary hypertension, but there is inadequate evidence from controlled trials.

Among adults with sickle cell disease, pulmonary hypertension is a significant cause of morbidity and appears to be a significant predictor of mortality, even with relatively modest elevations of pulmonary artery pressure. The pulmonary hypertension can be caused by widespread thrombosis of small arteries, although the cause is uncertain in many cases (Adedeji et al., 2001). Pulmonary hypertension complicates other chronic hemolytic anemias as well (Machado and Gladwin, 2005).

Malignant Disease

LUNG CANCER

Key Points

- Lung cancer is the leading cause of cancer deaths in U.S. men and women.
- Smoking is the most serious and prevalent risk factor for lung cancer.
- Any pulmonary symptoms persisting beyond 3 weeks are indications for diagnostic evaluation. Smokers and patients older than 40 years should receive a more aggressive workup.
- HRCT is more sensitive than chest radiography for diagnosing lung cancer. CT also provides anatomic detail for staging and operability.
- Patients with stage I, non–small cell carcinoma have 50% 5-year survival rate with appropriate surgical resection.
- The family physician plays a central role in facilitating family conversations about diagnostic and treatment options, advance directives, palliative care, and other end-of-life decisions.

Epidemiology and Risk Factors

Although not the most common cancer, lung cancer is the leading cause of cancer deaths in men and women in the United States. Lung cancer surpassed breast cancer as a cause of death among women in the 1990s because of increased smoking among women and better detection, treatment, and survival of breast cancer. Smoking is clearly the most serious and prevalent risk factor for the development of lung cancer. According to the CDC, from 2000 to 2004, smoking resulted in an estimated annual average of 269,655 deaths among men and 173,940 deaths among women in the United States. The top three smoking-attributable causes were lung cancer, ischemic heart disease, and COPD (CDC, 2008).

Clinical Presentation

Smokers are at significant risk for lung cancer, but other patients can develop lung cancers as well, especially if they have significant secondary exposure to tobacco smoke or other carcinogens. A history of asbestos exposure is a specific risk factor for the development of mesothelioma. Patients can present with respiratory symptoms such as a cough, hemoptysis, or shortness of breath, or they can present with constitutional symptoms such as fatigue and unexplained weight loss. In some cases, a chest radiograph done for other reasons reveals a pulmonary nodule or mass lesion. In patients with metastatic pulmonary lesions, the symptoms of the primary cancer may be predominant or occult.

Diagnosis

Any pulmonary symptoms persisting beyond 3 weeks are an indication for a more extensive evaluation, and smokers and patients older than 40 years should receive a more aggressive workup. Diagnostic evaluation can begin with chest radiograph, but negative results do not rule out lung cancer or provide tissue diagnosis or staging. HRCT scanning is a more sensitive test for identifying lung cancers even at asymptomatic stages. HRCT can also provide some anatomic detail for staging and determining operability of the cancer. Tissue diagnosis is essential not only for confirming the presence of malignancy but also for determining the histopathology. Fiberoptic bronchoscopy with biopsy brushings and washings is highly accurate for diagnosing centrally located bronchogenic carcinoma in the proximal bronchial tree. Transbronchial biopsy can reach deeper tissues for diagnosis of metastatic pulmonary nodules or even lymph node biopsy. Peripheral pulmonary lesions or pleural lesions can be reached by CT-guided needle biopsy or by surgical open-lung biopsy.

The combination of tissue biopsy and imaging studies yields both the histopathologic type and the stage of cancer. The non–small cell lung cancers may be further classified into various histopathologic cell types, such as adenocarcinoma and squamous cell carcinoma. Staging of non–small cell cancers is summarized in Table 16-13 (American Cancer Society, 2005).

Treatment

General treatment principles and guidelines provide a framework for primary care practitioners. Histopathology and stage at diagnosis drive treatment options. For example, surgical resection is not generally effective in treating small cell carcinomas of the lung, which may respond better to chemotherapy. On the other hand, a stage I, non–small cell

Table 16-13 Staging and 5-Year Survival Related to Lung Cancers

Clinical Stage	Defining Characteristics	Average 5-Year Survival Rate (%)
NON–SMALL CELL CANCERS		
I	Carcinoma confined to lung tissue; no spread to other organs or adjacent structures, and no lymph node involvement Substages A and B refer to size of tumor.	51
II	Carcinoma confined to lung tissue; no spread to other organs or adjacent structures but positive lymph node involvement Substages A and B refer to size of tumor.	26
III	Carcinoma with spread to adjacent structures, such as chest wall, diaphragm, mediastinum, or contralateral lung Stage IIIA may still be operable; IIIB is inoperable.	8 } 17
Stage IV	Metastatic to distant organs or tissue beyond the thoracic cavity	2
SMALL CELL CANCERS		
Limited	Limited to one lung or one side of the chest with no distant spread	10-20
Extensive	Spread beyond one lung to distant organs	1-2

From Lung and bronchus cancer: survival rates by race, sex, diagnosis-year, stage and age. SEER Statistics in Review, 1975–2003. National Cancer Institute. http://seer.cancer.gov/csr/1975_2003/results_merged/sect_15_lung_bronchus.pdf.

carcinoma might have as much as a 50% 5-year survival rate with appropriate surgical resection. The European Respiratory Society and European Society of Thoracic Surgeons have published extensive clinical guidelines for evaluating any lung cancer patient's fitness for combined surgery and chemoradiotherapy (Brunelli et al, 2009).

Treatment options in addition to surgery include radiation therapy and chemotherapy. Response to any therapy differs by cell type (e.g., squamous cell vs. adenocarcinoma), stage of disease, and whether the tumor is primary or secondary. Some genetic polymorphisms are associated with certain lung cancers in nonsmokers and can be responsive to more specific chemotherapeutic treatment regimens. Patients with metastatic pulmonary nodules from estrogen receptor–positive breast cancer may be treated quite differently from those with primary adenocarcinoma of the lung, although both generally receive some form of chemotherapy. The primary care practitioner must maintain a close working relationship with medical and surgical oncologists to help guide patients and families through various treatment options.

One specific role for the family physician is to help the patient and family address psychosocial needs in a proactive manner. The family physician may facilitate the first conversation between the patient and the patient's family in which the word "cancer" is mentioned or an ongoing conversation in which issues of death and dying can be addressed. The family physician must find the balance in encouraging the family to maintain hope but also in helping the family to develop contingency plans for potential crises, such as respiratory arrest or loss of function that leave the patient unable to live independently at home. Health care power of attorney and advance-directive documents are a much-needed complement to living wills, which cover only a narrow set of circumstances at the end of life. The family physician can help ensure that pain and other forms of discomfort are managed appropriately and can work closely with the patient, family, oncologist, nurses, hospice, and the patient's faith community to manage proactively the balance between preserving life and preventing suffering, especially in a patient with a terminal illness.

Prevention

Smoking causes lung cancer. Never smoking is the most important preventive measure available, but smoking cessation reduces the risk of all of the major histologic types of lung cancer (Khuder and Mutgi, 2001). Beta-carotene and vitamin E do not prevent lung cancer, and in therapeutic doses, beta-carotene might be associated with a slight increase in cancer (Albanes et al., 1995).

Regular chest radiography screening with or without sputum cytology does not improve mortality rates (Manser et al., 2003). Studies suggest that routine screening of smokers with spiral CT every 6 months does increase detection of early stage cancer and might improve mortality rates by increasing the percentage of non–small cell cancers that are operable (Gohagan et al., 2005). Patients with stage I, non–small cell lung cancers may have a 5-year survival rate of 50%, but only 15% of lung cancers are found at this stage without routine screening.

Another aspect of preventing lung cancer deaths is the rate at which patients of different racial and ethnic groups receive potentially curative surgery in stage I disease. African American patients, for example, have significantly lower rates of surgery and significantly higher mortality rates. Causes of these racial disparities include patient factors (locus of control, acceptability of surgery, health beliefs about risks of opening such cancers to air during surgery); provider factors (biased treatment recommendations or assumptions about what patients might want); systemic or institutional factors (lack of insurance, poverty); and perhaps most important, the patient–physician dyad (issues of respect, trust, and effective communication influence the outcome of negotiating the treatment plan).

KEY TREATMENT

- Smoking causes lung cancer. Never smoking is the most important preventive measure available, but smoking cessation also reduces the risk of all the major histologic types of lung cancer (Khuder, 2001) (SOR: A).
- Routine screening of smokers with chest radiography or sputum cytology does not improve survival. Use of frequent spiral CT suggests increased detection of early-stage cancer and improved mortality in non–small cell cancers (Gohagan et al., 2005; Manser et al., 2003) (SOR: A).
- Beta-carotene and vitamin E do not prevent lung cancer and in therapeutic doses might be associated with a slight increase in cancer (Albanes et al., 1995) (SOR: B).

Occupational Lung Disease

Key Points

- At least 10% of asthma cases in adults can be attributed to occupational causes.
- The two key questions are, "Have you ever been exposed to fumes, gases, or dusts?" and "Do your symptoms get better when you are away from work, such as during weekends and vacations?"
- Asbestosis passed coal miner's lung as the leading cause of death from occupational pneumoconiosis in the United States.
- Because most occupational masks or respirators are imperfect and workers often remove them, preventive strategies should focus on worksite air-quality improvement.

Exposure to fumes, gases, or dusts in the workplace are a common source of pulmonary symptoms and disease. Taking a good occupational history is essential. In the occupational history, ask the specific type of work the patient performs and other jobs the patient has performed in the past. Two key questions are, "Have you ever been exposed to fumes, gases, or dusts?" and "Do your symptoms get better when you are away from work, such as during weekends and vacations?" Clinically, occupational lung diseases can be divided into five major groups (National Institute for Occupational Health and Safety [NIOSH], 1999): work-related asthma, pneumoconiosis, hypersensitivity pneumonitis, acute irritant or inhalant toxicity, and work-related cancers.

WORK-RELATED ASTHMA

At least 10% of asthma cases in adults can be attributed to occupational exposures, so an occupational history should be obtained in every patient with asthma. Diagnostic criteria are the same as for other causes of asthma or airway obstruction, including spirometry (FEV_1/FVC ratio <0.7) and evidence of reversibility.

Chemical and natural agents can cause asthma or aggravate preexisting asthma. These include chemicals used in cleaning or manufacturing processes. Occupational exposures causing work-related asthma include dust exposures (e.g., cotton dust, wood sawdust, cement powder, bakery flour), organic exposures (e.g., molds and fungi in agricultural grains), chemical exposures (e.g., solvents, plastics, epoxies, ammonia, chlorine, petroleum vapors), and fumes from welding or other industrial sources (van Kampen et al., 2000), as shown in Figure 16-5 (NIOSH, 2004a). Peak-flow meter readings measured at the same time each day on workdays, weekends, and vacation days can help establish the occupational cause of disability for insurance purposes.

OCCUPATIONAL PNEUMOCONIOSES

The occupational pneumoconioses are diffuse parenchymal lung diseases caused by airborne exposure to inorganic materials such as asbestos, silica, and coal dust. In 1998 and 1999, asbestosis passed coal workers' pneumoconiosis (coal miner's lung) as the leading cause of death from occupational pneumoconiosis in the United States. Men accounted for 98% of these deaths. The rise in deaths caused by asbestosis is illustrated in Figure 16-6 (NIOSH, 2004b). Other occupational lung diseases are linked to heavy metal dust or fumes in specific syndromes such as berylliosis (beryllium) and stannosis (tin). Byssinosis, or brown-lung disease, occurs most often among workers in yarn, thread, and fabric mills from exposure to cotton dust.

Patients with occupational pneumoconioses may first develop symptoms of cough and dyspnea, with signs of small-airway disease or overt airway obstruction on pulmonary function testing. As the disease progresses, patients may also develop spirometric evidence of restrictive lung disease as well as chest radiography changes. Removing the patient from the exposure or workplace is the most important step for preventing progression of disease. These pneumoconioses respond poorly to corticosteroids. Smoking significantly worsens the progression of occupational pneumoconiosis (Wang and Christiani, 2000).

HYPERSENSITIVITY PNEUMONITIS

Exposure to organic materials such as fungi, plant proteins, animal danders, or other organic dust can cause a similar type of diffuse parenchymal lung disease known as

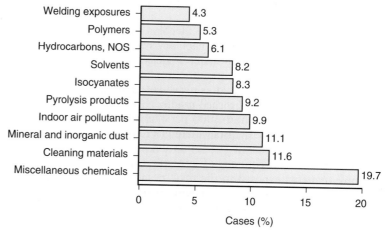

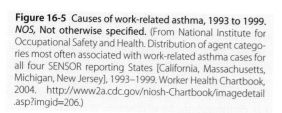

Figure 16-5 Causes of work-related asthma, 1993 to 1999. *NOS,* Not otherwise specified. (From National Institute for Occupational Safety and Health. Distribution of agent categories most often associated with work-related asthma cases for all four SENSOR reporting States [California, Massachusetts, Michigan, New Jersey], 1993–1999. Worker Health Chartbook, 2004. http://www2a.cdc.gov/niosh-Chartbook/imagedetail.asp?imgid=206.)

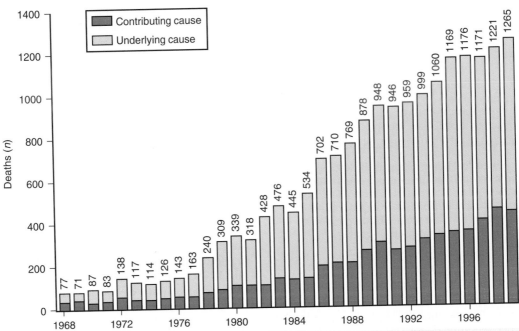

Figure 16-6 Asbestos as a contributing or underlying cause of death in the United States, 1968 to 1999. (From National Institute for Occupational Safety and Health: Number of deaths of U.S. residents aged 15 or older with asbestosis recorded as an underlying or contributing cause on the death certificate, 1968–1999. Worker Health Chartbook, 2004. http://www2a.cdc.gov/NIOSH-Chartbook/imagedetail.asp?imgid=217.)

hypersensitivity pneumonitis. Examples include farmers' lung, mushroom workers' lung, and bird fanciers' disease. Although fewer than 100 deaths per year in the United States are directly attributed to hypersensitivity pneumonitis, the number of cases and resulting short- or long-term disability are potentially much higher.

ACUTE IRRITANT OR INHALANT TOXICITY

A number of acute pulmonary exposures each year are related to inhaled exposures to irritant chemicals. For example, when certain household chemicals such as bleach and ammonia are mixed, chlorine gas can be produced. Chlorine and chlorinated chemicals cause direct injury to tissues throughout the respiratory tract, including the bronchial mucosa. Injury can fill the alveolar sacs with fluid in a noncardiac form of pulmonary edema, or "chemical pneumonitis."

The large surface area of the alveolar sacs in close approximation to the pulmonary capillary system also provides a portal of entry to systemic toxicity from certain inhaled agents. For example, organophosphate and carbamate chemicals, whether used as nerve gas or as agricultural pesticides, can be absorbed readily throughout the respiratory tract. More than 5000 persons died within 1 week after inhaling methyl isocyanate gas released from a factory in Bhopal, India, in 1984. Pulmonary toxicity can also occur as a consequence of systemic exposures. For example, patients exposed to the toxic pesticide paraquat through skin absorption or by ingestion through the GI tract often die from pulmonary hemorrhage or progressive pulmonary fibrosis.

WORK-RELATED CANCERS

The most obvious form of cancer associated with occupational inhalation exposures is mesothelioma, which is most often linked to asbestos exposure. Asbestos-related malignant mesothelioma accounted for an estimated 21,500 deaths in the United States from 1985 to 2009 (Lilienfeld et al., 1988). Persons with an occupational history of welding, pipefitting, shipbuilding, or other exposure to asbestos are at risk.

Lung cancers have also been associated with various occupational exposures, including welding or smelting fumes, coal dust, silica dust, and organic solvents. A more common exposure that has more recently been recognized as occupational is secondary exposure to tobacco smoke. Bartenders, restaurant staff, and others who work in smoke-filled environments are at significant risk for tobacco-related disease, including lung cancers, even if they have never personally smoked.

PREVENTION

Smoking significantly worsens the progression of occupational pneumoconioses such as black lung disease (coal miner's lung) and silicosis. Because most occupational masks or respirators are imperfect even when worn (and workers often remove masks intermittently for comfort), preventive strategies that rely on daily consistent use of respirators or masks in occupational settings are less effective than worksite air-quality improvement (e.g., increased ventilation, air filters, decreased dust or toxin production) in preventing occupational lung disease.

Granulomatous Diseases

SARCOIDOSIS

Sarcoidosis is the most common granulomatous disease of the lungs not attributed to a known infectious cause. Sarcoidosis is defined as a multisystem granulomatous inflammatory disease of unknown etiology, most likely caused by an aberrant immune response to an environmental or infectious agent in a genetically susceptible host. There may be multiple causes of sarcoidosis, based on specific arrangements of antigen, HLA molecules, and the T-cell receptor within individuals (Baughman, 2011; Spagnola, 2013).

Risk Factors

Sarcoidosis can be found worldwide, but regional and racial or ethnic variations in epidemiology and clinical manifestations are intriguing. For example, it affects persons of Scandinavian origin and African Americans at much higher rates than other populations, with an incidence of 35.5 per 100,000 in African Americans and a slight female predominance. Several occupational and environmental exposures have been studied as possible risk factors for sarcoidosis, but none has been conclusively identified. The Sarcoidosis Genetic Analysis (SAGA) study suggested specific genetic loci related to sarcoidosis susceptibility in African Americans (Gray-McGuire et al., 2006). Other studies show promise of characterizing susceptibility loci in a broader range of racial or ethnic groups (Iannuzzi, 2007).

Clinical Presentation

Sarcoidosis typically presents in early adulthood, between the ages 20 and 40 years. Although the disease is systemic, a spectrum of clinical manifestations may suggest the prognosis. The onset of fever; arthralgias; bilateral hilar adenopathy on chest radiography; and a raised, reddish skin lesion along the anterior tibial surfaces (erythema nodosum) characterize *Löfgren syndrome*, an acute, self-limiting form of sarcoidosis that often undergoes spontaneous remission and has a favorable prognosis. The insidious onset of dyspnea, dry cough, hilar adenopathy and infiltrates on chest radiography, new skin lesions of the trunk and extremities, and complaints of recent vision changes characterize a chronic progressive form of sarcoidosis marked by multiple flares of disease requiring repeated treatment throughout the patient's lifetime.

Symptoms that bring patients to medical attention most often emanate from the lungs, skin, or the eyes (uveitis and lacrimal gland enlargement). Diagnosis of sarcoidosis may be delayed when pulmonary symptoms present that are identical to more common lung diseases such as asthma or chronic bronchitis (Judson et al., 2003). The presence of airflow obstruction on pulmonary function testing and airway hyperreactivity have been identified in some subgroups of sarcoidosis patients, making differentiation from asthma difficult (Kalkanis, 2013; Young, 2012). Pulmonary symptoms may result from bronchial obstruction, either external compression caused by adenopathy or granulomas within the airways. Progressive disease may cause damage to the lung parenchyma, with a restrictive pattern of pulmonary function and decreased diffusion capacity consistent with progressive interstitial lung damage. Clinical features associated with a worse outcome include the presence of lupus pernio, chronic uveitis, hypercalcemia or nephrocalcinosis, nasal mucosal involvement, and bone cysts. Neurosarcoidosis and cardiac involvement, though not common, often carry increased morbidity and a more severe disease course for patients.

Diagnosis

The diagnosis of sarcoidosis is one of exclusion. The disease is established when clinical and radiographic findings are supported by a tissue biopsy specimen showing *noncaseating granuloma* (NCG). It is necessary to rule out known causes of NCG inflammation that may be seen in biopsies from fungal infection, foreign body inclusions, and other noninfectious granulomatous diseases such as Langerhans cell histiocytosis (also referred to as eosinophilic granulomatosis or pulmonary histiocytosis X) and Wegener granulomatosis. Tissue biopsy can usually be obtained from the lung, a palpable lymph node, a skin lesion, or the eye (conjunctiva or lacrimal gland). Percutaneous fine-needle aspiration specimen is less frequently obtained from the liver or from retroperitoneal or abdominal nodes by CT guidance. Biopsy from a CNS or cardiac location requires specialty consultation.

Along with clinical symptoms and biopsy, chest radiograph findings are added to support the diagnosis of sarcoidosis. The Scadding staging system classifies chest radiographs into stage 0 (normal), stage 1 (bilateral hilar adenopathy), stage 2 (adenopathy and infiltrates), stage 3 (infiltrates alone), and stage 4 (fibrosis and retractions). A chest radiograph showing bilateral hilar adenopathy in HIV-negative patients with negative skin test result and cultures for TB is suggestive, but lymphoma and other causes must be ruled out. HRCT can confirm the size and location of adenopathy as well as granulomas and early pulmonary fibrosis.

Transbronchial biopsy can document pathology and endobronchial involvement of the respiratory mucosa. Fine-needle aspiration of endobronchial lymph nodes is being used increasingly. Endobronchial ultrasonography to localize more peripheral adenopathy enhances accuracy. Analysis of BAL fluid showing a C4/C8 lymphocyte ratio greater than 3.5 has high specificity for sarcoidosis. Open-lung biopsy is usually not needed but can be diagnostic. Several biomarkers and cytokine profiles that may be helpful in the diagnosis and disease activity in sarcoidosis are under investigation (Bargagli et al., 2008). The serum ACE level has historically been used and is often elevated in initial cases, but it is not fully reliable as the disease progresses. A sarcoidosis assessment instrument has been developed to help clinicians better characterize organ involvement in patients with sarcoidosis (Judson et al., 1999).

Treatment

Some patients with sarcoidosis may require no treatment or only intermittent nonsteroidal antiinflammatory drugs for joint and constitutional symptoms. Topical corticosteroids may be effective for anterior uveitis and some skin lesions. ICSs and bronchodilators are often used when cough is a prominent symptom in patients with pulmonary involvement, but response has been equivocal. Systemic therapy is needed for the majority of patients. Systemic corticosteroids are first-line therapy and, for patients with pulmonary involvement, improve symptoms, pulmonary function, and chest radiographic signs of disease (Paramothayan, 2005a).

Second-line therapies include cytotoxic agents and other immunomodulating agents (Baughman et al., 2008). Methotrexate and hydroxychloroquine can be used as steroid-sparing agents. In patients with cardiac or neural sarcoidosis, treatment regimens that include cytotoxic therapy (e.g., cyclophosphamide) are needed. Other treatment strategies include agents that inhibit tumor necrosis factor α (infliximab, adalimumab, etanercept) (Nunes et al., 2005). Comorbid illnesses and multiorgan involvement are common in sarcoidosis (Cox et al., 2004; Westney et al., 2007), so health-related quality-of-life instruments should be used to monitor global response to therapy (DeVries and Drent, 2007), and multidisciplinary team–based care is recommended.

Interstitial Lung Diseases

The ILDs represent a broad range of acute and chronic lung disorders. The pathology may display varying degrees of pulmonary inflammation and fibrosis, leading ultimately to end-stage lung disease. ILDs are classified under the larger designation of *diffuse parenchymal lung disease*, which includes disorders from known causes (occupational and environmental exposures, as well as progressive infections) and unknown causes (sarcoidosis, lymphangioleiomyomatosis, pulmonary histiocytosis X, eosinophilic pneumonia, idiopathic ILDs). The idiopathic ILDs have been subclassified by the ATS and European Respiratory Society (2002) into the following clinicopathologic entities, in order of relative frequency: idiopathic pulmonary fibrosis (IPF), nonspecific interstitial pneumonia, cryptogenic organizing pneumonia, acute interstitial pneumonia, respiratory bronchiolitis-associated ILD, desquamative interstitial pneumonia, and lymphoid interstitial pneumonia.

EPIDEMIOLOGY AND RISK FACTORS

Occupational risk factors and specific occupational lung diseases are reviewed in previous sections. Various medications, chemotherapeutic agents, and radiation therapy can all cause diffuse parenchymal lung disease and may result in end-stage lung disease with pulmonary fibrosis. Other causes include autoimmune connective tissue disorders (SLE, RA), granulomatous diseases (sarcoidosis, pulmonary Langerhans cell histiocytosis, eosinophilic granuloma), and metabolic diseases (Gaucher disease, Niemann-Pick disease), congenital neoplasia (tuberous sclerosis, neurofibromatosis) malignancy (lymphangitic carcinomatosis, bronchoalveolar carcinoma, pulmonary lymphoma), and certain drugs (bleomycin, nitrofurantoin, amiodarone). Among the ILDs, idiopathic pulmonary fibrosis occurs more often in patients older than age 60 years and in men more than women. Cigarette smoking, chronic aspiration, various environmental exposures (metal and wood dust), and numerous viruses (Epstein-Barr, influenza, CMV) have been implicated as potential risk factors. The remaining ILDs rarely occur and are designated as separate disease entities based on specific clinicopathologic differences (Lynch et al., 2005).

CLINICAL PRESENTATION

The hallmark symptoms of ILDs are the insidious onset of progressive shortness of breath and exertional dyspnea with paroxysmal dry cough. A careful history may elicit symptoms of an earlier viral prodrome in patients that may also include cough with varying sputum production and systemic symptoms such as fever or weight loss. On physical examination, most patients can have the typical dry, end-inspiratory ("Velcro") crackles most appreciable in the lung bases. The finding of cyanosis and accentuated second heart sound, right ventricular heave, and lower extremity edema suggest late phases of the disease caused by chronic hypoxemia and pulmonary fibrosis.

DIAGNOSIS

The usual diagnostic approach for all ILDs is a thorough history and physical examination along with chest radiographic and pulmonary function studies. Assessment of serum antinuclear antibody titer with associated autoantibodies can implicate the presence of a connective tissue disease, which presages a better long-term survival than IPF (Cottin, 2013). The chest radiograph typically shows bilateral, often asymmetric reticular opacities in the peripheral and basal lung areas. A normal-appearing radiograph may rarely be encountered but does not exclude microscopic presence of an ILD. Often, radiographic abnormalities can be seen years before the development of symptoms, so past films should be reviewed. HRCT features of idiopathic pulmonary fibrosis may be distinct and include bibasilar subpleural honeycombing, traction bronchiectasis (as illustrated in Fig. 16-7), thick intralobular septa, and minimal ground-glass opacities. If the HRCT pattern shows a predominance of ground-glass opacification, especially located away from the subpleural areas, diagnoses such as

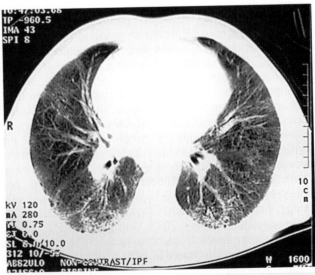

Figure 16-7 Computed tomography scan of a patient with idiopathic pulmonary fibrosis.

nonspecific interstitial pneumonia, bronchiolitis obliterans organizing pneumonia, or hypersensitivity pneumonitis should be considered. In some cases, fibrotic scarring and nodules create a mass lesion that must be distinguished from carcinoma or other neoplasm.

The typical PFT pattern is that of a restrictive ventilatory defect with decreased lung flow and volume, increased FEV_1/FVC ratio, and decreased DLco. Biopsy may be necessary to exclude malignancy or to rule in specific conditions such as sarcoidosis. Documenting pulmonary function, exercise capacity (6-minute walk test), and relationship of the ILD to any occupational or environmental exposure are all essential for helping patients receive appropriate worker's compensation or disability support when needed.

TREATMENT

Smoking cessation is essential, and pulmonary rehabilitation may improve quality of life and functional capacity for patients with any ILD. Pharmacologic options include single-agent or combination corticosteroid therapy and immunomodulating or antifibrotic agents (azathioprine, cyclophosphamide, colchicine, D-penicillamine). Overall, whereas these therapies have shown marginal to no benefit in cases of idiopathic pulmonary fibrosis, patients with other ILDs may have a better response (Davies et al., 2003). A meta-analysis of 390 patients with pulmonary fibrosis did find that interferon-γ-1b therapy significantly reduced the mortality rate (Bajwa et al., 2005). Causes of death identified for pulmonary fibrosis in one study included respiratory failure (39%), cardiovascular disease (27%), lung cancer (10%), and pulmonary infection or emboli (6%) (Panos, 1990).

Unilateral lung transplantation may enhance survival and functioning in patients with advanced interstitial fibrosis with chronic respiratory failure, but pulmonary fibrosis with pulmonary hypertension may require bilateral lung transplantation (Alalawi et al., 2005). The 1-year survival rate after lung transplantation is 75%, with 44% of patients surviving 5 years or longer (Trulock, 2001).

Lung Manifestations of Autoimmune Connective Tissue Disorders and Other Systemic Diseases

Many connective tissue diseases can have an impact on the lungs and pleura or on pulmonary function. RA, for example, can cause ILD because of a fibronodular inflammatory response or even larger rheumatoid nodules. Inflammation can also lead to pleural effusion or scarring, and pleural biopsy can reveal rheumatic nodules. Patients with RA can also develop one of several varieties of inflammatory interstitial pneumonia.

Systemic lupus erythematosus can affect the lungs. The inflammatory response of SLE is more vasculitic in nature, which can manifest as pulmonary hemorrhage, thromboembolic disease, or an inflammatory pleuritis with effusion.

Other autoimmune diseases with pulmonary manifestations include mixed connective tissue disease, Sjögren syndrome, and progressive systemic sclerosis (scleroderma). Progressive systemic sclerosis can manifest with thickening and tightening of the skin of distal extremities; sclerodactyly; Raynaud phenomenon; and multiorgan involvement of the lungs, skin, kidney, heart, and GI tract. Sixty percent of patients have shortness of breath; others have cough, pleuritic chest pain, or hemoptysis. Lung CT scan in progressive systemic sclerosis and other autoimmune conditions can show pleural scarring and ILD, especially a ground-glass fibronodular pattern and honeycombing.

Diseases of the Pleura and Extrapulmonary Space

Key Points

- In international settings, the most common cause of pleural disease is TB.
- More than 200 mL of pleural fluid may be detected by physical examination or by blunting of the costophrenic angles on upright chest radiography. Decubitus positioning of the patient can reveal as little as 10 mL of fluid on the dependent side.
- Thoracentesis may be done blindly if pleural fluid layers out to at least 1 cm on decubitus radiograph. Otherwise, ultrasound-guided thoracentesis may be indicated.
- An exudate is diagnosed in pleural fluid by finding a pleural/serum protein ratio greater than 0.5 and a pleural/serum LDH level greater than 0.6 (or pleural LDH > 200 IU/dL) or pleural protein greater than 3 g/dL.
- Purulent fluid in the pleural space is indicated by a high neutrophil count and pH less than 7.2, which can require a chest tube along with antibiotics.
- Rapid drainage of more than 1 L of fluid from large pleural effusions (or air from pneumothorax) can result in reexpansion pulmonary edema.

The lungs are lined by visceral pleura, and the inside of the thoracic cavity is lined by parietal pleura. Normally, these two are closely adjacent, with only enough fluid for lubrication in the space between them.

EPIDEMIOLOGY AND PRESENTATION

Outside the United States, the most common cause of pleural disease is TB. In the United States, TB is still significant, but other disorders, such as pneumonia, HIV-related infections, connective tissue disease (especially lupus), and malignancies (mesothelioma, peripheral lung cancer) must also be considered. Pleural effusions can be caused by systemic sources of transudate (CHF, hepatic failure with ascites, autoimmune disease) or by local inflammatory processes (parapneumonic effusion, pancreatitis, neoplasia).

Four major categories of pathology arise from the pleura or pleural space: pleural fluid (transudate, exudate, hemorrhage, or chylous effusion), pneumothorax, pleural scarring, and pleural mass.

DIAGNOSIS

Pleuritic disease is suggested by thoracic pain on inspiration. More than 200 to 300 mL of fluid in the pleural space may also be detected by physical examination. Decreased breath sounds with dullness to percussion could suggest pleural fluid or lung consolidation, but pleural effusion may be distinguished by the presence of decreased tactile and vocal fremitus. Often, there is a small (1-2 cm) zone at the top edge of the pleural effusion where traditional signs of consolidation may be heard, including egophony. A pleural rub may be heard in areas of inflammation but disappears when significant fluid cushions the movement of visceral pleura against parietal pleura. For pneumothorax, significant air must be present in the pleural space to detect hyperresonance, although breath sounds are often decreased on the affected side. In the 1% to 2% of cases producing *tension pneumothorax*, in which air is able to enter the space but not equilibrate with either extrathoracic or bronchial air pressures, the clinician may detect tracheal shift, cardiac shift, or decreased heart sounds.

Chest radiography reveals blunting of the costophrenic angles and visible fluid when about 200 mL of fluid has accumulated in the pleural space. Decubitus positioning of the patient can reveal as little as 10 mL of fluid on the dependent side on chest radiography. Thoracentesis may be done blindly if the fluid layers out to at least 1-cm thickness on decubitus radiography. Otherwise, ultrasound-guided thoracentesis may be indicated.

Pneumothorax is also visible on chest radiography, especially when it exceeds 10% or more than 100 mL of air is present in the pleural space. On radiographs, 2.5 cm of air space between the thoracic wall and the lung is equivalent to a 30% pneumothorax. This is best visualized on upright PA and lateral radiography or occasionally on the nondependent side when patients are in the decubitus position. Other imaging studies (CT, MRI) can give more anatomic detail in patients with mass lesions or scarring. These studies are also somewhat more sensitive than radiography in detecting small amounts of air in pneumothorax.

Diagnostic thoracentesis can help determine the type of fluid and potential causes. *Transudates* are serous fluids often associated with inflammatory conditions. Transudative fluid is thin and mildly yellow or straw colored, through which one can read newsprint. More specific laboratory criteria for differentiating exudate from transudate include a pleural/serum protein ratio greater than 0.5, pleural/serum lactate dehydrogenase (LDH) level greater than 0.6 (or measured pleural LDH >200 IU/dL), and pleural protein greater than 3 g/dL.

Exudates indicate the presence of WBCs and often a response to infection such as pleural abscess or TB. Parapneumonic effusions may be inflammatory transudates initially or may progress to exudative fluid as WBCs and even the infectious organism itself spread to the pleural space. Infectious exudates are suggested by pH higher than 7.2, which can be an indication for chest tube drainage. More specifically, TB may be suggested by an exudative pleural effusion with elevated WBC count, more lymphocytes than granulocytes, and pleural glucose/serum glucose ratio less than 0.5. Hemorrhage into the pleural space is indicated by the gross or microscopic presence of red blood cells, although poor technique can result in a bloody tap that is not diagnostic. For mass lesions or scarring, pleural biopsy may be obtained (revealing granulomas or malignancy) either percutaneously with needle or surgically in an open biopsy.

TREATMENT

Treatment most importantly targets the underlying condition. For example, the inflammatory pleural effusions of SLE may be treated with systemic corticosteroids or other antiinflammatory agents. Antibiotics treat pneumonia and parapneumonic effusions, although purulent fluid or abscess in the pleural space can require chest tube drainage in addition to antibiotics.

Other indications for chest tube placement include pneumothorax compromising ventilation, exceeding 25%, or recurring after initial needle thoracostomy. Trauma with hemorrhage into the pleural space can also require a chest tube or even open-chest surgery to identify and treat the source of bleeding. Some pleural effusions may be treated with therapeutic pleural tap rather than chest tube. In these cases, up to 1 L of fluid may be drained through a pleural needle and catheter. For these therapeutic taps, attaching the thoracostomy needle to a tube and vacuum bottle is an alternative to the traditional technique of using a large syringe and stopcock to remove 30 to 50 mL at a time. Rapid drainage of large pleural effusions or pneumothorax can result in reexpansion pulmonary edema.

Patients with recurrent pneumothorax may require surgery to repair a specific defect. Patients with malignant pleural effusion that has recurred after complete reexpansion may benefit from pleural sclerosis, instilling agents such as bleomycin or tetracycline. Pleural stripping is rarely used because of the high rate of complications.

Disorders of Breathing

Sleep apnea may be obstructive or central in origin or a combination of both. The effects of recurrent apnea extend well beyond simple fatigue or sleep deprivation, causing significant cardiovascular and neurologic disease. Patients with *obstructive* sleep apnea are often but not always obese. They experience episodes of intermittent apnea, often associated with snoring, especially during deeper stages of sleep. In addition to obesity, adenoidal or tonsillar enlargement, macroglossia, and laxity of the soft palate and pharyngeal tissue can contribute to sleep apnea. Stroke, brain tumors, trauma, cerebral edema, and other CNS disorders can affect breathing at the *central* level as well. Brainstem infarctions can lead to respiratory arrest and death. *Cheyne-Stokes respirations* describe an undulating pattern of breathing of increased depth and frequency alternating with waves of shallow, slower breathing and even apnea.

Many patients with obstructive sleep apnea have elements of central apnea as well. For example, alcohol and sedatives can exacerbate the respiratory depression and contribute to pharyngeal muscle laxity. In addition, patients with chronic obstructive sleep apnea can develop chronic CO_2 retention that further depresses respiration. Patients with the classic "pickwickian syndrome" (obesity and hypoventilation syndrome) have a constellation of signs, including morbid obesity, obstructive apnea, polycythemia, pulmonary hypertension, and right-sided heart failure. Patients can present with symptoms of daytime drowsiness, sleepiness, or feeling inadequately rested. Family members often bring the problem to the attention of the patient or the family physician, having observed loud snoring and interruptions in breathing during sleep. Sometimes a motor vehicle crash resulting from somnolence while driving brings the condition to light. Depression can also develop.

In addition to symptoms related to loss of sleep or upper airway obstruction, sleep apnea can contribute to other major causes of morbidity and mortality. Bradyarrhythmias are common, and hypoxia can lead to ventricular arrhythmias or even myocardial ischemia or stroke. When episodic hypoventilation becomes frequent or chronic, with resultant hypoxia and hypercapnia, a metabolic response may counteract the respiratory acidosis associated with hypoventilation; the kidneys retain bicarbonate to foster a compensatory metabolic alkalosis. Systemic and pulmonary hypertension may be intermediate outcomes that lead to more serious cardiac complications.

Formal diagnosis of sleep apnea can be made in a sleep laboratory using multichannel recording (polysomnography) of electroencephalography, ECG, airflow, upper airway muscle tone, and oximetry. Home oximetry alone might not be adequately sensitive. The most essential treatment is significant weight reduction to decrease obesity. Other behavioral treatments include avoiding supine sleep and avoiding alcohol and sedatives. Nasal CPAP is effective for patients who tolerate it. Various oral or dental devices are also available, but data on effectiveness are limited. Surgical procedures attempt to reduce airway obstruction at the palate or tonsillopharyngeal or adenoidal levels. The American Academy of Sleep Medicine has published clinical guidelines with evidence-based recommendations and algorithms for the evaluation, diagnosis, treatment, and follow-up of patients with sleep disorders (Epstein et al., 2009).

References

The complete reference list is available at www.expertconsult.com.

Videos

The following videos are available at www.expertconsult.com: Video 16-1 Chest Tube Placement

Web Resources

www.aafp.org/afp/2004/0301/p1107.html Interpretation of spirometry.

www.cdc.gov/flu/professionals/ and www.cdc.gov/vaccines/vpd-vac/pneumo CDC information on pneumococcal and influenza vaccines.

www.cdcnpin.org/scripts/tb/cdc.asp CDC tuberculosis information.

www.goldcopd.com Global Initiative for Chronic Obstructive Lung Disease (COPD); Global Strategy for the Diagnosis, Management, and Prevention of COPD (GOLD guidelines).

www.guidelines.gov Provides clinical guidelines for pulmonary function testing and treatment.

www.lungusa.org American Lung Association; community and patient resources.

http://meded.ucsd.edu/clinicalmed/lung.htm; www.med.ucla.edu/wilkes Physical examination and lung auscultation.

http://www.med-ed.virginia.edu/courses/rad/ On-line tutorials for reading chest x-rays and chest CT.

http://www.nhlbi.nih.gov/health-pro/resources/lung/naci/asthma-info/naepp.htm Clinical guidelines for asthma.

http://www.nlhep.org/pages/spirometry.aspx National Lung Health Education Program; spirometry information.

www.nlm.nih.gov/medlineplus National Institutes of Health MedlinePlus online service.

http://phil.cdc.gov/phil/quicksearch.asp Pulmonary imaging (e.g., chest radiograph, CT).

http://www.thoracic.org/statements American Thoracic Society guidelines on clinical areas such as TB, pneumonia, asthma, and COPD.

www.uams.edu/radiology/education/teaching_cases/default.asp University of Arkansas Medical Sciences, Department of Radiology Teaching Cases.

17 *Ophthalmology*

EARL R. CROUCH, Jr., ERIC R. CROUCH, and THOMAS R. GRANT, Jr.

Patients present to family physicians with a limited set of symptoms, often with subtle differences to indicate mild or serious ocular conditions. To decide when to treat patients and when to refer them to an ophthalmologist, family physicians must possess a complete appreciation of these subtle differences. Knowledge of the basic anatomy of the eye is essential in determining these diagnostic differences (Figure 17-1).

Red Eye

Family physicians frequently encounter patients who complain of "red eye." Usually, the condition causing the red eye is a simple disorder, such as conjunctivitis or subconjunctival hemorrhage. These conditions improve spontaneously or are readily treated. A red eye, however, may be a symptom of a more serious disorder, such as herpetic dendritic ulcer, iritis, acute angle-closure glaucoma, ophthalmia neonatorum, or congenital glaucoma. These conditions must be clearly distinguished from the much more common conjunctivitis and subconjunctival hemorrhage because *immediate referral* to the ophthalmologist is paramount. To evaluate the red eye, the family physician needs to have available a penlight, magnifying glasses, a visual acuity chart, fluorescein dye, anesthetic drops, and a tonometer.

EVALUATION

Symptoms and Signs

Patients who complain of a red eye generally can tell the physician whether the eye irritation occurred rapidly or progressed slowly. This information is important because a small foreign body, such as a grain of sand, lodged in the conjunctival sac produces a rapid hyperemia, but a viral or allergic conjunctivitis, or an iritis, generally produces a slowly progressive redness. Ocular pain is an important symptom (Table 17-1). Irritation of the superficial layer of the cornea, as caused by a small foreign body, is accompanied by a superficial "grain of sand" sensation in the eye. Deeper inflammatory processes, such as iritis or iridocyclitis, or a deeper penetrating foreign body in the cornea present with more severe, dull pain in the eye.

Abnormal light sensitivity (photophobia) is a third danger symptom that must be elicited by the family physician. Photophobia occurs with corneal inflammation, iritis, and angle-closure glaucoma. Patients who have conjunctivitis usually do not have abnormal light sensitivity (Table 17-2).

Patients who complain of a red eye often complain of discharge from the eye (Table 17-3). If they do not complain of eye discharge spontaneously, the physician must inquire about the presence, type, and quantity of discharge. Purulent (creamy white or yellow watery) discharge suggests a bacterial cause. A serous or clear discharge suggests a viral cause. Scanty, white, stringy exudate occurs most often with allergic conjunctivitis. The absence of discharge indicates an unusual cause for red eye, such as iridocyclitis, ultraviolet (UV) light keratitis (snow blindness), or acute angle-closure glaucoma. A complaint of diminished visual acuity is a serious danger sign and must be elicited in the history.

Physical Examination

It is important to examine both eyes because many patients with conjunctivitis in one eye have clear signs of early conjunctivitis in the other. The type of infection must be closely inspected; whereas *conjunctival* infection is characterized by individually visible vessels in the conjunctiva branching from the sclera toward the cornea, *ciliary* infection appears as a red ring surrounding the cornea in which individual vessels are not clearly visible. The significance of ciliary infection is that the deep ciliary vessels are involved, indicating a much more serious inflammatory condition of the eye, such as a deep corneal infection, iritis, or iridocyclitis. Inspect the palpebral conjunctiva carefully with magnification to determine whether lymphoid hyperplasia (cobblestone appearance) exists. The type and quantity of discharge are assessed by pulling down the lower eyelid. The appearance of the punctum should be examined to determine whether pus is coming out of the tear duct. Palpation of the tear sac on the upper portion of the nose (lacrimal crest) demonstrates tenderness in cases of acute dacryocystitis.

Carefully examine the cornea. Normally, the cornea is perfectly transparent. Excessive fluid within the stroma of the cornea results in partial opacification that can be observed by direct illumination with a penlight. A diffuse corneal haze can occur with congenital glaucoma and angle-closure glaucoma. After inspection with a penlight under magnification, corneal staining is performed with fluorescein using sterile filter paper strips. The stained part of the strip is moistened with water and touched to the conjunctiva away from the cornea. With blinking, the fluorescein spreads over the cornea. A UV light source

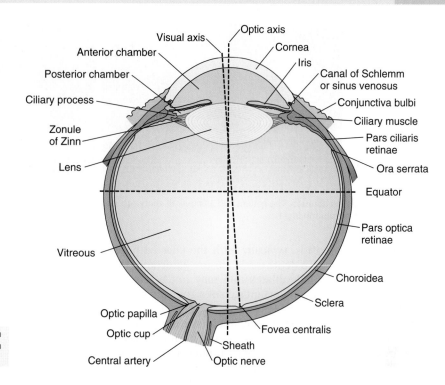

Figure 17-1 Anatomy of the right eyeball. (From Scheie HG, Albert DM. *Textbook of ophthalmology*, 9th ed. Philadelphia, Saunders, 1977.)

Table 17-1   Red Eye: Differential Diagnosis

Parameter	Conjunctivitis, Bacterial	Iritis	Keratitis	Acute Glaucoma
Vision	Normal	Blurred	Blurred	Marked blurring
Pain	None	Moderately severe; intermittent stabbing	Sharp, severe	Severe; sometimes nausea or vomiting
Photophobia	None	Moderate	Moderate	Moderate
Discharge	Usually significant with crusting of lashes	None	None to mild	None
Conjunctival injection	Diffuse	Circumcorneal	Circumcorneal	Diffuse
Appearance of cornea	Clear	Clear	Cloudy	Cloudy
Pupil size	Normal	Constricted	Normal	Dilated
IOP*	Normal	Normal or low	Normal	Elevated

*Caution: Do not measure intraocular pressure (IOP) with discharge present.
From American Academy of Ophthalmology. *The red eye.* San Francisco: AAO Professional Information Committee; 1986.

Table 17-2   Approach to a Patient Presenting with Red Eye (No History of Trauma)

1. Check for the following symptoms or signs:
   a. Reduced vision
   b. Pain
   c. Photophobia
   d. Corneal staining
   e. Corneal edema
   f. Unequal pupils
   g. Elevated intraocular pressure
2. Refer to ophthalmologist if any of these signals are present.
3. If none of the above is present, the diagnosis is probably conjunctivitis.
4. The triad of a red eye, pain, and loss of vision should *always* alert the examiner to a potentially blinding condition.

Table 17-3   Conjunctivitis Clues

Finding	Cause
Purulent discharge	Bacterial
Serous or clear discharge	Viral
Stringy, white discharge	Allergic
Preauricular lymph node enlargement	Viral

enhances fluorescence. Areas of bright-green staining denote absent or diseased epithelium. Corneal staining readily demonstrates a corneal abrasion and helps identify corneal foreign bodies and infectious epithelial defects, such as herpetic dendritic keratitis (Figure 17-2).

Examine the pupils carefully for size and shape. In most people, the pupils are of equal size; a small percentage have congenital variation in the size of the pupils (anisocoria). These patients are often aware that their pupils are unequal. In patients with previously equal pupils, inequality of the

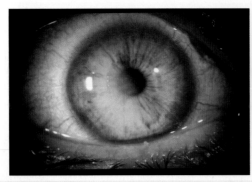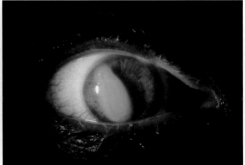

Figure 17-2 Corneal abrasion. The patient had a fingernail injury caused by the daughter *(left)*. Characteristic fluorescein staining is displayed in the adjacent photomicrograph *(right)*.

pupil may indicate iritis, typically with the affected pupil partially constricted. In acute angle-closure glaucoma, the pupil is usually partially dilated and may not be round. Unequal pupil size is an important sign of significant ocular trauma or third nerve palsies.

Estimate the anterior chamber depth by side illumination with a penlight. If the anterior chamber is normal or deep, the entire surface of the iris is well illuminated. When the anterior chamber is shallow, the iris on the more distant side of the pupil is in shadow. A shallow anterior chamber in a red eye may indicate acute angle-closure glaucoma or ocular trauma. The anterior chamber appears deep in patients with congenital glaucoma.

If the red eye does not have an obvious infection, the *intraocular pressure* (IOP) should be measured with a tonometer. IOP is normal in most patients with red eye, except for those with acute angle-closure glaucoma. With iritis and traumatic, perforating ocular injuries, IOP is generally low. Sterilize the tonometer before and after application to a red eye, preferably by heat sterilization.

Preauricular lymph node enlargement is a frequent sign of viral conjunctivitis and usually is not present with acute bacterial conjunctivitis (see Table 17-3).

RED EYE IN INFANTS

Key Points

- Red eye in infants requires special attention to differentiate ophthalmia neonatorum, congenital glaucoma, conjunctivitis, and dacryocystitis.
- Cultures should be obtained in neonates with symptoms suggestive of ophthalmia neonatorum.
- Febrile children with acute dacryocystitis should have cultures tested to direct management.
- Infants with symptoms of congenital glaucoma should be promptly referred to an ophthalmologist.
- For chronic dacryocystitis, the best age for surgical intervention is 6 to 12 months.
- Infants with a dacryocystocele require prompt ophthalmologist referral and systemic antibiotics.

Several conditions occur specifically during the first year of life. They include ophthalmia neonatorum, acute and chronic dacryocystitis, bacterial conjunctivitis, and congenital glaucoma.

Table 17-4   Management of Ophthalmia Neonatorum

Disease	Diagnosis	Treatment
Gonococcal conjunctivitis	Gram-negative intracellular diplococci *plus* Growth on chocolate agar or Thayer-Martin agar *plus* Fermentation glucose negative and maltose negative	Ceftriaxone, 125 mg IM single dose *plus* one of the following: Oral tetracycline, 500 mg qid Oral doxycycline, 100 mg bid Oral erythromycin, 500 mg qid Ophthalmology consultation
Other bacterial conjunctivitis	Gram stain *plus* Growth on blood agar or chocolate agar	Gram positive: erythromycin ointment qid, or fluoroquinolone qid for 2 wk Gram negative: gentamicin, tobramycin, or fluoroquinolone qid for 2 wk
Chlamydial conjunctivitis	Giemsa stain— basophilic intracytoplasmic inclusion bodies *plus* Chlamydial culture	Tetracycline, 500 mg qid for 3-4 wk Erythromycin, 250-500 mg for 3 wk bid Doxycycline, 100 mg bid for 2 wk Azithromycin, 1 g (one dose)

bid, Twice daily; *IM,* intramuscular; *qid,* four times daily.

Ophthalmia Neonatorum

Ophthalmia neonatorum is an infection or inflammation of the conjunctiva that occurs during the first 4 weeks of life. Possible causes include chemical conjunctivitis, *Neisseria gonorrhoeae,* and chlamydial infection. The increased incidence of venereal disease and shortcomings in silver nitrate prophylaxis are significant factors in the constantly evolving clinical picture. Ophthalmia neonatorum frequently is a manifestation of a systemic infection, requiring determination of the exact cause in all but the most transient cases. Table 17-4 outlines the management of the various types of ophthalmia neonatorum. At present, erythromycin is the medication of choice. Povidone–iodine ophthalmic solution (0.5%) is less toxic, inexpensive, and effective but is not generally used because of confusion over povidone solution versus povidone soap.

Silver nitrate has been replaced by erythromycin, so the incidence of chemical conjunctivitis has decreased significantly. Before the neonatal prophylaxis, gonorrhea was a common cause of ophthalmia neonatorum. Half of patients with *gonococcal* conjunctivitis develop corneal clouding, a major cause of blindness. Gonococcal conjunctivitis still occurs, despite erythromycin prophylaxis. Frequently, the infant with gonococcal conjunctivitis presents with swollen eyelids, purulent exudates, beefy-red conjunctiva, and conjunctival edema. The gonococcal organism can rapidly penetrate the intact corneal epithelium and produce corneal perforation if recognition and treatment are delayed. When gonococcal conjunctivitis is suspected, referral to an ophthalmologist is critical. Patients may also have systemic involvement, with associated central nervous system (CNS) signs. Both parents should be examined for venereal disease and treated, if necessary.

A recommended regimen for ophthalmia neonatorum prophylaxis is a single application of silver nitrate 1% aqueous solution, erythromycin 0.5% ophthalmic ointment, or tetracycline 1% ophthalmic ointment (Centers for Disease Control and Prevention [CDC], 2002b).

CHLAMYDIAL INFECTION

Chlamydial infections are a leading cause of ophthalmia neonatorum. There is a high incidence of this type of infection because of the frequent exposure to newborns during delivery and the lack of effective prophylaxis. The onset of infection can occur at any time. The typical picture is a mild unilateral or bilateral mucopurulent conjunctivitis with moderate eyelid edema, chemosis, and conjunctival injection. Systemic involvement may include rhinitis, vaginitis, and otitis media.

Treatment is with tetracycline ointment or erythromycin four times daily for 4 weeks. In addition, both parents should be treated with oral tetracycline or azithromycin. Alternative treatments include oral erythromycin or doxycycline for 3 weeks. Systemic tetracycline should be avoided in breastfeeding women with this infection.

Conjunctival cultures are indicated in all cases of suspected infectious neonatal conjunctivitis (CDC, 2002a).

Bacterial Conjunctivitis

The most common gram-positive bacteria that are causative agents of conjunctivitis include *Staphylococcus aureus*, *Streptococcus pneumoniae*, and group A and B streptococci (Figure 17-3). Gram-negative organisms include *Haemophilus influenzae*, *Escherichia coli*, and *Pseudomonas aeruginosa*. Bacterial conjunctivitis can occur at any age from the first day of life. Chemosis (edema of bulbar conjunctiva), purulent discharge, eyelid edema, and injection are common signs. Associated systemic septicemia can occur, especially with *Pseudomonas* infection. Cultures should be prepared on blood and chocolate agar.

A topical fluoroquinolone often provides effective treatment for severe cases before culture results (Leibowitz, 1991). Gram-negative organisms are best treated with tobramycin or a topical fluoroquinolone. Systemic antibiotics are recommended when there is evidence of systemic

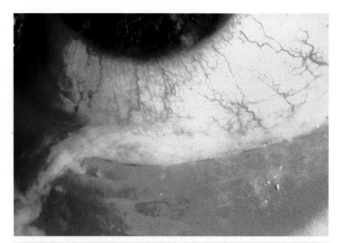

Figure 17-3 Purulent conjunctivitis may indicate infection with *Staphylococcus* spp., *Haemophilus influenzae, Streptococcus* spp., or *Pseudomonas* spp. (From American Academy of Ophthalmology. *The red eye.* San Francisco: AAO Professional Information Committee; 1986.)

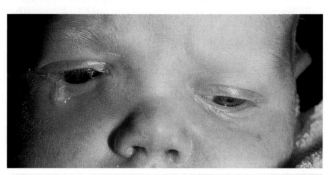

Figure 17-4 Acute dacryocystitis in a neonate with fever and malaise. Lacrimal sac massage and systemic antibiotics relieved the acute infection.

disease. Physicians should use caution with gentamicin, neomycin, and sulfacetamide eye medications because these drugs may cause a toxic chemical conjunctivitis and complicate management. Patients with mild conjunctivitis generally respond to erythromycin or bacitracin ointment.

Acute Dacryocystitis

Neonates may present with acute dacryocystitis, an inflammation of the lacrimal sac (Figure 17-4). Pain, tearing, redness, and discharge usually occur. If the child is febrile, culture testing and Gram staining should be done. *S. pneumoniae* and *S. aureus* are the most common pathogens. Systemic antibiotics are indicated for the acute stage. The ophthalmologist should be consulted immediately because irrigation and probing may be necessary to establish drainage as quickly as possible. Severe cases may progress to a dacryocystocele, sepsis, meningitis, or even death, especially in young infants.

Chronic Dacryocystitis and Nasolacrimal Duct Obstruction

Infants with chronic dacryocystitis usually present to the physician with a chronic history of tearing and crusting with a chronic yellow discharge. Topical antibiotics, such as

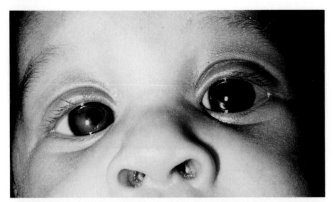

Figure 17-5 Congenital glaucoma in a 2-month-old infant who presented with a cloudy cornea involving the right eye. Intraocular pressure was elevated. The diagnosis was congenital glaucoma.

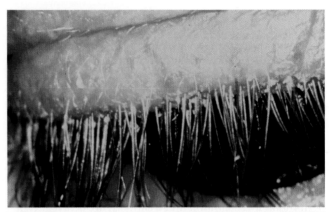

Figure 17-6 Seborrheic blepharitis is characterized by greasy, dandruff-like scales on the eyelashes. (From American Academy of Ophthalmology. *The red eye.* San Francisco: AAO Professional Information Committee; 1986.)

a fluoroquinolone four times daily, should be used. The parent should be taught to compress or massage the lacrimal sac four to six times daily. Approximately 80% of these inflammations resolve spontaneously by age 6 to 12 months. If treatment is not successful or if dacryocystitis persists, the patient should be referred and the nasolacrimal duct system irrigated between 6 and 10 months of age. Before age 14 months, a single probing is curative in about 90% of cases.

Congenital Glaucoma

Congenital glaucoma is a potentially blinding condition with an incidence of one per 10,000 births. It is often confused with chronic dacryocystitis. About two thirds of these cases are bilateral. These patients, similar to those with dacryocystitis, present with excessive tearing. The infants usually are light sensitive (photophobic) and frequently bury their heads in pillows or blankets. These infants often have intense blinking or eyelid spasms (blepharospasm). An enlarged cornea or corneal clouding can be detected clinically and measured with a plastic ruler (normal =12 mm) (Figure 17-5). Corneal edema is the result of elevated IOP, which causes breaks in the inner corneal layers (Desçemet membrane) and intrusion of anterior chamber fluid into the corneal stroma. Increased IOP causes significant optic nerve damage, which can lead to blindness. Whenever glaucoma is suspected, immediate consultation is indicated. Surgical treatment of congenital glaucoma is successful in approximately 90% of cases. These patients must be followed by an ophthalmologist for life as a precaution against recurrent IOP elevation and amblyopia.

KEY TREATMENT

- Newborns should be prophylactically treated with erythromycin 0.5% or tetracycline 1% ophthalmic ointment to reduce the risk of ophthalmia neonatorum (CDC, 2002a) (SOR: A).
- Ciprofloxacin 0.3% ophthalmic solution is effective empiric treatment of bacterial conjunctivitis (Leibowitz, 1991) (SOR: A).
- A broad-spectrum antibiotic for 5 to 7 days is generally effective for most cases of bacterial conjunctivitis (American Academy of Ophthalmology [AAO], 2008) (SOR: A).

- Children with nasolacrimal duct obstruction may undergo nasolacrimal duct surgery between 6 and 12 months of age or sooner if clinically indicated (Katowitz et al., 1987) (SOR: C).
- Children with congenital glaucoma should be promptly referred to a pediatric ophthalmologist or glaucoma specialist (AAO, 2008) (SOR: A).

RED EYE IN ADULTS AND OLDER CHILDREN

Key Points

- Red eye in adults and older children requires careful evaluation to differentiate the various causes of inflammation.
- Purulent conjunctival discharge warrants culturing and broad-spectrum antibiotics.
- Allergic conjunctivitis generally responds well to topical treatment; symptoms may manifest or worsen on initiation of systemic antihistamines.
- Orbital cellulitis requires prompt computed tomography and systemic antibiotics. Cultures should be obtained from the nasopharynx, conjunctiva, and blood.
- Iritis is characterized by pain, photophobia, miosis, and circumciliary injection and generally occurs after blunt trauma.
- A red eye in a contact lens wearer requires prompt evaluation for a corneal ulcer.
- Acute angle-closure glaucoma is an ocular emergency and requires immediate treatment by an ophthalmologist.

Blepharitis

Blepharitis is a chronic eyelid inflammation that involves abnormalities of the glands surrounding the eyelashes. The two most common types are chronic staphylococcal infections of the eyelid and seborrheic blepharitis (Figure 17-6). *Staphylococcal blepharitis* is the most common inflammation of the external eye. It is frequently asymptomatic initially, but as the disease progresses, the patient complains of

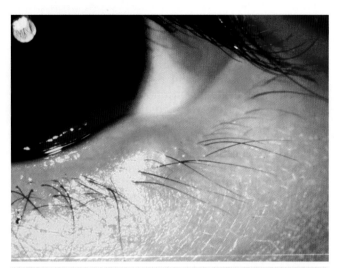

Figure 17-7 Acute hordeolum, or stye. The swollen, tender, red eyelid includes an acute, boil-like lesion. Treatment includes warm compresses and topical antibiotics. (From American Academy of Ophthalmology. *The red eye*. San Francisco: AAO Professional Information Committee; 1986.)

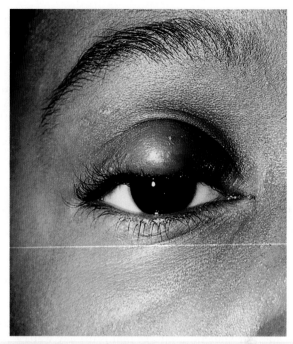

Figure 17-8 Chalazion of right upper eyelid in 10-year-old girl. (From American Academy of Ophthalmology. *The red eye*. San Francisco: AAO Professional Information Committee; 1986.)

foreign body sensation, matting of the lashes, and burning. Eyelid crusting, discharge, redness, and loss of the eyelashes are observed. *Seborrheic blepharitis* is associated with seborrhea of the scalp, lashes, eyebrows, and ears, characterized by greasy, dandruff-like scales on the eyelashes. Blepharitis is not associated with skin ulcerations. Treatment of both these conditions is long and laborious. Eyelid hygiene is recommended for both conditions. Topical antibiotics are prescribed for staphylococcal blepharitis. Both conditions are recurrent and require repeated therapy.

Stye

A stye is the most common localized infection of one of the glands of the eyelid margin (Figure 17-7). It is an acute boil-like lesion, and the patient usually has a swollen, tender, red eyelid. There may be a moderate amount of conjunctival injection. Treatment includes warm compresses for 15 minutes four times per day and topical antibiotics. Systemic antibiotics are usually not indicated unless there is a preseptal cellulitis component. Generally, the stye drains spontaneously within several days. If resolution does not occur within 2 weeks, the patient should be referred.

Chalazion

A chalazion is a chronic swelling of the eyelids not associated with conjunctivitis (Figure 17-8). The chalazion, a granulomatous inflammatory reaction, may persist for weeks or even months. Chalazia are generally not amenable to oral or topical antibiotics unless the lesion is secondarily infected. Chalazia are usually rubbery, cystic, and nontender on palpation. When the upper eyelid is involved, vision may be temporarily blurred. If the chalazion persists for more than 4 to 6 weeks, it may require incision and curettage. Recurrent chalazia may be caused by an underlying sebaceous carcinoma, so the lesion should be biopsied and sent for pathologic testing.

Bacterial Conjunctivitis

All common bacteria may cause acute conjunctivitis. Presently, *S. pneumoniae, H. influenzae, S. aureus,* and *P. aeruginosa* are the most common pathogens. The most frequent causes of hyperacute conjunctivitis are *N. gonorrhoeae* and *N. meningitidis.* Risk factors for bacterial conjunctivitis include contact lens wear, exposure to infectious persons, compromised immune systems, nasolacrimal duct obstruction, and sinusitis. In the presence of a severe purulent discharge, culture of the conjunctiva is mandatory (see Figure 17-3). Subconjunctival hemorrhage may occur with bacterial conjunctivitis and is especially common with *H. influenzae* conjunctivitis.

Treatment of conjunctivitis is with a topical antibiotic, such as erythromycin or bacitracin. Tobramycin ophthalmic ointment may be used for many gram-positive and gram-negative conjunctivitis cases. Ciprofloxacin and ofloxacin also provide effective broad coverage of most types of conjunctivitis. Gonococcal and *Haemophilus* conjunctivitis require systemic and topical therapy. If the conjunctivitis does not improve within 2 to 3 days or the worsening symptoms develop, the patient should be referred to an ophthalmologist.

Ciprofloxacin and ofloxacin provide effective broad coverage of most causative organisms. Newer fluoroquinolones such as gatifloxacin and moxifloxacin provide more potent coverage and better penetration for gram-positive organisms than earlier types of fluoroquinolones. Topical steroids or antibiotic–steroid combinations for conjunctivitis or other causes of red eye should not be used unless the patient is under the care of an ophthalmologist.

Topical corticosteroids have four potentially serious ocular side effects and are contraindicated for conjunctivitis, as follows:

1. Steroids can facilitate penetration of an undetected corneal herpetic infection to the deeper corneal layers and cause corneal perforation.
2. Prolonged local use of the corticosteroids (usually >2 weeks) can cause chronic open-angle glaucoma.
3. Prolonged use of topical corticosteroids can cause cataracts.
4. Topical corticosteroids are capable of potentiating the development of fungal corneal ulcers.

In general, topical steroids should be reserved for patients under the care of an ophthalmologist.

KEY TREATMENT

• Cultures of the conjunctiva are indicated in all cases of suspected infectious neonatal conjunctivitis (SOR: A).

Viral Conjunctivitis

Viral conjunctivitis, in contrast to bacterial conjunctivitis, has a less prominent discharge that is usually watery. The condition is highly contagious, and handwashing is important to avoid infection. When infected, hospital personnel, daycare workers, and institutional personnel should avoid contact with others. Palpable preauricular lymph nodes frequently are present with viral conjunctivitis and represent an important sign that can differentiate it from bacterial conjunctivitis. An associated upper respiratory infection may occur. In advanced cases, true photophobia and blurred vision caused by corneal involvement may be present and require consultation. However, most viral conjunctivitis is self-limiting, and no specific treatment is indicated. Topical steroids are contraindicated. Most viral infections resolve within 10 to 14 days, and specific serologic diagnosis is not necessary. If the conjunctivitis persists or there is any pain or change in vision, the patient should be referred.

Allergic Conjunctivitis

Allergic conjunctivitis is frequently found in pediatric patients and adults. It is usually seasonal, most often the spring and fall. Although often associated with allergic rhinitis, allergic conjunctivitis may occur without systemic symptoms. There is an increase in itching, redness, and swelling, which is variable from day to day. Seasonal allergic conjunctivitis is related to tree and grass pollens, each of which has a distinct season and severity. The condition may be asymmetric. Chronic allergic conjunctivitis is most often related to various indoor allergens, including dust mites, animal dander, molds, and cockroaches. Cats are especially irritating to the eye for the allergic patient.

Treatment for allergic conjunctivitis involves avoidance procedures for outdoor allergens, keeping windows closed at night during allergy season, and wearing eye protection (even sunglasses can reduce exposure to allergens). Washing the face after coming indoors, washing the hair when showering, and keeping the patient's hands away from the eyes can reduce allergen exposure. Bed linens should be washed weekly. Occasionally, allergy testing and allergy shots may be necessary in severe recalcitrant cases.

Symptomatic treatment of allergic conjunctivitis includes cool compresses, artificial tears, and nonprescription antihistamines. Topical antihistamine–decongestant combinations include naphazoline hydrochloride–antazoline phosphate (Vasocon-A) and naphazoline hydrochloride–pheniramine maleate (Naphcon-A), which are reasonably safe and effective. However, rebound vasodilation can occur and cause chronic hyperemia and conjunctival injection.

Cromolyn sodium 4% and olopatadine hydrochloride (Patanol) are effective mast cell stabilizers. Ketorolac tromethamine (Acular), azelastine hydrochloride (Optivar), and lodoxamide tromethamine (Alomide) are also reasonable options for managing allergic conjunctivitis. Systemic allergy medications may cause allergic conjunctivitis to manifest because of reduced tear film production.

Subconjunctival Hemorrhage

A patient may present with a bright-red eye, normal vision, and no pain. Usually, no obvious cause exists, but in some patients, there is a history of coughing, sneezing, or straining before the hemorrhage is present. The patient should be reassured that it is nothing more than hemorrhage of the conjunctiva. There is no therapy except reassurance that the blood will clear within 2 to 3 weeks. Hematologic blood coagulation studies are usually of limited value in patients with subconjunctival hemorrhages unless there is a history of recurrence. Additionally, it is unusual for a hemorrhage to involve the relatively avascular sclera. If trauma is suspected, the patient should be referred to an ophthalmologist to rule out more serious injuries, such as perforation, contusion, or occult rupture of the globe. Subconjunctival hemorrhage may indicate that the patient is a battered child or adult, and other signs of bodily trauma should be investigated.

Corneal Herpetic Infections

Herpetic infections of the eye can produce conjunctivitis, corneal inflammation (keratitis), and uveitis (inflamed iris, ciliary body, and choroid). The herpes simplex virus (HSV) is the most common cause of corneal opacification in temperate-zone countries. Humans are the only natural host for this DNA virus. Approximately 90% of the population has systemic antibodies to HSV. The incubation period of HSV infection is 2 to 12 days. HSV type 1 (HSV-1) is the most common cause of ocular infection, but transmission of HSV-2 also can occur. Although classically HSV-1 is the oral type and HSV-2 is the genital type, current epidemiologic studies indicate that either type may be the source of corneal infection, and therefore cultures and viral titers are often sent for both types.

Primary Herpes Simplex Infection. Primary ocular infection in a nonimmune subject usually presents as conjunctivitis with a clear watery discharge, skin vesicles on the eyelids, and preauricular nodes. Associated vesicles and ulcers on the oral mucosa and skin are common. Corneal involvement also may occur with single or multiple dendrites. If dendrites are present, the patient should be referred for treatment. Particular attention should be given to inspecting the nose for possible lesions. A lesion at the tip of the nose indicates involvement of the cornea through the nasociliary branch of cranial nerve V. Treatment generally

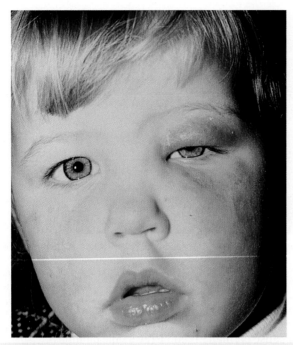

Figure 17-9 Orbital cellulites in 3-year-old patient. (From American Academy of Ophthalmology. *The red eye.* San Francisco: AAO Professional Information Committee; 1986.)

involves trifluridine 1% (Viroptic) drops five times daily for 10 to 14 days. If other regions are involved, oral acyclovir is added to trifluridine, as in eyelid or corneal involvement. These patients should be managed by an ophthalmologist.

Recurrent Corneal Herpetic Infections. At the time of the primary herpetic infection, the virus gains access to the CNS, where it resides in a latent state in the trigeminal and other ganglia. Recurrent attacks occur when the latent state is reversed. The virus travels via the sensory nerves to target tissues, one of which is the eye. Recurrent corneal involvement also includes the development of single or multiple dendritic ulcers. After a brief period, the plaque of epithelial cells desquamates to form a linear branching ulcer (dendrite). When a corneal dendrite is detected by corneal staining with fluorescein, the patient should be referred.

Preseptal Cellulitis. Preseptal cellulitis involves the eyelid and periorbital soft tissues and is characterized by acute eyelid erythema and edema. The infection usually occurs in the setting of an upper respiratory tract infection, external ocular infection, or trauma to the eyelids. Patients may have a mild fever and tend to complain of epiphora, conjunctivitis, and localized tenderness. However, the signs of orbital cellulitis are generally absent unless a preseptal cellulitis evolves into an orbital cellulitis. Treatment is initiated empirically in most cases with cefuroxime, ceftriaxone, or nafcillin.

Orbital Cellulitis

Orbital cellulitis, most frequently caused by an extension of infection from the ethmoid sinus, can occur in adults and children (Figure 17-9). It is the most common cause of exophthalmos in children. It may be difficult to differentiate a periorbital or anterior eyelid cellulitis from a true posterior orbital cellulitis. With a true orbital cellulitis, the child or adult has pain on movement of the eye, conjunctival edema, and limited extraocular movements. The most common causative organisms are *S. aureus, Streptococcus* spp., and *H. influenzae.* Cultures should be obtained from the nasopharynx, conjunctiva, and blood.

Immediate hospitalization and ophthalmic consultation are necessary. Emergent computed tomography (CT) should be performed to rule out orbital cellulitis. If orbital cellulitis is diagnosed, immediate hospitalization with intravenous (IV) antibiotics and ophthalmologic consultation should be undertaken. Appropriate systemic antibiotic treatment depends on the causative organism. Cavernous sinus thrombosis, meningitis, and blindness are serious complications of orbital cellulitis.

Iritis

Iritis is an inflammatory process of the anterior chamber, often associated with blunt trauma or infection. Redness, pain, and photophobia occur with iritis. No discharge is seen, and the pupil is constricted. Circumcorneal (ciliary) injection may occur. IOP is normal or low. Initial treatment may include dilation with homatropine and loteprednol etabonate (Lotemax) for patient comfort, with immediate referral to an ophthalmologist. Consultation should be obtained for all such patients as soon as possible.

Corneal Ulcers

The most common causes of corneal ulcers include gram-positive organisms, such as staphylococci and streptococci; and gram-negative organisms, such as *Pseudomonas aeruginosa* and *Enterobacteriaceae.* Less common gram-negative organisms include *Bacteroides.* Risk factors for corneal ulcers include patients with corneal erosions, persistent epithelial defects, impaired immunologic mechanisms, contact lenses, chronic topical or systemic steroid use, diabetes, and alcoholism. Corneal ulcers require consultation with an ophthalmologist for appropriate culture and antibiotic therapy.

Angle-Closure Glaucoma

Acute elevations in IOP can occur when the outflow of aqueous humor is suddenly blocked. The condition is more common in Asians but may occur in any patient. An acute angle-closure attack may follow an episode of emotional or physical stress; dilation of the pupil in dim lighting; or rarely, after instillation of dilating eyedrops. A patient having an acute attack usually has severe ocular pain, redness, blurred vision, rainbow-colored halos around lights, and sometimes nausea and vomiting. On examination, the eye is usually red, pupil mid-dilated and poorly reactive, and IOP greatly elevated. Generally, only one eye is affected at a time. Corneal clouding or corneal edema may be present in advanced cases.

An acute episode of angle-closure glaucoma is an ocular emergency and requires immediate treatment to lower IOP by medical treatment. After IOP is under control, yttrium-argon-garnet (YAG) or argon laser peripheral iridectomy is performed.

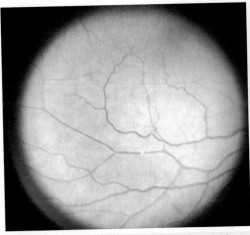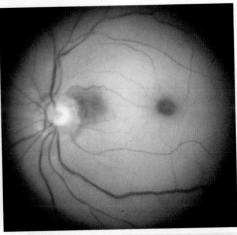

Figure 17-10 Central retinal artery occlusion of left eye with Hollenhorst plaque in the right eye. The patient has a characteristic cherry-red spot involving the macula of left eye *(left)*. Hollenhorst plaque with a retinal arcade in right eye suggests bilateral carotid disease and cardiovascular disease *(right)*.

Ocular Trauma and Other Emergencies

Key Points

- Chemical burns require immediate evaluation and treatment to stabilize the ocular surface.
- Central retinal artery occlusion requires immediate intervention to return oxygenation to the retina. Patients should be thoroughly evaluated to determine the source of the retinal artery occlusion.
- Hyphema should be carefully managed with bed rest, shielding the injured eye, and appropriate pharmacologic or surgical treatment to minimize potential complications. Patients with hyphema and angle recession require lifelong evaluation for possible glaucoma.
- Ocular foreign bodies of the surface can be conservatively managed with removal of the foreign material and appropriate antibiotic ointment. Care should always be taken to rule out an occult ruptured globe.
- The early signs of a retinal detachment include an increase in floaters or flashing lights. Retinal detachments warrant careful evaluation and prompt intervention.

EMERGENCIES

True emergencies can be classified as those for which therapy should be instituted within minutes. Two true emergencies in the eye are chemical burns of the cornea and central retinal artery occlusion.

Chemical Burns

Most acids produce the extent of their damage immediately on contact—the more concentrated the acid, the more severe the immediate effect. Alkali burns are more devastating to the eye because they continue to cause damage long after the initial chemical contact. Corneal melting can lead to perforation, and severe chronic glaucoma can occur as a later complication. Burns of the eye by acids or alkalis are true ocular emergencies. An alkaline substance, such as lye, can cause permanent and irreversible blindness.

The immediate treatment of chemical burns must be continual irrigation of the eyes, with up to 1000 mL of normal saline or lactated Ringer solution. If these solutions are not available, water from a shower, spigot, bathtub, or drinking fountain is appropriate. The conjunctival pH should be assessed after irrigation and again 30 minutes later to confirm stabilization of the ocular surface; pH value should be 7.5 to 8. If the pH remains abnormal, irrigation should be repeated until the pH is normal. Patients are managed with aggressive antibiotic ointment therapy and lubrication after a chemical burn. After the initial ocular irrigation, ophthalmologic consultation must be immediate.

KEY TREATMENT

- Chemical burns of the ocular surface should be washed with at least 1 L of fluid and tested until the pH returns to normal. An ophthalmologist should evaluate the affected eye within 24 hours after treatment (AAO, 2007) (SOR: C).

Central Retinal Artery Occlusion

With an incidence of about one in 10,000 people, central retinal artery occlusion is generally not the result of trauma. Risk factors include atrial fibrillation, mitral valve disease, atherosclerosis, a hypercoagulable state, and hypertension. Additionally, prolonged intraorbital swelling can cause occlusion of the central retinal artery. Such situations occur particularly in patients who are having surgery in the face-down position. The characteristic fundus appearance with central retinal artery occlusion is narrow arterioles and a pale optic disc. In addition, there is diffuse retinal whitening. A cherry-red spot occurs only several hours after the initial retinal artery occlusion (Figure 17-10).

Treatment of central retinal artery occlusion must be immediate, including breathing into a small paper bag to help increase the patient's carbon dioxide level. Emergency paracentesis is a rapid method to decompress the eye and may actually provide immediate restoration of vision. However, most physicians are reluctant to perform paracentesis on a patient within a few minutes. Ocular massage is another means of decompressing the eye. Some centers have hyperbaric oxygen available, which may also be helpful in restoring retinal perfusion for some patients. Treatment should be instituted within 90 minutes if any realistic hope of possible visual recovery can be expected. Patients with central retinal artery occlusion should be thoroughly evaluated for cardiac and carotid disease.

URGENT SITUATIONS

Urgent situations include those for which therapy should be instituted within minutes or a few hours. They include penetrating injuries of the globe, acute angle-closure glaucoma, papillary block, orbital cellulitis, corneal ulcer, corneal foreign body, gonococcal conjunctivitis, ophthalmia neonatorum, and acute iritis. In addition, trauma with retinal tears, vitreous hemorrhage, retinal detachment, and hyphemas constitute urgent situations.

Ocular Foreign Body and Other Eye Injuries

The most common eye injury encountered in family practice is a foreign body in the eye. The most common causes of a foreign body in the conjunctival sac or one embedded in the cornea are particles blown in by the wind; occupational or work-related injuries; and metallic foreign bodies that may fly into the eye, such as after a person hits a metal object with a hammer. It is important to evaluate the location of the foreign body and, in the case of corneal foreign bodies, the depth of penetration. Symptoms may be helpful; superficial foreign bodies in the cornea generally present with the complaint of a dust particle in the eye. Foreign bodies that have penetrated deeper into the corneal stroma produce a dull, aching pain perceived in or behind the eye.

On examination, it is important to look carefully at the inflammatory response of the eye. A purely localized conjunctival inflammation pattern is generally associated with superficial foreign bodies. Ciliary injection is a warning sign that a deep penetration may have taken place, and an ophthalmologic consultation should be sought immediately. Examine the eye after the instillation of ophthalmic local anesthetic to avoid blepharospasm and evasive eye movements. Inspect the cornea with a penlight or ophthalmoscope in a darkened room. Use of the slit on the ophthalmoscope can help visualize irregularities in the corneal surface. Staining with fluorescein demonstrates abrasions and helps identify otherwise transparent foreign bodies.

The family physician may elect to remove a foreign body in the conjunctival sac by irrigation with a sterile solution or after eversion of the upper eyelid with a moistened cotton swab. In the case of superficial corneal foreign bodies, a physician may attempt to remove it with a moist sterile swab, but embedded foreign bodies should be referred to an ophthalmologist.

Corneal Abrasions. Corneal abrasions are often caused by foreign bodies underneath the upper eyelid or inadvertent injury from a finger or small object. Evert the eyelid and examine for conjunctival foreign bodies. To evert the eyelid, the patient is seated and asked to look downward. The upper eyelid is grasped by its central eyelashes and pulled downward and slightly outward. The examiner then depresses the upper eyelid with a cotton applicator proximal to the upper tarsus margin. Gentle pressure is maintained until the upper eyelid is flipped into the everted position. Frequently, the foreign body is observed and can be removed with a cotton applicator or forceps. Corneal abrasions generally can be treated with an antibiotic ointment. Small abrasions often do not require patching. Large corneal abrasions may require pressure patching or a bandage contact lens.

If the conjunctival or corneal foreign body is not easily removed with a cotton applicator, the family physician should obtain ophthalmologic consultation. If the abrasion is not healed within 24 hours, an ophthalmic consultation should be obtained. Corneal abrasions should also be carefully inspected for other ocular injury. Any irregularity of the pupil in the presence of a corneal abrasion could signify an underlying occult penetrating injury. In such cases, the patient should be immediately directed to an ophthalmologist for further evaluation.

Contact Lens Overwear. Patients with contact lens overwear syndrome have worn their lenses longer than usual and typically awaken during the early-morning hours with severe pain and tearing. In response to prolonged wear, the cornea becomes swollen and develops epithelial defects. Patients need reassurance that the condition is usually not serious even though the pain is severe. However, occasional contact lens–induced corneal abrasions, especially those associated with soft lenses, can rapidly progress to severe corneal infection. Patients should be seen the next day and referred if they have not improved. Contact lens wear may be resumed only after the corneal epithelium is well healed.

Metallic Foreign Bodies. Metallic foreign bodies, if allowed to stay in the eye for a number of hours, frequently leave a "rust ring" that is clearly visible after removal of the foreign body. Rust rings irritate the cornea and result in long-lasting inflammatory changes in the eye. Follow-up should be done daily, with staining of the cornea to demonstrate the expected rapid healing. If healing does not take place over 24 to 48 hours, suspect an infection in the corneal stroma and obtain consultation. Topical antibiotic ointments are used after removal of foreign bodies in an attempt to prevent this complication.

Corneal and Scleral Lacerations

Corneal and scleral lacerations fall within the realm of the ophthalmologist and should be referred immediately after a shield is placed over the eye. Frequently, signs of corneal and scleral lacerations include unequal pupils, decreased IOP, iris prolapse, and hyphema, and a corneal laceration often also involves the lens. It is important to consider posterior injuries to the globe, including retinal detachment, retinal tear, and vitreous hemorrhage (Figure 17-11). Patients can often be managed as outpatients with oral antibiotics. Intravitreal antibiotics may be given at ruptured-globe repair. Some patients are hospitalized for IV antibiotics, although current intravitreal penetration of many antibiotics is often comparable. Corneoscleral

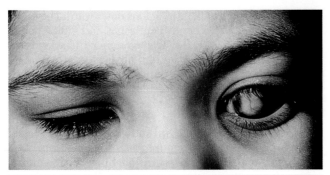

Figure 17-11 Corneal leukoma in 6-year-old boy. The diagnosis was ocular trauma and a penetrating corneal laceration.

lacerations should be principally repaired at the presenting institution when possible with available ophthalmology services. Hospital transfers delay wound closure or risk wound extension or prolapse of intraocular contents.

Blunt Eye Injuries

Blunt eye injuries are common and may result from relatively trivial injuries or high-velocity impact projectiles. An exact history of the trauma must be obtained to assess the velocity involved, which in turn may indicate the extent of ocular damage. Inquiry must be made to determine whether visual acuity changes occurred immediately after the injury. Flashing lights are often seen at the instant of injury and indicate irritation of the retina because any message to the brain from the retina is perceived as light. Persistent blurred vision is indicative of a more serious injury. It may indicate blood in the anterior chamber that is suspended in the aqueous humor. Free-floating blood in the anterior chamber is generally not appreciated by direct ophthalmoscopy. A slit-lamp examination is necessary to observe the suspended red blood cells in the anterior chamber.

Black Eye (Eyelid Contusion). A black eye may be serious or relatively minor. If accompanied by severe pain, bleeding, or constant blurred vision, more serious eye trauma must be considered. In such patients, orbital CT scan and ophthalmologic consultation may be necessary to rule out a ruptured globe.

Red Eye. Almost all ocular trauma cases include bleeding or dilation of blood vessels on the surface of the eye (subconjunctival hemorrhage). This may be observed with any degree of eye injury. For example, a subconjunctival hemorrhage may be spontaneous and often indicates minor injury. In the presence of other findings, a subconjunctival hemorrhage suggests more serious injury, particularly if a concomitant hyphema or vitreous hemorrhage is present.

Pupillary Change. Blunt trauma to the eye may result in lacerations of the sphincter muscle of the pupil. These are manifested by traumatic mydriasis. Unlike the unequal pupils seen with congenital anisocoria, traumatic mydriasis is characterized by recent onset of unequal pupils and by the irregularity of the dilated pupil. Although traumatic mydriasis by itself is not harmful, it suggests severe blunt trauma and is an indication for a careful assessment of other ocular structures, including the vitreous and retinal periphery.

Traumatic Hyphema. Blunt trauma to the eye may cause injury to the iris, angle structures, and other intraocular structures. Hemorrhage into the anterior chamber, or *hyphema*, is most often found in children. The agent producing the hyphema is usually a projectile that strikes the exposed portion of the eye. A great variety of missiles and objects may be responsible, including balls, rocks, projectile toys, air guns, paint balls, bungee cords, and human fists. With the increase of child abuse, fists and belts have started to play a prominent role. Boys are involved in 75% of cases.

Rarely, spontaneous hyphemas occur and may be confused with traumatic hyphemas. *Spontaneous* hyphemas are secondary to neovascularization, ocular neoplasms (retinoblastoma), and vascular anomalies (juvenile xanthogranuloma). Vascular tufts that exist at the pupillary border have been implicated in spontaneous hyphema. A *traumatic* hyphema may be graded by measuring the height of the layered hyphema in the anterior chamber in millimeters. A hyphema is an ocular emergency and should be referred immediately.

Cataract, choroidal rupture, vitreous hemorrhage, angle recession glaucoma, and retinal detachment are often associated with traumatic hyphema and compromise the final visual acuity prognosis. It is important to recognize that the prognosis for visual recovery from traumatic hyphema is directly related to three factors: (1) amount of associated damage to other ocular structures (e.g., choroidal rupture or macular scarring); (2) presence or absence of secondary hemorrhage; and (3) presence or absence of complications of glaucoma, corneal blood staining, or optic atrophy. With treatment, most hyphema patients have a good visual outcome. (See eAppendix 17-1 online for a discussion of hyphema grading and complications, treatment, and prognosis.)

KEY TREATMENT

- Hyphemas are generally well managed with bed rest, shielding of the injured eye, and medical control of the hyphema and IOP (Crouch, 2009) (SOR: A).
- If IOP remains elevated or hyphema occupies more than 50% of the anterior chamber, surgical evacuation of the clot may be required to lower IOP, preserve corneal clarity, and reduce optic atrophy (Sheppard et al., 2009) (SOR: A).

Nonaccidental Inflicted Neurotrauma (Formerly "Shaken Baby Syndrome")

The true incidence of nonaccidental inflicted neurotrauma is unknown because of the difficulty collecting statistical data. An estimated 1300 children in the United States experience fatal head trauma from child abuse annually. The findings of nonaccidental inflicted neurotrauma involve repetitive, violent, unrestrained, acceleration–deceleration head and neck movements. Neurotrauma can occur without blunt head trauma. Cases primarily occur in children younger than 3 years old, usually during the first year of life. Typically, patients present with fracture and intracranial or intraocular hemorrhages; not all findings are required to establish the diagnosis. An ophthalmologic consult should be obtained for all patients with suspected nonaccidental inflicted neurotrauma, with carefully documented retinal drawings or preferably fundus photography. Approximately 20% of cases are fatal within the first few days of presentation. Traumatic *retinoschisis*, if present, is highly specific for nonaccidental inflicted neurotrauma, particularly if the child is younger than 5 years.

Retinal Detachment

An increase in previous floaters or the onset of new floaters may occur in a retinal detachment. Traumatic detachment of the retina can be observed after blunt eye injury, especially in older adults. Retinal detachment may also occur spontaneously, especially in patients with high myopia. The patient may complain of reduced overall brightness in the involved eye or may have continuous light flashes, indicating retinal traction. After eye trauma, it is imperative to inspect not only the central portions of the retina but the peripheral portions as well. This examination should be performed in a darkened room after instillation of a short-acting mydriatic agent. Any questionable findings should be referred to an ophthalmologist immediately.

Other serious injuries are traumatic tears of the iris, subluxation or dislocation of the lens that occasionally displaces into the anterior chamber, and blowout fracture of the orbit, with impaired upward eye movement caused by entrapment of the inferior rectus muscle. These injuries are usually readily identified.

Pediatric Ophthalmology

Key Points

- Children should be screened at birth, birth to 3 months, 3 to 6 months, 6 to 12 months, 3 years, 5 years, and then every 1 to 2 years.
- Amblyopia and strabismus are distinct but may be associated. Children can have amblyopia without having strabismus. All children with amblyopia or strabismus should be referred to a pediatric ophthalmologist.
- Cataracts are an important cause of amblyopia in children and require prompt intervention.
- Pediatric cataracts may be a sign of a metabolic disorder, TORCH infection (toxoplasmosis, other agents, rubella, cytomegalovirus, herpes simplex), or chromosomal abnormality.
- Leukocoria warrants further investigation; significant causes include cataracts, *Toxocara canis* infection, retinal disease, and retinoblastoma.

EVALUATION OF VISION WITHIN FIRST 4 MONTHS OF LIFE

Parents may report that their baby does not appear to look at them. This statement requires the physician to document a history of prematurity, fetal distress, anoxia, or birth trauma carefully. A failure to reach developmental milestones may indicate neurologic abnormalities. A history of seizure disorder, cerebral palsy, or chromosomal abnormalities helps identify potentially serious causes. In these cases, visual acuity or the child's ability to fixate must be assessed. Normal newborns follow faces. By age 2 or 3 months, infants normally follow light and high-contrast objects. Assessment of vision can be achieved by using an optokinetic nystagmus drum. Oculomotor disturbances may be the underlying cause of the child's apparent visual inattention. Bilateral cranial nerve III palsy, congenital fibrosis syndrome, or partial cranial nerve III palsy may give this impression as well.

Searching or roving eye movements are a form of profound nystagmus, with little foveal perception. Nystagmus is an important sign of decreased vision, indicating visual acuity often in the range of 20/200. The onset is usually at birth or shortly thereafter. The nystagmus can be a jerk or pendular nystagmus. The direction should be characterized as horizontal, vertical, or rotary.

Abnormalities of the anterior portion of the eye can cause profound visual loss and are easily visible with a +10 magnification. They include corneal opacities (leukoma) caused by congenital glaucoma; *Peter's anomaly* (abnormal cornea and lens); and *leukocoria* (white pupil) related to congenital cataracts, inflammatory disease, or retinal disease.

Evaluation of the posterior aspect of the eye, including examination of the red reflexes, may indicate an early retinal detachment or retinoblastoma. Optic nerve abnormalities may be associated with midline CNS defects, such as an absent septum pellucidum, agenesis of the corpus callosum, or hypopituitarism. Optic nerve abnormalities such as optic nerve hypoplasia are associated with nystagmus. CT or magnetic resonance imaging (MRI) can identify these abnormalities. Electroretinography (ERG) may be helpful for determining the cause of decreased visual acuity. An abnormal ERG is seen with Leber's congenital amaurosis, congenital achromatopsia, and congenital stationary night blindness. Visual-evoked potential testing may be necessary to determine whether vision is intact.

Some infants who have completely normal eye examination results but demonstrate poor fixation may actually have a delay in maturation of the visual system. Normally, the initial visual system development matures by 4 to 6 months of age. Visual-evoked potential acuities are about 20/400 during the first few days of life and improve to about 20/40 by 6 months of age. In some patients, visual-evoked responses and clinically assessed visual function may be abnormal, only to improve between 4 and 12 months of age. Although incompletely defined, in delayed visual maturation, the vision is decreased, but the ocular examination appears normal, including brisk pupillary response to light. Typically, there is no nystagmus, and ERG results are normal.

VISION SCREENING AND OCULAR EXAMINATION

Appropriate vision screening is one of the most important factors in pediatric eye care. Because focused visual stimuli are critical to normal development, early detection and correction of visual problems reduce serious vision impairment or blindness. The AAO, American Academy of

Pediatrics (AAP), and American Association of Pediatric Ophthalmology and Strabismus (AAPOS) strongly support the goal of early detection and treatment of eye problems in children. In particular, vision screening is needed to detect four major conditions: strabismus, amblyopia, ocular disease, and refractive errors. Family physicians are ideal vision screeners because of their ability to detect abnormalities at an early age. Essential components of vision screening are age, testing format, testing procedures, efficacy, and referral criteria. On a practical level, vision screening must be cost effective and time efficient. The testing devices must be readily available and relatively easy to use. High sensitivity is essential to keep overreferrals and underreferrals to a minimum.

Four Stages of Screening

The AAO and AAPOS recommend that children be examined for eye problems in the following four stages (Table 17-5):

1. In the newborn nursery, physicians should examine all infants. Ophthalmologists should be consulted to examine patients at high risk for conditions such as retinopathy of prematurity (ROP), cataracts, congenital defects, and other ocular pathology.
2. At 6 months
3. At 3 years
4. At 5 years and older

The AAO statement recommends that family physicians establish a close working relationship with a local ophthalmologist who is familiar with children's eye problems. The collaboration can help clarify questions about vision screening and the need for referral. (See eAppendix 17-2 online for specific information on different stages of vision screening.)

Table 17-5 Recommended Vision Screening by Family Physicians

Age	Examination	Referral Criteria
Newborn	Penlight examination of cornea Rule out nystagmus Red reflexes	Any ocular pathology Nystagmus Abnormal red reflexes or white reflex
6 months	Fixation to light and small toys Penlight examination Corneal light reflex test, cover test Red reflexes	Object to occlusion Nystagmus; any ocular pathology Strabismus Abnormal red reflexes or white reflex
3 years	Visual acuity: Snellen letters, tumbling E, or HOTV wall chart Corneal light reflex test, cover test Fundus examination	Acuity of 20/40 or less in one or both eyes Strabismus Any ocular pathology
≥5 years	Visual acuity: Snellen letters, tumbling E, or HOTV wall chart (see online text) Corneal light reflex test, cover test Fundus examination	Acuity of 20/30 or less in one or both eyes Strabismus Any ocular pathology

Also, special groups may need additional vision screening. The following children should also be screened even if they are not due to be examined by their age: all children at high risk of having vision disorders, including those who are mentally retarded or who have trisomy 21 or cerebral palsy and all children who show signs or symptoms of visual problems, experience school failure, or have reading difficulties or other learning problems (e.g., dyslexia). It is important to note that children with learning disabilities such as dyslexia have the same incidence of ocular abnormalities (strabismus, refractive error) as children without such disabilities. Dyslexia involves interpretation by cortical processing centers and does not generally indicate any ocular pathology. Eye defects do not cause letter, number, or word reversal.

TESTING VISUAL ACUITY

Several diagnostic tests are used to detect strabismus, amblyopia, ocular disease, and refractive errors. These include visual acuity and fixation preference tests, corneal light reflex test, cover test, simultaneous red reflexes test, fundus examination, stereoscopic tests, and photorefractive techniques.

The best way to screen for possible visual loss caused by amblyopia is to measure the visual acuity or fixation preference of each eye separately. The covered eye should be firmly occluded during the assessment to avoid any peeking. When there is no apparent sign of amblyopia, the only clue to poor vision may be the child's objection to having the better eye occluded. Additionally, the child may demonstrate a fixation preference of the better-seeing eye, with an inability to fixate on distance objects in the amblyopic eye. Both are common signs of amblyopia that may be caused by a refractive error, media opacities, retinal or optic nerve abnormality, or cortical processing problem.

Equipment required for testing children older than 42 months consists of standard wall charts containing Snellen letters, Snellen numbers, tumbling Es, and HOTV wall charts, as well as some means of occluding the nontested eye, ideally, occluder patches (Opticlude, Coverlet).

Stereoscopic and Photorefractive Tests

The visual acuity test is the most widely used vision screening test, but use of this test alone will underrefer many patients with amblyopia and undiagnosed strabismus. Stereoscopic tests such as the random dot E stereogram are relatively inexpensive, fairly accurate, and easy to use. Stereopsis tests are complementary and offer additional information regarding a patient's visual health.

The use of photorefractive apparatus is relatively new. Reproducible results of photography of the red reflex can screen nonverbal infants and children. The sensitivity is high (95%) for refractive error in the range of 1.00 to 2.00 diopters. A problem with this technique is that cycloplegia is usually required to prevent obtaining false-positive results, especially for myopia. In addition, two photographs are needed to avoid missing an astigmatic refractive error. The technology offers great promise, but it must be cost effective. As newer, more rapid and accurate vision tests are developed, these may be incorporated into the screening process.

STRABISMUS AND AMBLYOPIA

Strabismus and amblyopia are two of the most common visual problems affecting children. Strabismus occurs in 4% and amblyopia in 4% of the population. Half of all amblyopia patients have a concomitant strabismus. Conversely, half of all amblyopia patients have no demonstrable strabismus.

Movements of the eyes horizontally and vertically are controlled by the six muscles attached to the sclera of each eye. Movement of both eyes in unison allows vision of singular images. Through a blending process called *fusion*, the brain combines the two images into a single, three-dimensional image. As long as the eye muscles are able to work together, the brain can process incoming visual information. When the eye muscles are not coordinated, one eye deviates inward, outward, or upward, and the other eye remains straight. When this occurs, the brain receives a different image from each eye and cannot combine the two disparate images into a single image frame.

Misalignment of the eye muscles results in strabismus. In addition to a breakdown or absence of fusion, the causes of strabismus may include refractive errors, anatomic anomalies, and abnormal tonic innervation. Adults with acquired strabismus frequently develop double vision, but children with strabismus quickly learn to ignore or suppress the image seen by the deviated eye. As a result of suppression, the straight eye takes over most of the work of seeing, and the crossed eye develops reduced central vision because of lack of use. There are various types of strabismus, including horizontal, vertical, or rotational (cyclotorsional). (See eAppendix 17-3 online for additional information on specific types of strabismus.)

Loss of vision in a relatively normal eye is called *amblyopia*. The phrase "lazy eye" should not be used in diagnosing patients because it can be confused with amblyopia and strabismus. As mentioned earlier, these two distinct clinical entities are associated with each other in only 50% of cases. In children younger than 4 years, amblyopia is the most frequent cause of unilateral vision loss (Figure 17-12). The condition is usually unilateral, although bilateral high myopia, hyperopia, or astigmatism may occur. Unless treatment begins early, loss of vision in the affected eye may be permanent. Amblyopia is usually treatable if detected at age 3 to 4 years but is generally considered irreversible after 13 years; however, treating amblyopia in patients older than 13 years has had some success. The earlier treatment

begins, the better the prognosis for the patient. The primary treatment of amblyopia includes the use of patches, glasses, or both. The better eye is occluded, and underlying conditions such as cataracts or refractive errors are treated.

Testing for Strabismus

The corneal light reflex test, cover test, red reflex, and extraocular rotations are four basic tests for strabismus. To perform the corneal light test, project a penlight onto the cornea of both eyes simultaneously while the child looks straight ahead. Compare the placement of the two corneal reflections. When the eyes are straight, the light appears at the same point on each cornea. If a muscle deviation is present, the reflected light appears slightly off center in one eye. Figure 17-13 illustrates the placement of corneal reflections as they would appear for each direction of deviation. In part *A*, note that the light is centered on the cornea of the left eye but is displaced laterally, or outward, on the right cornea, indicating that the right eye is turned inward, or is *esotropic*. In *B*, note that the light is centered again on the left cornea but is displaced medially, or inward, on the right cornea, demonstrating an outward-turning, *exotropia* of the right eye. In part *C*, the light indicates that the right eye is turned upward, or is *hypertropic*, and the left eye is straight.

The cover test is performed by having the child look straight ahead at an object 20 feet away (Figure 17-14). An eye chart is usually used to test children older than 3 years. For younger children, it is helpful to use a colorful, moving object or toy. As the child looks at the target, cover the

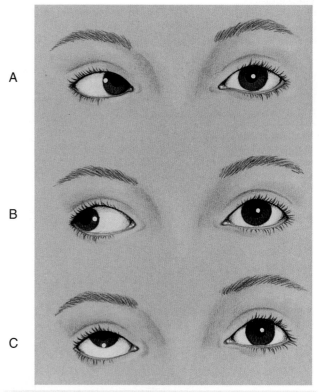

Figure 17-13 Strabismus of right esotropia (**A**), right exotropia (**B**), and right hypertropia (**C**). (From American Academy of Ophthalmology. *The child's eye: strabismus and amblyopia.* San Francisco: American Academy of Ophthalmology, Professional Information Committee; 1982.)

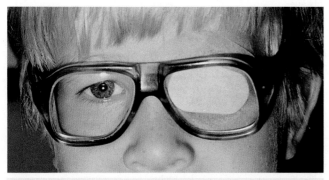

Figure 17-12 Amblyopia. This 5-year-old patient also required patching of the better-seeing eye to improve vision in the amblyopic eye.

child's right eye and look for movement of the uncovered eye. If the left eye moves to pick up fixation, it was deviated before placing the cover over the right eye. Repeat the procedure for the left eye and watch for any movement in the uncovered right eye. If the eye moves inward to pick up fixation, the eye is exotropic. If the eye moves outward to pick up fixation, the eye is esotropic.

The third test involves simultaneous examination of the pupillary red reflexes. This is a useful test to assess ocular alignment and rule out abnormal ocular media, such as cataracts. The test should be performed in a darkened room with the examiner approximately 18 to 24 inches from the patient. Both red reflexes should be simultaneously assessed and compared using the direct ophthalmoscope. If an abnormality exists in the ocular media, the red reflex will be asymmetric or a white reflex may be present. An abnormal reflex may also signify a high refractive error or a small strabismus. The red reflexes should be equal and symmetric. Ophthalmoscopy also permits direct visualization of the fundus and optic disc. The fourth test checks the extraocular movements in the cardinal positions of gaze (Figure 17-15). The results of these tests provide a good basis for determining whether there is any misalignment present. This is an important screening for all family physicians to learn because early intervention can help improve the overall visual and binocular status of the patient.

Table 17-6 lists several forms of strabismus. For congenital esotropia, surgery is the primary treatment for this condition and is performed between 6 and 12 months of age (Figure 17-16). Esotropia may also be related to refractive error and managed with spectacle correction (Figures 17-17 and 17-18). Large deviations of exotropia and hypertropia are also managed surgically (Figures 17-19 to 17-23). (See eAppendix 17-3.)

Pseudostrabismus

A common misconception is that children with cross-eye (esotropia) outgrow the condition, but this is generally not the case. This belief stems from confusion between true strabismus and what is known as pseudostrabismus, or false strabismus. A child with pseudostrabismus has broad folds of skin that partially cover the top of each eye and a flat nasal bridge that creates the illusion of crossed eyes. As the child ages and the skin fold becomes less apparent, the condition becomes less noticeable. When a child's eyes are truly crossed, it is always a serious condition and requires the care of an ophthalmologist.

Other Causes of Strabismus

Acute strabismus may be brought on by a viral upper respiratory tract infection, which can cause acute cranial nerve VI palsy. With the advent of antibiotics, middle ear infections with associated petrositis and cranial nerve VI palsies are relatively uncommon. Sudden-onset strabismus may also indicate underlying neurologic disease. Another cause is spasm of the near reflex. A hallmark of spasm of convergence is a constricted pupil. Paralytic or mechanical causes

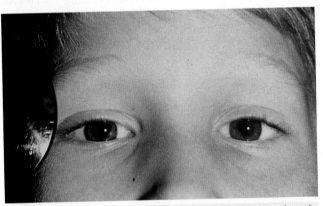

Figure 17-14 Cover–uncover test. The unoccluded eye is evaluated for strabismus. (From American Academy of Ophthalmology. *The child's eye: strabismus and amblyopia.* San Francisco: American Academy of Ophthalmology, Professional Information Committee; 1982.)

Table 17-6   Classification of Strabismus

Type	Cases (%)	Age of Onset
Congenital or infantile esotropia	20	Birth to 6 mo
Accommodative esotropia	45-50	6 mo to 7 yr (usually 2 yr)
Nonaccommodative (acquired) esotropia	10	Variable, depending on cause
Exotropia	20	Variable (usually during infancy to 4 yr)
Hypertropia	<5	Variable, depending on cause

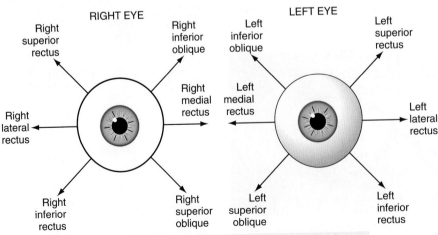

Figure 17-15 Ocular muscle movement in cardinal fields of gaze.

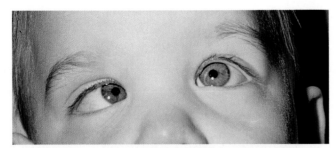

Figure 17-16 Clinical esotropia in 12-month-old infant. With the right eye fixing, there is a left esotropia.

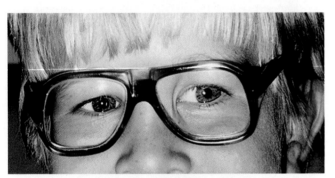

Figure 17-17 Accommodative esotropia and anisometropic amblyopia in 5-year-old patient who has unequal refractive errors between the two eyes as well as accommodative esotropia.

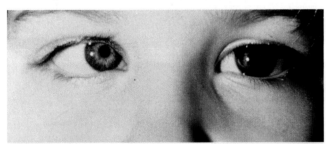

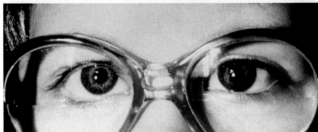

Figure 17-18 Accommodative esotropia in 3-year-old patient uncorrected *(top)* and corrected by hyperopic (farsighted) glasses *(bottom)*. (From American Academy of Ophthalmology. *The child's eye: strabismus and amblyopia.* San Francisco: American Academy of Ophthalmology, Professional Information Committee; 1982.)

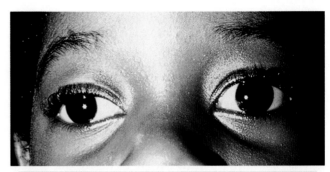

Figure 17-19 Exotropia in 8-year-old patient with right exotropia.

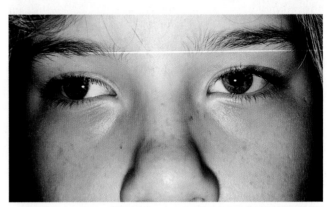

Figure 17-20 Positive angle kappa, which appears similar to exotropia, in 8-year-old patient. This patient has retinopathy of prematurity, with bilateral dragged maculas.

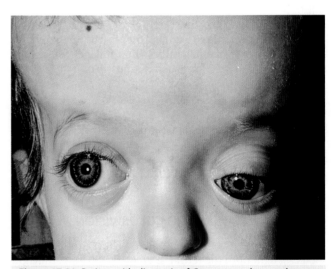

Figure 17-21 Patient with diagnosis of Crouzon syndrome who presented with proptosis, amblyopia, and left exotropia.

of strabismus occur with trauma and Duane syndrome. In addition, neurologic trauma accounts for paralysis to cranial nerves III, IV, and VI (Figure 17-24).

The proper corrective treatment for strabismus includes nonsurgical treatment, such as patching and glasses, and surgical treatment, when indicated. Eye muscle surgery is performed when nonsurgical methods cannot correct the misalignment, as well as with worsening misalignment, no effect on the deviation or stereopsis, or progressive loss of

fusion. Four aspects of strabismus surgery should also be stressed, as follows:

1. The surgery is safe and effective.
2. The eyeball is never removed from the orbit to perform the surgery.
3. More than one procedure may be required to establish alignment.
4. Both eyes may require surgery to correct the strabismus.

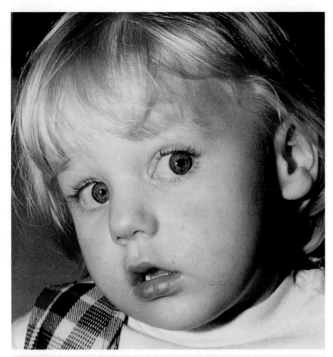

Figure 17-22 Positive head tilt in 4-year-old child could indicate a vertical deviation, especially superior oblique palsy. (From American Academy of Ophthalmology. *The child's eye: strabismus and amblyopia.* San Francisco: American Academy of Ophthalmology, Professional Information Committee; 1982.)

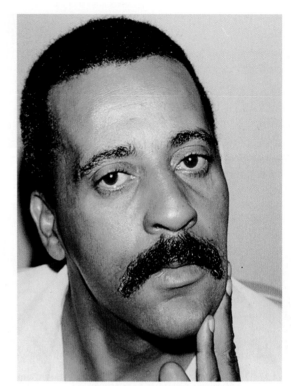

Figure 17-23 Ocular torticollis in 34-year-old patient. Note the abnormal head tilt.

The goals when treating strabismus include the ability to provide and maintain equal vision in both eyes, enable the eyes to work together rather than independently, and improve depth perception whenever possible.

KEY TREATMENT

• Surgical and nonsurgical treatment of strabismus is beneficial to appropriate visual development, reduction of amblyopia, and rehabilitation of sensorimotor function or depth perception (AAO, 2007) (SOR: A).

REFRACTIVE ERRORS AND COLOR VISION

Some eyes are either too long or too short and need help focusing light onto the retina. If an eye is too long, the light rays focus in front of the retina, and the image is blurred; the person can move things closer to see better or can wear glasses. This condition is called nearsightedness *(myopia).* With farsightedness *(hyperopia),* the light focuses behind the retina because the eye is too short and causes a blurred image. Both conditions are corrected by glasses or contact lenses. *Astigmatism,* another common error in the eye's focusing abilities, is caused by unequal curvature of the front surface of the cornea. Corrective glasses are necessary if it causes blurred vision or discomfort. Unless there is a marked amount of myopia (nearsightedness), hyperopia (farsightedness), or astigmatism, or a significant refractive difference between the eyes, eyeglasses can adequately

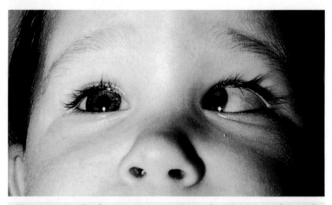

Figure 17-24 Chief presenting complaint of underaction of the left lateral rectus muscle and left esotropia after upper respiratory infection in 14-month-old patient, who had cranial nerve VI palsy related to the viral syndrome.

compensate for these problems. Refractive errors requiring eyeglasses affect almost 20% of the pediatric population before full growth is attained.

Color vision defects rarely result in significant visual difficulties. About 8% of white males have some red-green color deficiency, but fewer than 1% of females are affected. In isolation, this defect rarely results in any real drawback to normal function, especially during childhood. Although the identification of such defects can be helpful in a classroom situation, emphasis should not be placed on these minor abnormalities at this age. Color vision testing is not required unless a retinal dystrophy or optic nerve disease is suspected, the family history is positive, or the family specifically requests it.

HEADACHES

Headache is one of the most common conditions of humans, and children seem to complain less about headaches than adults. Most headaches are not serious and frequently are caused by tension. Many people believe incorrectly that eye strain and the need for glasses are common causes of headaches, although this is certainly possible. Headaches caused by eye disease are usually felt in the eye or in the eyebrow on the same side as the involved eye. Frequently, these headaches are associated with some other symptom, such as blurred vision, halos around lights, or extreme sensitivity to light. Most headaches are related to stress.

LEARNING DISABILITIES AND THE EYE

Although reading may be easier and faster when sight is clear, visual problems generally do not cause learning disabilities, and eye defects are not responsible for reversal of letters. In the past, reading problems were blamed on the eyes, although children with a learning disability have no greater incidence of eye problems than the rest of the population. Other issues, such as dyslexia, attention-deficit hyperactivity disorder, social issues, or family problems are often found to be contributing to a child's poor attention in class or learning difficulties.

It is important that a thorough medical eye examination be performed. The presence or absence of visual defects can be diagnosed and corrected. After vision is corrected, no other examinations or therapies involving the eyes diminish a learning disability. Meta-analysis shows that children with learning disabilities do not benefit from visual training, muscle exercises, perceptual training, or hand–eye coordination exercises (AAO/AAP/AAPOS Policy Statement, 2009). It may be difficult to diagnose a learning disability definitively before a child is 6 to 7 years old. However, after a diagnosis is made, educational assistance is needed promptly.

PEDIATRIC CATARACTS

Approximately 40% of acquired pediatric cataracts are secondary to trauma, and as many as approximately one third of pediatric cataracts are inherited. The basic approach to the patient with pediatric cataracts is to determine whether the cataract is an isolated finding, part of a systemic abnormality, or associated with ocular disease. When several members of the same family are affected by congenital cataracts, a hereditary origin may be assumed. Autosomal dominant hereditary patterns are the most frequent mode of transmission. X-linked cataracts are rare and occur primarily with the oculocerebrorenal syndrome. Congenital or infantile cataracts have been described in association with a large number of congenital anomalies. (See eTable 17-1, Pediatric Cataracts: Causes and Associated Conditions).

History and Ocular Examination

In patients with pediatric cataracts, the physician should determine the age when the cataract or decreased vision occurred. A detailed history of maternal intrauterine infections should include rubella, toxoplasmosis, herpes simplex, cytomegalovirus, and varicella. Drug and medication use during pregnancy and birth trauma should be ruled out.

A complete ocular examination should be performed, including visual acuity assessment using fixation and following responses. Infants with complete bilateral congenital cataracts usually demonstrate decreased visual interest and may have delayed development. Nystagmus results from early visual deprivation and is an ominous sign of poor vision. Ocular fixation and following movements may be decreased or absent. In some cases, strabismus is a presenting sign, especially in children with monocular cataracts.

Glaucoma and other ocular disorders must be ruled out. Examination of the red reflexes by retinoscopy can reveal even minute lens opacities. Direct ophthalmoscopy or retinoscopy through the child's nondilated pupil is helpful for estimating potential vision in an eye harboring a cataract. Any central opacity or surrounding cortical distortion larger than 3 mm can be visually significant. Generally, a more posterior lens opacity carries more visual significance. The presence of retinal detachment, retinoblastoma, or other ocular pathologies that preclude good visual outcome must be ruled out by indirect ophthalmoscopy or ultrasonography.

Most *anterior polar cataracts* are small, smaller than 1 to 2 mm, and are usually not progressive. Surgery is seldom required for small, anterior polar cataracts, and the visual prognosis is excellent. If the cataracts increase in size, visual acuity may be compromised and may require surgical intervention.

Nuclear cataracts are typically congenital, dense axial opacities 3 mm or larger. Nuclear cataracts are frequently associated with microphthalmos and are inherited as autosomal dominant traits. Visual results are generally only fair, even if surgery is done early, and poor if done late. Aphakic glaucoma has a much higher incidence in these patients. *Rubella cataracts* may occur as a manifestation of the classic rubella syndrome—the triad of cardiac defects, hearing impairment, and cataracts.

Partial Lens Opacities

The evaluation of partial lens opacities is related to the location of the cataract. *Anterior cataracts* include anterior lenticonus, polar cataracts, persistent pupillary membrane opacities, and those occurring with anterior segment dysgenesis. *Posterior cataracts* include posterior polar, posterior lenticonus, persistent hyperplastic primary vitreous, and posterior subcapsular lens opacities. Posterior subcapsular cataracts are typically associated with corticosteroid use, atopic dermatitis, or inflammatory diseases and are generally bilateral.

Traumatic and Posterior Lenticonus

Traumatic cataract, the most common cause of unilateral cataract in children, is caused by penetrating or blunt trauma. Posterior lenticonus cataracts are the second most common cause of unilateral acquired cataract in children. *Posterior lenticonus* is a circumscribed oval or round bulge in the infant's or child's posterior lens capsule and cortex, restricted generally to a 2×7–mm axial diameter. The bulge increases progressively, and cataractous changes occur in the cortex surrounding the posterior lenticonus. Generally, there is a reduced red reflex initially with posterior lenticonus, and cataractous changes occur in the surrounding cortex. In 21 patients with posterior lenticonus, only 2 had bilateral posterior lenticonus. The interval between the "oil droplet" posterior lenticonus and cataract development is variable. The eyes are normal in size, and visual results are good with surgery. Posterior lenticonus cataracts occur as early as 3 months of age or as late as 15 years. If the vision becomes worse than 20/70, the cataract should be removed by specialized instrumentation followed by contact lens fitting or an intraocular lens.

Complete Lens Opacities

Workup for complete cataracts includes systemic evaluation, ocular ultrasonography, metabolic evaluation, serum chemistry, and chromosomal analysis. Congenital cataract causes include intrauterine infection, metabolic disorders, chromosomal anomalies, and systemic syndromes. Workup for congenital cataracts includes urinalysis for reducing substances and amino acids. Serum chemistry for calcium, phosphorus, glucose, and blood urea nitrogen levels and TORCH titers should be obtained. When warranted, genetic and pediatric consultations should be requested. Radiologic imaging, including CT or MRI, may be needed.

Surgical Issues

Prompt clearing of the visual axis with immediate optical correction offers the best chance for visual recovery in pediatric patients with unilateral or bilateral cataracts. The surgical procedure recommended depends on the patient's age, risk of amblyopia and expected ocular growth, and reactivity to surgery. In patients younger than 6 months to 2 years old, the best option is to clear the visual axis and have it remain clear throughout the critical period of vision development with a lensectomy–vitrectomy procedure and 6-mm posterior capsulectomy with anterior vitrectomy. This procedure eliminates reopacification of the posterior capsule, which occurs in more than 90% of pediatric patients younger than 2 years. In children older than 2 years, lensectomy with vitrectomy and a 4-mm posterior capsulectomy are performed. Most of these children can be fitted with contact lenses, although an intraocular lens is indicated for some traumatic cataract patients. Traumatic unilateral cataracts present the least controversial situation in which intraocular lenses are considered in young children. Advances in intraocular lenses and surgical techniques have afforded significant improvements in pediatric cataract management.

The prognosis for children with monocular and binocular congenital and pediatric cataracts has improved markedly. Ongoing clinical studies will determine the best indications and procedures for use in pediatric cataract patients.

KEY TREATMENT

- The decision for cataract surgery with intraocular lens implantation depends on the degree of vision loss and potential for amblyopia. Among newborns and infants with cataracts, visually significant cataracts should be removed and corrected with intraocular lens, aphakic contact lens, or aphakic spectacles (AAPOS, 2007) (SOR: C).
- The decision for cataract surgery with intraocular lens implantation in older children depends on the degree of vision loss, comorbidities, and systemic disease (AAPOS, 2007) (SOR: C).

RETINOBLASTOMA

Retinoblastoma is the second most common primary intraocular malignancy in all age groups (melanoma is most common in adults) and is the most common intraocular malignancy of childhood. Its incidence is approximately 1 in every 14,000 births. Generally, there are 250 to 300 new cases in the United States annually.

The tumor occurs bilaterally in as many as 40% of cases. It is generally diagnosed between 14 and 18 months of age, and more than 90% of the tumors are diagnosed by the age of 3 years. Familial retinoblastoma accounts for 6% of patients, but 15% of unilateral cases are carriers for the retinoblastoma gene. The remaining 94% of cases are sporadic. Germinal mutations account for 25% of retinoblastoma cases and somatic mutations for 75%. Most bilateral cases are caused by germinal mutations. The disease is inherited through an autosomal recessive tumor suppressor gene; thus, the phenotype appears similar to that of autosomal dominant inheritance with incomplete penetrance. It is difficult, if not impossible, to differentiate the genetic mutations clinically and to determine which tumors will be passed on to offspring. There are occasional rare cases of retinoblastoma related to chromosomal abnormalities (partial deletion of long arm of chromosome 13). It has also been associated with trisomy 21.

The diagnosis of retinoblastoma is made by the patient presenting with a white pupil (leukocoria) in 61% of cases; strabismus in 22% of cases; and sometimes with a retinal detachment, red painful eye, or spontaneous hyphema (Figure 17-25). Generally, patients with small retinoblastomas have problems with vision or strabismus. More advanced lesions present with leukocoria and occasionally secondary glaucoma. The advanced lesions may metastasize to the orbit and produce proptosis through the orbital spread. In addition, patients with retinoblastoma may have systemic metastases to the CNS, skull bones, lymph nodes, and other organs.

The treatment of retinoblastoma is generally enucleation for patients with advanced retinoblastoma involving more than 50% of the eye. If the second eye is involved, treatment depends on the size of tumor and whether there is extraocular extension. External-beam irradiation treatment may be performed on the second eye or bilaterally, when necessary. Photocoagulation and cryotherapy are equally effective for small retinoblastomas confined to the retinal periphery. Newer modalities are incorporating chemoreduction and radioactive plaque therapy for localized retinoblastoma and possible vision preservation. Systemic chemotherapy may be indicated after enucleation for advanced unilateral or bilateral cases.

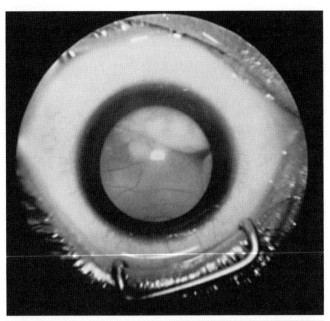

Figure 17-25 Total retinal detachment and advanced retinoblastoma in 23-month-old infant who presented with leukokoria (white reflex).

KEY TREATMENT

• Patients with retinoblastoma should receive long-term follow-up for evaluation of associated systemic cancers (Children's Oncology Group, 2006) (SOR: C).

• Surgery for retinoblastoma requires specialist services and should be referred to supraregional centers when possible (National Institute for Health and Clinical Excellence, 2005) (SOR: C)

Adult Ophthalmology

Key Points

▪ Refractive errors in adults may be corrected with glasses or contact lens or more recent advanced techniques in refractive surgery. Risks and benefits associated with each option vary considerably.

▪ Patients with an acquired unilateral ptosis should be evaluated for Horner syndrome, myasthenia gravis, and cranial nerve III palsy.

▪ Patients with recurrent anterior uveitis should be evaluated for ankylosing spondylitis, inflammatory bowel disease, sarcoidosis, juvenile rheumatoid arthritis, Reiter syndrome, herpetic keratitis, and Lyme disease. Patients should be seen by an ophthalmologist for further evaluation.

▪ Common causes of posterior uveitis include toxoplasmosis, sarcoidosis, cytomegalovirus, Epstein-Barr virus (EBV), Behçet disease, and *Bartonella* infection.

▪ Ocular medications, particularly antiglaucoma medications, are well known for having a variety of systemic side effects. Medications such as β-blockers may have implications for patients with heart or lung disease.

CORRECTION OF REFRACTIVE ERRORS

Contact Lenses

A major use of contact lenses is to correct myopia, aphakia, and astigmatism. It is critical to have a well-motivated patient who will wear contacts successfully. The many types of contact lenses mainly fall into four groups: (1) daily-wear hard lenses; (2) daily-wear soft lenses; (3) rigid, gas-permeable lenses; and (4) extended-wear soft lenses. Hard lenses have generally been constructed of polymethyl methacrylate. The material absorbs less fluid than soft contact lenses. Soft contacts may become 80% or more hydrated. New materials for hard and soft lenses continue to be developed. Complications of contact lenses, particularly extended-wear contacts, include infection, ocular allergies, follicular conjunctivitis, contact lens opacification, corneal edema, and corneal vascularization. Therefore, patients wearing contacts and complaining of red eyes require urgent evaluation.

Refractive Surgery

The latest treatment option for myopia, hyperopia, and astigmatism is laser refractive surgery with the excimer laser. Photorefractive keratectomy (PRK) and laser-assisted in situ keratomileusis (LASIK) use excimer lasers to remove corneal tissue to flatten the cornea or make it steeper. In the PRK procedure, the laser cuts through the surface cornea. Myopia of −1.00 to −10.00 diopters can be successfully corrected with PRK. This procedure does not involve a corneal flap, unlike LASIK, and has good visual recovery response. However, it is more painful than LASIK. The LASIK procedure is performed under a corneal flap. A 6-mm zone is cut with a microkeratome and the laser treatment directed to the exposed stromal tissue. LASIK is the preferred procedure for more than 6 to 8 diopters of myopia; its benefits are greater accuracy with the laser, reduced postoperative complications, quicker recovery of vision, and predictable healing. Some studies have suggested that LASIK has a slightly higher retreatment rate.

Hyperopia and astigmatism can now also be corrected with laser refractive surgery. The LASIK procedure is the preferred treatment for these conditions; PRK and LASIK are widely available. In the past several years, refractive surgery for myopia, hyperopia, and astigmatism has been considered instead of contact lenses or glasses. Recently, conductive keratoplasty has been advanced for treating presbyopia. However, there may be a compromise in balancing distance and near-vision postoperatively. Potential surgical complications include infections, epithelial ingrowth, halos, and loss of contrast sensitivity. In a patient with moderate cataracts, cataract surgery is more advisable than refractive surgery because the patient will often have only a few years of vision correction before needing cataract surgery.

Decisions regarding refractive surgery procedures should be based on surgeon expertise, patient refraction, and available equipment. The patient should be informed about the possible options. For patients who are not candidates for laser refractive surgery, other surgical methods can correct refractive error. For example, implantable collamer lenses are particularly useful for high myopic patients, are generally well tolerated, and have a lower incidence of postoperative symptoms (e.g., halos).

OCULAR MEDICATIONS

Ocular medications may have significant systemic side effects, such as many of the glaucoma medications. Glaucoma medications can generally be classified into β-blockers, prostaglandins and prostamides, carbonic anhydrase inhibitors, α-blockers, and older medications (e.g., epinephrine and pilocarpine).

Systemic absorption of β-adrenergic blockers, such as timolol (Timoptic), may exacerbate asthma. β-Blockers may also cause problems with breathing, bradycardia, and hypotension. These medications are contraindicated in patients with heart block, congestive heart failure, asthma, or obstructive lung disease.

Carbonic anhydrase inhibitors, such as methazolamide (Neptazane), lower IOP and decrease aqueous production. Carbonic anhydrase inhibitors, such as acetazolamide (Diamox), cause increased urination, decreased appetite, headache, nausea, malaise, and kidney stones. Additionally, these medications lower the serum potassium level, particularly in patients taking diuretics. Potassium supplements should be prescribed to prevent hypokalemia.

α-Adrenergic agonists, such as brimonidine tartrate (Alphagan), can lower blood pressure as well as IOP. Side effects include dry mouth and fatigue. Additionally, brimonidine can cross the blood–brain barrier and produce somnolence. Apraclonidine (Iopidine) induces allergy in 20% to 25% of patients and is found to be ineffective in about 25% of all patients.

A newer class of glaucoma medications includes the prostaglandins and prostamides. These medications, such as latanoprost (Xalatan), travoprost (Travatan), and unoprostone isopropyl (Rescula), are associated with increased eyelash growth and increased pigmentation of the iris, conjunctiva, and eyelids. Additionally, these medications can induce conjunctival hyperemia and can increase the risk of postoperative retinal edema.

Other ocular medications include antibiotics, antiinflammatory agents, and steroids. Patients are occasionally given an antibiotic–steroid combination, such as tobramycin–dexamethasone (TobraDex), that may increase IOP, cause cataracts, or potentiate fungal ulcers. Steroid glaucoma is a form of open-angle glaucoma. If the condition is undetected and the patient continues to refill the medication, damage may occur to the optic nerve, including glaucomatous optic atrophy. Generally, IOP is lowered after the steroids have been discontinued. However, it may take several months for IOP to return to a normal level. Vision loss that occurs during this period may be permanent. Because of the relative frequency of steroid glaucoma, cataract, and exacerbations of viral infections, topical corticosteroids should be avoided for minor ocular inflammations. Generally, ocular conditions that warrant the use of topical steroids also warrant consultation with an ophthalmologist.

OPHTHALMIC CONDITIONS IN OLDER ADULTS

The most important causes of central and peripheral visual impairment in older adults include glaucoma, cataract, diabetic retinopathy, and macular degeneration. Most of these conditions can be controlled or, as in the case of cataracts,

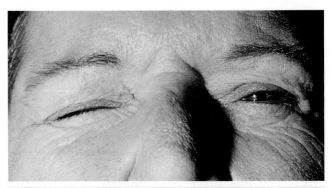

Figure 17-26 Blepharospasm in 68-year-old woman with a history of uncontrollable eyelid spasm resulted in her being unable to drive.

vision can be restored to a significant level to improve the quality of life. Glaucoma and macular degeneration progression may be slowed with proper treatment. Regular eye examinations for older adults can detect early signs of ocular abnormalities and ensure that proper treatment is initiated. Generally, adults older than 40 years should have a complete examination at least every 3 years. After age 65 years, the examination should be at 1- to 2-year intervals.

Diseases of the Eyelid

Entropion is a turning in of the eyelid margin so that there is a rubbing of eyelashes or cilia, with resultant ocular irritation. An *ectropion* is a turning out of the eyelid margin so that the eye builds up excessive tears and becomes inflamed. Both conditions are more common in the older adult population. Entropion and ectropion can cause symptoms of irritation and corneal changes.

Basal cell carcinoma is much more common in older adults. It occurs more often on the lower eyelid. Generally, basal cell carcinomas have pearly edges and a central depression that becomes ulcerated.

Dermatochalasis, or baggy eyelids, may interfere with vision, covering part of the eye. This condition is caused by atrophy of the eyelid skin and elasticity changes. Dermatochalasis causes no permanent damage to vision.

Blepharospasm is a chronic spasm of the eyelid in older adults (Figure 17-26). It may interfere with reading and driving. Botulinum toxin (Botox) injection in small doses is presently the treatment of choice.

Herpes Zoster and Herpes Simplex

Herpes zoster occurs more frequently in the older adult population. When the skin lesions involve the eyelids and tip of the nose, the ophthalmologist should be consulted for evaluation. Corneal dendrites and ulcers can occur with herpes zoster virus and HSV infection (Figure 17-27). HSV infection is more frequently associated with uveitis. Herpes simplex infection responds to trifluridine (Viroptic) eyedrops, whereas HSV infection requires topical steroids.

Ptosis

Ptosis can occur in a number of forms, including congenital ptosis, pseudoptosis, and acquired ptosis (Figure 17-28). Congenital ptosis can occur as a unilateral or bilateral ptosis. A Marcus Gunn jaw-winking ptosis results from a

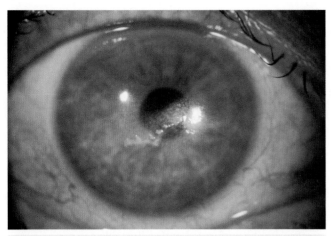

Figure 17-27 Herpes zoster keratitis. Photomicrograph shows pseudodendrites.

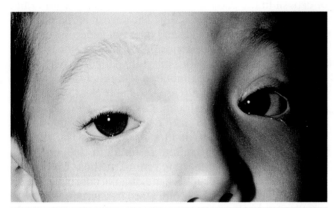

Figure 17-28 Congenital ptosis in 4-year-old patient with congenital bilateral ptosis.

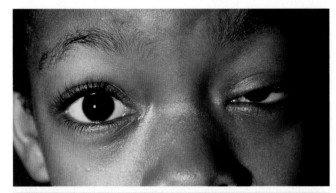

Figure 17-29 Ptosis of left upper eyelid in 8-year-old patient who had ocular myasthenia and subsequently developed ptosis of right upper eyelid and exotropia.

misdirected cranial nerve III. Acquired forms of ptosis include *myogenic* forms, such as myasthenia gravis and progressive external ophthalmoplegia, and *neurogenic* forms, such as Horner syndrome and cranial nerve III palsy (Figure 17-29). *Pseudoptosis* is caused by conditions giving the appearance of a ptosis. It is particularly common with

microphthalmia (small eye, or phthisis bulbi). Pseudoptosis may also be secondary to hypotropia.

Congenital ptosis generally is corrected with bilateral fascia lata brow suspension or a levator resection in patients with good levator function. Treatment of adult forms of ptosis includes correction with a tarsoconjunctival resection, strengthening of the levator aponeurosis, and levator resection.

Myasthenia Gravis

Myasthenia gravis is an autoimmune disease. It can occur at any age and is more common in women. There are some genetic associations, but usually it is sporadic. In myasthenia gravis, acetylcholine receptor antibodies decrease postsynaptic receptor activity at the neuromuscular junction. The muscle cannot receive the message propagated by the action potential. The clinical effect is muscle weakness, which may be variable, chronic, localized, or diffuse. The immunologic component (B and T cells produced in the thymus) plays a role. About 75% of patients have thymic abnormalities, and 10% have thymomas.

Common ocular findings include unilateral or bilateral ptosis, which is usually asymmetric eyelid fasciculations, and eyelid retraction. Patients with myasthenia gravis frequently have eye muscle deviations with double vision. Systemic manifestations include involvement of the jaw and neck, an inability to hold the body erect because of weakness of the spinal muscles, and limb weakness. In addition, symptoms may include choking on food and shortness of breath, which is considered a *myasthenic crisis.* Speech difficulties may also occur. A neurologist usually prescribes treatment for myasthenic patients. The prognosis is generally good in patients who present with ocular abnormalities initially.

Strabismus in Adults

Adult strabismus results in both visual and psychosocial disabilities. Adults with strabismus may not be offered appropriate surgical treatment because of misconceptions regarding surgical and nonsurgical correction. Successful strabismus surgery can relieve diplopia and visual confusion, restore or establish depth perception, expand the visual field, eliminate an abnormal head posture, and improve psychosocial function and employability.

Adults with strabismus should be referred to an ophthalmologist who specializes in surgical and nonsurgical correction of adults. Patients should understand the management of strabismus, if possible, and can be educated regarding the relative risks and benefits of surgery.

KEY TREATMENT

- The surgical and nonsurgical treatment of strabismus in adults results in improved binocular visual function, visual rehabilitation of the sensorimotor system, and improved psychosocial benefits (AAO, 2007) (SOR: A).

Dry Eye (Keratitis Sicca)

Tears, because of their lubricating and bacteriostatic properties, are essential for maintaining a healthy cornea and conjunctiva. A deficiency in tear production may result in a dry eye, also known as keratitis sicca. *Keratoconjunctivitis sicca* is an acquired disorder seen frequently during the fifth decade of life that occurs more often in women. Initial symptoms include a foreign body sensation, dryness, and burning, which often worsens as this condition progresses. Paradoxical tearing from reflex stimulation of the lacrimal gland occurs. Symptoms usually exceed the signs of this common condition. Examination reveals a lack of corneal and conjunctival luster, with punctate erosions. With a decrease in aqueous tears, there is an attempt to compensate by an increase in mucin production, leading sometimes to a stringy, ropelike discharge.

Some cases of keratoconjunctivitis sicca are related to an autoimmune cause, particularly in patients with dryness of other mucous membranes. It also often occurs with rheumatoid arthritis, systemic lupus erythematosus, and Sjögren syndrome. Initial treatment includes lubrication with artificial tears and ointments to supplement or replace the tear film deficit. In moderate or severe cases, an ophthalmologist may need to occlude the eyelid punctum surgically and perform a tarsorrhaphy to protect the corneal surface. Moisture chambers may also be prescribed. Topical antibiotics are required only if secondary infection occurs. Cyclosporine 0.05% (Restasis) is also useful in addressing inflammatory components of tear film insufficiency when other treatments are insufficient.

Exposure keratitis is a condition symptomatically similar to dry eyes that is caused by incomplete eyelid closure during blinking or with sleep. It may result from Bell palsy, scarred or malpositioned eyelids, or thyroid exophthalmos. Management involves the use of ophthalmic lubricating solutions and ointments. Mechanical measures designed to assist normal eyelid closure may be necessary, including frequent manual massage of the eyelids during the day to assist closure, forceful blinking exercises to elicit the Bell reflex, and taping the eyelids shut at night. Merely patching the eye should be avoided because of an increased risk of corneal abrasion if the eyelids do not cover the eye underneath the patch.

Thyroid Eye Disease (Thyroid Orbitopathy)

Hyperthyroidism may induce an orbitopathy in some patients. In such cases, there is diffuse hyperplasia of the thyroid and infiltrative ophthalmopathy. Thyroid eye disease is seen in association with thyroid dysfunction, although thyroid function test results may be normal. With thyroid orbitopathy, the extraocular muscle becomes infiltrated; this may occur even when the disease appears to be under good systemic control. The precise extraocular mechanism is unknown and the genetic predisposition uncertain.

Graves ophthalmopathy occurs in approximately 95% of patients with Graves thyroid disease but is only rarely seen with Hashimoto thyroid disease. The diagnosis of *euthyroid* Graves ophthalmopathy is primarily a clinical diagnosis, confirmed with orbital CT imaging. Clinical characteristics include hypotropia, esotropia, or a combination of vertical and horizontal strabismus. Many patients are euthyroid at diagnosis, but there may be a history of previous thyroid dysfunction. Thyroid myopathy is a common cause of acquired vertical deviation in adults but relatively uncommon in children. Werner has classified eye involvement in Graves' disease by the NO-SPECS mnemonic: *n*o signs of symptoms, *o*nly signs of eyelid retraction or gaze palsy with or without eyelid lag or proptosis, *s*igns and symptoms of soft tissue involvement, *p*roptosis, *e*xtraocular muscle involvement, *c*orneal involvement with corneal drying, and *s*ight loss with optic nerve involvement.

The total muscle volume of the extraocular muscles increases as the disease worsens. The volume can be computed by averaging serial CT sections. Indications for treatment of thyroid ophthalmopathy include diplopia, abnormal head position, a large horizontal or vertical strabismus, and loss of vision. Generally, the preferred treatment is orbital decompression if loss of vision is threatened. Nonsurgical management of the patient includes prisms to alleviate the diplopia in primary position. Eye muscle surgery can be performed with adjustable sutures.

Ocular Changes with Aging

Arcus senilis, or corneal arcus, is a hazy, white or yellow arc or deposit in the peripheral cornea. It has many causes and is more common in older adults. The deposit is composed of cholesterol and other lipids and does not generally indicate an underlying systemic abnormality. It does not interfere with vision or eye function. In white patients, this finding may indicate lipid abnormalities and an increased propensity for cardiovascular disease. No such clear correlation has been identified in African Americans, who are much more likely to have an arcus. The pupil becomes miotic and does not respond well to dilation or darkness. The vitreous body detaches from the retina, resulting in the perception of flashing lights secondary to retinal traction. The retinal pigment epithelium atrophies, making the choroidal vessels more visible. The lens becomes progressively stiffer with age. Symptoms begin in the mid-40s, with increasing difficulty in near-vision focusing. By age 60 years, most patients have had a major reduction in accommodative amplitudes. The universal stiffening of the lens with age causes the well-known symptoms of presbyopia, requiring the use of reading glasses.

Cataracts

A cataract is a condition that affects a large percentage of the population. As a result, cataract surgery is the most common U.S. surgery performed. Currently, cataracts affect approximately 40 million people in the United States. Generally, the normal aging and cataractous changes in the lens are related to its metabolic activity. *Acquired cataracts* may be caused by penetrating trauma, irradiation, heat, or blunt trauma. Metabolic cataracts occur particularly in association with diabetes. Changes in the blood glucose concentration may alter the refractive power of the lens. With hyperglycemia, glucose byproducts enter the lens, causing it to swell and inducing a myopic shift. *Nuclear sclerosis cataract* is the most common cause of lens opacity seen by ophthalmologists; an increased central density makes lens power stronger. As a result, frequent changes in the eyeglass prescription are necessary to correct the changing lens power. This type of cataract develops slowly, and surgery may not be necessary for several years.

The decision for cataract surgery with intraocular lens implantation depends on the degree of vision loss and the daily requirements of the patient. In patients with cataracts, indications for surgery include the patient's preference and needs, functional disability by Snellen visual acuity test and visual field testing, and concomitant ocular problems.

Cataract surgery involves removal of the cataractous lens and insertion of an intraocular lens. Generally, the procedure is performed under local anesthesia, although the patient may have general anesthesia. Modern cataract surgery primarily entails removing the lens through an extracapsular technique, which can be done en bloc or through a small corneal incision with phacoemulsification. In children, cataracts are generally soft and often require aspiration equipment.

Phacoemulsification is a technique that uses ultrasonic energy to break up the lens material so that it may be withdrawn through a small needle. Unfortunately, phacoemulsification has been confused with laser treatment for cataract removal. It is important to emphasize to patients that the laser is not used to remove the cataractous lens. Part of the confusion lies in the fact that secondary cataracts or opacification of the posterior capsule can be eliminated using the YAG laser. With the YAG laser, there is photodisruption of the capsule, which creates an opening and provides good visual acuity. Cataract removal is one of the most successful operations performed. Generally, adult patients are treated with intraocular lenses after cataract removal. If the patient has bilateral aphakia, contact lenses or cataract spectacles may be worn. However, moderate visual distortion occurs with aphakic spectacles, as well as restriction of peripheral vision. Routine preoperative testing does not improve clinical outcomes for healthy patients undergoing cataract surgery.

Uveitis

A red painful eye with photophobia and increased tearing often occurs with the presentation of anterior uveitis. In addition, the patient may have decreased vision. *Vascular injection,* a circumcorneal injection involving the deep vessels of the sclera, is one of the primary signs of anterior uveitis. Generally, patients with uveitis are moderately light sensitive. In addition, the inflammatory process may hinder aqueous production and reduce IOP.

Patients suspected of an *anterior uveitis* should be referred to an ophthalmologist for consultation and treatment. The most common cause of anterior uveitis is idiopathic; other common causes include ankylosing spondylitis, inflammatory bowel disease, sarcoidosis, juvenile rheumatoid arthritis, Reiter syndrome (urethritis, polyarteritis, and ocular inflammation), herpetic keratitis, and Lyme disease.

Patients with *posterior uveitis* usually present with a reduction in vision and vitreous floaters. They may have clinical signs of retinal vasculitis, retinal ischemia, optic nerve edema, and exudative retinal detachment. On careful inspection, cells may be visible floating in the vitreous. Common causes of posterior uveitis are toxoplasmosis, sarcoidosis, cytomegalovirus, EBV, Behçet disease, and *Bartonella* infection. *Toxoplasmosis* accounts for up to 30% of cases and may destroy the macula or other important visual structures. Characteristically, there is an exudation in the retina caused by an inflammatory process. *Toxocara canis* may also present as uveitis.

Diseases of the Retina and Optic Nerve

Key Points

- Glaucoma is a leading cause of blindness and is managed medically and surgically.
- Choroidal melanoma is the most common intraocular malignancy.
- Posterior vitreous detachment is a common cause of vitreous floaters but may present similar to retinal detachment.
- Age-related maculopathy represents a significant cause of central vision loss in older adults.
- Some patients with macular degeneration may benefit from advances in therapeutic laser treatments.
- Vitamin supplements have been shown to be beneficial for some patients with macular degeneration.
- Routine funduscopy should be performed to evaluate for hypertensive retinopathy and diabetic retinopathy.
- Diabetic retinopathy is the most common cause of blindness in Americans age 20 to 74 years.
- Giant cell arteritis generally occurs in patients 55 years and older, with headache, scalp tenderness, jaw claudication, malaise, fatigue, and amaurosis fugax.
- Carotid artery disease is an important cause of transient ischemic attacks; 50% of patients with transient ischemic attack (TIA) involving carotid artery disease have a major stroke within 1 month of the first attack.
- About 75% of women and 34% of men with optic neuritis will develop multiple sclerosis within 15 years.

Retinal diseases account for 10% to 15% of blindness. Common retinal diseases include macular degeneration, diabetic retinopathy, retinal detachment, and retinal vascular disease. Sudden loss of vision can have various causes; four common causes are retinal detachment, temporal arteritis, ischemic optic neuropathy, and optic neuritis (Table 17-7).

Vitreous Floaters. The vitreous gel degenerates during middle age and forms microscopic strands within the eye. An increase in previous floaters, acute flashing lights, or the appearance of a veil or curtain over a patient's vision may signify a retinal detachment. Posterior vitreous detachment is a common cause of vitreous floaters. The sudden onset of vitreous floaters can be alarming for the patient. Generally, they are simply the result of the normal aging process. Vitreous floaters may interfere with clear vision, particularly reading. Although generally benign, posterior vitreous detachments can create retinal hemorrhages and are associated with retinal tears and detachments.

Melanoma. Choroidal melanoma, a pigmented elevated mass in the choroid, is the most common intraocular malignancy. As the tumor spreads, it may produce a retinal detachment. In addition, retinal pigment epithelial alterations can occur in the form of *drusen* or *lipofuscin* (Figure 17-30). The differential diagnosis of choroidal melanoma includes choroidal nevus, retinal detachment, and metastatic tumor to the choroid. All patients with intraocular tumors should have an extensive physical examination and laboratory testing to exclude metastatic spread of

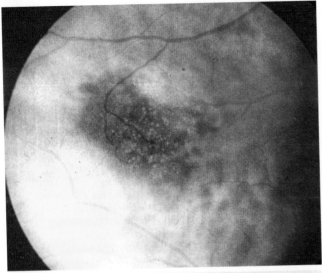

Figure 17-30 Choroidal melanoma. Increased pigmentation involves the choroid, with characteristic lipofuscin overlying the lesion, which is slightly elevated with bowing of the overlying vessels. This melanoma was locally treated.

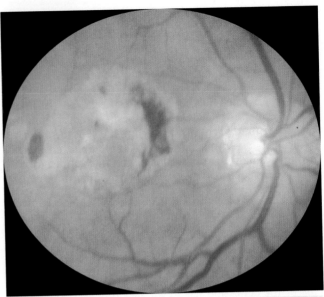

Figure 17-31 Age-related maculopathy in 73-year-old woman who demonstrated evidence of geographic atrophy with her macular degeneration.

Table 17-7   Systematic Approach to Patient Presenting with Rapid or Sudden Loss of Vision

Presentation	Symptoms	Signs	Treatment
Painful: Acute narrow, angle-closure glaucoma	Pain, tearing, headache Halos around light with intermittent blurring of vision Nausea, vomiting	Shallow anterior chamber Sudden rise of IOP Circumcorneal injection Cornea edematous and cloudy	**Refer immediately.** If no ophthalmologist available, begin oral glycerin (1 mL/kg), IM acetazolamide (500 mg) and topical pilocarpine (1%-4%) every 15 min
Painless: Central retinal artery occlusion	Sudden unilateral visual loss (may be preceded by transient blurring)	Cherry-red spot in macula Narrowed arteries Pale optic nerve head Edematous retina	Digital ocular massage Elevation of blood CO_2 level through rebreathing into paper bag or breathing 95% O_2 and 5% CO_2 (carbogen) if available
Painless: Cranial (giant cell) arteritis	Sudden unilateral visual loss preceded by vague migrating joint pains Low-grade fever, depressed appetite No localized pain in eyeball but scalp pain; severe, boring headaches	Enlarged and painful temporal artery Increased ESR is key to diagnosis	**Refer immediately.** Definitive treatment is high doses of systemic corticosteroids. Involvement of other eye in relatively short time; therefore, immediate referral is imperative
Retinal detachment	Usually rapid loss of vision but *may vary* Frequently preceded by flashing lights and floaters; more common in patients with myopia; after cataract extraction; after blunt trauma	Retinal elevation on ophthalmoscopic examination	Refer to ophthalmologist promptly

ESR, Erythrocyte sedimentation rate; *IM*, intramuscular; *IOP*, intraocular pressure.

the neoplasm. Many ocular melanomas have already metastasized at diagnosis. Treatment modalities generally involve radioactive plaques, and enucleation is performed less frequently. When a small, melanotic lesion is detected, observation is indicated in older adults with slow-growing lesions.

Macular Degeneration. *Age-related macular degeneration* (ARMD) is the most common form of breakdown in the macular area, accounting for 70% of all cases. *Age-related maculopathy,* formerly called "macular degeneration," leads to loss of fine or central vision but not side vision. Laser treatment is of benefit in select patients. Macular degeneration begins with nonexudative changes (Figure 17-31). However, many people with macular degeneration have an abnormal vascularization that is not always amenable to laser therapy (Figure 17-32). The condition occurs in the other eye within 1 year in 10% of cases. Another form of macular degeneration is *exudative macular degeneration,* which accounts for 10% of cases.

Normally, the macula is protected by thin tissue that separates it from the fine blood vessels that nourish the posterior aspect of the eye. When these blood vessels break or leak, scar tissue may form, often leading to abnormal

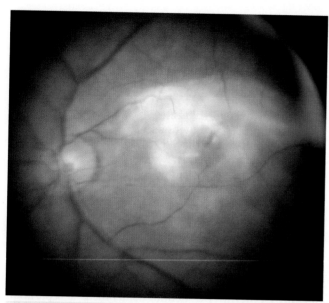

Figure 17-32 Age-related maculopathy with choroidal neovascularization. Abnormal blood vessels have formed in the area of macular degeneration and require further studies to determine whether laser treatment is indicated.

growth of new blood vessels (neovascularization). These new vessels are particularly fragile, and leakage and bleeding may occur. If macular degeneration involves both eyes, near activities become difficult. If an individual loses central vision related to macular degeneration, generally the peripheral vision is unaffected.

An ophthalmologist can confirm the diagnosis of macular degeneration; assessment includes color vision testing, ophthalmoscopy, and fluorescein angiography, when indicated. Examination reveals an accumulation of membranous debris on the posterior aspect of the retinal pigment epithelium, the presence of drusen, and atrophy of the retinal pigment epithelium. In addition, there may be detachment of the retinal pigment epithelium and choroidal neovascularization.

There is no cure for patients with ARMD. Ophthalmic laser surgery may be beneficial in reducing the spread of the exudative macular degeneration, but it is successful only in the early stages. Laser therapy and anti-VEGF (vascular endothelial growth factor) medications have been helpful in treating membranes and neovascularization. Advanced cases of macular degeneration have been treated with macular translocation with some success. At present, use of multivitamins with beta-carotene and vitamin E may delay progression for many patients with ARMD. However, beta-carotene supplements in smokers have been associated with an increase in lung cancer. Vitamin supplements have no impact on cataract formation.

KEY TREATMENT

- Patients with intermediate ARMD had a 25% reduction in the progression of ARMD with the following vitamin and mineral supplements: vitamin C (500 mg), vitamin E (400 IU), beta-carotene (15 mg [25,000 IU]), zinc oxide (80 mg), and cupric oxide (2 mg) (Age-Related Eye Disease Study Research Group, 2001) (SOR: A).

- Management options for macular degeneration include observation, antioxidant vitamin and mineral supplements, intravitreal injection of anti-VEGF agents, PDT, and laser photocoagulation surgery (AAO, 2008) (SOR: A).

Hypertensive Retinopathy. Routine ophthalmoscopy in patients with hypertension affords the physician a direct view of the arterioles and helps assess the long-term duration and severity of the hypertension as well as evidence of accelerated or malignant hypertension. In the vascular system, arterioles serve as the resistance vessels, and the overall cross-section of the arteriolar bed determines peripheral resistance. With the fundus examination, the physician can directly observe the degree of spasm in arterioles and the effects of long-term hypertension on the arteriolar wall. Severe hypertensive retinopathy can lead to profound vision loss, although usually the patient is completely asymptomatic.

The normal arteriolar wall is transparent, and the visible image is of the blood column as it passes through the arteriolar lumen. An additional anatomic consideration is that at the point of crossing of the arteriole and venule, the vasculature shares a common adventitial layer. Therefore, when arteriolar thickening occurs, the venule is compressed, resulting in arteriolar-venous nicking. It is practical to divide the changes in the fundus seen in hypertension into two scales: a hypertensive scale and an arteriolesclerotic scale (see eAppendix 17-4 online, Hypertensive Retinopathy Grading).

Diabetic Retinopathy. Diabetic retinopathy is the most common cause of blindness in Americans 20 to 74 years old. Patients with diabetes are at 25 times greater risk of becoming blind from diabetic retinopathy than nondiabetic persons of becoming blind from all other causes. Diabetic retinopathy is more common in women, but men appear to develop a more complicated and severe proliferative retinopathy. Findings have shown that in type 1 diabetes mellitus, it is unusual to detect diabetic retinopathy before 5 years after onset of disease. After 15 years from diagnosis, most patients with type 1 diabetes have some diabetic retinopathy, with incidence of proliferative disease greater than 40%. In type 2 diabetes, with onset after age 30 years, diabetic retinopathy is often detectable at the initial diagnosis. Diabetic patients requiring insulin have a higher incidence of diabetic retinopathy and proliferative disease.

The precise pathogenesis of diabetic retinopathy remains unclear, but the target tissue is the retinal capillary. Localized ischemia has been shown to increase levels of VEGF and result in a corresponding area of vascular proliferation. The vascular complications evolve through states defined by ophthalmoscopic findings.

The first stage is called *nonproliferative* or "background" retinopathy (Figure 17-33). Capillaries leak and later become occluded. The retinal findings include aneurysms, hard exudates, intraretinal hemorrhages, and macular edema. In the nonproliferative stage, patients only experience visual loss if there is macular involvement. Visual loss from macular edema is present in 5% to 20% of patients with diabetes, depending on the type and duration of disease. With progression, patients will develop *preprolifera- tive* diabetic retinopathy. This stage frequently progresses to proliferative diabetic retinopathy. The most readily recognized abnormality of preproliferative retinopathy is the cotton-wool spot, a white opacity with feathery edges indicative of localized retinal infarct of the nerve fiber layer.

Proliferative diabetic retinopathy (PDR) is responsible for most serious vision loss in patients with diabetes. As a result of continued retinal ischemia, new blood vessels form in the area of the optic disc or elsewhere on the retinal surface (Figure 17-34). Without laser photocoagulation, these vessels typically progress to retinal detachment and form vascularization within the vitreous cavity. Neovascularization results in vitreous hemorrhage and retinal traction. After fibrous proliferation has detached the retina, surgical repair can be challenging. Prophylactic laser photocoagulation is the best way to avoid this complication for diabetic patients with PDR.

SCREENING RECOMMENDATIONS
- Screening eye examinations for patients with type 2 diabetes reduce the chance of vision loss (Tubbs et al., 2004) (SOR: A, 1).
- Patients with type 1 diabetes should have their first eye examination 5 years after onset.
- Patients with type 2 diabetes should have their first eye examination at diagnosis.
- Patients with diabetes should have a baseline eye examination before becoming pregnant or early in the first trimester.
- On initiation of ophthalmic screening, all patients with diabetes should have annual dilated fundus examinations by an ophthalmologist or sooner if poor diabetic control or visual symptoms develop (AAO, 2007) (SOR: A, 1).

Retinal Detachment. Retinal detachment is separation of the retina from its blood supply. It usually follows a tear or hole in the retina. Retinal tears may be caused by trauma or retinal disease, but the cause of most tears is unclear. When the retina is detached, vision is lost from the involved area of the retina. If the macula detaches, irreversible loss of vision may occur unless the detachment is treated within 24 hours. Anatomic reattachment of the retina is successful in up to 90% of cases.

Giant Cell Arteritis (Temporal Arteritis)

Temporal arteritis is a systemic autoimmune disorder. Pathologically, there is a granulomatous inflammation of large and medium-sized arteries. It generally occurs in patients older than 55 years, with no gender predilection. Involvement may occur in any organ system. Ocular involvement is generally associated with inflammation of the posterior ciliary arteries. General symptoms include amaurosis fugax, headaches, scalp tenderness, jaw claudication, occasional ear pain or arthralgias, pain and tenderness on one or both temples, malaise, and intermittent fevers. Ocular symptoms include loss of vision, diplopia, pain, red eye, and ocular-ischemic syndrome. The workup

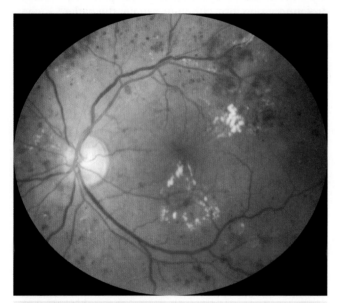

Figure 17-33 Nonproliferative diabetic retinopathy of left eye. There is extensive nonproliferative disease with macroaneurysms, hemorrhages, and exudates. Although there is no neovascularization, this patient is at risk of developing proliferative disease.

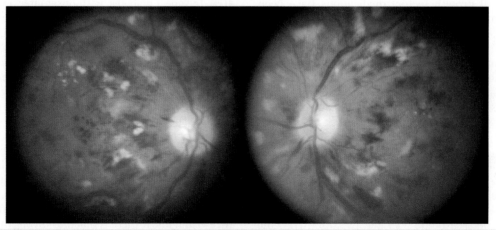

Figure 17-34 Proliferative diabetic retinopathy. The patient has severe disease, with diffuse retinal hemorrhages in all quadrants and evidence of neovascularization, and requires urgent panretinal photocoagulation. There is evidence of neovascularization of the optic disc in the left eye.

of patients suspected to have giant cell arteritis includes a careful history of nonvisual symptoms, examination, and laboratory studies to include erythrocyte sedimentation rate (ESR), C-reactive protein, and complete blood count with differential. Using the Westergren method, the value for a normal ESR is 30 mm/hr for a 60-year-old man; for women, top of normal range is age plus 10 divided by 2, so 35 mm/hr is the upper range of normal for a 60-year-old woman. The differential diagnosis of sudden vision loss also includes emboli, central retinal artery occlusion, and retinal detachment.

The visual loss of giant cell arteritis is caused by an ischemic process in the optic nerve. Central retinal artery occlusion may also occur with giant cell arteritis. It is important to diagnose giant cell arteritis as early as possible. Without corticosteroid treatment, patients often develop permanent vision loss bilaterally. When one eye is involved with giant cell arteritis, the second eye loses vision in 65% of untreated patients. Generally, involvement of the second eye occurs within 10 days of onset. When the diagnosis is suspected on the basis of clinical symptoms and signs, temporal artery biopsy is necessary to confirm the diagnosis. The ESR is often greatly elevated, although it may be normal for age. If there is any doubt regarding the diagnosis, a temporal artery biopsy is warranted.

After the diagnosis is established, steroid therapy should be instituted immediately. Up to 100 mg of prednisone (1.0-1.5 mg/kg/day) should be given orally if giant cell arteritis is suspected. Some physicians recommend IV steroids. Patients often require treatment for several months pending a positive biopsy or strong suspicion of giant cell arteritis. Steroids should not be delayed because of the temporal artery biopsy. Biopsy results will remain positive for up to 1 week after beginning steroid therapy. The patient can be monitored by symptoms occurring after institution of treatment and by ESR. Because of the severe systemic effects of giant cell arteritis, the patient should be followed closely.

KEY TREATMENT

- Giant cell arteritis should be promptly treated with oral or IV steroids before obtaining a temporal artery biopsy; treatment should not be delayed for laboratory confirmation (Turbin et al., 1999) (SOR: A).

Glaucoma

Glaucoma is responsible for at least 10% of cases of blindness in the United States. Glaucoma is four times more common in African Americans, who are also eight times more likely to develop blindness from glaucoma. Glaucoma appears to increase with age in the United States and decreases with age in Japan. Patients with diabetes also have an increased risk for developing glaucoma.

The most common form of glaucoma in the United States is primary *open-angle glaucoma*, which accounts for about two thirds of all cases. In Asia, the most common form of glaucoma is *angle-closure glaucoma*. Open-angle glaucoma tends to be genetically based, with multifactorial inheritance or as an autosomal recessive trait, with a high prevalence of carriers. Glaucoma is bilateral and occurs predominantly after age 50 years, although incidence is significant during the 30s and 40s, and it may even occur during the teenage years. Glaucoma is more severe in the African American population. Current incidence of glaucoma is 2% in the United States. The family physician can measure IOP using tonometry to detect elevated IOP. Tonometry can be performed with a Schiøtz tonometer, Perkins applanation tonometer, Tono-Pen XL tonometer, or Goldmann applanation tonometer held horizontally. This test should be performed at least every 3 years, beginning at age 35 years.

The damage to vision caused by glaucoma is irreversible. If the glaucoma can be detected early, it can usually be controlled and is curable by medical treatment, laser surgery, trabeculectomy, or some other filtering procedure. It is important to emphasize that glaucoma may occur at any age. Causes include congenital glaucoma, chronic open-angle glaucoma, narrow-angle glaucoma, or other forms of glaucoma, including pigmentary glaucoma.

One of the most common forms of secondary glaucoma is *steroid glaucoma*, which occurs in a substantial number of patients who use corticosteroid eyedrops or ointment for several weeks or longer. This condition also may occur with oral or systemic corticosteroid use, although it is rare. Steroid glaucoma is a form of open-angle glaucoma and, similar to primary open-angle glaucoma, can be effectively treated if detected early. If IOP is not lowered in time, there may be permanent damage to the optic nerve. Treatment for this type of glaucoma is discontinuation of corticosteroids and initiation of topical glaucoma medications. The IOP elevation is reversible after the steroids have been discontinued, but it may take 2 to 3 months or longer for pressure to return to a normal level. Any visual loss that occurs during this period may be permanent. There is no reliably safe dose of topical steroids that can ensure the prevention of steroid glaucoma. Even topical medications that consist of a combination of steroids and antibiotics or other type of medication can increase IOP. Because of the relative frequency of steroid glaucoma, as well as other ocular complications resulting from steroid use (e.g., cataract, exacerbation of viral infections), topical steroids should not be used for minor ocular inflammations, except in special circumstances.

Secondary glaucoma also may be caused by ocular trauma, intraocular inflammations, intraocular tumors, and carotid vascular disease. Regardless of cause, any patient suspected of having secondary glaucoma should be referred to an ophthalmologist as soon as possible for further evaluation and therapy. Management depends on the cause of the disease and character of the IOP elevation. Some medications can also result in glaucoma and include a warning related to developing angle-closure glaucoma. Additionally, topiramate (Topamax) is associated with an idiosyncratic acute glaucoma caused by uveal effusions.

With increased IOP, damage to the optic nerve and visual field abnormalities can occur. Almost all elevated pressures are caused by an obstruction to the outflow of aqueous humor. *Aqueous humor*, formed inside the eye in the ciliary body, circulates around the lens and through the pupil into the anterior portion of the eye. The aqueous humor exits through the anterior angle structures (trabecular

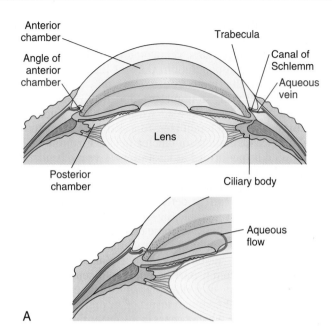

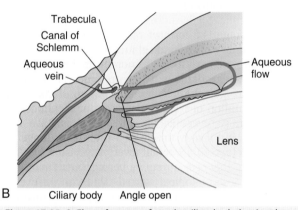

Figure 17-35 A, Flow of aqueous from the ciliary body, leaving the eye through the trabecula and canal of Schlemm via a normal, open, wide angle. **B,** Chronic open-angle glaucoma. (From Scheie HG, Albert DM. *Textbook of ophthalmology.* 9th ed. Philadelphia: Saunders; 1977.)

meshwork and Schlemm canal) (Figure 17-35). About 10% of glaucoma cases occur in the setting of normal IOP, suggesting that these eyes are particularly susceptible to pressure changes. Glaucoma management involves more than controlling IOP. Possible sources of damage to the optic nerve involve mechanical factors affecting the optic nerve, decreased optic nerve perfusion, and blockage of axoplasmic flow in the lamina cribrosa. Carotid artery stenosis can also cause problems because of decreased perfusion to the optic nerve. Occasionally, elevations result from impeded outflow caused by elevated venous pressure, such as in patients with Sturge-Weber syndrome.

The most serious consequence of elevated IOP is damage to the optic nerve (Figure 17-36). As IOP rises, retinal nerve fibers are destroyed at the optic nerve head, resulting in permanent visual loss. Peripheral vision is usually affected first, followed by progressive visual loss involving the entire visual field (Figure 17-37).

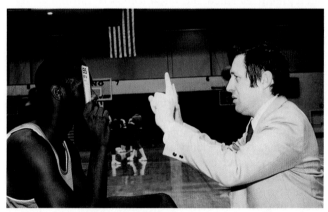

Figure 17-37 Testing peripheral fields by confrontation. (From American Academy of Ophthalmology. *The athlete's eye.* San Francisco: AAO Professional Information Committee; 1986.)

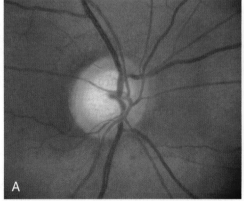
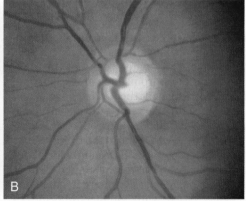

Figure 17-36 Bilateral glaucoma in 60-year-old man. The patient also had history of diabetes mellitus. The glaucoma is characterized by prominent optic nerve cupping. **A,** Enlarged optic nerve cup, right eye. **B,** Enlarged optic nerve cup, left eye. Note thinning of optic nerve rim.

- Long-term monitoring is essential for successful management of glaucoma (AAO, 2000) (SOR: A).
- For chronic open-angle glaucoma, initial treatment is topical medications (AAO, 2000) (SOR: C).
- For uncontrolled chronic open-angle glaucoma, surgical treatment should be considered (AAO, 2000) (SOR: C).
- For acute angle-closure glaucoma, medical treatment and surgery (laser or incision) should be implemented as soon as medically possible (SOR: A).

Anterior Ischemic Optic Neuropathy

The clinical characteristics of ischemic optic neuropathy include age at onset generally older than 60 years, painless vision loss, and afferent pupillary defect (Marcus Gunn pupil). These patients also usually have a visual field abnormality. Examination of the optic disc reveals edema in almost all cases. Pathology appears to be related to a diseased ciliary circulation. It is generally difficult to determine whether the disc edema will result in a mild peripheral (side) visual field defect and good visual acuity or reduced central acuity and a significant visual field defect. Giant cell arteritis must be ruled out in these patients. A general physical examination and associated blood work are indicated. No treatment prevents the progression of ischemic optic neuropathy, including steroids and anticoagulants.

Transient Ischemic Attacks in Carotid Artery Disease

Transient ischemic attacks are neurologic deficits lasting less than 24 hours and are reversible. The most common ophthalmologic TIA is *amaurosis fugax*, which is a fleeting monocular blindness caused by an embolic event. There is a sudden graying or reduction of vision, often moving from the peripheral vision to the center to cover the entire visual field within a few seconds. After 1 to 5 minutes, the central vision begins to return first. Other causes of TIAs include chronic disc edema (in which vision loss lasts seconds, not minutes), chronic papilledema with bilateral blackouts based on optic nerve disease (often also lasting a few seconds and caused by postural changes), and basilar artery insufficiency. TIAs related to basilar artery insufficiency are usually bilateral blackouts lasting seconds or minutes, often with changes in the posterior circulation.

The most important mechanisms involving carotid TIAs with stroke are embolization from the carotid artery or its branches, reduced perfusion caused by carotid stenosis or occlusion, or a combination of the two. In most patients (up to 90%), the site of the obstruction is the carotid sinus. Hollenhorst plaques are bright-yellow cholesterol emboli that may occlude the retinal arterioles (see Figure 17-10). Fibrin platelet emboli can occur near retinal arterioles and produce visual symptoms. A cholesterol or fibrin platelet embolus is indicative of ulcerative disease in the carotid arteries and is associated with a high incidence of ischemic heart disease, peripheral vascular disease, stroke, and aortic abdominal aneurysm. A rarer form of carotid TIA is related to valvular heart disease, particularly with a prolapsed mitral valve or cardiac arrhythmia. Approximately 30% to 50% of patients with TIAs and carotid artery disease have a major stroke within 1 month of the first attack.

Optic Neuritis

Optic neuritis is localized inflammation of the optic nerve sheath, resulting in reduced neuronal transmission and decreased visual acuity. Generally, there is a loss of color vision and red desaturation noticed by the patients. The symptoms generally worsen during the first few days and progressively improve over several weeks. In children, optic neuritis has various causes, typically associated with viral infections. In young adults, optic neuritis has a high association with multiple sclerosis (MS). Approximately 75% of women and 34% of men with optic neuritis will develop MS within 15 years of the onset of optic neuritis. Patients should undergo MR neuroimaging to investigate for plaque formations. They should be questioned regarding constitutional symptoms of fatigue, weakness, difficulty moving or seeing after strenuous activity, and previous attacks.

Intravenous methylprednisolone (1 g/day for 3 days) followed by oral prednisone (1 mg/kg/day for 11 days) reduced the rate of MS development for 2 years (Beck, 1988). Patients at high risk had a 44% reduction in the rate of developing MS when treated with interferon (Controlled High Risk Avonex Multiple Sclerosis Trial [CHAMPS]). Newer treatments with interferon-β-1a (Avonex) and interferon-β-1b (Betaseron, Copaxone) have shown significant improvement in quality of life for patients and reduction in relapses. The Optic Neuritis Treatment Trial recommendations included giving patients with optic neuritis IV methylprednisolone (1 g/day) for 3 days followed by 11 days of oral prednisone (1 mg/kg/day) (Beck et al., 1993). The dose is generally modified for children with 1 mg/kg/day whether using IV or oral steroids. Patients who receive oral rather than IV steroids for the first 3 days generally have more relapsing of their symptoms. Additionally, although corticosteroids hasten visual recovery, administration of steroids does not affect the overall visual acuity. The main benefit is delay of onset of multiple sclerosis.

Summary of Additional Online Content

The following content is available at www.expertconsult.com:

eAppendix 17-1 Hyphema

eAppendix 17-2 Vision Screening in Children

eAppendix 17-3 Specific Types of Strabismus

eTable 17-1 Pediatric Cataracts: Causes and Associated Conditions

eAppendix 17-4 Hypertensive Retinopathy Grading

References

The complete reference list is available at www.expertconsult.com.

Web Resources

www.aafp.org/afp/2007/1215/p1815.html *American Family Physician*; differential diagnosis of the swollen red eyelid.

www.aao.org AAO; includes education, practice guidelines, practice management tips, and news.

www.aapos.org AAPOS; focuses on research and training in pediatric ophthalmology and the advanced care of adults with strabismus.

www.ascrs.org American Society of Cataract and Refractive Surgeons; provides clinical and practice management information to members.

www.childrenseyefoundation.org Children's Eye Foundation; programs to help parents and physicians prevent vision loss and eye disease, especially related to amblyopia and strabismus.

emedicine.medscape.com/article/1217083-overview Summary of optic neuritis treatment.

www.eyecareamerica.org EyeCare America website, Foundation of AAO; includes information on cataracts, glaucoma, diabetic neuropathy, macular degeneration, and how patients can gain access to no-cost care.

www.nei.nih.gov/health/glaucoma/glaucoma_facts.asp Government site that includes many facts about glaucoma.

www.nei.nih.gov/health/maculardegen/nei_wysk_amd.PDF Age-related macular degeneration handout for patients.

www.nlm.nih.gov/medlineplus/maculardegeneration.html Macular degeneration reference for patients.

pediatrics.aappublications.org/cgi/content/extract/100/6/1021 AAP perinatal guidelines.

www.preventblindness.org Prevent Blindness America; volunteer eye health and safety organization to prevent blindness and preserve sight through vision screening and research.

telemedicine.orbis.org/learning/bins/login.asp?cid=740 Orbis CyberSight Telemedicine Learning of Ophthalmology.

18 Otorhinolaryngology

JOHN G. O'HANDLEY, EVAN J. TOBIN, and ASHISH R. SHAH

Emergencies

EPIGLOTTITIS

Epiglottitis (or "supraglottitis") is a condition that requires prompt attention by the physician. Epiglottitis results from bacterial (and rarely viral) infection of the supraglottic structures—that is, the epiglottis and arytenoid cartilages. A high level of suspicion is necessary to make a diagnosis and avoid significant morbidity. Rapid decompensation and complete loss of the airway are the sequelae of most concern. The physician should always be suspicious when a patient presents with fever, sore throat, and difficulty swallowing and when the severity of oropharyngeal physical findings is not in proportion to the symptoms. Croup, tonsillitis, peritonsillar abscess, and other neck infection may be incorrectly diagnosed in these patients. Epiglottitis occurs mainly in children age 2 to 7 years, although infants, older children, and adults can be affected. Mortality rates of 6% to 7% have been reported in adults.

Signs and symptoms of epiglottitis include a rapidly developing sore throat, high fever, restlessness, and lethargy. A "supraglottic," muffled voice is common. Many patients have difficulty with their saliva and drool. Classically, these patients are in a sitting position leaning forward because this position tends to alleviate obstructive symptoms from the supraglottic swelling. They may show signs of "air hunger" or may have stridor.

Key Points

- Drooling, posturing, and air hunger are classic signs of epiglottitis.
- Epiglottitis is much less common in the pediatric population with routine *Haemophilus influenzae* type b (Hib) vaccination and is now more often seen in adults. It is often more insidious in adults but can still progress to airway obstruction.
- A lateral neck radiograph showing a thumbprint sign can be diagnostic of epiglottitis, but visualization of the larynx is paramount.
- A high index of suspicion is required for the timely diagnosis of retropharyngeal abscess. The physical findings can be subtle.
- Sudden sensorineural hearing loss (SSNHL) should be considered in a patient who presents with a new complaint of hearing loss or tinnitus and no evidence of cerumen impaction or middle ear effusion.
- Acute onset of wheezing in a child with no history of asthma should alert the clinician to a possible airway foreign body.
- Esophageal foreign body in children often presents with drooling and refusal of oral intake and absence of signs of infection.
- Whereas esophageal foreign bodies are more often radiopaque on radiographs, airway foreign bodies are more likely to be radiolucent food material. With both, history and physical examination are paramount.

- Risk factors for epistaxis include nasal sicca, nasal trauma, hypertension, sinonasal neoplasia, and coagulopathy. Often the coagulopathy is iatrogenic and "therapeutic."
- Epistaxis can rarely progress to respiratory embarrassment or hypovolemic shock, especially in a patient with comorbid conditions.
- Adolescent boys with recurrent epistaxis may have a juvenile nasopharyngeal angiofibroma.
- Proper setup is necessary for effective treatment of epistaxis. This includes a headlight, suction, an epistaxis treatment kit, silver nitrate for cautery, and packing material.
- Nasal packing can cause toxic shock syndrome.
- Nasal packing can lead to hypoxemia, especially in a patient with cardiopulmonary disease or sleep apnea.
- Definitive diagnosis of an aerodigestive tract foreign body may require endoscopy.
- Suspicion of a disc battery esophageal foreign body requires emergent endoscopy because significant tissue necrosis can quickly occur.
- Epistaxis often responds to correction of risk factors (e.g. hypertension, sicca, and coagulopathy).
- If nasal packing is not effective, more invasive procedures may be necessary. These procedures include endoscopy with cautery, vessel ligation, and angiography and embolization.

Table 18-1 Distinguishing Features of Epiglottitis and Croup

Feature	Epiglottitis	Croup
Cause	Bacterial	Viral
Age	1 year to adult	1-5 years
Location of obstruction	Supraglottic	Subglottic
Onset	Sudden (hours)	Gradual (days)
Fever	High	Low grade
Dysphagia	Marked	None
Drooling	Present	Minimal
Posture	Sitting	Recumbent
Toxemia	Mild to severe	Mild
Cough	Usually none	Barking, brassy, spontaneous
Voice	Clear to muffled	Hoarse
Respiratory rate	Normal to rapid	Rapid
Larynx palpation	Tender	Not tender
Clinical course	Shorter	Longer

From Berry FA, Yemen TA. Pediatric airway in health and disease. *Pediatr Clin North Am.* 1994;41:153.

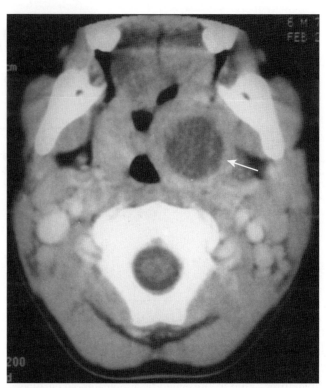

Figure 18-1 Large left peritonsillar abscess *(arrow)* that required surgical drainage.

The differential diagnosis includes tonsillitis, peritonsillar abscess, retropharyngeal abscess, airway foreign body, and croup. Physical examination with laryngoscopy is extremely useful in differentiating these diagnoses. Endoscopy should not be performed if there is concern of impending airway obstruction. Endoscopy typically shows erythema and edema of the epiglottis and arytenoid cartilages. Other findings include laryngeal tenderness on neck palpation, although palpation should be avoided when the diagnosis is being considered. Placement of a tongue depressor has been known to precipitate acute airway obstruction and should be avoided entirely if epiglottitis is strongly suspected.

Any time the diagnosis of epiglottitis is in question, otorhinolaryngologic (ear, nose, and throat [ENT]) and infectious disease consultations are warranted. Differentiation from croup can be difficult because there is considerable overlap of symptoms (Table 18-1) (Berry and Yemen, 1994). A lateral extended neck radiograph can help in the diagnosis. Radiographic evidence includes the classic "thumbprint" sign. If epiglottitis is suspected or lateral neck radiography is confirmatory, the patient should be taken to the operating room (OR) for orotracheal intubation in the presence of an anesthesiologist and an otorhinolaryngologist. In any case of airway obstruction, cricothyrotomy or tracheotomy can be lifesaving because orotracheal intubation can be difficult and sometimes impossible. Some patients, usually adults, may be treated expectantly with intravenous (IV) medications and intensive care unit (ICU) observation as long as personnel are available for control of the airway if necessary. If airway stability is questionable, observation is not recommended.

After control of the airway is achieved, cultures of the epiglottis should be obtained and directed antibiotics instituted. *Haemophilus influenzae* type b (Hib) is common and can be β-lactamase producing. The incidence of epiglottitis in children is decreasing since the introduction of the Hib vaccine in the late 1980s. However, the incidence has remained stable or slightly increased in adults. The relative incidence of *Staphylococcus aureus* has also increased since the widespread use of the Hib vaccine. Antibiotics should be administered parenterally; effective antibiotics include cefotaxime, ceftriaxone, ampicillin plus sulbactam, or ampicillin plus chloramphenicol. Steroids can be useful for edema and inflammation, but their effectiveness has not been proved in controlled studies.

PERITONSILLAR ABSCESS

A peritonsillar abscess is the accumulation of pus in the peritonsillar space that surrounds the tonsil. The same organisms responsible for common tonsillar infections—*Streptococcus* and *Staphylococcus* spp. and anaerobes—are also found in peritonsillar abscesses.

The typical signs and symptoms of peritonsillar abscess include fever, increasing sore throat, dysphagia, odynophagia, and a muffled "hot potato" voice. Trismus is extremely common. Examination confirms asymmetric tonsils and peritonsillar edema and erythema. The soft palate and uvula are swollen and displaced away from the side of the abscess. It is often difficult to distinguish between abscess and peritonsillar cellulitis. If possible, it is helpful to palpate because fluctuance indicates a loculation of pus. Diagnosis is often made by clinical impression, but computed tomography (CT) can be confirmatory and useful when the diagnosis is uncertain (Figure 18-1).

If untreated, a peritonsillar abscess may spontaneously drain, progress to involve the deep neck space or sepsis, or even lead to airway obstruction. The most important part of the treatment is drainage of the abscess cavity by needle aspiration, incision and drainage, or tonsillectomy. Cultures of the aspirate can be obtained, and broad-spectrum antibiotics should be started. Appropriate antibiotics include ampicillin–sulbactam (Unasyn) or clindamycin (Cleocin). Many patients present with dehydration, and parenteral fluids should be given if necessary. Analgesics should be prescribed as needed with careful monitoring of the airway and oxygenation. One or two doses of IV corticosteroids may be given to decrease inflammation and pain.

Children presenting with peritonsillar abscess should be admitted to the hospital. Treatment with IV hydration and parenteral antibiotics is appropriate initially. Patients with peritonsillar cellulitis/phlegmon or early abscess often demonstrate a rapid response to treatment, whereas those with a well-formed peritonsillar abscess do not typically improve. Drainage is necessary in nonresponders. Abscesses in cooperative adults can be drained under local anesthesia in the emergency department (ED) or office and treated in an outpatient setting. Children usually require general anesthesia for drainage, and a tonsillectomy may also be performed. Later, an elective tonsillectomy may be recommended to prevent recurrence, especially for patients with a history of recurrent tonsillitis, although few, if any, controlled studies support this recommendation.

SUDDEN SENSORINEURAL HEARING LOSS

Although most types of hearing loss are nonurgent problems, SSNHL deserves special note because it is considered an otologic emergency. Any patient complaining of sudden hearing loss requires prompt evaluation. An obvious cause such as cerumen impaction or middle ear fluid can be treated appropriately and routinely. If a cause is not identified, SSNHL should be suspected and prompt ENT referral arranged. SSNHL is thought to be secondary to vascular, thromboembolic, viral, or autoimmune causes. It may also be the result of ototoxicity. A viral etiology is thought to be the most common. Without treatment, hearing returns in one third of patients, partial hearing returns in one third, and there is no improvement in the remaining third. Early intervention with oral corticosteroids appears to improve outcomes and is recommended in patients without significant contraindications to oral steroids. Many steroid regimens are described. A 10- to 14-day course of prednisone beginning at 60 mg/day with a short taper is reasonable. The hearing loss needs to be followed. Finally, for patients who do not respond to systemic steroids, controlled studies do support the use intratympanic infusion of corticosteroids, demonstrating improved outcomes (Xenellis et al., 2006). Intratympanic steroids are also appealing for patients with contraindications to oral steroids (e.g., those with "brittle diabetes"). For patients who do not have complete return of hearing, magnetic resonance imaging (MRI) is necessary to rule out a vestibular schwannoma (acoustic neuroma), which can rarely present with sudden hearing loss.

FOREIGN BODIES

Swallowing or aspiration of objects is most common in children but also occurs in the adult population. These objects can become lodged anywhere in the upper aerodigestive tract.

Esophagus

The most common location for esophageal foreign bodies is at the level of the cricopharyngeal muscle. Other regions include the anatomic narrowings of the esophagus, such as the gastroesophageal junction, and the area of indentation of the esophagus by the left main stem bronchus and the arch of the aorta. Coins are by far the most common objects found in the esophagus in children. Chicken or fish bones are more common in adults.

The diagnosis of an esophageal foreign body is primarily based on the medical history and physical examination, with the aid of radiologic studies. Parents might witness ingestion of the foreign body and subsequent coughing, gagging, refusal to eat, or drooling. Often, however, the incident goes unwitnessed, and reliance on other diagnostic techniques is necessary.

Plain radiographs (including lateral radiographs) are often diagnostic in pediatric patients because most esophageal foreign objects are radiopaque (Figure 18-2). Other radiologic findings that can suggest a foreign body include increased soft tissue density in the prevertebral space, mediastinal widening, air-fluid levels in the esophagus, and paraesophageal air. Disk batteries *require a high index of suspicion* because they can cause significant tissue injury and lead to esophageal perforation *if they are not removed emergently.* They have a classic appearance when viewed laterally, approximating a dime resting on a nickel (similar to the appearance of Figure 18-2).

If there is sufficient evidence of an esophageal foreign body, consultation is indicated for esophagoscopy and removal. When radiolucent objects have been ingested, contrast esophagography might be indicated, although esophagograms can give a false-negative result and can also complicate visualization during rigid esophagoscopy.

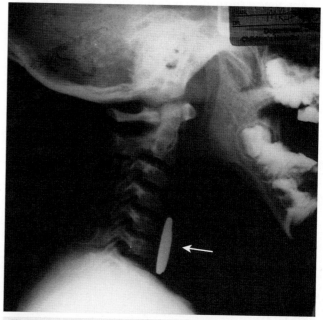

Figure 18-2 Lateral neck radiograph of a child presenting with gagging and drooling, showing two coins *(arrow)* in the esophagus near the cricopharyngeal junction.

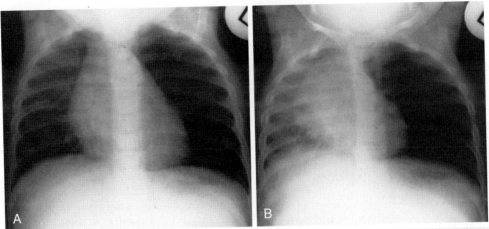

Figure 18-3 Inspiratory (**A**) and expiratory (**B**) radiographs of an 8-year-old boy with a left airway foreign body (peanut). No foreign object is visible on plain radiographs, but the expiratory radiograph shows overinflation of the left lung with mediastinal shift to the contralateral side.

Airway

As with esophageal foreign bodies, airway foreign bodies are much more common in infants and young children. Many deaths from foreign body aspiration occur in the home before medical intervention can be administered. The most frequently aspirated foreign bodies are foods, with nuts leading the list. Foreign bodies aspirated into the airway are usually found lodged in the bronchial tree but can also be found in the larynx or trachea. If the event is witnessed and results in complete airway obstruction, a Heimlich maneuver should be administered; however, the event is often not witnessed. Symptoms can include hoarseness, persistent cough, wheezing, or stridor if the foreign body is lodged in the trachea or larynx. Because the potential for morbidity and mortality is substantial, this condition requires urgent diagnosis and timely intervention to prevent catastrophe.

Any time a small child presents with wheezing or noisy breathing without a history of reactive airway disease, an airway foreign body should be included in the differential diagnosis. Typically, patients and parents recount a transient episode of coughing during eating that then subsided; the patient might even be symptom free for a time and then later have symptoms such as coughing or wheezing.

The most important diagnostic step for identifying a foreign body is a high index of suspicion. Careful auscultation of the lung fields is essential because subtle asymmetric differences may be found. Because most airway foreign bodies are radiolucent, chest radiographs can be normal, but abnormalities such as hyperinflation, atelectasis, or pneumonia can be present (Figure 18-3). If plain radiographs are equivocal or normal and the patient is in stable condition, airway fluoroscopy can be helpful.

Consultation with a physician experienced in foreign body removal is required. Definitive treatment of airway foreign bodies is direct laryngoscopy and rigid bronchoscopy to identify and remove the object.

EPISTAXIS

Although epistaxis is usually nothing more than a minor annoyance, some episodes are severe enough to require urgent medical attention and intervention. In rare cases, epistaxis can also be a life-threatening emergency.

Predisposing factors for epistaxis include trauma, frequent cleaning or picking, dry weather, hypertension, bleeding dyscrasias (factor deficiencies, hereditary hemorrhagic telangiectasia, lymphoproliferative disorders), anticoagulation therapy (e.g., acetylsalicylic acid, heparin, warfarin, clopidogrel), and intranasal tumors. Special consideration should be given to adolescent boys with recurrent epistaxis and nasal obstruction because these symptoms might be the result of a juvenile nasopharyngeal angiofibroma. These are benign but locally aggressive tumors. All of these potential risk factors should be considered because they must be addressed to treat the patient appropriately. If epistaxis is the result of significant trauma, this affects the algorithm for evaluation and treatment; this is discussed in the "Head and Neck Trauma" section of this chapter.

Epistaxis is classified according to its location. Bleeding from the anterior nasal cavity is most common and usually originates from a rich plexus of vessels at the anterior septum called the *Kiesselbach plexus* (Figure 18-4). Bleeding from this location, although troublesome, is less likely to be severe and is usually easier to control than posterior epistaxis. Posterior epistaxis originates from the posterior two thirds of the nasal cavity and can be quite severe and much more difficult to control.

Initial management of epistaxis includes assessment and stabilization of vital signs. Rarely, severe bleeding can lead to airway compromise, hemodynamic compromise, or both, especially in patients with underlying cardiopulmonary dysfunction. The airway should be assessed and stabilized, urgently if necessary. Hypertension, if severe, should be controlled, with care taken to avoid subsequent *hypotension*. Hematologic studies, including a complete blood count (CBC), prothrombin time, and partial thromboplastin time, should be ordered. IV access should be established, allowing administration of fluids as well as IV medications, if necessary, during treatment.

Treatment

Effective treatment requires adequate visualization and patient cooperation. The level of intervention by the primary

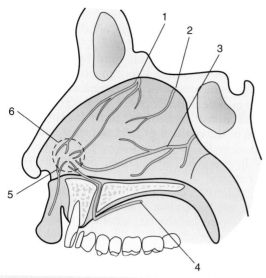

Figure 18-4 Kiesselbach plexus. *1* and *2*, Anterior and posterior ethmoid arteries; *3*, septal branch of the sphenopalatine; *4*, greater palatine; *5*, branch from superior labial; *6*, Kiesselbach plexus. (From Colman BH, Hall IS, eds. *Hall and Colman's diseases of the ear, nose and throat.* 15th ed. Philadelphia: Churchill Livingstone; 2000:82.)

care physician depends on level of experience, comfort level, and availability of appropriate supplies and equipment. ENT consultation should be considered when any of these prerequisites cannot be met. The patient should be reassured and given an explanation of the planned treatment. This results in better cooperation and decreases patient anxiety, improving treatment success. A bright headlight, nasal speculum, large nasal (Frazier tip) suction, and bayonet forceps are required. If the patient is monitored and stable, a small dose of IV narcotics titrated for analgesia and anxiolytic effect may be given. Extreme caution should be taken not to oversedate the patient. Also, instrumentation of the nose can lead to a significant vasovagal response that may be accentuated in a hypovolemic patient given narcotics. It is advised to err on the side of caution with regard to narcotic medication both during and after treatment.

All clots should be suctioned. They can be quite tenacious and require forceps for removal. The nasal cavity should next be topically anesthetized and decongested (a mixture of 4% lidocaine and phenylephrine applied with cotton balls or spray works well). If a bleeding site is easily identified, it may be cauterized with a silver nitrate stick.

Anterior Packing. If suction, decongestion, and cautery do not stop the bleeding and the site is still thought to be anterior, an anterior nasal pack should be placed. This can be done with 0.5-inch petroleum gauze coated in antibiotic ointment. A better option, if available, is to use a preformed pack. Merocel nasal packs or prepackaged inflatable packs are usually readily available and quite effective. Remembering that the nasal cavity extends *posteriorly* from the nostril and not *superiorly* facilitates placement. The pack should be coated in antibiotic ointment before placement. It is best to use the smallest pack that is effective.

Placement of the pack can be quite uncomfortable for the patient. Discomfort can be minimized by ensuring optimal decongestion and topical anesthesia of the nasal cavity. If using a Merocel pack, it is sometimes helpful to hydrate and expand the pack *before* placing it. This can be done with sterile saline or phenylephrine. Although the pack appears quite large after it is expanded, it decompresses readily and slides in easily when it is covered in antibiotic ointment. The entire length of the pack needs to be grasped with the bayonet forceps if this technique is used. Preexpansion of the pack also minimizes further abrasions and bleeding that can occur with placement of the firm, nonexpanded pack. This technique is especially advantageous if a septal deviation is on the bleeding side. Regardless of what type of pack is used, care must be taken not to distort or overstretch the nasal ala (nostril) when the pack is in place. This causes significant discomfort and can result in necrosis of the nostril.

After the pack is in place, the patient should be observed for further bleeding. If the patient remains stable, is tolerating the pack well, has no significant comorbid conditions, and has only a unilateral anterior pack, the patient may be discharged with mild narcotic pain medications and antibiotics for prophylaxis against toxic shock syndrome and sinusitis. If these conditions are not met, admission may be necessary. The pack should be removed 2 to 5 days later, with instructions to use nasal saline and nasal ointment liberally for the next 2 weeks. Recurrent bleeding should prompt an ENT consultation.

Posterior Packing. If the bleeding is not controlled with a smaller anterior pack, the origin of the bleeding may be posterior, requiring a larger anterior pack or *anteroposterior pack.* A very effective and commonly used pack is the Rapid Rhino (ArthroCare ENT) pack. The Rapid Rhino comes as a shorter *anterior* or a longer *anteroposterior* balloon tampon. It acts as a platelet aggregator and forms a lubricant upon contact with water. It has a cuff that is inflated by air. The prepackaged kit comes with detailed instructions for insertion. These packs are used in many EDs nationwide. They are effective for severe anterior as well as posterior nose bleeds. If a preformed anteroposterior pack is not available or not effective, a traditional anteroposterior pack may be placed. The posterior pack is necessary essentially to seal off the posterior nasal cavity and provide a buttress to prevent the anterior pack from slipping posteriorly.

Placement of a posterior pack requires experience, and even if it is successfully done, ENT consultation is indicated to assist with further bleeding, pack removal, and to monitor for pack complications. Anterior-posterior packs are associated with significant patient discomfort and potential complications during and after insertion. Local complications, including necrosis of the alae, septum, and palate, can occur, and close observation is required to prevent them. Hypoxemia can also result. Supplemental oxygen and monitoring of oxygen saturation is indicated. Patients with preexisting cardiopulmonary disease require closer observation, often in the ICU. The patient might require judicious doses of narcotics for pain and antibiotics for infection prophylaxis.

Other Techniques. Rarely, epistaxis cannot be controlled with packing, requiring further intervention. This can include intraoperative endoscopic cautery, endoscopic or open arterial ligation, or angiography with selective embolization of the offending vessel. There are advantages and disadvantages to each of these techniques. In general, the surgical techniques are usually favored over embolization if there are no significant contraindications to surgery. All of the surgical techniques have very high success rates. Embolization is also effective when performed by an experienced interventional radiologist, but it does carry the relatively low risk of inadvertent embolization of the internal carotid artery system and subsequent ischemic cerebral injury, which can be devastating.

KEY TREATMENT

- If there is ever concern about impending airway obstruction, steps should be taken rapidly to prepare to stabilize the airway (SOR: C).
- Interventions for airway obstruction include mask ventilation followed by endotracheal intubation or cricothyrotomy or tracheotomy (SOR: C).
- Patients with epiglottitis typically respond to IV steroids and IV antibiotics directed at *H. influenza* and *S. aureus*. Patients should be closely monitored for impending airway obstruction (SOR: B).
- Most peritonsillar abscesses should be drained, although patients with smaller or early abscesses may respond to medical therapy (SOR: C).
- Early treatment of SSNHL with corticosteroids appears to improve outcomes. The risks and contraindications of steroids need to be considered (SOR: B).

Head and Neck Trauma and Respiratory Embarrassment

Key Points

- The ABCs of trauma include *a*irway, *b*reathing, *c*irculation, and *c*ervical spine clearance.
- Laryngeal and pharyngoesophageal injuries must be suspected in blunt or penetrating neck injuries.
- Isolated facial injuries can result in significant bleeding and can be associated with orbital or central nervous system (CNS) injury.
- Overlooked facial fractures can result in long-term functional and cosmetic defects.

The ABCs of trauma should be remembered when treating a patient with cervicofacial trauma. This includes evaluation and treatment of *a*irway, *b*reathing, *c*irculation, and *c*ervical spine. The most pressing issue after significant face, head, or neck trauma is the potential for respiratory compromise secondary to several causes. Altered mental status can lead to aspiration of blood or secretions with or without central hypoventilation. Comminuted facial fractures (midface or mandibular) can distort the oral and pharyngeal airway sufficiently to cause obstruction. An undetected expanding pharyngeal or neck hematoma can cause airway obstruction by extrinsic compression of the trachea or pharynx. Blunt or penetrating neck injuries can cause laryngeal fracture, bleeding, or hematoma, leading to critical airway obstruction.

Potential airway obstruction must be addressed quickly because complete obstruction can progress rapidly. The diagnosis is clinical because hypoxemia and carbon dioxide retention are late signs. Extensive facial edema or ecchymosis should arouse concern for facial fracture. A muffled voice can be the result of expanding hematoma. Laryngeal or tracheal injury should be suspected if the patient has a change in the voice, hemoptysis, subcutaneous emphysema, or stridor.

Stabilization of a compromised airway should be accomplished as soon as possible. Endotracheal intubation may be attempted, with plans for emergent cricothyrotomy as necessary. If time permits, the on-call anesthesiologist, trauma surgeon, or otorhinolaryngologist should be consulted to assist in airway management. Blind intubation (especially nasotracheal) or insertion of a laryngeal mask airway is not recommended because this further compromises the already tenuous airway if intubation is unsuccessful. Although tracheotomy is the preferred procedure when endotracheal intubation is impossible or contraindicated, cricothyrotomy is also acceptable and can be lifesaving.

There is potential for significant blood loss after severe head and neck trauma. IV access should be established and volume replacement initiated quickly. Bleeding from facial wounds can be controlled with direct pressure and suture ligation of arterial bleeding. Management of epistaxis is discussed earlier. Bleeding from the neck or evidence of expanding hematoma implies a major vessel injury and requires immediate operative exploration by a trauma surgeon, vascular surgeon, or otorhinolaryngologist.

Unrecognized pharyngeal and esophageal injury can result in life-threatening infection. These injuries might not be obvious on initial evaluation and require a very high index of suspicion. Contrast studies and endoscopy are usually required to confirm the diagnosis. Treatment can include repair of the injury or external drainage to allow healing.

Isolated facial injuries are rarely life threatening but still can result in significant bleeding and, rarely, airway compromise and permanent disability. Significant facial trauma should be evaluated in the ED. The potential for intracranial and cervical spine injuries should be considered when major facial injuries are present. Trauma of the periorbital region requires ophthalmologic evaluation. All lacerations should be inspected, cleaned, and sutured. Antibiotics should be used if contamination is likely.

Deeper injuries can result in facial nerve transection. If facial nerve weakness is detected, plastic surgery or ENT consultation is necessary for expedient nerve exploration and repair. The parotid salivary duct can also be injured and requires repair over a stent. Facial fractures should be evaluated with CT (both axial and coronal images). Possible mandibular fractures should be evaluated with plain radiographs, including panographic (Panorex) films. Overlooked and untreated facial fractures can result in significant long-term functional and cosmetic deficits. Oral surgery consultation is sometimes required, especially with injury to the teeth or altered dental occlusion.

- If there is ever concern about impending airway obstruction, steps should be taken to secure the airway (SOR: B).
- If injuries prevent adequate visualization, intubation should not be attempted. In these cases, tracheotomy or cricothyrotomy should be performed (SOR: C).
- IV access should be established and volume replacement initiated quickly (SOR: C).
- Deep facial lacerations might require exploration to ligate vessels or repair an injury to the facial nerve or parotid salivary duct (SOR: C).

Nasal Trauma

Traumatic injuries to the nose are extremely common and usually of little long-term significance. In some patients, however, trauma can result in significant cosmetic and functional problems. In severe cases, nasal trauma can result in severe bleeding and cerebrospinal fluid (CSF) leakage and can even be life threatening.

Evaluation of a patient who has sustained nasal trauma requires a thorough history. The mechanism of injury must be understood. If the injury was recent, the patient must be examined for signs of cervical, mandibular, maxillary, orbital, and intracranial injury. Bleeding can be quite severe after isolated nasal trauma but usually stops spontaneously or with only digital pressure.

Initial evaluation includes assessment of the gross appearance of the face, with special attention to the possibility of other facial fractures (orbital, zygomatic, mandibular). Obvious deformity of the nose should be noted, although marked edema obscures this in some cases. Radiographs may be ordered, but their utility is variable because nondisplaced fractures usually require no treatment, and displaced nasal fractures are usually obvious on examination.

Intranasal examination is done to rule out the presence of a septal hematoma or CSF leakage. A septal hematoma results when bleeding occurs between the septal perichondrium and the underlying cartilage. The hematoma can be unilateral or bilateral. It results in a widened septum with nasal obstruction. Successful treatment requires prompt diagnosis followed by incision and drainage and packing to prevent reaccumulation. If untreated, and especially if bilateral, the hematoma leads to ischemic necrosis of the cartilage or can result in abscess formation. This can ultimately result in loss of enough septal cartilage to cause external nasal collapse, called *saddle nose deformity*. Because it is extremely difficult to repair, avoiding saddle nose deformity is paramount.

Severe bleeding after nasal trauma can result from a vascular injury of the ethmoidal, the sphenopalatine, or rarely the carotid arteries. Techniques for controlling epistaxis described in this chapter can be used, but ENT consultation should be obtained if the trauma is severe or if severe bleeding persists. *CSF leakage* is diagnosed when clear drainage is seen dripping from one or both sides of the nose. Leakage can increase in a more dependent position. Nasal CSF leakage requires urgent ENT and neurosurgical

consultation. It often resolves spontaneously but can lead to life-threatening problems such as pneumocephalus (air within the cranial vault), meningitis, and brain abscess.

Isolated nasal deformity after nasal trauma results from displacement of the nasal bones, the external nasal cartilages, or the septum. The nasal bones can often be repositioned with excellent results by performing a *closed reduction*. This is done under local or general anesthesia, usually after the initial edema has subsided and before the bones have set (7-10 days after injury). Sometimes an *open reduction*, which involves refracturing the nasal bones, is required. If the septum is significantly deviated, it can be repaired at the same time. If residual nasal deformity persists, a formal *rhinoplasty*, which more precisely addresses all aspects of the external nose, can be done later. In children with nasal fractures, closed reduction is usually recommended sooner than for adults because their fractures heal more quickly. Repair should be done within 7 days of the injury, if possible. Open reduction is generally not recommended in children because of concern for affecting future nasal growth. If necessary, rhinoplasty is delayed until nasal growth is complete, which is shortly after puberty.

The Ear

Key Points

- Otalgia may be from a referred source when the physical examination does not support an ear problem.
- In smokers with otalgia, the clinician should suspect laryngopharyngeal carcinoma when a presumed infection does not respond to antibiotics.
- Pneumatic otoscopy or tympanometry is most useful in confirming middle ear fluid.
- The most common cause of vertigo is a peripheral vestibular disorder (38%-56%).
- Benign paroxysmal positional vertigo (BPPV) is the most common cause of peripheral vertigo and is twice as common in women as in men.
- Unless the diagnosis of BPPV is uncertain, radiographic imaging and vestibular testing are not recommended.
- Pneumatic otoscopy can cause nystagmus and vertigo in the presence of a perilymph fistula.
- Tinnitus is primarily caused by sensorineural hearing loss (SNHL) but occasionally can be a symptom of a vascular abnormality, a hypermetabolic state, medications, or an intracranial mass.
- The most common infection in children seen in a physician's office is acute otitis media (AOM).
- Three criteria necessary for the diagnosis of AOM are acute onset, middle ear effusion, and signs and symptoms of middle ear inflammation.
- Severe AOM is defined as moderate to severe otalgia and fever greater than 39°C (102.2°F).
- Tympanic blistering (bullous myringitis) is simply a variant of AOM and should be treated as such.
- All traumatic perforations of the tympanic membrane require audiologic evaluation to rule out SNHL.
- SSNHL is an otologic emergency.

PHYSICAL EXAMINATION

See eAppendix 18-1 online.

OTALGIA

Although the vast majority of patients with otalgia have an otologic cause, the clinician must recognize that otalgia may be *referred*. Sensory innervation of the ear includes cranial nerves V, VII, IX, and X; therefore, disorders of structures with similar innervation can cause otalgia. It is imperative that the physician not simply attribute otalgia to an ear infection unless the physical examination supports this diagnosis. Otalgia can result from dysfunction of the nose, sinuses, oral cavity, pharynx, larynx, dentition, temporomandibular joints, and salivary glands. These structures must be thoroughly assessed, especially if the results from examination of the ear appears normal. This is especially true in smokers, whose initial symptom of laryngopharyngeal carcinoma may be otalgia. Otolaryngologic referral for laryngoscopy may be indicated with suspected referred otalgia. (See eTable 18-1 and eTable 18-2 online for the differential diagnosis of otalgia.)

TUMORS OF THE EAR

Tumors of the ear are rare. Classification is based on their location (external ear, middle ear, inner ear). A tumor of the external or middle ear is often easily diagnosed by visualizing a lesion on otoscopy. In some cases, symptoms may mimic infection (pain, otorrhea). Tumors of the inner ear can manifest with symptoms of hearing loss, tinnitus, disequilibrium, or facial weakness. (eTable 18-3 online lists tumors of the ear by location.)

VERTIGO

The sense of balance or equilibrium occurs when there is normal and harmonious function of several systems and organs in the body. These include the musculoskeletal system, the cardiovascular system, the CNS, the eyes, and the ears. Abnormal function of any of these can result in the sensation of dizziness or disequilibrium. The term *vertigo* is reserved to describe a perceived sensation of motion, usually spinning, of the person relative to the environment or vice versa. Causes of disequilibrium can be categorized into one of three groups: *peripheral* (inner ear or labyrinthine), *CNS*, or *systemic* (e.g., cardiovascular, metabolic). Although not pathognomonic of a labyrinthine disorder, true vertigo most often indicates aberrant function of the inner ear.

Because patients use "dizzy" to describe many sensations, the actual sensation is best clarified by a detailed history (Table 18-2). The major studies on the causes of persistent dizziness, from Drachman and Hart (1972) to Davis (1994), all describe four diagnostic categories: lightheadedness, presyncope, disequilibrium, and vertigo. The investigators all conclude that the most common cause of persistent dizziness is a peripheral vestibular disorder (38%-56% of cases) followed closely by a psychogenic disorder (6%-33%). In about 25% of patients, the complaint is the result of the combined effects of multiple sensory deficits, medications,

Table 18-2 History for "Dizziness"
Description of the sensation (including associated symptoms)
Onset (acute, gradual)
Duration (date sensation was first noted, length of time it lasts)
Intensity (how troubling is it?)
Exacerbations (activities, positions, circumstances that worsen the situation)
Remissions (activities, positions, circumstances that make sensation better)
Medications (prescription, herbal, over the counter)
Other medical problems (e.g., diabetes, hypertension, heart disease)
Psychosocial (any stressors?)

or orthostasis, leading to complaints of presyncope, lightheadedness, or disequilibrium. Finally, central vestibular etiologies are unusual and represent fewer than 10% of all causes.

A thorough medical history allows the physician to distinguish between true vertigo (a sensation of spinning) and other sensations, such as presyncope, lightheadedness, and unsteadiness. The physical examination and laboratory evaluation are guided by the accuracy of the history. A sensation of vertigo originates from within the vestibular system but can be either *peripheral* (vestibular nerve and inner ear) or *central* (cerebellum, brainstem, thalamus, and cortex).

Questions regarding hearing and neurologic deficits can help elicit which part of the vestibular system is involved (see eTable 18-4 online). Whereas peripheral vertigo tends to be episodic, central vertigo is constant. Neurologic symptoms or loss of consciousness do not occur with peripheral vertigo but are possible with central vertigo. Nystagmus, which is labeled by the direction of the fast component, can be present in both types of vertigo and can be horizontal or rotary; vertical nystagmus occurs only in central vertigo.

The physical examination should include assessment of orthostatic blood pressure changes, a complete ocular examination, tuning fork tests (Weber and Rinne), pneumatic otoscopy (elicits vertigo in patients with perilymphatic fistula), balance tests (Romberg), gait (including tandem walking), and cranial nerve evaluation. The Dix-Hallpike maneuver (see eFigure 18-3) is especially helpful in diagnosing BPPV. Head movement almost always worsens the feeling of true vertigo. If it does not, the dizziness may be attributed to a cause other than vestibular dysfunction.

Laboratory testing can include an audiogram if no specific cause of vertigo can be found after the medical history and physical examination. Electronystagmography (ENG) is an objective study of the vestibular system and can help localize a vestibular lesion. Electrodes placed about the eye sense the movements of nystagmus as either spontaneous or initiated by maneuvers such as caloric testing, positioning, optokinetics, and pendulum tracing. A brain MRI scan is indicated in patients with unilateral otologic symptoms and in those unresponsive to treatment. Blood tests, when necessary, can include CBC, rapid plasma reagin (RPR), vitamin B_{12} level, folate level, drug screens, and heavy metal testing when indicated.

Meniere Disease

Meniere disease is characterized by episodic severe vertigo lasting hours, with associated symptoms of unilateral roaring tinnitus, fluctuating low-frequency hearing loss, and aural fullness. The typical age of onset is in the fifth decade of life. The cause is uncertain but is speculated to result from allergic, infectious, or autoimmune injury. The histopathologic finding includes *endolymphatic hydrops*, which is thought to be caused by either overproduction or underresorption of endolymph in the inner ear.

Meniere disease is a clinical diagnosis mostly based on history. Testing may be obtained to support the diagnosis and rule out other disorders. Audiometry often demonstrates a low-frequency SNHL. An FTA-ABS (fluorescent treponemal antibody-absorption) test may be obtained to rule out syphilis. ENG may demonstrate a unilateral peripheral vestibular weakness on caloric testing. When the diagnosis is uncertain, a brain MRI with contrast is obtained to evaluate for a retrocochlear lesion. The differential diagnosis of Meniere disease includes acute labyrinthitis, neurosyphilis, labyrinthine fistula, autoimmune inner ear disease, vestibular neuronitis, and migraine-associated vertigo.

Although Meniere disease has a highly variable clinical course, most patients have long symptom-free periods between clusters of episodes. The majority of patients have an excellent prognosis, with symptoms burning out over several years. However, some patients have a disabling course with frequent and severe attacks. On average, a moderate SNHL is the end result. The disease may become bilateral in about 45% of cases (wide variability exists).

Treatment of an acute episode involves vestibular suppressants and antiemetics. As with any vestibular disorder, vestibular suppressants should be limited for use during acute symptoms because of their addictive potential and impairment of central compensation. Maintenance therapy includes reduction of sodium intake to less than 1500 mg/day and a diuretic such as hydrochlorothiazide–triamterene (Dyazide). Patients are also instructed to minimize caffeine, alcohol, nicotine, and chocolate. Allergy treatment may be helpful in some patients. Most patients have adequate control of symptoms with this regimen. Several studies have indicated that a short course of steroids is not likely to improve Meniere disease (Fisher et al., 2012).

Patients who fail conservative measures may be candidates for procedures and surgical treatment. Gentamicin, a vestibulotoxic aminoglycoside antibiotic, may be injected transtympanically into the middle ear to permeate into the inner ear. Control of vertigo may result in 90% of patients but with a risk of hearing loss. Endolymphatic sac decompression or shunting through a mastoidectomy appears to benefit most patients with minimal risk to hearing. Although a generally accepted procedure, adequate studies are lacking on its effectiveness. More invasive interventions, including vestibular nerve section and labyrinthectomy, are reserved for patients with severe disease who do not respond to other measures (Sajjadi and Paparella, 2008).

Vestibular Neuronitis

Acute vertigo associated with nausea and vomiting (but without neurologic or audiologic symptoms) that originates in the vestibular nerve is known as *vestibular neuronitis.* Vestibular neuronitis can occur spontaneously or can follow viral illness. Horizontal nystagmus shows the fast component beating away from the affected side. The symptoms peak within 24 hours and usually last for 3 to 4 days. Autopsy studies have shown cell degeneration of one or more vestibular nerve trunks, a finding similar to that seen in Bell palsy, which affects the facial nerve. A short course (3-5 days) of vestibular suppressants (e.g., meclizine [Antivert], diazepam [Valium]) and antiemetics such as promethazine (Phenergan) can provide symptomatic relief in the acute setting.

Distinguishing between vestibular neuronitis and bacterial labyrinthitis or labyrinthic ischemia is important. The diagnosis of *bacterial labyrinthitis is* based on hearing loss and otitis media or meningitis, and *labyrinthic ischemia* can be distinguished by hearing loss plus associated neurologic symptoms with a history of vascular disease.

Benign Paroxysmal Positional Vertigo

The most common cause of peripheral vestibular vertigo in adults is BPPV. BPPV occurs in all age groups but more often between ages 50 and 70 years. The incidence of BPPV is 11 to 64 per 100,000 persons per year and is twice as common in women as men (Froehling et al., 1991). It is caused when otoconia particles from the utricle or saccule lodge in the posterior semicircular canal and is also referred to as *canalithiasis.* This causes the canal to be a gravity-sensing organ, and head movement results in displacement of the otoconia and a sensation of vertigo.

The Dix-Hallpike maneuver reproduces this vertigo in the patient, resulting in nystagmus (see eFigure 18-3). Characteristics of the nystagmus of BPPV include fatigability, a latency period of 1 to 5 seconds before nystagmus begins after the head is moved, a short duration of nystagmus from 5 to 30 seconds, and reversal of the nystagmus components when the patient is returned to the sitting position. If these characteristics are not present and treatment is not successful, BPPV cannot be diagnosed. In such a case, a CNS lesion is possible. BPPV can be the residual effect of Meniere disease, ear surgery, vestibular neuronitis, or ischemia of the inner ear. Head trauma, even when it is minor, can lead to BPPV. However, one third of cases are idiopathic.

Treatment of BPPV consists of performing repositioning maneuvers with the goal of returning the otoconia to the utricle or saccule (Nguyen-Huynh, 2012). In addition, the patient may attempt to reposition the otoconia at home by sitting upright on the bed and rapidly lying supine with the affected ear facing downward. After 1 minute, the head should be repositioned with the opposite ear facing downward, and the patient should wait another minute. The patient should then return slowly to the upright seated position and repeat this exercise four more times. The entire process is completed twice daily until the symptoms have abated (Hilton and Pinder, 2010).

An expert panel convened by the American Academy of Otolaryngology–Head and Neck Surgery Foundation recommended against "routinely treating BPPV with vestibular suppressant medication such as antihistamines or benzodiazepines" (Bhattacharyya et al., 2008). Because of the variability of symptoms, the clinician must judge each case independently. Resolution occurs in a few weeks or months, and the condition is benign, although it can recur.

Perilymph Fistula

Rapid changes in air pressure (barotrauma), otologic surgery, violent nose blowing or sneezing, head trauma, or chronic ear disease may cause leakage of perilymph fluid from the inner ear into the middle ear and result in episodes of vertigo. Associated signs and symptoms are variable but can include a sudden pop in the ear followed by hearing loss, vertigo, and sometimes tinnitus. Diagnosis can be determined by a fistula test, in which negative and positive pressures are applied to the tympanic membrane using pneumatic otoscopy, causing nystagmus and vertigo.

Labyrinthitis

As with vestibular neuronitis, labyrinthitis causes sudden and severe vertigo. In contrast to vestibular neuronitis, the patient also has tinnitus and hearing loss. The hearing loss is sensorineural, is often severe, and can be permanent. Labyrinthitis is caused by inflammation within the inner ear. The cause is most often a viral infection but can be bacterial. Bacterial labyrinthitis usually results from extension of a bacterial otitis media into the inner ear. A noninfectious *serous* labyrinthitis can also occur after an episode of AOM. Other, less common causes include treponemal infections (syphilis) and rickettsial infection (Lyme disease).

Symptomatic treatment of labyrinthitis is similar to that for vestibular neuronitis. Antibiotics are recommended if a bacterial cause is suspected. As with AOM, bacterial labyrinthitis can, in rare cases, lead to meningitis. Few other conditions cause the constellation of hearing loss, tinnitus, and vertigo, but cerebrovascular ischemia, meningitis, brain abscess, and encephalitis should all be considered. Although the vertigo should resolve over days to weeks, hearing loss and tinnitus can persist.

Drugs known to be ototoxic can cause acute onset of hearing loss and disequilibrium, although this is not true labyrinthitis. These drugs include salicylates, aminoglycosides, loop diuretics, and various chemotherapeutic agents. This cause should be considered in patients who complain of hearing loss or dizziness while taking these medications.

TINNITUS

Tinnitus is a term used to describe an internal noise perceived by the patient. It is usually, but not always, indicative of an otologic problem. Tinnitus is most often subjective (that is, heard only by the patient). However, it can be objective and heard by the patient and the examiner. In most cases, tinnitus is secondary to bilateral SNHL and requires no further evaluation. In rare cases, tinnitus can be a symptom of a vascular abnormality (aneurysm or arteriovenous malformation), hypermetabolic state, or intracranial mass that, if not evaluated, could result in delayed treatment. Middle ear and rarely external ear pathology can also cause tinnitus, as can numerous medications (Table 18-3). The patient's medications should be reviewed.

Evaluation of tinnitus begins with a complete medical history, including duration of symptoms, possible inciting event (e.g., acoustic trauma), and accompanying symptoms (e.g., vertigo, hearing loss, headache, vision changes).

Table 18-3   Causes of Tinnitus

Subjective	Otologic: presbycusis, noise-induced hearing loss, Meniere disease, otosclerosis
	Metabolic: hyperthyroidism, hypothyroidism, hyperlipidemia, vitamin deficiency
	Neurologic: basilar skull fracture, whiplash injury, multiple sclerosis, meningitic effects
	Pharmacologic: aspirin, NSAIDs, aminoglycosides, TCAs, loop diuretics, heavy metals, oral contraceptives, caffeine, cocaine, marijuana
	Dental: temporomandibular joint syndrome
	Psychologic: depression, anxiety
Objective	Vascular abnormalities: AVM, glomus tumors, stenotic carotid artery, vascular loops, persistent stapedial artery, dehiscent jugular bulb, hypertension
	Tympanic muscle disorders: palatomyoclonus, idiopathic stapedial muscle spasm
	Patulous eustachian tube
	CNS anomalies: congenital stenosis of the sylvian aqueduct, type 1 Arnold-Chiari malformation

AVM, Arteriovenous malformation; *CNS,* central nervous system; *NSAID,* nonsteroidal antiinflammatory drug; *TCA,* tricyclic antidepressant.

Specific questions regarding the tinnitus are critical: Is it unilateral or bilateral? What is the quality of the tinnitus (pitch, volume)? Does it sound like a heartbeat or rushing blood? Does it change? A complete ENT evaluation should be performed, and audiometry is mandatory.

In general, if the tinnitus is bilateral, not particularly intrusive, not pulsatile, and associated with symmetric hearing loss, it is likely secondary to the hearing loss itself. The hearing loss requires further evaluation with MRI with contrast if it is asymmetric.

In cases of *pulsatile* tinnitus with normal otoscopy, magnetic resonance angiography (MRA) is performed to evaluate for vascular abnormalities. If otoscopy identifies a retrotympanic mass, temporal bone CT is obtained to evaluate for a vascular mass or abnormality. Blood tests can be performed to rule out anemia or hyperthyroidism, which can result in a hypermetabolic state and cause tinnitus secondary to increased blood flow near the cochlea. Auscultation of the neck, periauricular area, and chest may identify a bruit or murmur, indicating a need for a carotid duplex ultrasound study or echocardiogram, respectively. Most cases of arterial pulsatile tinnitus are secondary to atherosclerotic carotid artery disease. Venous pulsatile tinnitus often improves with digital pressure over the internal jugular vein. Etiologies include idiopathic venous hum, a high-riding jugular bulb, or benign intracranial hypertension.

Effective treatment of tinnitus is difficult and usually requires various approaches. Finding and eliminating potential causes (especially pharmaceutical) is imperative. Patients should be counseled to avoid caffeine and nicotine. A research review by the Agency for Healthcare Research and Quality's (AHRQ's) Effective Healthcare Program found that sertraline was the one selective serotonin reuptake inhibitor that consistently improved reducing loudness, improving quality of life and alleviating severity of tinnitus (Pichora-Fuller et al., 2013). IV lidocaine eliminates tinnitus in some patients but is not practical and has obvious potential side effects. Various homeopathic treatments and nutritional supplements are effective in some cases, but most have not been evaluated in controlled studies. Hearing aids are beneficial in *masking* the tinnitus if hearing loss exists. Tinnitus maskers can be purchased that essentially drown out the tinnitus with various distracting noises. Biofeedback and a technique called *tinnitus retraining therapy* are helpful for some patients. These techniques can be learned through various publications or at a tinnitus treatment center. All patients with obtrusive tinnitus are encouraged to join the American Tinnitus Association, the largest tinnitus support group and an excellent source of reliable information (Newman et al., 2011).

DISORDERS OF THE EXTERNAL EAR

Otitis Externa

The most common cause of pain in the external ear is acute otitis externa. It affects 3% to 10% of the patient population. The pain is caused by inflammation and edema of the ear canal skin, which is normally adherent to the bone and cartilage of the auditory canal. The inflammatory reaction can be caused by bacteria, fungi, or contact dermatitis (see eTable 18-5 online).

Cerumen protects the canal by forming an acidic coat that helps prevent infection. Factors that predispose to otitis externa include absence of cerumen, often from excessive cleaning by the patient; water, which macerates the skin of the auditory canal and raises the pH; and trauma to the skin of the auditory canal from foreign bodies or use of cotton swabs.

When a bacterial organism is suspected, treatment consists of cleaning the ear canal of any debris or drainage and then instilling antibiotic drops with or without steroids. Because the most common bacterial organisms in this infection are *Pseudomonas aeruginosa*, *Peptostreptococcus*, *Bacteroides fragilis*, and *S. aureus*, drops containing ciprofloxacin or neomycin–polymyxin B (Ciprodex, Cortisporin, Coly-Mycin, Pediotic) are effective against these pathogens, combined with a steroid to decrease inflammation, pain, and pruritus. A recent study found Ciprodex to be more effective against *P. aeruginosa* than neomycin–polymyxin B–hydrocortisone (Dohar et al., 2009).

The clinician must use judgment in assessing the severity of the infection and treat accordingly. If the infection spreads beyond the auditory canal, oral antimicrobials are indicated. If clinical improvement is not apparent after 48 hours, the patient needs to be reexamined for additional treatment or referral to an otorhinolaryngologist.

Fungal infections comprise fewer than 10% of external otitis cases. The most common fungi are *Aspergillus niger* and *Candida* spp. and are more prevalent in tropical climates. Itching is a more common complaint than pain in fungal ear infections. Thorough cleaning of the ear canal is the primary duty of the physician in this infection. Drops that are effective include 2% acetic acid with or without a steroid. Clotrimazole drops or powder can also be used to treat fungal infections of the ear canal (van Bolen et al., 2003).

Approximately 90% of necrotizing (malignant) otitis externa is seen in immunocompromised patients such as patients with diabetes, patients with acquired immunodeficiency syndrome (AIDS), and those receiving chemotherapy. Systemic antibiotics are mandatory in these cases. Antipseudomonal antimicrobial agents should be administered intravenously in the hospital setting, and surgical debridement is often necessary. Complications from necrotizing otitis externa include facial nerve palsy, mastoiditis, meningitis, and even death (Quick, 1999).

Other conditions that affect the external auditory canal include impacted cerumen, seborrheic dermatitis, psoriasis, contact dermatitis, and staphylococcal furunculosis. Symptoms and signs include pruritus, edema, scaling, crusting, oozing, and fissuring of the external auditory canal. Treatment of the underlying disease is the primary goal. Corticosteroid preparations are indicated for seborrheic dermatitis, psoriasis, and contact dermatitis. Oral antibiotics and sometimes incision and drainage are required for staphylococcal furunculosis.

Auricular Hematoma

Blunt auricular trauma, most commonly in wrestlers and boxers, may shear the perichondrium from the underlying cartilage, leading to a hematoma. The presence of a fluctuant swelling with loss of normal auricular landmarks helps to distinguish a hematoma from ecchymosis. If left untreated, an auricular hematoma may cause fibrosis and neocartilage formation, leading to a deformity of the auricle termed *cauliflower ear*. Therefore, treatment in a timely manner is recommended.

Although a Cochrane review could not define the best treatment for an acute auricular hematoma, a frequently successful treatment involves incision and drainage with dental rolls sutured to the anterior and posterior auricle (Figure 18-5). Needle aspiration alone often leads to recurrences. The bolster is usually left in place for 4 to 7 days, with the patient permitted to return to wrestling or boxing with headgear. Prophylactic antistaphylococcal antibiotics are given. For a long-standing hematoma or a cauliflower ear, debridement of fibrosis and cartilage is necessary (Jones and Mahendran, 2008).

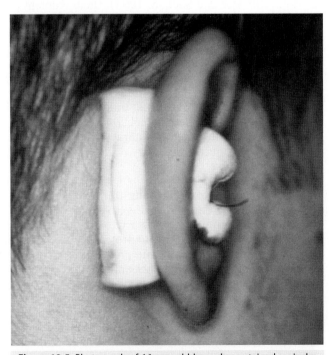

Figure 18-5 Photograph of 16-year-old boy who sustained auricular hematoma in a wrestling match. He underwent incision and drainage with placement of dental rolls.

External Auditory Canal Foreign Bodies

A common problem seen in family physicians' offices is a patient with an external auditory canal foreign body. A wide variety of objects can be found. In one study of 191 patients with aural foreign bodies, 27 different objects were discovered (Ansley and Cunningham, 1998). The most common were beads, plastic toys, pebbles, insects (especially cockroaches), popcorn kernels, earrings, paper, peas, cotton, pencil erasers, and seeds. When a patient presents with a chronic dry cough that has not responded to the usual measures, the physician should look for an aural foreign body (causing irritation of the ninth cranial nerve).

Removal of an external auditory canal foreign body is simplified if the object is in the lateral third of the external auditory canal. Objects within the medial two thirds pose a greater challenge. A variety of instruments can be used, depending on the object, including cerumen loops, alligator forceps, and otologic-tip suctions. Irrigation with body-temperature sterile water often dislodges the object. Hygroscopic objects such as vegetables, beans, and other food matter can swell and make the object even more impacted and should not be irrigated. Disk batteries should be removed immediately because of the possibility of lique-faction necrosis of the external auditory canal. Aural irrigation is contraindicated because wetting of the battery leads to leakage of electrolyte solution.

Smooth, round objects pose a difficult problem because, in trying to remove them, they are often pushed farther into the canal. Aural irrigation or even cyanoacrylate glue on the tip of a straightened paperclip is effective in removing objects that are difficult to retrieve. Methods to remove cockroaches or other insects include microscope immersion oil, mineral oil, or lidocaine. The effect of mineral oil or microscope immersion oil is to drown the insect, and lido-caine tends to make cockroaches crawl rapidly out of the ear canal (Bressler and Shelton, 1993). Otomicroscopy is often required for safe removal.

Depending on their age, fewer than 35% of patients should require anesthesia. The younger the patient, the more likely anesthesia will be required. Objects with sharp edges are best removed with an operating microscope with the patient under general anesthesia. Complications of foreign body removal include canal wall trauma and tympanic membrane perforation. Immobilization of the patient is the key to successful removal of aural foreign bodies, and at least two assistants are necessary.

Cerumen

Glandular secretions from the outer third of the external auditory canal and desquamated epithelium combine to form cerumen. Cerumen is necessary to provide a hydro-phobic and acidic environment to protect the underlying external ear canal epithelium and prevent infection. The external auditory canal is self-cleaning, with cerumen slowly pushed laterally to the external meatus.

Cerumen impaction is the symptomatic accumulation of cerumen in the external canal or an accumulation that prevents a needed assessment of the ear. Complete occlusion is not necessary. Symptoms may include hearing loss, tinnitus, pruritus, fullness, otalgia, cough, odor, and dizziness. Impaction often results from instrumentation with cotton-tipped applicators, which should be discouraged. Elderly patients with changes to external canal epithelium, patients with external canal abnormalities (e.g., osteomas, exostoses, stenosis), and users of hearing aids and earplugs are also at risk for impaction. Excessive cerumen production as a primary problem is relatively rare.

In most people, cleaning the external meatus with a finger in a washcloth while bathing is sufficient to maintain the ear canals. Treatment of cerumen impaction by the clinician may involve ceruminolytic agents, irrigation, or manual removal. Ceruminolytic agents include water-based; oil-based; and non–water-, non–oil-based solutions. A Cochrane review found that any type of ear drop (including water and saline) is more effective than no treatment, but the study quality was lacking (Burton and Glasziou, 2009). Office irrigations may be performed using a large syringe with a large angiocatheter tip. The type of irrigant solution used is probably not critical, although a tepid or warm temperature is important to prevent the patient from becoming vertiginous from a labyrinthine caloric response. Instilling a ceruminolytic 15 minutes before irrigation may improve the success rate. Irrigations should not be performed in those with tympanic membrane perforations or previous ear surgery. Of note, irrigation with tap water has been implicated as a causative factor in malignant otitis externa. Therefore, instilling an acidifying ear drop after irrigation in patients with diabetes is recommended. Manual removal requires knowledge of ear anatomy and special care to avoid trauma. A handheld otoscope with a curette and other instruments may be used. Otolaryngologists often use binocular microscopy to aid with visualization. Patients inquiring about ear candling should be informed that it has not been shown to be effective and presents a risk of thermal injury to the ear (Burton and Doree, 2008).

Frostbite

The ears, nose, and cheeks, in that order, are most at risk for frostbite. Exposure to subfreezing temperature is the main risk factor, but wind chill also greatly affects heat loss from the skin by convection. Protective clothing greatly diminishes the risk.

There are three grades: grade I frostbite, in which the skin is erythematous and edematous; grade II frostbite, in which the skin blisters and forms bullae; and grade III frostbite, which results in local necrosis of the dermis over 1 to 2 weeks. To assess the severity of frostbite, the physician must examine the tissue from several hours up to 2 days after the typical skin blanching occurs.

Treatment consists of quickly warming the ear with gauze soaked in saline at 38° to 40°C (100.4°-104.0°F). Any blisters that form should be allowed to reabsorb spontaneously. Topical antibiotic ointment can be applied, and viability of the tissue should be assessed periodically.

Lacerations

When there is trauma to the ear requiring suture closure, careful realignment is mandatory to maintain the auricular contour. The extent of the injury should be evaluated thoroughly with the tissue anesthetized with 1% lidocaine (without epinephrine). This allows a careful evaluation of the wound as well as a meticulous suture closure. Lacerations involving only the skin can be closed with everting nonabsorbable sutures. An earlobe that is torn from earring trauma can be closed in layers using absorbable chromic gut suture to close the dermis and nonabsorbable 5-0 or 6-0 suture to close the skin. Lacerations that involve cartilage, perichondrium, and skin must also be closed in layers but might best be referred to a specialist in otorhinolaryngology or to a plastic surgeon.

DISORDERS OF THE MIDDLE EAR

Bullous Myringitis

Bullous myringitis refers to painful inflammatory bullae on the tympanic membrane. The blebs appear hemorrhagic. It was formerly thought that bullous myringitis was caused by *Mycoplasma pneumoniae* infection. Roberts (1980), however, summarized six studies involving 858 patients with bullous myringitis, and *M. pneumoniae* was isolated from only one. The cause is usually viral but can be bacterial in some cases. Studies have confirmed that bacterial cultures from bullous fluid are similar to cultures from middle ear fluid taken from patients with AOM. The main isolates are *Streptococcus pneumoniae, H. influenzae,* and β-hemolytic streptococci. The tympanic blistering is probably a nonspecific reaction and simply a variant of AOM that should be treated as such.

It is important to distinguish bullous myringitis from acute otitis externa, which requires topical treatment, and from herpes zoster oticus, which can lead to cranial neuropathy and requires antiviral treatment. Neither of these conditions is usually limited to only tympanic membrane involvement.

Otitis Media

Acute Otitis Media. The most common infection for which children are seen in a physician's office is AOM. The annual cost of AOM in the United States is an estimated $2.88 billion (Ahmed et al., 2014). By age 7 years, 93% of children have had at least one episode of AOM, and 75% have had recurrent infections. AOM can occur at any age, but the highest incidence is between 6 and 24 months in the United States.

The primary cause of bacterial colonization of the middle ear is eustachian tube dysfunction. Abnormal tubal compliance in addition to delayed innervation of the tensor veli palatini muscle leads to collapse of the eustachian tube. Aerobic and anaerobic organisms, as well as viruses, can contribute to middle ear infection (Lieberthal et al., 2013). The three most common bacteria involved in AOM are *S. pneumoniae* (25%-40% of cases), *H. influenzae* (10%-30%), and *Moraxella catarrhalis* (2%-15%) (Klein, 2004). Risk factors most often associated with AOM are child care outside the home and parental smoking. Table 18-4 lists the common risk factors for AOM. A viral upper respiratory infection usually precedes an episode of AOM.

The criteria necessary to confirm the diagnosis of AOM are: acute onset of ear pain (holding, tugging, rubbing of the ear in a nonverbal child) or intense erythema of the TM, moderate to severe bulging of the TM, or new onset of otorrhea not due to OE. If there is no middle ear effusion (MEE), AOM may not be diagnosed (Lieberthal et al., 2013; Level of evidence [grade]: B). Middle ear effusion can be diagnosed by direct visualization of air-fluid levels behind the

Table 18-4 Common Risk Factors for Acute Otitis Media

Male gender

Bottle feeding, especially in the supine position

Exposure to upper respiratory tract infections (e.g., daycare setting, winter season)

Genetic factors

Ethnic factors (e.g., Inuit or Native American)

Parental smoking

Allergy

Craniofacial abnormalities (e.g., cleft palate)

Previous episode of acute otitis media, particularly during the preceding 3 months

Use of a pacifier

Table 18-5 Causes of Otalgia Other than Acute Otitis Media

Abscessed teeth

Cervical arthritis

Dental malocclusion

Nasopharyngeal carcinoma

Sinus infection

Sore throat

Temporomandibular joint disorders

tympanic membrane, a bulging drum, lack of movement on pneumatic otoscopy, or a flat tympanogram readout that indicates no tympanic membrane movement and therefore the presence of middle ear effusion. Redness of the tympanic membrane, pain, and fever are the most common signs and symptoms of middle ear inflammation (see eTable 18-6 online). Erythema of the tympanic membrane without middle ear effusion is myringitis or tympanitis and is a separate diagnosis from AOM. Ear pain in the presence of a normal-appearing, flaccid tympanic membrane indicates causes other than AOM (Table 18-5).

The standard of care for the treatment of AOM in children older than 6 months depends on the severity of the symptoms. Antibiotics should be prescribed for children 6 months and older with severe symptoms (moderate or severe otalgia or temperature 102.2°F or higher (Grade B). When the symptoms are nonsevere, the parents can be given the option of observation or antibiotics (Grade B). The decision either to begin antibiotics or to observe the patient without them is based on the certainty of diagnosis, severity of symptoms, and age of the patient (Lieberthal et al., 2013) (Table 18-6).

When the criteria for the diagnosis of AOM are met and the symptoms are bilateral, the diagnosis is certain, and antibiotic therapy is indicated for any child 2 years old or younger (Lieberthal et al., 2013). Observation is allowed for this age group if the symptoms are not severe and unilateral. For children older than 2 years, observation is an option if the illness is not severe and the parents can be relied on to report the patient's status and can obtain medication if necessary. Severe illness is defined as moderate to severe otalgia and fever higher than 39°C (102.2°F). When two or fewer diagnostic criteria are present, diagnosis is considered uncertain, and observation is allowed for children 6 months and older with nonsevere illness (Toll and Nuñez, 2012).

Table 18-6   Treatment of Acute Otitis Media

Features	Treatment
LOW-RISK PATIENTS	
Older than 6 yr, no antimicrobial therapy within past 3 mo, no otorrhea, not in daycare, and temperature <38°C (<100.5°F)	Amoxicillin: 40-50 mg/kg/day in divided doses for 5 days
HIGH-RISK PATIENTS	
Younger than 2 yr, in daycare, treated with antimicrobials within past 3 months, otorrhea, or temperature >38°C (>100.5°F)	Amoxicillin: 80-90 mg/kg/day in divided doses for 10 days
TREATMENT FAILURE	
Signs and symptoms persisting after 3 days	Amoxicillin–clavulanic acid (Augmentin): 80-90 mg/kg/day for 7-10 days Cefuroxime axetil (Ceftin): 20-30 mg/kg/day bid for 7-10 days Ceftriaxone (Rocephin): 50 mg/kg intramuscularly for 1 dose not to exceed 1 g for children <12 yr for 1-3 days or for >12 yr 1-2 g/day for 3-4 days depending on severity of symptoms
PENICILLIN-ALLERGIC PATIENTS	
Any	Cefuroxime axetil: 20 mo-5 yr, 30 mg/kg/day divided q 12 hr, max: 1000 mg/day Cefpodoxime: 2 mo-5 yr, 5 mg/kg/day, divided q 12-24 hr, max: 1000 mg/day; 6-12 yr, 10 mg/kg/day, max: 400 mg/day Ceftriaxone (see above)

bid, Twice a day; *q*, every;

Resistance of *S. pneumoniae* to penicillin is an increasing problem and ranges from 15% to 50% depending on the area. The mechanism of resistance is based on an alteration of penicillin-binding proteins rather than the production of β-lactamase, as occurs with *H. influenzae* and *M. catarrhalis* infections. Resistance rates are higher in children than in adults, especially if the children are in daycare or have received antimicrobial therapy in the previous 3 months.

The dose to treat AOM is 80 to 90 mg/kg/day in two divided doses (Lieberthal et al., 2013). This allows the drug to overcome resistance in the causative organism. For patients with a penicillin allergy or those who have been treated with amoxicillin in the past 30 days, alternative medications include cefuroxime, cefpodoxime, cefprozil, or ceftriaxone. A meta-analysis found that first-generation cephalosporins have cross-allergy with penicillin, although the cross-allergy with second- and third-generation cephalosporins is negligible (Pichichero and Casey, 2007). Macrolides are not recommended for AOM in children because *H. influenzae* is the dominant organism causing AOM in this age group. Middle ear fluid becomes sterile 3 to 6 days after starting treatment, so the duration of therapy for uncomplicated AOM in children older than 2 years of age is 5 to 7 days.

If the initial antibiotic fails to resolve symptoms in 72 hours (pain, fever, redness and bulging of the tympanic membrane, otorrhea), high-dose amoxicillin–clavulanic acid is recommended. Alternatives in penicillin-allergic patients include the antibiotics cited earlier. Patients who do not respond to amoxicillin–clavulanic acid therapy should be treated with intramuscular ceftriaxone for 3 days. This antibiotic in a single dose can also be used initially if the child is vomiting or unable to keep down oral medication. Doses of antimicrobials are given in Table 18-6.

Influenza vaccine has been shown to decrease the number of cases of AOM in immunized patients compared with control participants and is recommended for all children according to the Advisory Committee on Immunization Practices, AAP and AAFP. Breastfeeding should be

Table 18-7   Guidelines for Treatment of Otitis Media with Effusion in children 2 months to 12 years

Duration of Otitis Media with Effusion	Treatment
6 wk	Observation Hearing evaluation optional
3 mo	Hearing evaluation; if 20-dB hearing loss
4-6 mo	Referral for polyethylene tube if there is hearing loss

Adapted from Rosenfeld RM, Andes D, Bhattacharyya N, et al. Clinical practice guideline: adult sinusitis. *Otolaryngol Head Neck Surg.* 2007;137 (3 suppl):S1-S31.

encouraged for the first 6 months of life, and tobacco smoke should be avoided.

Otitis Media with Effusion. Otitis media with effusion (OME) is defined as persistent middle ear fluid without pain, fever, or redness of the tympanic membrane. It is often the result of AOM but can occur de novo. About 90% of children have OME before they reach school age. About 80% to 90% of cases resolve within 3 months and 95% within 1 year. Table 18-7 provides the AHRQ guidelines for treatment of OME.

Tympanometry can be used to judge the presence of middle ear fluid. It is important to document the affected ear, the duration of the effusion, and the presence and severity of symptoms associated with OME. The latter include a feeling of fullness in the ear, popping, mild pain, hearing loss, balance problems, and delayed language development.

If OME persists for 3 months, a comprehensive hearing evaluation should be performed. A 40-decibel (dB) loss (or worse) in hearing bilaterally mandates referral for evaluation for polyethylene (PE) tube placement. Management of hearing loss between 6 and 39 dB depends on parent or caregiver preferences and can include strategies to improve the listening and learning environment or referral for tube placement. If the hearing loss is 5 dB or less, repeat testing in 3 months may be performed if the middle ear effusion continues at that time. Follow-up testing is recommended every 3 to 6 months until the effusion resolves unless significant hearing loss occurs or there is evidence for structural abnormalities of the eardrum or middle ear. In these patients, PE tube placement is the preferred course.

When referring to a surgeon, the primary care physician must provide an adequate history of the duration of the middle ear effusion, developmental state of the child, and pertinent information such as a history of AOM. Physician and parental expectations for the referral should be clarified. Ultimately, the decision for PE tube placement should be based on a consensus among all parties involved. The possibility of repeat surgery after tube extrusion is 20% to 50%, and with reoperation, adenoidectomy is recommended in children with normal palates because it reduces the need for future surgery by 50%.

Recurrent Otitis Media. Three episodes of AOM within 6 months with complete resolution between episodes or four episodes in 12 months defines recurrent otitis media. Although the evidence is conflicting, a Cochrane review in 2006 showed only minimal improvement in recurrences, and this decrease in episodes only occurred when the antibiotic was continued. The authors recommended discouraging amoxicillin prophylaxis in children with recurrent otitis media not only because it is minimally effective but also to prevent antibiotic side effects and the acquisition of resistant pneumococci (Lieberthal et al., 2013). Pneumococcal vaccination has no beneficial effect on either health-related quality of life or functional health status in children 1 to 7 years old with recurrent AOM (Brouwer et al., 2005).

Tympanostomy tubes and also adenoidectomy may be offered to patients and may be beneficial in cases of recurrent AOM requiring multiple rounds of antibiotics within 6 to 12 months, especially if the episodes are severe.

Chronic Suppurative Otitis Media. Chronic suppurative otitis media (CSOM) is the presence of persistent purulent otorrhea through a perforated tympanic membrane or tympanostomy tube. A persistent tympanic membrane perforation may result from AOM, chronic eustachian tube dysfunction, or trauma. A cholesteatoma or rarely a tumor may also result in CSOM. Otorrhea may also be from chronic otitis externa, which may be difficult to distinguish from CSOM until treatment is initiated. Causes of otorrhea from the middle ear may not always be from middle ear bacterial infection (see eTable 18-7).

Associated symptoms often include hearing loss and tinnitus. Increasing pain, vertigo, or facial palsy imply a possible impending complication of CSOM (discussed later) and require urgent otolaryngologist consultation. Binocular otomicroscopy allows better visualization and suctioning of purulent material compared with routine otoscopy. Imaging is reserved for medical treatment failures or if a complication is suspected. CT is helpful to evaluate for bony erosion. MRI is indicated with suspicion of CNS involvement.

Initial management should include culture and sensitivity of the discharge to allow appropriate antibiotic selection.

If chronic otitis externa is suspected, the specimen should also be sent for fungal culture. Empiric antimicrobials should be started with coverage against the usual pathogens, which include *S. pneumoniae, H. influenzae, S. aureus, Pseudomonas* spp., and anaerobes. A Cochrane review demonstrated that ototopicals are superior to oral antibiotics. Quinolone ototopicals are safe for use in the middle ear. Topical aminoglycosides carry a risk of ototoxicity, but in some cases their use outweighs the risk. Systemic antibiotics may be required in severe cases or when copious drainage impairs administration of ototopicals. Aural toilet with an acetic acid solution (1 part distilled water, 1 part white vinegar) may be helpful to clear debris and provide antisepsis (Macfadyen et al., 2006a, 2006b).

If otorrhea resolves but a tympanic membrane perforation persists, the patient may be offered a tympanoplasty (tympanic membrane repair) to reduce the risk of recurrence and to improve hearing. If medical therapy fails to control inflammation, a tympanomastoidectomy may be indicated to eradicate infection, aerate the middle ear and mastoid, and repair the tympanic membrane. *Chronic tympanostomy tube otorrhea* is treated the same as typical CSOM. In recalcitrant cases, however, tube removal or replacement may be indicated. Also, adenoidectomy may be considered because chronic adenoiditis may act as a nidus for infection.

Complications. Although rare since the advent of antibiotics, complications of otitis media must be recognized early to avoid significant potential morbidity and mortality (Table 18-8). Chronic or recurrent otitis media can result in scarring of the tympanic membrane (*myringosclerosis* or *tympanosclerosis*), which alone is usually of no consequence. If scarring involves the ossicles, however, hearing loss can result. Tympanic membrane retraction or perforation can also occur.

INTRATEMPORAL COMPLICATIONS. Extension of the infection into the mastoid air cells can lead to *acute mastoiditis*. The signs and symptoms of acute mastoiditis are fever and postauricular tenderness, erythema, and edema. It is important to recognize that acute mastoiditis is a clinical and not a radiologic diagnosis. Therefore, inflammatory changes on a temporal bone CT must be correlated with examination findings to be called acute mastoiditis. Furthermore, acute mastoiditis must be distinguished from an auricular cellulitis secondary to acute otitis externa. *Facial paralysis* may result from AOM or CSOM because of inflammation along the facial nerve as it courses through the middle ear space.

Table 18-8 Complications of Otitis Media

Acute mastoiditis

Brain abscess

Epidural abscess

Facial nerve paralysis

Labyrinthitis

Meningitis

Sigmoid sinus thrombophlebitis

Subdural abscess

Subperiosteal abscess

Cholesteatoma

Treatment of acute mastoiditis and facial nerve paralysis includes IV antibiotics, insertion of a tympanostomy tube for drainage, and sometimes emergent mastoidectomy. Infection within the middle ear space can extend into the inner ear, leading to labyrinthitis. Symptoms may include vertigo, tinnitus, and SNHL. Expeditious initiation of broad-spectrum antibiotics and in some cases insertion of a tympanostomy tube may be necessary. *Petrositis* is a rare complication involving inflammation of the petrous apex mastoid air cells. *Gradenigo syndrome*, which includes retro-orbital pain, otorrhea, and cranial nerve VI palsy, may result. Treatment includes IV antibiotics and surgical drainage.

INTRACRANIAL COMPLICATIONS. The most serious complications of otitis media involve CNS extension of the infection and include sigmoid sinus thrombosis, meningitis, and brain abscess. Warning signs of an impending CNS complication include increasing pain, headache, spiking fever, or altered mental status. Evaluation may include MRI and lumbar puncture. Suspicion of CNS complication often requires urgent neurosurgical, ENT, and infectious diseases consultations. High-dose IV antibiotics and sometimes urgent surgery (mastoidectomy or craniotomy) are required to prevent significant morbidity or mortality. *Otitic meningitis* is a major cause of morbidity in the pediatric population. Fortunately, vaccines against Hib and *Pneumococcus* spp. (Prevnar) have decreased these occurrences.

A "cholesteatoma" is a destructive epithelial cyst in the middle ear that may extend to the mastoid air cells. The term is a misnomer because of the lack of cholesterol and presence of only squamous epithelium and keratin debris. The external ear canal and outer layer of the tympanic membrane are lined with squamous epithelium. Keratin debris is continuously sloughed as new epithelial cells mature. In a normal ear, the debris slowly migrates to the external meatus, where it is washed away. In contrast to the external ear, the middle ear space is lined with respiratory epithelium, which produces no keratin debris. Cholesteatomas form when squamous epithelium is abnormally located within the middle ear space, allowing the keratin debris to accumulate.

Cholesteatomas often result in CSOM with findings of purulent otorrhea, polyps, and granulation. However, some cholesteatomas are dry, with the finding of a white mass visible behind the tympanic membrane or a white mass or crusting on the tympanic membrane itself. A cholesteatoma must be differentiated from *myringosclerosis*, which is usually flat, white scarring on the tympanic membrane. Enzymatic properties, inflammation, and pressure may lead to bone erosion and hearing loss. If left untreated, serious problems may result, including facial nerve paralysis, labyrinthine fistula, and intracranial complications (see Table 18-8).

Congenital cholesteatomas occur without a history of tympanic membrane perforation or retraction and are postulated to result from congenital rests of epithelium in the middle ear space. These may occur in children with no significant history of otitis media and are usually diagnosed as an incidental white mass behind the tympanic membrane.

Primary acquired cholesteatomas result from prolonged eustachian tube dysfunction. Negative middle ear pressure results in a *retraction pocket* of the tympanic membrane, usually at the region of the pars flaccida. Squamous epithelium may become trapped and accumulate in the retraction pocket, resulting in a cholesteatoma. Any retraction pocket of the tympanic membrane requires further evaluation to prevent progression to cholesteatoma.

Secondary acquired cholesteatomas occur as a result of a tympanic membrane perforation. In some cases, a perforation of the tympanic membrane may allow the outer squamous epithelium to migrate into the middle ear space, leading to cholesteatoma formation.

Although aggressive medical treatment may reduce inflammation, surgical treatment is necessary for almost all cholesteatomas. In less advanced cholesteatomas, the external auditory canal is spared in surgery, a "canal wall up" tympanomastoidectomy. Close follow-up is required because of the risk of recurrence from microscopic disease or persistent eustachian tube dysfunction. In more advanced disease, the posterior canal is removed, termed a "canal wall down" tympanomastoidectomy (modified radical and radical mastoidectomy). The canal wall-down procedures are more likely to result in a conductive hearing loss (CHL), but the mastoid cavity becomes accessible through a larger external canal, thereby exteriorizing the cholesteatoma. Typically, semiannual mastoid bowl debridement is necessary to remove squamous and ceruminous debris to prevent inflammation.

Traumatic Tympanic Membrane Perforations

Traumatic perforation of the tympanic membrane may result from barotrauma (water skiing or diving injuries, blast injuries, blows to side of head), ear canal instrumentation (cotton-tipped applicators, bobby pins, paper clips, cerumen curettes), or otitis media (see earlier discussion). The patient usually complains of acute pain that subsides quickly, associated with bloody otorrhea. Severe vertigo can occur but is transient in most cases. Persistent vertigo suggests inner ear involvement (perilymphatic fistula). Hearing loss and tinnitus are also common.

Findings may include fresh blood in the canal and around the perforation. Any medial canal clots or debris should not be removed or irrigated except under microscopy. Secondary bacterial infection may require treatment with ototopical antibiotics. Topical fluoroquinolones are safe for use in the middle ear. Audiologic evaluation is necessary to rule out SNHL. If a tuning fork examination indicates SNHL or is unreliable, the patient should be referred for complete audiologic and ENT evaluation.

In uncomplicated cases, the perforation is expected to heal spontaneously over days to weeks. The patient should be instructed to keep the ear dry during this time. If the perforation has not healed after several weeks, a tympanoplasty to close the perforation and, if necessary, repair ossicles is indicated. Repair of the perforation may improve hearing, reduce infection, and prevent cholesteatoma formation.

Barotrauma and Barotitis

Changes in altitude while flying (or scuba diving) can lead to rapid changes in middle ear pressure, leading to accumulation of serous middle ear fluid or blood. Symptoms may include aural fullness, otalgia, and CHL. In most cases, the fluid is resorbed, although this may take several weeks. *Autoinflation* maneuvers (popping the ears) may hasten recovery. Oral and topical decongestants, nasal steroid sprays, or a short course of corticosteroids may be helpful. Antibiotics are indicated only if there are signs of infection. If fluid persists or is troublesome to the patient, a myringotomy allows the fluid to be drained. Tympanostomy tube insertion may be indicated for persistent middle ear fluid.

Rarely, a rapid change in middle ear pressure can lead to the creation of a *perilymphatic fistula* between the inner and middle ear. The patient complains of severe vertigo and hearing loss (sensorineural) (see "Vertigo"). Urgent ENT consultation is indicated.

HEARING LOSS

Hearing loss results from an interruption in the transmission of sound or subsequent nerve impulses in one or more areas of the ear. Recognition and treatment of hearing loss are imperative; unrecognized or untreated hearing loss may result in severe psychosocial ramifications in both adults and children. In the elderly population, hearing loss may lead to social withdrawal and depression. In the pediatric population, hearing loss may cause speech or cognitive delays. Hearing loss also has significant safety implications when it interferes with awareness of warning sounds (e.g., car horns, sirens, fire alarms). The four types of hearing loss are:

1. *CHL* occurs when there is a failure of normal propagation of acoustic energy through the conducting portions of the ear, which include the external auditory canal and the middle ear.
2. *SNHL* occurs from dysfunction of the inner ear, which may be caused by a failure of the generation of nerve signals in the cochlea by the cochlear hair cells or propagation of electrical signals along the cochlear division of the eighth cranial nerve.
3. *Mixed hearing loss (MHL)* occurs when hearing loss results from both CHL and SNHL.
4. *Central hearing loss* can result from ischemic or traumatic brain injuries.

Hearing loss may be subclassified according to whether it is *acquired* or *congenital*. Hearing loss is further classified based on its *severity* (mild, moderate, severe, profound), *sidedness* (right, left, bilateral), *stability* (stable, progressive, fluctuating), and *cause*.

Evaluation includes noting the onset and duration of the hearing loss, any inciting events, the subjective severity of the hearing loss, and any psychosocial impact. Associated ear symptoms, medical history, and a history of ototoxic medication exposure are also important. Although history and examination provide clues to the etiology of the hearing loss, comprehensive audiometric evaluation is essential to making a diagnosis. Table 18-9 lists the most common types of CHL and SNHL.

Otosclerosis

Otosclerosis is caused by sclerotic fixation of the stapes and is the most common cause of CHL in the adult population with no previous history of trauma or infection. It is autosomal dominant in inheritance and more common in women than in men. Otosclerosis is usually bilateral and progressive. Treatment options include no treatment, amplification (hearing aid), fluoride treatment (stabilizes

Table 18-9 Common Types of Conductive and Sensorineural Hearing Loss

Conductive Hearing Loss	Sensorineural Hearing Loss
Cholesteatoma	Acoustic neuroma
Cerumen impaction	Diabetes
Foreign body in ear canal	Hereditary (congenital) loss
Ossicular problems	Idiopathic loss
Otitis media with effusion	Meniere disease
Otosclerosis	Multiple sclerosis
Retracted tympanic membrane (eustachian tube dysfunction)	Noise-induced loss
	Ototoxicity
Tumor of the ear canal or middle ear	Perilymphatic fistula
Tympanic membrane perforation	Presbycusis
Tympanosclerosis	Syphilis

but does not improve hearing), and surgery (stapedectomy). Stapedectomy involves removing and replacing the stapes with a tiny prosthesis. This procedure has a success rate of greater than 95%. Risks of surgery, although rare, include worsened hearing, tympanic membrane perforation, changes in taste, and disequilibrium.

Sudden Sensorineural Hearing Loss

See "Emergencies."

Presbycusis

Presbycusis is an all-inclusive term to describe the process of hearing loss related to aging. An estimated 30% to 35% of adults age 65 to 75 years and 40% to 50% of adults older than 75 years have hearing loss. Symptoms of presbycusis include gradually decreasing hearing acuity, especially for higher pitch tones (women's and children's voices) and in certain situations (with background noise). Tinnitus is common.

The cause of presbycusis is likely multifactorial, but ultimately the loss of cochlear *hair cell* function is thought to be the cause in most cases. Hair cell damage or loss can result from chronic noise exposure, genetic predisposition, and ototoxic medications. The hearing loss may also be caused by neurovascular injury from chronic conditions such as hypertension or diabetes, which can affect the cochlea or cochlear nerve. Hormonal conditions such as hypothyroidism should be considered, as should unusual conditions such as tertiary syphilis. Central auditory problems might be the cause, from dementia, cerebrovascular disease, or cerebrovascular accident (cerebrovascular accident [CVA], stroke).

Although the term "presbycusis" implies sensorineural loss, CHL should also be considered, including cerumen impaction, chronic OME, and otosclerosis (see Table 18-9).

Acoustic Neuroma

An acoustic neuroma (or more precisely, *vestibular schwannoma*) is a benign tumor that arises from the Schwann cells of cranial nerve VIII. Acoustic neuromas account for about 10% of all intracranial tumors. They are most commonly diagnosed in middle age. They are slightly more common in women than men. They are usually sporadic but may be associated with neurofibromatosis 1 or 2 (NF-1, NF-2). Most patients with NF-2 will develop bilateral acoustic neuromas. Acoustic neuromas in NF-1 are much less common.

The primary symptoms of vestibular schwannoma are asymmetric hearing loss (sensorineural) and tinnitus. The hearing loss is usually gradual in onset and progressive but can occur suddenly. Disequilibrium is not usually the chief complaint on presentation, but patients often admit to mild unsteadiness. Larger tumors can cause dysesthesia around the ear, facial weakness, or both. If the neuroma is diagnosed late, patients can manifest cerebellar symptoms and symptoms of mass effect and obstructing hydrocephalus.

After a complete neuro-otologic examination and audiologic evaluation, an MRI scan of the brain with fine cuts through the internal auditory canal with gadolinium contrast is necessary for diagnosis.

Treatment options include observation, surgery, or stereotactic radiotherapy. Most vestibular schwannomas require treatment to prevent cerebral complications from future growth. If the patient is aged or infirm, watchful waiting may be considered. Very small tumors may be observed because the rate of growth is often slow. Surgical treatment involves either a translabyrinthine resection if hearing is poor or a craniotomy for hearing preservation. Stereotactic radiotherapy has the obvious advantage of avoiding major surgery. Success is similar to surgery for smaller tumors. Shortcomings of this treatment include delayed facial paresis, tumor recurrence (which requires routine monitoring), and the potential for radiation-induced malignancies in the future.

Hearing Loss from Acoustic Energy

Excessive noise exposure is an important and usually preventable cause of hearing loss. Hearing loss can result from chronic or acute noise exposure, usually causing injury at the level of the cochlear hair cells. However, acute acoustic trauma can also cause injury to the tympanic membrane and middle ear structures.

Chronic noise exposure may be recreational or vocational. The Occupational Safety and Health Administration (OSHA) has established guidelines for safe limits for acute and chronic noise exposure to prevent occupational noise-induced hearing loss. Exposure to noise of 90 dB or less is permissible for up to 8 hours per day. As the noise intensity increases, the permissible duration of exposure decreases. OSHA outlines procedures for hearing protection and monitoring. These standards also can help provide guidelines to minimize excessive recreational noise exposure. Recreational activities known to cause excessive noise include hunting or target shooting with firearms; use of power tools or power lawn equipment; attendance at sporting venues, motor racing events, action movies, or concerts; and listening to loud music on headphones. Hearing protection or avoidance is recommended for such activities.

Acute exposure to excessively loud noise can cause CHL or SNHL. CHL can result from a blast-type injury that leads to tympanic membrane perforation or ossicle injury. The conductive component of the hearing loss is usually reparable, but severe acoustic trauma can also cause sensorineural loss. SNHL from acute acoustic trauma is usually the result of temporary hair cell dysfunction or permanent injury, leading to transient or permanent *threshold shifts*, respectively. A concussive or blast injury (e.g.,

slap, airbag deployment to ear) can result in the formation of a labyrinthine fistula from the inner ear into the middle ear, which causes severe vertigo and SNHL. Most fistulas close spontaneously with bed rest, but some require middle ear exploration and repair. However, the SNHL is usually permanent.

Hearing Loss in the Pediatric Population

Congenital hearing loss is often hereditary but may be secondary to an intrauterine insult or infection. Of the hereditary variety, the majority are autosomal recessive and nonsyndromic. Risk factors for congenital hearing loss include a family history of hearing loss, facial abnormalities, ICU admission, history of meningitis, syndromes known to be associated with hearing loss, low Apgar scores at birth, medications known to cause hearing loss (e.g., aminoglycosides), elevated bilirubin, some prenatal maternal infections, or suspicion of hearing loss.

Universal newborn hearing screening using otoacoustic emissions and auditory brainstem response allows early identification of impaired children. Intervention by age 6 months appears to improve language development. A temporal bone CT is often obtained to evaluate for inner ear malformations that would predispose the patient to further hearing loss with even mild head trauma. A genetics evaluation and counseling may be indicated. Mutations of the Connexin-26 gene, an autosomal recessive disorder, account for a significant percentage of nonsyndromic hereditary hearing loss. Hearing loss may coexist with other conditions (e.g., renal, ophthalmologic, thyroid, infectious, cardiac), so other testing may be indicated based on clinical suspicion.

In children with a significant hearing loss, hearing aids are recommended. A cochlear implant may be indicated for those with hearing so poor to be considered unaidable. A cochlear implant is a surgically implanted device that receives sound, converts it to electrical signals, and directly stimulates the cochlea. Results are excellent in properly selected patients.

An important and often unrecognized cause of hearing loss in children is chronic OME. Children with either unilateral or bilateral middle ear effusions refractory to medical treatment for more than 3 months should have audiometric testing. Myringotomy with tube insertion is indicated if bilateral CHL is found and should be considered in some cases of unilateral loss as well.

Treatment of Hearing Loss

Individual treatments for specific causes of hearing loss vary greatly. This section gives a brief overview of options available to improve hearing in patients with the most common causes of hearing loss.

Surgery is often performed for CHL. Myringotomy with or without tube insertion corrects hearing loss in cases of OME. The procedure is performed under brief general anesthesia in children or under local anesthesia for most adults. A tympanoplasty is performed for tympanic membrane perforations and to reconstruct ossicles with a prosthesis. A stapedectomy with placement of a prosthesis is often a successful option in patients with otosclerosis.

Cochlear implantation is indicated for profound SNHL in patients who do not benefit from conventional hearing aids.

The procedure is indicated for adults and children as young as 12 months old.

A variety of styles of hearing aids are used to rehabilitate hearing loss in patients with SNHL and CHL. The simplest (and least expensive) are larger, behind-the-ear aids with analog amplification of sound. The most complex (and most expensive) are completely-in-the-canal aids with programmable digital amplification. Several other types of aids fall between these two extremes. A certified audiologist, under the supervision of an otorhinolaryngologist, assists the patient with proper selection of an appropriate hearing aid.

KEY TREATMENT

- Treatment of acute episodes of Meniere disease involves vestibular suppressants and antiemetics, and maintenance therapy consists of reduction in sodium chloride and the use of a diuretic (SOR: A) (Thirlwall and Kundu, 2006).
- A patient with Meniere disease who fails conservative treatment is likely to have improvement of vertigo with intratympanic gentamicin treatment (SOR: B).
- Patients with BPPV should be treated with an otoconia repositioning maneuver (SOR: B) (Herdman, 2013).
- Ciprofloxacin–dexamethasone 0.1% for acute otitis externa is more effective against *P. aeruginosa* (most common isolate) than neomycin–polymyxin B–hydrocortisone (SOR: A) (Dohar et al., 2009).
- Successful treatment of auricular hematoma is incision and drainage with dental rolls sutured to the anterior and posterior auricle (SOR: B) (Jones and Mahendran, 2008).
- In AOM, severity, laterality, and age of the patient determine whether to use antibiotics or close follow-up (SOR: B).
- Severe AOM is defined as moderate to severe otalgia and fever greater than 39°C (102.2°F) and should be treated with antibiotics.
- Second- and third-generation cephalosporins may be used to treat AOM in penicillin-allergic patients or in those who have received amoxicillin in the previous 30 days (SOR: A) (Pichichero and Casey, 2007).
- Antihistamines, decongestants, antibiotics, and corticosteroids are not recommended for routine management of OME (SOR: A) (van Zon et al., 2012).
- Tympanostomy tube insertion reduces recurrence frequency and total recurrence time in recurrent AOM (SOR: A) (Cheong and Hussain, 2012).

Facial Nerve Paralysis

Key Points

- Bell palsy is the most common cause of facial paralysis
- Lyme disease is often overlooked as a cause of facial paralysis.
- Audiometry is recommended in facial paralysis because of the proximity of the facial nerve to cranial nerves VII and VIII.

Table 18-10 Causes of Facial Paralysis in Order of Occurrence

Cause	Percentage	Characteristics
Idiopathic (Bell palsy)	60-85	Acute onset; viral prodrome (60% of cases)
Trauma	20-50	Acute-onset paralysis or paresis of previously functioning nerve
Herpes zoster	10-15	Ramsay Hunt syndrome with cranial nerve VII involvement, vestibular(vertigo), cochlear (hearing loss)
Tumor	10-15	Slow progression to complete paralysis
Birth	10-15	Part of congenital syndrome or birth trauma at delivery
Infection	4	Mastoiditis, otitis media, direct cranial nerve VII infection, Lyme disease
Brain lesion (central nervous system)	<10	Supranuclear or in brainstem

From Lucente FE, Har-El G. *Essentials of otolaryngology.* Philadelphia: Lippincott, Williams & Wilkins; 1999:131.

Facial paralysis occurs for various reasons. Possible causes are listed in Table 18-10. The eponym "Bell palsy" is reserved for cases of idiopathic facial paralysis. It has been shown, however, that many, if not most, cases of idiopathic facial paralysis are actually caused by reactivation of latent herpesvirus living in the facial nerve or geniculate ganglion.

Although the most common cause of facial paralysis is indeed Bell palsy, it is incumbent to rule out *other* potentially serious causes of facial paralysis before making this *diagnosis of exclusion*. Initially, a complete history and physical examination are required, including otologic and neurologic evaluation. The patient should be questioned regarding history of recurrent cold sores, which suggest herpetic involvement. Recent travel (especially camping) should be noted because Lyme disease is an often overlooked cause of facial paralysis. Involvement of facial nerves is a concern in patients with a history of chronic otitis media or cholesteatoma. Other symptoms should be noted. Otalgia is common with Bell palsy and does not always imply that the ear is involved. Of course, questions regarding risk factors for cerebrovascular disease or previous CVA should be obtained.

Evaluation of facial nerve function requires careful attention and comparison between the two sides of the face. The patient should be evaluated at rest and with voluntary movement. The patient should be asked to wrinkle the nose, raise the eyebrows, squeeze the eyes shut, and purse the lips to assess all branches of the facial nerve. The facial skin should be assessed because a rash can indicate *herpes zoster oticus* (Ramsay Hunt syndrome). The eyes should be inspected to rule out exposure keratitis from lack of eye closure and dryness. If keratitis is suspected, ophthalmologic consultation should be obtained to prevent loss of vision. A complete neurologic examination must be done. If other neurologic deficits are found, neurology consultation is indicated. Lesions in the auditory canal should raise suspicion of herpes zoster oticus or malignancy of the external auditory canal with facial nerve involvement.

Otitis externa and facial weakness can represent malignant otitis externa, especially if the patient has diabetes or is immunocompromised. Signs of otitis media imply involvement of the facial nerve as it courses through the middle ear. The parotid gland and the rest of the neck should be checked to rule out a parotid salivary gland mass that involves the facial nerve. Any of these associated ear findings should prompt ENT consultation because early intervention can improve outcome. Audiometry is recommended in the evaluation of facial paralysis because of the proximity of cranial nerves VII and VIII in the temporal bone.

In cases in which no identifiable cause is found, the diagnosis of Bell palsy is made (although this diagnosis is not certain until a facial or acoustic neuroma has been ruled out either with return of facial function or with MRI scan). In the past, Bell palsy was treated expectantly because the cause was not clear, making treatment difficult. Evidence now indicates that most Bell palsy cases are secondary to a reactivation of the herpes simplex virus (HSV) in the geniculate ganglion, causing neural edema and neurapraxia. On the basis of this research, treatment with antivirals and steroids are thought to improve outcomes. If no contraindications to steroids exist, prednisone (1 mg/kg, up to a maximum of 60 mg/day, over 7 days with a taper) is reasonable. In addition to steroids, an oral antiviral with activity against the herpesvirus is given (200 mg acyclovir [Zovirax] five times daily or valacyclovir [Valtrex] 500 mg twice daily for 7-10 days). Of the utmost importance is protection of the eye. Moisturizing eyedrops and nightly lubrication should be prescribed. Any signs of irritation should prompt an ophthalmology evaluation.

If the facial weakness is secondary to Ramsay Hunt syndrome, treatment is similar to that of Bell palsy, but the clinical course and expected outcomes differ. This syndrome is caused by herpes zoster (rather than herpes simplex) involvement of the facial (geniculate), vestibulocochlear, or trigeminal ganglia. The infection causes pain and eventually vesicular eruptions around the auricle and external ear canal. Vesicles may appear only in the pharynx or hard palate in some cases. Facial weakness and at times dense paralysis are common. Hearing loss, tinnitus, and persistent vertigo also occur in 20% to 30% of patients (Adour, 1994). As with Bell palsy, prompt initiation of oral steroids and acyclovir should begin when the diagnosis is suspected. This therapy can lessen vertigo and improve recovery of facial nerve function, although outcomes are not as favorable as for Bell palsy. Some patients struggle with persistent facial weakness, pain, and hearing loss (Robillard et al., 1988).

In cases of facial paralysis associated with otitis externa or otitis media, treatment differs. If malignant otitis externa is suspected, the patient requires hospital admission, control of diabetes, and infectious diseases and ENT consultation. IV antibiotics and sometimes surgical debridement are required. CNS complications are possible.

Facial weakness in the setting of AOM requires treatment with a broad-spectrum antibiotic covering the usual pathogens of otitis media. In addition, a myringotomy with or without tube insertion is thought to hasten resolution and improve outcomes by allowing decompression of the infection. This also allows a culture to be done and antibiotic sensitivities determined. If facial weakness occurs in the setting of chronic otitis media or known cholesteatoma, topical and systemic antistaphylococcal and antipseudomonal antibiotics should be started and an urgent ENT consultation obtained in hopes of preventing permanent facial paralysis and further complications.

Expected outcome for true Bell palsy is full return of function in 80% of patients. The remaining 20% have variable recovery. If recovery is incomplete, MRI is indicated to rule out neoplastic process (most likely a facial neuroma) that could mimic Bell palsy. Patients with diabetes mellitus have a higher incidence of Bell palsy and often have a poorer outcome. Permanent facial weakness is also more common after herpes zoster oticus. Outcomes of facial paralysis secondary to the other causes discussed are variable and depend on the severity of the pathology, the patient's general state of health, and the response to treatment.

In patients who have poor return of facial function, rehabilitation is necessary. The most important goal is protection of the eye followed by improved cosmesis. Ophthalmologic and ENT involvement is continued (Almeida et al., 2009).

KEY TREATMENT

- In Bell palsy, steroids are highly likely to increase the probability of recovery of nerve function (SOR: A) (Gronseth and Paduga, 2012).
- The addition of antivirals to steroids in the treatment of Bell palsy increases modestly (<7%) the functional recovery of the facial nerve (SOR: A) (Gronseth and Paduga, 2012).

The Nose and Paranasal Sinuses

Key Points

- Cigarette smoking and environmental allergies are important contributing factors to chronic nasal problems.
- Excessive use of decongestant nasal sprays can lead to rebound swelling and worsened nasal symptoms.
- A CT scan of the sinuses is not recommended to diagnose uncomplicated acute sinusitis in adults or children. CT should be considered when the diagnosis is uncertain, treatment has failed, or a complication or neoplasia is suspected. MRI is useful in evaluation of sinus tumors.
- Adenoid hypertrophy is a common cause of nasal symptoms in children but in an adult can indicate a lymphoproliferative disorder or HIV infection.
- A nasal foreign body should be suspected in a child who presents with recent unilateral nasal obstruction, rhinorrhea, and odor.
- Nasal polyps can be seen with asthma, cystic fibrosis, and rarely neoplasia. Nasal polyps always deserve further investigation.
- Unlike adults, children with sinusitis rarely complain of facial pain.
- The diagnosis of acute bacterial sinusitis should be considered when typical upper respiratory infection (URI) symptoms last longer than 10 days or symptoms worsen or fever occurs.

- Empiric antibiotic treatment for adult or pediatric acute sinusitis should provide coverage for the most common pathogens, *Pneumococcus* spp., *H. influenza*, and *M. catarrhalis*.
- Chronic and recurrent sinusitis leads to significant decrease in quality of life and can rarely lead to life-threatening complications.
- Sinonasal tumors often present with symptoms similar to sinusitis.
- An undiagnosed nasal septal hematoma can cause cartilage destruction and lead to disfigurement. Prompt diagnosis and treatment can prevent this.

HISTORY

Signs and symptoms of most nasal and sinus disorders include nasal congestion, rhinorrhea, bleeding, facial pressure, halitosis or pain, headache, cough, otalgia, facial or periorbital swelling, altered (diminished, absent, or distorted) sense of smell, or postnasal drainage. Initial evaluation of the patient with nasal complaints begins with a complete history, with specific questions directed at the timing and chronicity of the symptoms and modifying factors. The patient should be questioned specifically about previous nasal trauma.

Patients should be asked about prescription and over-the-counter (OTC) nasal, sinus, and allergy medications. Many patients try OTC remedies before seeking medical advice. Excessive use of decongestant nasal sprays can exacerbate and even cause nasal obstruction secondary to *rhinitis medicamentosa* and rebound nasal congestion. The patient should also be questioned about previous nasal surgery. Rarely, the patient admits to unorthodox self-treatment that may be significant (e.g., peroxide irrigation, overzealous nasal cleaning). This can explain continued symptoms and may indicate an underlying problem. The underlying problem may be true nasal pathology or rarely may be obsessive-compulsive disorder manifesting as repeated nasal cleaning.

Information about the patient's medical history and social history is also necessary. Knowledge of the patient's work environment may be relevant. Exposure to chemicals or fumes can cause nasal symptoms. Woodworkers are known to have a higher incidence of sinonasal carcinoma. A history of environmental allergies or immune dysfunction is relevant. Many medical conditions (e.g., asthma, autoimmune disorders) are associated with sinonasal dysfunction. Hypertension will limit the use of decongestants for treatment or predispose to epistaxis. A history of migraine is noteworthy because migraine headaches can be confused with sinus pain. Some prescriptions can exacerbate or even cause nasal dysfunction, especially medications that can lead to excessive nasal dryness (antihistamines, diuretics, antidepressants). Drug allergies should be noted. Previous nasal surgery, if done, may not have been successful or may even have led to increased problems. Cigarette smoking and excessive use of alcohol and caffeine have negative effects on mucociliary function that can lead to congestion. A history of nasal or facial trauma is important. Previous or current use of intranasal cocaine can lead to significant pathology and symptomatology.

PHYSICAL EXAMINATION

See eAppendix 18-2 online.

RADIOGRAPHY

Plain radiographs are often ordered in cases of facial trauma, especially isolated nasal trauma. The radiographs can be complementary to the physical examination.

Plain radiographs of the sinuses are still useful in certain circumstances. Plain sinus radiographs are reasonably accurate in assessing the maxillary and frontal sinuses in cases of *acute* sinusitis. Complete opacification or an air-fluid level in one of these sinuses usually indicates acute sinusitis. However, the relatively low sensitivity and specificity of plain radiographs, especially in evaluating the ethmoid sinuses, have limited their usefulness.

Computed tomography has become an invaluable diagnostic tool for evaluating chronic nasal and sinus problems and has essentially supplanted the use of plain sinus radiographs. CT of the sinuses allows unparalleled imaging of the complicated anatomy of the nose and paranasal sinuses. It has also increased understanding of the pathophysiology of sinusitis. CT scanning can show areas of mild mucosal thickening in the sinuses (indicating chronic sinusitis), complete opacification (seen in acute sinusitis, polyps, or sinus tumors), bone erosion, or abscess formation in adjacent critical structures such as the orbit or brain (Figure 18-6). CT can show whether the *ostiomeatal complex* (the "bottleneck" of normal sinus drainage) is patent or obstructed and shows the myriad nasal and sinus normal variants, some of which predispose to sinonasal pathology.

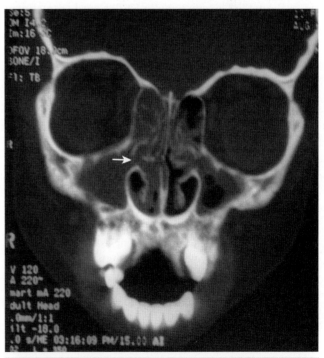

Figure 18-6 Coronal computed tomography scan showing complete opacification of the right maxillary and ethmoid sinuses with partial opacification of the left maxillary and ethmoid sinuses. *Arrow* indicates ostiomeatal complex.

Computed tomography of the sinuses should be ordered when the diagnosis of chronic sinusitis is suspected, medical treatment of sinusitis has failed and surgery is being contemplated, a complication of sinusitis is suspected, or a nasal or sinus mass is suspected. CT is not required as a confirmatory test in the treatment of uncomplicated acute sinusitis except in certain circumstances. The scan is helpful, however, in cases of *recurrent acute sinusitis* or when the diagnosis is not certain. Obtaining a scan during a patient's presumed infection allows the diagnosis to be confirmed or ruled out. Although some abnormalities require further treatment occasionally, the scan identifies abnormalities or variations of normal anatomy that require no intervention. Mucus retention cysts, for example, are seen in up to 20% of the population and are typically asymptomatic. Unless they are large or infection is suspected (the patient complains of pain in the vicinity of the cyst), treatment is not required. Recently, low radiation, cone-beam scanners have become common in ENT offices. This technology allows relatively inexpensive "point-of-care" imaging at a fraction of the radiation exposure and cost of helical CT scans.

Magnetic resonance imaging is not particularly helpful in evaluating sinusitis and has two main limitations in evaluating inflammatory sinus conditions. First, MRI often tends to be too sensitive, showing mucosal thickening that is often clinically insignificant. Second, MRI fails to show bony anatomy, which is critical in diagnosis and surgical planning in chronic sinusitis. MRI is useful in evaluating suspected sinonasal tumors and fungal infections of the sinuses. The limitations of MRI and its relatively high cost compared with CT do not justify its routine use in evaluating chronic sinusitis. If incidental sinusitis is noted on an MR image and the degree of sinusitis is severe, is asymmetric, or the patient is symptomatic, ENT referral or treatment is indicated.

CLINICAL PROBLEMS

Complaints related to the nose and sinuses are among the most common seen in a family medicine practice. Acute rhinitis (the common cold), allergic rhinitis, and sinusitis comprise the vast majority of these complaints and, taken together, result in an enormous socioeconomic impact in terms of missed workdays and schooldays and pharmaceutical costs. Nasal and sinus conditions can result in significant reduction in quality of life and can, rarely, be debilitating or even life threatening.

Epistaxis

See also the earlier section, "Emergencies." Epistaxis can be caused by trauma, dry weather, hypertension, bleeding dyscrasias, anticoagulation therapy, and intranasal tumors. Adolescent boys with recurrent epistaxis and nasal obstruction might have juvenile nasopharyngeal angiofibroma. Intranasal hemangioma can affect any age group. Epistaxis typically responds to conservative treatment, including nasal hydration with saline mist, nasal ointment, environmental humidification, avoidance of digital trauma, and control of hypertension if present. If bleeding continues to be a problem, the patient should be referred to an ENT consultant for a complete evaluation of the nasal cavities and possible cautery. Screening blood studies for coagulopathy or imaging may be necessary.

Nasal Obstruction

The sensation of unilateral or bilateral nasal obstruction is relatively common and can range from mildly annoying to extremely frustrating to the patient. Nasal obstruction may be associated with other symptoms such as rhinorrhea, lost or altered sense of smell, or facial discomfort. Nasal obstruction may result from pathology of the nasal cavity or nasopharynx. (eTable 18-8 online summarizes the most common causes, associated signs and symptoms, and treatment for nasal obstruction.)

Physical Examination. See eAppendix 18-3 online.

Treatment. Successful treatment of nasal obstruction depends on making a correct diagnosis. After the diagnosis has been established, a treatment plan should be developed. If the nasal obstruction is secondary to one of the various types of rhinitis, it is treated medically. This includes nasal steroids, antihistamines, leukotriene inhibitors, mucolytics, oral decongestants, topical decongestants, and nasal saline. These medications may be used alone or in various combinations. The choice of medications is determined by the severity of symptoms and the patient's medical history, response to treatment, and wishes. Oral steroids can be used in select severe cases but are associated with potential significant side effects. Nasal decongestant sprays are very effective for treating severe nasal congestion but should be used sparingly and never for longer than 3 days to prevent rebound nasal obstruction (rhinitis medicamentosa). Allergy testing is done when allergies are suspected and the standard regimen is largely ineffective. Antibiotics are administered if a bacterial infection is suspected (acute rhinosinusitis).

Adenoid Hypertrophy

Adenoid hypertrophy is common in children. If identified in an adult, adenoid hypertrophy could indicate a lymphoproliferative disorder or HIV infection. The patient may present with nasal symptoms or symptoms of eustachian tube dysfunction. In the pediatric population, adenoid hypertrophy causes chronic or recurrent nasal obstruction, rhinorrhea, snoring, cough, or otitis media. The diagnosis is usually clinical but can be confirmed with lateral neck radiography. If symptoms are severe or persistent, adenoidectomy should be considered. Improvement in properly selected patients is usually significant, although well-controlled studies demonstrating efficacy are few (Aardweg, 2010).

Foreign Body

A nasal foreign body should be suspected in a child with or without a history of previous nasal problems who presents with recent unilateral nasal obstruction, rhinorrhea, and odor. The nasal foreign body might not be visible secondary to the presence of mucosal edema, mucus, or pus.

If the foreign body is identified, removal may be attempted in a cooperative child. If removal is not possible or the diagnosis is uncertain, ENT consultation should be obtained. The ENT evaluation may be done in the office setting or in the OR, depending again on patient cooperation and degree of suspicion. The nasal cavity is suctioned, decongested, and anesthetized with topical lidocaine. Endoscopy may be done. If the foreign body is seen, removal is undertaken.

If the child is old enough, asking him or her to blow the nose after decongestion might remove the foreign body or at least move it anteriorly. Removal can be difficult, and experience helps. Problems that can hinder removal include bleeding that obscures visibility. The foreign body can also be inadvertently pushed posteriorly. Softer foreign bodies, such as food matter and tissue paper, can disintegrate, requiring piecemeal removal.

A headlight and bivalve nasal speculum are recommended. Suction should be available. A small alligator or bayonet forceps is sometimes used but may simply push the foreign body posteriorly. In many cases, a useful instrument is a small, ball-tipped, right-angle probe, actually an otologic surgical instrument called an "attic hook." This can be gently passed posterior to the foreign body, turned 90 degrees, and then used to pull the foreign body anteriorly and out of the nose.

After the foreign body is removed, the nasal cavity should be reinspected for retained, more distal foreign bodies. The other nasal cavity and ears should also be inspected because the child may have introduced foreign bodies into multiple orifices. Retained foreign bodies for years have been described. If the foreign body might be a disc battery, emergent removal is necessary to prevent significant tissue injury. Antibiotics are recommended if there is evidence of obvious infection or complete removal is not certain and reexamination is planned.

Nasal Vestibulitis

A low-grade infection of the anterior nasal vestibule will cause chronic irritation, crusting, and sometimes bleeding. The examination typically shows mild erythema, cracking, and yellow crusting just inside the nostril, but it may also appear fairly normal. The cause is usually *S. aureus* infection but may be fungal. Herpetic infections are typically more severe and not as protracted. Treatment is with OTC topical antibiotic ointment (without neomycin because of possible sensitivity) and avoidance of irritating the area. If symptoms continue, methicillin-resistant *S. aureus* (MRSA) infection is possible and should respond to mupirocin ointment. Sometimes an oral antibiotic may be necessary. Obtaining a culture may be helpful. Continued symptoms require ENT consultation to evaluate for other possible causes, including chronic sinusitis, anatomic problems such as deviated nasal septum, or even a neoplastic etiology.

Choanal Atresia

Choanal atresia is a common cause of nasal obstruction in children but can also be seen in adults. If bilateral, it manifests shortly after birth as an airway emergency because neonates are "obligate nasal breathers" and cannot tolerate nasal obstruction. Typically, they oxygenate well while crying but become cyanotic when crying stops and they cannot feed. This condition requires urgent ENT consultation. The airway is stabilized and the atresia repaired shortly thereafter. If unilateral, the atresia can go undiagnosed until later in childhood or even adulthood. The patient will report a lifelong history of nasal obstruction and

rhinorrhea. Diagnosis is made with endoscopy and CT. Treatment is surgical.

Nasal Polyps

Nasal polyps are the result of nasal mucosal inflammation and edema. On examination, nasal polyps are usually silver-gray in color and may be translucent. If there is associated infection, polyps can appear erythematous or may be obscured by mucus. Polyps cause significant and sometimes complete nasal obstruction but are painless and insensate. Nasal polyps predispose the patient to sinusitis and often cause anosmia.

The exact cause of nasal polyps is unclear. Polyps are often associated with chronic sinusitis, reactive airway disease, and less often with environmental allergies. In children, the presence of polyps should prompt testing for cystic fibrosis. Nasal polyps always require investigation because sinonasal tumor or fungal involvement is possible, especially if the polyps are unilateral. If polyps are identified, further evaluation includes allergy and asthma testing and CT scan. Medical treatment is initially offered but is often inadequate. Initial treatment includes topical steroids, allergy treatment, and treatment of sinusitis. In many patients, endoscopic sinus surgery (ESS) is an important adjunct to medical treatment and results in significant improvement in symptoms. Polyps almost always recur after removal without continued medical treatment. Appropriate postoperative treatment can dramatically slow, and sometimes halt, the rate of polyp regrowth. Symptom improvement after polyp removal with sinus surgery is usually dramatic.

Deviated Septum

Most patients have some degree of asymptomatic septal deviation, but in some patients, it is severe enough to cause symptoms of obstruction. Septal deviation is usually the result of previous nasal trauma. The trauma might have seemed relatively minor at the time or might have resulted in a nasal fracture. Deviated septum may be congenital. Physical examination clearly demonstrates an anterior septal deviation. If more posterior, nasal endoscopy or CT may be necessary to make the diagnosis. Any patient complaining of persistent nasal obstruction deserves further evaluation, especially if the cause is not immediately evident. Symptomatic septal deviation is readily treatable with outpatient surgery.

Septoplasty is done through an intranasal incision, allowing deviated portions of cartilage and bone to be replaced to the midline or removed, resulting in a symmetrically patent nasal airway. Septoplasty is often combined with a turbinate reduction procedure. The procedures are usually well tolerated. Postoperative pain, formerly a greater problem, usually resulted from the need for nasal packing and removal. Newer devices such as soft-silicone (Silastic) splints now cause much less postoperative discomfort than traditional packing.

In pediatric patients, septoplasty is not usually recommended because of concern about disrupting nasal and facial growth, although this risk appears to be low. Chronic mouth-breathing can also negatively affect facial growth, so for this reason, "limited" septoplasty may be considered in pediatric patients with severe or congenital deviation.

Hypertrophied Turbinates

Inferior turbinate hypertrophy is relatively common in adults and children. This usually occurs with chronic inflammation, usually resulting from allergy or rhinosinusitis. Turbinate hypertrophy usually responds to medical treatment addressing the primary problem. If the turbinates remain significantly hypertrophied despite medical treatment, turbinate reduction is offered, using cautery, radiofrequency treatment, fracture, excision, laser treatment, or cryotherapy. Submucosal resection of a portion of the conchal bone and reactive stromal tissue seems to provide the greatest improvement. It is important to preserve functional turbinate tissue. The turbinates are reactive structures that allow the nose to filter, warm, and humidify inspired air. Overly aggressive removal of turbinate tissue can leave the nasal cavity too vacuous, leading to nasal sicca, discomfort, bleeding, and infection. This is referred to as the "empty nose syndrome." Because this condition is very difficult to treat, avoidance with conservative surgery is paramount.

Rhinitis

Acute Viral Rhinitis, the Common Cold, and Upper Respiratory Infection. The symptoms of "the common cold" are well known to all. Many viruses are known to be pathogenic to the upper respiratory tract, the most common being rhinovirus. The infection typically causes damage to the respiratory epithelium, leading to symptoms of sore throat, cough, low-grade fever, malaise, rhinorrhea, ear fullness, hoarseness, and nasal congestion. Symptom control is the patient's primary concern, and there are myriad OTC medications available to control cough, nasal congestion, and rhinorrhea. These include oral and topical decongestants, saline mist or irrigations, cough suppressants or mucolytics, and analgesics and antipyretics. Topical decongestants are very effective treatment for nasal congestion but must be stopped after 3 days of use to prevent rebound swelling ("rhinitis medicamentosa"). Saline mist and saline irrigations are useful for thinning and washing away thick nasal secretions. Unless a bacterial infection is suspected, antibiotics are not indicated to treat an uncomplicated URI.

Although many treatments are available for viral URI, few have been well studied. The Cochrane Collaboration has made specific statements on the following treatments for URIs (The Cochrane Collaboration. Published by John Wiley & Sons, Ltd):

- Vitamin C with regular supplementation has been shown to reduce the severity and duration of the common cold. It is recommended that patients try vitamin C to see if it is helpful on an individual basis. Further studies are necessary.
- Antihistamine–decongestant–analgesic combinations have "some general benefit" in adults and older children.
- Intranasal ipratropium bromide spray appears to be effective in decreasing rhinorrhea with little effect on nasal congestion with tolerable side effects.
- Zinc lozenges at 75 mg/day or more administered within 24 hours of onset of symptoms reduces the duration of common cold symptoms, although there is heterogeneity of the data. Zinc has a bad taste and can cause nausea. The effect of prophylactic use of zinc is less clear.
- Current evidence does not support the use of oral corticosteroids in the treatment of URI.
- Routine use of antibiotics is contraindicated in the treatment of the common cold in children and adults.
- There is a lack of evidence supporting the use of vaccines for the common cold.
- Garlic supplementation has not been proven effective in the treatment of URI.

The main concern of primary care physicians is to help patients with symptom relief and to determine which patients need more close follow-up or treatment. As a result of temporary mucociliary dysfunction, impaired local immunity, and epithelial damage from a viral URI, the patient's infection can progress to AOM, bacterial pharyngitis, bronchitis or pneumonia, or acute bacterial rhinosinusitis (ABRS). Further evaluation is necessary if clinical suspicion of any of these exists. The determination of when a cold has progressed to bacterial sinusitis can be especially challenging and frustrating to both the patient and the clinician. It is estimated that 1% to 2% of colds will progress to bacterial sinusitis. A reasonable guide to make this determination is persistence of symptoms past 10 to 14 days or significant worsening of symptoms earlier (Figure 18-7). Preexisting medical conditions and the patient's smoking history should also be considered. There must be a balance of listening to the patient's concerns and recommending appropriate symptomatic treatment but not prescribing unnecessary treatment such as antibiotics or oral steroids, which can be counterproductive or even dangerous.

Allergic Rhinitis. See Chapter 19, Allergy.

Vasomotor Rhinitis and Idiopathic Rhinitis. When a cause for rhinitis cannot be made, the diagnosis of vasomotor or idiopathic rhinitis may be given. The primary symptoms are a feeling of nasal congestion and rhinorrhea. Table 18-11 lists some of the conditions that are included in the category of vasomotor rhinitis. Allergy skin test results in patients with vasomotor rhinorrhea are negative, with less than 25% eosinophils present on a nasal swab. These patients do not fully respond to topical or systemic corticosteroids. The condition suggests hyperactivity of parasympathetic tone, blockage of sympathetic tone with vasodilation of submucosal venous sinusoids, and excessive seromucous secretions from the mucous glands. A good analogy to vasomotor rhinorrhea is functional bowel disease. Treatment is with systemic decongestants and antihistamines or topical anticholinergic agents such as ipratropium bromide (Atrovent 0.06% nasal spray). Because of the persistence of symptoms, patients should be warned about excessive use of OTC nasal sprays, which can lead to rhinitis medicamentosa.

Rhinitis Medicamentosa. The prolonged use of topical decongestants for the nose can itself induce nasal stuffiness. The condition is caused by *rebound swelling* after dissipation of the decongestive effect of the nasal spray. Increasing the dose of the spray is the patient's response to the rebound

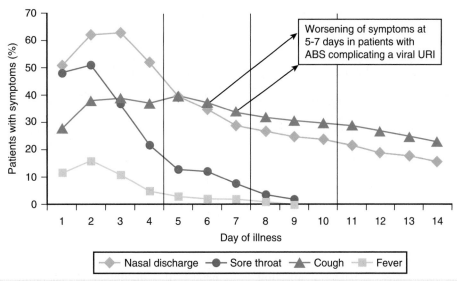

Figure 18-7 Time course of symptoms during an upper respiratory (viral) illness. *ABS,* Acute bacterial sinusitis; *URI,* upper respiratory infection. (From McCoul ED. Upper respiratory infections. American Rhinologic Society, 2011. http://care.american-rhinologic.org/upper_respiratory_infections.)

Table 18-11 Conditions Included Under Vasomotor Rhinitis

Drug-induced rhinitis (reserpine, nonselective β-blockers, antidepressants, oral contraceptives)
Irritant rhinitis (smoke, gases)
Temperature- and humidity-induced rhinitis
Emotion- and stress-induced rhinitis
Hormonal rhinitis (pregnancy, premenstrual, hypothyroidism)
Idiopathic rhinitis

swelling, and the vicious cycle is difficult to break without education and medical help.

To treat rhinitis medicamentosa, the patient must stop using the topical decongestant to allow recovery of the damaged nasal mucosa. To relieve the subsequent rebound mucosal swelling, topical and oral corticosteroids are recommended. The length of time needed to successfully treat rhinitis medicamentosa varies depending on the duration the patient has used nasal decongestants. It takes at least 2 weeks to reverse the edema and histamine sensitivity. Other forms of treatment include systemic antihistamines or decongestants, corticosteroid injection into the inferior turbinate, and nocturnal sedation. Many patients begin using these sprays because of underlying pathology such as deviated septum, turbinate hypertrophy, or chronic sinusitis. Surgery may be helpful in these cases. Graf and colleagues (1995) achieved a 100% success rate at the end of 6 weeks of nasal corticosteroid therapy and avoidance of nasal decongestants. It takes time and patience to educate the patient about rhinitis medicamentosa, and both are essential for the treatment to be successful.

Atrophic Rhinitis. Elderly patients are more prone to develop atrophic rhinitis, which leads to nasal congestion, crusting, and foul odor. Although the Cochrane Collaboration found insufficient evidence for any consistently effective treatment for atrophic rhinitis, improvement can be seen

with moisturizing the nose with saline nose sprays (combinations of saline, aloe vera, oils) or saline irrigations with culture-directed topical antibiotics (Mirshra et al., 2012).

Atrophic rhinitis can also result from previous nasal surgery (referred to as "empty nose syndrome"), use of cocaine, and autoimmune or systemic inflammatory disorders (e.g., lupus, Wegener granulomatosis). In the case of a systemic disease, appropriate medical treatment of that condition will often help the associated nasal symptoms. If the cause of the patient's atrophic rhinitis is unclear, further workup, including biopsy, is indicated.

Sinusitis and Rhinosinusitis

Symptoms of rhinitis and sinusitis are often very similar and even difficult to differentiate in many cases. Sinusitis implies inflammation of the mucosa of one or more of the paranasal sinuses. This usually coexists with rhinitis and is actually more accurately referred to as *rhinosinusitis.* Studies have shown that CT scans of patients with uncomplicated viral URIs have mucosal thickening and opacification of the sinuses. For this reason, most URIs are technically considered *viral rhinosinusitis.* In most cases, these changes resolve with time and symptomatic treatment. The terms *rhinosinusitis* or *sinusitis* are typically used when a bacterial infection of the sinuses is suspected. About 2% of viral URIs will progress to bacterial rhinosinusitis. An estimated 20 million cases of bacterial sinusitis occur in the United States annually, accounting for 9% and 21% of all pediatric and adult antibiotic annual prescriptions, respectively (Anon et al., 2004).

Inflammatory conditions of the paranasal sinuses cause significant socioeconomic impact annually secondary to considerable medical expense and missed workdays. Chronic sinusitis can be quite debilitating. Studies have shown that quality-of-life scores of patients with chronic sinusitis are often similar to those of other, more severe conditions (congestive heart failure, chronic obstructive pulmonary disease). Chronic sinusitis can also exacerbate coexisting medical conditions, most notably reactive airway disease.

Sinusitis represents one of the most common disorders requiring antibiotic treatment in adults. The challenge to the clinician in evaluating a patient with possible sinusitis is to differentiate viral URI, allergic rhinitis, and even a migraine headache, which do not require antibiotics, from bacterial sinusitis, which does respond to antibiotic treatment. There still seems to be a public perception that antibiotics hasten recovery from the common cold. Some physicians prescribe antibiotics in these situations, not wanting to disappoint the patient and seeing no significant risk. In fact, evidence suggests that there is a greater likelihood of *harming rather than benefiting* the patient with inappropriate use of antibiotics (Scott and Orzano, 2001). The emergence of bacteria highly resistant to broad-spectrum antibiotics has forced the medical community to modify its behavior regarding the treatment of URIs. More recently, there is concern that antibiotics may harm the patient's own protective "microbiome." For these reasons, antibiotics should not be prescribed unless a bacterial infection is certain or at least probable. The patient should be educated about the rationale for this.

The underlying cause of most cases of sinusitis is mucociliary dysfunction and sinus obstruction. The maxillary sinuses, anterior ethmoid sinuses, and frontal sinuses all drain through small ostia that converge into a small channel called the *ostiomeatal unit*, which then empties into the middle meatus beneath the middle turbinate. Obstruction at the ostiomeatal unit leads to obstruction of these sinuses and secondary infection. The posterior ethmoid sinuses and sphenoid sinuses are usually affected later. Sinusitis most often follows a viral URI or an episode of allergic rhinitis. Mucosal edema, impaired local immunity, and ciliary dysfunction lead to impaired sinus drainage and mucus stasis followed by bacterial infection.

Sinusitis is classified into *acute* (symptoms up to 3 weeks), *subacute* (symptoms from 3 to 6 weeks), and *chronic* (symptoms longer than 6 weeks) cases. Cases of acute sinusitis that clear completely only to develop again quickly are referred to as *recurrent acute sinusitis*. Although the types of sinusitis share many characteristics, there are several critical differences in pathogenesis and treatment.

The most important risk factor for the development of sinusitis is rhinitis (e.g., viral, allergic). Other risk factors include anatomic abnormalities (abnormality within the sinuses, septal deviation, choanal atresia, foreign body, adenoid hypertrophy), nasal polyps (which can also occur secondary to chronic sinusitis), conditions of local or systemic immunodeficiency, cystic fibrosis, primary ciliary dysfunction (Kartagener syndrome), secondary ciliary dysfunction (cigarette smoking, nasal decongestant abuse, cocaine abuse), gastroesophageal reflux disease (GERD), systemic inflammatory conditions (sarcoidosis, Wegener granulomatosis), dental disease, and nasal or sinus tumors. Any of these conditions can mimic or cause rhinosinusitis. Further workup or referral is indicated if a patient continues to struggle with nasal or sinus symptoms despite medical therapy.

The diagnosis of sinusitis is initially clinical. Imaging and cultures are not initially indicated unless symptoms are severe or become chronic or if a complication is suspected (Reider, 2003). A CT scan may also be helpful when the diagnosis of acute sinusitis has been made multiple times but is still not certain. In 1996, the Task Force on Rhinosinusitis sponsored by the American Academy of Otolaryngology–Head and Neck Surgery developed diagnostic criteria for sinusitis. The signs and symptoms of sinusitis are divided into major and minor. *Major* signs and symptoms include facial pain and pressure, nasal congestion and obstruction, nasal discharge, discolored posterior discharge, anosmia or hyposmia, fever (acute only), and purulence on intranasal examination. *Minor* signs and symptoms include headache, otalgia or ear pressure, halitosis, dental pain, cough, and fever (nonacute) and in children, fatigue and irritability. The diagnosis of sinusitis is *probable* if the patient has two or more major factors *or* one major and two or more minor factors. A *suggestive* history is indicated by the presence of one major factor or two minor factors.

Microbiology of sinusitis varies according to its chronicity. Acute sinusitis is most often *initially* viral. If symptoms persist, the likelihood of bacterial infection increases. The bacteria most often involved in acute sinusitis are *Pneumococcus* spp., *H. influenzae,* and *M. catarrhalis,* with β-lactamase production common in all these. Chronic sinusitis is caused by the same bacteria as in acute sinusitis, but anaerobic bacteria, *Pseudomonas* spp., and staphylococci become involved more often. The incidence of antibiotic-resistant bacteria, including MRSA and multidrug-resistant *Pneumococcus* spp., seems to be increasing. Polymicrobial infections are not uncommon.

Sinusitis can also be caused by fungi. *Invasive* fungal sinusitis (caused most often by *Aspergillus* or *Mucor* spp.) can be seen in patients with impaired immune function and poorly controlled diabetes. It is life threatening even with aggressive medical and surgical treatment. Much more common is a more indolent fungally mediated sinusitis. *Allergic fungal sinusitis* is seen in patients with normal immune function. This is often seen in association with nasal polyps and is thought to be the result of an aberrant immune response to the fungus rather than a true infection. Patients do not always have type I hypersensitivity to fungi. Secondary bacterial infection is often associated with this problem.

Rarer causes of sinusitis are secondary to mycobacterial or parasitic infection.

Complications of Sinusitis. Most cases of sinusitis would resolve with or without medical treatment. Sinusitis is usually treated, however, to avoid potential complications and hasten recovery. The proximity of the paranasal sinuses to the orbits and brain potentially allows infection to spread to these locations. Orbital and CNS involvement of sinusitis can lead to loss of vision and can be life threatening and therefore requires early recognition and treatment. Table 18-12 lists the potential complications of sinusitis and treatment recommendations. A high degree of clinical suspicion is required in cases of possible complicated sinusitis, especially in young children. Patients with a recent URI who present with periorbital erythema, vision change, increasing or severe headache, high fever, or altered mental status require *urgent evaluation* and treatment. Ophthalmologic, infectious disease, and ENT consultations are obtained in cases of orbital complication. Periorbital and orbital cellulitis usually can be managed with IV antibiotics.

Table 18-12 Complications of Sinusitis

Complication	Physical Findings	Treatment
Periorbital cellulitis	Periorbital erythema, edema	Antibiotics: PO or IV
Orbital cellulitis	Erythema, edema, proptosis ± vision loss	IV antibiotics, close observation
Orbital abscess	Erythema, edema, proptosis ± vision loss	IV antibiotics + drainage, FESS
Cavernous sinus thrombosis	Erythema, edema, proptosis + vision loss	IV antibiotics + FESS
Meningitis	Headache, altered mental status, nuchal rigidity, fever	IV antibiotics ± FESS
Intracranial abscess	Headache, altered mental status, high fever	IV antibiotics + drainage, FESS
Mucocele or pyocele	Facial swelling ± fever ± pain	Drainage

FESS, Functional endoscopic sinus surgery; *IV,* intravenous; *PO,* oral.

The more severe orbital complications, however, usually require drainage procedures in combination with IV antibiotics. Surgical drainage also allows cultures to be obtained. Recovery from orbital complications is usually complete with prompt and aggressive treatment. Permanent vision impairment can occur even after appropriate treatment.

The CNS complications require neurosurgical, ENT, and infectious disease consultation. High-dose IV antibiotics are administered. Surgical drainage of the sinuses is sometimes recommended to treat the nidus of the infection and identify the exact pathogen. Recovery from CNS complications is more variable and depends on the patient's age and medical history, severity of the infection, and response to treatment.

Although not always complicated infections, sphenoid and frontal sinusitis deserve special mention because of their proximity to adjacent, critical structures. In some cases, drainage of the frontal sinuses is compromised. Chronic and recurrent frontal sinusitis can lead to both intracranial and ophthalmologic complications if untreated. Large *mucoceles* or *mucopyeloceles* or frontal bone osteomyelitis can also occur, causing disfigurement and diplopia. These conditions usually require surgical drainage. Similarly, sphenoid sinusitis can rarely be aggressive. The carotid artery and optic nerves traverse the lateral walls of the sphenoid sinuses. The sphenoid sinus occupies a space inferior and anterior to the cranial vault. Acute or long-standing sphenoid sinusitis can progress to CNS or eye complications or both. If frontal or sphenoid sinus involvement is noted on CT scan, ENT evaluation is usually indicated.

Medical Treatment of Acute Sinusitis. Treatment of acute sinusitis is almost always medical. Medical treatment of sinusitis is intended to restore normal mucociliary function, eradicate infection, and improve patient symptoms. Treatment to restore mucociliary function is critical and is as important as antibiotic treatment. Improved mucociliary function allows the patient's local immunity to function better and often leads to resolution of the infection.

The patient's medical history must be considered. Patients with poorly controlled hypertension or coronary artery disease may not tolerate decongestants. In acute cases of sinusitis, mucociliary function can be improved by a combination of medications, including oral or topical decongestants (topically for less than 3 days), mucolytics (guaifenesin), and nasal saline mist or irrigations. Nasal saline irrigations are available OTC or can be homemade. Both 0.9% isotonic saline and hypertonic saline irrigations are extremely beneficial. Although nasal steroids are *not indicated* for acute sinusitis, they have been shown to decrease symptoms and hasten recovery in patients. Antihistamines are usually not helpful unless there is a strong allergic component, and they can actually be counterproductive by increasing mucus viscosity and mucosal dryness. Oral steroids are usually not indicated in acute sinusitis, but they may be helpful in select patients.

Antibiotics are typically prescribed when acute bacterial sinusitis is suspected. Even an appropriate course of antibiotics can lead to significant side effects or complications. According to Cochrane Collaboration recommendations for treatment of acute sinusitis, antibiotics provide a minor improvement in simple, acute (uncomplicated) sinus infections. However, eight of 10 patients improve without antibiotics within 2 weeks. The Cochrane Collaboration states, "The potential benefit of antibiotics in the treatment of clinically diagnosed acute rhinosinusitis needs to be seen in the context of a high prevalence of adverse events. Taking into account antibiotic resistance and the very low incidence of serious complications, we conclude that there is no place for antibiotics for the patient with clinically diagnosed, uncomplicated acute rhinosinusitis." This leaves the clinician the task of using good judgment regarding when to prescribe antibiotics. With proper counseling, some patients may choose to avoid antibiotics. These patients need close follow-up.

A rapid assay to detect specific pathogens in acute sinusitis may be available in the future, but antibiotics are empirically chosen based on the expected pathogens and local antibiotic resistance patterns. The high incidence of β-lactamase–producing strains of *H. influenzae* and *M. catarrhalis* and the penicillin-resistant pneumococci must be considered. More prudent use of antibiotics seems to have resulted in a plateau of the emergence of antibiotic resistance of these pathogens. The incidence of MRSA seems to be increasing, especially in chronic sinusitis.

Many antibiotics are indicated for the treatment of ABRS. In addition, some antibiotics do not have Food and Drug Administration (FDA) approval for treatment of sinusitis but are still appropriately used.

Anon et al. (2004) made the following comprehensive recommendations regarding the treatment of acute rhinosinusitis:

1. A bacterial infection should be suspected if symptoms of a viral URI do not improve after 10 days or if symptoms worsen after 5 to 7 days.
2. Antibiotic resistance is common. Specifically, intermediate resistance of *S. pneumoniae* to penicillin is 15%, and complete resistance is estimated at 25%. Resistance of *S. pneumoniae* and *H. influenzae* to trimethoprim–sulfamethoxazole (TMP-SMX) is common, as is

resistance of *S. pneumoniae* macrolides. β-Lactamase production of *H. influenzae* and *M. catarrhalis* is 30% and 100%, respectively.

3. Selection of an antibiotic should be based on severity of symptoms, whether the patient has received an antibiotic in the past 4 to 6 weeks, and the response to current antibiotic therapy after 72 hours. Mild symptoms include rhinorrhea and fatigue. Moderate symptoms include congestion, low-grade fever, and facial pain.

4. The widespread use of fluoroquinolones for mild sinusitis may promote resistance to this class of antibiotics.

5. Antibiotic choices for adults with mild disease and no recent antibiotics include amoxicillin (1.75-4 g/day, with or without clavulanate), cefpodoxime proxetil, cefuroxime axetil, or cefdinir. TMP-SMX, doxycycline, azithromycin, erythromycin, and clarithromycin may be considered in penicillin-allergic patients, but the failure rate may be as high as 20% to 25%. Failure of therapy should prompt reevaluation of the patient or a switch in therapy.

6. Antibiotic choices for adults with moderate disease or with mild disease who have received recent antibiotics include amoxicillin–clavulanate (4 g/day) or a respiratory fluoroquinolone (levofloxacin or moxifloxacin). Ceftriaxone (1-2 g parenterally for 5 days) or combination therapy for gram-positive and gram-negative bacteria may also be considered. Failure of therapy should prompt reevaluation of the patient, CT scan, endoscopy with culture, or a switch in therapy.

7. Antibiotic choices for children with mild disease and no recent antibiotics include amoxicillin (90 mg/kg/day, with or without clavulanate), cefpodoxime proxetil, cefuroxime axetil, or cefdinir. TMP-SMX, doxycycline, azithromycin, erythromycin, and clarithromycin may be considered in penicillin-allergic patients (especially immediate type I hypersensitivity), but the failure rate may be as high as 20% to 25%. If the patient has a true type I hypersensitivity to β-lactams, desensitization, sinus culture, CT scan, or other intervention may be necessary. Less severe reaction may allow use of another β-lactam antibiotic. Failure of therapy should prompt reevaluation of the patient or a switch in therapy.

8. Antibiotic choices for children with moderate disease or with mild disease who recently received antibiotics include amoxicillin–clavulanate (90 mg/kg/day). Cefpodoxime proxetil, cefuroxime axetil, or cefdinir may be used if there is a nonsevere penicillin allergy (rash). Cefdinir is preferred because of high patient acceptance. Ceftriaxone (50 mg/kg/day parenterally for 5 days) or combination therapy for gram-positive and gram-negative bacteria may also be considered. Failure of therapy should prompt reevaluation of the patient, CT scan, endoscopy with culture, or a switch in therapy.

As recurrence or severity of the infection increases, broader spectrum antibiotics are indicated. Macrolides, fluoroquinolones, augmented penicillins, and cephalosporins are useful in these cases. Culture-directed antibiotic treatment may be indicated in more refractory cases. Obtaining a culture usually requires an ENT referral because simply swabbing the nasal cavity is not reliable.

Cultures can be obtained from an endoscopically guided middle meatus swab. Maxillary sinus aspiration can also be done but is more invasive and not much more accurate than a middle meatal culture. DNA swabs allowing for rapid identification of pathogens and resistance may be available in the near future. Adjunctive treatment to help improve mucociliary function becomes more important as recurrence increases.

TREATMENT

KEY TREATMENT

The American Academy of Otolaryngology–Head and Neck Surgery produced a consensus statement of Clinical Practice Guidelines for Treatment of Presumed Sinusitis (Rosenfeld et al., 2007). The following summary guidelines are for acute viral sinusitis (VRS), presumed ABRS, and chronic rhinosinusitis (CRS). The key symptoms of sinusitis were rhinorrhea, nasal obstruction, and facial pressure or pain.

Strongly Recommended Treatment
The quality of data supporting the benefits of treatment outweighing the potential harm is strong (Grades A, B):
- Clinicians should attempt to differentiate between viral and bacterial sinusitis.
- The level of pain should be assessed when treating ABRS.

Recommended Treatment
The benefits of treatment outweigh the risks, but the data are not as strong (grades B, C):
- Imaging studies are not recommended for cases of uncomplicated VRS.
- If a decision is made to treat ARS, amoxicillin should be used as first-line therapy if the patient does not have a penicillin allergy.
- If the condition worsens or fails to improve in 7 days, antibiotics should be started or changed.
- The clinician should attempt to differentiate CRS from recurrent ARS.
- The clinician should assess the patient with CRS or recurrent ARS for conditions or anatomic abnormalities that would predispose the patient to these conditions.
- The clinician should obtain a CT scan when evaluating a patient with recurrent ARS or CRS.
- The patient should be educated on control measures for ARS and CRS.

Optional Treatment
There is only weak evidence that the benefit of treatment outweighs the risk (grade D):
- Symptom relief should be offered when treating VRS.
- Symptom relief should be offered when treating ARS.
- Observation without use of antibiotics may be done in cases of uncomplicated ARS with temperature less than 101°F (<38.3°C).
- Diagnostic nasal endoscopy should be used in the evaluation of recurrent ARS or CRS.
- Testing should be done for allergy and immune system dysfunction in patients with recurrent ARS or CRS. (SOR: B).

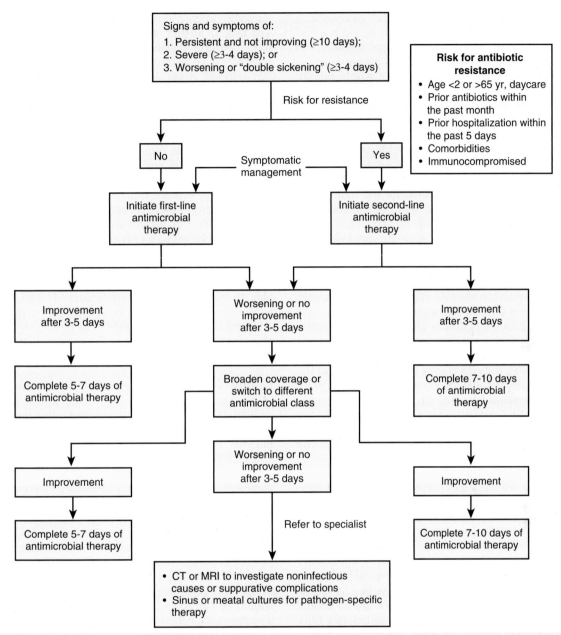

Figure 18-8 Algorithm for the management of acute bacterial rhinosinusitis. *CT,* Computed tomography; *MRI,* magnetic resonance imaging. (Reprinted with permission from Chow AW, Benninger MS, Brook I, et al. IDSA clinical practice guideline for acute bacterial rhinosinusitis in children and adults. *Clin Infect Dis.* 2012;54(8):e72-e112.)

In 2012, The Infectious Disease Society of America (IDSA) published a practice guideline for the treatment of ABRS in adults and children. The multidisciplinary panel addressed several issues in the management of ABRS, including (1) the difficulty of accurately differentiating bacterial from viral acute rhinosinusitis, leading to inappropriate antimicrobial therapy; (2) lack of consensus regarding the use of empiric antimicrobial therapy for ABRS; (3) changing bacterial isolates and antimicrobial susceptibility profiles associated with ABRS; and (4) impact of the conjugated vaccines for *S. pneumoniae* and the emergence of nonvaccine serotypes associated with ABRS. A useful algorithm for subsequent management based on risk assessment for

antimicrobial resistance and evolution of clinical responses was offered (Figure 18-8).

Medical Treatment of Chronic Sinusitis. Medical treatment of CRS is based on the same principles as for acute sinusitis: improvement of mucociliary function and eradication of bacteria. Treatment of chronic sinusitis requires more aggressive therapy, with potential side effects. If chronic sinusitis is suspected, CT scan of the paranasal sinus should be ordered to confirm the diagnosis before further treatment is initiated. This contrasts with acute sinusitis, for which CT is not necessary before treatment. In addition to confirming the diagnosis and severity of the infections, CT can identify abnormalities that can predict a poorer response to medical treatment. This includes a posterior septal deviation, polyps, allergic fungal sinusitis, and various sinus abnormalities. The scan may also arouse suspicion of sinonasal mass or tumor, which would require earlier ENT evaluation.

It is noteworthy that there are *no* medications with FDA indications for treatment of chronic sinusitis. Despite this, several medical options are effective in improving symptoms in patients with CRS. Nasal saline irrigations for the symptoms of CRS are effective and well tolerated. Although minor side effects are common, the beneficial effect of saline appears to outweigh these drawbacks for the majority of patients. The use of topical saline could be included as a treatment adjunct for the symptoms of CRS. Additionally, a Cochrane Collaboration review in 2011 concluded that the topical nasal steroids were likely beneficial in the treatment of CRS, and the adverse affects were mild (Snidvongs et al., 2011).

Topical and systemic steroids can be used to improve drainage in cases of chronic sinusitis by decreasing mucosal inflammation, edema, and mucus production. Most topical nasal steroids must be used daily for several weeks to have significant benefit. Although oral steroids significantly improve symptoms, the effects may be short lived, and the potential side effects must be considered. Patients with known allergies should be treated. It should be remembered, however, that antihistamines cause mucosal drying and mucus stasis. Other allergy and asthma medications such as leukotriene inhibitors and IgE antagonists can also benefit coexisting sinusitis.

Although it is common to use antibiotics, the efficacy in treating chronic sinusitis has not been validated in controlled studies in adults. Two consensus statements do report that antibiotic treatment is likely beneficial in adults but not in children (Duiker, 2004; grade B). Because of the apparent benefit, antibiotics are typically used to treat chronic sinusitis in adults. An antibiotic with activity against staphylococci, as well as the more typical pathogens (with predicted antibiotic resistance), must be chosen. In cases of nasal polyps, an antibiotic with antipseudomonal activity may be necessary. Although no antibiotics have FDA indications for "chronic sinusitis," appropriate choices include macrolides, broader spectrum cephalosporins, fluoroquinolones, and augmented penicillin. "Older" antibiotics, such as TMP-SMX, clindamycin, doxycycline, and linezolid, may be quite useful in documented staphylococcal infections. Also, the addition of rifampin may be useful in treating documented staphylococcal infections. ENT evaluation, including diagnostic nasal endoscopy, will allow for a swab and culture of the middle meatus. Middle meatal culture has been shown to be a reliable substitute to an invasive maxillary puncture and aspiration. Typically, longer courses of antibiotics are used (3-6 weeks) to treat chronic sinusitis. Few controlled studies are available to support this, and side effects may be significant. An oral probiotic should be considered because it may offer gastrointestinal (GI) protection.

In the past, studies demonstrated successful treatment of patients with CRS using systemic, topical antifungals, or both. This was based on a theory that environmental fungi incited an intense immune response in predisposed patients. The lack of further studies supporting this theory has led the Cochrane Collaboration to recommend against the routine use of antifungals in the treatment of CRS. There are selected cases in which this treatment should be considered.

Otolaryngologists have begun to use a variety of medications topically to treat chronic sinusitis. Some of this is off-label use or compounded (usually antibiotics and steroids). The vast number of topical medications for the treatment of nasal and sinus conditions (and the paucity of well-controlled comparison studies) makes it very difficult to make recommendations about which treatment to use. In general, topical medications are appealing because the medication is deposited where the pathology exists and not subjected to GI breakdown and metabolism. Side effects and complications are rare, and many of these medications are indicated in children (some as young as 2 years old). For any topical medication to be effective, it must be able to reach the nasal epithelium. If pathology such as deviated nasal septum or polyps exists, this must be addressed. FDA indications for most of these sprays are for allergic rhinitis but also have efficacy for nonallergic causes of rhinitis.

Failure of Medical Treatment of Sinusitis. When medical treatment of recurrent acute sinusitis or chronic sinusitis is not successful, further evaluation and treatment are indicated. An ENT consultation should be obtained for patients unresponsive to medical treatment of chronic sinusitis. The risk factors listed previously should be considered and modified if possible. Allergy and immune system testing should be arranged. Pulmonary evaluation may be helpful if the patient has poorly controlled reactive airway disease.

If CT has not been done, a scan of the sinuses should be ordered to evaluate the anatomy of the sinuses. If CT has already been done and symptoms have changed or significant time has elapsed since the first scan, a repeat scan may be helpful. Before repeating the scan, ENT consultation should be considered because the consultant might have a preference for the type of scan ordered. A standard sinus CT scan often contains only coronal views; more detailed scans may be necessary for surgical planning. Low-radiation sinus scanners are now in many ENT offices, and these are typically much less expensive than a hospital scan.

The CT scan will show any evidence of chronic mucosal edema of the sinuses or even complete opacification. Partial or complete bilateral sinus opacification is typically seen in cases of long-standing chronic sinusitis or polyposis. Unilateral opacification or bony erosion is more worrisome for neoplastic disease or fungal sinusitis. The size of the turbinates and position of the nasal septum can also be assessed. In cases of medical failure or intolerance to continued aggressive medical treatment, surgery should be considered. ESS or *functional* ESS (FESS) has become the mainstay of surgical intervention for chronic sinusitis. Although earlier external surgical techniques are still occasionally indicated, FESS has the advantage of leaving no external scars and specifically addresses the critical area within the sinuses: the ostiomeatal unit. The procedure is typically done under general anesthesia but can also be done under local anesthesia. Success rates of greater than 90% are expected and have been reported in many studies. Some patients experience relapse of their condition, especially if they had nasal polyps. Revision surgery is offered in these cases and is usually quite successful.

Successful sinus surgery often results in fewer and less severe infections and improved response to future medical treatment. The procedure is often done with septoplasty and turbinate surgery and is well tolerated. Advancements in minimally invasive surgical techniques have allowed preservation of more normal tissue and less surgical morbidity. Nasal packing is often not necessary. When used, resorbable packs are typically applied, obviating the need and discomfort of pack removal. Potential complications of ESS include bleeding, scarring leading to further sinus blockage, loss of smell, and rare orbital and CNS injury. For this reason, surgery is undertaken only after appropriate medical treatment and careful patient consideration.

According to Cochrane Collaboration recommendations for CRS, FESS as currently practiced is a safe procedure. The limited evidence suggests that FESS has not been demonstrated to confer additional benefit to that obtained by medical treatment (with or without sinus irrigation) in CRS. It is important to note that FESS should be viewed as an adjunct to medical therapy and not as a stand-alone procedure in most cases. After surgery, the sinuses should be much more receptive to topical therapy, including saline, steroid, or antibiotic rinses. The open sinus cavities also allow for direct endoscopic culture and more tailored antibiotic treatment. With this in mind, FESS has been shown to be a viable treatment option for patients who fail medical treatment. More randomized controlled trials comparing FESS with medical and other treatments are required, with long-term follow-up.

Advances in medical and surgical treatment deserve mention. Newer allergy and asthma medications (leukotriene inhibitors and IgE antagonists) show promise in the future treatment of chronic sinusitis. New antibiotics continue to be released to treat antibiotic-resistant bacteria. Compounding pharmacies have made available topical antibiotic and antifungal formulations that are quite effective in some patients. Topical treatment is appealing because it delivers extremely high concentrations of medication to the target area, minimizing systemic side effects and, theoretically, development of resistance. Topical treatment seems more effective in patients with sinus surgery that created open sinuses, allowing antibiotic delivery. Research into the genetics of sinusitis continues and should lead to further advances in treatment.

Surgical advances include improved power surgical debriders that spare normal mucosa, have more efficient surgery, and reduce blood loss. Packing materials have improved and often are resorbable or impregnated with medication. Image-guided surgery has become more common. Balloon techniques allow dilation of the sinus ostia without tissue removal but do not treat the ethmoid sinuses, which are most commonly involved. Balloon dilation can be done in the office on selected patients. Although not a substitute for an experienced surgeon, these advances often allow more focused and possibly safer surgery.

Pediatric Sinusitis. Although the sinuses are not completely developed until adolescence, children can still develop sinusitis, usually involving the ethmoid and maxillary sinuses. Young children can have 5 to 10 episodes of acute rhinitis (viral URI) in a year. The usual symptoms of a URI lasting longer than 2 weeks can indicate development of bacterial sinusitis. Other symptoms indicating sinusitis in children include nighttime cough and foul breath. Children rarely complain of facial pain, which is common in adults.

Diagnoses other than sinusitis should also be considered in children with prolonged URI-type symptoms. Previously undiagnosed choanal atresia or stenosis can be present. Unilateral or bilateral nasal foreign bodies can also cause these symptoms. Environmental allergies should be considered, as should immunodeficiency, GERD, ciliary dyskinesia, and cystic fibrosis. Many children with asthma also have coexisting sinusitis, which can complicate asthma management. Recurrent sinusitis can cause or worsen asthma exacerbations.

Chronic adenoid hypertrophy or chronic adenoiditis can mimic sinusitis in children. Adenoid hypertrophy can also *cause* sinusitis secondary to nasal obstruction, mucus stasis, and subsequent infection. This can occur with or without the presence of tonsil hypertrophy. Adenoid hypertrophy can lead to facial changes caused by chronic mouth breathing. Children with long-standing nasal obstruction tend to have elongated, narrow faces with open-mouth breathing, the "adenoid facies." Differentiating chronic adenoiditis from sinusitis can be difficult because the symptoms may be identical, and the disorders often coexist.

According to Cochrane Collaboration recommendations, limited evidence suggests that *intranasal corticosteroids* may significantly improve nasal obstruction symptoms in children with moderate to severe adenoidal hypertrophy. This improvement may be associated with a reduction of adenoid size.

Medical treatment of pediatric acute sinusitis is similar to that for adults: decongestants, nasal saline irrigations or mist, and antibiotics (Duiker, 2004). The pathogens are similar to those of adults: pneumococci, *H. influenzae,* and *M. catarrhalis.* Coexisting problems (e.g., allergies) should be controlled. Diligence on the part of the parents is required because children might not tolerate nasal saline sprays willingly. If compliance is ensured, medical treatment should result in improvement in the vast majority of patients.

Children who fail medical therapy should be referred to an otorhinolaryngologist. Often, adenoidectomy, sometimes combined with a turbinate reduction procedure. is recommended. In properly selected patients, this procedure has a high success rate in greatly improving symptoms. For children unresponsive to medical treatment and adenoidectomy, a CT scan should be obtained. If significant sinusitis exists, the child likely has chronic sinusitis. Medical treatment should be reattempted because it might be more effective after the obstructing adenoids have been removed. If not previously done, the child should be screened for allergies, immune deficiency, and cystic fibrosis.

The efficacy of antibiotics in the treatment of pediatric chronic sinusitis has not been validated. Unlike adults with chronic sinusitis who likely benefit from longer courses of antibiotics, evidence-based research indicates that this is not the case for children (Duiker, 2004).

If symptoms persist, ESS is considered. The surgery targets the ostiomeatal unit in hope of improving sinus drainage and aeration. A ciliary biopsy may also be done to evaluate for ciliary dyskinesia. Cultures should also be obtained to tailor postoperative antibiotics. In properly selected patients, sinus surgery has an extremely high success rate. Although rare, significant risks, including bleeding and orbital and intracranial injury, must be considered. Surgery may be especially beneficial in children with coexisting pulmonary disease (asthma or cystic fibrosis).

Sinonasal Tumors

Intranasal and sinus tumors often manifest with symptoms identical to those of more benign sinonasal conditions. Nasal obstruction, facial pressure or pain, and bloody rhinorrhea are common symptoms of a neoplastic process within the nasal cavity or sinuses. Because these symptoms are also common with sinusitis, a high index of suspicion is required, and diagnosis is often delayed.

Tumors of the external nose are usually related to prolonged exposure to the sun. Basal cell carcinoma and squamous cell carcinoma (SCC) are most common (see Chapter 33). Intranasal tumors can be benign or malignant. The most common growth within the nasal cavity is *benign squamous papilloma*, caused by human papillomavirus (HPV). This typically appears as an exophytic lesion within the nose, often at a junction between squamous and respiratory epithelium, and causes irritation and bleeding. Treatment consists of simple excision, and recurrence is uncommon. Malignant degeneration is extremely unlikely.

A much more aggressive papillary lesion is an *inverted papilloma*. These tumors often manifest as unilateral polyps and can cause symptoms of nasal obstruction, bleeding, and sinusitis. These lesions require excision because they can be locally destructive, and malignant degeneration can occur. Endoscopic excision is usually possible, although external approaches are sometimes required.

The *juvenile nasopharyngeal angiofibroma* is a tumor that occurs exclusively in adolescent boys. The tumor is located within the nasopharynx but typically causes nasal symptoms. Patients present with nasal obstruction and recurrent epistaxis. Because nosebleeds and nasal obstruction are both common problems, a high index of suspicion is required to make a timely diagnosis. These tumors can be extremely aggressive, and surgical excision is required. Recurrences are possible, and radiation therapy is recommended for some patients.

Malignant tumors of the nose and sinuses include SCC, adenocarcinoma, adenoid cystic carcinoma, hemangiopericytoma, osteosarcoma, and malignant melanoma. Again, early symptoms are similar to those of sinusitis, which often results in a delayed diagnosis. The prognosis ranges from extremely good to extremely poor, depending on tumor type and stage. Orbital and intracranial extension often occurs. Both regional and distant metastases result in poorer prognosis. Aggressive treatment is required and involves combined treatment with surgery and radiation, sometimes with chemotherapy.

KEY TREATMENT

- Nasal saline sprays or irrigations are a very effective treatment for both rhinitis and sinusitis (SOR: B).
- Nasal steroids sprays are an important treatment for chronic sinusitis (SOR: B).
- Treatment to restore mucociliary function in sinusitis is likely as important as antimicrobial therapy (SOR: C).

Oral Cavity and Pharynx

Key Points

- The IDSA now recommends the rapid antigen test alone to confirm the presence of group A β-hemolytic streptococcal (GABHS) pharyngitis in adults.
- Back-up throat cultures for those with a negative rapid antigen detection test (RADT) are not necessary in adults because of the low incidence of GABHS and low risk for rheumatic fever. Antistreptococcal antibody titers are not recommended to diagnose acute GABHS because they indicate past infection.
- Whereas motor disorders of the esophagus are more likely to cause difficulty swallowing liquids, mechanical obstruction produces dysphagia with both solids and liquids.
- From 23% to 60% of patients presenting with a globus sensation have GERD.
- Snoring is the most common symptom of obstructive sleep apnea (OSA) and is more common in men than women.

PHYSICAL EXAMINATION AND RADIOGRAPHY

See eAppendix 18-4 online.

ACUTE PHARYNGITIS AND TONSILLITIS

Viral agents cause the majority of sore throats. Even when exudates are present, fewer than 15% of children and 10% of adults have documented GABHS as the cause. In children younger than 3 years, the predominance of a viral cause is even higher than in school-age children.

Pharyngitis caused by GABHS (*Streptococcus pyogenes*) has its peak incidence in late winter and early spring. The incubation phase is 2 to 5 days and leads to sudden onset of sore throat, painful swallowing, fever, and chills. Less frequent symptoms include headache, abdominal pain, and nausea. On physical examination, a purulent white exudate is often seen on the tonsils, and the anterior cervical nodes are tender and enlarged. There is sometimes a scarlet fever rash (a diffuse, erythematous, macular, rough rash that tends to coalesce) and soft palate petechiae. Scarlet fever is the result of exotoxin-producing strains of GABHS. Pastia lines are caused by prominence of the rash in the flexor creases of the antecubital space or axilla. A strawberry tongue is another sign of GABHS.

A throat culture is the "gold standard" for diagnosing GABHS infection. A 5% sheep blood agar plate is used to plate the throat swab and can be read in 24 hours (sensitivity, 96%). Serologic tests (antistreptolysin O [ASO] titer) are accurate but not practical to use in diagnosing an acute infection because of the time involved in obtaining results and the fact that an elevated titer could just indicate a past infection. RADTs or optical immunoassays (OIAs) are the most popular tests for detection of GABHS. Although most manufacturers claim 95% to 97% true negatives (specificity), clinical trials suggest a lower figure of 90%. True positives (sensitivity) are claimed to be 90% to 95%, but again, clinical trials show closer to 60% to 80% sensitivity (Shulman et al., 2012).

Scoring systems based on features of sore throat have been developed. The McIsaac Decision Rule is a modification of the Centor criteria for diagnosing GABHS (McIsaac et al., 2000). McIsaac allots points to specific criteria. One point is given for each of the following criteria: temperature higher than 38°C, no cough, tender anterior cervical adenopathy, tonsillar swelling or exudates, and age 3 to 14 years. No points are given for age 15 to 44 years, and −1 point is taken away for age older than 45 years. The number of points provides a predictive percent of the probability of having GABHS A score of 0 means 2% to 3% of patients have GABHS; 1 point, a 4% to 6% incidence; 2 points, a 10% to 12% incidence; 3 points, a 27% to 28% incidence; and 4 points, a 38% to 63% incidence of GABHS. When the score is less than 2, no treatment is recommended. When the score is 2 or 3, cultures or OIAs are recommended. When the score is 4 or 5, treatment is the best option. The IDSA now recommends the use of the rapid antigen test alone to confirm the presence of GABHS in adults (Bisno et al., 2002).

A study comparing five management strategies (no treatment or testing, empiric treatment with penicillin, throat culture, OIA with culture if results negative, OIA alone) found empiric therapy the least cost effective and culture the most cost-effective strategy when the GABHS prevalence was 10%. OIA alone was as effective as OIA followed by throat culture when the OIA result was negative (Neuner et al., 2003). After a test result is positive, treatment with penicillin or a cephalosporin is recommended because there has been no incidence of in vitro resistance to these drugs.

Treatment for GABHS is penicillin VK, 250 mg two or three times daily in children and 500 mg twice daily in adolescents and adults for 10 days. Intramuscular penicillin G benzathine, 600,000 U for a child weighing less than 60 lb (27 kg) or 1.2 million U for patients weighing more than 60 lb, can be used if compliance is a problem or if the child cannot swallow or is vomiting. Mixing the benzathine penicillin with 300,000 U of procaine penicillin alleviates some of the discomfort. Penicillin-allergic patients can use erythromycin, 40 mg/kg in two or four divided doses daily for 10 days. In recurrent disease, cephalexin, 12.5 mg/kg or 500 mg twice daily for 10 days, can be prescribed. Alternative antibiotics include cefpodoxime (Vantin), cefprozil (Cefzil), cefuroxime axetil (Ceftin), cefixime (Suprax), ceftibuten (Cedax), azithromycin (Zithromax), clarithromycin (Biaxin), and amoxicillin–clavulanic acid (Augmentin). Cephalosporins appear to be superior to penicillin in terms of bacterial eradication and clinical cure (Pichichero and Brixner, 2006).

After treatment, 15% of throat cultures remain positive for GABHS. This is considered a carrier state. One effective way to eliminate the carrier state is to use clindamycin (Cleocin), 20 mg/kg/day in three divided doses (maximum,

450 mg/day) for 10 days (Tanz et al., 1998). Contagiousness to others is inversely proportional to the length of time that GABHS is carried. Culturing contacts is indicated only when the contact is symptomatic. Pets have been considered a reservoir for GABHS, but some evidence casts doubt on this supposition (Wilson et al., 1995).

Although antimicrobial treatment is believed to decrease the suppurative (peritonsillar abscess) and immunologic (acute rheumatic fever, acute glomerulonephritis [AGN]) sequelae of GABHS infection, much is not known. *Acute rheumatic fever* had become rare until 1986, when its incidence increased; any explanation is mere speculation. Good evidence indicates that antimicrobial treatment shortens the symptomatic period of GABHS and plays a part in preventing acute rheumatic fever. However, acute rheumatic fever can still occur in the presence of appropriately diagnosed and treated cases of GABHS pharyngitis and even in the absence of a symptomatic infection.

Only specific serotypes of GABHS (12, 49, 55, 57, Red Lake strain) cause AGN because of an antigen–antibody deposition on the kidney glomerular membrane. When a patient does have GABHS infection caused by one of these strains, only 15% develop AGN. Edema, hypertension, and rusty urine are the hallmarks of AGN and occur 10 days after the infection. Prompt treatment of GABHS pharyngitis with penicillin does not appear to prevent AGN. Treatment is symptomatic to control the blood pressure and edema.

The indications for tonsillectomy after GABHS infections are six episodes within 1 year or three to four episodes within each of 2 years (Pichichero, 2004). The severity of the infections and the total number of missed workdays or schooldays should also be taken into account when considering tonsillectomy. Sleep-disordered breathing is another indication for tonsillectomy and runs the gamut from snoring to sleep apnea.

Viral causes of pharyngitis include rhinovirus (20% of all pharyngitis) and coronavirus, adenovirus, and parainfluenza virus (5% of all pharyngitis) (Middleton, 1996). Coxsackievirus A can cause 1- to 2-mm red-ringed vesicles on the tonsils, uvula, and soft palate and is known as *herpangina*. Coxsackievirus A16 is the major cause of hand, foot, and mouth disease, a 1-week illness with 4- to 8-mm ulcers on the tongue and buccal mucosa and vesicles on the palms and soles. The incubation time for this illness is 4 to 6 days.

A type of pharyngitis similar to coxsackievirus A16 pharyngitis is caused by HSV. Painful, shallow, red-bordered ulcers develop on the soft palate, gums, lips, or buccal mucosa and cause fever, pain, and lymphadenopathy. Acyclovir (Zovirax), 200 mg five times daily for 5 days; famciclovir (Famvir), 125 mg twice daily for 5 days; or valacyclovir (Valtrex), 500 mg twice daily for 5 days, can be used in severe cases of herpes stomatitis and lessen the duration of symptoms and viral shedding.

Epstein-Barr virus (EBV) as a cause of pharyngitis can mimic GABHS infection. It can also occur concurrently with GABHS infection. Studies have shown the two infections occurring together in 2% to 33% of cases. Prodromal symptoms to severe sore throat include malaise, anorexia, chills, and headache. Fatigue, lymphadenopathy, and hepatosplenomegaly can follow in 5 to 14 days. Pharyngitis with tonsillar hypertrophy and a membranous white tonsillar exudate lasts 5 to 10 days. Lymphadenopathy and hepatosplenomegaly can persist for 3 to 6 weeks. Contact sports should be avoided for 6 weeks because of the possibility of splenic rupture. Complications that occur in fewer than 2% of patients with EBV infection include thrombocytopenia, hemolytic anemia, Guillain-Barré syndrome, Bell palsy, transverse myelitis, and aseptic meningitis. Hepatitis can be seen in 20% to 50% of patients with EBV infection.

The diagnosis is made on clinical grounds, supported by positive antibody test results. A CBC shows atypical lymphocytes, and a monospot test is positive in 95% of cases of infectious mononucleosis (Middleton, 1996). Steroids (and rarely urgent tonsillectomy) are indicated when the tonsillar hypertrophy causes pharyngeal obstruction or when other life-threatening complications occur. Amoxicillin should be avoided because it often causes a rash in patients with infectious mononucleosis.

When the symptoms point to infectious mononucleosis but the monospot test or EBV titer result is negative, the patient may be infected with cytomegalovirus (CMV). The illness lasts 2 to 6 weeks and is characterized in older patients by a higher fever and greater malaise but milder pharyngitis than with infectious mononucleosis. A CMV-specific immunoglobulin M (IgM) antibody test is the best means of diagnosing this infection. In immunocompromised patients, ganciclovir (Cytovene) or foscarnet (Foscavir) can control the infection. Bacterial causes of pharyngitis other than GABHS are shown in Table 18-13.

KEY TREATMENT

- Although current treatment guidelines recommend oral penicillin V or intramuscular penicillin G benzathine as drugs of choice for GABHS, strong evidence supports cephalosporins as a first choice for this infection (SOR: A) (Casey and Pichichero, 2007).
- In countries with low rates of rheumatic fever, 3 to 6 days of oral cephalosporins to treat GABHS has comparable efficacy to the usual 10-day oral penicillin regimen (SOR: A) (Altamimi et al., 2009).
- Once-daily amoxicillin (750 mg to 1 g) for 10 days is as good as twice-daily or three-times-daily dosing (SOR: A) (Lennon et al., 2008).

Table 18-13   Bacterial Causes of Pharyngitis Other Than Group A β-Hemolytic Streptococci

Anaerobes (*Peptostreptococcus, Fusobacterium,* and *Bacteroides* spp.)
Arcanobacterium haemolyticum
Chlamydia pneumoniae
Corynebacterium diphtheriae
Corynebacterium haemolyticum
Francisella tularensis (tularemia)
Group C β-hemolytic streptococci
Group G β-hemolytic streptococci
Haemophilus influenzae (epiglottitis)
Mycoplasma pneumoniae
Neisseria gonorrhoeae
Yersinia enterocolitica

Bisno AL, Gerber MA, Gwaltney JM Jr, et al: Practice guidelines for the diagnosis and management of group A streptococcal pharyngitis, *Clin Infect Dis* 35:113-115, 2002.

ABNORMALITIES OF THE ORAL REGION
(eTable 18-9)

Swallowing Disorders

Patients who experience difficulty swallowing solids or liquids have *dysphagia.* About 7% of Americans experience dysphagia in their lifetimes, and 30% to 40% of nursing home residents have swallowing disorders. Whereas motor disorders of the esophagus are more likely to cause difficulty in swallowing liquid, mechanical obstruction causes dysphagia with both solids and liquids.

Pharyngeal muscle weakness or CNS disease can lead to difficulty beginning the act of swallowing. The proximal third of the esophagus is composed of striated or voluntary muscles, the middle third is a combination of striated and smooth muscles, and the distal third is entirely smooth muscle tissue. The two sphincters involved in swallowing are the upper and lower esophageal sphincters (UES and LES).

Food sticking in the throat is known as *oropharyngeal dysphagia,* and 80% of the cases are the result of neuromuscular disease (see eTable 18-10 online for causes) (Trate et al., 1996). An inability to move solids from the esophagus to the stomach is referred to as *esophageal dysphagia,* which is more common than oropharyngeal dysphagia (see eTable 18-11 online for causes). The history is extremely important in determining the cause of the dysphagia. If dysphagia is associated with chest pain, especially difficulty swallowing cold liquids, diffuse esophageal spasm is the most likely diagnosis.

A constant sensation of a lump in the throat is known as *globus hystericus* and is not necessarily associated with the act of swallowing. This diagnosis can be made only by ruling out anatomic or motor abnormalities of the pharynx, larynx, or esophagus. From 23% to 60% of patients presenting with a globus sensation have GERD as the origin (Ahuja et al., 1999). eTable 18-12 online lists head and neck symptoms related to GERD versus gastroesophageal symptoms.

If the food bolus sticks in the distal esophagus, a stricture, malignancy, or ring is most likely the cause. Achalasia or degeneration of the nerve cell bodies of the myenteric plexus leads to esophageal dilation and food retention associated with increased tone of the LES.

Motor disorders of the esophagus cause progression of dysphagia over months to years. A carcinoma should be suspected when there is a rapid progression of dysphagia for solids in an older person with anorexia and weight loss; a history of smoking and alcohol use makes this diagnosis more likely. Medication-induced esophagitis is characterized by acute retrosternal pain exacerbated by swallowing. The most common medications associated with this syndrome are the tetracyclines (doxycycline, minocycline), potassium chloride pills, iron preparations, quinidine and its derivatives, aspirin, and nonsteroidal antiinflammatory drugs.

Another mechanical reason for dysphagia is an *esophageal web,* a thin diaphragm most often in the proximal esophagus. When associated with iron-deficiency anemia, the condition is known as *Plummer-Vinson syndrome. Pulsion diverticula* are usually seen at the level of the cricopharyngeal muscle and occur predominantly in men older than

50 years. Regurgitation of food and liquid immediately after swallowing is the hallmark of this condition, with large diverticula that can cause almost complete obstruction. A *Zenker diverticulum* originates from the posterior aspect of the esophagus and is bounded superiorly by the cricopharyngeal muscle and inferiorly by the inferior pharyngeal muscle. Treatment is usually surgical.

Dysphagia in the pediatric population is often secondary to tonsillar hypertrophy or an esophageal foreign body. Diagnostic studies include a barium esophagram with views of the pharynx, esophagus, and stomach. To detect rings and early strictures, a barium-coated tablet or marshmallow can reveal the site of narrowing. When there is radiographic evidence of a lesion, esophagogastroscopy is indicated.

If no abnormality is found, esophageal manometry should be performed. The goal of esophageal manometry is to assess the characteristics of esophageal contractions and to define the LES and the UES and their response to swallowing. Only about 50% of patients show a definitive abnormality with this test. Provocative testing with manometry involves infusion of edrophonium, esophageal balloon dilation, or acid perfusion into the esophagus. Recording esophageal pH in an ambulatory setting can indicate if acid reflux episodes are present at the same time as the patient's symptoms.

The management of swallowing difficulties is directed toward the specific cause involved. eTable 18-13 lists the treatments for the various causes of dysphagia.

Snoring and Obstructive Sleep Apnea

Snoring is extremely prevalent but is also the most common symptom of OSA. OSA occurs when the upper airway collapses during sleep, leading to obstruction, hypoventilation, and hypoxemia. OSA has been associated with development or exacerbation of hypertension, coronary artery disease, pulmonary hypertension, poor concentration, impotence, obesity, depression, and increased risk of motor vehicle crashes. It is a potentially serious medical condition that can be overlooked if not specifically sought.

Men have OSA more than women, and children can also be affected. Adults with OSA are often overweight or stocky. They are told that they snore loudly, and episodes of respiratory obstruction or gasping might be witnessed by a family member. Symptoms of OSA include loud snoring, daytime fatigue, morning headache (secondary to hypoxemia), restless sleeping habits, and frequent catnaps (often unintentionally, sometimes while driving).

Physical examination should be performed with attention to the patient's body habitus. The oral cavity should be inspected for tonsillar hypertrophy and evidence of excess soft palate tissue. The size and position of the tongue should be noted. The nose should be inspected for nasal obstruction. The size and position of the mandible and its relationship to the neck should be evaluated.

Strong suspicion of sleep apnea should be confirmed with an overnight sleep study or polysomnogram. The sleep study measures intensity of snoring, presence of apnea or hypopnea (partial apnea), oxygen saturation, sleep efficiency, and cardiac rhythm. The data are compiled and analyzed by a sleep specialist. A numeric value of the total number of apneas and hypopneas is derived, called the apnea-hypopnea index or *respiratory distress index* (RDI). An RDI of less than 5 is considered normal. An RDI greater than 5 with or without oxygen desaturation indicates sleep apnea. Some patients are found to have normal RDI values but have snoring with disrupted sleep. This condition has been described as "upper airway resistance syndrome."

Treatment. Treatment for OSA is either nonsurgical or surgical. Nonsurgical methods are always attempted first and include weight loss and assisted nighttime ventilation by continuous positive airway pressure (CPAP). CPAP essentially splints the collapsed airway open with positive pressure, given as the patient initiates inhalation. It is generally well tolerated, safe, and extremely effective in compliant patients. Unfortunately, some patients either do not tolerate CPAP or choose not to use it. Surgery is a potential option in these patients.

Numerous surgical procedures exist for the treatment of OSA. The gold standard is tracheotomy, which bypasses the upper airway obstruction and is almost always successful in eliminating sleep apnea. Obviously, most patients do not see this as an appealing solution. For patients with severe OSA and morbid obesity, however, a tracheotomy can give extremely satisfying results. More popular procedures have been devised to try to eliminate (rather than bypass) the upper airway anatomic obstruction. Uvulopalatopharyngoplasty is used most often and entails removal of redundant oropharyngeal tissue, including the tonsils, the uvula, and a strip of soft palate. Its success depends on the severity of the OSA and the patient's anatomy. Other procedures use laser or radiofrequency tissue ablation to eliminate excess pharyngeal tissue. If nasal obstruction exists, it is corrected. In severe cases, procedures directed at the tongue base and facial skeleton have been effective in properly selected patients.

The Larynx

Key Points

- Most cases of acute stridor are secondary to inflammatory disorders such as croup, epiglottitis, and tracheitis.
- Parainfluenza virus is the most common cause of croup.
- Neoplasia must be considered in adults with voice or swallowing complaints.
- Visualization of the laryngopharynx is required to evaluate any patient with persistent or severe stridor or with voice or throat symptoms.
- Laryngomalacia is the most common cause of chronic stridor in neonates.
- Vocal cord nodules are always bilateral; polyps and cysts are usually unilateral.
- It is essential to elicit smoking and alcohol histories in patients with voice complaints because of the association with cancer.
- Although often idiopathic or iatrogenic, vocal cord paralysis requires thorough investigation.
- Vocal cord dysfunction is often misdiagnosed as asthma.

INITIAL EVALUATION

Hoarseness, stridor, foreign body (globus) sensation, and dysphagia are all symptoms of laryngeal or hypopharyngeal pathology. When a patient presents with any of these persistent symptoms, a complete past medical and social history is essential. In addition, if hoarseness has persisted, laryngoscopy is indicated. Laryngoscopy can be performed indirectly using a mirror. If the hypopharynx and larynx are not adequately visualized with the mirror because of an excessive gag reflex, direct flexible fiberoptic laryngoscopy can be performed. A topical vasoconstrictor (e.g., 0.5% ephedrine) with a topical anesthetic (e.g., topical lidocaine) can be applied in the nose to improve patient comfort; however, this is not always necessary. The flexible fiberoptic nasopharyngoscope is then passed through the pharynx to visualize the larynx.

RADIOGRAPHY

Indications for imaging the larynx include evaluation of laryngeal tumors and traumatic laryngeal injuries. CT or MRI is performed to evaluate depth of invasion with tumors. CT is the preferred method for imaging malignant and non-malignant disease, although MRI has certain indications. Traumatic injuries are best evaluated by CT scan. The modalities to assess stridor are directed by the history and physical examination. Available imaging techniques include chest radiography (posteroanterior [PA] and lateral radiographs), neck radiography (PA and lateral radiographs), and fluoroscopy. Contrast esophagography may be necessary to evaluate for vascular anomalies that can cause airway and esophageal compression or to rule out tracheoesophageal fistulas.

SPECIAL STUDIES

Airway fluoroscopy is useful for evaluating pediatric stridor. Fluoroscopy provides a dynamic picture of the entire airway from the nasopharynx to the carina. This facilitates the identification of obstructive lesions or foreign bodies during both phases of respiration.

A more specialized examination called video laryngeal stroboscopy (VLS) is performed by a speech-language pathologist. This technique allows highly detailed views of the larynx and evaluation of the gross movement of the vocal cords and their vibratory motion. VLS is an excellent modality to photodocument lesions of the laryngopharynx. VLS is also helpful to voice therapists in identifying and following patients with voice disorders, including hoarseness and paradoxical vocal cord dysfunction (see later discussion).

Finally, direct laryngoscopy using a rigid laryngoscope can be performed, usually in the OR. Indications include the need for further evaluation and biopsy of pathology of the larynx.

LARYNGITIS

Laryngitis is the most common cause of acute hoarseness. It is secondary to diffuse swelling of the larynx. Viral infections are the most common cause and are often associated with other upper respiratory tract symptoms. Treatment is conservative, and recommendations include relative voice rest and avoidance of inhalational substances such as cigarette smoke or other irritating substances. Humidification may be helpful. Symptoms from viral laryngitis usually improve within days. Consider other causes if symptoms persist. A Cochrane review concluded that the risks of antibiotics outweigh the benefits in treatment (Reveiz & Cardona, 2013).

Fungal infections can also localize to the larynx. Of these, *Candida albicans* is the most common and is found in immunocompromised patients; patients using inhaled steroids; and those using long-term, broad-spectrum antibiotics. Characteristic findings on examination include a diffuse reddened mucosa covered by white patches. Topical treatment includes nystatin, miconazole, or clotrimazole; systemic therapy includes fluconazole or ketoconazole. Other uncommon infectious causes of laryngitis include tuberculosis and syphilis.

STRIDOR

Stridor is noisy breathing. Stridor is a symptom, not a definitive diagnosis. It results from turbulent airflow and some degree of airway obstruction, usually at the level of the laryngopharynx or trachea. Stridor can affect both adults and children, but children present special diagnostic and therapeutic challenges because the antecedent history may be limited, physical examination is more challenging, and their small airways are more susceptible to critical obstruction. Because of the small airway diameter in infants and children, even small and subtle abnormalities can cause stridor and obstruct the airway.

It is helpful to localize stridor in the respiratory cycle. In general, whereas *inspiratory* stridor typically is caused by an obstruction at or above the level of the true vocal cords, *expiratory* stridor is usually localized to the more distal tracheobronchial tree. Biphasic stridor is usually caused by an obstruction at the true vocal cords, typically at the immediate subglottic level.

The medical history provides valuable information in the evaluation of stridor. In the pediatric population, a history should include questions about cyanosis, feeding difficulty, failure to gain weight, and retractions. Time of onset of stridor, birth history, prematurity, and need for immediate intubation at birth may help to identify the cause of stridor. A past medical history of smoking or ethanol abuse in an adult patient should raise the suspicion of a neoplastic process. Factors that tend to exacerbate the stridor are noted. These include change of intensity of stridor when in different positions, when crying, and when feeding. Previous intubation or laryngotracheal trauma can lead to acquired subglottic or tracheal stenosis. The presence of fever and a history of acute onset may be significant for an infectious process, including epiglottitis, croup, or tracheitis. New-onset stridor or increased stridor may portend impending airway distress, which would require more immediate workup, close monitoring, and possibly the need to stabilize the airway.

The severity of the obstruction and the need for intervention are sometimes difficult to determine. A child with a partially obstructed airway can have stridor but may not appear to be in respiratory distress. Intervention might or might not be needed. Examination should include documentation of stridor in the phase of respiration and whether suprasternal or intercostal retractions are present. The patency of the nose, oral cavity, and oropharynx should be noted. Large tonsils and adenoids can contribute to obstruction of the airway. The neck should be palpated for any masses that can cause extrinsic compression. Significant obstruction can cause signs of tachycardia, tachypnea, confusion, restlessness, or obtundation. Visualization of the larynx is paramount. Flexible fiberoptic laryngoscopy is the most useful modality in the workup of stridor. This usually requires an ENT consultation. It is easily performed in infants and adults.

There are many causes of stridor in the adult and pediatric population. The differential diagnosis includes lesions affecting various parts of the airway (see eTable 18-14 online). Pediatric patients are more likely to have congenital causes of stridor, but any age group may have stridor secondary to trauma; inflammation; neoplasia, polyps, or papillomas; and foreign bodies. Common congenital anomalies include laryngomalacia, true vocal cord paralysis, subglottic stenosis, laryngeal webs and clefts, subglottic hemangiomas, anomalous great vessels, and complete tracheal rings. Most cases of acute stridor are caused by inflammatory disorders, including croup, epiglottitis, and tracheitis. Chronic causes of stridor are more likely to be congenital, neoplastic, or from airway stenosis.

The most common cause of acute stridor in the pediatric population is *croup* (laryngotracheobronchitis). The parainfluenza virus is the most common cause and affects primarily the subglottic area but can also affect other portions of the laryngotracheal complex. Stridor can be inspiratory or biphasic and is often associated with a barking cough. Radiographs usually show the typical subglottic narrowing caused by edema. The typical age group is 6 months to 2 years, but the condition can be seen in children up to 5 years. The infection and inflammation are usually self-limiting, and conservative management is recommended. Evidence supports the routine use of corticosteroids in most children with croup (Husby et al., 1993). Intervention at an earlier phase of the illness reduces the severity of symptoms and the rates of return to a health care practitioner for additional medical attention, ED visits, and hospital admissions. Many children respond to a single oral dose of dexamethasone. For those who do not tolerate the oral preparation, nebulized budesonide or intramuscular dexamethasone is a reasonable alternative.

According to Cochrane Collaboration recommendations regarding glucocorticoids for croup, dexamethasone and budesonide are effective in relieving the symptoms of croup as early as 6 hours after treatment. Fewer return visits and (re)admissions are required, and hospital stay is shortened. Dexamethasone is also effective in patients with mild croup (Russell et al., 2011).

Severe cases of croup can manifest with significant respiratory distress or even obstruction. Therapy in these patients requires hospitalization (ICU in some cases); treatment includes corticosteroids, supplemental oxygen, fluids, humidification, nebulized racemic epinephrine aerosols, heliox, and occasionally intubation. A Cochrane review concluded benefit of symptoms at 30 minutes with nebulized epinephrine (Bjornson et al., 2013). Complications from croup include airway obstruction, pneumonia, pulmonary edema, and cardiac failure.

Laryngomalacia is the most common cause of chronic stridor in neonates and is characterized by high-pitched inspiratory stridor that can be intensified with agitation, feeding, and placement in the supine position. The disorder is caused by immaturity of the laryngeal cartilages and is typically seen on examination as an omega-shaped epiglottis and floppy aryepiglottic folds that partially obstruct the laryngeal inlet on inspiration. The key to the diagnosis lies in the history and typical findings on flexible fiberoptic laryngoscopy. Airway fluoroscopy provides a dynamic evaluation of the laryngotracheal complex and often shows a component of tracheomalacia as well (laryngotracheomalacia). Treatment is rarely needed because the problem is self-limiting and resolves by 18 months of age. Gastroesophageal reflux is extremely common because the increased pressure gradient needed for adequate ventilation causes an increase in acid reflux into the esophagus. This exacerbates the condition by causing a component of reflux laryngitis. Rarely, failure to thrive because of feeding problems, cor pulmonale, or persistent desaturations while asleep can indicate the need for surgical intervention to improve the airway. Even if uncomplicated laryngomalacia is suspected, ENT evaluation is still recommended to confirm the diagnosis.

True *vocal cord paralysis* is another common cause of congenital stridor and usually occurs at birth to 2 months of age. In newborns, the cause is usually injury to the vagus nerve sustained at birth, or it can be secondary to CNS abnormalities. Unilateral paralysis is more common than bilateral paralysis. The diagnosis is confirmed by flexible fiberoptic laryngoscopy. Workup also includes barium swallow, neck and chest radiography, and cardiology consultation to rule out a cardiothoracic cause of vagal paralysis. Treatment is rarely necessary because most patients improve or compensate adequately with the opposite vocal cord. On the other hand, bilateral vocal cord paralysis manifests with a high-pitched stridor and upper airway obstruction. MRI of the brain should be included in the workup to rule out hydrocephalus and Arnold-Chiari malformation. Emergent airway intervention by intubation or tracheotomy might be necessary.

Adults may also be affected by vocal cord paralysis, either unilateral or bilateral. Possible etiologies include neoplastic processes, traumatic injuries to the recurrent laryngeal nerve, or idiopathic causes. If the cause is known (e.g., occurring after cervical surgery resulting in recurrent laryngeal nerve injury), further workup may not be recommended. If the cause is not clear, imaging of the brain, neck, and chest is ordered to rule out a compressive lesion affecting the recurrent laryngeal nerve.

Recurrent respiratory papillomatosis occurs in all ages but is more common in children. It is the most common benign tumor of the airway and is usually found on the true vocal cords and supraglottic and subglottic areas. The causative agent is HPV, typically subtypes 6 and 11. In juvenile onset cases, the virus is thought to be acquired through the birth canal. Adult cases are thought to be sexually transmitted. Symptoms usually begin with hoarseness or aphonia and progress to stridor and dyspnea at a later stage of disease.

The disease can progress to complete airway obstruction and eventually death. There is no cure, but some patients eventually go into remission. Treatment includes endoscopic debulking with various lasers or laryngeal shaver, but recurrence and multiple procedures are common. Intralesional cidofovir is often used for recalcitrant cases, but adequate studies are lacking (Chadha, 2012). Intralesional bevacizumab is a promising new treatment. Hopefully, the HPV vaccination program will lead to a reduced incidence of respiratory papillomatosis.

Subglottic tracheal stenosis is caused by cicatricial scarring of the subglottic trachea and can be congenital or acquired. This area is often affected because the cricoid cartilage is the only complete ring in the trachea and is the narrowest segment in the airway. Acquired subglottic stenosis is most frequently a result of long-term intubation, with traumatic injury to the subglottic segment causing pressure necrosis and subsequent scarring. It may be idiopathic. Subglottic stenosis can occur in adults or children. Patients with severely stenotic segments causing significant respiratory symptoms usually require surgical intervention that includes splitting the subglottis with short-term stents, use of cartilage grafts, or placement of long-term stents.

Although many of the etiologies previously listed may also cause stridor in the adult population; most often an adult who presents with stridor will have this symptom secondary to subglottic tracheal stenosis, inflammation or edema of the larynx, neoplasia, or vocal cord paralysis. The workup is tailored to the history and endoscopic findings. In general, treatment of stridor depends on the etiology. The critical issue is stabilizing the airway in hopes of preventing catastrophe. Some conditions may respond to medical treatment, but any patient with stridor should be treated as having an impending airway obstruction until proved otherwise. ICU observation may be required, with personnel available to stabilize the airway by intubation or tracheotomy. ENT consultation is recommended for further evaluation and more definitive treatment.

LARYNGEAL TRAUMA

Injury to the airway is an important cause of death in patients with head and neck trauma. Laryngeal trauma must be recognized early to avoid catastrophic sequelae. Securing the airway is the most important initial step in the management of these injuries to preserve life. The most preventable factor in morbidity and mortality is likely a delay in diagnosis. Less severe laryngeal injuries may initially go undiagnosed, but major injuries can lead to early death.

Blunt trauma is a common cause of death in motor vehicle crashes. The mechanism of blunt laryngeal trauma is typically caused by a hyperextension of the neck (i.e., against the dashboard) with compression and fixation of the larynx against the cervical spine, which leads to fracture or comminution of cartilage with associated soft tissue injury. Laryngotracheal disruption can occur from "clothesline" injury, which can occur with motorcycle and snowmobile accidents.

Penetrating trauma is becoming more common with an increase in civilian violence. Knife and gunshot wounds are the most common cause of death in homicide cases. Other traumatized structures in the neck can include the great vessels, the esophagus, and the cervical spine.

Signs of laryngotracheal trauma include tenderness over the larynx, anterior neck contusion, subcutaneous emphysema, palpable fractures or crepitus, loss of thyroid prominence, tracheal deviation, and hemoptysis. Symptoms include hoarseness, shortness of breath, inability to tolerate the supine position, and dysphagia.

Examination should include flexible fiberoptic laryngoscopy in every patient, if possible, to evaluate the anatomy and function of the larynx. Diagnostic imaging includes cervical spine films, chest radiographs, and CT scan. Unless physical examination and flexible fiberoptic laryngoscopy are normal, CT should be done in most cases. The decision to take a patient to the OR is based on history, physical examination, flexible fiberoptic laryngoscopy, and CT scanning.

As with any trauma patient, management of the airway is of primary importance. Some controversy still exists on the optimal management of the airway. Most authors recommend awake local tracheotomy as the safest and least traumatic method of securing the airway in an adult patient with laryngeal trauma. Some reports recount the disastrous outcome of a lost airway after attempted oral or nasal intubation in patients with laryngeal trauma. However, many still advocate intubation as the initial method of securing the airway. Emergency cricothyroidotomy can be performed if time does not permit a formal tracheotomy.

HOARSENESS

All patients who present with hoarseness should be questioned about the history, the duration, and the progression of symptoms. Hoarseness may be categorized as chronic or acute. Acute hoarseness is rarely secondary to a malignant process. Acute hoarseness usually results from vocal abuse, laryngitis, or smoking. Malignancy should be considered in patients with chronic hoarseness, but the differential also includes GERD, polyps, nodules, neurologic disorders, papillomas, and functional voice disorders (see eTable 18-15 online).

Other symptoms can coexist with hoarseness. Cough can be secondary to irritation of the vocal cords from acute or chronic inflammation but can also indicate cancer of the larynx or lung. Dysphagia or odynophagia can be present from disorders of the pharynx and esophagus. Hemoptysis with hoarseness should be considered secondary to a malignancy until proved otherwise. A history of smoking and vocal abuse is an important consideration. Clear visualization of the larynx by indirect or direct laryngoscopy is absolutely necessary for all patients who present with hoarseness that does not resolve on its own or with medical therapy. This can require referral to an otorhinolaryngologist unless the family physician has training and experience in the procedures.

An unusual cause of voice problems is *spasmodic dysphonia* (or laryngeal dystonia). The exact cause is unknown but is thought to be a CNS condition classified under "focal dystonias." It typically causes a harsh staccato voice but may cause breathiness. Spasmodic dystonia responds poorly to voice therapy but has been shown to respond very well to botulinum toxin injections into the larynx, which is done endoscopically or externally. The treatment weakens the muscles and lessens the symptoms for several months. Repeat injections are usually done, and response to treatment can decrease over time.

VOCAL CORD PARALYSIS

Vocal cord paralysis can manifest itself as hoarseness. However, many patients are able to maintain a relatively normal voice because of compensation from the opposite vocal cord. Patients can present with shortness of breath while conversing, cough when swallowing, aspiration, or recurrent pneumonia. They may complain of the inability to hold a breath while exerting against a closed glottis (Valsalva maneuver). Visualization of the larynx by indirect or flexible fiberoptic nasolaryngoscopy usually reveals an immobile, sluggish vocal cord in a paramedian position.

Paralysis can result from peripheral (recurrent laryngeal or vagus) nerve involvement or a CNS disorder (e.g., CVA). Approximately 90% of vocal cord paralyses result from dysfunction of the peripheral nerve. Most causes of paralysis are found after a careful history and physical examination (see eTable 18-16 online). Because of the course of the recurrent laryngeal nerve around the arch of the aorta on the left and around the subclavian artery on the right, imaging, typically with CT, includes the skull base to mediastinum to evaluate the entire extent of the nerve. VLS is very useful and often yields further diagnostic and prognostic information.

Surgical trauma from thyroidectomy, carotid artery surgery, or transcervical spine procedures is the most common cause of unilateral vocal cord paralysis. Idiopathic or a presumed viral etiology is another common cause. Neoplastic processes, including thyroid, lung, and esophageal cancers, must always be ruled out as a cause of either compression or invasion. Skull base tumors and mediastinal lesions are less common causes of paralysis. Careful palpation of the neck to rule out masses and evaluation of other cranial nerves help identify these problems.

Bilateral vocal cord paralysis typically manifests with significant respiratory distress caused by obstruction of the glottis from bilateral medialization of vocal cords. Many of these patients need emergent establishment of the airway by intubation or tracheotomy. Causes of bilateral vocal cord paralysis include thyroid or cervical spine surgery or CNS disorders. Hydrocephalus or an Arnold-Chiari malformation can cause bilateral paralysis via brainstem herniation with stretching of the vagus nerves. Treatment in these circumstances is aimed at stabilizing the airway and treating the underlying problem, with the paralyzed cord usually returning to normal function after a few months.

Numerous surgical techniques can improve vocalization. Endoscopic injection of autologous, allogenic, or alloplastic substances can provide temporary and even permanent improvement by medializing the weak vocal cord so that the mobile vocal cord can make contact. Open surgical approaches can also be performed for permanent unilateral paralysis, with excellent results. Medialization of the vocal cord with the use of alloplastic materials is now common. Surgical options to correct permanent bilateral vocal cord paralysis include removal of a portion of the arytenoids or

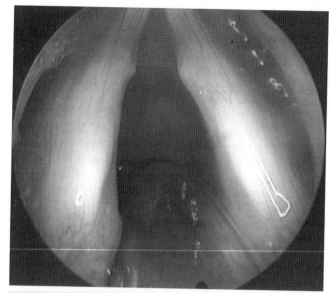

Figure 18-9 Intraoperative photograph of true vocal cords with nodules in 25-year-old teacher.

vocal cords to open the airway; permanent tracheotomy is a last resort.

VOCAL CORD NODULES

Vocal cord nodules result from long-term vocal overuse or abuse. Nodules are typically seen as symmetric raised areas at the anterior aspect of each vocal cord. These occur more often in women, boys, lecturers, coaches, and professional singers. The most common symptom is hoarseness and a persistent raspy voice. Smoking, allergies, and GERD tend to aggravate the condition and can prevent healing.

Nodules are always bilateral and classically occur at the junction of the anterior third and posterior two thirds of the vocal cords (Figure 18-9). Nodules must be distinguished from polyps, which are smooth and often unilateral, and granulomas, which tend to be located more posteriorly on the vocal cord. Treatment is initially conservative. The patient is referred for voice therapy, which consists of counseling, vocal reeducation, relative voice rest, and psychotherapeutic rehabilitation. Most patients respond after several sessions of voice therapy, but satisfactory improvement can take up to 12 to 18 months. Measures to control acid reflux and avoidance of irritating substances such as cigarette smoke are also routinely recommended. Surgery is reserved for rare patients who do not respond to voice therapy and consists of endoscopic removal. Postoperative voice therapy and acid reflux control are always indicated after surgical removal of nodules.

REFLUX LARYNGITIS

Reflux laryngitis, also known as *laryngopharyngeal reflux* (LPR), is a relatively common condition. Many patients do not have the classic symptoms of GERD, including heartburn, and the correct diagnosis is often initially overlooked. Constant throat clearing may be the only presenting symptom. Other manifestations include a feeling of a lump in the throat with a choking sensation *(globus pharyngeus)*, odynophagia, dysphagia, chronic cough, and hoarseness. The patient may also complain of postnasal drainage. Spicy foods, fats, caffeine, chocolate, beer, milk, and orange juice are known to exacerbate the condition by lowering LES pressure. Several medications increase reflux of acid into the esophagus, such as β-blockers, calcium channel blockers, diazepam, and progesterone. Obesity and sleep apnea also predispose the patient to GERD and reflux laryngitis.

A careful history and examination allow the diagnosis to be made. Findings on indirect or flexible fiberoptic laryngoscopy are nonspecific and include edema, erythema, and redundancy of the mucosa around the arytenoids and postcricoid area. Occasionally, small granulomas are present posteriorly near the vocal processes of the arytenoids. Studies that help confirm the diagnosis of GERD include barium swallow, pH probe, esophageal manometry, and esophagoscopy. Gastroenterology consultation may be necessary.

Often the diagnosis of reflux laryngitis cannot be confirmed or excluded without a trial of empiric therapy. The treatment for reflux laryngitis consists of diet and lifestyle modifications and acid-reducing medications. Diet modification includes avoidance of foods and substances known to increase acid reflux. Lifestyle modifications include avoidance of eating near bedtime, elevation of the head of the bed 6 to 10 inches (15-25 cm), weight loss, and avoidance of tight-fitting clothing. Medical therapy usually begins with a trial of H_2 blockers or preferably daily dosing of proton pump inhibitors (PPIs). Refractory or severe cases usually respond well to twice-daily PPI therapy. Although most patients respond to treatment, resolution of symptoms can take several months after initiating proper treatment. It is critical that visualization of the larynx be obtained early if the patient's symptoms persist to rule out more serious pathology such as neoplasia.

CANCER OF THE LARYNX

Squamous cell carcinoma is by far the most common malignancy of the larynx. Laryngeal cancer accounts for 1% to 4% of all malignancies detected every year. The peak age group is between 60 and 65 years old, and it is more prevalent in men than in women (8 : 1), although the incidence in women is rising. Malignancies of the larynx are most common in smokers and alcohol abusers. When both these factors are present, the risk of developing cancer becomes 50% greater than the additive risk of each. Only 2% to 5% of laryngeal cancer patients have no history of smoking. Thus, it is extremely important to elicit smoking and alcohol histories in patients with head and neck complaints.

Hoarseness can be a very early symptom, making most cancers of the larynx curable because they are detected early. For this reason, hoarseness should never be simply attributed to "laryngitis" without proper evaluation. Other symptoms, including sore throat and referred otalgia, can exist without hoarseness. These patients are often treated incorrectly with antibiotics for an extended period, and referral is delayed, thereby increasing morbidity and mortality.

Detection of cancer requires visualization of the larynx. Indirect or direct laryngoscopy usually shows a discrete,

well-circumscribed exophytic lesion in the endolarynx, most frequently on one of the true vocal cords. A critical concern is potential airway obstruction in bulky tumors; emergent airway intervention is fairly common. The neck should be palpated to evaluate for cervical lymphadenopathy. Metastasis to the lungs or brain is also possible.

Several modalities of treatment exist for laryngeal cancer. Carcinoma in situ and leukoplakia can be treated with laser vaporization. Stage I carcinoma is treated with external-beam radiation or partial laryngectomy techniques. Stage II carcinoma may be treated with radiation therapy, partial laryngectomy, or total laryngectomy. Stage III disease may be treated with single or combined modality treatments. Single modality treatment includes radiation or surgery. Combined modality includes chemoradiation or surgery and radiation. Stage IV treatment includes total laryngectomy with radiation or chemoradiation with or without total laryngectomy. Specific treatment depends on the location and extent of the tumor. Radiation and chemoradiation are often used in organ-sparing protocols to preserve function. Speech restoration is still possible after total laryngectomy with a tracheoesophageal prosthesis. Neck dissection is required in patients with cervical metastases. Stage I glottic carcinoma has a 90% 5-year survival with treatment because a tumor on the vocal cord presents early as hoarseness and the vocal fold has less lymphatics to allow tumor to metastasis. Unfortunately, tumors at other laryngeal locations often cause symptoms only when large or when regional metastases develop. Therefore, the prognosis of these tumors is much worse.

KEY TREATMENT

The American Academy of Otolaryngology–Head and Neck Surgery produced a consensus statement of clinical practice guidelines for hoarseness (dysphonia).

Strongly Recommended Treatment
The quality of data supporting the benefits of treatment outweighing the potential harm is strong (grades A, B):
- Clinicians should not routinely prescribe oral antibiotics to treat hoarseness.
- Voice therapy should be employed for patients with hoarseness that affects voice-related quality of life.

Recommended Treatment
The benefits of treatment outweigh the risks, but the data are not as strong (grades B, C):
- Hoarseness should be diagnosed in a patient with an altered quality of voice.
- Patients with hoarseness should be assessed with history or physical examination with attention to previous factors or treatments that may have affected the recurrent laryngeal nerve or larynx. This may include neck or chest surgery or radiation therapy, endotracheal intubation, tobacco use, or occupational vocal overuse.
- The clinician may perform laryngoscopy (or refer) if hoarseness persists at a maximum of 3 months or sooner if suspicion of serious illness is high. A general rule of thumb is to refer for laryngoscopy after 3 weeks as this is the time frame that a viral laryngitis should have resolved.

- CT or MRI should not be performed until the larynx has been visualized (these tests may not be necessary).
- Antireflux medications should not be prescribed in the absence of other signs or symptoms of reflux.
- Clinicians should not routinely prescribe oral corticosteroids to treat hoarseness.
- Laryngoscopy should be performed before recommending voice therapy.
- Clinicians should advocate for surgery as an option in cases of suspected malignancy, soft tissue lesion, or glottic insufficiency.
- Patients should be referred for possible treatment with botulinum toxin in cases of spasmodic dysphonia.

Optional Treatment

There is only weak evidence that the benefit of treatment outweighs the risk (grade D):
- The clinician may perform laryngoscopy (or refer) at any time after diagnosis of hoarseness.
- Antireflux medications may be prescribed in patients with hoarseness if there are signs of chronic laryngitis with laryngoscopy.
- Patients with hoarseness should be educated on control and prevention methods (SOR: A; B).

The Neck

Key Points

- Knowledge of anatomy is critical in the diagnosis of a neck mass.
- In the pediatric population, a neck mass is by far most commonly infectious or inflammatory.
- In adults, a neck mass is neoplastic until proven otherwise.
- Imaging may be necessary in the evaluation and can include CT with contrast, ultrasonography, or MRI.
- Tissue sampling in the form of fine needle biopsy or excisional biopsy may be necessary when the examination and imaging are not diagnostic.
- Avoid core biopsy and incisional biopsy in cases of suspected neoplasm other than lymphoma as to avoid seeding tumor into surrounding tissue.

PHYSICAL EXAMINATION

See eAppendix 18-5 online.

NECK MASSES

Proper evaluation of a neck mass includes obtaining a complete history and performing a thorough examination of the neck and all mucosal surfaces. Knowledge of anatomy is critical in narrowing the differential diagnosis because the list of possible diagnoses for a neck mass is extensive. History should include duration; growth rate; and associated symptoms such as pain, sore throat, voice change, dysphagia, fever, weight loss, night sweats, and otalgia. Aspects of the social history, such as tobacco use or exposure, alcohol use, ill contacts, and recent travel, should be obtained. The clinician should ascertain characteristics of the mass on examination, such as whether the mass is soft, firm, mobile, fixed, pulsatile, fluctuant, tender, or overlying skin change. Imaging options include CT with contrast, MRI with contrast, and ultrasonography, which may assist in the diagnosis and help define the extent of a lesion. Tissue sampling is often necessary to determine the etiology of a neck mass. Usually a fine-needle biopsy is recommended as the first-line option for biopsy. This test is sometimes necessary to obtain under image guidance. Excisional biopsy is performed when needle biopsy is inconclusive or if further pathologic assessment is necessary. Core needle biopsy and incisional biopsy should be avoided when there is a concern for neoplasm other than lymphoma to avoid seeding surrounding tissue with neoplastic cells. Classification includes congenital, inflammatory, and neoplastic disorders. In general, pediatric neck masses are usually inflammatory followed by congenital lesions. Neoplasia occurs less often in pediatric patients. In adults, neoplasia is by far the most common entity, with inflammatory causes less common and congenital masses rare.

Congenital Neck Masses

Congenital neck masses are common in children but can occur in any age group. These are the most common cause of noninflammatory neck masses in the pediatric population. Classifying these into midline or lateral location helps in the workup because congenital neck masses occur in consistent anatomic sites (see eTable 18-17 online).

Midline Neck Masses

Thyroglossal duct cysts are the most common anterior midline neck masses in children. They are remnants of the descending tract of the thyroid gland from the foramen cecum at the base of the tongue to its normal position in the lower neck. Cysts or fistulas can occur anywhere along this tract and can intermittently become infected. Physical examination usually reveals a 2- to 4-cm mass in the anterior neck that moves with swallowing and elevates with tongue protrusion (Figure 18-10). Treatment is surgical excision of the cyst and the tract, including the midhyoid bone, to the base of the tongue (Sistrunk procedure). There have been reports of neoplastic transformation of these cysts. Recurrence is possible.

Dermoid cysts typically develop along midline embryonic fusion planes and are composed of ectodermal and mesodermal embryonic remnants. Their usual location in the neck is in the submental area. They are also found along the dorsum of the nose. Dermoid cysts tend not to move with swallowing or elevate with tongue protrusion, unlike thyroglossal duct cysts. Treatment is surgical excision.

Ranulas are cystic lesions that are usually present in the floor of the mouth. They can become "plunging" and extend through muscle planes into the upper midneck area. Plunging ranulas are thought to occur from mucus extravasation from a blocked salivary duct. Physical examination of a plunging ranula reveals a cystic mass in the submental area with or without a cystic mass in the floor of the mouth.

Lateral Neck Masses

Branchial cleft cysts are common congenital abnormalities found in the lateral neck area and are caused by failure of

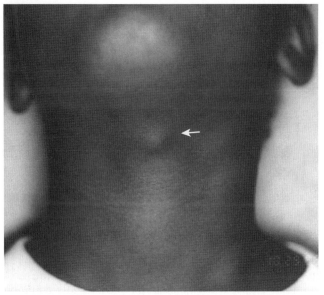

Figure 18-10 Photograph of 9-year-old child with midline neck mass *(arrow)* near the hyoid bone. Swallowing produced movement in the mass. Surgical excision with pathologic evaluation demonstrated a thyroglossal duct cyst.

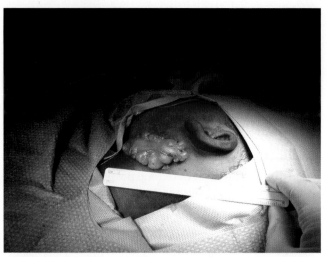

Figure 18-11 Intraoperative photograph of a large lipoma of the left upper neck.

obliteration of the embryonic branchial clefts during development. Abnormalities can also manifest as sinus tracts or fistulas in the skin. These can become intermittently infected, especially after URIs.

Second branchial cleft abnormalities are by far the most common. These usually manifest as masses anterior to the sternocleidomastoid muscle with or without a fistulous opening. The sinus tract passes between the external and internal carotid arteries and ends in the tonsillar fossa. Treatment is complete surgical excision of the cyst and sinus tract after control of infection with appropriate antibiotics. First branchial cleft cysts are less common and manifest as a duplication abnormality of the external auditory canal (type I) or as an infected mass near the angle of the mandible with a sinus tract passing superiorly through the parotid salivary gland (type II).

Lymphangiomas (cystic hygromas) are congenital lymphatic masses often found in the neck. They usually manifest during the first year of life and often enlarge after a URI. They can also increase in size after hemorrhage into the cystic cavities. Lymphangiomas form from a failure of complete development and subsequent obstruction of the lymphatic system. They are most frequently found as an asymptomatic mass in the posterior triangle of the neck but can also be found anteriorly, causing airway or swallowing problems. Physical examination reveals a nontender, fluctuant, soft, spongy mass without discrete margins. Surgery is the mainstay treatment for lymphangiomas, although other modalities of treatment include intralesional injection sclerotherapy and systemic interferon.

Hemangiomas are the most common congenital malformations. Most are cutaneous, but they can also be found in deep tissues. The most common deep location in the head and neck is the masseter muscle. Hemangiomas are characterized by appearance at or after birth followed by a rapid proliferative phase at 6 to 18 months of age. The

lesion then reaches a plateau phase followed by a slow, involutional phase over 6 to 8 years. Even large, uncomplicated lesions left untreated usually undergo almost complete resolution. Conservative management is almost always recommended.

Certain locations, including the nasal tip, lips, and eyelids, can cause severe functional or cosmetic deformities, and referral for removal may be appropriate. Massive lesions can cause high-output heart failure or a consumptive coagulopathy (Kasabach-Merritt syndrome); others can become ulcerated, infected, or hemorrhagic. Treatment of hemangiomas includes surgical excision, pulsed-dye laser therapy, β-blockers, interferon-α-2ab and -2b, and corticosteroids.

Neoplastic Neck Masses

Benign lesions in the head and neck include *lipomas* and *fibromas* and require no treatment unless they cause significant functional or cosmetic deformity (Figure 18-11).

All neck masses in adults should be presumed to be malignant until proved otherwise. The most common malignant neck mass in adults is metastatic SCC. Primary tumors are usually found in the upper aerodigestive tract or skin and metastasize to cervical lymph nodes according to identifiable lymphatic drainage patterns. Smoking and alcohol abuse are major etiologic factors. However, base of tongue and tonsil SCCs related to HPV subtypes 16 and 18 are becoming more common. Careful examination of all mucosal surfaces of the head and neck is crucial to identify the primary tumor site. Endoscopy with biopsies is the first step in the diagnosis. Treatment may include any combination of surgical resection of the primary site neck dissection, radiation, and chemotherapy, depending on the location and extent of the primary tumor and the extent of cervical metastasis. HPV-related SCC has high cure rates in contrast to tobacco-related carcinoma and is often treated with chemoradiation.

Lymphomas are one of the most common malignancies of the neck in children but can occur at any age. Patients can present with lymphadenopathy associated with constitutional symptoms (night sweats, fever, weight loss), hilar adenopathy, or hepatosplenomegaly. Diagnosis is confirmed by excisional biopsy. Most head and neck lymphomas are treated with a combination of radiation and chemotherapy.

Rhabdomyosarcoma is a common childhood neoplasm with peak incidence at age 5 years. Early symptoms include a painless, enlarging mass or symptoms related to obstruction by tumor. Approximately 35% of rhabdomyosarcomas manifest in the head, neck, and orbit. Embryonal rhabdomyosarcoma and botryoid sarcoma (a variety of embryonal rhabdomyosarcoma) are most common in the head and neck, accounting for 75% of cases. Other forms include alveolar and pleomorphic. Diagnosis is made by excisional biopsy, and treatment is multimodal, including surgery, radiation, and chemotherapy.

Carotid body tumors are paragangliomas that arise from the adventitia of the common carotid bifurcation. They are thought to arise from derivatives of neural crest cells and are members of the diffuse neuroendocrine system. They can be associated with other tumors of similar origin, including medullary thyroid carcinoma, parathyroid adenoma, and pheochromocytoma, in up to 7% of cases. Familial incidence is 8% to 10%, and inheritance is autosomal dominant. A high incidence of bilateral carotid body tumors occurs in familial paraganglioma syndromes, and 1% to 3% of these tumors actively secrete substances such as catecholamines or serotonin. Symptoms of catecholamine secretion include headache, perspiration, palpitations, pallor, and nausea. Screening for blood and urinary catecholamines should be performed to rule out a secreting tumor or pheochromocytoma. Symptoms of serotonin secretion are carcinoid syndrome, including diarrhea, flushing, severe headaches, and hypertension.

Other tumors of the head and neck arise from neurogenic tissue. These include schwannomas, neurofibromas, neurofibrosarcomas, and neuroblastomas. These tumors can manifest with associated cranial nerve deficits. Treatment is surgical excision.

Inflammatory Neck Masses

Whereas *reactive lymph nodes* from a viral infection should be treated expectantly, bacterial infections such as streptococcal tonsillitis or pharyngitis should be treated with appropriate antibiotics. Infectious mononucleosis is an important cause of extensive cervical lymphadenitis. An association with tonsillopharyngitis, fever, and malaise should raise suspicions. Monospot or EBV serology can be obtained for diagnosis. In general, a CBC with differential and ESR or CRP can aid in determining if lymph node enlargement is inflammatory. In some cases, inflamed lymph nodes can suppurate and become abscessed, requiring incision and drainage. Masses thought to be reactive lymph nodes not responding to conservative management (antibiotics) after approximately 4 to 6 weeks often need referral for further evaluation to obtain a definitive diagnosis.

Cervical lymphadenitis can be caused by *atypical mycobacteria*, which may appear as a subcutaneous abscess with erythematous overlying skin (Figure 18-12). Treatment includes excisional biopsy and appropriate antibiotics according to culture sensitivities. Incisional drainage is contraindicated and can cause chronic fistulization.

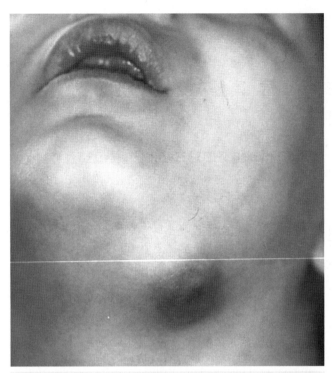

Figure 18-12 Photograph showing cervical adenitis with overlying skin erythema in a young child. Cultures revealed atypical mycobacteria.

Cat-scratch disease is another pediatric infection that can manifest with lymphadenopathy. Most patients recount exposure to a cat, and many have a cutaneous lesion representing an inoculation site. The diagnosis is made by serologic testing for *Bartonella henselae.* The disease is self-limited.

Tuberculous cervical lymphadenitis (scrofula), caused by *Mycobacterium tuberculosis,* can manifest with bilateral lower lymph node enlargement. It is usually associated with pulmonary involvement, and treatment is with a multidrug regimen. Nodes not responding to treatment should be excised.

Patients infected with *human immunodeficiency virus* (HIV) can present with asymptomatic lymph node enlargement. Persistent lymphadenopathy in AIDS patients is common, and most are followed if the nodes remain stable. Because of the higher incidence of non-Hodgkin lymphoma and Kaposi sarcoma in these patients, any suspicious neck masses with other constitutional symptoms should be referred for biopsy and tissue diagnosis. Fine-needle aspiration biopsy is appropriate, with indeterminate cytology requiring open excisional biopsy. Other possible causes of neck lymphadenopathy in immunocompromised patients include histoplasmosis, tuberculosis, atypical mycobacterial infections, and toxoplasmosis.

Sarcoidosis is a granulomatous disease that causes cervical lymphadenopathy and may be the presenting sign in 10% to 15% of cases. This disorder typically affects the African American population. Other findings include fever, sinusitis, parotid swelling, and hilar adenopathy on chest radiographs. Diagnosis is classically made by tissue biopsy showing noncaseating granulomas. A high angiotensin-converting enzyme level is common but not diagnostic.

Other studies include cytoplasmic antineutrophil cytoplasmic antibody (c-ANCA) to rule out other granulomatous diseases, purified protein derivative and acid-fast bacillus stains to rule out tuberculosis, and Venereal Disease Research Laboratory and RPR tests to exclude syphilis.

Sebaceous cysts and epidermal inclusion cysts are also common and usually need to be excised because of the high incidence of recurrent infection.

DISORDERS OF THE SALIVARY GLANDS

The salivary glands consist of the paired parotid, submandibular, and sublingual glands and the minor salivary glands. Disorders of the salivary glands can be categorized into inflammatory, metabolic, and neoplastic problems (see eTable 18-18 online). The history and physical examination facilitate differentiation among these categories.

Inflammatory Disorders

Acute sialoadenitis is a common cause of painful enlargement of the parotid and submandibular glands. The organism is usually *S. aureus,* but it can also be caused by *S. pneumoniae* and other bacteria. The infection is secondary to salivary stasis caused by decreased production (dehydration, poor oral hygiene) or intrinsic or extrinsic obstruction (stones, strictures, masses). Patients present with exquisite tenderness over the gland, fever, and sometimes skin erythema. Purulence can be expressed from the duct with manual massage of the gland. Treatment includes antistaphylococcal antibiotics, adequate hydration, massage of the gland, sialogogues, and warm compresses. Abscess can occur and requires incision and drainage.

Mumps is a relatively common cause of painful unilateral or bilateral parotid gland enlargement in children. It is caused by a paramyxovirus, and the diagnosis is confirmed by elevation of antibodies to the S and V virus antigens or by isolation of the virus in the urine. The incubation period is 2 to 3 weeks, and infection lasts 7 to 10 days. Treatment is conservative, with close follow-up to observe for possible complications such as pancreatitis, meningitis, orchitis, and hearing loss.

Sialolithiasis is a cause of intermittent salivary gland enlargement and is usually associated with eating. Most calculi occur in the submandibular duct, and most are radiopaque. Calculi arising in the parotid duct are less common and tend to be radiolucent. Symptoms include recurrent, unilateral, tender salivary enlargement that subsides within 24 to 48 hours. Physical examination usually reveals a palpable stone in the duct of the gland. Sialography is successfully diagnostic if a calculus is not palpable. CT scan and ultrasonography are also effective in identifying calculi. Treatment depends on the location of the obstruction. Calculi near the terminal orifice are easily removed transorally. Symptomatic calculi located near the hilum of the gland usually require excision of the gland. Sialoendoscopy is a novel method often used successfully to remove sialoliths.

Patients with HIV infection can present with enlargement of salivary glands. Glands can become infiltrated with benign lymphoid tissue or *lymphoepithelial cysts.* The cystic lesions often occur in the tail of the parotid gland, and aspiration can provide temporary relief of symptoms. These patients are treated conservatively because cysts tend to recur after excision or aspiration procedures. The differential diagnosis of salivary gland enlargement in HIV-infected patients includes non-Hodgkin lymphoma and Kaposi sarcoma. Fine-needle aspiration or excisional biopsy of suspicious masses is performed for diagnosis of malignancy.

Included in the differential diagnosis of inflammatory lesions of the major salivary glands are tuberculosis, cat-scratch disease, CMV infection, and first branchial arch cysts and sinuses.

Autoimmune Disorders

Sjögren's syndrome is characterized by xerostomia (dry mouth) with or without parotid gland enlargement. Chronic inflammatory cells and lymphocytes infiltrate the glands, leading to fibrosis and atrophy of the parenchyma. Xerophthalmia suggests involvement of the lacrimal gland and causes a gritty or painful sensation of the eye. Primary Sjögren syndrome involves the exocrine glands, only without association with other connective tissue disorders. Secondary Sjögren syndrome is often associated with rheumatoid arthritis and other autoimmune disorders.

The SS-A and SS-B autoantibodies are positive in most cases of primary Sjögren syndrome. Other useful laboratory tests include rheumatoid factor, antinuclear antibody, thyroid globulin antibody, and thyroid antimicrosomal antibody titers. Lip biopsy can confirm the diagnosis of Sjögren syndrome, and referral to a rheumatologist is appropriate. Treatment includes proper oral hygiene, mouth rinses, and medications that stimulate salivary flow. Steroids are useful for severe cases.

Other causes of xerostomia include surgery and irradiation of the head and neck. Several common classes of medications can cause mouth dryness as a side effect. These include antihistamines, analgesics, anticonvulsants, antidepressants, and antihypertensives. Systemic disorders that can be associated with xerostomia include dehydration, diabetes, anemia, and overall debilitation.

Neoplastic Disorders

Most salivary gland neoplasms arise in the parotid gland, and most are benign. Approximately 80% of parotid gland tumors are benign, with *pleomorphic adenoma* (mixed tumor) being the most common in adults. *Hemangiomas* are the most common benign tumor in children, but malignancy in children is more likely than in adults when a solid mass is found in the salivary gland. Other benign tumors include Warthin tumors (papillary cystadenoma lymphomatosum) and oncocytomas. The most common malignancy in adults and children is *mucoepidermoid carcinoma.* Other malignancies include adenoid cystic carcinoma, malignant mixed tumor, and SCC. Treatment of salivary gland neoplasms is surgical excision.

THYROID MASSES

Careful examination for thyroid abnormalities should be performed on each patient in routine office visits. *Thyroid nodules* occur in about 5% to 10% of the population; of these, approximately 10% are malignant. The differential

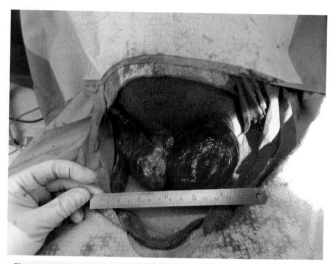

Figure 18-13 Intraoperative photograph of a massive multinodular goiter.

Table 18-14   Thyroid Masses

Degenerative	Graves disease
	Nontoxic multinodular goiter
Thyroiditis	Acute thyroiditis
	Chronic lymphocytic throiditis (Hashimoto)
	Fibrous thyroiditis (Riedel)
	Subacute thyroiditis (granulomatous, lymphocytic)
Neoplastic	**Benign**
	Follicular adenoma
	Malignant
	Anaplastic carcinoma
	Follicular carcinoma
	Lymphoma
	Medullary carcinoma
	Papillary carcinoma

diagnosis of thyroid masses is presented in Table 18-14. Risk factors for malignancy include exposure to radiation and family history of medullary carcinoma. Factors that increase the possibility of carcinoma include hoarseness; age younger than 20 years or older than 45 years; male gender; presence of a firm, hard nodule; and vocal cord paralysis.

The most common disorder in patients who present with a thyroid nodule is *nontoxic multinodular goiter.* The presence of multiple nodules is helpful in diagnosis, but only one dominant nodule may be apparent on physical examination. Nontoxic multinodular goiter may be endemic in iodine-deficient areas or sporadic. Nodularity is thought to be secondary to repeated episodes of deficiency of thyroid hormone, causing increased levels of thyroid-stimulating hormone (TSH), which results in hyperplasia of the gland. Symptomatic compression on the trachea or esophagus can occur. Surgery is reserved for functional problems caused by compression or to rule out malignancy. Chest radiography and CT are helpful in evaluating substernal extension of goiter (Figure 18-13).

Graves disease is an autoimmune disease that causes diffuse thyroid enlargement, hyperthyroidism, infiltrative ophthalmopathy, and myxedema. It is the most common cause of hyperthyroidism and is more common in women age 20 to 50 years. Treatment modalities include antithyroid medications, radioactive iodine ablation, or surgical excision when medical treatment fails.

Thyroiditis can cause nodular enlargement of the thyroid gland. Subacute thyroiditis may be a cause of intermittent hyperthyroidism from the release of stored thyroid hormone. Chronic lymphocytic (Hashimoto) thyroiditis can cause diffuse nodular enlargement of the thyroid. Measurement of antithyroid microsomal antibodies is helpful but not specific for this disorder. Fibrous (Riedel) thyroiditis is a rare cause of thyroid enlargement, and distinction from neoplasia can be difficult.

Neoplasms of the thyroid are classified as malignant or benign tumors. Follicular adenoma is the most common benign tumor. Malignancies include papillary (65%), follicular (20%), medullary (5%), and anaplastic (10%) carcinomas. Medullary carcinoma is associated with an elevated calcitonin level, with pheochromocytoma and parathyroid hyperplasia in multiple endocrine neoplasia (MEN) IIA, and with pheochromocytoma, mucosal neuromas, ganglioneuromatosis, and marfanoid body habitus in MEN IIB. Measurement of urinary catecholamines, vanillylmandelic acid, and metanephrine levels is necessary to aid in the diagnosis of pheochromocytoma, which must be treated before surgery for medullary thyroid carcinoma. Hypercalcemia is diagnosed by measuring serum calcium levels.

Initial evaluation of a suspected or palpable nodule includes a thyroid ultrasound and TSH level. If the TSH level is low, a radioiodine scan is obtained. If the nodule corresponds to an area of increased uptake, a biopsy is not necessary because almost all "hot" nodules are benign. Ultrasonography will define the number and size of nodules and identify characteristics suggesting malignancy.

Fine-needle aspiration biopsy (FNAB) is indicated for nodules larger than 1 cm or with suspicious ultrasound or examination features. Ultrasound guidance may be used to improve the diagnostic yield for difficult-to-palpate nodules (see eFigure 18-9). FNAB is highly accurate. Results are reported as benign, indeterminate or unsatisfactory, suspicious for follicular cancer, suspicious for cancer, or malignant. Benign nodules should be followed with serial examination and ultrasonography. Repeat FNAB is indicated with a significant size change. An indeterminate diagnosis may represent a follicular lesion. Follicular neoplasms are not distinguishable as benign or malignant because fine-needle aspiration fails to identify the critical factor of vascular or capsular invasion. Therefore, a thyroid lobectomy may be necessary for diagnosis. Alternatively, a radioiodine scan may be obtained and surgery performed if the nodule is "cold." Indeterminate aspirates should undergo repeat FNAB. A malignant diagnosis often requires a total thyroidectomy with central compartment lymphadenectomy. Postoperative radioactive iodine is often given. Risks of thyroid surgery include recurrent laryngeal injury and hypoparathyroidism.

The prognosis for patients with papillary thyroid carcinoma is excellent, especially for younger patients. The prognosis is good for those with medullary and follicular carcinoma and universally poor for those with anaplastic carcinoma (Cooper et al., 2006).

- The Sistrunk procedure (removal of the central portion of the hyoid) leads to less than 5% recurrence rate of thyroglossal duct cysts (SOR: A).
- Chemoradiation offers greater than 90% 5-year survival rate for HPV-related oropharyngeal SCC with neck metastasis (SOR: A).
- Ultrasonography and TSH are recommended in the evaluation of a suspected thyroid nodule (SOR: A).
- If needle biopsy cytology is suspicious or diagnostic for papillary thyroid carcinoma, surgery is recommended (SOR: A).

Summary of Additional Online Content

The following content is available at www.expertconsult.com.

eAppendix 18-1, Ear: Physical Examination (with eFigures 18-1 to 18-7)

eTable 18-1 Differential Diagnosis of Otogenic Otalgia

eTable 18-2 Possible Sources of Referred Otalgia

eTable 18-3 Tumors of the Ear

eTable 18-4 Comparative Features of Peripheral Vestibular Disorders

eTable 18-5 Otorrhea from the External Ear Canal

eTable 18-6 Common Signs and Symptoms of Inflammation and Fluid in the Middle Ear

eTable 18-7 Otorrhea from the Middle Ear

eAppendix 18-2, Nose and Paranasal Sinuses: Physical Examination (with eTable 18-8)

eAppendix 18-3, Nasal Obstruction: Physical Examination

eAppendix 18-4, Oral Cavity and Pharynx: Radiography

eTable 18-9 Some Disorders of the Oral Regions by Predominant Site of Involvement

eTable 18-10 Causes of Oropharyngeal Dysphagia

eTable 18-11 Causes of Esophageal Dysphagia

eTable 18-12 Gastroesophageal Reflux Disease–Related Head and Neck Symptoms

eTable 18-13 Treatment of Dysphagia

eTable 18-14 Causes of Stridor

eTable 18-15 Common Causes of Hoarseness

eTable 18-16 Causes of Vocal Cord Paralysis

eAppendix 18-5, Neck: Physical Examination

eTable 18-17 Differential Diagnosis of Neck Mass

eTable 18-18 Salivary Gland Enlargement

eFigure 18-9 Algorithm for the diagnosis and treatment of thyroid nodules

References

The complete reference list is available at www.expertconsult.com.

Web Resources

www.ahrq.gov The Association for Healthcare Research and Quality provides updated comparative effectiveness reviews of various interventions for many otolaryngology problems.

www.cochrane.org The Cochrane Collaboration. Contains reviews of the latest literature in the field of otolaryngology.

www.entnet.org The American Academy of Otolaryngology–Head and Neck Surgery. Contains resources for physicians seeking information on ENT topics, as well as a section on patient education.

www.medlineplus.com A service from the National Library of Medicine. Contains the most accurate database of the scientific medical literature plus a guide to more than 9000 prescription and OTC medications.

www.nidcd.nih.gov The National Institute on Deafness and Other Communication Disorders. Contains information about hearing, balance, smell, taste, voice, speech, and language.

www.UTMB.edu/otoref/ Dr. Quinn's Online Textbook of Otolaryngology, The Texas Nasal and Sinus Center, The Centers for Cancers of the Head and Neck, The Center for Audiology and Speech Pathology. Contains up-to-date information on all aspects of otolaryngology.

19 *Allergy*

VIVIAN HERNANDEZ-TRUJILLO, ELLY RILEY, and CHAD RUDNICK

An allergic patient differs from a nonallergic patient in several ways (Table 19-1). The cause is unknown, but these abnormalities clearly are associated with abnormal cytokine production (Table 19-2). The result of these abnormalities is that allergic persons have diseases such as allergic rhinitis and allergic asthma.

It must always be remembered, however, that these diseases are defined by their *phenotype*, and for each allergic disease, there is an almost identical phenotypic expression unrelated to allergy, such as allergic and nonallergic (intrinsic) asthma, allergic and nonallergic rhinitis, and IgE-mediated and non–IgE-mediated anaphylactic events. Thus, when approaching the patient, the physician must always consider the mechanism of production of the symptoms because subtle differences may exist in treatment between allergic and nonallergic forms of disease, often with significant differences in prognosis.

The most important aspect of establishing the diagnosis of each of these illnesses is the history. The distinction between the allergic and nonallergic forms can only be conclusively determined by allergy testing. The most sensitive and least expensive (per test) means of assessing the presence of allergy is the allergy skin test. In vitro testing is often helpful, however, as a screening procedure.

The other important phenomenon to recognize is that the major allergic diseases (allergic rhinitis, allergic asthma, and anaphylaxis) are all increasing in incidence. The cause is unknown, but several hypotheses have been proposed. The *hygiene hypothesis* postulates that the rise in allergic disease is related to infection control in infants and children (e.g., through vaccination) and improved public health (e.g., through hygienic measures). Another hypothesis is that the allergic response is the same response used to defend against parasites. With a reduction in parasitic disease in more technically developed countries, a population has arisen that is free from exposure to parasites but still maintains a vigorous antiparasitic immune response that is aberrantly directed against the normally harmless organic substances such as pollen, animal dander, and food. Regardless of the mechanism, the burden of allergic disease in developed countries has increased rapidly since the 1970s.

Allergic Rhinitis

Key Points

- Symptoms of allergic rhinitis include allergic shiners, allergic salute, pale nasal mucosa, loss of taste or smell, nasal speech, eustachian tube dysfunction, and disrupted sleep.
- Ophthalmologist referral should be provided to prevent cornea complications.
- Treatment of acute rhinitis includes environmental control, medications, and immunotherapy.
- Use environmental controls such as air conditioning with change of filters, high-efficiency particulate air (HEPA) filters, and masks with microfoam filters for dust allergy.
- Wash linens in hot water using impermeable encasings for pillows and mattresses.
- Avoid fans and cool-mist vaporizers and remove carpets.
- Oral second-generation antihistamines provide less sedation than previous drugs.
- Medications include intranasal steroids, topical antihistamines, and leukotriene modifiers.
- Immunotherapy is directed at specific allergens with possible resolution of allergy.

Allergic rhinitis is a symptom complex caused by airborne antigens. After initial sensitization, exposure to airborne antigens causes activation of allergen-specific T cells, which activate and increase other factors, leading to production of allergen-specific IgE (Rosenwasser, 2011). It occurs as *seasonal rhinitis* (hay fever) when pollens are in high concentration in the air. When it is intermittent or continuous without seasonal variation, it is termed *perennial allergic rhinitis* (Orban et al., 2009). Often occurring in families with an allergic history, perennial allergic rhinitis and mixed perennial and seasonal rhinitis were found to be twice as common as seasonal allergic rhinitis (Skoner, 2001).

Table 19-1 Abnormalities Described in Allergic Patients

Predisposition to manufacture large amounts of IgE directed against formerly harmless substances (e.g., pollen and food)
Abnormalities in the autonomic nervous system
Hyporesponsive β-adrenergic system
Hyperresponsive α-adrenergic system
Hyperactive cholinergic responses in the airways
Hyperreleasability of mast cells and basophils

Table 19-2 Cytokine Production Abnormalities and Effects in Allergic Patients

Cytokine	Effects
Increased production of IL-4	Enhanced IgE production
Increased production of IL-13	Enhanced IgE production
Increased production of IL-5	Enhanced eosinophil activity and prolongation of the life of eosinophils
Increased production of IL-9	Bronchial hyperreactivity

Ig, Immunoglobulin; *IL,* interleukin.

MANIFESTATIONS

In seasonal allergic rhinitis, exposure is followed by complaints of paroxysmal sneezing, a watery nasal discharge with congestion, and nasal pruritus. Conjunctival and pharyngeal itching often occurs. Less specific symptoms are postnasal drainage or fullness or aching in the frontal areas.

The patient might exhibit an *allergic salute,* an upward thrust of the palm against the nares to relieve itching and open the nasal airways and a gaping expression from mouth breathing. *Allergic shiners* or Dennie lines are wrinkles beneath the lower eyelid. Speech can have a nasal quality. In children, nasal irritation can result in nose picking and recurrent epistaxis. Sleep disruption is often associated with nasal obstruction and mouth breathing. Patients might have sleep apnea–like symptoms, including restless sleep, snoring, or nighttime coughing, associated with postnasal mucus drainage and mild hoarseness. The nasal mucosa is typically moist, with enlarged, pale turbinates and serous discharge. Because the sense of smell is impaired, appetite may be decreased. Maxillomandibular alignment problems (overbite or underbite) result from chronic symptoms.

In perennial allergic rhinitis, nasal congestion, itching, obstruction, and frequent sniffing may be associated with a loss of sense of taste or smell, with decreased hearing and a popping sensation in the ears. A lower sneezing threshold often occurs with altered autonomic reflexes in perennial allergic rhinitis. Paroxysms of sneezing and rhinorrhea can result from changes in ambient temperature, odors from perfume, tobacco smoke, irritants, alcohol, and exposure to small quantities of antigen. Exercise reverses nasal congestion temporarily, from minutes to hours.

The turbinates are usually swollen and edematous and may be mistaken for nasal polyps, which are pearl-gray gelatinous masses and unusual in uncomplicated allergic rhinitis. Below the turbinates, the floor of the nostril is often prominent as a result of mucosal edema. One third to half of children with allergic rhinitis have eustachian tube obstruction and resultant serous otitis. Otoscopy reveals a retracted or bulging tympanic membrane, impaired mobility, or fluid level. In patients with intact tympanic membranes, tympanometry to measure middle ear pressures provides an indirect measure of eustachian tube function (Lazo-Saenz et al., 2005). The edematous nasal mucosa can obstruct the ostia, resulting in congestion or sinusitis with pressure symptoms or headache that is particularly notable with bending forward. Up to one third of patients have a lower respiratory tract component, including exercise-induced and mild persistent asthma.

DIAGNOSIS

A seasonal history or an association with an inhaled allergen is helpful. It is often difficult to associate specific allergens with perennial rhinitis, although late-evening or early-morning symptoms may be seen with dust allergy. Occasionally, improvement of symptoms with a change in environment, such as a vacation, indicates the presence of environmental allergens. A nasal smear, stained with Hansel's stain to identify eosinophils, can support a diagnosis of nasal allergy, but it is not itself diagnostic. An elevated peripheral eosinophil count may be helpful; however, marked allergic symptoms can occur in the absence of blood eosinophilia.

Along with clinical history, the diagnosis of allergic rhinitis can be supported by skin prick testing. This involves passing a fine needle through a drop of allergen extract and into the skin. Positive results are indicated by the wheal response with wheal diameters ≥ 3 mm considered positive. Surrounding erythema may be present, but its appearance or size is not indicative of a positive or negative test result (Bousquet et al., 2012). Skin prick testing is more sensitive than specific IgE assays for identifying sensitization to inhalant allergens and confirming clinical allergy. IgE assays with defined quantifiable threshold levels can also predict positive respiratory responses after allergen exposure (Bernstein et al., 2008).

TREATMENT

Nonspecific Measures

Removing known allergens is of prime importance because it can eliminate symptoms. When exposure is unavoidable, environmental control should reduce symptoms and prevent exacerbations. The patient or the family must assume responsibility for environmental control, so an understanding of the allergens to which the patient is sensitized is helpful. Commonly, inhaled allergens can lead to allergic rhinitis, allergic conjunctivitis, and asthma. Allergenic pollens come from trees, grasses, and weeds (Platts-Mills, 2003; Shiekh et al., 2004). Pollens from flowering plants are insect borne and are not important allergens. Pollen prevalence is usually determined by gravity slides, which sample pollen fallout without regard to wind direction, speed, and turbulence, so that daily reports of pollen prevalence often do not reflect the true concentration in the air or individual exposure.

Inhaled fungal allergens in fungus-sensitive subjects can produce seasonal symptoms during situations that promote fungal growth, such as humid and rainy weather and exposure to hay, mulch, commercial peat moss, and compost. Indoors, areas of spore formation can be identified at sites of water condensation such as shower curtains, window moldings, and damp basements. In addition, cool-mist vaporizers can serve as sources of fungal contamination.

A prime role for the patient and family is controlling house dust. House dust is a heterogeneous mixture of bacteria, fibrous matter of plant and animal origin, human epidermis, food remnants, fungi, insect debris, and animal dander and contains one major source of antigen: dust mites. Mites are ubiquitous in households and are most prevalent in bedding, mattresses, carpeting, and upholstered furniture, particularly where warmth and humidity are high. Air conditioners and dehumidifiers are useful for these patients. HEPA filters are effective in removing dust and animal dander. Fans should not be used so that these lightweight particles can settle. Minimizing clutter and removing carpets are also effective measures. Linens should be washed in hot water (130°F or 55°C). Impermeable cases can be used for pillows and mattresses. The use of a mask over the nose and mouth with replaceable microfoam filters significantly reduces the effects of temporary exposure to inhaled allergens such as dust or pollens.

Animal allergens are derived from dried saliva on shed cat fur, rodent urine, and epidermal material from farm animals. The allergic respiratory reactions produced by animal allergens are species specific. Finished furs and wools are not allergenic. Feathers are often nonallergenic when fresh, and they produce allergic symptoms only after degradation. A careful history to identify environmental allergens is important for advising avoidance and treatment.

Control of Symptoms

Antihistamines are effective for symptomatic control of allergic rhinitis, whether it is seasonal or perennial (Bousquet et al., 2008; Brozek et al., 2010; Simons and Adkis, 2009; Wallace et al., 2008; SOR: A). For optimal results, antihistamines should be used before exposure to the known allergen. Complete control might not be achieved when patients use antihistamines only sporadically. During the implicated season, around-the-clock administration provides maximal symptomatic relief. Because compliance is always an issue, the new second-generation antihistamines offer a convenient dosing regimen because the half-lives of these medications are longer (see eTable 19-1 online). These groups of drugs, with specific binding properties, allow little to no penetration into the central nervous system (CNS), greatly reducing their side effects, primarily sedation. The second-generation antihistamines also have antiinflammatory effects.

Fexofenadine (Allegra), an analog of terfenadine, is safe and effective. Through its effects on T cells, fexofenadine can decrease airway inflammation. Loratadine (Claritin) is available as a once-daily product (Gelfand et al., 2002). It provides safe and effective control of most symptoms of allergic rhinitis if taken regularly. Desloratadine (Clarinex), also a once-daily medication, is a metabolite of loratadine. In murine models, desloratadine inhibits bronchial hyper-responsiveness and airway inflammation (Bryce et al., 2003). Cetirizine (Zyrtec), a metabolite of hydroxyzine, is available in once-daily dosing. Cetirizine has antiinflammatory properties and may be effective in patients with allergic rhinitis and reactive airway disease. Cetirizine's chemical properties, however, allow greater CNS penetration, and

sedation is its chief side effect (16% vs. 4% for fexofenadine and loratadine). Levocetirizine (Xyzal), also a once-daily medication, is a metabolite of cetirizine. Less sedation is associated with it than cetirizine.

Herbal medications have been used with effectiveness in treating perennial and seasonal allergic rhinitis. Butterbur (32 mg daily) was effective in treating seasonal allergic rhinitis when compared with cetirizine (10 mg daily) in 125 patients. After 2 weeks, patients treated with butterbur had improved vitality, general health, and physical activity as well as less sedation (Schapowal, 2002; SOR: A).

Second-generation antihistamines are available in combination with α-adrenergic decongestants and might be more effective in this form than antihistamines alone. α-Adrenergic drugs are also effective applied topically. Topical vasoconstrictors (sprays and drops) are best restricted to temporary use, such as when taking an airplane trip or during a severe flare-up of symptoms. Unfortunately, the side effect profile increases in these combinations. Intranasal antihistamines have the most rapid onset of action and are as effective as oral second-generation antihistamines in the treatment of seasonal allergic rhinitis (SOR: A). Azelastine (Astelin, Astepro), available in a nasal spray formulation, decreases nasal airway resistance and is an effective treatment for rhinitis. Olopatadine (Patanase) is another topical antihistamine with effectiveness against symptoms of rhinitis. Leukotriene receptor antagonists, such as montelukast (Singulair), are also effective for the treatment of perennial and seasonal allergic rhinitis (Wallace et al., 2008).

Topical intranasal glucocorticoids—beclomethasone, fluticasone, mometasone, triamcinolone, flunisolide, ciclesonide, and budesonide—are the most effective medication in the treatment of allergic rhinitis (Wallace et al., 2008; SOR: A). Their effectiveness is directly related to proper and daily use, posing problems with patient compliance. Side effects are related primarily to nasal dryness and epistaxis, which may improve when using saline as a moisturizer. The therapeutic effects are generally not immediate, and some patients must take these medications for 1 to 3 weeks before they achieve maximum benefit.

When symptoms are severe and not responsive to trials of topical therapy, oral glucocorticoid therapy can be used as a last resort and only for limited duration. The rationale for glucocorticoid therapy for allergic rhinitis is that the condition, although mediated by immunoglobulin E (IgE), has a dual component: the immediate phase of edema and hypersecretion and a late inflammatory phase (Castro-Rodriguez et al., 2005; Ciprandi et al., 2005). This dual reaction occurs in asthma as well.

Specific Immunotherapy

When skin tests identify sensitivity to an unavoidable inhalant allergen, immunotherapy may be indicated for treating allergic rhinitis. Its efficacy has been shown to be 80% for controlling pollen symptoms and 60% for controlling mold and house dust symptoms. Immunotherapy is therefore more effective in seasonal allergic rhinitis than perennial allergic rhinitis. When considering immunotherapy, the ease of control of other therapies should be weighed against the frequency and severity of symptoms as well as the possibility of complete resolution of allergy with immunotherapy (Cox, et al., 2011).

KEY TREATMENT

- Oral antihistamines, including fexofenadine, cetirizine, loratadine, levocetirizine, and desloratadine, improve symptoms (e.g., runny nose, nasal pruritus, sneezing, and quality of life) in patients with seasonal allergic rhinitis compared with placebo (SOR: A).
- Herbal medications have been used with effectiveness in treating perennial and seasonal allergic rhinitis (SOR: A).
- Inhaled corticosteroids were more effective than oral antihistamines in treating most nasal symptoms of seasonal allergic rhinitis, including nasal congestion, runny nose, pruritus, and sneezing (SOR: A).
- Immunotherapy is effective against allergic rhinitis and can prevent the development of asthma in children (SOR: A).

Nonallergic Rhinitis

Key Points

- Symptoms of nonallergic rhinitis include chronic nasal obstruction and eosinophils on nasal smear, in the absence of allergy.
- Topical glucocorticoid steroid therapy is useful in treatment of nonallergic rhinitis with eosinophilia (NARES).
- Aggravating factors include physical changes or irritants for vasomotor rhinitis.
- Ipratropium bromide is best for controlling symptoms of vasomotor rhinitis.

Some patients with perennial rhinitis are not atopic by history or skin testing. Chronic nasal obstruction is the predominant symptom, and the condition may be associated with sinus disease and nasal polyps. Although there is no evidence of allergy by skin testing, numerous eosinophils are present, and the diagnosis is readily made by examining the nasal secretions for eosinophils and eosinophilic cationic protein (Kramer et al., 2004). The condition is also called NARES. A substantial number of patients have chronic rhinitis with rhinorrhea, postnasal drainage, and chronic or intermittent nasal obstruction. Symptoms are aggravated by many physical or irritant factors, such as cold air, odors, and smoke. Skin test results are negative, and no eosinophils are present in the tissue or secretions.

Topical glucocorticoid therapy is much more effective than antihistamines or decongestants for NARES. As with patients with asthma, patients with associated sinus disease and nasal polyps are at risk for adverse reactions to aspirin and nonsteroidal antiinflammatory drugs (NSAIDs). Patients with NARES are also at risk for obstructive sleep apnea (Wallace et al., 2008). Ipratropium bromide (0.03%) spray solution, fluticasone, and azelastine nasal sprays have all been shown to be effective treatments. Some patients benefit from antihistamine–decongestant combinations. The regular use of buffered saline lavage can also provide satisfactory symptomatic relief.

Allergy in the Eye

Key Points

- Symptoms of eye allergy include pruritus, erythema, and lacrimation.
- Treatment includes oral antihistamines plus topical medications such as mast cell stabilizers or H_1 blockers.

Allergic conjunctivitis is the usual ocular reaction to airborne allergens. As in other forms of allergic inflammation, the mast cell plays a key role. Itching is the first symptom and may be associated with lacrimation. Dilation of the conjunctival blood vessels produces a "red" eye. Transudation of fluid through vessel walls results in edema of the conjunctiva, and exuded cells with increased glandular mucus secretions result in ocular discharge. In most atopic patients, conjunctivitis and allergic rhinitis occur together, but some patients are bothered only by eye symptoms. In contrast to other forms of conjunctivitis, the secretions contain eosinophils.

Vernal conjunctivitis is so called because of its occurrence in spring and summer. It is characterized by a bilateral recurrent inflammation of the conjunctiva. Vernal conjunctivitis typically occurs between ages 5 and 20 years. It often spontaneously resolves in 10 years. More than 50% of children with vernal conjunctivitis also have an atopic disorder such as allergic rhinitis, eczema, or asthma. Signs and symptoms include acute itching, tearing, photophobia, and excess mucus production.

The topical conjunctival appearance establishes the diagnosis, which is confirmed by cytologic smears showing numerous eosinophils. In the tarsal (palpebral) form, there are flat-top cobblestone papillae; in the limbal form, there may be gelatinous hypertrophy and limbal papillary hypertrophy often associated with white dots (Trantas dots). Although vernal conjunctivitis is usually self-limiting, corneal complications can occur, and ophthalmology consultation should be obtained (Bozkurt, et al., 2009). Although conjunctivitis is typically seasonal and common in atopic patients, no allergens have been identified as causal or aggravating factors.

The usual therapy for allergic conjunctivitis is an oral antihistamine with a topical medication (see eTable 19-2 online). Cromolyn (Opticrom) and lodoxamide 0.1% (Alomide) are mast cell stabilizers. Topical H_1 histamine blockers are also effective for treating allergic conjunctivitis. Ophthalmic histamine blocker solutions include emedastine (Emadine) and levocabastine (Livostin). Azelastine (Optivar), epinastine (Elestat), ketotifen (Zaditor, Claritin Eye, Zyrtec Itchy Eye), and olopatadine (Patanol, Pataday) are dual-acting drugs, preventing mast cell release and exerting antihistamine activity as well. Ketorolac (Acular) is an NSAID. Regular daily use is necessary to obtain maximum positive results with all topical agents. In severe cases and in vernal conjunctivitis, a soluble steroid such as fluorometholone ophthalmic solution (0.1%) is effective. The dose should be titrated to the minimum required to control symptoms. Use should be intermittent because glucocorticoids can lead to the development of cataracts, potentiate a secondary bacterial infection or a herpes simplex keratitis, and increase intraocular pressure. Steroid eyedrops should always be used under supervision by an ophthalmologist.

Asthma

Key Points

- The diagnosis is based on presence of reversible airway obstruction, airway inflammation, and increased airway responsiveness to a variety of stimuli.
- Identification and avoidance of allergens or triggers are essential.
- Control of rhinitis symptoms is often necessary to improve the control of asthma.
- An action plan is needed to aid the patient in identifying a possible exacerbation.
- Therapy is based on presence of certain clinical features, as well as spirometric values.

The definition of asthma has undergone many changes over the years, but three elements are key to the diagnosis: reversible airway obstruction, airway inflammation, and increased airway responsiveness to a variety of stimuli. Physicians must remember that not all wheezing is asthma, and not all asthma has wheezing. Asthma is a chronic inflammatory disorder of the airways in which many different cells play a role. In patients with asthma, this inflammation causes breathlessness, chest tightness, recurrent episodes of wheezing, and cough, particularly at night. These symptoms are usually associated with variable airflow limitation that is partly reversible with treatment or sometimes spontaneously. This inflammation causes an associated increase in airway responsiveness to a variety of stimuli (Busse et al., 2007). Data from the Centers for Disease Control and Prevention (CDC) have shown an increase in the prevalence of asthma in the United States from 1980 to 2010. However, there has been no increase in mortality and hospitalization rates since 1997, and the number of asthma deaths has declined steadily since 2001 (cdc.gov/asthma).

DIAGNOSIS

Because of the lack of any specific symptom or sign to define asthma by history or physical examination, some patients are mistakenly thought to have asthma. Numerous other diseases must be considered in the differential diagnosis of asthma (Table 19-3; eBox 19-1 and eBox 19-2). Although parental history of asthma is present in half of children with asthma, the positive predictive value of this history ranges from 11% to 37% (Burke et al., 2003). The diagnosis of asthma should occur in three stages. First, suggestive symptoms referable to the chest with precipitating factors should raise the possibility of asthma. Second, further testing should be performed to confirm the diagnosis. Third, the patient should have symptomatic improvement with the appropriate asthma therapy (see

Table 19-3 Differential Diagnosis of Asthma

Infants and Children	Adults
Allergic rhinosinusitis	ACE inhibitor–induced cough
Cystic fibrosis	COPD
Foreign body	Congestive heart failure
GERD	Eosinophilic pulmonary infiltration
Heart disease	GERD
Paradoxical vocal cord motion	Mechanical obstruction of the airway
Tumor	Paradoxical vocal cord motion
Viral bronchiolitis	Pulmonary embolism

ACE, Angiotensin-converting enzyme; *COPD,* chronic obstructive pulmonary disease; *GERD,* gastroesophageal reflux disease.

Table 19-4 Factors That Can Precipitate Asthma

Environmental allergens such as pollen, molds, house dust mites, cockroach excreta, and animal danders
Environmental changes or climate change
Exercise
Exposure to irritants (e.g., tobacco smoke), strong odors, and air pollutants
Exposure to medication: salicylates, NSAIDs, or β-blockers
Exposure to occupational chemicals or allergens
Exposure to some food additives
GERD
Menses
Pregnancy
Sinusitis
Strong emotional feelings
Viral respiratory infections

GERD, Gastroesophageal reflux disease; *NSAID,* nonsteroidal antiinflammatory drug.

"Classification"). When all the stages have been performed and meet the criteria, the diagnosis of asthma can be made.

Precipitating Factors

All patients suspected of having asthma should be questioned about early warning signs and precipitating factors. Early warning signs of an attack include symptoms such as cough, a scratchy throat, and nasal stuffiness, especially if an attack follows an upper respiratory tract infection. Many other precipitating factors can provoke asthma symptoms or an acute attack (Table 19-4). Identification of these precipitating factors can help patients manage their asthma by learning their early warning signs and avoiding any exposure that triggers an exacerbation. These symptoms and identification of triggers are the first stages of diagnosis of asthma.

Confirmatory Testing

Pulmonary function testing is the "gold standard" for the diagnosis and management of asthma and is the second stage in the diagnosis of asthma. The only exclusion for obtaining pulmonary function tests should be the lack of an ability to perform the testing, most often determined by the patient's age (usually <4 years).

Spirometry is the most useful test in the diagnosis of asthma. Spirometry includes measuring the forced expiratory volume of air in 1 second (FEV_1) and forced vital capacity (FVC), the amount of air one can expel during

Table 19-5 Severity of Any Spirometric Abnormality Based on FEV$_1$

Degree of Severity	FEV$_1$ (% Predicted)
Mild	>70
Moderate	60-69
Moderately severe	50-59
Severe	35-49
Very severe	<35

FEV$_1$, Forced expiratory volume in 1 second.
From Brusaco V, Crapo R, Viegi G. Interpretative strategies for lung function tests. *Eur Respir J.* 2005;26:948-968. American Thoracic Society.

forced expiration. FEV$_1$ is the most important value for the assessment of airflow obstruction. It declines in direct and linear proportion of worsening airway obstruction and increases with successful treatment of airway obstruction. Degrees of airway obstruction are defined according to the percentage of predicted FEV$_1$ achieved by the patient (Table 19-5) (Brusaco et al., 2005).

Administration of a bronchodilator such as albuterol is indicated when performing spirometry. Improvement of FEV$_1$ by 12% or 200 mL after administering a bronchodilator suggests significant reversibility of the airway obstruction. Another useful value is the FEV$_1$/FVC ratio. A reduced ratio below the fifth percentile of the predicted value suggests obstructive airway disease. A reduced FVC with a normal or increased FEV$_1$/FVC ratio (>5% of predicted value) suggests a restrictive pattern of lung disease (Brusaco et al., 2005). Additional testing by bronchoprovocation may be considered if one suspects a patient has asthma but spirometry testing results are normal. The only absolute contraindications to methacholine bronchoprovocation testing are severely reduced airflow (FEV$_1$ <50%), acute coronary syndrome or stroke in the past 3 months, uncontrolled hypertension, or known aortic aneurysm.

PEAK-FLOW MONITORING

The home use of peak-flow meters is helpful in the self-management of asthma but not in the diagnosis. The National Asthma Education and Prevention Program (Brusaco et al., 2005) recommends daily monitoring for patients with moderate to severe persistent asthma; for those with severe exacerbation history; and for patients who have poor perception of their worsening asthma, including children. There is no evidence that peak-flow monitoring improves patient outcomes over self-monitoring of symptoms. However, if a practitioner provides a peak-flow meter, the patient should be properly instructed in its use (Busse et al., 2007). The patient should establish a baseline peak flow in the absence of asthma symptoms. Three zones on the meter are then set—green, yellow, and red. The green zone is 80% to 100% of the patient's "personal best" and reassures the patient to continue the current regimen. The yellow zone is 50% to 80% of personal best and should signal the patient to change the measurement plan according to the clinician. The red zone is less than 50% of the personal best and should signal the patient to

seek medical attention. The use of the peak-flow meter can help give some patients objective findings of the severity of their asthma.

TREATMENT

Classification

Asthma is classified into four categories based on subjective symptoms of frequency and severity and objective measurements of pulmonary function (Figures 19-1 and 19-2). Classification is initially based on the highest step at which any feature occurs, realizing that clinical features for individual patients can overlap. An individual patient's classification can and should change over time so the patient can move to a lower classification with adequate therapy.

The goal of asthma therapy is to maintain control of asthma with the least amount of medication and the least risk for adverse side effects. Obtaining control of asthma can be difficult to define for the patient and the clinician. Several keys to the definition of controlled asthma are prevention of troublesome symptoms (cough or wheezing), maintenance of normal pulmonary function, maintenance of normal activity levels, prevention of recurrent exacerbations, and meeting patients' and families' expectations of asthma care.

Classification of asthma is the last stage in the diagnosis of asthma. Patients with asthma should respond to traditional treatment based on the stage of asthma. The National Heart, Lung and Blood Institute (NHLBI) provides the current clinical guidelines (Figures 19-3 and 19-4) (Busse et al., 2007). The physician should keep the following points in mind when using the NHLBI guidelines:

1. The stepwise approach is intended to assist, not replace, the clinical decision making required to meet individual patient needs.
2. Classify severity; assign the patient to the most severe step in which any feature occurs.
3. Gain control as quickly as possible (a course of short systemic corticosteroids may be required); then step down to the least medication necessary to maintain control.
4. Minimize the use of short-acting inhaled β$_2$-agonists. Overreliance (e.g., use of short-acting inhaled β$_2$-agonist every day, increasing use or lack of expected effect, or use of approximately one canister a month even if not using it every day) indicates inadequate control of asthma and the need to initiate or intensify long-term-control therapy.
5. Provide parent education on asthma management and controlling environmental factors that make asthma worse at all points of care (e.g., allergens, irritants).
6. Consultation with an asthma specialist is recommended for patients with moderate or severe persistent asthma. Consider consultation for patients with mild persistent asthma.

Management of Asthma in Children

More than half of children with asthma develop symptoms before their fifth birthday. However, diagnosis can be difficult because there are no reliable tests for children at this age, and diagnosis must rely solely on clinical presentation.

Components of severity		Classifying Asthma Severity and Initiating Therapy in Children							
		Intermittent		Persistent					
				Mild		Moderate		Severe	
		Ages 0-4 yr	Ages 5-11 yr	Ages 0-4 yr	Ages 5-11 yr	Ages 0-4 yr	Ages 5-11 yr	Ages 0-4 yr	Ages 5-11 yr
Impairment	Symptoms	≤2 d/wk		>2 d/wk but not daily		Daily		Throughout the day	
	Nighttime awakenings	0	≤2x/ mo	1-2x/ mo	3-4x/ mo	3-4x/ mo	>1x/wk but not nightly	>1x/ wk	Often 7x/wk
	Short-acting β$_2$-agonist use for symptom control	≤2 d/wk		>2 d/wk but not daily		Daily		Several times per day	
	Interference with normal activity	None		Minor limitation		Some limitation		Extremely limited	
	Lung function • FEV$_1$ (predicted) or peak flow (personal best) • FEV$_1$/FVC	N/A	Normal FEV$_1$ between exacerbations >80% >85%	N/A	>80% >80%	N/A	60%-80% 75%-80%	N/A	<60% <75%
Risk	Exacerbations requiring oral systemic corticosteroids (consider severity and interval since last exacerbation)	0-1/yr (see notes)		≥2 exacerbations in 6 months requiring oral systemic corticosteroids or ≥4 wheezing episodes/1 yr lasting >1 d AND risk factors for persistent asthma	≥2x/yr (see notes) Relative annual risk may be related to FEV$_1$	→			→

Recommended step for initiating therapy (See "Stepwise Approach for Managing Asthma" for treatment steps.) The stepwise approach is meant to assist, not replace, the clinical decision making required to meet individual patient needs.	Step 1 (for both age groups)		Step 2 (for both age groups)		Step 3 and consider short course of oral systemic cortico-steroids	Step 3: medium-dose ICS option and consider short course of oral systemic cortico-steroids	Step 3 and consider short course of oral systemic cortico-steroids	Step 3: medium-dose ICS option OR step 4 and consider short course of oral systemic cortico-steroids
	In 2-6 wk, depending on severity, evaluate level of asthma control that is achieved. • Children 0-4 yr old: If no clear benefit is observed in 4-6 wk, stop treatment and consider alternative diagnoses or adjusting therapy. • Children 5-11 yr old: Adjust therapy accordingly.							

Figure 19-1 Classifying asthma severity and initiating therapy in children. *FEV$_1$*, Forced expiratory volume of air in 1 second; *FVC*, forced vital capacity; *ICS*, inhaled corticosteroid; *N/A*, not applicable. (From Busse WW, Boushey HA, Camargo CA, et al. *Guidelines for the diagnosis and management of asthma.* National Asthma Education and Prevention Program, Expert Panel Report 3. NIH Pub No 08-5846, October 2007.)

Among children younger than 5 years, the most common cause of asthma symptoms is a viral upper respiratory tract infection. Based on expert opinion, daily long-term control therapy should be initiated in young children who consistently require symptomatic treatment more than twice per week and those who experience severe exacerbations that occur less than 6 weeks apart. Therapy is recommended for children who had more than four episodes of wheezing in the past year that lasted more than 1 day and affected sleep and who have a positive asthma predictive index (Busse et al., 2007). A positive asthma predictive index is at least three episodes of wheezing in a years' time during the first 3 years of life and either one of two major risk factors

(parental history of asthma or physician diagnosis of atopic dermatitis) or two of three minor risk factors (wheezing apart from colds, peripheral blood eosinophilia higher than 4%, or evidence of sensitization of foods) (Castro-Rodriguez, 2011). Therapy may be given by metered-dose inhalers with a spacer; evidence suggests they are as good as or better than nebulizers for children with asthma (SOR: A) (Hsu et al., 2004).

Management of Asthma Exacerbation

Asthma exacerbations consist of episodes of progressively worsening shortness of breath, cough, wheezing, or chest tightness. These exacerbations are characterized by

Components of severity		Classification of Asthma Severity ≥12 years of age			
		Intermittent	Persistent		
			Mild	Moderate	Severe
Impairment Normal FEV₁/FVC: 8-19 yr 85% 20-39 yr 80% 40-59 yr 75% 60-80 yr 70%	Symptoms	≤2 d/wk	>2 d/wk but not daily	Daily	Throughout the day
	Nighttime awakenings	≤2x/mo	3-4x/mo	>1x/wk but not nightly	Often 7x/wk
	Short-acting β₂-agonist use for symptom control (not prevention of EIB)	≤2 d/wk	>2 d/wk but not daily and not more than 1x on any day	Daily	Several times per day
	Interference with normal activity	None	Minor limitation	Some limitation	Extremely limited
	Lung function	• Normal FEV₁ between exacerbations • FEV₁ >80% predicted • FEV₁/FVC normal	• FEV₁ >80% predicted • FEV₁/FVC normal	• FEV₁ >60% but <80% predicted • FEV₁/FVC reduced 5%	• FEV₁ <60% predicted • FEV₁/FVC reduced 5%
Risk	Exacerbations requiring oral systemic corticosteroids	0-1/yr (see note)	≥2/yr (see note) ⟶		
		⟵ Consider severity and interval since last exacerbation. Frequency and severity may fluctuate over time for patients in any severity category. ⟶ Relative annual risk of exacerbations may be related to FEV₁.			

Recommended step for initiating therapy (See "Stepwise Approach for Managing Asthma" for treatment steps.)	Step 1	Step 2	Step 3 and consider short course of oral systemic corticosteroids	Step 4 or 5
	In 2-6 wk, evaluate level of asthma control that is achieved and adjust therapy accordingly.			

Figure 19-2 Classification of asthma severity. *EIB,* Exercise-induced bronchospasm; *FEV₁,* forced expiratory volume of air in 1 second; *FVC,* forced vital capacity. (From Busse WW, Boushey HA, Camargo CA, et al. *Guidelines for the diagnosis and management of asthma.* National Asthma Education and Prevention Program, Expert Panel Report 3. NIH Pub No 08-5846, October 2007.)

decreases in FVC and FEV₁. Peak-flow monitoring can help grade the severity of an exacerbation. Early treatment is the best strategy for effective treatment of asthma exacerbations. Patients should receive a written action plan to guide self-management of exacerbation, especially patients with persistent asthma or any history of a severe exacerbation. Patients should be able to recognize the early indicators of an exacerbation, such as a decline in peak expiratory flow rate (PEFR). There should be prompt communication between the clinician and patient during any abrupt worsening of asthma, as well as availability of a short course of systemic corticosteroids even before this communication takes place. The goals of treating an exacerbation are correction of any significant hypoxemia, rapid reversal of airflow obstruction, and reduction of the likelihood of recurrence of severe airflow obstruction by intensifying therapy.

The NHLBI expert panel recommends increasing the frequency of inhaled β₂-agonists and initiating or increasing oral corticosteroid treatment. The panel does not recommend drinking large volumes of liquids or breathing warm, moist air. They also discourage the use of over-the-counter products such as antihistamines, cold remedies, or bronchodilators. For patients who present to emergency departments (EDs), the clinician should obtain a brief targeted history as well as objective data such as peak-flow measurement and pulse oximetry. Clinicians should be aware of risk factors for asthma-related deaths: previous intubation or intensive care unit admission for asthma, two or more hospitalizations, or more than three ED visits in the past year; use of more than two canisters of short-acting β₂-agonist per month; low socioeconomic status; illicit drug use; major psychosocial problems; and comorbidities such as cardiovascular or chronic lung disease.

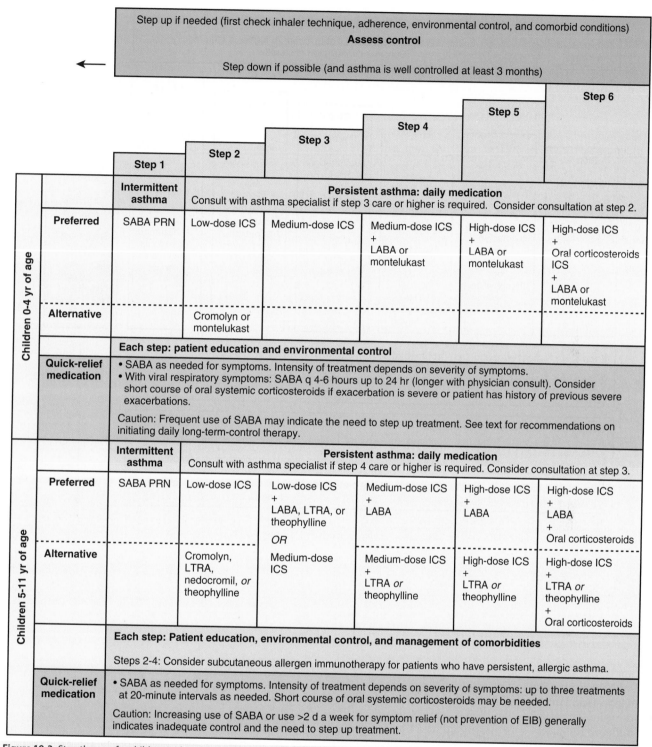

Figure 19-3 Step therapy for children with asthma. *EIB*, Exercise-induced bronchospasm; *ICS*, inhaled corticosteroid; *LABA*, long-acting β-agonist; *LTRA*, leukotriene receptor antagonist; *PRN*, as needed; *q*, every; *SABA*, short-acting β-agonist. (From Busse WW, Boushey HA, Camargo CA, et al. *Guidelines for the diagnosis and management of asthma.* National Asthma Education and Prevention Program, Expert Panel Report 3. NIH Pub No 08-5846, October 2007.)

Chest radiographs should be obtained only in patients suspected of having a more complicated process such as pneumothorax, pneumonia, or congestive heart failure. Treatment of exacerbations in the ED should include nebulizer therapy with short-acting β₂-agonists and nebulized anticholinergics such as ipratropium bromide (SOR: A)

(Busse et al., 2007). However, the NHLBI does not recommend continued use of nebulized anticholinergics during hospitalization. In general, patients should be discharged if their FEV₁ or PEFR has returned to greater than 70% of their predicted personal best and they are in no respiratory distress.

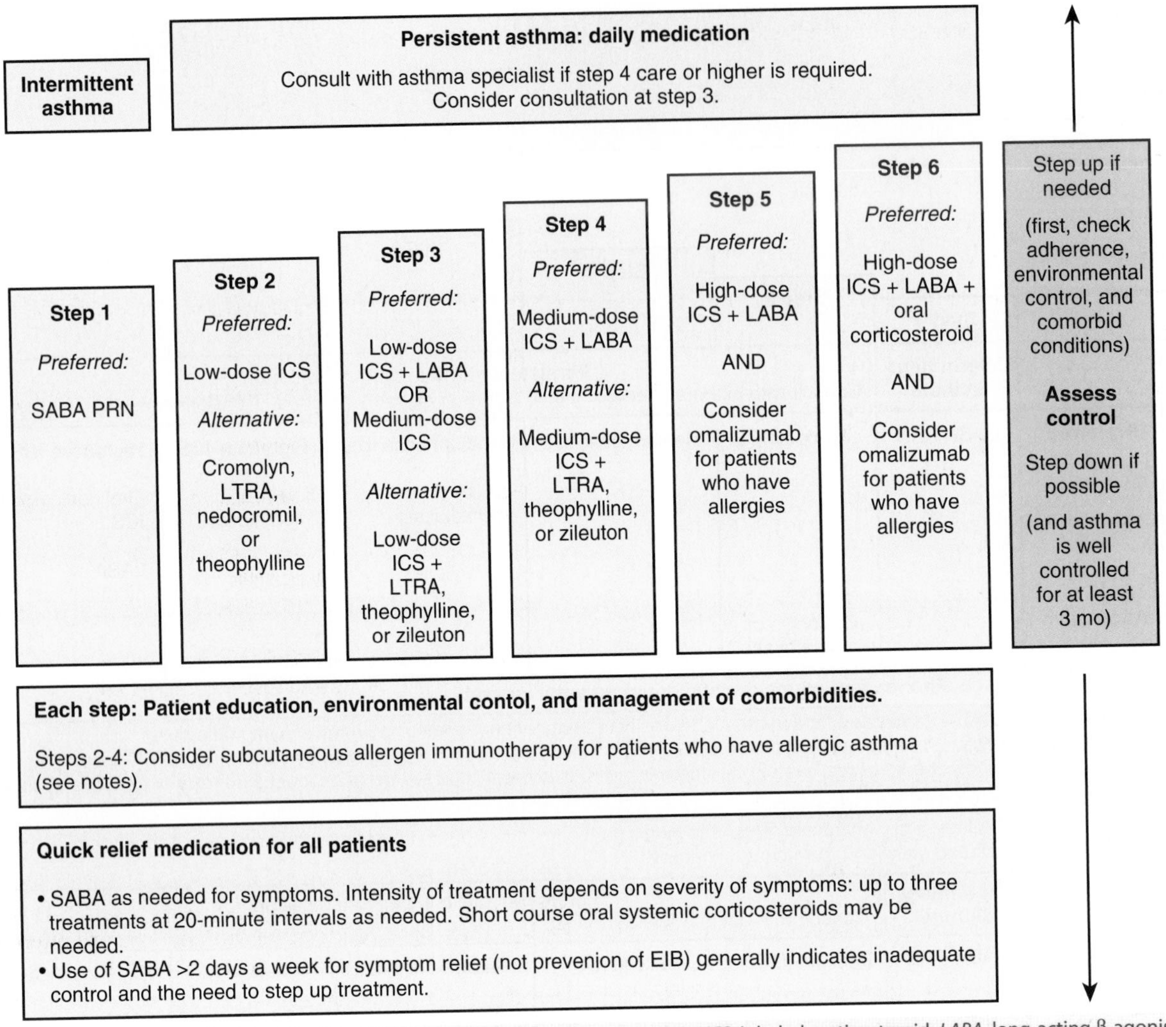

Figure 19-4 Step therapy for adults with asthma. *EIB,* Exercise-induced bronchospasm; *ICS,* inhaled corticosteroid; *LABA,* long-acting β-agonist; *LTRA,* leukotriene receptor antagonist; *PRN,* as needed; *SABA,* short-acting β-agonist. (From Busse WW, Boushey HA, Camargo CA, et al. *Guidelines for the diagnosis and management of asthma.* National Asthma Education and Prevention Program, Expert Panel Report 3. NIH Pub No 08-5846, October 2007.)

KEY TREATMENT

- Pulmonary function testing is the "gold standard" for the diagnosis and management of asthma and should be performed in all patients older than 4 years of age (SOR: C).
- Minimize the use of short-acting inhaled β₂-agonists for asthma patients (SOR: C).
- Short-acting inhaled β₂-agonists should be used less than twice a week for asthma, or step therapy should be increased (SOR: C).
- Inhaled corticosteroids are the preferred therapy for all patients with persistent asthma (SOR: A).
- Asthma exacerbations should be treated with oral corticosteroids (SOR: A).
- Nebulized ipratropium can be used for asthma exacerbation in the ED setting but should not be used in the inpatient setting (SOR: A).

Anaphylaxis

Key Points

- Anaphylaxis is a severe allergic reaction that can result in death.
- Increasing numbers of patients with anaphylaxis are reported.
- Identification of the signs and symptoms is necessary to prevent mortality.
- Diagnostic testing can aid the clinician in identifying the allergen responsible.
- Physicians should have intramuscular (IM) epinephrine readily accessible at all times for these patients.

Table 19-6 Signs and Symptoms of Anaphylaxis and Frequency of Occurrence

Signs and Symptoms	Frequency (%)
CUTANEOUS	**90**
Urticaria and angioedema	85-90
Flushing	45-55
Pruritus without rash	2-5
RESPIRATORY	**40-60**
Upper airway angioedema	60-60
Dyspnea, wheeze	45-50
Rhinitis	15-20
ABDOMINAL	
Nausea, vomiting, diarrhea, cramping abdominal pain	25-30
MISCELLANEOUS	
Dizziness, syncope, hypotension	30-35
Headache	5-8
Substernal pain	4-6
Seizure	1-2

Table 19-7 Diagnosis of Anaphylaxis*

Acute onset of an illness (minutes to hours) with involvement of skin and mucosal tissue (e.g., hives, generalized itch and flush, swollen lips, tongue, and uvula)

and

Airway compromise (e.g., dyspnea, wheeze or bronchospasm, stridor, reduced lung functions)

or

Reduced blood pressure or associated symptoms (e.g., hypotonia, syncope)

Two or more of the following after exposure to known allergen for that patient (minutes to hours):

History of severe allergic reaction

Skin or mucosal tissue involvement (e.g., hives, generalized itch or flush, swollen lips, tongue, uvula)

Airway compromise (e.g., dyspnea, wheeze/bronchospasm, stridor, reduced lung function)

Reduced blood pressure or associated symptoms (e.g., hypotonia, syncope)

In suspected food allergy: gastrointestinal symptoms (e.g., cramping abdominal pain, vomiting)

Hypotension after exposure to known allergen for that patient (minutes to hours)

Infants and children: low systolic blood pressure (age specific)

Adults: systolic blood pressure less than 100 mm Hg

*Caution: These criteria describe classic cases of anaphylaxis. Other presentations can also indicate anaphylaxis. Physicians must remember the potential for false-positive symptoms or signs resulting from panic, vasovagal episodes, and other causes.

Anaphylaxis has been traditionally defined as an acute, systemic, immediate hypersensitivity reaction produced by IgE-mediated degranulation of mast cells and basophils (Lieberman, 2006). The term *anaphylactoid* has referred to a clinically similar event not mediated by IgE-induced mast cell and basophil degranulation. An alternative classification by the World Allergy Organization (Johansson et al., 2004) eliminates the term *anaphylactoid* and refers to all events as *anaphylactic,* subdividing them into immunologic and nonimmunologic episodes. Immunologic episodes are then further subdivided into those caused by IgE-mediated mast cell and basophil degranulation and those resulting from other immunologic processes. An example of a non-IgE immunologically mediated event is a transfusion reaction. An example of a nonimmunologic event is a reaction to the administration of radiocontrast media (RCM) that can directly degranulate mast cells and basophils without intervening IgE. In the case of anaphylaxis to RCM, patients should be premedicated with steroids and antihistamines if its use is clinically indicated (Lieberman, 2009; Lieberman et al., 2010; eTable 19-3 online).

MANIFESTATIONS

Almost all patients with anaphylaxis express cutaneous symptoms, the most common of which are urticaria and angioedema. However, anaphylactic events can occur without any cutaneous manifestation. The most common cause is probably the rapid onset of hypotension and shock, which diverts blood flow from the skin. Anaphylaxis can clearly be the cause of syncope without any other manifestation and therefore must be considered as a cause of any syncopal episode. Table 19-6 lists signs and symptoms of anaphylaxis and their frequency (Sampson et al., 2005).

Criteria have been established for the diagnosis of anaphylaxis (Table 19-7) (Sampson et al., 2005). Anaphylaxis usually requires at least two-system involvement; in most cases, the skin is involved, and respiratory, vascular, or gastrointestinal symptoms accompany skin involvement. Patients with gastrointestinal anaphylaxis are often misdiagnosed. Single-system involvement (usually the skin) may be sufficient when this symptom appears after exposure to a known allergen (e.g., a person known to be allergic to shellfish who develops urticaria within 30 minutes of shellfish ingestion); the diagnosis of anaphylaxis can be made without two-system involvement. This concept is important because rapid administration of epinephrine in such a patient might prevent further manifestations. The earlier the symptoms are recognized, the more likely the patient will respond to the epinephrine. The risk of death exists in patients who either do not receive epinephrine or epinephrine is not administered promptly during an anaphylactic reaction (Simons et al., 2011, Simons et al., 2013).

The differential diagnosis and most common causes of anaphylaxis are shown in Tables 19-8 and 19-9. The most frequent cause of anaphylaxis is foods, and the next most common is drugs. The most common food to cause anaphylaxis in adults is shellfish. In infants, cow's milk is the most common food allergen; in older children, peanuts are the most common offenders. As many as 50% of cases of anaphylaxis occur without a known cause despite intense investigative efforts (Webb et al., 2004). Recently, delayed anaphylaxis to a carbohydrate in red meat (α-1,3-galactose) has been reported (Simons et al., 2011). Laboratory testing can be useful to establish a diagnosis of anaphylaxis and to rule out other causes of symptoms caused by conditions that mimic anaphylaxis (Table 19-10). The most common test to confirm a diagnosis of anaphylaxis is serum tryptase, with high specificity but low sensitivity.

Table 19-8   Differential Diagnosis of Anaphylaxis

Anaphylaxis
Vasodepressor and vasovagal reactions
Other forms of shock
Hemorrhagic
Hypoglycemic
Cardiogenic
Endotoxic
Flushing syndromes
Carcinoid
Red man syndrome caused by vancomycin
Postmenopausal
Alcohol induced
Vasointestinal peptide and other vasoactive peptide–secreting
   gastrointestinal tumors
Nonorganic diseases such as panic attacks

Table 19-9   Most Common Causes of Anaphylaxis

Foods	Shellfish
	Peanuts
	Tree nuts
	Fish
Drugs	Antibiotics (especially β-lactams)
	NSAIDs
Physical	Exercise
	Cold
	Heat
	Sunlight
	Idiopathic

NSAID, nonsteroidal antiinflammatory drug.

TREATMENT

Special equipment is necessary to deal with anaphylactic events that occur in the office (Table 19-11). An algorithm for the management of the acute episode is shown in Figure 19-5.

On suspicion that an anaphylactic event has occurred, therapy should be initiated immediately (Table 19-12). The airway, circulation, and level of consciousness should immediately be assessed. Oxygen should be started and the patient placed in the recumbent position with the feet elevated. The recumbent position is important because death has been associated with the upright position. The upright position allows decreased venous return to the heart, resulting in pulseless ventricular contractions and arrhythmias.

Simultaneous with assessment, epinephrine should be administered (Working Group of the Resuscitation Council, 2008). IM injection in the lateral thigh gives a more rapid peak level than subcutaneous or deltoid IM injection; therefore, the lateral thigh is the preferred site of injection. For adults, the dose is 0.2 to 0.5 mL of a 1 : 1000 aqueous epinephrine preparation. For children, the dose is 0.01 mg/kg to a maximum of 0.3 mg. A more precise dosage regimen has been recommended by the Resuscitation Council of the United Kingdom (Table 19-13). If symptoms do not improve, this dose can be readministered at 5-minute intervals (or more frequently if the physician deems necessary). After several injections, if there is no response, an intravenous (IV) infusion of epinephrine may be considered. An infusion

Table 19-10   Tests Used to Confirm a Diagnosis of Anaphylaxis

Test	Comment
TESTS USED TO RULE IN ANAPHYLAXIS	
Serum tryptase	Peaks at 60-90 minutes after onset of symptoms. May be elevated up to 6 hours. Ideal time to obtain blood is 1-2 hours after symptoms begin.
Plasma histamine	Begins to rise 5 to 10 minutes after onset of symptoms but remains elevated only up to 60 minutes.
24-hour urinary N-methylhistamine	May be assayed in urine for up to 24 hours after initiation of histamine metabolite symptoms.
TESTS USED TO RULE OUT OTHER CONDITIONS	
Serum serotonin	Rules out carcinoid
Urinary 5-hydroxyindoleacetic acid	Rules out carcinoid
Serum vasointestinal hormonal polypeptide panel*	Rules out vasoactive polypeptide–secreting gastrointestinal tumor or medullary carcinoma of thyroid
Plasma-free metanephrine and urinary vanillylmandelic acid	Rules out paradoxical response to pheochromocytoma

*For example, pancreastatin, pancreatic hormone, vasointestinal polypeptide, and substance P.

Table 19-11   Equipment and Medication for Therapy of Anaphylaxis in the Office

PRIMARY

Epinephrine solution (aqueous) 1 : 1000 (1-mL ampules and multidose vials)
Epinephrine solution (aqueous) 1 : 10,000 (commercially available preloaded in a syringe)
Tourniquet
1-mL and 5-mL disposable syringes
Oxygen tank and mask or nasal prongs
Diphenhydramine injectable
Ranitidine or cimetidine injectable
Injectable corticosteroids
Ambu bag, oral airway, laryngoscope, endotracheal tube, no. 12 needle
IV setup with large-bore catheter
IV fluids: 2000 mL of crystalloid solution, 1000 mL of hydroxyethyl starch
Aerosol β-II bronchodilator and compressor nebulizer
Glucagon
Electrocardiogram
Normal saline: 10-mL vial for epinephrine dilution

SUPPORTING

Dopamine
Suction apparatus
Sodium bicarbonate
Aminophylline
Atropine
IV setup with needles, tape, and tubing
Nonlatex gloves

OPTIONAL

Defibrillator
Calcium gluconate
Neuroleptic agents for seizures
Lidocaine

IV, Intravenous.

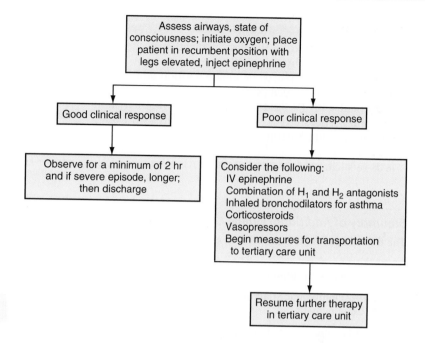

Figure 19-5 Algorithm for managing an episode of anaphylaxis. *IV,* Intravenous.

Table 19-12 Therapy for Anaphylaxis

Immediate Action	Treatment
Assessment	Epinephrine
Check airway and secure if needed	Supine position, legs elevated
Rapid assessment of level of consciousness	Oxygen
	Tourniquet proximal to injection site
Vital signs	
DEPENDENT ON EVALUATION	**HOSPITAL MANAGEMENT**
Start peripheral IV fluids	MAST
H₁ and H₂ antagonist	Continued therapy with
Vasopressors	above agents and
Corticosteroids	management of
Aminophylline	complications
Glucagon	
Atropine	
Electrocardiographic monitoring	
Transfer to hospital	

IV, Intravenous; *MAST,* medical antishock trousers.

Table 19-13 Dosing Recommendations for Intramuscular Epinephrine in Anaphylaxis*

ADULTS

0.5 mg (0.5 mL of 1:1000 concentration)

CHILDREN

Age > 12 yr: 0.5 mg (0.5 mL of 1:1000 concentration)
or
0.3 mg (0.3 mL of 1:1000 concentration) if child is small or prepubertal

6-12 yr: 0.3 mg (0.3 mL using a 1:1000 concentration)†

6 mo to 6 yr: 0.15 mg (0.15 mL of 1:1000 concentration)

Age <6 mo: 0.15 mg (0.15 mL of 1:000 concentration)

*Dosing in pediatrics depends on weight of child, not age. In the office/hospital setting, 0.5 mg of 1:1000 concentration is recommended dose in adults. Current autoinjector devices for patient use come in 2 doses: 0.15 mg is the lower dose and 0.3 mg is the higher dose.
†If the child is small, use the 0.01 mg/kg dose.

can be prepared by adding 1 mg (1 mL of 1:1000 dilution of epinephrine) to 250 mL of D5W, yielding a concentration of 4.0 µg/mL. This solution is infused at a rate of 1 to 4 µg/min (15-60 drops/min with microdrop apparatus), increasing to a maximum of 10.0 µg/min for adults and adolescents. For children, the dose is 0.01 mg/kg (0.1 mL/kg of 1:10,000 solution up to 10 µg/min); the maximum recommended dose is 0.3 mg.

Epinephrine is mandated and is the drug of choice for anaphylaxis. Other drugs include H₁ and H₂ antagonists; a combination of both is more effective than an H₁ antagonist alone for vascular manifestations. Antihistamines, however, should only be considered as part of treatment after epinephrine has been administered. Diphenhydramine, 25 to 50 mg for adults and 1 mg/kg for children, can be given by slow IV infusion. Ranitidine can be administered in a dose of 1 mg/kg in adults and 12.5 to 50 mg in children, infused over 10 to 15 minutes. No controlled studies have demonstrated efficacy of corticosteroids, but they should help in prolonged reactions. Although there is no established dose, the suggested dose equivalent is 1 to 2 mg/kg of methylprednisolone every 6 hours.

For persistent hypotension, fluids or other vasopressors (or both) should be administered. For adults with persistent hypotension, 1 to 2 L of normal saline can be administered at rates of 5 to 10 mg/kg in the first 5 minutes. After resolution of symptoms, patients should be observed because biphasic reactions can occur in up to 23% of cases (Scranton et al., 2009). The observation period should range from 6 to 24 hours, depending on the severity of the reaction (Tole and Lieberman, 2007).

Patients who have experienced episodes of anaphylaxis and who are at further risk of future events (e.g., insect sting hypersensitivity, food allergy) should have a prescription for an epinephrine autoinjector and should be instructed in its use. Medical alert bracelets can benefit these patients. In addition, such patients should not take, if at all possible, drugs that might increase the severity of any future event or interfere with the use of epinephrine to treat such an event (eTable 19-3 online).

KEY TREATMENT

- Epinephrine should be the first medication used in the treatment of anaphylaxis (SOR: A).
- Patients should be placed in supine position and oxygen administered, if needed (SOR: A).
- Treatment with IV fluids, antihistamines (both H_1 and H_2), and corticosteroids should be considered only after epinephrine administration (SOR: A).
- Glucagon or atropine should be considered in anaphylaxis recalcitrant to treatment (SOR: A).

Summary of Additional Online Content

The following content is available at www.expertconsult.com:

eTable 19-1 Second-Generation Oral Antihistamines for Treatment of Allergic Rhinitis

eTable 19-2 Ophthalmic Solutions Useful in the Treatment of Allergic Conjunctivitis

eBox 19-1 Exercise-Induced Bronchospasm

eBox 19-2 Paradoxical Vocal Cord Motion

eTable 19-3 Drugs That Can Worsen or Complicate Therapy in Anaphylaxis

References

The complete reference list is available at www.expertconsult.com.

Web Resources

www.aaaai.org American Academy of Allergy, Asthma and Immunology website; includes information on the diagnosis and treatment of allergic diseases.

www.acaai.org American College of Allergy, Asthma and Immunology website; includes information on the diagnosis and treatment of allergic diseases.

www.cdc.gov/nchs/fastats/asthma.htm and www.cdc.gov/ASTHMA/healthcare.html Centers for Disease Control and Prevention statistics.

www.nhlbi.nih.gov/guidelines/asthma/asthgdln.pdf National Heart, Lung and Blood Institute and National Asthma Education and Prevention Panel: Expert Panel Report 3: Guidelines for the diagnosis and management of asthma, 2007.

http://www.thoracic.org/statements/resources/pft/pft5.pdf American Thoracic Society information for interpretative strategies for lung function tests.

20 *Obstetrics*

DAVE ELTON WILLIAMS and GABRIELLA PRIDJIAN

Key Points

- The United States ranks 31th in infant mortality.
- The causes of infant mortality are preterm birth, birth defects, sudden infant death syndrome, respiratory distress syndrome, and maternal pregnancy complications.

The American Academy of Family Physicians (AAFP) describes the specialty of family practice as the enhanced expression of general medical practice that is uniquely defined within the context of the family. Providing care across the continuum of the family life cycle, the family physician provides care to the pregnant woman as part of the full expression of the field. The family physician incorporates a comprehensive approach to maternity care that includes the assessment and management of psychosocial and biomedical risk factors. The family physician provides care to patients with low-risk pregnancies and equips them to birth their children without unnecessary interventions.

The family physician brings a unique approach to the management of the pregnant woman, who is often a healthy individual undergoing a natural process. This approach is patient centered, prevention oriented, educational, and noninterventional. Nationwide, approximately 29.6% of all family physicians provide routine obstetric services as part of their hospital care (AAFP, 2011). This number has been steadily declining, with regional variations reflecting the needs of the population and local attitudes (AAFP, 1998). The majority of family physicians do not desire to practice obstetrics because of lifestyle issues, increasing costs of malpractice insurance, and difficulty obtaining hospital privileges. However, the family physician may be asked to counsel or care for the pregnant woman even if not part of daily practice. It becomes incumbent on the individual practitioner to have a fundamental knowledge and appreciation of the field of obstetrics, including the obstetric emergency. Given that the family physician may be the sole provider of obstetric services, particularly in rural or underserved areas, the need to maintain the knowledge and skills to treat the problems and emergencies unique to obstetrics becomes increasingly important. The Advanced Life Support in Obstetrics (ALSO) course developed in 1990 effectively incorporates the techniques of other established life support courses as it applies to obstetric care.

For the successful practice of obstetrics, it is imperative for the family physician to practice in concert with an obstetric specialist. A collaborative relationship among obstetricians; family physicians; and in some cases, nurse midwives is essential for provision of consistent, high-quality care to pregnant women. Access to reliable consultation and suitable referral facilities for complicated patients will optimize patient care and outcomes.

The integration of prenatal care into the clinical practice of the family physician not only reflects the full scope of the field but also provides a continuous infusion of pediatric patients into the practice. It serves as a model for the training of medical students and residents interested in the practice of obstetric care in the context of family practice.

This chapter provides an overview of the field of obstetrics, which includes prenatal, intrapartum, and postpartum care of the pregnant woman. An evidence-based approach to areas of controversy and empiric practice is used while addressing the unique needs of family physicians, emphasizing their contribution and role in the research and development of the obstetrics literature.

Woman and Child Health

The health of a nation is often reflected in the health of its mothers and newborns. The World Health Organization (WHO) often uses a nation's maternity and neonatal morbidity and mortality statistics as a proxy for the health status of its population. It is an important summary reflecting social, political, health care delivery, and medical outcomes in a geographic area. The United States, despite its economic wealth and medical resources, consistently ranks poorly in such measures as maternal and infant mortality rates (IMRs).

The most recent data available (2008) in the United States record that 28,059 infants died before reaching their first birthdays, an IMR of 6.6 per 1000 live births. Despite a decline from an IMR 6.9 in 2005 and an historical low rate, the United States still ranks 31st, after such countries as Japan, the Scandinavian countries, and Canada, as ranked by the Organization for Economic Cooperation and Development (OECD), as shown in Table 20-1. This number reflects in part the continuing disparities in health access and delivery for U.S. citizens.

The causes of infant death are multiple, with birth defects being the leading cause, with a 2008 rate of 20.1% of the infant deaths in the first year of life. Preterm birth (birth at <37 completed weeks of gestation) or low birth weight (LBW) is the second leading cause of infant mortality in the United States. Preterm birth rates differ by race in the United States; the rates were highest for black infants (13.3) followed by Native Americans (8.4), whites (5.7), and Asians (4.8). This persistent disparity contributes to the relative high IMR in the United States compared with similarly developed countries. Other causes of infant mortality include sudden infant death syndrome, respiratory distress syndrome, and maternal pregnancy complications. The top 10 causes of infant mortality account for nearly 70% of the total (Figure 20-1). Despite gains in the overall IMR, the rates of preterm birth, birth defects, and LBW remain relatively constant. This indicates a need for further health initiatives to address the health needs of pregnant women and unborn fetuses.

Preconception Counseling

Key Points

- Preconception care is an integral part of prenatal care and permits health promotion and early identification of risk factors that can then be treated before pregnancy.
- Folic acid supplementation should be started before conception, if possible, or immediately on diagnosis of pregnancy.

Table 20-1 Infant Mortality Rates (Infant Deaths per 1000 Live births) and Rankings for OECD and Other Selected Countries, 2008

Country	IMR	Rank
Luxembourg	1.8	1
Slovenia	2.1	2
Iceland	2.5	3
Sweden	2.5	3
Japan	2.6	5
Finland	2.6	5
Norway	2.7	7
Greece	2.7	7
Czech Republic	2.8	9
Ireland	3.0	10
Portugal	3.3	11
Belgium	3.4	12
Germany	3.5	13
Spain	3.5	13
Austria	3.7	15
Italy	3.7	15
France	3.8	17
Israel	3.8	17
Netherlands	3.8	17
Denmark	4.0	20
Switzerland	4.0	20
Australia	4.1	22
OECD Average	4.6	-
Korea	4.7	23
United Kingdom	4.7	23
New Zealand	4.9	25
Estonia	5.0	26
Hungary	5.6	27
Poland	5.6	27
Canada	5.7	29
Slovak Republic	5.9	30
United States	6.6	31
Chile	7.0	32
Mexico	15.2	33
Turkey	17.0	34

OECD, Organisation for Economic Co-operation and Development.
Adapted from Organization for Economic Cooperation and Development. *OECD Health Data,* 2010. http://www.oecd.org/dataoecd/4/36/46796773 .pdf. U.S. 2008 data from Ariadi M, Minino MPH, Sherry L, et al. *National Vital Statics Reports: deaths: final data for 2008.* Hyattsville, MD: National Center for Health Statistics 59(10), December 7, 2011.

Ideally, women should plan pregnancy and discuss this plan with their physicians. Often, however, this option is not considered. It becomes the task of the physician to anticipate the potential and discuss preparation for pregnancy just as for methods of birth control. Primary care physicians are in the best position to anticipate the need for this counseling, being most aware of ongoing medical problems and social concerns of the women in their care. Indeed, the practice of preconception care has been formally recommended since at least 1989 (Caring for Our Future, 1989). However, we believe that preconception care, in particular

education, should begin at the time a woman reaches reproductive age, not only when she announces the desire to become pregnant.

The preconception period is an ideal time for education and counseling regarding cessation of cigarette, alcohol, or drug use. Often, the incentive of a healthier pregnancy is sufficient impetus for a change in behavior. Although many women are able to cease cigarette, alcohol, or drug use during pregnancy, the majority resume use after delivery or breastfeeding. This is an opportune time for the family physician to reinforce further health-conscious behavior. Tobacco is a known carcinogen that can harm developing

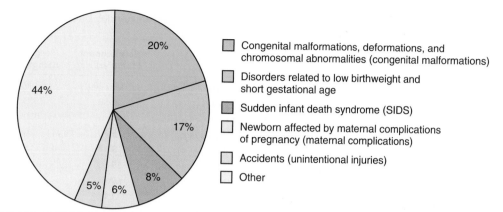

Figure 20-1 Six leading causes of U.S. infant deaths, 2008. (Data from Ariadi M, Minino MPH, Sherry L, et al. *National Vital Statics Reports: Deaths: Final Data for 2008.* Hyattsville, MD: National Center for Health Statistics 59(10), December 7, 2011.)

fetuses. Women who quit smoking before pregnancy or in early pregnancy significantly reduce the risk of adverse outcomes, including preterm birth, LBW, and infant mortality. However, smoking cessation therapies also carry risks in pregnant women. Using nicotine replacement therapies during the early stages of pregnancy may increase the risk of birth defects, according to a study of 77,000 pregnant Danish women (Morales-Suárez-Varela et al., 2006).

Other pharmacologic aids have not been tested for safety and effectiveness in treating tobacco dependence in pregnant women. Therefore, pregnant smokers should be offered intensive person-to-person interventions that exceed minimal advice to quit, such as behavioral support and problem solving, counseling, and referral to support organizations (Fiore et al., 2008).

The preconception use of folic acid supplementation was formally recommended by the U.S. Centers for Disease Control and Prevention (CDC) in 1991 and later by others (American Academy of Pediatrics, Committee on Genetics, 1999). Evidence supports a reduction in neural tube defects by 50% when folic acid stores are replenished before pregnancy (Milunsky et al., 1989). It is now recommended that all reproductive-age women take 0.4 mg of folic acid daily (CDC, 1992). This is easily accomplished by prescribing prenatal vitamins before pregnancy as well as throughout gestation. Alternately, over-the-counter (OTC) vitamins can also be used because many now contain this higher amount of folic acid. For couples with one or more children with a neural tube defect or a family history, there should be a referral for specific counseling. From 2 to 4 mg of folic acid daily is recommended for these women at least 1 month before pregnancy and during the first 3 months of pregnancy.

Many genetic disorders are now amenable to prenatal diagnosis through direct analysis of the underlying mutations, analysis of their protein products, or abnormal metabolites. Genetic counseling should include a systematic assessment of the family history of both parents. This can be done through a targeted questionnaire or formal genetic counseling by a genetic counselor or geneticist (Table 20-2). The family physician should be aware of the ethnic makeup of the practice and be especially familiar with disorders in these groups (Table 20-3). When targeted screening reveals an area of potential concern, formal

Table 20-2 Genetic Screening and Teratology Counseling

1. Will you be 35 years old or older at the time of your baby's birth?
2. What medications—prescribed, herbal, or over the counter—have you taken since your last menstrual period?
3. How much alcohol, cigarettes, or street drugs have you used since your last menstrual period?
4. Have you had miscarriages or stillborns? How many?
5. Do you have any metabolic disorders (e.g., diabetes or phenylketonuria)?
6. Have you been ill or had any infections since your last menstrual period?
7. What are the ethnic backgrounds of you and the baby's father? Are you related in any way?
8. Do you, the baby's father, or anyone in either of your families have:
   a. Neural tube defects (meningomyelocele, spina bifida, or anencephaly)?
   b. Congenital heart defects?
   c. Down syndrome?
   d. Tay-Sachs disease (Jewish, Cajun, or French Canadian)?
   e. Sickle cell disease or trait (African American)?
   f. Thalassemia (mean corpuscular volume <80 fL/red cell) (Italian, Mediterranean, Asian, or African American)?
   g. Muscular dystrophy?
   h. Cystic fibrosis?
   i. Huntington's chorea?
   j. Fragile X, mental retardation, or autism?
   k. Other chromosomal or inherited disorders or birth defects?

genetic counseling should be obtained. With advances in discovery of the genetic basis for many diseases, the list of disorders amenable to prenatal diagnosis grows daily.

KEY TREATMENT

- Folic acid supplementation is 0.4 mg for women without risk factors and up to 4 mg for those with risk factors (USPTF, 2009) (SOR: A).

Nutrition

There are sufficient data to confirm that poor nutrition during the prenatal period is associated with adverse pregnancy outcomes, specifically *fetal growth restriction* (FGR)

Table 20-3 Genetic Screening and Teratology Counseling and Risk

Ethnic Group	Higher Risk	Carrier Frequency
White	Cystic fibrosis	1 in 25
African American	Sickle cell disease β-Thalassemia	1 in 12
Southeast Asian	α-Thalassemia	1 in 20
Mediterranean (Italian, Greek)	β-Thalassemia	1 in 25
Ashkenazi Jewish	Tay-Sachs disease	1 in 30
	Gaucher disease type 1	1 in 12
	Canavan disease	1 in 40
	Cystic fibrosis	1 in 25

Table 20-4 Recommended Total Weight Gain for Pregnant Women

		Weight Gain	
Phenotype	BMI	lb	kg
Underweight	<18.5	28-40	13.7-18.2
Normal weight	18.5-24.9	25-35	11.4-15.9
Overweight	25-29.9	15-25	6.8-11.4
Obese (all classes)	≥30	11-20	5-9.1

BMI, Body mass index.
Modified from Institute of Medicine, National Academies of Science: Weight gain during pregnancy: reexamining the guidelines. *Curr Opin Obstet Gynecol* 21(6):521-526, 2009.

Table 20-5 Recommended Dietary Allowances for Women

	Nonpregnant (15-50 yr)	Pregnant (Singleton)	Lactating (first 6 mo)
Energy, kcal	1900-2200	+300	+500
Protein, g	44-50	60	65
Vitamin A, µg RE	800	800	1300
Vitamin D, µg*	5-10	10	10
Vitamin E, mg TE	8	10	12
Vitamin K, µg	55-65	65	65
Vitamin C, mg	60	70	95
Thiamin, mg	1.1	1.5	1.6
Riboflavin, mg	1.3	1.6	1.8
Niacin, mg NE	15	17	20
Vitamin B_6, mg	1.5-1.6	2.2	2.1
Folate, µg	400	400	400
Vitamin B_{12}, µg	2.0	2.2	2.6
Calcium, mg	800-1200	1200	1200
Phosphorus, mg	800-1200	1200	1200
Magnesium, mg	280	300	355
Iron, mg	15	30	15
Zinc, mg	12	15	19
Iodine, µg	150	175	200
Selenium, µg	50-55	65	75

*As cholecalciferol.
NE, Niacin equivalents; *RE*, retinal equivalents; *TE*, α-tocopherol equivalents.
Data from Report of the Subcommittee on the Tenth Edition of the RDAs, Recommended Dietary Allowances, National Academy of Sciences, with modifications from ACOG Committee Opinion #196, 1998; and Centers for Disease Control. Use of folic acid for the prevention of spina bifida and other neural tube defects. *MMWR Morb Mortal Wkly Rep.* 1991;40:513-516.

and preterm delivery. Specific nutritional guidelines have been developed based on a woman's prepregnancy weight or, more specifically, her body mass index (BMI) (Table 20-4). Caloric intake of an extra 300 kcal/day is sufficient for adequate maternal weight gain and fetal growth.

The practice of prenatal supplementation of vitamins and minerals is widespread, although many nutritionists believe it is unnecessary. Only the following two supplements are recommended in an adequately nourished woman with a singleton pregnancy:

1. Iron, 30 mg/day, in the second and third trimester to meet the fetal demands for erythropoiesis
2. Folic acid, 400 µg/day, in the preconception period and during the first trimester for prevention of birth defects

However, because many U.S. women do not consume adequate vitamins and minerals (Block and Adams, 1993) and specific assessment of nutritional intake is often difficult, supplements are now widely used. Recommended daily allowances for pregnant women have been established and continue to be reevaluated (Table 20-5). Care must be taken to avoid toxicity of the fat-soluble vitamins, in particular vitamin A (retinol), because more is not necessarily better. Daily doses of retinol greater than 10,000 IU, approximately 3000 retinol equivalents, have been associated with birth defects (American College of Obstetrics and Gynecologists, 2008; Rothman et al., 1995). Women who do not consume sufficient milk products may benefit from calcium supplementation. This can easily be accomplished by prescribing an antacid that is made of calcium

carbonate, most easily taken in chewable form. This will not only replenish calcium stores but also treat reflux esophagitis, which often occurs in the latter half of pregnancy.

Recent data suggest that supplementation with omega-3 fatty acids, specifically docosahexaenoic acid (DHA) plus eicosapentaenoic acid (EPA), may be beneficial (Dunstan et al., 2008). Both DHA and EPA may be beneficial for fetal brain development and are found in large amounts in wild fish. However, increased fish intake in pregnancy is not recommended because of the risk of increased mercury ingestion. Therefore, supplementation is required. Large, well-controlled studies are needed before recommendation in pregnancy, but supplementation may be considered on an individual basis. The U.S. Food and Drug Administration has formally warned women of childbearing age, pregnant and lactating women, and young children to avoid eating swordfish, shark, king mackerel, and tilefish and to consume no more than one 6-oz can of albacore tuna per week. In all pregnant women, nutritional risk factors should be addressed, including low starting BMI, prior LBW infants, adolescence, religious and cultural dietary restrictions, medical illnesses requiring dietary manipulation, substance abuse, and eating disorders (Kolasa and Weismiller, 1995). Certain woman may benefit from formal dietary counseling from a dietician or nutritionist.

- Iron (30 mg/day) is recommended in the second and third trimesters (SOR: A).
- Folic acid (400 µg/day) is recommended in the preconception period and the first trimester (SOR: A).

Medical Risk Assessment

The preconception period is the ideal time to assess and counsel the prospective pregnant woman regarding medical disorders or risks she may encounter during the pregnancy. Of medical problems that have substantial impact on the fetus, hypertensive disorders and diabetes are among the most common.

Hypertension may have many effects on the pregnancy depending on the degree of abnormality. Fetal effects range from none to increased miscarriage, FGR, abruptio placentae, and fetal death. Underlying blood pressure (BP) disorders should be treated appropriately before pregnancy. Some hypertensive, reproductive-age women are treated with angiotensin-converting enzyme (ACE) inhibitors. This class of therapeutics can cause significant risk to the developing fetus. These medications should be stopped and alternate medications started if needed. Women with preexisting hypertension should be referred for concurrent care with a physician experienced in managing hypertension in pregnancy.

Diabetes can also have many effects on a developing fetus. The preconception control of the maternal metabolism, reflected as normal blood glucose values before and after meals and normal hemoglobin A_{1c}, has been shown to decrease the incidence of diabetes-associated embryopathy to almost that of a nondiabetic pregnant woman (Mills et al., 1988). Women with preexisting diabetes should be referred for specialized care if pregnancy is contemplated.

Less attention is directed to emotional and psychiatric disorders. Pregnancy may be a stressor that precipitates an acute event or worsens ongoing anxiety or depression. This is more likely in the postpartum period.

- Preconception care is an integral part of prenatal care and permits health promotion and early identification of risk factors that can then be treated before pregnancy, such as diabetes or hypertension (SOR: A).
- Women with preexisting diabetes should be referred for specialized care if pregnancy is contemplated (SOR: C).

Routine Prenatal Care

In most Western countries, women attend between 7 and 11 prenatal visits, although recent data suggest that a reduced number of antenatal visits could be introduced into clinical practice without adverse effect to the mother and child (Carroli et al., 2001). Obstetric care provided by obstetricians, family physicians, and midwives has been found to be equally effective; however, patients were slightly more

satisfied by the care provided by midwives and family physicians (Villar et al., 2004). Prenatal care services typically include screening and treatment for medical conditions and identification and interventions for behavioral risk factors associated with poor birth outcomes (e.g., smoking, poor nutrition).

One of the most important goals of prenatal care is recognizing which women have high-risk pregnancies and triaging these women to appropriate care (Kontopoulos and Vintzileos, 2004). It is important to identify the women at risk for adverse outcomes and refer them to appropriate specialty care. Adequate prenatal care has been shown to increase the chances that a woman has a healthy pregnancy and baby.

FIRST PRENATAL VISIT

The first prenatal visit is one of the most important, particularly if the woman has not had preconception care (Table 20-6). The first prenatal visit should occur shortly after the woman discovers she might be pregnant and should be viewed as a continuation of preconception counseling. Home pregnancy test kits have a sensitivity and specificity of at least 95%; many can detect pregnancy by the fifth menstrual week. The most important aspects of the first prenatal visit include education, risk assessment, appropriate laboratory testing, and establishment of gestational age.

Education is an important component of prenatal care, particularly for women who are pregnant for the first time. The frequency of prenatal visits should be explained, with information about the physiologic changes that occur during pregnancy. Preparation for the birthing process is a key theme around which to discuss care issues and choices such as breastfeeding. Structured educational programs to promote breastfeeding have unclear effectiveness. Pregnant women should be counseled about the risks of possible teratogens, including smoking, alcohol, drug use, and exposure to medications, prescriptions, OTC drugs, and herbal remedies. Good hand washing is always encouraged because this is one of the best ways to avoid community-acquired infectious diseases. Appropriate immunizations such as influenza and novel influenza A (H1N1) virus should be offered. Common exposures such as workplace conditions and use of hot tubs and saunas should be explored. Exercise should also be encouraged if there is no obstetric contraindication (ACOG, 1994) (Table 20-7). Intercourse during pregnancy should be actively addressed because some women are reluctant to discuss this topic even with their physicians. Sexual activity can generally continue during pregnancy except for few situations, such as placenta previa and preterm labor. Counseling regarding sexually transmitted diseases (STDs) and their avoidance should occur. Nutrition should be individualized, with an estimate of desirable weight gain given to the pregnant woman.

The estimated date of delivery (EDD) should be calculated by accurate determination of the last menstrual period (LMP). The first day of the LMP is a good clinical sign from which to calculate the EDD, remembering that it must be adjusted for cycles shorter or longer than 28 days. The EDD can be calculated by Nagle's rule, that is, subtracting 3 months and adding 7 days to the first day of the LMP. The

Table 20-6 Expert Panel Recommendations for First Prenatal Visit

RISK ASSESSMENT FOR ALL

Medical History

Medical and surgical update
Nutrition update
Current pregnancy to date*

Psychosocial History

Smoking
Alcohol
Drugs
Social support
Extremes of physical work, exercise, and other activity
Stress

Physical Examination

Blood pressure*
Weight
Breast examination*
Pelvic examination for uterine size, dating, and abnormalities*

Laboratory Tests

Recommended for all:

Hemoglobin and hematocrit
Urine culture

Recommended for some:

Rh screen
Syphilis test
Blood glucose level
Gonococcal culture

HEALTH PROMOTION ACTIVITIES AND INFORMATION FOR ALL

Avoidance of teratogens
Safer sex*
Physical and emotional changes in pregnancy*
Sexuality*
Self-help strategies for discomforts (for some)
Fetal growth and development
Classes on nutrition, physical changes, exercise, and psychological adaptation
Nutritional counseling (some or all)
Preparation for screening and diagnostic tests
Content and timing of visits*
Need to report danger signs*

*From Rosen M, Merkatz I, Hill J. Caring for our future: a report by the expert panel on the content of prenatal care. *Obstet Gynecol* 77:785, 1991.

Table 20-7 Recommendations for Exercise in Pregnancy

1. Established exercise routines can be continued with mild to moderate intensity.
2. High-intensity or high-impact routines should be avoided or reduced.
3. The supine position should be avoided in the second and third trimesters.
4. Hyperthermia should be avoided.
5. Weight-bearing exercise should minimize strain because joints are more lax.
6. Routines should be designed to minimize the risk of maternal trauma (falling).
7. Adequate nutritional intake to compensate for pregnancy should be assured.
8. Resumption of prepregnancy routines in the postpartum period should be gradual.

A history and directed physical examination should be performed to detect conditions associated with increased maternal and perinatal morbidity and mortality. The first prenatal examination provides an opportunity for cervical cancer screening with a Papanicolaou (Pap) test in women who have not been screened recently. However, Pap tests performed in pregnant women may be less reliable. Risk factors should then identify other testing that might be done at this time, including blood glucose, sickle cell screening, Tay-Sachs screening, and surveillance for other infectious diseases.

Routine fetal heart auscultation; urinalysis; and assessment of maternal weight, BP, and fundal height generally are recommended, although the supportive evidence varies (Kirkham et al., 2005). Women should be offered ABO and Rh blood typing and screening for anemia during the first prenatal visit. Genetic counseling and testing should be offered to couples with a family history of genetic disorders, a previously affected fetus or child, or a history of recurrent miscarriage. All women should be offered prenatal serum marker screening for neural tube defects and aneuploidy. Women at increased risk for aneuploidy should be offered amniocentesis or chorionic villus sampling (CVS). Counseling about the limitations and risks of these tests, as well as their psychologic implications, is necessary. Folic acid supplementation beginning in the preconception period and early pregnancy reduces the incidence of neural tube defects. Laboratory testing during the first prenatal visit consists of assessment of hemoglobin and hematocrit to identify anemia, blood D(Rh) type, serologic tests for syphilis and rubella immunity, hepatitis B, and urinalysis. Testing for human immunodeficiency virus (HIV) infection should be offered and highly recommended because perinatal transmission can be decreased with appropriate medical intervention. During the pelvic examination, a Pap smear (if indicated) as well as cultures for *Neisseria gonorrhoeae* and *Chlamydia* should be taken.

FOLLOW-UP PRENATAL VISITS

According to the report of the Expert Panel on Prenatal Care (Rosen et al., 1991), low-risk primigravid women should have at least 10 prenatal visits; low-risk multiparous women should have at least eight visits. Again, however,

EDD should then be extended by the number of days longer than a 28-day cycle or shortened by the number of days shorter. This approach should be considered if there is uncertainty about the LMP.

The physical examination during the first prenatal visit should include careful assessment of uterine size. If there is a discrepancy between menstrual age and uterine size, ultrasonography should be considered early in the pregnancy to resolve the issue of dating. Recent evidence suggests that early ultrasonography provides more accurate dating, which is important for timing screening tests and interventions and for optimal management of complications such as postterm pregnancies (Neilson, 2004). Late ultrasonography, after 24 weeks, is not as sensitive for confirming gestational age. Additionally, any irregular bleeding or abdominal pain should prompt the practitioner to obtain ultrasonographic confirmation of viability of the pregnancy as well as its normal intrauterine location.

Table 20-8 Expert Panel Recommendations for Visits Throughout Pregnancy

Activity	Week/Trimester
Check for any exposure to infection*	
Physical Examination	
Blood pressure	24†
Weight	Each visit
Fundal height and growth	16†
Fetal lie, presentation, engagement, and heart rate*	24†
Cervical examination	41*
Laboratory Tests	
Hemoglobin and hematocrit	24-28
Rh sensitivity‡	26-28
Diabetic screen	26-28
Repeat syphilis‡	Third trimester
Repeat gonococcal and HIV‡	36
Serum α-fetoprotein	14-16
Ultrasonography*	When indicated
Health Promotion Activities	
Teratogen avoidance	Each visit
Safer sex*	Each visit
Maternal seatbelt use	Each trimester
Smoking cessation‡	Each trimester
Work and nutrition counseling‡	Each visit
Signs of preterm labor	Second and third trimesters
Physical and emotional changes*	First and third trimesters
Sexuality counseling*	Last half of pregnancy
Fetal growth and development	Each visit
Self-help for discomforts‡	Each visit
General health habits	Each visit
Breastfeeding	26†
Infant car seat safety	Each visit
Childbirth and parenting classes	32
Family roles adjustment	38
Information about laboratory tests*	Before testing
Birth plan*	Third trimester
Labor (when to call/where to go)*	Third trimester

*Accepted by panel but not specifically reviewed.
†That week and each week thereafter.
‡For some.
HIV, Human immunodeficiency virus.
From Rosen M, Merkatz I, Hill J. Caring for our future: a report by the expert panel on the content of prenatal care. *Obstet Gynecol.* 1991;77:785.

data suggest that antenatal visits could be reduced without adverse effect to the mother and child (Carroli et al., 2001). Women with psychosocial issues or pregnancy complications should be seen more frequently. In the first two trimesters, prenatal visits may be 5 to 6 weeks apart if no problems have been ascertained. The frequency of visits should increase after 30 weeks, with weekly visits after 37 weeks. Specific recommendations are noted in Table 20-8. Routine visits for low-risk women should be scheduled at times that recommended laboratory testing could be accomplished. Prenatal screening for chromosomal abnormalities is available in the first trimester between 10 weeks, 2 days and 13 weeks, 6 days. Structural defects of the fetus (in particular neural tube defects) and karyotypic abnormalities in the form of α-fetoprotein (AFP)–based tests (quad screen; see later discussion) can be obtained at 16 to 18 weeks. Screening for gestational diabetes (GDM) is

recommended at 26 to 28 weeks of gestation, as well as screening for anemia with a hemoglobin or hematocrit. Antibody screening, $Rh_0(D)$ immune globulin (RhoGAM) prophylaxis for D-negative mothers, and repeat testing for infectious diseases for at-risk mothers are recommended at this time.

Group B streptococcus (GBS) is the leading cause of early-onset neonatal sepsis in the United States. At 35 to 37 weeks' gestation, rectocervical cultures for GBS should be obtained in all pregnant women. The CDC recently updated its guideline for the prevention of early-onset neonatal GBS disease (2010). If cultures are positive or the patient tests positive for GBS bacteriuria, antibiotic prophylaxis during labor is indicated. For women without a penicillin allergy, penicillin (5 million units; then 2.5 million units intravenously [IV] every 4 hours) is administered during labor. Ampicillin (2 g IV initial dose; then 1 g IV every 4 hours until delivery) is an acceptable alternative. If there is a penicillin allergy, sensitivities to clindamycin and erythromycin should be obtained. If the GBS is sensitive to both antibiotics, clindamycin can be used. If the GBS is resistant to either clindamycin or erythromycin or if time does not permit testing, women with a serious penicillin allergy should receive vancomycin. Women with a minimal reaction from penicillin (e.g., rash) should receive a first-generation cephalosporin such as cefazolin IV during labor (American College of Obstetricians and Gynecologists [ACOG], 2002a; CDC, 2009; Schrag et al., 2002; Verani et al., 2010). A patient with a severe allergy is defined as one with a history of developing angioedema, anaphylaxis, urticaria, or respiratory distress after receiving penicillin or a cephalosporin. Women with GBS bacteriuria or a prior child affected with GBS sepsis should be treated during labor without screening cultures. Intrapartum antibiotic prophylaxis is not indicated if an elective cesarean delivery is planned and there is no labor or rupture of membranes.

KEY TREATMENT

- Universal screening at 35 to 37 weeks of gestation and intrapartum treatment of colonized women are the most effective approaches in reducing GBS sepsis of the newborn (ACOG, 2011) (SOR: A).

The clinical components of routine prenatal visits are controversial. Most guidelines recommend routine assessment with fundal height and maternal weight and BP measurements, fetal heart auscultation, urine testing for protein and glucose, and questions about fetal movement. The assessment of uterine growth and size should be performed at every prenatal visit. Documentation of fetal heart tones is also recommended with each prenatal visit. Before 12 weeks' gestation, the size of the uterus is estimated by bimanual pelvic examination. The ability to assess the presence of fetal heart tones using Doppler ultrasonography before 12 weeks is variable. After 12 weeks and before 20 weeks, adequate uterine growth is assessed by location of the uterine fundus in the lower abdomen (Figure 20-2). Fetal heart tones should be reliably heard during this period. At 20 weeks of gestation, most women have a palpable fundus at the umbilicus. After 20 weeks, fundal height is measured using the distance from the top of the symphysis

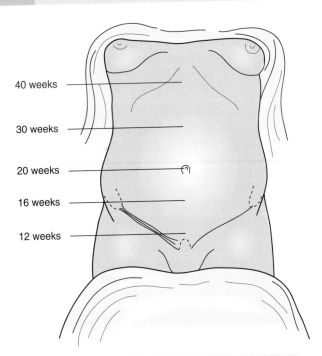

Figure 20-2 Fundal growth at various weeks of gestation.

40 weeks

30 weeks

20 weeks

16 weeks

12 weeks

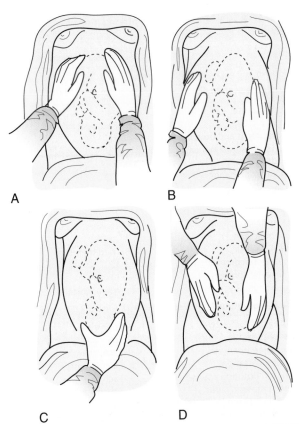

A   B

C   D

Figure 20-3 Leopold's maneuvers for determination of fetal position. **A,** First maneuver: palpation of the uterine fundus to identify the fetal part. **B,** Second maneuver: location of the fetal back. **C,** Third maneuver: cupped hands to determine the presenting part and station. **D,** Fourth maneuver: palpation of the cephalic prominence to determine the degree of flexion.

pubis to top of the fundus. The number of completed weeks of gestation should equal this measurement in centimeters (±2 cm). This measurement should be performed as accurately as possible. The most common reasons for inconsistency between menstrual age and fundal height is an inaccurate menstrual-age assignment and inaccurate measurements caused by maternal obesity. Larger-than-expected fundal height may also be caused by multiple gestation, uterine fibroids, polyhydramnios, or a large-for-gestational-age (LGA) fetus. Smaller-than-expected fundal height should warrant an exploration for etiologies such as oligohydramnios, FGR, and fetal demise.

By 30 weeks' gestation, the fetus is large enough that it can be palpated through the maternal abdomen. The position of the fetus should be documented at this and subsequent visits. This is easily done in most women by Leopold's maneuvers (Figure 20-3). The first maneuver involves palpation of the uterine fundus to identify the fetal part that is there. The palpating hands then glide downward laterally to perform the second maneuver, location of the fetal back. In the third maneuver, the hands are cupped around the presenting part at the level of the symphysis pubis to determine the presenting part as well as its degree of descent into the pelvis. If the presenting part is cephalic, the fourth maneuver will determine its degree of flexion. The examiner now turns 180 degrees to face the mother's legs, and the cephalic prominence is palpated. Another aid in ascertaining the position of the fetal back is the location of the fetal heart tones by Doppler sonography or auscultation. These sounds are best heard through the fetal back; in the left lower uterus in left occiput anterior, transverse, and posterior positions of the fetal head; and in the right lower uterus in right occiput positions. The evidence supporting the previous practices is variable but continues as the standard of care (Kirkham et al., 2005).

By the end of gestation, the practitioner as well as the woman should know the presentation of the fetus. This avoids emergent management when she presents in labor with a nonvertex presentation. Internal digital cervical examination can also verify presentation of the fetus and may be done when needed. Unless indicated, however, routine cervical examination to determine cervical readiness for labor need not be done until 41 weeks' gestation.

Prenatal Screening and Diagnostic Testing

Prenatal screening for fetal abnormalities should be offered to all pregnant women. If specific risk factors for fetal abnormalities are identified in the mother, appropriate counseling and specific diagnostic testing should be offered (CVS or amniocentesis). The most common reason to offer prenatal genetic diagnosis is advanced maternal age (maternal age at birth of 35 years or older); a somewhat linear increase in nondisjunction in meiosis increases the risk of a liveborn infant with aneuploidy (abnormal chromo-

Table 20-9   Second Trimester Quadruple-Screen Results

	Biochemical Results			
	α-Fetoprotein	Estriols	β-HCG	Inhibin A
Down syndrome	Decreased	Decreased	Increased	Increased
Trisomy 18	Decreased	Decreased	Decreased	No change to decreased
Open neural tube defect*	Increased	†	†	†

	Capabilities Statistics		
	Detection Sensitivity (%)	False-Positive Rate (%)	Positive Predictive Value (%)
Down syndrome	77-79	3-5	3.7
Trisomy 18	60	2-4	2.2
Open neural tube defect*	90	4.0	2.5

*Most sensitive at 16 to 18 weeks of gestation.
†Not used for neural tube defect screening.
hCG, Human chorionic gonadotropin.

some number), most commonly Down syndrome, as well as an increased risk of first trimester miscarriage or fetal abnormalities.

Low-risk women can be offered screening for genetic abnormalities of the fetus by biochemical testing in the first or second trimester and ultrasound nuchal translucency screening (first trimester) and targeted ultrasound evaluation of fetal anatomy, best done at 18 to 20 weeks' gestation. Traditionally, biochemical testing was used for screening. Measurement of certain chemicals found in the mother's blood is predictive of fetal abnormality. The quadruple screen is a maternal blood test in which one maternal sample drawn at 15 to 20 weeks (but most sensitive at 16 to 18 weeks) is assayed for AFP, estriols, and β subunit of human chorionic gonadotropin (hCG). Normal ranges vary for each gestational week. Maternal serum α-fetoprotein (MSAFP) elevations can result from open neural tube defects such as spina bifida or anencephaly, when the protein leaks from the fetal tissue into the amniotic fluid through the amniochorion and into the maternal system. A lower-than-expected MSAFP suggests Down syndrome. The addition of β subunit of hCG and estriols has improved sensitivity for the detection of chromosomal abnormalities (Table 20-9). This test should be offered to all pregnant women with appropriate counseling regarding sensitivity and specificity. Women with abnormal test results should be referred for targeted ultrasonography and possible amniocentesis.

First trimester ultrasound and biochemical screening are now available for clinical use in all women. Specifically, the "first trimester screen" is performed between 10 weeks, 2 days and 13 weeks, 6 days of gestation. Testing involves an ultrasound measurement of the nuchal translucency (lymphatic fluid at fetal neck) (Figure 20-4) and laboratory measurement of pregnancy-associated plasma protein A (PAPP-A) and β subunit of hCG. The first trimester screen has about 85% sensitivity for Down syndrome detection at a 4% false-positive rate. Several tests are also available that combine a first trimester screen with a second trimester screen for even higher sensitivity. Physicians should become familiar with the sensitivity, specificity, and availability of the test most suitable for their practices.

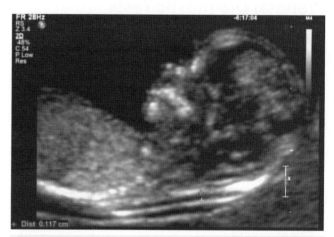

Figure 20-4 Transabdominal ultrasound assessment of nuchal translucency (NT). The measurement in this figure is normal. An increased measure (>3 mm) is associated with an increased risk of chromosomal abnormalities, complex congenital heart disease, and other genetic syndromes.

Newly developed cell-free fetal DNA (cffDNA) in maternal blood screening tests have improved the sensitivity of aneuploidy screening while having a very low false-positive rate (Chiu et al., 2011). For example, these tests detect Down syndrome with 99% sensitivity and trisomy 18 with 98% sensitivity. The basis of these tests, which can be performed any time after 10 weeks of gestation, is determination of the relative quantity of cffDNA fragments in the maternal blood, which are thought to be derived from placental cell apoptosis. The relative quantities of cell-free fragments form each chromosome can predict a trisomy or monosomy for a particular chromosome. Cell-free fetal DNA based screening is recommended for women with advanced maternal age, a history of aneuploidy, an abnormal finding on fetal ultrasonography, or an abnormal serum biochemical based screening test result. This testing modality is currently being studied for use in low-risk women and is expected to replace biochemical-based screening in the future.

Any abnormality in cffDNA in maternal blood testing should be confirmed by CVS or amniocentesis.

- First trimester screening between 10 weeks, 2 days and 13 weeks, 6 days of gestation using both nuchal translucency measurement and biochemical markers is an effective screening test for Down syndrome in the general population (SOR: A).
- Women found to have increased risk of aneuploidy with first trimester screening should be offered genetic counseling and the option of CVS or second trimester amniocentesis (SOR: A).
- Cell-free fetal DNA screening in maternal blood is a newly developed screening test with high sensitivity and low false positive rate which is currently available for high risk women. Any abnormality should be confirmed with more definitive testing, CVS, or amniocentesis (SOR: A) (Wilson et al., 2013).

Prenatal Diagnostic Tests

AMNIOCENTESIS

Genetic amniocentesis is typically performed at 15 to 20 weeks of gestation but can also be done any time after 20 menstrual weeks. After ultrasound examination of the fetus and placenta, an area of skin overlying a pocket of amniotic fluid is cleaned with iodine solution. With ultrasound guidance throughout the procedure, a 22-gauge spinal needle is used to remove 20 mL of amniotic fluid. Special care is taken to avoid the fetus, the umbilical cord, and the large placental vessels. In experienced hands, the pregnancy loss rate attributed to the procedure is about one in 300. The entire testing time for a chromosomal analysis is about 10 to 12 days. Alternately, the supernatant may be assayed for metabolites to diagnose other disorders that run in the family if identified on counseling. Earlier amniocentesis (at 11 to 13 weeks) has been successfully performed but is not recommended any longer because of the recent initial reports regarding a slightly higher rate of clubfoot in these newborns.

CHORIONIC VILLUS SAMPLING

In CVS, another technique for obtaining fetal tissue for genetic evaluation, the chorionic villi, or placental cells, are aspirated. With ultrasound guidance, CVS can be performed at 10 to 13 menstrual weeks transabdominally with a spinal needle or transvaginally with a catheter designed and approved for this purpose. Chromosomal analysis of the villous cells can be completed in 7 days. Thus, the advantage to CVS is the early gestational time of the procedure and availability of the results. The procedure-related fetal loss rate is approximately one in 125 tests (Jackson et al., 1992).

- Early amniocentesis performed before 14 completed weeks of gestation is not considered a safe alternative to second trimester amniocentesis or CVS (SOR: A).
- CVS should *not* be performed before 10 completed weeks of gestation (SOR: B).
- CVS should always be performed under direct ultrasound control (SOR: B).
- Third trimester amniocentesis does not appear to be associated with significant risk of complications leading to emergency delivery (SOR: B).

Drug and Chemical Exposures in Pregnancy

Pregnant women frequently ask about the effect of drug and other chemical exposures on the unborn infant, whether environmental, OTC, or prescription. Many of these are everyday exposures at the workplace, in the community, or as a result of medical treatment and management. The consequences can range from the most innocuous to actually jeopardizing the pregnancy. The physician should be prepared to answer these pregnancy-related questions and advise their patients appropriately.

The consequences of a chemical exposure may be related to the nature of the agent and the timing, dose, and duration of the exposure. The effect can range from minor morphologic abnormalities and growth deficiency to severe malformation and loss of the pregnancy. Thalidomide has obvious effects on the fetus, causing one third of fetuses to have limb reduction defects. Furthermore, the effect of a drug may be subtle or delayed (Welch et al., 1993). Diethylstilbestrol (DES) is associated with the development of uterine structural abnormalities and clear cell carcinoma of the vagina in daughters whose mothers took this medication.

Much of the knowledge about chemical exposures and effects on reproduction and fetal development comes from research on experimental animals. This poses great uncertainty given genetic variability and species-specific responses. Given these limitations, the health care provider must carefully weigh the evidence before using a drug. To help practitioners classify a drug for use, the U.S. FDA developed a risk factors index. The abbreviated definitions of these categories are as follows:

- **Category A:** Controlled studies in women fail to demonstrate a risk to the fetus.
- **Category B:** Animal reproduction studies have not demonstrated a fetal risk, but there are no controlled studies in pregnant women, or animal reproduction studies have shown adverse effect that was not confirmed in controlled human studies.
- **Category C:** Studies in animals have revealed adverse effects on the fetus, and there are no controlled studies in women. Drugs should be given only if the potential benefit justifies the potential risk to the fetus.
- **Category D:** There is positive evidence of human fetal risk, but the benefits from use in pregnant women may be acceptable.
- **Category X:** Studies in animals or humans have demonstrated fetal abnormalities, or there is evidence of fetal risk based on human experience. The drug is contraindicated in women who are or who may become pregnant.

Table 20-10 Drugs and Exposures in Pregnancy

Agent	Recommendation	Comments
Antihistamines	Acceptable	Most are category B
Decongestants	Acceptable	Pseudoephedrine preferred
Cough medication with guaifenesin	Acceptable	—
Acetaminophen	Acceptable	Preferred analgesic and antipyretic
Aspirin	Avoid	Increases risk of bleeding; no benefit in preeclampsia; may be prescribed in low doses for specific conditions
NSAIDs	Avoid	Premature closure of ductus arteriosus
Cephalosporins	Acceptable	—
Sulfonamides	Avoid in third trimester	Kernicterus in newborn
Tetracyclines	Avoid	Discoloration of teeth
ACE inhibitors	Avoid	Stillborn, renal abnormalities, renal failure in newborn
Immunizations	Avoid live, attenuated viruses	Measles, mumps, rubella
Allergy shots	Acceptable	Alteration in maintenance dose may be necessary

ACE, Angiotensin-converting enzyme; *NSAID,* nonsteroidal antiinflammatory drug.
Modified from Hueston WJ, Eolers GM, King DE, McGlaughlin VG. Common questions patients ask during pregnancy. *Am Fam Physician.* 1995;51: 1465-1470.

This classification is an oversimplification, and the individual practitioner will need to weigh the available data in the management of the pregnant woman. Few absolutes are possible in the field of human teratology; however, current recommendations for common drug categories in pregnancy are summarized in Table 20-10 (Briggs et al., 1994). It is important to emphasize that it is difficult to demonstrate an actual cause-and-effect relationship between a specific drug and an adverse pregnancy outcome. At no time, however, should a drug be considered safe because no data exist.

Infections in Pregnancy

Although a woman is subject to many of the same infections during pregnancy as when not pregnant, specific infectious diseases have implications on fetal development and complications of pregnancy, such as premature labor and premature rupture of membranes. Certain infections in pregnancy can be teratogenic to the fetus, particularly if infections occur in the first trimester. These agents have been given the acronym of TORCH for toxoplasmosis, other (e.g., syphilis), rubella, cytomegalovirus (CMV), and herpesvirus. Although not teratogenic, HIV may be transmitted to the fetus and may be lethal in the child.

TOXOPLASMOSIS

The causative agent of toxoplasmosis is *Toxoplasma gondii,* a parasite that usually infects rodents. Based on serologic studies, approximately one third of reproductive-age women have had toxoplasmosis. In the United States, maternal infection is thought to occur in about 0.5%. Congenital toxoplasmosis can only occur when active infection occurs during pregnancy. Recognizable damage to newborns is estimated to occur in about one in 10,000 births; the incidence of infected but asymptomatic newborns is unknown. Maternal infections that occur in the first trimester are more likely to cause abortion and significant fetal damage. Infections later in pregnancy tend to be asymptomatic at birth.

A pregnant woman can contract toxoplasmosis by eating raw meat containing the cysts of the organism or by fecal–oral transmission of the oocytes from an infected cat. Cats that are fed cooked or canned food are most often not infectious. Those that obtain rodents from the wild are more at risk. Pregnant women should avoid changing cat litter and handling cats, particularly cats allowed to roam outdoors. Maternal toxoplasmosis may be asymptomatic or may present as a mononucleosis-like syndrome. Congenital disease ranges from overwhelming, including seizures, microcephaly or hydrocephaly, chorioretinitis, hepatosplenomegaly, jaundice, microphthalmia, and cataracts, to less symptomatic, which usually involves chorioretinitis. Prenatal ultrasonography or postnatal brain scan can also show intracranial calcifications. The placenta should be examined pathologically for cysts of *T. gondii* (Beazley and Egerman, 1998).

The diagnosis of toxoplasmosis is serologic, looking for immunoglobulin G (IgG) and IgM by enzyme-linked immunosorbent assay (ELISA). Some assays have a high level of false-positive results. Laboratories well versed in performing these serologic tests should be used. Pyrimethamine and sulfadiazine can treat women who acquire the infection prenatally. Effectiveness of treatment protocols for prevention of congenital infection appears variable (Wallon et al., 1999). Screening of all pregnant women is not recommended at this time.

SYPHILIS

Syphilis is a treatable infection caused by *Treponema pallidum,* a motile spirochete. In pregnant women, infection is most often sexually transmitted. The infection is described in four stages: primary, secondary, latent, and tertiary or late. It is rare to see pregnant women with tertiary or late syphilis (Sheffield and Wendel, 1999).

Pregnancy has little effect on the course of syphilis, but syphilis has a substantial effect on pregnancy and the fetus. Stages with spirochetemia are the most deleterious for the fetus. This is most often seen in late primary syphilis and in secondary syphilis. An increase in miscarriage, hydrops fetalis, stillborn, and preterm delivery of an infected fetus can be seen. Penicillin is the only antibiotic currently recommended for syphilis treatment in pregnancy because of its safety, efficacy, and transplacental passage to treat the fetus (CDC, 1999). Penicillin-allergic women should undergo desensitization first. Whenever treatment adequacy is questioned in pregnancy, repeat therapy should occur because congenital syphilis is a preventable disorder. All women with syphilis should be carefully evaluated for other STDs, in particular HIV, because the treatment and surveillance is different in co-infection and the possibility of neurosyphilis must be carefully evaluated.

RUBELLA

Congenital rubella was first recognized in 1941, when after a rubella epidemic, a large number of children born to infected mothers were noted to have cataracts. Immunization against the rubella virus in the United States, Canada, and many European countries has decreased maternal rubella and thus congenital rubella. In the United States, only a few cases of congenital rubella are reported per year. Attention is now directed at its eradication in developing countries (Banatvala, 1998).

Although maternal infection can be subclinical, it usually presents 14 to 21 days after exposure with a maculopapular rash that begins on the face and spreads to the neck, trunk, arms, and legs. It is associated with lymphadenopathy, malaise, arthralgias, and petechiae. There is no therapy other than supportive. Pregnant women found not to have immunity to rubella should be instructed to avoid individuals who have viral illnesses. Suspected infection should be documented by specific rubella IgG and IgM measurement or by viral culture of the mother.

Maternal rubella acquired in the first trimester of pregnancy has a high risk of conferring damage to the developing fetus, and documented cases should be counseled and pregnancy interruption offered. In congenital rubella syndrome, many abnormalities can be found, such as cataracts, chorioretinitis, microphthalmia, congenital heart disease, myocarditis, microcephaly, deafness, mental retardation, and bone lesions, as well as signs of systemic infection (pneumonitis, hepatosplenomegaly, hepatitis, thrombocytopenia) (Stamos and Rowley, 1994).

CYTOMEGALOVIRUS

Two percent of pregnant women develop primary CMV infection, obtained by direct contact or respiratory aerosol from an infected individual. They are most often asymptomatic or have mild generalized symptoms such as fatigue, malaise, fever, lymphadenopathy, and pharyngitis. Approximately 50% of fetuses whose mothers seroconvert during pregnancy will develop CMV infection, but only 10% to 15% of these fetuses will have damage from the infection. Hearing loss is the most common manifestation.

Fetal infection and damage are more likely in the first and second trimesters. Although hearing loss is the most common presentation, congenital CMV can also present with microcephaly or hydrocephalus, microphthalmia, mental retardation, and brain calcifications. Overwhelming fetal infection at birth, known as cytomegalic inclusion disease, is uncommon, is most often caused by maternal primary infection late in gestation, and is often fatal.

Recurrent CMV infection in pregnancy can also cause infection of the fetus but rarely fetal damage (Stagno, 1982). Thus, documented immunity to CMV with serologic studies performed before a pregnancy can be reassuring to women at risk of exposure, such as child care providers or health care workers. General screening for CMV in pregnancy is not recommended at present. Suspected CMV infection should be documented by serology or cultures of the cervix, amniotic fluid, or maternal urine.

HERPESVIRUS

Herpes simplex virus type 2 (HSV-2) is the causative agent in most cases of genital herpes, with a few cases caused by HSV-1, which most often causes oropharyngeal herpes. Primary infection is most deleterious for both mother and fetus and can present as fever, malaise, inguinal lymphadenopathy, and urinary retention. At 2 to 10 days after exposure, vesicles containing numerous viral particles painfully erupt on the cervix, vagina, perineum, or rectum; ulcerate; and remain open for 1 to 3 weeks. Herpetic lesions in recurrent disease last a shorter period and are most often not associated with systemic symptoms.

Fetuses are most susceptible to herpesvirus infection and damage during viremia, which most often occurs in primary herpes. At that time, herpes-specific maternal IgG is not adequate for transplacental passage and protection of the fetus from serious disease. The fetus may also acquire a herpetic infection from delivery through an infected vaginal canal. If this occurs during a primary episode, the risk of congenital infection is about 50%; if during a recurrent infection, the risk is less than 8%. Congenital herpes may be localized to skin, eyes, and oral cavity and may involve the central nervous system (CNS). Congenital infection may be disseminated and is often fatal or entirely asymptomatic (Riley, 1998).

Various surveillance protocols have been attempted to decrease perinatal transmission at delivery. At present, at labor and delivery, a careful evaluation of the genital tract for ulcers is performed. If any active lesions are found, the baby is delivered by cesarean section (Roberts et al., 1995). Prenatal use of acyclovir is controversial, but it has been used with informed consent in pregnant women with systemic disease or frequent episodes of recurrent disease.

HUMAN IMMUNODEFICIENCY VIRUS

Human immunodeficiency virus is a retrovirus transmitted through infected secretions, most often sexually. The most serious consequence of HIV infection in pregnancy is transmission to the fetus, resulting in the birth of an HIV-congenitally infected newborn. Maternal HIV is not teratogenic or associated with increased fetal loss (except end-stage disease). The goal in pregnancy is identification of HIV disease and prevention of perinatal transmission. At-risk women include those with hemophilia, IV drug users, prostitutes, and female partners of infected men. Although most often seen in urban areas, HIV infection in women is rising throughout the United States.

Screening for HIV is recommended and should be offered to all pregnant women. At-risk women should be screened more than once during the pregnancy. Testing for IgG antibody with ELISA is the basis of screening for an HIV infection. Western blot or another, more specific test confirms all positive test results. If a pregnant woman is found to have HIV infection, specific counseling should be given, which is often best done in a center familiar with treatment and management. Specific therapy should be instituted to prevent perinatal transmission.

Zidovudine administration in HIV-infected pregnant women from 14 to 34 weeks' gestation decreased perinatal HIV transmission from 25.5% to 8.3% (Connor et al., 1994). Presently, highly active retroviral therapy (HART) or combination anti-retroviral therapy, which includes zidovudine, is recommended for HIV-infected pregnant women. HIV-infected pregnant women should be referred for consultation to a center with experience in management of HIV in pregnancy. In the intrapartum period, women who have any detectable viral load should receive at least 4 hours of IV zidovudine before delivery, specifically 2 mg/kg body weight IV over 1 hour, then 1 mg/kg/hr until delivery. IV zidovudine is no longer required for HIV-infected women receiving combination antiretroviral regimens who have an HIV viral load of less than 400 copies/mL.

Zidovudine is given to newborns (2 mg/kg orally every 6 hours for 6 weeks). This therapeutic regimen is currently used in pregnancy. However, combination therapy, including reverse-transcriptase inhibitors, is recommended by some experts (Rose, 1998).

Pregnant women on zidovudine therapy must be followed for bone marrow suppression and liver toxicity on a monthly basis. Although long-term studies are not available, the drug appears safe for the fetus. The quantity of viral load (HIV-1 RNA) in the mother appears to be a significant risk factor to fetal infection (Mofenson et al., 1999). The mode of delivery is controversial, with many experts recommending cesarean section to those women with high viral load. During vaginal delivery, artificial rupture of membranes and placement of a scalp electrode onto the fetal head are contraindicated. Amniocentesis and breastfeeding are also contraindicated in HIV-infected women.

EVIDENCE-BASED SUMMARY

• Pregnant women should be offered screening for HIV infection early in pregnancy because appropriate antenatal interventions can reduce maternal-to-child transmission (SOR: A).
• Women diagnosed as HIV positive during pregnancy should be informed that interventions such as antiretroviral therapy, cesarean section, and avoidance of breastfeeding can reduce the risk of mother-to child HIV transmission (SOR: A).
• Amniocentesis and breastfeeding are contraindicated in HIV-infected pregnant patients (SOR: A).

IINFLUENZA AND NOVEL INFLUENZA A (H1N1) VIRUS

The influenza virus poses a particular threat to the pregnant patient. The majority of pregnant women with novel influenza A (H1N1) or the regular seasonal influenza virus infection present with typical acute upper respiratory, influenza-like illness (e.g., cough, sore throat, rhinorrhea), and fever. Other symptoms can include body aches, headache, fatigue, vomiting, and diarrhea. Most pregnant women have an uncomplicated disease course. However, pregnant women appear to be at higher risk for severe complications from influenza infection, and for some, illness might progress rapidly and be complicated by secondary bacterial infections, including pneumonia and evidence of fetal distress. Case reports of adverse pregnancy outcomes and maternal deaths have been associated with severe illness and death. Ideally, pregnant women who have suspected novel influenza A (H1N1) virus infection should be tested for influenza, although commercially available rapid-testing kits have limited sensitivity.

Treatment should not be delayed pending results of testing or withheld in the absence of testing. Antiviral treatment is most effective when started as early as possible after the onset of symptoms (i.e., within first 2 days). The highest priority is to treat pregnant women with influenza-like symptoms as soon as possible. The currently novel influenza A (H1N1) virus is sensitive to the neuraminidase inhibitor antiviral medications zanamivir (Relenza) and oseltamivir (Tamiflu). Pregnancy should not be considered a contraindication to oseltamivir or zanamivir use. Because pregnant women may be at higher risk, the benefits of treatment or chemoprophylaxis with oseltamivir or zanamivir outweigh the theoretic risks of antiviral use. The Advisory Committee on Immunization Practices recommends that H1N1 monovalent flu and the seasonal flu vaccine be given to all pregnant women at any time during pregnancy. The ACOG and AAFP also recommend routine vaccination of all pregnant women. The nasal spray vaccine is not approved for use by pregnant women. Pregnant women should not receive nasal spray vaccine for either seasonal flu or H1N1 flu.

KEY TREATMENT

• Pregnant women with confirmed, probable, or suspected novel influenza A (H1N1) infection should receive antiviral therapy with oseltamivir (Tamiflu) (CDC, 2009) (SOR: C).

IMMUNIZATIONS IN PREGNANCY

Tetanus, Diphtheria, and Pertussis (Tdap) and Tetanus and Diphtheria (Td)

Health-care personnel should administer a dose of Tdap during each pregnancy irrespective of the patient's prior history of receiving Tdap (CDC, 2013). To maximize the maternal antibody response and passive antibody transfer to the infant, optimal timing for Tdap administration is between 27 and 36 weeks of gestation, although Tdap may be given at any time during pregnancy.

The risk to a developing fetus from vaccination of the mother during pregnancy is theoretical. Immunizations that are not live, attenuated virus are not contraindicated in pregnancy. No evidence exists of risk to the fetus from vaccinating pregnant women with inactivated virus or bacterial vaccines or toxoids. Live vaccines administered to a pregnant woman pose a theoretical risk to the fetus; therefore, live, attenuated virus and live bacterial vaccines generally are contraindicated during pregnancy. The measles, mumps, and rubella (MMR) are the most common vaccines with live attenuated viruses and should be

Table 20-11   General Recommendation for Use of Vaccines in Pregnant Women

Vaccine	Recommendation	Comments
Hepatitis A	Recommended if otherwise indicated	Recommended if another high-risk condition or other indication is present.
Hepatitis B	Recommended if otherwise indicated	Available vaccines contain noninfectious HBsAg and should cause no risk of infection to the fetus.
Human papillomavirus	Not recommended	If a woman is found to be pregnant after initiating the vaccination series, the remainder of the three-dose series should be delayed until completion of pregnancy.
Influenza (inactivated)	Recommended	Routine influenza vaccination is recommended for all women who are or will be pregnant (in any trimester) during influenza season.
Influenza (LAIV)	Contraindicated	
MCV4 (MenACWY)	May be used if otherwise indicated	
MMR	Contraindicated	Women should be counseled to avoid becoming pregnant for 28 days after vaccination with measles or mumps vaccines or MMR or other rubella-containing vaccines.
PCV13	Inadequate data for recommendation	ACIP has not published pregnancy recommendations for PCV13 at this time.
Polio	May be used if needed	
PPSV23	Inadequate data for recommendation	
Rabies	May be used if otherwise indicated	
Td	Should be used if otherwise indicated	
Tdap	Recommended	Administer a dose of Tdap during each pregnancy irrespective of the patient's history of receiving Tdap.
Varicella	Contraindicated	Nonpregnant women who are vaccinated should avoid becoming pregnant for 1 month after each injection.
Zoster	Contraindicated	Women should avoid becoming pregnant for 4 weeks after zoster vaccination. If a pregnant woman is vaccinated or becomes pregnant within 1 month of vaccination, she should be counseled about potential effects on the fetus.

ACIP, Advisory Committee on Immunization Practices; *MCV4*, meningococcal conjugate vaccine; *MMR*, measles, mumps, and rubella; *PCV13*, pneumococcal conjugate vaccine; *PPSV23*, pneumococcal polysaccharide vaccine; *Td*, tetanus and diphtheria, and pertussis; *Tdap*, tetanus, diphtheria, and pertussis.
Adapted from Centers for Disease Control and Prevention. General Recommendation on immunization: recommendations of the Advisory Committee on Immunization Practices (ACIP). *MMWR.* 2011;60(2):26.

avoided during pregnancy, although assessment of risks to the fetus has not been documented as a significant risk. The benefits of vaccinating pregnant women usually outweigh the potential risks when the likelihood of disease exposure is high, when infection would pose a risk to the mother or fetus, and when the vaccine is unlikely to cause harm (CDC, 2011). A clear example of the benefits of vaccination is the new recommendations to administer a dose of Tdap during each pregnancy, irrespective of the patient's immunization history. Optimally administered between 27 weeks and 36 weeks, this is done to minimize the significant burden of pertussis disease in the vulnerable newborn (CDC, 2011). Please see Table 20-11 for a more complete list.

Medical Disorders in Pregnancy

Many medical disorders can be seen in pregnant women; few are incompatible with pregnancy. In the management and care of a pregnant woman with a medical illness, it is important to understand the normal physiology of pregnancy and the effect of the disorder on the pregnancy and vice versa. Common medical problems in pregnancy include anemia, asthma, hypertension, diabetes, and pyelonephritis. Women with moderate to severe preexisting medical illness should be referred for evaluation to a physician experienced in managing the disorder in pregnancy.

VENOUS THROMBOEMBOLISM

Venous thromboembolism (VTE) is the leading cause of maternal death in the United States. Pregnancy increases the risk of VTE four to fivefold over that of the nonpregnant state. The risk is further increased if there is a personal or family history of thrombosis or thrombophilia. The two manifestations of VTE are deep vein thrombosis (DVT) and pulmonary embolus (PE). Although most reports suggest that VTE can occur at any trimester in pregnancy, some studies suggest that VTE is more common during the first half of pregnancy. The sequelae of DVT and PE include complications such as pulmonary hypertension, postthrombotic syndrome, and venous insufficiency. Studies in this area suggest that the anatomic distribution of DVT in pregnant women differs from that for nonpregnant patients. Left-sided DVT is more common in pregnancy, and furthermore, it appears that proximal DVT is restricted to the femoral or iliac veins, where they are more likely to embolize and are also more common (Chan, 2010). This can occur without involvement of the calf vasculature.

The symptoms of DVT are nonspecific as in the nonpregnancy state and can include unilateral leg pain and swelling. The Homan sign (unilateral pain with dorsiflexion) is neither sensitive nor specific in the diagnosis of this disorder. PE disease more often presents in the postpartum period and after a cesarean section. The signs and symptoms of a PE are equally nonspecific and include shortness of breath, chest pain, and even cardiopulmonary collapse. Both disorders require a high level of suspicion on the part of the clinician.

Diagnostic testing can be equally challenging in the pregnancy state. D-Dimer testing, which is routinely used in the clinic setting for risk stratification, progressively increases during pregnancy, and there are no universally accepted values for pregnancy. However, a low D-dimer with a low clinical suspicion has a high negative predictive value. The current initial test of choice in the evaluation of VTE is compression ultrasonography (CUS) of the lower extremity veins. However, if the CUS study is equivocal, if Doppler testing results are abnormal, or if suspicion of pelvic DVT is high, further evaluation with magnetic resonance imaging (MRI) is recommended. MRI has been shown to have 97% sensitivity and 95% specificity for pelvic DVT in nonpregnant patients. The spiral computed tomography pulmonary angiography (CT-PA) is the recommended study for the evaluation of PE in pregnancy, particularly in the presence of known pulmonary disease or abnormal chest radiography findings (Michiels, 2000). In a pregnant patient with no known pulmonary disease and normal chest radiograph findings, ventilation/perfusion (V/Q) scanning is an acceptable alternative if a spiral CT is not available.

Anticoagulation at a therapeutic dose is indicated when either DVT or PE is diagnosed. Anticoagulation options include low-molecular-weight heparins (LMWHs), unfractionated heparin (UFH), and warfarin. Warfarin is a known teratogen and its use should be restricted to the postpartum period. Warfarin is safe during breastfeeding. LMWHs have replaced UFH as the first-choice medications for VTE treatment and prophylaxis in pregnancy. Compared with UFH, LMWHs have lower rates of adverse effects, including heparin-induced thrombocytopenia, symptomatic osteoporosis, bleeding, and allergic reactions.

ANEMIA

Iron-deficiency anemia during pregnancy has been associated with an increased risk of LBW, preterm delivery, and perinatal death. Normal physiologic changes in intravascular volume cause a physiologic anemia of pregnancy. However, severe anemia with maternal hemoglobin (Hb) levels less than 6 g/dL has been associated with abnormal fetal oxygenation, resulting in nonreassuring fetal heart rate (FHR) pattern, reduced amniotic fluid volume, fetal cerebral vasodilatation, and fetal death. In normal singleton pregnancy, blood volume increases approximately 36%, plasma volume 47%, and red blood cell (RBC) mass 17%, causing a relative hemodilution throughout pregnancy, but most pronounced after 28 weeks' gestation. Thus, Hb, hematocrit (Hct), and RBC count will be lower than normal, but RBC indices, specifically the mean corpuscular volume (MCV), mean corpuscular hemoglobin (MCH), and mean corpuscular hemoglobin concentration (MCHC), remain normal. Iron, iron-binding capacity, and ferritin remain unchanged. Hb less than 15 mg/dL and Hct less than 33% are generally considered nonphysiologic anemia in pregnancy.

The most common nonphysiologic anemia encountered in pregnancy is iron deficiency. *Iron-deficiency anemia* is suspected when the RBC indices are low and there are microcytic, hypochromic RBCs on the peripheral blood smear. This anemia is confirmed by a low serum iron concentration, high total iron binding capacity, and low ferritin. Risk factors for iron-deficiency anemia in otherwise healthy women include poor nutrition, menstrual loss, and short interconceptual period. Reproductive-age women have low-normal to abnormal iron stores for this reason. Iron requirements in pregnancy put an increased demand on maternal iron stores because iron is actively transported across the placenta to the fetus regardless of maternal stores. Iron supplementation decreases the prevalence of maternal anemia at delivery, and without iron supplementation in pregnancy, many women will become iron deficient. The recommendation is 30 mg of elemental iron in the form of simple salts such as ferrous sulfate, gluconate, or fumarate. Iron-deficiency anemia should be treated with 60 to 120 mg of elemental iron in two or three divided doses daily, which can cause gastric irritation and constipation. More frequent administration has not been shown to improve absorption. Because iron demands in pregnancy are highest after 20 weeks' gestation, depending on the degree of anemia, full-dose iron therapy can be delayed until that time, when pregnancy-associated nausea and vomiting should have subsided. Dietary modifications or stool softeners may be required when pregnant women take large doses of iron.

The failure to respond to appropriate iron therapy should prompt further investigation and may suggest an incorrect diagnosis, coexisting disease, malabsorption (sometimes caused by enteric-coated tablets or concomitant antacids), patient noncompliance, or ongoing blood loss. Hypochromic, microcytic RBCs with an MCV of less than 80 femtoliters suggest thalassemia. Hemoglobin electrophoresis should also be performed when evaluating hypochromic, microcytic anemia. Iron-deficiency anemia and β-thalassemia can coexist. Megaloblastic anemia from folic acid deficiency is unlikely in the pregnant woman because many reproductive-age women take at least 400 μg of folic acid daily. Any other anemia may occur in pregnancy. Its diagnosis and therapy should be prompt to ensure a healthy outcome for the fetus. Hereditary anemias have the additional implication of possible inheritance by the fetus that should be addressed with the pregnant woman.

EVIDENCE-BASED SUMMARY

- Iron supplementation decreases the prevalence of maternal anemia at delivery (SOR: A).
- Iron-deficiency anemia during pregnancy has been associated with an increased risk of LBW, preterm delivery, and perinatal mortality (SOR: B).
- Severe anemia with maternal hemoglobin levels less than 6 g/dL has been associated with abnormal fetal oxygenation; thus, maternal transfusion should be considered for fetal indications (SOR: B).

ASTHMA

Asthma is caused by reversible airway obstruction from bronchial smooth muscle contraction, excessive secretions, and edema in response to various stimuli, most often

Table 20-12   Pulmonary Function Changes in Pregnancy

Parameter	Nonpregnant Value	Pregnant Value
Tidal volume (V_T) (amount of air moved in one respiratory cycle)	450 mL	600 mL
Respiratory rate (breaths/min)	16-18	Same
Minute ventilation (volume of air moved/min)	7.2 L	9.6 L
Forced expiratory volume in 1 second (FEV_1)	80%-85% of VC	Same
Peak expiratory flow rate (PEFR)	380-550 L/min	Same
Forced vital capacity (FVC) (largest amount of air that can by exhaled after maximum filling of lungs)	3.5 L	Same
Residual volume (RV) (amount of air left in lungs after maximum expiration)	1000 mL	800 mL

Modified from Cugell DW, Frank NR, Gaensler EA, Badger TL. Pulmonary function in pregnancy. I. Serial observations in normal women. *Am Rev Tuberc*, 1953;67:568.

Table 20-13   Normal Arterial Blood Gas Values in Pregnancy

	pH	PCO_2 (mm Hg)	PO_2 (mm Hg)
Normal	7.40	35-40	75-100
Pregnancy	7.45	27-32	90-108

Table 20-14   Classification of Hypertensive Disorders in Pregnancy

Chronic hypertension
Preeclampsia or eclampsia
Preeclampsia superimposed on chronic hypertension
Gestational hypertension
   Transient hypertension of pregnancy if preeclampsia is not present at delivery and blood pressure returns to normal by 12 weeks postpartum
   Chronic hypertension if the elevation persists

infectious or allergic. Airway obstruction is most severe in expiration, making breathing difficult and fatiguing. Asthma is a chronic illness with acute exacerbations.

Approximately 4% of pregnant women will have asthma with severity varying from mild to life threatening. One third of pregnant patients with asthma will experience exacerbations of their disease (Stenius-Aarnaila et al., 1988). Women with severe asthma are more likely to have disease exacerbation while pregnant. Additionally, moderate to severe asthma can have a significant effect on pregnancy, including an increase in preterm labor, LBW, perinatal death, and preeclampsia.

In normal pregnancy, progesterone causes an increase in tidal volume and thus minute ventilation to make more oxygen available for the fetus (Table 20-12). These changes result in a mild respiratory alkalosis that should be taken into account when interpreting blood gas values (Table 20-13).

Evaluation and management of acute asthma should include objective assessment of maternal lung function and fetal well-being, avoidance or control of environmental precipitating factors, pharmacologic therapy, and patient education (Clark, 1993). The best respiratory parameter to measure for assessment of the degree of obstruction in asthmatic patients is forced expiratory volume in 1 second (FEV_1) (see Table 20-12). This requires formal pulmonary function testing, so it is not a practical tool for monitoring. However, this value can be estimated by measuring the peak expiratory flow rate (PEFR) using an inexpensive portable peak-flow meter. Women with moderate to severe asthma should monitor their PEFR several times daily while pregnant. Normal PEFR for pregnant as well as nonpregnant women is 380 to 550 L/min. PEFR can be used to diagnose an exacerbation early, as well as for evaluation of therapy.

Pharmacologic therapy in pregnant patients with asthma is similar to that in nonpregnant women. The main goal of therapy is to maintain adequate oxygenation for the mother and fetus. The arterial oxygen partial pressure (PaO_2) should be kept above 60 mm Hg and oxygen saturation (SO_2) at least 95%. In acute exacerbations during pregnancy, the clinician should have a lower threshold for hospital admission and intubation. Women in the late second trimester and the third trimester should also have fetal monitoring.

Ultrasonography to detect FGR of the fetus in patients with moderate to severe asthma is warranted. If FGR is diagnosed, antenatal testing should be performed. During labor and delivery, the F-series prostaglandins (PGs), in particular prostaglandin $F_2\alpha$ (Hemabate), should be avoided because they stimulate bronchial smooth muscle to constrict. Instead, PGE_2 (Prostin E_2), which causes bronchodilation, should be used.

CHRONIC HYPERTENSION

Historically, there have been many classifications of hypertension in pregnancy with no apparent consensus. In this chapter, we use the now-accepted classification as developed by the National Institutes of Health (Report of the National High Blood Pressure Education Program Working Group on High Blood Pressure in Pregnancy). Hypertension during pregnancy is categorized as (1) preeclampsia or eclampsia, (2) gestational hypertension, (3) chronic hypertension, or (4) preeclampsia superimposed on chronic hypertension (Table 20-14). These categories identify different disorders that at times overlap but with different epidemiologic characteristics, pathophysiology, and risks for the mother and baby. Pregnancy-induced hypertensive disorder is an older, less specific term no longer in general use.

Preexisting hypertension often complicates pregnancy. A diagnosis of chronic hypertension is made when hypertension precedes pregnancy or is diagnosed before 20 weeks of gestation. In normal pregnancy, arterial BP and peripheral vascular resistance (PVR) decrease shortly after implantation of the conception. Normal first trimester and early second trimester BP ranges from 92 to 114 mm Hg systolic, 46 to 66 mm Hg diastolic sitting, 103 to 123 mm Hg systolic, 47 to 67 mm Hg diastolic supine. At 28 to 30 weeks' gestation, BP in normal pregnant women increases to near prepregnancy range. It is generally accepted that BP greater than 130/80 mm Hg at any time during pregnancy is abnormal.

Fetal effects of chronic or essential hypertension depend on severity of hypertension and range from none to FGR, fetal distress, abruptio placentae, prematurity, and fetal death (Haddad and Sibai, 1999). Women with preexisting hypertension have approximately a 20% chance of developing superimposed preeclampsia. The maternal and fetal morbidity and mortality rates are higher in chronic hypertension with superimposed preeclampsia than in each disorder alone.

Most women with chronic hypertension present at their first prenatal visit with the diagnosis. As many as one third of pregnant women with essential hypertension become normotensive in the first half of pregnancy. Often, their antihypertensive medications can be discontinued and only restarted when elevations recur, typically after 28 weeks. Controversy exists as to whether medical treatment of essential hypertension in pregnancy improves fetal outcome or decreases the risk of superimposed preeclampsia. However, maternal complications can occur when diastolic BP is persistently elevated. Thus, it is generally accepted that therapy to decrease maternal BP be instituted or modified to keep maternal diastolic BP lower than 100 to 105 mm Hg. A profound drop in maternal BP over a short period should be avoided to prevent decreased cardiac output to the placenta and fetus.

α-Methyldopa (Aldomet), a central-acting, α-adrenergic, false neurotransmitter, and labetalol, an α- and β-blocker, are the two most commonly used drugs for treatment of chronic hypertension in pregnancy. The initial starting dose for methyldopa is 250 mg every 8 hours. This dose can be increased to 2 g/day if needed. The initial starting dose of labetalol is 200 mg orally, twice a day, for a maximum 800 mg three times a day.

If adequate control cannot be obtained, a second drug, most often nifedipine or hydralazine, can be added. ACE inhibitors and diuretics for BP control are contraindicated in pregnancy (Witlin and Sibai, 1998).

Obstetric management includes baseline laboratory studies early in pregnancy that will later help in diagnosis of superimposed preeclampsia. Specifically, in addition to routine prenatal testing, this includes renal function studies, liver enzymes, platelets, uric acid, and 24-hour urine test for protein and creatinine clearance. If chronic hypertension is a new diagnosis, pheochromocytoma should be ruled out by catecholamine levels in serum or 24-hour urine (Keely, 1998). Early ultrasonography to confirm dating and intermittently to evaluate fetal growth will aid in the diagnosis of FGR. Women with moderate to severe hypertension benefit from more frequent prenatal visits as well as home BP monitoring. Antenatal testing should be performed at least for women with superimposed preeclampsia or FGR. Preterm delivery may occur.

KEY TREATMENT

- Monotherapy with α-methyldopa (Aldomet), a central-acting α-adrenergic, false neurotransmitter, or labetalol, an α- and β-blocking agent, is the treatment of choice of chronic hypertension in pregnancy (SOR: C).

GESTATIONAL DIABETES

Gestational diabetes, or diabetes diagnosed in pregnancy, affects 3% to 5% of pregnant women. Pregnancy is a state of increasing insulin resistance predominantly caused by placentally produced hormones, in particular human placental lactogen, which increases with placental mass and gestational age. Although most women can compensate, a small subset of pregnant women cannot. Early impairment of glucose metabolism may have no maternal signs or symptoms but can have fetal effects that include macrosomia, fetal distress, and fetal demise.

Screening for GDM by a glucose challenge is recommended at 26 to 28 weeks of gestation. There is little evidence supporting earlier screening. The USPSTF recommends screening for gestational diabetes mellitus (GDM) in asymptomatic pregnant women after 24 weeks of gestation (B recommendation). The USPSTF concludes that the current evidence is insufficient to assess the balance of benefits and harms of screening for GDM in asymptomatic pregnant women before 24 weeks of gestation (I statement). Discussions should include information about the uncertainty of benefits and harms as well as the frequency of positive screening test results. Women who are obese, older than 25 years of age, have a family history of type 2 diabetes or GDM, or are members of certain ethnic groups (i.e., Hispanics, Native Americans, Asians, and African Americans) are at increased risk for GDM.

The initial screening test is performed in a nonfasting state. The pregnant woman is asked to drink a mixture containing 50 g of glucose; 1 hour later, a plasma glucose level is performed. If the result is 140 mg/dL or greater, the more definitive 100-g 3-hour glucose challenge is performed. The pregnant woman should have at least 3 days of adequate carbohydrate intake, fast the night before the test, and receive 100 g of glucose. Venous blood glucose is determined fasting and at 1, 2, and 3 hours after the glucose challenge. Two abnormal values make the diagnosis of GDM (Table 20-15). Different studies have various thresholds for making the diagnosis, and clinicians should review their institutional norms (Carpenter and Coustan, 1982) (Table 20-16). Women at high risk for GDM, such as those with glucosuria, prior GDM, obesity, or a strong family history, should be screened earlier in pregnancy. If the test result is negative, testing should be repeated in the latter half of pregnancy. The evidence supporting this practice is variable.

Table 20-15 Screening for Gestational Diabetes*

Test	Abnormal Glucose Level (mg/dL)
50-g glucose, 1-hr challenge	≥140
100-g glucose, 3-hr challenge*	
Fasting	≥105
1 hour	≥190
2 hour	≥165
3 hour	≥145

*Two abnormal values needed for diagnosis of gestational diabetes. From National Diabetes Data Group. Classification and diagnosis of diabetes mellitus and other categories of glucose intolerance. *Diabetes.* 1979;28: 1039-1057.

Table 20-16   Diagnosis of Gestational Diabetes Mellitus

OGTT	NDDG*	Carpenter[†]
Fasting	105	95
1 hour	190	180
2 hour	165	155
3 hour	145	140

*National Diabetes Data Group. Classification and diagnosis of diabetes mellitus and other categories of glucose intolerance. *Diabetes*. 1979;28: 1039-1057.

[†]Carpenter MW, Coustan DR. Criteria for screening tests for gestational diabetes. *Am J Obstet Gynecol*. 1982;144:768-773.

Initial therapies of GDM are diet and, if not contraindicated in the pregnancy, exercise in the form of walking, as well as support from diabetes educators and nutritionists and increased surveillance in prenatal care. The daily recommendation is 30 to 35 kcal/kg lean body weight. If fasting blood sugar cannot be maintained below 105 and 2-hour postprandial blood sugars below 120 mg/dL, insulin therapy is begun. Hemoglobin A_{1c} can be performed every 4 to 6 weeks but will not be elevated unless there is fasting hyperglycemia. At least weekly, evaluation of blood sugar is recommended because insulin resistance increases with advancing gestation. Ultrasonography to assess fetal size should be performed every 4 to 6 weeks. Women requiring insulin should have antenatal testing in the third trimester. Good blood sugar control is also important to decrease the incidence of metabolic newborn complications such as hypoglycemia, hypocalcemia, polycythemia, and hyperbilirubinemia.

The family physician should remember that women who have had GDM have a 30% to 60% chance of developing type 2 diabetes mellitus in their lifetimes (O'Sullivan, 1979). Postpartum and yearly glucose tolerance testing is recommended in these women. Weight loss and exercise have been shown to decrease their risk.

EVIDENCE-BASED SUMMARY

- The USPSTF recommends screening for gestational diabetes mellitus (GDM) in asymptomatic pregnant women after 24 weeks of gestation (SOR: B).
- The USPSTF concludes that the current evidence is insufficient to assess the balance of benefits and harms of screening for GDM in asymptomatic pregnant women before 24 weeks of gestation (I statement).

PYELONEPHRITIS

Asymptomatic bacteriuria can be found in 3% to 5% of pregnant women and up to 10% of those with sickle cell trait. Asymptomatic bacteriuria is most often caused by *Escherichia coli*. Antibiotic therapy is similar to that in the nonpregnant state. Cephalosporins, ampicillin, and nitrofurantoin (Macrodantin) are frequently used medications that are safe in pregnancy. It appears best to treat asymptomatic bacteriuria in pregnancy for 5 to 7 days. If they are untreated, 30% of women with asymptomatic bacteriuria will progress to pyelonephritis. Hormonal and anatomic changes of pregnancy causing hydronephrosis and

hydroureter are responsible for the higher incidence of pyelonephritis in the pregnant woman. A urinary pathogen count of at least 100,000 colonies/mL is considered significant, although pyelonephritis also occurs at counts as low as 20,000 to 50,000 colonies/mL (Cunningham and Lucas, 1994). Periodic cultures for screening should be performed in women with sickle cell trait, recurrent urinary tract infection, recurrent asymptomatic bacteriuria, or urine dipstick suggesting bacterial growth (e.g., positive nitrite).

Pyelonephritis in pregnancy requires hospitalization because of frequently associated dehydration, nausea, vomiting, and premature labor, as well as the uncommon but serious risk of endotoxic shock and endotoxin damage of alveolocapillary membranes leading to pulmonary edema and a clinical picture of adult respiratory distress syndrome (Gurman et al., 1990). Pregnant women with pyelonephritis require hospitalization for aggressive hydration and parenteral antibiotics. Antibiotic treatment is similar to those of other adult regimens. IV antibiotic therapy with a cephalosporin or an extended-spectrum penicillin until symptoms improve and the fever has completely resolved is usually sufficient for initial therapy. Because 25% of patients with mild acute pyelonephritis who are pregnant have a recurrence, these patients should have monthly urine cultures or antimicrobial suppression with oral nitrofurantoin (Macrodantin), 100 mg/day, until 4 to 6 weeks postpartum. Fluoroquinolones should be avoided because of concerns about their teratogenic effects on the fetus. Oral antibiotics are then prescribed for 7 to 10 additional days. For seriously ill women, the addition of an aminoglycoside at the onset of therapy may be warranted until sensitivities of the offending organism are available. Renal function as well as peak and trough aminoglycoside levels should be followed.

Complications of Early Pregnancy

ECTOPIC PREGNANCY

An ectopic pregnancy occurs when the fertilized ovum implants on any tissue other than the endometrial lining of the uterus. Overall, 95% of all ectopic pregnancies are tubal, 1.5% abdominal, 0.5% ovarian, and 0.03% cervical (Breen, 1970). A *heterotopic pregnancy* is a coexisting intrauterine and extrauterine pregnancy. Historically, there is an increasing incidence reported in the literature to a current rate of about one in 4000 pregnancies. This increased rate is thought to be associated with the use of ovarian stimulation and with assisted reproductive technologies. Ectopic pregnancies are responsible for more than 10% of all maternal deaths in the United States (Koonin et al., 1997).

The rate of ectopic pregnancy in women with known history of pelvic inflammatory disease (PID) is six to 10 times higher than in women with no history of PID. PID usually results from invasion by either gonorrhea or Chlamydia from the cervix into the uterus and tubes. The infection in these tissues causes an intense inflammatory reaction. Bacteria, white blood cells, and other fluids fill the tubes as the body combats the infection. During the healing process, however, the delicate tubal mucosa is permanently scarred. The fimbriated end of the fallopian tube as well as the lumen may become partially or completely blocked with scar tissue. If PID is treated very early and aggressively with IV antibiotics, the tubal damage might be minimized and fertility preserved. Other conditions associated with ectopic pregnancies include progestin-bearing intrauterine devices (IUDs), previous tubal surgery, and tubal ligation.

Diagnosis

A common clinical presentation of a woman with an ectopic pregnancy is the classic triad of amenorrhea, abdominal pain, and irregular vaginal bleeding. All women with these symptoms should be evaluated for possible ectopic gestation.

Serum quantitative hCG is often used to help identify those women with ectopic pregnancies. An isolated hCG level is not of much use unless it is above the threshold where one should visualize an intrauterine pregnancy with ultrasound. This threshold may vary depending on type of hCG assay used and the sonographic technique (Peisner and Timor-Tritsch, 1990). Two hCG levels drawn 48 hours apart are more informative. The general rule is a doubling of values in 48 hours. However, one must be careful to give pregnancies with a slow hCG rise every chance possible because they may turn out to be normal. A plateauing of hCG is consistent with an ectopic gestation or abnormal intrauterine pregnancy; ultrasonography can be used to differentiate the two.

Serum progesterone levels are of some value in making the diagnosis of ectopic pregnancy (Stovall et al., 1989). A progesterone level less than 15 ng/mL is seen in 81% of ectopic, 93% of abnormal intrauterine, and 11% of normal intrauterine pregnancies. Fewer than 2% of ectopic pregnancies and fewer than about 4% of abnormal intrauterine pregnancies will have progesterone levels of 25 ng/mL or greater. Therefore, a single progesterone value less than 15 ng/mL is probably an abnormal pregnancy and should prompt further evaluation. A single value greater than 25 ng/mL probably indicates a normal pregnancy.

Ultrasound

> **Key Point**
>
> ■ Routine screening ultrasonography in low-risk pregnancies is not associated with a decrease in perinatal death, birth weight, or preterm birth (Bernard et al., 1993).

With high-resolution vaginal sonography, a normal singleton pregnancy can be seen by 5.5 to 6 weeks of pregnancy (1.5 to 2 weeks after the missed period). By this time, the quantitative hCG level has reached the *discriminatory zone,* or the level above which a gestational sac is always visualized. The discriminatory zone may vary from institution to institution because of differences in equipment and assays, but ranges from 800 to 1000 IU/L (Second International Standard) or 1000 to 2000 IU/L (First International Reference Preparation) (Nyberg et al., 1985; Peisner and Timor-Tritsch, 1990).

As many as 20% to 30% of ectopic gestations have no detectable sonographic abnormality (Figure 20-5, *A*). The typical ultrasound findings for ectopic pregnancy are a unilateral mass, fluid in the cul de sac, and no evidence of intrauterine pregnancy (Figure 20-5, *B* and *C*). Conclusive diagnosis of an ectopic gestation by sonography can only be made if a fetus or fetal cardiac motion is seen outside the uterus. With vaginal ultrasonography, this only occurs in about 20% of ectopic pregnancies.

Management

Treatment for ectopic pregnancy can be medical or surgical. Methotrexate, a folate antagonist, is often used in the medical management of ectopic gestation. It inhibits the rapidly growing trophoblast cells of the early placenta. Several treatment protocols are accepted (Buster and Pisarska, 1999). Most side effects seen with low-dose methotrexate therapy are mild and transient. Resolution of the ectopic state has been reported in about 70% to 95% of cases treated, depending somewhat on selection criteria.

The surgical approaches for ectopic pregnancy include laparoscopy for both confirmation and treatment and occasionally, laparotomy. The procedure of choice is salpingostomy, reserving salpingectomy for women not wanting future fertility.

SPONTANEOUS ABORTION

First trimester miscarriage is a common event. All women with clinically recognized pregnancies have approximately a 15% chance of spontaneous pregnancy loss in the first 3 months of pregnancy (Evans and Beischer, 1970). The risk is lower for younger women and higher for older mothers. Because women can present with symptoms of spontaneous miscarriage even before they are aware of pregnancy, all family physicians should be well versed in its assessment and management.

There are many causes of spontaneous pregnancy loss in the first trimester; sporadic chromosomal aneuploidy accounts for about 60%. The remaining 40% have various etiologies, including chronic maternal illness (e.g., diabetes, connective tissue disorder), uterine structural malformations, certain infections, inadequate progesterone production, and possibly other less-well-understood causes such as immunologic "rejection" and environmental factors.

Diagnosis

First trimester miscarriage can be further defined according to the stage of pregnancy loss and associated symptoms.

Threatened abortion is diagnosed when the pregnant woman presents with vaginal bleeding, lower back discomfort, or midline pelvic cramping. On examination, the cervical os is closed, and the pregnancy is viable (by Doppler ultrasonography). About 25% of women will have some degree of bleeding in the first trimester, about half of whom will miscarry. The remaining women may have a slightly higher risk of perinatal complications, such as preterm labor and FGR. The risk of congenital malformations is not increased.

Inevitable abortion occurs when there is profuse bleeding requiring surgical intervention or overt rupture of membranes. Although the cervical os may be initially closed and tissue has not passed, the miscarriage is inevitable.

Incomplete abortion is diagnosed when products of conception have passed the level of the cervical os. The woman

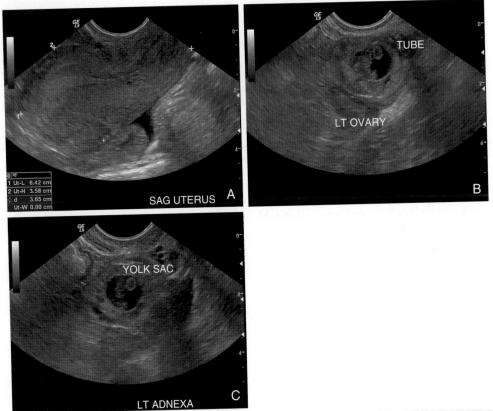

Figure 20-5 A, First trimester scan for ectopic pregnancy. The uterus is small and empty, suspicious for an ectopic pregnancy. This could also be a very early intrauterine pregnancy that is too early to be seen by transvaginal scan. However, further ultrasound assessment makes the diagnosis. **B,** Cross-section of the left fallopian tube shows an early pregnancy with a yolk sac (fetal heart motion was also seen). The left ovary is separate from the tube and pregnancy. **C,** Same tubal pregnancy with a normal-appearing yolk sac.

often has heavy vaginal bleeding, midline cramping, and an open cervical os.

Complete abortion occurs when all the gestational products have passed. This is ascertained by examination of the passed products of conception, pelvic ultrasonography to ascertain emptiness of the uterus, and at times retrospectively with falling quantitative hCG levels.

"Missed abortion" is a poor term still in use to describe retention of a nonviable pregnancy for longer than 4 weeks. Ultrasound scans of these women provide a more specific and usually earlier diagnosis, such as an empty sac or an embryonic gestation or fetal demise.

Septic abortion is diagnosed when there is infection of the uterus and products of conception. This occurs most often with incomplete abortions. Fever, uterine tenderness, foul discharge, and leukocytosis should aid the practitioner in making this diagnosis.

Recurrent spontaneous abortion is reserved for women who have had three or more first trimester losses. This diagnosis should prompt further evaluation for etiology.

Management

The goal of management of early miscarriage is assurance of complete emptying of the uterus in the least traumatic manner, avoidance of excessive blood loss, prevention of infection, and administration of adequate emotional support. Women with threatened abortions are reassured somewhat that the loss is neither imminent nor inevitable.

Bed rest is encouraged, but no evidence supports its value in prevention of miscarriage.

When there is profuse bleeding or sepsis, women with inevitable, incomplete, or septic abortions require prompt surgical treatment in the form of dilation and curettage (D&C), or in some, curettage alone. IV antibiotics should be used when appropriate. Rarely, blood transfusion is required. Certain women may benefit from oral antibiotics and methylergonovine (Methergine) on discharge.

When the diagnosis is missed abortion or incomplete abortion without hemorrhage or infection, the choice is surgical intervention versus natural spontaneous completion of the miscarriage. In well-selected women, no convincing evidence suggests one method is preferable. Many practitioners give these patients the option of D&C or spontaneous resolution. D&C has risks of anesthesia, cervical trauma, uterine scarring, and perforation; spontaneous resolution has risks of infection and hemorrhage. If products of conception for karyotype analysis are required for the evaluation of recurrent losses, the surgical approach is more successful in producing uncontaminated tissue for culture.

Women who are Rh(D) negative and at less than 13 weeks' gestation should receive 50 µg of D immune globulin intramuscularly (IM) when the abortion is diagnosed to prevent sensitization. If they are beyond 13 weeks' gestation, 300 µg is used. This treatment can be omitted if the father is known to be D negative as well. Iron therapy should

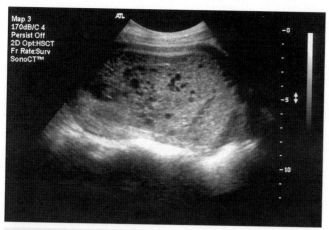

Figure 20-6 Hydatidiform mole (complete mole) at 12 weeks of gestation (transabdominal scan); the ultrasound shows a distended endometrial cavity containing numerous anechoic cysts of various sizes. No fetus is seen.

Table 20-17 Risk Factors for Preterm Labor

Low socioeconomic status
Uterine anomalies
African American ethnic group
Uterine leiomyoma
Poor nutritional state
Bacterial vaginosis
Low maternal weight (<50 kg)
Multiple gestation
Poor pregnancy weight gain
Bacteriuria or urinary tract infection
Prior preterm labor
Placenta previa or abruptio
Cocaine use
Polyhydramnios
Nicotine use
Poor prenatal care

be given to women when heavy bleeding occurs or is anticipated.

MOLAR PREGNANCY

A molar pregnancy, or *hydatidiform mole*, is uncommon. A *gestational trophoblastic disease* (GTD), it occurs predominantly in older women. In the United States, molar pregnancy occurs in about one in 1800 pregnancies (Grimes, 1984). Molar pregnancy can be classified as complete or incomplete, which are two distinct entities etiologically and pathologically. A *complete* or hydatidiform mole has no fetal components, consists entirely of hydropic placental villi, is frequently associated with medical complications, and has a 15% to 20% risk of GTD (Jones, 1987) (Figure 20-6). In an *incomplete* mole, a fetus, usually abnormal, is often present. The placenta may be hydropic or small, and there is a 5% to 10% risk of GTD.

A hydatidiform mole is most often diagnosed in the first trimester because of symptoms of excessive nausea and vomiting, vaginal bleeding, uterine size larger than expected, and sonographic findings of no fetus but a large placenta with numerous small cysts. These findings should prompt quantitative hCG evaluation, which is often elevated. Evacuation of the uterus with careful attention to levels of hCG postevacuation is important to detect GTD, usually an invasive mole and occasionally choriocarcinoma. Pregnancy is avoided for 1 year after a complete mole.

An incomplete mole is most often diagnosed in the second trimester and occasionally the third trimester. There may be an abnormal placenta, fetal growth and structural abnormalities, or signs and symptoms of preeclampsia.

Complications of Late Pregnancy

PRETERM LABOR

Preterm labor is defined as uterine contractions occurring before 37 weeks of gestation that cause cervical change.

Cervical change can be diagnosed if an initial examination reveals a cervix that is at least 2 cm dilated or 80% effaced or if interval cervical examinations document progression of effacement or dilation. Preterm contractions without cervical advancement can also occur; these do not require intervention. The distinction may be difficult, in particular at the onset of contractions.

Certain women are at higher risk of developing preterm labor (Table 20-17). These women should be assessed more frequently in the prenatal period and instructed on signs and symptoms of premature labor. Although many tests to identify women at risk of preterm labor have been proposed and evaluated, only ultrasonography for cervical length and fetal fibronectin have been shown to be effective (ACOG, 2001; Iams et al., 1996). A short cervix by transvaginal ultrasonography and positive cervicovaginal fetal fibronectin test is predictive of an increased risk of preterm delivery in the index pregnancy.

Assessment of patients thought to be in premature labor involves monitoring for premature contractions as well as FHR while they are in the right or left lateral recumbent position. Complete history and physical examination should be performed to find any treatable causes of premature labor as well any contraindications to tocolytic therapy. Urinalysis and culture are obtained and antibiotic therapy instituted if the urinalysis is suspicious. If there is a possibility of rupture of membranes, a sterile speculum examination of the cervix should be performed and vaginal fluid for nitrazine and ferning obtained. Cultures for GBS, *Chlamydia*, and possibly herpesvirus and *N. gonorrhoeae* are often performed in this setting. If there is no historical or physical evidence of rupture of membranes, digital examination of the cervix with careful assessment of consistency as well as dilation and effacement is performed. Chorioamnionitis should be ruled out by assessing the degree of uterine tenderness, leukocytosis, maternal fever, and fetal well-being.

In a woman at 22 to 35 weeks' gestation, before digital examination, assessment of the presence of fetal fibronectin can be determined. *Fetal fibronectin* is released from the interface of the chorion and decidua in women likely to deliver preterm. Fetal fibronectin can be determined in 1 hour by most hospital laboratories and is used predominantly for its high negative predictive value. Thus, if the fetal fibronectin result is negative, the woman will likely not deliver for at least 7 to 10 days; if positive, closer surveillance or treatment is warranted.

Management

Hydration appears to decrease the frequency of preterm contractions, but it does not decrease the rate of preterm birth. Intermittent digital cervical examinations should be performed either to confirm the diagnosis of preterm labor or to monitor progression. The frequency of these examinations has not been established and should be based on the clinical situation. However, a digital examination should always be performed at discharge to assess any cervical change.

If preterm delivery is a possibility, antibiotic prophylaxis for GBS should be administered (ACOG, 2002a). Betamethasone is also recommended, 12 mg IM every 24 hours for two doses, to accelerate fetal lung maturity in patients between 24 and 34 weeks of gestation (Liggins and Howie, 1972).

If a diagnosis of preterm labor is made and contractions do not subside with bed rest and hydration, pharmacologic therapy is considered. Contraindications to stopping labor include chorioamnionitis, abruptio placentae, heavy vaginal bleeding, severe or chronic hypertension, and fetal demise. Although many tocolytic drugs are available, terbutaline and magnesium sulfate are used often.

Historically, terbutaline has been administered subcutaneously in an effort to prolong pregnancy; however, the FDA is now warning the public that *injectable* terbutaline should not be used in pregnant women for prevention or prolonged treatment (beyond 48-72 hours) of preterm labor in either the hospital or outpatient setting because of the potential for serious maternal heart problems and death. Through β-1 receptors, β-agonists increase heart rate and thus stroke volume, increase fat breakdown, drive intravascular potassium into cells, and decrease gastrointestinal motility. Through β-2 receptors, bronchial and uterine smooth muscle relaxation and glycogenolysis occurs. Women taking β-adrenergic agonists experience tachycardia, jitteriness, and occasionally nausea and vomiting. A maternal heart rate of 120 beats/min or greater is a contraindication for further dosing, and the interval or quantity may need modification. Although it may be clinically deemed appropriate based on the health care professional's judgment to administer terbutaline by injection in urgent individual obstetrical situations in a hospital setting, the prolonged use of this drug is discouraged to prevent recurrent preterm labor. FHR elevations can also be seen. Oral or injectable terbutaline should not be used in the outpatient setting.

Intravenous magnesium sulfate therapy can also be used for preterm labor. There is no clear-cut greater efficacy of one tocolytic versus another. Magnesium sulfate relaxes uterine smooth muscle by competitive inhibition of the action of calcium. The dose should be adjusted so that contractions are decreased or abolished but maternal toxicity is not reached. This can be done by frequent examination of deep tendon reflexes, which should be present but depressed. Complete loss of deep tendon reflexes can herald further toxicity, and dosing should be decreased. Plasma magnesium levels can also be performed and should be kept between 5 and 8 mg/dL. Because it is excreted predominantly by the kidneys, the plasma magnesium level is influenced by urine output as well as infusion rate. Calcium gluconate should be readily available in case of magnesium toxicity. Women receiving IV magnesium experience warmth, flushing, and poor muscle tone; some develop diplopia, nausea, and vomiting. The majority of these side effects occur with the loading dose. Magnesium sulfate therapy is typically used for 24 hours and then discontinued. Long-term tocolytic therapy has not been shown to be efficacious.

EVIDENCE-BASED SUMMARY

- There are no clear "first-line" tocolytic drugs to manage preterm labor; clinical circumstances and physician preferences should dictate treatment (SOR: A).
- Antibiotics do not appear to prolong gestation and should be reserved for GBS prophylaxis in patients in whom delivery is imminent (SOR: A).
- Neither maintenance treatment with tocolytic drugs nor repeated acute tocolysis improves perinatal outcome; neither should be undertaken as a general practice (SOR: A).
- Tocolytic drugs may prolong pregnancy for 2 to 7 days, which may allow for administration of steroids to improve fetal lung maturity and consideration of maternal transport to a tertiary care facility (SOR: A).
- Cervical ultrasound examination and fetal fibronectin testing have good negative predictive value; thus, either approach or both combined may be helpful in determining which patients do not need tocolysis (SOR: B).
- Amniocentesis may be used in women in preterm labor to assess fetal lung maturity and intraamniotic infection (SOR: B).
- Bed rest, hydration, and pelvic rest do not appear to improve the rate of preterm birth and should not be routinely recommended (SOR: B).

INTRAUTERINE GROWTH RESTRICTION

Fetuses with FGR are those that fall below the 10th percentile for weight for a given gestational age. FGR occurs when a fetus does not meet its growth potential (Vandenbosche and Kirchner, 1998). Some below-10th-percentile fetuses are not growth restricted but constitutionally small, have reached their growth potential, and are healthy. Often, it is difficult to differentiate the two states.

Although mild growth abnormalities are generally tolerated well by the fetus, more severe growth abnormalities can be associated with poor outcome, including fetal distress, fetal demise, and postnatal developmental abnormalities (Botero and Lifshitz, 1999). Growth-restricted fetuses should be identified so that appropriate management can be instituted to ensure the best outcome. Factors that influence fetal growth can be divided into the following three categories:

1. Maternal factors affecting nutrient availability to the fetus, such as poor nutrition and cigarette smoking (Chomitz et al., 1995)

2. Maternal factors influencing placental growth and function, such as maternal hypertension, diabetes with vascular involvement, and connective tissue disorders
3. Fetal factors interfering with adequate utilization of nutrients despite their availability, such as fetal infection or a genetic disorder

Growth restriction has also been described as asymmetric and symmetric. *Asymmetric* or "head-sparing" FGR occurs because of fetal autoregulation of blood flow. The initial response to a lack of adequate delivery of oxygen and nutrients to the fetus results in shunting of blood flow to important organs such as the brain and adrenal glands. Muscle and other viscera such as the kidneys are somewhat underperfused, resulting in a smaller body than head, smaller muscle mass, and oligohydramnios caused by underperfusion of the fetal kidneys and decreased fetal urine output. If inadequate delivery of oxygen and nutrients is early, persistent, or profound, all organs and tissues of the body will be affected, and *symmetric* FGR ensues. FGR from fetal infection or genetic disorder is often symmetric as well because all of the tissues of the body are often affected.

Diagnosis

The physician can suspect FGR based on lack of appropriate growth of the uterine fundus. Poor fundal growth with or without risk factors for FGR should prompt ultrasound evaluation. Women at risk for FGR should have early sonography to confirm their estimated day of delivery to aid in diagnosis. For example, a woman at 30 weeks' gestation has her first ultrasound examination for possible FGR. The fetus is found to be 27 weeks by all parameters measured. It would be difficult to decide if the fetus is symmetrically growth restricted or just due 3 weeks later. Overall, ultrasonography for diagnosis of FGR is 80% to 90% sensitive, depending on the measurements used. The abdominal circumference, a soft tissue measurement, is the first routinely measured parameter to fall behind normal growth in FGR. Estimation of fetal weight, calculated using the abdominal circumference, can be plotted on fetal growth curves to evaluate its percentile for a specific gestational age.

Management

The only treatment modality thought to be of benefit for FGR is bed rest in a lateral recumbent position. This position prevents vena caval compression by the gravid uterus and allows maximal venous return to the heart, maximizing cardiac output and uteroplacental perfusion. Certain fetuses with growth restriction caused by significant maternal illness may benefit from improvement of the maternal condition. Antenatal testing is recommended for FGR fetuses. If antenatal testing results are abnormal or persistent oligohydramnios is present, delivery may be warranted before term. Otherwise, these fetuses are delivered at 38 to 40 weeks of gestation, depending on the degree of growth restriction.

PREECLAMPSIA

Preeclampsia is one of the most common causes of perinatal morbidity and mortality. The etiology for preeclampsia remains unknown. However, placental dysfunction may initiate systemic vasospasm, ischemia, and thrombosis that eventually damage maternal organs and cause placental infarction, FGR, and death. Preeclampsia complicates 5% to 10% of all pregnancies. It occurs at both extremes of reproductive age but is greatest in women younger than 20 years of age. Risk factors for preeclampsia include extremes of maternal age, nulliparity, African American race, multiple gestation, molar pregnancy, preexisting medical conditions (hypertension, diabetes, renal disease, connective tissue disorders, vascular disease), and prior or family history of preeclampsia or eclampsia.

The disorder is typically suspected in the presence of hypertension and proteinuria in the pregnant woman without history of preexisting chronic hypertension. Edema is no longer considered a reliable clinical sign and is often seen after the 20th week of gestation without signs of a hypertensive disorder. Historically, mild preeclampsia was diagnosed with a systolic BP rise of 30 mm Hg or diastolic BP rise of 15 mm Hg. Consensus statements now describe mild preeclampsia as an absolute reading of 140/90 mm Hg or greater in a pregnant woman with proteinuria greater than 0.3 g in a 24-hour urine collection. Again, nondependent edema is no longer considered a diagnostic criterion. Severe preeclampsia consists of a systolic BP greater than 160 mm Hg or diastolic BP greater than 110 mm Hg complicated by significant proteinuria (>5.0 g/day) and evidence of end-organ damage. Signs and symptoms indicating severe preeclampsia include headache, visual disturbances, confusion, right upper quadrant (RUQ) or epigastric pain, impaired liver function, proteinuria, oliguria (<500 mL/24 hr), pulmonary edema, microangiopathic hemolytic anemia, thrombocytopenia, oligohydramnios, and FGR.

Pregnant women with hypertension documented before pregnancy may develop preeclampsia. Chronic hypertension with superimposed preeclampsia is responsible for 15% to 30% of hypertensive disease in pregnancy. Treatment for mild preeclampsia involves bed rest and surveillance to assess development of complications. Delivery is carefully delayed until fetal maturity, development of severe preeclampsia, or other complications occur. In most cases, treatment of severe preeclampsia is delivery.

During labor and delivery, women with preeclampsia should receive IV magnesium sulfate for seizure prophylaxis, with a loading dose of 4 g infused over 15 to 20 minutes, then continuous infusion at 2 g/hr, similar to the preterm-labor magnesium therapy protocol (Table 20-18). BP should be carefully evaluated and treated with IV hydralazine if levels are persistently above 110 mm Hg diastolic. Women with severe preeclampsia should generally deliver within 24 hours. Postpartum therapy with magnesium sulfate is recommended for 12 to 24 hours depending on the degree of severity.

HELLP SYNDROME

If unrecognized, preeclampsia can progress to a syndrome of hemolysis, elevated liver enzymes, and low platelets (HELLP syndrome). This is another complication in seemingly stable patients. The HELLP syndrome is noted in 5% to 10% of patients with preeclamptic symptoms. Such patients often present with RUQ and epigastric pain and a

Table 20-18 Magnesium Sulfate Protocol for Preterm Labor

Continuous electronic fetal and contraction monitoring
Patient in lateral recumbent position
Nothing by mouth initially; then clear liquids if muscle tone adequate to prevent aspiration
Intravenous fluids begun with lactated Ringer 5% dextrose solution
Four g (range, 2-6 g) of $MgSO_4 \cdot 7H_2O$ in 500 mL of 5% dextrose administered over 15 minutes as loading dose
Continuous infusion of 1 to 3 g/hr of $MgSO_4 \cdot 7H_2O$ after initial load
Calcium gluconate readily available
Accurate intake and output
Frequent assessment of deep tendon reflexes
Frequent examination of lungs for early signs of pulmonary edema
Plasma magnesium levels monitored as clinically indicated
Continue protocol for 24 hours; change to oral β-adrenergic agent if needed

peripheral blood smear consistent with a microangiopathic hemolytic anemia. There may be decrements in the platelet count and increments in the transaminase (aspartate aminotransferase, alanine aminotransferase) and lactic acid dehydrogenase enzymes. This is a life-threatening emergency that requires prompt delivery of the baby.

ECLAMPSIA

Another serious complication of preeclampsia is development of seizures or coma. This is known as eclampsia. Eclampsia occurs in approximately 0.2% of pregnancies and terminates one in 1000 pregnancies. The seizures and mental status changes of eclampsia are thought to result from hypertensive encephalopathy. The perinatal mortality rate is 2.0% to 8.6% (Sibai et al., 1981). The maternal mortality rate is less than 2%, with intracranial hemorrhage the major cause.

GESTATIONAL HYPERTENSION

Gestational hypertension is defined as systolic BP of 140 mm Hg or greater or a diastolic BP of 90 mm Hg or greater in the absence of proteinuria in a previously normotensive pregnant woman at or after 20 weeks of gestation. Gestational hypertension is considered severe with sustained elevations in systolic BP of 160 or diastolic of 110 mm Hg or greater. Women with BP greater than 140/90 mm Hg without proteinuria or end-organ damage may ultimately develop preeclampsia. These initially normotensive women usually become hypertensive late in pregnancy, during labor, or within 24 hours postpartum and note a return to normal BP within 10 days postpartum. If preeclampsia does not develop, the diagnosis of gestational hypertension is made. The diagnosis of gestational hypertension is a temporary one and should be used during pregnancy only in women who do not meet criteria for preeclampsia or chronic hypertension.

ABRUPTIO PLACENTAE

Abruptio placentae (placental abruption) refers to separation of a normally located placenta before the birth of the fetus. This event occurs in 1 in 129 births. Severe abruption results in a fetal mortality rate of 0.2%. Bleeding into the decidua basalis leads to separation of the placenta. Hematoma formation further separates the placenta from the uterine wall and compresses these structures, compromising the blood supply to the fetus, leading to increased intrauterine pressure, uterine tenderness, frequent uterine contractions, fetal distress, and demise. The severity of fetal distress correlates with the degree of placental separation.

When the abruption is extensive, retroplacental blood may penetrate the thickness of the uterine wall into the peritoneal cavity because of increased intrauterine pressure. This phenomenon is called "couvelaire uterus." The myometrium becomes weakened and rarely may rupture, leading immediately to a life-threatening obstetric emergency. In near-complete or complete abruption, fetal death is inevitable unless immediate delivery by cesarean section is performed. Abruptio placentae received renewed awareness with the causal relationship to cocaine (Kline et al., 1997).

Abruptio placentae is a clinical diagnosis. Painful vaginal bleeding in the third trimester is the hallmark. Because ultrasonography for this disorder has a high false-negative rate, this complication is diagnosed primarily on the findings of vaginal bleeding, abdominal pain, uterine tenderness, uterine contractions, and fetal distress. In one prospective study, almost 80% of patients with abruptio placentae presented with vaginal bleeding, 66% with uterine or back pain, and 60% with fetal distress (Hurd et al., 1983). Other evidence of abruptio placentae can include idiopathic preterm labor, uterine hypertonicity, and fetal demise. The monitoring of uterine contractions may reveal a high baseline pressure with concurrent contractions often 1 to 2 minutes apart.

Etiology

From 40% to 50% of women with abruptio placentae have underlying hypertension. Maternal trauma is the cause in 1.5% to 9.4%. The remainder can be associated with excessive alcohol consumption, cocaine use, sudden decompression of the uterus (as in delivery of a first twin), retroplacental bleeding from needle puncture after amniocentesis, and possibly tobacco use. In a small group, no underlying association is found; abnormalities of uterine blood vessels and decidua likely exist in this idiopathic group.

Management

The management of abruptio placentae is primarily supportive and entails both aggressive hydration and monitoring of maternal and fetal well-being, with the expeditious delivery of the fetus if indicated (Turner, 1994). Maternal and fetal death may result from hemorrhage and coagulopathy. Coagulation studies should be performed to look for disseminated intravascular coagulation (DIC). Packed RBCs should be typed and held. If the fetus appears viable but compromised, urgent cesarean delivery should be considered. Recommended laboratory testing includes complete blood count (CBC) with platelets, prothrombin and partial thromboplastin time, fibrinogen, fibrin degradation products, D-dimer, blood type, and Kleihauer-Betke acid elution. D(Rh)-negative mothers benefit from administration of D immune globulin (Pearlman et al., 1990).

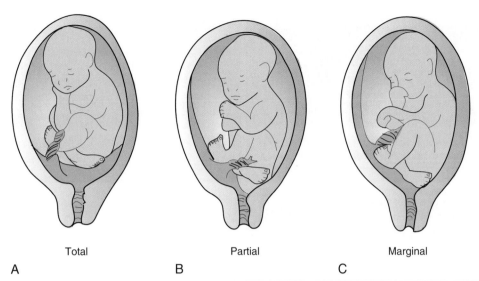

Total	Partial	Marginal
A	B	C

Figure 20-7 Various types of placenta previa. **A,** The cervical os is completely covered by the placenta. **B,** The cervical os is partially covered by the placenta. **C,** The placenta extends to the edge of the cervical os.

PLACENTA PREVIA

Placenta previa is a life-threatening condition that presents in three forms (Figure 20-7). When the cervical os is completely covered with placenta, it is classified as a *complete* or *total* placenta previa. *Partial* placenta previa occurs when the placenta covers a portion of the cervical os. A *marginal* placenta previa is one that extends just to the edge of the cervix. Placental implantation in the lower uterine segment is termed *low-lying placenta.* The incidence of placenta previa is about 1 in 200 to 250 pregnancies and is associated with potentially serious consequences from hemorrhage, separation of the placenta, or emergency cesarean delivery (Iyasu et al., 1993).

Placenta previa is usually diagnosed when the patient complains of painless vaginal bleeding in the third trimester. A smaller number of patients present with excessive bleeding in labor. Usually the initial bleeding is not profuse enough to be fatal and spontaneously ceases, only to recur later. The average first bleed occurs at 27 to 32 weeks of gestation. Women with a centrally implanted placenta previa tend to have earlier episodes of bleeding, which are more severe. Another suspicious aspect of the history includes an abnormal lie, in particular transverse or breech presentation.

Risk Factors

There are a few predisposing factors for placenta previa. They include advanced maternal age, increased parity, uterine abnormalities, multiple gestation, tobacco abuse, prior placenta previa, and previous uterine surgery.

Ultrasonography

Transabdominal ultrasonography is a simple, precise, and safe method to visualize the placenta. It has an accuracy of 93% to 98% (Bowie et al., 1978). False-positive results can result from focal uterine contractions or bladder distention. The accurate assessment of placental position can also be difficult with a placenta implanted on the posterior uterine wall. In a patient whose placental edge is not well visualized and is not actively bleeding, the transvaginal approach may be used (Laing, 1981). The bladder should be empty, and initially the vaginal transducer should be inserted into the vagina to visualize the cervix. After the closed cervix is visualized, deeper insertion of the probe aids in visualization of the placenta. The use of the vaginal approach is safe and accurate in diagnosis of a placenta previa (Figure 20-8).

During routine second trimester ultrasonography, placenta previa is frequently diagnosed. Typically, at 16 weeks' gestation, the placenta occupies 25% to 50% of the uterine surface area. As the third trimester approaches, growth of the lower uterine segment outflanks growth of the placenta, allowing apparent "migration" of the placenta (placental migration) away from the cervical os. For this reason, although 5% of pregnancies are diagnosed with complete previa by second trimester ultrasonography, 90% of these resolve by term (Rizos et al., 1979). When second trimester ultrasonography suggests a placenta previa, transvaginal ultrasonography can be helpful in making a more accurate diagnosis before term.

VASA PREVIA

Vasa previa is a rarely reported condition in which fetal blood vessels unsupported by the umbilical cord or placental tissue traverse the fetal membranes below the presenting part, covering the cervical os. It almost always coexists with a velamentous insertion of the umbilical cord. Vasa previa leads to fetal exsanguination from tearing of the large-caliber fetal vessels when the membranes rupture spontaneously or artificially. This event has an associated fetal mortality rate of 33% to 100% (Bright and Becker, 1991).

When pulsatile vessels are palpated preceding the fetal vertex during digital examination, vasa previa should be considered along with cord presentation. Vasa previa must be included in the differential diagnosis of all cases of third trimester bleeding. The blood that is lost can be tested for the presence of fetal hemoglobin, but often there is insufficient time to accomplish this. Vasa previa is often a retrospective diagnosis made after emergent cesarean delivery

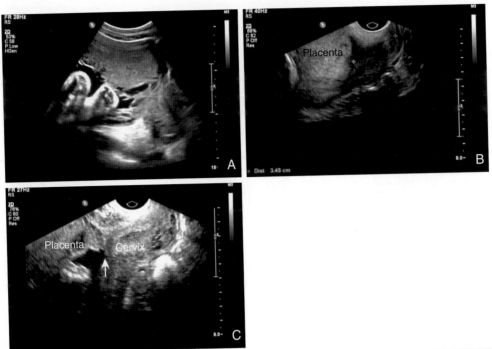

Figure 20-8 A, Complete placenta previa from transabdominal midline sagittal scan. The anterior wall implanted placenta covers the cervix completely. **B,** Complete placenta previa from transvaginal scan. The endocervical canal is measured in the image with (+). Note that the placenta covers the entire endocervical canal. **C,** Marginal placenta previa. The anterior uterine wall-implanted placenta covers just to the internal cervical os.

for fetal distress. Fetal mortality and morbidity from vasa previa may be reduced if there are a high index of suspicion, reliable method of diagnosis, and prompt surgical intervention (Messer et al., 1987).

PLACENTA ACCRETA, INCRETA, AND PERCRETA

These three conditions are forms of abnormal placental attachment in which the trophoblasts invade beyond the normal location into the uterine muscle to varying degrees. Abnormal blood supply to the inner lining of the uterus and prior trauma to both the endometrium and myometrium (the muscle layer) appear to alter lower uterine physiology and influence placental implantation. The most common risk factor is a previous cesarean delivery or prior uterine surgery.

The risk of maternal death is 3%. In cases of bladder involvement with a placenta percreta, the risk of maternal death increases to 20%. The leading immediate causes of death are uterine bleeding and DIC. Placenta accreta, increta, or percreta is often the etiology of retained placenta (Breen et al., 1997). During manual extraction, the placenta fragments without complete separation, resulting in uncontrolled hemorrhage.

The major factor affecting outcome is the degree of placental invasion. A minimally invasive placenta (accreta) can often be removed manually or by curettage. Invasion deeper in the myometrium (increta) or through the myometrium (percreta) more often requires hysterectomy. The increased rate of cesarean deliveries is making abnormalities of placental attachment more frequent, particularly if the placenta is attached in the area of the prior uterine incision.

Multiple Gestation

At least 1 in 80 births is a twin gestation. With assisted reproductive technologies, this rate has now increased to almost 1 in 50 to 60. Approximately two thirds to three quarters of twins are dizygotic.

Twin gestation presents unique challenges. Monozygotic twins have twice the anomaly rate of dizygotic twins or singletons. Women with twin gestations are more likely to miscarry early in gestation and more likely to deliver prematurely. Half of mothers of twins experience premature labor. Bed rest is often recommended after 5 months of gestation to aid in preterm labor prevention. Education regarding associated signs and symptoms is important in this group. The average gestational age of delivery for a twin gestation is 36 menstrual weeks.

Women with twin gestations are also at higher risk for chronic hypertension, pyelonephritis, GDM, and placenta previa. They should take supplemental iron, particularly in the latter trimesters, even if they are not iron deficient. Growth discordance can also occur, from twin–twin transfusion syndrome or more often simply from different placental implantation and different accessibility to nutrients. Serial ultrasound studies for growth approximately every 6 weeks is recommended. Twin fetuses with growth discordance should have antenatal testing.

The majority of twins will present both head first, cephalic–cephalic (Figure 20-9, *A*), or first one cephalic and second one breech (cephalic–breech; Figure 20-9, *B*). Any other combination can be seen, although cephalic–transverse (Figure 20-9, *C*) and breech–cephalic are the most likely in this remaining group. When well into the

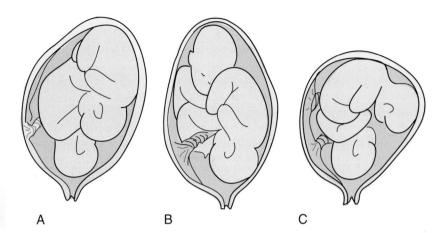

Figure 20-9 Three common twin presentations: cephalic–cephalic (**A**). cephalic–breech (**B**), and cephalic–transverse (**C**).

A   B   C

third trimester, the first presenting fetus most often stays in its position; the second fetus often changes position, occasionally even during early labor. Twins who are cephalic–cephalic can be delivered vaginally. Those who are cephalic–breech and cephalic–transverse can also be attempted vaginally by skilled operators in carefully chosen women. When the first fetus is presenting other than cephalic, delivery is often best accomplished by cesarean section. Breastfeeding has been successful in many women with twins and should be encouraged.

Antepartum Fetal Surveillance

The three most common methods used to evaluate fetal well-being in utero are the nonstress test (NST), contraction stress test (CST), and biophysical profile (BPP) (Babbitt, 1996). Vibroacoustic stimulation and fetal movement counts are also useful adjunctive tools in the evaluation of fetal well-being.

The indications for antepartum fetal surveillance are multiple and reflect conditions that are associated with increased fetal morbidity and mortality (Smith-Levitin et al., 1997). Conditions that lead to fetal hypoxia, utero-placental insufficiency, and death are all indications for increased fetal surveillance. There are no absolute protocols for increased fetal surveillance, but there are certain accepted practices for given maternal–fetal risks. For example, weekly antenatal testing beginning in the 32nd week of gestation is often performed in women with low to moderate risk (e.g., GDM, chronic hypertension, mild pre-eclampsia). For women with a higher risk of an abnormal outcome, earlier and more frequent antenatal testing is indicated, requiring an individualized approach.

NONSTRESS TEST

Most often the NST is used as the primary tool in antepartum fetal surveillance. It has been used to document second and third trimester fetal well-being for the past 40 years. It serves as a surrogate measure of the developing fetal autonomic nervous system and the adequacy of the uteroplacental function (Myrick and Harper, 1996).

The NST is more specific than sensitive and thus a better indicator of fetal health than fetal illness. The test itself is read as reactive or nonreactive and may be repeated at intervals as a screen for high-risk maternal conditions. A reactive or reassuring NST is defined as one with at least two accelerations above a baseline FHR of 15 beats/min for 15 seconds in a 20-minute period. If a reactive pattern is not present at the end of the first 20 minutes, attempts may be made to arouse the fetus. Fetal rest periods, reportedly 30 to 40 minutes in duration, must be excluded for the fetus to demonstrate a reactive NST. Because fetuses can have normal sleep cycles lasting up to 40 minutes, NST might require more than 1 hour to complete if it is initially nonreactive. It is important to differentiate whether a nonreactive tracing truly represents a compromised fetus versus a temporary behavioral state (Knuppel et al., 1982).

The absence of fetal accelerations with the exclusion of a fetal sleep state denotes a nonreactive test. There are no contraindications to the NST as a primary screening tool, and it is easily reproducible, relatively inexpensive, and acceptable to most patients. Maternal narcotics, extreme prematurity, and fetal cardiac or CNS anomalies may also be responsible for a nonreactive NST. A nonreactive NST does not indicate fetal jeopardy but should be viewed as an indication for further evaluation. This evaluation may take the form of a BPP or CST.

BIOPHYSICAL PROFILE

The BPP is an ultrasound assessment of fetal well-being. It was originally designed to mimic the Apgar score for postnatal assessment. The BPP is technically more difficult to perform and interpret but provides a greater degree of certainty of fetal well-being. During a 30-minute examination, certain behavioral patterns associated with a healthy fetus are documented. The test is scored with five components, each worth 2 points (Table 20-19). Indicators such as amniotic fluid volume, fetal breathing, FHR, movement, and tone are evaluated. A score of 8 or 10 is reassuring; a score of 6 is suspicious and indicates a need for further evaluation; and a score of 4 or less is ominous, indicating the need for immediate intervention. A low score may also reflect the fetus's behavioral state during the test, such as normal sleep or sedation from maternal use of narcotics or CNS depressants. However, a decreasing score has been well correlated with a poor outcome and with increasing degrees of fetal acidemia.

Table 20-19   Components of the Biophysical Profile*

Parameter	Normal (Score = 2)	Abnormal (Score = 0)
Nonstress test	Two or more accelerations of at least 15 beats/min above baseline for at least 15 sec	Less than two accelerations of sufficient height and duration
Amniotic fluid volume	At least one amniotic fluid pocket is ≥2 × 2 cm in perpendicular plane	No 2 × 2-cm pockets *or* AFI <5.0
Fetal breathing movements	Sustained fetal breathing for at least 30 sec	<30 seconds of fetal breathing
Fetal body movements	At least three limb or gross body movements	Less than three limb or body movements
Fetal tone	Extremities in flexion at rest and at least one episode of extension of extremity or spine with return to flexion	Extension at rest or no return to flexion after movement

*Scoring of the latter four components is done sonographically in 30-minute observation period. A total score of 8 to 10 is reassuring, a score of 6 is suspicious, and a score of 4 or less is ominous.
AFI, Amniotic fluid index (sum of largest vertical pocket in each of four quadrants of uterus).
Modified from Norman LA, Karp LE. Biophysical profile for antepartum fetal assessment. *Am J Fam Physician.* 1986;34:83-89.

MODIFIED BIOPHYSICAL PROFILE

The modified BPP consists of the NST and the amniotic fluid index. It has proved to be an excellent means of fetal surveillance and identifies a group of patients at increased risk for poor perinatal outcome and small-for-gestational-age (SGA) infants. It has proved to be as effective as a full BPP in assessing fetal well-being.

CONTRACTION STRESS TEST

With the increasing popularity of the NST, the CST, also known as the *oxytocin challenge test* (OCT), is most often used as a supplementary tool in fetal surveillance. The CST is more cumbersome to perform, is difficult to interpret, and has several contraindications. This test is used to assess the reserve of the marginally compromised fetus when subjected to the stress of several uterine contractions (Collea and Holls, 1982; Lagrew, 1995). The goal of the CST or OCT is to achieve three contractions in a 10-minute period through oxytocin infusion or nipple stimulation and look for late decelerations.

The CST result is considered to be negative if no late decelerations are noted. A negative (normal) CST result is a good indication of adequate fetal well-being as judged by fetal distress in labor, Apgar scores, and absence of meconium. The CST result is considered positive if late decelerations accompany 50% or more of contractions. A positive CST result is predictive of fetal compromise and distress in labor in up to 80% of cases and in specific clinical situations indicates need for delivery of the fetus. The presence of fewer decelerations indicates a suspicious study. The latter two conditions mandate need for further evaluation. Contraindications to a CST include risk of preterm labor, placenta previa, classic uterine scar or full-thickness scar from previous uterine surgery, incompetent cervix, and multiple gestation (Babbitt, 1996).

VIBROACOUSTIC STIMULATION

Vibroacoustic stimulation is an artificial burst of noise produced by a handheld battery-powered artificial larynx (Birnholz and Benacerraf, 1983). This device is portable and easy to apply to the maternal abdomen and provides a stimulation that combines both sound and vibration. The goal is to alter the fetal behavioral state, waken a sleeping fetus, and provoke accelerations in the heart rate. Use of this device is associated with a significant increase in the number of reactive NSTs and a significant decrease in overall testing time. The use of vibroacoustic stimulation in achieving FHR accelerations has been found to be equally predictive of a favorable fetal outcome as spontaneously generated FHR accelerations (Smith et al., 1986).

Normal Labor and Delivery

Labor, whether preterm or term, is defined as the presence of sufficient uterine contractions in frequency, intensity, and duration to bring about effacement and dilation of the cervix. Control of normal labor is complex and, despite advances in medical science, poorly understood. Evidence supports PG involvement, in particular PGE_2 and $PGF_2\alpha$, as well as other mediators (Ulmsten, 1997).

Before the onset of labor, the fetal head may descend into the pelvis, and the height of the fundus will diminish. This lightening may occur acutely and may be very obvious to the pregnant woman, or it may occur over several weeks. An increase in pelvic pressure is experienced at this time. *False labor,* or irregular, short contractions that occur often before true labor, may in fact aid in cervical effacement and shortening of the cervical canal that begins as funneling at the internal cervical os. With impending true labor, cervical effacement and early dilation may allow the passage of a blood-tinged mucous, termed "bloody show." Most women go into true labor within 3 days of a bloody show. Bleeding described as "heavy as the beginning of a menstrual period" may be pathologic, and the pregnant woman should be evaluated for placenta previa, abruptio placentae, and other causes of vaginal bleeding.

Contractions of active labor most often occur every 2 to 3 minutes, last about 1 minute, and have a mean of 40 mm Hg in intensity. However, some women successfully deliver babies with less frequent and intense uterine contractions. Frequent contractions of 1 to 2 minutes apart may be a sign of the increased intrauterine pressure associated with abruptio placentae. Adequate relaxation between contractions is imperative to allow oxygenated blood to enter the intravillous spaces and transfer to the fetal compartment. During the course of labor, uterine contractions cause cervical effacement and then dilation to a full 10 cm

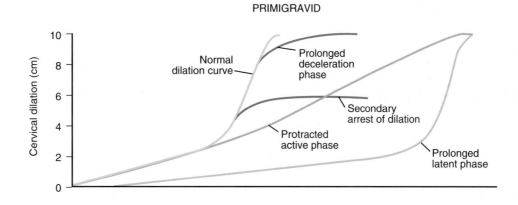

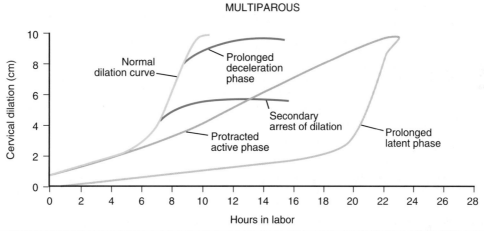

Figure 20-10 Composite curves of normal and abnormal labor progress. (From Scherger J, Levitt C, Acheson L: Teaching family-centered perinatal care in family medicine. Part 2. *Fam Med*. 1992;24:369.)

Table 20-20   Stages of Labor

Stage	Onset	Completion
First (latent and active phases)	Active labor	Complete dilation
Second	Complete dilation	Delivery of baby
Third	Delivery of baby	Delivery of placenta
Fourth*	Delivery of placenta	Contracted uterus

*Not always considered a stage.

to allow passage of the fetal head, the largest diameter of the fetus to pass through the birth canal.

PROGRESS OF LABOR

The degree and rate of cervical dilation measures the progress of labor. Labor can be divided into stages that are somewhat predictable in nulliparous and multiparous women (Table 20-20 and Figure 20-10). The first stage of the labor course can be subdivided into the latent phase and the active phase.

First Stage of Labor

Latent Phase
The latent phase of the first stage of labor is variable in length but is usually less than 20 hours for a nullipara and 14 hours for a multipara. Little cervical dilation is seen, but cervical preparation for labor occurs with changes in consistency caused by changes in collagen and connective tissue. An increase in effacement as well as the anterior positioning of the cervix is also noted. Conduction anesthesia given in this phase may prolong or arrest progress. In normal pregnant women, latent phase labor is best experienced at home. Clear liquids instead of heavy meals are encouraged during this time. Instructions for coming to the hospital include vaginal bleeding similar to a period, rupture of membranes, painful contractions at least 3 to 4 minutes apart, and decreased fetal movement. A subset of women may have a prolonged latent phase that can be treated with morphine in a hospital setting. Often this treatment accelerates transition to the active phase.

Active Phase
The active phase of the first stage of labor is the segment of rapid dilation, the progress of which is not affected by

sedation or conduction anesthesia. This phase usually occurs at about 4 to 5 cm of cervical dilation. In general, nulliparous women dilate at least 1.2 cm/hr and multiparous 1.5 cm/hr (Friedman, 1978). Progress of the active phase depends on the strength and frequency of uterine contractions; size, position, and attitude of the fetal head; and the size and shape of the bony pelvis. Because of the different diameters of the pelvic inlet, midplane, and outlet, the fetal head must turn at different times of descent to negotiate the bony structure. Flexion of the fetal head during this process is crucial because this diminishes its anteroposterior diameter and permits easier descent. The cardinal movements of the fetal head during labor include engagement, descent, flexion, internal rotation, extension, external rotation, and expulsion.

Either continuous electronic fetal monitoring (EFM) or intermittent auscultation can be used to monitor the fetus in the active phase of labor (ACOG, 1995a). Instead of continuous EFM in this phase, in low-risk mothers with normal labor, the fetal heart may be auscultated after a contraction and recorded every 30 minutes; the frequency should be increased to every 15 minutes in higher risk labors. FHR decelerations should prompt even more frequent auscultation or continuous EFM. Auscultation rather than continuous EFM will allow mobility during labor, which may improve maternal comfort. IV fluids in a normal gravida can be reserved for women with long labor who become dehydrated despite oral liquids, those who require conduction anesthesia or large doses of pain medication, and those in whom complications develop or are suspected.

Second Stage of Labor

The second stage of labor involves maternal expulsive forces during uterine contractions to aid in the descent and ultimate delivery of the fetus. Instead of continuous monitoring, the fetal heart should be auscultated and recorded every 15 minutes in normal, low-risk pregnancies and every 10 minutes in higher risk pregnancies. The second stage of labor averages 20 minutes for multiparas and 50 minutes for nulliparas. Although pushing for longer than 2 hours without an epidural or 3 hours with an epidural in a nullipara should alert the practitioner to possible cephalo-pelvic disproportion (CPD), pushing can continue longer in cases of adequate FHR and continued progress in descent.

Third Stage of Labor

The third stage of labor begins with the delivery of the baby. Appropriate equipment for resuscitation should be available. Maternal pushing with contractions will cause the fetal head to bulge the perineal tissues with increasing pressure to distend the opening of the vaginal canal and allow the fetal head to deliver. It is only when the head is stretching these tissues should the decision for episiotomy be made. The fetal head delivers with extension, after which the practitioner suctions the fetal mouth, pharynx, and nose. If meconium is present, wall suction to a DeLee trap is used for suctioning, and the fetus is not stimulated to breathe before a laryngoscope is used to assess the presence of meconium below the cords. After delivery of the fetal head and suctioning are complete, the neck of the fetus is explored for nuchal cords, which are preferably reduced if possible.

If too tight to reduce, the cord must be clamped and then cut. The anterior shoulder of the fetus is then delivered with gentle downward traction but predominantly with maternal expulsive forces to avoid excessive pulling on the fetal neck, which can be associated with brachial plexus injury. Hyperflexion of the legs at the hip joint will allow the anterior shoulder to deliver more easily. After delivery of the anterior shoulder, the posterior shoulder is delivered usually quite easily with gentle upward traction. Excessive maternal efforts at this point can cause perineal lacerations. Thus, the mother is instructed to push hard for the delivery of the anterior shoulder and gently for the posterior shoulder. After the shoulders are delivered, the remainder of the body escapes easily. The baby can then be placed on the mother's abdomen where warm towels await. The timing of clamping of the cord is controversial. As long as the baby is kept on the maternal abdomen, excessive blood shifts through an unclamped cord will usually not occur. The cord can then be clamped. Cord blood is obtained, as well as cord pH if desired.

The placenta should then be allowed to separate spontaneously. During this time, inspection of the vaginal canal and cervix for tears can be started, but adequate inspection for lacerations should be done after delivery of the placenta. Signs of placental separation include lengthening of the cord, a gush of blood, and a change in the contour of the uterine fundus. Separation of the placenta from the maternal decidua is most likely from shearing forces as the now-smaller uterus contracts. After separation, uterine contractions decrease the size of the implantation site to arrest bleeding from this area. Maternal expulsive forces may be required to deliver the placenta along with gentle traction on the cord. Uterine massage and immediate breastfeeding will aid in maintaining a contractile state of the uterus and decrease uterine atony. In some cases, oxytocin may be required to maintain uterine contractility. After separation of the placenta, the episiotomy (if cut) and any lacerations should be repaired.

Fourth Stage of Labor

Some consider the first hour after delivery of the placenta the fourth stage of labor. Risk of uterine atony is highest during this period. The patient should be watched carefully for excessive vaginal bleeding, an enlarging boggy fundus, and hypotension. Massage of the uterine fundus most often is sufficient to return it to a contracted state and stop bleeding. Oxytocin may be added to the IV fluids in doses of 20 or 40 units/L of fluid and the IV rate increased, or if no IV fluid is needed, 20 units of oxytocin can be given IM. Alternatively, methylergonovine (Methergine), 0.2 mg, can be given IM every 20 minutes if the mother is not hypertensive. Finally, if there is no resolution to bleeding, 250 μg of $PGF_2\alpha$ (Hemabate) can be given IM every 15 to 20 minutes as needed for up to three doses. Misoprostol is a PG that is now widely used despite its "off-label" indication that has demonstrated to increase uterine tone and decrease bleeding in the postpartum period. It can be administered via the oral, sublingual, vaginal, and rectal routes in doses ranging from 200 to 1000 μg. It has no known contraindication but should be used with caution in cardiovascular disease and is associated with nausea, vomiting, pyrexia, and diarrhea in high doses.

Table 20-21 Bishop Pelvic Scoring for Elective Induction of Labor

Score	Dilation	Effacement (%)	Station	Position	Consistency
0	Closed	0-30	−3		
1	1-2 cm	40-50	−2	Posterior	Firm
2	3-4 cm	60-70	−1, 0	Midposition	Moderately firm
3	5+ cm	80+	+1, +2	Anterior	Soft

The Bishop score generally follows this scale:

Modifiers

A point is added to the score for each of the following:
Preeclampsia
Each prior vaginal delivery
A point is subtracted from the score for:
Postdates pregnancy
Nulliparity
Premature or prolonged rupture of membranes
Interpretation

Indications for Cervical Ripening with Prostaglandins

1. Bishop score <5
2. Membranes intact
3. No regular contractions

Indications for Labor Induction with Pitocin

1. Bishop score ≥5
2. Rupture of membranes

Cesarean Rates	First-Time Mothers (%)	Women with Past Vaginal Deliveries (%)
Scores of 0-3	45	7.7
Scores of 4-6	10	3.9
Scores of 7-10	1.4	0.9

Points for each parameter are added. A score of 9 or greater is favorable for induction.
Modified from Bishop EH. Pelvic scoring for elective induction. *Obstet Gynecol*. 1964;24:266.

INDUCTION OF LABOR

Physicians have turned to induction of labor as a means of preventing complications from conditions such as prolonged rupture of membranes, fetal demise in utero or severe preeclampsia, or a postterm pregnancy. For example, postterm delivery beyond 42 weeks' gestation poses risks to both mothers and babies, including increased perinatal death, increased cesarean deliveries, perineal injuries from macrosomia, and labor dystocias (Gülmezoglu et al., 2006). The onset of labor can be stimulated in different ways. Less interventional approaches, such as stripping of the amniotic membranes, may be effective but not predictable and thus may not be sufficient in women who need prompt delivery. Stripping of the membranes requires the cervix to be dilated sufficiently to introduce the examining finger. Potential risks include rupture of membranes, infection, and bleeding. However, this technique appears safe particularly for gravidas approaching postdates (El-Torkey and Grant, 1992).

In most cases, the pharmacologic induction of pregnancy should be reserved for a medical or obstetric indication, such as hypertension, diabetes, premature rupture of membranes, postdates, fetal demise, and FGR. Logistic and psychosocial factors, such as distance from the hospital and rapid labors, are also indications. Absolute contraindications for induction of labor are similar to those for spontaneous labor and vaginal delivery. Before an induction, accurate dating and if necessary, fetal maturity should be confirmed. Gestational age of at least 39 weeks should be confirmed by early positive pregnancy test, early ultrasonography, or early fetal heart tone auscultation. In some cases, fetal lung maturity studies from amniotic fluid may be required.

Successful induction is mainly a factor of parity and cervical readiness at the time of induction. A scoring system developed by Bishop in 1964 to assess the cervix has become popular (Table 20-21). A Bishop score of 9 or greater is favorable for induction. Women with low scores benefit from cervical ripening with PGs before induction.

Prostaglandin E_2 is now approved by the FDA for cervical ripening. Dinoprostone (Prepidil) is 0.5 mg of modified PGE_2 in 2.5 mL of gel that is placed intracervically and repeated once in 6 to 12 hours if the Bishop score does not change appreciably. Intracervical dinoprostone may or may not cause uterine contractions. Its effect on cervical consistency appears unrelated to the number of contractions. Alternately, dinoprostone (Cervidil) may be given intravaginally as a slow-release, 12-hour vaginal insert that may be removed if uterine hyperstimulation occurs. Previous cesarean section is not a contraindication for use. If spontaneous labor does not ensue, an oxytocin infusion may then be used.

Misoprostol (Cytotec), a synthetic PGE_1 FDA approved for prevention of gastric ulcers, has been used off label for cervical ripening and labor induction. Several protocols have been developed. It is a potent uterotonic agent that may be associated with an increased incidence of uterine rupture. Misoprostol is best not used in women with prior cesarean section or uterine surgery.

Oxytocin has been available for labor induction for 40 years. Administered appropriately, it is as safe as spontaneous labor. Many protocols are available for IV oxytocin infusion for induction of labor, from low-dose constant infusion (Mercer et al., 1990) to higher dose incremental infusion (Muller et al., 1992; Satin et al., 1994). Steady-state levels after IV infusion occur about 40 minutes after the start of infusion. Starting doses range from 0.5 to 2 mU/min with incremental increases of 1 to 2 mU/min every 30 to 60 minutes (ACOG, 1995b). The goal is to achieve two to four uterine contractions in 10 minutes. All protocols share certain precautions. Continuous FHR and uterine contraction monitoring is mandatory. Hyperstimulation can occur even after a stable infusion rate has been established. Often, contraction intensity and frequency will increase spontaneously after the pregnant woman reaches the active phase or if the amniotic membranes rupture, necessitating a decrease in the oxytocin infusion rate. Hyperstimulation associated with FHR decelerations requires discontinuing or lowering of the infusion until recovery. Prolonged use of high doses of oxytocin can cause water intoxication because of its biochemical similarity to antidiuretic hormone.

Amniotomy alone or in conjunction with oxytocin has been shown to decrease the length of labor. In some cases, amniotomy alone can stimulate normal labor, omitting the need for oxytocin. The risks of early amniotomy include cord prolapse and chorioamnionitis. In clinical practice, the decision between induction and expectant management should include favorability of the cervix, maternal parity, and complicating medical or obstetric issues, as well as patient or physician convenience and preferences.

EVIDENCE-BASED SUMMARY

- Patients should be counseled that walking during labor does not enhance or improve progress in labor and that it is not harmful (SOR: A).
- Continuous support during labor from caregivers should be encouraged because it is beneficial for women and their newborns (SOR: A).
- Active management of labor may shorten labor in nulliparous women, although it has not consistently been shown to reduce the rate of cesarean delivery (SOR: B).
- Amniotomy may be used to enhance progress in active labor but may increase the risk of maternal fever (SOR: B).
- Intrauterine pressure catheters may be helpful in the management of dystocia in select patients, such as obese women (SOR: C).
- Women with twin gestations may undergo augmentation of labor (SOR: C).

KEY TREATMENT

- PGE analogs are effective for cervical ripening and inducing labor (SOR: A).
- Low- or high-dose oxytocin regimens are appropriate for women in whom induction of labor is indicated (SOR: A).
- Before 28 weeks' gestation, vaginal misoprostol appears to be the most efficient method of labor induction regardless of Bishop score, although high-dose oxytocin infusion is also acceptable (SOR: A).

- Approximately 25 µg of misoprostol should be considered as the initial dose for cervical ripening and labor induction; the frequency of administration should be no more than every 3 to 6 hours (SOR: A).
- Intravaginal PGE$_2$ for induction of labor in women with premature rupture of membranes appears to be safe and effective (SOR: A).
- The use of misoprostol in women with prior cesarean delivery or major uterine surgery has been associated with an increase in uterine rupture and therefore should be avoided in the third trimester (SOR: A).
- Misoprostol (50 µg every 6 hours) to induce labor may be appropriate in some situations, although higher doses are associated with an increased risk of complications, including uterine tachysystole with FHR decelerations (SOR: B).

Abnormalities of Labor and Delivery

DYSFUNCTIONAL LABOR

A dysfunctional pattern of labor is defined as a deviation from the norm for the different phases of labor described earlier (see Figure 20-10). In the latent phase of the first stage of labor, a prolonged or protracted course can be seen. In the active phase of the first stage of labor, both a protracted course and an arrested course can be seen (O'Brien and Cephalo, 1991). The disorders for each of these phases are examined separately.

PROLONGED LATENT PHASE

The latent phase of the first stage of labor is variable in length but usually less than 20 hours for a nullipara and 14 hours for a multipara. It is defined by the onset of regular contractions and is terminated by the onset of the active phase. The rate of dilation is usually 0.6 cm/hr or less. This phase is considered prolonged if it falls outside these parameters. The possible etiologies include an unripe cervix, false labor, sedation, and uterine inertia. The management of this condition is primarily conservative unless there is an expeditious need to deliver the fetus. This includes rest, observation, and possibly oxytocin augmentation. Maternal rest can be induced by a therapeutic dose of morphine to provide a respite from the stresses of early labor and to promote sleep. The vast majority of these patients will declare themselves and either progress into labor or cease contractions, and then the diagnosis of false labor can be made. Amniotomy should be avoided in this phase because it increases the risk for chorioamnionitis. A prolonged latent phase in itself is not an indication for cesarean section.

PROTRACTED ACTIVE PHASE

The active phase of labor is defined as dilation of the cervix occurring at a rate of at least 1.2 cm/hr for nulliparous women and 1.5 cm/hr for multiparous women. A slower rate of dilation is known as protracted active phase or *primary dysfunctional labor.* The etiologies of a protracted active phase include fetal malposition (e.g., occiput posterior), relative CPD, inadequate uterine contractions, and anesthesia. Historically, debate has surrounded its management. The current trend is active management with oxytocin to optimize uterine contractions. A protracted active phase is a frequent predecessor of secondary arrest of cervical dilation and is associated with an increased risk of operative delivery.

SECONDARY ARREST OF CERVICAL DILATION

The cessation of cervical dilation for 2 hours with a history of previously normal dilation is termed *secondary arrest.* The management of this condition varies considerably; however, an initial assessment and examination of the patient (including vaginal) are probably warranted to document cervical dilation, fetal station, presentation, and position. Placement of an intrauterine monitor should be considered to assess the adequacy of uterine contractions. Alternative measures include ambulation, amniotomy, and oxytocin augmentation if the uterine contractions are judged inadequate. There is a high association with CPD, and a significant number of these patients will need operative delivery.

ABNORMALITIES OF THE SECOND STAGE OF LABOR

The second stage of labor is defined as the interval between the complete dilation of the cervix to the delivery of the infant. As with previous stages of labor, abnormalities in this stage include a protracted rate or a complete "arrest of descent," or the more common term *failure of descent,* used to describe an unchanged station. The evaluation of descent disorders should include maternal and fetal well-being, adequacy of contractions, obstructive etiologies (e.g., distended bladder), and cephalopelvic relationships. Other mitigating factors include maternal exhaustion, ineffective pushing, conduction anesthesia, and perineal resistance. There is also a high incidence of CPD with this condition and an increased risk of operative deliveries.

A *protracted descent* is more difficult to gauge but is defined by a rate of less than 1 cm/hr in nullipara women and less than 2 cm/hr in multiparous women. This diagnosis should prompt an evaluation for such causes as CPD, macrosomia, and inadequate pushing.

SHOULDER DYSTOCIA

Shoulder dystocia is defined as the impaction of the anterior shoulder against the pubic symphysis after the delivery of the head and occurs when the breadth of the shoulder is greater than the biparietal diameter of the head (Figure 20-11). It is a life-threatening event associated with significant morbidity and mortality that needs to be recognized early and managed promptly. The overall incidence of shoulder dystocia is 0.3% to 1% but increases to 5% to 7% for newborns with macrosomia (birth weight >4500 g). Although a number of factors are associated with its occurrence, their predictive values are low, making it incumbent on the practitioner to be ever vigilant.

Several maternal and fetal complications are associated with shoulder dystocia (Carlan et al., 1991). Maternal

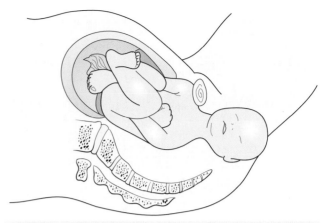

Figure 20-11 Shoulder dystocia. Impaction of the anterior shoulder against the pubic symphysis.

complications are usually a consequence of soft tissue damage. The attempt to deliver the baby can result in an extension of an episiotomy to a fourth-degree laceration, with disruption of the anal sphincter and rectal mucosa. Other complications include hemorrhage secondary to uterine atony, vaginal lacerations, and, rarely, uterine rupture.

Fetal complications tend to be more profound. Brachial plexus injury can occur. Most resolve within 6 months with adequate physical therapy. However, the injury may persist as a source of lingering disability. Erb palsy is the most common brachial plexus injury and involves the fifth and sixth cervical roots. Klumpke palsy involves injury to the eighth cervical root and the first thoracic fibers. Clavicular fracture may occur spontaneously or intentionally and may rarely result in damage to the underlying tissue. Prolonged fetal hypoxia secondary to a delay in the delivery can result in severe neurologic damage and even death.

Conditions that predispose to development of shoulder dystocia are related to either a macrosomic fetus or a contracted pelvis. Importantly, however, approximately half of all shoulder dystocias occur with normal-weight fetuses and are unanticipated. Predisposing conditions include prepregnancy weight of greater than 180 lb, excessive maternal weight gain, a history of diabetes or abnormal glucose tolerance, advanced maternal age, or a postterm pregnancy.

The key to management of this condition is anticipation and preparation. Warning signs include a prolonged second stage of labor or use of a vacuum or forceps. When shoulder dystocia becomes apparent, a number of maneuvers can be used to disimpact the shoulder (Figure 20-12). The McRoberts maneuver is a time-honored and proven technique that is ideal in initial management (Gherman et al., 1997). It involves the flexion of the maternal thighs onto the abdomen, which increases the inlet diameter, straightens the lumbosacral lordosis, and removes the sacral prominence as a possible obstruction to delivery. This procedure is often done with suprapubic pressure to dislodge the offending shoulder from behind the maternal pubic symphysis. In contrast to suprapubic pressure, fundal pressure, which often serves to exacerbate the condition, should not be exerted. Other measures include the Woods

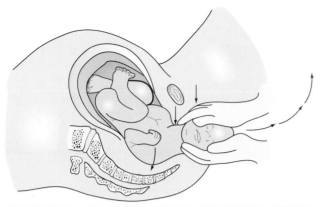

Figure 20-12 Shoulder dystocia. Release of the anterior shoulder from behind the pubic symphysis.

screw maneuver, an attempt to apply pressure to the back of the posterior shoulder to rotate the fetus, free the anterior shoulder, and attempt delivery obliquely. Alternately, delivery of the posterior arm can be attempted. Finally, as a measure of last resort, the Zavanelli maneuver, the cephalic replacement of the fetus followed by cesarean delivery, can be attempted.

Electronic Fetal Monitoring

Electronic fetal monitoring, developed at Yale University in the 1960s, was introduced into clinical practice in the early 1970s as an indirect measure of fetal oxygenation. EFM allowed the early detection of abnormal FHR patterns potentially associated with hypoxia and metabolic acidosis. Use of EFM has quickly become the standard of care for the management of high-risk pregnancies and a standard practice for low-risk pregnancies. In 2002, the National Center for Health Statistics estimated that approximately 85% of women in labor had EFM. When used, EFM is predictive of a good outcome but not accurate or predictive of a bad outcome. In other words the false-positive rate of EFM is high for predicting adverse fetal outcomes. Recognizing the limitations of this technology, the ACOG (2005) concurred that EFM appears to have no inherent benefit over auscultation properly performed in low-risk women. Furthermore, the USPSTF (1996) could not recommend its routine use for the management of low-risk deliveries.

The use of EFM is associated with an increase in the rate of surgical interventions (vacuum, forceps, cesarean delivery), increased cost, and possibly increased legal risk; however, it is not associated with a decrease in the incidence of cerebral palsy. If the monitoring is done internally, there is increased risk of uterine perforation and scalp abscess in the neonate.

The multiple reasons for EFM may be subdivided into maternal and fetal indications (Table 20-22). EFM is indicated mainly for the monitoring of high-risk patients in labor, as well as for abnormalities in structured intermittent auscultation and when inadequate staffing is available to maintain the protocol for intermittent auscultation.

Table 20-22   Indications for Electronic Fetal Monitoring

Maternal	Fetal
Hypertension	Premature rupture of membranes
Insulin-dependent diabetes	Abnormal presentation
Asthma	Prematurity
Other maternal diseases	Postdates pregnancy
Advanced maternal age	Oxytocin use
Epidural analgesia	Intrauterine growth restriction
Absence of prenatal care	Meconium
Multiple gestations	

INTERPRETATION OF FETAL HEART RATE RECORDINGS

A systematic approach in evaluation of FHR recordings is recommended to optimize interpretation. Studies have demonstrated poor reliability and consistency among various expert interpreters even in controlled settings. The initial recommendations in 1997 by a National Institute of Child Health and Human Development (NICHHD) work group have been revised and updated by a 2008 work group cosponsored by the Society for Maternal-Fetal Medicine, in part to simplify and standardize FHR interpretation (ACOG, 2009; Macones et al., 2008). Five features of the FHR that need to be assessed are baseline, variability, accelerations, decelerations and their subclassifications, and corresponding contractions. As of 2008, FHR recordings can be considered as belonging to one of three categories: normal (NICHHD category I), indeterminate (category II), and abnormal (category III). *Normal* tracings are associated with a normal pH and fetal well-being, and current management should continue. *Indeterminate* tracings and *abnormal* tracings suggest the need for further evaluation and possible intervention. This evaluation may include vaginal examination, checking maternal vital signs, giving oxygen, changing maternal position, administering fluids, scalp stimulation, and determination of scalp pH measurement. An NICHHD category II tracing represents a significant fraction of those encountered in clinical care and includes all tracings that do not belong in categories I and III. An abnormal (NICHHD III) tracing usually indicates the need for the previous measures and consideration of expedited delivery.

Baseline Fetal Heart Rate

Normal baseline FHR ranges from 110 to 160 beats/min. A baseline change is interpreted as one that persists for 10 minutes or more and occurs between or in the absence of contractions. An FHR of less than 110 beats/min is considered *bradycardia*. FHR is a function of the autonomic nervous system. Whereas the vagus nerve provides an inhibitory affect, the sympathetic nervous system provides an excitatory influence. As the gestation advances, the vagal system gains dominance, resulting in a gradual decrease in the baseline. Stressful events such as hypoxia, uterine contractions, and head compression evoke a baroreceptor reflex, with resulting peripheral vasoconstriction and hypertension causing bradycardia. Stimulation of peripheral nerve receptors can cause acceleration of FHR (Figure 20-13). An FHR baseline greater than 160 beats/min is defined as *tachycardia*. This is seen with certain

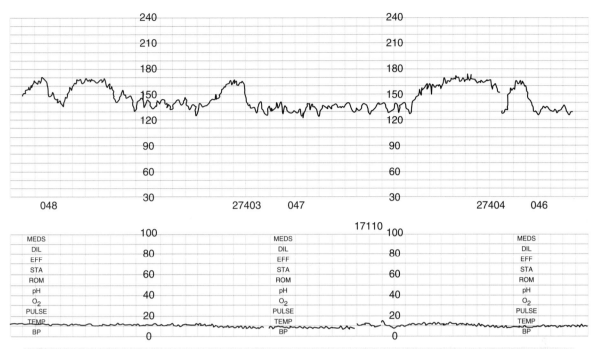

Figure 20-13 Accelerations of the fetal heart rate above a baseline rate of 130 to 140 beats/min. Good variability is present.

maternal and fetal conditions, such as chorioamnionitis, maternal fever, and fetal tachyarrhythmias.

Variability of Fetal Heart Rate

The baseline FHR fluctuates constantly under normal conditions, described as its *variability*. This variability is often a good indicator of a healthy nervous system. Variability is the oscillation of the FHR around the baseline with amplitude of 6 to 25 beats/min. Variability reflects vagal efferent impulses only. Uncomplicated loss of variability is often caused by fetal quiescence (sleep state), CNS depressants (e.g., diazepam, morphine, magnesium sulfate), or parasympatholytic agents (e.g., atropine). The uncomplicated loss of variability is associated with no risk or minimal risk of acidosis and low Apgar scores. The presence of decreased variability in combination with late or severe variable deceleration is an ominous finding. Clinically, variability is one of the most important indicators of fetal well-being, and the majority of babies with good variability do well regardless of the presence of decelerations.

Recent guidelines do not recommend the use of or differentiation between short-term and long-term variability in the assessment of fetal well-being (NICHHD, 2008). In the assessment of variability, the following categories are now recommended, reflecting the amplitude of the FHR tracing around the baseline (Figure 20-14):

- *Absent:* Amplitude range is undetectable.
- *Minimal:* Amplitude range is detectable, but 5 beats/min or less.
- *Moderate:* Amplitude is 6 to 25 beats/min.
- *Marked:* Amplitude range is greater than 25 beats/min.

Bradycardia

Bradycardia is defined as FHR less than 110 beats/min for at least 10 minutes. *Mild* bradycardia ranges between 100 and 110 beats/min. Mild bradycardia with normal variability is not associated with fetal acidosis and is considered reassuring. *Moderate* bradycardia of 80 to 100 beats/min is considered a nonreassuring pattern. Bradycardia less than 80 beats/min is considered ominous and is often a terminal event (Figure 20-15). There are numerous etiologies for fetal bradycardia (Table 20-23).

Tachycardia

Fetal tachycardia is defined as a baseline FHR of greater than 160 beats/min for at least 10 minutes. *Mild* tachycardia is a FHR of 160 to 180 beats/min; in *severe* tachycardia, the FHR is greater than 180 beats/min. Fetal tachycardia greater than 200 beats/min is usually caused by fetal tachyarrhythmia or rarely a congenital anomaly and seldom results from fetal hypoxia. There are numerous etiologies of fetal tachycardia (Table 20-24).

Accelerations

Accelerations are transitory increases in FHR associated with fetal movement, scalp or acoustic stimulation, and uterine contractions. Accelerations are considered reassuring and are associated with fetal well-being. Accelerations form the basis of a reactive NST, defined as the presence of two or more accelerations of 15 beats/min above baseline for at least 15 seconds (see Figure 20-13).

Early Decelerations

Early decelerations are caused by a vagal response to fetal head compression resulting in a slowing of FHR. These decelerations have a smooth, uniform shape that is a mirror image of the corresponding contraction. They begin with the onset of a contraction, nadir at the peak of the contraction, and promptly return to baseline. Early decelerations are considered reassuring and are associated with a good outcome.

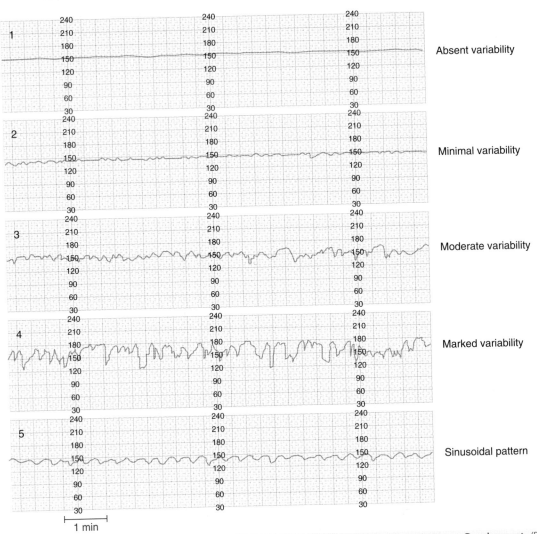

Figure 20-14 Variability in fetal heart rate (FHR). Definitions from National Institute of Child Health and Human Development. (Redrawn from Cunningham FG, Leveno KL, Bloom SL, et al. *Williams obstetrics*. 2nd ed. New York: McGraw-Hill; 2005).

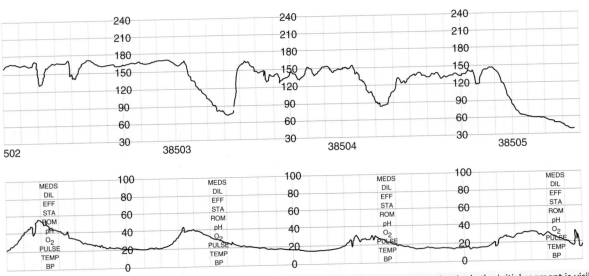

Figure 20-15 Fetal heart rate decelerations with contractions. Bradycardia occurred after the last contraction (only the initial segment is visible).

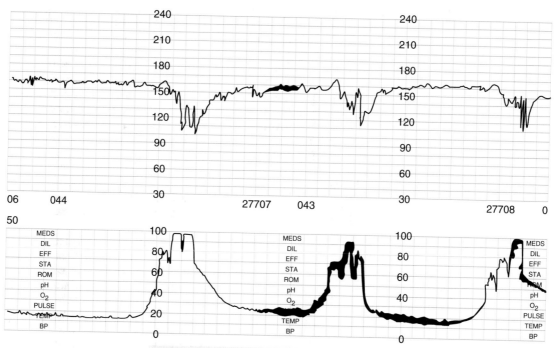

Figure 20-16 Variable decelerations of fetal heart rate.

Table 20-23	Etiology of Fetal Bradycardia

Prolonged cord compression or cord prolapse
Hypothermia
Tetanic uterine contractions
Paracervical block
Epidural and spinal analgesia
Maternal seizure
Rapid descent
Vigorous vaginal examinations
Congenital heart disease
Fetal heart block
Severe hypoxia

Table 20-24	Etiology of Fetal Tachycardia

Chorioamnionitis
Hyperthyroidism
Parasympatholytic drugs (atropine, Atarax)
Sympathomimetic drugs (terbutaline)
Fetal tachyarrhythmia
Maternal anxiety
Maternal fever
Fetal infection
Prematurity
Fetal hypoxia
Idiopathic

Variable Decelerations

Variable decelerations are characterized by an acute fall in FHR with a rapid down slope and a variable recovery. These have variable shapes, at times described as being "v," "u," or "w" (Figure 20-16). They also have a variable relationship with contractions. Variable decelerations may be classified according to their depth and duration as *mild* when the depth is greater than 80 beats/min and duration less than 30 seconds. Variable decelerations are considered *moderate* when the depth is 70 to 80 beats/min and duration is 30 to 60 seconds. Variable decelerations are *severe* when the depth is less than 70 beats/min and duration longer than 60 seconds.

Variable decelerations are the most commonly encountered pattern, occurring in 50% to 80% of all deliveries. They are almost always caused by umbilical cord compression. Variable decelerations are noted to be common with nuchal cord, a short or prolapsed cord, or when the membranes have been ruptured. Segments of FHR accelerations just before and after the variable deceleration (shoulders) indicate a healthy response.

Late Decelerations

Late decelerations are consistent with NICHHD category III, abnormal FHR tracing, and are associated with uteroplacental insufficiency. These are provoked by uterine contractions and are associated with decrease in uterine blood flow or placental dysfunction. A late deceleration is a symmetric, gradual fall in FHR beginning at or after the contraction peak, with a slow return to baseline only after the contraction has passed (Figure 20-17). Postdate gestation, preeclampsia, chronic hypertension, and diabetes mellitus are among the many causes of placental dysfunction. The management of late decelerations include turning the patient on her side to physiologically increase cardiac output and uterine blood flow, administering IV fluids to correct hypotension, discontinuing oxytocin infusion, and administering oxygen.

Sinusoidal Patterns

Sinusoidal patterns are rare but particularly ominous, belong to the NICHHD category III, and are associated with a high rate of fetal morbidity and mortality.

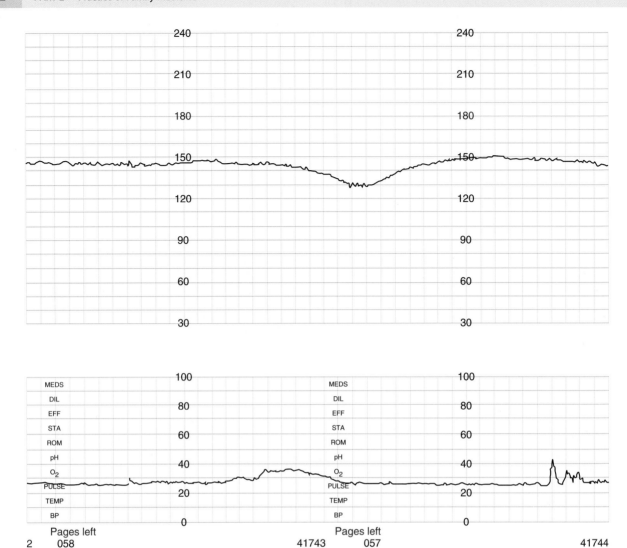

Figure 20-17 Late deceleration of fetal heart rate.

Sinusoidal patterns are characterized by a smooth, undulating, sine-wave pattern of 2 to 5 cycles/min and amplitude of 5 to 15 beats/min, with a notable absence of variability (Figure 20-18). They occur with fetal anemia or severe hypoxia and need to be differentiated from a "pseudosinusoidal" pattern, which is a benign, uniform variability pattern with the preservation of beat-to-beat variability. Sinusoidal patterns are often ominous but are occasionally seen after the administration of narcotics to the mother.

CONTRACTIONS

Contractions are classified as *normal* (no more than five contractions in a 10-minute period) or *tachysystole* (more than five contractions in a 10-minute period, averaged over a 30-minute window). The term *hyperstimulation* is no longer accepted and should be discontinued. Tachysystole is qualified by the presence or absence of decelerations, and it applies to both spontaneous and stimulated labor.

EVIDENCE-BASED SUMMARY

- The false-positive rate of EFM for predicting adverse outcomes is high (SOR: A).
- The use of EFM is associated with an increase in the rate of surgical interventions (SOR: A).
- Compared with structured intermittent auscultation, continuous EFM shows no difference in overall neonatal mortality (SOR: A).
- Continuous EFM reduces neonatal seizure rates (SOR: A).
- Fetal pulse oximetry has not shown a reduction in cesarean delivery rates (SOR: A).
- The use of EFM does not result in a reduction of cerebral palsy rates (SOR: A).
- The labor of women with high-risk conditions should be monitored continuously (SOR: B).
- Reinterpretation of the FHR tracing, especially knowing the neonatal outcome, is not reliable (SOR: B).
- The use of fetal pulse oximetry in clinical practice cannot be supported at this time (SOR: B) (East et al., 2007).

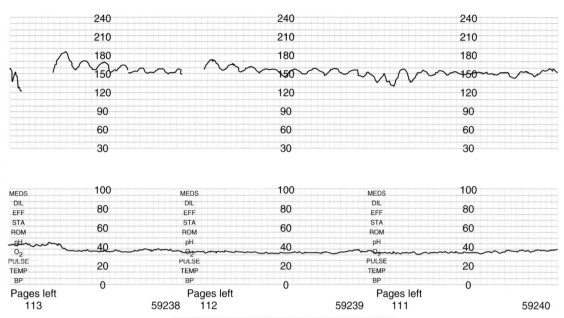

Figure 20-18 Sinusoidal fetal heart rate pattern.

Vaginal Birth after Cesarean Section

A trial of vaginal birth after a previous cesarean delivery (VBAC) is an accepted method of delivery for most women with a prior low-transverse cesarean delivery. Factors that increase morbidity in VBAC should be understood so that practical decisions can be made regarding the best route of delivery for each patient. The ACOG (2004) suggests the following criteria for selection of appropriate candidates: one previous cesarean delivery, adequate pelvis, no uterine scars, and immediate availability of both a physician to perform an emergency cesarean delivery and facilities and anesthesia to support an immediate cesarean delivery. Use of PG cervical ripening is discouraged in these women because of the small increased risk of uterine rupture associated with these medications when used with a scarred uterus.

The AAFP (2005) reviewed a trial of labor after cesarean (TOLAC) and compared TOLAC with elective repeat cesarean section (ERCS) and formulated the following recommendations:

- Most women with one previous cesarean delivery with a low-transverse incision are candidates for VBAC and should be counseled about VBAC and offered a trial of labor; epidural anesthesia may be used for VBAC (SOR: A).
- Women with a vertical incision within the lower uterine segment that does not extend into the fundus are candidates for VBAC (limited or inconsistent scientific evidence; SOR: B).
- The use of PGs for cervical ripening or induction of labor in most women with a previous cesarean delivery should be discouraged. Because uterine rupture may be catastrophic, VBAC should be attempted in institutions equipped to respond to emergencies with physicians immediately available to provide emergency care. After thorough counseling that weighs the individual benefits

and risks of VBAC, the ultimate decision to attempt this procedure or undergo a repeat cesarean delivery should be made by the patient and her physician. This discussion should be documented in the medical record. VBAC is contraindicated in women with a previous classic uterine incision or extensive transfundal uterine surgery (primarily consensus and expert opinion; SOR: C).

After careful patient selection, preparation, and management, seven or eight of 10 women with uterine scars deliver vaginally. The strongest predictor of the safety of VBAC is the location of the previous uterine scar. Safety of TOLAC in women with history of one cervical low-transverse cesarean has been documented. Rupture of these incisions is low at 0.5% (Pridjian, 1992). Information is insufficient to determine whether TOLAC is safe for VBAC candidates with two or more prior low-transverse cesarean sections, previous low-vertical incision, multiple gestation, breech presentation, or suspected macrosomia.

Oxytocin use and epidural anesthesia are not contraindicated in women attempting VBAC, although they should be used cautiously in this setting. An internal uterine pressure monitor is recommended when labor is enhanced or induced medically. The most common signs and symptoms of uterine rupture are fetal decelerations and distress, heavy vaginal bleeding, decreasing station or complete loss of the presenting part, loss of contraction intensity as documented by internal pressure monitor, uterine or pelvic pain in between contractions, and bloody urine.

Women who are most likely to have a successful VBAC are younger than 40 years old, have had one prior cesarean delivery, undergo spontaneous labor, have a baby weighing no more than 4000 g, and had a prior cesarean section that was not for failure to progress or CPD in the active phase of labor. Based on the available data, the overall outcomes from TOLAC and ERCS are so similar that the two birthing methods appear medically equivalent. As a consequence, women's preferences for the method of delivery must be explored and respected throughout pregnancy and during the delivery process. Women should be encouraged to undergo a TOLAC, but they should also have the opportunity to weigh the potential harms and benefits of TOLAC versus ERCS. A decision to have a cesarean delivery should be supported.

EVIDENCE-BASED SUMMARY

- Most women with one previous cesarean delivery with a low-transverse incision are candidates for VBAC and should be counseled about VBAC and offered a trial of labor (SOR: A).
- Epidural anesthesia may be used for VBAC (SOR: A).
- Women with a vertical incision within the lower uterine segment that does not extend into the fundus are candidates for VBAC (SOR: B).
- The use of misoprostol in women with prior cesarean delivery or major uterine surgery has been associated with an increase in uterine rupture and therefore should be avoided in the third trimester (SOR: A).
- After thorough counseling about benefits and risks of VBAC, the decision to attempt this procedure or undergo a repeat cesarean delivery should be made by the patient and her physician (SOR: C).
- VBAC is contraindicated in women with a previous classic uterine incision or extensive transfundal uterine surgery (SOR: C).

Intrapartum Procedures

OBSTETRIC ANESTHESIA

At present, many pregnant women are choosing to receive analgesia to relieve the pain of childbirth through several methods. More than 50% of women in labor are reported to choose intrapartum epidural analgesia at many U.S. institutions. This probably reflects changing societal expectations and increasing participation in the birth process on the part of both anesthesiologists and certified registered nurse anesthetists.

Pain during the first stage of labor is attributable to uterine contractions and cervical dilation. Afferent impulses from the cervix and uterus are transmitted to the spinal cord via the tenth thoracic to first lumbar (T10-L1) segments. Pain is conducted along the paracervical and inferior hypogastric plexus. During the second stage, pain also occurs from distention and stretching of pelvic structures and the perineum. Second-stage pain is principally somatic in nature and is transmitted through the spinal second to fourth sacral (S2-S4) segments.

Therapeutic modalities to manage the pain of childbirth include systemic narcotics, local anesthesia, and psychological methods (Howell, 2000). Systemic narcotics used to manage pain during labor include meperidine (Demerol, 25 mg IM or IV) and nalbuphine (Nubain, 10 mg IV). Narcotics should be avoided at or near delivery because they can cause nausea, vomiting, decreased gastric motility, and respiratory depression and can interfere with the mother's ability to concentrate and cooperate. Fetal effects include respiratory and CNS depression and temperature instability. Naloxone (0.01 mg/kg) can be administered to depressed newborn as an IV bolus for counteracting the effect of narcotics.

A pudendal block provides analgesia to the vaginal introitus and perineum. Usually done in the second stage of labor, 5 mL of 1% lidocaine is injected into the pudendal canal, the location of the pudendal nerves and vessels. Care is taken to aspirate for blood before instilling the anesthetic solution. It takes approximately 10 minutes for anesthesia to establish. Infection at the injection site, intravascular injection, and maternal overdose are the major potential complications.

Neuraxial or epidural analgesia is popular among both physicians and patients (Vincent and Chestnut, 1998). The anesthesiologist's goal for epidural analgesia during the first stage of labor is to provide segmental sensory anesthesia of the T10 to L1 dermatomes. The dose of anesthetic necessary to achieve effective labor analgesia will depend on the intensity and location of the patient's pain. These in turn depend on the amount and rate of cervical dilation; the strength, frequency, and duration of uterine contractions; and the position of the fetal head at the time epidural analgesia is placed. Typically, bupivacaine (Marcaine) or ropivacaine (Naropin), with or without a small dose of a lipid-soluble opioid such as fentanyl (Sublimaze) or sufentanil (Sufenta), establishes effective analgesia with minimal motor block. Maintenance of epidural analgesia may be achieved with intermittent bolus injections, continuous infusion, or patient-controlled dosing frequency.

Although epidural analgesia provides superior pain relief during labor, much controversy surrounds its drawbacks. These include the increased duration of labor, increased need for oxytocin augmentation, and increased rate of cesarean section for failure to progress. The most common complications, however, are maternal hypotension and headache from inadvertent puncture of the dura.

Contraindications to epidural analgesia include patient refusal, active maternal hemorrhage, maternal septicemia or untreated febrile illness, infection at or near needle insertion site, and maternal coagulopathy.

Psychological methods of pain relief include Lamaze, natural-childbirth methods, acupuncture, biofeedback, and self-hypnosis. These techniques are useful in decreasing maternal anxiety and may reduce the amount of analgesia needed.

EPISIOTOMY

An episiotomy is a surgical incision in the perineum to enlarge the introitus at delivery. Episiotomy is one of the most common medical procedures performed in the United States. There are two types of episiotomies (Figure 20-19). The midline or *median* episiotomy is the most common in the United States. It involves an incision from the posterior aspect of the vagina downward, directly toward the anus, approximately half the length of the perineum. The *mediolateral* episiotomy is a diagonal incision toward either side of the midline that is done to prevent tearing into the rectum. The mediolateral incision may serve to decrease the incidence of third- and fourth-degree extensions but is more difficult to repair and is associated with more blood

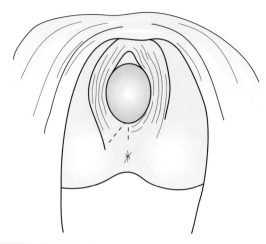

Figure 20-19 Crowning fetal head distending the perineal tissues. *Broken lines* depict the location of the incision for a midline (median) or mediolateral episiotomy.

Table 20-25 Categories of Perineal and Vaginal Lacerations

First degree	Confined to the superficial skin or mucosa; repair usually not required unless extensive or bleeding
Second degree	Involves the mucosa and deeper tissues of the vagina and perineum
Third degree	Involves the anal sphincter
Fourth degree	Involves the rectal mucosa and usually transects the anal sphincter

loss, pain, slow healing, and dyspareunia. It is performed when the fetal head is crowning 3 to 4 cm. An average incision extends 5 to 6 cm into the vagina. Lacerations and extensions of episiotomies are described according to the extent of tissue involvement (Table 20-25).

Historically, episiotomies were performed for a number of indications. These include the substitution of an anticipated ragged spontaneous laceration for a more controlled straight surgical incision, reduction in the second stage of a labor, and reduction in subsequent pelvic relaxation and trauma to pelvic musculature.

The literature since 1980 does not substantiate the alleged benefits of episiotomy (Argentine Episiotomy Trial Collaborative Group, 1993), as supported by more recent review by the Agency for Healthcare Research and Quality (Viswanathan et al., 2005). The reputed long- and short-term benefits have not been substantiated. Episiotomy is used in approximately one third of vaginal deliveries to hasten birth and prevent tearing of the perineum during delivery, but in fact it fails to accomplish any of the other maternal or fetal benefits traditionally ascribed to it (Klein, 1995). Episiotomies fail to prevent perineal damage, pelvic floor relaxation, reduction of the second stage of labor, and protection of the newborn from either intracranial hemorrhage or intrapartum asphyxia (Klein, 1995). Also, episiotomy does not protect women against urinary or fecal incontinence, pelvic organ prolapse, or difficulties in sexual function in the first 3 months to 5 years after delivery. Furthermore, in primigravid women, episiotomy appears to be causally associated with third- and fourth-degree lacerations.

In summary, episiotomy is an unproven, controversial surgical procedure best restricted to specific fetal and maternal indications. Most data do not support its routine application, making its use a decision best left to the individual physician and patient (Sleep et al., 1984).

The repair of an episiotomy should be approached with standard surgical principles. After appropriate positioning of the patient and with adequate lighting, the practitioner should determine the extent of the wound. Efforts should be made to assess the adequacy of the anesthesia. Sites of uncontrolled bleeding should be identified and hemostasis ensured. In the repair, the practitioner should aim to use the least amount of suture material possible and achieve wound approximation without dead space. Several techniques of repair are accepted. Typically, an anchoring, hemostatic stitch of an absorbable or delayed-absorbable material such as 2-0 chromic catgut or polyglycolic acid is placed at the apex of the vaginal incision, and the vaginal mucosa is approximated in a continuous interlocking fashion to the hymenal ring (Figure 20-20, A). Polyglycolic acid sutures may be superior to chromium catgut for episiotomy suturing. Compared with surgical repair using catgut or chromic suture, repair using 3-0 polyglactin 910 (Vicryl) suture results in decreased wound dehiscence and less postpartum perineal pain. This suture can then be tied or brought through to repair the deep layer of the perineum (Figure 20-20, B). The deep perineal tissues are then approximated with interrupted or continuous stitches in the muscle and fascia. Finally, the skin is approximated with a subcuticular stitch, knotted, and buried inside the vagina above the hymenal ring (Figure 20-20, C).

DIAGNOSTIC ULTRASONOGRAPHY

Ultrasonographic examination with the appropriate indication is a skill that enhances the diagnostic and therapeutic capabilities of family physicians who practice obstetrics. Even physicians who do not deliver babies are faced with clinical questions for which diagnostic ultrasonography is indicated. Studies do not support the routine use of ultrasonography in low-risk prenatal care; however, societal expectations and the relative ease of access to this technology have made it an established aspect of obstetric care. The Radius study group evaluated the use of screening ultrasonography in 15,151 low-risk pregnancies and found no difference in perinatal mortality, birth weight, or preterm birth. The study did not evaluate its use in high-risk pregnancy (Bernard et al., 1993).

Obstetric ultrasonography has numerous indications and benefits in prenatal care (Table 20-26). Benefits include estimation of fetal age through biometry (accurate to within 1 week before 20 weeks, ±2 weeks at 20-28 weeks, and ±4 weeks after 28 weeks). In the hands of an experienced ultrasonographer, the gestational sac size or the crown–rump length has proved a reliable measure of gestational age (Figure 20-21). Again, early ultrasonography may provide more accurate dating, which is important for timing screening tests and interventions and for optimal management of complications such as postterm pregnancies (Neilson, 2004). Prenatal diagnosis and evaluation of fetal anomalies, growth anomalies (e.g., size vs. date discrepancies), fetal assessment (e.g., BPP, confirmation of

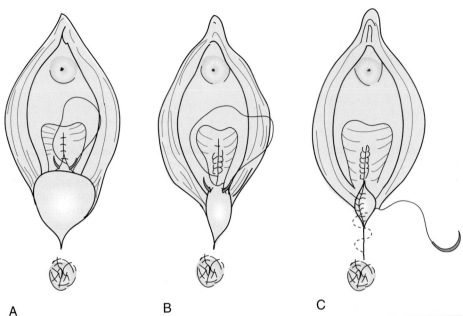

Figure 20-20 Episiotomy repair. **A,** Placement of the vaginal portion of the sutures. **B,** Deep perineal repair. **C,** Superficial perineal repair.

Table 20-26	Indications for Obstetric Ultrasound
Determination of gestational age	
Diagnosis	Suspected miscarriage or fetal demise
	Vaginal bleeding
	Pelvic pain
	Suspected multiple gestation
	Suspected hydatidiform mole
	Suspected ectopic pregnancy
	Size–date discrepancy
	Uterine or pelvic mass or abnormality
	Congenital anomalies
	Fetal presentation
Antenatal monitoring	Biophysical profile
	Intrauterine growth retardation
	Fetal macrosomia
Adjunct to obstetric procedures	Chorionic villus sampling
	Amniocentesis
	Cephalic version
ACOG recommends ultrasonography at 18 weeks for all patients	Confirm dates and fetal survey

ACOG, American College of Obstetricians and Gynecologists.

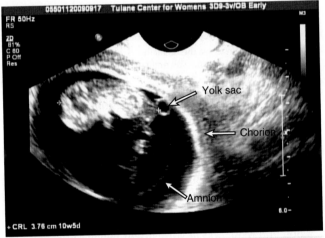

Figure 20-21 The crown–rump length (CRL) is denoted by *crosses.* Care should be taken to view the entire fetus in the midsagittal plane so as not to undermeasure. Conversely, the yolk sac is not a part of the CRL, so its inclusion will falsely increase the measurement.

fetal demise), maternal factors (e.g., diagnosis of ectopic pregnancy), and uterine anomalies are other indications and benefits.

The overuse or recreational use of ultrasound technology may pose a medical-legal risk, particularly in the hands of an inexperienced provider.

OPERATIVE VAGINAL DELIVERIES

Safe reduction of the rate of primary cesarean deliveries can be achieved by adjustments on how we manage labor and the threshold for intervention. For example, it may be necessary to revisit the definition of labor dystocia because recent data show that contemporary labor progresses at a rate that is substantially slower than what was historically taught. Additionally, improved and standardized FHR interpretation and management may have an effect. Increasing women's access to nonmedical interventions during labor, such as continuous labor and delivery support, also has been shown to reduce cesarean birth rates. External cephalic version for breech presentation and a trial of labor for women with twin gestations when the first twin is in cephalic presentation are other of several examples of interventions that can contribute to the safe lowering of the primary cesarean delivery rate.

Indications for operative vaginal delivery in a low-risk mother are nonreassuring FHR, maternal exhaustion, and prolonged second stage, which is generally 3 hours for a nulliparous woman and 2 hours for a parous woman.

Essential for safe operative vaginal delivery is optimal readiness. The laboring woman should understand the reasons why operative delivery has been chosen, with documentation in the chart. She should then be placed in a position in which her legs are maximally open, preferably in stirrups, with the perineum at the edge of the bed. Usual washing and draping are performed. The bladder is emptied. Adequate anesthesia makes placement of instruments easier and improves maternal cooperation. Pudendal block is often adequate for procedures when the fetal head is at the outlet. However, conduction anesthesia is often used. The cervix should be completely dilated and the membranes ruptured. Station, position, and attitude of the fetal head should be known. The fetal head should be engaged. Palpation, maternal sensation, or contraction monitoring can help identify the timing of contractions. Facilities for cesarean section should be available. Decision to use forceps or vacuum is based on operator skill; availability of instruments; and fetal-maternal considerations, including pelvic shape and size, fetal head position, and availability of anesthesia.

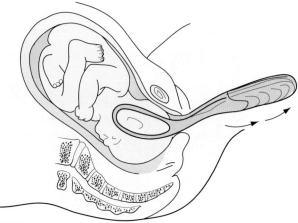

Figure 20-22 Outlet forceps delivery. The direction of traction is first downward so that the fetal head negotiates the pubic symphysis and then upward to deliver in extension.

FORCEPS DELIVERY

Currently, forceps deliveries are divided into outlet, low, mid, and high forceps, determined by the station of the fetal head. In an *outlet* forceps delivery, the fetal head has reached the pelvic floor and is seen at the introitus without separating the labia. The fetal head may be right, left, or straight occiput anterior or posterior, and delivery is accomplished without rotation of greater than 45 degrees. A *low* forceps delivery is one in which the fetal head is at least +2 cm (on a 0 to +5 cm scale of station) but not on the pelvic floor. Rotation may be greater than or less than 45 degrees. A *mid* forceps delivery occurs when the head is engaged but less than +2 cm station. A *high* forceps delivery, when the fetal head is unengaged, is no longer performed in modern obstetrics.

The choice of forceps to use is based on the operator's training and the type of forceps delivery. Typically, Simpson (or Simpson-DeLee) or Elliot forceps are used for low and outlet deliveries. After requirements for operative vaginal deliveries are met, the operator faces the maternal perineum with forceps held in the position desired. The left blade is generally placed first. The operator's right hand is fitted between the fetal head and the left vaginal side wall, and the left blade is placed by holding the handle at 12 o'clock and rotating counterclockwise as the blade slips between the fetal head and the operator's right hand. After adequate placement, the majority of the blade is no longer visible. In a similar fashion, the operator's left hand then aids in placement of the right blade. When properly placed, the handles should come together easily. Appropriate placement is then ascertained. The sagittal suture should be equidistant from both blades and perpendicular to the shanks, with the posterior fontanelle exactly between the two blades. The posterior fontanelle should be palpable about 1 fingerbreadth above the interdigitated shanks. Failure to apply the forceps symmetrically will increase risk of injury and failure of the technique.

Holding the handles together with moderate pressure, the operator rotates the fetal head if needed so that the occiput is directly anterior or posterior (sagittal suture is perpendicular to the floor). This rotation should be done during uterine muscle relaxation just before a contraction. A mild degree of flexion of the fetal head during rotation will make rotation easier. With a contraction and additional expulsive forces from the mother, the operator applies traction. Traction direction should be guided by the maternal pelvis. Initial traction is downward (toward the floor) until the fetal head clears the symphysis pubis. Then traction is directed more upward as the fetal head delivers with extension (Figure 20-22). Although in some cases early episiotomy is beneficial to forceps delivery, most often episiotomy should be cut if needed when the fetal head is bulging the perineal tissues. In many cases, removal of the forceps at this time will preclude the need for episiotomy. Removal of the forceps before delivery of the head should be in the opposite direction and order of placement. Maternal expulsive forces during a contraction can then often deliver the remainder of the fetal head. The vagina and cervix should be carefully inspected for lacerations.

VACUUM EXTRACTION

Vacuum extractors currently in widespread use in the United States are those with a soft cup made of silicone or plastic. They are smaller and more flexible than the classic Malstrom metal cup. Vacuum can be easily applied. Although these cups tend to dislodge somewhat more frequently than the Malstrom metal cup, less scalp trauma is noted with their use. Often, vacuum delivery can be performed with little to no anesthesia. However, requirements of operative vaginal delivery still apply. For the best results, the vacuum cup should be placed over the sagittal suture about 3 cm from the posterior fontanelle. This can be difficult in fetal heads descending with asynclitism (lateral deflection). After placement of the cup, an examining finger is used to ascertain that no cervical, vaginal, or perineal tissue is trapped in the cup. With a contraction, after adequate vacuum is generated, downward and then upward traction should be applied to the fetal head (Figure 20-23). The fetal head should be allowed to rotate if needed during descent. Forceful rotation of the fetal head using the suction

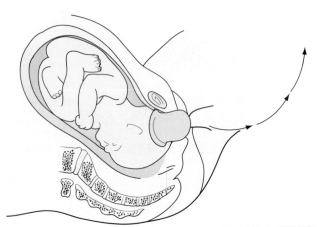

Figure 20-23 Vacuum extraction with J-shaped direction of traction, similar to forceps delivery.

cup is generally not recommended because of the increased risk of scalp injury. Removal of the cup is easily accomplished after suction is discontinued. The cervix and vagina should be examined carefully for lacerations.

The Puerperium

The postpartum period, or puerperium, is the time during which the mother's altered anatomy, physiology, and biochemistry return to the nonpregnant state. This process has its onset at the third stage of labor and is completed 6 weeks after delivery. These changes are normal and should not be confused with a pathologic condition. The woman undergoes physiologic and emotional changes that need to be monitored by her primary care physician.

Within the first 24 hours, the mother's pulse rate drops, and her temperature may be slightly elevated. Generally, the white blood cell count increases during labor, with a marked leukocytosis (to 20,000/μL) occurring in the first 24 hours postpartum. The vaginal discharge is grossly bloody (lochia rubra) for the first 3 or 4 days. During the next few to 10 days, the lochia becomes more serous and pinkish brown and decreases in amount (lochia serosa). Finally, 7 to 10 days postpartum, the lochia becomes pale yellow–white and decreases even more in volume. Urine output temporarily increases and might contain protein and sugar, reflecting a maternal diuresis. This loss of fluid with the accompanying decrease in intravascular volume artificially elevates the hematocrit for a few days. The uterus involutes progressively; after 5 to 7 days, it should be firm and nontender, extending midway between the symphysis and umbilicus. By 2 weeks, the uterus should no longer be palpable abdominally. Contractions of the involuting uterus are often painful and can require analgesics. Care should be exercised in choice of analgesia so as not to interfere with the maternal–infant bond or breastfeeding.

The mother is observed for 1 hour after completing the third stage of labor and given periodic uterine massage to make sure that the uterus contracts and remains contracted, preventing excess bleeding. If desired, breastfeeding can be initiated at this stage to promote uterine contraction, minimize bleeding, and promote involution of the uterus. If the uterus does not remain contracted with massage alone, oxytocin can be administered, either 10

units IM or dilute oxytocin with IV drip (10 or 30 U/1000 mL of IV fluid) at 125 to 200 mL/hr for 1 to 2 hours. Recent trends in the active management of labor encourage the administration of oxytocin before delivery of the placenta. This has been found to promote the delivery of the placenta and decrease the incidence of uterine atony and postpartum hemorrhage (PPH) (Prendiville et al., 2000). If general anesthesia was used for operative delivery, the mother is monitored (preferably in a recovery room or a labor, delivery, recovery, and postpartum room); oxygen and blood are tested for compatibility, and IV fluids must be readily available after delivery.

After the first 24 hours, postpartum recovery is rapid. A regular diet after a normal vaginal delivery can be offered as soon as the patient requests food. Full ambulation is encouraged as soon as possible. Showers can be encouraged, but vaginal douching is prohibited during the early postpartum period. Discomfort from an episiotomy can be relieved with hot sitz baths several times a day and analgesia. Drugs may be offered for pain as necessary but should be limited in breastfeeding mothers because most drugs are secreted in breast milk. Meperidine (Demerol) is not the preferred analgesic for use in breastfeeding women because of the long half-life of its metabolite in infants. Repeated exposure to analgesics, especially meperidine, can result in drug accumulation and toxic effects in young or compromised infants because of their underdeveloped hepatic conjugation.

Bladder care is important. Urine retention, bladder overdistention, and catheterization should be avoided if possible. Rapid diuresis can occur, especially when oxytocin is discontinued. The woman must be encouraged to void and must be monitored to prevent asymptomatic bladder overfilling. The woman should be encouraged to defecate before leaving the hospital, although with early discharge, women often leave before a bowel movement has occurred. Laxatives may be needed for constipation. If a bowel movement has not occurred within 3 days, a mild cathartic may be given. Hemorrhoids can be minimized by maintaining an appropriate diet and good bowel function and can be treated with warm sitz baths. Regional anesthesia (spinal or epidural) delays ambulation and can delay spontaneous urination. Catheterization is recommended if significant urine output is not achieved by 12 hours and a distended bladder is apparent.

A CBC should be performed before discharge to verify that the woman is not significantly anemic. Women who have been determined to be seronegative should be immunized against rubella on the day of discharge. If the woman has Rh-negative blood, is not sensitized, and has an infant with Rh-positive blood, she should be given Rh₀D immune globulin 300 μg within 72 hours of delivery to prevent sensitization.

Rh(D) blood typing and antibody testing are strongly recommended for all pregnant women during their first visit for pregnancy-related care. The USPSTF found good evidence that Rh(D) blood typing, anti-Rh(D) antibody testing, and intervention with Rh(D) immunoglobulin are appropriate, prevent maternal sensitization, and improve outcomes for newborns. The USPSTF found good evidence that Rh (D) blood typing, anti-Rh (D) antibody testing, and intervention with Rh (D) immunoglobulin, as appropriate, prevents maternal sensitization and improves outcomes for newborns. The benefits substantially outweigh any potential harms (USPSTF, 1996).

The breasts might become painfully engorged during early lactation, when the amount of milk is beginning to increase. If the mother is not going to breastfeed, lactation can be suppressed by firmly supporting the breasts because gravity stimulates the letdown reflex and encourages milk flow. Many mothers find that tight binding of the breasts and restriction of oral fluid intake followed by firm support are effective, with symptoms lasting only 3 to 5 days.

The postpartum period can be complicated by the "baby blues," a common, self-limited mood disorder. This is characterized by mild depressive symptoms, tearfulness (often for no discernible reason), anxiety, irritability, mood lability, increased sensitivity, and fatigue. The "blues" typically peak 4 to 5 days after delivery, can last hours to days, and usually resolve by the 10th postnatal day.

The "blues" is distinct from postpartum major depression, which occurs in approximately 10% of childbearing women (O'Hara et al., 1990). It can begin from 24 hours to several months after delivery. Its onset can be abrupt and symptoms severe, and it can be associated with a lack of interest in the infant, suicidal or homicidal thoughts, hallucinations, or psychotic behavior. True psychosis probably reflects the exacerbation of preexisting mental illness in response to the physical and psychological stress of pregnancy and delivery. Psychotherapy or pharmacotherapy is indicated, alone or in combination. Selective serotonin reuptake inhibitors may be associated with congenital heart anomalies and should be used with caution in pregnancy. All women should be routinely assessed during the antenatal period for a history of depression.

Prevention of pregnancy for several months to allow complete recovery is in the woman's best interest. *Rubella immunization mandates a delay of 3 months before a woman becomes pregnant.* Therefore, although intercourse may be resumed as soon as desired and comfortable, contraception is required because pregnancy is possible. Oral contraceptives may be started at discharge. A low-dose estrogen or progesterone-only preparation is desirable. A diaphragm should be fitted only after complete involution of the uterus at 6 to 8 weeks; meanwhile, foams, jellies, and condoms may be used. In mothers who are not breastfeeding, earliest ovulation usually occurs about 4 weeks postpartum, 2 weeks before the first menses. However, conception has been reported as early as 2 weeks postpartum, so ovulation can occur earlier. Breastfeeding mothers tend to ovulate and then menstruate, usually at 10 to 12 weeks postpartum. The duration of anovulation is influenced by the frequency of breastfeeding, the duration of feedings, and the proportions of supplemental feeding.

Postpartum Hemorrhage

Traditionally, PPH was defined as blood loss greater than 500 mL in a vaginal delivery and greater than 1000 mL in a cesarean delivery. However, studies have revealed that an uncomplicated delivery often results in blood loss of more than 500 mL without any compromise of the mother's condition (Pritchard et al., 1962). Clinically, these findings led some authors to adopt a broader definition for PPH. Any bleeding that results in signs and symptoms of hemodynamic instability or bleeding that could result in hemodynamic instability if untreated is considered PPH. The loss of these amounts within 24 hours of delivery is termed *early* or *primary* PPH, and such losses are termed *late* or *secondary* PPH if they occur 24 hours after delivery or later. This section focuses primarily on early PPH.

The most common causes of PPH are uterine atony and lacerations of the vagina and cervix. Other causes include retained placental fragments, lower genital tract lacerations, uterine rupture or inversion, placenta accreta, and hereditary coagulopathy. Causes of late PPH (24 hours to 6 weeks after delivery) include infection, placental site subinvolution, retained placental fragments, and hereditary coagulopathy (ACOG, 1998a).

Risk factors for uterine atony include uterine overdistention secondary to hydramnios, multiple gestation, use of oxytocin, fetal macrosomia, high parity, rapid or prolonged labor, intraamniotic infection, and use of uterine-relaxing agents (Combs et al., 1991). Uterine rupture occurs in approximately one in 2000 deliveries. Previous uterine surgery is a significant risk factor for uterine rupture, placenta accreta, and PPH. Other risk factors include obstructed labor, multiple gestations, abnormal fetal lie, and high parity.

Risk factors for hemorrhage at the time of cesarean delivery include preeclampsia, disorders of active labor, a history of previous hemorrhage, obesity, use of general anesthesia, and intraamniotic infection.

Adequate intravascular access should be obtained in women who have significant risk factors for PPH. Active management of the third stage of labor has been shown to decrease the incidence of PPH. Early administration of oxytocin, early cord cutting and clamping, and controlled cord traction have been shown to decrease PPH by two thirds (Soriano et al., 1996).

In the event of hemorrhage, supplemental oxygen should be administered to enhance cellular oxygen delivery. Heart rate and BP should be monitored closely. Initial laboratory evaluation includes a CBC with platelet concentration. Blood type and crossmatch should be performed if not previously obtained. Fibrinogen, fibrin split products, prothrombin time, and partial thromboplastin time should be measured (ACOG, 1998a).

Excessive vaginal bleeding after placental delivery should prompt vigorous fundal massage while the patient is rapidly given 10 to 30 units of oxytocin in 1 L of IV fluid. If the fundus does not become firm, uterine atony is the presumed (and most common) diagnosis. Uterine atony should be initially managed by bimanual uterine massage and compression in addition to the oxytocin. If IV or IM oxytocin proves ineffective, other uterotonic agents, such as methylergonovine and PG derivatives (15-methyl PGF$_2\alpha$), may be used as second-line treatment (ACOG, 1998a). Methylergonovine may be administered at 0.2 mg IM every 2 to 4 hours. Methylergonovine can cause cramping, headache, and dizziness. This agent is contraindicated in hypertensive disease states because it induces vasoconstriction, which can lead to severe hypertension.

15-Methyl PGF$_2\alpha$ (Hemabate), may be given in a dose of 0.25 mg IM every 15 to 90 minutes (no more than eight doses). PGF$_2\alpha$ may also be given by intramyometrial injection at cesarean delivery or transabdominally after vaginal delivery. PGE$_2$ can cause vasodilation and exacerbation of hypotension; therefore, 15-methyl PGF$_2\alpha$ is preferred. Because oxygen desaturation has been reported with use of PGF$_2\alpha$, patients should be monitored by pulse oximetry.

Continuing hemorrhage in a patient with a firm uterine fundus can indicate a hidden vaginal or cervical laceration. This type of injury is usually easy to identify and repair with adequate lighting, exposure, and assistance. If no laceration is present and the fundus is firm, the uterus requires gentle but thorough manual exploration for retained placenta, which should be removed. Uterine rupture is occasionally evident and requires immediate surgery.

An occult uterine inversion might also be discovered on vaginal examination, or it can manifest frankly. Uterine inversion is somewhat more common in primiparas and has no clear association with the mismanagement of labor. Because uterine inversion can quickly lead to shock, the physician should order brisk IV hydration and grasp the uterus in the palm, with the thumb anterior. The uterus is then firmly pushed back up into the abdominal cavity and held in place for several minutes (Brar et al., 1989). Magnesium sulfate, 0.25 mg IV, has been reported to assist in the repositioning of the uterus (Catanzarite et al., 1986).

If uterine and vaginal exploration is nondiagnostic, uterine inversion is excluded, and the fundus is firm, rarer causes of hemorrhage should be considered. Puerperal *hematomas* typically cause a vulvar or vaginal mass, and an occult retroperitoneal hematoma can manifest with severe abdominal pain and shock after delivery. The diagnosis is confirmed on laparotomy. Visible hematomas smaller than 4 cm and not expanding may be managed with ice packs and observation. Larger or expanding hematomas must be incised, irrigated, and packed, and any obvious bleeding vessels must be ligated. If venipuncture sites are oozing, coagulopathy should be considered.

Surgical intervention is undertaken for direct indications, such as uterine curettage for suspected retained placental tissue or for hemostasis if medical therapy fails. The most common indications for emergency hysterectomy include uterine atony, placenta accreta, uterine rupture, and the extension of a low-transverse uterine incision.

KEY TREATMENT

- Uterotonic agents should be the first-line treatment for PPH caused by uterine atony (SOR: C).
- Management of PPH may vary greatly among patients, depending on the etiology and available treatment options, and often a multidisciplinary approach is required (SOR: C).
- When uterotonics fail after vaginal delivery, exploratory laparotomy is the next step (SOR: C).
- In the presence of conditions known to be associated with placenta accreta, the obstetric care provider must have a high clinical suspicion and take appropriate precautions (SOR: C).

Videos

The following videos are available at www.expertconsult.com:

Video 20-1 Repair of Vaginal Tears: 1st and 2nd Degree

Video 20-2 Repair of Vaginal Tears: 3rd and 4th Degree

References

The complete reference list is available online at https://expertconsult.inkling.com.

Web Resources

www.aafp.org American Academy of Family Physicians. Includes continuing medical education opportunities, clinical information, and links to the American Family Physician, Family Practice Management, and the Annals of Family Medicine.

www.ahrq.gov Agency for Healthcare Research and Quality. Contains clinical information, research findings, survey data, and funding opportunities.

www.guideline.gov U.S. federal health guidelines. Contains links to a variety of medical care and evidence-based guidelines for many clinical problems, in addition to obstetrics.

www.marchofdimes.com/peristats Excellent source of free access to national, state, and city maternal and infant health data; includes graphs, quick facts, maps, and state summaries.

www.uptodate.com Subscription program offering clinical information focused on primary care but also including a variety of other clinical specialties.

21 Care of the Newborn

SHERIN E. WESLEY, ERIN ALLEN, and HEATHER BARTSCH

The birth of a child is an exciting and, at times, overwhelming experience for parents. Family physicians are in a unique position because they have the opportunity to care for both the expectant mother and the newborn. They are able to provide anticipatory guidance to the mother early in the pregnancy and continued support after delivery of the newborn. They are familiar with the details of the mother's pregnancy and delivery as well as the family environment that the newborn will enter. The physician will have established rapport with the expectant parents, which will be useful when giving advice in the care of the newborn. In a world where health care is increasingly fragmented, parents will be relieved to know their doctor can provide comprehensive and integrated medical care to all family members.

Care at Delivery

Key Points

- For most infants, the transition to the extrauterine environment involves little resuscitation. Infants who are premature, born via cesarean section, or have congenital anomalies may have difficulty transitioning and have increased resuscitation needs.
- Airway, breathing, and circulation are the key principles of neonatal resuscitation.
- A term, vigorous infant is one who is breathing and crying at birth with a strong respiratory effort, has a heart rate greater than 100 beats/min, and has good muscle tone.
- Fetal and maternal factors can predict a high-risk delivery where a practitioner trained in neonatal care and resuscitation should be present.
- Intramuscular vitamin K is administered to all newborns at birth to prevent hemorrhagic disease of the newborn.
- Erythromycin 0.5% ophthalmic ointment is applied to the eyes of all newborns to prevent gonococcal ophthalmia neonatorum.
- If a two-vessel umbilical cord is detected after birth, the infant should be carefully examined for syndromic features and anatomic abnormalities.

PHYSIOLOGIC TRANSITION

At birth, a newborn undergoes a rapid physiologic transition to the extrauterine environment. This transition is a complex interaction among multiple organ systems, including the cardiovascular, pulmonary, neurologic, and endocrine systems.

The placenta is responsible for oxygenation of fetal blood. The fetal circulation acts in parallel through three shunts: the ductus venosus, the ductus arteriosus, and the foramen ovale. Figure 21-1 illustrates the fetal circulation. The umbilical vein returns oxygenated blood from the placenta to the liver of the fetus. A portion of the blood from the umbilical vein is shunted directly to the inferior vena cava away from the liver via the ductus venosus. From the inferior vena cava, oxygenated blood flows into the right atrium. Because the pressure in the right atrium is greater, most of this blood is shunted through the foramen ovale into the left atrium to be distributed to the brain and coronary arteries via the aorta. Blood returns from the head by way of the superior vena cava to the right atrium. It flows into the pulmonary artery from the right ventricle, and via the ductus arteriosus, most of this blood reenters the descending aorta, where it is distributed to the body and lower extremities. Deoxygenated blood containing waste products and carbon dioxide then leaves the fetus via the umbilical arteries to be disposed of by the mother.

As the neonate takes his or her first breath at delivery, pulmonary vascular resistance falls, pulmonary blood flow increases, and the oxygen saturation of the blood increases. Clearance of fetal lung fluid and surfactant production is important for the expansion of the lungs. Surfactant production, which begins at 24 to 28 weeks of gestation, decreases surface tension in the alveoli and allows for lung expansion. The mechanism and timing of the clearance of fetal lung fluid is not entirely understood. Previously, mechanical forces such as vaginal squeeze and Starling's forces were hypothesized to be the major factors in clearing fetal lung fluid (Jain et al., 2006). Studies have shown that clearance of fetal lung fluid is also dependent on termination of the chloride-mediated channels that secrete fluid and activation of the basal Na-K+ ATPase channels on type II cells of airway epithelium to resorb fluid (Jain et al., 2006). Elevated levels of cortisol, thyroid hormones, and

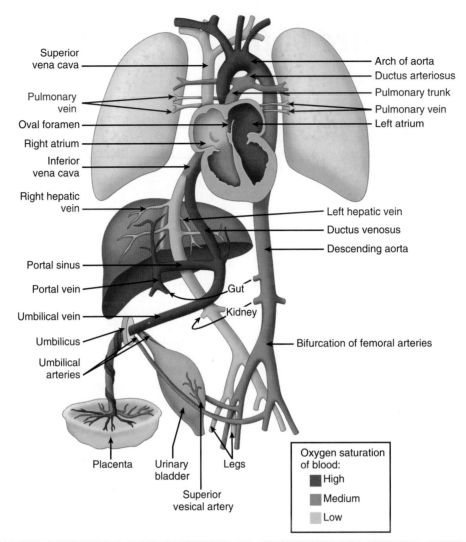

Superior
vena cava

Pulmonary
vein

Oval foramen

Right atrium

Inferior
vena cava

Right hepatic
vein

Portal sinus

Portal vein

Umbilical vein

Umbilicus

Umbilical
arteries

Arch of aorta

Ductus arteriosus

Pulmonary trunk

Pulmonary vein

Left atrium

Left hepatic vein

Ductus venosus

Descending aorta

Gut

Kidney

Bifurcation of femoral arteries

Placenta

Urinary
bladder

Legs

Superior
vesical artery

Oxygen saturation
of blood:
High
Medium
Low

Figure 21-1 **Prenatal and postnatal circulation.** (Used with permission from Florin T, Ludwig S, Aronson PL, Werner HC, eds. *Netter's pediatrics*. Philadelphia: Elsevier; 2011.)

catecholamines in the fetus and neonate also play a role in clearing fluid from the lungs (Hillman et al., 2012; Jain et al, 2006; Liggins, 1994). In addition, initiation of continuous breathing by activation of the respiratory center in the brainstem is critical to survival of the neonate.

With the cutting of the umbilical cord, the peripheral vascular resistance of the neonate increases, and without a blood supply, the ductus venosus closes functionally within minutes after birth and structurally within the first week of life. As pulmonary vascular resistance decreases secondary to the expansion of the lungs and oxygenation of blood, the pulmonary blood flow to the left atria increases, which in turn increases left atrial blood pressure. Because the left atrial pressure now exceeds that of the right atria, the foramen ovale closes. The ductus arteriosus constricts after birth secondary to increased oxygen saturation of the blood as well as in response to decreased blood flow. With the closure of the fetal cardiac shunts, the circulation functions like that of an adult.

For a full term, normal newborn, this transition occurs rapidly with little resuscitation required aside from standard drying, stimulation, and clearance of the airway.

Preterm infants, infants with congenital anomalies of the heart or lungs, infants of mothers with diabetes, and infants born via cesarean section may struggle with the transition to the extrauterine environment and have increased resuscitation needs.

RESUSCITATION OF THE NEONATE

After delivery, evaluating the neonate's airway, breathing, and circulation will allow the practitioner to determine the resuscitation needs of the newborn. At every delivery, a staff member trained in the resuscitation of neonates should be designated to care for the neonate. Supporting staff members, who will aid in resuscitating the neonate, should also be trained. The American Heart Association (AHA) and American Academy of Pediatrics (AAP) offer a course in the resuscitation of neonates called the Neonatal Resuscitation Program (NRP). The algorithm in Figure 21-2 provides a brief summary of the steps needed to resuscitate a neonate, but it does not replace taking the course and becoming certified in neonatal resuscitation. Resuscitation equipment should be easily accessible, and if

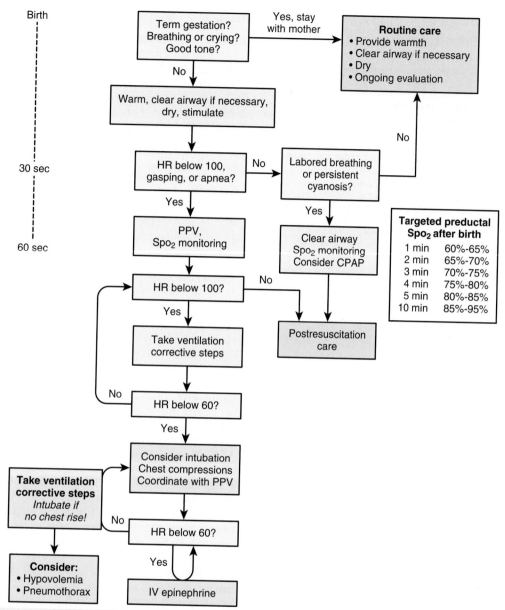

Figure 21-2 Algorithm for neonatal resuscitation. (Used with permission from Kattwinkel J, Perlman JM, Aziz K, et al; American Heart Association. Neonatal resuscitation: 2010 American Heart Association Guidelines for Cardiopulmonary Resuscitation and Emergency Cardiovascular Care. *Pediatrics.* 2010;126:e1400-e1413. American Academy of Pediatrics. 2010.)

a neonate is at high risk for complications, the equipment should be assembled and tested before delivery (Table 21-1).

ASSESSMENT OF THE NEONATE

A term infant with clear amniotic fluid who is vigorous (breathing or crying at birth with a strong respiratory effort, heart rate greater than 100 beats/min, and good muscle tone) can be returned to the mother after being dried for skin-to-skin contact and to breastfeed. Breastfeeding should start as soon as possible after birth, preferably within the first hour after delivery.

If the infant is not breathing or crying, the infant is placed under a warmer on his or her back with the neck slightly extended. This position facilitates air entry by aligning the posterior pharynx, larynx, and trachea (Kattwinkel,

2011). Next, the airway is cleared using bulb suction or a large-bore suction catheter. Simultaneously, the newborn is dried. The act of drying and suctioning also provides stimulation to the infant. Additional techniques for providing tactile stimulation include using the fingers to flick the soles of the feet and rubbing the newborn's back, trunk or extremities gently with the hand. Heart rate, respiratory rate, and color of the newborn are then assessed, and the resuscitation algorithm is followed as outlined in Figure 21-2.

NEONATE WITH MECONIUM-STAINED FLUID

Infants with meconium-stained fluid who are not vigorous (poor muscle tone, heart rate less than 100 beats/min, and poor respiratory effort) should be temporarily intubated

Table 21-1   Neonatal Resuscitation Supplies and Equipment for Delivery of a Term Infant

Suction equipment	Bulb syringe Mechanical suction and tubing Suction catheters 8-Fr feeding tube and 20-mL syringe Meconium aspirator
Bag and mask equipment	Neonatal resuscitation bag with a pressure-release valve or pressure manometer Face masks, newborn and premature sizes Oxygen source with flow meter and tubing
Medications and supplies to be immediately available if necessary	Epinephrine 1:10,000 Isotonic crystalloid for volume expansion Sodium bicarbonate 4.2% Naloxone hydrochloride (0.4 mg/mL) Dextrose 10% Normal saline for flushes Umbilical vessel catheterization supplies Syringes and needles
Miscellaneous	Gloves and appropriate personal protection Radiant warmer or other heat source Firm, padded resuscitation surface Clock Warmed linens and dry blankets Stethoscope Oropharyngeal airways
Intubation equipment	Laryngoscope with straight blades, no. 1 Extra bulbs and batteries for laryngoscope Endotracheal (ET) tubes, sizes 2.5, 3.0, 3.5, and 4.0 mm Materials to secure ET tube in place CO_2 detector

Modified from Kattwinkel J, ed. *Textbook of neonatal resuscitation.* 6th ed. Elk Grove Village, IL: American Academy of Pediatrics and American Heart Association; 2011.

Table 21-2   The Apgar Score*

Sign	Score*		
	0	**1**	**2**
Heart rate	Absent	<100 beats/min	≥100 beats/min
Respirations	Absent	Irregular and slow	Strong breaths, crying
Muscle tone	Limp	Some flexion	Good flexion, active motion
Reflex irritability to tactile stimulation	No response	Grimace	Cough, sneeze, cry,
Color	Blue or pale	Blue extremities, pink body	Completely pink

*The infant's Apgar score should be assessed at 1 and 5 minutes. A score of 7 to 10 is considered normal. A score of less than 7 should be repeated at 5-minute intervals up to 20 minutes while resuscitation efforts continue. Resuscitation of the neonate should not be interrupted to assign the Apgar score.

Modified from Kattwinkel J, ed. *Textbook of neonatal resuscitation.* 6th ed. Grove Village, IL: American Academy of Pediatrics and American Heart Association; 2011.

with an endotracheal tube and meconium should be aspirated from the airway if present. If an infant with meconium-stained fluid is vigorous, the mouth and nose should be cleared of meconium using bulb suction or a large-bore catheter. The infant can then be dried and returned to the mother for bonding and breastfeeding.

HIGH RISK DELIVERIES

Fetal and maternal factors can predict a high-risk delivery. Fetal factors include prematurity, gestational age greater than 42 weeks, multiple gestations, meconium-stained fluid, nonreassuring fetal heart tones, abnormal presentation (e.g., breech), and congenital anomalies. Maternal factors include diabetes, hypertension, substance abuse, advanced maternal age, placental anomalies, and chorioamnionitis (Kattwinkel, 2011). A team of health care providers who are trained in neonatal resuscitation and competent in resuscitating and stabilizing a neonate should be present at high-risk deliveries. If a high-risk delivery is anticipated, transfer to a hospital with a perinatal center is recommended before delivery.

THE APGAR SCORE

The Apgar score, devised by Virginia Apgar in 1952, is a tool that provides a standard method to assess the physical condition of newborns immediately after birth. It can also be used to assess an infant's response to resuscitation. The heart rate, respiratory effort, muscle tone, response to stimuli, and color are assessed at 1 and 5 minutes. Zero to two points are awarded in each category (Table 21-2). A score of 7 to 10 is considered normal. A score of less than 7 should be repeated at 5-minute intervals up to 20 minutes (AAP, 2006). Assessment of the newborn's airway, breathing, and circulation should not be delayed for calculation of the Apgar score. The Apgar score can be affected by gestational age, maternal medications, neurologic and cardiorespiratory conditions, trauma, infection, and ongoing resuscitation efforts (Freeman et al., 1988). A low Apgar score (0-3) has not been shown to predict neurologic outcome nor can a low score be used to determine if a hypoxic event occurred in utero (AAP, 2006). Some evidence suggests that a score of 0 to 3 at 5 minutes may correlate with neonatal death (Casey et al., 2001).

ASSESSMENT OF GROWTH PARAMETERS AND GESTATIONAL AGE

The length, weight, and head circumference of the infant should be measured and plotted on growth charts. The infant is then characterized as large, small, or appropriate for gestational age based on these measurements. The length, weight, and head circumference of appropriate for gestational age infants (AGA) fall between the 10th and 90th percentiles for age. Infants with growth parameters less than the 10th percentile for age are classified as small for gestational age (SGA) and may have complications after birth, including temperature instability and hypoglycemia. Large-for-gestational-age (LGA) infants whose growth parameters are greater than the 90th percentile for age are often born to mothers with uncontrolled diabetes, and these infants are also at risk for hypoglycemia after birth.

Gestational age is assessed using the new Ballard score. In the new Ballard score (Figure 21-3), the neuromuscular

NEUROMUSCULAR MATURITY

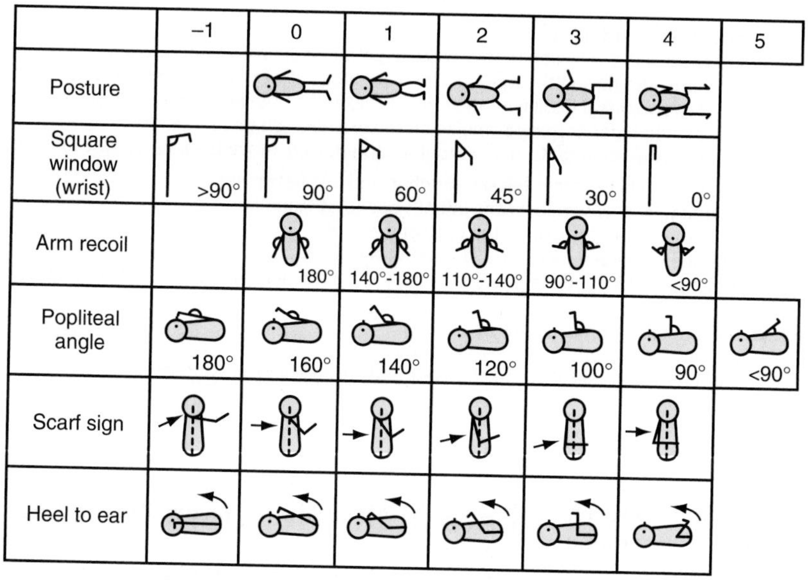

	−1	0	1	2	3	4	5
Posture							
Square window (wrist)	>90°	90°	60°	45°	30°	0°	
Arm recoil		180°	140°-180°	110°-140°	90°-110°	<90°	
Popliteal angle	180°	160°	140°	120°	100°	90°	<90°
Scarf sign							
Heel to ear							

MATURITY RATING

Score	Weeks
−10	20
−5	22
0	24
5	26
10	28
15	30
20	32
25	34
30	36
35	38
40	40
45	42
50	44

PHYSICAL MATURITY

Skin	Sticky; friable; transparent	Gelatinous; red; translucent	Smooth; pink; visible veins	Superficial peeling and/or rash; few veins	Cracking; pale areas; rare veins	Parchment; deep cracking; no vessels	Leathery; cracked; wrinkled
Lanugo	None	Sparse	Abundant	Thinning	Bald areas	Mostly bald	
Plantar surface	Heel-toe 40-50 mm: -1 <40 mm: -2	>50 mm; no crease	Faint red marks	Anterior transverse crease only	Creases ant. 2/3	Creases over entire sole	
Breast	Imperceptible	Barely perceptible	Flat areola; no bud	Stippled areola; 1-2 mm bud	Raised areola; 3-4 mm bud	Full areola; 5-10 mm bud	
Eye/ear	Lids fused loosely: -1 tightly: -2	Lids open; pinna flat; stays folded	Sl. curved pinna; soft; slow recoil	Well-curved pinna; soft but ready recoil	Formed & firm; instant recoil	Thick cartilage; ear stuff	
Genitals male	Scrotum flat; smooth	Scrotum empty; faint rugae	Testes in upper canal; rare rugae	Testes descending; few rugae	Testes down; good rugae	Testes pendulous; deep rugae	
Genitals female	Clitoris prominent; labia flat	Prominent clitoris; small labia minora	Prominent clitoris; enlarging minora	Majora & minora equally prominent	Majora large; minora small	Majora covers clitoris & minora	

Figure 21-3 Maturational assessment of gestational age using the new Ballard score. See Table 21-3 for a description of the new Ballard examination technique. (From Ballard JL, Khoury JC, Wedig K, et al. New Ballard score, expanded to include extremely premature infants. *J Pediatr.* 1991;119:417-423.)

and physical maturity of the neonate is evaluated. The scores for each are summed, and a table is used to determine the gestational age based on the score. Table 21-3 explains the examination for the new Ballard score in detail. If there is a discrepancy of greater than 1 week between the gestational age by dates versus the gestational age by exam, the earlier gestational age should be used. A head-to-toe examination of the neonate should be performed within 24 hours of delivery. Detailed information on this examination is provided in the next section, "Care in the Newborn Nursery."

ROUTINE CARE AT DELIVERY

After delivery, the umbilical cord is clamped and cut. The timing of cord clamping after delivery is not standardized. Current evidence is insufficient to support early (within 15-20 seconds after birth) versus delayed (30-60 seconds after birth) clamping in term infants (American College of Obstetricians and Gynecologists [ACOG], 2012). The number of arteries and veins in the umbilical cord should be counted after the cord is clamped. The umbilical cord normally contains two arteries and one vein. A single

Table 21-3 Examination for the New Ballard Score

Neuromuscular maturity	*Posture:* Assign score when infant is relaxed and quiet. *Square window:* Measure the angle of the wrist in flexion between the hypothenar eminence and the forearm. *Arm recoil:* Score the position of the arm after flexing the forearms for 5 seconds, fully extending the arm and releasing quickly. *Popliteal angle:* Measure the angle of the popliteal fossil with the hip fully flexed and the knee extended with gentle pressure. *Scarf sign:* Maneuver arm over opposite shoulder keeping scapulae on the examination table. *Heel to ear:* Keeping the pelvis on the examination table and without forcing the leg, move the infant's foot toward the head.
Physical maturity	*Skin:* With increasing gestational age, the skin becomes thicker, tougher, and less transparent. *Lanugo:* Describe the fine, downy lanugo hair as seen over the infant's back and scapulae. *Plantar surface of foot:* Measure from the tip of great toe to the back of the heel. *Breast tissue:* Describe nipple size, stage of development, and amount of breast tissue. *Eyes and ears:* Loosely fused eyelids open with gentle traction; the pinna in a term infant is well formed and quickly recoils after bending. *Genitalia:* Describe the development of the external genitalia.

Modified from Tureen PJ, Deacon J, Hernandez JA, et al. *Assessment and care of the well newborn.* 2nd ed. Philadelphia: Saunders; 2005.

umbilical artery typically is an isolated finding; however, it has been associated with chromosomal and anatomic abnormalities (Granese et al., 2007). If a two-vessel cord is detected with a prenatal ultrasonography, the heart and kidneys should also be imaged (Dagklis et al., 2010; Pursutte and Hobbins, 1995). If anomalies are present, the mother should be offered fetal karyotype analysis. If a two-vessel cord is detected after delivery, the infant should be carefully examined for syndromic features and anatomic abnormalities.

Additional measures taken at birth to care for the newborn include administration of vitamin K and prophylactic ocular topical medication. At birth, newborn infants are given 0.5 to 1.0 mg of vitamin K intramuscularly to prevent early and late hemorrhagic disease of the newborn. All infants are born vitamin K deficient (Zipursky, 1999). Additional factors that place newborns at risk for hemorrhagic disease include lower stores of vitamin K in the liver, low levels of vitamin K in breast milk, and the short half-life of vitamin K (Loughnan et al., 1996). Intramuscular vitamin K has been shown to be more effective at preventing late hemorrhagic disease than oral administration of vitamin K (Zipursky, 1999).

To prevent gonococcal ophthalmia neonatorum, erythromycin 0.5% ophthalmic ointment is routinely applied to both eyes of all newborns. Gonococcal ophthalmia neonatorum can result in corneal scarring, ocular perforation, and blindness. Gonococcal ophthalmia neonatorum develops in 28% of infants born to women infected with gonorrhea (U.S. Preventive Services Task Force [USPSTF], 2012). Silver nitrate 1.0% solution and tetracycline 1.0% ointment can also be used but are no longer available in the United States. Prophylaxis should be applied within the first 24 hours of life.

KEY TREATMENT

- Intramuscular vitamin K administered to all newborns at birth prevents hemorrhagic disease of the newborn (Zipursky, 1999) (SOR: A).
- Erythromycin 0.5% ophthalmic ointment applied to the eyes of all newborns prevents gonococcal ophthalmia neonatorum (USPSTF, 2012) (SOR: A).

Care in the Newborn Nursery

INITIAL NEWBORN EVALUATION AND COMMON PHYSICAL EXAMINATION FINDINGS

Key Points

- A complete head-to-toe examination of the newborn should be completed within the first 24 hours of life to identify any potential physical abnormalities or medical problems.
- Periodic breathing is a normal finding in the newborn, characterized by an irregular breathing pattern.
- Grunting may be present during the first hour of life as fetal lung fluid is cleared, but persistent evidence of respiratory distress requires further evaluation.
- Soft systolic murmurs may be present in the first 24 hours of life because of delayed closure of the ductus arteriosus or peripheral pulmonary stenosis.
- Molding and overriding sutures are common findings in newborns because of the compression of the head through the birth canal.
- Milky, white, or blood-tinged vaginal discharge is common in the first few weeks of life because of withdrawal of maternal hormones.
- The hips should be carefully examined with the Ortolani and Barlow maneuvers for signs of dislocation.
- Benign skin lesions are common and require appropriate education and reassurance of the parent.

Within the first 24 hours of life, a complete history and physical examination of the infant should be completed. The newborn history should review all components of the pregnancy, labor, and delivery. Gathering a complete maternal history, including a review of the mother's medical problems; past obstetric history; medications, drug, alcohol, or tobacco use during pregnancy; and prenatal serologies is important. Delivery complications and neonatal resuscitation measures should also be noted. The examination is best performed if the infant is quietly resting and should begin with an assessment of the infant's general appearance followed by auscultation of the heart and lungs. The examination should then proceed from head to toe in a systematic

Table 21-4 Vital Signs in the First Days of Life

Vital Sign	Normal Value
Heart rate	100-180 beats/min
Respiratory rate	24-60 beats/min
Systolic blood pressure	65-90 mm Hg
Diastolic blood pressure	50-70 mm Hg
Temperature	<100.4°F (38.0°C) and >96.8°F (36.0°C)

Data from Gunn VL, Nechyba C. *The Harriet Lane handbook*. 16th ed. St Louis: Mosby; 2002; Rudolph AM, Kamei RK, Sagan P. *Rudolph's fundamentals of pediatrics*. 2nd ed. Norwalk, CT: Appleton & Lange; 1998.

fashion. The following sections describe how to perform each portion of the physical examination in an infant as well as normal and abnormal findings that may be present in the examination.

General Appearance

The examination should begin with a general assessment of the infant's respiratory effort, position, level of activity, and color. A healthy infant should breathe comfortably with no respiratory distress. *Periodic breathing* is characterized by an irregular breathing pattern consisting of rapid breaths intermixed with short pauses lasting 5 to 10 seconds and is considered a normal finding in newborns. A normal newborn rests with his or her extremities flexed and should appear pink. A bluish discoloration of the hands and feet, known as *acrocyanosis*, is common. Central cyanosis, pallor, jaundice, or a ruddy complexion signals underlying medical problems. Table 21-4 lists normal vital signs for a term infant. An infant's weight, length, and head circumference should also be reviewed and plotted on standard growth charts.

Head and Face

Examination of the head should include observation of the head shape and size and palpation of the anterior and posterior fontanels and cranial sutures. The anterior fontanel is located at the juncture of the metopic, sagittal, and coronal sutures, and the posterior fontanel is located at the juncture of the sagittal and lambdoid sutures. Both fontanels should be soft and flat when palpated. A bulging or tense fontanel in an otherwise calm neonate may be an indication of raised intracranial pressure and should be further evaluated. The anterior fontanel size is typically 4 to 6 cm in diameter, and the posterior fontanel is usually smaller than 1 cm in diameter (Bickley, 2012). Large fontanels are often associated with congenital hypothyroidism. Molding and overriding sutures are common findings in newborns caused by the compression of the head through the birth canal. Asymmetry caused by molding is temporary and should resolve in the first few days of life. Persistent asymmetry, however, should be further evaluated for craniosynostosis. Delivery can also cause extracranial complications such as caput succedaneum and cephalohematoma. *Caput succedaneum*, an area of edema on the scalp, is present at birth, crosses suture lines, and resolves within days (Figure 21-4). A *cephalohematoma* develops from bleeding in the subperiosteal space, is not evident until a few hours of age, does not cross suture lines, and can take weeks or months to resolve (Figure 21-5).

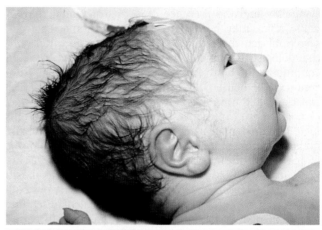

Figure 21-4 Caput succedaneum in a newborn infant. (Used with permission from Brozanski BS, Riley MM, Bogen DL. Neonatology. In Zitelli BJ, McIntire SC, Nowalk AJ, eds. *Atlas of pediatric physical diagnosis*. 6th ed. Philadelphia: Elsevier; 2012:45-77.)

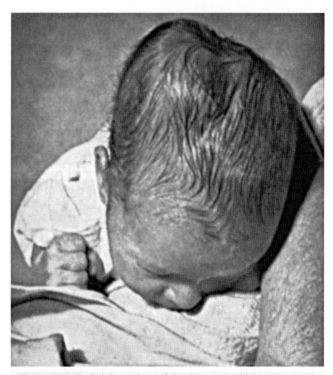

Figure 21-5 Cephalohematoma of the right parietal bone. (Used with permission from Carlo WA. Nervous system disorders. In Kliegman RM, Stanton BF, St. Geme JW, et al, eds. *Nelson textbook of pediatrics*. 19th ed. Philadelphia: Elsevier; 2011:565-574.)

The face should be examined for symmetry. Asymmetry may be attributable to facial palsies from birth trauma or congenital abnormalities. Transient skin lesions may be present on the face from delivery, especially if forceps were used.

Eyes

The eyes should initially be inspected to evaluate for spacing and symmetry and normal extraocular movement. Intermittent crossing of the eyes is a normal finding in the first few months of life. The pupils should be evaluated for symmetry and the presence of a *red reflex* bilaterally. A white reflex may be a sign of retinoblastoma, cataract, or retinal detachment and requires a referral to an ophthalmologist for further evaluation. The sclera, iris, and conjunctiva of both eyes should also be examined. Subconjunctival hemorrhages may be present from trauma experienced during birth. *Congenital nasal lacrimal duct obstruction* may present shortly after birth. Symptoms include persistent tearing and collection of debris on the eyelashes. In most infants, symptoms resolve by 6 months of age with gentle massage to the area and watchful waiting (Pediatric Eye Disease Investigator Group, 2012; Takahashi et al., 2010). Discharge from nasal lacrimal duct obstructions needs to be differentiated from purulent discharge caused by neonatal conjunctival infections, which require urgent medical attention. Because newborns keep their eyes closed most of the time, examining the eyes may be difficult. Holding the infant upright while slowly rotating him or her in a darkened room may stimulate eye opening.

Ears, Nose, and Throat

Ears should be evaluated for position and appearance. Malpositioned, rotated, or poorly formed ears can be a sign of underlying medical problems. The ear canal should be inspected for patency. Visualization of the tympanic membrane is difficult because of the small size of the canal and presence of vernix obscuring the tympanic membrane. Hearing can be assessed by monitoring for startling and blinking in response to a sudden noise.

The shape of the nose should be inspected, and patency of the nares should be verified. Obstructed nares may be due to anatomic problems such as choanal atresia, which can be tested by attempting to pass a small feeding tube or suction catheter through each nare.

The mouth should be both inspected and palpated for abnormalities. Small white retention cysts may be present on the gums, known as *Bohn nodules*, or the hard palate, known as *Epstein pearls*, and resolve within a few months (Figure 21-6). Occasionally, natal teeth are noted. They are typically an isolated finding but may be associated with other congenital abnormalities. The palate should be palpated to ensure it is intact and that no submucosal clefts are present. *Ankyloglossia* occurs if the frenulum is short and limits protrusion of the tongue. Most infants with ankyloglossia experience no symptoms. Some infants may have difficulty breastfeeding and future articulation problems

and therefore may benefit from surgical intervention (Buryk et al., 2011; Lalakea and Messner, 2003).

Chest and Lungs

The chest wall should be inspected for abnormalities in symmetry and structure. Gynecomastia may be present in male and female infants because of the effects of maternal estrogen and can be accompanied by a white, milky discharge referred to as "witch's milk." The clavicles should be palpated for smoothness and symmetry. An asymmetric Moro response, crepitus, or tenderness with palpation may be signs of a clavicle fracture. Infants who present with shoulder dystocia are at risk of clavicle fracture during delivery.

The lung examination is best performed if the newborn is quietly resting. Before auscultation, the infant's respiratory effort should be observed for signs of respiratory distress, including tachypnea, nasal flaring, grunting, or retractions. Tachypnea is defined as a respiratory rate greater than 60 breaths/min. Auscultation should then be performed to assess for quality of breath sounds and accessory noises. Grunting without tachypnea or other symptoms of respiratory distress may be present during the first hour of life as fetal lung fluid is cleared from the lungs. Persistent grunting or retractions are signs of respiratory distress and require further evaluation.

The most common cause of tachypnea in the newborn is *transient tachypnea of the newborn (TTN)*, which occurs from delayed clearing of fetal lung fluid. The most prominent symptom of TTN is tachypnea, but retractions, grunting, and cyanosis may also be present. Infants with TTN should be closely monitored and may need respiratory support with oxygen. Symptoms typically resolve by 12 to 24 hours but may persist for up to 72 hours.

Cardiovascular

Before auscultation, capillary refill should be noted, and the point of maximal impulse (PMI) of the heart should be palpated. Auscultation of the heart is best done along the left sternal border and should reveal clear, regular first and second heart sounds. Dextrocardia may be diagnosed by the presence of heart sounds or the PMI in the right chest. Murmurs are common in the first 24 hours of life. They are often caused by delayed closure of the *ductus arteriosus* or *peripheral pulmonary stenosis* and are considered transient and benign. Murmurs that are harsh, pansystolic, grade III/IV or greater in intensity, and associated with abnormal

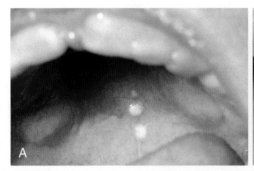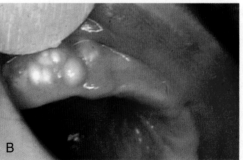

Figure 21-6 A, Epstein pearls located along the midpalatine raphe. **B,** Bohn nodules located on the alveolar ridges. (Used with permission from Martin B, Baumhandt H, D'Aleslo A, et al. Oral disorders. In Zitelli BJ, McIntire SC, Nowalk AJ, eds. *Atlas of pediatric physical diagnosis.* 6th ed. Philadelphia: Elsevier; 2012:775-802.)

second heart sounds require further evaluation. Femoral pulses should be palpated to assess for adequate perfusion. Absent or asymmetric femoral pulses may indicate the presence of coarctation of the aorta.

Abdomen

The abdomen in a normal newborn is soft, symmetric, and slightly protuberant. A scaphoid abdomen or distended abdomen requires further investigation. *Diastasis recti* or an *umbilical hernia* may be present. Both can be closely monitored for spontaneous resolution. Most umbilical hernias resolve by 1 year of age, and nearly all resolve by 5 years of age unless a large defect is present (Katz, 2001; Kelly and Ponsky, 2013; Snyder, 2007). The umbilical cord should be dry and clamped. Erythema of the skin surrounding the umbilicus or a foul-smelling discharge may indicate omphalitis or an infection of the umbilicus.

The abdomen should be auscultated for the presence of bowel sounds in all quadrants. The abdomen should then be palpated to assess the liver, spleen, and kidneys. The liver edge can be palpated 1 to 2 cm below the right costal margin and should be smooth. A spleen tip may be present. Palpation of additional masses requires further evaluation.

Genitalia

In female newborns, the labia majora, labia minora, clitoris, urethral orifice, and vaginal opening should be inspected. The labia majora should be opened to ensure that they are completely separate from each other, and the vaginal opening should be inspected for imperforate hymen. Vaginal or hymenal tags may be present. *Milky, white, or blood-tinged vaginal discharge* is common in the first few weeks of life because of withdrawal of maternal hormones.

In male newborns, the penis, urethral opening, scrotum, and testes should be examined. The length of the penis should be evaluated by measuring the stretched penis. The mean length of a full term infant's penis is 3.5 cm (Feldman and Smith, 1975). The urethral meatus should be midline and central on the glans. Ventral placement of the urethra is known as *hypospadias,* and dorsal placement is known as *epispadias* (Figure 21-7). Circumcision should not be performed in infants with an abnormally placed urethral meatus. The scrotum should be palpated for the presence of both testes. *Hydroceles* and *inguinal hernias* are common scrotal masses in newborns (Figure 21-8). Hydroceles are caused by a fluid collection around the testes and resolve spontaneously by 1 year of age. They can be differentiated from inguinal hernias on examination because they are not reducible and can be transilluminated. Inguinal hernias should be referred for surgical correction.

Back and Spine

The spine should be inspected and palpated for signs of a neural tube defect, including soft tissue masses, sacral cleft or dimple, tuft of hair, or skin abnormalities (e.g., hemangioma). *Sacral dimples* are very common, and those with an intact base typically do not warrant further imaging. Dimples that occur more than 2.5 cm from the anus, are deep and large, are associated with skin abnormalities, or that do not have an intact base should be further evaluated with a spinal ultrasound (Zywicke et al., 2011).

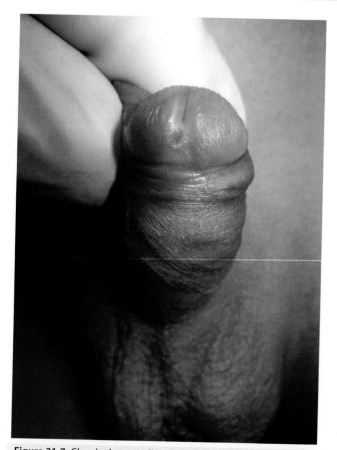

Figure 21-7 Glanular hypospadias, the most common form, in which the urethral opening is found near the head of the penis. (Used with permission Elder JS. Anomalies of the penis and urethra. In Kliegman RM), Stanton BF, St. Geme JW, eds. *Nelson textbook of pediatrics.* 19th ed. Philadelphia: Elsevier; 2011:1852-1858.)

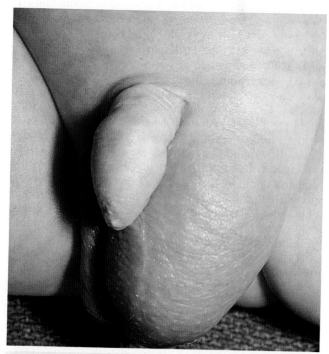

Figure 21-8 Inguinal hernia produces a bulge in the left groin. (Used with permission from Davenport KP, Kane TD. Surgery. In Zitelli BJ, McIntire SC, Nowalk AJ, eds. *Atlas of pediatric physical diagnosis.* 6th ed. Philadelphia: Elsevier; 2012:643-692.)

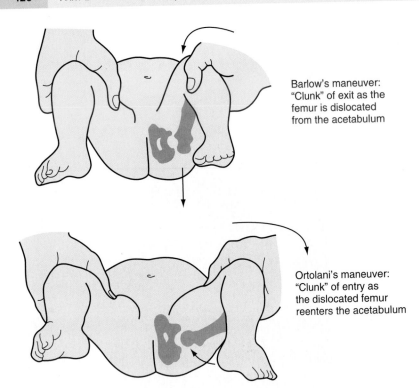

Barlow's maneuver:
"Clunk" of exit as the
femur is dislocated
from the acetabulum

Ortolani's maneuver:
"Clunk" of entry as
the dislocated femur
reenters the acetabulum

Figure 21-9 Physical examination maneuvers for developmental dysplasia of the hip.

Hips

The hips should be carefully examined for signs of dislocation. Dislocation may be present in infants with *developmental dysplasia of the hips (DDH)*. The Ortolani and Barlow maneuvers should be used to assess hip stability (Figure 21-9). The *Ortolani maneuver* tests for the presence of a posteriorly dislocated hip and is performed by abducting the hips while firmly pressing on the greater trochanter of each femur. The test is result positive if a "clunk" is palpated as the femoral head moves back into place. The *Barlow maneuver* tests for subluxation of an intact but unstable hip by pressing down on flexed and adducted hips while applying pressure to the greater trochanter. A positive Barlow sign occurs if the head of the femur is felt slipping posteriorly out of the acetabulum. Risk factors for DDH include female gender, breech presentation, and family history. All infants should be evaluated by physical examination for DDH at well-child visits until they are walking. Newborns with a positive examination should be referred to an orthopedic specialist. If the examination is equivocally positive, the infant should be reexamined at the 2-week visit. Infants with a breech presentation but normal physical examination and female infants with a positive family history of DDH should receive a screening hip ultrasonography at 6 weeks of age (Committee on Quality Improvement, 2000; Shipman et al., 2006).

Neurologic

The neurologic examination of the infant includes assessment of the infant's general state, tone, posture, and primitive reflexes. The infant's level of alertness should be documented. Tone should be assessed by monitoring a newborn's posture at rest and testing his or her resistance to passive movements. Tone varies depending on gestational age. A full-term infant should have strong flexion and symmetric movement of all extremities. Hypotonic infants are limp and lie in a frog-legged position with their arms flexed and hands positioned near the ears. Hypertonic infants may have spasticity or rigid movements. All newborns should exhibit innate reflexes called *primitive reflexes* that develop during gestation and are present at birth (Table 21-5). Asymmetry of movements, localized neurologic findings, or failure to elicit primitive reflexes are indicators of neurologic disease.

Brachial plexus injuries may occur because of pulling on the arm during delivery. These injuries result from stretching or tearing the nerve or hemorrhage within the nerve. *Erb's palsy* is an upper brachial plexus injury (C5-C6) that leads to adduction and internal rotation of the shoulder and pronation of the forearm. *Klumpke's palsy* is a lower plexus injury (C7-C8 and T1) that leads to isolated hand paralysis. Both conditions typically resolve within 1 to 3 months and leave no lasting neurologic deficit.

Skin

During the newborn period, common benign rashes may develop that often require education and reassurance to the parent. The skin of newborns is thinner and has less hair and sweat and sebaceous gland production. These benign lesions are typically self-limited to the newborn period (Treadwell, 1997).

Erythema toxicum neonatorum (ETN) is a common benign skin lesion occurring in 31% to 72% of full-term infants (Figure 21-10) (Treadwell, 1997). ETN is characterized by multiple erythematous macules and papules that rapidly progress to pustules on an erythematous base. The lesions are distributed over the trunk and proximal extremities, sparing the palms and soles. They typically first appear

Table 21-5 Primitive Neurologic Reflexes in Newborns

Primitive Reflex	Maneuver	Ages present
Stepping reflex	Hold the infant in a vertical position with the feet in contact with a flat surface. The infant will make alternating stepping movements.	Birth to 1-2 months
Galant reflex	Stroke the paravertebral region of the back from the shoulder to the buttocks. The infant's trunk will move to the side of stimulation.	Birth to 2 months
Asymmetric tonic neck reflex	Turn the infant's head to one side. The upper and lower extremities on that side will extend while the contralateral extremities will flex.	Birth to 2-4 months
Rooting reflex	Stroke the skin near the mouth of the newborn. The newborn will open his or her mouth and turn toward the direction of stimulation.	Birth to 3-4 months
Palmar and plantar grasp reflex	Press against the palmar or plantar surface. The infant will curl his or her fingers or his or her toes around the examiner's finger.	Birth to 3-4 months
Moro reflex	Hold the newborn in a supine position and abruptly lower his or her body. The infant's arms abduct and extend and the hands open followed by immediate flexion of the arms and closure of the fists.	Birth to 4-6 months

Adapted from Bickley L. *Bates' guide to physical xxamination and history taking.* 11th ed. Philadelphia: Lippincott Williams & Wilkins; 2012.

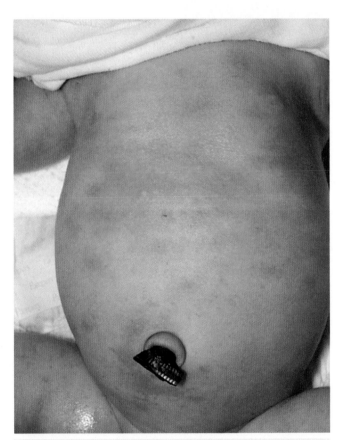

Figure 21-10 Erythema toxicum neonatorum. (Used with permission from Cohen BA, Davis HW, Gehris RP. Dermatology. In Zitelli BJ, McIntire SC, Nowalk AJ, eds. *Atlas of pediatric physical diagnosis.* 6th ed. Philadelphia: Elsevier; 2012:299-368.)

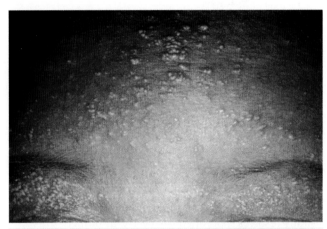

Figure 21-11 Transient neonatal pustular melanosis. (Used with permission from Muniz AE. Neonatal skin disorders. In Baren JM, Rothrock SG, Brennan JA, Brown L, eds. *Pediatric emergency medicine.* Philadelphia: Elsevier; 2008:345-349.)

within 24 to 48 hours of life and resolve within 5 to 7 days. Most physicians are able to diagnose ETN from its clinical appearance, but it can be confirmed by microscopic examination. A Wright-stained smear of the contents of a pustule will demonstrate a predominance of eosinophils. ETN resolves spontaneously without intervention or treatment.

Transient neonatal pustular melanosis (TNPM) is another benign skin lesion seen less commonly than ETN (Figure 21-11). It mostly affects full-term infants with darker skin pigmentation but can be seen in all races. TNPM is characterized by three different lesions that occur at various stages. Initially, small superficial white pustules erupt on a nonerythematous base and may be present at birth. These pustules later unroof to reveal well-circumscribed erythematous macules with a surrounding collarette of scale that may persist for weeks to months. Last, hyperpigmented macules occur and gradually fade over several weeks to months. TNPM can also be confirmed by microscopic examination of a Wright-stained smear, which will show a predominance of neutrophils. TNPM also resolves without treatment.

Neonatal acne occurs in approximately 20% of infants and does not appear to run in families (Figure 21-12) (Treadwell, 1997). The neonate can have multiple papules and pustules distributed primarily on the forehead, cheeks, and upper chest. It is thought to be exacerbated by stimulation of sebaceous glands by maternal and endogenous androgens. Neonatal acne usually starts around 2 or 3 weeks of life. In most cases, no additional treatment is needed because these lesions usually resolve spontaneously within 4 to 6 months

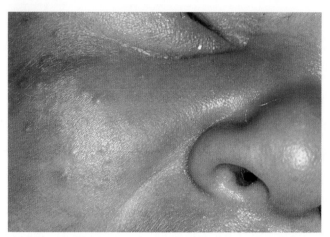

Figure 21-12 Neonatal acne. (Used with permission from Burch JM, Aeling JL. Acne and acneiform eruptions. In Fitzpatrick JE, Morelli JG, eds. *Dermatology secrets plus.* 4th ed. Philadelphia: Elsevier; 2011:148-155.)

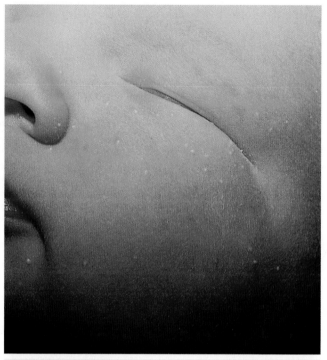

Figure 21-13 Milia. (Used with permission from Cohen BA, Davis HW, Gehris RP. Dermatology. In Zitelli BJ, McIntire SC, Nowalk AJ, eds. *Atlas of pediatric physical diagnosis.* 6th ed. Philadelphia: Elsevier; 2012:299-368.)

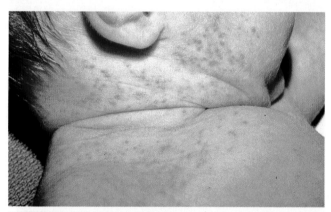

Figure 21-14 Miliaria rubra. (Used with permission from Cohen BA. *Pediatric dermatology.* 4th ed. Philadelphia: Elsevier; 2013:14-67.)

without scarring. Affected newborns do not appear to have a greater risk of acne in adolescence, which can be reassuring to parents.

Infantile acne is different from neonatal acne in that it presents at 3 to 4 months of age. The presentation is often more severe and consists of typical acneiform lesions, including comedones, inflammatory papules, pustules, and occasionally nodules on the face. Infantile acne also results from hyperplasia of sebaceous glands secondary to androgenic stimulation and is more common in boys (Treadwell, 1997). If lesions are severe and cause scarring, treatment by a specialist may be required. Otherwise, infantile acne usually resolves spontaneously by 1 year of life.

Milia are also benign skin lesions consisting of white pinpoint papules that are usually scattered on the nose and cheeks (Figure 21-13) (Zitelli et al., 2007). These epithelial-lined papules are caused by retention of keratin and sebaceous material in the pilosebaceous follicles. These lesions also resolve in the first few weeks of life without any treatment. In fact, parents should be educated to not attempt to denude these lesions because that may lead to scarring.

Miliaria is a common finding in newborns, especially in warm climates (Figure 21-14). It is caused by an accumulation of sweat beneath eccrine sweat ducts that are obstructed by keratin. A common form of this is miliaria rubra or "heat rash" or "prickly heat." Groups of erythematous papules and pustules erupt over the face, upper trunk, and the folds of the neck when the obstructed sweat leaks into the dermis and causes a localized inflammatory response. Miliaria is another self-limited rash that requires no specific treatment. Lesions usually resolve rapidly when the infant is placed in a cooler environment. Parents should be advised to take measures that reduce sweating, such as using light, loose clothing and cool water baths.

Congenital dermal melanocytosis, also called Mongolian spot, is the most frequently encountered benign pigmented lesion in newborns (Figure 21-15). There is a significant racial disparity in the prevalence of these benign lesions, with Asian neonates having the highest prevalence at greater than 85% (Treadwell, 1997). Congenital dermal melanocytosis typically appears as a blue-grey pigmented,

flat patch with irregular borders. The diameter of the lesion may be as large as 10 cm or more. The most common location is the sacral-gluteal region, but these lesions can appear anywhere on the body. Congenital dermal melanocytosis usually fades during the first or second year of life and most resolve completely by 7 to 10 years of age without any intervention or treatment (Treadwell, 1997). Although the distinctive clinical appearance of these blue-grey patches is usually diagnostic, there are reports of false accusations of child abuse when these lesions are misinterpreted as bruises (Cohen, 1987). Therefore, it is important to document the presence of these benign lesions on the newborn record and to educate the parents of the benign, self-limited nature of these lesions.

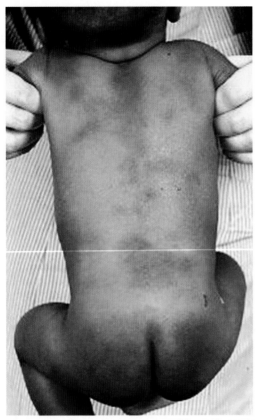

Figure 21-15 Congenital dermal melanocytosis (Mongolian spot). (Used with permission from Lissauer T, Clayden G. *Illustrated textbook of paediatrics.* 4th ed. Philadelphia: Elsevier; 2012:133-153.)

SCREENING

Key Points

- Routine glucose screening is not recommended in healthy term infants.
- Physiologic jaundice is the most common cause of hyperbilirubinemia and typically resolves in the first week of life.
- A total bilirubin should be obtained and plotted on the phototherapy nomogram before discharge from the hospital.
- Pulse oximetry screening is becoming an increasingly common practice to screen for congenital heart disease.
- Universal hearing screen is recommended for all infants before discharge.

Glucose

Routine glucose screening is not recommended in healthy term infants after a normal pregnancy and delivery. Blood glucose levels should be measured in infants at risk of developing hypoglycemia and those displaying symptoms of hypoglycemia. Risk factors include infants who are SGA, LGA, born to mothers with diabetes, or late preterm infants (34-36⅚ weeks' gestation). Infants with clinical symptoms of hypoglycemia should be immediately screened with a blood glucose level. Clinical symptoms of hypoglycemia

are nonspecific and include jitteriness, decreased tone, irritability or lethargy, tachypnea, apnea, bradycardia, cyanosis, poor feeding, hypothermia, seizures, or weak cry. Hypoglycemia itself can be a sign of more serious medical problems, such as sepsis or inborn errors of metabolism.

The definition of hypoglycemia is controversial. A 2011 AAP report recommends using 45 mg/dL as a target; however, each hospital system may define hypoglycemia differently (AAP, 2011). Bedside glucose testing can be used as a rapid screening method. Because these measures are less accurate than laboratory testing, abnormal blood glucose concentrations should be confirmed by laboratory testing, but confirmation should not delay treatment.

Management of hypoglycemia should be tailored to the needs of the infant depending on the presence or absence of signs of hypoglycemia (AAP and ACOG, 2012). Infants at risk of developing hypoglycemia should be encouraged to feed in the first hour of life, and the initial blood glucose level should be obtained 30 minutes after feeding. Screening should continue every 2 to 3 hours for the first 12 to 24 hours of life or until the infant is feeding well and blood glucose levels are normal. Intravenous (IV) glucose should be initiated in symptomatic infants or infants with severe hypoglycemia. Asymptomatic infants with hypoglycemia should be fed breast milk or formula and have a glucose level repeated in 1 hour. If the blood glucose level has not increased at that time, IV glucose is recommended.

Bilirubin

Predischarge bilirubin screening is recommended to prevent acute bilirubin encephalopathy or kernicterus because jaundice is a common finding in newborns. Kernicterus occurs when toxic levels of bilirubin cross the blood–brain barrier, leading to devastating and permanent neurologic defects. Jaundice results from increased levels of conjugated (direct) or unconjugated (indirect) bilirubin in the blood (Table 21-6). In most infants, jaundice is secondary to unconjugated hyperbilirubinemia, which occurs because of increased production of bilirubin, decreased clearance of bilirubin, or increased enterohepatic circulation. The most common cause of unconjugated hyperbilirubinemia in infants is physiologic jaundice (Kliegman et al., 2007). *Physiologic jaundice* is a result of increased turnover of red blood cells; transient deficiency of the enzyme UDP glucuronosyltransferase (UGT), which is responsible for bilirubin clearance in the liver; and increased enterohepatic circulation. Physiologic jaundice typically resolves in the first week of life without need for intervention. In infants with persistent or severe jaundice (jaundice in the first 24 hours of life or total bilirubin level greater than the 95th percentile), a direct and total bilirubin level should be measured to differentiate between conjugated and unconjugated hyperbilirubinemia, and the infant should be further evaluated for pathologic causes of jaundice.

Bilirubin screening identifies infants at risk of developing severe levels of hyperbilirubinemia (Subcommittee on Hyperbilirubinemia, 2004). Major risk factors include predischarge total bilirubin level in the high-risk zone, jaundice in first 24 hours of life, blood group incompatibility, gestational age of 35 to 36 weeks, sibling requiring phototherapy, cephalohematoma or bruising, exclusive breastfeeding and excessive weight loss, and East Asian race. A

Table 21-6   Causes of Hyperbilirubinemia in Newborns

Conjugated hyperbilirubinemia	Sepsis
	Infection (toxoplasmosis, cytomegalovirus, rubella, herpes, syphilis)
	Paucity of bile ducts
	Disorders of bile acid metabolism
	Severe hemolytic disease
	Biliary atresia
	Giant cell hepatitis
	Choledochal cyst
	Cystic fibrosis
	Galactosemia
	α_1-Antitrypsin deficiency
	Tyrosinemia
Unconjugated hyperbilirubinemia	Increased production of bilirubin
	▪ Isoimmune-mediated hemolysis (ABO blood group incompatibility, Rh incompatibility)
	▪ Inherited red blood cell membrane defects (spherocytosis, elliptocytosis)
	▪ Erythrocyte enzyme defects (glucose-6-phosphate dehydrogenase deficiency, pyruvate kinase deficiency)
	▪ Sepsis
	▪ Polycythemia
	▪ Extravascular hemorrhage (cephalohematoma, extensive bruising)
	Decreased bilirubin clearance
	▪ Crigler-Najjar syndrome
	▪ Gilbert syndrome
	▪ Infant of mother with diabetes
	▪ Congenital hypothyroidism
	Increased enterohepatic circulation
	▪ Physiologic jaundice
	▪ Breast milk jaundice
	▪ Functional or anatomical obstruction

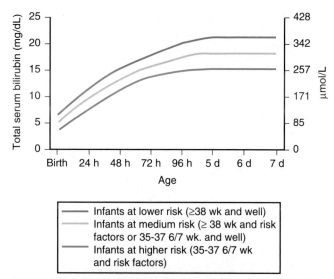

Figure 21-16 Phototherapy nomogram for infants of 35 or more weeks' gestation. Risk factors include isoimmune hemolytic disease, glucose-6-phosphate dehydrogenase deficiency, asphyxia, significant lethargy, temperature instability, sepsis, acidosis, or albumin less than 3.0 g/dL. (From AAP Subcommittee on Hyperbilirubinemia. Management of hyperbilirubinemia in the newborn infant 35 or more weeks of gestation. *Pediatrics.* 2004;114:297-316.)

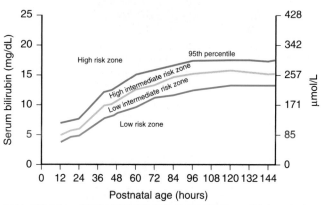

Figure 21-17 Nomogram for designation of risk of hyperbilirubinemia in well newborns. The serum total bilirubin level should be obtained before discharge. The zone in which the value falls predicts the likelihood of subsequent bilirubin level exceeding the 95th percentile (high-risk zone) and should determine the timing of follow-up. (From AAP Subcommittee on Hyperbilirubinemia. Management of hyperbilirubinemia in the newborn infant 35 or more weeks of gestation. *Pediatrics.* 2004;114:297-316.)

total bilirubin level should be obtained before discharge and plotted on the phototherapy nomogram (Figure 21-16). Treatment with phototherapy is initiated when the total bilirubin level exceeds the threshold level on the phototherapy nomogram based on the infant's age in hours and risk level (see Figure 21-16). The infant's risk level is determined by the presence or absence of the following risk factors: isoimmune hemolytic disease, glucose-6-phosphate dehydrogenase (G6PD) deficiency, asphyxia, significant lethargy, temperature instability, sepsis, acidosis, or albumin less than 3.0 g/dL. BiliTool is an excellent online resource that can be used to assist in assessing need for phototherapy (http://www.bilitool.org).

While receiving phototherapy, infants may continue to breastfeed but may require supplementation with expressed breast milk or formula if weight loss is excessive (greater than 12% of birth weight) or intake is inadequate. Hydration with IV fluids is reserved for infants with significant hypovolemia and does not need to be initiated in all infants. Phototherapy should be discontinued when total bilirubin levels decrease to safe levels. Total bilirubin levels should be reassessed 18 to 24 hours after discontinuing phototherapy to ensure that levels have not rebounded.

In infants whose bilirubin levels do not indicate need for treatment before discharge, the need for and timing of repeat evaluation depends on the zone in which the total bilirubin level falls and the age of the infant (Figure 21-17). Timing of follow-up is important, and a follow-up appointment should be secured with the infant's primary care provider before discharge.

Critical Congenital Heart Disease

Screening for critical congenital heart disease with pulse oximetry is becoming an increasingly common practice. Pulse oximetry can detect mild levels of hypoxemia in infants with congenital heart disease who do not have obvious examination findings, such as a murmur or cyanosis (Thangaratinam et al., 2012). Screening is directed at identifying hypoplastic left heart syndrome, pulmonary atresia, tetralogy of Fallot, total anomalous pulmonary venous return, transposition of the great arteries, tricuspid atresia, and truncus arteriosus. Screening should be done after 24 hours of life by placing a pulse oximetry probe on the right hand and either foot. A positive screening test result meets the following criteria: (1) SaO_2 less than 90% in either extremity, (2) SaO_2 less than 95% in both upper and lower extremities on three measurements with each measurement separated by 1 hour, or (3) SaO_2 difference of greater than 3% between the upper and lower extremities (Mahle et al., 2012). Positive screening warrants referral to the specialist for an echocardiogram.

Newborn Screen

The goal of newborn screening programs is to detect disease before the onset of symptoms to initiate early treatment and prevent complications. Newborn screening programs test for various congenital disorders, including metabolic disorders, endocrinopathies, hemoglobinopathies, cystic fibrosis, and immunodeficiencies. They are mandated by law and are implemented at the state level. Blood specimens should be collected between 24 and 48 hours of life via heel prick (AAP and ACOG, 2012). Some states mandate that a repeat specimen be obtained at 10 to 14 days of life to reduce the chance of missed diagnosis.

Hearing

Universal hearing screening is recommended for all infants. Hearing impairment occurs in approximately one to three per 1000 live births and has a significant impact on a child's language and social development and academic performance (USPTF, 2008). The USPTF recommends that all infants be screened before 1 month of age. Infants who fail a screening test should receive audiologic assessment by 3 months of age, and infants diagnosed with hearing loss should receive intervention by 6 months of age. Otoacoustic emissions (OAEs) and auditory brainstem response (ABR) are both appropriate screening tests. In OAEs, a microphone placed near the infant's ear produces stimulus noises and detects sound waves produced from the infant's cochlea. In ABR screening, electrodes placed on the forehead, neck, and mastoid measure waveforms generated by the auditory brainstem response to stimuli. The ABR must be completed when the infant is asleep. OAEs are most often used because they are quick, easy to administer, inexpensive, and can be performed when then infant is awake or asleep. Many hospitals use a two-step approach to screening. OAEs are administered first followed by an ABR if the infant fails the first test. Infants who fail hearing screening should be referred to a pediatric audiologist for further evaluation.

DISCHARGE FROM THE NEWBORN NURSERY

Discharge home optimally occurs when the newborn has been observed for a long enough period of time to identify medical problems and when the family is able and prepared to care for the newborn at home. If either the mother or the newborn requires a longer stay, all efforts should be made to keep the newborn and mother together to promote bonding if possible. Before discharge, the infant should have normal and stable vital signs for at least 12 hours, including a normal temperature in an open crib (Committee on Fetus and Newborn, 2004). The infant should have urinated and passed stool at least once and fed successfully twice. Feeding should be observed to document that the infant is able to coordinate sucking, swallowing, and breathing and has an appropriate latch if breastfeeding. Parents of the newborn should be given appropriate anticipatory guidance (covered in the section, "Care at the Primary Care Office") to confidently provide adequate care. Most mother–newborn dyads meet discharge criteria after 48 hours of care. All infants should have follow-up scheduled with a medical home within 2 to 3 days after discharge.

Care at the Primary Care Office

Key Points

- The infant should be assessed for appropriate weight gain, voiding and stooling patterns, and jaundice at the initial visit in the primary care office.
- The AAP recommends the prompt assessment of a breastfed infant with greater than a 7% loss from birth weight.
- A normal newborn should pass urine and meconium stool within the first 24 hours of life.
- It is important to reassure parents that there may be occasional variations in the color and consistency of the stools.
- Breastfed infants may develop breast milk jaundice or physiologic jaundice that persists past the first week of life.

ASSESSMENT AND EVALUATION

A newborn will visit his or her physician in the first year of life more than at any other time. The schedule usually starts with the newborn examination at the time of delivery and then transitions to the first visit in the primary care office. This occurs as early as 3 to 5 days of life. At this initial visit in the primary care office, the provider will perform a similar comprehensive newborn examination as outlined earlier in this chapter. The physician should also evaluate the infant for weight gain or loss, difficulty with feeding, abnormal voiding or stooling patterns, and jaundice. Infants should have a second ambulatory visit at 2 to 3 weeks of age so the physician can monitor weight gain and provide additional support and encouragement to the mother during this critical period (Wenner Van Vleet, 2012).

Growth

The initial assessment of the newborn in the office includes a measurement of the weight, length, and fronto-occipital circumference (FOC). These measurements are plotted on the growth curve. Weight loss is normal after delivery, and the expected loss is 5% to 7% of birth weight (Paul et al., 2006). Term, healthy infants usually stop losing weight by 5 days of life and typically regain their birth weight by 2 weeks of age. After breastfeeding or formula feeding is well established, infants should gain 15 to 30 g/day. Excessive weight loss is a loss of greater than 10% of the birth weight. Weight loss beyond this normal expected amount may be an indication of poor intake that requires medical attention and intervention. The AAP recommends prompt assessment of a breastfed infant if there is more than a 7% loss from birth weight (Section on Breastfeeding, 2012).

The physician should also get a detailed history of the voiding and stooling pattern. Voiding increases from one void in the first 24 hours to two or three in the second 24 hours, four to six during the third and fourth day, and six to eight on day 5 and thereafter.

Infants who are successfully feeding from the breast or bottle should pass a meconium stool in the first 48 hours of life and then have transitional stools within approximately 3 days of birth. After day 4 or 5, the majority of infants have three or more stools per day, which is often timed with feeding episodes. After the dark, thick meconium stool passes, normal infant stool will turn yellow-green, soft, and almost runny with seedlike particles (Wenner Van Vleet, 2012).

It is important to reassure the parents that there may be occasional variations in the color and consistency of the stools. The gastrocolic reflex of newborns is a physiologic reflex controlling the motility, or peristalsis, of the gastrointestinal tract. It involves an increase in motility of the colon in response to stretch in the stomach. This can be used to explain the increased frequency of stools, especially in breastfed infants. By 1 month of age, it is normal for some infants to have less frequent stools. Some infants may only have one bowel movement per week. If the infant is feeding well, making appropriate urine-filled diapers, and producing soft stools, the parents need to be reassured that this stooling pattern may still be within normal limits.

In breastfed infants, stool may appear green and frothy. This occurs in infants of mothers who produce copious milk and switch the infant from one breast to the other before most of the hind milk is completely extracted from the first breast. The high fat content in the hind milk usually slows gut motility enough that the majority of milk lactose digestion occurs in the small intestine. If the infant does not completely empty one breast, he or she will have less hind milk to slow motility, and high concentrations of lactose will reach the large bowel. This in turn causes excess gas and frothy stool production by the bacterial flora in the large intestine. Mothers should be advised to allow the infant to finish nursing on one breast before switching to the other even if the child does not take the second breast (Section on Breastfeeding, 2012).

Hyperbilirubinemia

An important component of the early follow-up visit is to reassess the infant for jaundice because hyperbilirubinemia is the most common cause of readmission to the hospital (Paul et al., 2006). Physicians should use their clinical judgment to determine if the infant requires a serum or transcutaneous bilirubin measurement. Need for treatment should again be based on the phototherapy nomogram (see Figure 21-16). Infants requiring treatment with phototherapy will likely require readmission to the hospital.

Breastfed infants may develop *breast milk jaundice* or physiologic jaundice that persists past the first week of life. Breast milk jaundice is a mild unconjugated hyperbilirubinemia caused by a factor in breast milk that promotes increased intestinal absorption of bilirubin. Infants with jaundice past the first week of life should be evaluated with a total and direct bilirubin level to ensure that pathologic causes of jaundice are not present. After the diagnosis of breast milk jaundice has been established, the infant can be closely monitored to ensure the concentration of bilirubin is not increasing to a level requiring phototherapy. These infants can continue to receive breast milk until the jaundice resolves.

Parental Education and Anticipatory Guidance

Key Points

- Breastfeeding should be recommended for all infants, unless contraindicated, and is most successful if initiated within the first few hours of life.
- Supplements of water, glucose water, or formula should not be given to breastfed infants unless medically indicated.
- All breastfed infants should receive vitamin D drops daily during the first 2 months of life.
- The umbilical cord should be kept clean and dry without the repeated use of antiseptic agents.
- Infants should be placed in a supine position on a firm sleeping surface to reduce the risk of sudden infant death syndrome (SIDS).
- AAP car seat recommendations, updated in 2011, include the use of a rear-facing car seat until the child is 2 years of age.
- The Edinburg Postnatal Depression Scale is a useful and validated tool to screen for postpartum depression.

BREASTFEEDING

Successful breastfeeding requires support and education for both parents during pregnancy, throughout the postpartum hospitalization, and during the early newborn period. Immediately after delivery, the mother should be encouraged to make skin-to-skin contact with her newborn. At that time, it is important to support the mother in holding the infant in a comfortable position at the breast and in establishing a good latch (Figure 21-18). The mother should be encouraged to feed her newborn on demand and whenever the infant shows early signs of hunger, such as mouthing, rooting, or increased alertness or physical activity. During the initiation of breastfeeding, infants typically feed every 2 to 3 hours, or 8 to 12 times in a 24-hour period (AAP Committee on Nutrition, 2009). Mothers should be encouraged to offer both breasts at each feeding, but the first breast offered should be alternated so that both breasts receive equal stimulation and draining. Milk production is established in the first 2 to 4 days of life during which time the infant receives colostrum. On day 3 to 5 of life, milk production will dramatically increase. Mothers should be reassured that milk production is based on the demand of the infant and that formula supplementation is not necessary unless there is a medical indication. Similarly, water, glucose water, or other fluids should not be given to a newborn. Breastfed infants should be closely followed after hospital discharge to ensure weight gain is adequate and to provide support to the mother as breastfeeding is being

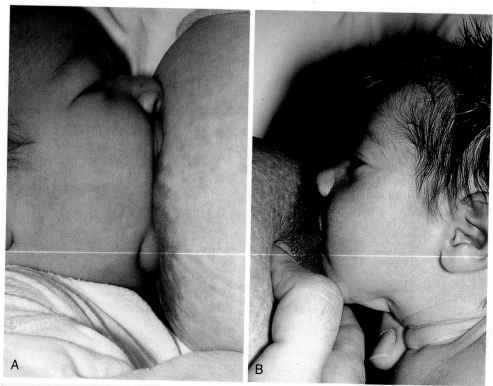

Figure 21-18 A, An appropriate latch for breastfeeding is characterized by a wide-open mouth, everted lips, and a high position on the mother's areola. **B,** An inadequate latch is characterized by a partially closed mouth with the lips near the base of the mother's nipple and little of the mother's areola in the infant's mouth. (Used with permission from Brozanski BS, Riley MM, Bogen DL. Neonatology. In Zitelli BJ, McIntire SC, Nowalk AJ, eds. *Atlas of pediatric physical diagnosis.* 6th ed. Philadelphia: Elsevier; 2012:45-77. Courtesy Susan Costanza, RN, IBCLC, Rochester General Hospital, Rochester, NY.)

established. Using a lactation consultant or trained obstetric nurse to establish breastfeeding can provide comfort and confidence to the mother, as well as evaluation of the infant's position, latch, suck, and swallow while feeding.

Parents should be made aware that exclusive breastfeeding is sufficient to support optimal growth and development for the first 6 months of life (Section on Breastfeeding, 2012). Continued breastfeeding with complementary foods should be encouraged for at least the first year of life and beyond as long as it is beneficial and desired by the mother and child. Complementary foods rich in iron should be introduced gradually beginning around 6 months of age. During the first 6 months of age, water and juice are not recommended because it offers no nutritional benefit to the infant (Gartner et al., 2005).

Although human milk contains small amounts of vitamin D, it is not enough to prevent hypovitaminosis D or rickets. All breastfed infants should receive 200 IU of oral vitamin D drops daily during the first 2 months of life (AAP Committee on Nutrition, 2009). Vitamin D should be continued in breastfed infants until the daily consumption of vitamin D–fortified formula or milk is at least 500 mL (about 16 oz) per day. Supplementary fluoride should not be provided during the first 6 months of life. From 6 months to 3 years of age, the decision whether to provide fluoride supplementation should be made on the basis of whether there is adequate fluoride concentration in the water supply.

Many mothers experience problems while breastfeeding, including concern for decreased supply, nipple problems, engorgement, plugged ducts, and mastitis. In most women, milk supply can be augmented by increasing breast stimulation through increased feeding time or pumping. Adequate rest, hydration, and nutrition are also important to ensure an adequate milk supply. Nipple pain commonly occurs in the immediate postpartum period, and cracked or blistered nipples often develop from incorrect breastfeeding technique. The infant–mother dyad should be observed while breastfeeding to ensure that a proper latch is being achieved. Nipple injury can be treated with cool or warm compresses, hydrogel pads, antibiotic ointments or other barrier ointments (e.g., lanolin), and mild analgesics. Nipple shields may also be used to assist with pain during feeding. Engorgement occurs when more milk than needed is produced. Engorgement typically resolves over time, but symptoms may be managed with warm or cold compresses, mild analgesics, and application of cool green cabbage leaves. Manual expression or pumping may be necessary to provide relief from pain. Plugged ducts present as painful lumps and may progress to infection or mastitis. Mothers should be encouraged to frequently feed or pump to help drain the plugged area. Breastfeeding should not be stopped as cessation will worsen the problem. Applying warm compresses and massage to the area may facilitate removal of the blockage (AAP and ACOG, 2012).

Physicians should recommend breastfeeding or expressed breast milk for all infants in whom human milk is not specifically contraindicated. There are few true contraindications to breastfeeding. These include (1) maternal infection with HIV, human T-cell lymphotrophic virus, herpetic breast lesions, or active tuberculosis; (2) maternal substance abuse; and (3) newborns with galactosemia who require a non–lactose-based formula. Most maternal medications are compatible with breastfeeding, but medications should be reviewed for potential contraindications before use (see LactMed in Web Resources) (AAP and ACOG, 2012).

UMBILICAL CORD CARE

In the hospital, aseptic care of the cord involves clamping and cutting of the umbilical cord. These measures have been incorporated as part of routine care to minimize the risk of omphalitis. In a meta-analysis of trials conducted in hospital settings, there was no reported difference in the risk of omphalitis between routine dry cord care and the addition of any antiseptic topical agent, including triple dye, alcohol, chlorhexidine, salicylic sugar powder, or green clay powder (Imdad et al., 2013). Anticipatory guidance to parents should include the importance of keeping the cord clean and dry.

Cord separation normally occurs within the first few weeks of life. Umbilical cord separation is initiated by thrombosis and contraction of the umbilical vessels followed by phagocyte-mediated tissue breakdown and epithelialization of the cord stump (Imdad et al., 2013). Stump colonization by bacteria acquired from the maternal genital tract or the environment can potentially cause umbilical infections, and it is imperative to keep the cord clean and dry. Until the cord has separated, physicians should advise parents to sponge bathe the infant rather than submersing his or her body in a tub of water. Keeping the diaper folded below the cord and exposing the cord to air may help to keep the area dry. Cleaning the cord too often and using rubbing alcohol may prevent normal leukocyte adhesion from occurring. There is a large variation in the time of normal cord separation; therefore, delayed cord separation does not have a specific definition. In general, any cord that persists after 4 to 6 weeks probably represents delayed cord separation. Delayed cord separation can be associated with an underlying immunodeficiency, infection, or urachal abnormality. Neutrophil function should be evaluated in infants with delayed cord separation and signs of umbilical infection because infants with leukocyte adhesion defects often present with these findings (Imdad et al., 2013).

SLEEP SAFETY

The AAP released its recommendation in 1992 that infants be placed for sleep in a nonprone position. Since the release of this recommendation, there has been a major decrease in the incidence of SIDS, but this decline has plateaued in recent years. In addition to prone sleeping, several other causes of sudden unexpected infant death (SUID) were published in the AAP's latest statement on SIDS issued in 2005 (Task Force on Sudden Infant Death Syndrome, 2011). Many of these risk factors are also modifiable, such as soft sleep surfaces, loose bedding, secondhand smoke exposure, overheating the infant, and bed sharing. It has become increasingly important to address these other causes of sleep-related infant death. The AAP expanded its recommendations from focusing only on SIDS to ensuring that parents always provide a safe sleep environment that can reduce the risk of all sleep-related infant deaths, including SIDS. Although the side position is safer than the prone position, it still remains a risk for SIDS and should not be recommended. Supine positioning is preferred and still highly recommended. Physicians should also recommend that parents use a firm sleep surface such as crib mattress covered by a fitted sheet. A bassinet or portable crib or play yard that conforms to the safety standards of the Consumer Product Safety Commission can also be recommended. The infant should sleep in an area free of dangling cords, electric wires, and window-covering cords because they might present a strangulation risk. Sitting devices, such as car safety seats, strollers, swings, infant carriers, and infant slings, are not recommended for routine sleep in the hospital or at home. Soft objects, such as pillows, stuffed animals, and large blankets, should be kept out of the area where an infant is sleeping. The AAP does not recommend bumper pads or similar products that attach to crib slats or sides because there is no reliable evidence that these products prevent injury in young infants (Task Force on Sudden Infant Death Syndrome, 2011). In addition, these products do pose a risk for potential suffocation, entrapment, and strangulation. Parents should be advised that they can reduce the infant's risk of SIDS by not smoking when pregnant and not smoking in the home or around the infant. It is also important that the sleep clothing for an infant is light and does not promote overheating.

Since the Back to Sleep National Campaign recommendations, there has been an increase in cranial asymmetry and positional plagiocephaly. It is very important that anticipatory guidance regarding "tummy time" be given to parents as early as the 2-week well-child examination and repeated at subsequent visits (Task Force on Sudden Infant Death Syndrome, 2011).

CAR SEAT

In March 2011, the AAP released its revised Child Passenger Safety recommendations. The statement increased the minimum age that children should remain rear facing in infant and convertible seats from 1 to 2 years of age. Young children should ride in car safety seats with a harness until at least age 4 years, and school-aged children should ride in belt positioning booster seats until at least age 8 years or until the seat belt fits correctly, as described by the AAP and National Highway Traffic Safety Administration. The policy also included a change that children should remain in the rear seat of the car until 13 years of age (Committee on Injury, Violence and Poison Prevention, 2011). Physicians should review these new recommendations with the parents at every visit and remind them that a car seat should never be placed in the front seat of a car with a passenger side air bag. In addition, a car seat that has been involved in a motor vehicle accident should never be reused (Lincoln, 2005).

BATHING

Bathing an infant can eventually be a fun time for both the infant and parent; however, initially it can be a very daunting experience. Accidental drowning causes more than 600 deaths annually among children younger than 5 years of age. Bathtubs are one of the leading sites for such drowning for children younger than 2 years of age according to the Consumer Products Safety Commission Report (2011).

Physicians should remind parents that an infant should never be left alone in the bathtub and always advise the parent to have all of the supplies prepared before starting the bath. Parents should ensure that the temperature of the water in the home is set no hotter than 120°F to avoid burns (Simon et al., 2003).

An infant does not need be bathed daily because frequent bathing may promote drying of the infant's skin. However, physicians should remind parents that it is important that parents wash or clean the diaper area thoroughly with each diaper change. Physicians should also advise parents to use fragrant-free, hypoallergenic products that are intended for infants when bathing and when applying lotions or cream (AAP, 2009).

FEVER AND SIGNS OF ILLNESS

Anticipatory guidance given to the parents of an infant should always include the discussion of fever and how to appropriately and accurately take a temperature. The AAP no longer recommends the use of glass mercury thermometers because of the potential for these thermometers to break and lead to inhalation toxicity. The AAP does recommend the use of digital thermometers. If the infant feels warm to touch, parents are advised to take the temperature with a clean thermometer. Feeling the skin is a subjective measure and may be highly inaccurate. The rectal temperature is the most accurate and preferred method in infants. If parents are not familiar or are not comfortable with this technique, then suggest taking an axillary temperature. Physicians should advise parents to avoid pacifier thermometers and forehead strips that gauge temperature. Fever in an infant is a rectal temperature of 100.4°F or 38°C or higher. Parents should be informed that if an infant younger than 3 months of age were to develop a fever, the physician should be immediately notified. Current guidelines recommend that physicians take a cautious approach to neonates (0-28 days) and young infants (29-90 days) with fever because of the risk and potentially adverse consequences of an unrecognized or untreated serious bacterial infection (Ishimine, 2006). Approximately 12% of febrile neonates may have a serious bacterial illness, and group B streptococcus is a common pathogen in this age group. The current guidelines suggest that all neonates with a rectal temperature greater than or equal to 100.4°F or 38°C have blood, urine, and cerebrospinal fluid cultures performed regardless of the infant's clinical appearance. In addition, chest radiography may be added to this workup if the neonate is also having evidence of respiratory distress (Lissauer, 2011).

POSTPARTUM DEPRESSION

After giving birth, most women and their friends and families expect the postpartum period to be a very pleasant period with the arrival of a healthy newborn. The reality, though, is that many women will experience mood disturbances that may be acute or chronic in nature. *Postpartum blues* refers to a transient condition characterized by mild and rapid mood changes. About 40% to 80% of postpartum women develop these mood changes, which may include extremes of elation, sadness, irritability, anxiety, insomnia, forgetfulness, tearfulness, and even crying spells. This usually occurs within 2 to 3 days of delivery and resolves within 2 weeks of delivery (Cox et al., 1987). *Postpartum depression*, on the other hand, refers to a diagnosis of depressed mood or loss of interests that is present most of the day, occurs almost every day, and lasts for at least 2 weeks at a time.

It is imperative that physicians caring for newborns inquire about the mental health of the postpartum mother. The Edinburgh Postnatal Depression Scale (EPDS) is a 10-item self-report questionnaire designed specifically for the detection of depression in the postpartum period. It has been validated and is available in more than 12 different languages (Cox et al., 1987). Responses are scored 0, 1, 2, or 3, with a maximum score of 30. Mothers who score above 13 are likely to have a depressive illness of varying severity (Cox et al., 1987). When scoring the EPDS, the physician must also pay particular attention to question number 10 regarding a mother's intention to harm herself. Regardless of the total EPDS score, if the answer to this question is not zero, the test result is considered abnormal. The EPDS score should not override clinical judgment and should not prevent the physician from engaging the mother in a conversation about how she feels and determining what level of support she has. A mother identified as having postpartum blues or depression should be offered support, counseling, and a referral to a specialist.

References

The complete reference list is available online at https://expertconsult.inkling.com.

Web Resources

bilitool.org An online tool designed to help providers assess the risk of hyperbilirubinemia.

pediatrics.aappublications.org/content/114/1/297.full The full clinical practice guideline regarding the management of hyperbilirubinemia from the American Academy of Pediatrics.

toxnet.nlm.nih.gov LactMed is an online database of drugs and their interactions with breastfeeding.

www.cdc.gov/vaccines Updated childhood immunization schedule from the Centers for Disease Control and Prevention as well as information about vaccines and preventable diseases.

www.childrenshealthnetwork.org/CRS/CRS/pa_index.htm Updated patient information and handouts from Barton Schmitt's Pediatric Advisor. Handouts are available in six other languages.

www.dermatlas.net Collection of dermatology images.

www.healthychildren.org An American Academy of Pediatrics–sponsored parenting website with ample information related to child health and guidance on parenting issues.

www.nichd.nih.gov/sts/Pages/default.aspx Information provided by the National Institute of Child Health and Human Development about sudden infant death syndrome and safe sleep practices for infants.

www.pediatriccareonline.org/pco/ub A website offering multiple resources, including Point-of-Care Quick Reference, AAP Textbook of Pediatric Care, Bright Futures, Antimicrobial Therapy Guide, and a Visual Library. Other tools include Pediatric Care Updates, Algorithms, a Signs and Symptoms Search, and Patient Handouts.

www.seatcheck.org Provides locations for parents to have car seats inspected for proper installation.

www2.aap.org/nrp/index.html Information on the Neonatal Resuscitation Program from the American Academy of Pediatrics and American Heart Association.

22 Growth and Development

SANFORD R. KIMMEL and KAREN RATLIFF-SCHAUB

Children are distinguished from people in other age groups by physical growth and developmental changes that are ongoing, normative, and expected. These changes usually proceed in an orderly progression that allows for individual variation. The family physician must be familiar with the range of normal physical and developmental changes that occur in the process of providing health supervision to children.

Growth is a dynamic process in which increasing cell size and number in various tissues result in a physical increase in the size of the body as a whole. Simultaneously, development occurs as tissues differentiate in form and mature in function, reflecting the person's genetic heritage and environmental interaction. Nutritional, family, emotional, sociocultural, and community influences as well as physical factors play a role in shaping the child's psychological and physiological development (Vaughan and Litt, 1992). The child responds emotionally to a particular stimulus in an apparently innate and characteristic style that reflects his or her temperament.

Knowledge of normal as well as abnormal patterns of growth and development enables the physician to assist the child in maximizing his or her fullest potential. Growth in height and weight is a sensitive reflection of a child's general health. Deviations from normal can reflect the presence of physical illness or a disturbance in the child's environment. Table 22-1 lists some significant causes of growth abnormalities.

Care of Children in Family Medicine

Family physicians have the opportunity to provide family-centered pediatric care in the context of the child's family and community. The office should be "child friendly" and child safe, with at least one room equipped to evaluate children's physical growth. Blood pressure (BP) cuffs should be available to measure children's BP, at least from age 36 months and older. Electrical outlets and cords should be secured, and potentially hazardous chemicals and biohazard bins stored either out of reach or under lock and key from curious young toddlers. Guidelines for the frequency of "well-child" or "well-teen" visits are available from the American Academy of Pediatrics (AAP) *Bright Futures:*

Guidelines for Health Supervision of Infants, Children, and Adolescents (Hagan et al., 2008).

Initial history for a new infant or child includes the birth history, nutritional history (e.g., breastfed vs. bottle fed), developmental milestones achieved, immunization record, and environmental history (e.g., do parents smoke?). Later, the physician or staff will also perform anticipatory guidance, including injury prevention and the need to immunize against vaccine-preventable diseases.

Observation of the parent–child interaction informs the physician about the relationship between parent(s) and the child, especially with infants and young children. A parent sitting in a chair reading a magazine while her young infant teeters on an examination table engenders more concern than a parent who is standing next to the child or has him in her lap. Observation of the child's appearance, alertness, muscle tone, state of hydration, and respiratory status also raise or lower the index of concern about a child. Whereas the cardiorespiratory examination is often done best if the child is sitting or lying on a parent's lap, examination of the abdomen, genitalia, and hips is generally done on the examination table. The HEENT (head, eyes, ears, nose, and throat) examination is often done last because it is the most likely to provoke discomfort.

Blood Pressure Monitoring

Hypertension has become increasingly common in children and adolescents. Since 1988, the prevalence of high BP has increased, especially for certain populations, such as Mexican Americans and blacks (Din-Dzietham et al., 2007). The rising rate of obesity, particularly truncal obesity, at least partly accounts for this. Because of potential end-organ damage and cardiovascular risk in adulthood, auscultatory monitoring of BP is recommended during health care visits for all children 3 years and older and for younger children with certain high-risk features (Table 22-2). Automatic devices may be needed to measure BP in young infants. Elevated BP should be confirmed on repeat visits. The guidelines define *hypertension* as average systolic or diastolic BP of 95% or higher for gender, age, and height on three or more occasions. *Prehypertension* is defined as values of 90% or greater and less than 95%. For

Table 22-1 Significant Causes of Growth Abnormalities in Children

Short Stature

Familial	Constitutional growth delay
	Familial (genetic) short stature
Genetic	Down syndrome
	Noonan syndrome
	Russell Silver syndrome
	Skeletal dysplasia (dwarfism)
	Turner's syndrome
	Virilizing congenital adrenal hyperplasia (tall child, short adult)
Systemic disorders	AIDS
	Asthma (poorly controlled)
	Cancer, caused by poor nutrition, chemotherapy, or radiotherapy
	Celiac disease
	Chronic heart failure
	Congenital heart disease
	Cushing's syndrome
	Cystic fibrosis
	Diabetes mellitus (poorly controlled)
	Endocrine disease
	Gastrointestinal disease
	Growth hormone deficiency, congenital or acquired
	Heart disease
	Hypopituitarism
	Hypothyroidism
	Immunologic diseases
	Inflammatory bowel disease (Crohn's disease)
	Malabsorption syndromes
	Pulmonary disease
	Renal disease, chronic renal failure, renal tubular acidosis
	Severe combined immunodeficiency
Environmental	Malnutrition
	Psychosocial deprivation
	Toxin or drug exposure (e.g., lead)

Tall Stature*

Familial	Constitutional acceleration of growth
	Familial tall stature
Genetic	Beckwith-Wiedemann syndrome
	Cerebral gigantism (Soto's syndrome)
	Homocystinuria
	Marfan syndrome
Systemic disorders	Endocrine disease
	Pituitary gigantism (acromegaly)
	Thyrotoxicosis

*Data from Bell J. Tall stature. In Finberg L, ed. *Saunders manual of pediatric practice*. Philadelphia: Saunders; 1998:728-730.

adolescents, BP greater than or equal to 120/80 mm Hg but less than 95% is defined as prehypertensive. Because of the inclusion of a diverse population, these guidelines and tables appear applicable to all ethnic groups (see eTable 22-1 and eTable 22-2 online or at www.nhlbi.nih.gov/files/docs/guidelines/child_tbl.pdf).

The approach to confirmed hypertension in children should be individualized and should consider variables such as comorbidities and family history. In overweight or obese children, the possibility of metabolic syndrome should be investigated. Lifestyle changes, including diet and exercise, may be sufficient for overweight children with stage 1 hypertension (BP at 95% to 99% plus 5 mm Hg). Children with stage 2 hypertension (BP >99% plus 5 mm Hg) and those with end-organ damage likely require medical therapy

Table 22-2 Indications for Blood Pressure Measurement in Children Younger Than 3 Years Old

History of prematurity, very low birth weight, or other neonatal complication requiring intensive care
Congenital heart disease (repaired or nonrepaired)
Recurrent urinary tract infections, hematuria, or proteinuria
Known renal disease or urologic malformations
Family history of congenital renal disease
Solid-organ transplant
Malignancy or bone marrow transplant
Treatment with drugs known to raise blood pressure
Other systemic illnesses associated with hypertension (e.g., neurofibromatosis, tuberous sclerosis)
Evidence of elevated intracranial pressure

Data from National High Blood Pressure Education Program Working Group on High Blood Pressure in Children and Adolescents: The Fourth report on the diagnosis, evaluation, and treatment of high blood pressure in children and adolescents. *Pediatrics*. 2004;114:555-576.

(National High Blood Pressure Education Program Working Group, 2004).

Measuring Physical Parameters of Growth

Key Points

- Measure height and weight at all well-child visits.
- Measure head circumference in children up to 24 months of age and BP in children 3 years and older.
- Plot measurements on National Center for Health Statistics (NCHS) growth charts to demonstrate normal growth.
- Investigate significant deviations if the child's growth crosses multiple percentile lines on the growth chart.

Weight, length, and head circumference are the most useful routine measurements in infants. Total body length in children up to age 2 years is obtained most accurately by placing them in the recumbent position and measuring from the crown to the heel. The child's head is placed perpendicular to the surface touching a fixed plate, the hips and knees are fully extended, and the soles of the feet are placed against a sliding board. Older children should have their shoeless standing height measured with a stadiometer with their heels and back touching the wall. Regardless of age, the head should be positioned so that the outer canthus of the eye is aligned with the external auditory canal and perpendicular to the measuring surface (Halac and Zimmerman, 2004). Children should ideally be weighed on the same scale at each visit. Infants should preferably be weighed nude; older children may wear light clothing but not shoes. Height and weight are then plotted on age- and gender-appropriate growth charts developed by the NCHS (see eFigure 22-1) or downloaded from http://www.cdc.gov/growthcharts/clinical_charts.htm.

Body mass index (BMI) is a reliable indicator of body fatness for most children and teenagers that is age and gender specific. A BMI less than the 5th percentile for age is *underweight*, from the 5th to 85th percentiles is *healthy weight,* from the 85th up to 95th percentiles is *overweight,* and the 95th percentile or greater is considered *obese* (Centers for Disease Control and Prevention [CDC], 2009). BMI charts are also available from the same website.

Head circumference reflects the growth of the cranium and its contents. It should be determined and recorded at all routine physical examinations during the first 2 years of life. This also may be done as part of the initial examination at any age. A nonstretchable measuring tape (usually paper or flexible plastic) is used to obtain the greatest circumference encompassing the occipital, parietal, and frontal prominences. A small head circumference (microcephaly) may be familial; caused by craniosynostosis, congenital viral infections, fetal drug syndromes, or underlying structural abnormalities; or secondary to trauma, infection, or dysmorphic syndromes. A large head circumference (macrocephaly) most often is caused by hydrocephalus, but it may be familial, caused by intracranial bleeding or masses or thickening of the skull, or associated with fragile X syndrome and other conditions (Green, 1986).

PROPER USE AND INTERPRETATION OF GROWTH CHARTS

The growth charts shown in eFigure 22-1 online were revised by NCHS (2000) from surveys of generally well-nourished children representing a cross-section of ethnic and economic groups in the United States. These graphs provide a normal range of weight and length or height for a given chronologic age. Recumbent length is recorded on the chart for children from birth to 36 months, and standing height is recorded on the chart for children from 2 to 18 years. Premature infants should have their chronologic age adjusted according to their degree of prematurity up to age 2 years because most catch-up growth is complete by this time. Although a height or weight above the 95th percentile or below the fifth percentile should alert the physician to a possible problem, these can represent the outer fringe of the normal range.

Linear growth in infants has been shown to occur in incremental bursts rather than continuously (Lampl et al., 1992). A growth curve constructed by a series of heights and weights taken over time allows the physician to compare current growth with the child's previous pattern. The *linear growth velocity,* or rate of gain in height, decreases from 25 cm/yr during the first year of life to a prepubertal rate of 5 to 6 cm/yr by age 6 or 7 years (Miller and Zimmerman, 2004). The rate accelerates during puberty. A child whose growth curve parallels the normal curve regardless of the child's absolute percentile has a normal rate of growth for that particular child. In comparison, a child whose height or weight crosses multiple percentile lines or whose linear growth rate drops below 4 cm/yr requires further evaluation for nutritional, psychosocial, or organic problems that could impede or accelerate growth (Lipsky and Horner, 1988). Children with familial short stature have normal length and weight at birth, but their growth percentiles decline within the first 2 to 3 years of life as they reach their genetic potential (Halac and Zimmerman, 2004).

Although careful measuring and plotting of growth parameters is the most accurate method by which to follow a child's physical growth, approximate growth guidelines

Table 22-3 Approximate Growth Guidelines for Children

Age	Length or Height (ht)	Weight (wt)
Newborn	50 cm (20 in) average	3.4 kg (7.5 lb) average
Newborn to 3 mo	—	1 kg/mo (1 oz/day) average weight gain
3-12 mo	—	Wt (kg) = [Age (mo) + 9] ÷ 2 Wt (lb) = Age (mo) + 11*
12 months	75 cm (30 in) average	Triples birth weight
12-24 mo	Increases by >10 cm/yr	0.25 kg/mo
>5 yr	>5 cm (2 in)/yr until adolescent growth spurt	2.3 kg (5 lb)/yr until adolescent growth spurt
2-12 yr	Ht (cm) = [Age (yr) × 6] + 77 Ht (in) = [Age (yr) × 2.5] + 30* (e.g., 4-year-old child = 40 in)	Ages 1-6 yr: Wt (kg) = [Age (yr) × 2] + 8 Wt (lb) = [Age (yr) × 5] + 17* Ages 7-12 yr: Wt (kg) = [Age (yr) × 7 − 5] ÷ 2 Wt (lb) = Age (yr) × 7 + 5*
Puberty	8-14 cm/yr	

*Modified from Needleman RD. The first year. In Behrman RE, Kliegman RM, Jenson HB, eds. *Nelson textbook of pediatrics.* 17th ed. Philadelphia: Saunders; 2004:31.
Ht, Height; *wt,* weight.

are helpful to the physician in remembering and forming an overall impression of the child's progress (Table 22-3).

FAMILIAL SHORT STATURE AND CONSTITUTIONAL GROWTH DELAY

Each child has a different rate of maturation, or what Boas termed "tempo of growth" (Tanner, 1986). Persons with *short stature* are more than 2 standard deviations (SD) below the mean in height and constitute approximately 2.5% of children (Miller and Zimmerman, 2004). If a child's growth falls outside the range of normal, it is useful to obtain a bone-age radiograph, usually of the left hand and wrist, and compare it with age-specific standards. Children must be at least 2 years of age to reliably identify epiphyseal ossification centers. Table 22-4 lists some causes of retarded or accelerated bone age. Calculation of mean predicted adult height is also useful in determining whether a child is fulfilling her or his genetic potential. The mean predicted adult height is calculated as follows (Rogol, 2004):

Boys mean height =
  [Father's height + (Mother's height + 13 cm)] /2
Girl's mean height =
  [(Father's height − 13 cm) + Mother's height]/2

Children and adolescents of short stature whose bone age is delayed relative to their chronologic age have more growth potential than do children with a skeletal age appropriate for their chronologic age. If an organic cause of short stature has been excluded, children with delayed bone age are likely to have *constitutional growth delay.* The majority of these children are boys who were of normal length and weight at birth. Their growth rate decelerates during the first 2 years of life and subsequently returns to normal.

The children then follow a lower percentile on the growth curve until the onset of their pubertal growth spurt and development, which often occurs later than their peers. There is usually a family history of delayed growth and development (Bareille and Standhope, 1998). The bone age of these children equals their height age, which is the age at which their height plots on the 50th percentile of the growth chart.

Children with familial short stature usually have parents or close relatives who are short. They often have normal birth weight and length, but their growth rate declines during the first 2 to 3 years of life. Their growth curve subsequently parallels the normal curve but falls below the fifth percentile (Bareille et al., 1998). Their bone age is approximately equal to their chronologic age but less than their height age. These children usually enter puberty at the appropriate age. The U.S. Food and Drug Administration (FDA) has approved the use of recombinant growth hormone for the treatment of idiopathic short stature. This can result in an increase of predicted height of more than 7 cm (Miller and Zimmerman, 2004). Because of potential side effects and the high cost, treatment should be undertaken in consultation with a specialist in pediatric growth disorders.

PUBERTAL GROWTH AND DEVELOPMENT

All children grow at a different tempo, with some maturing earlier than others and some later. This difference is most apparent during puberty. The NCHS growth charts now extend to age 20 years. Tanner and Davies (1985) took the earlier NCHS data and constructed height and weight velocity curves for American boys and girls that account for those groups who mature earlier and later. These charts also allow for notation of the various stages of puberty described by Tanner (1986) (Table 22-5).

The onset of puberty generally occurs at age 9 in American girls, with the peak height velocity occurring at age 11.5 years (range, 9.7 to 13.5 years for early to late maturers). American boys have onset of puberty at age 11 and peak height velocity at 13.5 years (range, 11.7-15.3 years) (Tanner and Davies, 1985). Because boys have two additional years of prepubertal growth and a peak height velocity greater than that of girls, their ultimate height is usually taller. Head, hands, and feet are first to reach their adult size followed by leg length, trunk length (which accounts for much of the spurt), and body breadth. Pubertal boys develop greater shoulder breadth than do pubertal girls, who develop wider hips. Adolescents can be reassured that their bodies eventually will become more proportionate with their hands and feet. Boys ultimately gain greater muscle size and strength than do girls while losing limb fat. This results from their increased secretion of testosterone,

Table 22-4 Causes of Short Stature and Relationship to Bone Age and Growth Rate

Bone age less than chronologic age	**Growth Rate Normal or Slightly Decreased**
	Constitutional growth delay
	Growth Rate Decreased
	Endocrine disorders
	Cushing's syndrome
	Growth hormone deficiency
	Chronic systemic disease
	Crohn's disease
	Heart failure
	Renal failure
	Severe malnutrition
	Severe psychosocial deprivation
Bone age equals chronologic age	**Growth Rate Normal or Slightly Decreased**
	Familial short stature
	Skeletal dysplasias
	Rickets
	Growth Rate Decreased
	Chromosomal disorders
	Down syndrome
	Turner's syndrome
Bone age greater than chronologic age	**Growth Rate Initially Increased But Short Adult**
	Congenital adrenal hyperplasia
	Exogenous androgenic steroids
	Precocious puberty

Table 22-5 Sexual Maturity Stages in Boys and Girls

Stage	Male Genitalia	Pubic Hair	Female Breasts
1	Preadolescent: testes, scrotum, and penis are childlike in size	None; may be vellus hair, as over abdomen	Preadolescent: elevation of papilla only
2	Slight enlargement of scrotum with reddening of skin; little or no enlargement of penis	Sparse growth of long, slightly pigmented, downy hair, straight or slightly curled, primarily at base of penis or along labia	Breast bud stage; breast and papilla form a small mound; areolar diameter enlarges
3	Further enlargement of scrotum; penis enlarges, mainly in length	Hair considerably darker, coarser, and more curled; spreads sparsely over junction of pubes	Further enlargement of breasts and areola with no separation of their contours
4	Further enlargement and darkening of scrotum; penis enlarges, especially in breadth; glans develops	Adult-type hair that does not extend onto thighs, covering a smaller area than in adults	Areola and papilla project to form a secondary mound above the contour of the breast; stage 4 development of the areolar mound does not occur in 10% of girls and is slight in 20%; when present, it may persist well into adulthood
5	Adult in size and shape	Adult in quantity and type with extension onto thighs but not up linea alba	Mature female; papilla projects and areola recesses to general contour of breast
6	—	Spreads up linea alba (80% of men, 10% of women)	—

Modified from Tanner JM. Normal growth and techniques of growth assessment. *Clin Endocrinol Metab.* 1986;15:436.

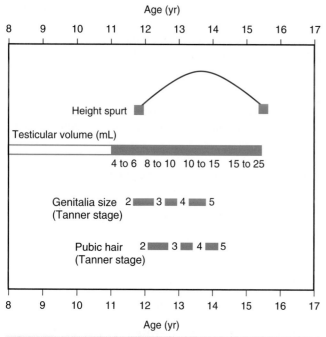

Figure 22-1 Sequence of pubertal events in average American boys. (Modified from Brookman RR, Rauh JL, Morrison JA, et al. The Princeton maturation study; 1976, unpublished data for adolescents in Cincinnati, Ohio. In Copeland KC, Brookman RR, Rauh JL, eds. *Assessment of pubertal development.* Columbus, OH: Ross Products Division, Abbott Laboratories; 1986:4.)

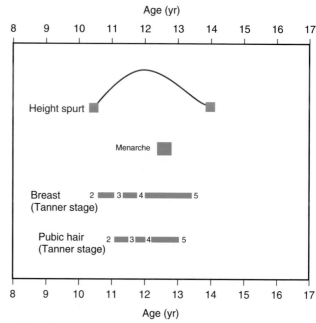

Figure 22-2 Sequence of pubertal events in average American girls. (Modified from Brookman RR, Rauh JL, Morrison JA, et al. The Princeton maturation study; 1976, unpublished data for adolescents in Cincinnati, Ohio. In Copeland KC, Brookman RR, Rauh JL, eds. *Assessment of pubertal development.* Columbus, OH: Ross Products Division, Abbott Laboratories; 1986:4.)

which also increases red blood cell mass and hemoglobin (Tanner, 1986).

The adolescent growth spurt in skeletal and body dimensions is associated closely with the development of the reproductive system. Although the onset and rate of maturation vary according to the individual, the sequence is usually the same within genders (Figures 22-1 and 22-2). Girls who demonstrate signs of puberty before 7 to 8 years of age and boys who show signs before 9 years should be evaluated for *precocious puberty.* Conversely, girls who do not show signs of puberty by age 13 years and boys by age 14 years should be evaluated for *pubertal delay* (Plotnick, 1999).

The first sign of puberty in boys is an increase in growth of the testes and scrotum, with reddening and wrinkling of the scrotal skin. Pubic hair appears within 6 months followed by phallic enlargement in 12 to 18 months and peak height velocity 2 to 2.5 years after testicular enlargement (Copeland, 1986). Axillary hair usually appears 2 years after the beginning of pubic hair growth (stage 4 pubic hair), but there is considerable variability. Some boys may have enlargement of the breasts midway through adolescence. After the attainment of peak height velocity, boys develop mature spermatozoa, full facial hair, and voice change. However, breaking of the voice is a late and often gradual process.

In girls, the breast buds are the first sign of puberty, and the pubertal growth spurt typically occurs concurrently, peaking at stage 3 breast and pubic hair. The uterus and vagina develop simultaneously with the breasts, but menarche usually does not occur until stage 4 breast and pubic hair. Although the peak height velocity has been passed, girls may grow an average of 6 cm more after menarche. Early cycles may be irregular and anovulatory, but early sterility should never be presupposed (Tanner, 1986).

Screening Healthy Children

Key Points

- All newborns should have a hearing screen within the first month of life.
- Examine eyes at all well care visits; screen vision beginning at age 3 years.
- Provide anticipatory guidance regarding discipline starting at 15 months of age.

Preventive care services for children often include screening for health conditions in which early detection and early treatment can prevent or ameliorate more serious disease in the future. Screening tests should detect most persons with the condition *(sensitivity)* while excluding most persons who do not have the condition *(specificity)* in a cost-effective manner. In an inner-city Medicaid population, high continuity of care in infancy was associated with improved screening for anemia, lead, and tuberculosis (TB) (Flores et al., 2008).

HEARING AND VISION SCREENING

Early detection and intervention for hearing and vision deficits are important for maximal long-term functioning. Without appropriate opportunities to learn language, children with significant hearing deficits fall behind peers in terms of communication, cognition, reading, and social-emotional development, with long-term effects on educational attainment and adult employment (AAP Joint Committee on Infant Hearing, 2007). All infants should be screened for hearing loss by 1 month of age, regardless of risk factors. Those who do not pass the screening should have a complete audiologic evaluation by 3 months of age, and those with confirmed hearing loss should receive appropriate treatment by 6 months to ensure optimal outcome. Regardless of the outcome of newborn screening, ongoing surveillance of hearing status is recommended. Developmental delays and other risk factors (Table 22-6), particularly in language, as well as the presence of parental concern about hearing, should prompt referral for a complete audiologic evaluation, even if the newborn screening results were normal and there are no risk factors for hearing impairment (Hagan et al., 2008). Gradations of hearing loss are presented in Table 22-7.

Eyesight evaluation is a recommended part of routine health maintenance examinations in children beginning in the newborn period. In young children (<3 years), the evaluation, besides the actual eye examination, is somewhat subjective and based on parental history. Children with risk factors, such as prematurity, family history of retinoblastoma or glaucoma, or significant developmental delays or neurologic difficulties, should be referred to an experienced pediatric ophthalmologist. The U.S. Preventive Services Task Force (USPSTF) recommends vision screening for all children at least once between the ages of 3 and 5 years, especially to detect amblyopia or its risk factors (e.g., strabismus), which occurs in 2% to 4% of preschool children (USPSTF, 2011, grade B evidence). Testing of children at this age may use standardized systems such as the Allen Cards, which have easily recognized pictures. Normal visual acuity is in the 20/30 to 20/40 range for children 3 to 4 years old but increases to 20/20 by early school age. Eye-specific screening should be attempted in an effort to detect amblyopia (more than one line difference on the chart) (SOR: B). The suspicion of amblyopia or strabismus requires further evaluation to prevent long-term visual loss. Routine screening should be done at least through early school age, at puberty, and whenever there are other signs, such as squinting or complaints of inability to see the board at school (Hagan et al., 2008).

SCREENING FOR IRON-DEFICIENCY ANEMIA

The USPSTF (2006) currently has found insufficient evidence to recommend for or against routine screening of asymptomatic infants age 6 to 12 months for iron-deficiency anemia (IDA). Hemoglobin determines red blood cell mass and the presence of anemia but is neither sensitive nor specific. Serum ferritin is more sensitive and may be used as a confirmatory test for iron deficiency as long as inflammation is absent (Baker et al., 2010). True iron deficiency is much more common than IDA. In addition, there is evidence that even children with severe anemia who are treated with iron supplementation continue to demonstrate behavioral and developmental deficits 10 years afterward (Lozoff et al., 2000). Nevertheless, the AAP Committee on Nutrition recommends universal screening for anemia at about 1 year of age. This should include an assessment of risk factors, including history of prematurity or low birth weight, exclusive breastfeeding beyond 4 months of age without supplemental iron, or weaning to whole milk or foods that are low in iron. If these risk factors are present, selective screening can be done at any age (Baker et al., 2010).

SCREENING FOR LEAD TOXICITY

Because lead is neurotoxic and affects both intellectual and behavioral function, the CDC defines a blood lead level (BLL) of 5 μg/dL or greater as a high BLL (CDC, 2013). This is based on the 97.5th percentile in the 2007 to 2010 National Health and Nutrition Examination Survey (NHANES), which demonstrated that the percentage of children with BLLs of 5 μg/dL or higher was 2.6% overall for children age 1 to 5 years, with 5.6% in black, non-Hispanic; 2.6% in Mexican American; and 2.4% in white non-Hispanic children. However, approximately 7% to 40% of immigrant and refugee children, especially from the Near East, Africa, Asia, and Central American or Caribbean countries, have high BLLs. Therefore, these children 6 months to 16 years old should be screened for lead within 30 to 90 days of arrival in the United States (CDC, 2013). Screening for IDA should also be done because this is a significant risk factor for elevated BLL. Targeted screening of specific groups of children may be recommended by state mandate or third-party

---

Table 22-6 Risk Factors for Delayed Onset of Hearing Loss in Young Children

Caregiver concern regarding hearing, speech, language, or developmental delay

Family history of permanent childhood hearing loss

Neonatal intensive care longer than 5 days

In utero infections (e.g., cytomegalovirus)

Craniofacial anomalies (e.g., ear pits, ear canal defects)

Syndromes known to be associated with hearing loss (e.g., neurofibromatosis)

Neurodegenerative disorders (e.g., Friedreich ataxia)

Postnatal infections (e.g., meningitis)

Head trauma (e.g., basal skull/temporal bone fracture)

Chemotherapy

Modified from Hagan JF, Shaw JS, Duncan PM, eds. *Bright futures: guidelines for health supervision of infants, children, and adolescents.* 3rd ed. Elk Grove Village, IL: American Academy of Pediatrics; 2008:232.

Table 22-7 Hearing Loss Scale

Hearing Impairment	Hearing Threshold (dB)
None	10-25
Mild	26-40
Moderate	41-55
Moderate to severe	56-70
Severe	71-90
Profound	>91

payers (e.g., Medicaid). Specific state information can be obtained at http://www.cdc.gov/nceh/lead. Children considered at risk who require screening include (1) those suspected by a parent or health care provider to be at risk for exposure; (2) those with a sibling or frequent playmate with an elevated BLL; (3) those with a parent or caregiver who works professionally or recreationally with lead; (4) those with a household member who uses traditional folk or ethnic remedies or cosmetics; or (5) those designated at increased risk for lead exposure by the health department because of local risk factors for lead exposure, such as residing in a high-risk zip code (Wengrovitz and Brown, 2009).

SCREENING FOR TUBERCULOSIS

In 2007, there were approximately 10 million cases of new and recurrent TB and 1.8 million deaths worldwide, with the highest rates occurring in low-income countries (Marais et al., 2009). The incidence of active TB is much lower in the United States, but an estimated 10 to 15 million persons have *latent tuberculosis infection* (LTBI). Six groups considered at high risk are children, foreign-born persons, HIV-infected persons, homeless persons, detainees and prisoners in correctional facilities, and close contacts of infectious persons (CDC, 2005). Targeted rather than universal testing of children for TB is now recommended. Risk factors for LTBI include (1) previous positive tuberculin skin test result, (2) birth in foreign country with high prevalence of TB (e.g., China, India, Mexico, Philippine Islands, Vietnam, certain African countries), (3) nontourist travel to a high-prevalence country for more than 1 week, (4) contact with a TB-infected person, and (5) presence in the household of another person with LTBI (CDC, 2005). The Mantoux TB skin test is recommended for children because its correlation with results of interferon-γ release assays is often discordant in children (Connell et al., 2008).

Discipline

Parents frequently ask their primary care physicians about discipline. Discipline should be a priority topic for anticipatory guidance when the child is 15 months and 18 months (Hagan et al., 2008). Effective discipline requires three essential components: (1) a positive, loving relationship between the parent(s) and child; (2) positive reinforcement strategies to increase desired behaviors; and (3) punishment or removal of reinforcement to reduce or eliminate undesired behaviors. Although often confused with punishment, discipline actually means to *teach*. All children benefit from guidance and structure, and most children require occasional discipline. The best discipline is consistent and considers the child's developmental level as well as the child's point of view. Effective strategies include environmental modifications (e.g., childproofing the house), distraction, redirection, giving appropriate choices, and time-outs. Although many parents spank (Regalado et al., 2004), corporal punishment is controversial and has potential long-term negative effects (Smith, 2006). Other methods of discipline are more effective over time and should be used. Some families may require more intensive assistance,

and clinicians should be aware of local resources for teaching parents.

Nutrition

Key Points

- Breast milk is the recommended food for infants and the standard to which infant formulas are compared.
- Give vitamin D supplements to all breastfed infants and those taking less than 1 L of vitamin D–fortified milk or formula per day.
- Begin iron-fortified cereal for infants older than 4 to 6 months or low-birth-weight (LBW) infants older than 2 weeks.
- Obtain a fasting lipid profile in children with a family history of dyslipidemia; premature atherosclerotic vascular disease; or personal risk factors such as overweight, hypertension, smoking, and diabetes mellitus.

INFANCY THROUGH ADOLESCENCE

Proper physical growth and appropriate cognitive development depend on adequate nutrition. Infants and young children with severe IDA were found to have significantly lower verbal and full-scale IQ scores and lower achievement test scores in arithmetic and writing than infants without iron deficiency, even 10 years after treatment (Lozoff et al., 2000). An increase in behavioral problems was also reported, although this could not be directly linked to the preceding iron deficiency. In NHANES III (1988-1994), 7.2% of 12- to 16-year-old girls had iron deficiency, but only 1.5% demonstrated anemia (Halterman et al., 2001). Adolescent iron-deficient girls scored significantly lower math scores compared with non–iron-deficient girls. Vitamin D deficiency and insufficiency in children and adolescents has been reported worldwide, including in North America (Wagner and Greer, 2008). Mealtimes also represent times for social interaction within the family unit, whether it is the bonding of mother and child during breastfeeding or discussion of the day's events during dinnertime.

Although malnutrition is still a problem in the United States, *inappropriate nutrition*, especially calorie-nutrient imbalance leading to overweight and obesity, has become commonplace. Recent NHANES studies demonstrate that the prevalence of overweight (BMI ≥95%) in girls 2 to 19 years old increased from 13.8% in 1999 to 2000 to 16% in 2003 to 2004, and the prevalence of overweight in boys 2 to 19 years old increased from 14% to 18.2% (Ogden et al., 2006). Increased pediatric BMI is associated with high BP, sleep apnea, asthma, polycystic ovarian syndrome, type 2 diabetes, gastroesophageal reflux, and orthopedic problems (Benson et al., 2009). A nationwide survey of more than 6000 children and adolescents found that at least 30% consumed "fast food" on a typical day. These children consumed more total fat, total carbohydrate, and added sugars and sugar-sweetened beverages, less milk, and fewer fruits

Table 22-8 Comparison of Common Milks and Infant Formulas

Milk or Formula	kcal/ 30 mL	Protein (g/dL)	CHO (g/dL)	CHO Type	Fat (g/dL)	Iron (mg/L)	Comments
Human milk	20	1.0	6.9	Lactose (primary), glucose, oligosaccharides	4.4	<0.1	Small flocculent curd is easily digestible, and iron is absorbed.
Whole cow's milk	19	3.3	4.7	Lactose	3.7	Trace	Curd is less easy to digest. Can cause intestinal blood loss. Do not use before age 12 mo.
Evaporated whole milk	43	6.9	10.0	Lactose	7.6	Trace	Curd is softer, smaller, and may be less allergenic. Dilute and add dextrose to make 20 kcal/oz formula.
Prepared formula, cow's milk based	20	1.4-1.7	6.9-7.5	Lactose	3.4-3.8	4.7-12.2*	AAP recommends only iron-fortified formulas.
Prepared formula, soy based	20	1.7-1.8	6.8-7.4	Corn syrup, corn syrup solids, sucrose, corn maltodextrin	3.4-3.7	12-12.2	May use if lactase-deficient vegetarian, galactosemic, or allergic to cow's milk.†

*Iron-fortified formula; †However, cross-reactivity with cow's milk protein sometimes occurs.
AAP, American Academy of Pediatrics; CHO, carbohydrate.
Modified and compiled from Kleinman RE, ed. *Pediatric nutrition handbook.* 6th ed. Elk Grove Village, IL: American Academy of Pediatrics; 2008:1250-1265.

and nonstarchy vegetables than children who did not eat fast food (Bowman et al., 2004). The odds of having a BMI of 85th percentile or higher was more than four times that for 10- to 15-year-old children viewing more than 5 hours of television per day compared with those watching for 0 to 2 hours (Gortmaker et al., 1996). A survey of low-income preschool children in New York State found that children with TV sets in their bedrooms watched 4.6 hours per week more TV and videos than those without bedroom TVs. In this group, the prevalence of child overweight (BMI >85%) was associated with an odds ratio of 1.06 for each additional hour per day of TV or videos viewed (Dennison et al., 2002). Frequent television viewing can lead to decreased activity, excessive snacking on high-calorie junk foods, and subsequent obesity (Dietz and Gortmaker, 1985). In contrast, dieting in pursuit of the media's representation of the ideal woman can lead to eating disorders, such as bulimia or anorexia. The CDC has proposed 24 strategies to prevent obesity in the United States, including increasing the availability of healthier food and beverage choices, restricting the availability of less healthy foods and beverages in public service areas, and increasing the amount of physical activity in schools (Khan et al., 2009).

INFANTS AND TODDLERS

Infants require approximately 120 kcal/kg/day to meet basal metabolic requirements and the energy demands of growth and activity during the first 6 months of life. LBW newborns may require 130 to 150 cal/kg/day for catch-up growth. Weight gain should be 25 to 30 g/day during the first 3 months of life, decrease to 15 to 20 g/day between 3 and 6 months of age, and decrease to 10 to 15 g/day between 6 and 12 months (AAP, 2009). Energy requirements are increased by greater physical activity, stress imposed by disease processes (e.g., cystic fibrosis), or symptoms (e.g., fever). Fever can increase the fluid requirements of infants younger than 6 months beyond the usual 130 to 190 mL/kg/day (Barness and Curran, 1996).

The composition of human milk varies by time, day, and maternal nutrition and from woman to woman. Infant formulas contain about 50% more protein than human milk and, similar to breast milk, provide 40% to 50% of energy as fat (Table 22-8). Beginning at 2 years of age, fat calories should decrease to approximately 30% of total energy consumption, with less than 10% of calories from saturated fat, and dietary cholesterol less than 300 mg/day (AAP, 2009).

The ideal food for full-term infants during the first 12 months of life is human milk. Oliver Wendell Holmes once noted, "A pair of substantial mammary glands has the advantage over the two hemispheres of the most learned professor's brain in the art of compounding a nutritious fluid for infants" (Cone, 1979, p. 138). Human milk is fresh, readily available at the proper temperature, and generally free of contaminating bacteria. Its acid-resistant whey proteins include secretory immunoglobulin A (sIgA); α-lactalbumin; and lactoferrin, a whey protein that transports iron and inhibits the growth of a range of organisms in the intestine. The protein in human milk consists predominantly of whey proteins that are of higher nutritional quality and digested and absorbed more easily than cow's milk proteins (AAP, 2009).

Commercial cow's milk and soy-based formulas must contain higher levels of protein to compensate for their lower quality (see Table 22-8). However, they are quite acceptable for mothers who are unable to nurse their infants or for parents who wish to bottle feed their children. Soy formulas are recommended for infants with hereditary lactase deficiency or galactosemia and may be tried in infants intolerant to cow's milk, but soy formula should not be used in preterm infants. Because some infants allergic to cow's milk protein will develop an allergy to soy protein, it is advisable to use an extensively hydrolyzed protein formula in cases of true milk allergy or malabsorption. These are lactose free and may contain medium-chain triglycerides to improve fat absorption (AAP, 2009).

Human breast milk or iron-fortified infant formula is recommended for the first 12 months of life. Cow's milk is not suitable for infants because the higher intake of protein, sodium, potassium, and chloride increases renal solute load. In addition, the lower concentrations of iron, zinc, essential fatty acids, vitamin E, and other micronutrients can result in deficiencies. Significant intestinal blood loss can occur in infants younger than 12 months of age receiving cow's milk. Very-low-fat milks lack adequate calories for growth despite promoting excessive volume ingestion. Breastfed full-term infants seldom develop IDA before 4 to 6 months of age because the iron present in breast milk is well absorbed. Iron-fortified infant cereal or meats are then good sources of the 1 mg/kg/day of elemental iron required by full-term infants. All preterm or LBW infants should receive at least 2 mg/kg/day of elemental iron from 2 weeks until 12 months of age (AAP, 2009). Parents should be warned that iron is toxic in excessive amounts, and appropriate precautions should be taken.

Children 6 months to 3 years old who do not drink fluoridated water or other beverages may be given 0.25 mg/day of supplemental fluoride. Human milk contains only small amounts of biologically active vitamin D, and rickets has been reported in breastfed infants, infants with darker skin pigmentation, and even older children with minimal exposure to sunlight. Consequently, all breastfed infants, partially breastfed infants, nonbreastfed infants, and older children ingesting less than 1000 mL/day of vitamin D–fortified formula or milk should receive 400 IU/day of supplemental vitamin D daily beginning within the first few days of life until the infant or child is ingesting 1000 mL/day of vitamin D–fortified formula or milk (AAP, 2009). Higher doses of vitamin D may be required in children with chronic fat malabsorption. Vitamin B_{12} supplementation should be given to breastfed infants whose mothers are strict vegetarians.

Both the World Health Organization and AAP promote exclusive breastfeeding for the first 6 months of life. However, safe, nutritious solid foods may be introduced between 4 and 6 months of age when the infant is developmentally ready. The order of introduction of solid foods is generally not critical; however, single-ingredient foods should be tried for 1 week at a time to observe for possible allergic reactions before introducing another food or mixtures of foods. Single-grain infant cereals such as rice (which lacks gluten) are usually well tolerated and provide a source of fortified iron. Homemade infant foods should not have added salt or sugar. Honey is associated with infant botulism and should not be given to infants younger than 1 year. Teething biscuits or finely chopped foods may be given by 8 to 10 months of age. However, foods such as popcorn, nuts, and rounded candies should not be offered to infants or toddlers because of the risks of choking, aspiration, and even death. Potentially hazardous foods such as hot dogs and grapes must be cut into small pieces, and the caregiver should always be present during mealtimes. Children should be weaned from the bottle to a cup by 12 to 15 months of age and bedtime bottles discouraged because they are associated with dental caries (AAP, 2009).

A toddler's food intake may be quite variable from day to day or even meal to meal. Because young children cannot choose a well-balanced diet, parents must provide nutritious, safe, developmentally appropriate foods at regular meals and snacks. Children should sit in a designated area for mealtimes, without distractions such as television (AAP, 2009). Small portions of food should be offered to preschool children, allowing the child to determine how much he or she will eat and offering more as necessary. Excessive portion sizes can contribute to obesity later in life. Guidelines about types and quantities of foods from the basic food groups are available from the U.S. Department of Agriculture's Choose My Plate website (http://www.choosemyplate.gov), which provides recommendations on the amount of grain products, vegetables, fruits, and milk products based on the person's age, gender, and activity level.

Parents should be counseled that toddlers and preschool children are often picky eaters but generally grow well despite this. Parents need to guide children in their selection of food by offering a variety of nutritious items such as fruits and vegetables, keeping in mind that it can require eight to 10 exposures to a new food before a child accepts it (AAP, 2009). Mealtimes should not turn into a battleground because forcing a child to clean the plate can lead to specific food dislikes or promote obesity in later life. Snacking or eating while watching television should be discouraged, and physical activity should be encouraged.

Healthy children eating a varied diet usually do not require a multivitamin supplement. Children who do not eat dairy products, meat, or eggs require supplemental vitamin B_{12} and are at risk for vitamin D deficiency, especially if they lack adequate sunlight exposure or have darkly pigmented skin. Children following strict vegetarian diets often have low intakes of iron and calcium that can require supplementation. They often have a low intake of zinc that may be obtained from zinc-fortified infant and adult cereals. The recommended fiber intake is 19 g/day for children 1 to 3 years old and 25 g/day for those 4 to 8 years old. Excessive fiber consumption may decrease the intake of energy-dense foods and inhibit the absorption of some minerals (AAP, 2009).

Children with malabsorption or hemolytic anemia can require additional folic acid. Parents who insist on using a vitamin supplement without any obvious deficiency on the part of the child should be counseled to use a preparation that does not exceed the dietary reference intakes established by the Institute of Medicine and the National Academy of Sciences. In particular, vitamins A and D can produce toxicity if given in excessive doses.

ADOLESCENTS

Adolescents are at greater risk than other age groups for nutritional deficiencies because they may skip meals, snack more, eat more fast foods, and follow fad diets for reasons ranging from weight loss to cultural differentiation. Teenage boys and girls often replace milk and juice with soft drinks, coffee, tea, and alcoholic beverages, thereby lowering their intake of calcium as well as vitamins A and C. Adolescents' iron intake may be lower than required for their rapid increases in lean body mass and hemoglobin mass in addition to menstrual blood loss in girls. Zinc is also required for growth and sexual maturation. Most teenagers do not ingest the recommended 1300 mg of calcium daily (AAP, 2009).

Energy requirements vary greatly in teenagers, depending on their gender, activity, and stage of adolescence.

Sedentary adolescent girls require 1600 to 1800 cal/day and sedentary boys 1800 to 2200 kcal/day. As much as 200 kcal/day may be added for moderate physical activity and 200 to 400 kcal/day added for those who are very active (Daniels and Greer, 2008). Healthy pregnant women of normal BMI should tailor their prenatal diet to achieve a total weight gain of 11.5 to 16 kg (26-35 lb), or an additional 300 kcal/day during the second and third trimesters. Additional protein requirements are about 15 and 27 g/day during the second and third trimesters, respectively. Most require some form of iron supplementation, about 30 mg/day during the second and third trimesters. Because zinc deficiency has potential teratogenic effects, pregnant adolescents should receive about 13 mg/day of zinc supplementation along with 1 mg/day of copper supplementation. All women of childbearing potential should take 400 to 600 μg of folic acid supplement per day in addition to 400 μg of dietary folate to decrease the risk of giving birth to children with neural tube defects. Pregnant women also require 1300 mg/day of calcium in their diets (AAP, 2009).

Cholesterol Recommendations

Universal screening for hypercholesterolemia in children is not currently recommended. A fasting lipid profile should be obtained in children who have a family history of dyslipidemia or premature (men ≤55 years, women ≤65 years) coronary heart disease or peripheral vascular or cerebrovascular disease. Children for whom the family history is not known or who have other risk factors such as overweight (BMI ≥85% and <95%), obesity (BMI ≥95%), hypertension (BP ≥95%), cigarette smoking, or diabetes mellitus should also be screened. This screening should be done between 3 and 10 years of age. The National Cholesterol Education Program guidelines indicate that a total cholesterol less than 170 mg/dL is acceptable, 170 to 199 mg/dL is borderline, and 200 mg/dL or greater is high. Similarly, a low-density lipoprotein (LDL) level less than 110 mg/dL is acceptable, 110 to 129 mg/dL is borderline, and higher than 130 mg/dL is elevated (Daniels and Greer, 2008). The American Heart Association has designated triglyceride levels greater than 150 mg/dL and high-density lipoprotein (HDL) level less than 35 mg/dL as abnormal. If initial lipid values are within acceptable levels, retesting should be done in 3 to 5 years.

It is recommended that all healthy children older than 2 years follow a diet in which a wide variety of foods provide adequate caloric intake to achieve proper growth and development as well as desirable weight. Total fat and saturated fat intake should be no more than 30% and 10%, respectively, of total calories; dietary cholesterol should be less than 300 mg/day. Children who are overweight or obese and have a high triglyceride or low HDL level should be counseled regarding proper diet and increased physical activity. Children at especially high risk based on familial hyperlipidemias or premature cardiovascular disease may undertake a diet restricting saturated fat to 7% of total calories and cholesterol to 200 mg/day (Daniels and Greer, 2008). Children 10 years and older may be considered for pharmacologic therapy with LDL of 190 mg/dL or higher without additional risk factors, 160 mg/dL or greater with a family history of early heart disease or two or more other

risk factors, or 130 mg/dL or higher if diabetes mellitus is present (AAP, 2009).

KEY TREATMENT

- Ensure vitamin D intake of at least 400 IU/day, either by diet or supplementation (Wagner and Greer, 2008) (SOR: A).
- Children 2 years and older should follow a diet with less than 30% of calories from total fat and 10% from saturated fat (Daniels and Greer, 2008) (SOR: B).
- Communities should improve the availability of affordable healthier food and beverage choices and restrict the availability of less healthy choices in public service areas by decreasing the cost of healthy foods and increasing the cost of less healthy foods (Khan et al., 2009) (SOR: B).

Behavior and Neurodevelopment

Key Points

- Development is a product of factors intrinsic and extrinsic to the child.
- Basic knowledge of child development enables clinicians to guide and educate families.
- Development proceeds in a basic sequence.
- Delays in one area of development may affect another.
- In preterm infants, correct for prematurity until age 2 years.

One of the rewards of providing primary care for a child is sharing with the family in the development of cognitive, motor, social, and language skills. Clinicians need to understand the theoretic framework on which the scientific understanding of child development is based to individualize the approach to the unique needs and concerns of each family. Physicians should develop strategies for clinically assessing child development and managing identified developmental abnormalities.

THEORIES OF DEVELOPMENT

Child development was widely studied in the 20th century. A general understanding of the common theories can enrich the clinician's relationship with young patients. Most researchers in child development believe that developmental outcomes are a product of intrinsic child factors, including genetic potential and temperament, and extrinsic environmental factors, such as intrauterine, infectious, traumatic, chemical, and sociocultural factors (Vaughan and Litt, 1992). The relative weights of each of these factors vary considerably among persons, thus frustrating the attempts of researchers to develop a formula for predicting developmental outcome for any individual person.

A clinician who is familiar with the key elements of theoretic models can develop expertise in applying them appropriately to meet the needs of countless clinical scenarios. For example, a physician might use Erikson's theory

Table 22-9   Summary of Developmental Theories of Child Development

Theory (Proponents)	Key Features	Potential Clinical Applications
Normative approach: development as maturation (Gesell)	Behavior depends on neurologic and physical maturation. Universal progression of developmental sequence. Minimal role of environment and temperament.	Basis for age norms for developmental milestones typically used in clinical setting.
Psychosexual and psychoanalytic theory: development as resolution of conflict (Freud, Erikson)	Emotional life exerts a strong influence on development and behavior. Unconscious conflicts between biologic drive and social expectations continuously shape behavior and self-concept. Parents exert primary influence on child, affecting behavior into adulthood. Mastery of major developmental tasks at different stages is required for emotional growth.	Interpersonal relationships, especially with primary caregivers, influence present and future adjustment, functioning, and self-concept. Importance of "bonding."
Behaviorism and social learning: development as learning (Pavlov, Skinner, Bandura)	Behavior, but not its underlying influences and motives, can be studied and changed. Environmental stimuli are the major forces shaping development and behavior. Environmental stimuli act as positive and negative reinforcements to existing behavior.	Children imitate what they see, so environmental models are important to learning (e.g., influences of media). Basis for behavioral management approaches.
Constructivist views: development as cognitive change (Piaget)	Cognitive development depends on both nature and nurture. Child uses physical and mental abilities to observe and act on the environment. Observation and action advance cognitive development. Child's mental processing develops with age, influencing how child perceives and interacts with the world.	Children possess an innate drive to learn. Play is the medium by which children learn and develop. Parents can be guided in choosing appropriate playthings and settings to allow their children to learn.
Ecologic system: development as cultural and ecologic adaptation (Bronfenbrenner)	A set of interrelated systems (e.g., family, school, community, health services) influences development. These systems exert reciprocal influence on one another. Development is determined by interactions of child and family.	Children's needs must be considered in context of the family and the environment.

of psychosocial stages to explain to a vexed parent of a 2-year-old child that the child's constant temper tantrums represent a normal expression of the child's need to exert autonomy over the environment. In the next room, the physician might refer to Piaget's concept of concrete operational thought to explain why a 10-year-old child might not be capable of considering remote consequences of present actions (e.g., "If I don't study for my science test, I might not meet my goal of becoming an astronaut").

Features of the most widely accepted developmental theories are found in many pediatric references (Dixon and Stein, 2000). A summary of the salient features of each theory and potential clinical applications is presented in Table 22-9.

Erikson's psychosocial stages theory is particularly relevant (Table 22-10). According to his theory, at each discrete life stage, persons are confronted with a crisis requiring integration of personal needs with sociocultural demands. Successful integration of needs and development indicates normal adaptation. A practitioner who is familiar with these stages can counsel families about the emotional needs of children at different ages and explain the appropriateness of challenging but normal childhood behavior.

The concept of temperament is also clinically relevant for primary care. *Temperament* is a set of consistent, inborn characteristics that influence how people interact with and learn from their environments (Thomas et al., 1968). A person's temperament characteristics are innate to his or her personality. Three basic temperament profiles based on nine separate infant characteristics are outlined in Table 22-11. These are broad generalizations, and not all infants fit easily into one of these three categories.

Each family's personal value system influences their reaction to a child of a particular temperament. For

Table 22-10   Using Erikson's Psychosocial Stages to Guide Development

Psychosocial Stage	Guidance
Basic trust and mistrust (0-2 yr; infancy)	Parent can provide consistent nurturing to aid development of attitude of trust.
Autonomy vs. shame and doubt (2-4 yr)	Parent should allow safe exploration of environment and encourage decision making.
Initiative vs. guilt (5-7 yr)	Limits on child should be for protection of child, family, and society and not random or condemning.
Industry vs. inferiority (8-12 yr)	Caregiver must work with the school to ensure that child is achieving to his or her abilities and feeling a sense of competence vs. inferiority.
Identity vs. role confusion (13-17 yr)	Selection of career goals; establishment of relationships with the gender of attraction; independence from family should be encouraged by caregiver; failures to adapt in previous stages make this stage more difficult.
Intimacy vs. isolation (18-22 yr)	Need to make personal and occupational commitment.

example, a highly competitive, athletically oriented family may view high-energy, high-intensity characteristics more positively than a family who values studiousness. Qualities such as introversion or extroversion are often based on characteristics of temperament and are not modified readily by the environment. In a family in which "goodness of fit" between individual members' temperaments does not exist, knowledge of the inborn nature of temperament can

Table 22-11 Temperament Characteristics and Profiles

Feature	Description
Characteristics	
Activity	Frequency and speed of involvement
Rhythmicity	Regularity of physiologic functions (e.g., hunger, sleep, elimination)
Approach and withdrawal	Immediate reaction of child to new stimuli
Adaptability	Degree of ease or difficulty with which child adjusts to new stimuli
Intensity	Energy level of responses, without regard to positive or negative quality of the response
Mood	Predominance of pleasant and friendly versus unfriendly behavior during waking
Attention span and persistence	Length of time the child will engage in a single activity with or without interruption
Distractibility	Degree of ease with which extraneous stimuli interfere with child's task performance
Sensory threshold	Amount of external stimulation required to evoke a response
Profiles	
Easy (40% of children)	Regularity of biologic functions; positive approach responses to new stimuli; high adaptability to change; mild to moderately intense mood that is predominantly positive
Difficult (10% of children)	Irregularity of biologic functions; negative withdrawal responses to new stimuli; no or slow adaptability to change; intense expressions of mood that are predominantly negative
Slow to warm up (15% of children)	Negative responses of mild intensity to new stimuli, with slow adaptability with repeated contact; mild intensity of reactions

Modified from Chess S, Thomas A. Dynamics of individual behavior development. In Levine MD, Carey WB, Crocker AC, eds. *Developmental-behavioral pediatrics*. Philadelphia: Saunders; 1992:86.

help the family accept a child's unique characteristics. Anticipatory guidance can then focus on achieving a better relationship between family and child.

Guidelines for Clinical Assessment

Although individual children develop at their own rate, with great variability in the normal range, general rules for neurodevelopmental maturation can serve as guidelines to help practitioners formulate a developmental trajectory for each child (Sturner and Howard, 1997). The developmental trajectory can be envisioned as an individualized growth chart of anticipated developmental progress based on normal neurodevelopmental milestones and moderated by child, parent, and environmental factors such as temperament, parental mental health, and exposure to lead.

Development usually is categorized into the domains of language, fine motor, gross motor, personal-social, and cognitive. Delays can occur in one or any combination of these domains. For example, a child with intellectual disability is likely to have delays in multiple domains, although gross motor skills may be fairly well preserved. Conversely, a child with cerebral palsy may have normal or near-normal cognitive development with significant delays in gross and fine motor function. Many of the neurodevelopmental rules of thumb address the relationships among these domains.

Children acquire developmental tasks in a predictable sequence. For example, children typically do not learn to walk until they have mastered crawling and then standing. Although most children are able to crawl by 9 months of age and walk by 14.5 months, even severely delayed children follow the sequence of crawl, stand, and walk (Milani-Comparetti and Gidoni, 1967). This predictable sequence is dictated by building on previously learned skills, as well as by maturation of the central nervous system (CNS) (Springate, 1981). Before a critical stage in the maturation of the CNS, certain skills cannot be learned regardless of the intellectual potential or will of the child or parent. For example, because CNS control of the external anal sphincter is incomplete before 18 to 24 months of age, it is impossible to toilet train even the most precocious toddler before this age.

Responses to stimuli proceed from generalized, symmetric, whole-body reflexes to discrete, cortically controlled, voluntary actions. Newborn reflexes can be thought of in terms of their role in survival of the individual; an example is the rooting reflex, which helps the newborn seek out nutrition. Voluntary movements develop as the child learns to control the environment.

Development proceeds in head-to-toe (cephalocaudal) and proximal-to-distal directions. Therefore, an infant bears weight on the arms before bearing weight on the legs. As proximal-to-distal progression occurs, the infant becomes more precise in fine tuning the smaller muscles involved in reaching, grasping, and manipulating an object with his or her hand. Vocalization skills follow this pattern as well. A newborn infant vocalizes with "grunts" originating in the chest. As proximal-to-distal maturation develops, vocalizations originate more distally in the larynx (cooing), glottis (guttural syllables, "ga"), tongue ("da"), and lips ("ba").

Delays in one developmental domain can impair development in another domain. For example, an 18-month-old infant with motor impairments secondary to spina bifida lacks the freedom to explore the environment to learn how two pieces of furniture are oriented in space. Likewise, delays in one developmental domain can impair the practitioner's ability to evaluate skills in other domains. A 4-year-old toddler with cerebral palsy might understand the concept of sorting by shape but lack the motor control to manipulate the shapes to pass a standardized test.

An outline of salient features of development in each domain based on age is presented in Table 22-12. This guide to normal development should be considered by the physician along with past history, parental concerns, clinical observations, and developmental screening in the ongoing surveillance of child development. Until chronologic age 2 years, the development of a premature infant should be judged on corrected age (i.e., the chronologic age minus the number of weeks premature).

Table 22-12   Developmental Milestones in Young Children

Age	Gross Motor	Fine Motor and Reflex Motor	Social, Adaptive, and Cognitive	Language
Neonate	Flexed attitude, turns head side to side when prone without lifting, head sags if unsupported, body sags on ventral suspension	*Reflex:* moro symmetric, grasp reflex, stepping reflex, suck reflex, placing reflex	Fixates on face or light, moves in cadence with sound	Alerts to voice
1 mo	Extends legs more, holds chin up briefly when prone, head lag persists	*Reflex:* persistence of neonatal reflexes, tonic neck posture	Watches person, visually tracks to midline, begins to smile, body moves in cadence with voice	Throaty noises, range of cries to signal hunger, pain
2 mo	Raises head from prone position, sustains head in plane with body or ventral suspension, head lag on pull to sit	*Reflex:* stepping reflex fades	Smiles on social contact, attracts to voice	Coos
4 mo	Head up to vertical axis in prone position, bears weight on arms, extends legs, symmetric posture with hands in midline in supine position, no head lag on pull to sit, pushes with feet in standing position, holds head erect in sitting position	*Fine:* grasps and attains object, brings to mouth *Reflex:* grasps, Moro, tonic neck fade; downward parachute present	Laughs out loud, voices displeasure if contact is broken, excites at sight of food, regards a small pellet	Vowel sounds, visually searches for speaker
6 mo	Sits alone with rounded back, rolls over, pivots, creeps	*Fine:* rakes at pellet, transfers, turns body to reach *Reflex:* sideways parachute present	Prefers mother, responds to emotion, imitates banging, visually follows dropped objects	Polysyllabic babble, blows bubble ("raspberry"), laughs
9 mo	Sits with erect back, crawls, walks holding both hands, pulls to stand, can get to sitting position	*Fine:* pokes with forefinger, uses assisted pincer grasp *Reflex:* forward (7 mo) and backward parachute present, plantar grasp fades	Plays "peekaboo," "pat-a-cake"; waves bye-bye; finds an object after watching it hidden; may cry at sight of unfamiliar person	Responds to some verbal commands: "no"; imitates some sounds; uses "mama," "dada" nonspecifically
12 mo	Cruises holding on, stands alone, may take several steps, walks holding hand	*Fine:* neat pincer grasp, releases on request; puts 2 cubes in cup, pellet in bottle	Plays ball, adjusts posture when dressing, drinks from a cup, imitates activity (talks on toy phone)	1-2 true words, symbolic gestures (e.g., shakes head "no"), points to indicate wants
15 mo	Walks alone, crawls up stairs, walks backward, rises after stooping	*Fine:* dumps pellet from bottle or draws line with crayon when demonstrated, scribbles spontaneously, stacks 2 cubes	Feeds self with utensils, performs simple household tasks (pick up toys), hugs parent	Points to body parts, jargons, follows one-step command without gestures
18 mo	Runs stiffly, sits on small chair, walks up stairs with hand holding rail	*Fine:* tower of four cubes, dumps pellet on request, imitates line with crayon	Feeds self with utensils; kisses parent with pucker; explores drawers, wastebaskets; removes garments; seeks help when in trouble	10 words, says "no," names pictures, points to one body part
24 mo	Runs well; walks up and down stairs, one at a time; jumps in place, climbs on furniture; kicks ball	*Fine:* tower of seven cubes, "train" of four cubes; imitates vertical and circular crayon stroke; imitates folding paper	Listens to story with pictures, helps to undress, dresses with help, parallel play, uses spoon well	30-50 words; two- or three-word sentences; uses pronouns, sometimes incorrectly; relates recent experience; speech 50% intelligible
36 mo	Alternates feet climbing stairs, stands on one foot briefly, broad jumps with both feet, pedals tricycle, throws ball overhand	*Fine:* tower of 10 cubes, imitates "bridge" of 3 cubes, imitates cross, copies circle, attempts to draw person	Knows age and gender, counts three objects, repeats three serial numbers, understands turn-taking, washes and dries hands, helps with dressing	States full name; uses complete sentences; speech 75% intelligible to stranger; uses plurals, past tense, pronouns correctly
48 mo	Hops on one foot, throws ball overhand, balances on each foot 2-3 seconds	*Fine:* uses scissors to cut out pictures; copies cross, square; draws man with head and two to four body parts (pairs count as 1 part); tells a story	Counts four objects correctly, group play with role playing, toilets independently, dresses with little supervision	—
60 mo	Skips, balances on each foot 4-5 seconds	*Fine:* copies triangle, eight- to 10-part person	Counts 10 objects, prints first name, domestic role playing, asks meaning of words, dresses and undresses independently	Uses complete sentences, names four colors, repeats 10-syllable sentence, follows three-stage command

Compiled from Vaughn VC, Litt IF. Growth and development. In Behrman RE, Kliegman RM, Nelson WE, Vaughn VC, eds. *Nelson textbook of pediatrics.* 14th ed. Philadelphia: Saunders; 1992:41-42.

Table 22-13 Developmental Screening Tools

Tool	Age Range	Time	Source
Ages and Stages Questionnaire	0-60 mo	~7 min	Paul H. Brooks Publishers, www.pbrookes.com
Child Development Inventories	3-72 mo	~10 min	Behavior Science Systems*
Parents' Evaluations of Developmental Status (PEDS)	Birth-8 yr	~2 min	Ellsworth & Vandermeer, www.pedstest.com

*PO Box 580274, Minneapolis, MN 55458.

DEVELOPMENTAL SCREENING IN YOUNG CHILDREN

Key Points

- Always refer the child to audiology if language is delayed.
- Never ignore parents' concerns.
- Suspect delays and refer early.
- Developmental screening, using standardized parent report measures, is more accurate than clinical judgment.
- Autism usually manifests as language delay.

Every encounter between a physician and child involves developmental and behavioral issues. Attention to such matters can benefit every child. By monitoring development, the primary care physician has the opportunity to customize anticipatory guidance based on the child's current abilities and temperament (Sturner and Howard, 1997).

Additionally, the family physician has a responsibility to identify children with delayed development. Federal law (Individuals with Disabilities Education Act [IDEA]) mandates physicians to refer children with suspected delays to early intervention (birth to 3 years) or early childhood services (3 to 5 years). The specifics of these services vary from state to state but are free and individualized according to the child's and family's needs (AAP Committee on Children with Disabilities, 1999). As the professional with the most frequent—and sometimes only—contact with young children, the family physician is in the ideal position to detect possible developmental problems. Additionally, parents may feel more comfortable sharing concerns and seeking advice from a trusted physician.

Early detection of delays is important because brain development is most malleable in the early years of life (Shonkoff and Phillips, 2000). Early intervention has been shown to be cost effective, resulting in better intellectual, social, and adaptive behavior; increased high school graduation and employment rates; and decreased criminality and teen pregnancy (Gomby et al., 1995; Reynolds et al., 2001). Unfortunately, fewer than half of children with developmental difficulties are identified before kindergarten (Pelletier and Abrams, 2002).

Research shows that clinical impression alone is quite poor at detecting developmental delays (Glascoe, 2000). This has led the AAP to recommend routine monitoring (surveillance) at all preventive care visits and use of standardized developmental screening tests at 9, 18, and 24 or 30 months of age, with the addition of autism-specific screening at 18 and 24 or 30 months (AAP Council on Children with Disabilities, 2006). Newer screening tools based on parent report can facilitate fulfilling this recommendation. Parent report has been found to be a reliable way to identify children in need of further developmental assessment, particularly if the concerns are elicited and interpreted in a standardized manner (Glascoe and Macias, 2003).

Parent report measures can be used in a variety of ways. They can be completed in the waiting room; sent out to be returned at the next appointment; or completed via an interview, either in person or by telephone with a staff member. It is helpful to have a staff member routinely inquire if the parents would like someone to go over the measure with them; this ensures that literacy or language issues are not barriers to screening. Even if staff administer the parent report, parent report measures are the most accurate, time-effective, and cost-efficient method of developmental screening currently available. Accurate screening tools with acceptable sensitivity and specificity (70%-80%) are listed in Table 22-13. Physicians can bill for screening, although reimbursement varies widely (Glascoe and Macias, 2003). More information regarding developmental screening, including coding and billing aspects, can be found at http://www.dbpeds.org.

EVALUATION OF DEVELOPMENTAL DELAY

Developmental disabilities are common, affecting approximately 15%, or one in six children in the United States (Boyle et al., 2011). Although this includes attention-deficit hyperactivity disorder (ADHD), which is often not manifest until school age, many children present with other developmental delays. Some children present with delays in multiple areas, or global developmental delay. *Global developmental delay* is defined as significant delay in two or more areas of development (gross or fine motor, speech and language, cognition, social and personal, and activities of daily living). The more severe the delay, the more likely a cause can be determined (Roberts et al., 2004). When a significant delay is recognized, parents are often eager to know the cause. The family physician can be instrumental in referring for appropriate intervention, as well as overseeing an initial workup.

Although many physicians refer to specialists (e.g., developmental pediatricians, neurologists) for further evaluation, these specialists may have long waiting lists. Some aspects of the workup can easily be ordered by the family physician. Guidelines from the American Academy of Neurology and Child Neurology Society for the workup of the child with global developmental delay are shown in Table 22-14 (Michelson et al., 2011; Shevell et al., 2003). The guidelines listed in the table are evidence based and

Table 22-14   Evaluation of Global Developmental Delay

Indication	Workup
Everyone	
First-line workup	Comprehensive history and physical examination
	Hearing and vision screening
	Metabolic studies and thyroxine (if newborn screen results not known)
	EEG if symptoms of seizures
	Screen for autism if language delayed
Positive Family History	
Genetic, metabolic, or CNS disorder	Test for specific condition
Nonspecific developmental delays	Microarray and fragile X
Signs or Symptoms Present	
Specific genetic disorder	Specialized genetic testing
Hypothyroidism	Thyroid studies
CNS abnormality	MRI
Other	
Possible lead exposure	Lead level
Regression of skills or parental consanguinity	MRI, microarray, fragile X, metabolic testing, EEG, genetics evaluation
No specific signs or symptoms (stepwise in order)	MRI, microarray, fragile X, metabolic testing, Rett syndrome testing
Motor delays	Low muscle tone-CK, thyroid studies
	High muscle tone-MRI

CK, Creatinine kinase; *CNS,* central nervous system, *EEG,* electroencephalogram; *MRI,* magnetic resonance imaging; *T₄,* thyroxine.
Data from Roberts G, Pafrey J, Bridgemohan C. A rational approach to the medical evaluation of a child with developmental delay. *Contemp Pediatr.* 2004;21:76-100; Shevell M, Asheval S, Donley D, et al. Practice parameter: evaluation of the child with global developmental delay. *Neurology.* 2003;60:367-380; Michelson D, et al. Evidence report: genetic and metabolic testing on children with global developmental delay. *Neurology.* 2011:77:1629-1635; and Noritz G, Murphy NA; Neuromotor Screening Expert Panel. Motor delays: early identification and evaluation. *Pediatrics.* 2013:131:e2016.

Table 22-15   Red Flags and Absolute Indications for Immediate Evaluation

Age	Sign
12 mo	No babbling
	No pointing
	No gestures
16 mo	No single words
24 mo	No two-word phrases
Any age	Loss of language or social skills

Modified from Filipek PA, Accardo PJ, Ashwal S, et al. Practice parameter: screening and diagnosis of autism. *Neurology.* 2000;55:468-479.

could be readily used by family physicians to start the workup while waiting for a specialist appointment. Results of the workup may facilitate more specific referrals. Even if not globally delayed, all children with language delays should have a formal audiology assessment to rule out hearing impairments.

AUTISM SCREENING

Autism is a developmental disability involving difficulties with communication and social interaction as well as unusual and restricted behavior. The prevalence of autism appears to be rapidly increasing, for reasons not yet clear (Fombonne, 2003; Yeargan-Allsopp et al., 2003). The latest prevalence estimates are one in 68 children (Autism and Developmental Disabilities Monitoring Network Surveillance, 2014). This makes it essential that all primary care physicians seeing children be able to recognize the signs and symptoms suggesting autism and refer for further evaluation promptly. Early diagnosis allows earlier initiation of

intensive behavioral intervention, which has been shown to be very helpful (Butter et al., 2003). Table 22-15 lists "red flags" that should prompt referral for further evaluation (Filipek et al., 2000). A formal audiology evaluation is also indicated, as well as lead screening if the child has pica. It is important to keep in mind that most young children with autism are presented to their physicians with the chief complaint of language delay. The physician should consider autism in the differential diagnosis for a child with language delay.

ASSESSING DEVELOPMENT IN THE SCHOOL-AGE CHILD

Developmental surveillance in a school-age child should focus on identification of unsuspected learning problems, including ADHD, mild mental retardation, and learning disabilities, as well as detection of emotional problems such as anxiety, depression, or school phobia. Emotional problems can be screened for using the Pediatric Symptom Checklist (PSC). The PSC is a one-page questionnaire that is relatively easy to administer and interpret during routine well-child care. Positive results should prompt the physician to probe further with questions regarding school, friends, family, moods, and activities. Referrals to other professionals can then be made if necessary. More information regarding the PSC is available on the Massachusetts General Hospital's PSC website.

Asking the child and parent about school progress and reviewing report cards and standardized testing results are simple ways for the physician to monitor school progress. Checklists completed by the parent and teacher can provide further information about specific issues (e.g., attention) or behavior in general (Table 22-16).

Federal law (IDEA) mandates a free and appropriate education for all children, regardless of handicapping condition. Therefore, if a child is suspected to have a learning disability, the school is obligated to evaluate and provide necessary services free of charge. The parent should be advised to request the evaluation, called the Multi-Factored Evaluation (MFE), in writing. Federal law requires the MFE be done within 60 days. The MFE consists of standardized assessments of various aspects of learning. After the MFE is completed, school personnel meet with the parents to review testing results and determine if the child is eligible for special education services. These services may occur in the regular classroom or in a separate one, although the

Table 22-16 School-Age Checklists

Purpose	Ages	Description	Website/Contact
Pediatric Symptom Checklist			
Brief screening for behavioral concerns	4-16 yr	35 items completed by parents	www.brightfutures.org/mentalhealth/pdf/professionals/ped_symptom_chklst.pdf
Child Behavior Checklist			
In-depth screening for behavioral/emotional problems	Separate forms for 1-5 yr and 6-18 yr	Parents, teachers, caregivers, youth (11-18 yr); 99-118 items depending on form used	www.aseba.org
Conners Scales			
More specific for ADHD and learning difficulties	3-17 yr	Parent, teacher, youth (12-17 yr); short and long forms, 27-87 items	www.pearsonassessments.com
Clinical Attention Problem Scale			
Brief, specific for attention and overactivity symptoms	6-12 yr	24-item checklist Teacher version	www2.aap.org/sections/dbpeds/screening.asp
Vanderbilt			
Symptoms of ADHD; common comorbidities	6-12 yr	Teacher and parent; initial (43-55 items) and follow-up (26 items) forms	www.nichq.org/NIaCHQ/Topics/ChronicConditions/ADHD/Tools/

ADHD, Attention-deficit hyperactivity disorder.

law requires that services be provided in the least restrictive environment. The goal is to keep children with their typical peers as much as possible.

After a child is deemed eligible for services, an Individualized Education Plan (IEP) is developed. Parent input is required as part of the process. If the parent disagrees with the suggested IEP, the parent has the right to due process. An explanation of due process must be given to all parents at the beginning of the MFE/IEP process. After it has been developed, the IEP is updated annually. Parents should receive progress reports throughout the school year. They may request interim changes to the IEP if needed. Reevaluations are conducted at least every 3 years (Henderson, 2001).

All of this is often overwhelming for families. The physician can assist by providing simple explanations of the process as well as periodically reviewing the IEP and helping parents understand it. The physician should also encourage parents to become knowledgeable advocates for their child.

Some children have conditions that can benefit from extra assistance but that do not qualify as disabilities according to the IDEA. Conditions such as ADHD are covered by Section 504 of the Rehabilitation Act of 1973 (Henderson, 2001). The qualifications are broader under this law, allowing children with less serious issues to still receive special services. This assistance, although helpful, is often less extensive than if the child qualified for an IEP.

Regardless of the issues, communication with school personnel is often helpful. Teacher rating scales (general or specific for certain concerns) may be useful, as well as direct communication, either verbally or in writing. Such dialogue also illustrates for families the advantages of cooperative teamwork with school personnel. It is always important for physicians to follow the Health Insurance Portability and Accountability Act (HIPAA) guidelines, obtain written permission from parents, and show discretion ("need to know") when sharing information with schools.

Immunizations

Key Points

- Avoid missed opportunities to vaccinate by reviewing the child's immunization record at every visit.
- Schedule adolescents for an immunization visit at age 11 to 12 years to catch up on missed vaccines and administer new ones.
- Provide current vaccine information statements to parents or guardians for each vaccine given during the visit.

INDICATIONS AND CONTRAINDICATIONS

Routine immunizations are essential for the control and prevention of previously common childhood infectious diseases. During 2012, approximately 90% of U.S. children age 19 to 35 months received one or more doses of measles, mumps, and rubella (MMR) vaccine, three or more doses of poliovirus vaccine, three or more doses of hepatitis B vaccine (Hep B), and one or more dose of varicella vaccine. Although below the Healthy People 2020 objectives of 90% coverage, approximately 80% of young children received four or more doses of diphtheria, tetanus toxoids, and pertussis (DTaP) vaccines; four or more doses of pneumococcal conjugate vaccine (PCV), and the full series of *Haemophilus influenzae* type b (Hib) vaccine (CDC, 2013). However, there is still considerable disparity in immunization rates among states and communities. Young children might not be immunized at the recommended age because of missed opportunities to vaccinate, deficient health care delivery in the public sector, lack of insurance, inadequate access to medical care, lack of public awareness about the necessity for immunizations, or concern about potential or alleged adverse effects of immunizations. Both the AAFP and AAP endorse the Recommended Immunization Schedule for Persons Aged 0 Through 18 years—2014 (see http://www.cdc.gov/vaccines/schedules for a full set of schedules, including catch-up schedule) (SOR: A).

Parents and guardians should be questioned about possible contraindications, precautions, and any previous adverse events in response to vaccine administration (see eTable 22-3 online). They should be informed about the potential benefits and risks of the vaccine and the risks of the natural disease if the immunization is not given. Health care providers administering any vaccine covered by the National Vaccine Compensation Injury Act or purchased by federal contract must provide the most current *vaccine information statements* (VISs) detailing the potential benefits and risks of each vaccine to the parents or guardians each time that vaccine is given (AAP Red Book, 2012, 7-8). Copies of VISs may be obtained from the CDC (http://www.cdc.gov/vaccines/pubs/VIS/default.htm), the Immunization Action Coalition (http://www.immunize.org), or state health departments.

Vaccines have become "victims of their own success" (Cooper et al., 2008). Because they no longer are confronted with the presence of vaccine-preventable diseases, some individuals, parents, and groups have become more concerned about the alleged adverse effects of immunization. A Danish study is one of many that confirmed the effectiveness of vaccines such as Hib and pertussis and did not find an association of MMR or thimerosal-containing vaccines with autism spectrum disorders (Hviid, 2006). Physicians serve as the primary source of information about immunizations, and family physicians should explain the potential benefits and risks of immunizations to parents and older patients such as adolescents (Gellin et al., 2000). If parents still do not wish to have their child vaccinated, further information and documentation may be obtained at http://www2.aap.org/immunization/pediatricians/pdf/RefusaltoVaccinate.pdf.

Before administering vaccines, the physician should ask about the child's current state of health, as well as that of other family members. Pregnancy or immunosuppression of a household member usually does not contraindicate the administration of most routine live-virus vaccines, such as MMR, varicella, or rotavirus vaccines. Nasal live, attenuated influenza vaccine (LAIV) should not be given to close contacts of immunosuppressed people who require a protective environment (e.g., recipients of stem cell transplants) but may be given to others. Minor febrile illnesses are not contraindications to vaccine administration. General contraindications are a previous anaphylactic reaction to the specific vaccine or a severe hypersensitivity reaction to vaccine constituents such as gelatin or antibiotics such as neomycin, streptomycin, or polymyxin B. Latex allergy may also be a contraindication if the vaccines are supplied in vials or syringes containing natural rubber (AAP Red Book, 2012, pp. 49-53).

VACCINE ADMINISTRATION

Most immunizations must be given by deep intramuscular (IM) or subcutaneous (SC) injection. IM injections should be given in the anterolateral thigh for infants or the deltoid muscle of the arm for older children. The sciatic nerve may be injured by deep intragluteal injections. Although acetaminophen (paracetamol) administered for 24 hours has been demonstrated to decrease mild to moderate reactions, such as temperature of 38°C (100.4°F) or greater, it may reduce antibody responses to some vaccine antigens (Prymula et al., 2009). Topical local anesthetics, sweet-tasting solutions, and breastfeeding may decrease injection pain for childhood immunizations (HELPinKIDS, 2009).

Immune responses may be impaired if two live-virus vaccines are given within 28 days of each other. Live-virus vaccines must be given simultaneously or at least 4 weeks apart (AAP Red Book, 2012, 25). If immune globulin is given, live-virus vaccine administration should be delayed for up to 3 to 6 months to allow optimal antibody production (AAP Red Book, 2012, pp. 37-38). An even longer period may be required if high doses of intravenous (IV) gamma globulin have been given.

SCHEDULE OF IMMUNIZATIONS

The recommended schedule for childhood and adolescent immunizations for ages 0 to 18 years are shown at http://www.cdc.gov/vaccines/schedules, including a catch-up schedule. A lapse in the immunization schedule does not require starting over the entire series. Doses of any vaccine should not be divided or reduced because this can result in an inadequate response. Premature infants should receive the same vaccine dose, usually at the same chronologic age as full-term infants. Most vaccines can be administered simultaneously using separate syringes at separate sites (AAP Red Book, 2012, 33-34).

POLIOVIRUS VACCINE

The last indigenous case of wild-type poliomyelitis in the United States occurred in 1979, and the last identified imported case occurred in 1993. From 1980 to 1996, there were approximately eight cases per year of vaccine-associated paralytic poliomyelitis (VAPP) caused by oral poliovirus vaccine (OPV) in the United States. In 2000, inactivated poliovirus vaccine (IPV) was recommended for all routine childhood polio vaccinations in the United States. In 2005, one case of VAPP was identified in a symptomatic, unimmunized, immunodeficient child and subsequently in seven other unimmunized children in the same community (AAP Red Book, 2012, 588).

MEASLES, MUMPS, AND RUBELLA VACCINE

The MMR vaccine should be given to children 12 to 15 months of age. The second MMR or measles, mumps, rubella, and varicella (MMRV) vaccine is recommended before school entry at 4 to 6 years of age, but it can be given earlier in the event of an outbreak or as a requirement for travel, provided the second dose is given at least 28 days after the first. The recommended interval between varicella doses for children 12 years old or younger is 3 months, but a minimum interval of at least 4 weeks is acceptable for children 7 to 12 years for catch-up purposes. When MMRV is given to 12- to 23-month-old children, there is a slight increase in the risk of febrile seizures (about one in 2500), and parents should be apprised of this. All children should receive the second MMR or MMRV before school entry at ages 4 to 6 years (AAP Red Book, pp. 493-495). Many colleges require documentation of immunity to MMR, either by immunization or serologically. Children may be immunized with MMR even if there is a pregnant or immunosuppressed family member because the vaccine viruses are not transmitted (AAP Red Book, 2012, p. 50).

HAEMOPHILUS INFLUENZAE TYPE B CONJUGATE VACCINE

The use of Hib conjugate vaccines has lowered the U.S. incidence of invasive Hib disease in children younger than 5 years of age by 99%. Vaccines currently available in the United States, such as PRP-OMP (PedvaxHIB) and PRP-T (ActHIB), are given beginning at age 2 months. PRP-T (Hiberix) is licensed for use as a booster in children 15 months through 4 years of age (CDC, 2009); PRP-OMP-HepB (Comvax) is administered at 2, 4, and 12 to 15 months of age; DTaP-IPV+PRP-T (Pentacel) is given at 2, 4, 6, and 15 to 18 months of age (AAP Red Book, 2012, pp. 346-351). If indicated, Hib-MenCY (MenHibrix) is given at 2, 4, and 6 months of age with a booster dose at age 12 to 15 months.

The schedule of administration varies according to the type of vaccine (visit http://www.cdc.gov/vaccines/schedules, which also includes a catch-up schedule). Children age 12 to 15 months of age who received the primary series need one dose of any Hib conjugate vaccine given at least 2 months after the last dose. If the child is 15 months of age or older, only one dose is needed. Children who have received a primary Hib series with a booster dose at 12 months of age or older do not need further immunization if they have hyposplenia or asplenia. However, children undergoing scheduled splenectomy may be given a booster dose of Hib 7 to 10 days beforehand. It is not known whether children with human immunodeficiency virus (HIV) infection, who are receiving chemotherapy for malignancies, or who have other immunologic impairment benefit from a booster dose of Hib. At-risk children who are unimmunized or only received one dose of Hib before age 12 months should receive two doses of Hib separated by 2 months. Children 59 months of age or older who are unimmunized with Hib and potentially at risk because of diseases such asplenia, leukemia, or HIV should receive one dose of HiB vaccine (AAP Red Book 2012, pp. 349-351).

ACELLULAR PERTUSSIS VACCINE

Acellular pertussis vaccines combined with DTaP are used in the United States for the primary and booster doses in children. These vaccines (DAPTACEL, Infanrix) are immunogenic and produce fewer adverse local and systemic reactions, such as fever and irritability, than do whole-cell pertussis vaccines. Whenever possible, the same DTaP vaccine should be used throughout the entire vaccination series because there are no data on safety or efficacy when different formulations of these vaccines are interchanged. However, if the previously used vaccine is not known or is unavailable, any of the DTaP vaccines licensed for use in children may be given to complete the

immunization series. Combination vaccines such as DTaP-IPV-HepB (Pediarix) and DTaP-IPV-Hib (Pentacel) are licensed for use as the first three doses and first four doses, respectively, of their components, but DTaP-IPV (Kinrix) is licensed only as the booster fifth dose of DTaP and fourth dose of IPV at ages 4 to 6 years (AAP Red Book, 2012, pp. 557-566).

Two vaccines containing reduced concentrations of diphtheria toxoid and pertussis antigens combined with tetanus toxoid (Tdap) are now licensed for use in adolescents and adults (Boostrix and ADACEL). The vaccines are recommended for adolescents 11 to 18 years of age in place of the Td booster to decrease the reservoir of *Bordetella pertussis* in this population. Increasing reported cases of pertussis in the United States (>42,000 in 2012) has led to the recommendation to give one dose of these vaccines to children 7 to 10 years of age who are incompletely immunized against pertussis. In addition, one dose of Tdap should be given to pregnant women, preferably after 20 weeks of gestation, during each pregnancy and to adolescents and adults likely to have close contact with infants younger than 12 months old.

ROTAVIRUS VACCINE

Rotavirus is responsible for up to 500,000 deaths from diarrhea worldwide and 20 to 60 U.S. deaths each year. Before the introduction of rotavirus vaccines (RV1 or Rotarix, RV5 or RotaTeq), rotavirus caused 3 million infections per year in the United States, resulting in more than 400,000 physician visits and 55,000 to 70,000 hospitalizations per year (CDC *Pink Book*, 2012, pp. 263-274). RV1 is given as two oral doses at 2 and 4 months of age, and RV5 is given as three oral doses at 2, 4, and 6 months of age. The minimum interval between doses of either vaccine is 4 weeks. Neither vaccine should be started for infants age 15 weeks, 0 days of age or older, and all doses must given by 8 months, 0 days of age. The vaccine-specific package insert should be seen for full prescribing indications and contraindications.

VARICELLA VACCINE

Two SC doses of monovalent varicella zoster virus (VZV) vaccine or MMRV are indicated in children age 12 months through 12 years. The doses should be separated by at least 3 months, with the second dose routinely recommended at age 4 to 6 years before kindergarten or first grade. Parents should be counseled that MMRV carries a slightly higher risk for febrile seizures when given as the first dose to young children and should be given a choice of MMRV or separate MMR and VZV vaccine injections. MMRV may then be used for the second dose. Persons age 13 years or older who do not have evidence of immunity to varicella should receive two doses of monovalent VZV vaccine at least 28 days apart. A second dose of varicella vaccine should be given to people who previously received only one dose. In children age 7 to 12 years, a minimum interval of at least 4 weeks is acceptable for catch-up purposes. The vaccine is generally contraindicated in pregnant women, immunodeficient persons, and those receiving high doses of systemic corticosteroids (≥20 mg/day of prednisone or equivalent) for 14 days or more. However, VZV vaccine may be considered for

HIV-infected patients with a CD4+ T-lymphocyte count of 15% or greater. Vaccine-strain VZV has been rarely transmitted, and vaccinated patients who develop a rash should avoid contact with immunocompromised persons (AAP Red Book, 2012, pp. 786-788). Zoster vaccine is not interchangeable with varicella vaccine and is not used in children.

HEPATITIS A VACCINE

Hepatitis A virus (HAV) is usually transmitted person to person through the fecal–oral route and by ingestion of contaminated food or water, but it has rarely been transmitted by transfusion of blood or blood products. Two HAV inactivated vaccines, HAVRIX and VAQTA, are licensed in the United States for use in children age 1 year and older. TWINRIX is a combined hepatitis A and hepatitis B vaccine licensed for use in persons at least 18 years old. Physicians should consult the package insert for proper dosing because there are different formulations of these vaccines.

Childhood vaccination against HAV is recommended for all U.S. children 12 to 23 months of age and should be considered for unimmunized children ages 2 to 18 years old. Indications for immunization with hepatitis A vaccine include travel to or residence in countries or areas endemic for hepatitis A; close contacts of newly arriving international adoptees; persons who receive clotting-factor concentrates; persons with chronic liver disease; injection (IDU) and noninjection drug users; men who have sex with men (MSM); and people at risk of household, sexual, and occupational exposure (e.g., handlers of primates) (AAP Red Book, 2012, pp. 364-367).

HEPATITIS B VACCINE

Hepatitis B virus (HBV) is endemic in Southeast Asia, the Pacific Islands, China, Africa, parts of the Middle East, and the Amazon Basin. More than 350 million people worldwide have chronic HBV infection. Although transmission in U.S. children is less likely because of high coverage with Hep B vaccine, the risk of perinatal transmission of HBV from an infected mother to her infant varies from 10% to as high as 90%, depending on whether the mother is negative or positive for hepatitis B e antigen (HBeAg) (CDC *Pink Book*, 2012, pp. 115-138).

The pediatric formulations of Hep B vaccine should be given to all infants soon after birth or before hospital discharge. Hep B vaccine should be given within 12 hours to all newborns of mothers positive for hepatitis B surface antigen (HBsAg) or infants of mothers whose HBsAg status is unknown. An infant born to an HBsAg-positive mother should receive an initial dose of 5-µg RecombivaxHB or 10-µg Engerix-B and 0.5 mL of hepatitis B immune globulin (HBIG) IM at separate sites within 12 hours of birth. Repeat vaccine doses should be given at ages 1 month and 6 months. If the maternal HBsAg status remains unknown, HBIG may be given within 7 days of birth. For infants of HbsAg-negative mothers, the combination DTaP-HBV-IPV (Pediarix) or PRP-OMP-HBV vaccine (Comvax) may then also be used, beginning at 6 to 8 weeks of age. Practitioners should consult the package insert for the appropriate dose according to the formulation and intended use. Any adolescent who has not yet received Hep B vaccine should also be immunized with two doses at least 4 weeks apart, with a third dose 4 to 6 months after the second dose. An alternative schedule using two 10-µg doses of RecomivaxHB separated by at least 4 to 6 months may be used only in adolescents 11 through 15 years old (CDC *Pink Book*, 2012, pp. 115-138).

Hepatitis B vaccine should be given to all children, but especially susceptible high-risk children or adults who are institutionalized; those who have end-stage renal disease, chronic liver disease, or HIV infection; those who receive clotting-factor concentrates; household or sexual contacts of HBsAg-positive people; MSM; IDUs; and adoptees from or long-term travelers to countries endemic for hepatitis B. Unimmunized victims of sexual assault or inmates in juvenile detention centers or adult correctional facilities as well as people ages 19 through 59 years of age with diabetes mellitus should be immunized (AAP Red Book, 2012, pp. 377-390).

CONJUGATE PNEUMOCOCCAL VACCINE

In 2008, more than 500,000 children younger than age 5 years died worldwide from pneumococcal disease (O'Brien, 2013). In 2010, the FDA licensed the 13-valent conjugate pneumococcal vaccine (PCV13) for use in children 6 weeks to 71 months old. The vaccine stimulates functional antibodies to all 13 serotypes in more than 90% of recipients and is given to infants at 2, 4, 6, and 12 to 15 months of age. Children 7 to 11 months old require two doses 2 months apart followed by a third dose at 12 to 15 months of age (two or more months later). Children 12 to 23 months old require two doses 2 months apart. One dose of PCV13 is required for all healthy children 24 to 59 months of age even if they previously received the 7-valent PCV. Children age 24 to 71 months and those age 6 to 18 years with conditions placing them at high risk for invasive pneumococcal disease (e.g., immunocompromising conditions, anatomic or functional asplenia including sickle cell disease, HIV, cochlear implants) should receive one dose of PCV13 vaccine. This should be followed 8 weeks later by the 23-valent polysaccharide vaccine (PPSV23) (AAP Red Book, 2012, pp. 578-580; CDC, 2013). PCV13 and PPSV23 have more recently been recommended for use in adults 19 years of age and older with immunocompromising conditions (CDC, 2012).

INFLUENZA VACCINE

Routine annual immunization with influenza vaccine is recommended for all persons 6 months of age and older, including those with high-risk conditions such as HIV or chronic pulmonary (including asthma) or cardiac, renal, or metabolic diseases; those receiving immunosuppressive or long-term aspirin therapy; those who have hemoglobinopathies; and those with any condition (e.g., cognitive dysfunction, seizure disorder, neuromuscular disorder) that could compromise respiratory function. Pregnant women and persons who are household contacts of high-risk patients, including health care workers, should also be vaccinated. Multiple inactivated influenza vaccines (IIVs) are now available, including the trivalent vaccine containing 2 influenza A viruses and 1 B virus and the newer quadrivalent vaccines containing 2 influenza A and 2 influenza B viruses. Providers should read the prescribing information regarding the appropriate age and dosing of these vaccines. In general, children 9 years of age and older need only one dose of influenza vaccine. Children 6 months to 8 years old need two doses of vaccine separated by 4 weeks unless they have received two doses of influenza vaccine since July 1, 2010. The live, attenuated influenza vaccine (LAIV4) is now a quadrivalent vaccine approved for use in healthy people ages 2 through 49 years who are not pregnant. LAIV4 should not be used in persons with asthma or those in close contact with severely immunosuppressed hospitalized patients receiving care in a protected environment. Although most IIV and LAIV4 vaccines are produced in eggs, only a history of severe egg allergy (e.g., anaphylaxis involving cardiorespiratory or gastrointestinal symptoms or those requiring the use of epinephrine) is now considered a true contraindication to immunization. However, observation of the vaccinee for 30 minutes afterward is recommended, and appropriate resuscitative equipment must be available. A trivalent inactivated cell culture–based vaccine and a recombinant vaccine are now available for persons 18 years and older (AAP Committee on Infectious Diseases, 2013). These are not produced using eggs.

CONJUGATE MENINGOCOCCAL VACCINE

Two quadrivalent meningococcal polysaccharide–protein conjugate vaccines (MCV4-D [Menactra, Sanofi Pasteur] and MCV4-CRM [Menveo, Novartis]) have been licensed in the United States for use in persons 9 months and 2 months of age, respectively, through 55 years old. Routine immunization of all children age 11 to 12 years old with either MCV4 followed by a booster dose at 16 years is recommended. Persons receiving the first dose at 13 to 15 years old should receive a one-time booster at age 16 to 18 years. The vaccines contain serogroups A, C, Y, and W-135 that cause 75% of all cases of meningococcal disease in persons older than 11 years in the United States (Bilukha and Rosenstein, 2005). Neither vaccine is protective against serogroup B, which accounts for most of the remaining cases. Children 9 to 23 months old with persistent complement deficiency or traveling to or residing in countries where meningococcal disease is hyperendemic should receive two doses of MCV4 3 months apart. Because MCV4-D may interfere with immunity to PCV13, it is recommended not to give this vaccine until 4 weeks after the PCV13 series is completed. In children younger than 19 months with anatomic or functional asplenia, MCV4-CRM or HibMenCY (MenHibrix) is given at 2, 4, 6, and 12 to 15 months of age. In unimmunized children ages 19 to 23 months, primary doses of MCV4-CRM are given at least 3 months apart. Unimmunized children 2 to 18 years old with persistent complement deficiency or anatomic or functional asplenia should receive two doses of either MCV4 vaccine 8 weeks apart. In asplenic children, MCV4-D should not be given until 4 weeks after completion of all PCV13

doses. Children with continued risk for meningococcal disease may be given a booster in either 3 years or 5 years depending on whether they received their initial immunization series at either 2 to 6 years of age or 7 years or older, respectively (AAP Red Book, 2012, pp. 505-508). Persons age 2 years of age or older traveling to or residing in countries with hyperendemic or epidemic *Neisseria meningitidis* (e.g., sub-Saharan Africa, Mecca during the Hajj) should also be immunized with one dose of MCV4 (CDC *Pink Book*, 2012, pp. 200-201). Previously unimmunized college freshman living in dormitories also have a higher risk of meningococcal infection and should be given a single dose of MCV4.

A vaccine containing meningococcal serogroups C and Y and Hib tetanus toxoid (Hib-MenCY [MenHibrix]) is licensed for use in infants 6 weeks through 18 months old who are at increased risk for meningococcal disease. It may be given in a four-dose series to infants with complement component deficiencies or functional asplenia such as sickle cell disease. It does not prevent disease against serogroup B, which causes about 60% of disease among children ages 0 to 59 months. Because it does not contain serogroup A, infants 9 to 23 months old traveling to the Hajj or the "meningitis belt" of sub-Saharan Africa should be given two doses at least 8 weeks apart of either MCV4 vaccine before travel. If MenACWY-D is used, then it should be given at least 4 weeks after completion of the PCV13 series. Children 2 to 10 years old and adolescents who travel or reside in countries where meningococcal disease is hyperendemic should receive one dose of MCV4 (AAP Red Book, 2012, pp. 505-508).

HUMAN PAPILLOMAVIRUS VACCINE

Although most human papillomavirus (HPV) infections spontaneously resolve, high-risk HPV types are found in 99% of cervical cancers with types 16 and 18, accounting for about 70% of cervical cancers worldwide. HPV is also believed to account for 90% of anal cancers; 40% of vulvar, vaginal, or penile cancers; and 12% of oral and pharyngeal cancers. Types 6 and 11 HPV account for 90% of genital warts in addition to laryngeal papillomatosis. The bivalent HPV2 (types 16 and 18) vaccine (Cervarix) and the quadrivalent HPV4 (types 6, 11, 16, and 18) vaccine (Gardasil) are recommended for routine vaccination of girls at ages 11 or 12 years and are ideally given before onset of sexual intercourse. They are also recommended for unimmunized girls and women 13 through 26 years old. HPV4 is now recommended for routine immunization of boys at ages 11 to 12 years and for unimmunized boys and men ages 13 to 21 years. Men ages 22 to 26 years may also be immunized (AAP Red Book, pp. 529-530). Both vaccines are given in a three-dose series and are prophylactic only for the HPV types they contain and do not treat preexisting infection with these HPV types. They may be given at the same visit at different sites with the MCV4 and Tdap vaccines.

SPECIAL CLINICAL SITUATIONS

Children who are immunocompromised or infected with HIV usually should not be given live-virus vaccines.

However, measles can cause severe disease and death in symptomatic HIV-infected patients. MMR (but not MMRV) is recommended at age 12 months for HIV-infected children with CD4+ T-lymphocyte counts of 15% or greater. The second dose can be given 28 days later to improve the immune response. Children with age-specific low CD4+ counts should not be given measles virus–containing vaccine (AAP Red Book, 2012, pp. 86-87). HIV-infected children are also at increased risk from complications of chickenpox and zoster, and children with CD4+ counts of at least 15% should receive two doses of varicella vaccine 3 months apart. The MMRV vaccine is not used in this situation (AAP Red Book, 2012, pp. 86-87).

Most new cases of measles in the United States are imported from abroad, including European countries. Therefore, infants 6 through 11 months old traveling to foreign countries should receive one dose of MMR. This dose should be repeated when they become 12 months of age. Children 12 months of age or older should have two doses of MMR separated by 28 days before traveling abroad (AAP Red Book 2012, pp. 103-106).

Children with anatomic or functional asplenia have a 350-fold higher rate of septicemia than children without asplenia (AAP Red Book, 2012, p. 88). PCV13 is recommended for all children younger than 60 months and children 24 to 71 months old who have high-risk conditions such as sickle cell disease, functional or anatomic asplenia, HIV infection, other immune deficiencies or immunosuppressive therapies, chronic cardiac or pulmonary disease, chronic renal insufficiency, diabetes mellitus, cerebrospinal fluid leaks, or cochlear implants. High-risk children who have received four doses of PCV13 should also receive one dose of the 23-valent polysaccharide pneumococcal vaccine (PPSV23, Pneumovax-23) at 24 months. Children 24 to 71 months old who have received less than three doses of PCV13 should receive two doses of PCV13 followed by one dose of PPSV23 8 weeks later. PCV13 is now recommended for unimmunized children ages 6 to 18 years who are at risk because of anatomic or functional asplenia, HIV, cochlear implant, cerebrospinal fluid leak, or other immunocompromising conditions. PPSV23 should then be given 8 weeks later. All immunosuppressed children and those with anatomic or functional asplenia should receive a second dose of PPSV23 vaccine 5 years after the first dose (ACIP, CDC, pp. 521-524).

NATIONAL CHILDHOOD VACCINE INJURY ACT

The National Childhood Vaccine Injury Act of 1986 was passed to provide compensation for children inadvertently injured by any of the routinely recommended childhood vaccines and to provide liability protection for manufacturers and for health care providers who administer the vaccines. The intent of the law is to ensure a stable supply of vaccine and allow routine immunizations to continue. The physician or other health care provider must maintain permanent documentation of the date, vaccine type, manufacturer, lot number, and name, address, and title of the person administering the vaccine. A list of reportable but not necessarily compensable events is available from the Health Resources and Services Administration. Significant adverse events should be reported to the Vaccine Adverse Event Reporting System (VAERS) at 800-822-7967 or http://www.vaers.hhs.gov.

KEY TREATMENT

• Administer all recommended or required immunizations, except when true contraindications or precautions are present or the immunizations are refused by the parent or patient (AAP Red Book, 2012; Hviid, 2006) (SOR: A).

Acknowledgment

This chapter incorporates some material that was written by Lorraine M. Fay, MD, for this chapter in the 6th edition of *Textbook of Family Practice*.

Summary of Additional Online Content

The following content is available at www.expertconsult.com:

eTable 22-1 Blood Pressure Levels for Boys by Age and Height Percentile

eTable 22-2 Blood Pressure Levels for Girls by Age and Height Percentile

eTable 22-3 Guide to Contraindications and Precautions for Immunizations

eFigure 22-1 Growth charts for boys and girls.

References

The complete reference list is available at www.expertconsult.com.

Key Resource

Centers for Disease Control and Prevention, Atkinson W, Wolfe S, Hamborsky J, McIntyre L, editors: *Epidemiology and prevention of vaccine-preventable diseases. Pink book*, ed 12, Washington, DC, 2012, Public Health Foundation. Inexpensive reference from the CDC that is updated yearly, covering the nuts and bolts of vaccine-preventable diseases and immunizations.

Web Resources

www.aan.com American Academy of Neurology. Practice parameters for screening and diagnosis of autism and evaluation of developmental delay.

www.aap.org American Academy of Pediatrics. Good general information regarding health care for children and access to guidelines for developmental screening and other topics.

www.brightfutures.org/mentalhealth/pdf/professionals/ped_symptom_chklst.pdf Massachusetts General Hospital, Pediatric Symptom Checklist. Free access and instructions for use and scoring.

www.cdc.gov/growthcharts/clinical_charts.htm National Center for Health Statistics' growth charts for female and male development.

www.cdc.gov/growthcharts Centers for Disease Control and Prevention's developmental screening for health care providers. Provides excellent information about child development and screening with helpful links and patient material.

www.cdc.gov/vaccines/pubs/VIS/default.htm Centers for Disease Control and Prevention, National Immunization Program. Vaccine information statements.

www.choosemyplate.gov U.S. Department of Agriculture's MyPyramid allows development of a personalized meal plan based on age, gender, and activity level.

www.dbpeds.org Developmental Behavioral Pediatrics. Provides a wealth of information about developmental screening and other topics related to child development and behavior.

www.hhs.gov/ocr/hipaa US Department of Health and Human Services, Office for Civil Rights, Health Insurance Portability and Accountability Act (HIPAA).

www.hrsa.gov/vaccinecompensation/vaccineinjurytable.pdf Health Resources and Services Administration, National Vaccine Injury Compensation Program, National Childhood Vaccine Injury Act. A vaccine injury table lists potentially compensable vaccine adverse events.

www.immunize.org/vis Immunization Action Coalition. Includes vaccine information statements.

www.vaers.hhs.gov Vaccine Adverse Event Reporting System (VAERS). Individuals, health care providers, and manufacturers may report vaccine-associated adverse events; this does not prove causation.

23 Behavioral Problems in Children and Adolescents

SCOTT E. MOSER and KELLI L. NETSON

Primary care physicians are generally the first point of contact with a family when questions arise about a child's health and development. The onus is on the physician to allay unnecessary fears when development is progressing appropriately but also to act quickly when problems arise because early intervention is a key piece of treatment for behavioral disorders or abnormalities. Childhood behavioral problems are a complex assortment of individual mental disorders, genetic and medical disorders, family interaction difficulties, social and school problems, and combinations of these. The rates of many psychosocial problems in children and adolescents, including depression, suicide, conduct disorders (CDs), and drug and alcohol abuse, have been rising in recent years throughout Western culture (Fombonne, 1998). This increase is only partly explained by changes in diagnostic criteria and reporting. The trend is particularly troubling when the economic conditions and physical health of the population have been improving. The implication for office physicians is that psychosocial problems will encompass a growing proportion of patient care both as presenting problems and as cofactors in other medical conditions.

This chapter is arranged in problem-focused fashion along a developmental continuum from infancy through adolescence based on when various problems are most frequently encountered in practice. For conditions encountered at different developmental stages, discussions include similarities and differences in recognition and treatment at different ages. Management focuses on early, brief interventions the physician can make with the patient and family as well as suggestions about referrals.

Regardless of the behavioral concern or the child's age, general principles for evaluation and management include the following:

1. Obtain specific examples of the problem behaviors rather than general conclusions. For example, "Child is out of his seat, walking around the classroom every few minutes," rather than "Disruptive in class" and "Screams inconsolably at 2 AM" rather than "Doesn't sleep well."

2. Obtain as complete information from as many observers as possible. Unusual seizure disorders and other neurologic problems are included in the differential diagnosis of many behavioral disorders. Keys to their diagnosis are found in a careful history, including neurologic and age-appropriate mental status examination.

3. Emotional stressors and abuse, whether physical, verbal, or sexual, can be important precipitants of behavioral problems or can exacerbate existing behavioral problems. Therefore, explore these, including an interview of the child apart from their parents when the child is verbal.

4. Consider multiple diagnoses simultaneously. Multifactorial etiologies are common for many behavioral complaints, and many psychiatric diagnoses carry a high risk of comorbid conditions. Therefore, avoid a linear approach of working up one potential diagnosis at a time.

5. Use a multidimensional treatment approach. Many behavioral problems respond best to combinations of psychotherapy, medication, parent and teacher education, and other therapies rather than only one of these at a time.

Many times, a referral to a behavioral or psychiatric specialist is warranted. Knowing the resources within the community, the differences among providers, and the state statutes governing what various providers are qualified to do will help providers steer patients in the appropriate direction. For cases of psychological or behavioral difficulty that warrant counseling or psychotherapy, a referral to a licensed clinical psychologist, psychological counselor, marriage and family therapist, or clinical social worker is appropriate. Each of these professionals is qualified (in most states) to provide individual or family therapy to address specific behavioral or mood-related concerns. When a potential intellectual or developmental disorder may be causing behavioral problems, the child should be referred to a licensed clinical psychologist or neuropsychologist for evaluation. Although school psychologists can often provide assistance with academic difficulties, they are not licensed to diagnose in many states; therefore, a private clinical evaluation is likely to be most helpful. Many primary care physicians are comfortable prescribing psychoactive medications for their well-known patients. In cases of complicated psychiatric problems with multiple comorbid complaints or in cases that have been refractory to treatment, a referral to a child and adolescent psychiatrist may be indicated. Local community mental health agencies are often helpful sources of information for patients seeking assistance.

Sleep Problems

Key Points

- Many sleep problems can be prevented with good sleep hygiene.
- Sleep disorders have important interactive and bidirectional effects with many medical and mental disorders.
- For obstructive sleep apnea syndrome (OSAS), criteria to order a sleep study in the evaluation of a child are similar to criteria for adults, but interpretation of the results requires special pediatric expertise.
- The most common cause of obstructive sleep apnea in children is adenotonsillar hypertrophy, and the treatment of choice is surgery.

Normal sleep has a well-characterized pattern of rapid eye movement (REM) and non-REM sleep that changes with age. Non-REM sleep is further categorized into stages 1, 2, 3, and 4 on the basis of electroencephalographic (EEG) characteristics, with the deepest non-REM sleep occurring in stages 3 and 4. A normal nighttime sleep cycle is about every 90 minutes, with multiple brief arousals and quick returns to sleep without memory of having awakened. Deep non-REM sleep predominates in the first several hours of sleep, and REM is most prominent in the last few hours. Children have substantial periods of very deep sleep that lessen with age. There is a gradual decrease in the amount of REM sleep and a significant decrease in deep non-REM sleep, especially in adolescence.

Children and adolescents in American society sleep less than those in other societies and less than children in the past (Dahl, 1998). This has serious implications for family physicians because short sleep duration is predictive of poor cognitive performance; increased behavior problems, including hyperactivity; and development of obesity and metabolic syndrome (Kelly et al., 2013; Scharf, et al., 2013; Xi et al., 2014). Because of the wide variations in normal sleep patterns and development, physicians should avoid rigid expectations in counseling parents, but the following are some useful guidelines. A typical infant is able to sleep 6 to 8 hours through the night by age 2 months and 10 to 12 hours by age 6 months. A child usually no longer requires a morning nap by about 1 year of age and outgrows the afternoon nap around age 3. The total daily sleep requirement decreases with age, from $16\frac{1}{2}$ hours at 1 week of age to 14 hours by age 1 year, 13 hours by age 2 years, 12 hours by age 3 years, 11 hours by age 5 years, and 10 hours by age 9 years (Blum and Carey, 1996).

Table 23-1 Good Sleep Hygiene

Environment	Dark
	Quiet
	Cool
Schedule	Regular morning waking time
	Consistent nap length
	Regular bedtime
Activities	Morning sunlight exposure
	No late day caffeine
	No frightening TV or stories in the evening
	No late evening electronic media (TV, computer, video games)
	Daily physical exercise but no vigorous physical activities in the hour before bedtime
	Consistent bedtime routine
	Consistent soothing methods
	Child put into bed awake

From Blum NJ, Carey WB. Sleep problems among infants and young children. *Pediatr Rev.* 1996;17(3):87-92.

An important aspect of preventing sleep problems is guidance regarding good sleep hygiene (Table 23-1), the conditions that are most conducive to healthy, restorative sleep. Some children are reassured by a low-wattage nightlight but more light than that may disturb sleep. Parents of newborns should be counseled to put their infant to sleep supine rather than prone unless there is a specific medical indication to the contrary. This results from the association of the prone sleeping position with sudden infant death syndrome (SIDS) in young infants (Guntheroth and Spiers, 1992) (SOR: A). Many children rest better with a "transitional object," a favorite blanket or toy. However, parents should avoid putting the child to bed with a bottle left in the mouth because it may lead to severe dental caries. Finally, the child should be put to bed awake, so that the child develops self-soothing skills to initiate sleep and resume sleep after nighttime disruptions.

About 20% to 30% of children and adolescents have sleep problems that are a serious concern to them and their families (Dahl, 1998). Problems with sleep initiation and nighttime awakenings are most common during infancy. Parasomnias and OSAS are most common in the 3- to 8-year-old group. Sleep deprivation, delayed sleep-phase syndrome, and narcolepsy are important considerations in the adolescent age group (Carskadon and Roth, 2000).

Sleep problems have a serious negative impact on many aspects of physical, mental, and social well-being. Also, many medical problems, such as conditions that cause nighttime pain or nocturia, and mental disorders, such as bipolar disorder (BD), can lead to sleep problems. Changes made in the *Diagnostic and Statistical Manual of Mental Disorders*, 5th edition (DSM-5) from the DSM-IV acknowledge these bidirectional and interactive effects. Sleep problems early in life are predictive of many later behavioral and emotional problems (Dahl, 1998). Children with frequent nighttime awakenings are at increased risk for physical abuse, perhaps because the parents of these children show increased levels of fatigue, irritability, and depression. The assessment and management of sleep problems in general should include consideration of potential sleep interrupters as primary causes or as exacerbators. One important category of interrupters is conditions that cause pain or itching (e.g., juvenile rheumatoid arthritis, migraine, atopic dermatitis). Another category is problems that lead to respiratory symptoms, including nocturnal asthma, gastroesophageal reflux, and obstructive sleep apnea.

SLEEP REFUSAL

Toddlers often resist going to bed when their parents want them to. Parents may have difficulty recognizing whether the resistance is related to true needs and fears or whether it is attention seeking or oppositional. The resistance often takes the form of repeated requests for a snack, a drink, or a trip to the toilet and may include fears of noises, shadows, or imaginary monsters.

A sleep diary can be helpful to sort out the etiology for the sleep refusal and direct management efforts. The parents record bedtimes and waking times for 2 weeks and indicate specific problem behaviors and their responses to each situation. Parents are often able to recognize patterns and problems themselves as they review the diary.

Many common refusal patterns can be addressed by focusing on the problem aspects of good sleep hygiene (see Table 23-1). If the problem seems to be oppositional, the best approach is for parents to ignore it. If the child gets out of bed, a parent should place the child back in bed without conversation other than a firm, "It's time for bed." When the parents actively ignore their child's efforts to get attention, the behaviors often get worse before they improve. However, even persistent children eventually respond (Blum and Carey, 1996). If standard ignoring is too stressful on the family, a "gradual ignoring" technique is also effective (Reid et al., 1999) (SOR: B). This involves briefly checking on the child every few minutes until he or she is asleep and gradually lengthening the interval between checks.

For a child who is fearful, having parents ignore them may make the fears worse. A gradual withdrawal of the parent's presence after the bedtime routine works better. The parent may sit in the room while the child falls to sleep but should avoid lengthy discussion of the child's fears. After the child is able to get to sleep without fear, the parent begins to move their chair closer to the child's door and eventually outside the bedroom. Fearful children who do not respond to this technique should be considered for referral for more intensive treatment similar to that applied toward phobias.

NIGHT WAKING

Most children wake up in the night but are able to get back to sleep without arousing their parents. The exceptions can have a serious impact on the entire family, as previously noted. As with sleep refusal, a sleep diary can help, and parent education regarding good sleep hygiene is beneficial. However, two common problems deserve particular attention: night terrors and nightmares (Table 23-2).

Night terrors come about as a sudden partial arousal from the deepest non-REM sleep. Essentially, part of the brain snaps into wakefulness, but part remains soundly asleep. Because deep non-REM sleep predominates in the first 4 hours of sleep, night terrors usually happen during the early part of the night. The child bolts upright in bed, screaming, sweating, tachycardic, and tachypneic. The episodes usually last only a few minutes, ending as abruptly as they began, with the child falling back to sleep quickly

Table 23-2   Diagnostic Features of Night Terrors versus Nightmares

Feature	Night Terrors	Nightmares
Time of night	Early; usually within 4 hours of bedtime	Late
State on waking	Disoriented or confused	Upset or scared
Response to parents	Unaware of presence; not consolable	Comforted
Memory of event	None unless fully awakened	Vivid recall of dream
Return to sleep	Usually rapid unless fully awakened	Often delayed by fear
Sleep stage	Partial arousal from deep non-REM sleep	REM sleep

REM, Rapid eye movement.
From Blum NJ, Carey WB. Sleep problems among infants and young children. *Pediatr Rev.* 1996;17(3):87-92.

unless fully awakened by the parents. Not fully awake, these children do not respond to the parents' efforts to comfort them. The child appears disoriented and confused, often with a blank stare, and has no recall of the event the next morning. Night terrors usually occur in children ages 2 to 6 years and are more common during times of illness, stress, or sleep deprivation. A nocturnal seizure should be considered in the differential diagnosis if the events are more likely right at sleep onset or if there is a personal or family history of seizures (Dahl, 1998).

Nightmares, on the other hand, are frightening dreams that awaken the child from REM sleep. Therefore, they tend to occur during the second half of the night, leaving the child upset or scared with a vivid recall of the dream. The child responds to comforting efforts by the parent but may be slow to go back to sleep because of fear. As with night terrors, nightmares occur most often during the toddler to preschool years and are more common during stressful times.

Management

In general, sedative medications are not indicated for night waking. Instead, behavior management techniques similar to those outlined for sleep refusal are appropriate for most cases.

There is no specific treatment for night terrors. Parents should be reassured with the explanation that the problem is common and self-limited. They should not try to wake the child up because this may only frighten the child or slow the child's return to sleep. For children who thrash violently, the parent should take precautions to provide protection for them. If the child sleepwalks into potentially dangerous situations, the parents can hang a bell or electronic movement alarm on the child's bedroom door to warn them. Because overtiredness is a major factor in the tendency to have night terrors, increasing the total amount of sleep and keeping a consistent sleep–wake cycle should be emphasized.

Because nightmares tend to occur at times of emotional stress, the focus of treatment should be on assisting parents with effective ways to manage the underlying stress. When a nightmare has occurred, the child is awake and frightened. The parent should comfort the child *without* a detailed review of the nightmare contents or "flashlight searches for monsters" (Blum and Carey, 1996), which can further increase the child's fears.

OBSTRUCTIVE SLEEP APNEA SYNDROME

Habitual snoring occurs in 3% to 12% of preschool-age children. The childhood incidence of OSAS is estimated to be 2%. The American Academy of Pediatrics (AAP) has published an evidence-based guideline for the diagnosis and management of OSAS (Marcus et al., 2012).

In children, OSAS is most often associated with large adenoids or tonsils, as well as specific facial features such as micrognathia, macroglossia, and Down syndrome. Unlike adults with sleep apnea, children can be affected without large drops in blood oxygen levels because children can have frequent brief awakenings to quickly reestablish their airway. Thus, the primary clinical issue may be sleep fragmentation. In the context of a child with snoring and restless sleep, OSAS should be considered any time there are symptoms or signs suggesting sleep deprivation, such as difficulty paying attention, emotional lability, partial arousals during the night (night terrors, sleepwalking), or difficulty waking up in the morning (AAP, 2012).

Because only a portion of children with snoring and adenotonsillar hypertrophy have OSAS, a sleep study is recommended to avoid unnecessary surgery. A caution, however, is that sleep studies in children require special expertise that may not be available at an adult sleep center.

Treatment of a child with OSAS on the basis of adenotonsillar hypertrophy is surgery. Continuous positive airway pressure (CPAP) is effective in children but is reserved for when adenotonsillectomy is contraindicated or unsuccessful (AAP, 2012) (SOR: A).

SLEEP DEPRIVATION AND DELAYED SLEEP-PHASE SYNDROME

Sleep deprivation and delayed sleep-phase syndrome are common problems in adolescents for several reasons. The total sleep requirement is as much or more in adolescence as in preadolescence (Carskadon and Roth, 2000), but adolescents tend to attain less sleep for both biologic and cultural reasons. School-age children are more likely to be "larks," preferring to wake up early even if they are up late at night. At puberty, a circadian rhythm change occurs that results in a switch from larks to "owls," the preference for a late-night bedtime and late-morning awakening. This biologic tendency is encouraged by the availability of stimulating activities late into the night, whether social events, part-time jobs, or technologic advances (e.g., TV, Internet). Stimulants such as caffeine and tobacco also act to delay sleep. Despite these factors that act to delay sleep, school schedules often require the adolescent to awaken early. Thus, sleep deprivation develops. Also, jet lag–like shifts often develop between the weekday and weekend or holiday schedule. These schedule shifts probably play a role in the most common adolescent sleep problem: delayed sleep-phase syndrome (Dahl, 1998).

The assessment is by history. The main differential diagnosis to consider from delayed sleep-phase syndrome is a teenager who is choosing a late-night schedule for some secondary gain. This person is not distressed by the dysfunctional sleep pattern and is unmotivated to change it. Therefore, the adolescent with secondary gain requires treatment directed at the underlying school or family issues rather than the sleep disturbance.

Treatment of the cooperative adolescent involves attempting a schedule shift and consistently maintaining it. Those with marked difficulty initiating timely sleep may respond to staying awake through an entire night and then reestablishing a regular schedule. Mindell and Owens (2009) provide a practical clinical guide for sleep in children.

NARCOLEPSY

Although rare, narcolepsy is an important cause of daytime sleepiness because it can affect personal safety and school performance, but it is readily treatable. Normally, REM sleep only occurs when a person has been asleep for 60 to 90 minutes and follows all four stages of non-REM sleep. Narcoleptic patients, on the other hand, experience sudden episodes of REM sleep in the middle of a wakeful state or immediately after falling asleep.

The key feature of narcolepsy is recurrent *sleep attacks:* sudden, unintentional, irresistible bouts of sleep that occur in inappropriate situations, such as during conversations or while driving. Other common findings include *cataplexy* (sudden bilateral loss of muscle tone without loss of consciousness), *hypnagogic hallucinations* (vivid dreamlike imagery just before falling asleep), and *sleep paralysis* (inability to move or speak just after morning awakening). Any child or adolescent with unexplained daytime sleepiness who does not respond to initial management with good sleep hygiene or who has a family history of narcolepsy should be considered for evaluation. A sleep study is required to make the diagnosis.

Narcolepsy treatment combines behavioral approaches with medications. The patient should adhere to good sleep hygiene. Therapeutic naps enhance daytime alertness and reduce the necessary dose of stimulants. Stimulant medications, such as methylphenidate, dextroamphetamine, or modafinil, are very helpful for daytime sleepiness (Vgontzas and Kale, 1999) (SOR: A). The antidepressants are REM suppressants that help prevent cataplexy or hypnagogic hallucinations. The nonsedating antidepressants, especially the selective serotonin reuptake inhibitors (SSRIs), work synergistically when combined with stimulants (Vgontzas and Kale, 1999) (SOR: B).

Autism

Key Points

- Autism spectrum disorder (ASD) has an onset before age 3 years and is characterized by impaired social interaction; impaired communication; and repetitive, stereotyped patterns of behavior.
- Autism is not caused by thimerosal-containing vaccines.
- Standard developmental screening tests have poor sensitivity for autism.
- Early intervention with a multidisciplinary approach improves autism outcomes.

Autism spectrum disorder describes a constellation of symptoms in two primary categories: (1) impaired social interaction and communication and (2) repetitive, stereotyped patterns of behavior. It is estimated that one in 88 children are diagnosed with ASD with a higher prevalence in boys (CDC, 2008). Children diagnosed with ASD under the DSM-5 criteria experience difficulty in social-emotional reciprocity, use and interpretation of nonverbal gestures, and maintaining relationships. They must also experience symptoms in at least two of the following areas: stereotyped or repetitive use of speech, movement, or objects; excessive adherence to rituals, resistance to change, or ritualized patterns of behavior; restricted interests unusual in their intensity or focus; or unusual sensory interests or reactions (American Psychiatric Association [APA], 2013). The DSM-5 also removes the requirement that symptoms are fully evident before age 3 years, instead using the criterion that symptoms may manifest when social demands exceed the capacity of the child or adolescent. Thus, children whose social deficits do not emerge until middle school or high school, when social interactions become more complex and require greater skill, may still qualify for a diagnosis of ASD if all criteria are met. Qualifying statements may be added to the ASD diagnosis in cases of accompanying intellectual impairment; language impairment; association with medical, genetic, and environmental factors; or association with another neurodevelopmental, mental, or behavioral disorder (e.g., attention-deficit hyperactivity disorder [ADHD]).

Former related disorders including Asperger disorder and pervasive developmental disorder, not otherwise specified (PDD, NOS) have been removed from the diagnostic profile of the DSM-5. A lack of scientific evidence distinguishing among the disorders drove members of the revision committee to join these disorders under one spectrum because of the clinical practice of inconsistently interchanging diagnoses of high-functioning autism and Asperger disorder. Whereas some children with prior diagnoses of Asperger disorder or PDD, NOS may no longer qualify for an ASD diagnosis, others may meet diagnostic criteria for a new category of social (pragmatic) communication disorder (without repetitive or stereotyped behaviors). The impact of this categorical change on eligibility for community-based and educational services is currently unknown.

Evidence is mounting that both genetic and environmental factors influence the etiology of autism (Kolevzon et al., 2007; Schaefer and Mendelsohn, 2008). Approximately 15% of autism cases are related to known genetic mutations; however, specific gene contributions vary among families, and it is suspected that more than 100 genetic loci may contribute independently to the ASD phenotype (APA, 2013). Assertions that autism is caused by thimerosal-containing vaccines have been discounted by a comprehensive meta-analysis (Parker et al., 2004; Thompson, 2013).

ASSESSMENT

Developmental screening should be part of each well-child examination. Physicians should take parental concerns about delayed speech and language development seriously, especially beyond 18 months of age. In addition to delayed speech development, the other common presenting symptom is *challenging behavior*. The behaviors may include a violent reaction to minor changes in the environment or routine, stereotypic movements such as clapping or rocking, and preoccupation with narrow interests or inanimate objects. The AAP released a policy statement on developmental surveillance in primary care, offering an algorithm for determining when specialized assessment is needed (AAP, 2006). Frequently used general screening measures include the Denver II Developmental Screening Test (Frankenburg et al., 1992) and the Ages and Stages Questionnaire (ASQ; Bricker and Squires, 1999), although these measures are not specific for ASD. ASD-specific measures appropriate for primary care include the Modified Checklist for Autism in Toddlers (M-CHAT), a brief, freely available screener that quickly identifies children in need of more intensive assessment (Robins et al., 2001).

When autism is suspected, a thorough evaluation should be performed, including appropriate intellectual testing, speech-language assessment, and assessment of behaviors specific to ASD. The gold standard evaluation tools include the Autism Diagnostic Interview–Revised (ADI-R; Rutter et al., 2008) and the Autism Diagnostic Observation Schedule, Second Edition (ADOS-2; Lord et al., 2012), although these are not required for an accurate diagnosis of ASD. Referral to a multidisciplinary clinic, developmental behavioral pediatrician, clinical psychologist, or clinical neuropsychologist may be appropriate. Because hearing loss can mimic autism, the evaluation should also include formal audiologic testing. Common comorbidities include anxiety, depression, and obsessional behavior (Prater and Zylstra, 2002).

MANAGEMENT

Early intervention is critical in improving outcomes in children with ASD (Rogers and Vismara, 2008). The landmark autism treatment study by Lovaas (1987) suggests intensive, individualized behavioral intervention with massed practice is key in improving outcomes. Currently, the most successful programs use a multidisciplinary approach that includes behavior modification, development of social communication, active involvement of parents and families, and use of psychotropic medications for dangerous behaviors that do not respond to behavior modification (Myers and Johnson, 2007). Referral to an established program is recommended. Early intensive behavioral interventions (EIBIs) are conducted with the goal of improving intellectual, social, behavioral, and emotional outcomes using empirically supported, consistently implemented, data-driven behavioral interventions across a range of the child's environments (LeBlanc and Gillis, 2012), and these EIBIs are the only autism interventions with consistent demonstration of efficacy. Despite anecdotal reports on the effectiveness of alternative and complementary treatments (e.g., dietary changes), none has shown consistent benefit in clinically controlled trials. Young adults with autism have persistent difficulties functioning in the community, with just more than one third achieving any level of postsecondary education and approximately half maintaining any level of paid employment (Shattuck et al., 2012). Clear gains in language by age 5 years is the most important predictor of adult outcomes (Bryson et al., 2003).

- Comprehensive EIBIs that address the child and parents across settings (e.g., home, school, community) hold the most research evidence of efficacy (LeBlanc and Gillis, 2012).
- Risperidone effectively treats irritability, repetition, and social withdrawal in individuals with autism, with weight gain as the most prominent side effect (Jesner et al., 2007).

Encopresis and Enuresis

See eAppendix 23-1 online at www.expertconsult.com.

Attention-Deficit Hyperactivity Disorder

Key Points

- Consider ADHD in a child presenting with hyperactivity, impulsivity, inattentiveness, academic underachievement, or behavior problems.
- Use the DSM-5 diagnostic criteria when assessing for ADHD.
- Obtain information from the parents, child, and teacher using standardized behavior reports, if possible.
- When planning treatment, recognize that ADHD is a chronic condition for which medication only temporarily decreases symptoms and improves functioning.
- Stimulants are the first and second lines of medication treatment.

Attention-deficit hyperactivity disorder is the most frequently diagnosed behavioral disorder of childhood. The prevalence among school-age children is at least 5%, with a 2:1 ratio of boys to girls (DSM-5 2013). ADHD is a chronic disorder persisting from childhood into adolescence and adulthood in the majority of cases. Obvious hyperactivity usually subsides, but inattention and impulsivity persist, leading to potentially serious consequences. ADHD should be considered and assessed in any child age 4 to 18 years who presents with symptoms of inattention, hyperactivity, or impulsivity and academic or behavior problems related to these (AAP, 2011).

The heritability of ADHD appears to be about 77% with a polygenic mechanism of inheritance. Thus, children who are diagnosed with the disorder very often have parents who are also affected. Environmental factors with a positive evidence of association with ADHD include maternal smoking, fetal exposure to alcohol, pregnancy and delivery complications, psychosocial adversity, and exposure to environmental toxins such as PCBs or pesticides. Widely held public beliefs blaming food additives or television viewing have not been supported when studied scientifically (Banerjee et al., 2007; Bouchard et al., 2010).

Comorbidity is common in ADHD, including oppositional defiant disorder (ODD) (54%-84%), smoking (19%), language or learning disorder (25%), anxiety (up to 33%), and depression (up to 33%) (Dobie et al., 2012).

ASSESSMENT

There is no independent valid test to determine that a child has ADHD. The diagnosis can only be obtained reliably by using a combination of established diagnostic criteria and comprehensive evaluation methods. The recently published DSM-5 made only minor revisions to the criteria set forth in the DSM-IV (Table 23-3). Instead of the prior "types" of ADHD, the DSM-5 refers to three "presentations": (1) combined, (2) predominantly inattentive, and (3) predominantly hyperactive and impulsive. The individual criteria for each presentation are unchanged from the DSM-IV except that more behavioral examples are given for each, including examples that apply to adults. Also, a diagnosis in adults requires the presence of just five of nine criteria under each category instead of six of nine as required for children. The biggest change in the DSM-5 is that symptoms must be present before age 12 years (rather than age 7 years). The potential these changes have to increase the prevalence of ADHD will be a matter of future study.

Comprehensive diagnostic evaluation for ADHD includes obtaining information from the child, parents, teacher(s), and other caregivers. The process is greatly facilitated by the use of standardized behavior reports, such as the Conners Rating Scales (1997 revision), National Institute for Children's Health Quality (NICHQ) Vanderbilt forms, or the Swanson, Nolan, and Pelham (SNAP) checklist. Broadband behavioral rating scales, such as the Child Behavior Check List (CBCL, Achenbach), do not effectively discriminate between ADHD and non-ADHD children but do assist in identifying comorbid disorders (Dobie, 2012). Because of the significant prevalence of comorbid psychiatric disorders, the assessment should include inquiring about these conditions. In addition to psychiatric symptoms, the ability of the child to function normally in different domains must also be assessed, including family relationships with adults and siblings, peer social relationships, community behavior, school academic performance, school behavior, interests and play activities, and subjective psychological distress.

The physician should conduct a medical screening examination, including hearing and vision tests. Other diagnostic tests, including laboratory screening tests for lead intoxication, abnormal thyroid function, neuroimaging for brain tumor, or seizure disorder, should be conducted when indicated by the history and physical examination (Dobie, 2012). Computerized continuous performance tests and a full psychological evaluation are not required for diagnosis of ADHD. In fact, most straightforward cases can be diagnosed in a primary care setting using standardized parent and teacher questionnaires and a careful clinical history.

MANAGEMENT

The clinician should establish a comprehensive management program that recognizes ADHD as a chronic

Table 23-3   DSM-5 Diagnostic Criteria for Attention-Deficit/Hyperactivity Disorder

A. A persistent pattern of inattention and/or hyperactivity-impulsivity that interferes with functioning or development, as characterized by (1) and/or (2):

  1. Inattention: six (or more) of the following symptoms of inattention have persisted for at least 6 months to a degree that is inconsistent with developmental level and that negatively impacts directly on social and academic/occupational activities:

    Note: The symptoms are not solely a manifestation of oppositional behavior, defiance, hostility, or failure to understand tasks or instructions. For older adolescents and adults (age 17 and older), at least five symptoms are required.

    (a) Often fails to give close attention to details or makes careless mistakes in schoolwork, at work, or during other activities (e.g., overlooks or misses details, work is inaccurate).

    (b) Often has difficulty sustaining attention in tasks or play activities (e.g., has difficulty remaining focused during lectures, conversations, or lengthy reading).

    (c) Often does not seem to listen when spoken to directly (e.g., mind seems elsewhere, even in the absence of any obvious distraction).

    (d) Often does not follow through on instructions and fails to finish schoolwork, chores, or duties in the workplace (e.g., starts tasks but quickly loses focus and is easily sidetracked).

    (e) Often has difficulties organizing tasks and activities (e.g., difficulty managing sequential tasks; difficulty keeping materials and belongings in order; messy, disorganized work; has poor time management; fails to meet deadlines).

    (f) Often avoids, dislikes, or is reluctant to engage in tasks that require sustained mental effort (e.g., schoolwork or homework; for older adolescents and adults, preparing reports, completing forms, reviewing lengthy papers).

    (g) Often loses things necessary for tasks or activities (e.g., school materials, pencils, books, tools, wallets, keys, paperwork, eyeglasses, mobile telephones).

    (h) Is often easily distracted by extraneous stimuli (for older adolescents and adults, may include unrelated thoughts).

    (i) Often forgetful in daily activities (e.g., doing chores, running errands; for older adolescents and adults, returning calls, paying bills, keeping appointments).

  2. Hyperactivity and impulsivity: six (or more) of the following symptoms of hyperactivity-impulsivity have persisted for at least 6 months to a degree that is inconsistent with developmental level and that negatively impacts directly on social and academic/occupational activities:

    Note: The symptoms are not solely a manifestation of oppositional behavior, defiance, hostility, or failure to understand tasks or instructions. For older adolescents and adults (age 17 and older), at least five symptoms are required.

    (a) Often fidgets with or taps hands or feet or squirms in seat.

    (b) Often leaves seat in situations in which remaining seated is expected (e.g., leaves his or her place in the classroom, in the office or other workplace, or in other situations that require remaining in place).

    (c) Often runs about or climbs in situations where it is inappropriate (Note: in adolescents or adults, may be limited to feeling restless).

    (d) Often unable to play or engage in leisure activities quietly.

    (e) Is often "on the go," acting as if "driven by a motor" (e.g., is unable to be or uncomfortable being still for extended time, as in restaurants, meetings; may be experienced by others as being restless or difficult to keep up with).

    (f) Often talks excessively.

    (g) Often blurts out an answer before a question has been completed (e.g., completes people's sentences; cannot wait for turn in conversation).

    (h) Often has difficulty waiting his or her turn (e.g., while waiting in line).

    (i) Often interrupts or intrudes on others (e.g., butts into conversations, games, or activities; may start using other people's things without asking or receiving permission; for adolescents and adults, may intrude into or take over what others are doing).

B. Several inattentive or hyperactive-impulsive symptoms were present prior to age 12 years.

C. Several inattentive or hyperactive-impulsive symptoms are present in two or more settings (e.g., at home, school, or work; with friends or relatives; in other activities).

D. There is clear evidence that the symptoms interfere with, or reduce the quality of, social, academic, or occupational functioning.

E. The symptoms do not occur exclusively during the course of schizophrenia or another psychotic disorder and are not better explained by another mental disorder (e.g., mood disorder, anxiety disorder, dissociative disorder, personality disorder, substance intoxication or withdrawal).

DSM-5, Diagnostic and Statistical Manual of Mental Disorders, 5th edition.
Adapted from American Psychiatric Association. *Diagnostic and statistical manual of mental disorders.* 5th ed. Arlington, VA: American Psychiatric Publishers; 2013.

condition and works with the parents, child, and teachers to identify the most important problems as targets of treatment. Indications for referral to a specialist include (1) children with ADHD plus a comorbid psychiatric disorder and (2) children with ADHD who do not respond to initial treatment. More specific guidance in assessment and management may be obtained by consulting practice guidelines or parameters (American Academy of Child and Adolescent Psychiatry [AACAP], 2007; AAP, 2011; Dobie, 2012). An initial effort must be made to educate the parents and child about ADHD (see Web Resources).

Psychosocial Therapy

The physician or staff should review techniques of parent behavioral management to assess how well they are understood and effectively implemented. This includes the proper use of positive reinforcers and punishment. A structured and standardized system, called the "token economy," can

be very effective but requires considerable time and effort by the parents. Common mistakes made by parents include too much punishment versus positive reinforcement, too long a delay in receiving a reward, making the system too difficult initially so the child never achieves success, inconsistent implementation, and poor supervision.

Assessing for proper educational placement is important. At a minimum, the parents should consult with the child's classroom teacher and confirm close supervision of the child, a structured classroom, good behavioral management, and good communication with parents. If this effort is not sufficient, the parents can request educational accommodations under Section 504 of the 1973 Rehabilitation Act. This federal law provides for special accommodations and services in a person with a chronic disabling condition, including psychiatric disorder. The request must be accompanied by a physician statement documenting the disabling condition and directed to the building principal or school

Table 23-4 Stimulant Medications Used in Treatment of Attention-Deficit Hyperactivity Disorder

Drug	Brand Name	Dosage Forms	Duration of Behavioral Effects	Suggested Dosage
Methylphenidate, plain	Ritalin regular Methylin	5-, 10-, 20-mg tablet Methylin is also available in chewable tablet and solution	1-4 hr	0.3-2.0 mg/kg/day in divided doses FDA approved for use in children age ≥6 yr Maximum dose, 60 mg/day
Methylphenidate, extended release	Ritalin SR	20-mg tablet	3-9 hr	Titrate quickly up to 0.5 mg/kg in a single dose. Observe for benefit and titrate to maximum dose if necessary (2 mg/kg/day up to 60 mg).
	Ritalin LA	10-, 20-, 30-, 40-mg tablet	10-12 hr	—
	Metadate ER	20-mg tablet	8 hr	—
	Metadate CD	10-, 20-, 30-, 40-, 50-, 60-mg capsule	8-12 hr	—
	Concerta	18-, 27-, 36-, 54-mg capsule	12 hr	Start all patients at 18 mg/day and titrate up prn. Child: up to 54 mg/day Adolescent and adult: up to 72 mg/day
	Quillivant XR	5 mg/mL extended release liquid	12 hr	0.3-2 mg/kg/day, single dose
	Daytrana skin patch	10-, 15-, 20-, 30-mg/9-hr patch	9 hr while patch applied	—
Dexmethyl-phenidate	Focalin	2.5-, 5-, 10-mg tablet	4-6 hr	0.3-1.0 mg/kg/day to a maximum of 20 mg/day
	Focalin XR	5-, 10-, 15-, 20-, 30-, 35-, 40- mg capsule	12 hr	30 mg maximum daily dose
Amphetamine salts	Adderall	5-, 7.5-, 10-, 12.5-, 15-, 20-, 30-mg scored tablet	6-8 hr	0.3-1.0 mg/kg/day to a maximum of 40 mg/day
	Adderall XR	5-, 10-, 15-, 20-, 25-, 30-mg capsule	10-12 hr	10 mg/day to a maximum of 30 mg/day for child or 40 mg/day for adolescent or adult
Dextroamphetamine, plain	Dexedrine	2.5-, 5-, 7.5-, 10-, 15-, 20-, 30-mg tablet	1-8 hr	0.3-1.0 mg/kg/day FDA approved for use in children age ≥3 yr
Dextroamphetamine, extended release	Dexedrine ER	5-, 10-, 15-mg spansule	8-9 hr	Maximum dose, 60 mg/day
	Procentra	5 mg/5 mL ER liquid	10-12 hr	3-5 yr old: start 2.5 mg/day single dose; maximum dose, 40 mg/day ≥6 yr old: start 5 mg/day single dose; maximum dose, 60 mg/day
Lisdexamfetamine	Vyvanse	20-, 30-, 40-, 50-, 60-, 70-mg capsule	10-13 hr	Maximum dose, 70 mg/day

ER, Extended release; *FDA,* U.S. Food and Drug Administration; *PDR, Physicians' Desk Reference; prn,* as needed.

district "Section 504 compliance officer." If this is not enough and the child is failing in one or more subjects, the parents can request a comprehensive evaluation by the Child Study Team for possible Special Education placement ("Other Health Impaired" eligibility condition—Federal Public Law 94-142, currently the Individuals with Disabilities Education Act [IDEA]). The request should be in writing and directed to the building principal. The evaluation may take up to 85 school days but could result in an *Individualized Education Program* (IEP), a description and contract of what special services the school will provide.

For children with ADHD alone, other psychosocial treatments have not been shown to be more effective than aggressive use of stimulant medication or even to provide an additional benefit (MTA Cooperative Group, 1999). However, psychosocial treatments are beneficial in children with ADHD and other comorbid disorders or those from families with chaotic functioning.

Pharmacotherapy

The stimulants are the medications of first choice at any age unless comorbid factors take precedence (Dobie, 2012).

Methylphenidate was also shown to be beneficial for very young children with ADHD through the National Institutes of Mental Health (NIMH) Preschoolers with ADHD Treatment Study (PATS); however, the benefit was not as robust as in older children, and adverse effects were more prominent (Abikoff et al., 2007; Gleason et al., 2007). Table 23-4 lists specific dosing recommendations. Of children with ADHD, 70% show a significant improvement on the first trial of a stimulant, and 85% to 90% improve significantly taking at least one of the listed stimulants. When the medication is in effect, motor activity decreases, certain cognitive processes improve, motivation improves, academic performance improves, and oppositional and aggressive behaviors decrease. However, the medication works only for as long as it is given, with no long-lasting or curative effect.

The physician should use a systematic approach. If the first stimulant is not effective after an adequate trial of maximum doses, a sequential trial of each available stimulant is appropriate before moving to another class of medication. At a minimum, at least one methylphenidate preparation and one amphetamine preparation should be tried. Follow-up appointments should be regular and scheduled and should include information from the parents, teachers, and child (Dobie, 2012). Adverse effects are similar for all stimulants and can affect up to 20% of children. Important side effects include anorexia, weight loss, irritability (more likely in younger children), abdominal pain, insomnia (only if given after 5 PM), dysphoria (more likely in younger children), "behavioral rebound" after wearing off, impaired cognitive performance on laboratory tests (methylphenidate at single doses >1 mg/kg), tachycardia, and increased tic symptoms (if the patient has a tic disorder). In general, growth suppression is not a concern except in children with dramatic anorexia. There is no evidence that the legitimate prescribed use of stimulants by children and adolescents with ADHD leads to future drug abuse, and proper use may actually have a protective effect (Biederman, 1999). Sudden death in children taking stimulant medication has been raised as a potential concern to the point that the U.S. Food and Drug Administration (FDA) issued a communication in 2009 recommending caution but not stopping the use of stimulants for ADHD. Physicians should screen patients via history and physical examination for conditions that would put them at increased risk for cardiac complications, but current evidence does not support routine electrocardiography for all patients (Dobie, 2012).

The third line of treatment (after two trials of stimulants) is atomoxetine. It is initially given at 0.5 mg/kg/day, either in the early morning or as a divided dose (morning and late afternoon). It is titrated up to a maximum dose of 1.4 mg/kg/day (or 100 mg maximum). The full benefit may not be seen for 4 weeks (Dobie, 2012). Atomoxetine is not a U.S. Drug Enforcement Administration scheduled medication, has no potential for abuse, and therefore can be written with refills. Common adverse effects include nausea, vomiting, gastrointestinal pain, anorexia, headache, fatigue, and sleepiness. Potentially serious side effects include liver injury and suicidal thinking.

Extended-release clonidine (Kapvay) and extended-release guanfacine (Intuniv) are available as adjunctive therapy to stimulants for ADHD. They can be especially useful for oppositional symptoms (Dobie, 2012).

Bupropion, the tricyclic antidepressants (TCAs, e.g., imipramine, nortriptyline), and the α-adrenergic agent clonidine do not have an official FDA indication for the treatment of ADHD. The evidence for their benefit is based on randomized controlled trials (RCTs) and nonrandomized trials with control participants (Dobie, 2012). A variety of other psychoactive medications have been studied for use in ADHD, but these generally go beyond the scope of primary physicians.

KEY TREATMENT

- The stimulants are the medications of first choice for ADHD at any age (Dobie, 2012) (SOR: A).
- Although not a first-line drug, atomoxetine is effective for treatment of ADHD (Hammerness et al., 2009) (SOR: A).
- Behavioral treatments for children with ADHD are effective adjuncts to pharmacologic therapy (Fabiano et al., 2009) (SOR: A).

Oppositional Defiant Disorder

Key Points

- The provider must establish a therapeutic alliance with both the child and the family to be successful in treating ODD.
- The diagnosis of ODD is based on reports from the parents and child; the possibility of comorbid conditions should be carefully considered.
- The best treatment of ODD usually is parent training in behavior management techniques.
- Medication may be helpful in treating the symptoms of comorbid conditions.

The prevalence of ODD in children younger than 18 years old is 1% to 11% (APA, 2013). Before puberty, rates in boys outnumber girls, but after puberty, the rates are more equal. ODD is a chronic persistent disorder marked by a pattern of angry or irritable mood, argumentative or defiant behavior, or vindictiveness with interaction patterns occurring with at least one individual other than a sibling (APA, 2013). The severity of the disorder depends on the pervasiveness of behaviors. Often, children and adolescents with ODD do not behave in an overtly defiant manner with teachers or strangers but exhibit marked behavioral difficulty in the home setting. Characteristics of headstrong and irritable behavior at age 13 years are correlated with increased callousness, depression, and delinquency in later adolescence and early adulthood (Whelan et al., 2013).

The characteristics predisposing to ODD are biologic, social, and psychological, involving the parents and child. The parents usually use poor, ineffective, inconsistent, and indiscriminate behavioral management methods, which are often combined with unusually harsh but inconsistent discipline and poor monitoring of activities. These children are usually temperamental, impulsive, active, and inattentive. The parents themselves are frequently immature, temperamental, and impulsive. The family members usually experience significant marital, financial, health, and personal distress (Barkley, 1997). Physiologic markers may include decreased skin conductance reactivity and lower resting heart rate, as well as reduced basal cortisol reactivity, although these may be more generalized to other disruptive behavior disorders (APA, 2013).

ASSESSMENT

There are two periods of developmentally normal oppositional behavior: the "terrible twos," between 18 and 24 months of age, when toddlers behave negatively as an expression of developing autonomy, and sometimes in adolescence, when teenagers try to separate from their parents and establish autonomous identities. Unlike ODD, these stages usually last less than 6 months (Table 23-5).

A child with ODD reported by the parents may not show much oppositional behavior while being examined in the office. The symptoms of ODD that these children display are much more evident in interactions with people and situations that they know well. The child takes a self-defeating

Table 23-5 DSM-5 Diagnostic Criteria for Oppositional Defiant Disorder

A. A pattern of angry/irritable mood, argumentative/defiant behavior, or vindictiveness lasting at least 6 months with at least four of the following symptoms:

Angry/Irritable Mood
1. Often loses temper
2. Is often touchy or easily annoyed
3. Is often angry and resentful

Argumentative/Defiant Behavior
4. Often argues with authority figures or, for children and adolescents, with adults
5. Often actively defies or refuses to comply with requests from authority figures or with rules
6. Often deliberately annoys others
7. Often blames others for his or her mistakes or misbehavior

Vindictiveness
Has been spiteful or vindictive at least twice within the past 6 months

B. The disturbance in behavior is associated with distress for the individual or caregivers or negatively impacts social, educational, occupational, or other important areas of functioning.

C. The behaviors do not occur exclusively during the course of a psychotic, substance use, depressive, or bipolar episode. Criteria are not met for Disruptive Mood Dysregulation Disorder.

Severity:
Mild: Symptoms confined to one setting
Moderate: Some symptoms are present in at least two settings
Severe: Some symptoms are present in three or more settings

Adapted from American Psychiatric Association. *Diagnostic and statistical manual of mental disorders.* 5th ed. Arlington, VA: American Psychiatric Publishers; 2013.

position in arguments with adults. The struggle becomes more important than the reality of the situation, such that the child may be willing to risk losing the object or activity rather than lose the argument. Even a significant delay by the child in complying with a parental request is seen as a victory by the child. The assessment of ODD should include direct information from the child and parents regarding symptoms, age of onset, duration, and degree of functional impairment.

If oppositional behavior is confined mostly to school and not much at home (except as it relates to schoolwork), additional diagnoses must be considered in the differential, including mental retardation; borderline intellectual functioning; a specific developmental disorder (e.g., learning disability); and, most often, ADHD. No specific laboratory tests or pathologic findings can assist the clinician in making the diagnosis of ODD.

MANAGEMENT

With methodologically sound RCTs lacking and recommendations based on clinical consensus, the appropriate psychosocial interventions for ODD include parenting training in behavior management techniques, including an improved parent–child relationship, positive reinforcement, closer supervision, giving more effective commands, time-outs, and token economies. When implemented before age 6 years, there is a 50% to 67% response rate to structured behavioral interventions (Barkley, 1997). Despite the usually chaotic family situation and high emotions involved, the family physician needs to establish a therapeutic alliance with both the child and the family to have the best

chance of success (Steiner and Remsing, 2007). Interventions should be family based, targeted to specific concerns, and oriented to problem solving. Traditional individual psychotherapy, unstructured or nondirected family therapy, or short-term treatment is usually not helpful. Psychoactive medications are used to treat comorbid conditions and targeted symptoms but have not demonstrated benefit for ODD alone. Intense and prolonged treatment may be necessary for severe and persistent ODD. One-time crisis interventions (e.g., "scared straight" attempts) are not effective.

Conduct Disorder

Key Points

- A poorer prognosis for CD is associated with an earlier age at onset, lower IQ, more conduct symptoms, and greater frequency and severity of symptoms.
- Alcohol and drug use should be suspected in a teenager with CD.
- Talking to the adolescent who has CD is not sufficient; collateral sources of information (parents, teachers, courts) are essential.
- Physicians should diligently search for another, more treatable condition if it exists because CD does not have an effective treatment.
- Involvement by the juvenile court or placement outside the home may be the best option for some patients.

Conduct disorder is seen in approximately 4% of children younger than 18 years of age (APA, 2013). At all ages, rates in boys outnumber girls. Whereas boys usually exhibit more aggression, girls usually commit more covert crimes and prostitution. CD is more common in urban than rural settings and is one of the most frequent diagnoses in outpatient and inpatient psychiatric facilities for children. The mortality rate for seriously disturbed delinquents is elevated relative to non–conduct disordered youth, and misconduct in childhood may predispose individuals to poor lifestyle choices and chronic health conditions well into adulthood (von Stumm et al., 2011). Adolescents with CD are more likely to die by homicide, suicide, violent accident, or drug overdose and are more likely to engage in substance abuse behaviors and injuries inflicting persistent effects on health.

Generally, the natural history of children with severe CD is marked by the development of ADHD at a very early age followed by ODD and then finally the onset of CD. In adolescence, alcohol and substance abuse occur. The factors that determine a poorer prognosis in a patient with CD are an early age of onset of symptoms, greater number of symptoms, and greater frequency of expression of these CD symptoms. The factors that determine a better prognosis are a minimum number of CD symptoms, absence of comorbid psychiatric diagnoses, and normal intellectual functioning. Characteristics more common in childhood-onset versus adolescent-onset CD are greater frequency of neuropsychiatric disorders, lower IQ, higher levels of aggression, male gender, and greater frequency of externalizing behavior disorders in other family members. Just more than half of individuals with childhood-onset CD, versus only 15% of those with adolescent-onset CD, go on to develop *antisocial personality disorder,* a chronic pattern of lawlessness (Burt et al., 2007).

Current views posit an interaction among genetic, biologic, and environmental factors (i.e., parental, sociocultural, psychological, prolonged abuse). No single factor accounts for more than 50% of the variance in the occurrence of CD, and no combination of factors accounts for more than 70% of the variance. Many children with risk factors do not develop CD.

ASSESSMENT

The diagnostic criteria for CD are summarized in Table 23-6. The clinician should not quickly accept the diagnosis of CD in a youth because no specific effective treatment exists and instead should diligently search for other, more treatable psychiatric conditions. Other psychiatric diagnoses that should be considered as the primary disturbance in a child presenting with CD symptoms include ADHD, ODD, intermittent explosive disorder, psychoactive substance use disorder, mood disorders (bipolar and depressive disorders), posttraumatic stress disorder (PTSD), dissociative disorder, borderline personality disorder, and adjustment disorder with disturbance of conduct. A manic episode must be seriously considered in a teenager presenting with frequent lying, physical aggression against others, impulsive sexual activity, stealing, sneaking out in the middle of the night, grandiosity, and persistent pervasive irritability.

The interview of an adolescent with CD is not sufficient, in itself, for the psychiatric evaluation. Lying is a common problem for these teenagers, as is conscious and unconscious underreporting of their problem behaviors. Other sources of information, including parents, teachers, other professionals, past records, and court personnel, are essential to obtain a valid evaluation. Complications seen in association with CD symptoms include impairment in school performance, poor social and family relationships, problems with the legal system, poor work performance, physical injuries from fighting or carelessness, sexually transmitted diseases, teenage pregnancy, drug problems, suicide, and homicide. Common examples of interpersonal impairment in these children include suspiciousness or paranoia, misperception of others' actions as hostile, difficulty relating to peers and adults, lack of guilt, and lack of empathy.

Children with CD respond differently to punishment than normal children. Whereas the frequency of negative behavior of normal children decreases when they are punished, the negative behavior of children with CD increases when they are punished.

No specific laboratory tests can assist in making the diagnosis of CD. However, the differential diagnosis for CD symptoms includes conditions for which tests may be important. These include head trauma, seizure disorder, birth injury to the brain, and encephalitis.

MANAGEMENT

One-time interventions affecting a single domain are ineffective in treating patients with CD. Interventions need to target all affected domains in a naturalistic setting for a long

Table 23-6   DSM-5 Diagnostic Criteria for Conduct Disorder

A. A repetitive and persistent pattern of behavior in which the basic rights of others or major age-appropriate societal norms or rules are violated, as manifested by the presence of at least three of the following 15 criteria in the past 12 months, with at least one criterion present in the past 6 months.

Aggression to People and Animals
1. Often bullies, threatens, or intimidates others
2. Often initiates physical fights
3. Has used a weapon that can cause serious physical harm to others (e.g., a bat, brick, broken bottle, knife, gun)
4. Has been physically cruel to people
5. Has been physically cruel to animals
6. Has stolen while confronting a victim (e.g., mugging, purse snatching, extortion, armed robbery)
7. Has forced someone into sexual activity

Destruction of Property
1. Has deliberately engaged in fire setting with the intention of causing serious damage
2. Has deliberately destroyed others' property (other than by fire setting)

Deceitfulness or Theft
1. Has broken into someone else's house, building, or car
2. Often lies to obtain goods or favors or to avoid obligations (i.e., "cons" others)
3. Has stolen items of nontrivial value without confronting a victim (e.g., shoplifting, but without breaking and entering; forgery)

Serious Violations of Rules
1. Often stays out at night despite parental prohibitions, beginning before age 13 years
2. Has run away from home overnight at least twice while living in the parental or parental surrogate home, or once without returning for a lengthy period
3. Is often truant from school, beginning before age 13 years

B. The disturbance in behavior causes clinically significant impairment in social, academic, or occupational functioning.

C. If the individual is age 18 years or older, criteria are not met for antisocial personality disorder.

Specifiers:

Childhood-onset type: Individuals show at least one symptom characteristic of conduct disorder prior to age 10 years.

Adolescent-onset type: Individuals show no symptom characteristic of conduct disorder prior to age 10 years.

Unspecified onset: Criteria for a diagnosis of conduct disorder are met, but there is not enough information available to determine whether the onset of the first symptom was before or after age 10 years.

With limited prosocial emotions: The individual displays at least two of the following over at least 12 months and in multiple relationships and settings:

Lack of remorse or guilt

Callous—lack of empathy

Unconcerned about performance

Shallow or deficient affect

Adapted from American Psychiatric Association. *Diagnostic and statistical manual of mental disorders.* 5th ed. Arlington, VA: American Psychiatric Publishers; 2013.

period in a consistent manner. Multisystemic family interventions (parenting training and guidance, functional family therapy) and social skill training with a behavioral approach seem to be the most effective treatments for patients with CD (von Sydow et al., 2013). Individual therapy that focuses on problem-solving skills and empathy training can also be useful. An environment with consistent rules and consequences is helpful. Proper school placement using behavioral techniques to encourage prosocial behavior and discourage antisocial incidents is appropriate.

Factors that can cause a treatment program to fail include the following: the situation is "too hot to handle," the youth is "too brittle," the parents covertly support the youth's behavior, the parents have given up on the youth, the parents are inconsistent and are unable to supervise adequately, the program is poorly designed, rewards are too costly, or the parents have little social support. Factors that can interfere with limit setting of the child or adolescent at home include parental conflict, parental absence, parental psychiatric illness, inconsistent discipline, and vague or minimal expectations regarding appropriate behavior.

Several legal options are available if parents are unable to control their children. Most state laws have a special status that can be petitioned by the county district attorney to the juvenile court judge (i.e., child or person in need of care laws) that can allow the court to supervise the child by having hearings, placing a child on probation, mandating treatment and monitoring, or eventually taking the child away from the parents and placing the child in a residential treatment facility. However, some dangers must be kept in mind when teenagers with CD are confined to a juvenile detention facility. These patients prefer to be unrestricted and active; they can become depressed and at risk for impulsively attempting suicide when placed in confinement. Inpatient psychiatric hospitalization can be used to assess and initiate treatment for comorbid psychiatric disorders. A homicidal or suicidal patient can be stabilized and then moved to a less restrictive long-term setting. However, the stay is usually too brief to effectively treat CD itself.

Medications used as the sole treatment for CD have not been demonstrated to be effective. Psychoactive medications are used for the treatment of concurrent psychiatric disorders and concurrent target symptoms (aggression, impulsiveness, mood instability). Some of these medications are lithium, antidepressants, carbamazepine, propranolol, stimulants, clonidine, and antipsychotics (usually haloperidol). The physician should be cautious when prescribing medication to a youth with CD. Medication can be "cheeked," sold or traded, hoarded, and taken all at once in an impulsive suicide attempt.

Eating and Feeding Disorders

Key Points

- When considering a diagnosis of feeding disorder, consultation with a physician familiar with growth problems in children may be necessary because of the extensive differential diagnosis.
- The long-term mortality rate for individuals with anorexia nervosa is 6% to 20%, the highest rate for any psychiatric disorder.
- The most useful measure to assess for extreme weight loss in adolescents is age-adjusted body mass index (BMI) less than the fifth percentile.
- For anorexia nervosa, vomiting is a poor prognostic feature, as is purgative use for bulimia nervosa.
- Patients with eating disorders should be managed by a multidisciplinary team that includes a primary physician, mental health professional, and nutritionist.

Good nutrition is vital to good health, so feeding problems and eating disorders have important consequences for multiple organ systems and child development. The most serious eating disorders, anorexia nervosa and bulimia nervosa, typically have their onset in adolescence, but a variety of eating problems are common in infants and children. These include several disorders that were classified under "disorders usually diagnosed in infancy, childhood, or adolescence" in the DSM-IV and have been reclassified to "feeding and eating disorders" in the DSM-5 in recognition that they can develop at any time in life.

FEEDING AND EATING DISORDERS OF INFANCY AND EARLY CHILDHOOD

Most feeding difficulties in infants and young children are minor and self-limited and can be addressed through education and reassurance of caregivers. However, physicians must be alert for specific feeding and eating disorders that can lead to malnutrition or chronic toxicity from ingested substances. "Avoidant/restrictive food intake disorder" (ARFID) is the new term used in DSM-5 that replaces former terms of "feeding disorder of infancy or early childhood," "psychosocial failure to thrive," and "psychosocial dwarfism." To warrant this diagnosis, the child must show evidence of inability to take adequate calories or nutrition through their diet beyond what can be explained by a concurrent medical condition or another mental disorder. Of children admitted to the hospital for failure to thrive, as many as half have a psychosocial etiology. Because the differential diagnosis for ARFID is complex, the nutritional consequences serious, and the social implications of potential abuse or neglect are challenging, early consultation with an experienced team is advised.

The other important consideration in young children is *pica*, the persistent eating of nonnutritive substances, such as hair, soil, paint, animal droppings, or sand. Pica can result in vitamin deficiencies, lead or other heavy metal intoxication, phytobezoars, and other complications. The prevalence of pica is not certain, but it is probably fairly common in preschool children, especially those with mental impairment. Pica can be differentiated from developmentally normal oral exploration when it occurs after approximately 24 months of age. Persistent or obsessive chewing (e.g., fingernails, clothing, straws) *without* ingestion should also be distinguished from pica. The important aspect to assessment of pica is to *ask*. Evaluation and treatment then depend on the specific substance ingested and symptoms the child exhibits, if any.

The most important aspect in assessing feeding difficulties in infants and children is tracking height and weight with each office visit. Children who are not maintaining expected gains should be observed more closely and evaluated for psychosocial causes in addition to medical conditions.

ANOREXIA NERVOSA AND BULIMIA NERVOSA

In adolescent girls, eating disorders are the third leading chronic illness, after obesity and asthma. The number of young people diagnosed with eating disorders (anorexia nervosa or bulimia nervosa) and eating disturbances (some but not all criteria for diagnosis of a "disorder") is increasing, the result of a combination of improved recognition and reporting as well as an apparent true increased incidence. About 95% of cases are girls or women, and the prevalence of eating disorders has been directly correlated to the rates of dieting behavior. High-risk groups include female athletes and patients with diabetes. Some patients with eating disorders find a social network online that encourages maladaptive eating behaviors. Parents and physicians should be wary of online activity related to "Ana" (anorexia) and "Mia" (bulimia) characters because these are often used to conceal discussions about dangerous eating behavior. Frequent posting of nude or nearly nude photos to these websites is also a common practice among patients who wish to compare visible evidence of weight loss.

The three essential features of anorexia nervosa are (1) persistent energy intake restriction, (2) intense fear of gaining weight or of being fat or persistent behavior that interferes with weight gain, and (3) disturbance in self-perceived weight or shape (APA, 2013). Amenorrhea, although common, is no longer required for the diagnosis in DSM-5. The long-term mortality rate for those with anorexia nervosa is 6% to 20%, the highest rate for any psychiatric disorder (Roerig et al., 2002), often as an acute suicidal act rather than slow bodily destruction alone (Pompili et al., 2006). Bulimia nervosa is characterized by binge eating and inappropriate compensation attempts to avoid weight gain, such as self-induced vomiting, misuse of laxatives or diuretics, fasting, or excessive exercise. The prevalence of bulimia nervosa is 1% to 1.5% in adolescent and young adult women, more common but less often fatal than anorexia nervosa (APA, 2013). The DSM-5 also recognizes "binge-eating disorder," typically in obese individuals who meet the binge eating criteria for bulimia but without the subsequent purging behaviors.

Assessment

A prime objective in assessment is to distinguish "normal dieters" from individuals with eating disorders. In addition to the characteristics outlined in Table 23-7, patients with eating disorders have a pathologic reaction to weight gain. To explore this possibility, a useful question to ask is, "What would it be like to find you weighed 1 lb more next week when you get on the scale?" This may provoke an overly emotional response in a person with an eating disorder (Selzer et al., 1995).

Another important aspect to evaluation is to exclude certain medical conditions in the differential diagnosis as the primary cause of the symptoms. This includes such diverse problems as inflammatory bowel disease, hyperthyroidism, chronic infections, diabetes mellitus, and Addison's disease. The erythrocyte sedimentation rate (ESR) and serum albumin tend to remain normal in patients with eating disorders, so an elevated ESR or a reduced albumin suggest an organic cause for weight loss (Selzer et al., 1995).

It is important to assess the acuteness and severity of malnutrition or fluid and electrolyte abnormalities. Indications for immediate referral include any patient with abnormal findings on physical examination or laboratory studies because these indicate severe and entrenched eating disorders. Laboratory studies should include a complete blood count, electrolytes, magnesium, calcium, phosphorus, urea nitrogen, creatinine, glucose, albumin, and electrocardiography (Walsh et al., 2000).

The diagnosis of anorexia nervosa no longer requires specific evidence of "extreme weight loss" but uses BMI percentile in children and adolescents to define severity from mild to extreme. For anorexia nervosa, the presence of vomiting is a poor prognostic feature, as is the use of purgatives for bulimia nervosa (Wilhelm and Clarke, 1998).

Management

Indications for inpatient management include "extremely low weight (≤75% of expected body weight) or rapid weight loss; severe electrolyte imbalances, cardiac disturbances, or other acute medical disorders; severe or intractable purging; psychosis or a high risk of suicide; and symptoms refractory to outpatient treatment" (Becker et al., 1999).

Patients with eating disorders should be managed by an experienced multidisciplinary team that includes a primary physician, mental health professional, and nutritionist. Family physicians should be aware of the resources available in their area and should be prepared to refer any adolescent suspected of an eating disorder or with abnormal eating behaviors who does not respond to initial efforts at diet education. A valuable resource for developing a treatment plan is a practice guideline published by the APA (Yager, 2006).

Various antidepressants are effective for treatment of bulimia nervosa but have not shown definite benefit for anorexia nervosa. Cognitive-behavioral therapy (CBT) has been shown to be the most effective psychological approach to bulimia nervosa (Berkman et al., 2006).

Table 23-7   Characteristics of Normal Dieting versus Eating Disorders

Feature	Normal Dieting	Eating Disorder
Communication with others	Dieters tell those around them that they are dieting, seeing it as "something to be proud of."	Dieters are reluctant to discuss their diets even when it is obvious to those around them that they are restricting their intake.
Intake regulation	They use internal cues and the rules of their diet plan.	They often use external cues, such as eating less than the person at the table who eats the least, to avoid feeling selfish or gluttonous.
Behavior	When weight loss goal is achieved, they want to show off their "new body," often in new and more revealing clothes or situations (e.g., new swimsuit, sunbathing).	They usually avoid exposing their bodies, often with baggy clothing, or regard their physical dimensions with disgust, no matter how much weight they lose.
Self-esteem	They exhibit a feeling of accomplishment and increased self-esteem when they achieve planned weight loss.	They tend to become self-critical, often depressed or irritable, and avoid social occasions.

- Primary prevention programs have greatly improved knowledge but with "small net effects on reducing maladaptive eating attitudes and behaviors." Studies targeted at high-risk groups produced greater benefits. "Concerns about iatrogenic effects of including psychoeducational material on eating disorders were not supported by the data" (Fingeret et al., 2006) (SOR: A).
- Anorexia nervosa (AN): "The literature regarding medication treatments for AN is sparse and inconclusive. ... Cognitive behavioral therapy may reduce relapse risk for adults with AN after weight restoration. Family therapy focusing on parental control of renutrition is efficacious in treating AN in adolescents" (Berkman et al., 2006) (SOR: B).
- Bulimia nervosa (BN): "Fluoxetine (60 mg/day) reduced core bulimia symptoms in the short term. ... The optimal duration of treatment is unknown. Cognitive behavioral therapy is effective in both short and long term" (Berkman et al., 2006) (SOR: A).

Mood Disorders

Key Points

- Physicians should attempt to define a timeline of discrete mood "episodes" to distinguish them from stable behavior patterns (e.g., ODD, ADHD).
- Careful identification of manic symptoms distinguishes among disorders.
- Suicidal ideation and impulsive attempts are not specific to any one mood disorder.

Mood dysregulation in children and adolescents has been a controversial diagnostic issue, and one that has been addressed with changes in the DSM-5. Children can present with a range of mood symptoms, including sadness, irritability, elation, anger, and temper tantrums, which can be short-lived and developmentally appropriate or can signal more enduring and maladaptive patterns of coping. Children with other behavior disorders (e.g., ADHD, ODD) are at greater risk for mood disturbance; therefore, comorbid conditions must be carefully considered. In general, when children experience mood dysregulation of any kind, a referral to a psychotherapist and consideration of psychoactive medications may be warranted.

ASSESSMENT

Assessment of patients with mood disorders should include a careful history of symptom onset, triggering stressors or events, symptom duration, and pattern or consistency of symptoms. Determining whether the child has episodic or persistent symptoms can help differentiate among disorders by elucidating which symptoms are a change from baseline functioning (e.g., episodic psychomotor agitation concurrent with a manic episode versus hyperactivity related to ADHD). Parent, child, and teacher questionnaires

(e.g., Conners, Third Edition; *Behavior Assessment System for Children*, Second Edition; Achenbach Child Behavior Checklist) can provide standardized evaluation of a range of diagnostic dimensions correlating with DSM categories. Free tools such as the Centers for Epidemiological Studies Depression Scale for Children (CES-DC), Young Mania Rating Scale (YMRS), and Disruptive Behavior Checklist can also be useful tracking instruments; however, results should only be interpreted in the context of symptoms reported by the patient, parent, and other sources of information such as teachers.

MAJOR DEPRESSIVE DISORDER

Major depressive disorder (MDD) remains a significant risk for children and adolescents, with an 11% lifetime prevalence between 13 and 18 years of age (National Institutes of Mental Health, 2013). Diagnostic criteria have remained relatively stable in the DSM-5, including duration (at least 2 weeks) and symptom requirement (five of nine: sad or depressed mood, diminished interest or pleasure in enjoyed activities, significant weight fluctuation, sleep disturbance, psychomotor agitation or retardation, fatigue or low energy, feelings of worthlessness or guilt, inability to concentrate or make decisions, and recurrent thoughts of death). Specifiers now available include anxious distress, mixed (e.g., hypomanic) features, psychotic features, and seasonal pattern. Diagnostic criteria have also removed the bereavement exclusion, recognizing that grief is a triggering event for many major depressive episodes, even in children.

Management

Nearly all adolescents (>90%) recover fully from an initial depressive episode, although more than half experience recurrent episodes (Melvin et al., 2013). Fluoxetine became the first FDA-approved drug for treating childhood depression in 2003, and by 2005, the FDA required a black box warning on antidepressant drugs for children. A possible safety risk of increased suicidal ideation was identified, suggesting a need for increased monitoring and more careful follow-up with assessment of suicidal ideation, thoughts about death, and intent for self-harm. Despite these risks, SSRIs remain a first line of treatment for childhood and adolescent depression. Meta-analysis suggests that TCAs are not effective in treating childhood and adolescent depression (Hazell and Mirzaie, 2013). Either in combination with medication or alone, psychotherapy is also an efficacious depression treatment with evidence-based therapies, including CBT and interpersonal therapy, holding the strongest support (Curry, 2001). The combination of CBT and fluoxetine was found to be superior to either treatment alone in the Treatment for Adolescents with Depression Study (TADS; March et al., 2004).

BIPOLAR DISORDER

Pediatric BD is a controversial diagnosis with current estimates suggesting a 3% prevalence for bipolar spectrum disorders in children younger than 18 years of age ((NIMH, 2013). Diagnostic criteria for adult BD are questionable for diagnosing children with the disorder. It is generally agreed that the presence of mania or a hypomanic episode be required for a diagnosis of pediatric BD. Proposed criteria for a "broad phenotype" (i.e., more lax diagnostic criteria) suggest that presence of four of eight DSM criteria be present, which *must* include (1) elation, (2) grandiosity, or (3) racing thoughts (Staton et al., 2008). Many clinicians do not require the episodic course criteria for diagnosis in pediatric populations because many children with a BD diagnosis are noted to "cycle" or switch moods several times within one day. The AACAP, however, recommends using the DSM criteria for purposes of clinical and research consistency, resulting in more stringent criteria for a "narrow phenotype" of the disorder. Given the frequent absence of episodic criteria (e.g., 4 days for a hypomanic episode and 7 days for a manic episode), children may meet the criteria for BD, not otherwise specified (Leibenluft and Rich, 2008).

Management

Medication with mood stabilizing agents such as lithium or anticonvulsants is often the first line of treatment of pediatric BD, although few RCTs exist to demonstrate efficacy (Leibenluft and Rich, 2008). Lithium has demonstrated effective suicide prevention in adult meta-analyses, although its effect in children and adolescents has not been well researched (Cipriani et al., 2013). Psychotherapeutic interventions should aim to (1) provide education about the disorder to children and families, (2) manage symptoms, (3) improve coping skills, (4) address social and family relationships, (5) improve academic and vocational functioning, and (6) address relapse prevention (AACAP, 2007; McClellan et al., 2007).

DISRUPTIVE MOOD DYSREGULATION DISORDER

Disruptive mood dysregulation disorder (DMDD) is a new disorder introduced in the DSM-5 consisting of a pattern of chronic, severe, persistent irritability with superimposed temper outbursts that are not developmentally appropriate. DMDD was conceptualized as an alternative explanation for behaviors that were often classified (or misclassified) as pediatric BD, with research instead suggesting that DMDD is more closely aligned with a unipolar mood disorder in adulthood (Copeland et al., 2013). These children exhibit temper tantrums three or more times per week for a period of at least 1 year. They must be at least 6 years old at the time of diagnosis and not older than 10 years at time of symptom onset. An initial community study examining the feasibility of DMDD diagnostic criteria suggested an overall prevalence between 1% and 3%; however, there was a high degree of symptom overlap with other psychiatric diagnoses, most notably ODD and depressive disorders (Copeland et al., 2013). Yet, current diagnostic criteria suggest that DMDD may not be diagnosed in the presence of ODD or BD. As a result of high rates of overlap in both community and clinical samples, the utility of the diagnosis as a separate entity has been called into question (Axelson et al., 2012).

Management

Given the status of DMDD as a new diagnosis, treatment studies are almost completely absent from the literature. Anecdotal evidence suggests symptom management as a primary target, combining treatment approaches for similar disorders such as ODD, ADHD, depression, and BD. Parent training and behavior management can target many of the aggressive, explosive, and defiant behaviors accompanying DMDD. Patients with underlying depressive or irritable symptoms can be treated with antidepressant medications and psychotherapy. At the present time, the primary treatment approach appears to be mood stabilization with atypical antipsychotics or anticonvulsants in combination with improvement of impulsivity with stimulants or α-agonists. Controlled treatment trials will be forthcoming as clinicians and research centers begin using the diagnosis more frequently.

Summary of Additional Online Content

The following content is available at www.expertconsult.com:

eAppendix 23-1 Encopresis and Enuresis

References

The complete reference list is available at www.expertconsult.com.

Web Resources

www.dshs.state.tx.us/mhprograms/adhdpage.shtm Texas Children's Medication Algorithm Project. The most recent algorithms are from May 2006.

Sleep Disorders

www.aasmnet.org Sponsored by the American Academy of Sleep Medicine, a professional society, with public access to patient information and referral centers.

www.nlm.nih.gov/medlineplus/sleepdisorders.html National Institutes of Health–sponsored patient-oriented site with extensive background information and links to recent research and ongoing clinical trials.

www.sleepfoundation.org Sponsored by the National Sleep Foundation, an advocacy group. This is a patient-oriented site with direct answers to frequently asked questions.

Autism

www.autism-society.org Sponsored by the Autism Society of America, a national advocacy group, with good general information and networking opportunities.

www.autismspeaks.org Advocacy and funding agency supporting research and dissemination of information, as well as support networks for families.

www.ninds.nih.gov/disorders/autism/detail_autism.htm National Institutes of Health–sponsored patient-oriented site with extensive background information and links to other valuable sites.

Encopresis and Enuresis

familydoctor.org/familydoctor/en/kids/toileting/enuresis-bed-wetting.html Sponsored by the American Academy of Family Physicians, with general patient recommendations; less commercialized than many other sites.

www.lpch.org/diseaseHealthInfo/healthLibrary/growth/encopres.html Sponsored by the Lucile Packard Children's Hospital at Stanford, answers patients' frequently asked questions, including diet and activity recommendations.

Attention-Deficit Hyperactivity Disorder

www.add.org Resources from the ADD Association, a national ADHD adult support group.

www.chadd.org Resources from the national support group for children and adults with ADHD.

www.nichq.org/adhd_tools.html#adhd_parent Resources for clinicians and parents on ADHD from the National Initiative for Children's Healthcare Quality, including a number of assessment forms.

www.nimh.nih.gov/health/topics/attention-deficit-hyperactivity-disorder-adhd/index.shtml Information on ADHD from the National Institutes of Mental Health, including a link to current ADHD clinical trials.

Oppositional Defiant and Conduct Disorders

jamesdauntchandler.tripod.com/ODD_CD/oddcdpamphlet.htm Detailed assessment and treatment information on ODD and CD from a physician; includes case examples.

www.aacap.org/cs/ODD.ResourceCenter Resource Center on ODD by the American Academy of Child and Adolescent Psychiatry.

Eating Disorders

www.anad.org Sponsored by the National Association of Anorexia Nervosa and Associated Eating Disorders, an advocacy group with general information and networking opportunities.

www.nationaleatingdisorders.org Sponsored by the National Eating Disorders Association, an advocacy group, with general information and networking opportunities.

Book Resources

Attention-Deficit Hyperactivity Disorder

Taking Charge of ADHD by Russell A. Barkley. Book recommending environmental changes to structure the schedule and behavior of children with ADHD.

Smart but Scattered by Peg Dawson and Richard Guare. Book recommending routines and study skills to maximize functioning in children with ADHD.

Oppositional Defiant and Conduct Disorders

Barkley RA, Benton CM: *Your Defiant Child: Eight Steps to Better Behavior,* 2nd ed, The Guilford Press, 2014, New York.

Barkley RA, Robin A, Benton CM: *Your Defiant Teen: Ten Steps to Resolve Conflict and Rebuild Your Relationship,* .2nd ed, The Guilford Press, 2014, New York.

24 Child Abuse

ROBERT SHAPIRO, KAREN FARST, and CAROL L. CHERVENAK

Our brains are sculpted by our early experiences. Maltreatment is a chisel that shapes a brain to contend with strife, but at the cost of deep, enduring wounds.

TEICHER, 2000.

A 6-month-old male infant is seen in his physician's office for decreased appetite and irritability. The physician notes that the infant's upper lip is swollen on the left and that there is a small bruise of the right temple. The physician accepts the offered explanation from the mother, that the infant had "slipped in the bathtub" the previous evening. One week later, the infant is dead from abusive head trauma (AHT). The father of the child admitted that he shook the baby and hit his face and head, resulting in his death.

"Child maltreatment is a deceptive and easily disguised entity" (Jenny et al., 1999), the diagnosis of which is very challenging. Many of these children are seen by health care providers in the weeks leading up to their deaths; often the injuries they present with are diagnosed as "accidental" (King et al., 2006). The early recognition of child abuse is critical to preventing further injury or death of a child. The risk of recurrence of abuse is approximately 50% (Alexander et al., 1990; McDonald, 2007), neglect being the type of maltreatment associated with the highest risk for future abuse (Hindley et al., 2006).

Child abuse and neglect are major causes of morbidity and mortality in the United States (U.S. Department of Health and Human Services [HHS], 2012).

- In 2011, the national estimate of child abuse and neglect victims determined by child protective services (CPS) was 681,000 (9.1 victims per 1000 children).
- A total of 79% were victims of neglect, 18% of physical abuse, and 9% of sexual abuse.
- More than 1500 children died from abuse and neglect in 2011.
- A total of 82% of all the fatalities were in children younger than 4 years old, and the majority (78%) were caused by one or more parents.
- Child abuse is the leading cause of injury-related deaths among infants and the second leading cause of injury deaths in older children (Jenny and Isaac, 2006).

- The total lifetime economic burden of child maltreatment in the United States is approximately $124 billion (Fang et al., 2012).

As the family's health care provider, family medicine physicians are in an ideal position to detect, assess, diagnose, and intervene for children experiencing child abuse and neglect. When suspicions of child maltreatment arise, many physicians are uncomfortable confronting or blaming parents and possibly disrupting the family unit. Understanding the devastating effects of child maltreatment, becoming familiar with evidence-based indicators of abuse and neglect, and adopting strategies for assessment and management can help the physician have a positive, meaningful impact on the lives of children and families.

Physicians are required by law to report suspected or confirmed child abuse and neglect to CPS or law enforcement or both. Table 24-1 defines the different types of child abuse.

Implications and Long-Term Outcomes

The long-term impact of traumatic childhood stressors on health risk behaviors, disability, disease, and premature mortality has been extensively studied (Felitti et al., 1998). The Adverse Childhood Experiences (ACE) Study assessed more than 17,000 adult members of an HMO and collected histories of various forms of child maltreatment, exposure to domestic violence, parental substance abuse and mental illness, and parental loss. (A complete bibliography of ACE Study publications listed by topic area is available at http://www.cdc.gov/ace.) "Adverse childhood experiences" are common, highly interrelated, and strongly associated with multiple enduring health and social problems impacting adolescents and adults (Anda et al., 2006; Larkin et al., 2012), including ischemic heart disease, cancer, chronic lung disease, liver disease, multiple mental health diagnoses, and premature death.

Experiences during infancy and early childhood affect brain development and create the basis for the expression of intelligence, emotions, and personality (Butchart et al., 2006). Children who have suffered chronic abuse and neglect during the first few years may experience

Table 24-1 Definitions of Child Maltreatment

	Definition	Comments
Child maltreatment (Leeb et al., 2008)	Any act of commission or omission by a parent or other caregiver that results in harm, potential for harm, or threat of harm to a child; harm does not need to be intended	More than 80% of perpetrators were parents (Child Welfare Information Gateway, 2013)
Physical abuse	The intentional use of physical force against a child that results in or has the potential to result in physical injury Includes acts that do not leave a physical mark as well as those causing permanent disability, disfigurement, or death (Barnett et al., 1993)	Physical acts can include hitting, kicking, punching, beating, stabbing, biting, pushing, shoving, throwing, pulling, dragging, dropping, shaking, strangling or choking, smothering, burning, scalding, and poisoning
Sexual abuse	Any completed or attempted sexual act, sexual contact with, or exploitation (i.e., noncontact sexual interaction) of a child by a caregiver	Includes substitute caregivers (e.g. teachers, coaches, clergy, and relatives) **Sexual acts:** involve penetration, no matter how slight, between the mouth, penis, vulva, or anus of the child and another individual; also penetration of anal or genital opening by a hand, finger, or other object **Sexual contact:** includes intentional touching, either directly or through clothing, of the genitalia, anus, breast, or buttocks (excluding contact required for normal care) **Noncontact sexual abuse:** exposure to sexual activity, filming, or commercial sexual exploitation
Psychological (or emotional) abuse	Intentional behavior that conveys to a child that he or she is worthless, flawed, unloved, unwanted, endangered, or valued only in meeting another's needs (APSAC, 1995)	Continual or episodic (e.g., associated with caregiver substance abuse) May include blaming, belittling, degrading, intimidating, terrorizing, isolating, restraining, confining, corrupting, exploiting, spurning, or otherwise behaving in a manner that is harmful, potentially harmful, or insensitive to the child's developmental needs or that can potentially damage the child psychologically or emotionally
Neglect	Failure to meet a child's basic physical, emotional, medical or dental, or educational needs; failure to provide adequate nutrition, hygiene, or shelter; or failure to ensure a child's safety	Includes failure to provide adequate food, clothing, or accommodation; not seeking medical attention when needed; allowing a child to miss large amounts of school; and failure to protect a child from violence in the home or neighborhood or from avoidable hazards

APSAC, American Professional Society on the Abuse of Children.
Adapted from Gilbert R, Widom CS, Browne K, et al. Burden and consequences of child maltreatment in high-income countries. *Lancet.* 2009;373:68-81.

hyperarousal or dissociation, difficulty with attachment, limited capacity for empathy, and various mental health problems, including depression, posttraumatic stress disorder (PTSD), attention-deficit hyperactivity disorder, and sensory integration disorder (National Clearinghouse on Child Abuse and Neglect Information, 2001).

Neglect

> ## Key Points
>
> - Neglect is the most common form of child maltreatment.
> - Child neglect has been associated with worse outcomes and the highest risk for future abuse compared with other forms of child maltreatment.
> - There is a strong association of substance abuse with child maltreatment.
> - Child maltreatment commonly occurs in homes with domestic violence.

Child neglect is common, complex, and insidious. Although difficult to clearly define and identify, neglect is the most common form of child maltreatment, accounting for 78%

of substantiated cases in 2011. Neglect has been associated with worse outcomes than other forms of child abuse over a range of cognitive, developmental, psychosocial, and physical parameters (American Professional Society on the Abuse of Children, 2008; Perez and Widom, 1994; Teicher, 2000).

Child neglect is often defined by child welfare agencies and in state law as an act of omission by a parent or caretaker, specifically the failure to provide for a child's basic physical, emotional, or educational needs or to protect a child from harm or potential harm (Table 24-2). Neglect includes isolated incidents as well as a pattern of failure over time by a parent or caretaker (Butchart et al., 2006).

A broader *child-centered* view of child neglect, however, describes neglect as occurring when a child's basic needs are not met; recognizing that multiple factors contribute, including individuals, families, communities, and society; and focusing interventions on multiple levels (DePanfilis, 2006; Dubowitz, 2009) (Table 24-3).

The approach toward neglect management is varied and depends on the identified causes of the neglect as well as an assessment of urgency. The goal of management is to assist the family in providing a safe and healthy environment for their children. A review of these management principles and steps can be found in the article by Dubowitz (2013).

Table 24-2 Types of Neglect

Types of Neglect	Definition	Comments
Failure to Provide		
Physical neglect	Caregiver fails to provide adequate nutrition, hygiene, or shelter; fails to provide clothing that is adequately clean, of appropriate size, or adequate for the weather; includes abandonment or expulsion from the home	Inadequate food may present as failure to thrive or repeated hunger Inappropriate food or poor nutrition may present as obesity Other examples: Child may be dirty or smell bad; living arrangements unstable for 2 weeks or more; home may be infested with insects or vermin; animal feces on floor and bedding; unsafe, dirty sleep environment
Emotional neglect	Caregiver ignores the child or denies emotional responsiveness or adequate access to mental health care	Includes constantly belittling the child, withholding affection; exposing the child to domestic violence; allowing the child to use drugs or alcohol
Medical or dental neglect	Failure to provide appropriate health care for a child (although financially able to do so), thus placing the child at risk of being seriously disabled or disfigured or dying	Includes nonadherence with health care recommendations; delay or failure in getting health care Religious beliefs: the AAP strongly opposes these exemptions for medical care
Educational neglect	Failure to provide access to adequate education	Includes chronic truancy; failure to enroll a child in school, to provide adequate home schooling, or to attend to special education needs
Failure to Supervise		
Inadequate supervision	Failure to ensure that the child engages in safe activities and uses appropriate safety devices; to ensure that the child is not exposed to unnecessary hazards; or to ensure appropriate supervision by an adequate substitute caregiver	Includes lack of supervision appropriate for developmental needs (e.g., infant left unattended in bathtub; toddler left home alone) Inappropriate caregiver: knowingly leaving child in the care of a sexual offender Abandonment is an extreme form
Exposure to a violent environment	Caregiver fails to take available measures to protect the child from pervasive violence within the home, neighborhood, or community	Exposure of child to criminal activities (e.g., illicit drug trade, allowing bullying of child without intervention). Exposure to domestic violence is associated with psychological harm, increased risk of abuse, and neglect.
Inadequate protection from environmental hazards	Avoidable exposure to environmental hazards in and out of the home	Examples include toxic substances in reach of children; smoking in the presence of children with asthma; and access to loaded firearms
Drug-exposed newborns and older children	In utero exposure to substance abuse; direct and indirect (e.g., ingestion, passive inhalation) exposure of older children	Includes exposure of children to illicit manufacturing of drugs, drug trafficking, parental alcohol and substance abuse, and prescription narcotic abuse or misuse

AAP, American Academy of Pediatrics.
Adapted from Leeb RT, Paulozzi L, Melanson C, et al. *Child maltreatment surveillance. Uniform definitions for public health and recommended data elements.* Version 1.0. Atlanta: Centers for Disease Control & Prevention; 2008.

DRUG-EXPOSED NEWBORNS AND OLDER CHILDREN

A strong association of substance abuse with child maltreatment has been well documented (Wells, 2009). Children in homes with adults who abused drugs and alcohol were found to have a nearly threefold increased risk for child abuse and fourfold risk for neglect (U.S. Department of HHS, 1998).

Prenatal substance exposure increases the vulnerability of the infant to poor caretaking, partly because of the cognitive and behavioral effects on the newborn (Zuckerman and Bresnahan, 1991). Additionally, studies have shown that children exposed prenatally to illicit substances have two to three times increased risk for abuse and neglect compared with children in the same socioeconomic class and neighborhood (Jaudes et al., 1995).

Drug-endangered children have a markedly increased exposure to interpersonal violence, traumatic events, child maltreatment, toxic chemicals in their immediate environment, and significantly higher rates of PTSD compared with other children (Sprang et al., 2008). Passive inhalation, accidental ingestion, and exposure of drugs and alcohol through breast milk or intentional administration are all risk factors for children in homes with substance abuse.

DOMESTIC VIOLENCE AND CHILDREN

Assaultive, aggressive, coercive, or threatening behavior within the home between intimate partners victimizes not only the adult target of the violence but the child witnesses as well, whether the violence is seen or overheard. Co-occurrence rates of domestic violence and child maltreatment have been found to be between 30% and 60% (Appel and Holden, 1998; Edleson, 1999). A study of at-risk parents with firstborn children revealed that domestic violence during the first 6 months of child rearing more than tripled the likelihood of physical abuse and more than doubled the likelihood of psychological abuse and neglect occurring during the child's first 5 years of life (McGuigan and Pratt, 2001). Children exposed to domestic violence are at risk for difficulties with behavioral, emotional, and cognitive functioning, as well as dysfunctional attitudes about violence and conflict resolution (Edleson, 1999).

Table 24-3   Risk Factors for Child Maltreatment

Individual factors	Child Characteristics	Caregiver or Parent Characteristics
	Low birth weight Prematurity Chronic disability or illness Genetic abnormalities Personality or temperament perceived by parents as difficult (e.g., infant cries persistently, not easily soothed; child hyperactive, impulsive, aggressive) Child with symptoms of mental ill health	Substance abuse Mental health problems, especially depression Cognitive delay Impulsive, poor judgment Lack of nurturing or empathy toward child Involved in criminal activity Unrealistic expectations of child Poor parenting skills
Family characteristics and relationship factors	Parent–child relationship adversarial or lacks attachment Domestic violence Social isolation Criminal involvement Chaotic lifestyle (e.g., frequent moves, unstable housing) High levels of stress (e.g., poverty, unemployment)	
Community factors	Tolerance of violence Inadequate housing Poverty Few resources or support services Poor access to health care Easy availability to alcohol; illicit drug trade	
Societal factors	Poverty Limited access to health care Poor access to mental health care for adults or children Inadequate educational system Social and cultural norms that promote violence; support rigid gender roles; diminish the status of the child Conditions that enable commercial sexual exploitation of children	

Adapted from American Professional Society on the Abuse of Children. *Psychosocial evaluation of suspected psychological maltreatment in children and adolescents. Practice guidelines*. Chicago: American Professional Society on the Abuse of Children; 1995 and Ondersma SJ. Predictors of neglect within low-SES families: the importance of substance abuse. *Am J Orthopsychiatry*. 2002;72(3)383-391.

Physical Abuse

Key Points

- Children from all socioeconomic groups may become victims of physical child abuse.
- Child abuse should be considered in all preambulatory children with injuries.
- Dating of bruises is often an inexact practice in the absence of history.
- A skeletal survey can provide key information regarding the likelihood of child abuse in children younger than the age of 3 years.

Recognizing physical abuse can be lifesaving and will prevent further trauma to the child. Recognizing children at risk before abuse has occurred offers an opportunity to prevent child abuse through early intervention. The family physician can support parents by helping them become more effective at parenting, advocating for their basic living needs such as food and shelter, and encouraging quality childcare.

PRESENTATIONS OF PHYSICAL ABUSE

Bruises

The most common presentation of child physical abuse is bruising. Although accidental bruising is common in ambulatory children, it is rare in the nonambulatory infant and when found should trigger an evaluation for nonaccidental injury. Bruising in the ambulatory child is suspicious for abuse if the history does not explain the location, number, or pattern of bruising; if the history is developmentally inconsistent with the child's abilities; or if the bruising patterns or locations indicate that abusive trauma is likely. Bruising found over the trunk, abdomen, cheeks, ears, and buttocks are all concerning for abusive injury, although this list is not exclusive. Patterns of injury caused by belts, cords, hands, and paddles must be recognized. Dating of bruises is very inaccurate because of the tremendous variability in healing, from 1 day to many weeks. Bruises that are raised, tender, and abraded are likely recent, but color change within the bruise is an inaccurate method of dating. Bites are a common abusive injury in children, and recognition requires a high index of suspicion. Look for impressions of individual teeth and upper and lower arch-shaped trauma. The most common bruise mimics include coagulopathies (e.g., von Willebrand disease, vitamin K deficiency, leukemia, and hemophilia); Mongolian spots; traditional therapies such as cupping, coining, and moxibustion; Henoch-Schönlein purpura; idiopathic thrombocytopenic purpura; and accidental bruising.

Fractures

Fractures are a strong indicator of current or past child abuse. Abusive fractures are most often identified through the skeletal survey or those with fractures for which there is no satisfactory explanation. Similar to bruises, fractures in nonambulatory children are always concerning for abuse. Multiple occult fractures, fractures demonstrating different ages of healing, rib fractures, classic metaphyseal lesions (CMLs or corner fractures), and vertebral compression fractures are most often associated with child abuse. Abusive fractures can involve any bone. The clinical signs of fracture may be absent when abuse has occurred because of a delay or absence in seeking care. In addition, the history of trauma may be withheld and a history of pain or disability not disclosed. Rarely is there bruising over the site of fracture after accidental or abusive injury. It is possible to determine if a fracture is recent or healing based on the clinical presentation and radiographic appearance, but exact dating is difficult. Signs of radiographic callous are expected to first appear at about 10 days after the fracture, although the appearance may be a few days earlier in very young infants. Lack of immobilization after fracture may result in an exaggerated callus response. Skull and vertebral fractures heal without callus formation. Remodeling may take up to 2 years to complete. The most common fracture mimics include accidental fracture, bone fragility, osteopenia, birth trauma, Menkes syndrome, neoplasms, infection, rickets, and normal radiographic variants.

Burns

Hot water burns are most often diagnosed in abusive burns, but cigarette burns, burns from irons, and lighters are also frequently seen. Hot water scalding is often associated with toileting accidents and punishment. The pattern of scald burns, coupled with a detailed history of the incident from which the burn occurred, is usually required to differentiate abusive from accidental burns. The depth of burn depends on the temperature of the water or object, the length of contact time, and the degree of skin thickness. Young children sustain deeper burns than adults; areas of thick skin such as the palms and soles may demonstrate more superficial burning. As the burn evolves over a few days, the burn pattern and depth may change, which should be considered when differentiating accidental from inflicted burns. The most common burn mimics include diaper rash, accidental burn, impetigo, and varicella.

Abusive Head Trauma

Abusive head trauma can result in serious mortality and morbidity. Terminology for AHT includes shaken baby syndrome, shaken impact syndrome, inflicted head injury, and nonaccidental head injury. Severe shaking is often involved in AHT, but even when there is no sign of contact injury to the scalp or skull, impact cannot be excluded. Victims of AHT are most often younger than 1 year old, and a history of crying is often identified as an important reason for the escalation to shaking. AHT can occur in any socioeconomic group, although it is seen more often when the social risks factors for abuse are present (see earlier discussion). The most common anatomic injury is subdural hemorrhage (SDH), although skull fractures, subarachnoid hemorrhage, and intraparenchymal injuries are also seen. The most common locations for SDH are frontoparietal and interhemispheric. Dating of SDH is difficult and should only be estimated. A mixed-density subdural density does not necessarily indicate two separate injuries because acute bleeding frequency causes this radiographic picture. Surgical intervention is not commonly required. In addition to other physical indications of child abuse, retinal hemorrhages are seen in about 85% of AHT cases. Retinal hemorrhages are also caused by birth trauma, hypertension,

vasculitis, and increased intracranial pressure. Symptoms of AHT include altered mental status, difficulty breathing or apnea, seizures, vomiting, and irritability. The clinical presentation is varied and includes mild vomiting or irritability on one end of the spectrum to cardiac arrest on the other. A history to explain the child's abusive intracranial injury is typically absent or minor, such as a fall from a couch or bed. Some reports include "rescue trauma" in which the child is shaken in response to choking or a seizure. The most common perpetrators of AHT are the child's father or the mother's boyfriend. Outcomes are typically poor and include death, significant developmental delay, seizures, or vision and hearing impairment. Some children, however, have a relatively good outcome after AHT. The most common head injury mimics include accidental injury, birth trauma, vascular malformations, and glutaric aciduria type I.

DIAGNOSIS AND EVALUATION OF SUSPECTED CHILD PHYSICAL ABUSE

A careful history and physical examination direct the assessment and often determine whether child physical abuse should be considered. When abuse is suspected, a *skeletal survey* should be obtained in all children younger than 2 years old (Duffy et al., 2011). Recent studies suggest that the age for skeletal survey should be extended to age 3 years. The skeletal survey includes 19 images of the entire skeleton (Table 24-4). A "babygram" is not sufficient for evaluation (Figure 24-1). After the evaluation is completed, if abuse is confirmed or still suspected, a follow-up skeletal survey should be obtained in 2 weeks (Harper et al., 2013). The follow-up survey often identifies fractures not recognized on the initial survey or clarifies questionable findings. Children younger than 6 months of age should have intracranial imaging even when neurologic symptoms are absent. A *head computed tomography (CT) scan* is typically most readily available, but in the asymptomatic child, brain magnetic resonance imaging is an acceptable alternative. In children for whom a diagnosis of AHT is being considered, a *dilated retinal examination* should be completed using indirect ophthalmoscopy. Retinal photography should be obtained whenever possible to document findings. The location, depth, and number of any retinal hemorrhages should be recorded. *Photographs* of any cutaneous findings should be obtained along with documentation showing the locations and measurement of injuries. When bruising or

Table 24-4   Complete Skeletal Survey

Appendicular Skeleton Views	Axial Skeleton Views
Humeri (AP)	Thorax (AP, lateral, right and left oblique to include ribs, thoracic, and upper lumbar spine)
Forearms (AP)	Pelvis
Hands (PA)	Lumbosacral spine (lateral)
Femurs (AP)	Cervical spine (lateral)
Lower legs (AP)	Skull (frontal and lateral)
Feet (AP)	

Adapted from the American College of Radiology. *Society of Pediatric Radiology practice guideline for skeletal surveys in children.* 2011, available at http://www.acr.org/~/media/9bdcdbee99b84e87baac2b1695bc07b6.pdf.

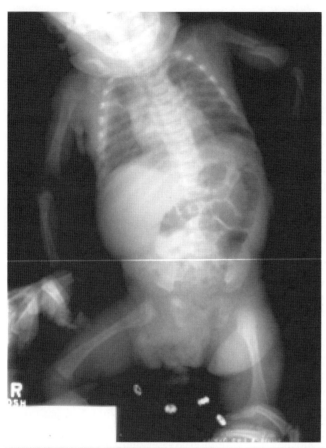

Figure 24-1 Babygram. This should never be obtained to substitute for a full skeletal survey (see Table 24-4).

bleeding is present, serum should be obtained to *rule out a coagulopathy*. In addition, abdominal trauma is often occult in children, and an *abdominal CT* should be obtained whenever abdominal bruising is present or *liver function test* results are elevated (Lindberg et al., 2013). When bites are present, *swabs for DNA analysis* should be collected from the center of the bite mark. Siblings and household contacts of abused children should be evaluated for abuse (Lindberg et al., 2012).

Sexual Abuse

Key Points

- The majority of children and adolescents who have been sexually abused have no findings of physical trauma on examination.
- The medical evaluation for suspected child sexual abuse (CSA) should occur urgently if there was sexual contact in the past 72 to 96 hours that might have left biologic material such as semen or blood or the child is having symptoms of injury or infection.
- In most cases, the person responsible for sexually abusing a child is known to the child and family. Delays in disclosure of CSA are common because of manipulation, coercion, deception, and threats by the abuser.

The prevalence of CSA in the United States may be as high as 7.5% in boys and 25% in girls (Pereda et al., 2009). The term *child sexual abuse* is often used to describe acts in which a child is used for sexual stimulation by an adolescent or adult and includes exposure to pornography, sexual fondling, or penetration. *Sexual assault* is a term usually reserved for acute cases in which the offender is not a caretaker of the victim. *Rape* refers to either an acute or past act(s) in which there was oral, vaginal, or anal penetration (whether the victim is a child, adolescent, or adult).

There are several important differences between CSA and adolescent or adult sexual assault, but overlap does occur. Knowledge of these differences is helpful to understanding why the disclosure of CSA is often delayed and why there are typically no physical examination findings in cases of CSA. CSA typically involves a period of "grooming" when the offender builds trust with the child by spending time with the child, providing gifts, and making the child feel special. This grooming then progresses to sexual contact. Because the child trusts the perpetrator, the sexual contact may be permitted without any physical or emotional violence. However, as the sexual advances continue, coercion, manipulation, and threats of harm to the child or the child's family may occur (U.S. Department of HHS, 2006). Disclosure of the abuse by the child victim is frequently delayed because of intimidation or guilt. Furthermore, when children do finally disclose it, their disclosure is frequently not believed. This is particularly true when a child is abused by a relative or other adult with a respected community position. Children who are abused by a relative, compared with children abused by strangers or acquaintances, are more likely to blame themselves for the abuse (Ullman, 2007) and may have more significant psychological distress. Almost one third of CSA victims reach adulthood without disclosing it, and almost half delay their disclosure for more than 5 years (Smith et al., 2000).

CLINICAL EVALUATION OF SEXUAL ABUSE

History

Best practice in the evaluation of alleged or suspected CSA involves a multidisciplinary (MDT) response that includes the local child protection agency, law enforcement, and medical team operating collaboratively. This team approach minimizes the child's psychological trauma from the time of disclosure through prosecution and therapy. Children's Advocacy Centers (CACs) are community-based MDT entities that work to promote a coordinated, trauma-focused approach to child abuse (National Children's Alliance, 2014). CAC protocols minimize the number of times a child will be interviewed about his or her abuse, use forensic interview techniques to increase the validation of a child's disclosure, and may video record the interview for future investigative uses. The CAC MDT model has been shown to result in more effective investigations, increased satisfaction by the caregiver and child, and higher referral rates for victim medical and mental health services (Farst, 2013).

The specific history regarding CSA includes the type of contact (what body parts contacted by what object or body part); under or over clothing; history of ejaculation, licking, or kissing; where the abuse occurred; the time since last contact; the identity of the alleged perpetrator(s); and the relationship to the victim. In older children, the last menstrual period and any history of consensual intercourse should be asked. The history should include an assessment for changes such as diet, sleeping, school performance, bowel or bladder symptoms, and behavioral changes. Although physical injury is uncommon in evaluations for sexual abuse, behavioral changes are common after the trauma of CSA. The child should be asked open-ended, nonleading questions during the interview, such as: "Tell me how that felt to you" rather than "Did it hurt?" Documentation of the interview should be precise. In CACs, the interview is often audio or video recorded. If recording is not possible, the documentation should include the exact questions asked as well as the child's responses.

Examination

The medical examination should occur emergently if there was sexual contact in the past 72 to 96 hours that might have left semen, saliva, blood, or other biologic material on the child or child's clothing. In this situation, the examination must include collection of forensic evidence specimens while maintaining the chain of custody, and most typically is completed in the emergency department or a facility equipped for this procedure. Other factors that dictate the need for an emergent or urgent evaluation include symptomatology or assessment of child safety (Table 24-5). Most disclosures present beyond this 72- to 96-hour time frame

Table 24-5 Timing of the Medical Evaluation for Suspected Child Sexual Abuse

Emergent (without delay)	The alleged assault may have occurred within the previous 72-96 hr (or other state-mandated time interval), and the transfer of trace evidence may have occurred, which will be collected for later forensic analysis (i.e., a sexual assault evidence kit should be collected because of suspected transfer of semen, blood, saliva or other DNA material).
	The need for emergency contraception (morning-after pill)
	The need for postexposure prophylaxis for STIs, including HIV (antibiotic or antiviral therapy)
	The child complains of pain in the genital or anal area.
	There is evidence or complaint of anogenital bleeding or injury.
	The child is experiencing significant behavioral or emotional problems and needs evaluation for possible suicidal ideation or plan.
Urgent (scheduled within 1-2 days)	None of the emergent criteria are met, but there was suspected or reported sexual contact occurring within the previous 2 weeks.
Non-urgent (scheduled)	None of the emergent or urgent criteria are met, but the child has disclosed abuse or sexual abuse is suspected by MDT or there is a family concern for abuse.

MDT, Multidisciplinary; *STI,* sexually transmitted infection.
Floyed RL, Hirsch DA, Greenbaum VJ, et al. Development of a screening tool for pediatric sexual assault may reduce emergency-department visits. *Pediatrics.* 2011;128:221-226 and Christian CW. Timing of the medical examination. *J Child Sex Abus.* 2011;20:505-520.

and should be scheduled with an experienced provider in a timely manner after safety issues are addressed.

The physical examination for CSA, in addition to an overall assessment of the child, includes the collection and documentation of forensically significant findings. An examiner must be knowledgeable in anogenital anatomy, examination techniques, interpretation of examination findings, and the diagnosis of sexually transmitted infections (STIs). Although primary care providers may not have the time, expertise, or equipment available to perform an in-depth assessment, they should know what local recourses are available to them for referral. The examination is well tolerated by most children when performed by an experienced clinician (Marks et al., 2009; Palusci and Cyrus, 2001). The two factors that have been shown to positively correlate with accuracy in interpreting examination findings are experience within the field of CSA and participation in expert peer review of examination findings (Adams et al., 2012). Studies have demonstrated that inexperienced clinicians are unable to identify normal female genital structures and misinterpret examination findings as indicative of abuse (Hornor and McCleery, 2000; Ladson et al., 1987; Makoroff et al., 2002).

The adolescent female anogenital examination is performed in the customary fashion using stirrups and, if indicated, a speculum. The prepubertal female genitourinary examination is always limited to an external-only examination. The most typical prepubertal examination position is supine with the soles of the feet approximated and thighs abducted. The genital area is visualized by placing gloved fingertips on the labia majora and inguinal area and gently separating the labia majora ("supine separation"). If the hymen orifice is not well visualized by this maneuver, then the labia majora are grasped by the examiner's thumb and forefingers, and traction is applied out toward the examiner and downward toward the medial thighs ("labial traction"). If further techniques are needed to better visualize the inferior hymen, the knee–chest position can be used (Berkoff et al., 2008). A cotton-tipped swab can be used to assist with visualization of an estrogenized hymen (postpubertal), but not before puberty because touching an unestrogenized hymen is very painful. A speculum may be needed to identify a source of vaginal bleeding or to assess for a vaginal foreign body in a prepubertal girl, but only when used with sedation. The anogenital examination should be photodocumented with magnified digital still or video capture for the purposes of peer or forensic review (Figure 24-2).

EXAMINATION FINDINGS OF SEXUAL ABUSE

Fewer than 10% of CSA victims have physical findings present on examination that can be attributed to acute or healed trauma (Anderst et al., 2009; Berkoff et al., 2008; Heger et al., 2002; Kellogg et al., 2004). Examples of specific findings diagnostic of healed genital trauma in girls include transections and missing segments of hymen in the posterior rim (inferior to the 3 to 9 o'clock locations). Many nonspecific findings (seen in studies of both abused and nonabused children) such as variations in hymen configuration, "gaping" of the hymen orifice, and reflexive anal dilation are not indications of sexual abuse but if misinterpreted as such are misleading and potentially harmful to

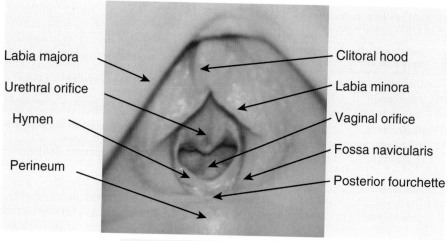

Figure 24-2 Female genitourinary anatomy.

Table 24-6 Classification of Anogenital Findings ("Adams Classification")

Normal variants and conditions mistaken for abuse	Congenital variations in hymen configurations (annular, crescent, redundant) Hymen notch or cleft in superior hymen (above 3 to 9 o'clock in the supine position) Hymen bumps or mounds Erythema of anogenital tissues Labial adhesions Perianal venous pooling Diastasis ani Urethral prolapse Failure of midline fusion and perineal grooves
Indeterminate findings (no expert consensus)	Deep notches or clefts at the 3 and 9 o'clock position of the hymen in postpubertal girls Anogenital condyloma Anogenital herpes simplex virus
Diagnostic of trauma or sexual contact	Acute lacerations of the anogenital tissues Healed transection of the hymen between the 4 and 8 o'clock positions Missing segment of hymen tissue Confirmed diagnosis of gonorrhea, Chlamydia, trichomonas, or syphilis (when perinatal transmission excluded) Confirmed diagnosis of HIV (when perinatal, blood product, or needle-stick transmission has been excluded) Pregnancy Sperm from child's body

Adapted from Adams JA, Kaplan RA, Starling SP, et al. Guidelines for medical care of children who may have been sexually abused. *J Pediatr Adolesc Gynecol.* 2007;20:163-172.

the child and family (Adams, 2011) (Table 24-6). For a more detailed description of the medical evaluation of CSA, please refer to the Guidelines by Adams et al. (2007, 2011).

SEXUALLY TRANSMITTED INFECTION TESTING FOR SEXUAL ABUSE

Testing for STIs should be considered in all cases of sexual abuse and assault of children when mucosal skin contact between the alleged perpetrator and victim has occurred (Centers for Disease Control and Prevention [CDC], 2010). Although symptoms such as discharge or dysuria may be present in the infected child, genital *Trichomonas vaginalis* and *Chlamydia trachomatis* are well known to reside in infected individuals without causing overt symptoms, and cases of asymptomatic genital gonorrhea have been documented. Whereas testing by culture methods for trichomonas, gonorrhea, and Chlamydia provides direct identification of the involved organism, nonculture testing by nucleic acid amplification tests (NAATs) offers advantages in test sensitivity (especially for Chlamydia) and patient comfort (CDC, 2010). All positive test results should be confirmed by use of a method different than the first test, either by culture or a second NAAT that uses an alternate or different genetic target (Hammerschlag, 2011) if the infection will be significant in investigative or legal proceedings. This can be expected to occur if the test results are positive in a young child or an adolescent who has had no peer-consensual sexual activity. In prepubertal children, unless clinical indications prohibit waiting, confirmatory testing should be obtained before they are treated with antibiotics. Serologic testing for HIV, syphilis, and hepatitis should be obtained when indicated (Table 24-7).

MANAGEMENT OF SEXUAL ABUSE

Medical management for CSA and sexual assault victims is directed toward treatment or prophylaxis for conditions that could result from the sexual contact (infection and pregnancy), referral for other medical issues discovered in the course of the evaluation, mental health intervention, and reporting and collaboration with law enforcement and protective services. Postpubertal girls who have been acutely assaulted and have had genital-to-genital contact should receive antibiotic prophylaxis for gonorrhea, Chlamydia, and trichomonas after the assault because of their risk for ascending pelvic infection (CDC, 2010). Oral gonorrhea transmission as well as postexposure prophylaxis for HIV, hepatitis, and syphilis should be considered. Emergency contraception should be offered to postpubertal girls. Prepubertal girls and boys should have follow-up testing in 2 to 3 weeks after the assault without provision of postassault prophylaxis when indicated.

Table 24-7   Relationship of Sexually Transmitted Infections to Diagnosis of Child Sexual Abuse

STI Confirmed	Relationship to Sexual Abuse*	Suggested Action by Provider
Gonorrhea	Diagnostic	Report
Chlamydia	Diagnostic	Report
Trichomonas	Diagnostic	Report
HIV	Diagnostic	Report
Syphilis	Diagnostic	Report
Condyloma acuminata (anogenital warts)	Suspicious[†]	Report[‡]
Anogenital herpes simplex virus	Suspicious[†]	Report[‡]
Bacterial vaginosis	Inconclusive	Medical follow-up

*If transmission by perinatal or peer age, consensual encounters are excluded.

[†]Transmission can occur from perinatal spread, sexual contact, or nonsexual skin-to-skin contact.

[‡]Nonsexual transmission is more feasible in young children, but a thorough medical evaluation by a provider experienced in evaluation of child sexual abuse is still needed.

Adapted from Kellogg N; American Academy of Pediatrics Committee on Child Abuse and Neglect. The evaluation of sexual abuse in children. *Pediatrics.* 2005;116:506-512.

Although management focuses on the needs of the child, many cases of CSA involve trauma and stress to the entire family unit and should be addressed. Many caregivers of children who have been sexually abused have been victims of abuse themselves and never disclosed or had the opportunity to have treatment. The abuse of their child can trigger posttraumatic stress symptoms. Other sources of stress and trauma in the child's home should also be screened for and addressed at this time. Domestic violence, caregiver substance abuse, and depression should be recognized as significant adverse childhood experiences that, if left unaddressed, may have cumulative long-term negative health effects on the child's physical and emotional well-being (Felitti et al., 1998). Evidence-based or evidence-informed treatment should be offered to all victims of CSA.

Finally, CSA must be reported to the local mandated agencies. The report should be made immediately by phone and followed by a written report. Health Insurance Portability and Accountability Act (HIPAA) exclusions provide for the sharing of relevant information with children's services and law enforcement if child abuse is suspected.

SEXUAL ABUSE MYTHS

Cultural myths and societal expectations create an expectation that examination findings will prove penetration after sexual abuse and assault or that the lack of findings proves abuse did not occur. However, the majority of CSA victims have no physical evidence of the abuse. There are several reasons for this: (1) Delays in disclosure make it less likely to discover superficial injuries that heal quickly, (2) the mucosal skin of the anus and genitalia is elastic and can accommodate penetration without tearing, (3) injuries and tears to mucosal skin heal quickly and typically without scars, (4) a young girl's description of painful genital

Table 24-8   Common Myths and Misconceptions About Child Sexual Abuse

Children usually tell right away after abuse has occurred.
Physical or laboratory findings should be abnormal if penetration has occurred.
The hymen is commonly injured by activities such as gymnastics and bicycle riding.
Something has to "pop," break, or bleed the first time a girl has a sexual encounter.
Sexually transmitted infections in young children are common from casual contact or fomite spread.
Family members do not sexually abuse their own children.

penetration may reflect painful contact with her unestrogenized hymen without further penetration, and (5) it is uncommon to recover trace biologic evidence from the bodies of young children but more likely to recover biologic evidence from clothing and bedding (Anderst et al., 2009; Heppenstall-Heger et al., 2003; Thackeray et al., 2011) (Table 24-8).

Summary

KEY TREATMENT

- Health care workers are mandated reporters and must report all reasonable concerns for child maltreatment to county authorities. Early recognition of child abuse can be lifesaving.
- Child neglect can result in serious developmental deficits and must be treated by placing the child in an attentive and supportive environment.
- Treatment for certain STIs should be delayed until confirmatory testing has been completed.
- Children who have been abused or neglected should be screened for the need for referral for trauma-focused cognitive-behavioral therapy.

References

The complete reference list is available at www.expertconsult.com.

Web Resources

developingchild.harvard.edu Center on the Developing Child. Discusses reducing toxic stress.

emedicine.medscape.com/article/915664-overview Child abuse review, including an image library of injury patterns.

nrepp.samhsa.gov/Index.aspx U.S. Department of Health and Human Services Substance Abuse and Mental Health Services Administration. Evidence-based interventions to use after trauma.

purplecrying.info Newborn abuse prevention program.

theinstitute.umaryland.edu/seek Safe Environment for Every Child (SEEK) model of prevention.

www.cdc.gov/ace Centers for Disease Control and Prevention Adverse Childhood Experience (ACE) Study.

www.cdc.gov/std/treatment/2010 The Centers for Disease Control and Prevention's sexually transmitted disease treatment guidelines.

www.childwelfare.gov/pubs/usermanual.cfm *Child Neglect: A Guide for Prevention, Assessment, and Intervention.*

www.dontshake.org National Center on Shaken Baby Syndrome. Includes resources and references.

www2.aap.org/connectedkids Child abuse prevention materials.

25 Gynecology

SARINA B. SCHRAGER, HEATHER L. PALADINE, and KARA CADWALLADER

Patient-Centered Approach to the Well-Woman Examination

The well-woman examination is an opportunity for the family physician to promote health, prevent disease, and strengthen the physician–female patient relationship. Although women have traditionally been advised to see their doctors for an "annual examination," which includes a Papanicolaou smear, new screening guidelines have widened the scope of the visit and deemphasized the Pap smear (which may not be needed on an annual basis). Building a trusting relationship is important because women may be more likely to volunteer sensitive problems with a physician they trust. In addition, some women may have had previous negative experiences with pelvic examinations.

EVIDENCE-BASED SCREENING GUIDELINES

Screening guidelines published by the U.S. Preventive Services Task Force (USPSTF) provide an evidence-based guide for family physicians to follow. Recommendations with A and B levels of evidence for adult women are included in Table 25-1. Unfortunately, many established components of the well-woman examination are not supported by evidence. Testing for lipid disorders in average-risk women, type 2 diabetes screening, and physical activity counseling are examples of "uncertain" recommendations, according to the USPSTF. A physician may choose to cover these areas in a well-woman visit, but it is important to ensure that the areas with stronger evidence of benefit are thoroughly discussed. The USPSTF also lists areas of screening that have the potential to cause harm and therefore are not recommended. These include cervical cancer screening in women with previous hysterectomy for benign causes, screening for gonorrhea in low-risk women, teaching breast self-examination, and screening for ovarian cancer.

Immunizations are an important part of well-woman care. All patients benefit from disease prevention, and women are often caregivers for children or elderly persons, who are at higher risk from vaccine-preventable illnesses. Vaccines recommended by the U.S. Centers for Disease Control and Prevention (CDC) Advisory Committee on Immunization Practices (ACIP) include tetanus, diphtheria, and pertussis (Tdap); influenza; herpes zoster for adults older than age 50 years; pneumococcal vaccine for adults older than age 65 years; and human papillomavirus (HPV) vaccine for women 26 years of age and younger.

PAP SMEAR GUIDELINES

Key Points

- Pap screening should begin at age 21 years. Women should have Pap smears every 3 years. Women age 30 years and older may have co-testing with the Pap smear and HPV testing, which can be done together every 5 years.
- Women who have had a hysterectomy for benign disease should not have Pap smear screening.
- Women are not required to have a Pap smear before starting hormonal contraception.
- Women do not need a pap smear after age 65 years if they have had normal results in the past.

Although the Pap smear is still the mainstay of cervical cancer screening, recent advances in the understanding of HPV have revolutionized this field. HPV is the most common sexually transmitted infection (STI), with its highest prevalence among the 20- to 24-year-old age group (53.8%) (Hariri et al., 2011). Although HPV is typically spread through sexual activity, 15% of women in this study who reported that they had never had sex were infected with HPV. Physicians should keep in mind that some of these women may have been uncomfortable disclosing their sexual activity, even on an anonymous survey, but others may have had sexual contact they did not consider intercourse. Risk factors for HPV infection include low socioeconomic status, number of sexual partners in the past year, lifetime number of sexual partners, age at first intercourse, and marital status.

Strength of recommendation (SOR) taxonomy level A recommendations for cervical cancer screening include starting Pap test screening at age 21 years and repeating every 3 years. A screening option for women age 30 years and older is to perform Pap smear and HPV testing together, with repeat co-testing every 5 years if results of both are

Table 25-1   USPSTF Level A and B Recommendations for Adult Women

Condition	Recommendation	SOR
Alcohol misuse	Screening and behavioral counseling	B
High blood pressure	Screening every 2 yr if blood pressure is less than 120/80 mm Hg; yearly in women with blood pressure of 120-139/80-89 mm Hg	A
Breast cancer	Mammography every 2 yr for women age 50-74 yr	B
Pap smear	Screening every 3 yr from age 21-65 yr or every 5 yr from age 30-65 yr in combination with HPV testing	A
Chlamydia	Women age 24 yr and younger who have ever been sexually active	A
Lipid disorders	Women age 45 yr and older at increased risk for heart disease	A
	Women age 20-44 yr at increased risk for heart disease	B
Colorectal cancer	Adults age 50-75 yr, using fecal occult blood testing, sigmoidoscopy, or colonoscopy	A
Depression	Screening in adults when staff-assisted depression supports are in place	B
Type 2 diabetes	Adults with blood pressure >135/80 mm Hg	B
Obesity	Screening adults; intensive behavioral and counseling interventions	B
Osteoporosis	Screening of women age 65 yr and older and younger women at increased risk	B
Tobacco use	Screening adults; cessation interventions	A
HIV testing	Screening ages 15-65 yr; other ages if high risk	A
Hepatitis C	Screening in adults born between 1945 and 1965	B
Intimate partner violence	Screening in women of childbearing age	B

HPV, Human papillomavirus; *SORT,* strength of recommendation taxonomy (level of evidence).
U.S. Preventive Services Task Force (USPSTF) recommendations available at http://www.ahrq.gov/clinic/uspstfix.htm.

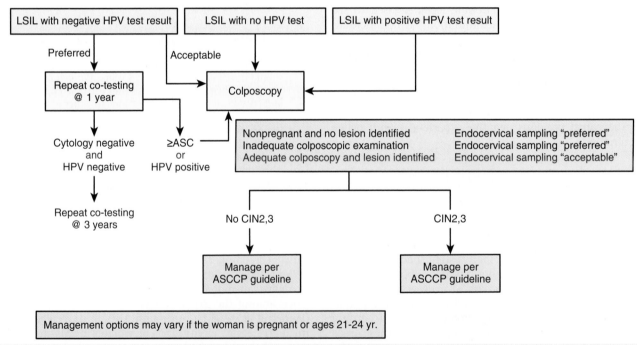

Figure 25-1 Management of women with low-grade squamous intraepithelial lesions (LSILs). *ASC,* Atypical squamous cells; *ASCCP,* American Society for Colposcopy and Cervical Pathology; *CIN,* cervical intraepithelial neoplasia; *HPV,* human papillomavirus. (Used with permission from American Society for Colposcopy and Cervical Pathology © Copyright 2013.)

normal. The recommendations for fewer Pap tests in women younger than 21 years and older than 30 years are consistent with the epidemiology of HPV. Younger women acquire HPV infections more frequently, but most clear the infection without intervention. Older women are less likely to develop new HPV infections, and only persistent HPV is a concern for cervical cancer. Women are not required to have a Pap smear before starting hormonal contraception. Physicians can use visits when a Pap test is not needed as an opportunity to educate female patients about STIs and reproductive health, as well as perform the other, evidence-based

screening recommendations previously cited (American College of Obstetricians and Gynecologists [ACOG], 2012a).

Abnormal Pap Smear Management

Guidelines for management of abnormal Pap test results have also been updated to reflect understanding of the epidemiology of HPV infection (Figure 25-1) (Saslow et al., 2012). These guidelines include recommendations for the management of special populations, such as adolescents, pregnant women, and postmenopausal women, and are available online at the American Society for Colposcopy and

Cervical Pathology (ASCCP) at http://www.asccp.org. Most women with low-grade squamous intraepithelial lesions (LSIL), atypical squamous cells of undetermined significance (ASCUS) with positive HPV test results, and high-grade SIL (HSIL) should have colposcopy.

Abnormal Vaginal Bleeding

Key Points

- Anovulation is common in adolescents for the first 18 months after menarche.
- Bleeding disorders typically present as menorrhagia in adolescence.
- Anovulation is the most common cause of abnormal vaginal bleeding in reproductive-age women.
- The four most common causes of secondary amenorrhea are pregnancy, hyperprolactinemia, thyroid disorders, and iatrogenic.
- Evaluation of abnormal bleeding in women older than age 45 years should include an endometrial biopsy.
- Anovulatory women are at risk for endometrial hyperplasia or carcinoma from unopposed estrogen and should have regular progesterone-induced withdrawal bleeds.
- Any bleeding after menopause in a woman who is not taking hormone therapy (HT) is abnormal.
- Evaluation with an endometrial biopsy or pelvic ultrasonography can exclude endometrial cancer in postmenopausal women.

Normal menstrual bleeding is defined as regular vaginal bleeding that occurs at intervals from 21 to 35 days. A normal menstrual cycle begins with the follicular phase before ovulation and then the luteal phase after ovulation. Abnormal vaginal bleeding is a common complaint in primary care. The prevalence of some type of abnormal bleeding is 10% to 30% among women of reproductive age. The estimated annual direct and indirect costs of abnormal bleeding are $1 billion and $12 billion, respectively (Liu et al., 2007). Abnormal bleeding is also a common reason for women to be referred to gynecologists and is an indication for up to 25% of all gynecologic surgery (Goodman, 2000). The ACOG has recently described a classification system for abnormal vaginal bleeding in women of reproductive age—polyp, adenomyosis, leiomyoma, malignancy and hyperplasia, coagulopathy, ovulatory dysfunction, endometrial, iatrogenic, not yet classified (PALM COEIN) (Table 25-2) (ACOG, 2012b).

A life cycle approach to abnormal vaginal bleeding is helpful in determining etiology and treatment options.

ADOLESCENTS

In adolescents, the three most common presentations of abnormal vaginal bleeding are anovulation, menorrhagia, and amenorrhea. It is normal for menstrual cycles to be anovulatory for an average of 18 months after menarche while the hypothalamic-pituitary axis matures. *Menorrhagia* (heavy bleeding) is quite common in adolescent patients and is most often caused by anovulation (Rimsza, 2002). In

Table 25-2 American College of Obstetricians and Gynecologists Classification System for Abnormal Bleeding in Reproductive-Age Women

PALM (Structural Causes)	COEIN (Nonstructural Causes)
Polyp	**C**oagulopathy
Adenomyosis	**O**vulatory dysfunction
Leiomyoma	**E**ndometrial
Malignancy and hyperplasia	**I**atrogenic
	Not yet classified

From American College of Obstetricians and Gynecologists. Diagnosis of abnormal uterine bleeding in reproductive-aged women. Practice Bulletin No. 128. *Obstet Gynecol.* 2012;120(1):197-206.

some young women, however, menorrhagia at menarche can be a sign of a bleeding disorder. Up to 24% of adolescents with menorrhagia may have an undiagnosed bleeding disorder (Strickland, 2004). Evaluation of menorrhagia in adolescents includes a complete blood count, coagulation profile, and von Willebrand disease screening test if clinically indicated. Treatment of both anovulation and menorrhagia in adolescents is usually hormonal contraception for cycle control.

The most common causes of primary amenorrhea include pregnancy; chromosomal abnormalities (e.g., Turner or Sawyer syndrome); hypothalamic hypogonadism; congenital absence of the uterus, cervix, or vagina; and structural abnormalities (e.g., transverse vaginal septum or imperforate hymen). Evaluation of primary amenorrhea includes a careful history, pelvic examination, pelvic ultrasonography to document the presence of pelvic organs, and chromosome analysis if clinically indicated.

REPRODUCTIVE-AGE WOMEN

The most common causes of abnormal bleeding in reproductive-age women are pregnancy complications, anovulatory disorders, and benign pelvic pathology. Characteristics of ovulatory cycles include regular cycle length, presence of premenstrual syndrome symptoms, and changes in cervical mucus. In contrast, anovulatory cycles tend to be unpredictable, with varying bleeding amounts and intervals.

Abnormal bleeding in ovulatory cycles includes menorrhagia, polymenorrhea, oligomenorrhea, and intermenstrual bleeding. Menorrhagia can be associated with structural lesions (uterine leiomyomas, endometrial polyps or hyperplasia), coagulation disorder, liver failure, or chronic renal failure. *Polymenorrhea* (bleeding at short intervals) can be caused by a luteal-phase disorder (not enough progesterone is produced after ovulation to stabilize the endometrium) or a short follicular phase. *Oligomenorrhea* (infrequent bleeding) is usually caused by a prolonged follicular phase. Intermenstrual bleeding can be caused by cervical pathology (dysplasia or infection) or an intrauterine device (IUD). Evaluation of a woman with abnormal bleeding is based on the type of bleeding (Table 25-3).

Anovulation is the most common cause of abnormal vaginal bleeding in reproductive-age women. The majority of anovulation is related to hypothalamic abnormalities or polycystic ovarian syndrome (PCOS) (Table 25-4). By

Table 25-3   Clinical Evaluation of Reproductive-Age Woman with Abnormal Bleeding

Ovulatory abnormal bleeding	History, physical examination, pregnancy test
Menorrhagia
Consideration of liver function tests, BUN/Cr, CBC, coagulation profile
Pelvic ultrasonography to exclude uterine fibroids
Endometrial biopsy (especially if older than 35 yr) to exclude endometrial hyperplasia
Intermenstrual bleeding
Pap smear, cervical cultures
Basal body temperature chart to determine length of follicular and luteal phases
Anovulatory bleeding	History, physical examination, pregnancy test
Laboratory studies
TSH level
Prolactin level
CBC (if acute bleeding episode or frequent heavy bleeding)
Fasting glucose and insulin levels
Screening for eating disorder, stress, and female-athlete triad

BUN/Cr, Blood urea nitrogen/creatinine; *CBC,* complete blood count; *TSH,* thyroid-stimulating hormone.

Table 25-4   Causes of Anovulatory Cycles

HYPOTHALAMIC

Weight loss
Eating disorders
Female athlete triad
Chronic illness
Stress
Excessive exercise

POLYCYSTIC OVARIAN SYNDROME

Thyroid disorders
Hyperprolactinemia
Idiopathic chronic anovulation
Medication induced (discontinuation of hormonal contraceptives)

Table 25-5   Treatment Options for Abnormal Vaginal Bleeding

Pregnancy desired	Ovulation induction with clomiphene citrate
Referral to gynecologist
Contraception desired	Cycle control with estrogen/progestin method, depot medroxyprogesterone acetate, or levonorgestrel IUD
Acute bleeding episode	**OUTPATIENT**
Administration of high-dose OCs, up to 4 pills daily for 5 to 7 days, with subsequent continuous OC cycling for at least 1 mo
Administration of oral estrogen or oral progesterone to stop the bleeding acutely

INPATIENT
IV fluids, supportive care, IV estrogen therapy
Consultation for surgical intervention |
| Contraception regimen used | **ESTROGEN/PROGESTIN**
Supportive care for first 3 mo
Assessment of adherence to OC regimen
Add supplemental estrogen
Change to method with higher dose of estrogen or different class of progestin

PROGESTIN ONLY
Add supplemental estrogen or combination OC
Administer NSAID to decrease bleeding |

IUD, intrauterine device; *IV,* intravenous; *NSAID,* nonsteroidal antiinflammatory drug; *OC,* oral contraceptive.
Modified from Ely JW, Kennedy CM, Clark EC, Bowdler NC. Abnormal uterine bleeding: a management algorithm. *J Am Board Fam Med.* 2006;19:590-602 and Schrager S. Abnormal uterine bleeding associated with hormonal contraception. *Am Fam Physician.* 2002;65:2073-2080.

definition, anovulatory cycles are unpredictable and cannot be classified by any one type of vaginal bleeding pattern. A woman may experience 14 days of heavy bleeding one month, light spotting intermittently for the next month, and then go for 3 months without a cycle. The pathologic abnormality in these cycles is a lack of ovulation, which produces an unopposed-estrogen state. The lack of progesterone production resulting from no ovulation contributes to irregular endometrial growth and nonuniform bleeding. In a normal cycle, the entire endometrium sloughs off during menstruation. In an anovulatory cycle, different sections of endometrium outgrow their blood supply at different times and bleed erratically.

Treatment of women with either ovulatory bleeding or anovulatory bleeding is not necessary unless the woman wants to become pregnant, is bothered by her bleeding pattern, or has systemic symptoms from anemia. However, anovulation is an unopposed-estrogen state, and treatment with some type of progesterone is necessary to reduce the risk of endometrial hyperplasia or carcinoma. *Unopposed estrogen* is a risk factor for endometrial cancer, along with obesity, diabetes, nulliparity, and age after 35 years. To protect against the development of endometrial hyperplasia, a precursor to endometrial cancer, all women with

chronic anovulation should have a progesterone-induced withdrawal bleed at least four times a year (Albers et al., 2004). Women may take medroxyprogesterone acetate, 10 mg/day for 10 days, and then expect a withdrawal bleed within a few days of stopping the medication.

Treatment of abnormal bleeding consists of ovulation induction if pregnancy is desired or cycle control with hormonal contraceptives if it is not. In women who are not candidates for estrogen-containing contraceptives, a monthly cycling of progesterone or continuous administration of progestin contraception (e.g., depot medroxyprogesterone acetate or levonorgestrel IUD) can also be an effective treatment. For women who do not want to take hormonal medications, nonsteroidal antiinflammatory drugs (NSAIDs) can decrease the amount of bleeding (Ely et al., 2006) (Table 25-5).

Another common presentation of abnormal bleeding is an *acute bleeding* episode. In this situation, a woman is most likely anovulatory. Evaluation in an acute bleeding episode should include hemoglobin (Hb) and hematocrit (Hct), assessment of volume status, and an endometrial biopsy in women older than age 45 years.

If a woman presents with heavy bleeding and exhibits any signs or symptoms of *hypovolemia,* she should be admitted to the hospital and either treated with intravenous (IV) estrogen to stop the bleeding or have a surgical procedure, such as dilation and curettage. If the woman is stable and her Hb and Hct are near normal, outpatient treatment with high-dose oral contraceptives (OCs), estrogen, or progesterone may be attempted (Ely et al., 2006).

A woman may also present with *amenorrhea*. The four most common causes of secondary amenorrhea (when a woman who previously had normal menses stops having menses for at least 6 months) are pregnancy, hyperprolactinemia, thyroid disorders, and iatrogenic (from medications). Other reasons for amenorrhea include outflow obstruction (e.g., Asherman syndrome, caused by scarring of uterus from instrumentation, or cervical stenosis) and primary ovarian failure. Evaluation of a woman with amenorrhea begins with a history and physical examination. Laboratory studies should include a pregnancy test and thyroid-stimulating hormone and prolactin levels. The next step is an induced withdrawal bleed after administering progesterone for 10 to 14 days. If a woman has a menstrual bleed after taking progesterone, outflow obstruction and low estrogen state (as in primary ovarian failure) are excluded as the causes of amenorrhea. If a woman does not have a withdrawal bleed after progesterone administration, a trial of estrogen supplementation for 3 weeks should be given before another course of progesterone is attempted. In this situation, if a woman has a withdrawal bleed, the diagnosis of primary ovarian failure is considered, and levels of gonadotropins (follicle-stimulating hormone [FSH], luteinizing hormone [LH]) should be obtained. If a woman does not have a withdrawal bleed after estrogen and progesterone administration, a hysterosalpingogram (radiograph of uterus and ovaries after dye injection) should be obtained to evaluate for outflow obstruction.

PERIMENOPAUSAL WOMEN

Abnormal bleeding in the 5 to 10 years before menopause is very common. The most common pathology is anovulation caused by declining numbers of ovarian follicles and decreasing inhibin B levels (Jain and Santoro, 2005). Perimenopausal women may also bleed from structural lesions (most often uterine fibroid tumors or polyps) or bleeding disorders. Evaluation of a perimenopausal woman with abnormal bleeding should include an endometrial biopsy to exclude endometrial hyperplasia or cancer. The risk of endometrial cancer increases in women who are nulliparous, diabetic, or obese (Espindola et al., 2007). Nonsmoking women in this age group can be effectively managed with hormonal contraception for cycle control. Smokers who should avoid estrogen because of a thrombotic risk can use cyclic progestin to provide a monthly withdrawal bleed.

POSTMENOPAUSAL WOMEN

Menopause is defined as 12 months without a menstrual period. After that 12-month period, any bleeding is abnormal. A large Danish study found a 10% prevalence of postmenopausal bleeding (Astrup, 2004). Bleeding episodes decreased as the time since menopause increased. The main concern in a postmenopausal woman with bleeding is endometrial carcinoma. Between 10% and 20% of all postmenopausal bleeding is caused by malignancy (Hale and Fraser, 2007). Evaluation of postmenopausal bleeding can be done effectively with either pelvic ultrasonography or an office endometrial biopsy. A pelvic ultrasound can assess the thickness of the endometrium, the *endometrial stripe*. A stripe less than 4 mm in diameter is the cutoff to exclude endometrial cancer (ACOG, 2009). An office endometrial biopsy is an excellent diagnostic test to evaluate endometrial tissue (Dijkhuizen et al., 2000). In some postmenopausal women, however, cervical stenosis precludes a successful biopsy. In this situation, if ultrasonography is nonreassuring, a surgical procedure may be indicated.

KEY TREATMENT

- Unstable women with acute heavy vaginal bleeding should be admitted to the hospital for IV estrogen therapy or surgical intervention (ACOG, 2012b) (SOR: C).
- Treatment of abnormal bleeding includes ovulation induction if a woman desires pregnancy and hormonal cycle control if she does not (ACOG, 2012b) (SOR: C).
- To protect against the development of endometrial hyperplasia, a precursor to endometrial cancer, all women with chronic anovulation should have a progesterone-induced withdrawal bleed at least four times a year (Albers et al., 2004) (SOR: C).
- If Hb and Hct are near normal, outpatient treatment with high-dose oral contraceptives, estrogen, or progesterone may be attempted (Ely et al., 2006) (SOR: C).

Pelvic Mass

Key Points

- Pelvic examination is not sensitive or specific for the diagnosis of a pelvic mass.
- Initial evaluation of a pelvic mass should include a focused history, physical examination, pelvic ultrasonography, and CA-125 level in postmenopausal women.
- Pelvic ultrasonography with cyst morphology and Doppler flow studies can distinguish benign cysts from ovarian carcinoma, especially in postmenopausal women.
- Although combination oral contraceptives can reduce the risk of functional ovarian cysts, OCs are not useful for treatment.

DIAGNOSIS

A patient may report a symptomatic pelvic mass, or it may be discovered as part of a pelvic examination or ultrasonography done for other reasons. A pelvic mass can be associated with the uterus, ovaries, or nongynecologic organs. The first step in evaluation is to review the patient's age, history, and risk factors. For example, an ovarian cyst is more likely to be a functional cyst in a younger woman, but it has a higher potential to be ovarian cancer in postmenopausal women. Additional historical details include menopausal status, menstrual history, family history, STI risk, symptoms of hyperandrogenism, and dysmenorrhea.

Pelvic examination is not sensitive or specific for diagnosis of a pelvic mass, especially as body mass index increases (Myers et al., 2006). However, pelvic examination can

Table 25-6   Differential Diagnosis of Pelvic Mass

Diagnosis	Features
UTERUS	
Uterine fibroid	Pelvic pressure, heavy vaginal bleeding
Intrauterine pregnancy	Positive pregnancy test result, amenorrhea
FALLOPIAN TUBES	
Ectopic pregnancy	Positive pregnancy test result, adnexal pain or tenderness, hemodynamic instability
Tubo-ovarian abscess	STI risk, pelvic pain, cervical motion tenderness, vaginal discharge, fever
OVARIES	
Simple cysts	More common in premenopausal women; sharp, may have pelvic pressure
Endometriomas	Dysmenorrhea
Dermoid cysts (teratomas)	Pelvic pressure
Ovarian carcinoma	Postmenopausal women
Polycystic ovarian syndrome	Hyperandrogenism, irregular menses, multiple cysts on ultrasonography
Germ cell tumors	Pelvic pressure, chromosomal abnormalities, younger women (teens and 20s)
INTESTINES	
Appendicitis	Anorexia, right lower quadrant pain or tenderness, elevated WBC count, fever
Diverticulitis	Left lower quadrant pain or tenderness, cramping, constipation, older age, fever
URINARY TRACT	
Bladder tumor	Hematuria
Pelvic kidney	Usually asymptomatic

STI, Sexually transmitted infection; *WBC,* white blood cell.

provide other information helpful in the diagnosis, such as location of the mass, mobility of the mass, cervical motion tenderness, pelvic tenderness, and vaginal discharge. The initial evaluation of a pelvic mass should include pelvic ultrasonography, which can be transabdominal or transvaginal, depending on the size and location of the mass. Premenopausal women should be tested to exclude pregnancy. Doppler ultrasonography, cyst morphology, and CA-125 testing are useful in ruling out ovarian cancer in a postmenopausal woman with an adnexal mass. Table 25-6 lists the differential diagnosis and common features of pelvic masses.

UTERINE FIBROIDS

Clinically significant uterine fibroids are present in approximately one third of reproductive-age women (Viswanathan et al., 2007). Although often asymptomatic, fibroids may cause pelvic pain, pressure, and heavy or irregular vaginal bleeding and are the most common reason for hysterectomy in the United States. Treatment options for fibroids include watchful waiting because most fibroids will decrease in size after menopause. Although hysterectomy is definitive treatment, it carries the risks of major surgery. Myomectomy and other uterine-sparing procedures have a high rate of symptom recurrence (up to 50% within 5 years) and may

be more effective for symptom control in perimenopausal women. Women with fibroids are more likely to be infertile, although it is not clear if the association is causative. Removal of fibroids has not been shown to improve fertility (Metwally et al., 2012). Medical treatments such as NSAIDs and OCs have not been well studied. The levonorgestrel intrauterine system (Mirena) has been shown to decrease menstrual bleeding in women with fibroids when compared with OCs (Sayed et al., 2011). Mifepristone (ru 486) has been shown to reduce heavy menstrual bleeding and improve fibroid-related quality of life (Tristan et al., 2012).

OVARIAN CYSTS AND CARCINOMA

As mentioned, the initial evaluation of an ovarian cyst includes transvaginal ultrasonography. Simple cysts are very likely to be benign, but complex cysts (with thick walls, irregularity, papillations, septa, and echogenicity) and cysts that are larger than 10 cm have a higher risk of malignancy (Modesitt, 2003). Malignant neoplasms also display increased vascularity on Doppler ultrasonography (ACOG, 2007). The Society of Gynecologic Oncologists and the American College of Obstetrics and Gynecology have developed criteria for referral to a gynecologic oncologist. Premenopausal women should be referred if they have a CA-125 level greater than 200 U/mL, ascites, evidence of metastases, or a first-degree relative with breast or ovarian cancer. Postmenopausal women should be referred if they have an elevated CA-125 level, ascites, a nodular or fixed pelvic mass, evidence of ascites, or a family history of breast or ovarian cancer in a first-degree relative (Liu and Zanotti, 2011). Although combination OCs can reduce the occurrence of functional ovarian cysts, OCs are not helpful for treatment (Grimes et al., 2011).

KEY TREATMENT

- Most simple ovarian cysts can be managed expectantly (ACOG, 2007) (SOR: B).
- The levonorgestrel intrauterine system can reduce heavy menstrual bleeding in women with uterine fibroids (ACOG, 2007) (SOR: B).
- Low-dose mifepristone decreases symptoms and improves quality of life (ACOG, 2007) (SOR: B).

Vaginal Discharge

Key Points

- Douching is not helpful for prevention or treatment of vaginitis.
- Signs and symptoms of vaginitis are not specific, but a cause can usually be diagnosed on office microscopy.
- Speculum examination is not necessary for diagnosis of vaginitis; a blind swab in the vaginal vault is equally sensitive.
- Self-diagnosis of vaginal infection by the patient is unreliable.

Table 25-7 Comparison of Findings for Vaginitis

Type	Symptoms	Signs	pH	KOH	Saline Wet Mount
Bacterial vaginosis	Malodorous discharge	Thin, gray adherent discharge	>4.5	Amine or fishy odor	Clue cells
Vulvovaginal candidiasis	Itching, burning pain	Curdlike discharge, vulvar erythema	3.8-4.5	Pseudohyphae; budding yeast	Occasional hyphae; yeast
Trichomoniasis	Fish-odor discharge	Erythema, tenderness	6-7	Negative	Trichomonads, many WBCs
Atrophic vaginitis	Dryness, pain	Pale, friable	>4.5	Negative	RBCs, WBCs; many bacteria
Aerobic vaginitis	Foul odor	Heavy purulent discharge	>4.5	Negative	Cocci or coarse rods
Irritant or allergic vaginitis	Itching, swelling	Erythema	Any	Negative	Negative

KOH, Potassium hydroxide; *RBCs,* red blood cells; *WBCs,* white blood cells.

Table 25-8 Differential Diagnosis of Vaginal Discharge: Vaginitis

Candida spp. (*Candida albicans, Candida glabrata*)
Bacterial vaginosis (anaerobic bacteria: *Gardnerella vaginalis, Bacteroides* spp.)
Desquamative inflammatory vaginitis: aerobic bacteria
Trichomonas vaginalis
Allergic vaginitis or contact dermatitis
Chlamydial infection or gonorrhea
Erosive lichen planus vaginitis
Actinomyces Behçet syndrome (associated with IUC use)
Vulvar vestibulitis
Physiologic (leukorrhea)
Atrophic vaginitis

IUC, Intrauterine contraception.

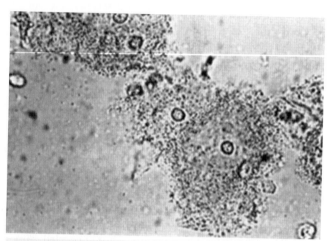

Figure 25-2 Bacterial vaginosis. Typical clue cells of vaginal epithelium are heavily covered by coccobacilli, with loss of distinct cell margins (magnification ×400). (From Holmes KK. Lower genital tract infections in women: cystitis/urethritis, vulvovaginitis, and cervicitis. In Holmes KK, Mårdh PA, Sparling PF, et al, eds. *Sexually transmitted diseases.* New York: McGraw-Hill; 1984.)

Vaginitis is the most common gynecologic diagnosis made in the primary care setting. Common symptoms include increased vaginal discharge without pelvic pain or systemic symptoms, vulvar itching and burning, dysuria, and possible odor. Physiologic leukorrhea varies and may change with a woman's menstrual cycle. If purulent cervicitis is present on examination, testing for *Chlamydia* and *Neisseria gonorrhoeae* should be performed (French et al., 2004). In postmenopausal women, vaginal irritation, dryness, and superficial bleeding are often caused by atrophic vaginitis (see the section titled "Menopause"). A medication history is important because isotretinoin and some contraceptives may also cause dryness and itching. Personal hygiene habits of excessive washing with soap and use of highly absorbent panty liners may cause irritation. If a woman has self-diagnosed and treated with an antifungal agent and symptoms persist, a clinical examination should be encouraged (ACOG, 2006). Tables 25-7 and 25-8 review the differential diagnosis and findings in vaginitis.

Office microscopy is used most often to make a diagnosis of vaginitis. A finding of many leukocytes is uncommon in candidiasis or bacterial vaginosis (BV) and suggests trichomoniasis. If trichomonads are not present, consider gonorrhea or chlamydial infection (Anderson et al., 2004). Fem V, an over-the-counter (OTC) diagnostic kit, can be used; a positive test result suggests BV or trichomoniasis; a negative test result is likely a yeast infection (Prescriber's Letter, 2006).

BACTERIAL VAGINOSIS

Bacterial vaginosis is caused by a shift from the normal lactobacilli-dominated vaginal flora to a polymicrobial flora dominated by gram-positive anaerobes. Although BV is the most common cause of vaginal discharge and foul odor, more than half of women with BV are asymptomatic (CDC, 2010). BV is associated with postoperative infection, pelvic inflammatory disease (PID), premature delivery in women with certain risk factors (French et al., 2004), and an increased risk of human immunodeficiency virus type 1 (HIV-1) transmission (Oduyebo et al., 2009). Risk factors for acquisition of BV include tobacco use; intrauterine contraception (IUC) use; new male sexual partner; sex with another woman; and use of vaginal foreign bodies, perfumed soaps, or douching (Allsworth and Peipert, 2007).

The diagnosis of BV can usually be made by history and laboratory microscopy (Figure 25-2). Self-diagnosis by the patient is unreliable (ACOG, 2006). A strong "musty cheese" odor predicts BV, but a lack of a perceived odor makes BV unlikely (Anderson et al., 2004). Use of Gram stain or the Amsel criteria on a vaginal (not cervical) sample can be used to diagnose BV in clinical practice (Table 25-9).

There are many effective options for the treatment of BV. A 2009 Cochrane review states that clindamycin and metronidazole have equivalent efficacy, regardless of regimen. The standard oral dose of metronidazole for BV is 500 mg twice daily for 7 days. Both metronidazole gel and clindamycin vaginal cream are dosed daily. Clindamycin 2% cream has lower adverse event rates. Intravaginal

Table 25-9 Amsel Criteria for Bacterial Vaginosis*

1. Vaginal pH >4.5 (most sensitive) (89% sensitivity, 74% specificity)
2. Clue cells >20% on wet-mount (74% sensitivity, 86% specificity)
3. Homogeneous discharge, gray, adherent, but wipes off easily (79% sensitivity, 54% specificity)
4. Whiff test (amine odor when KOH added; 67% sensitivity, 93% specificity)

*A score of 3 of 4 is diagnostic.
KOH, Potassium hydroxide.
Modified from Gutman RE et al. Evaluation of clinical methods for diagnosing bacterial vaginosis. *Obstet Gynecol.* 2005;105:551-556.

lactobacilli gelatin tablets are also effective (Oduyebo et al., 2009). Tinidazole is effective with no serious side effects but is more expensive (Livengood et al., 2007). The Food and Drug Administration (FDA) approved metronidazole, 750 mg/day for 7 days, and a single dose of intravaginal clindamycin for treatment of BV, but only limited data are available on efficacy (CDC, 2010). Hydrogen peroxide douching and triple-sulfonamide cream are considered ineffective (Oduyebo et al., 2009).

Recurrent BV can present a treatment challenge. If recurrence is suspected, the diagnosis should be confirmed, risk factors identified and controlled, and other causes considered while retreating BV (Alfonsi et al., 2004). Metronidazole gel used twice weekly reduces recurrences of BV but is offset by increased vaginal candidiasis and pain complaints (Sobel et al., 2006). If retreatment fails, suppressive therapy with metronidazole 0.75% gel for 10 days, then twice weekly for 4 to 6 months, should be tried. There is no evidence that treatment of sexual partners is effective to prevent recurrence (CDC, 2010). Using vaginal suppositories or consuming yogurt with *Lactobacillus* may decrease recurrences of BV (Jurden et al., 2012) (SOR: B).

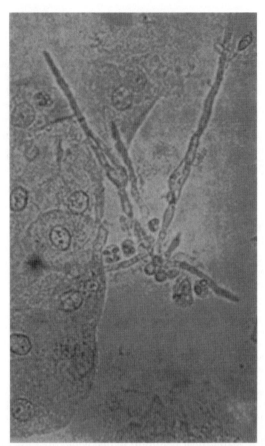

Figure 25-3 Candidal vaginitis (vulvovaginal candidiasis). Candidal organisms in a saline wet-mount preparation clearly demonstrate hyphae and conidia under high-power magnification. (From Kaufman RH, Faro S: *Benign disease of the vulva and vagina.* 4th ed. St. Louis: Mosby; 1994.)

KEY TREATMENT

- All symptomatic women with BV should be treated (CDC, 2010) (SOR: B).
- Asymptomatic women undergoing abortion should be treated to decrease the risk for infectious complications (British Association for Sexual Health and HIV [BASH]H, 2012) (SOR: A).
- Oral or vaginal metronidazole (BASHH, 2012) and vaginal clindamycin are effective and equivalent in non-pregnant women (Kane, 2001) (SOR: A).
- Treatment of male partners does not decrease relapse rates (CDC, 2010) (SOR A).
- Tinidazole is effective with no serious side effects but is more expensive than metronidazole (Livengood et al., 2007) (SOR: A).
- In recurrent BV, suppressive therapy with metronidazole 0.75% gel for 10 days and then twice weekly for 4 to 6 months may be successful (Alfonsi et al., 2004) (SOR: C).

CANDIDAL VAGINITIS

Vulvovaginal candidiasis (VVC) is the second most common cause of vaginitis after BV, with a lifetime prevalence in women of 70% to 75% (Spence, 2007). *Candida albicans* is the most common cause (80%-90%). Type 1 diabetes is the strongest risk factor for VVC; other risk factors include recent antibiotic use, condom and diaphragm use, spermicide use, receptive oral sex, OC use, pregnancy, hormone replacement therapy, and immunosuppression. Patient self-diagnosis of VVC is incorrect 50% of the time and is therefore unreliable. Asymptomatic treatment of VVC is *not* recommended even in women who have a positive swab for *Candida* (Spence, 2007). Because VVC is not sexually transmitted, routine partner treatment is also not recommended. Recurrent VVC is defined as four or more symptomatic episodes in a year. Rare complications of VVC include vulvar vestibulitis and chorioamnionitis (French et al., 2004).

The most common complaint associated with culture confirmed VVC is burning or pruritus. A thick, curdled-appearing discharge, signs of inflammation, and lack of odor all have high positive predictive value for diagnosing VVC (Anderson et al., 2004). In one study, however, a thin discharge was present in about half of women later found to have VVC (French et al., 2004).

Although office microscopy is the first line for diagnosis of VVC, culture is the "gold standard" (Figure 25-3) (ACOG, 2006). With *C. albicans*, the vaginal pH is usually 5.0 or less but may be higher with non-*albicans* species. A wet mount should be performed to exclude trichomoniasis or BV. Potassium hydroxide (KOH) examination should also be performed, but it has a wide range of sensitivity. Thus, if candidiasis is suspected in a patient with persistent or recurrent symptoms and wet mount and KOH results are negative, a culture should be performed (French et al., 2004). The use of rapid antigen testing to detect vaginal yeast is more sensitive than a wet mount and is feasible for office practice. However, a negative result lacks sensitivity to rule out yeast, and a culture needs to be sent (Chatwani et al., 2007).

The imidazoles are the cornerstone of VVC treatment. Intravaginal OTC imidazoles (e.g., clotrimazole, miconazole, tioconazole) come in 1-, 3-, and 7-day therapy regimens and are equivalent to oral therapies for treatment, and single-dose therapy seems as efficacious as multidose therapy over days (Nurbhai et al., 2007). *Lactobacillus*, administered vaginally, orally, or both, does not prevent postantibiotic-associated vaginal candidiasis (Pirotta et al., 2004).

Recurrent VVC occurs in 5% to 8% of women. The Infectious Diseases Society of America recommends treating recurrent VVC for 10 to 14 days followed by suppressive therapy using fluconazole, a single 150-mg dose weekly for 6 months (Pappas et al., 2009). It is unclear if oral regimens are better than intravaginal administration. In preventing recurrence, there is no evidence of benefit with intravaginal boric acid, tea tree oil, garlic, douching, or treating a woman's male sexual partner. *Lactobacillus*, in the form of suppositories or oral yogurt, does not appear to prevent recurrence (Jurden et al., 2012) (SOR: B). Douching is associated with increased pelvic infections (Spence, 2007). For specific treatment regimens, see http://www.cdc.gov/std/treatment/.

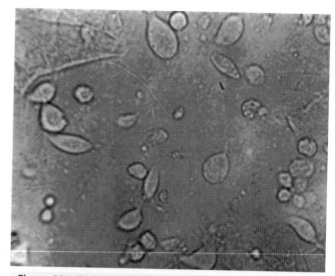

Figure 25-4 Trichomoniasis. Trichomonads are seen under high-power magnification in a wet mount prepared with physiologic saline. Usually, more immature epithelial cells are seen in the secretions of active trichomoniasis. (From Kaufman RH, Faro S. *Benign disease of the vulva and vagina.* 4th ed. St Louis, Mosby, 1994.)

KEY TREATMENT

- Oral fluconazole and itraconazole are both effective for VVC (Spence, 2007) (SOR: A).
- Oral and intravaginal regimens are equivalent, so cost and patient preference should guide choice (Nurbhai et al., 2007) (SOR: B).
- Intravaginal imidazoles are equivalent to oral therapies for VVC treatment, and single-dose seems as efficacious as multidose therapy (Spence, 2007) (SOR: B).
- Treat recurrent VVC for 10 to 14 days followed by suppressive therapy using fluconazole, single 150-mg dose weekly for 6 months (Pappas et al., 2009) (SOR: A).

TRICHOMONIASIS

Trichomoniasis is caused by a motile protozoan and affects 120 million women worldwide every year. It is usually sexually transmitted and is associated with transmission of other STIs (Forna, 2003). Risk factors for acquisition include multiple sexual partners and possibly a decrease in the normal vaginal acidity. Men are usually asymptomatic carriers, but 10% of nongonococcal urethritis in men is caused by *Trichomonas* (French et al., 2004).

Up to 50% of women with trichomoniasis are asymptomatic. Symptomatic women may complain of a yellow-green, malodorous discharge; vaginal burning; and dysuria. On physical examination, hemorrhagic, punctate cervical lesions are pathognomonic but are only present in 2% of

cases (French et al., 2004). More common signs are foul-smelling purulent discharge, vaginal tenderness, vulvar erythema, and edema. The vaginal pH is usually basic. Office microscopy is first line for diagnosis of trichomoniasis (ACOG, 2006). The sample should be taken from the posterior vault, diluted in 2 drops of saline, and assessed quickly because motility of the protozoa diminishes rapidly (Figure 25-4). Although microscopy has good specificity (99%), motile trichomonads are seen in only 50% to 80% of culture-proven cases. Both the OSOM Trichomonas Rapid Test and the AFFIRM VP III are FDA-approved point-of-care tests for trichomoniasis and have higher sensitivity but more false-positives results (CDC, 2010). Thus, culture is the gold standard. Trichomonads can be reported on a Pap smear, but it is not recommended as a diagnostic test because of the low sensitivity (58%) (French et al., 2004). In men, the wet prep has poor sensitivity, so culture of a urethral, urine, or semen sample or NAAT testing on urine can increase the diagnostic rate.

Metronidazole or tinidazole single-dose therapy is effective for treatment of trichomoniasis. An alternative effective regimen is metronidazole, 500 mg orally twice daily for 7 days. Metronidazole gel is less effective (<50% cure rate) compared with oral metronidazole (CDC, 2010). Desensitization is recommended for patients who are allergic to metronidazole. Avoidance of alcohol is important with all nitroimidazoles. Metronidazole is not teratogenic in the first trimester (BASHH, 2007). Because most male sexual partners have asymptomatic trichomoniasis, simultaneous treatment is recommended.

If treatment fails with a 2-g single dose of metronidazole, a trial of metronidazole, 500 mg twice daily for 7 days, or a single 2-g dose of tinidazole is recommended (CDC, 2010). If this fails, a trial of tinidazole or metronidazole, 2 g orally once daily for 5 days, is recommended. Referral is advised for persistent failure. A test of cure is unnecessary if symptoms resolve (BASHH, 2007).

- A women with trichomoniasis should abstain from intercourse until both she and her partner have been treated and are asymptomatic (ACOG, 2006) (SOR: A).
- A single dose of a nitroimidazole can achieve parasitologic cure; tinidazole as a single 2-g dose may be most efficacious (CDC, 2010; Forna, 2003) (SOR: A).
- If treatment fails with a single 2-g dose of metronidazole, a trial of metronidazole, 500 mg twice daily for 7 days, or a single 2-g dose of tinidazole is recommended (CDC, 2010) (SOR: B).

OTHER FORMS OF VAGINITIS

Aerobic vaginitis is characterized by purulent vaginal discharge with a dominant abnormal aerobic flora. Patients experience a foul-smelling nonfishy discharge, and examination may reveal erythema, inflammation, and ulcers of the posterior fornix. Although culture is the gold standard, the diagnosis is usually one of exclusion, with pH greater than 6.0, white blood cells (WBCs) on microscopy, and absence of hyphae or clue cells. Treatment with topical clindamycin has a good response (French et al., 2004). The addition of a topical estrogen may increase treatment success.

Irritant and allergic vaginitis should be considered in the differential diagnosis of vaginal complaints. Common etiologies include spermicidal products, douching solutions, diaphragms, latex condoms, and topical medications. The treatment is discontinuation of intravaginal products (French et al., 2004).

Cytolytic vaginitis is caused by an overgrowth of lactobacilli and cytolysis of squamous epithelial cells. Although it may be related to intravaginal products or other medication use, its etiology remains unclear. It can mimic VVC with a white, curdled-cheese discharge, and the pH range is typically 3.5 to 5.5. Treatment is discontinuation of intravaginal medications. Baking soda douches or sitz baths have been used, but minimal data exist to support this recommendation (French et al., 2004).

Desquamative inflammatory vaginitis is characterized by copious purulent discharge with squamous epithelial cell exfoliation. The etiology is unclear but likely multifactorial. Some cases may be linked to lichen planus spectrum. Laboratory evaluation reveals a negative wet mount, KOH, and cultures. Treatment options include a trial of local or systemic corticosteroids (French et al., 2004) or clindamycin suppositories.

Vulvar Lesions

Key Points

- Visible condyloma should be treated. (SOR: C).
- Biopsy is indicated for treatment-resistant warts; chronic symptomatic lesions; and nevus-like, pigmented lesions. (SOR: B).
- Biopsy of lichen sclerosus is recommended to rule out vulvar squamous cell carcinoma. (SOR: B).

- Topical corticosteroids are the cornerstone of management for non-neoplastic epithelial disorders of the vulva. (SOR: C).

The differential diagnosis of vulvar lesions includes external genital warts (EGWs), *Candida,* herpes simplex, lichen sclerosus et atrophicus, lichen planus, psoriasis, and eczema. EGWs are caused by HPV (90% by HPV 6 or 11), which is primarily transmitted through sexual contact. Although exophytic warts are usually diagnosable with the naked eye, application of acetic acid can make flat warts visible. Biopsy is indicated for treatment-resistant warts; chronic symptomatic lesions; and nevus-like, pigmented lesions. For EGWs, treatment is divided into patient-applied (podofilox, imiquimod, and sinecatechins) and provider-administered (cryotherapy, podophyllin resin, trichloroacetic acid, and surgical removal) modalities. Cryotherapy is as effective as trichloroacetic acid and more effective than podophyllin. Podophyllotoxin and podophyllin are equally effective for clearance of EGWs and useful for small, solitary lesions. Imiquimod cream is also effective and should be applied to intact skin. Sinecatechin ointment is effective but should be avoided in immunocompromised patients (CDC, 2010). Topical interferon is effective and preferable to systemic interferon. Electrosurgery is at least as effective as cryotherapy and more effective than podophyllin (Buck, 2006). The quadrivalent vaccine is effective protection against the types of HPV that cause 90% of genital warts (CDC, 2010).

Non-neoplastic epithelial lesions of the vulva include lichen sclerosus, lichen planus, and lichen simplex chronicus (Figure 25-5). *Lichen sclerosus* is most common in postmenopausal women and presents with intense vulvar pruritus (see Figure 25-5, *A*). Physical examination initially reveals thickened, white skin not involving the vagina, which progresses to a thin, wrinkled, "cigarette paper" appearance. High-potency topical steroids are effective in alleviating symptoms and preventing progressive architectural damage. *Lichen planus* is an autoimmune disorder that may involve the vagina as well as vulva. High-potency topical steroids or hydrocortisone suppositories are effective for treatment. *Lichen simplex chronicus* presents as lichenified, erythematous plaques resulting from chronic itching and scratching (see Figure 25-5, *B*). Breaking the itch–scratch cycle is the cornerstone of treatment (O'Connell et al., 2008).

- For external warts, cryotherapy is as effective as trichloroacetic acid and more effective than podophyllin; electrosurgery is at least as effective as cryotherapy and more effective than podophyllin (Buck, 2006) (SOR: B).
- For lichen sclerosus, high-potency topical steroids are effective in alleviating symptoms and preventing progressive architectural damage (O'Connell et al., 2008) (SOR: B).
- For lichen simplex chronicus, breaking the itch–scratch cycle is primary treatment (O'Connell et al., 2008) (SOR: C).

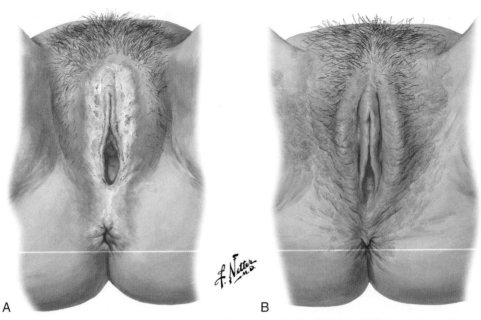

Figure 25-5 A, Lichen sclerosus. **B,** Lichen simplex chronicus. (Used with permission from Anderson BE. *The Netter collection of medical illustrations. Vol. 4, integumentary system.* Philadelphia: Elsevier; 2012.)

Acute Pelvic Pain

Key Points

- Acute pelvic pain can be related to multiple organ systems.
- Gynecologic pain typically includes pregnancy complications, infection, and ovarian cysts.
- Clinicians should have a low threshold for treating PID because of the potential for long-term complications.

Acute lower abdominal pain can be caused by multiple organ systems. Urinary tract infections are often associated with pain over the bladder related to dysuria, frequency, and urgency of urination. Gastrointestinal (GI) causes of lower abdominal pain include acute appendicitis, diverticulitis, irritable bowel syndrome, and ischemic bowel.

Gynecologic causes of acute pelvic pain are usually related to complications of pregnancy, infections, or ovarian pathology. *Ectopic pregnancy* is a serious cause of acute pain in the context of an early pregnancy. Ectopic pregnancy should be suspected when the quantitative human chorionic gonadotropin (hCG) level does not increase appropriately or if the hCG level is greater than 1500 mIU and transvaginal ultrasonography does not show an intrauterine gestational sac. The dilation of the fallopian tube caused by the growing embryo is the etiology of the pain. Emergent treatment with either medication or surgery is necessary to prevent rupture of the tube. Ectopic pregnancy is usually diagnosed by ultrasonography. Treatment of an ectopic pregnancy can be surgical or medical. Single-dose methotrexate is the most frequently used regimen, 50 mg/m^2 of body surface intramuscularly, but no studies have compared efficacy between single-dose and multidose therapies (ACOG, 2008). Degenerating fibroid tumors may also cause pain as a result of ischemia during pregnancy, usually in the second trimester.

Pelvic infections such as acute cervicitis and PID can cause pain associated commonly with abnormal vaginal discharge and systemic symptoms of infection. On examination, most affected women will have a purulent cervicitis, a tender uterus, and cervical motion tenderness. Both outpatient and inpatient treatment options are available from the CDC's STI treatment guidelines (2010). Outpatient treatment of PID usually includes intramuscular (IM) ceftriaxone and doxycycline for 10 days to cover both *Neisseria gonorrhoeae* and *Chlamydia* spp. Oral cephalosporins are not indicated in treatment of PID because of the increased national resistance of gonorrhea (CDC, 2010). Untreated PID can lead to an abscess or scarring that can cause infertility. The clinical diagnosis of PID has a positive predictive value of 65% to 90% (BASHH, 2005). Therefore, clinicians should have a low threshold for treating women with suspected PID.

Ovarian cysts are common and often cause no pain. When cysts rupture, however, women experience acute pelvic pain from peritoneal irritation. Large ovarian cysts are more likely to undergo torsion and can cause pain from ischemia.

KEY TREATMENT

- Medical and surgical treatments for ectopic pregnancy are equivalent when patient selection is appropriate (ACOG, 2008) (SOR: B).
- Single-dose methotrexate is the most common regimen (50 mg/m^2 body surface IM) for ectopic pregnancy (ACOG, 2008) (SOR: C).
- Clinicians should have a low threshold for treating women with suspected PID because of potential long-term consequences (BASHH, 2005) (SOR: C).

CHRONIC PELVIC PAIN

Key Points

- Chronic pelvic pain is an indication for up to 40% of the laparoscopies in the United States.
- The four most common causes of chronic pelvic pain are endometriosis, pelvic adhesions, interstitial cystitis, and irritable bowel syndrome.
- Up to 70% of women with chronic pelvic pain have more than one cause for their pain.
- Up to half of all women with chronic pelvic pain have a history of abuse or trauma.

Chronic pelvic pain is defined as noncyclic pain that lasts longer than 6 months. It occurs frequently, affecting up to 15% of all women at some point in their reproductive years. Chronic pelvic pain is a diagnosis associated with up to 10% of all outpatient gynecologic consultations, 40% of all laparoscopies, and 18% of all hysterectomies performed each year in the United States (Zondervan and Barlow, 2000). In 1996, the estimated cost of services related to chronic pelvic pain was $880 million (Yunker et al., 2012).

Almost half of all women with chronic pelvic pain have a history of past sexual abuse or depression (Latthe et al., 2006). Women with a history of trauma have more severe symptoms (Meltzer-Brody et al., 2007). A meta-analysis of women with a history of abuse found an increased prevalence of functional bowel disorders, nonspecific chronic pain, and chronic pelvic pain (Paras et al., 2009). Drug and alcohol abuse are associated with an increased likelihood of pain (Latthe et al., 2006). There is no difference in prevalence based on race, ethnicity, education, or socioeconomic status (ACOG, 2004).

The etiology of chronic pelvic pain is frequently multifactorial and comes from multiple organ systems. Up to 70% of women have more than one cause of pain (Butrick, 2007). The most common gynecologic causes of chronic pelvic pain are endometriosis and pelvic adhesions. The most common GI cause is irritable bowel syndrome, and the most common urologic cause is interstitial cystitis (Bordman and Jackson, 2006). In addition, many women who have chronic pelvic pain also have some myofascial pain from the pelvic floor muscles (Table 25-10).

The initial evaluation of a woman with chronic pelvic pain includes a careful history to determine any pattern of the pain that would lead to a possible diagnosis. For example, a history of abdominal surgery increases the risk of pelvic adhesions. A complete medical, surgical, family, sexual, and psychological history should also be completed. It is important to determine how the pain is affecting the woman's daily life. The physical examination should include a general examination in addition to a thorough pelvic assessment. Every effort should be made to replicate the pain through a bimanual or rectovaginal examination.

Laboratory evaluation is focused on the likely diagnosis. Many women have pelvic ultrasonography for further evaluation of the pelvic anatomy. Ultimately, many women undergo a diagnostic laparoscopy to evaluate the etiology of the pain. Laparoscopy is normal in 35% to 40% of these women. Endometriosis is diagnosed in about 30% of women

Table 25-10   Common Causes of Chronic Pelvic Pain

Gynecologic	Endometriosis
	Pelvic adhesions
	Pelvic congestion
	Pelvic inflammatory disease
	Adenomyosis
	Vulvodynia
	Uterine myomas
Gastrointestinal	Irritable bowel syndrome
	Inflammatory bowel disease
	Chronic constipation
	Colitis
	Diverticulitis
Urologic	Interstitial cystitis
	Chronic urinary tract infections
	Urethral syndrome
	Radiation cystitis
	Urinary calculi
Musculoskeletal	Myofascial pain (abdominal wall or pelvic floor muscles)
	Fibromyalgia
	Coccygeal or low back pain
	Nerve pain

Modified from Bordman R, Jackson B. Below the belt: approach to chronic pelvic pain. *Can Fam Physician.* 2006;52:1556-1562 and Reiter RC. Chronic pelvic pain. *Clin Obstet Gynecol.* 1990;33:117-118.

at laparoscopy, and adhesions are diagnosed in about 25% (Howard, 2000).

Treatment of a woman with chronic pelvic pain should be multimodal to address the multifactorial nature of her pain (ACOG, 2004; Stones et al., 2009). A strong physician–patient relationship is imperative as a basis for successful treatment. First-line treatment includes pain control with nonnarcotic medication. Hormonal manipulation with medroxyprogesterone acetate, combined hormonal contraception, or gonadotropin-releasing hormone (GnRH) analogues can be effective treatments for endometriosis-related pain. GnRH analogues can only be used for up to 6 months because of side effects (e.g., menopausal symptoms, osteoporosis).

Laparoscopic treatment of endometriosis and lysis of dense adhesions are helpful in a subset of women. Lysis of adhesions that are not severe has not consistently decreased pain (ACOG, 2004). Hysterectomy is performed in women with untreatable pain and is most effective if accompanied by bilateral oophorectomy. Hysterectomy is major surgery with many potential complications but can cure some cases of pain related to endometriosis. Uterosacral nerve ablation is not an effective method for treating idiopathic chronic pelvic pain (Daniels et al., 2009).

None of the listed treatment modalities addresses the *physiology* of chronic pain. Several newer anticonvulsants (gabapentin, topiramate, valproic acid, pregabalin) and antidepressants, such as tricyclic antidepressants and selective serotonin reuptake inhibitors, have been successful in treating neuropathic pain from other sources. However, limited data are available in women with pelvic pain. Trigger point injections and botulinum toxin (Botox) injections in pelvic floor muscles show promise for treating myofascial pain (Gomel, 2007). Multidisciplinary treatment teams should include mental health professionals and physical therapists as well as physicians.

- Treatment of chronic pelvic pain should be multidisciplinary and include a mental health professional (Stones et al., 2009) (SOR: A).
- Uterosacral nerve ablation is **not** an effective method for treating idiopathic chronic pelvic pain (Daniels et al., 2009) (SOR: A).
- First-line treatment includes pain control with nonnarcotic medication (ACOG, 2004) (SOR: A).
- Hormonal manipulation with medroxyprogesterone acetate, combined hormonal contraception, or GnRH analogues can be effective treatments for endometriosis-related pain (ACOG, 2004) (SOR: A).

Menopause

Key Points

- The average age of menopause is 52 years.
- Vasomotor symptoms are the most common menopausal sign.
- The Women's Health Initiative (WHI) showed that hormone replacement therapy did not prevent cardiovascular disease in postmenopausal women and in fact increased the risk of breast cancer.

Menopause is defined as the cessation of menstruation. It is a retrospective diagnosis that comes after a woman has not menstruated for 12 months. The menopausal transition occurs over several years as the number of ovarian follicles slowly decreases. This period in a woman's life can include menstrual cycles of variable lengths and durations, called the *perimenopause.* Because of the waxing number of follicles, the ovaries require higher levels of estrogen to stimulate a LH surge and subsequent ovulation. Consequently, serum levels of estrogen can vary substantially from one cycle to the next. The first physiologic change noted is a decrease in inhibin B levels (Burger et al., 1999). Subsequently, FSH level will increase in response to lower estrogen levels. An FSH level greater than 40 U/L on two separate occasions at least 1 month apart is diagnostic of menopause. The main pathologic cause of abnormal vaginal bleeding during this period is anovulation in those cycles when estrogen did not reach target levels.

The average age of menopause in the United States is 52 years old. The majority of women will go through menopause between ages 40 and 58 years. Menopause before age 40 years is defined as premature ovarian failure and may be related to other autoimmune disease. Factors associated with age at menopause include smoking and family history (Nelson, 2008).

Vasomotor symptoms, including hot flashes and night sweats, are the most common symptoms of menopause. Some women may begin to experience these symptoms years before their final menstrual period, during the months where their estrogen levels are lower. Many women experience symptoms for several years. Up to 10% of women continue to experience vasomotor symptoms into their 70s (Politi et al., 2008). Symptoms are worse in women who experience premature ovarian failure, have a premenopausal oophorectomy, are overweight or obese, or are depressed (Hendrix, 2005). Treatment of vasomotor symptoms begins with lifestyle changes and can also include pharmacologic treatment with hormonal or nonhormonal medications. Women may be able to manage their vasomotor symptoms by wearing natural-fiber clothing in layers, avoiding spicy foods, avoiding hot environments (e.g., saunas, hot tubs), avoiding alcohol, exercising, and maintaining a healthy weight.

Pharmacologic treatment of vasomotor symptoms includes HT at the lowest effective doses orally or transdermally (Bachmann et al., 2007). HT should include both estrogen and progestin in women who have a uterus and estrogen alone in women who have had a hysterectomy. HT should be used in women at the lowest possible doses to treat symptoms for as short a time as possible (North American Menopause Society [NAMS], 2012). Transdermal HT has a lower risk of thromboembolism (ACOG, 2013). In women for whom HT is contraindicated or who are worried about the risks, several nonhormonal options have been studied. Antidepressant medications such as fluoxetine, paroxetine, and venlafaxine have been shown to be better than placebo. Gabapentin, 900 mg/day (dosed either as 300 mg three times a day or 900 mg at night), is also better than placebo in treating hot flashes (Grady, 2006).

Many women use complementary therapies to treat vasomotor symptoms. Various herbal preparations (e.g., black cohosh) have been used to treat vasomotor symptoms with varying success. Many women also obtain relief from soy products or other isoflavones. However, none of these treatments has consistently been more effective than placebo in randomized trials (Nelson et al., 2006). Stress management and meditation show promise in controlling these troublesome symptoms (Tremblay et al., 2008).

Atrophic vaginitis, or thinning of the vaginal epithelium caused by a lack of estrogen stimulation after menopause, is common, affecting 10% to 40% of all postmenopausal women. Women complain of vaginal dryness, irritation, and pain with intercourse. Unlike vasomotor symptoms, atrophic vaginitis does not develop immediately after menopause but causes symptoms months to years after the withdrawal of estrogen. Left untreated, atrophic vaginitis is progressive and is unlikely to improve spontaneously. Treatment of atrophic vaginitis begins with use of appropriate water-based lubricants to make intercourse more comfortable. The mainstay of treatment is vaginal estrogen (NAMS, 2013). Several preparations of vaginal estrogen are available in the United States. Estrogen cream, tablets, and a slow-release silicone ring are all well tolerated and are equally effective in reducing symptoms of atrophic vaginitis. Because the vaginal estrogen has limited systemic absorption, a concomitant dosing with progestin is not necessary, although safety studies are not available for more than 1 year of therapy (NAMS, 2013). The FDA recently approved a dedicated product for treating atrophic vaginitis and associated dyspareunia. Ospemifine is a selective estrogen receptor modulator and is effective at reducing symptoms related to atrophic vaginitis. Its main side effect is hot flashes (Portman et al., 2013).

Other common menopausal changes include memory difficulty (mostly with word finding), mood lability, and decreased libido (from decreased testosterone levels after menopause).

Before the WHI, HT was used for prevention of heart disease and osteoporosis. The WHI was a large (>16,000 participants) population-based study of women between 50 and 79 years studying the effectiveness of estrogen plus progestin on congestive heart disease (CHD) prevention. The trial was stopped early because of excess cardiovascular and breast cancer events. There was an excess of seven CHD events, eight strokes, eight breast cancers, and 14 venous thromboembolic events per 10,000 women. The estrogen-only arm of the study was stopped 2 years later because of excess strokes (12 per 10,000 women). There was no statistically significant increase in breast cancer incidence in the estrogen-only group (Manson et al., 2013). The HT group in both arms of the study had fewer hip fractures.

KEY TREATMENT

- HT can be used for treatment of menopausal symptoms but should be used at the lowest possible dose for the shortest time possible with consideration of non-oral routs (NAMS, 2013) (SOR: C).
- Atrophic vaginitis is treated most effectively by vaginal estrogen cream or tablets, usually three times a week initially and titrated down based on symptoms (NAMS, 2013) (SOR: A).

- Antidepressant medications (fluoxetine, paroxetine, venlafaxine) are better than placebo in treating hot flashes (Grady, 2006) (SOR: A).
- Gabapentin (900 mg/day—dosed either 300 mg three times a day or 900 mg at bedtime) is also better than placebo in treating hot flashes (Grady, 2006) (SOR: A).
- Stress management and meditation show promise in controlling troublesome menopausal symptoms (Tremblay et al., 2008) (SOR: B).

References

The complete reference list is available at www.expertconsult.com.

Web Resources

http://www.uspreventiveservicestaskforce.org/recommendations.htm U.S. Preventive Services Task Force screening recommendations. Includes the Electronic Preventive Services Selector (enter a patient's age and gender and receive a list of evidence-based recommendations) and the option to sign up for e-mail updates on preventive services.

http://www.asccp.org/Portals/9/docs/ASCCP%20Management%20 Guidelines_August%202014.pdf American Society for Colposcopy and Cervical Pathology guidelines for management of abnormal Pap test results. Provides detailed algorithms describing how to manage each specific Pap smear abnormality.

www.cdc.gov/std/treatment The 2006 sexually transmitted infection treatment guidelines provide detailed recommendations for treatment of all sexually transmitted diseases as well as other types of vaginitis.

http://www.cdc.gov/vaccines/schedules/ Centers for Disease Control and Prevention and Advisory Committee on Immunization Practices immunization guidelines, including tables for adults, adolescents, and pregnant women; e-mail updates are also available.

26 *Contraception*

DIANE M. HARPER, LAUREN E. WILFLING, and CHRISTOPHER F. BLANNER

Key Points

- Estrogen and progestin dosing often needs to be changed over time from the adolescent to perimenopausal years as a woman ages.
- There are multiple choices of estrogen and progestin contraceptives that will meet the ever-changing needs of most women.
- Progestin-only contraception creates an estrogen deficiency state, leading to early cycle bleeding or continuous bleeding throughout the cycle.
- Copper intrauterine devices (IUDs) are the most effective emergency contraception.
- Low dose progestin IUDs are recommended for early adolescence to avoid noncompliance.

Healthy People 2020 aims to reduce unintended pregnancy from 49% of pregnancies to 44% of pregnancies over the next 10 years (Guttmacher Institute, 2013). Nearly half of these pregnancies result in abortion (Figure 26-1). The youngest adolescent females have the highest rate of unintended pregnancy (Figure 26-2). This results in delayed independent social development, such as being less likely to graduate from high school or attain a GED before 30 years of age or receiving more federal aid for longer time frames than those who do not have an unintended pregnancy (Hoffman 2006; Hoffman and Maynard, 2008).

Regardless of whether the pregnancy is intentional or not or whether the mother and child are socially dependent or not, birth-related deaths are real and occur at all ages, more frequently as women age (Figure 26-3). The use of low-dose hormonal contraceptives in the form of pills, implants, IUDs, rings, and patches has significantly reduced the risk of death from hormone-related side effects in all age groups except women 40 years and older, in whom only oral contraceptive pills (OCPs), regardless of tobacco use, carry a higher death risk. The social use of contraceptives is thus twofold: to prevent premature deaths of women of childbearing age and to provide choice about conception.

The Centers for Disease Control and Prevention (CDC, 2010) has published a pictorial guide of all contraceptive methods and their failure rates (Figure 26-4). Among those 15 to 44 years old in the United States who use contraception, OCPs are the most common method used (27.5%) followed closely by female sterilization (26.6%). Male condom (16%) and male sterilization (10%) constitute the next largest share of the contraceptive burden, with IUDs and withdrawal (coitus interruptus) each sharing about 5% of the burden (Mosher and Jones, 2010).

This chapter describes the decision-making process that has the potential to minimize side effects and maximize compliance among adolescents and women of all ages who choose to take OCPs on a daily basis. The method relies on an understanding of the side effects of estrogen and progestin and the subtle change in hormonal concentrations that may make the difference between compliance and noncompliance. The effects of the hormones on the hypothalamic–pituitary–ovarian (HPO) axis and their effects on each other cannot be separated as cleanly, as these tables represent. The metabolic activity of progestins varies widely, and the attempt to convert all compounds to a norethindrone equivalent is limited by extrapolation from animal data. But the hallmarks of this decision-making methodology, which include categorization of symptoms of each of the hormonal components, flexibility in preparations available for prescribing, and patience with trying new formulations, allow practicing physicians to find the hormonal formulations that match women's ever-changing bodies.

Combined Oral Contraceptive Pills

Key Points

- Modern OCPs have multiple mechanisms by which they cause infertility and risks that must be weighed against the risk of pregnancy.
- Ethinyl estradiol, the estrogen component of all combined OCPs except for one, is a key driver of pill-related symptoms, and the dose should be adjusted to the particular woman's needs.
- There are four generations of progestins currently in use in the United States, with each generation having unique symptoms and side effects leading to unique medical, social, and legal issues (Davtyan, 2012).
- OCPs can both mask and enhance androgenic symptoms in individual women, and these affects can be a key part of comprehensive contraceptive management.
- The initial selection of an OCP should be individual specific, but for those with no prior menstrual difficulties, no risk factors, and no experience with using OCPs, any preparation up to 735 μg of ethinyl estradiol per 28-day cycle is appropriate.

Exogenous hormones of sufficient concentration alter the HPO axis and inhibit ovarian cycling, thus causing temporary infertility. Low-dose combined OCPs, however, rely more on the progestational component to cross-link the cervical mucus, making it impenetrable to sperm, than on the estrogen to inhibit follicular maturation. This nuance allows personal sensitivities to hormone concentrations to direct pill-prescribing patterns.

The risk of taking estrogen-containing contraceptives must be weighed against the risk of pregnancy. Those at increased risk of side effects from combined OCPs are women who smoke more than 15 cigarettes a day; who are 35 years old or older; or who have cardiac disease, hypertension, cerebrovascular disease, renal disease, diabetes with end-organ damage or a family history of diabetes, sickle cell disease (hemoglobin SS or SC), systemic lupus erythematosus, active gallbladder disease, congenital hyperbilirubinemia (Gilbert's disease), history of death of a parent or sibling from myocardial infarction before age 50 years (especially if it was a mother or sister), family history

of hyperlipidemia, risk for deep vein thrombosis or pulmonary embolism, or migraine headaches.

No OCP should be used in women with undiagnosed abnormal genital bleeding, liver tumors, or breast cancer or other estrogen- or progestin-sensitive cancer or who are pregnant.

ESTROGEN

Prior OCP formulations used high-dose mestranol as the estrogen component of OCPs, but because of the serious side effects of mestranol, as well as other high-dose estrogens, a low-dose ethinyl estradiol is currently used in all pill formulations except for one quadriphasic pill.

The metabolism of ethinyl estradiol varies significantly from individual to individual and from one population to another population (Goldzieher, 1990) with the same single dose able to create side effects of excessive systemic estrogen in one woman and side effects of estrogen deficiency in another (Table 26-1). Individual effects of the hormones cannot be precisely defined, but the effects of estrogen are often a predominant driver of symptom expression. This decision-making guide allows changes in OCPs to trend with the woman's needs. There are six pills with ethinyl estradiol content per 28 days below 500 µg, four below 600 µg, eight below 700 µg, 10 below 800 µg, two below 900 µg, and four with ethinyl estradiol content per 28 days above 1000 µg.

PROGESTIN

There are four generations of progestins used in OCPs. The first-generation progestins (e.g., norethindrone and norethindrone acetate) were formulated for ovarian suppression. Second-generation progestins are mainly used alone in the depomedroxyprogesterone acetate (DMPA) formula or as the progestin for hormone therapy in postmenopausal women. Third- (e.g., levonorgestrel, desogestrel, gestodene) and fourth- (e.g., drospirenone) generation

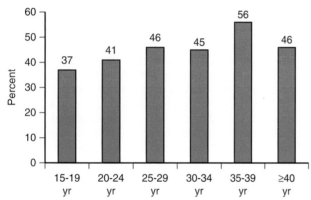

Figure 26-1 Percentage of unintended pregnancies ending in abortion by age group. (Data from Finer LB, Zolna MR. Shifts in intended and unintended pregnancies in the United States, 2001-2008. *Am J Public Health.* 2014;104(suppl 1):S43-S48.)

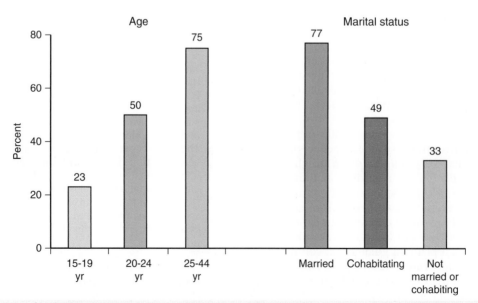

Figure 26-2 Percentage of births that were intended at conception, by mother's age and marital status at birth: United States, 2006 to 2010. (Data from Mosher WD, Jones J, Abma JC. Intended and unintended births in the United States: 1982-2010. *Natl Health Stat Report.* 2012;(55):1-28.)

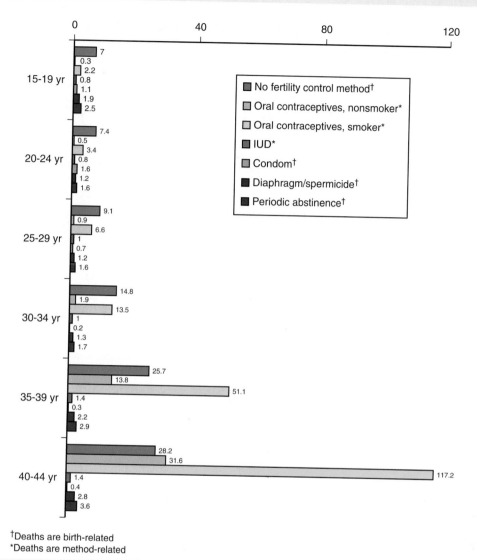

†Deaths are birth-related
*Deaths are method-related

Figure 26-3 Birth-related and method-related deaths per 100,000 nonsterile women per year by age group and contraceptive choice. (Data from Ory HW. Mortality associated with fertility and fertility control: 1983. *Fam Plann Perspect.* 1983;15:50-56.)

progestins were developed for the antiestrogenic properties in the endometrium, making it inhospitable for implantation, in addition to addressing the systemic effects of estrogen excess (bloating and cyclic weight gain) and androgenic excess (acne, hirsutism, and oily skin). These progestins have minimal androgenic and increased mineralocorticoid effects (Table 26-2). Although increasing doses of estrogen in OCPs are associated with increased risk of arterial thrombotic events, an increased threefold risk of venous thrombotic events occurs equally with the first three generations of progestins (Stegeman et al., 2013).

The only fourth-generation progestin used in OCPs in the United States is drospirenone. This progestin is derived from 17 α-spironolactone rather than from the 19-nortestosterone associated with prior generations of progestins. Over time, studies have shown a doubling of the risk of venous thromboembolism in OCPs containing drospirenone than in those containing levonorgestrel, and a sixfold increase over those not using any OCP (Wu, 2013). More than $1.6 billion has been paid in lawsuits to Yaz and

Yasmin users. Use of contraceptives containing drospirenone has plummeted for this reason.

The progestin content converted to norethindrone equivalents per 28 days ranges from less than 5 mg to more than 35 mg of norethindrone with a single formulation below 5 mg for those exquisitely sensitive to progestin excess, three formulations below 10 mg, eight at or below 15 mg, four below 20 mg, seven below 25 mg, and four above 30 mg norethindrone equivalents per 28 days.

ANDROGEN

Androgenic symptoms (Table 26-3) are only expressed when androgen is overabundant. To decrease androgen production, combined OCPs can act to suppress the ovarian testosterone production as well as increase the quantity of sex hormone–binding globulin, which binds whatever free testosterone there is available. With the lower dose contraceptive combinations, ovarian suppression is less likely to occur, allowing the exogenous progestin formulations in

Effectiveness of Family Planning Methods

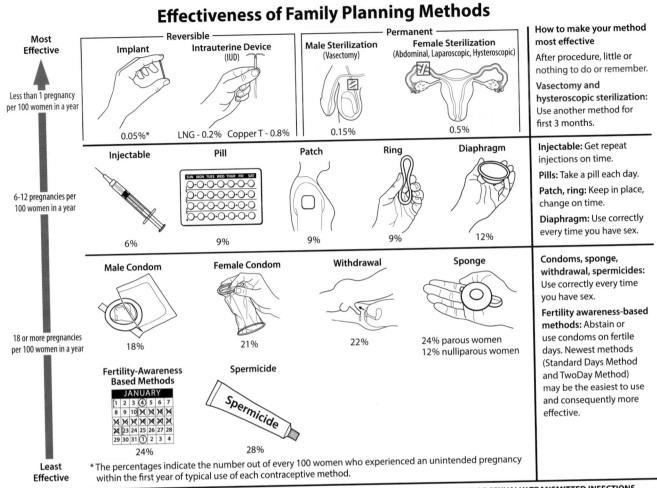

				How to make your method most effective
Most Effective ↑ Less than 1 pregnancy per 100 women in a year	Reversible — Implant 0.05%* / Intrauterine Device (IUD) LNG - 0.2% Copper T - 0.8%	Permanent — Male Sterilization (Vasectomy) 0.15%	Female Sterilization (Abdominal, Laparoscopic, Hysteroscopic) 0.5%	After procedure, little or nothing to do or remember. **Vasectomy and hysteroscopic sterilization:** Use another method for first 3 months.

Less than 1 pregnancy per 100 women in a year

6-12 pregnancies per 100 women in a year

Injectable 6%   Pill 9%   Patch 9%   Ring 9%   Diaphragm 12%

Injectable: Get repeat injections on time.
Pills: Take a pill each day.
Patch, ring: Keep in place, change on time.
Diaphragm: Use correctly every time you have sex.

18 or more pregnancies per 100 women in a year

Male Condom 18%   Female Condom 21%   Withdrawal 22%   Sponge 24% parous women 12% nulliparous women

Fertility-Awareness Based Methods 24%   Spermicide 28%

Condoms, sponge, withdrawal, spermicides: Use correctly every time you have sex.
Fertility awareness-based methods: Abstain or use condoms on fertile days. Newest methods (Standard Days Method and TwoDay Method) may be the easiest to use and consequently more effective.

Least Effective   * The percentages indicate the number out of every 100 women who experienced an unintended pregnancy within the first year of typical use of each contraceptive method.

CS 242797

CONDOMS SHOULD ALWAYS BE USED TO REDUCE THE RISK OF SEXUALLY TRANSMITTED INFECTIONS.

<u>Other Methods of Contraception</u>
Lactational Amenorrhea Method: LAM is a highly effective, temporary method of contraception.
Emergency Contraception: Emergency contraceptive pills or a copper IUD after unprotected intercourse substantially reduces risk of pregnancy.

Adapted from World Health Organization (WHO) Department of Reproductive Health and Research, Johns Hopkins Bloomberg School of Public Health/Center for Communication Programs (CCP). Knowledge for health project. Family planning: a global handbook for providers (2011 update). Baltimore, MD; Geneva, Switzerland: CCP and WHO; 2011; and Trussell J. Contraceptive failure in the United States. Contraception 2011;83:397–404.

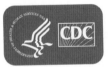

U.S. Department of Health and Human Services
Centers for Disease Control and Prevention

Figure 26-4 Failure rates of family planning methods. (From Centers for Disease Control and Prevention. U.S. Medical Eligibility Criteria for Contraceptive Use, 2010. Adapted from the World Health Organization Medical Eligibility Criteria for Contraceptive Use, 4th edition, May 28, 2010. http://www.cdc.gov/mmwr/preview/mmwrhtml/rr59e0528a1.htm.)

---

the contraceptives to contribute to androgenic side effects. The side effects are again individual in expression and can be managed by changing pills.

CHOOSING A COMBINED ORAL CONTRACEPTIVE PILL

Table 26-4 lists the contraindications to OCPs. Table 26-5 lists the OCPs currently approved in the United States by the Food and Drug Administration (FDA), with their estrogen, progestin, and androgen content per 28-day cycle (Dickey and Dickey, 2010; Harper, 2001). Many competing products have the same composition. Of note, generics may not always be cheaper than brand-name drugs and by law need to be only 80% as effective (bioequivalent; CDC, 2014; Hupila and Smith, 2008) as the brand-name product.

Selection of the initial pill formulation should take into account the patient's body mass index because obese women require, in general, higher doses of estrogen and progestin to induce infertility without bleeding side effects (Reifsnider et al., 2013). Other patient characteristics to consider are acne, depression, and propensity to gain weight, all of which can be modified by a change in hormonal dose. A physical examination, including blood pressure, lipid levels, liver and renal function, query about pregnancy status, and documentation of current bleeding patterns, is recommended before a woman starts OCPs.

For women with no prior menstrual difficulties, no risk factors, and no experience with using OCPs, any preparation up to 735 µg of ethinyl estradiol per 28-day cycle is appropriate. Pills with lower androgen levels may be less likely to cause acne and other adverse cosmetic effects.

A 3-month trial is necessary to understand how the body will respond to any new hormonal regimen. If this will be the patient's first experience with OCPs, warnings about breast tenderness and nausea increasing over the first

Table 26-1 Estrogen Side Effects

	Excess	Deficiency
General	Bloating (fluid retention)* Edema Irritability* Weight gain (cyclic)*	Nervousness
Cardiovascular	Capillary fragility Cerebrovascular accident Deep vein thrombosis Pulmonary emboli Telangiectasia Thromboembolic disease	
Gastrointestinal	Hepatocellular adenomas Hepatocellular cancer Nausea and vomiting	
Urinary		Pelvic relaxation symptoms
Gynecologic	Cervical extrophy* Cystic breast changes Dysmenorrhea* Hypermenorrhea, menorrhagia* Increase in breast size (ductal and fatty tissue) Leukorrhea or mucorrhea Uterine enlargement Uterine fibroid growth	Absence of withdrawal bleeding Atrophic vaginitis Hypomenorrhea Breakthrough bleeding and spotting: 1. Early cycle (pill days 1-9) 2. Continuous spotting (throughout cycle)
Neurologic	Dizziness Headaches (cyclic: vascular [migraine]) Visual changes (cyclic)	Vasomotor symptoms
Musculoskeletal	Leg cramps	
Dermatologic	Chloasma	

*Most common.
Based on information in Dickey R, Dickey RP. *Managing contraceptive pill/ drug patients*. 14th ed. Durant, OK: Essential Medical Information Systems; 2010.

Table 26-2 Progestin Side Effects

	Excess	Deficiency
General	Decreased libido Depression* Increased appetite (noncyclic weight gain)* Fatigue*	
Cardiovascular	Hypertension	
Metabolic	Decreased carbohydrate tolerance (diabetogenic) Decreased HDL cholesterol Increased LDL cholesterol	
Gynecologic	Cervicitis Decreased flow length Candidiasis* Increased breast size (alveolar tissue) Withdrawal bleeding delayed	Dysmenorrhea Breakthrough bleeding (pill days 10-21) Hypermenorrhea, menorrhagia Vaginal bleeding and spotting
Dermatologic	Neurodermatitis, pruritus	

*Most common.
HDL, High-density lipoprotein; *LDL*, low-density lipoprotein.
Based on information in Dickey R, Dickey RP. *Managing contraceptive pill/ drug patients*. 14th ed. Durant, OK: Essential Medical information Systems; 2010.

Table 26-3 Androgen Symptoms

Excess
Acne* Cholestatic jaundice Edema Hirsutism* Increased libido Oily skin and scalp* Pruritus Rash

*Most common.
Based on information in Dickey R, Dickey RP. *Managing contraceptive pill/ drug patients*. 14th ed. Durant, OK: Essential Medical information Systems; 2010.

Table 26-4 Contraindications to Oral Contraceptive Pills

Absolute contraindications	Acute phase mononucleosis
	History of
	    Cerebrovascular accident
	    Coronary artery disease
	    Known or suspected breast carcinoma
	    Known or suspected estrogen-dependent neoplasia
	    Liver neoplasia, malignant or benign
	    Thrombophlebitis or thromboembolic disorder (also factor V Leiden mutation carriers)
	Pregnancy

Relative contraindications	Completion of term pregnancy within previous 3 weeks Hypertension of 140/90 mm Hg at three visits Diastolic hypertension of >110 mm Hg at one visit Impaired liver function Lactation Major injury or immobilization of lower extremities Major surgery planned in next 4 weeks Previous cholestasis during pregnancy Undiagnosed abnormal vaginal bleeding

month of hormone use are necessary to prevent premature cessation ("I can't take pills; they don't agree with me."). If the patient has adverse effects after 3 months, they are valid and should be addressed. She should be assured that continuing problems can likely be corrected by switching to a different pill. Only about 16% of women are unable to take OCPs for medical reasons (Shortridge and Miller, 2007). Most women quit using OCPs because of side effects that remain unaddressed by providers who lack knowledge of the 34 different hormonal combinations possible.

New pill regimens should be started at the end of a 28-day cycle of prior hormones and can be done based on patient symptomatology rather than requiring an office visit (Guttmacher Institute, 2008). Dispensing three packages at a time allows uninterrupted dosing. Symptom-based adjustments can be managed in a stepwise fashion: (1) identify the most significant adverse effects and the hormone most likely to be the cause, (2) determine the content of the current pill formulation, (3) keep the level of the components that are not causing problems stable, and (4) find a pill with a greater or lesser amount of the component responsible for the side effect (see Table 26-5).

Table 26-5   Oral Contraceptive Pills: Estrogen, Progestin, and Androgen Content Per 28 Days

Estrogen (µg Ethinyl Estradiol)	Progestin (mg Norethindrone)*	Androgen (mg Methyl-Testosterone)†	Number of Days: Ethinyl Estradiol Dose	Number of Days: Progestin Dose	Brand Name‡ (Phasic)
420	11.1	0.39	21:20 µg	21:0.10 mg LN	Alesse (mono) *Aviane* (mono) *Falmina* (mono) *Lutera* (mono) *Orsythia* (mono)
420	11.1	0.39	21:20 µg	21:0.10 mg LN	Loestrin 1/20 (mono) *Junel* (mono) *Microgestin* (mono)
420	11.1	0.39	21:20 µg	21:0.10 mg LN	Levlite (mono) *Lessina* (mono) *Sronyx* (mono)
470	12.6	0.42	21:20 µg 5:10 µg	21:0.15 mg DG	Mircette (bi) *Azurette* (bi) *Kariva* (bi) *Jenest-28* (bi)
480	no data	0	24:20 µg	24:3 mg DRSP	Yaz (mono) *Loryna* (mono) *Vestura* (mono) *Gianvi* (mono)
480	no data	0	24:20 µg	24:3 mg DRSP	Beyaz (mono)
525	4.5	0.09	7:25 µg 7:25 µg 7:25 µg	7:0.18 mg NORG 7:0.215 mg NORG 7:0.25 mg NORG	Ortho Tri-Cyclen Lo
525	10.5	0.35	7:25 µg 7:25 µg 7:25 µg	7:0.1 mg DG 7:0.125 mg DG 7:0.15 mg DG	Cyclessa (mono) *Caziant* (mono) *Cesia* (mono) *Velivet* (mono)
560	14.8	0.52	84:20 µg 7:10 µg	84:0.10 mg LN 7:0 mg LN	LoSeasonique (mono) *Camrese Lo* (mono) *Amethia Lo* (mono)
560	14.8	0.52	28:20 µg	28:0.09 mg LN	Lybrel (mono) *Amethyst* (mono)
625	21	0.42	5:20 µg 7:30 µg 9:35 µg	21:1 mg NE	Estrostep (tri)
630	12.6	0.42	21:30 µg	21:0.15 mg DG	Desogen (mono) Ortho-Cept (mono) *Apri* (mono) *Enskyce* (mono) *Reclipsen* (mono) *Emoquette* (mono) *Solia* (mono)
630	16.4	0.59	21:30 µg	21:0.3 mg NG	Lo/Ovral (mono) *Low-Ogestrel* (mono) *Cryselle* (mono) *Elinest* (mono)
630	16.7	0.59	21:30 µg	21:0.15 mg LN	Nordette (mono) *Levlen* (mono) *Levora 0.15/30* (mono) *Altavera* (mono) *Kurvelo* (mono) *Portia* (mono)
630	37.8	1.01	21:30 µg	21:1.5 mg NG	Loestrin 1.5/30 (mono) *Altavera* (mono)
630	no data	0	21:30 µg	21:3 mg DRSP	Yasmin (mono) *Ocella* (mono) *Syeda* (mono) *Zarah* (mono)
680	10.2	0.87	6:30 µg 5:40 µg 10:30 µg	6:0.05 LN 5:0.075 LN 10:0.125 LN	Triphasil (tri) Tri-Levlen (tri) *Trivora* (tri) *Enpresse* (tri) *Levonest* (tri) *Myzilra* (tri)

Table 26-5 Oral Contraceptive Pills: Estrogen, Progestin, and Androgen Content Per 28 Days (Continued)

Estrogen (μg Ethinyl Estradiol)	Progestin (mg Norethindrone)*	Androgen (mg Methyl-Testosterone)†	Number of Days: Ethinyl Estradiol Dose	Number of Days: Progestin Dose	Brand Name‡ (Phasic)
704	21	0.42	21:50 μg	21:1 mg NE	Ortho-Novum 1/50 (mono) *Norinyl 1+50 (mono)* *Necon 1/50 (mono)* Genora 1/50 (mono) Nelova 1/50 (mono) Norethin 1/50M (mono)
735	5.4	0.17	7:35 μg 7:35 μg 7:35 μg	7:0.18 mg NORG 7:0.215 mg NORG 7:0.25 mg NORG	Ortho Tri-Cyclen (tri) *Trinessa (tri)* *Tri-Sprintec (tri)* *Tri-Privifem (tri)* *Tri-Linyah (tri)* *Tri-Estarylla (tri)*
735	6.3	0.2	21:35 μg	21:0.25 mg NORG	Ortho-Cyclen (mono) *Estarylla (mono)* *Mono-Linyah (mono)* *MonoNessa (mono)* *Previfem (mono)* *Sprintec (mono)*
735	8.4	0.17	21:35 μg	21:0.4 mg NE	Ovcon 35 (mono) *Briellyn (mono)* *Balziva (mono)* *Zenchent (mono)* *Philith (mono)*
735	10.5	0.21	21:35 μg	21:0.5 mg NE	Brevicon (mono) 0.5/35 Modicon (mono) *Necon 0.5/35 (mono)* *Nortrel 0.5/35 (mono)* *Wera (mono)* Genora 0.5/35 (mono) Modicon (mono) Nelova 0.5/35E (mono)
735	15	0.3	7:35 μg 9:35 μg 5:35 μg	7:0.5 mg NE 9:1 mg NE 5:0.5 mg NE	Tri-Norinyl (tri) *Aranella (tri)* *Leena (tri)*
735	15.8	0.3	7:35 μg 7:35 μg 7:35 μg	7:0.5 mg NE 7:0.75 mg NE 7:1 mg NE	Ortho-Novum 7/7/7 (tri) *Alyacen 7/7/7 (tri)* *Necon 7/7/7 (tri)* *Nortrel 7/7/7 (tri)* *Cyclafem 7/7/7 (tri)* *Dasetta 7/7/7 (tri)* *Pirmella 7/7/7 (tri)*
735	16	0.032	21:35 μg	21:1 mg NE	Ortho-Novum 1/35 (mono) *Necon 1/35 (mono)* *Norinyl 1+35 (mono)* *Nortrel 1/35 (mono)* *Cyclafem 1/35 (mono)* *Alyacen 1/35 (mono)* *Dasetta 1/35 (mono)* *Pirmella 1/35 (mono)* Genora 1/35 (mono) Nelova 1/35 (mono) Norethin 1/35E (mono)
735	21	0.42	10:35 μg 11:35 μg	10:0.5 mg NE 11:1 mg NE	Ortho-Novum 10/11 (bi) *Necon 10/11 (bi)* *Nelova 10/11 (bi)*
735	29.4	0.25	21:35 μg	21:1 mg ED	Demulen 1/35 (mono) Zovia 1/35E (mono)
840	22.3	0.56	84:30 μg	84:0.15 mg LN	Seasonale (mono) *Daysee (mono)* *Quasense (mono)* *Jolessa (mono)* *Introvale (mono)*
840	22.3	0.79	84:30 μg 7:10 μg	84:0.15 mg LN 7:0 mg LN	Seasonique (mono) *Amethia (mono)* *Camrese (mono)*

Continued on following page

Table 26-5 Oral Contraceptive Pills: Estrogen, Progestin, and Androgen Content Per 28 Days (Continued)

Estrogen (µg Ethinyl Estradiol)	Progestin (mg Norethindrone)*	Androgen (mg Methyl-Testosterone)†	Number of Days: Ethinyl Estradiol Dose	Number of Days: Progestin Dose	Brand Name‡ (Phasic)
1050	21	0.17	21:50 µg	21:1 mg NE	Ovcon 50 (mono)
1050	27.3	0.99	21:50 µg	21:0.5 mg NORG	Ovral (mono) Ogestrel (mono)
1050	29.4	0.25	21:50 µg	21:1 mg ED	Demulen 1/50 (mono) Zovia 1/50 (mono)
1050	29.4	0.25	21:35 µg	21:1 mg ED	Demulen 1/35 (mono) Zovia 1/35 (mono) Kelnor (mono)
–	4.9	0.10	—	28:0.075 mg DG	Cerzette
–	9.8	0.20	—	28:0.35 mg NE	Nor-QD Camila Heather Nora-BE
–	9.8	0.33	—	28:0.35 mg NE	Ortho-Micronor Errin Jencycla Jolivette

*Androgen levels have been calculated from progestin potency based on Dickey and Dickey 2010.
†All progestins have been converted to norethindrone equivalents based on Dickey and Dickey 2010.
‡Italicized drugs are generic products.
DG, Desogestrel (third-generation progestin); DRSP, Drospirenone (fourth-generation progestin); ED, ethynodiol diacetate (first generation); LN, levonorgestrel (third-generation progestin); MDPA, medroxyprogesterone acetate (second-generation progestin); NE, norethindrone (first-generation progestin); NORG, norgestimate (third-generation progestin).
Adapted from Harper DM. A practical approach to managing oral contraceptive pills in adolescents. *Family Practice Recertification.* 2001;23(11):47-57.

EXAMPLES OF MANAGING COMBINED ORAL CONTRACEPTIVE PILL SIDE EFFECTS

Key Points

- Changing the estrogen-to-progestin ratios to prevent breakthrough bleeding early in the cycle before ovulation requires changing to a pill with more estrogen while keeping the progestin dose similar. Breakthrough bleeding late in the cycle after ovulation (when more progestin is needed) requires changing to a pill with more progestin while keeping the estrogen dose similar.
- Heavy bleeding with periods and bloating requires changing to a pill with a lower estrogen-to-progestin ratio, accomplished by decreasing the estrogen dose. Estrogen builds up the endometrium, leading to hypermenorrhea.
- Breakthrough bleeding throughout the cycle requires changing to a pill with more estrogen without changing the progestin dose.
- Elevated blood pressure and depressed mood require changing to a pill with less progestin.

Menstrual Irregularities

A college-age female on the cross-country team has taken Apri for the past 2 years. She reports over the past 6 months, she has 3 days of a light period followed by 4 days without bleeding and then 3 days of spotting. This breakthrough bleeding, which is distressing to her, is caused by estrogen deficiency. A pill with more estrogen and a similar amount of progestin would be ideal. Tri-Norinyl or Ortho Novum 7/7/7 is a good choice, with a sufficient increase in estrogen and almost the same amount of progestin.

A 16-year-old young woman taking Tri-Sprintec complains of brown blood spotting her underwear beginning 3 to 5 days before her period and numerous soaked pads during her period. Because she is a competitive swimmer, the heavy bleeding is particularly troublesome, leaking around tampons. Her late cycle (days 10-21) breakthrough bleeding and hypermenorrhea are probably attributable to a progestin deficiency. Tri-Sprintec has very low progestin but a common estrogen content, so there is an abundant choice for an alternative. She is switched to Necon 0.5/35. Three months later, the spotting has resolved, but her heavy periods have continued. She also reports bloating the week before her period, which she says interferes with her swimming performance. Hypermenorrhea and bloating are symptoms of estrogen excess, so she should be given a pill with less estrogen. Cyclessa, a good alternative, might work well for her.

A 42-year-old woman not yet experiencing perimenopausal symptoms has been using Mircette. Recently, she has experienced 2 days of bleeding with brown spotting every other day of her cycle. Because breakthrough bleeding is occurring continuously throughout the cycle, her endometrium needs more estrogen than Mircette provides. Desogen would increase the estrogen level while keeping her progestin and androgen levels constant. The Necon 0.5/35 group, with more estrogen, slightly less progestin, and half the androgen, is also a good candidate.

Weight Gain and Depression

An 18-year-old woman with polycystic ovarian syndrome (PCOS) was not well controlled on a low-estrogen pill and was switched to Demulen 1/35. At the 3-month follow-up, her blood pressure was mildly elevated (140/92 mm Hg), she had gained 30 lb, and she complained of a "blue mood."

She would like to stay with the pill because it has helped her PCOS symptoms, but she needs a different one. The problem appears to be a progestin excess. Many OCPs, such as Genora 1/35, have 735-μg ethinyl estradiol and less progestin. She is given a 3-month supply and scheduled for monthly blood pressure monitoring.

COMBINED PHASIC FORMULATIONS AND EXTENDED CYCLE PILLS

Initial formulations were monophasic, with no variation of estrogen and progestin doses throughout the first 21 days of the 28-day cycle, with inert placebo or iron supplementation added to the last 7 days of the cycle. Subsequent biphasic formulations attempted to reduce breakthrough bleeding and other side effects by more closely mimicking the initial estrogen peak followed by the progestin peak of the menstrual cycle.

Triphasic formulations initially varied only the progestin component to increase the dose in three steps over the course of 21 days within the cycle. Later triphasic formulations kept the progestin component constant and increased the estrogen content over the 21 days of the cycle. One set of formulations maximizes the estrogen content midcycle (low, high, low), and the progestin content progressively increases over the 21 day cycle.

Extended-cycle pills were created to minimize the risk of anemia and reduce withdrawal bleeding blood loss to four times a year. Three cycles of 28 days were combined followed by a 7-day withdrawal period. The initial extended cycle was monophasic 30 μg of ethinyl estradiol with 0.15 mg of levonorgestrel for 84 days (e.g., Seasonale, Introvale, Quasense, Jolessa). Estrogen deficiency symptoms of early cycle bleeding or continuous spotting throughout the 84-day cycle were experienced, leading to the next extended-phase formulation that remained the same for the initial 84 days but added 10 μg of ethinyl estradiol to the original 7 placebo days (e.g., Seasonique, Amethia, Camresse, Daysee). Finally, a lower estrogen and lower progestin formulation for reduced thromboembolism risk has been approved using 20 μg of ethinyl estradiol with 0.10 mg of levonorgestrel for 84 days followed by 10 μg of ethinyl estradiol for the remaining 7 days of the extended cycle (e.g., LoSeasonique, AmethiaLo, CamresseLo).

Quadriphasic pills are the most recent formulation meant to more closely mimic the menstrual cycle and reduce metrorrhagia or irregular cyclic bleeding. The 28-day cycle formulation (Figure 26-5, A) contains four different combinations of estrogen and progestin. The new estrogen formulation (estradiol valerate) initiates at the highest dose and decreases to zero over the cycle. The fourth-generation progestin (dienogest) is separated into two different doses, with the higher dose for 17 days over the midcycle.

The extended quadriphasic formulation (Figure 26-5, B) contains four doses of estrogen and a single dose of progestin. The first 42 days contain 20 μg of ethinyl estradiol and 0.15 mg of levonorgestrel in a monophasic attempt to stabilize the endometrium. There is no monophasic pill combination that contains this low dose of estrogen balanced with the highest approved dose of levonorgestrel. The next two 21-day segments increase the estrogen dose to 25 μg of ethinyl estradiol and then to 30 μg all with the same high dose of 0.15 mg levonorgestrel. The final 7 days of the extended period reduce the estrogen dose to 10 μg of ethinyl estradiol without any progestin.

Altering the phasic component of the pill formulation should be considered after finding the best range of 28-day cycle hormone doses.

Progestin-Only Contraception

> ### Key Points
>
> - Unlike combined estrogen–progestin options, progestin-only options are useful for breastfeeding women in the initial postpartum period.
> - Progestin-only options include pills, an injection, and a subdermal implant, all of which work by thickening cervical mucus and thinning the endometrium.
> - Progestin-only pills must be taken at the same time every day to be effective.
> - The loss of bone mineral density with the use of DMPA must be considered when prescribing, especially in adolescent and perimenopausal women.

Progestin-only contraceptives are useful for women who wish to immediately start breastfeeding postpartum. CDC recommendations support immediate use of progestin-only pills, DMPA injections, or progestin implants (CDC, 2011) despite some who recommend a 3-week hormone-free period because of increased risks of venous thrombosis (Marik and Plante, 2008; Rodriguez and Kaunitz, 2009). The progestin-only pills available in the United States have one dose, which is 0.35 mg norethindrone for a total of 9.8 mg per 28-day cycle. This dose of progestin causes cervical mucus thickening to be impenetrable to sperm and thinning of the endometrium to reject implantation. The short half-life of this progestin and its mechanism of action requires the woman to take the pill at the same time every day without more than 3 hours' variance (Wright et al., 1970). A European progestin-only pill contains 75 μg of desogestrel and allows up to 12 hours variance in the daily dose (Korver et al., 2005).

The most common side effects associated with the progestin-only pills are irregular bleeding, depression, and acne outbreaks (McCann and Potter, 1994; St-André et al., 2012). These symptoms are worse with the DMPA (150-mg) intramuscular shot given every 90 days and with the subdermal implants proven effective through 3 years (68 mg of etonogestrel, Nexplanon) (Hoggart et al., 2013). Of note is the bone mineral density loss that occurs within 2 years of continuous DMPA use (Isley and Kaunitz, 2011). This is especially troublesome among adolescents who have not completed their bone mass accumulation and among perimenopausal women who have started to actively lose bone mass. In 2004, the FDA added a black box warning to DMPA, but the World Health Organization (WHO) and American College of Obstetricians and Gynecologists (ACOG) have not included this risk in their recommendations (ACOG Committee on Gynecologic Practice, 2008; FDA, 2014; WHO, 2007).

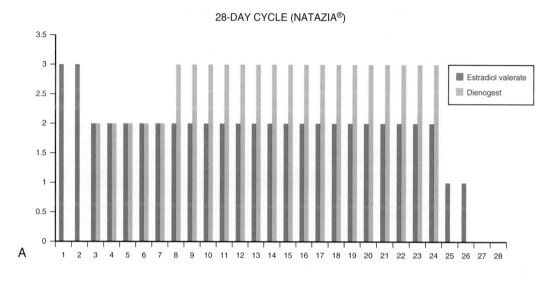

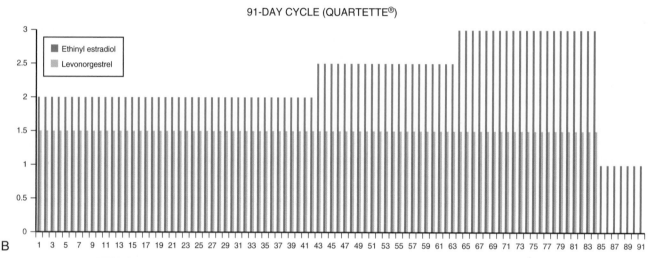

Figure 26-5 Quadriphasic design. **A,** Twenty-eight-day cycle (Natazia). **B,** Ninety-one-day cycle (Quartette).

Additional Contraceptive Choices

Key Points

- A flexible, vaginally inserted plastic ring and a transdermal patch are additional contraceptive options; both have an estrogen component and the third-generation progestin, levonorgestrel, which has been associated with venous thrombosis.
- Options for emergency contraception, when used within 5 days of intercourse, are the copper IUD and hormonal options, including estrogen and progestin pills and progestin-only pills.
- Hormonal emergency contraceptives are currently sold over the counter in the United States for women 17 years of age and older.
- IUDs prevent fertilization by creating a sterile inflammatory reaction in the uterus.
- The copper-containing and levonorgestrel-containing IUD options are among the most effective reversible contraceptive options, with irregular bleeding and cramping being the most common reasons for removal.

CYCLIC HORMONAL CHOICES

Nuvaring, the only flexible plastic ring that is inserted intravaginally, has the lowest ethinyl estradiol content at 315 μg per 28-day cycle. Ortho-Evra, the only transdermal contraceptive patch, contains 420 μg per 28-day cycle. The progestin is third generation for etonogestrel and norelgestromin, respectively. These progestins have resulted in significant numbers of venous thrombotic events for which the manufacturers of Nuvaring (Merck) and Ortho-Evra (Ortho McNeil) have reached multimillion dollar settlements (Feeley and Voreacos, 2014; Voreacos, 2008). As with any contraceptive choice, a discussion with individual patients about the risks and benefits of Nuvaring or Ortho-Evra should be undertaken before its initiation, and any symptoms should be reported immediately.

EMERGENCY CONTRACEPTION

Hormonal emergency contraception has received over-the-counter approval in the United States for women age 17 years and older within 5 days of intercourse for purposes of preventing unintended pregnancies. A total of 11%

of sexually experienced women 15 to 44 years old in the United States have used hormonal emergency contraception, with the largest proportion of users 20 to 24 years of age (Daniels et al., 2013). Nine times as many women choose to use oral hormonal emergency contraception as the copper IUD (Belden et al., 2012) despite evidence of superior efficacy of the copper IUD (risk reduction of 99.2% vs. 89% and 74% with progestin-only and estrogen–progestin pills, respectively [Cheng et al., 2008; Trussell et al., 2003; Zhou and Xiao, 2001]). This is assumed to be attributable to the need for a health care professional to insert the copper IUD within 5 days of intercourse; the false impression that one cannot remove the IUD for 10 years; and, depending on the clinic, a need for upfront payment.

INTRAUTERINE CONTRACEPTIVE DEVICES

Intrauterine devices prevent fertilization, not implantation. A foreign body within the uterus causes a sterile inflammatory reaction that is toxic to sperm, causing inhibition of sperm motility, reduced sperm capacitation and survival, and sperm phagocytosis (Ammälä et al., 1995; Patai et al., 2003).

There are two types of IUDs. One contains copper as described in the emergency contraception section, with 380 mm^2 copper surface that remains effective for up to 20 years (ParaGard). The mechanism of action of the IUD is augmented by copper salts. The other contains levonorgestrel in two dosage forms. The 52 mg of levonorgestrel (LNg20) releases 20 μg of levonorgestrel daily, declining to 10 to 14 μg at 5 years (Mirena), and is the same size as the copper IUD. The 13.5-mg levonorgestrel dose (LNg14) releases 14 μg daily, decreasing to 5 μg at 3 years (Skyla), and is smaller for adolescents and those with a stenotic os. Both the copper and LN IUDs cause irregular bleeding and cramping, which are the most common reasons for early removal (Teal and Sheeder, 2012). The LN IUD can result in amenorrhea in some women.

Adolescent Concerns

Key Points

- Adolescents have the highest rate of unintended pregnancy at 77% for 15- to 19-year old young women in the United States.
- Discontinuation rates of all forms of contraception except IUDs and subdermal implants is highest in adolescents among all age groups; rates are greater than 50% at 24 months.
- The ACOG recommends that IUDs be considered as a first-line contraceptive option in sexually active adolescents.

Adolescents have the highest rate of unintended pregnancy and the highest discontinuation rate with any form of contraception (ACOG, 2012; Finer & Zolna, 2014; Mosher

et al., 2012). Although many adolescents chose a contraceptive method initially, they discontinue them by 24 months at the following rates: 23% for IUD (no difference between copper or LN), 31% for subdermal implants, 57% for OCPs, 60% for the patch, 59% for the ring, and 62% for DMPA (O'Neil-Callahan et al., 2013). The ACOG has recently asserted the most cost-effective method for adolescents is the long-acting reversible contraceptive choice of an IUD either with or without hormone (ACOG, 2012). The risk of infertility caused by multiple sexual partners seen in a prior generation of IUDs is vastly diminished because of the monofilament tail on this generation of IUDs.

Additional Information

Key Points

- Considering all contraceptive options except abstinence, male and female condoms offer the most protection against sexually transmitted infections.
- Sterilization methods are some of the most effective family planning methods, but failures do occur.
- Estrogen- and progestin-containing pills are one of the most commonly used contraceptive methods, with management of formulations being a key part of individualization.

The new 10th revision of the *International Statistical Classification of Diseases and Related Health Problems* (ICD-10) billing codes for reimbursement around contraceptive issues are included in Table 26-6.

No method of contraception protects completely against STIs. Barrier methods, such as the male and female condom, offer the highest protection after abstinence. Spermicides such as nonoxynol-9 are no longer recommended because of their facilitative effect for human papillomavirus and HIV infections (Gupta and Nutan, 2013). If a lubricant is desired, saline-based lubricants are safest. Diaphragms, cervical caps, and sponges offer other barrier methods that may appeal to some women.

Fertility awareness methods have the greatest failure rate but are often methods of choice because there are no exogenous hormones or devices to which side effects may occur (Gribble et al., 2008).

Sterilization is meant to be permanent, but failures do occur. Female sterilization by tubal disruption is associated with a 2 to 10 in 1000 failure rate; male sterilization by vasectomy has an 11 in 1000 failure rate (ACOG, 2013; Jamieson et al., 2004). Essure, a hysteroscopically placed nickel-containing coil, fails to scar the fallopian tubes, resulting in pregnancy in 2 or 3 of 1000 procedures (Bradley et al., 2008), and is associated with nickel allergies.

The most commonly used contraceptive methods are those using the combination of estrogen and progestin in varying proportions with monthly withdrawal bleeding. Designing the doses in the combination to result in the least amount of monthly bleeding and the fewest side effects is possible with dedication and patience.

Table 26-6 ICD-10 Codes Used for Contraception Reimbursement

Z30.0 Encounter for general counseling and advice on contraception
Z30.0.1 Encounter for initial prescription of contraceptives
Z30.011 Encounter for initial prescription of contraceptive pills
Z30.012 Encounter for initial prescription of emergency contraception
Z30.013 Encounter for initial prescription of injectable contraceptive
Z30.014 Encounter for initial prescription of intrauterine contraceptive device
Z30.018 Encounter for initial prescription of other contraceptives
Z30.019 Encounter for initial prescription of contraceptives, unspecified*
Z30.02 Counseling and instruction in natural family planning to avoid pregnancy
Z30.09 Encounter for other general counseling and advice on contraception*
Z30.2 Encounter for sterilization
Z30.4 Encounter for surveillance of contraceptives
Z30.40 Encounter for surveillance of contraceptives, unspecified*
Z30.41 Encounter for surveillance of contraceptive pills
Z30.42 Encounter for surveillance of injectable contraceptive
Z30.43 Encounter for surveillance of intrauterine contraceptive device
Z30.430 Encounter for insertion of intrauterine contraceptive device
Z30.431 Encounter for routine checking for intrauterine contraceptive device
Z30.432 Encounter for removal of intrauterine contraceptive device
Z30.433 Encounter for removal and reinsertion of intrauterine contraceptive device
Z30.49 Encounter for surveillance of other contraceptives*
Z30.8 Encounter for other contraceptive management including post-vasectomy sperm count
Z31.4 Encounter for procreative investigation and testing
Z31.41 Sperm count for fertility testing
Z31.42 Sperm count following sterilization
Z30.9 Encounter for contraceptive management, unspecified*
Z31 Encounter for procreative management
Z31.61 Procreative counseling and advice using natural family planning
Z32.0 Encounter for pregnancy test
Z32.01 Encounter for pregnancy test, result positive
Z32.02 Encounter for pregnancy test, result negative

*Code is unlikely to be reimbursed.
ICD-10, International Statistical Classification of Diseases and Related Health Problems, 10th ed.

KEY TREATMENT

- OCPs are the most commonly used method of contraception and the most commonly abandoned method because of side effects (SOR: A).
- Long-acting reversible contraceptives, such as copper IUDs and levonorgestrel IUDs, are recommended for adolescents seeking contraception (SOR: C).
- Progestin-only OCPs are useful in women who wish to breastfeed in the postpartum period (SOR: C) or are otherwise unable to tolerate an estrogen component of contraception. The short half-life of this medication requires women to take it at the same time every day, within 3 hours.
- Hormonal emergency contraception is available in both oral and intrauterine forms. Although more women are choosing to use the oral formulations, copper IUDs are the most effective in preventing unwanted pregnancies (SOR: A).

References

The complete reference list is available at www.expertconsult.com.

Video

The following videos are available at www.expertconsult.com:

Video 26-1 Vasectomy

Web Resources

www.cdc.gov/mmwr/preview/mmwrhtml/rr5904a1.htm and http://www.cdc.gov/mmwr/pdf/rr/rr5904.pdf Describe the U.S. and World Health Organization medical eligibility criteria to use different contraceptive formulations.

www.guttmacher.org/statecenter/adolescents.html Describes the laws concerning confidentiality of providing contraceptive care to adolescents with or without parental consent.

www.menopause.org/for-women/sexual-health-menopause-online/reminders-and-resources/contraception-you-need-it-longer-than-you-may-think Describes the methods of contraception as women age into the perimenopausal years.

27 *Cardiovascular Disease*

PETER P. TOTH, NICOLAS W. SHAMMAS, BLAIR FOREMAN, J. BRIAN BYRD, and ROBERT D. BROOK

Cardiovascular disease (CVD) is the leading cause of morbidity and mortality for both men and women in the United States and most other parts of the developed world. In recent decades CVD has become a leading cause of death and disability in most regions of Asia. Enormous efforts continue to be expended to stem the physical, emotional, and socioeconomic costs attributable to CVDs throughout the world. Significant progress is being made. Between 2000 and 2010, death rates associated with CVD and stroke decreased by 31% and 35.6%, respectively (Go et al., 2014). The total costs associated with CVD and stroke is approximately $315 billion annually in the United States alone. In the United States, one person sustains a coronary event every 34 seconds.

Considerable progress in detecting and managing CVD is being made. With the introduction of new pharmacologic interventions, development of numerous percutaneous approaches to managing cardiac valvular disease, aneurysms, and peripheral vascular disease, and innovative approaches for correcting arrhythmias, cardiovascular medicine changes rapidly. The molecular defects characterizing many forms of CVD are being brought into sharper focus, which increases the potential to develop novel therapies for preventing or managing a broad variety of cardiovascular abnormalities.

Detailed guidelines by professional societies and national commissions are being issued and continuously reevaluated and updated so as to optimize the management of risk factors and established forms of disease. Despite these efforts, compliance with guidelines remains relatively low throughout the world. In addition, although randomized clinical trials have firmly established the efficacy of numerous drug classes to reduce cardiovascular morbidity and mortality, many of these drugs are underused or are not used at appropriate doses. As populations age worldwide; as more patients survive acute cardiovascular and cerebrovascular events; and as the incidence of hypertension (HTN), dyslipidemia, metabolic syndrome, diabetes mellitus (DM), obesity, and other risk factors continues to increase, the burden on family physicians to identify and effectively manage CVD will continue to escalate dramatically.

Atherosclerosis

Atherosclerosis is a complex, multifactorial disease that is highly prevalent throughout the world. Atherosclerotic disease is etiologic for acute coronary syndromes (ACS) such as myocardial infarction (MI) and unstable angina (UA), carotid artery disease and ischemic stroke, renal arterial stenosis, and peripheral vascular disease (Libby, 2001). The development and progression of atherosclerosis is driven by a variety of risk factors, including dyslipidemia, HTN, impairments in glycemic control, age, family history, cigarette smoking, obesity, and systemic inflammation. Novel risk factors are being recognized, and their utility for identifying patients at risk for disease are being tested in epidemiologic and clinical trial settings. Evaluating patients for global cardiovascular risk burden and aggressively treating modifiable risk factors is a significant focus of any primary care setting.

Atherogenesis is no longer viewed as an inevitable consequence of passive, progressive lipid accumulation within the arterial wall gradually resulting in symptomatic reductions in blood flow and oxygen delivery. Instead, atherosclerosis is a dynamic process encompassing a diverse array of biochemical and histologic changes that continuously modulate the establishment and evolution of atheromatous plaque (Hansson, 2005; Libby et al., 2002). Atheromatous plaque is modifiable, and therapeutic interventions can stabilize and even regress plaque, resulting in reductions in risk for cardiovascular morbidity and mortality.

Endothelial cell dysfunction is an early hallmark of atherogenesis (Toth, 2009). The endothelium is as an organ system. Endothelial cells line the luminal surface of blood vessels and mediate vascular tone and molecular trafficking into the vessel wall. When endothelium is stressed by rheological disturbances, increased inflammatory or oxidative insult, glycemic injury, hyperlipidemia, and HTN, its functional characteristics change. Dysfunctional endothelium has less vasodilatory capacity, is more thrombogenic, and upregulates the expression of a variety of cell adhesion molecules, such as vascular cell adhesion molecule-1 (VCAM-1) and intercellular adhesion molecule-1 (ICAM-1) (Lusis, 2000). These adhesion molecules promote the binding of monocytes, T cells, and mast cells to the endothelial surface. Bound inflammatory white blood cells (WBCs) then follow a gradient of monocyte chemoattractant protein-1 and other cytokines by intercalating between endothelial cells and ultimately transmigrate into the subendothelial space. In the subendothelial space, these WBCs take up residence, where they create an inflammatory nidus. Monocytes can convert to macrophages in response to macrophage colony-stimulating factor. Inflammatory WBCs are potent sources of oxygen free radicals such as superoxide anion, peroxide, and hydroxyl. These reactive oxygen species can oxidize phospholipids and fatty acids within lipoproteins, rendering them more proinflammatory and atherogenic. When exposed to oxidatively modified atherogenic lipoproteins, macrophages upregulate the expression of cell surface scavenger receptors (e.g., CD36 and scavenger receptor A), which promote the internalization of cholesterol and cholesterol esters resulting in the formation of foam cells. Foam cells coalesce to form fatty streaks, the histologic precursor to atheromatous plaques. Resident macrophages, T cells, and mast cells facilitate additional WBC recruitment and progression of atherosclerotic disease by producing a variety of cytokines, interleukins (ILs), and oxidative enzymes that adversely impact endothelial, smooth muscle cell, and fibroblast function and proliferation.

With disease progression, the molecular and histologic dynamics of atheromatous plaque remain in continuous flux. As foam cells die, cellular debris accumulates and further potentiates the inflammatory response (Tabas, 2005). Matrix metalloproteinases (MMPs) are expressed, which degrade the collagen, elastin, and proteoglycan extracellular matrix of plaque. When this occurs in the shoulder region of a plaque, acute rupture or plaque fissuring can result. Sudden plaque rupture exposes collagen, tissue factor, and the thrombogenic lipid core to platelets and coagulation factors, ultimately resulting in overlying thrombus formation, luminal obstruction, acute ischemia, and possible infarction if tissue blood flow is not rapidly reestablished. Atheromatous plaques that are highly inflamed and contain concentrated macrophage infiltrates or large lipid cores are particularly vulnerable to architectural destabilization and acute plaque rupture. Plaque can also suddenly distend and reduce coronary luminal diameter from intraplaque hemorrhaging if the delicate vasa vasorum feeding the surrounding vascular tissue is injured from vasospasm.

In the majority of cases, culprit lesions giving rise to acute MI are not flow limiting before rupture or fissuring. Any atheromatous plaque identified on coronary angiography should be viewed as a potential cause of an ACS. Patients with evidence of atherosclerotic disease in any portion of the vascular tree require rigorous evaluation of all risk factors and the appropriate institution of lifestyle and pharmacologic intervention to reduce the risk for both disease progression and cardiovascular morbidity and mortality.

Dyslipidemia

Key Points

- Patients undergoing screening for dyslipidemia should have a complete fasting lipid profile.
- The new American College of Cardiology/American Heart Association (ACC/AHA) guideline on the treatment of blood cholesterol has shifted to a risk-centric model.
- Statin therapy is indicated for all patients in secondary prevention and patients with a 10-yr risk for atherosclerotic cardiovascular disease (ASCVD) of 7.5% or greater.
- The intensity of statin therapy is based on risk level. Secondary causes of dyslipidemia should also be ruled out.
- Therapeutic lifestyle changes are an important component of any regimen designed to treat dyslipidemia.

Although it is pathogenic, cholesterol is also an important modulator of cell membrane fluidity and is a substrate for hormone biosynthesis by steroidogenic organs. There is an unequivocal relationship between dyslipidemia and risk for atherogenesis within the coronary, peripheral, renal, and cerebral vasculature. Dyslipoproteinemias develop in response to genetic and environmental factors and are modifiable through lifestyle modification and pharmacologic intervention. As demonstrated in the Framingham Study, Multiple Risk Factor Intervention Trial, and the Seven Countries Study, as serum levels of cholesterol increase, the risk for developing coronary artery disease (CAD) increases. The identification and treatment of dyslipidemia lower the risk for developing atherosclerotic disease and its various clinical manifestations.

Serum very-low-density lipoprotein (VLDL) and low-density lipoprotein (LDL) particles deliver cholesterol and triglycerides to peripheral tissues and blood vessel walls. These lipoproteins can cross the endothelial barrier and induce atherogenesis. Atherogenic lipoproteins not taken up by peripheral tissues are cleared from the circulation by hepatic LDL receptors. Lipid-lowering therapies that upregulate hepatic LDL receptors are antiatherogenic by virtue of their ability to reduce circulating levels of atherogenic lipoproteins.

Dyslipidemia can be the result of abnormalities in gastrointestinal (GI) nutrient absorption, serum and intracellular enzyme activities, and/or cell surface receptor expression. A complete fasting (12-14 hours) lipoprotein profile (including LDL cholesterol [LDL-C], triglyceride, and high-density lipoprotein cholesterol [HDL-C]) should be obtained on anyone screened for dyslipidemia. Because of the relationship between specific lipoprotein fractions and risk for CAD, measuring total cholesterol levels has little clinical relevance.

The National Cholesterol Education Program Adult Treatment Panel III (NCEP ATPIII) recommendations are now replaced by the ACC/AHA Guideline on the Treatment of Blood Cholesterol to Reduce Atherosclerotic Cardiovascular Risk in Adults (Stone et al., 2013). The new guideline has prompted considerable debate, and not all specialty societies have endorsed it. The new recommendations are summarized in Figure 27-1 and Table 27-1. The new guideline has shifted emphasis away from LDL-C and non-HDL-C thresholds and targets and is now basing the decision on whether or not to treat with statin therapy on overall risk for acute cardiovascular events. The Framingham risk equation is not a part of the new guideline. For patients in primary prevention, use of the new Pooled Cohort Equation is recommended for estimating 10-year risk for ASCVD, which can be downloaded at http://my.americanheart.org/professional/Statements Guidelines/PreventionGuidelines/Prevention-Guidelines _UCM_457698_SubHomePage.jsp. ASCVD includes ACS, history of MI, stable or unstable angina, coronary or other arterial revascularization, stroke, transient ischemic attack (TIA), or peripheral arterial disease (PAD) presumed to be of atherosclerotic origin.

The 10-year risk threshold for initiating statin therapy for patients in the primary prevention setting is 7.5% or greater irrespective of gender or race or ethnicity. The definitions for high-, moderate-, and low-intensity statin therapies are summarized in Table 27-2. There are no recommendations for treating non–HDL-C or low HDL-C. When estimating risk, consideration can also be given to LDL-C level of 160 mg/dL or greater or other evidence of genetic hyperlipidemias; family history of premature ASCVD with onset before 55 years of age in a first-degree male relative or before 65 years of age in a first-degree female relative; high-sensitivity C-reactive protein (CRP) greater than 2 mg/L; coronary artery calcium score 300 Agatston units or greater or 75 percentile or greater for age, sex, and ethnicity; ankle-brachial index (ABI) less than 0.9; or elevated

Table 27-1 ACC/AHA Guideline Recommendations for the Treatment of Blood Cholesterol

Recommendations	NHLBI Grade	NHLBI Evidence Statements	ACC/AHA COR	ACC/AHA LOE
TREATMENT TARGETS				
1. The panel makes no recommendations for or against specific LDL-C or non–HDL-C targets for the primary or secondary prevention of ASCVD.	N (no recommendation)	1-4	—	—
SECONDARY PREVENTION				
1. High-intensity statin therapy should be initiated or continued as first-line therapy in women and men ≤75 years of age who have *clinical ASCVD** unless contraindicated.	A (strong)	1, 6-8, 10-23, 26-28	I	A
2. In individuals with *clinical ASCVD** in whom high-intensity statin therapy would otherwise be used, when high-intensity statin therapy is contraindicated,† or when characteristics predisposing to statin-associated adverse effects are present, moderate-intensity statin should be used as the second option if tolerated.	A (strong)	13-22, 24, 27, 28	I	A
3. In individuals with *clinical* ASCVD >75 years of age, it is reasonable to evaluate the potential for ASCVD risk-reduction benefits, adverse effects, and drug–drug interactions, and to consider patient preferences when initiating a moderate- or high-intensity statin. It is reasonable to continue statin therapy in those who are tolerating it.	E (expert opinion)	—	IIa	B (16,20-43)
PRIMARY PREVENTION IN INDIVIDUALS ≥21 YEARS OF AGE WITH LDL-C ≥190 MG/DL				
1. Individuals with LDL-C ≥190 mg/dL or triglycerides ≥500 mg/dL should be evaluated for secondary causes of hyperlipidemia	B (Moderate)	75	I‡	B (44,45)
2. Adults ≥21 years of age with primary LDL-C ≥190 mg/dL should be treated with statin therapy (10-year ASCVD risk estimation is not required): • Use high-intensity statin therapy unless contraindicated. • For individuals unable to tolerate high-intensity statin therapy, use the maximum tolerated statin intensity.	B (Moderate)	6, 19, 28, 33-35, 37, 38	I§	B
3. For individuals ≥21 years of age with an untreated primary LDL-C ≥190 mg/dL, it is reasonable to intensify statin therapy to achieve at least a 50% LDL-C reduction.	E (expert opinion)	—	IIa	B (20,46-50)
4. For individuals ≥21 years of age with an untreated primary LDL-C ≥190 mg/dL, after the maximum intensity of statin therapy has been achieved, addition of a nonstatin drug may be considered to further lower LDL-C. Evaluate the potential for ASCVD risk reduction benefits, adverse effects, and drug–drug interactions and consider patient preferences.	E (expert opinion)	—	IIb	C (51)

Continued on following page

Table 27-1 ACC/AHA Guideline Recommendations for the Treatment of Blood Cholesterol (Continued)

Recommendations	NHLBI Grade	NHLBI Evidence Statements	ACC/AHA COR	ACC/AHA LOE
PRIMARY PREVENTION IN INDIVIDUALS WITH DIABETES MELLITUS AND LDL-C 70-189 MG/DL				
1. Moderate-intensity statin therapy should be initiated or continued for adults 40-75 years of age with diabetes mellitus.	A (strong)	19, 29-34, 40	I	A
2. High-intensity statin therapy is reasonable for adults 40-75 years of age with diabetes mellitus with a ≥7.5% estimated 10-year ASCVD risk‖ unless contraindicated.	E (expert opinion)	—	IIa	B (49,52)
3. In adults with diabetes mellitus who are <40 or >75 years of age, it is reasonable to evaluate the potential for ASCVD benefits, for adverse effects, and for drug–drug interactions and to consider patient preferences when deciding to initiate, continue, or intensify statin therapy.	E (expert opinion)	—	IIa	C (53-62)
PRIMARY PREVENTION IN INDIVIDUALS WITHOUT DIABETES MELLITUS AND WITH LDL-C 70-189 MG/DL				
1. The pooled cohort equations should be used to estimate 10-year ASCVD‖ risk for individuals with LDL-C 70-189 mg/dL without *clinical ASCVD** to guide initiation of statin therapy for the primary prevention of ASCVD.	E (expert opinion)	—	I	B (11)
2. Adults 40-75 years of age with LDL-C 70-189 mg/dL, without *clinical ASCVD** or diabetes and an estimated 10-year ASCVD‖ risk ≥7.5% should be treated with moderate- to high-intensity statin therapy.	A (strong)	28, 34-36, 38, 42-44, 47, 49-56, 76	I	A
3. It is reasonable to offer treatment with a moderate-intensity statin to adults 40-75 years of age, with LDL-C 70-189 mg/dL without *clinical ASCVD** or diabetes and an estimated 10-year ASCVD‖ risk of 5% to <7.5%.	C (weak)	28, 34-36, 38, 42-44, 47, 49-56, 76	IIa	B
4. Before initiating statin therapy for the primary prevention of ASCVD in adults with LDL-C 70-189 mg/dL without *clinical ASCVD** or diabetes, it is reasonable for clinicians and patients to engage in a discussion that considers the potential for ASCVD risk reduction benefits and for adverse effects and for drug–drug interactions and patient preferences for treatment.	E (expert opinion)	—	IIa	C (63)
5. In adults with LDL-C <190 mg/dL who are not otherwise identified in a statin benefit group or for whom after quantitative risk assessment a risk-based treatment decision is uncertain, additional factors¶ may be considered to inform treatment decision making. In these individuals, statin therapy for primary prevention may be considered after evaluating the potential for ASCVD risk reduction benefits, adverse effects, drug–drug interactions, and discussion of patient preferences.	E (expert opinion)	—	IIb	C (11,13)
HEART FAILURE AND HEMODIALYSIS				
1. The Expert Panel makes no recommendations regarding the initiation or discontinuation of statins in patients with NYHA class II-IV ischemic systolic heart failure or in patients on maintenance hemodialysis.	N (no recommendation)	71, 72	—	—

Clinical ASCVD includes acute coronary syndromes, history of MI, stable or unstable angina, coronary or other arterial revascularization, stroke, TIA, or peripheral arterial disease presumed to be of atherosclerotic origin.

†Contraindications, warnings, and precautions are defined for each statin according to the manufacturer's prescribing information (64-70).

‡Individuals with secondary causes of hyperlipidemia were excluded from the RCTs reviewed. Triglycerides >500 mg/dL were an exclusion criteria for almost all RCTs. Therefore, ruling out secondary causes is necessary to avoid inappropriate statin therapy.

§No RCTs included only individuals with LDL-C ≥190 mg/dL. However, many trials did include individuals with LDL-C ≥190 mg/dL, and all of these trials consistently demonstrated a reduction in ASCVD events. In addition, the cholesterol treatment trialists meta-analyses have shown that each 39–mg/dL reduction in LDL-C with statin therapy reduced ASCVD events by 22%, and the relative reductions in ASCVD events were consistent across the range of LDL-C levels. Therefore, individuals with primary LDL-C >190 mg/dL should be treated with statin therapy.

‖Estimated 10-year or "hard" ASCVD risk includes first occurrence of nonfatal MI, congestive heart disease death, and nonfatal and fatal stroke as used by the Risk Assessment Work Group in developing the Pooled Cohort Equations.

¶These factors may include primary LDL-C >160 mg/dL or other evidence of genetic hyperlipidemias, family history of premature ASCVD with onset <55 years in a first-degree male relative or <65 years in a first-degree female relative, high sensitivity-C-reactive protein >2 mg/L, CAC score ≥300 Agatston units or ≥75 percentile for age, sex, and ethnicity (for additional information, see http://www.mesa-nhlbi.org/CACReference.aspx.), ABI <0.9, or lifetime risk of ASCVD. Additional factors that may aid in individual risk assessment may be identified in the future.

—, Not applicable; *ABI,* ankle-brachial index; *ACC,* American College of Cardiology; *AHA,* American Heart Association; *ALT,* alanine transaminase; *ASCVD,* atherosclerotic cardiovascular disease; *AST,* aspartate aminotransferase; *CAC,* coronary artery calcium; *CK,* creatine kinase; *COR,* class of recommendation; *HDL-C,* high-density lipoprotein cholesterol; *LDL-C,* low-density lipoprotein cholesterol; *LOE,* level of evidence; *MI,* myocardial infarction; *NHLBI,* National Heart, Lung, and Blood Institute; *NYHA,* New York Heart Association; *RCT,* randomized controlled trial; *TIA,* transient ischemic attack; *ULN,* upper limit of normal.

Used with permission from Stone NJ, Robinson J, Lichtenstein AH, et al. 2013 ACC/AHA guideline on the treatment of blood cholesterol to reduce atherosclerotic cardiovascular risk in adults: a report of the American College of Cardiology/American Heart Association Task Force on Practice Guidelines, *Circulation* 2014;129(25, Suppl 2):S1-S45.

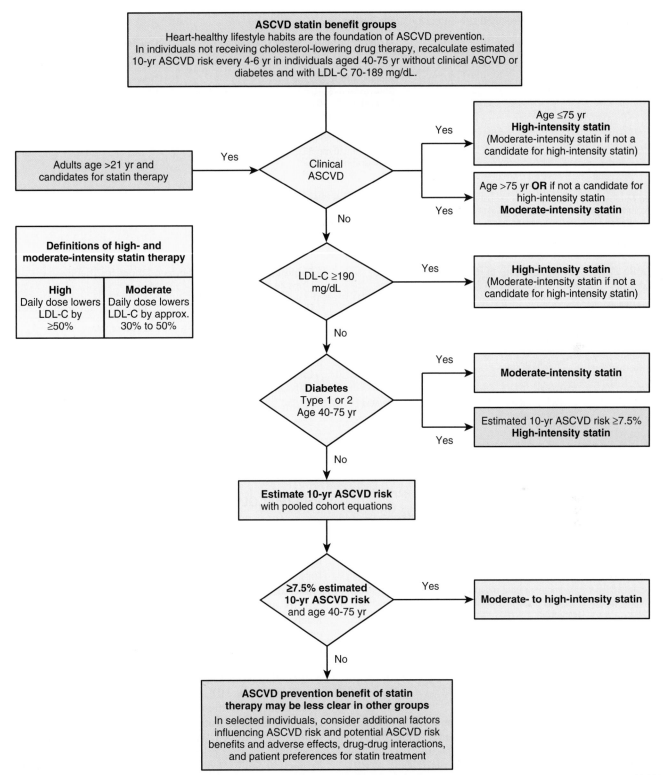

Figure 27-1 Recommendations for statin treatment of blood cholesterol to reduce atherosclerotic cardiovascular risk in adults. (Used with permission from Stone NJ, Robinson J, Lichtenstein AH, et al: 2013 ACC/AHA guideline on the treatment of blood cholesterol to reduce atherosclerotic cardiovascular risk in adults: a report of the American College of Cardiology/American Heart Association Task Force on Practice Guidelines, *Circulation* 2014;129(25, Suppl 2):S1-S45.

Table 27-2   High-, Moderate-, and Low-Intensity Statin Therapy

High-Intensity Statin Therapy	Moderate-Intensity Statin Therapy	Low-Intensity Statin Therapy
Daily dose lowers LDL-C by approximately ≥50%	Daily dose lowers LDL-C by ≈30% to <50%	Daily dose lowers LDL-C by <30%
Atorvastatin 40 mg or 80 mg Rosuvastatin 20 mg or 40 mg	Atorvastatin 10 (20) mg Rosuvastatin (5) 10 mg Simvastatin 20-40 mg[†] Pravastatin 40 (80) mg Lovastatin 40 mg Fluvastatin XL 80 mg Fluvastatin 40 mg BID Pitavastatin 2-4 mg	Simvastatin 10 mg Pravastatin 10-20 mg Lovastatin 20 mg Fluvastatin 20-40 mg Pitavastatin 1 mg

BID, Twice a day; *LDL-C,* low-density lipoprotein cholesterol.
Used with permission from Stone NJ, Robinson J, Lichtenstein AH, et al. 2013 ACC/AHA guideline on the treatment of blood cholesterol to reduce
 atherosclerotic cardiovascular risk in adults: a report of the American College of Cardiology/American Heart Association Task Force on Practice Guidelines,
 Circulation 2014;129(25, Suppl 2):S1-S45.

Table 27-3   Secondary Causes of Hyperlipidemia Most Commonly Encountered in Clinical Practice

Secondary Cause	Elevated LDL-C	Elevated Triglycerides
Diet	Saturated or trans-fats, weight gain, anorexia	Weight gain, very low-fat diets, high intake of refined carbohydrates, excessive alcohol intake
Drugs	Diuretics, cyclosporine, glucocorticoids, amiodarone	Oral estrogens, glucocorticoids, bile acid sequestrants, protease inhibitors, retinoic acid, anabolic steroids, sirolimus, raloxifene, tamoxifen, β-blockers (not carvedilol), thiazides
Diseases	Biliary obstruction, nephrotic syndrome	Nephrotic syndrome, chronic renal failure, lipodystrophies
Disorders and altered states of metabolism	Hypothyroidism, obesity, pregnancy*	Diabetes (poorly controlled), hypothyroidism, obesity, pregnancy*

*Cholesterol and triglycerides increase progressively throughout pregnancy;
 treatment with statins, niacin, and ezetimibe is contraindicated during
 pregnancy and lactation.
LDL-C, Low-density lipoprotein cholesterol.
Used with permission from Stone NJ, Robinson J, Lichtenstein AH, et al.
 2013 ACC/AHA guideline on the treatment of blood cholesterol to
 reduce atherosclerotic cardiovascular risk in adults: a report of the
 American College of Cardiology/American Heart Association Task Force
 on Practice Guidelines, *Circulation* 2014;129(25, Suppl 2):S1-S45.

lifetime risk of ASCVD. Secondary causes of dyslipidemia to be evaluated and treated are summarized in Table 27-3.

Therapeutic lifestyle change is first-line therapy for patients at risk for cardiovascular events (NCEP ATPIII, 2001). Patients who smoke should stop. The amount of daily-consumed cholesterol should be less than 200 mg. The distribution of calories from nutrients is summarized in Table 27-4. Reduced saturated fat and increased consumption of mono- and polyunsaturated fats promote serum LDL-C reduction. The ingestion of viscous fiber and plant stanols decrease cholesterol absorption. Ideally, patients should exercise for 20 to 30 minutes five times per week. Regular exercise promotes weight loss and relieves visceral adiposity and insulin resistance.

Table 27-4   Dietary Recommendations for Therapeutic Lifestyle Change

Dietary Component	Recommendation Allowance
Polyunsaturated fat	≤10% of total calories
Monounsaturated fat	≤20% of total calories
Total fat	25%-35% of total calories
Carbohydrate	50%-60% of total calories
Dietary fiber	20-30 g/day
Protein	≈15% of total calories
Dietary cholesterol	<200 mg/day

PHARMACOLOGIC INTERVENTIONS

Statins

The statins are reversible, competitive 3-hydroxy-3-methylglutaryl coenzyme A (HMG-CoA) reductase inhibitors. HMG-CoA reductase is the rate-limiting step for cholesterol biosynthesis in the liver and systemic tissues. Statins are the most potent agents for reducing serum levels of LDL-C. The statins augment the elimination of atherogenic apoB100-containing lipoproteins (VLDL, VLDL remnants, and LDL) from plasma by upregulating the LDL receptor on the surface of hepatocytes. The statins also reduce VLDL secretion and stimulate apoprotein A-I expression and hepatic HDL secretion.

In a large number of prospective, placebo-controlled clinical trials, the statins have been shown to significantly reduce rates of MI, stroke, and coronary and all-cause mortality in the primary (Downs et al., 1998; Heart Protection Study Group, 2002) and secondary prevention settings (Cannon et al., 2004; LaRosa et al., 2005; Scandinavian Simvastatin Survival Study Group, 1994) (Table 27-5). Statins reduce the frequency of stable and unstable angina and decrease atheromatous plaque progression, and based on intravascular ultrasonographic measurements (Nissen et al., 2004), quantitative coronary angiography, and high-resolution magnetic resonance imaging (MRI) (Corti et al., 2002), even stimulate some degree of plaque resorption. The statins reduce cardiovascular events in men and women, blacks and Hispanics,

Table 27-5 Prospective Randomized Statin Trials in Both Primary and Secondary Prevention

PRIMARY PREVENTION STUDIES

Study	Drug	Design	Outcomes
AFCAPS/ TexCAPS	Lovastatin, 20 mg/d to 40 mg/d vs placebo	6605 men and women	40% reduction in fatal and nonfatal MI; 37% reduction in first ACS; 33% reduction in coronary revascularizations; and 32% reduction in unstable angina
ASCOT	Atorvastatin 10 mg/d vs placebo	10,305 hypertensive men (n = 8463) and women (n = 1942) with treated high BP and no previous CAD	36% reduction in total CHD/nonfatal MI; 27% reduction in fatal and nonfatal stroke; and total coronary event reduced by 29%
CARDS	Atorvastatin 10 mg/d vs placebo	2838 patients with type 2 diabetes mellitus and ≥1 CHD risk factor(s)	37% reduction in major cardiovascular events; 27% reduced total mortality; 13.4% reduction in acute CVD events; 36% reduction in acute coronary events; 48% reduction in stroke
Heart Protection Study	Simvastatin 40 mg/d vs placebo	20,536 high-risk (previous CHD, other vascular disease, hypertension among men aged > 65 yr, or diabetes)	25% reduction in all-cause and coronary death rates and in strokes; 24% reduction in need for revascularization; 25% reduction in fatal and nonfatal stroke; 38% reduction in nonfatal MI; 18% reduction in coronary mortality; 13% reduction in all-cause mortality; 24% reduction in cardiovascular event rate
PROSPER	Pravastatin 40 mg/d vs placebo	5804 men (n = 2804) and women (n = 3000) aged 70 to 82 yr	15% reduction in combined endpoint (fatal/nonfatal MI or stroke); 19% reduction in total/nonfatal CHD; no effect on stroke (but 25% reduction in TIA)
WOSCOPS	Pravachol therapy 40 mg/d vs placebo	6595 men	31% reduction in CHD death from nonfatal MI; 32% reduction in CVD death; 22% reduction in total mortality

SECONDARY PREVENTION STUDIES

Study	Drug	Design	Outcomes
4S	Simvastatin 20 mg/d vs placebo	4444 patients with angina pectoris or history of MI	42% reduction in coronary mortality; 37% reduction in myocardial revascularization; 30% reduction in all-cause mortality; 34% reduction in nonfatal major coronary event; 30% reduction in fatal and nonfatal stroke
AVERT	Atorvastatin 80 mg/d vs angioplasty + usual care	341 patients with stable CAD	36% reduction in ischemic event; 36% reduction in delayed time to first ischemic event
CARE	Pravastatin 40 mg/d vs placebo	3583 men and 576 women with history of MI	24% reduction in death from CHD or non-fatal MI; 37% reduction in fatal MI; 27% reduction in CABG or PTCA
IDEAL	Atorvastatin 80 mg/d vs simvastatin 20-40 mg/d	8888 men and women with CHD	13% reduction in major cardiac events; 17% reduction in nonfatal MI; 23% reduction in revascularization; 24% reduction in peripheral arterial disease
JUPITER	Rosuvastatin 20 mg/d vs placebo	17,802 men (>50 yr) and women (>60 yr) with no history of CAD or DM, entry LDL <130 mg/dl and CRP >2.0 mg/L	44% reduction in primary endpoint of major coronary events; 65% reduction in nonfatal MI; 48% reduction in nonfatal stroke; 46% reduction in need for revascularization; 20% reduction in all-cause mortality
LIPID	Pravachol 40 mg/d vs placebo	9014 patients	24% reduction in coronary mortality; 19% reduction in stroke; 24% reduction in fatal CHD or nonfatal MI; 29% reduction in fatal or nonfatal MI
LIPS	Fluvastatin 40 mg/d vs placebo	1667 men and women aged 18-80 yr post-angioplasty for CAD	22% lower rate of major coronary events (i.e., cardiac deaths, nonfatal MI, or reintervention procedure)
MIRACL	Atorvastatin 80 mg/d vs placebo	3086 patients with ACS	16% reduction in composite endpoint; 26% reduction in ischemia; 50% reduction in stroke
PROVE IT	Atorvastatin 80 mg/d vs pravastatin 40 mg/d	4162 patient with ACS	16% reduction of composite endpoint; 14% reduction in CHD death, MI, or revascularization; 14% reduction in revascularizations; 29% reduction in unstable angina
REVERSAL	Atorvastatin 80 mg/d vs pravastatin 40 mg/d	654 patients with CAD	Atheroma: atorvastatin −0.4%, pravastatin 2.7%, difference of −3.1%, P = 0.02
TNT	Atorvastatin 10 mg/d vs 80 mg/d	10,003 patients with CHD and LDL cholesterol 130-250 mg/dL	22% reduction in composite endpoint; 22% reduction in MI; 25% reduction in stroke

ACS, Acute coronary syndrome; *AFCAPS/TexCAPS*, the Air Force/Texas Coronary Atherosclerosis Prevention Study: Implications for Preventive Cardiology in the General Adult US Population; *ASCOT*, Anglo-Scandinavian Cardiac Outcomes Trial-Lipid Lowering Arm; *AVERT*, Atorvastatin versus Revascularization Treatment Investigators; *CABG*, coronary artery bypass grafting; *CAD*, coronary artery disease; *CARDS*, Collaborative Atorvastatin Diabetes Study; *CARE*, Cholesterol and Recurrent Events Trial; *CHD*, coronary heart disease; *4S*, the Scandinavian Simvastatin Survival Study; *IDEAL*, Incremental Decrease in End Points Through Aggressive Lipid Lowering Study; *JUPITER*, the Justification for the Use of Statins in Prevention: an Intervention Trial Evaluating Rosuvastatin; *LDL*, low-density lipoprotein; *LIPID*, Long-Term Intervention with Pravastatin in Ischemic Disease; *LIPS*, Lescol Intervention Prevention Study; *MI*, myocardial infarction; *MIRACL*, Myocardial Ischemia Reduction with Aggressive Cholesterol Lowering Study; *PROSPER*, pravastatin in elderly individuals at risk of vascular disease; *PROVE IT*, Pravastatin or Atorvastatin Evaluation and Infection Therapy study; *PTCA*, percutaneous transluminal coronary angioplasty; *REVERSAL*, The REVERSing Atherosclerosis with Aggressive Lipid Lowering study; *TNT*, Treating to New Targets Trial; *WOSCOPS*, West of Scotland Coronary Prevention Study. Used with permission from Toth, PP. Management of Dyslipidemia. In Comprehensive Cardiovascular Medicine in the Primary Care Setting (Toth, PP and Cannon CP, editors) Humana-Springer, Philadelphia. 2010.

individuals with HTN or diabetes, smokers, and patients older than 70 years of age. In addition, based on meta-analyses performed by the Cholesterol Treatment Trialists Collaboration, statins provide benefit largely independent of baseline LDL-C levels and Framingham risk score and are not associated with increased risk for any type of malignancy (Cholesterol Treatment Trialists, 2012a, 2012b).

Seven statins are currently available. These drugs differ by potency and a number of pharmacokinetic properties. The choice of statin and its dosing depend on the magnitude of LDL-C and non-HDL-C reduction required (baseline vs. risk-stratified NCEP target). The LDL-C lowering efficacy of the statins is as follows: rosuvastatin (Crestor), 45% to 63% (5-40 mg/day); atorvastatin (Lipitor), 26% to 60% (10-80 mg/day); simvastatin (Zocor), 26% to 47% (10-80 mg/day); lovastatin (Mevacor), 21% to 42% (10-80 mg/day); fluvastatin (Lescol), 22% to 36% (10-20 mg/day); pitavastatin (Livalo), 32% to 43% (1-4 mg/day); and pravastatin (Pravachol), 22% to 34% (10-80 mg/day) (e.g., Jones et al., 2003). Each doubling of a statin's dose yields an additional 6% reduction, on average, in serum LDL-C (the so-called "rule of 6s"). Patients who are heterozygous or homozygous for familial hypercholesterolemia frequently require high-potency statins at their highest doses coupled with stringent restriction in dietary lipid ingestion and the addition of one or more other lipid-lowering agents. The statins induce significant reductions in serum triglyceride levels (typically 10%-25%) and modest elevations in serum HDL-C (2%-14%). Unlike the other statins, atorvastatin therapy is associated with decreasing capacity for raising HDL-C as a function of increasing dose. In patients with high baseline serum triglyceride levels (>300 mg/dL), simvastatin and rosuvastatin raise HDL-C up to 18 and 22%, respectively.

The statins display significant differences in their pharmacokinetic profiles. Due to their relatively short half-lives (1-4 hours), lovastatin, fluvastatin, pravastatin, and simvastatin should be taken after the evening meal to intercept the peak activity of HMG-CoA-reductase, which occurs around midnight. Rosuvastatin and atorvastatin can be taken at any time during the day or night because of their long half-lives (≈19 hours and 14 hours, respectively). The coadministration of drugs or compounds that inhibit cytochrome P450 3A4 (macrolide antibiotics [erythromycin, clarithromycin], azole-type antifungals [ketoconazole, itraconazole], cyclosporine, HIV protease inhibitors, nefazodone, >1 qt of grapefruit juice daily) with atorvastatin, simvastatin, and lovastatin is contraindicated because these statins are dependent on this P450 isozyme for oxidative modification and elimination (Neuvonen et al., 1998). P450 3A4 inhibition is associated with increased risk for myopathy and hepatotoxicity. The dose of simvastatin should be 20 mg/day or less in patients being treated with amiodarone, amlodipine, or verapamil.

Although there is some concern about the potential toxicity of statins, their benefits significantly outweigh their risks. Moreover, because the risk of true hepatotoxicity from a statin is quite low, the Food and Drug Administration (FDA) issued an advisory stating that in general, the monitoring of liver enzymes in patients treated with statins is no longer necessary given the low yield of findings. The majority of cases of elevated transaminases in these patients are caused by hepatic steatosis.

Liver toxicity is defined as an alanine aminotransferase (ALT) elevation ≥ 3 the upper limit of normal (ULN) on two occasions at least 1 month apart. Mild elevations in serum transaminase levels early during the course of therapy are observed and usually resolve spontaneously. If hepatotoxicity develops, statin therapy should be discontinued until transaminase levels normalize and therapy with a different statin can be initiated. There is no documented evidence that the statins increase risk for liver failure.

The most important adverse events associated with statin therapy are rhabdomyolysis, myoglobinuria, and renal failure. The risk for rhabdomyolysis is less than 0.1%. Symptoms of rhabdomyolysis include worsening muscle pain, proximal weakness, nausea and vomiting, and brownish-red discoloration of urine. The statins can cause myalgia. If a patient develops myalgia or muscle weakness, a serum creatine kinase level can be obtained. The diagnosis of myopathy is made when creatine kinase levels exceed 10 times ULN. When assessing myalgia, it is important to evaluate patients for pain that is caused by arthritis, tendinopathy, thyroid dysfunction, electrolyte disturbances, fibromyalgia, polymyalgia rheumatica, blunt muscle trauma, and muscle strain induced by exertion. There are no large, convincing randomized studies demonstrating that coenzyme Q or vitamin D supplementation reduces statin-associated muscle pain or weakness.

A newly elucidated potential adverse event associated with statin therapy is new-onset DM. It is not yet established how statins cause DM. Meta-analyses suggest that the risk of new-onset DM with statin therapy is approximately 1 per 1000 patients treated per year (Sattar et al., 2010). Patients treated with maximum doses of statin therapy have a risk of approximately one per 500 patients treated per year (Preiss et al., 2011). It appears that the patients at increased risk for new-onset DM are the ones who have established impaired glucose tolerance or one or more other components of the metabolic syndrome. All major guideline-writing bodies throughout the world recommend that statin therapy not be withheld out of concern that it may cause DM. The benefits of statin therapy still outweigh its risks, and statin therapy is highly efficacious for reducing risk of cardiovascular events in patients with DM.

Ezetimibe (Zetia)

Dietary and biliary sources contribute significantly to serum levels of cholesterol (Figure 27-2). Although plant sterols and stanols block GI cholesterol absorption, ezetimibe is the first member of a class of lipid-lowering drugs known as cholesterol absorption inhibitors. Mechanistically, ezetimibe inhibits the Niemann-Pick C1-like-1 protein, which mediates cholesterol and phytosterol transport along the brush border of the jejunal enterocyte (Altmann et al., 2004; Davis et al., 2004). After undergoing glucuronidation, ezetimibe undergoes enterohepatic recirculation with negligible systemic exposure. The half-life of ezetimibe is approximately 22 hours. When dosed at 10 mg once daily, ezetimibe reduces serum LDL-C on average by 20%, but up to 24% of patients experience a reduction of 25% or greater (Ballantyne et al., 2004; Davidson et al., 2002). Ezetimibe also decreases triglycerides by up to 8% and raises

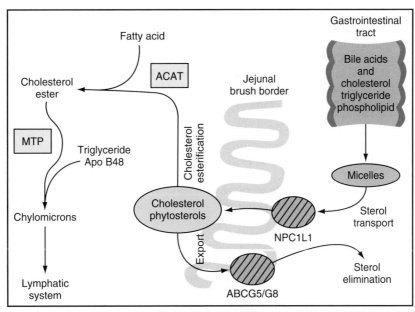

Figure 27-2 Gastrointestinal (GI) absorption of dietary and biliary lipid and cholesterol. In the GI tract, cholesterol and triglycerides arising from biliary and dietary sources are assimilated with bile salts and phospholipids to form micelles. Micelles transport cholesterol and lipid to the jejunal brush border. Along the enterocyte surface, the sterol transporter known as Niemann Pick C1–like 1 (NPC1L1) protein is responsible for importing cholesterol and phytosterols into the neurocyte. After being internalized, the cholesterol is esterified to cholesterol esters via the activity of acyl-CoA acyltransferase (ACAT). The esterified cholesterol is packaged with triglycerides, phospholipids, and apoprotein B48 (ApoB48) to form chylomicrons in an assimilation reaction catalyzed by microsomal transfer protein (MTP). The chylomicrons are released into GI lacteals, which conduct these lipoproteins into the central circulation. Excess intracellular sterols can be excreted back into the GI tract via the activity of the sterol exporter complex ABCG5/G8 (ATP-binding membrane cassette transporter G5/G8). (Reproduced with permission from Toth PP, Davidson MH. Cholesterol absorption blockade with ezetimibe. *Curr Drug Targets Cardiovasc Haematol Disord.* 2005;5:455-462.)

HDL-C by up to 4%. Ezetimibe does not decrease the absorption of bile acids; steroid hormones (ethinyl estradiol, progesterone); or such fat-soluble vitamins as vitamins A, D, E, or α- and β-carotenes. In addition to its indication for reducing LDL-C, ezetimibe is approved for use in patients with β-sitosterolemia, a rare genetic disorder that gives rise to severe elevations in serum levels of plant sterols (campesterol, β-sitosterol, and others) and premature onset CAD.

The risk of hepatotoxicity with ezetimibe is nearly identical to placebo (0.5% vs. 0.3%), and there is no documented evidence of increased risk for myopathy. Fixed-dose ezetimibe is also available in combination with increasing doses of simvastatin (Vytorin; 10/10; 10/20; 10/40; 10/80 mg/day) and atorvastatin (Liptruzet). Ezetimibe can also be safely used in combination with other statins (Toth, 2005). Ezetimibe provides additive changes in lipoprotein levels to that observed with statin therapy. The addition of ezetimibe to a statin provides incremental LDL-C reduction equivalent to three titration steps of a statin.

Bile Acid Binding Resins

The bile acid sequestration agents (BASAs) are orally administered anion exchange resins that bind bile acids in the GI tract and prevent them from being reabsorbed into the enterohepatic circulation. These drugs reduce serum LDL-C by two mechanisms: (1) increased catabolism of cholesterol secondary to the upregulation of 7-α-hydroxylase, the rate-limiting enzyme for the conversion of cholesterol into bile acids, and (2) increased expression of LDL receptors on the hepatocyte surface, which augments the clearance of apoB100-containing lipoproteins from plasma. At maximum doses, the BASA can reduce serum LDL-C by 15% to 30% and increase HDL-C by 3% to 5%. It is recommended that these drugs be used in conjunction with a statin whenever possible because BASA therapy increases HMG-CoA reductase activity in the liver, which leads to increased hepatic biosynthesis of cholesterol, thereby offsetting the effects of the BASA over time. The BASA are contraindicated in patients with serum triglycerides greater than 400 mg/dL because they can exacerbate hypertriglyceridemia.

There are currently three different BASAs available. These include cholestyramine (Questran; 4-24 g/day in 2-3 divided doses daily), colestipol (Colestid; 5-30 g in two or three divided doses daily), and colesevelam (Welchol; 1250 mg two to three times daily). The development of constipation, flatulence, and bloating are relatively frequent, but colesevelam has the most favorable side effect profile of the three available BASAs. Increasing water and soluble fiber ingestion ameliorates some of the difficulty with constipation. The BASAs bind negatively charged molecules in a nonspecific manner. Consequently, they can decrease the absorption of warfarin, phenobarbital, thiazide diuretics, digitalis, β-blockers, thyroxine, statins, fibrates, and ezetimibe. These medications should be taken 1 hour before or 4 hours after the ingestion of BASA. The BASA can reduce the absorption of fat-soluble vitamins. Colesevelam also has an indication to reduce serum glycated hemoglobin levels in patients with DM.

Fibrates

The fibrates are fibric acid derivatives that exert a number of effects on lipoprotein metabolism. These agents reduce serum triglycerides by 25% to 50% and raise HDL-C by 10% to 20%. Fibrates activate lipoprotein lipase by reducing levels of apoprotein CIII (an inhibitor of this enzyme) and increasing levels of apoprotein CII (an activator of lipoprotein lipase) (Andersson et al., 2011). This stimulates the hydrolysis of triglycerides in chylomicrons and VLDL. Fibrates increase HDL-C by two mechanisms. First, the fibrates are peroxisome proliferator-activated receptor α (PPAR-α) agonists and stimulate increased hepatic expression of apoproteins AI and AII. Second, by activating lipoprotein lipase, surface coat mass derived from VLDL is ultimately used to assimilate HDL in serum. In some patients, fibrate therapy may be associated with an increase in serum LDL-C (the so-called "β" effect) secondary to increased enzymatic conversion of VLDL to LDL. This effect may diminish over time as the patient increases the expression of hepatic LDL receptors.

The fibrates are particularly valuable for treating dyslipidemia in patients with a combination of hypertriglyceridemia and low HDL-C levels. In this patient type, post hoc evaluations of data from three studies (Helsinki Heart Study, Fenofibrate Intervention and Event Lowering in Diabetes, and the Bezafibrate Infarction Prevention Study) have demonstrated substantial cardiovascular event rate reductions using fibrate therapy (Bezafibrate Infarction Prevention Study Group, 2000; Manninen et al., 1988). In the Veterans Affairs High-Density Lipoprotein Intervention Trial (VA-HIT), men with CAD and low HDL levels (mean, 31 mg/dL) were treated with either gemfibrozil (600 mg orally twice a day) or placebo over a 5-year follow-up period (Robins et al., 2001). With a 6% elevation in HDL, no change in LDL, and a 31% decrease in triglycerides, gemfibrozil therapy resulted in a 22% reduction in the composite end point of all-cause mortality and nonfatal MI compared with placebo (Rubins et al., 1999). Gemfibrozil therapy also reduced the risk of stroke and TIAs by 31% and 59%, respectively (Rubins et al., 2001). Among the patients with diabetes in VA-HIT treated with gemfibrozil, there was a 32% reduction in the combined end point (41% in coronary heart disease [CHD] death and 40% in stroke) (Rubins et al., 2002). Fibrates have been shown to exert many of the same pleiotropic effects as statins and reduce atheromatous plaque progression in native coronary vessels and in coronary venous bypass grafts (Diabetes Atherosclerosis Intervention Study Investigators, 2001; Ericsson et al., 1996).

Similar to the statins, fibrates are associated with a low incidence of myopathy and mild elevations in serum transaminases. Fibrate therapy can increase the risk for cholelithiasis and can increase the prothrombin times by displacing warfarin from albumin binding sites. The periodic monitoring of serum transaminases (6-12 weeks after initiating therapy and twice annually thereafter) is recommended. The two most commonly used fibrates are gemfibrozil (Lopid; 600 mg twice daily) and fenofibrate (Tricor; 54 or 160 mg/day). Bezafibrate is available in Europe and is dosed at 400 mg/day. The use of therapies combining a statin and fibrate is becoming more common in clinical practice, especially as the incidence of complex dyslipidemias increases (Davidson and Toth, 2004). Gemfibrozil significantly reduces the glucuronidation of statins, which decreases their elimination (Backman et al., 2002; Prueksaritanont et al., 2002a, 2002b). This

increases the risk for myopathy or rhabdomyolysis and hepatotoxicity. When used in combination with gemfibrozil, the doses for simvastatin and rosuvastatin should not exceed 10 mg/day. In general, when embarking on combination therapy, fenofibrate is a safer choice because it does not adversely impact the glucuronidation of the statins (Bergman et al., 2004).

In both Fenofibrate Intervention and Event Lowering in Diabetes (FIELD) and Action to Control Cardiovascular Risk in Diabetes (ACCORD) trials (Ginsberg et al., 2010), fenofibrate reduced the risk of progression of retinopathy in patients with diabetes by approximately one third. Fenofibrate has also been shown to reduce microalbuminuria. Reducing the risk of blindness and progression of albuminuria are important therapeutic considerations in patients with DM. Among patients with low HDL-C and high triglycerides, post hoc subgroup analyses demonstrate that fenofibrate reduces risks for the primary composite end point of cardiovascular events by 27% and 31% in the FIELD and ACCORD trials, respectively. Although post hoc findings must be considered hypothesis-generating only, there is remarkable consistency of benefit in patients given fibrate therapy when triglycerides are high and HDL-C is low.

Among patients in whom serum triglycerides do not normalize in response to a low-fat diet and fibrate therapy, consideration should be given to the addition of other agents. Patients with severe hypertriglyceridemia frequently possess mutations in lipoprotein lipase, which reduce the lipolytic activity of this enzyme. In this scenario, the addition of orlistat (Xenical; 120 mg with meals) can reduce the absorption of dietary fat and hence the circulating levels of chylomicrons and triglycerides. The addition of fish oil (see next section) should also be considered.

Fish Oils

Fish oil capsules enriched with ω-3 (eicosapentaenoic acid) and ω-6 (docosahexaenoic acid) fatty acids can reduce serum triglyceride and VLDL levels and raise HDL-C in a dose-dependent manner. The ω-3 fatty acids inhibit the enzyme diacylglycerol acyltransferase-2, thereby reducing intrahepatic triglyceride biosynthesis. They also stimulate mitochondrial β-oxidation of fatty acids, decrease VLDL production and biosynthesis, and stimulate triglyceride hydrolysis by lipoprotein lipase. Dietary supplementation with the n-3 polyunsaturated fatty acids (PUFAs) eicosapentaenoic acid (EPA) and docosahexaenoic acid (DHA) has also been shown to lower the risk of death, nonfatal coronary events, and stroke after MI (GISSI-Prevenzione Investigators, 1999). In several clinical trials, PUFAs have been shown to reduce triglyceride levels by 20% to 30% and up to 50% in patients with severe hypertriglyceridemia (triglyceride level > 500 mg/dL) (O'Keefe and Harris, 2000).

The Japan EPA Lipid Intervention Study (JELIS) evaluated whether the addition of fish oils to patients already taking a statin would provide incremental risk reduction. Approximately 19,000 Japanese men and women with hypercholesterolemia were prospectively randomized to statin therapy with or without 1800 mg/day of EPA (Yokoyama et al., 2007). Combination therapy resulted in an additional 19% reduction in major coronary events at 4.6 years of follow-up compared with statin monotherapy.

Niacin

Niacin or nicotinic acid is a B vitamin that exerts multiple beneficial effects on lipoprotein metabolism. In contrast to statins and fibrates, niacin does not stimulate hepatic biosynthesis of HDL. Niacin appears to block HDL particle uptake and catabolism by hepatocytes without adversely impacting reverse cholesterol transport. This helps to increase circulating levels of HDL. Niacin reduces hepatic VLDL and triglyceride secretion according to two mechanisms: (1) it decreases the flux of fatty acids from adipose tissue to the liver by inhibiting lipase activity, and (2) it inhibits triglyceride formation within hepatocytes by inhibiting diacylglycerol acyltransferase. Niacin also reduces serum LDL-C concentrations by increasing the catabolism of apoB100. Consequently, niacin beneficially impacts all components of the lipoprotein profile.

When used as monotherapy at 3.0 g/day, crystalline niacin significantly reduced the incidence of MI and stroke in patients with established CAD in the Coronary Drug Project (Coronary Drug Project Research Group, 1975). In the HDL-Atherosclerosis Treatment Study (HATS), patients (baseline LDL-C, 124 mg/dL; HDL-C, 34 mg/dL) treated with combinations of high-dose niacin (2-4 g) with simvastatin reduced cardiovascular morbidity and mortality by up to 90% compared with those given placebo (Brown et al., 2001). This combination therapy also induced atheromatous plaque stabilization over a 3-year follow-up period. Two more recent clinical trials demonstrate that when atherogenic lipoprotein burden in serum is low, niacin therapy provides no incremental benefit over and above background therapy with a statin or statin–ezetimibe. In the Atherothrombosis Intervention in Metabolic syndrome with low HDL/high triglicerides: Impact on Global Health outcomes (AIM-HIGH) trial, patients with CAD and exquisitely well-controlled lipids (baseline LDL-C, 70 mg/dL; non-HDL-C, 106 mg/dL; and apoprotein B, 80 mg/dL) derived no benefit from the addition of 1.5 to 2.0 g of niacin (Boden et al., 2011). However, in the subgroup with HDL-C less than 32 mg/dL and triglycerides greater than 200 mg/dL, niacin therapy was associated with a significant 37% incremental reduction in the primary composite end point (Guyton et al., 2013). In the HPS2-THRIVE trial, the addition of niacin and laropiprant (an agent that reduces the flushing associated with niacin therapy) provided no incremental benefit in patients with CAD and remarkably well-controlled baseline levels of lipoproteins (LDL-C, 63 mg/dL; HDL-C, 44 mg/dL; and triglycerides, 125 mg/dL) (http://www.thrivestudy.org).

In patients with mixed dyslipidemia whose lipids are not adequately controlled on statin therapy, the addition of niacin can be considered as adjuvant therapy. Niacin should be started at a low dose and gradually titrated upward based on the results of follow-up lipid panels. When evaluated as a function of dose (500-2000 mg/day), Niaspan induces the following changes in serum lipid levels: LDL-C, 3% to 16% reduction; triglycerides, 5% to 32% reduction; and HDL-C, 10% to 24% elevation (Capuzzi et al., 1998).

Niacin therapy is associated with a number of side effects. The most common side effect with niacin is cutaneous flushing. Taking a 325-mg tablet of aspirin 1 hour before taking niacin can reduce the incidence of this. The flushing is prostaglandin mediated. Limiting fat intake for 2 to 3 hours before taking niacin also helps as fat is a source of arachidonic acid, the substrate for cyclooxygenase. Niaspan is a sustained-release preparation of niacin associated with less flushing. Other side effects include bloating, pruritus, acanthosis nigricans, transient disturbances in glycemic control, and increased serum concentrations of uric acid. Niacin appears to increase rates of proximal tubular reuptake of urate from the glomerular ultrafiltrate. Niacin is available as a combination pill with lovastatin (Advicor; 500/20 mg, 1000/20 mg, and 2000/40 mg) or simvastatin (Simcor; 500/20 mg, 750/20 mg, and 1000/20 mg), with the two drugs in each combination pill providing additive changes in the levels of serum lipoproteins.

KEY TREATMENT

- Statins, fibrates, niacin, ω-3 fish oils, and bile acid sequestration are highly efficacious agents for treating dyslipidemia (SOR: A).
- Statins are the most efficacious drugs currently available for reducing serum levels of LDL-C and significantly impact the risk for both cardiovascular morbidity and mortality (SOR: A). The ω-3 fish oils also appear to impact cardiovascular mortality, although the evidence is not as strong as with statins.
- Fibrates have the greatest capacity to reduce serum triglycerides (SOR: A). The fibrates have not yet been shown to beneficially impact mortality as an independent end point in clinical trials. The fibrates have been shown to reduce rates of atherosclerotic disease progression in both individuals with diabetes and without diabetes who have CAD. Fenofibrate reduces the risk of progression of retinopathy and albuminuria. Gemfibrozil as monotherapy reduces the risk for cardiovascular events in men in both the primary and secondary prevention settings as demonstrated in the Helsinki Heart Study and VA-HIT trial, respectively (SOR: A).
- Niacin raises serum levels of HDL-C significantly better than other currently available antilipidemic medications, and it also reduces LDL-C, triglycerides, and lipoprotein (a) (SOR: A). As demonstrated in both AIM-HIGH and HPS2-THRIVE, niacin does not provide incremental benefit if the atherogenic lipoprotein burden is already well controlled with other lipid lowering agents.
- Therapy with combinations of drugs (statin–fibrate, statin–niacin, fibrate–niacin, statin–ezetimibe) is frequently required in patients with mixed forms of dyslipidemia and increases the likelihood of improving multiple abnormal components of the lipid profile. However, incremental reductions in primary cardiovascular outcomes have not yet been demonstrated in trials testing combination therapy (SOR: C). In the ACCORD trial, the addition of fenofibrate to ongoing statin therapy in patients with diabetes with LDL-C of 100 mg/dL, HDL-C of 39 mg/dL, and normal triglyceride levels did not provide incremental benefit. The impact of ezetimibe adjuvant therapy with a statin is currently being evaluated in the IMPROVE-IT trial in patients who are status post an ACS.
- Antilipidemic agents can induce myalgia and myopathy and, rarely, hepatotoxicity (SOR: A).
- It is common for statins and fibrates to induce transient elevations in serum transaminases. If this occurs, these

Continued

drugs should be discontinued if levels exceed three times the ULN (SOR: A). However, if levels are below this threshold, it is acceptable to monitor liver function tests (LFTs) because transaminase levels usually decrease and trend toward normal spontaneously. Often, these drugs are discontinued prematurely, to the detriment of patient care. If LFTs do elevate, it is important to rule out drug interactions and evaluate the patient for baseline hepatic dysfunction (e.g., viral hepatic infection, structural injury, steatosis).

- When combining a statin with a fibrate, the use of gemfibrozil should be discouraged because it impairs the glucuronidation and elimination of the statins to varying degrees (SOR: A). This can result in increased risk for hepatotoxicity and rhabdomyolysis. Fenofibrate and fenofibric acid are safer choices in this context.
- Patients complaining of myalgias or weakness, especially if escalating, should be monitored for myopathy. The statins and fibrates should be discontinued if serum creatine kinase levels exceed 10 times the ULN (SOR: A). However, myalgias are common and not necessarily attributable to statin and fibrate usage. Other etiologies for myalgia and myopathy (fibromyalgia, polymyalgia rheumatica, muscle injury, electrolyte disturbances) should be investigated as appropriate.
- In patients presenting with rhabdomyolysis, antilipidemic medications should be discontinued immediately. Patients should be hospitalized and hydrated with intravenous (IV) fluids and provided with all manner of supportive care (SOR: A).

Hypertension

Key Points

- Hypertension is highly prevalent, affecting one third of the adult population.
- Undertreatment is common, with only 50% of people achieving goals in the United States.
- Attention to proper technique for office blood pressure (BP) measurement is mandatory to accurately characterize BP levels and HTN control.
- Most patients should use proper home BP monitoring to aid in the proper diagnosis and management of HTN.
- The goal BP is a matter of considerable controversy. The panel members appointed to the Eighth Joint National Committee (JNC 8) suggest a goal of less than 140/90 mm Hg in patients under 60 years of age and 150/90 mm Hg in patients older than 60 years. Other influential guidelines suggest a more general application of 140/90 mm Hg as BP goal.
- Goal home BP averages are less than 135/85 mm Hg. Goal 24-hour ambulatory BP levels are less than 130/80 mm Hg.
- In uncomplicated HTN without compelling indications because of comorbidities, the specific choice of drug is less important than the attainment of goal BP. However, most patients should avoid monotherapy with a β-blocker or an α-blocker, given clinical trial evidence demonstrating their inferiority.
- If BP is more than 20/10 mm Hg above target level, then starting two antihypertensive medications (e.g., a combination pill) should be strongly considered.
- The use of combination therapy to treat HTN allows for the interruption of multiple mechanisms etiologic for this disorder and increases the likelihood of therapeutic success. Most recent evidence suggests that the majority of patients (perhaps 75%) will require two or more medications to obtain goals.
- The most compelling evidence suggests that if two agents are required, a combination of an angiotensin-converting enzyme (ACE) inhibitor plus a calcium channel blocker (CCB) (amlodipine) should be used first line based on the Avoiding Cardiovascular Events through Combination Therapy in Patients Living with Systolic Hypertension (ACCOMPLISH) study. Other combination agents, such as an ACE inhibitor plus a thiazide diuretic, are acceptable alternative regimens.
- The combination of two or more agents that block the renin–angiotensin system (e.g., ACE inhibitor angiotensin receptor blocker [ARB]; ARB + renin inhibitor) is almost always contraindicated.
- The Seventh Report of the Joint National Committee on Prevention, Detection, Evaluation, and Treatment of High Blood Pressure (JNC 7) encouraged the use of specific antihypertensive agents in the setting of HTN complicated by congestive heart failure (CHF), CAD, MI, and nephropathy, among other forms of CVD. Although more recent guidelines focus less on selecting specific agents, the importance of the "compelling indications" for an ACE inhibitor (or ARB) as the first-line treatment should still be considered, particularly among patients with CHF or proteinuria. The report of the panel members appointed to JNC 8 presents several additional considerations regarding compelling indications.
- Assuring adherence and persistence with medications and the institution of proven lifestyle modifications are important components of successful HTN management.
- Resistant HTN is common, affecting approximately 10% of the hypertensive population. Numerous approaches to obtain BP control have been shown to be helpful, including the empirical usage of aldosterone blockade (spironolactone 25-50 mg/day).
- In difficult cases, referral to an HTN expert may be warranted.
- Health care providers may believe that diastolic blood pressure (DBP) impacts CVD risk more than systolic blood pressure (SBP). The opposite is true among people older than 50 years of age.
- Therapeutic inertia (e.g., underaggressive dosing, underuse of combination medications, infrequent follow-up) is common and a prevalent cause of uncontrolled HTN.
- Suboptimal patient education about high BP and incomplete adherence to medical therapy are common causes of poorly controlled HTN.
- Underuse of diuretics, in particular chlorthalidone (a longer acting and more potent thiazide), is a frequent cause of uncontrolled HTN.
- The CCBs (both dihydropyridines and nondihydropyridines) tend to be underused because of peripheral edema. Combining these drugs with a low dose of an ACE inhibitor reduces the incidence of edema.
- ACE inhibitors and ARBs tend to be withheld in patients with mild to moderate renal insufficiency. However, such patients benefit significantly from these drugs. An increase in serum creatinine of up to 30% to 40% is

- not unexpected and is acceptable (if it stabilizes), and patients should be monitored for hyperkalemia.
  - β-Blockers are often overprescribed given the belief that they prevent MIs more than other agents in primary prevention. This is untrue, and given their inferior prevention of strokes, they should not be given as first-line agents in most patients for the treatment of HTN.
  - Thiazide diuretics and β-blockers can antagonize glycemic control in patients with insulin resistance and impaired glucose tolerance and are associated with an increased risk for diabetes. ACE inhibitors and ARBs are metabolically beneficial and should be prescribed in most situations among such patients.

Hypertension is defined as persistently elevated BP 140 mm Hg or greater SBP or 90 mm Hg or greater DBP (Chobanian et al., 2003; James et al., 2014). It is a common and increasingly prevalent disorder affecting roughly one third of adults in the United States (Go et al., 2013) and at least one fourth of adults around the globe (Kearney et al., 2005). A higher than ideal BP (i.e., >115/75 mm Hg) is a well-established risk factor for CAD, MIs, left ventricular hypertrophy (LVH), CHF, PAD, aneurysmal diseases, strokes, chronic kidney disease (CKD), and sudden death. Approximately half of all strokes and ischemic heart disease (IHD) worldwide are attributable to HTN (Lawes et al., 2008). The Global Burden of Disease study has demonstrated that HTN is the single leading cause of morbidity worldwide (Lim et al., 2012). Moreover, there is a well-established log-linear relationship between the severity of HTN and cardiovascular risk. Data from 1 million adults demonstrate that every 20/10 mm Hg elevation in BP leads to an approximate doubling of risk of death from IHD and other vascular causes (Lewington et al., 2002). Even "pre-HTN" (120-139/80-89 mm Hg) is associated with an approximate doubling of cardiovascular risk (Mancia et al. 2013). In this context, the standard definition of HTN is arbitrary from a cardiovascular health standpoint. Nevertheless, a definition of HTN based on 140/90 mm Hg has been widely accepted because of a lack of large-scale randomized trials proving that treatment of BP initially below this threshold reduces morbidity and mortality (Law et al., 2009; Mancia et al., 2013).

RISK FACTORS FOR HYPERTENSION

The incidence of HTN increases as a function of age (Egan et al., 2010). Patients who are normotensive at age 55 years have a 90% risk of developing HTN at some point in their lives (Vasan et al., 2002). Some of the most important environmental risk factors predicting its incidence are obesity (≈1 mm Hg increase per kilogram of weight gain) (Staessen et al., 1988), excess sodium (>1.5-2.3 g/day) and alcohol intake (>10-20 g/day), lack of physical activity, and use of several over-the-counter (OTC) and prescription medications (e.g., stimulants, decongestants, estrogen-containing birth control pills, nonsteroidal antiinflammatory drugs [NSAIDs]) (Chobanian et al., 2003; Mancia et al., 2013). These risks are compounded in the setting of an underlying genetic predisposition. Although monogenic abnormalities exist (most typically affecting the kidney and

renal sodium handling; Simonetti et al., 2012), the genetic underpinning of the vast majority of "primary" HTN is attributable to the inheritance of multiple genes (Munroe et al., 2013). As such, a history of HTN doubles the risk for developing abnormal BP levels in other first-degree family members. Several common genetic variants (≈29 independent alleles have been identified) associate with HTN in genome-wide association studies (Munroe et al., 2013). The effect of each of these common variants on the risk of developing HTN appears to be small, although the cumulative effect of many risk-causing variants might be clinically important (i.e., altering BP by 4-6 mm Hg) (Mancia et al., 2013).

Hypertension is rarely caused by mutations in a single gene. However, in these uncommon scenarios, the onset of HTN is often observed during childhood and typically with other pertinent signs (e.g., low potassium) or characteristic phenotypes (e.g., Turner syndrome) (Simonetti et al., 2012). It is important for primary care physicians to be aware that some uncommon genetic disorders can lead to early-onset (and often severe) HTN that strongly clusters in families. Well-defined conditions include Liddle syndrome, the syndrome of apparent mineralocorticoid excess, congenital adrenal hyperplasia, and several familial syndromes of early-onset hyperaldosteronism or pheochromocytomas. However, by far the majority of HTN cases in children and adolescents are attributable to "primary" polygenic-environmental HTN, largely caused by increasing rates of obesity in the population (Koebnick et al., 2013). Guidelines for the management of HTN in special situations such as in children and adolescents have been published (Mancia et al., 2013).

THE ASSESSMENT OF HYPERTENSION IN ADULTS

The JNC 7 provides a comprehensive framework for defining and managing HTN among adults older than 18 years of age in the United States (Chobanian et al., 2003). However, these guidelines are now more than 10 years old and do not account for the findings of several important clinical trials published in the interim. The recently published report by the JNC 8 panel members highlights the lack of placebo-controlled trials targeting a BP less than 150/90 mm Hg in patients older than the age of 60 years (James et al., 2014). The panel members recommend that in the general population age 60 years of age and older, a BP of 150/90 mm Hg should be threshold for treatment and the treatment goal. In addition, the JNC 8 panel members placed less emphasis on thiazide-like diuretics as initial therapy for HTN compared with the JNC 7 recommendations. A comprehensive current set of guidelines has been published by the European Society of HTN (Mancia et al., 2013) The JNC 7 classifications of BP were not addressed by the JNC 8 panel members, and they remain valid (Table 27-6) (Chobanian et al., 2003). The importance of following careful methods and scrupulous attention to proper technique for the clinic measurement of BP cannot be overstated. Numerous patient and health care provider factors are involved as outlined by the AHA in detail (Pickering et al., 2005). A few of the most critical issues are to assure adequate patient rest time (5 minutes) in a seated position with the feet and back fully

Table 27-6 JNC 7 Blood Pressure Classification*

BP Classification	SBP (mm Hg)	DBP (mm Hg)	Lifestyle Modification	Drug Therapy
Normal	<120	and <80	Yes	Usually no treatment
Prehypertension	120-139	and 80-89	Yes	Yes, for compelling JNC 7 indications
Stage 1 hypertension	140-159	or 90-99	Yes	Yes
Stage 2 hypertension	≥160	or ≥100	Yes	Yes

*This classification is based on blood pressure (BP) levels being measured in at least duplicate readings on two or more separate occasions in a stable situation. This represents the "average" prevailing BP. Single elevations, sporadic, or transient increases in BP, such that might occur during pain, stress, illness, or anxiety, do not represent hypertension and should not be used to classify BP. The ESH 2013 classifies patients with systolic blood pressure (SBP) ≥180 or diastolic blood pressure (DBP) ≥110 mm Hg as having "stage 3" hypertension.
JNC, Seventh Report of the Joint National Committee on Prevention, Detection, Evaluation, and Treatment of High Blood Pressure.
From *The Seventh Report of the Joint National Committee on Prevention, Detection, Evaluation, and Treatment of High Blood Pressure.* Washington, DC: U.S Department of Health and Human Services. National Institute of Health Publication No. 04-5230. August 2004.

supported before measurement, a properly supported arm with the brachial artery at heart-level (defined as the fourth intercostal space), use of an appropriate size cuff for the arm circumference (the length and width of the bladder should be 80% and 40% arm circumference, respectively), the averaging of duplicate-to-triplicate BP recordings obtained 30 to 60 seconds apart, and assuring that the sphygmomanometer is routinely validated as being accurate (Mancia et al., 2013). Under most circumstances, a well-trained medical assistant or nurse should measure BP in a clinical setting given that most epidemiologic studies and clinical trials have been based on BP measurements obtained by nonphysicians. BPs are higher when measured by a physician because of an exaggerated "white coat" effect (Mancia et al., 1987). Several validated oscillometric office-based automated BP devices are currently available. These monitors can be programmed to measure multiple BP recordings while health care providers are absent from the clinic room, thus substantially reducing the "white coat" effect; studies have shown them to provide readings closer to BP levels obtained by home and ambulatory BP monitoring (Pickering et al., 2005) and to be superior predictors of cardiovascular morbidity (Pickering et al., 2008).

Both the JNC 7 and ESH 2013 guidelines outline standard recommendations for the assessment of patients with elevated BP levels (Chobanian et al., 2003; Mancia et al., 2013). These include an evaluation of HTN-related target organ status (TOS) and other concomitant cardiovascular risk factors (i.e., absolute global CVD risk estimation) and obtaining basic laboratory tests. A standard evaluation of TOS involves a funduscopic, neurologic, cardiac, and vascular physical examination and history looking for evidence of prior HTN-related disease(s) (e.g., MI, CHF, PAD, carotid stenosis, stroke, abdominal aneurysm) that might affect subsequent management decisions, including the use of specific medications or treatment targets. At a minimum, a resting electrocardiogram (ECG) and urinalysis for protein should also be obtained. Basic laboratory tests include a metabolic panel (creatinine, potassium, glucose, and estimated glomerular filtration rate [GFR]), thyroid-stimulating hormone, complete blood count, and a lipoprotein profile. An evaluation for other cardiovascular risk factors (e.g., diabetes, hyperlipidemia, low HDL-C, tobacco smoking, family history of HTN and CVDs) should be performed. Further testing (e.g., novel risk factors) and the evaluation of TOS in greater detail (e.g., echocardiography, stress testing, carotid or renal ultrasonography, coronary artery

calcium) should be performed on a case-by-case basis (Chobanian et al., 2003).

"SECONDARY" HYPERTENSION

It has been suggested that up to about 10% of HTN cases are attributable to "secondary" causes (Omura et al., 2004); however, the true prevalence is unknown and varies depending on the population assessed (Mancia et al., 2013). There are no well-adjudicated factors guiding clinicians when and how to evaluate for secondary or correctable causes of high BP. Although numerous rare causes exist, both JNC 7 and ESH 2013 provide outline recommendations regarding some of the most common scenarios (Chobanian et al., 2003; Mancia et al., 2013). It is suggested that patients with "resistant" HTN (BP uncontrolled on three or more medications, including a diuretic), those with sudden or severe alterations in BP levels, people with a paucity of risk factors for "primary" HTN, individuals without prior pre-HTN, patients admitted for hypertensive emergencies, and those with new HTN at extremes of age (<35-40 years or >70 years) should be considered for secondary HTN evaluation.

Pathological signs that suggest a certain etiology might also warrant specifically directed investigation. Common conditions to consider and their symptoms and signs include CKD (anemia, low GFR, small kidney), hypothyroidism (high TSH), renovascular HTN (abdominal bruit, elevated plasma renin activity, asymmetric kidney sizes, >30% elevation of creatinine after starting BP-lowering agents), hyperparathyroidism (high calcium), and obstructive sleep apnea (OSA) (excessive daytime somnolence, snoring, witnessed apnea) (Mancia et al., 2013). Although OSA is extremely common among patients with HTN, treatment with continuous positive airway pressure (CPAP) provides only a modest reduction in BP (≈2-4 mm Hg SBP) on average among patients with HTN and OSA (Martinez-Garcia et al., 2013). Nonetheless, there are some individuals with severe OSA and refractory HTN in whom CPAP can be extremely helpful in achieving BP control. Similarly, several recent studies (e.g., Cardiovascular Outcomes in Atherosclerotic Renal Disease [CORAL]) demonstrate that under most circumstances, renal artery stenting, even with significant stenosis, provides on-average minimal benefit in regards to protection of kidney function and BP lowering (Cooper et al., 2014). As a general rule, the limited number of patients that might benefit from renal revascularization should be considered carefully when evaluating patients for renovascular HTN. Several reviews of the evaluation and management of renal artery stenosis have been published (Meier, 2011).

Although frequently suspected, pheochromocytoma is extraordinarily uncommon (<0.1-0.5% of cases of HTN; Omura et al., 2004). The classic symptoms include the "5 Ps," which are palpitations, pain (headache), pressure (high BP), perspiration, and pallor (skin blanching) (Callender et al., 2011). The optimal screening test is the plasma free metanephrines, which have a negative predictive value greater than 98% (Vaclavik et al., 2007). This test is minimally altered by medications, and results are constantly elevated in affected individuals given its continuous non-cyclic release from tumors. However, given the rarity of this disorder, most patients with this symptom constellation or borderline abnormal blood test results (two to three times elevated plasma free metanephrines) will have other etiologies (e.g., pseudopheochromocytoma, panic disorder, migraines, arrhythmias, autonomic failure, baroreceptor failure). Confirmatory tests (e.g., clonidine suppression testing) and imaging (e.g., computed tomography [CT], MRI, nuclear medicine functional tests [metaiodobenzyl-guanidine or MIBG]) for tumor localization may be required if repeat testing is abnormal, symptoms persist, paroxysmal HTN episodes continue, or BP remains elevated. Guidelines for the evaluation and management of pheochromocytomas are available (Pacak et al., 2007).

Finally, the past decade has witnessed a resurgence of evidence suggesting the importance of primary aldosteronism in the etiology of HTN in up to about 5% to 10% of patients (Fardella et al., 2000; Schwartz and Turner 2005). An inappropriate elevation of aldosterone from adrenal hyperplasia or an adenoma ("Conn disease") may be the single most common secondary etiology of HTN, and primary care physicians should have a low threshold for its consideration among difficult-to-control patients. Contrary to common thought, classic signs such as hypokalemia actually occur in fewer than 50% of patients (Funder et al., 2008). A screening seated ratio of serum aldosterone (ng/dL)/plasma renin activity (ng/mL/hr) obtained in an ambulatory setting is a reasonable first test. A ratio greater than 25 to 30 warrants further evaluation, and if hyperaldosteronism is confirmed, then localization with imaging studies is warranted. Whether or not to manage medically with aldosterone-blocking agents or with surgical removal (if an adenoma is found) should be considered on a case-by-case basis. Endocrine Society recommendations for the management of primary aldosteronism have been published (Funder et al., 2008).

GENERAL MANAGEMENT OF HIGH BLOOD PRESSURE IN ADULTS

The management of high BP in adults has been outlined in the ESH 2013 guidelines (Mancia et al., 2013). Recently, the AHA along with the ACC and the Centers for Disease Control and Prevention (CDC) released a science advisory outlining an "effective approach to high blood pressure control" (Go et al., 2014). This document provides recommendations for achieving BP targets, including a practical algorithm for pharmacological therapy (Figure 27-3).

In rare circumstances when BP is found to be severely and persistently elevated (e.g., >180-200/110-120 mm Hg) by accurate clinic readings or symptoms or signs of acute HTN-related target organ damage are reported (e.g., acute stroke or TIA, encephalopathy, CHF, aortic dissection, acute MI, rapid deterioration in renal function), patients may require urgent (within 1 week) or emergent (immediate hospital admission) evaluation and treatment. Management of HTN "emergencies," defined as a severe elevation in BP with the presence of new or ongoing target organ damage, are outlined in the JNC 7 and ESH 2013 guidelines (Mancia et al., 2013).

DIETARY AND LIFESTYLE TREATMENT

All guidelines agree that most patients with BP values above ideal should be educated about the lifestyle modalities proven effective to lower BP. Given that drug treatment of pre-HTN is not recommended at this point in time unless patients have compelling indications because of other comorbidities (e.g., CHF), people with BP levels between 120 to 139/80 to 89 mm Hg are ideal candidates for aggressive dietary and lifestyle changes to lower BP and prevent the onset of overt HTN. The AHA, American Society of HTN, and ESH 2013 have promulgated several dietary-lifestyle changes, including a low sodium diet (<1.5 to 2.3 g/day), a diet consistent with the Dietary Approaches to Stop Hypertension (DASH) eating pattern, weight reduction if the body mass index (BMI) is greater than 25 kg/m^2, alcohol restriction to less than 10-20 g/day, and aerobic exercise (target of 150 min/wk) (Mancia et al., 2013). Although not proven to reduce hard CVD events, each of these lifestyle treatments is well established to lower BP on average by 4 to 6 mm Hg SBP in a dose-response and additive manner. As such, most patients with pre-HTN and many with stage I HTN (without compelling indications for a specific BP-lowering medication) can be successfully managed and reach BP targets using one or more of these nonpharmacologic interventions. More recently, the AHA also published recommendations regarding the use of other nonpharmacologic alternative approaches to help manage HTN (Brook et al., 2013). For select individuals, it was concluded that some alternative treatments, notably resistance and isometric exercise, device-guided slow breathing, and certain meditation techniques, can serve as effective and helpful adjuvants to lower BP. Whether or not patients are able to adhere to these nonpharmacologic lifestyle treatments to control BP over several years remains uncertain. Primary care physicians should carefully monitor BP and healthy lifestyle patterns among such individuals.

CLINICAL TRIAL EVIDENCE GUIDING PHARMACOLOGIC THERAPY

The pharmacologic reduction of BP using most classes of antihypertensive drugs reduces the risk for cardiovascular events (strokes, CHF, CKD, MIs) and end-organ injury (LVH, microalbuminuria) and prevents the onset of more severe forms of HTN (Mancia et al., 2013). The latest comprehensive meta-analysis demonstrates a consistent reduction in CVD events by antihypertensive treatment whereby a 10/5–mm Hg reduction produces an approximate 40% and

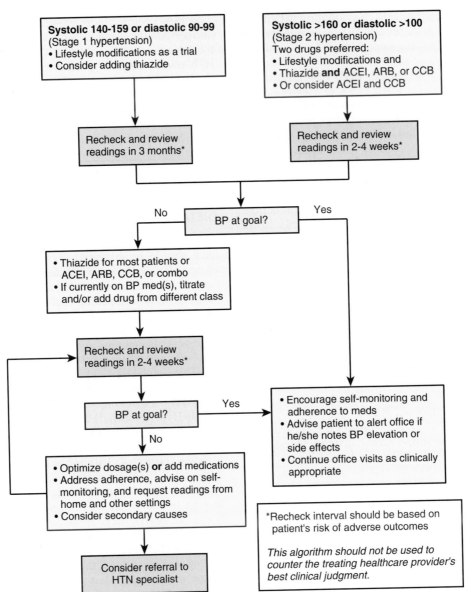

Figure 27-3 Practical approach for blood pressure control. (Used with permission from Go AS, Bauman M, King SM, et al. An effective approach to high blood pressure control: a science advisory from the American Heart Association, the American College of Cardiology, and the Centers for Disease Control and Prevention. *Hypertension.* 2014;63(4):878-885.)

20% reduction in strokes and IHD events, respectively (Law et al., 2009). Importantly, this improvement in outcomes occurs rapidly within 1 year of treatment and, based on modern medical therapy, is a health benefit consistent with what would be expected by prospective cohort studies.

Numerous clinic trials have been performed over the past several decades. Several key points from these trials as summarized in the most recent meta-analyses are as follows. Achieving BP goal target is of preeminent importance. The antihypertensive agents used are of secondary importance (Mancia et al., 2013). Prevailing expert opinion contends that unless there are compelling indications for the use of a specific drug class because of background cardiovascular or renal disease, it makes little difference which agent is first prescribed in the setting of uncomplicated HTN (SOR: A) (Julius et al., 2004; Law et al., 2009; National Institute for Clinical Excellence 2004; Pepine et al., 2003; Turnbull 2003; Williams 2005). As supported by the most recent

comprehensive meta-analysis, risk reduction is predominately driven by the magnitude of BP reduction rather than the specific mechanism by which it is achieved (SOR: A) (Law et al., 2009). If a single agent can be used to obtain goals, recent data support that monotherapy with a β-blocker (in particular atenolol because of excess risks of strokes) or an α-blocker (caused by excess risks of CHF events by doxazosin in the Antihypertensive and Lipid-Lowering Treatment to Prevent Heart Attack [ALLHAT] study) should be discouraged because they are less effective than most other agents (Law et al., 2009). Although β-blockers might be effective in the secondary prevention of IHD, they are no more effective than other agents (in particular thiazides) in the primary prevention of MIs. Meta-analyses suggest that β-blockers are inferior in the prevention of strokes (Bangalore et al., 2007). In the past, thiazides were recommended as first-line drugs for most patients based on their low costs and abundant clinical trial evidence (Chobanian et al., 2003). However, given the reduction in costs and generic formulation availability for all classes of antihypertensive agents, there is no compelling evidence against starting as a first-line agent any of the following: thiazides, CCBs, ACE inhibitors, and ARBs. There are marginal differences in outcomes among these agents observed in trials and meta-analyses (Law et al., 2009). Nevertheless, if a diuretic is chosen, the longer acting and more potent agent chlorthalidone should be considered as first-line treatment given that it has the highest level of clinical trial evidence supporting its use. Many experts recommend it over other thiazides (e.g., hydrochlorothiazide); however, head-to-head outcome trials have not been performed (Beckett et al., 2008; Mancia et al., 2013).

It is also important to highlight that "isolated systolic HTN" (i.e., SBP >160 mm Hg with DBP <90 mm Hg) is a potent risk factor for strokes and CVDs (Mancia et al., 2013). Among patients older than 50 years, SBP levels are more strongly related to CVD and renal disease than DBP (Leonetti et al., 2000; Nielsen et al., 1997). Treatment of isolated systolic HTN leads to improved CVD outcomes regardless of achieved DBP levels on treatment (Berl et al., 2005). Although there have been long-standing concern and debate about the risks of the "J-curve," whereby excessive reductions in DBP may lead to increased risk for CHD events, the overall evidence supports that this effect is limited largely to high-risk patients with established CAD. Treatment-induced reduction in SBP to less than 140 mm Hg typically provides a greater overall event reduction than is offset by any adverse effect of excessive lowering of DBP (Mancia et al., 2013). Nevertheless, careful monitoring of certain individuals in this scenario is warranted, including those older than 80 years, patients with active angina worsened by BP lowering, and people with excessively low DBP (<65 mm Hg) or orthostatic hypotension.

ALGORITHM FOR ANTIHYPERTENSIVE MEDICATION PRESCRIPTION

A large number of antihypertensive medications are available. These medications, along with their dosing regimens, are summarized in Table 27-7. Despite the recognized dangers of HTN and the large number of available medications, only about 50% of patients with this disorder are treated to target BP levels in the United States (Go et al., 2013). Given this public health shortcoming and the lack of clear evidence that any single BP-lowering medication is the most effective in reducing cardiovascular events in any subgroup of individuals, more practical approaches for controlling HTN have been advocated recently compared with past guidelines. The ESH 2013, AHA 2013, and JNC 8 documents outline straightforward algorithms for prescribing antihypertensive regimens based on the most recent level of evidence from clinical trials (Go et al., 2013; James et al., 2014; Mancia et al., 2013). We agree with the approach offered by the AHA 2013 statement; it is a reasonable recommendation applicable to most patients (see Figure 27-3).

Although recommendations regarding the selection of the first drug class have figured less prominently in recent guidelines (ESH 2013, AHA 2013), most experts agree that starting or rapidly intensifying treatment to combination antihypertensive therapy among most patients who have BP levels greater than 20/10 mm Hg above goals is important. Given that a majority of patients will ultimately require two or more BP-lowering medications to achieve goals (Hansson et al., 1998), elucidating the optimal combination of agents is becoming more important to determine. There has only been one clinical trial in HTN with hard cardiovascular outcomes that based treatment limbs on differing initial combination regimens. The Avoiding Cardiovascular events through COMbination therapy in Patients LIving with Systolic Hypertension (ACCOMPLISH) trial (Jamerson et al., 2008) demonstrated a significant 20% reduction in combined cardiovascular events in patients treated with a combination of an ACE inhibitor plus CCB (benazepril + amlodipine) compared with patients treated with an ACE inhibitor plus a thiazide diuretic (benazepril + hydrochlorothiazide) (Jamerson et al., 2008). This occurred in the overall population and in the subsets of patients with diabetes, CAD, and CKD. All subsets of outcomes evaluated were reduced by a greater extent by the ACE inhibitor–CCB combination except CHF, which was neutral. This includes the prespecified outcome of hard CKD end points. Thus, we have previously suggested that most patients who require dual antihypertensive therapy should strongly consider starting with an ACE inhibitor plus a CCB (Brook and Weder, 2011). In this manner, our recommendations slightly differ from the official AHA 2013 and ESH 2013 guidelines that suggest an ACE inhibitor plus either a CCB or thiazide is reasonable.

Table 27-7 Oral Antihypertensive Drugs

Drug	Trade Name	Usual Dose Range, Usual Milligrams Per Dose (Usual Frequency of Doses Per Day)	Selected Side Effects and Comments
DIURETICS (PARTIAL LIST)			Short term: increase cholesterol and glucose levels; biochemical abnormalities; decrease potassium, sodium, and magnesium levels
THIAZIDE AND THIAZIDE-LIKE DIURETICS			Increase uric acid and calcium levels; rare: blood dyscrasias, photosensitivity, pancreatitis, hyponatremia
Chlorthalidone (G)	Thalitone	12.5-50 (1)	
Hydrochlorothiazide (G)	Microzide	12.5-50 (1)	
Indapamide (G)		1.25-2.5 (1)	Less or no hypercholesterolemia

Continued on following page

Table 27-7 Oral Antihypertensive Drugs (Continued)

Drug	Trade Name	Usual Dose Range, Usual Milligrams Per Dose (Usual Frequency of Doses Per Day)	Selected Side Effects and Comments
Loop Diuretics			
Bumetanide (G)		0.5-2 (1-2)	Short duration of action; no hypercalcemia
Ethacrynic acid	Edecrin	25-100 (1-2)	Only nonsulfonamide diuretic, ototoxicity
Furosemide (G)	Lasix	20-80 (2)	Short duration of action, no hypercalcemia
Torsemide (G)	Demadex	5-10 (1-2)	
Potassium-Sparing Agents			**Potentially fatal hyperkalemia**
Amiloride hydrochloride (G)	Midamor	5-10 (1)	
Spironolactone (G)	Aldactone	12.5-100 (1)	More gynecomastia
Eplerenone (G)	Inspra	25-50 (1-2)	Less gynecomastia
Triamterene (G)	Dyrenium	50-100 (1)	Hypertension is an unlabeled use
ADRENERGIC INHIBITORS			
Peripheral Agents			
Reserpine (G)		0.05-0.25 (1)	Nasal congestion, sedation, depression, activation of peptic ulcer
Central α-agonist			Sedation, dry mouth, bradycardia, withdrawal hypertension
Clonidine hydrochloride, oral (G)	Catapres	0.1-0.8 (2-3)	More withdrawal
Clonidine, transdermal patch (G)	Catapres-TTS	0.1-0.3 mg/24 hour patch replaced every 7 days	
Guanfacine hydrochloride, immediate release (G)	Tenex	1-2 (1)	Less withdrawal
Methyldopa (G)		250-500 (2)	Hepatic and "autoimmune" disorders
α-Blockers			Can elevate HDL
Doxazosin mesylate, immediate release (G)	Cardura	2-16 (1)	
Prazosin hydrochloride (G)	Minipress	1-10 (2)	
Terazosin hydrochloride (G)	Hytrin	1-20 (1)	
β-Blockers			Increased risk of diabetes mellitus, bronchospasm, bradycardia, heart failure; may mask insulin-induced hypoglycemia, hypoglycemia unawareness; impaired peripheral circulation, insomnia, fatigue, decreased exercise tolerance, hypertriglyceridemia (except agents with intrinsic sympathomimetic activity), reduced HDL
Acebutolol (G)	Sectral	200-400 (1-2)	
Atenolol (G)	Tenormin	25-100 (1-2)	
Betaxolol hydrochloride (G)		10-20 (1)	
Bisoprolol fumarate (G)	Zebeta	2.5-10 (1)	
Metoprolol tartrate (G)	Lopressor	25-200 (2)	
Metoprolol succinate (G)	Toprol XL	25-300 (1)	
Nadolol (G)	Corgard	40-80 (1)	
Nebivolol	Bystolic	5-20 (1)	Vasodilating agent with less metabolic abnormalities
Penbutolol sulfate	Levatol	10-20 (1)	
Pindolol (G)		5-15 (2)	
Propranolol immediate release (G)	Inderal	40-120 (2)	
Propranolol extended release (G)	Inderal LA	80-160 (1)	
Timolol maleate (G)		10-20 (2)	
Combined α- and β-Blockers			Postural hypotension, bronchospasm
Carvedilol, immediate release (G)	Coreg	6.25-25 (2)	
Carvedilol, extended release	Coreg CR	20-40 (1)	
Labetalol (G)		100-400 (2-3)	
Direct vasodilators			Headaches, fluid retention, tachycardia

Table 27-7 Oral Antihypertensive Drugs (Continued)

Drug	Trade Name	Usual Dose Range, Usual Milligrams Per Dose (Usual Frequency of Doses Per Day)	Selected Side Effects and Comments
Hydralazine hydrochloride (G)		10-100 (4)	Lupus-like syndrome, myocardial ischemia
Minoxidil (G)		2.5-40 (1)	Hirsutism, edema, pericardial effusion
CALCIUM ANTAGONISTS			
Nondihydropyridine			Conduction defects, worsening of systolic dysfunction, gingival hyperplasia
Diltiazem hydrochloride (G)	Cardizem CD, Cardizem LA, Dilacor XR, Tiazac	120-360 (1)	Nausea, headache
Verapamil hydrochloride (G)	Calan SR, Verelan, Covera-HS	90-240 (2) 120-480 (1)	
Dihydropyridines			Edema of the ankle, flushing, headache, gingival hypertrophy
Amlodipine besylate (G)	Norvasc	2.5-10 (1)	
Felodipine (G)	Plendil	2.5-10 (1)	
Isradipine (G)	Dynacirc	2.5-10 (2)	
Nicardipine hydrochloride, sustained release (G)	Cardene SR	30-60 (2)	
Nifedipine (G)	Procardia XL, Adalat CC	30-60 (1)	
Nisoldipine (G)	Sular	20-40 (1)	
ANGIOTENSIN-CONVERTING ENZYME INHIBITORS			Common: cough, hyperkalemia; rare: angioedema, rash, loss of taste, leukopenia
Benazepril hydrochloride (G)	Lotensin	5-40 (1)	
Captopril (G)	Capoten	25-50 (2-3)	
Enalapril maleate (G)	Vasotec	5-40 (1)	
Fosinopril sodium (G)	Monopril	10-40 (1)	
Lisinopril (G)	Prinivil, Zestril	5-40 (1)	
Moexipril hydrochloride (G)	Univasc	7.5-30 (1)	
Quinapril hydrochloride (G)	Accupril	5-80 (1)	
Ramipril (G)	Altace	1.25-20 (1)	
Trandolapril (G)	Mavik	1-4 (1)	
Angiotensin II Receptor Blockers			Hyperkalemia, angioedema (very rare [association with ARBs is controversial])
Losartan potassium (G)	Cozaar	25-100 (1-2)	
Valsartan (G)	Diovan	80-320 (1)	
Irbesartan (G)	Avapro	150-300 (1)	
Telmisartan	Micardis	40-80 (1)	
Olmesartan	Benicar	40-40 (1)	
Azilsartan	Edarbi	40-80 (1)	
Candesartan (G)	Atacand	4-32 (1)	
Direct Renin Inhibitor			Hyperkalemia, hypotension, angioedema, diarrhea, cough, seizures, rash, gout, and renal stones. Contraindicated in patients with diabetes who are treated with an ARB or ACE inhibitor; avoid use with ARB or ACE inhibitor in patients with moderate to severe renal impairment
Aliskiren	Tekturna	150-300 (1)	

G indicates that a generic formulation is currently available.
ACE, Angiotensin-converting enzyme; ARB, angiotensin receptor blocker; HDL, high-density lipoprotein.

Combinations of drugs that are efficacious and those associated with undesirable side effect profiles are summarized in Table 27-8. The most important recent observation from clinical trials is that under most circumstances, combination blockade of the renin–angiotensin system is not warranted and may be dangerous. The Ongoing Telmisartan Alone and in Combination with Ramipril Global Endpoint Trial (ONTARGET) study demonstrated that combined ACE inhibitor–ARB therapy does not prevent cardiovascular events more than monotherapy (Yusuf et al., 2008). However, renal outcomes were worsened by this combination. The Aliskiren Trial in Type 2 Diabetes Using Cardiorenal Endpoints (ALTITUDE) study also showed that combined ARB plus direct renin inhibition is not protective to renal

Table 27-8   Antihypertensive Drug Combinations

Desirable or Acceptable	Not Desirable
THIAZIDE OR THIAZIDE-LIKE DIURETIC PLUS:	**β-BLOCKER PLUS:**
ACE inhibitor*	Central adrenergic inhibitor
Aldosterone antagonist	Rate-lowering CCB (NDHPCCB)
Angiotensin receptor blocker*	ACE inhibitor/ARB: less effective
β-Blocker	CCB plus:
CCB	Diuretic: less effective
Direct renin inhibitor	ACE inhibitor plus:
CCB plus:	ARB‡
ACE inhibitor†	ARB plus:
ARB*	Direct renin inhibitor‡
β-Blocker (if DHPCCB)	

*Acceptable alternative (second-line) combination regimens.
†Considered most effective combination based on blood pressure–lowering efficacy and should be strongly considered first-line treatment or most patients based on evidence from outcome trials (Avoiding Cardiovascular Events through Combination Therapy in Patients Living with Systolic Hypertension [ACCOMPLISH] trial).
‡These combinations should be avoided under most circumstances.
ACE, Angiotensin-converting enzyme; *ARB,* angiotensin receptor blocker; *CCB,* calcium channel blocker; *DHPCCB,* dihydropyridine calcium channel blocker; *NDHPCCB,* nondihydropyridine calcium channel blocker.

function among patients with diabetes and poses excess side effect risk (Parving et al., 2012). Recommendations for attaining BP targets in the more challenging patients who often require multiple BP-lowering agents are summarized in Table 27-9. There are numerous benefits to prescribing combination agents to achieve control of HTN. Comprehensive recommendations regarding combination antihypertensive regimens have been published (Gradman et al., 2011).

COMPELLING INDICATIONS FOR MEDICATIONS

JNC 7 guidelines recommended tailoring first-line antihypertensive therapy choices in the context of other comorbidities (Chobanian et al., 2003). Certain medication choices may be appropriate initial selections and more strongly considered for subsets of individuals based on ancillary benefits (e.g., reduction in proteinuria by ACE inhibitor and ARBs). On the other hand, other agents may be avoided because of potential side effects (e.g., worsening glycemic control by thiazides and β-blockers). Prior recommendations for "compelling indications" based on JNC 7 guidelines are summarized in Table 27-10. Nevertheless, the most important considerations that remain valid are in relation to the following disease states. Individuals with heart failure (HF) with reduced ejection fraction (EF) should receive either an ACE inhibitor or ARB, with the careful addition of a β-blocker (e.g., metoprolol or carvedilol). Many patients with CHF should thereafter have an aldosterone blocker added if tolerated (Pitt et al., 2003). Diabetic and nondiabetic patients with overt proteinuria and CKD should receive either an ACE inhibitor or ARB as part of their BP-lowering regimen (Brenner et al., 2001; Lewis et al., 1993; Lewis et al., 2001). Whether or not patients with CKD or diabetes must receive these agents in the absence of frank proteinuria remains a matter of debate; however, given their ability to reduce microalbuminuria and their beneficial metabolic profile, these drugs remain excellent selections for BP control (Mancia et al., 2013).

Table 27-9   Ten Tips for Attaining Goal Blood Pressure

1. If BP ≥20/10 mm Hg above goal, monotherapy is unlikely to be effective, so consider a combination antihypertensive agent. The strongest evidence is for an ACE inhibitor or ARB + CCB based on outcome studies (ACCOMPLISH). A combination with ACE inhibitor or ARB + thiazide is an acceptable alternative.
2. In most situations, allow for 2-4 weeks of treatment before titrating BP medications upward (or adding additional drugs) to establish the full efficacy of the medication(s). However, a longer delay can lead to "therapeutic inertia" and should be avoided in most scenarios if BP remains above target.
3. Realize that most hypertensive patients (≈75%) will ultimately require two or more drugs to attain goal BP, especially persons with diabetes, obesity, decreased kidney function, or proteinuria. Use of one or more combination antihypertensive agents is effective for achieving BP targets.
4. Initiate lifestyle modifications for most patients: DASH diet, low sodium (<1.5-2.3 g/day) and alcohol intake (<2 drinks/day); aerobic exercise; and weight loss (if indicated). Ask about adherence and assure persistence with diet, lifestyle, and prescribed medications if BP remains elevated.
5. To avoid falsely high BP measurements (pseudo-HTN, pseudo-resistance, white coat HTN), careful attention to BP measurement technique is critical to obtain accurate readings in the clinical setting.
6. Minimize exposure to medications known to raise BP such as NSAIDs. Ask about all recreational and OTC medications and prescription medications that can elevate BP.
7. A diuretic appropriate to the level of kidney function is essential to the multidrug regimen when three or more antihypertensives are prescribed. Thiazide diuretics are typically more effective BP-lowering agents than loop diuretics unless stage IV or V CKD is present. Chlorthalidone is more potent and longer acting than hydrochlorothiazide and has more clinical trial outcome evidence, so it should be considered as the first diuretic choice in most patients.
8. Self-measured blood pressure and 24-hour ABPM can be useful adjuncts, especially when white coat hypertension or white coat worse hypertension are suspected or when BP appears to be refractory to treatment. If discordant from clinic BP values, the ABPM readings are typically more accurate estimates of true BP levels and future CVD risk.
9. Diuretic doses may need to be relatively high (e.g., furosemide 160 mg/day in divided doses or metolazone 10-20 mg/day) when kidney function is <30 mL/min/1.73 m². Combination loop + thiazide diuretics can be effective in this scenario to achieve BP targets with severe CKD.
10. In "resistant hypertension," if BP remains above goal on three or more antihypertensives (one of which is a diuretic) at near-maximal doses, consider referral to a hypertension specialist. Empirical treatment with an aldosterone antagonist (spironolactone 25-50 mg/d) may be highly effective in difficult-to-control HTN and should be strongly considered. Novel treatments (e.g., renal sympathetic nerve ablation) and evaluation for secondary HTN (e.g., primary aldosteronism) are warranted.

ABPM, Ambulatory blood pressure monitoring; *ACCOMPLISH,* Avoiding Cardiovascular Events through Combination Therapy in Patients Living with Systolic Hypertension; *ACE,* angiotensin-converting enzyme; *ARB,* angiotensin receptor blocker; *BP,* blood pressure; *CCB,* calcium channel blocker; *CKD,* chronic kidney disease; *DASH,* Dietary Approaches to Stop Hypertension; *HTN,* hypertension; *NSAID,* nonsteroidal antiinflammatory drug; *OTC,* over-the-counter.
Adapted from Flack JM, Nasser SA. *Hypertension Pocket Guide.* New York: McMahon Pub; 2005.

BLOOD PRESSURE TARGETS

Prior guidelines, including JNC 7, emphasized lower BP goals (<130/80 mm Hg) for certain individuals, including those with CKD and diabetes. Recent outcome trials have tested the benefits of more aggressive treatment among

Table 27-10 JNC 7–Defined Compelling Indications for Use of Specific Antihypertensive Agents in Complicated Hypertension

	Diuretic	BB	ACE Inhibitor	ARB	CCB	MRA
Heart failure	✓	✓	✓	✓		✓
Post-MI		✓	✓			✓
CAD risk	✓	✓	✓		✓	
Diabetes mellitus	✓	✓	✓	✓	✓	
Renal disease			✓	✓		
Recurrent stroke prevention	✓		✓			

ACE, angiotensin-converting enzyme; *ARB,* angiotensin receptor blocker; *BB,* β-blocker; *CAD,* coronary artery disease; *CCB,* calcium channel blocker; *JNC 7,* Seventh Report of the Joint National Committee on Prevention, Detection, Evaluation, and Treatment of High Blood Pressure; *MI,* myocardial infarction; *MRA,* mineralocorticoid receptor antagonist.
From *The Seventh Report of the Joint National Committee on Prevention, Detection, Evaluation, and Treatment of High Blood Pressure.* Washington, DC: U.S Department of Health and Human Services. National Institute of Health Publication No. 04-5230. August 2004.

patients with diabetes. The ACCORD trial demonstrated that aggressive reduction of BP (target <120/80 mm Hg) did not reduce combined cardiovascular and renal outcomes compared with usual care (target BP <140/90 mm Hg) (Cushman et al., 2010). Among secondary outcomes, strokes were reduced by the lower BP goals but at the expense of twice as many serious side effects. Several meta-analyses have demonstrated that lowering BP to below 130 mm Hg systolic does not reduce mortality rates or most cardiovascular outcomes (Mancia et al., 2013). The exception to this rule is that a lower BP level below 130/80 mm Hg may be protective against strokes in both primary and secondary prevention (Benavente et al., 2013; Weber et al., 2013). There is little evidence to support more aggressive BP targets even among individuals with CKD in the absence of overt proteinuria (>500 mg/day) (Mancia et al., 2013). In the latter case with significant levels of proteinuria, tighter BP control to below 130/80 mm Hg or lower might be helpful; however, compelling evidence from clinical trials is still lacking.

The ideal BP level remains questionable; however, few studies support lowering BP below a value of 140/90 mm Hg in most patients. Hence, the old JNC 7 targets among patients with diabetes and those with CKD have not been promulgated by more recent ESH 2013 and JNC 8 guidelines (James et al., 2014; Mancia et al., 2013). In rare circumstances (prevention of strokes) and among complicated patients (e.g., aortic aneurysms, recurrent cardiovascular events), lower BP targets can be selected on an individual basis.

EMERGING MANAGEMENT STRATEGIES, RESISTANT HYPERTENSION, AND CONTROVERSIES

Emerging strategies for assessment of BP include use of self-measured home BP and 24-hour ambulatory blood pressure monitoring (ABPM) (O'Brien et al., 2013; Pickering et al., 2008). Home BP is a useful adjunct to clinic BP measurements, which are often affected by the "white coat effect." ABPM can rule out "white coat" HTN and "white coat worse" HTN and has the added benefit of assessing nocturnal BP, which may be a more important predictor of cardiovascular events than daytime BP (Clement et al., 2003). Both techniques may also uncover "masked HTN,"

a scenario when clinic BP is controlled in the setting of high out-of-office BP readings (Yano and Bakris, 2013). Although white coat HTN is not associated with excess cardiovascular risk (Fagard et al., 2000), masked HTN conveys an equal risk as sustained elevations in BP observed in the clinic. The availability of ABPM is more limited than the availability of home BP, which depends primarily on the patient's ability to obtain an automated oscillometric BP cuff and to follow detailed instructions. A normal home BP is lower than a normal clinic BP, with 135/85 mm Hg suggested by some authorities as differentiating normal from HTN (Hodgkinson et al., 2011). ABPM values for a 24-hour average greater than 130/80 mm Hg are considered elevated. Although there is compelling evidence that both home and ABPM levels are more strongly related to cardiovascular morbidity and mortality than traditional clinic readings, few data support tailoring treatment goals based on these values. Guidelines for both home and ABPM have been published (O'Brien et al., 2013; Pickering et al., 2008). Several expert societies now support that home BP monitoring should be performed in most (if not all) patients with HTN (Pickering et al., 2008).

To tailor drug therapy and reduce the number of people requiring more than one or two medications, several strategies have been proposed. The most well-known algorithm suggests selecting drug therapy based on ambulatory measurement of plasma renin activity (Mulatero et al., 2007). Those defined as "low-renin" (<0.65 ng/mL/hr) patients are treated with diuretics or CCBs; others are treated with ACE inhibitors, ARBs, or β-blockers. Although this approach can improve the rates of BP control in selected patients and clinical trials, the usefulness of this strategy in real-world clinical setting remains unclear. Other strategies based on hemodynamic monitoring (e.g., cardiac bioelectrical impedance), demographic profiling, and pharmacogenetics have been proposed. It has also been proposed to start most patients with combination medications (even in stage I) given that more than 50% to 75% of people will inevitably require two or more drugs. Whether or not these approaches will be effective in a broad clinical setting remains to be proven. For the time being, following the clinical strategies outlined in guideline documents is recommended (Go et al., 2013) (see Figure 27-3).

The optimal treatment of HTN "emergencies" remains unproven (Mancia et al., 2013). The standard guidelines

Table 27-11   Parenteral Drugs for Treatment of Hypertensive Emergencies

Drug	Dose	Onset of Action	Duration of Action	Adverse Effects	Special Instructions
Sodium nitroprusside	0.25-10 μm/kg/min as IV infusion (maximal dose for 10 min only)	Immediate	1-2 min	Nausea, vomiting, muscle twitching, sweating, thiocyanate and cyanide intoxication	Most hypertensive emergencies; caution with high ICP or azotemia
Nicardipine hydrochloride	5-15 mg/hr IV	5-10 min	1-4 hr	Tachycardia, headache, flushing, local phlebitis	Most hypertensive emergencies except acute heart failure; caution with coronary ischemia
Fenoldopam mesylate	0.1-0.3 μm/kg/min as IV infusion	<5 min	30 min	Tachycardia, headache, nausea, flushing	Most hypertensive emergencies; caution with glaucoma
Nitroglycerin	5-100 μm/min as IV infusion	2-5 min	3-5 min	Headache, vomiting, methemoglobinemia, tolerance with prolonged use	
Enalaprilat	1.25-5 mg every 6 hr IV	15-30 min	6 hr	Precipitous fall in pressure in high-renin states; response variable	Acute LV failure; avoid in acute MI
Hydralazine hydrochloride	10-20 mg IV 10-50 mg IM	10-20 min 20-30 min	3-8 hr	Tachycardia, flushing, headache, vomiting, aggravation of angina	Eclampsia; caution with coronary ischemia
Labetalol hydrochloride	20-80 mg as IV bolus every 10 min 0.5-2.0 mg/min as IV infusion	5-10 min	3-6 hr	Vomiting, scalp tingling, burning in throat, dizziness, nausea, heart block, orthostatic hypotension	Most hypertensive emergencies except acute heart failure
Esmolol hydrochloride	250-500 μm/kg/min for 1 min, then 50-100 μm/kg/min for 4 min; may repeat sequence	1-2 min	10-20 min	Hypotension, nausea	Aortic dissection; perioperative
Phentolamine	5-15 mg IV	1-2 min	3-10 min	Tachycardia, flushing, headache	Catecholamine excess
Clevidipine	1-2 to 16 mg/hr	2-4 min	5-15 min	Hypotension, tachycardia	Avoid with hyperlipidemia No use with egg or soy allergy

IM, Intramuscular; *IV*, intravenous; *ICP*, intracranial pressure; *LV*, left ventricular; *MI*, myocardial infarction.

are to lower mean arterial pressure by 20% to 25% within hours and to avoid overaggressive treatment, which may worsen outcomes, particularly cerebrovascular function when cerebral perfusion pressures may be altered. Few trials have compared the effectiveness of various medications and treatment approaches. Nonetheless, numerous agents are available (Table 27-11). The optimal management of HTN in the setting of an acute ischemic or hemorrhagic stroke in particular has undergone many recent clinical trials; however, the optimal treatment goals and timing of medications remain unclear (Mancia et al., 2013). At present, the most recent clinical trials do not support early or aggressive BP lowering in most patients with ischemic strokes or TIAs (He et al., 2013).

Patients with resistant HTN are defined as having a BP above target (usual >140/90 mm Hg) despite taking three or more BP-lowering agents (one of which is a diuretic appropriate for renal function). Its prevalence is estimated at approximately 10% of the HTN population. The AHA has published guidelines outlining management approaches in these difficult-to-control patients (Calhoun et al., 2008). The evidence outlined suggests that close to 85% to 95% of all patients with HTN can achieve BP goals despite the U.S. national control rate of only 50%. One important strategy with some clinical evidence is the empirical usage of add-on aldosterone blockade (e.g., spironolactone 25-50 mg/day; eplerenone 25-50 mg twice a day) while watching potassium and creatinine closely. Even in the absence of overt hyperaldosteronism, this approach has proven effective in

helping to control BP among those with resistant HTN (Calhoun et al., 2008). A common error in the effective treatment of resistant HTN is underuse of diuretic therapy. Changing less potent diuretics (e.g., hydrochlorothiazide) to a more potent, longer acting thiazide-like diuretic such as chlorthalidone has also proven effective in further lowering BP (Matthews et al., 2013). Furthermore, several triple-drug combination pills are available that combine a thiazide, an ARB, and amlodipine. Finally, the addition of a fourth and fifth agent may be necessary in rare individuals; however, there are few data to support an evidence-based approach. Empiric addition with dose titration of an α-blocker (e.g., doxazosin), a direct vasodilator such as minoxidil (typically in conjunction with a loop diuretic to control volume status and a heart rate–slowing agent), or a central sympatholytic (e.g., guanfacine, clonidine) may be effective approaches.

The prevalence of patients uncontrolled on more than four or five medications who are truly adherent to the regimen is unknown. What does the future hold for managing the most difficult cases? Several novel treatment strategies are undergoing clinical trials for patients with truly "refractory HTN," which includes BP levels greater than 160 mm Hg systolic despite taking three or more appropriately dosed antihypertensive agents, including a diuretic. Primary care physicians should be aware that endovascular radiofrequency ablation of the renal artery sympathetic nerves and baroreceptor activation therapy (via electrical stimulation from an implanted pacemaker) are emerging interventions that may be therapeutic options for select patients in the near future. The completion of ongoing trials will determine the usefulness of these interventional approaches.

SUMMARY

Hypertension is the leading risk factor for premature morbidity and mortality in the world. Successful treatment of an elevated BP to target goals requires a concerted effort on the part of the health care provider and patient alike. Comprehensive approaches involving home BP monitoring that involve patients in their own care in conjunction with diet and lifestyle changes, alternative approaches (in select individuals), medications, and combination regimens are generally successful. However, among the truly refractory HTN cases, several novel approaches may soon be available.

Metabolic Syndrome

Key Points

- Metabolic syndrome is an insulin-resistant state associated with visceral adiposity, HTN, hyperglycemia, dyslipidemia, and a proinflammatory and pro-oxidative state.
- Metabolic syndrome is not a CAD risk equivalent but is associated with a heightened risk for CVD and DM. Comprehensive risk factor evaluation should be undertaken in all of these patients.
- Patients with metabolic syndrome should be treated with aggressive lifestyle modification, including weight loss, exercise, smoking cessation, and dietary modification. As shown in the Diabetes Prevention Project, lifestyle modification can reduce risk of developing DM by 58%.
- Weight loss can be achieved through caloric restriction; exercise; and, when indicated, pharmacologic intervention or bariatric surgery.
- The dyslipidemia and HTN of metabolic syndrome should be treated pharmacologically if lifestyle modification does not help to normalize these risk factors.

The incidence of obesity is rising worldwide. With increased mechanization and changes associated with increased food availability and lower average daily caloric expenditure, people are experiencing continuous weight gain with aging. Being overweight and the development of obesity now constitute the second most important preventable cause of mortality. Among Americans 20 years and older, 154.7 million are overweight or obese, including 79.9 million men and 74.8 million women (AHA, 2013). The incidence of obesity is rising among both genders as well as all racial and ethnic groups. One very important consequence of obesity is the development of insulin resistance and the metabolic syndrome (Haffner et al., 2003; Haffner and Taegtmeyer, 2003). The metabolic syndrome is defined by a constellation of cardiovascular risk factors and is associated with heightened risk for new onset DM as well as cardiovascular

Table 27-12 NCEP ATP III Criteria for Diagnosing the Metabolic Syndrome*

Risk Factor	Defining Level
Abdominal obesity	Men, waist >40 in Women, waist >35 in
Triglycerides	≥150 mg/dL
HDL-C	Men <40 mg/dL Women <50 mg/dL
Blood pressure	≥130/≥ 85 mm Hg
Fasting glucose	≥100 mg/dL

*Patients having any three of the above five risk factors meet criteria for the diagnosis of the metabolic syndrome.
HDL-C, High-density lipoprotein cholesterol; NCEP ATP III, National Cholesterol Education Program Adult Treatment Panel III.
From Third Report of the National Cholesterol Education Program (NCEP) Expert Panel on Detection, Evaluation, and Treatment of High Blood Cholesterol in Adults (Adult Treatment Panel III) final report, *Circulation* 2012;106: 3143-3421.

morbidity and mortality. A variety of definitions of the metabolic syndrome have been developed, but the one with the greatest clinical utility is that defined by the NCEP ATPIII (Eckel et al., 2005; Grundy et al., 2004a, 2004b). Waist circumference, BP, fasting blood sugar, and serum triglyceride and HDL-C levels are used to make the diagnosis (Table 27-12). When three of the five criteria are met, the diagnosis of metabolic syndrome can be made. Based on data from the third National Health and Nutrition Examination Survey, the incidence of metabolic syndrome increases in a linear fashion in both men and women as a function of age (Ford et al., 2002; see also Alexander et al., 2003). Hispanic and Native Americans are disproportionately affected. Current estimates suggest that 32% of the population in the United States has metabolic syndrome. In the Kuopio Ischaemic Heart Disease Risk Factor Study, patients with metabolic syndrome experienced a 3.77- and 2.43-fold increase in risk for CHD mortality and all-cause mortality, respectively, over a 12-year period of follow-up compared with patients without the metabolic syndrome (Lakka et al., 2002).

As waist circumference increases, visceral adiposity increases. Visceral adipose tissue is metabolically highly active. An important conceptual shift has occurred in recent years with respect to how adipose tissue is viewed. It is no longer seen as a passive storage site for excess caloric ingestion. Instead, it is clear that visceral adipose tissue displays many features of an endocrine organ (Bradley et al., 2001; Toth, 2005a) (Figure 27-4). Visceral adipose tissue produces a variety of inflammatory cytokines (tumor necrosis factor [TNF], transforming growth factor-β), ILs (IL-1, IL-6), and effector molecules that regulate appetite (leptin) as well as insulin sensitivity and resistance (adiponectin and resistin, among others). As the mass of visceral adipose tissue increases, adiponectin production decreases, which is associated with increased insulin resistance in adipose tissue, skeletal muscle, and the hepatic parenchyma (see Figure 27-4). As adipose tissue becomes more insulin resistant, its capacity to regulate the catabolism of stored triglycerides becomes progressively more dysregulated and unresponsive to systemic tissue needs. Serum levels of free fatty acids (FFA) rise. The portal circulation becomes flooded with FFAs. This results in both increased triglyceride

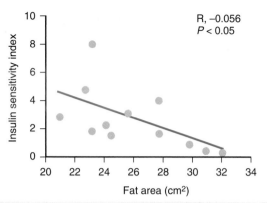

Figure 27-4 Insulin sensitivity and degree of adiposity. (From Fujimoto WY, Abbate SL, Kahn SE, et al. The visceral adiposity syndrome in Japanese-American men. *Obes Res.* 1994;2:364-371.)

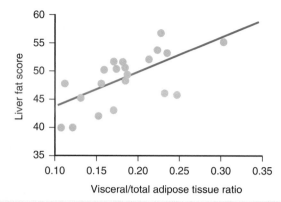

Figure 27-6 Severity of hepatic fat deposition as visceral adiposity worsens. (From Banerji MA, Buckley MC, Chaiken RL, et al. Liver fat, serum triglycerides and visceral adipose tissue in insulin-sensitive and insulin-resistant black men with NIDDM. *Int J Obes.* 1995;19:846-850.)

KAPLAN-MEIER SURVIVAL CURVE

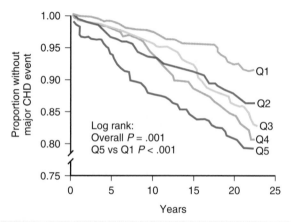

Figure 27-5 Risk of major coronary heart disease (CHD)–related event associated with quintile of insulin levels in nondiabetic men enrolled in the Helsinki Policemen Study. (From Pyorala M, Miettinen H, Laakso M, Pyorala K. Hyperinsulinemia predicts coronary heart disease risk in healthy middle-aged men: the 22-year follow-up results of the Helsinki Policemen Study. *Circulation.* 1998;98:398-404.)

deposition within the liver (nonalcoholic steatohepatitis [NASH] or fatty liver) (Banerji et al., 1995) and increased VLDL secretion, resulting in hypertriglyceridemia. A fatty liver in the absence of excessive alcohol intake is an important marker for insulin resistance and is highly correlated with the magnitude and severity of adiposity; it is also associated with ectopic fat deposition in skeletal muscle, myocardium, and the pancreas (Figure 27-5). Elevations in FFA induce progressive deterioration in glycemic control by (1) interfering with normal phosphorylation of the insulin receptor, resulting in less expression of a glucose transporter (GLUT 4) necessary for the internalization and oxidation of serum glucose (Dresner et al., 1999), and (2) the induction of "lipotoxicity," the process by which FFAs induce premature apoptosis and dropout of pancreatic β-islet cells. Patients experiencing concomitant worsening insulin resistance and progressive loss of insulin-producing capacity experience a continuum of glycemic disturbances, beginning with impaired fasting glucose, then impaired glucose tolerance, and ultimately DM. As serum levels of insulin rise, the risk for CAD-related events increases

precipitously (Pyorala et al., 1996) (Figure 27-6). Patients with metabolic syndrome have a three- to fivefold increased risk for developing diabetes compared with patients without metabolic syndrome.

Insulin resistance and increased visceral adiposity in the setting of metabolic syndrome are associated with changes in multiple risk factors (Lamon-Fava et al., 1996; Figure 27-7). Insulin-resistant adipose tissue is a potent source of angiotensinogen, the precursor to vasoconstrictor angiotensin II. The BP in these patients also increases because (1) insulin stimulates increased sodium reabsorption at the level of the proximal tubular epithelium, increasing intravascular volume; (2) there is reduced endothelial nitric oxide production (Caballero, 2003); and (3) there is increased vascular sympathetic tone. In the face of insulin resistance, obesity can steadily worsen because of dysregulation of central centers transducing the signals for appetite and satiety in the hypothalamus. Serum levels of HDL decrease for three principal reasons (Figure 27-8). First, as the liver becomes insulin resistant, the capacity for insulin to stimulate the hepatic production of apo AI and AII is compromised. This results in less HDL secretion. Second, in patients with insulin resistance, lipoprotein lipase is relatively inhibited. This reduces the hydrolysis of triglycerides in VLDL and chylomicrons. These large lipoproteins remain incompletely catabolized and form atherogenic remnant particles. Unless they are broken down further, they cannot release many of the surface coat constituents that can be used to assimilate HDL in serum. Third, as HDL particles become more enriched with triglycerides, they become a better substrate for hepatic lipase, an enzyme that catabolizes HDL and promotes its clearance from serum (Toth, 2005b). Patients with metabolic syndrome also tend to have smaller, denser LDL particles. These small LDL particles are believed to be more atherogenic than the larger, more buoyant variety because they are more easily oxidized and have reduced affinity for the hepatic LDL receptor, resulting in less systemic clearance, and they appear to more easily access the subendothelial space because of their smaller volume (St. Pierre et al., 2001). Visceral adipose tissue promotes increased systemic inflammation by secreting inflammatory mediators and by stimulating hepatic production of CRP via IL-6. As serum levels of such acute

METABOLIC SYNDROME

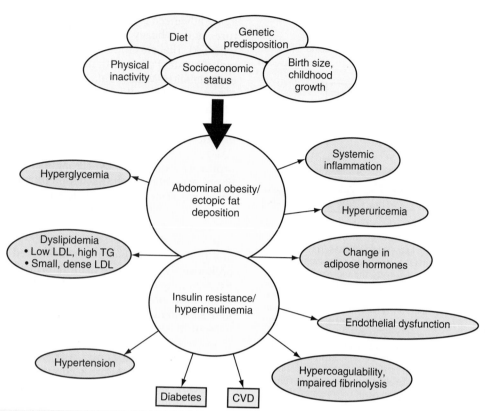

Figure 27-7 Complex interactions among genetic, environmental, and socioeconomic factors increase the risk for developing visceral adiposity; insulin resistance with risk factor generation and clustering; and, ultimately, diabetes mellitus with atherosclerotic disease. *CVD,* Cardiovascular disease; *LDL,* low-density lipoprotein; *TG,* triglyceride.

phase reactants as fibrinogen, CRP, and plasminogen activator inhibitor-1 (PAI-1) rise, the risk for metabolic syndrome and diabetes increases (Dandona et al., 2005; Festa et al., 2002). As shown in the Women's Health Study, as serum CRP levels increase in women with metabolic syndrome but no prior history of CAD, the risk for an acute cardiovascular event increases significantly (Ridker et al., 2003). As insulin resistance worsens, risk for NASH increases steadily (see Figure 27-7).

Metabolic syndrome is not defined by NCEP as a CAD risk equivalent. It is crucial that these patients undergo comprehensive evaluation of their global cardiovascular risk factor burden. Aggressive lifestyle modification with weight loss, increased exercise and physical activity, smoking cessation, and reductions in carbohydrate and saturated fat intake constitute front-line therapy for patients with the metabolic syndrome (Grundy et al., 2004b; Liu and Manson, 2001; Salmeron et al., 2001). Referral to a dietitian is frequently helpful. Weight loss and aerobic exercise are associated with improved insulin sensitivity and significant improvements in BP and lipid levels (DeFronzo et al., 1987; Franssila-Kallunki et al., 1992). As shown in the Diabetes Prevention Project, aggressive lifestyle modification reduces the risk for new-onset DM in obese middle-aged patients by 58% (Tuomilehto et al., 2001). In motivated patients unable to achieve adequate weight loss, pharmacologic intervention is an option. Orlistat (Xenical) is a GI lipase inhibitor that reduces the absorption of dietary fat from the gut. It facilitates weight reduction and should be taken with meals. The major side effect of the medication is fatty, oily stools that can precipitate diarrhea. Newer drugs such as lorcaserin and extended-release phentermine–topiramate can also be considered. Bariatric surgery for morbidly obese patients has been shown to relieve insulin resistance, promote substantial weight loss, reduce BP, and improve dyslipidemia. The Mediterranean diet (increased consumption of fish, legumes, whole grains, and olive oil) is associated with weight loss and improvements in lipid, insulin sensitivity, and inflammatory indices.

Diabetes Mellitus

Key Points

- DM is a CAD risk equivalent.
- More than three quarters of people with diabetes will die of complications of macrovascular disease.
- Tight control of glycemia, dyslipidemia, and HTN to nationally defined standards is tantamount for aggressive risk reduction.
- Nephropathy increases risk for CVD and should be screened for and treated when discovered with ACE inhibitors, ARBs, or both (SOR: A).

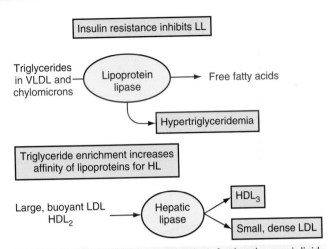

Figure 27-8 Molecular mechanisms etiologic for the atherogenic lipid triad in patients with insulin resistance. As a patient becomes insulin resistant, the activity of lipoprotein lipase (LL) decreases. This can occur secondary to reduced apoprotein CII or increased apoprotein CIII production. With reduced capacity to hydrolyze the triglycerides in such large lipoproteins as very-low-density lipoprotein (VLDL) (derived from the liver) and chylomicrons (derived from the gut), triglycerides, and large remnant particles accumulate in serum. In this scenario, low-density lipoprotein (LDL) levels in serum tend to be relatively low because less VLDL is being converted to LDL. As high-density lipoprotein (HDL) and LDL particles become progressively more enriched with triglycerides, these lipoproteins become better substrates for the enzyme hepatic lipase. Hepatic lipase catabolizes these lipoproteins to form small, dense LDL and HDL. The small HDL particles can be further degraded to their phospholipid and apoprotein constituents, thereby reducing circulating levels of this beneficial lipoprotein. (Based on Toth PP, Davidson MH. Comparative effects of lipid-lowering therapies. *Prog Cardiovasc Dis*. 2004;47:73-104.)

According to statistics compiled by the American Diabetes Association, approximately 1.9 million new cases of DM were diagnosed in people age 20 years and older in 2010. A total of 25.8 million people have DM in the United States, and 79 million have prediabetes. One third of people with the disease are undiagnosed and usually have multiple other risk factors for CVD (http://www.diabetes.org/diabetes-basics/diabetes-statistics/). Nearly all adult patients with DM (90%-95%) have the type II or non-insulin dependent form. However, as the disease progresses and pancreatic islet cell mass is progressively lost, many will become insulin dependent over time. The World Health Organization (WHO) estimates that by the year 2025, there will be more than 350 million people with diabetes throughout the world (King et al., 1998; see also Amos et al., 1997). Diabetes significantly magnifies the risk for MI, sudden death, stroke, CHF, adult-onset blindness, loss of lower extremities, and end-stage renal disease. Given the burgeoning incidence of this disease, the complications stemming from DM will likely incur a level of human suffering that is unprecedented outside of wartime. This is an issue that must be addressed head on by family physicians throughout the world.

Diabetes induces diffuse atherosclerotic disease throughout the vascular tree. Nearly 80% of people with diabetes will die of CVD. The hyperglycemic, insulin-resistant milieu of type 2 DM initiates a broad-ranging cascade of pathophysiology that accelerates atherogenesis. Unfortunately, because of increasing obesity and metabolic syndrome in adolescents and young adults, type 2 DM is becoming relatively common in those younger than 21 years of age. Diffuse endothelial dysfunction, the accumulation of damaging advanced glycation end products within the vasculature, and a heavy risk factor burden typify the patient with DM. Diabetes induces a pro-oxidative and proinflammatory state. People with diabetes also tend to have hypercoagulability (Meigs et al., 2000). This likely results from (1) increased hepatic production of coagulation factors; (2) increased platelet reactivity and aggregability; and (3) as endothelial dysfunction progresses, the endothelium produces less tissue plasminogen activator (tPA), and more PAI-1, rendering the surface of the vascular lumen more prothrombotic. This hypercoagulability and disordered fibrinolysis increase the likelihood that if a person with diabetes experiences acute plaque rupture, it will result in greater and perhaps complete vascular luminal obstruction with acute ischemia and infarction.

It is critical for people with diabetes to be diagnosed early and that their risk factors are evaluated and treated comprehensively. In addition to monitoring indices of glycemia, BP, serum lipids, smoking and obesity status, and baseline renal function should be evaluated. HTN, dyslipidemia, and albuminuria or proteinuria require aggressive management. Based on the East-West (Haffner et al., 1998) and Organization to Assess Strategies for Ischemic Syndromes (OASIS) (Malmberg et al., 2000) studies, the NCEP has defined DM as a CAD risk equivalent. As shown in the European Prospective Investigation of Cancer (EPIC)-Norfolk Study, as hemoglobin A1c (HgbA1c) levels steadily rise above 5.0, the risk for coronary events rises continuously (Khaw et al., 2004). The American Diabetes Association recommends that HgbA1c be below 7.0% (American Diabetes Association, 2013), but the American College of Endocrinology endorses a level below 6.5%. With more aggressive diabetes management, the risk for vascular disease development decreases, but the risk for episodic hypoglycemia increases (Diabetes Control and Complications Trial Research Group, 1995). If a patient tolerates an HgbA1c level that is below 6.5% without undue risk for hypoglycemia, then more aggressive control should be encouraged. In contrast, if an insulin-dependent diabetic patient has CAD and is prone to hypoglycemia, then an HgbA1c level of 7.5 or 8.0% may be more appropriate. The intensity of glycemic control should be balanced against the risks of hypoglycemia. The United Kingdom Prospective Diabetes Study (UKPDS) 35 demonstrated that for every 1% drop in HgbA1c, people with diabetes experience a 21% reduction in any diabetes-related end point, a 14% drop in MI, a 12% reduction in stroke, and a 37% reduction in risk of microvascular disease (Stratton et al., 2000). In the STENO-2 Study, intensive therapy of blood sugars, BP, and serum lipids resulted in a 50% lower incidence of the primary composite cardiovascular end point compared with "conventional" therapy, which was substantially less aggressive (Gaede et al., 2003). In the UKPDS, it was shown that metformin therapy reduces the risk for acute cardiovascular events by 38%. Unless there is a contraindication, individuals with diabetes should take prophylactic aspirin therapy.

Patients with diabetes should be treated with a statin. In such studies as the Collaborative Atorvastatin Diabetes Study (Colhoun et al., 2004) and Scandinavian Simvastatin Survival Study (Dunstan et al., 2002; Pyorala et al.,

1998), statin therapy was associated with a 37% and 42% reduction in the risk of cardiovascular events among people with diabetes in the primary and secondary prevention settings, respectively. Fibrate therapy has also been shown to reduce risk for cardiovascular events and rates of atheromatous plaque progression in patients with DM.

Cigarette Smoking

Key Points

- Cigarette smoking is the single most preventable cause of mortality in the United States.
- Cigarette smoking cessation reduces the risk for MI and death by 36%.
- Smoking cessation is facilitated by patient education about the dangers of smoking and pharmacologic intervention with nicotine replacement products, bupropion, and varenicline.
- Relapse rates are high in the absence of education, encouragement, and individualized courses of therapy and follow-up.

According to the CDC, 19% of U.S. adults were cigarette smokers in 2011 (http://www.cdc.gov/mmwr/preview/mmwrhtml/mm6144a2.htm). Unfortunately, the incidence of smoking among adolescents and teenagers continues to rise despite legislation limiting some forms of advertising and the sale of cigarettes to minors. Smoking is the single most *preventable* cause of death in the United States. In addition to increasing the risk for developing pulmonary, oral, laryngeal, and bladder neoplasms, cigarette smoking significantly raises the risk for developing all forms of atherosclerotic disease and potentiates myocardial ischemia, adverse structural damage to the lung parenchyma, and arterial aneurysm formation. More than 440,000 Americans succumb annually from tobacco-related disease.

Cigarette smoke contains more than 4000 exogenous chemicals. Cigarette smoking is associated with increased intravascular oxygen free radical production and induces diffuse endothelial dysfunction, resulting in marked reductions in nitric oxide and tPA production (Chia and Newby, 2002). These changes result in increased oxidative injury to cells and lipoproteins, vasoconstriction, and reduced capacity for fibrinolysis in the setting of plaque rupture and overlying thrombus formation. In addition to accelerating rates of atherogenesis in native arteries, continued smoking reduces rates of arterial and venous graft patency in the heart and peripheral vasculature. Cigarette smoking is associated with increased serum levels of multiple emerging risk factors, including CRP, fibrinogen, and homocysteine compared with nonsmokers (Bazzano et al., 2003).

Achieving lifelong smoking cessation in patients who have or are at risk for CVD is a critical therapeutic goal. Smoking cessation results in a 36% reduction in risk for MI and mortality (van Berkel et al., 1999). Bupropion (Zyban 150-300 mg/day orally) reduces the intensity of withdrawal symptoms in patients trying to quit smoking by inhibiting the neuronal reuptake of norepinephrine, serotonin, and dopamine. These neurotransmitters are associated with central centers modulating addiction and craving or appetitive behaviors. After taking Zyban for approximately 2 weeks, patients can begin to wean themselves from cigarette smoke according to a plan established with their providers. Sustained smoking cessation is facilitated by continuing Zyban for 3 to 6 months after the patient smokes his or her last cigarette. Continued counseling and encouragement are important. Smoking cessation classes are also usually available as part of community health awareness programs. Another approach involves the use of nicotine replacement therapies, such as NicoDerm CQ or Habitrol (transdermal delivery systems) and Nicorette gum. These therapies also control withdrawal and craving by providing an alternative source of nicotine that can be progressively weaned over the course of weeks to months. One recommended regimen for the nicotine patch is to wear each dose (21, 14, and 7 mg) for 1 month in a stepped-down fashion. Patients wearing the patch should be counseled not to smoke because this can induce headache, nausea, flushing, and even angina. If a patient cannot achieve smoking cessation on single-agent therapy, the combination of Zyban and a transdermal nicotine patch has been shown to increase success rates compared with the use of either agent alone. Varenicline therapy is another pharmacologic option for controlling withdrawal and promoting smoking cessation (Rollema et al., 2006). Patients can smoke while taking varenicline and can wean themselves from cigarettes gradually. Smoking cessation success rates are approximately doubled by this drug compared with placebo. Patients should be cautioned about the possibility of new-onset depression, anxiety, and suicidal ideation, although in general it is well tolerated. Varenicline therapy can also increase the vividness and intensity of dreams, which some patients find unpleasant.

Coronary Artery Disease

STABLE ISCHEMIC HEART DISEASE

Chronic stable ischemic heart disease (SIHD) affects 17 million Americans, 10 million of whom have chronic angina. This disease is more prevalent with age, affecting approximately one third of men and one fourth of women older than 80 years of age (Fihn et al., 2012). SIHD can be asymptomatic or present with typical angina (definite), atypical angina (probable), and noncardiac chest pain. Definite angina meets the following criteria: (1) chest pain with characteristic quality and duration that is (2) provoked by stress and (3) resolved with rest or nitroglycerin. Probable angina meets two of these criteria, and noncardiac pain meets none or one of these criteria (Fihn et al., 2012). Angina is classified by the Canadian Cardiovascular Society Classification into four classes: class I, no chest pain with ordinary activity or exertion; class II, chest pain with moderate exertion (e.g., walking more than 2 blocks or flight of stairs); class III, angina with mild exertion (e.g., walking 1-2 blocks or 1 flight of stairs); and class IV, angina with no or minimal activity.

Angina is a symptom of myocardial ischemia. Stable angina is caused by a mismatch between coronary blood supply and myocardial oxygen demand. The latter is determined by several factors, including heart rate and left ventricular (LV) wall stress and contractility (Braunwald, 2000). Coronary supply is determined by oxygen transport capacity and delivery and conditions that regulate the coronary circulatory system, such as endothelial secretory products (e.g., nitric oxide, endothelin), the autonomic nervous system, metabolic activity, neural control, and perfusion pressure. Several pharmacologic interventions, such as adrenergic receptor activation or blockade, adenosine, and acetylcholine, also affect the coronary circulation. Most coronary flow occurs during diastole; only 25% of flow occurs in systole (Feigl, 1998; Yada et al.,1999).

In stable angina, blood flow cannot meet myocardial oxygen demands because of an obstructive atherosclerotic plaque in one or more coronary arteries. Atherosclerosis develops early in life, with progression depending on age and the severity of one or more risk factors as established by such longitudinal cohorts as the Framingham Heart Study. As the volume of atherosclerotic plaque increases, there is a compensatory outward bulging of the vessel that maintains the diameter and patency of the arterial lumen. This generally is not appreciated on an angiogram and can be seen best using intravascular ultrasonography (Figure 27-9). This is referred to as the Glagov phenomenon. It is not until atherosclerotic plaque reaches almost 40% of the plaque surface area before compensatory mechanisms start to fail and the plaque starts to impinge on the lumen. Coronary blood flow starts to decline when the lumen becomes narrowed at about 70% or more. An early clinical manifestation of this pathophysiologic change is the occurrence of chest pain or dyspnea with exertion that resolves within minutes of rest. This "stable angina" pattern does not usually occur at rest. Nonatherosclerotic obstructive CAD may also cause angina. Although infrequent, it could be mediated by myocardial bridging, vasculitis, or congenital malformation of the coronary arteries. In addition,

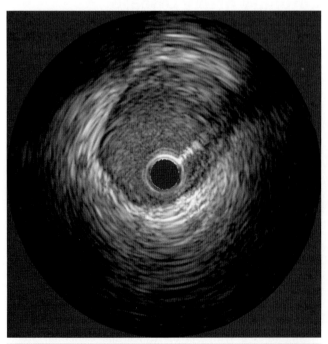

Figure 27-9 Glacov remodeling of the coronary lumen in response to early plaque formation.

conditions without obstructive coronary disease such as cardiomyopathies or valve disease can also trigger angina (Lee, 2002).

Symptoms of stable angina differ among patients. Angina can be perceived as a pressure, tightness, squeezing, or heaviness in the chest. This can radiate to the arm, jaw, shoulders, back, or abdomen. The pain can be associated with an increase in shortness of breath, a feeling of nausea, diaphoresis, or occasional vomiting. Lightheadedness and anxiety may accompany these symptoms. Chest pain or angina may not be present in patients with IHD. Myocardial ischemia with no chest pain is commonly present in people with diabetes secondary to glycemic injury to pain-sensing fibers in the myocardium. Also, dyspnea without chest pain can be an anginal equivalent. Ischemia can induce stiffness in the myocardium and reduces ventricular relaxility, which in return raises LV end-diastolic pressure and leads to dyspnea. Angina or anginal-equivalent symptoms typically resolve with rest or the administration of nitroglycerin.

Noncardiac chest pain typically occurs with certain maneuvers, such as taking a deep breath (e.g., pleuritic sharp pain, pneumothorax, pneumonitis), palpation of the chest wall (as in musculoskeletal pain, costochondritis, rib fracture, fibrositis), after ingestion of certain types of food (esophagitis, gastroesophageal reflux, pancreatitis, gallbladder disease), or as a clinical manifestation of the reactivation of a latent varicella-zoster virus (shingles) (Ma et al., 2007) generally occurring before the appearance of the rash. Other causes of noncardiac pain may also need to be considered, such as pulmonary embolism (Lee, 2002; Lee and Goldman, 2000), aortic dissection (Collins et al., 2004), pericarditis, or psychiatric (anxiety, panic) disorder. When a clear diagnosis explains noncardiac chest pain, additional cardiac evaluation may not be necessary and likely depends on whether the presenting symptom continues after addressing the primary etiology.

Several signs can be noted on examination in a patient with angina. Paradoxical splitting of the second heart sound, systolic murmurs, or S3 or S4 sounds can be appreciated during an anginal episode. Findings of cardiomyopathy or valvular disorders can also be present and might help in establishing the diagnosis of a noncoronary cause of chest pain. Patients can also have hypertension, signs of hyperlipidemia (corneal arcus, periorbital xanthelasma, tendinous xanthomas), or findings of DM (peripheral neuropathy or diabetic retinopathy).

Noninvasive Testing

Electrocardiography. The ECG quite often does not show ischemic changes in patients with stable angina who are at rest and have no symptoms. The resting ECG might show, however, nonspecific ST segment and T-wave abnormalities in a patient with known severe CAD. False-positive results are common in patients with LVH, digoxin intake, electrolyte imbalances, or electrical conduction anomalies such as bundle branch blocks or preexcitation syndromes.

Electrocardiograms need to be compared with old ones. Quite often, new Q-wave abnormalities or the emergence of conduction disturbances might indicate an interval change in the patient's cardiac status. The ECG can be helpful during an episode of chest pain in which more than 50% of patients with normal resting ECGs show new changes.

Typically, these changes include the presence of ST segment depression or elevation in two contiguous leads, new T-wave inversions, or pseudonormalization of already inverted T waves.

At present, it is considered reasonable to obtain a 12-lead ECG on patients with SIHD at 1-year or longer intervals. Performing an ECG, however, should be performed in patients with new or worsening symptoms.

Echocardiography. Echocardiography is currently not indicated in SIHD patients with stable symptoms or no symptoms. However, echocardiography should be done in patients with new or worsening HF or new MI to assess LV function and regional wall motion.

Noninvasive Stress Testing in Patients with Stable Ischemic Heart Disease

Exercise Treadmill Testing. Exercise stress testing uses different protocols (Bruce, modified Bruce, and Naughton) based on a patient's ability to exercise. The patient exercises at different inclines and speeds until achieving 85% of peak predicted heart rate for age ([220 − Age] × 85%). The test provides information about the presence of ischemic ST segment changes, reproducibility of chest pain, arrhythmias, changes in BP and heart rate, and functional capacity. The mean sensitivity of this test is 68% and specificity is 77% (Gibbons et al., 2002). Some studies indicate that, when selection bias is removed, the sensitivity can be as low as 40% to 50% but specificity as high as 85% to 90% (Detrano et al., 1989; Gianrossi et al., 1989; Gibbons et al., 2002). Despite this reduced accuracy, patients with good functional capacity generally have a good prognosis. An early positive stress test result (in the first two stages of exercise) can indicate a worse prognosis and denotes a high risk finding. Furthermore, if a patient experiences chest pain and 1-mm ST segment depression during exercise, the test can be 90% predictive of the presence of CAD. A 2-mm ST segment depression accompanied by chest pain is almost pathognomonic of the presence of obstructive CAD.

The test specificity is reduced when baseline ECGs are abnormal with LVH, preexcitation syndrome, or a bundle branch block or if the patient is taking digoxin (Sketch et al., 1981; Sundqvist et al., 1986) or has electrolyte abnormalities (Froelicher et al., 1999; Gibbons et al., 2002). Also, if a patient cannot reach target heart rate, the diagnostic accuracy of the test is diminished. It should be noted that the presence of antiischemic agents (nitrates, β-blockers, and CCBs) can reduce the sensitivity of the test and should be withheld for 2 to 3 days before the procedure for long-acting drugs and 24 hours for short-acting drugs if the intent is for the test to diagnose the presence of obstructive disease (Gibbons et al., 2002).

The absolute contraindications to stress testing are decompensated CHF, symptomatic severe aortic valve stenosis, ongoing rest chest pain, a recent MI (within the past week), severe HTN, and intractable arrhythmias. When patients have conditions that reduce the specificity of a stress test, an imaging stress test (nuclear or echocardiographic) can be an alternative, more accurate means by which to evaluate for CAD.

Stress Myocardial Perfusion Imaging. Myocardial perfusion imaging (99mTc-sestamibi, 99mTc-tetrofosmin, or thallium-201) (Figure 27-10) provides a more accurate

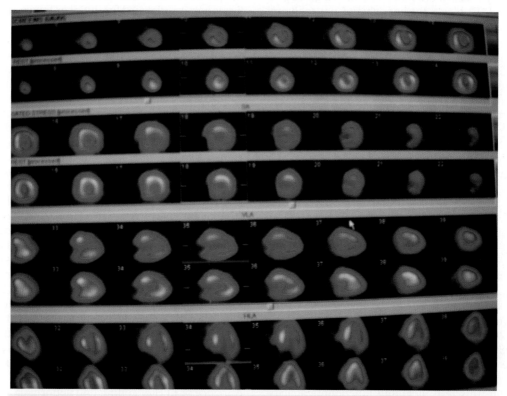

Figure 27-10 Myocardial perfusion scan shows reversible ischemia in the anterior wall, apex, and inferior wall.

modality to diagnose the presence of obstructive CAD than a treadmill ECG alone. The sensitivity and specificity of this test have been reported to be 88% and 72%, respectively. When referral bias is accounted for, the specificity of this test is as high as 90%. In addition to myocardial perfusion, the test provides information about EF and wall motion abnormalities and is very valuable to predict a patient's prognosis (Klocke et al., 2003).

Nuclear stress testing is useful in patients with a low-specificity treadmill ECG. Nuclear imaging can provide information about prognosis and myocardial viability in regions of wall motion abnormalities and can help localize the area of myocardium in jeopardy. Similar to most stress tests, they are best ordered in patients with an intermediate likelihood of obstructive CAD.

Myocardial perfusion imaging also can be performed with the induction of pharmacologic stress. Adenosine and dobutamine are the most commonly used pharmacologic agents. Adenosine is a vasodilator and stresses the heart by a "steal phenomenon." Adenosine and dipyridamole dilate normal coronaries, shunting blood away from abnormal regions of the myocardium and creating a discrepancy in perfusion between normal and abnormal regions. Dobutamine increases heart rate and contractility and therefore increases myocardial oxygen demand.

Adenosine is typically infused over 4 or 6 minutes, depending on the protocol used. The infusion rate of 140 µg/kg/min starts with ECG monitoring. Usually halfway through the infusion, sestamibi ("Myoview") or thallium is injected. Adenosine causes flushing, shortness of breath, nausea, chest pain, and a "strange" feeling in most patients, and this does not reflect the presence of CAD. Adenosine can also cause bradycardia and a high-degree atrioventricular (AV) block. Patients should not take any caffeinated beverages for at least 12 to 24 hours before the test. Also, adenosine can precipitate asthma and should not be used in patients with hyperreactive airway disease. Adenosine is an excellent choice for a test in patients who cannot exercise on a treadmill. The sensitivity and specificity of adenosine stress imaging are 90% and 82%, respectively (Klocke et al., 2003).

Dobutamine is infrequently used and is reserved for patients who cannot exercise on a treadmill and have a contraindication to taking adenosine. Dobutamine is infused at 10 µg/kg/min for 3 minutes and then increased by increments of 10 µg/kg/min every 3 minutes to a maximum of 50 µg/kg/min or if target heart rate has been achieved. If despite this high dose of dobutamine, target heart rate is not achieved, atropine is administered to a maximum of 1 to 2 mg. Cardiolite is injected typically at target heart rate, and the infusion is then terminated. Patients are generally observed for at least 10 minutes after the test or until the heart rate is below 100 beats/min. Dobutamine can cause a shaky feeling, nausea, and arrhythmias. In general, it is well tolerated.

Although pharmacologic nuclear stress imaging provides similar diagnostic accuracy to treadmill nuclear stress testing for the presence of obstructive CAD, patients are best exercised on a treadmill because more information can be obtained from this test, including functional capacity, which is a strong predictor of prognosis, the presence of

arrhythmias with exercise, and the hemodynamic response to physical exertion.

Stress Echocardiography. Stress echocardiography (Cheitlin et al., 2003) is an alternative imaging stress test to a nuclear stress test. However, the sensitivity is slightly lower with an increase in specificity, making the overall accuracy of this test similar to that of stress nuclear imaging. Stress echocardiography is performed by obtaining an initial resting echocardiogram to assess a patient's left ventricular ejection fraction (LVEF), wall motion characteristics, and cavity size. In about 25% of patients, it may be difficult to obtain optimal echocardiographic images for adequate interpretation of the test, and therefore an alternative form of stress testing is needed. This is particularly true in patients with severe chronic obstructive pulmonary disease (COPD) and patients with severe obesity. Patients are exercised on a treadmill using a symptom-limited protocol. Patients need to achieve the minimum target heart rate for age (85% of maximum predicted) but preferably a higher rate to allow ample time for the sonographer to obtain immediate post-stress echocardiographic images while the heart rate is still over target for age. Typically, the sonographer needs about 20 to 30 seconds to obtain these images. In patients who cannot exercise, dobutamine can be used as described earlier to achieve target heart rate, and the infusion is discontinued when all echocardiographic images are acquired.

Choice of the Stress Test or Imaging Modality. The choice of the stress test depends on several factors, including the patient population being tested (whether SIHD is suspected or known); the ability of the patient to exercise; the presence of an interpretable 12-lead ECG; whether the test is being performed for initial or follow-up risk stratification; and whether the patient has SIHD with stable symptoms, is asymptomatic, or has new, recurrent, or worsening symptoms (that do not meet the definition of moderate- or high-risk UA). Table 27-13 summarizes level A choices as recommended by the ACC/AHA recent guidelines (Fihn et al., 2012).

The main goal of noninvasive stress testing in patients with stable symptoms or asymptomatic SIHD is risk stratification to guide revascularization and to improve hard outcomes. Symptomatic patients with SIHD who continue to be limited in their daily activity despite guideline-directed medical therapy need to undergo coronary angiography and revascularization for symptom control and to restore normal activities irrespective of risk stratification.

As a general rule, if a patient is able to exercise and has an interpretable baseline ECG, a regular treadmill stress test is recommended for initial evaluation of suspected SIHD. If the ECG is noninterpretable, myocardial perfusion imaging (MPI) can be added to the exercise stress test. Pharmacologic MPI is preferred in patients who are unable to exercise. If patients with known SIHD have a change in symptoms, the same recommendations hold for repeat testing. It is highly discouraged in these patients to perform pharmacologic MPI if they are able to exercise and have a baseline interpretable ECG. An interpretable baseline ECG should have no evidence of LVH or conduction abnormalities, there should be no electrolyte disturbances, and the patient should not

Table 27-13   Choice of Stress Testing in Patients with Stable Ischemic Heart Disease*

Patients with suspected (not yet documented) SIHD: initial evaluation	Exercise ECG if patient is able to exercise and ECG is interpretable Exercise with nuclear MPI or echocardiography if patient is able to exercise and ECG is uninterpretable Avoid exercise with nuclear MPI or echocardiography in patients who are able to exercise and who have an interpretable ECG but have a low pretest probability for disease; could consider regular ECG testing Pharmacologic stress test with MPI, echocardiography, or CMR should be avoided in patients who are able to exercise and with an interpretable ECG Pharmacological stress with nuclear MPI or echocardiography should be performed as the first choice in patients who are unable to exercise If a patient is unable to undergo stress testing, has an inconclusive stress test, or has symptoms despite normal stress test, consider coronary CTA
Patients with SIHD and stable symptoms or asymptomatic for risk stratification	Exercise ECG if is patient able to exercise and ECG is interpretable. Can consider exercise with nuclear MPI or echocardiography (less evidence) Exercise with nuclear MPI or echocardiography if patient is able to exercise and ECG is uninterpretable Pharmacologic stress test with MPI, echocardiography or CMR, or CCTA should be avoided in patients who are able to exercise and with an interpretable ECG Pharmacologic stress with nuclear MPI or echocardiography should be performed as the first choice in patients who are unable to exercise; pharmacologic stress CMA or CCTA can be considered (less evidence) Nuclear MPI, echocardiography or CMR with exercise, or pharmacologic stress test or CCTA is not recommended for follow-up assessment in patients with SIHD if performed more frequently than at 5-year intervals after CABG or 2-year intervals after coronary angioplasty
Patients with SIHD and new, recurrent, or worsening symptoms (not unstable angina)	Exercise ECG if patient is able to exercise (at least moderate physical functioning with no disabling comorbidity) and ECG is interpretable Exercise with nuclear MPI or echocardiography if patient is able to exercise and ECG is uninterpretable Consider exercise with nuclear MPI or echocardiography in patients at high risk for multivessel disease or who have had prior requirement for imaging with exercise Pharmacologic stress test with MPI, echocardiography or CMR, or CCTA should be avoided in patients who are able to exercise and with an interpretable ECG Pharmacological stress with nuclear MPI or echocardiography should be performed as first choice in patients who are unable to exercise; pharmacologic stress CMA can be considered (less evidence) CCTA should not be performed if a patient has severe calcification or a prior stent

*Level A, American College of Cardiology/American Heart Association guidelines (Fihn et al., 2012).
CABG, Coronary artery bypass graft; *CCTA*, cardiac computed tomography angiography; *CMA*, cardiac magnetic angiography; *CMR*, cardiac magnetic resonance; *CTA*, computed tomography angiography; *ECG*, electrocardiography; *MPI*, myocardial perfusion imaging; *SIHD*, stable ischemic heart disease.

be taking digoxin (Melin et al., 1985). When adjusting for the pretest probability of disease, women have only a slightly reduced specificity on a regular stress test compared with men. In addition, a baseline borderline ST segment depression of less than 1 mm is not an exclusionary criterion to perform a treadmill stress test.

For stable or asymptomatic patients with SIHD, there is currently no SOR: A evidence defining the frequency of risk stratification on follow-up. Current guidelines by the ACC/AHA recommend nuclear perfusion imaging, echocardiography, or cardiac mitral regurgitation (MR) with exercise or pharmacologic stress testing at longer than 2-year intervals in patients with SIHD and with prior evidence of silent ischemia or at high risk for recurrent event *and* who meet one of the following criteria: (1) unable to exercise to an adequate workload, (2) have an uninterpretable ECG, or (3) have a history of incomplete revascularization (Fihn et al., 2012). These tests, however, should not be performed at more than 5-year or longer intervals after bypass surgery or 2-year or longer intervals after coronary angioplasty. In this patient population, the use of routine periodic follow-up imaging stress testing is preferred over regular stress testing.

Irrespective of the modality of stress testing, a test should be terminated when a patient displays significant arrhythmias, lightheadedness, a symptomatic drop in BP, or significant ischemic changes on the ECG, particularly if associated with anginal symptoms. Also a stress test should not be performed in patients with unstable rest symptoms, frequent arrhythmia, known severe left main (LM) disease,

severe symptomatic valvular disease, or decompensated CHF. The test needs to be closely monitored at all times by the technician, and a provider needs always to be in the immediate vicinity while the test is being conducted. Providers or supervising staff need to be trained in advanced cardiac life support.

PHARMACOLOGIC MANAGEMENT OF THE PATIENT WITH STABLE ANGINA

Patients with stable angina have an imbalance between coronary blood supply and demand. They are at increased risk of MI and arrhythmias. The management of these patients is predominantly medical with intensive guideline-based therapy focusing on alleviating angina, reducing plaque progression and risk of rupture, and restoring a patient's functional capacity. Some reversible causes of angina need to be evaluated, such as conditions that increase myocardial oxygen demand. These include fever, thyrotoxicosis, anemia, and cardiac stimulants such as cocaine or amphetamines. Severe valvular dysfunction and CHF might be also precipitating factors. Interventional therapies in stable angina are reserved for patients with continued limiting symptoms despite optimal medical therapy and those patients with high-risk findings on their noninvasive evaluation.

Nitrate Therapy

Nitrate therapy reduces myocardial oxygen demand by increasing venous capacitance and, therefore, reducing venous return and ventricular wall stress. Also, nitrates increase coronary blood supply by dilating the coronary arteries (Parker, 1993; Parker et al., 1995; Parker and Parker, 1998). Administering nitrates to patients with stable angina increases their symptom-free walking distance and reduces the frequency and severity of their anginal episodes. Nitrates are not known to significantly reduce risk for MI or prolong survival. On a chronic basis, nitrates can be administered orally or transdermally. Irrespective of the mode of administration, it is important to have 8 to 10 hours of a nitrate-free period to avoid tolerance to this drug (Parker et al., 1995). IV nitroglycerin is reserved for the UA patient to reduce anginal pain and intracardiac filling pressures and to improve symptoms of HF.

β-Blockade

β-Blockers reduce myocardial oxygen demand primarily by reducing heart rate and contractility. β-Blockers are essential in patients with stable angina and a history of prior MI or reduced LV function. In these conditions, β-blockers can prolong survival and should be administered to these patients unless absolutely contraindicated (Gottlieb et al., 1998). In patients with normal LV systolic function after MI or other ACS, β-blockers should be continued for 3 years. If, however, LV function remains reduced at 40% or less in patients with a history of MI or who have CHF, β-blockers need to be continued indefinitely. β-Blockers are best limited to those with data that have shown reduction in mortality. These include metoprolol XL, carvedilol, and bisoprolol.

It is unclear whether β-blockers improve survival or serious arrhythmias in patients with stable angina and no prior infarction or LV dysfunction. Relative or absolute contraindications to β-blocker therapy include patients with severe hyperreactive airway disease, heart block, severe bradycardia, or severe symptomatic peripheral vascular disease.

Calcium Channel Blockers

Long-acting CCBs are potent antiischemic drugs and can also be used to treat patients with stable angina (Braunwald, 1982). Generally, short-acting calcium blockers need to be avoided because they could potentially increase adverse events. Dihydropyridines (e.g., amlodipine or nifedipine XL) do not alter heart rate significantly and are primarily vasodilators. Whereas diltiazem reduces heart rate but also increases coronary blood supply, verapamil reduces oxygen demand primarily by reducing heart rate with less vasodilatory effects. The CCBs are generally used as a second-line treatment if there is inadequate response to β-blockers. Also, nondihydropyridine CCBs may be used as first-line treatment in patients intolerant of β-blockers.

Ranolazine (Ranexa)

Ranolazine is indicated to treat chronic stable angina. It can be used in conjunction with other antiischemic drugs, including β-blockers, nitrates, and CCBs. Also, in patients intolerant to β-blockers, ranolazine can be an effective substitute.

Ranolazine is metabolized through the CYP3A cytochrome system. Therefore, it should not be administered to patients taking strong CYP3A inhibitors (e.g., ketoconazole, clarithromycin, and some antiretroviral drugs) or

CYP3A inducers (e.g., rifampin, phenobarbital, phenytoin, St. John's wort) or with a history of hepatic cirrhosis. Ranolazine has been shown to increase the QTc interval in a dose-dependent manner, but no increase in arrhythmia or sudden death has been demonstrated. Ranolazine has been shown to increase exercise duration and delay anginal onset and ST depression on treadmill testing in severe chronic angina patients. The number of anginal attacks and the need for sublingual nitroglycerin are reduced with ranolazine (Chaitman et al., 2004; Stone et al., 2006). The most common side effects of ranolazine are dizziness, headache, constipation, and nausea. The starting dose is 500 mg orally twice a day, which is increased to 1000 mg twice a day as needed. In patients on moderate CYP3A inhibitors (e.g., diltiazem, verapamil, erythromycin, fluconazole, and grapefruit juice) the dose is limited to 500 mg twice a day. The advantage of ranolazine is its lack of effect on BP and heart rate; therefore, it can be used in patients with a low rate-pressure product as an add-on antiischemic drug.

Antiplatelet Agents

In high-risk patients, aspirin (81 mg) reduces vascular events by approximately 35% and is a primary therapy in patients with stable angina (Antiplatelet Trialists Collaboration, 1994). Aspirin is very effective in reducing MI in healthy subjects with elevated serum CRP levels (Ridker et al., 1997).

Aspirin resistance has been reported recently and can be present in approximately 25% of patients. Also, aspirin hypersensitivity is common and primarily related to GI side effects. The side effects (including bleeding and dyspepsia) of aspirin can be reduced without compromising the effectiveness of this drug with the use of enteric-coated aspirin. The dose of aspirin is best limited to 81 mg with no compromise to its effectiveness and with a reduced bleeding risk compared with a full aspirin dose (325 mg).

Clopidogrel (Plavix) is an adenosine diphosphate (ADP) receptor antagonist and a potent, irreversible antiplatelet drug. In the Clopidogrel versus Aspirin in Patients at Risk of Ischaemic Events [CAPRIE] study (CAPRIE Steering Committee, 1996), clopidogrel was slightly but statistically more effective than aspirin in reducing cardiovascular events in high-risk patients with a history of stroke, MI, or peripheral vascular disease (8.7% relative risk reduction; $P = 0.043$). Clopidogrel is an effective alternative to patients who are unable to tolerate aspirin.

Dipyridamole is not recommended as an antiplatelet therapy in patients with stable IHD because it has not been shown to be beneficial. Also, there are no data to substitute aspirin with NSAIDs, which should be avoided in general in patients with SIDH.

The combination of clopidogrel (75 mg/day) and aspirin (81 mg/day) (i.e., dual antiplatelet therapy) is required in patients with recent percutaneous intervention. For patients receiving a bare-metal stent or balloon angioplasty alone without stenting, clopidogrel may be administered for 3 to 4 weeks. For patients receiving a drug-eluting stent, dual antiplatelet therapy needs to be continued for a minimum of 1 year. The optimal duration of this dual antiplatelet therapy after a drug-eluting stent is currently unknown and is being evaluated in large-scale studies. There is no evidence that continuing clopidogrel and aspirin combination beyond 1 year after the deployment of a drug-eluting stent carries an added advantage. Aspirin alone, on the other hand, should be continued indefinitely (Bhatt and Topol, 2004).

Angiotensin-Converting Enzyme Inhibitors

In patients with SIHD, ACE inhibitors are recommended in patients with concomitant LV systolic dysfunction, HTN, DM, and CKD unless contraindicated. In patients with severe renal insufficiency (creatinine clearance <30 mL/min), ACE inhibitors are generally avoided. Providers should expect a slight rise in creatinine with the initiation of an ACE inhibitor. A rise of creatinine of 0.5 is not unusual and should not be a reason to stop this medication. If a patient develops a cough from ACE inhibitor therapy, consideration can be given to the use of ARBs as a substitute (Fihn et al., 2012).

Influenza Vaccination

All patients with SIHD, unless they have a clear contraindication, should receive an annual influenza vaccination. The purpose of this treatment is to reduce cardiovascular events. Data suggest that the influenza virus may precipitate plaque rupture, and vaccination against this virus can prevent the onset of ACS and death.

In addition to these measures, aggressive management of dyslipidemia, weight, HTN, impaired glucose control, and smoking cessation are essential interventions to reduce future cardiovascular events in the stable angina patient. Cardiac rehabilitation is a critical therapeutic modality in patients with CAD, particularly after revascularization. It is advisable that patients have 30 to 60 minutes of moderate-intensity aerobic activity at least 5 and preferably 7 days per week. Identifying and managing depression are also important steps in the management of patients with SIHD. The initiation of hormone replacement therapy in postmenopausal women is not indicated for cardiovascular risk reduction.

MECHANICAL AND REVASCULARIZATION STRATEGIES FOR TREATING STABLE ANGINA PATIENTS

Coronary Angioplasty and Bypass Surgery

Revascularization in SIHD can be performed for improving survival or for improving symptoms when unacceptable angina remains despite optimal medical therapy.

Revascularization for Improving Survival

Patients with unprotected left main disease are best treated with bypass surgery. Current guidelines (Fihn et al., 2012), however, support the treatment of LM disease with angioplasty and stenting for improvement of survival if the LM anatomy is favorable and surgery is high risk, a decision that will be made by the cardiac care team. Also, patients with three-vessel CAD or two-vessel disease that include the proximal left anterior descending (LAD) artery are best treated with bypass surgery to improve survival. Also, there is evidence that one-vessel proximal LAD treated with the left internal mammary artery (LIMA) provides a long-term survival benefit. Bypass surgery is also preferred for patients with three-vessel disease and reduced LV function

(35%-50%) or patients with three-vessel disease and those with diabetes even in the absence of disease in the LM or proximal LAD. Bypass surgery or angioplasty is indicated in survivors of sudden cardiac death with presumed ischemia-mediated ventricular tachycardia (VT).

Revascularization for Improving Symptoms

Both bypass surgery and angioplasty can be considered as first-line treatment in symptomatic patients with one or more significant stenoses (LM ≥50%, non LM ≥70%, or physiologic fractional flow reserve ≤0.8) and optimized on medical treatment or who cannot tolerate additional medications or if the patient's preference is to not take medications. Angioplasty is preferred for symptom control in patients with prior bypass surgery and unacceptable angina despite good medical treatment (Fihn et al., 2012).

Angioplasty should be avoided in patients with low-risk findings on noninvasive testing who have only one- or two-vessel, nonproximal LAD disease or one chronically occluded vessel who are asymptomatic or minimally symptomatic without medications. Angioplasty is not indicated in patients who are asymptomatic on no treatment and have only one- or two-vessel nonproximal LAD disease or one chronically occluded vessel and intermediate findings on noninvasive testing. The value of revascularization in this same patient population is unclear even if high-risk findings are seen on noninvasive imaging. In general, however, it is acceptable to revascularize the majority of patients with high-risk findings on noninvasive testing, particularly those who are symptomatic on medical treatment and have proximal LAD involvement or three-vessel disease (Patel et al., 2012).

NONPHARMACOLOGIC OR REVASCULARIZATION STRATEGIES TO TREAT CHRONIC STABLE ANGINA

Mechanical interventions such as enhanced external counterpulsation (EECP) can be effective in the treatment of patients with stable angina who are not candidates for revascularization and have continued chest pain despite medical therapy (Michaels et al., 2005). This therapy requires approximately 32 sessions each of about 1 hour duration for 5 days weekly. The functional mechanism of EECP is largely unknown. EECP, however, improves exercise tolerance, reduces exercise-induced myocardial ischemia, and improves LV diastolic filling (Urano et al., 2001) in patients with CAD. *Spinal cord stimulation* and *laser transmyocardial revascularization (laser-TMR)* can also be considered with possible benefits. *Acupuncture* has no role in the treatment of patients who are refractory to conventional pharmacologic and revascularization means.

KEY TREATMENT

- In symptomatic SIHD, regular treadmill stress testing is the preferred modality in patients who are able to exercise and have an interpretable baseline ECG. If the baseline ECG cannot be interpreted, then treadmill exercise imaging tests are preferred. Pharmacologic testing is best reserved for patients who cannot exercise (SOR: A, ACC/AHA guidelines).

- β-Blockers are recommended as initial therapy in the absence of contraindications in patients with prior MI or ACS and should be continued for at least 3 years in patients with normal LV systolic function or indefinitely in patients with EF less than 40% (SOR: A, ACC/AHA guidelines).
- Aspirin (75-162 mg/day) is strongly recommended in patients with stable angina and should be continued indefinitely in the absence of contraindications (SOR: A, ACC/AHA guidelines).
- All patients with SIHD, unless they have a clear contraindication, should receive the annual influenza vaccination (SOR: A, ACC/AHA guidelines, 2012).
- Comprehensive risk factor management and cardiac rehabilitation are essential in the management of patients with stable angina (SOR: A, ACC/AHA guidelines).
- Several OTC medications or vitamins should not be used to treat SIHD. These include vitamins C, E, B_6, B_{12}, β-carotene, folate, CoQ10, chromium, selenium, garlic, chelation, and estrogen therapy in postmenopausal women (SOR: A, ACC/AHA guidelines, 2012).

ACUTE CORONARY SYNDROMES

The ACS occur as a result of sudden atheromatous plaque rupture. Plaques with heightened inflammation, irrespective of severity, can rupture, leading to overlying platelet and fibrin mesh formation, resulting in abrupt reduction or cessation of coronary blood flow secondary to luminal obstruction (Ikeda, 2002; Zhou, 1999). Patients might experience UA or MI depending on whether myocardial necrosis occurs. In the United States, 2.3 million people have ACS annually.

Several crucial facts need to be considered by the practicing family physician. First, a large percentage of angiographically "normal" coronaries have significant plaque burden by intravascular ultrasonography or MRI, particularly in patients older than the age of 40 years (St Goar, 1992). Second, more than 60% of MIs are induced by culprit lesions that initially obstruct less than 50% of the arterial lumen. These lesions are generally not detected by stress testing. Third, when an ACS occurs, multiple vulnerable plaques generally coexist at the same time throughout the vascular tree. In an inadequately managed patient, any one of these lesions could suddenly rupture and precipitate an ACS. Therefore, a normal stress test result does not necessarily exclude the possibility of underlying CAD and risk for ACS. The prevention of MI should focus on reducing the chance of plaque rupture by controlling and normalizing as much as possible multiple cardiac risk factors, including HTN, uncontrolled diabetes, insulin resistance or metabolic syndrome, dyslipidemia, obesity, lack of routine exercise, a heightened inflammatory state, and smoking.

Unstable Angina and Non–ST Segment Myocardial Infarction

Patients with UA or a non–ST segment elevating myocardial infarction (NSTEMI) experience a partial occlusion to coronary flow as a result of plaque rupture and thrombus formation, microembolization, or the release of vasoactive substances, leading to localized spasm. UA is defined as class IV rest angina of at least 20 minutes in duration occurring at rest (within 1 week of presentation), new-onset class III angina occurring within 2 months of presentation, or previously diagnosed chronic angina increased by more or equal 1 class in severity in the 2 months before presentation (Fihn et al., 2012). Prolonged rest angina (generally >30 minutes to 1 hour) typically leads to myocardial necrosis and NSTEMI. Patients are generally at high risk of developing ST segment elevation MI (STEMI) and sudden death. Data from the Thrombolysis in Myocardial Infarction III (TIMI III) registry indicate that death and MI could occur in these patients at a rate of 7.3% to 18.5%, depending on the severity of their symptoms, with postinfarction angina carrying the highest risk (Sharis et al., 2002). Patients may have ECG changes to indicate ischemia, mostly ST segment depression in contiguous leads, T-wave inversion, or pseudonormalization of T waves. However, the ECG could also be silent in UA/NSTEMI. Comparing the ECG with a previous one can be very helpful for detecting subtle but significant new changes.

Patients with suspected UA should be referred to the emergency department (ED) or a specialized chest pain unit as soon as possible. They should be encouraged to call 911 and not drive themselves to the ED. A complete evaluation of their chest pain, including a comprehensive physical examination and history; obtaining an ECG within 10 minutes of arrival; chest radiography; and cardiac enzymes, including troponin I and creatinine kinase with MB fraction (CKMB), needs to be performed. Patients should be admitted to the hospital if they have a suspicion of UA and one or more of these high-risk features: elderly (>70 years of age), have had history of SIHD or revascularization, have ischemia on the ECG (ST segment deviation or new T-wave abnormalities or left bundle branch block), ongoing chest pain (>20 minutes or accelerating), abnormal cardiac biomarkers, or developing CHF or hemodynamic instability. Patients who do not have these high-risk UA features may be treated medically and then risk stratified on an elective basis either in the chest pain unit or shortly after discharge from the ED. If they do not have high-risk features on noninvasive imaging, they can continue to be treated medically. If high-risk noninvasive features are detected, then angiography and revascularization are indicated.

Abnormal cardiac enzymes allow a definite diagnosis of MI. The most frequently used cardiac markers are myoglobin, CK and CKMB fractions, and troponins T (TT) and I (TI). Myoglobin becomes abnormal in the first 1 to 2 hours after myocardial necrosis and remains abnormal for at least 7 to 12 hours. Its sensitivity is high for myocardial injury (sensitivity of 83% within 6 hours of onset of symptoms), but it has a lower specificity. A positive myoglobin can be due to muscle trauma, muscle disorders, rigorous exercise, and certain drugs such as statins. A more sensitive and specific marker than myoglobin is CK and its cardiac isoform, CKMB. This marker is 90% accurate for the diagnosis of MI at 6 hours from symptom onset. CK reaches its peak at about 24 hours of symptom onset and returns to normal or near normal by 72 hours. Troponin I is a very sensitive test for the diagnosis of MI at about 10 to 14 hours after the onset of chest pain. Its sensitivity and specificity at 6 hours are approximately 58% and 94%, respectively, and 92% and 95%, respectively, at 10 hours. Troponin I levels remain abnormal for several days after myocardial injury.

Table 27-14* High-Risk Indicators in Patients with Unstable Angina*

New or presumably new ST segment depression
Elevated troponin T or I
Recurrent angina at rest
Reduced LV function (EF <40%)
Heart failure or new or worsening MR
Sustained ventricular arrhythmias
Hemodynamic instability
History of bypass surgery
History of recent angioplasty within the past 6 months
High risk based on noninvasive stress testing
High-risk score (e.g., TIMI or Grace)

*Level A, American College of Cardiology/American Heart Association guidelines (Braunwald et al., 2002).
EF, Ejection fraction; *LV,* left ventricular; *MR,* mitral regurgitation; *TIMI,* Thrombolysis in Myocardial Infarction.

Table 27-15 Acute Pharmacologic Therapy of Patients with Unstable Angina/Non–ST Elevation Myocardial Infarction*

Aspirin (or clopidogrel in patients who cannot take aspirin) should be administered as soon as possible after onset of symptoms and continued indefinitely.
Antithrombin therapy with UFH, fondaparinux, or enoxaparin (preferred over UFH unless bypass surgery is planned within 24 hours) should be started in conjunction with aspirin.
Clopidogrel should then be added to antithrombin and aspirin in hospitalized patients and continued for 1 year whether the patient is treated medially, with bare-metal stent, or with drug-eluting stent.
Fondaparinux should not be used when patient is undergoing PCI procedures (catheter and wire thrombosis have been described).
The use of upstream intravenous GP 2b/3a inhibitors such as tirofiban (Aggrastat) or eptifibatide (Integrilin) may be considered in patients with early recurrent ischemic discomfort, delay to revascularization, or high-risk features.
If bivalirudin is planned as the antithrombin of choice during the procedure, GP 2b/3a inhibitors are not used except as a bail-out treatment.
Fibrinolytics are contraindicated in patients with unstable angina NSTEMI.

*Level of evidence: A, American College of Cardiology/American Heart Association guidelines (Braunwald et al., 2002).
GP, Glycoprotein; *NSTEMI,* or non–ST segment elevation myocardial infarction; *PCI,* percutaneous coronary intervention; *UFH,* unfractionated heparin.

Depending on the time of onset of chest pain, these markers have different levels of utility in the diagnosis of MI. For instance, the diagnosis of MI in a patient who had chest pain more than 72 hours after presentation is best made with TI because the CK enzymes could have normalized on presentation. CK enzymes should not be used as the sole markers to assess the presence of an acute coronary event in the ED. A negative TI result after 8 to 12 hours of chest pain indicates a low chance for a cardiac event in the immediate near future. Therefore, patients who present with chest pain and have a negative TI result at 8 to 12 hours after the onset of chest pain and no ECG changes to indicate ischemia can undergo a stress test either in the ED or within 72 hours of discharge (Anderson et al., 2013).

Patients with definite UA/NSTEMI benefit significantly from early aggressive intervention with angiography and revascularization, particularly when early high-risk indicators exist (Table 27-14). The early invasive strategy can be immediate or at 12 to 48 hours after hospital admission, depending on the patient's hemodynamic stability and continued symptoms. An early conservative treatment can be adopted in patients with no high-risk features. Angiography can then be performed if high-risk features reappear or based on the presence of moderate to high risk findings on noninvasive imaging.

The Treat Angina with Aggrastat and Determine Cost of Therapy with an Invasive or Conservative Strategy (TACTICS TIMI-18) study (Cannon et al., 2001) randomized UA/NSTEMI patients to an early aggressive therapy with revascularization (within 48 hours of presentation) versus an early conservative therapy in which patients were treated medically and then risk stratified with exercise stress testing. In this study, a significant reduction in the primary combined end point of death, MI, and rehospitalization for ACS was noted at 6 months (odds ratio, 0.78; 95% CI [0.62, 0.97]; $P=0.025$). Other high-risk features include advanced age (>70 years); history of vascular disease; diabetes; and elevated high-sensitivity C-reactive protein (hsCRP), WBC count, and B-type natriuretic peptide (BNP). Furthermore, based on data for the TIMI11B trial (Antman et al., 1999), Antman and coworkers (2000) predicted that the risk of death, reinfarction, or recurrent severe ischemia requiring revascularization increased from 5% to 41% depending on the sum of the following individual prognostic variables: age older than 65 years, more than three coronary risk

factors, prior angiographic coronary obstruction, ST segment deviation, more than two angina events within 24 hours, use of aspirin within 7 days, and elevated cardiac markers. These variables have been incorporated into the TIMI score to assess the risk of death and MI and need for urgent revascularization in patients with UA.

Although most ACS are caused by plaque rupture, thrombosis, and superimposed spasm, rapidly progressive plaques can infrequently lead to an unstable syndrome. In addition, UA can be precipitated by secondary causes such as thyrotoxicosis, severe HTN or valvular stenosis, tachycardia, anemia, hypotension, and hypoxia.

Pharmacologic Therapy of Unstable Angina or Non–ST Segment Myocardial Infarction

Pharmacologic management of patients with UA or NSTEMI can be divided into *acute* and *chronic* therapy. In the *acute* phase (Table 27-15; SOR: A, ACC/AHA guidelines), patients are typically treated with an antithrombin drug (unfractionated heparin [UFH] or low–molecular-weight heparin), aspirin, clopidogrel, β-blockers, statins, IV nitrate therapy, ACE inhibitors (in patients with LV dysfunction and continued HTN or in those with diabetes), and supplemental oxygen therapy (in patients with respiratory distress and hypoxemia). The use of upstream IV glycoprotein (GP) IIb/IIIa inhibitors such as tirofiban (Aggrastat) or eptifibatide (Integrilin) may be considered in patients with early recurrent ischemic discomfort, delay to revascularization, or high-risk features. If bivalirudin (Angiomax) is planned as the antithrombin of choice during the procedure, GP IIb/IIIa inhibitors are not used except as a "bail-out" intervention.

Low-molecular-weight heparin (e.g., Lovenox) has been shown to have some advantages over UFH. These include more reliable anticoagulation with predictable pharmacokinetics, resistance to inhibition by platelet factor 4, a lower risk of causing heparin-induced thrombocytopenia, greater anti-Xa activity, and possibly greater efficacy in reducing risk for ACS. In the Efficacy and Safety of Subcutaneous Enoxaparin in Non-Q-Wave Coronary Events (ESSENCE) trial (Cohen et al., 1997), enoxaparin (Lovenox) plus aspirin was more effective than UFH plus aspirin in reducing the incidence of the combined end points of death, MI, and recurrent angina (19.8% vs. 23.3%, respectively; *P* = 0.016) in patients with UA or NSTEMI at 1 month of follow-up. A recent meta-analysis of 22,000 patients also demonstrated that enoxaparin is more effective than UFH in preventing the combined end point of death or MI (Petersen et al., 2004). Currently, enoxaparin 1 mg/kg given subcutaneously twice a day is preferred over UFH (70 units/kg bolus IV, then 1000 units/hour adjusted every 6 hours with partial thromboplastin time checks) in patients who present with UA/NSTEMI and in whom a conservative approach has been the initial management therapy. Both enoxaparin and UFH, however, have level A evidence to support their use in these patients.

Continued chest pain despite optimal medical therapy indicates that the patient should be brought to the cardiac catheterization laboratory for emergent angiography and revascularization to minimize the chance of irreversible myocardial injury and loss of function. As noted earlier, even in a pain-free UA patient with high-risk features, an aggressive approach to therapy is indicated and needs to be implemented within 48 hours of symptom onset. Morphine sulfate can be used to treat acute pain unresponsive to antiischemic therapy.

Adenosine Diphosphate Receptor Antagonists. Optimal antiplatelet treatment is needed with antithrombin drugs in the management of the patients with ACS. Vascular injury leads to platelet activation and aggregation with subsequent fibrin deposition and thrombosis. Antithrombin therapy alone without optimal platelet inhibition leads to an inferior outcome during percutaneous coronary intervention (PCI). Early experience with PCI was performed with UFH in patients pretreated with aspirin. Aspirin is only partially effective as an antiplatelet drug by inhibiting cyclooxygenase and therefore partially blocking thromboxane A2 and collagen-mediated platelet activation and aggregation (Shammas, 2005).

Platelet inhibition with clopidogrel (Plavix) is dose and time dependent. After a single loading dose of 600 mg of clopidogrel, inhibition of platelet aggregation reaches steady state in 2 to 3 hours. In contrast, 75 mg/day of clopidogrel requires 5 to 7 days to reach the same level of inhibition of platelet aggregation. In patients with ACS, blocking the ADP receptor on platelets with clopidogrel is an important step to reduce the combined end point of cardiovascular death, nonfatal MI, or stroke, whether they have been treated aggressively with bare-metal stents or drug-eluting stents or managed conservatively. In the Clopidogrel for the Reduction of Events During Observation (CREDO) study (Steinhubl et al., 2002), pretreatment of patients with 300 mg of clopidogrel at least 15 hours before intervention reduced long-term adverse events. In the Intracoronary Stenting and Antithrombotic Regimen Rapid Early Action for Coronary Treatment (ISAR-REACT) trial (Kandzari, 2004), pretreatment with 600 mg of clopidogrel

provided similar outcomes in low- to intermediate-risk patients irrespective of whether they were assigned to abciximab or placebo, with maximum antiplatelet effect seen within 2 to 3 hours of treatment before intervention. In the Antiplatelet therapy for Reduction of MYocardial Damage during Angioplasty (ARMYDA-2) study (Patti et al., 2005), 600 mg of clopidogrel was more effective in reducing cardiac events than 300 mg of clopidogrel when given at a mean time of 6 hours before PCI in both arms. ARMYDA-2 also did not exclude patients from receiving GP IIb/IIIa inhibitors, thereby supporting the hypothesis that optimal ADP receptor antagonism before PCI might be essential even when intraprocedural inhibition of platelet aggregation is achieved with GP IIb/IIIa inhibitors.

Currently, clopidogrel is given to all patients with an ACS with an oral loading dose of 600 mg followed by 75 mg/day. Clopidogrel is generally administered after initiating treatment with aspirin and antithrombin and as part of a conservative management strategy or preceding PCI.

Prasugrel (Effient) is also a thienopyridine and oral ADP receptor antagonist. It is indicated in ACS patients undergoing PCI. It is not indicated in patients with stable angina or those not undergoing PCI. Prasugrel is also absolutely contraindicated in patients with any prior history of stroke or TIA. It is relatively contraindicated in older patients older than the age of 75 years and in patients who weigh less than 60 kg. In the TRITON TIMI-38 study, Prasugrel was shown to be superior to clopidogrel in reducing the primary end point of cardiovascular death, nonfatal MI, or stroke and reducing acute stent thrombosis. However, it did have a higher incidence of major and minor bleeding than clopidogrel, including fatal bleeding. Prasugrel is reserved for patients when their coronary anatomy becomes known in the cardiac catheterization laboratory and it has become clear that they will be undergoing PCI. It can, however, be administered to patients with STEMI in the ED because these patients are predominantly managed by PCI. The loading dose of prasugrel is 60 mg with a maintenance dose of 10 mg/day orally or 5 mg/day orally (for patients weighing less than 60 kg) (Wiviott et al., 2007).

Ticagrelor (Brilinta) is the most recently introduced ADP receptor antagonist. It is indicated in patients with ACS who are treated either medically or who undergo PCI. The loading dose is 180 mg orally followed by a maintenance dose of 90 mg twice daily. Ticagrelor was compared with clopidogrel in the Ticagrelor versus Clopidogrel in Patients with Acute Coronary Syndrome (PLATO) trial (Wallentin et al., 2009). It was shown to be superior to clopidogrel in reducing the composite end point of cardiac death, nonfatal MI, and stroke and in reducing acute stent thrombosis. It increases the risk of non–coronary artery bypass graft major bleeding compared with clopidogrel. The PLATO trial excluded patients with sick sinus syndrome (SSS) or heart block. Ticagrelor inhibits adenosine reuptake and can worsen bradycardia and heart block. Also, it can cause dyspnea that leads to cessation of the drug in 0.9% of patients. Patients receiving ticagrelor should not receive more than 100 mg/day of aspirin because doses that exceed this appear to attenuate the efficacy of ticagrelor. In addition, they should not receive drugs that are potent inhibitors (e.g., ketoconazole, clarithromycin, and some antiviral drugs) or inducers (e.g., rifampin, antiseizure drugs) of the CYP3A system.

In the *chronic* phase, typically after a revascularization procedure, the mainstay of therapy is aspirin indefinitely, clopidogrel (or prasugrel–ticagrelor) for 12 months, statins, ACE inhibitors, and β-blockade. In the Heart Outcomes Prevention Evaluation (HOPE) (Yusuf et al., 2000) trial, ramipril (10 mg/day) was shown to reduce cardiovascular events significantly, including cardiovascular and total mortality and strokes. In HOPE, patients were 55 years or older, and the majority had a history of vascular disease (80% history of CAD and 42% with PAD). Similar results were obtained in the European Trial on Reduction of Cardiac Events with Perindopril in stable CAD (EUROPA) (Fox, 2003). In the EUROPA trial, 13,655 patients were included with previous MI (64%), angiographic evidence of CAD (61%), coronary revascularization (55%), or a positive stress test result only (5%). The mean age was 60 years, and patients had no CHF or stable CAD. In this study, 10% of placebo and 8% of perindopril (8 mg once daily) patients experienced the combined primary end point of cardiovascular death, MI, or cardiac arrest (20% relative risk reduction; $P = 0.0003$ favoring perindopril therapy) at a mean follow-up period of 4.2 years.

Patients also need to quit smoking; exercise; adhere to a low-fat and low-carbohydrate diet; lose weight if obese; enroll in cardiac rehabilitation; and, if they have diabetes, achieve aggressive control of their blood sugar to keep their HbA_{1c} below 7%.

KEY TREATMENT

- Patients with definite ACS should be evaluated for immediate reperfusion therapy based on the presence of high-risk features (SOR: A, ACC/AHA guidelines).

- Whether an invasive or conservative strategy is chosen, aspirin (or clopidogrel if aspirin intolerant) needs to be initiated. In conservatively managed patients, enoxaparin or fondaparinux (first choice) or UFH (second choice) needs to be initiated. In aggressively managed patients, UFH, enoxaparin, or bivalirudin needs to be initiated. Fondaparinux should be avoided in the setting of angioplasty. Clopidogrel is then initiated before angiography in the aggressively managed group and in all patients managed conservatively (SOR: A; ACC/AHA, 2007).

- In patients with UA/NSTEMI, aspirin (81 to 162 mg/day) and clopidogrel 75 mg/day for preferably 1 year should be administered in patients treated conservatively (SOR: A, ACC/AHA guidelines, 2012).

- In patients with UA/NSTEMI receiving bare-metal stents, aspirin 162 to 325 mg/day should be administered for 1 month followed by 81 to 162 mg/day indefinitely and clopidogrel 75 mg/day orally for at least 1 year (SOR: A, ACC/AHA guidelines, 2012).

- In patients with UA/NSTEMI receiving drug-eluting stents, aspirin 162 to mg/day should be administered for 3 to 6 months followed by 81 to 162 mg/day indefinitely and clopidogrel 75 mg/day orally for at least 1 year (SOR: A, ACC/AHA guidelines).

ST ELEVATION MYOCARDIAL INFARCTION

STEMI occurs secondary to a sudden interruption of coronary blood supply (Figure 27-11) to a part of the myocardium as a result of a complete thrombotic occlusion of a coronary artery (DeWood et al., 1980). Plaque rupture is the predominant mechanism of STEMI, with subsequent platelet and fibrin deposition. It is estimated that there are 0.5 million STEMI events in the United States annually.

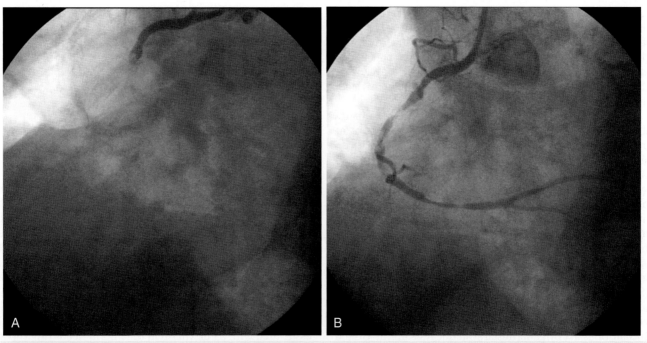

Figure 27-11 Acute inferior myocardial infarction. **A,** Sudden occlusion of the right coronary artery with a filling thrombus at the occlusion site. **B,** The same vessel after initial angioplasty showing multiple filling defects, indicating thrombus.

Emergent and complete revascularization is the most important goal in the acute therapy of STEMI. Current guidelines indicate that a patient with symptoms and signs of STEMI should undergo emergent revascularization with primary angioplasty if possible within 90 minutes of arrival to the ED (door to balloon) (Antman et al., 2004). Currently, angioplasty is considered the first choice of therapy because it leads to overall superior results (Magid et al., 2000), primarily reducing the rate of nonfatal MI, and leading to fewer intracranial bleeds compared with thrombolysis. Stronger evidence exists for primary angioplasty in STEMI because the risk of fibrinolysis increases (Hochman et al., 2001; Kent et al., 2002; Wu et al., 2002). If angioplasty is not available or if transfer to a nearby facility with primary angioplasty is not possible to achieve with first medical contact to revascularization occurring at less than 120 minutes, then fibrinolysis needs to be administered in the absence of contraindications. Even after lytic therapy is administered, it is recommended that patients be transferred to a facility with primary angioplasty capability. This ensures that patients who fail lysis can be treated with rescue angioplasty in a timely manner. The door-in, door-out, or the time from arrival to transfer to a primary PCI facility, should be less than 30 minutes. It is currently acceptable to pursue an early elective angioplasty between 3 and 24 hours of successful lysis (O'Gara et al., 2013).

Patients with cardiogenic shock (Hochman et al., 2001) or severe CHF (Wu et al., 2002) benefit more from primary angioplasty. Irrespective of the delay time for door to balloon, it is recommended that patients with cardiogenic shock be treated immediately or transferred for primary angioplasty. Fibrinolysis is not recommended in cases of cardiogenic shock except in patients unsuitable for angioplasty or bypass surgery.

Primary angioplasty is best done in intermediate- and high-volume centers (Canto et al., 2000) with an experienced catheterization team and interventional cardiologists on call and an approved hospital process that has been agreed upon by various disciplines involved in the care of the patient. This MI "alert system" should be capable of effectively mobilizing all resources available to stay within the 90-minute timeframe to first balloon inflation from arrival to the ED.

Thrombolytic therapy has been shown to reduce mortality rates in patients with STEMI. Thrombolytics are contraindicated in patients with NSTEMI because they have been shown to have no clinical benefit and carry unwarranted risks. Thrombolysis enhances the body's own fibrinolytic system by accelerating the formation of plasmin from plasminogen (Shammas et al., 1993). Plasmin degrades fibrin and several plasma proteins, including fibrinogen, prothrombin, and factors V and VIII, leading to a defective hemostasis. Thrombolytic agents are classified as clot-specific (alteplase [tPA], retavase [recombinant-PA], and tenecteplase [TNK-tPA]) or non–clot specific (streptokinase [SK], urokinase [UK], and anisoylated plasminogen activator complex [APSAC]). Whereas clot-specific thrombolytics activate plasminogen at the site of the clot, non–clot-specific ones act by generalized systemic lysis. In the United States, clot-specific thrombolytics are most commonly used. The different dosages and mode of administration

Table 27-16   Thrombolytics Commonly Used in the Treatment of Acute Myocardial Infarction

Drug	Dose	Cautions
Streptokinase	1.5 million IU IV Give infusion over 60 min	Watch for hypotension, anaphylaxis, severe bleeding, and stroke.
Retavase	10 U IV over 2 min Give second dose of 10 U IV 30 min after first dose if no complications	Watch for intracranial hemorrhage, arrhythmia, and hemorrhage.
Activase	15 mg bolus IV; then 0.75 mg/Kg (maximum, 50 mg) over 30 min; then 0.5 mg/kg (maximum, 35 mg) over 60 min; give with heparin	Watch for intracranial hemorrhage, arrhythmia, severe bleeding, and anaphylaxis.
Tenecteplase	Wt <60 kg: 30 mg IV; maximum, 50 mg Wt 60-69 kg: 35 mg IV; maximum, 50 mg Wt 70-79 kg: 40 mg IV; maximum, 50 mg Wt 80-89 kg: 45 mg IV; maximum, 50 mg Wt >90 kg: 50 mg IV; maximum, 50 mg	Watch for intracranial bleeding, anaphylaxis, and reperfusion arrhythmias.

IV, Intravenous.

Table 27-17   Contraindications to Fibrinolytic Therapy*

Absolute	History of intracranial hemorrhage Known intracranial neoplasm or vascular lesions Active bleeding or known bleeding disorder (exclude menses) Embolic stroke within 3 mo (exception: embolic stroke within 3 hr) Suspected aortic dissection Significant facial or head trauma within 3 mo
Relative	Uncontrolled severe hypertension (>180 mm Hg systolic; >110 mm Hg diastolic) Prolonged CPR (>10 min), recent surgery (<3 wk), or noncompressible vascular puncture Recent internal bleeding or active peptic ulcer disease Pregnancy Currently anticoagulated with high INR For streptokinase: prior exposure to the drug or history of allergic reaction

*American College of Cardiology/American Heart Association guidelines (Antman et al., 2004).
CPR, Cardiopulmonary resuscitation; *INR*, international normalized ratio.

of these thrombolytics are provided in Table 27-16. Contraindications for fibrinolysis are listed in Table 27-17.

Upon arrival to the ED, patients with chest pain should get ECG done within 10 minutes of arrival. If the ECG does not show ST segment elevation, it is advised that the ECG be repeated within 5 to 10 minutes in patients with continued chest pain to rule out the possibility of late appearance STEMI. It should be noted that ST segment depression in the anterior leads with early precordial transition could indicate ST elevation posterior wall MI, particularly if associated with ST elevation in the inferior leads (inferoposterior MI). Right-sided precordial leads can be helpful in patients with acute inferior wall MI to determine right

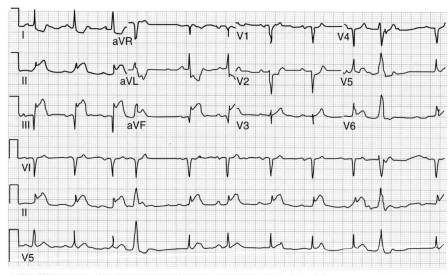

Figure 27-12 Acute inferior myocardial infarction with ST segment elevation in the inferior leads.

Table 27-18 Acute Pharmacologic Therapy of Patients with ST Elevation Myocardial Infarction*

Chewable aspirin 162-325 mg in patients not previously on aspirin

UFH (with or without GP IIb/IIIa inhibitors) or bivalirudin

Clopidogrel (600 mg PO), prasugrel (60 mg PO), or ticagrelor (180 mg PO) load as soon as possible or at time of PCI

Oral β-blockers within 24 hr of STEMI; IV β-blockers should be reserved for patients with severe hypertension or ongoing ischemia.

ACE inhibitor should be administered to patients as soon as possible after STEMI, particularly those with reduced LVEF (<40%) or heart failure and those with anterior MI. If intolerant to ACE inhibitor, ARBs are to be used.

Aldosterone antagonist should be given to patients with STEMI who are already receiving an ACE inhibitor and a β-blocker and have an EF <40% and have either symptomatic heart failure or DM.

High-intensity statin therapy should be administered to patients with STEMI.

Treatment of pericarditis in the setting of STEMI should be high-dose aspirin and if not tolerated, colchicine or a narcotic analgesic. Glucocorticoids and NSAIDs should be avoided.

*Strength of recommendation: A (American College of Cardiology/American Heart Association guidelines, Antman et al., 2004).

ACE, Angiotensin-converting enzyme; *ARB,* angiotensin receptor blocker; *DM,* diabetes mellitus; *EF,* ejection fraction; *GP,* glycoprotein; *IV,* intravenous; *LVEF,* left ventricular ejection fraction; *MI,* myocardial infarction; *NSAID,* nonsteroidal antiinflammatory drug; *PCI,* percutaneous coronary intervention; *PO,* oral; *STEMI,* ST segment elevation myocardial infarction; *UFH,* unfractionated heparin.

ventricular (RV) involvement (ST elevation will be seen in the right precordial leads) (Figure 27-12).

Patients with STEMI should receive supplemental oxygen, morphine sulfate for pain control, IV nitrate therapy if they do not have hypertension and have not ingested a phosphodiesterase inhibitor for erectile dysfunction, 162 mg of chewable aspirin, β-blockade, a statin, an ACE inhibitor (particularly in patients with CHF, reduced LV function, hypertension, or diabetes), and an ADP receptor antagonist (Table 27-18). At present, β-blockers are recommended in the first 24 hours of a STEMI when there are no contraindications to their use. IV β-blockers are reasonable to administer at the time of presentation if the patient is hypertensive or has ongoing ischemia. The general use of IV β-blockers at the time of presentation has not been shown to alter the combined end point of death, MI, and stroke in STEMI patients (Chen et al., 2005).

Hemodynamic instability should be aggressively treated with pressor agents (typically dopamine started at 5 µg/kg/min and titrated every 5 minutes to keep the systolic pressure >90 mm Hg). Normal saline fluid boluses can be helpful, particularly in patients with inferoposterior MI with right-sided involvement. In these patients, bradycardia also needs to be aggressively treated if associated with hypotension with either atropine (1 mg IV, which can be repeated twice), or with a temporary pacemaker if there is inadequate response to atropine. Patients with RV involvement usually respond well to a fluid challenge, correcting the bradycardia, administering dopamine, and maintaining sinus rhythm because they rely on a normal atrial kick for increasing their end-diastolic volume and cardiac output. If hypotension does not respond well to these conservative measures, patients need to have an intraaortic balloon pump inserted. Typically, these patients should be brought emergently to the cardiac catheterization laboratory for more definitive management because their mortality rate is excessively high without immediate revascularization (Hochman et al., 2001).

Induced hypothermia is highly recommended in comatose patients and out-of-hospital cardiac arrest caused by ventricular fibrillation (VF) or pulseless VT, including patients who undergo angioplasty (O'Gara et al., 2013).

The long-term management of these patients is similar to that for those with UA/NSTEMI with aggressive preventive measures and continued long-term aspirin, β-blockers, ACE inhibitor, statins, exercise, and a low-fat diet. Smoking cessation, control of HTN and diabetes, and achieving ideal body weight are of paramount importance to prevent further progression of disease and recurrent MI. Preferably, ADP receptor antagonists need to be continued for 12 months irrespective of whether the patient received a revascularization procedure with drug-eluting stents or bare-metal stents or was conservatively managed.

Valvular Heart Disease

AORTIC STENOSIS

Aortic stenosis is defined as an obstruction that impedes blood flow from the LV to the aorta and is mostly secondary to aortic valvular disease. Other less common causes of AS include supravalvular and membranous subvalvular stenosis, which are generally congenital.

Aortic valvular stenosis is the most common valvular abnormality in the United States. It can be congenital, rheumatic, or calcific or degenerative. Whereas calcific aortic valve stenosis (Figure 27-13) is most prevalent in patients older than 70 years of age, congenital, mostly bicuspid valve disease (Figure 27-14) is more common in younger patients. A bicuspid aortic valve leads to flow turbulence and valve trauma, which in return precipitates fibrosis, stiffness, and calcification. One third of bicuspid valves will become stenotic between the fourth and sixth decades of life and account for half of all surgical cases. In age-related calcific valves, the valve is affected by the same risk factors as atherosclerosis, in which inflammatory cells (macrophages and T lymphocytes), lipid and calcium deposits, and the development of fibrosis are seen. To date, statin therapy has not been shown to reduce rates of progression of aortic valve stenosis or reduce the need for aortic valve replacement. Rheumatic aortic valve stenosis is now uncommon in developed countries and is mediated by adhesion and the fusion of cusps after streptococcal infection.

The aortic valve surface area is normally 3.0 to 4.0 cm². Symptoms typically do not appear unless the valve is narrowed to at least one fourth of its normal surface area. Stenosis is graded as mild (valve area >1.5 cm²), moderate (>1.0-1.5 cm²), or severe (≤1 cm²) (Rahimtoola, 1989). The valve area narrows at an average rate of 0.12 cm² per year (Otto et al., 1997). As the valve narrows, cardiac output remains stable at rest but diminishes with exercise. As disease progresses, LV mass increases, and diastolic dysfunction becomes evident with an increase in LV filling pressure. Myocardial oxygen demand typically increases, and even in the absence of CAD, patients may experience angina. Patients with AS have a good prognosis if they do not have symptoms of angina, CHF, or syncope or near syncope, particularly with activity. Surgical management of the valve becomes necessary in symptomatic patients because the incidence of sudden cardiac death increases in these patients.

Patients with severe aortic valve stenosis describe progressive dyspnea; chest pain and syncope with exertion; and symptoms of HF, including orthopnea, paroxysmal nocturnal dyspnea, and edema. Syncope at rest is typically arrhythmia induced. Patients with severe aortic valve stenosis have an approximate 5% history of sudden cardiac death. In addition, these patients may give a history of rheumatic fever or rheumatic heart disease, TIAs from calcium deposit systemic embolization, and intermittent GI bleeding from an increased incidence of arteriovenous malformations.

The typical physical signs of severe aortic valve stenosis are diminished carotid pulses (delayed and weak); a sustained apical impulse; a single second heart sound; an S4 gallop; and a midsystolic crescendo–decrescendo murmur with late peaking best heard at the base of the heart, although in elderly patients, it might be heard only at the

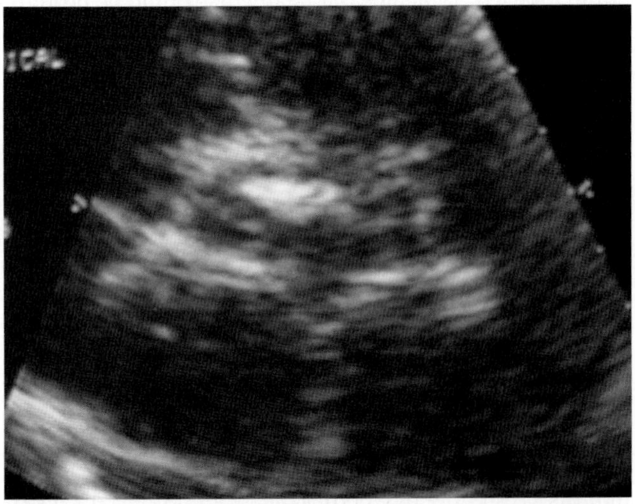

Figure 27-13 Aortic valve stenosis with calcification as seen with two-dimensional Doppler echocardiography.

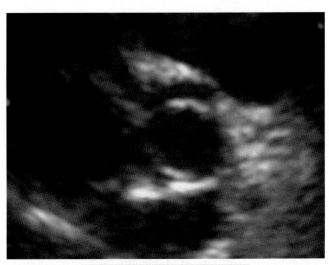

Figure 27-14 Bicuspid aortic valve.

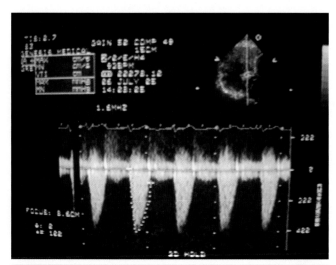

Figure 27-15 Velocity gradient across a calcified stenotic aortic valve, as seen with Doppler echocardiography.

apex. Aortic valve stenosis can be distinguished clinically from dynamic left ventricular outflow tract (LVOT) obstruction such as in hypertrophic obstructive cardiomyopathy (HOCM) by certain clinical maneuvers at the bedside. An HOCM murmur tends to increase during the strain phase of the Valsalva maneuver and during standing up from a squatting position. In both maneuvers, the preload of the LV is reduced, leading to a smaller cavity size and an increase in the LVOT obstruction.

Diagnostic tests include chest radiography, which could show a calcified valve, pulmonary venous congestion, or an increase in ascending aortic root size secondary to poststenotic dilation. Also, a 12-lead ECG may show LVH and conduction abnormalities. An echocardiogram typically confirms the diagnosis. Valve structure can be assessed, including the presence of calcification, reduction in cusp motion, and congenital abnormalities such as a bicuspid or abnormal tricuspid valve. A gradient can be measured across the valve (Figure 27-15), and the valve area can be determined using Doppler flow with reasonable accuracy (Currie et al., 1986). The presence of concomitant aortic valve insufficiency can also be visualized using color Doppler flow characteristics. Other important findings on echocardiography include the presence or absence of LVH and assessment of LV compliance, atrial size, and associated other valvular abnormalities. If noninvasive findings support the diagnosis of severe AS and the patient is symptomatic, then diagnostic angiography is indicated to confirm the presence of severe aortic valve stenosis and assess the coronary arteries. Also, it is important to recognize low-gradient severe aortic valve stenosis (<1 cm²) in patients with EFs less than 40%. In these patients, it is unclear whether the severity of the aortic valve stenosis is overestimated because of a low cardiac output state or if it is true severe AS. Obtaining baseline hemodynamics with echocardiography and then repeating them with dobutamine stress will help in distinguishing true severe AS from pseudo AS. If the gradient across the aortic valve increases and the valve area worsens, this indicates that the stenosis of the aortic valve is truly severe. Stress testing is contraindicated in the setting of symptomatic, severe aortic valve stenosis.

The treatment of aortic valve stenosis depends on the presence or absence of symptoms. Symptomatic severe aortic valve stenosis carries a poor prognosis, with an average life expectancy of 2 to 3 years (Ross and Braunwald, 1968). The 5- and 10-year mortality rates are approximately 52% to 80% and 80% to 90%, respectively (Horstkotte and Loogen, 1988; Turina et al., 1987). Aortic valve surgery with or without coronary artery bypass grafting is the treatment of choice (Lund, 1990; Schwarz et al., 1982). Aortic valvuloplasty carries a poor outcome and is reserved as a palliative therapy for inoperable patients. Typically, the improvement in the aortic valve gradient is mild with valvuloplasty, and a recurrence of severe stenosis can be expected within 6 months (Block and Palacios, 1988; Davidson et al., 1990). Surgery is typically not advised for patients with asymptomatic severe valvular stenosis. Patients with dyspnea and progressive LV dysfunction need to be considered for valve replacement. Most patients with asymptomatic, severe aortic valve stenosis will, however, develop symptoms within 5 years of follow-up. The 1-, 2-, and 5-year event-free probabilities were 80%, 63%, and 25%, respectively. Independent predictors of all-cause mortality include age, chronic renal failure, inactivity, and aortic valve velocity (Pellikka et al., 2005). A low threshold to intervene in patients with asymptomatic severe AS may be considered, particularly when peak systolic velocity (PSV) is 4.5 m/sec or greater on Doppler echocardiography (Pellikka et al., 2005; Rosenheck, 2000) if associated with moderate or severe valvular calcification (Rosenheck, 2000). Predictors of survival in asymptomatic AS include a PSV across the valve of more than 4 m/sec, the rate of change of the PSV over time, and functional class (Otto et al., 1997). It is currently recommended that patients with severe AS undergo aortic valve replacement if they have symptoms (chest pain, syncope, or HF), if EF is less than 50%, or in conjunction with another valve surgery or bypass surgery (even if the aortic valve is moderate in severity). Furthermore, European guidelines currently favor aortic valve replacement in patients with severe AS with a valve area less than 0.6 cm² (irrespective of symptoms), rapidly progressing valve area severity, or an abnormal response to exercise testing (Vahanian et al., 2012).

Patients need to be advised about antibiotic prophylaxis to prevent endocarditis, especially with rheumatic valve disease (Dajani et al., 1997) (Table 27-19). Patients with moderate to severe aortic valve stenosis need to avoid moderate to severe physical exertion (Cheitlin et al., 1994). Arrhythmias need to be corrected promptly in patients with severe AS. Follow-up echocardiography is indicated every year in patients with asymptomatic severe AS and every other year in those with moderate stenosis (Bonow et al., 1998).

Aortic valve replacement can be performed with a mechanical valve or a tissue valve. Mechanical valves are more durable than bioprosthetic valves but require lifetime anticoagulation. The choice of the valve depends on the patient clinical situation but takes into consideration the patient's age, need for future pregnancies, ability to take anticoagulants, compliance, and preference. For instance, patients who have a contraindication to anticoagulation with warfarin should receive a bioprosthetic valve. These valves typically do not require anticoagulation with

Table 27-19 Prophylaxis for Bacterial Endocarditis*

Drug	Adult Dose	Pediatric Dose*	Time before Procedure
GENERAL PROPHYLAXIS			
Amoxicillin	2 g	50 mg/kg PO	1 hr
	2 g IV or IM	50 mg/kg IM or IV	30 min
PENICILLIN-ALLERGIC PATIENTS			
Clindamycin	600 mg	20 mg/kg PO	1 hr
Clarithromycin	500 mg	15 mg/kg PO	1 hr
Azithromycin	500 mg	15 mg/kg PO	1 hr
Clindamycin	600 mg	20 mg/kg IV	30 min
Cefazolin	1 g	25 mg/kg IM or IV	30 min

*Pediatric dose should not exceed adult dose.
IM, intramuscular; *IV*, intravenous; *PO*, oral.
From Dajani AS, Taubert KA, Wilson W, et al. Prevention of bacterial endocarditis: recommendations by the American Heart Association. *Circulation.* 1997;96:358-366.

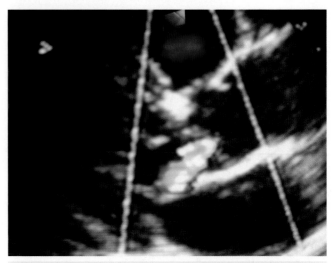

Figure 27-16 Aortic valve regurgitation, as seen with color Doppler echocardiography. Note the blue turbulent jet into the left ventricle in diastole.

warfarin, and patients are generally put only on an aspirin subsequent to the procedure. Younger patients and those with no contraindication to Coumadin are best served with mechanical valves because they are more durable and hopefully will obviate the need for another valve surgery in the future. Very elderly patients (in their 80s) are typically given a tissue valve to obviate the need for anticoagulation. Antibiotic prophylaxis to prevent endocarditis is strongly recommended in patients with prosthetic valves.

Transcatheter aortic valve replacement (TAVR) using a stent valve has recently emerged as a less invasive procedure to replace severe aortic valve stenosis in patients who are deemed inoperable or are at high risk for conventional aortic valve surgery. In the Placement of Transcatheter Aortic Valve (PARTNER) trial (cohort B), patients with severe symptomatic aortic valve stenosis and an estimated high likelihood of death with conventional aortic valve surgery (>50%) were randomized to receive the Edwards SAPIEN valve versus standard therapy (Leon et al., 2010). At 1 year, the rate of death from any cause was 30.7% with the SAPIEN valve versus 50.7% with conservative treatment (*P* <0.001). Also, the rate of the composite end point of death from any cause or repeat hospitalization was 42.5% with TAVR versus 71.6% with conservative treatment (*P* <0.001). In cohort A of the PARTNER trial, patients with high operative surgical risk (>15% mortality rate) were randomized to open aortic valve surgery versus TAVR (Smith et al., 2011). No difference in mortality was seen with both modalities, but there was more bleeding and atrial fibrillation (AF) with surgery and more vascular complications with TAVR. TAVR is approved at this time for both inoperable and high-risk patients for open aortic valve replacement.

KEY TREATMENT

- Aortic valve replacement is indicated in symptomatic patients with severe AS (SOR: A, ACC/AHA 2008 guidelines).
- Aortic valve replacement is indicated in patients with severe AS and LV dysfunction (SOR: A, ACC/AHA 2008 guidelines).

AORTIC VALVE REGURGITATION

Key Points

- Echocardiography is indicated to confirm the presence and severity of aortic insufficiency (SOR: A, ACC/AHA 2008 guidelines).
- Periodic echocardiography is recommended to evaluate LV function and cavity size in patients with asymptomatic severe aortic insufficiency (SOR: A, ACC/AHA 2008 guidelines).
- Coronary angiography is indicated before valve surgery in patients with severe aortic insufficiency if there is suspicion of CAD (SOR: A, ACC/AHA 2008 guidelines).

Aortic valve regurgitation (AR) is defined as blood flow from the aorta to the LV in diastole because of an incompetent aortic valve (Figure 27-16). Aortic valve insufficiency is generally acquired because of valve infection, dilation and dissection of the aortic root, trauma, or long-term degenerative change of the valve, particularly in the setting of HTN. Patients with a history of prosthetic valves (Figure 27-17) can also have aortic valve insufficiency. Aortic insufficiency can also be caused by a congenital bicuspid aortic valve.

Aortic valve regurgitation leads to volume overload of the LV and an increase in LV end-diastolic pressure. In chronic AR, symptoms might not appear before LV cavity dilation, and a reduction in LV function develops. Patients will have a long diastolic murmur, a wide pulse pressure, and bounding pulses. In acute AR, a sudden rise of LV end-diastolic pressure occurs because of the inability of the LV to acutely dilate in response to a sudden volume overload. Patients are generally acutely symptomatic with HF. Patients have a short diastolic murmur and a soft S1 with tachycardia.

Patients with severe AR will eventually become symptomatic, displaying symptoms of dyspnea and CHF. Angina is less common, but it can occur as a result of reduction in

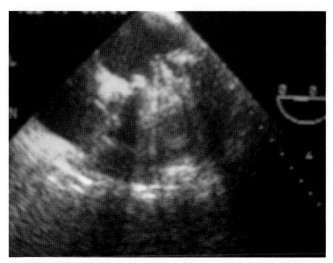

Figure 27-17 Mechanical prosthetic valve. Note the acoustic shadowing generated by the mechanical prosthesis.

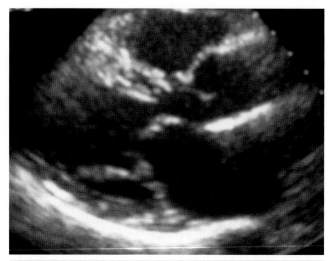

Figure 27-18 Rheumatic mitral valve stenosis. Note the doming of the stenotic mitral valve with thickening of the anterior leaflet.

coronary perfusion pressure. Physical signs of severe AR include a rapid and quick arterial pulse (Corrigan pulse); a wide pulse pressure; an early high-pitched, blowing diastolic murmur heard best over the left sternal border; an S3 gallop; and a low-pitched diastolic murmur at the apex (Austin-Flint murmur).

The ECG shows LVH and possibly conduction abnormalities. Echocardiography can help make the diagnosis accurately and provides information about LV function and cavity size. Other associated valvular abnormalities can also be assessed by the echocardiogram. Aortic root size and left atrial size can also be measured (Zoghbi et al., 2003). Echocardiographic findings of severe AR include a color jet width of more than 60%, vena contracta of more than 6 mm, half-time AI of less than 200 msec, regurgitant volume of more than 60 mL, and an effective regurgitant orifice of greater than 30 mm². Stress testing can provide information about functional capacity and hemodynamic response to exercise. Diagnostic angiography allows the verification of the severity of the AR and helps in the assessment of the aortic root size, cavity size, and the presence or absence of CAD.

The surgical treatment of AR is indicated in symptomatic patients with dyspnea, angina, or CHF (Bonow, 2000). Asymptomatic patients should undergo surgery if the LVEF is 50% or less, LV end-systolic dimension approaches 5.5 cm, or there is an LV end-diastolic dimension of more than 75 mm. Patients also should be advised on prophylaxis against infective endocarditis (Dajani et al., 1997) (see Table 27-19). Patients with moderate to severe AR should avoid competitive sports, heavy workloads, and weight lifting. Patients with severe AR do not benefit from chronic long-acting vasodilators such as nifedipine XL or enalapril (Evangelista et al., 2005). After valve replacement for AR, the use of β-blockers may improve cardiac performance (Matsuyama et al., 2000).

Patients with AR may have a dilated ascending aortic root. Patients with bicuspid aortic valve and (1) ascending aortic root size of larger than 5 cm or (2) increasing aortic root size of more than 0.5 cm per year need to be considered for ascending aortic root repair. Also, if patients with bicuspid aortic valve need to undergo aortic valve repair for severe AS or AR, an ascending root of larger than 4.5 cm should be corrected at the same time (Bonow et al., 2008).

KEY TREATMENT

- Vasodilator therapy is indicated in patients with symptomatic severe aortic insufficiency when surgery is not an option (SOR: A, ACC/AHA 2008 guidelines).
- Aortic valve replacement is recommended for severe symptomatic aortic valve insufficiency irrespective of LV function (SOR: A, ACC/AHA 2008 guidelines).
- Aortic valve replacement is recommended in asymptomatic patients with chronic severe aortic insufficiency and LV systolic dysfunction and in patients undergoing bypass surgery or aortic surgery (SOR: A, ACC/AHA 2008 guidelines).

MITRAL STENOSIS

Key Points

- Echocardiography should be performed in patients with mitral stenosis (MS) to assess hemodynamic severity, concomitant valvular lesion, and assessment of valvular morphology (SOR: A, ACC/AHA 2008 guidelines).
- Echocardiography should be performed in patients with MS and prior embolic event (SOR: A, ACC/AHA 2008 guidelines).

Mitral stenosis is defined as the reduced ability of blood to move from the left atrium to the LV in diastole. It is mostly caused by dysfunction in the mitral valve, which lacks the ability to open its leaflets in diastole. MS (Figure 27-18) is predominantly caused by rheumatic carditis and is more prevalent in females (Bonow et al., 1998). Acute rheumatic carditis leads to valvular disease in approximately 50% of affected patients. The mitral valve is the most commonly affected by rheumatic heart disease, followed by the aortic valve, and then combined aortic and mitral valves. MS is considered severe if the valve area is less than 1 cm^2 (normal mitral valve area is 4 to 6 cm^2). A valve area of 1.5 cm^2 or smaller associated with severe dyspnea (class III or IV New York Heart Association [NYHA] class C) or severe pulmonary HTN (pulmonary pressure of >50 mm Hg at rest and ≥60 mm Hg with exercise) is also considered clinically significant and warrants therapy.

The main symptom of MS is slowly progressive dyspnea and fatigue. In advanced MS, left atrial pressure and a redistribution of blood to the chest occurs. Patients might complain of orthopnea and paroxysmal nocturnal dyspnea. Pulmonary HTN can become severe, and right-sided ventricular failure can then lead to dependent edema, hepatomegaly, and right upper quadrant pain. An increase in left atrial size can lead to palpitations secondary to AF as well as subsequent cardioembolic strokes if not recognized in a timely fashion.

Most auscultatory signs of MS are missed if not performed in the left lateral decubitus position. Typically, the first heart sound, S1, is accentuated. A low-pitched diastolic rumble, heard with the bell of the stethoscope over the apex, is also present. The high-pitched *opening snap* (OS), caused by the abrupt stopping of the domed mitral valve into the LV, is also appreciated in most patients midway between the left sternal border and apex. A shorter A2–OS distance indicates a more severe MS. Signs of pulmonary HTN such as a loud P2 and right ventricular hypertrophy (RVH) can also be present as MS becomes more severe.

The ECG findings in MS might show a biphasic P wave in V1, a large P wave in lead II, and possibly AF. Chest radiography could show evidence of an enlarged left atrium and an increase in pulmonary congestion with interstitial edema. An echocardiogram can accurately diagnose MS and assess valvular and subvalvular structure and valve area (Rahimtoola et al., 2002). In addition, an echocardiogram can help distinguish the cause of MS, whether it is valvular or from different causes such as tumors, vegetations, extreme calcification of the annulus, left atrial myxoma, cor triatriatum, or presence of a large thrombus. An echocardiogram can also help estimate pulmonary pressures and assess for right-sided enlargement. Typically, LV function is preserved in MS. In addition, echocardiography can help in calculating a mitral valve score that takes into account leaflet mobility, thickening, valve calcification, and distortion of the subvalvular apparatus. The interventional cardiologist typically uses the valve score to determine the feasibility of balloon valvuloplasty. A score of less than 8 generally indicates a good prognosis from mitral valvuloplasty. Furthermore, because a transthoracic echocardiogram is not well suited to see the left atrial appendage, a transesophageal echocardiogram becomes necessary to rule out the presence of an atrial thrombus before valvuloplasty because this can be a significant risk factor for an embolic stroke. Finally, a left and right heart catheterization remains the best modality to assess mitral valve severity and full hemodynamics and determine coronary anatomy before contemplated corrective surgery.

Treatment of Mitral Stenosis

All patients with rheumatic mitral valve disease require bacterial endocarditis prophylaxis before dental, genitourinary,

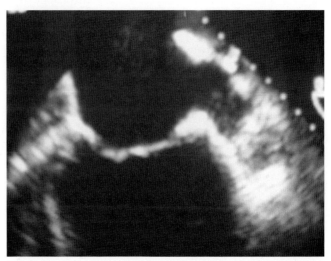

Figure 27-19 Left atrial appendage thrombus seen on transesophageal echocardiography.

or GI procedures. Increasing diastolic filling time is important in the treatment of moderate to severe MS. Therefore, drugs such as β-blockers or verapamil might be used. Maintaining sinus rhythm can also reduce symptoms as loss of atrial contraction reduces ventricular emptying. Patients with AF need to be aggressively treated with rate control and anticoagulation with warfarin to reduce embolic strokes. Chemoversion (with amiodarone or other antiarrhythmics) or cardioversion can be performed after the patient has been anticoagulated for at least 3 or 4 weeks before the procedure. Anticoagulation should be maintained after the procedure for a minimum of 1 month. Generally, anticoagulation is maintained long term because the recurrence of AF can be unpredictable. Transesophageal echocardiography can be performed before cardioversion to rule out the presence of a left atrial thrombus (Figure 27-19). Even when a thrombus is excluded, patients need to be heparinized for at least 48 to 72 hours before cardioversion then maintained on warfarin afterwards. The target international normalized ratio (INR) in patients with AF needs to be 2.0 to 3.0.

Patients with moderate to severe symptoms (NYHA class II to IV) or asymptomatic patients with severe MS (valve area <1.5 cm^2) and pulmonary HTN (pulmonary pressure >50 mm Hg at rest and ≥60 mm Hg with exercise) require percutaneous valvuloplasty, mitral valve repair, or mitral valve replacement.

Balloon valvuloplasty leads to commissural separation as the main mechanism that leads to an improvement in valvular function. Mitral valvuloplasty is currently the preferred method of treating severe MS when no contraindications exist (Table 27-20). The procedure carries an exceedingly low risk of death, with an acute success rate greater than 95% and very good long-term results similar to results for surgical commissurotomy (Rahimtoola et al., 2002). Patients who are qualified for valvuloplasty (favorable valve score) can undergo valve repair if balloon valvuloplasty is not available or left atrial thrombus persists despite anticoagulation. Mitral valve surgery is reserved for those patients with a calcified valve and a high valve score

Table 27-20 Common Contraindications for Mitral Balloon Valvuloplasty

Presence of left atrial thrombus seen on transesophageal echocardiography
Associated severe mitral regurgitation
Associated coronary artery disease that requires bypass surgery
A high valve score as determined by echocardiography (unfavorable valve morphology)
Associated other valvular pathology or aortic pathology that will require surgical interventions
Difficulty in obtaining access

on echocardiography who are essentially excluded from balloon valvuloplasty.

KEY TREATMENT

- Percutaneous mitral balloon valvotomy is effective for symptomatic patients with moderate to severe MS and favorable valve morphology when no left atrial thrombus or moderate to severe MR is present (SOR: A, ACC/AHA 2008 guidelines).
- Mitral valve surgery is indicated in patients with moderate to severe MS when mitral balloon valvotomy is not available or not feasible or in patients with concomitant moderate to severe mitral insufficiency (SOR: A, ACC/AHA 2008 guidelines).

MITRAL REGURGITATION

Key Points

- Echocardiography is indicated in symptomatic patients with suspected MR (SOR: A, ACC/AHA 2008 guidelines).
- Echocardiography is indicated annually or semiannually in asymptomatic patients with severe mitral insufficiency to assess LV cavity size and EF (SOR: A, ACC/AHA 2008 guidelines).
- Transesophageal echocardiography is indicated to evaluate the mitral valve apparatus before surgery to determine the feasibility of repair or replacement (SOR: A, ACC/AHA 2008 guidelines).
- In patients with suspected CAD and severe MR, coronary angiography is indicated before surgery (SOR: A, ACC/AHA 2008 guidelines).

Mitral regurgitation is defined as an abnormal blood flow into the left atrium in systole as a result of an abnormal closing of the mitral valve. In chronic mitral insufficiency, the LVEF and cavity size may remain preserved for several years. However, LV remodeling eventually occurs, cavity size begins to dilate, EF becomes reduced, and patients enter a decompensated state. In acute MR, the left atrium and LV have no chance for gradual dilation and, therefore, a sudden rise in LV and pulmonary venous pressure occurs, leading to pulmonary edema.

Chronic MR is generally asymptomatic or associated with minimal symptoms of dyspnea or generalized fatigue. When

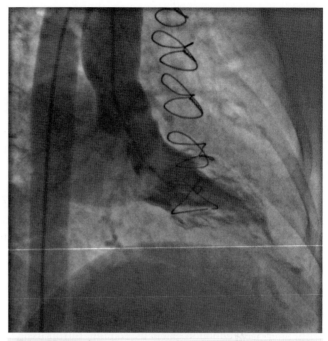

Figure 27-20 Left ventriculogram in the right anterior oblique projection showing severe mitral insufficiency.

LV function declines severely, patients can become symptomatic, with symptoms and signs of HF. Patients might provide a history of rheumatic fever, endocarditis, CAD, or CHF. Acute MR needs to be in the differential diagnosis of a patient with a sudden onset of pulmonary edema.

On examination, patients display a systolic murmur, most often holosystolic, high pitched, and present at the apex with radiation to the axilla, left scapula, midback, or left sternal border, depending on the direction of the regurgitant jet. A midsystolic click is often heard if associated mitral valve prolapse (MVP) is seen. Occasionally, a low-pitched diastolic rumble and an S3 sound can be heard.

The ECG often displays an enlarged left atrium (biphasic P wave in V1), large QRS complex secondary to LV enlargement, and possible AF, and, in ischemic MR, evidence of old or acute inferior infarcts can be seen. The chest radiograph may show an enlarged cardiac silhouette, a calcified mitral valve, or increased pulmonary vascular congestion. Echocardiography provides the diagnosis by assessing the presence of the MR; its severity; and its cause, such as severe prolapse, endocarditis, calcification, papillary muscle or chordae rupture, or a degenerative valve. Regurgitant volume (30-59 mL is moderate; ≥60 mL is severe) and effective regurgitant orifice (20-39 mm^2 is moderate; ≥40 mm^2 is severe) can be calculated. Left and right heart catheterization is indicated before corrective surgery to determine the presence of CAD and confirm the diagnosis of MR with the use of left ventriculography. MR is graded based on the amount of contrast seen in the left atrium in systole: grade I, contrast does not opacify entire left atrium; grade II, contrast opacifies all left atrium but less dense than the contrast in the LV; grade III, contrast equally opacifies left atrium and LV; grade IV, contrast in the left atrium is darker than the LV with opacification of pulmonary veins (Figure 27-20). Also, the angiogram can quantitatively determine the regurgitant fraction (RF). RF greater than 50% generally indicates severe MR that requires corrective surgery.

Treatment of Mitral Regurgitation

Patients with a history of mitral insufficiency need to have bacterial endocarditis prophylaxis. Those with chronic MR benefit from long-term afterload reduction, although this remains controversial. Aggressive treatment of AF with rate control and warfarin anticoagulation is needed. Patients with moderate to severe MR need to be closely monitored for EF and LV cavity size. A lower threshold for surgical intervention is generally agreed upon when compared with AR. Symptomatic patients (NYHA class II-IV) or asymptomatic patients with a LV end-systolic dimension approaching 4.0 cm or LVEF of 60% or less should undergo intervention. Patients with lower EF and a bigger cavity size carry a poorer outcome after surgery. However, those with an EF of 30% to 50% and a LV cavity size in systole between 50 mm and 55 mm may also benefit from surgery. Asymptomatic patients with preserved LV function and cavity size but with AF might benefit from surgery.

Patients with acute MR should be treated aggressively with afterload reduction such as sodium nitroprusside. These patients generally require immediate surgery but do best if they can be initially treated medically and enter a compensated state before surgery. Most regurgitant mitral valves can now be repaired instead of replaced. Techniques for percutaneous repair of the mitral valve are now being tested and hold significant promise.

MITRAL VALVE PROLAPSE

Mitral valve prolapse is described as bulging of one or more of the mitral leaflets into the left atrium in systole (see Figure 27-20). Although it is a common cause of significant MR (Cheng and Barlow, 1989), it can be isolated without valvular insufficiency. MVP carries a benign course (Freed et al., 2002). In rare occasions, it can be associated with significant arrhythmias and sudden cardiac death. When associated with MR, patients need to be carefully monitored for progressive left atrial and LV cavity dilation and AF.

Primary MVP might be familial and is inherited as an autosomal dominant trait with different rate of penetrance and commonly found in patients with connective tissue disease, cardiomyopathies, and Marfan syndrome (Pyeritz and Wappel, 1983). Secondary MVP is generally seen in patients with CAD and rheumatic heart disease.

Patients with MVP are often asymptomatic. However, some patients describe palpitations, chest pain, dyspnea, and fatigue with or without MR. Although previously thought that strokes occur more frequently in patients with MVP, recent data do not support this conclusion (Gilon et al., 1999). Panic attacks have been frequently described. A high-pitched midsystolic click is often heard that occurs shortly after the first heart sound and can be associated with a systolic murmur. Baseline ECG is quite often unrevealing, and routine stress testing carries a high false-positive rate. Stress imaging is more accurate in evaluating these patients for myocardial ischemia. An echocardiogram is the most helpful methodology for making the diagnosis of MVP. A displacement of the leaflets beyond the mitral

annulus on a parasternal short-axis view is strongly suggestive of MVP. Cardiac catheterization is generally not needed for diagnostic purposes.

Asymptomatic patients with MVP generally do not require treatment unless they have severe associated MR (Devereux et al., 1989). Symptomatic patients with MVP can be treated with β-blockers. Flail mitral leaflets caused by chordae rupture or severe MR associated with MVP needs to be followed, and mitral valve repair becomes indicated if patients develop symptoms of dyspnea (NYHA class III or IV), the EF and cavity size become adversely affected, or AF appears.

TRICUSPID VALVE DISEASE

Tricuspid regurgitation (TR) is commonly present on echocardiography in the majority of patients and therefore, when mild, is considered a normal variant. Severe TR can occur, however, and can create significant symptoms of right-sided CHF (cor pulmonale) and dyspnea. Isolated TR is commonly seen in drug addicts secondary to tricuspid valve endocarditis but can also be caused by carcinoid syndrome, trauma, RV infarction, and certain congenital anomalies. The most common etiology of TR is, however, annular dilation caused by RV cavity dilation.

Patients with TR present with various symptoms depending on the etiology of the valvular abnormalities. Typically, dyspnea, right- and left-sided failure, and in the case of endocarditis, fever and night sweats can be present. The RV is generally dilated, and a precordial lift is present. The jugular veins are pulsatile and increased. A systolic murmur is generally heard along the left sternal border that increases with respiration.

Patients with severe TR are treated with diuretics and digitalis to treat the associated right-sided failure. ACE inhibitors are indicated if LV dysfunction is present. It is recommended that tricuspid valve replacement or repair be performed if severe TR is present and the patient is undergoing simultaneous mitral valve surgery or if severe TR is present as a primary disorder in a symptomatic patient.

Tricuspid valve stenosis (TS) is mostly caused by rheumatic heart disease and is typically associated with other valvular involvement. TS can also be caused by the carcinoid syndrome (most commonly causes TR) and certain connective tissue diseases. Secondary causes of TS such as tumors or thrombi can also precipitate secondary TS.

In TS, patients can be dyspneic with activity. Typically, there is an increase in the jugular vein, with a large a wave indicating atrial contraction against a stiff tricuspid valve. TS is typically treated with percutaneous valvular commissurotomy unless it is unfeasible. Open commissurotomy is then performed, or valve replacement is then performed if the leaflets and subvalvular structures are not repairable. Bioprosthetic valves are typically used, and patients are generally prescribed warfarin after tricuspid valve replacement.

PULMONIC VALVE DISEASE

Pulmonary valve regurgitation (PR) is typically acquired because of increased pulmonic pressures (pulmonary HTN). Primary valve abnormalities caused by endocarditis can also cause PR. PR due to pulmonary HTN causes a diastolic murmur along the left sternal border (Graham Steel murmur). Surgery on acquired PR is rarely performed.

Pulmonic valve stenosis (PS) is mostly congenital, but secondary causes such as tumors, endocarditis, or carcinoid can also cause PS. PS is best treated with percutaneous valvuloplasty with good long-term results.

ENDOCARDITIS

Endocarditis is defined as an oscillating intracardiac mass without alternate anatomic classification, the presence of an abscess, or dehiscence of a new prosthetic valve (Durack et al., 1994). Endocarditis is treated with a prolonged course of IV antibiotics. Surgical management can be considered in patients who develop HF or LV dysfunction, damage to the valve annulus with an abscess or perforation of the leaflet, or isolating a resistant organism to antibiotics after 1 week of treatment. Large vegetations, particularly those that are increasing in size and recurrent emboli, are to be considered as indications for valve surgery. Prophylaxis for endocarditis is now limited to patients with prosthetic valves or rings, a history of prior endocarditis, congenital heart disease, or transplant with valvular heart disease.

PROSTHETIC VALVES

Echocardiography (transthoracic, transesophageal, or both) is indicated to evaluate stenotic or regurgitant prosthetic valves. Prosthetic valves are associated with several complications, including infective endocarditis, a paravalvular leak, thrombosis and embolization, pannus formation, and hemolytic anemia.

Prosthetic valve thrombosis requires surgery if it is a left-sided valve and is associated with advanced HF (class III and IV NYHA) and there is large clot burden. Lytic treatment for these valves is not recommended because of the associated high stroke risk. On the other hand, lysis can be considered for right-sided valve thrombosis when a large thrombus burden or advanced HF is present (Bonow et al., 2008).

Heart Failure

Heart failure is a clinical syndrome resulting from the inability of the heart to meet the metabolic requirements of the body at normal filling pressures. Although HF can be precipitated by LV systolic dysfunction, it can also be secondary to diastolic dysfunction. HF with preserved EF (HFpEF) is nearly equally common to HF with reduced EF (HFrEF). HFpEF is characterized with EF more than 45% to 50% and impaired LV filling or relaxation. HFrEF is characterized with EF less than 45% to 50% with reduced LV contraction. Fluid retention and pulmonary congestion are hallmarks of HF but are not universally present. In fact, patients may describe dyspnea and a reduction in exercise capacity with no fluid overload. Because pulmonary congestion may be absent in HF patients, the term *heart failure* is preferred over *congestive heart failure*.

Heart failure is highly prevalent in the United States. More than 650,000 new cases are diagnosed annually. Also, the mortality rate remains very high, with more than

300,000 people dying every year from this syndrome (Hunt et al., 2001). The mortality rate from HF remains at about 50% within 5 years of diagnosis. Hospitalization for HF in the United States is rising in both men and women at a prohibitively high cost to the health care system (O'Connell and Bristow, 1993). One-month rehospitalization after discharge has remained at about 25%. HF costs have reached $39.2 billion in 2010 (Roger et al., 2012). It is important for family physicians to understand the pathophysiology of HF and apply known effective therapies.

PATHOPHYSIOLOGY OF HEART FAILURE

The hemodynamic model of HF has been largely abandoned and replaced by the concept of LV remodeling (Francis, 1998; Francis, 2001). Remodeling of the LV indicates stretching and dilation with subsequent reduction in LV function. The remodeling process can be triggered by a multitude of potential injuries (Kannel et al., 1994; Levy et al., 1996), including CAD, MI, HTN, valvular heart disease, diabetes, congenital heart defects, anemia, and alcoholism. Remodeling is a reversible process with appropriate therapy.

Irrespective of the precipitating injury, neurohormonal mechanisms are activated and promote the remodeling process. These include the renin–angiotensin–aldosterone (RAAS) system and the sympathetic nervous system (SNS). A rise in endothelin-1 production, a product of dysfunctional endothelium, also occurs and contributes to vasoconstriction. In addition, inflammatory markers and cytokines are increased, thereby further exacerbating endothelial dysfunction (Blum and Miller, 2001; Francis, 1998). At the cellular level, MMPs and tissue inhibitors of MMP are increased, leading to cardiac fibrosis and collagen deposition. Also, alterations in calcium fluxes, β-adrenergic receptors, and cardiac metabolism with dependence on glycolysis instead of oxidation of FFAs occur (Braunwald et al., 1976).

Pharmacologic interventions that block neurohormonal activation can reduce mortality and morbidity in patients with HF (Figure 27-21). A rise in angiotensin II (AII) promotes cardiac myocyte programmed cell death (apoptosis), hypertrophy, and ventricular fibrosis. AII also causes an increase in aldosterone secretion (Figure 27-22), which in return augments the harmful effects of AII on the myocardium and promotes adverse remodeling. Aldosterone, however, "escapes" angiotensin suppression (McKelvie et al., 1999); therefore, selective aldosterone blockade is needed in addition to therapy with ACE inhibitors or ARBs (Pitt et al., 1999, 2001). A rise in circulating levels of catecholamines in response to SNS activation can lead to the suppression of adrenergic receptors (Bristow, 1993) and has direct toxic effects (Mann et al., 1992) on the myocardium. Catecholamines mediate toxicity as a result of β-adrenoceptor–mediated cyclic adenosine monophosphate-dependent calcium overload of cardiac myocytes (Mann, 1998). Also, catecholamines increase myocardial oxygen consumption and coronary blood flow requirements and decrease myocardial mechanical efficiency (Nikolaidis et al., 2004). Catecholamines also induce LVH and can precipitate potentially debilitating and fatal arrhythmias.

Inappropriate high cardiac output (>4 L/min/m^2) can precipitate HF. Causes include hyperthyroidism, Paget

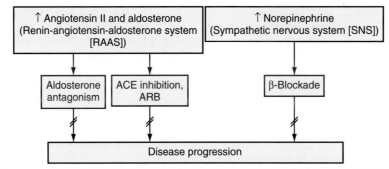

Figure 27-21 The renin–angiotensin–aldosterone system and the sympathetic nervous system are currently the target for treating patients with congestive heart failure. *ACE,* Angiotensin-converting enzyme; *ARB,* angiotensin receptor blocker.

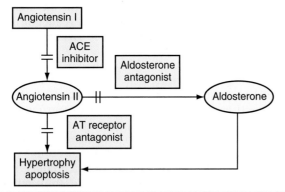

Figure 27-22 Various pharmacologic interventions to block the renin–angiotensin–aldosterone system; *ACE,* Angiotensin-converting enzyme; *AT,* angiotensin.

disease, thiamine deficiency (beriberi), anemia, multiple myeloma, and arteriovenous malformations.

ACC/AHA CLASSIFICATION OF CONGESTIVE HEART FAILURE

A relatively new classification for HF was proposed by the ACC/AHA (Hunt et al., 2001), which takes into account the risk factors for developing HF in addition to the presence of LV dysfunction and symptoms. This classification complements the NYHA classification and takes into account recent advances in pharmacologic and nonpharmacologic approaches to evaluate and treat the HF patient (Ahmed, 2003). Four stages have been proposed:

Stage A describes patients who are at risk of HF but are asymptomatic and have no LV dysfunction. More than 60 million people fall into this category and include those with IHD, HTN, DM, and a family history of cardiomyopathy. Stage A is an additional classification that was not present in the prior NYHA class.
Stage B describes patients with LV dysfunction but who are asymptomatic. This is equivalent to class I of the NYHA classification. This includes about 10 million people in the United States.
Stage C describes patients with LV dysfunction who are symptomatic with exertion. This is equivalent to the NYHA class II and III. This includes about 5 million people in the United States.

Stage D describes patients with symptoms at rest. This is equivalent to class IV of the NYHA classification. This includes about 200,000 people in the United States.

This classification reliably allows the physician to follow patients as their HF progresses from one stage to the next and offers a unique set of treatments appropriate to each stage. Patients with advanced class III and IV HF are now further classified into seven different profiles using the Interagency Registry for Mechanically Assisted Circulatory Support (INTERMACS) database (Stevenson et al., 2009). INTERMACS was developed in a joint effort by the National Heart Lung and Blood Institute, Centers for Medicare and Medicaid Services, FDA, clinicians, scientists, and industry representatives for the purposes of following patients receiving mechanical circulatory support device therapy. Patients presenting with very advanced HF symptoms INTERMACS 1 to 3 (on IV inotropes whether stable or not) have a poorer survival outcome compared with those with INTERMACS 4 and 5 (on oral therapy at home or with symptoms with minimal activity) after mechanical assist device implantation or transplantation, likely reflecting a more advanced degree of end-organ damage in these patients.

EVALUATION OF PATIENTS WITH CONGESTIVE HEART FAILURE

Patients with symptoms and signs of HF need to have ECG, chest radiography, and, when available, natriuretic peptides. Abnormalities seen on these tests should trigger a structural heart evaluation with echocardiography. If LV dysfunction is documented, testing for the etiology and initiating treatment are indicated (Swedberg et al., 2005). Patients with HF (Hunt et al., 2001) need to have a complete history and physical examination with a focus on cardiovascular risk factors that lead to progression of failure. A careful documentation of their NYHA stage, history of hospitalizations, medications, and a full review of systems is indicated. A comprehensive physical examination should also include volume status and weight. Diagnostic tests should include a complete blood count; serum electrolytes; kidney and liver functions; urinalysis; blood glucose; thyroid function test; iron saturation test and ferritin; sedimentation rate; antinuclear antibodies to rule out connective tissue disease; sleep apnea testing (if suspected); 12-lead ECG; an echocardiogram; and coronary angiography, particularly in those with significant reduction in LV function and a suspicion of obstructive CAD.

Routine myocardial biopsy and Holter monitoring are not recommended. Biopsy is recommended, however, in patients with new-onset HF (<2 weeks) with (1) a normal-sized or dilated LV and hemodynamic compromise, (2) new-onset HF (2 weeks to 3 months) with dilated LV and new ventricular arrhythmias, or (3) heart block or failure to respond to therapy (Cooper et al., 2007). Levels of catecholamines might be obtained if clinically indicated in patients with severe episodic HTN and tachycardia. MRI can be considered if available to evaluate for infiltrative disease or scar. The rapid development of HF with reduced LV function in the absence of a clear etiology should raise suspicion of a viral cardiomyopathy, especially in younger patients. This can be suspected if the patient had a recent viral syndrome over the past several weeks followed by a progression of dyspnea and HF. Therapy for viral cardiomyopathy and HF consists of supportive therapy and the use of β-blockers, diuretics, ACE inhibitors, and, if failure is advanced (class III and IV), administration of spironolactone. Patients with fulminant myocarditis with hemodynamic instability may require support with a mechanical assist device.

RISK FACTOR MODIFICATION

Patients with HF should have their cardiovascular risk factors modified aggressively. HTN is strongly linked to the development of HF and should be aggressively treated (Vasan and Levy, 1996). The target BP should be 130/85 mm Hg or less except in patients with diabetes in whom the target is lowered to 125/85 mm Hg or less.

Control of dyslipidemia and diabetes is also very important in the management of patients with HF. Screening for sleep apnea and thyroid disease and aggressively treating these conditions if present needs to be done. The avoidance of alcohol, illicit drugs, and smoking is strongly advised. Losing weight and establishing a routine exercise program are also important preventive measures. Patients with a history of heart palpitations need to be evaluated for tachycardia because this is a well-established risk factor for cardiomyopathy and HF. If patients have daily palpitations, then a 24-hour Holter monitor is sufficient to help establish the type of arrhythmia. On the other hand, if palpitations occur infrequently (a few times per month), then an event care monitor is more useful because patients can keep this type of monitor with them at home for a longer time and record the arrhythmia as it occurs. Newer monitors have the ability to be autotriggered when arrhythmias are detected and can be useful in some asymptomatic patients. If palpitations are very infrequent, it is unlikely that they contribute to tachycardia-induced cardiomyopathy, but their diagnosis can be made with an implantable loop recorder, typically done by an electrophysiologist.

PHARMACOLOGIC THERAPY OF CONGESTIVE HEART FAILURE

Diastolic Dysfunction

Diastolic dysfunction is typically diagnosed by echocardiography. It is characterized by normal LV systolic function but impaired relaxation. Conditions that increase LV stiffness include CAD, HTN, diabetes, valvular heart disease, and age (Ewy, 2004).

Currently, the term *HF with preserved LVEF (HFpEF)* is used for patients with symptoms of HF in the setting of normal LV systolic function. These patients are typically treated with aggressive BP control and with the use of diuretics, β-blockade, or nondihydropyridine CCBs (diltiazem or verapamil). ACE inhibitors or ARBs can have long-term value in reducing LVH and, theoretically, may improve LV compliance (Mandinov et al., 2000).

Left Ventricular Systolic Dysfunction. Patients with *asymptomatic* LV dysfunction (stage B, ACC/AHA classification) benefit significantly from ACE inhibitors and β-blockade. The correction of anatomic abnormalities that are linked to LV systolic dysfunction, including severe mitral or aortic insufficiency and AS, is also important. Periodic follow-up of these patients is indicated with serial assessment of LV function using echocardiography or isotope ventriculography. Patients with familial LV systolic dysfunction need to have their immediate family members screened for asymptomatic cardiomyopathy.

Symptomatic LV systolic dysfunction (stage C, ACC/AHA classification) requires intensive pharmacologic treatment and close follow-up. Echocardiography or isotope ventriculography (IVG) are typically done to monitor LVEF over time when new symptoms or changes in therapy have been introduced. An IVG provides a more accurate assessment of EF (within ±3% variability in reading) than an echocardiogram but is more expensive and subjects the patient to radiation exposure. Whether an echocardiogram or an IVG is ordered depends on the patient's clinical presentation and history and the management approach of the treating physician. Diuretics are important in patients with hypervolemia, and digoxin improves symptoms in patients with clinical evidence of systolic HF in the setting of severely reduced LV function. There are no data, however, to support that diuretics or digoxin alter a patient's long-term survival. Current therapies known to impact a person's mortality are summarized below (Cohn, 1996; Hunt et al., 2001; Packer et al., 1999). Drugs and their dosages in treating patients with HF are summarized in Table 27-21.

Although there is no one way to start pharmacologic therapy for HF patients, it is advisable that patients be started on a small dose of β-blockers, ACE inhibitor, or both. Diuretics are generally reserved for patients with fluid overload. Caution needs to be exerted when a diuretic and an ACE inhibitor are started simultaneously because hypotension could occur, and serum creatinine levels can rise markedly. β-blockers (Hori et al., 2004) and ACE inhibitors (Majumdar et al., 2004) need to be titrated to the maximum tolerated dose to achieve maximal therapeutic efficacy.

Angiotensin-Converting Enzyme Inhibitors

Angiotensin-converting enzyme inhibitors reduce the mortality rate by an absolute 4% and relative 15% to 20% in patients with LV systolic dysfunction (EF <40%). In addition, ACE inhibitors reduce the combined end point of morbidity (HF hospitalizations) and mortality by 30% to 35%. Despite the benefits of ACE inhibitors (Wong et al., 2004), the mortality rate from HF remains at 50% within 5 years

Table 27-21   Selected Drugs and Their Dosages Currently Used in the Treatment of Congestive Heart Failure

Drug	Dosage
ANGIOTENSIN-CONVERTING ENZYME INHIBITORS	
Enalapril	2.5-20 mg PO BID; maximum, 40 mg/day; start at 2.5 mg QD
Captopril	12.5-50 mg PO TID; maximum, 150 mg/day; start at 6.25-12.5 mg PO TID
Ramipril	5 mg PO BID; maximum, 10 mg/day; start at 2.5 mg PO BID
Lisinopril	5-20 mg PO QD; maximum, 40 mg/day; start at 2.5 to 5 mg PO QD
Perindopril	4-16 mg PO QD; maximum, 16 mg/day; start at 2 mg PO QD
Monopril	10-40 mg PO QD/BID; maximum, 80 mg/day; start at 10 mg PO QD
ANGIOTENSIN RECEPTOR BLOCKERS (FOR ACE INHIBITOR–INTOLERANT PATIENTS)	
Losartan	25-100 mg PO QD; maximum, 100 mg/day; start at 25-50 mg PO QD*
Candesartan	8-32 mg PO QD; maximum, 32 mg/day; start at 16 mg PO QD*
Valsartan	40-160 mg PO BID; maximum, 320 mg/day; start at 40 mg PO BID
Irbesartan	75-300 mg PO QD; maximum, 300 mg/day; start at 75 mg PO QD*
β-BLOCKERS	
Carvedilol	3.125-25 mg PO BID; maximum, 50 mg PO QD; start at 3.125 mg PO BID
Metoprolol succinate	12.5-200 mg PO QD; maximum, 200 mg/day; start at 12.5 mg PO QD
Metoprolol	12.5-100 mg PO BID; maximum, 100 mg PO BID; start at 12.5 mg PO BID*
ALDOSTERONE ANTAGONISTS	
Spironolactone	12.5-25 mg PO BID; maximum, 50 mg/day; start at 12.5 mg PO BID
Eplerenone	50 mg PO QD; maximum, 50 mg/day; start at 25 mg PO QD†

*Off-label use.
†For heart failure patients after myocardial infarction.
ACE, Angiotensin-converting enzyme; *BID*, twice a day; *PO*, oral; *QD*, once a day; *TID*, three times a day.

of the diagnosis, and 30% of patients are rehospitalized within 3 months.

Several trials have noted a mortality reduction with ACE inhibitors in patients with clinical evidence of HF after sustaining an MI (Acute Infarction Ramipril Efficacy Study [AIRE] Study Investigators, 1999; Kober et al., 1995). The AIRE showed a 27% ($P = 0.002$) reduction in the 30-month cumulative mortality rate with ramipril over placebo in post-MI HF patients. Furthermore, trandolapril reduced the mortality rate by 22% ($P = 0.01$) in patients with reduced LV function after an MI (Kober et al., 1995). Guidelines also emphasize the use of ACE inhibitors in patients with asymptomatic LV dysfunction and a history of MI. These patients are at high risk of developing LV remodeling and CHF several months after the initial insult (Jessup and Brozena, 2003).

Angiotensin Receptor Blockers

Early studies comparing ARBs and ACE inhibitors in the management of HF patients suggested that an ARB was as safe, effective, and tolerable as an ACE inhibitor. In the Randomized Evaluation of Strategies for Left Ventricular Dysfunction (RESOLVD) pilot study (McKelvie et al., 1999), 768 patients in NYHA classes II to IV and EF less than 40% received candesartan, candesartan plus enalapril, or enalapril alone for 43 weeks. LV cavity size increased less and BNP levels decreased more with combination therapy compared with an ARB or ACE inhibitor alone. In the Losartan Heart Failure Survival Study ELITE II (Pitt et al., 2000), 3152 patients age 60 years or older with NYHA class II to IV and EF of less than 40% were randomly assigned to losartan ($n = 1578$) titrated to 50 mg once daily or captopril ($n = 1574$) titrated to 50 mg three times daily. There were no differences in all-cause mortality or sudden death between the two groups. In a subset of the Val-HeFT (Valsartan in Heart Failure Trial) trial of patients intolerant to ACE inhibitors, valsartan (titrated to 160 mg twice daily) reduced both all-cause mortality and combined mortality and morbidity compared with placebo (17.3% vs. 27.1%, $P = 0.017$ and 24.9% vs. 42.5%, $P <0.001$, respectively) (Maggioni et al., 2002). In this trial, adding an ARB (Valsartan) to an ACE inhibitor in HF patients with EF below 40% did not reduce mortality further, but the combined end point of mortality and morbidity was reduced by about 27.5%, mostly because of a reduction in HF hospitalizations (Cohn et al., 2001).

In the Candesartan in Heart Failure Assessment of Reduction in Mortality and morbidity (CHARM) study, candesartan (titrated to 32 mg once daily) significantly reduced cardiovascular deaths and hospital admissions for HF (Pfeffer et al., 2003). In the "overall programme" of this study, which included both preserved and reduced LV function, total mortality was not reduced compared with placebo. However, in a subset analysis, in patients with symptomatic HF and reduced LV function (<40%), candesartan significantly reduced all-cause mortality, cardiovascular death, and HF hospitalizations when added to standard therapies, including ACE inhibitor, β-blockers, and aldosterone antagonists (Young et al., 2004). These patients should have their BP, creatinine, and serum potassium carefully monitored. The Valsartan in Acute Myocardial Infarction Trial (VALIANT) randomized patients 0.5 to 10 days after an acute MI with reduced LV function to valsartan (4909 patients) titrated to 160 mg twice a day, valsartan (80 mg twice a day) plus captopril (50 mg three times a day) (4885 patients), or captopril (4909 patients) titrated to 50 mg three times a day in addition to standard therapy (Pfeffer et al., 2003). Valsartan was equally effective to captopril in reducing all-cause mortality. For reasons that remain unclear, combining valsartan with captopril did not improve survival compared with either captopril or valsartan alone but did increase adverse events.

Currently, the recommendation is to use an ACE inhibitor as first-line therapy to treat HF patients. However, a growing body of evidence suggests that an ARB could be as effective as an ACE inhibitor in the treatment of HF patients with reduced LV function.

Aldosterone Blockers

Aldosterone is secreted by the zona glomerulosa of the adrenal gland and is induced by AII, adrenocorticotropic hormone, and potassium. Aldosterone leads to sodium and water absorption and the excretion of potassium. Although AII is a dominant stimulus of aldosterone secretion (Weber, 2001), ACE inhibitors used as monotherapy are not sufficient to therapeutically block aldosterone secretion (McKelvie et al., 1999; Schjoedt et al., 2004). Until recently, the role of aldosterone blockade in the management of patients with HF has been unclear.

Two large trials investigated the role of aldosterone antagonists in HF management. The Randomized Aldactone Evaluation Study (RALES) (Pitt et al., 1999) randomized patients with advanced HF and EF less than 35% to spironolactone 25 mg/day or placebo in addition to standard therapy. After a mean follow-up period of 24 months, spironolactone reduced the mortality rate by 30% caused by a reduction of progression of HF and sudden cardiac death. In addition, patients who received spironolactone had a significant improvement in the symptoms of HF as assessed by the NYHA functional class ($P < 0.001$). Recurrent hospitalization caused by worsening HF was also reduced by 35% ($P < 0.001$). The Eplerenone Post-AMI Heart Failure Efficacy and Survival Study (EPHESUS) (Pitt et al., 2001) randomized patients with HF and an EF less than 40%, 3 to 14 days after MI, to eplerenone (25 mg-50 mg/day) or placebo. At a mean follow-up period of 27 months, eplerenone, a competitive, relatively selective mineralocorticoid receptor antagonist, reduced the total mortality rate by 15% ($P = 0.008$), cardiovascular mortality or cardiovascular hospitalizations by 13% ($P = 0.002$), and sudden cardiac death by 21% ($P = 0.03$). Based on these trials, aldosterone antagonists are now considered to be a primary therapy in patients with LV dysfunction and HF.

β-Blockade in Heart Failure

The activation of the SNS in patients with HF leads to excess catecholamine secretion, which adversely affects the myocardium and contributes to LV remodeling and HF. Multiple β-blockers have been tested in patients with HF. β-Blockers have been shown to reduce the mortality rate by approximately 35% when added to an ACE inhibitor in mild to moderate (MERIT-HF with metoprolol succinate, US Carvedilol trials with carvedilol and CIBIS-II trial with bisoprolol) (CIBIS-II, 1999; MERIT-HF study group, 1999; Packer et al., 1996) or in very advanced HF (Copernicus trial with carvedilol) (Packer et al., 2001). β-Blockers also reduce hospitalizations by 33% to 38% (Fowler et al., 2001; MERIT-HF study group, 1999; Packer et al., 1996) and work synergistically with ACE inhibitor to reduce cardiac remodeling, reduce cavity size, and improve EF (Remme et al., 2004).

There are differences in the antiadrenergic actions of β-adrenergic blocking drugs. The ratio of β_2- and α_1-adrenergic receptors in the damaged heart changes compared with normal myocardium (Bristow, 1993). β1 receptors are reduced, and α1 receptors are increased with little change in the β2 receptors. Almost 50% of the adrenergic receptors on the failing myocardium are β2 and α1, which are typically not affected by selective β1 blockade. Norepinephrine is known to exert negative effects through β_1-, β_2-, and α_1-receptors. The theory whether a nonselective β1, β2, and α1 blocker yields better mortality reduction than a β1 blocker alone was recently tested in the Carvedilol Or Metoprolol European Trial (COMET trial) (Poole-Wilson et al., 2003; Torp-Pedersen et al., 2005). In this study, 3029 patients with class II to IV HF were recruited at 317 centers in 15 European countries. At 58 months, there was a 17% reduction in mortality rate with carvedilol compared with metoprolol tartrate ($P = 0.0017$). Despite the controversy about the adequacy of β-blockade and the use of the shorter-acting metoprolol tartrate instead of the long-acting metoprolol succinate in this study, the data seem to favor the theory that the nonselective adrenergic blockade is superior to the selective short-acting β1 receptor blockade in reducing mortality in HF patients.

Carvedilol (6.25-25 mg twice daily) was shown in The Glycemic Effects in Diabetes Mellitus: Carvedilol-Metoprolol Comparison in Hypertensives (GEMINI) study not to alter glycemic control in patients with diabetes compared with metoprolol tartrate (50-200 mg twice a day). Also, it did improve some components of the metabolic syndrome such as insulin sensitivity (Bakris et al., 2004). Carvedilol appears to be a favorable drug in patients with diabetes, in contrast to other selective β-blockers.

Aggressive titration of β-blockers is needed in patients with HF. Higher levels of β-blockade are associated with better improvement of EF and greater reductions in cardiovascular hospitalizations (Bristow et al., 1996; Hori et al., 2004). A stepwise approach in titration of β-blockade is generally followed with an increase in the dose every 2 weeks as tolerated until achieving the maximum tolerable dose. Current β-blockers approved for treatment of systolic HF in the United States are carvedilol, metoprolol XL, and bisoprolol. β-Blockade should be used in asymptomatic patients with a recent MI regardless of EF. Also, β-blockade should be used in all stable stage C patients unless contraindicated (SOR: A, ACC/AHA guidelines).

Miscellaneous Therapy

In addition to pharmacologic therapy, HF patients should be instructed on dietary salt restriction (2 g/day of sodium), daily weight monitoring (with reporting of 3 lb per week weight increase to their doctors), free water restriction to 1 L daily, smoking cessation, regular exercise, avoidance of alcohol intake, and aggressive treatment of HTN and lipid disorders. Supplemental oxygen is needed in patients with oxygen saturation of less than 92% on room air after ambulation. Finally, sleep apnea has been associated with HF, and these patients need to be screened and aggressively treated for moderate to severe apnea. Patients with symptomatic HF are best treated within an HF clinic that ensures that appropriate therapy is administered by a specialized provider, might increase patients' compliance, and reduces the chance of recurrent hospitalizations. An HF clinic will also ensure that national benchmarks in the management of HF patients are met. These include the optimal use of ACE inhibitor and β-blockers, documentation of LV function, and smoking cessation.

- Two-dimensional echocardiography with Doppler should be performed during initial evaluation of patients presenting with CHF to assess LVEF, LV size, wall thickness, and valve function (SOR: A) (Hunt et al., 2009).
- Control of systolic and diastolic HTN in accordance with established guidelines is strongly indicated in HF patients (SOR: A, ACC/AHA guidelines).
- ACE inhibitors are recommended in all patients with HF and LV dysfunction unless a contraindication exists (SOR: A, ACC/AHA guidelines).
- ACE inhibitors should be used in all patients with history of MI and reduced LV function (SOR: A, ACC/AHA guidelines).
- Angiotensin receptor blockade can be used in patients who are being treated with digitalis, diuretics, and a β-blocker and who cannot be given an ACE inhibitor because of cough or angioedema (SOR: A, ACC/AHA guidelines).

Myocardial and Pericardial Diseases

CARDIOMYOPATHIES

Key Points

- The following elements of a good history need to be obtained in patients with cardiac dysfunction: family history, duration of illness, weight loss or gain, anorexia, severity and triggers of dyspnea and fatigue, presence of edema, palpitations or difficulty breathing at night, prior hospitalizations, current and past medications, and diet (ACCF/AHA 2013 Heart Failure Guidelines).
- The physical examination needs to focus on BP and heart rate, BMI, recent change in weight, presence of jugular vein distention, orthostatics, extra heart sounds, presence of RV heave, apical displacement, presence of organomegaly or edema, lung auscultation, and peripheral extremity temperature (ACCF/AHA 2013 Heart Failure Guidelines).

Cardiomyopathy is defined as a disorder of the heart muscle and has been classified by the WHO/International Society and Federation of Cardiology into dilated, restrictive, hypertrophic, arrhythmogenic right ventricular (ARVC), and unclassified (Richardson et al., 1996). Cardiomyopathy is a common cause of HF but is not HF. HF is a clinical diagnosis characterized by fatigue and dyspnea in the setting of normal or compromised LV systolic function and may occur with or without pulmonary congestion. A thorough history and examination are important in the initial evaluation of patients with suspected cardiomyopathy.

DILATED CARDIOMYOPATHY

Strictly speaking, cardiomyopathy is a primary disorder of the heart muscle that is not secondary to ischemia, HTN, or valvular, congenital, or pericardial disease. In this section, both primary and secondary dilated cardiomyopathy (DC) are addressed. DC is characterized by enlargement (increase in both end-systolic and end-diastolic volumes) and weakness of the LV (i.e., remodeling). Multiple risk factors can lead to DC, including the presence of CAD, HTN, connective tissue disease (lupus, scleroderma, juvenile rheumatoid arthritis, dermatomyositis), infiltrative diseases (amyloidosis, sarcoidosis), glycogen storage disease, hemochromatosis, vasculitis, sleep apnea, viral infections, valvular disease, metabolic abnormalities (endocrine, nutritional, electrolytes, obesity), hypersensitivity myocarditis (sulfa, penicillin, methyldopa, tetanus toxoid, hydrochlorothiazide, dobutamine, phenytoin, amphotericin B), tachycardia, anemia, various toxins (including alcohol, doxorubicin, and anthracycline), muscular dystrophies, and peripartum or unknown causes (idiopathic or primary DC). Irrespective of the etiology, the reduction in systolic heart function leads to neurohormonal activation, including activation of the sympathetic and RAAS systems, endothelial dysfunction, inflammation (Pankuweit et al., 2004), endothelin production, vasoconstriction, and sodium and fluid retention. Common cardiomyopathies encountered in a primary care practice are ischemic, valvular, hypertensive, and idiopathic.

Patients with DC have progressive dyspnea, fatigue, and occasional chest pain even in the absence of CAD. They could display signs of both left- and right-sided HF. Arrhythmias are encountered and could be supraventricular, such as AF or atrial flutter (AFL), or ventricular. Patients with AF or AFL need to be anticoagulated with warfarin to reduce risk for thromboembolic events. Electrocardiographic findings are nonspecific. Nondiagnostic ST/T changes, conduction abnormalities, and supraventricular or ventricular arrhythmias can be seen. Echocardiography generally confirms the diagnosis, revealing enlarged and dilated cardiac chambers with a reduced LVEF. Echocardiography can also help define the presence of valvular pathology and rule out the presence of a thrombus in the left-sided chambers of the heart. Isotope ventriculography is used to determine LVEF and therapeutic efficacy. Cardiac catheterization is important in patients in whom there is a suspicion of CAD, intracardiac shunts, or severe valvular abnormalities. Determining the presence of IHD with angiography is important because noninvasive imaging has a lower sensitivity in patients with severe three-vessel CAD or LM disease, conditions known to reduce LV function. Cardiac catheterization is also important in patients in whom cardiac transplantation is contemplated to assess pulmonary pressures and pulmonary vascular resistance and to test whether vasodilators can reduce elevated pulmonary resistance.

Secondary Cardiomyopathies

Ischemic Cardiomyopathy. Ischemic DC is caused by obstructive CAD and a history of MI. A small injury to the myocardium can precipitate remodeling with subsequent weakness in cardiac function. In fact, up to 40% of patients with anterior MI display remodeling within 12 months. Therapy of ischemic CM is the same as described in the CHF section of this chapter and consists mostly of β-blockers, ACE inhibitors or ARBs, and aldosterone antagonists. Digoxin is for symptomatic patients and appears to improve symptoms but has no effect on mortality. Diuretics are reserved for patients who are fluid overloaded. Revascularization is necessary in patients with ischemic, hibernating myocardium in whom viability can be demonstrated. Viability tests might include rest–redistribution thallium-201 scanning, low-dose dobutamine echocardiography, positron emission tomography, or cardiac MRI.

Hypertensive Cardiomyopathy. Hypertension initially leads to LVH of the myocardium. Eventually, untreated HTN leads to dilation and weakness of the LV and subsequent DC. The initial stage of hypertensive cardiomyopathy is diastolic dysfunction with no LVH followed by diastolic dysfunction and LVH, then CHF with normal LV systolic function, and finally DC with reduced LV systolic function (Iriarte et al., 1995). HTN is a significant risk factor for developing cardiomyopathy and should be aggressively managed (Vasan and Levy, 1996). The presence of LVH on ECG doubles the chance of developing HF. Several mechanisms have been implicated in the development of HF in patients with hypertension, including collagen deposition in the interstitial space impairing the diffusion of oxygen and nutrients to myocytes (Verdecchia, 2000). ACE inhibitors, diuretics, and β-blockers are important therapies for the treatment of hypertensive DC.

Valvular Cardiomyopathy. Mitral insufficiency and aortic insufficiency are the most common valvular abnormalities that precipitate DC. A severe reduction in LV function can occur in mitral insufficiency that remains silent until significant remodeling of the LV occurs. Early diagnosis and mitral valve repair or replacement is particularly important when LV function is still preserved (≥60%). The lower the EF, the worse the immediate and long-term surgical results. The mortality rate is excessively high in patients with severely reduced LVEF (<25%).

Aortic insufficiency is poorly tolerated over time. Surgical repair, however, leads to significant improvement in LV function and symptoms, even with a reduced EF. Surgery needs to be considered, however, if the EF is 55% or less. Aortic valve stenosis leads to LVH and subsequent DC if not treated. MS generally does not affect ventricular function and size. Tricuspid insufficiency and pulmonic insufficiency, if severe, can lead to RV fluid overload and dilation and failure of the right-sided chambers of the heart. A pattern of right HF becomes apparent, including jugular venous distention, pulsatile and enlarged liver, ascites, and lower extremity edema.

Primary Cardiomyopathies

Viral Cardiomyopathy. Viral DNA was found in 67.4% of patients with DC within the genome of myocardial cells (Kuhl et al., 2005). Evidence of prior viral infection in these patients suggests a causal relationship. Viral cardiomyopathy is postulated to be the most common cause of DC.

Familial Dilated Cardiomyopathy. It is estimated that 30% of patients with idiopathic DC have a genetic cause, although familial DC remains clinically underappreciated. Familial DC is an inherited autosomal dominant condition; the symptom onset varies with different families. Obtaining a family history of DC is important in all patients who

present with cardiomyopathy, including a history of unexplained sudden death (Schmidt et al., 1988). The diagnosis is suspected if two or more affected individuals are in the same family or if sudden death has occurred in a first-degree relative before the age of 35 years (Mestroni et al., 1999). The family of patients with suspected familial cardiomyopathy should undergo periodic serial echocardiography at least every 3 to 5 years in conjunction with genetic counseling as needed (Yancy et al., 2013).

Alcoholic Cardiomyopathy. Alcohol cardiomyopathy (Piano, 2002) is likely due to a direct toxic effect of alcohol on muscle cells with variable genetic vulnerability. Other mechanisms include a potential increase in norepinephrine and acetaldehyde. Alcohol consumption of several drinks per day for approximately 10 years or more increases the risk of alcoholic cardiomyopathy (10 oz of whiskey, 32 oz of wine, 64 oz of beer). Abstinence from alcohol is essential in all patients with DC, including alcoholic cardiomyopathy.

Tachycardia-Induced Cardiomyopathy. Prolonged rapid heart rate can induce DC and is generally reversible upon controlling the arrhythmia (Cruz et al., 1990). The main treatment of this cardiomyopathy is in the control of the rapid heartbeat. This condition is frequently seen in patients with unrecognized AF with rapid ventricular response but also can be caused by sinus tachycardia and ventricular arrhythmias.

Takotsubo Cardiomyopathy. Apical ballooning syndrome, or Takotsubo cardiomyopathy, typically occurs in women older than 50 years of age, precipitated by emotional or physiologic stress with subsequent LV dysfunction (involving the apex and typically sparing the base of the ventricle). Patients present with acute ischemia and have normal coronaries. Wall motion abnormality extends beyond a single coronary territory. In the majority of patients, the cardiomyopathy resolves within weeks of presentation. The long-term prognosis of patients is good with no further deterioration of heart muscle on follow-up (Sharkey et al., 2011).

Drug-Induced Cardiomyopathy. Dilated cardiomyopathy has been well described with several antineoplastic agents such as anthracyclines (doxorubicin), high-dose cyclophosphamide, trastuzumab (Herceptin), and tyrosine kinase inhibitors (sunitinib). Doxorubicin-induced myopathy is dose dependent and is generally irreversible (Lipshultz et al., 1995; Steinherz et al., 1991). Other drugs that can induce cardiomyopathy include cocaine (Felker et al., 1999), ecstasy (3,4-methylenedioxymethamphetamine) (Mizia-Stec et al., 2008), ma huang (Ephedra) (Samenuk et al., 2002), and amphetamine (Crean and Pohl, 2004).

Peripartum Cardiomyopathy. Peripartum cardiomyopathy occurs in one in 1300 to one in 1400 births. Etiologic factors remain unknown but likely include autoimmune factors, myocarditis, toxemia, nutritional deficiencies, and tocolytics. Risk factors include age older than 30 years, African American race, multiparity, HTN and preeclampsia, cocaine use, and pregnancy with multiple fetuses.

Patients with history of peripartum cardiomyopathy should be advised against future pregnancies.

Idiopathic Dilated Cardiomyopathy. The presence of DC without an identifiable cause is called idiopathic dilated cardiomyopathy (IDC). The cardiac chambers are enlarged, and LV function is reduced. Myocytes can be hypertrophied or atrophied with interstitial fibrosis present. It is unclear what precipitates IDC, but an autoimmune mechanism has been hypothesized.

The treatment of DC consists of diuretics, digoxin, ACE inhibitors, and β-blockade. Aldosterone antagonists are reserved for patients with advanced symptoms (class III or IV) or those with ischemic cardiomyopathy and a history of prior MI. Mechanical therapies with biventricular pacing and cardiac resynchronization therapy can be very helpful to improve symptoms in patients with a wide QRS on ECG and an abnormal, asynchronous septal wall motion.

Patients with DC and a prior history of sustained ventricular arrhythmias have a high risk of sudden cardiac death. The implantation of an internal defibrillator is associated with improved mortality outcomes in these patients (Moss et al., 2002, 2004; Moss 2003). Defibrillator therapy is also indicated for patients with asymptomatic depressed LV systolic function regardless of the etiology (Bardy et al., 2005). Empiric antiarrhythmic therapy to prevent sudden death in patients with DC did not show a mortality benefit. Internal defibrillators are now advised for patients with an LVEF 35% or less at least 40 days from an MI and revascularization or 3 months from initiation of optimal medical treatment in noninfarct patients.

Hypertrophic Cardiomyopathy. Hypertrophic cardiomyopathy (HCM) is characterized by inappropriate LV wall thickness larger than 15 mm in the setting of normal cavity size, impaired diastolic filling, and, in some patients, LV outflow obstruction. Patterns of hypertrophy are variable in HCM (Klues et al., 1995) and depend on the phenotypic expression of the autosomal dominant mutations in genes encoding protein components of the sarcomere (chromosomes 1, 11, 14, and 15) and its myofilaments (Alcalai et al., 2008; Ly et al., 2005). LVH can be concentric, apical (Yamaguchi disease), or involving the free wall of the LV in 75% of HCM patients. In the remaining 25%, it is septal (idiopathic hypertrophic subaortic stenosis or asymmetric septal hypertrophy). HCM affects 0.2% of the population (Zou et al., 2004) and is the leading cause of nonviolent death among young people in the United States.

Hypertrophic cardiomyopathy is sometimes characterized by normal systolic function with asymmetric LVH and variable degrees of LV outflow obstruction. The LV outflow in HCM is caused by the asymmetric hypertrophy of the LV septum and the systolic anterior motion (SAM) of the anterior leaflet of the mitral valve. Patients with HCM can have abnormal intramural coronary arteries that contribute to fibrosis and myocardial ischemia even in the absence of obstructive atherosclerotic lesions.

Patients can be asymptomatic (10%-15%) or more typically present with dyspnea or pulmonary congestion (90%), chest pain (75%), occasional dizziness, and syncopal events, and in young athletes with a significant LV outflow obstruction, sudden death can be the first manifestation of the disease (1%-3% annual incidence and can be as high as 6% in childhood). HCM is quite often first uncovered on physical examination when a systolic ejection murmur is first appreciated along the lower left sternal border that is made worse with Valsalva maneuver or standing up from a squatting position. Patients might also have a bisferiens carotid pulse and an S4 gallop. These signs are mostly present in patients with a significant LV outflow obstruction and can be absent in nonobstructive HCM.

The ECG in patients with HCM might show LVH, deep inferior and lateral Q waves, poor R wave progression across the precordium, left anterior fascicular block, and an enlarged left atrium. The echocardiogram is generally diagnostic. Asymmetric LVH can be seen along with SAM of the anterior leaflets and secondary mitral insufficiency. LV outflow obstruction can be measured with Doppler flow and its severity to provocative maneuvers can be assessed, including inhalation of amyl nitrite and Valsalva maneuver. A gradient of 30 mm Hg or more at rest or with provocative measures indicates the presence of obstructive HCM (Panza et al., 1992; Sasson et al., 1988). The resting gradient is associated with progression to severe CHF and death from HF but does not correlate with sudden cardiac death or correlate with overall prognosis. Cardiac catheterization might be necessary in some patients to confirm the diagnosis and to assess gradients accurately. Cardiac MRI is helpful in establishing the diagnosis of HCM in patients in whom echocardiography is inconclusive and can provide information about the pattern of hypertrophy. The accuracy of myocardial perfusion nuclear imaging is reduced in HCM and may lead to high false-positive findings.

The natural history of HCM is variable, with an annual mortality rate of 1% to 2% (Hess and Sigwart, 2004). Patients at high risk of premature sudden cardiac death include young patients (30 years of age or younger) irrespective of the degree of obstruction of the LVOT, history of syncope or prior cardiac arrest, massive LVH (wall thickness >29 mm), nonsustained VT on Holter monitoring, sustained ventricular arrhythmias, abnormal BP response to exercise, or family history of sudden cardiac death. Certain gene defects are also associated with sudden cardiac death (α-tropomyosin) in younger patients. A 12-lead ECG is recommended for all athletes involved in organized competitive sports in addition to a detailed history and physical examination to screen for HCM and other potential lethal cardiac diseases (Corrado et al., 2005).

In patients with stable mild to moderate symptoms, pharmacologic therapy is indicated, including β-blockers to a heart rate of 60 beats/min and the CCB verapamil if the patient remains symptomatic. Patients with progressive symptoms might benefit from the addition of disopyramide to a β-blocker (with or without verapamil). In general, physicians need to avoid the use of dihydropyridine CCBs, digoxin, inotropes, or disopyramide with no β-blockers.

Patients with severe symptoms and a LV gradient of 50 mm Hg or greater at rest need to be considered for dual-chamber pacing, alcohol septal ablation (Hess and Sigwart, 2004), or septal myotomy or myectomy and consideration for an implantable cardioverter-defibrillator (ICD), particularly in those at high risk of sudden cardiac death (Maron et al., 2000). Mitral valve replacement is generally not indicated in those with HCM with an obstructive gradient over 50 mm Hg.

Patients with symptomatic HCM should avoid participation in competitive sports. Low-intensity exercise is reasonable in patients with asymptomatic HCM (bowling, golfing, brisk walking, modest biking). Patients should not be involved in competitive sports or sports that require systematic training.

In the setting of acute hypotension in patients with LVOT obstruction, increasing afterload with the use of IV phenylephrine or another selective vasoconstrictor is an important step to reduce the LV outflow obstruction.

Restrictive Cardiomyopathy. Restrictive cardiomyopathy (RC) is a disease of the heart muscle characterized by reduced relaxation (diastolic impairment) and restrictive filling in the presence of normal or nearly normal ventricular function and cavity size. It can be idiopathic or familial or caused by infiltrative or storage diseases. Secondary causes of RC are many and include amyloidosis, sarcoidosis, hemochromatosis, glycogen storage disease, and Fabry disease. Certain connective tissue diseases, including scleroderma and pseudoxanthoma elasticum, can also lead to RC. Endomyocardial diseases such as hypereosinophilic (Loeffler) syndrome, endomyocardial fibrosis, carcinoid, and malignant infiltration can also lead to RC.

Idiopathic RCM is equally present in males and females. A familial pattern is present in some cases. One third of patients may have thromboembolic complications. LVH and interstitial fibrosis are present to varying degrees. Amyloidosis-induced RCM is secondary to extracellular amyloid protein deposition throughout the heart and can be diagnosed with biopsy. There are four types of amyloidosis that depend on the amyloid protein composition: (1) primary amyloidosis caused by myeloma protein fibrils diffusely deposited throughout the myocardium, (2) secondary amyloidosis, (3) senile amyloidosis, and (4) familial amyloidosis. Amyloidosis should be suspected if patients complain of peripheral neuropathy, carpal tunnel syndrome, difficulty swallowing, hoarseness, macroglossia, hepatomegaly, autonomic neuropathy, and nephrotic syndrome. Patients frequently have elevated jugular venous pressure. Kussmaul sign is generally not present. Pleural effusions, hepatomegaly, and peripheral edema are present. Echocardiography may show a granular, sparkling appearance with biventricular thickening and biatrial enlargement. EF is typically normal. Serum and urine immunofixation electrophoresis looking for free light chains and tissue amyloid deposits on biopsy (apple-green birefringence when stained with Congo red and viewed under polarizing microscopy) are tests that can be performed to establish the diagnosis.

Sarcoidosis-induced RCM is characterized by the formation of granulomas in multiple organs with cardiac involvement in about 25% of patients (2% clinically). It is frequently seen in African Americans, women, and patients between the age of 25 and 50 years. Patients can present with heart block and ventricular arrhythmias. Sarcoid is diagnosed by biopsy. Clinically cardiac sarcoidosis is suspected if there is an extracardiac manifestation of the disease and there are two major or one major and one minor cardiac criteria met.

Major cardiac criteria include heart block, EF less than 50%, positive gallium scan, and basal thinning of the ventricular septum. Minor criteria include abnormal ECG, abnormal echocardiogram, perfusion defects on myocardial perfusion imaging tests, and abnormal MRI with delayed enhancement and presence of fibrosis (Soejima and Yada, 2009).

Patients with RC typically present with dyspnea and signs of left and right-sided failure. The jugular venous pulse is elevated with a prominent X and Y descent. The ECG is nonspecific and might show low voltage, conduction abnormalities, and increase in atrial sizes. Echocardiography will show diastolic dysfunction and might help in the diagnosis of infiltrative diseases such as amyloidosis. It can also help exclude the diagnosis of other causes of HF and assess valvular function. In addition, tissue Doppler and color M-mode Doppler can facilitate the diagnosis of RC.

Restrictive cardiomyopathy might be difficult to distinguish from constrictive pericarditis. The distinction between these two entities is important because RC has no cure, but constrictive pericarditis can be cured surgically by pericardial stripping. Several parameters can be used in the angiography suite to help distinguish between these entities. Typically, RC patients have a higher end-diastolic pressure in the LV compared with the RV (>5 mm Hg), a RV pressure that exceeds 50 mm Hg, and a RV end-diastolic pressure to RV systolic pressure ratio less than 1 : 3. The overall predictive accuracy of these parameters independently is 85%, 70%, and 76%, respectively, but if all were concordant in one patient, the diagnostic accuracy can reach 90% (Vaitkus and Kussmaul, 1991). Imaging modalities such as MR and CT scanning can help in determining whether pericardial thickening is present as in the case of constrictive pericarditis. Endomyocardial biopsies can be helpful in determining the presence of infiltrative disease.

Treatment of RC is mostly palliative and symptom directed. Small doses of diuretics can be helpful, but caution should be taken not to dehydrate the patient because cardiac output heavily relies on adequate preload volumes in these patients.

Arrhythmogenic Right Ventricular Dysplasia. Arrhythmogenic right ventricular dysplasia (ARVD) is a form of cardiomyopathy caused by either a replacement of the RV myocardium with fat or a genetically susceptible RV to environmental agents leading to myocarditis (Fontaine et al., 1999). ARVD is autosomal dominant in 50% of patients; therefore, first-degree relatives should be screened. Clinically, ARVD can present with VTs with a left bundle branch block pattern or VF (Corrado et al., 2001). ARVD can cause sudden cardiac death in young, otherwise healthy persons and athletes. Multiple modalities can be used to assist in the diagnosis, including ECG (inverted T waves in V1-V3 with epsilon waves in V1-V3), echocardiography, MRI, and contrast ventriculography. MRI is emerging as an important technique for assisting in the diagnosis and follow-up of these patients (Kayser et al., 2002). On MRI, the RV appears thin (<2 mm) with focal regions of hypertrophy, dilated with regional dysfunction, enlarged right ventricular outflow tract (RVOT), and with abnormal morphology (trabecular disarray). Therapy of ARVD consists of antiarrhythmic drugs, catheter ablation, and implantable defibrillators (McRae 3rd, 2001). In cases of refractory HF, cardiac transplantation should be considered.

- Endomyocardial biopsy is indicated in: (1) patients with recent onset HF (<2 weeks) in the presence of normal or dilated LV and hemodynamic compromise and in (2) patients with HF onset between 2 weeks and 3 months and with dilated LV and new ventricular arrhythmias, heart block, or not responding to medical treatment in 1 to 2 weeks (SOR: A) (Cooper, 2007).
- Patients with HCM should undergo yearly ECG, Holter at baseline, echocardiography at baseline, repeat echocardiography for children 12 years of age or younger every 12 to 18 months if history of sudden cardiac death or playing sports, MRI if echocardiography is inconclusive, and cardiac angiography if chest pain and intermediate to high risk of CAD. There is no indication to perform an echocardiogram more than once per year (SOR: A) (Gersh et al., 2011).
- ICD therapy is indicated in patients with prior cardiac arrest or VT or fibrillation and should be strongly considered in patients with a family history of sudden cardiac death, severe wall thickness (≥30 mm), syncope, nonsustained VT on Holter monitoring, or a drop in BP with exercise and in high-risk children (SOR: A) (Gersh et al., 2011).

MYOCARDITIS

Myocarditis is an acute injury to the myocardium with subsequent autoimmune and inflammatory response leading to further damage to the myocardium (Blauwet and Cooper, 2010). Myocarditis can be triggered by several agents, most commonly the coxsackie B virus. Other viruses can precipitate myocarditis, including echovirus, human immunodeficiency virus (HIV), influenza, cytomegalovirus, adenovirus, respiratory syncytial virus, varicella zoster, and arbovirus. Various nonviral agents, including bacterial, fungal, and parasitic (toxoplasmosis and schistosomiasis) agents, can also trigger myocarditis. Noninfectious etiologies are also numerous and include systemic diseases (sarcoidosis, celiac disease), drugs and toxins (anthracyclines, cocaine), autoimmune disease (giant cell myocarditis, lupus), radiation, genetic, environmental (carbon monoxide, lead), endocrine, and metabolic.

A variety of clinical presentations can be encountered, from minimal symptoms and a very benign course to severe symptoms and cardiogenic shock. Damage to the myocardium can be a direct result of the injurious insult to the myocardium or secondary to an autoimmune reaction against the invading agent. Patients can give a history of a viral infection several weeks before the onset of cardiac symptoms, which include dyspnea, chest pain, and CHF. Palpitations, dizzy spells, syncope, and even sudden cardiac death can occur as a result of arrhythmias. Patients display signs of CHF with S3 gallops and rales in their lungs. A pericardial rub can be heard in some when the pericardium is also involved. An elevated erythrocyte sedimentation rate (ESR), WBC count, and cardiac enzymes can be seen. ECG changes are nonspecific but can show ST/T changes diffusely, sinus tachycardia, a prolonged QT interval, conduction delays, and low voltage. Echocardiography shows a reduced LV function and possibly segmental wall motion abnormalities and ventricular thrombus. RV dysfunction is a poor prognostic indicator in acute myocarditis (Mendes, 1994). The value of endomyocardial biopsy is questionable except in recent unexplained HF in the setting of fulminant myocarditis with normal or dilated LV and in suspected giant cell myocarditis (Blauwet and Cooper, 2010).

Treatment of myocarditis is the same as treatment of CHF. Steroids and other immunomodulatory agents are not known to be helpful. Recovery is generally the rule with a good long-term prognosis. NSAIDs should be avoided in those with acute myocarditis (Khatib et al., 1990). Mechanical hemodynamic support in the acute phase may be needed when hemodynamic compromise is present. Patients should avoid aerobic exercise for 6 months. Patients with giant cell myocarditis may require transplantation as a definitive therapy.

PERICARDIAL DISEASE

The pericardium consists of two layers: the outer fibrous pericardium and the inner double-layer serous pericardium that consists of the visceral epicardium (covers the heart and great vessels) and the parietal pericardium (covers the fibrous pericardium). The pericardium contains from 15 to 50 mL of plasma ultrafiltrate. Pericardial disease can present itself as pericarditis (acute or chronic recurrent), pericardial effusion (with or without hemodynamic consequences), or constrictive disease (Khandaker et al., 2010).

Pericarditis

Acute pericarditis is an inflammatory process involving the pericardium. It occurs in 0.1% of hospitalized patients and up to 5% of noncoronary chest pain patients presenting to the ED (Spodick, 2003). Acute pericarditis is mostly idiopathic with no identifiable cause. Several factors, however, can cause acute pericarditis, including infectious (bacterial, viral, fungal, parasites, HIV), neoplastic (primary or metastatic), inflammatory, metabolic (uremia, hypothyroidism), traumatic, pharmacologic, and iatrogenic caused by instrumentation and radiation.

Acute pericarditis is diagnosed if at least two of four criteria are met: (1) chest pain characteristic of pericarditis, (2) pericardial rub, (3) characteristic ECG changes, and (4) a new or worsening pericardial effusion. Patients with pericarditis for the first time should be admitted to the hospital for inpatient observation. In multivariable analysis, being female, having large effusion or tamponade, and failure of aspirin or of NSAIDs are predictors of poor outcome in acute pericarditis (Imazio et al., 2007).

The symptoms of pericarditis include sharp retrosternal pain, localized or radiating to the neck, shoulder, or arms, that is made worse with lying down and improves with sitting up. The pain is sharp in nature and is worse with a deep breath. Patients can have associated dyspnea, cough, hiccups, and dysphagia (Hoit, 1991). A pericardial friction rub may be heard in both systole and diastole and is best heard at the left lower sternal border with the diaphragm of the stethoscope.

The ECG typically shows diffuse ST segment elevation that lasts for days followed by T-wave inversions with normal ST segments that then normalizes within 2 weeks. The chest radiograph can show an enlarged heart if a pericardial effusion is present. The echocardiogram confirms typically the presence of the effusion and helps in assessing whether hemodynamic compromise is present. Blood tests generally show an elevation of ESR and possibly cardiac enzymes if myopericarditis is present. Finally, serology is of low yield in the diagnosis of acute pericarditis. Antiviral titers in general will not alter the management of the patient (Permanyer-Miralda, 2004; Zayas, 1995).

The mainstay of treatment of acute pericarditis is NSAIDs for approximately 3 weeks (Maisch et al., 2004). Aspirin is preferred as first-line therapy. If symptoms persist, colchicine (Adler et al., 1998; Imazio et al., 2005) is then recommended for 4 to 6 weeks if the patient has no severe hepatic or renal impairment. Treatment with steroids needs to be avoided unless all other treatments have failed because it is associated with relapse of pericarditis. Steroids may be used as first-line treatment, however, in cases of autoimmune disease or uremic pericarditis (Imazio et al., 2004). Pericardiectomy is reserved for patients with recurrent pericarditis who are unresponsive to aggressive medical treatment. Pericardiectomy, however, may not always eliminate the symptoms of recurrent pericarditis.

Pericardial Effusion

Pericarditis can lead to pericardial effusion and subsequent cardiac tamponade. In this condition, there is an equalization of pressures in the right atrium, left atrium, wedge pressure, and the pulmonary end-diastolic pressure with a blunted or absent y descent on the right atrial tracing. Typically, pulsus paradoxus is present in which there is a more than 10–mm Hg drop in systolic BP with inspiration. Tachycardia is the first compensatory mechanism to increase cardiac output, and when it fails, hypotension occurs. The most common cause of pericardial effusion is malignancies, particularly of the breast and lung, lymphomas, and melanomas. An aortic dissection can cause a hemorrhagic pericardial effusion, and avoiding pericardiocentesis in this case is important to minimize rapid blood loss. Treatment should be disease-specific. For instance, bacterial pericarditis and effusion should be treated with appropriate antibiotics and surgical drainage; myxedematous pericardial effusions respond to thyroid hormone replacement; and uremic pericardial effusion responds to steroids (Hoit, 2002).

When pericardial fluid develops acutely, tamponade physiology can result with less than 150 cc of fluid because the pericardium has not had a chance to expand to accommodate the fluid in the pericardial space, and the intrapericardial pressure rises sharply. Chronic pericardial effusion that has developed slowly, however, can accumulate without hemodynamic compromise with up to 2 to 3 L of fluid. Eventually, the pressure in the pericardial space rises over the intracardiac pressures with subsequent diminished venous return and reduced cardiac output and hypotension. Cardiac tamponade can occur in the setting of a localized effusion, generally postoperatively, or because of gas-producing bacteria (pneumopericardium) after penetrating chest trauma.

The ECG findings in tamponade are low voltage or electrical alternans. Echocardiography can make the diagnosis of tamponade when clinically suspected. Typically, the right-sided chambers of the heart show collapse with an increase in the size of the inferior vena cava. The presence of both right atrial and RV collapse has a positive predictive value of 74% for tamponade physiology (Mercé, 1999). Mitral inflow variability by the Doppler flow is also seen and exceeds 25% with respiration. Fluid in the pericardial space can be identified and its quantity estimated. These echocardiographic findings are reversible after the fluid is removed from the pericardial space.

The preferred treatment of hemodynamically significant tamponade is pericardiocentesis. A needle is directed under local anesthetic into the pericardial space, typically guided by echocardiography, and the fluid is aspirated. In the case of a malignant effusion, a drainage catheter is left in the pericardium for 24 to 48 hours to drain most of the accumulating fluid. Surgical drainage offers an advantage over pericardiocentesis in recurrent pericardial fluid when a complete drainage can be achieved and the creation of a pericardial window prevents reaccumulation of fluid. Fluid removed from the pericardium needs to be sent for detailed analysis, including cell count, chemistries, cultures (bacterial and fungal), and cytology. Pericardial tissue also needs to be sent for pathologic and microbiologic analyses to assist in identifying the etiology of the pericardial fluid.

Chronic Constrictive Pericarditis

Pericarditis can result in a thickened and scarred pericardium that impairs cardiac filling. Patients have a normal systolic function and a small cavity size. The most common etiologies of constrictive pericardial disease are idiopathic, iatrogenic secondary to surgeries and radiation therapies, inflammatory, infectious, and secondary to neoplasms and renal failure.

Patients have high intracardiac filling pressures and pulmonary HTN and complain of dyspnea and fatigue. They display signs of right-sided HF, including hepatosplenomegaly, central venous congestion and ascites, lower extremity edema, and an elevated jugular venous pressure with a deep Y descent. Patients may have a pericardial knock in diastole. Kussmaul sign, a paradoxical rise in venous pressure with inspiration, is also present. When constrictive pericarditis presents acutely, patients will have agitation; tachycardia; or the Beck triad of elevated jugular veins, hypotension, and a small quiet heart. The ECG may display a low QRS voltage and the presence of supraventricular arrhythmias. Pericardial thickening can be seen on CT or MRI and assists in the diagnosis. Pericardial thickening may not be present in almost 18% of patients. As noted earlier, distinguishing between restrictive and constrictive pericardial disease is challenging but very important because constrictive pericardial disease can be effectively treated with pericardiectomy. Cardiac catheterization is an important procedure to help in distinguishing between these two diagnoses.

Patients with mild to moderate symptoms can be treated initially with diuretics and digoxin. A trial of antiinflammatory drugs and possibly steroids has been suggested in patients with acute symptoms before considering surgery, as 15% of these patients could have a reversible course. Pericardiectomy is associated with more than 6% mortality

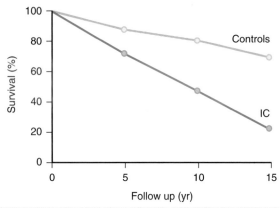

Figure 27-23 Survival of patients with intermittent claudication and matched controls. (Reprinted with permission from the Society of Vascular Surgery. Dormandy JA, Rutherford RB. Management of peripheral arterial disease (PAD). TransAtlantic Inter-Society Consensus (TASC). *J Vasc Surg.* 2000;31(suppl):S1-S296.)

rate, particularly in elderly patients or those with advanced HF, prior radiation treatment, pulmonary HTN, and renal insufficiency (Bertog et al., 2004; DeValeria et al., 1991).

Peripheral Arterial Disease

EPIDEMIOLOGY

Atherosclerotic PAD is an underdiagnosed, undertreated, age-dependent disease that profoundly impacts patient quality of life and is an independent predictor of mortality (Criqui et al., 1992; Nikolsky et al., 2004; Vogt et al., 1993a). On average, the mortality rate of claudicant patients is 2.5 times higher than nonclaudicant patients (Figure 27-23). Atherosclerosis is a ubiquitous process that affects the entire arterial tree in the coronary, cerebral, visceral, and upper and lower extremity. Patients with PAD are at increased risk of cardiovascular and cerebrovascular events, including death, MI, and ischemic stroke. The clinical continuum of PAD ranges from asymptomatic stenosis to limb-threatening ischemia. Intermittent claudication (IC) is defined as ischemic limb pain in one or both legs that occurs with exertion and is alleviated with rest. IC is associated with marked limitations in walking ability, which translates into a considerable negative impact on occupational, social, and leisure activities (Olsen et al., 1988; Regensteiner et al., 1990; Vogt et al., 1994).

Atherosclerosis begins in childhood and evolves over decades (Freedman et al., 1988), affecting more than 85% of adults older than the age of 50 years old (Tuzcu et al., 2001). However, many patients remain entirely asymptomatic; thus, estimating the true prevalence of PAD is difficult and highly dependent on the definition of disease. Most epidemiologic studies only report symptomatic disease; therefore, the true incidence of PAD is not accurately known and is underestimated. In addition, published reports on the incidence and prevalence of PAD vary greatly because the true occurrence of disease is directly related to the risk group of the population studied and the sensitivity and specificity of the diagnostic testing methodology (Criqui et al., 1985).

INTERMITTENT CLAUDICATION

Intermittent claudication is only a symptom of PAD and can be misleading in measuring the prevalence of PAD. For example, a patient with advanced PAD may not have significant IC because of functional decline and inactivity, but someone who is very active may have significant IC even if he or she only has mild disease. Several questionnaires, such as the WHO/Rose Questionnaire, the Edinburgh Claudication Questionnaire, and the Walking Impairment Questionnaire, have been developed to identify patients with IC. The prevalence of IC based on the Rose criteria ranged from 0.4% to 14% of the adult population (Dormandy and Rutherford, 2000). Although these questionnaires are typically highly specific in excluding healthy patients, as assessed by a physician, they are only moderately sensitive in detecting disease. Only approximately one third of patients with PAD have typical symptoms of IC (Schroll and Munck, 1981; Zheng et al., 1997). Furthermore, asymptomatic patients are not at all detected by questionnaire screening. These individuals can only be diagnosed via noninvasive or invasive imaging. Therefore, epidemiologic studies based solely on the use of questionnaires significantly underestimate the true prevalence of disease.

ASYMPTOMATIC DISEASE

More than 50% of patients with PAD are asymptomatic and only identified by noninvasive testing, such as the ABI. Most epidemiologic studies have used a resting ABI less than 0.9 as the criteria for the diagnosis of PAD. However, this definition has several limitations and leads to an underestimation of the true prevalence of disease. For example, this definition will miss mild to moderate disease in patients who have normal resting ABIs but may have a considerable ischemic drop in the ABI with exercise. Furthermore, heavily calcified vessels, particularly in people with diabetes, will have falsely elevated ABIs because of an inability to compress the vessel. Nonetheless, the Systolic Hypertension in the Elderly Program (SHEP) found a prevalence of asymptomatic PAD in 25.5% of 1537 patients (Newman et al., 1993) using a resting ABI less than 0.9 as the diagnostic criterion. The Peripheral Arterial Disease Detection, Awareness and Treatment in Primary Care (PARTNERS) program was a nationwide cross-sectional study that screened patients for PAD in a primary care setting. A total of 6979 patients age 70 years of age or older or age 50 to 69 years old with a history of either diabetes or cigarette smoking were evaluated by history and ABI. The diagnosis of PAD was made based on a resting ABI less than 0.9, a documented medical history of PAD, or a prior lower extremity revascularization. The PARTNERS program found a prevalence of PAD in 29% of patients. However, more concerning is that 83% of patients with a known prior history of PAD were aware of their diagnosis, but only 49% of their physicians were aware of this diagnosis (Hirsch et al., 2001).

CRITICAL LIMB ISCHEMIA

Critical limb ischemia (CLI) is defined by the presence of ischemic resting pain in the distal foot, ischemic nonhealing ulcerations, or gangrene and represents fewer than 10% of patients with PAD (Hiatt, 2001). Although this subset represents the smallest percentage of patients with PAD, these patients have tremendous disease burden and are clearly the highest risk subset for morbidity and mortality, with up to 73% to 95% progressing to limb loss or death at 1 year if left untreated (Wolfe and Wyatt, 1997). Each year, there are approximately 150,000 to 200,000 nontraumatic lower extremity amputations in the United States, and it has been estimated that 85% to 90% of these could be avoided through early revascularization and aggressive risk factor management. Amputation carries a high rate of long-term morbidity and mortality. The fate of those with amputations is poor, particularly in elderly individuals. The level of amputation also dictates the overall prognosis, but two to three times as many below-the-knee (BK) amputees achieve full mobility compared with above-the-knee (AK) amputees, the initial rehabilitation may take up to 9 months. In addition, 5 years after a BK amputation, 30% of patients will have had a major contralateral amputation, 50% will be dead, and only 20% will be alive with one leg intact (Dormandy and Rutherford, 2000).

PATHOPHYSIOLOGY

Peripheral arterial insufficiency is caused by hemodynamically significant narrowing of the arterial lumen usually caused by atherosclerosis, which clinically reduces blood flow to the affected limb. Longitudinal, epidemiologic studies such as the Framingham Heart Study (Murabito et al., 1997) and the INTERHEART (Yusuf et al., 2004) study have defined the risk factors for PAD.

TRADITIONAL RISK FACTORS

Age

The prevalence of PAD increases with age. The incidence of IC in five large population-based studies is four times higher, and the prevalence is eight times higher comparing the 35- to 39-year-old age group with the 70- to 74-year-old age group (Dormandy and Rutherford, 2000).

Smoking

Smoking is a very strong independent risk factor of atherosclerotic PAD. The severity of PAD increases with the number of cigarettes smoked (Cronenwett et al., 1984; Powell et al., 1997) and the amount of exposure to second-hand smoke (Barnoya and Glantz, 2005). In a series of epidemiologic studies, the incidence of developing IC among smokers is approximately two- to threefold higher than nonsmokers (Dormandy and Rutherford, 2000). Smokers develop IC approximately a decade before nonsmokers (Kannel and Shurtleff, 1973), and the association between smoking and PAD may be stronger than the association between smoking and CAD (Fowkes et al., 1992; Kannel et al., 1994). Moreover, smokers are much more likely to progress to CLI than nonsmokers. Smokers with IC have an 11-fold greater amputation rate than nonsmokers (Dormandy et al., 1999).

Smoking cessation slows the progression of disease, improves the symptoms of IC, decreases the likelihood of amputation, improves the patency of revascularization

procedures (Krupski, 1991), and improves overall longevity (Taylor et al., 2002). Finally, all-cause mortality is significantly reduced by smoking cessation but not by smoking reduction (Godtfredsen et al., 2002). It is imperative that patients entirely cease smoking and not just reduce their consumption of tobacco products.

Diabetes

Diabetes or glucose intolerance is one of the most powerful independent modifiable risk factors that contribute to the development of PAD, IC, and CLI (Fowkes et al., 1992; Kannel and McGee, 1979; Murabito et al., 1997). The incidence of IC in patients with diabetes is approximately two times higher than those without diabetes (Dormandy and Rutherford, 2000). Diabetes not only has a significant effect on the larger vessel arterial circulation but also causes microangiopathy as well. Therefore, in conjunction with diabetic peripheral neuropathy, these patients are particularly vulnerable to amputation.

Approximately 60% of all nontraumatic amputations performed in the United States each year are in patients with diabetes (American Diabetes Association Fact Sheet, 2005). A patient with diabetes with PAD has approximately a 10-fold higher amputation rate than a patient without diabetes (Da Silva et al., 1979). There does not appear to be any significant difference in microvascular or macrovascular comorbidity between type 1 and type 2 diabetes (Zander et al., 2002). However, there is a dose-response relationship between the HgbA$_{1C}$ level and the risk of amputation (Lehto et al., 1996). Therefore, patients with diabetes should be aggressively treated to normalize glycemic control. In addition, patients with diabetes should be instructed on good foot care, such as properly fitting shoes and foot hygiene, to avoid skin breakdown and ulcer formation.

Hyperlipidemia

As in CAD, LDL-C and triglyceride levels are directly related, but HDL-C levels are indirectly related to the progression of PAD, and the observed risk seems to demonstrate a linear relationship (Fowkes et al., 1992; Murabito et al., 2002). The majority of the data on lipid-lowering therapy is in patients with CAD. However, several studies have specifically demonstrated an improvement in the relative risk of an abnormal ABI, walking distance on a treadmill, frequency and severity of claudication, and limb loss (Blankenhorn et al., 1991; Buchwald et al., 1996; Mohler et al., 2003; Pedersen et al., 1998), suggesting that all patients with PAD should be treated with statin therapy irrespective of baseline LDL-C.

Hypertension

Hypertension is a major risk factor for PAD and carries a 2.5-fold age-adjusted risk for men and a 3.9-fold age-adjusted risk for women (Kannel and McGee, 1985; Murabito et al., 1997). There have been concerns, based on early case reports, that β-blockade therapy may worsen the symptoms of IC. A meta-analysis on this subject and critical review of these studies concluded that β-blockers are safe and do not worsen IC (Radack and Deck, 1991). ACE inhibitors may offer significant benefits for the prevention of atherosclerotic vascular disease beyond that expected from a reduction in BP alone (Fox, 2003; The Heart Outcomes Prevention Evaluation Study Investigators, 2000). However, there remains considerable debate as to whether or not the data from the HOPE study and the EUROPA study can be generalized to all ACE inhibitors.

Gender

The initial data from Framingham suggested that men develop IC approximately 10 years before women (Kannel et al., 1970). More recent data do not support this observation (Hirsch et al., 2001; Murabito et al., 2003; Reunanen et al., 1982). In light of these data, patients should be screened for PAD regardless of gender.

Obesity

Obesity, as measured by an increased BMI greater than 30, has long been recognized as a risk factor for atherosclerotic disease. It is now recognized that adipocytes, particularly visceral adipocytes, contribute to a pro-inflammatory state by generating a variety of cytokines such as IL-6, TNF-α, and CRP, which play a direct role in the development of atherosclerosis (Hansson, 2005). This theory is further supported by the fact that liposuction does not seem to lower risk for CAD because liposuction reduces subcutaneous fat mass but has no effect on reducing visceral fat mass (Klein et al., 2004).

NONTRADITIONAL RISK FACTORS

High-Sensitivity C-Reactive Protein

Atherosclerosis is a disease of chronic low-grade inflammation. hsCRP is a nonspecific marker of inflammation that is emerging as a simple yet powerful marker of atherosclerotic risk. Prospective data from the Physicians' Health Study demonstrate that baseline levels of hsCRP independently predict a future risk of developing symptomatic PAD (Ridker et al., 1998).

Lipoprotein(a)

Lipoprotein(a) [Lp(a)] is an atherogenic subspecies of LDL that is covalently linked to apoprotein(a). Apo(a) is homologous to plasminogen. Lp(a) may exacerbate risk for ACS by inhibiting endogenous fibrinolysis (Hajjar et al., 1989). Furthermore, Lp(a) may augment the release of endothelial PAI-1, which further impairs fibrinolysis (Etingin et al., 1991). The net result is that Lp(a) contributes to atherogenesis and a prothrombotic or hypercoagulable state.

Lipoprotein(a) has been implicated as an independent predictor of PAD (Cheng et al., 1997; Prior et al., 1995); however, many of these studies are cross-sectional or retrospective and cannot establish causal relationships between risk factors and disease. Prospective data from the Physicians' Health Study did not show a significant relationship in baseline Lp(a) levels and the future development of PAD (Ridker et al., 2001). Widespread screening of Lp(a) levels in the general population is not recommended. However, this should be considered in patients who present with premature vascular disease and few or no traditional risk factors. Niacin can modestly reduce Lp(a) levels. There is no clinical trial evidence to prove that reducing serum levels of Lp(a) reduces risk for the development or progression of PAD.

Fibrinogen

Fibrinogen has been implicated in atherogenesis by early epidemiologic studies (Kannel et al., 1987). However, fibrinogen is an acute phase reactant, and there is considerable intrapatient variability in its expression over time. Other markers of inflammation, such as hsCRP, have a more powerful association in predicting PAD. Furthermore, fibrinogen levels are directly related to age, obesity, cigarette smoking, diabetes, and LDL-C and inversely related to HDL-C, physical activity, alcohol use, and estrogen levels. There is controversy regarding the independent predictive value of hyperfibrinogenemia. Therefore, routine fibrinogen level screening is not recommended unless there is suspicion of a hypercoagulable state.

NATURAL HISTORY OF DISEASE

Atherosclerosis is an age-dependent disease that begins in childhood and progresses throughout adulthood, particularly if the risk factors are left unchecked. Yet early studies suggested that PAD led a contrary, benign course that was not progressive (Imparato et al., 1975; McAllister, 1976). However, in most of these studies, IC was used as an end point rather than ABI or even a patient functional assessment. IC is a relatively insensitive marker of PAD. Those studies typically reported a stabilization or improvement in IC over time, which does not necessarily indicate stabilization or improvement in the disease process, ability to ambulate, or functional status. Early authors suggested that relief of IC over time was a sign of improved collateral flow, yet to experience IC, a patient must be physically active. McDermott et al. (2004) demonstrated that the stabilization or improvement of IC was strongly related to functional decline (i.e., patients walked at a slower pace and for shorter distances to avoid experiencing IC). Thus, PAD is a progressive disorder that leads to a significant decline in quality of life.

COEXISTING VASCULAR DISEASE

The most important fact regarding the diagnosis and management of PAD is that PAD is a powerful, independent predictor of mortality (Criqui et al., 1992). IC and CLI can have a significant impact on quality of life. Many patients may accept their physical limitations as a consequence of aging and tolerate this morbidity. Fewer than 5% of patients with IC will ever progress to amputation. Much more significant, however, is that PAD is a systemic disorder, and it has considerable overlap with CAD and cerebrovascular disease, ultimately leading to an increase in mortality. Approximately 40% of patients with atherosclerotic vascular disease manifest symptoms in more than one vascular bed (Figure 27-24) (Ness and Aronow, 1999). Compared with people without PAD, patients with PAD have an approximately fourfold higher likelihood of having an MI (Criqui et al., 1992), and a two- to threefold higher likelihood of having a stroke (Wilterdink and Easton, 1992). The all-cause mortality rate in patients with PAD is approximately equal between men and women and is elevated even in asymptomatic patients (Hiatt, 2001). The lower the ABI is, the greater the risk for cardiovascular events. Patients with CLI, who typically have the lowest ABIs, have an annual

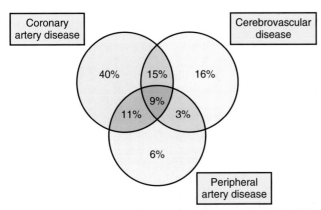

Figure 27-24 Overlap of atherosclerotic disease. Patients often manifest symptoms in more than one vascular bed. (Modified from Ness J, Aronow WS. Prevalence of coexistence of coronary artery disease, ischemic stroke, and peripheral arterial disease in older persons, mean age 80 years, in an academic hospital-based geriatrics practice. *J Am Geriatr Soc.* 1999;47:1255-1258.)

mortality rate of 25% (Dormandy et al., 1999; McKenna et al., 1991; Vogt et al., 1993b).

DIAGNOSIS

A thorough history and physical examination can accurately suggest a diagnosis of PAD 80% to 90% of the time.

History

The vast majority of disorders related to the peripheral vascular system are (1) atherosclerosis involving the arterial tree or (2) thrombophlebitis involving the venous circulation, both predominantly affecting the lower extremities more so than the upper extremities or viscera. Patients with suspected vascular disease typically present for evaluation with (1) varying types of limb pain or discomfort, (2) ulcerations or gangrene of the extremities, or (3) swelling of the affected limb.

The majority of limb pain or discomfort typically falls into three etiologies: (1) vascular, (2) musculoskeletal, or (3) neuropathic. The majority of limb swelling is caused by (1) venous obstruction or insufficiency; (2) increased venous pressure, such as HF; (3) decreased oncotic pressure, such as hypoproteinemia or hypoalbuminemia; (4) lymphedema; or (5) lipoedema. Many patients, particularly elderly patients, have multifactorial etiologies of pain or swelling, which can usually be distinguished by a thorough history and physical examination. Using a systematic approach with key pointed questions, a presumptive diagnosis can often be deduced on clinical grounds and subsequently confirmed with noninvasive testing. The history should focus on identifying risk factors for atherosclerosis. The past medical history should concentrate on prior vascular events such as MI; stroke; amputation; deep vein thrombosis; and revascularizations in any vascular bed, either percutaneously or surgically, as well as, but not limited to, a history of HF; back problems; osteoarthritis; inflammatory conditions such as rheumatoid arthritis, plantar fasciitis, or polymyalgia rheumatica; gout; varicose veins; and lymphatic obstruction, such as that after surgery or radiation therapy.

The cause of leg pain can be determined by the characteristics, severity, location, duration, frequency, and precipitating or alleviating factors of the discomfort. Claudication is typically described as a cramping or aching discomfort in the muscle associated with exertion and alleviated with rest. Most often this occurs in the calf, but it can also occur in the hip and buttocks if there is occlusive disease in the aortoiliac segment. Nocturnal cramping of the calf and foot is not typically vascular in etiology and is most likely caused by an exaggerated neuromuscular response to stretch that occurs while sleeping.

Critical limb ischemia can cause resting pain that is constant throughout the day and night. Nocturnal pain from CLI is a moderate to severe aching paresthesia or dysesthesia while lying horizontal that is alleviated by dangling the leg over the side of the bed. Pain from CLI can be so severe that it may not be relieved by narcotic analgesia. On the other hand, patients with diabetes with severe peripheral neuropathy may be completely insensate despite significant tissue loss. Distinguishing the etiology of constant resting limb pain between a vascular and nonvascular etiology can be done by physical examination and noninvasive testing. Pain that occurs at rest may be caused by CLI if there are other findings in the history and physical examination that support the diagnosis of advanced atherosclerosis. Otherwise, pain that occurs at rest, with change in position, or simply standing without exertion is more typically musculoskeletal or neuropathic in nature. Tables 27-22 and 27-23 list the distinguishing features and differential diagnosis of the most common types of leg pain and swelling, respectively.

For example, acute loss of motor or sensory function in the distal extremities, particularly with associated acute severe pain, pallor, and coolness of the limb, is a sign of acute arterial occlusion. However, chronic motor or sensory loss may be vascular in etiology but more likely is neuropathic. Several standardized classification schemes exist for categorizing the severity of both acute and chronic limb ischemia. Table 27-24 is the revised Rutherford-Becker classification for acute limb ischemia and Table 27-25 is the combined Fontaine classification, which is more popular in Europe, and the Rutherford-Becker scheme for chronic limb ischemia (Dormandy and Rutherford, 2000; Rutherford et al., 1997).

Physical Examination

The physical examination in patients with PAD should consist of inspection, palpation, auscultation, and even percussion. Observations should note any asymmetry between the limbs, joint deformities, varicose veins, skin discoloration, absence of hair, swelling, ulcerations, tissue loss, and gangrene. Acute CLI from embolism or thrombosis typically causes pallor with decreased capillary refill that eventually leads to mottling unless adequate collateral flow can be recruited. Patients with chronic ischemia may have a normal skin color with relatively normal or slightly delayed capillary refill, particularly if collateral flow has developed. Chronic advanced CLI can lead to dependent rubor caused by chronic dilation of the postcapillary venules. The toes of the dependent limbs can become red with brisk capillary refill. This is often mistaken for hyperemia rather than a sign of severe ischemia. A cadaveric pallor on elevating the

Table 27-22 Differential Diagnosis of Claudication

Diagnosis	Location of Discomfort	Characteristic of Discomfort	Onset Relative to Exertion	Onset Relative to Standing	Effect of Rest	Effect of Body Position	Miscellaneous Characteristics
Arterial claudication	Depends on level of stenosis or occlusion: aortoiliac disease affects hip, thigh, or buttock or can affect the entire limb; infrainguinal disease affects the calf and foot	Aching, cramping, weakness	Consistently reproduced with same degree of activity	Unrelated to standing	Relieved promptly	None	Gradual onset of discomfort with exercise Very reproducible
Venous claudication	Entire limb; usually worse in thigh and groin	Tight, tense sensation	After exercise	Unrelated to standing	Relieved slowly	Relieved more quickly with elevation	History of DVT, edema, or venous congestion
Chronic critical limb ischemia	Always involves foot; symptoms may be more proximal with more proximal disease	Severe burning, aching but may be asymptomatic in patients with profound neuropathy	Worse with minimal activity	Unrelated to standing	Improved but incompletely	Symptoms may be improved with dangling foot over side of bed while sleeping	Gradual or subacute onset Dependent rubor Elevation pallor Gangrene
Acute critical limb ischemia	Always involves foot; symptoms may be more proximal with more proximal disease	Severe aching, cramping, painful	Worse with minimal activity	Unrelated to standing	Improved but incompletely	Symptoms may be improved with dangling foot over side of bed while sleeping	Acute onset Pale, cold Loss of motor or sensory function is an emergency
Arthritis	Joints	Aching; may be sharp with position change	Variable	Weight bearing reproduces pain	Variable; may be present at rest	Less pain in non–weight-bearing position	Variable; may be related to weather May have effusion
Lumbar back pain (e.g., herniated disc, nerve root compression)	Lumbar region; may radiate down dermatomes if there is nerve root compression	Sharp, stabbing, shooting	Immediate	Weight bearing reproduces pain	Variable; may be present at rest	Certain positions exacerbate or alleviate pain	History of back problems Worse with lifting May have motor or sensory deficits Reproducible with percussion
Sacroiliitis	Sacroiliac region	Sharp, stabbing, shooting	Immediate	Weight bearing reproduces pain	Variable; may be present at rest	Certain positions exacerbate or alleviate pain	Inflammatory disorder Reproducible with palpation
Plantar fasciitis	Plantar region	Sharp, stabbing, searing	Immediate	Weight bearing reproduces pain	Immediate relief with non–weight bearing	Less pain in non–weight-bearing position	Reproducible with palpation
Peripheral neuropathy	Stocking glove distribution	Paresthesia, dysesthesia; may be quite severe	Unrelated to activity	Unrelated to standing	Usually a constant sensation, unrelated to rest	Unrelated to change in position	Common in people with diabetes Present 24 hr a day; may interrupt sleep
Myopathy	In the muscle groups, may be systemic	Dull, aching, weakness	Immediate	Variable	Improved with less physical activity	May exacerbate discomfort	Reproducible with palpation Statin myopathy common Inflammatory disorders are rare

DVT, Deep vein thrombosis.

Table 27-23 Differential Diagnosis of Chronic Leg Swelling

Clinical Feature	Venous	Lymphatic	Cardiac Orthostatic	"Lipedema"
Consistency of swelling	Brawny	Spongy	Pitting	Noncompressible (fat)
Relief by elevation	Complete	Mild	Complete	Minimal
Distribution of swelling	Maximal in ankles and legs; feet spared	Diffuse; greatest distally	Diffuse; greatest distally	Maximal in ankles and legs; feet spared
Associated skin changes	Atrophic and pigmented, subcutaneous fibrosis	Hypertrophic, lichenified skin	Shiny, mild pigmentation, no trophic changes	None
Pain	Heavy, ache, tight or bursting	None or heavy ache	Little or none	Dull ache, cutaneous sensitivity
Bilaterality	Occasionally but usually unequal	Occasionally but usually unequal	Always but may be unequal	Always

From Rutherford RB: Basic approaches to vascular problems. In Rutherford RB, editor: *Vascular surgery*, vol 1, ed 5, Philadelphia, 2000, WB Saunders Company, pp 1–13.

Table 27-24 Clinical Categories of Acute Limb Ischemia

		Findings		Doppler Signals	
Category	Description and Prognosis	Sensory Loss	Motor Weakness	Arterial	Venous
I. Viable	Not immediately threatened	None	None	Audible	Audible
II. Threatened					
a. Marginally	Salvageable if promptly treated	Minimal (toes) or none	None	Inaudible	Audible
b. Immediately	Salvageable with immediate revascularization	More than toes; associated with rest pain	Mild, moderate	Inaudible	Audible
III. Irreversible	Major tissue loss or permanent nerve damage inevitable	Profound, anesthetic	Profound, paralysis (rigor)	Inaudible	Inaudible

From Rutherford RB, Baker JD, Ernst C, et al. Recommended standards for reports dealing with lower extremity ischemia: revised version. *J Vasc Surg.* 1997;26:517-538, Table 1. Reprinted with permission from The Society of Vascular Surgery.

Table 27-25 Clinical Categories of Chronic Limb Ischemia: Fontaine's Stages and Rutherford's Categories

Fontaine		Rutherford		
Stage	Clinical	Grade	Category	Clinical
I	Asymptomatic	0	0	Asymptomatic
IIa	Mild claudication	I	1	Mild claudication
IIb	Moderate to severe claudication	I	2	Moderate claudication
		I	3	Severe claudication
III	Ischemic rest pain	II	4	Ischemic rest pain
		III	5	Minor tissue loss
IV	Ulceration or gangrene	III	6	Major tissue loss

From Dormandy JA, Rutherford RB. Management of peripheral arterial disease (PAD). TransAtlantic InterSociety Consensus (TASC). *J Vasc Surg.* 2000;31(suppl):S1-S296, Table 9. Reprinted with permission from The Society of Vascular Surgery.

limb to greater than 45 degrees above the horizontal for 1 to 2 minutes followed by slow venous filling with rubor after returning to a dependent position (Buerger sign) is also a sign of advanced CLI.

Ulcerations may be caused by chronic venous insufficiency or edema or arterial insufficiency. Chronic venous disease typically causes pigmentation of the lower legs due to extravasation of red blood cells with superficial ulcers in the calves, more often medially than laterally. Arterial ulcerations are characteristically distal, involving the toes and even forefoot in advanced disease.

Palpation of the pedal pulses should be a mandatory part of the routine physical examination. It should be noted that even in healthy individuals, the dorsalis pedis (DP) pulse, the posterior tibial (PT) pulse, or both are unable to be palpated 8.1%, 2.9%, and 0.7% of the time, respectively (McGee and Boyko, 1998). This is because of normal anatomic variations. Wide and prominent femoral or popliteal pulses may be a sign of an aneurysm. A significant temperature gradient from proximal to distal and between ipsilateral and contralateral limbs often is a sign of advanced disease. The abdomen should be palpated to assess for the presence of an abdominal aortic aneurysm (AAA). Reproduction of pain with palpation over joints is not due to vascular disease and is thought to be a sign of such orthopedic conditions as degenerative joint disease, sacroiliitis, gout, trauma, or plantar fasciitis. Reproduction of pain with palpation of muscle groups may be vascular in etiology if there is severe ischemia, but one should also consider other causes of myopathy such as fibromyalgia, polymyalgia rheumatica, drug-induced myalgia, and trauma.

The carotid arteries, abdomen, and femoral arteries should be auscultated for bruits. Only gentle pressure should be applied with the stethoscope over the carotid and femoral arteries because pseudobruits can be created by compression of the underlying vessel. Finally, percussion over the lumbar spine may be useful in eliciting pain caused by sacroiliitis, lumbar disk disease, or nerve root compression.

Noninvasive Testing

Noninvasive vascular testing is useful to confirm clinical suspicion of PAD in patients with leg discomfort or screen asymptomatic patients who are at risk for vascular disease, particularly individuals with diabetes. Noninvasive testing is also very helpful for the surveillance of vessel patency after percutaneous or surgical intervention.

Noninvasive Vascular Study. A complete noninvasive vascular study (NIVS) consists of the ABI, segmental BPs, and pulse-volume recordings (PVRs) obtained at rest. When physically possible, the ABIs should also be ordered with exercise to assess for an ischemic response. A normal NIVS is shown in Figure 27-25.

The ABI is defined as the highest SBP of either the DP artery or PT artery divided by the higher of the SBP from either the right or left brachial artery. Segmental BPs provide more specific information as to the location of the stenosis or obstruction. BP readings are obtained at the high thigh, low thigh, calf, ankle, metatarsal, and toe level, specifically looking for pressure gradients proximally to distally. PVRs are plethysmographic measurements that detect changes in the blood volume flowing through the limb. A normal PVR tracing resembles a normal arterial pulse wave tracing with a rapid upstroke, prominent dicrotic notch, and rapid down stroke. As the severity of the disease increases, the waveforms become more blunted, the dicrotic notch disappears, and ultimately the waveforms become flat.

The standard exercise protocol of Rutherford (walking on a treadmill for 5 minutes at 2 mph at a 12% grade) (Rutherford et al., 1997) is quite modest compared with the workload involved in a routine Bruce protocol that is typically used for cardiac stress testing. The purpose of the Rutherford protocol is not to induce coronary ischemia and thus is typically well tolerated from a cardiopulmonary standpoint. Relative contraindications to walking on a treadmill include severe symptomatic CAD (i.e., Canadian Cardiovascular Society class 3 or 4), severe decompensated CHF (i.e., New York Heart Association class 3 or 4), severe symptomatic COPD, orthopedic or balance disorders that preclude safe ambulation on a treadmill, or severely depressed resting ABIs (i.e., ABI < 0.5). If patients are unable to walk on a treadmill, then other means of exercise may suffice, such as stationary bicycling, walking in the hallway, or toe lifts. However, these alternative forms of exercise are not standardized and may impact the diagnostic sensitivity and specificity of the study.

Commonly, patients with mild PAD may have an ABI that is actually normal at rest yet may be significantly decreased with exercise, as shown in Figure 27-26. In fact, comparing angiography, which is the gold standard for diagnosing PAD, with ABIs, there actually needs to be a rather severe single stenosis or moderate diffuse multilevel disease to have a depression in the resting ABI. Even a mildly depressed resting ABI implies that there is a considerable burden of disease. Therefore, ABIs that are done at rest only and not

with exercise will have a relatively high false-negative rate, and many patients with a normal resting ABI will be misdiagnosed as having nonvascular limb pain when indeed the true etiology of their discomfort is PAD. A corollary to this is that many epidemiologic studies use only resting ABIs as a diagnostic criteria for PAD, which leads to underestimation of the true incidence of PAD. It should be noted, however, that a recent update of the 2005 U.S. Preventive Services Task Force (USPSTF) recommendation on screening for PAD concluded that the current evidence does not support the use of resting ABI as a sole screening method in asymptomatic, unselected patients with no known PAD, CAD, severe CKD, or diabetes (Moyer, 2013).

Another potential pitfall of ABIs is vascular calcification. Severe calcification of the arterial wall eventually leads to an inability to compress the blood vessels despite cuffs inflated to suprasystolic pressures. Consequently, ABIs can be falsely elevated, and caution should be used in interpreting an ABI greater than 1.4. This is particularly common in patients with diabetes and patients on chronic hemodialysis. In this instance, the toe-brachial index has been established as an adequate surrogate to the ABI (Sahli et al., 2004).

A NIVS can provide a general region (e.g., the femoropopliteal segment) that is diseased. Yet a NIVS is not precise enough to determine the exact location of the stenosis or occlusion. In other words, a NIVS provides physiologic information with limited anatomic localization of disease. Arterial duplex Doppler ultrasonography, computed tomography angiography (CTA), and magnetic resonance angiography (MRA) are studies that are more suited to proved detailed anatomic information and complement the data obtained with a NIVS.

Doppler Ultrasonography. Arterial duplex Doppler ultrasonography uses high-frequency sound waves, typically in the 5.0- to 7.5-MHz range, to provide real-time vascular images that can accurately localize atherosclerotic disease. Color-flow encoding is useful to quickly localize vessels and determine the presence or absence of blood flow. Doppler technology uses the physical principles of the reflected sound wave frequency in relation to the transmitted frequency to determine the velocity of blood flow. As the severity of stenosis increases, the PSV of flow increases. By using established criteria of the absolute PSV and the ratio of PSV in the proximal normal reference segment compared with the PSV in the diseased segment, the overall range of stenosis can be determined. A peak systolic velocity ratio (PSVR) of 2.4 or higher is considered indicative of obstructive disease. A PSVR of 3.0 or higher is likely to indicate functionally significant obstruction.

Ultrasonography is particularly useful for assessing stent or graft patency after a revascularization procedure. Potential pitfalls of ultrasonography include visualizing the tibial vessels, which are relatively small and deep in the calf, as well as visualizing highly calcified vessels, which are acoustically shadowed by the calcium.

Computed Tomography and Magnetic Resonance Angiography. Computed tomographic angiography (CTA) and MRA are noninvasive imaging modalities that have essentially replaced traditional invasive diagnostic

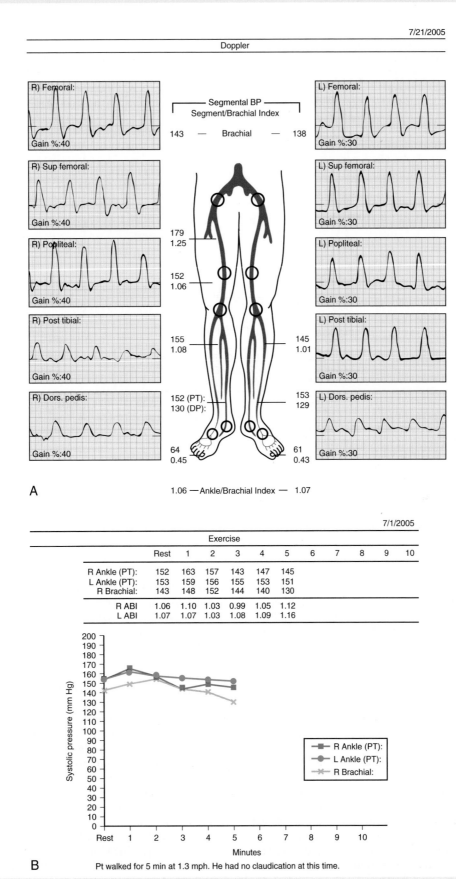

Figure 27-25 A, Normal pulse volume recording demonstrates triphasic waveforms with normal segmental pressures. No pressures were obtained in the left thigh because of previously placed stent. **B,** Normal ankle-brachial indexes at rest, with a normal response to exercise. The *red lines* and *green lines* are essentially flat throughout exercise.

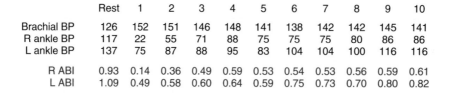

	Rest	1	2	3	4	5	6	7	8	9	10
Brachial BP	126	152	151	146	148	141	138	142	142	145	141
R ankle BP	117	22	55	71	88	75	75	75	80	86	86
L ankle BP	137	75	87	88	95	83	104	104	100	116	116
R ABI	0.93	0.14	0.36	0.49	0.59	0.53	0.54	0.53	0.56	0.59	0.61
L ABI	1.09	0.49	0.58	0.60	0.64	0.59	0.75	0.73	0.70	0.80	0.82

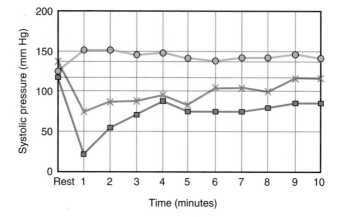

■ = R ankle BP ISCHEMIC WINDOW; 444
X = L ankle BP ISCHEMIC WINDOW; 393
◉ = Brachial BP

Figure 27-26 Normal noninvasive vascular study at rest. The right ankle-brachial index (ABI) is 0.93, and the left ABI is 1.09. However, there is a marked ischemic response to exercise. Note the pronounced drop of the *red* and *blue lines* with exercise and the severe drop of the right ABI to 0.14 and the left ABI to 0.49. This patient had bilateral, focal, 95% to 99% stenoses in the superficial femoral arteries, which were successfully stented. This example clearly demonstrates the importance of obtaining ABIs at rest and with exercise. Failure to obtain ABIs with exercise, particularly when the resting values are normal, often fails to diagnose the disease. *BP,* Blood pressure.

angiography. Both CTA and MRA produce similarly accurate anatomic information and provide highly detailed images that can be used to plan revascularization procedures, assess the size and location of aneurysms, and occasionally find incidental pathology such as occult malignancy. These two technologies are fundamentally very different.

Traditional CT has evolved by the addition of multiple detectors, now up to 320 slices per machine. Multidetector CT allows much shorter acquisition times and submillimeter resolution; thus, an entire body scan can be performed in seconds to minutes with excellent spatial resolution. By adding three-dimensional reconstruction software, the bone, soft tissue, and organs can be virtually removed and the vasculature reconstructed and viewed from multiple projections. An example of a normal and abnormal CTA is shown in Figure 27-27.

CTA uses ionizing radiation and iodinated contrast. Therefore, multiple scans (because of accumulative radiation dose) and renal insufficiency are relative contraindications to CTA. Other limitations in CTA imaging include severe vascular calcifications and prosthetic joints, which cause scatter artifact. The lumen of a stented vessel can be visualized with CTA, although there will be a mild to moderate degree of scatter artifact that makes accurate assessment of in-stent restenosis difficult.

Traditional MRI has also evolved through the development of more powerful magnets and improved scanning algorithms. Similar to CTA, MRA can produce

submillimeter spatial resolution. In contrast to CTA, the scanning time for MRA can be up to 1 hour per patient. In a busy practice or hospital, this can lead to problems with patient throughput. Software can also reconstruct MRA images into three dimensions.

MRA uses magnetic fields and variable frequency radiowaves to detect changes in alignment and distribution of protons in a given tissue. The obvious advantage over CTA is that MRA does not use ionizing radiation or iodinated contrast. Thus, there is practically no risk of stochastic injury or iodine contrast nephropathy. However, MRA often uses gadolinium-based contrast, a paramagnetic metal ion, to provide an improved image of body organs, tissues, and blood vessels. Nephrogenic systemic fibrosis has been reported with gadolinium-based contrast, which is listed as a boxed warning to the label of these agents. Although gadolinium is not FDA approved for MRA (only approved for MRI), it is often used by radiologists for better visualization of the blood vessels. MRA can be performed without gadolinium, and the ordering provider may want to specify avoiding this contrast, particularly in patients with renal insufficiency. Patients with pacemakers or defibrillators cannot undergo MRA because the magnet can interfere with device function. Recently, MRA-compatible pacemakers have become available. Finally, severely calcified vessels can be adequately imaged with MRA, but stents appear as voids and thus falsely give the impression of a totally occluded artery even if the stent is widely patent.

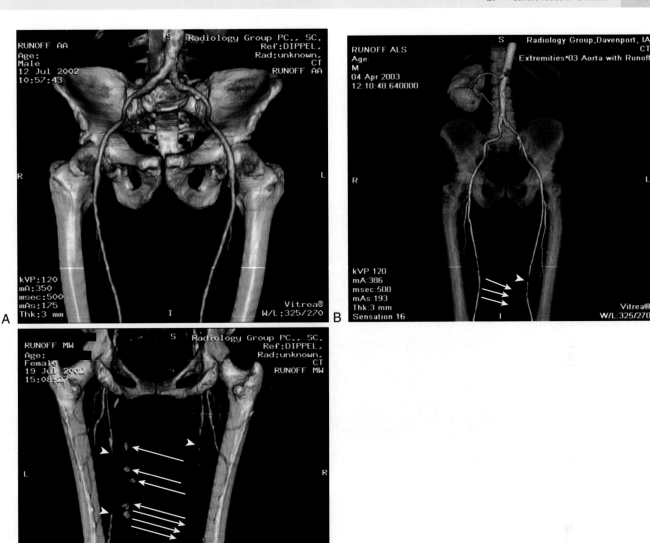

Figure 27-27 A, Anteroposterior (AP) view of a multidetector computed tomography angiogram (CTA) reconstructed with three-dimensional imaging software. This image shows the distal aorta, iliac arteries, common femoral arteries, and proximal superficial femoral arteries. There are minimal plaques in the distal aorta, common iliac arteries, and superficial femoral arteries. **B,** AP view of a multidetector CTA demonstrating a short total occlusion of the distal left superficial femoral artery *(arrowhead)*. Note surgical clips from prior saphenous vein harvest *(arrows)*. Note absence of the left kidney. **C,** Posterior view of a multidetector CTA demonstrating a long total occlusion of superficial femoral arteries (between *arrowheads*). These were successfully stented. Again, note vascular clips from prior saphenous vein harvest *(arrows)*.

The false-positive rate for detecting a hemodynamically significant stenosis is considerably higher with MRA than CTA. With CTA, the lumen of the vessel that is visualized is essentially a column of contrast; thus, a precise assessment of the degree of stenosis is usually possible. However, MRA technology requires flow through the vessel to determine where the lumen exists. The pitfall occurs when the vessel runs through the same plane as the frequency of the radiowave. This leads to flow voids, which appear as gaps in the vessel and are frequently overdiagnosed as stenoses. This phenomenon is particularly common at the origin of the renal arteries and throughout the tortuosity of the carotid arteries.

Invasive Imaging

Traditional invasive diagnostic angiography has been the gold standard for diagnosing PAD since the 1950s. This technique involves the percutaneous placement of catheters within the vessel, injecting iodinated contrast through the catheters, and recording fluoroscopic and cineographic images. Similar to CTA, conventional angiography uses ionizing radiation, and the same relative risks apply. The potential complications include vascular access site injury, pseudoaneurysm or arteriovenous fistula formation, bleeding, dissection, and atheroembolization. For these reasons, angiography is mostly reserved for patients in whom a revascularization procedure is anticipated.

THERAPY

Therapy for PAD should involve a patient care plan consisting of (1) patient education as to the pathophysiology of atherosclerosis, the risk factors that contribute to the disease, and the prognosis of the condition; (2) encouragement of lifestyle changes that emphasize risk factor modification and routine exercise; (3) pharmacologic therapy both for the relief of symptoms and treatment of risk factors; and (4) revascularization procedures to relieve IC and limb salvage in the case of CLI. The goals of therapy are to (1) improve the patient's functional status by relieving symptoms, improving the quality of life, and improving exercise capacity; (2) preserve the limb via revascularization and decrease or limit the extent of amputation; (3) prevent the progression of atherosclerosis by aggressive risk factor modification; and (4) reduce cardiovascular and cerebrovascular mortality and nonfatal events such as MI and stroke.

Risk Factor Management

The most important therapy for prevention of PAD is aggressive management of the risk factors for atherosclerosis. Both the AHA and the NCEP recommend the same level of risk factor modification in patients with PAD as in patients with known CAD (Grundy et al., 2004c; Smith et al., 2001). Despite the growing recognition that PAD is associated with a higher mortality rate, the risk factors in patients with PAD have historically been grossly undertreated. This is exemplified by data from Rehring et al. (2005), who reported on a cohort of 1733 patients with known PAD and no overt CAD. Of these patients, only 33.1% were receiving β-blockade therapy, 28.9% were receiving ACE inhibitors, and 31.3% were treated with a statin. Furthermore, 92% had a recent BP measurement, but 56% had a SBP greater than 130 mm Hg, 45.5% had a DBP greater than 80 mm Hg, and 13.6% had a DBP greater than 90 mm Hg. In addition, only 62.6% had a screening lipid profile, yet 56% had an LDL-C greater than 100 mg/dL and 21% had an LDL-C greater than 130 mg/dL. Finally, in patients with diabetes, HbA_{1c} was greater than 7.0% in 54.2% of patients (Rehring et al., 2005). Current practice patterns should markedly improve on these statistics. The risk factors of atherosclerosis must be aggressively identified and treated to reduce the risk for disease progression.

Exercise

Routine aerobic exercise is recommended for all patients with PAD. The benefit of walking programs has been clearly established to increase time to claudication and maximal walking distance (Hiatt and Regensteiner, 1990; Hiatt et al., 1994). Regular exercise has a strong impact on improving functional capacity and quality of life. A minimum of 30 to 45 minutes of exercise is recommended preferably daily but at least three times per week. This should be supplemented by an increase in daily lifestyle activities, such as walking breaks at lunch, gardening, or household chores (Smith et al., 2001).

Weight Management

Obesity is at epidemic levels, which ultimately contributes to the progression of atherosclerosis. Patients should be counseled on weight loss strategies with a target BMI of 18.5 to 24.9 kg/m^2 (Smith et al., 2001).

Pharmacologic Therapy

Pharmacologic treatment can be divided into two separate but important components: (1) therapy for the control of risk factors and (2) therapy for the relief of symptoms of ischemia or claudication.

Pharmacologic therapy for risk factor modification is the same as for any other forms of atherosclerotic vascular disease, such as coronary or cerebrovascular disease. The most important thing to keep in mind is that the mortality rate of patients with PAD is high; thus, these patients should be treated aggressively. Current national guidelines exist and should be adhered to for the primary and secondary prevention of atherosclerotic vascular disease (American Diabetes Association, 2005; Grundy et al., 2004c; The Seventh Report, 2004; Smith et al., 2001). The four primary categories of pharmacologic therapy are (1) antiplatelet therapy, (2) lipid-lowering therapy, (3) antihypertensive therapy, and (4) glycemic control. Specific therapies and therapeutic targets are listed elsewhere in this chapter. It should be kept in mind that these therapies are complementary and confer additive benefit. From a practical standpoint, patients with several comorbidities can end up taking multiple medications a day, and thus to ensure compliance, the patients should be repeatedly educated as to the importance of risk factor control.

The only FDA-approved pharmacologic therapy that has a consensus of benefit for the relief of claudication is cilostazol. Cilostazol is a phosphodiesterase III inhibitor, which increases the intracellular concentration of cAMP (cyclic adenosine monophosphate), leading to significant antiplatelet and vasodilatory properties and possibly antiproliferative properties (Tsuchikane et al., 1999). Cilostazol undergoes extensive metabolism by the hepatic cytochrome $P450_{3A4}$ (CYP3A4) isoform enzyme and to a lesser extent the 2C19 and 1A2 isoforms. Although cilostazol does not inhibit the CYP450 system, drugs that inhibit CYP3A4, CYP2C19, and CYP1A2 can lead to increased levels of cilostazol in serum.

Pentoxifylline is another drug that was approved by the FDA for claudication in 1984. However, no randomized data demonstrate it to be any better than placebo. Therefore, there is no recommendation to use this agent for the treatment of claudication.

There have been eight randomized trials comparing cilostazol with placebo and pentoxifylline (Smith, 2002). In all eight studies, cilostazol demonstrated a statistically significant improvement in objective and subjective end points compared with placebo. In one study comparing cilostazol 100 mg twice a day with pentoxifylline 400 mg three times a day or placebo, the maximal walking distance on a treadmill increased by 54% from baseline in the cilostazol group compared with a 30% increase in the pentoxifylline group ($P < 0.001$) and a 34% increase in the placebo group (Figure 27-28) (Dawson et al., 2000).

Revascularization

Peripheral arterial revascularization is indicated for relief of ischemic symptoms, including IC and resting ischemic pain, and limb preservation in the setting of CLI. Historically,

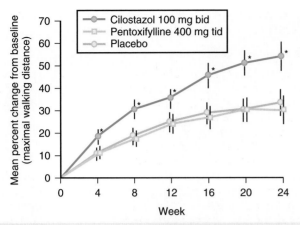

Figure 27-28 Mean percentage change from baseline maximum walking distance on a treadmill for patients with intermittent claudication randomly assigned to cilostazol, pentoxifylline, or placebo. *Asterisk* indicates *P* <0.05 at each 4-week point for cilostazol versus placebo and pentoxifylline. (Reprinted with permission from Exerpta Medica. Dawson DL, Cutler BS, Hiatt WR, et al. A Comparison of cilostazol and pentoxifylline for treating intermittent claudication. *Am J Med.* 2000;109:523-530.)

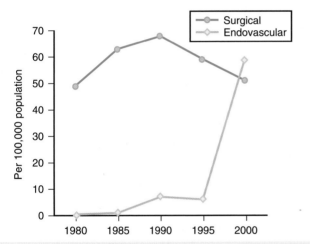

Figure 27-29 Volume trends for percutaneous revascularization and surgical revascularization for the lower extremities from 1980 through 2000. Data were obtained by reviewing *International Classification of Diseases*, edition 9, codes for all vascular procedures using the National Hospital Discharge Survey of nonfederal U.S. hospitals. (Modified from Anderson PL, Gelijns A, Moskowitz A, et al. Understanding trends in inpatient surgical volume: vascular interventions, 1980-2000. *J Vasc Surg.* 2004;39:1200-1208.)

revascularization has been performed surgically; however, with advances in endovascular technology, a percutaneous approach is now being performed as a first-line therapy. From 1995 to 2000, there was a nearly 1000% increase in the number of percutaneous revascularizations performed in the United States compared with approximately a 30% to 35% decrease in the number of surgical revascularizations (Figure 27-29) (Anderson et al., 2004).

An endovascular approach confers a similar acute procedural success rate with considerably less periprocedural morbidity, shorter recovery time, shorter hospitalization time, and less pain than a surgical procedure. On the other hand, restenosis by neointimal hyperplasia of an endovascular procedure is a well-documented, slow process that occurs over weeks to months, and thus a higher rate of repeat revascularization is needed, particularly over an intermediate follow-up range. Surgery, on the other hand, carries a higher initial risk of morbidity and mortality, but a less frequent need for repeat revascularization is anticipated. Surgery, however, can only be repeated a limited number of times because dissection planes, surgical targets, and anastomosis sites become obliterated by repetitive surgery and conduit becomes exhausted. An endovascular procedure can be repeated as often as necessary to maintain vessel patency.

The attractiveness of a minimally invasive approach for revascularization is that it significantly lowers the threshold of when patients are treated. Because of the higher initial risk with surgery, the traditional surgical dogma has reserved revascularization until there is a limb-threatening situation. However, this leaves many patients left to face debilitating IC inadequately treated. Endovascular therapy offers a paradigm shift in this philosophy. Because it is safer, effective, and reproducible, patients can be treated earlier in the disease process when they are in the claudication stage, with significant improvement in their quality of life (Dippel et al., 2004). An example of an artery before and after an endovascular revascularization is shown in Figure 27-30.

There are approximately 150,000 to 200,000 nontraumatic amputations done annually (American Diabetes Association Fact Sheet, 2005). The alarming statistic is that 40% to 50% of limbs are amputated without doing an angiogram beforehand. It is estimated that more than 90% of these limbs could be salvaged or converted to a lesser amputation with revascularization. Another advantage of an endovascular approach over a surgical approach is that totally occluded arteries can be revascularized endovascularly with a high acute procedural success rate even when there are no distal targets available to bypass and surgery is not technically feasible. Therefore, it is recommended that patients with CLI or symptom-limiting claudication that is not adequately alleviated with medical therapy be referred for endovascular revascularization. If an endovascular approach is not viable, then surgical therapy should be considered as a second-line alternative.

CONCLUSIONS

Peripheral vascular disease is an underdiagnosed, undertreated, highly prevalent, age-dependent condition that is associated with a high mortality rate caused by cardiac and cerebrovascular events. PAD has a very strong negative impact on quality of life, and patients have a functional status similar to NYHA class 3 symptoms of CHF. Clinicians must be more diligent in diagnosing and treating PAD. The diagnosis consists of a goal-directed history and physical examination, noninvasive vascular studies, and CTA or MRA imaging. Therapy consists of routine exercise, smoking cessation, treating the appropriate risk factors to their target goals, and relief of ischemic symptoms either pharmacologically or via a revascularization procedure. Patients with CLI, with or without tissue loss, should be referred urgently for revascularization. An algorithm for management is shown in Figure 27-31.

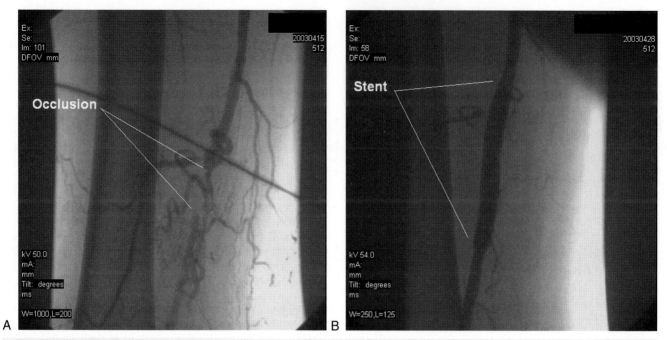

Figure 27-30 A, Baseline angiogram of the right superficial femoral artery demonstrates a short, chronic total occlusion. **B,** Angiogram of the same artery 2 weeks after stent placement.

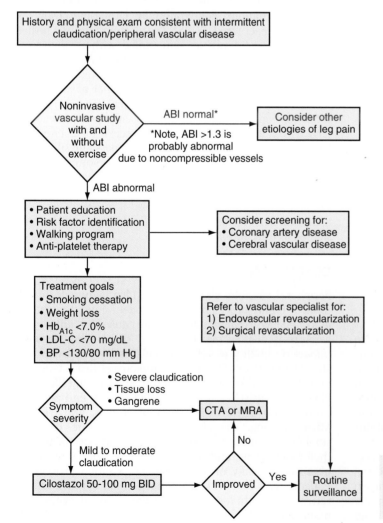

Figure 27-31 Management algorithm for patients with peripheral vascular disease. *ABI,* Ankle-brachial index; *BID,* twice daily; *BP,* blood pressure; *CTA,* computed tomographic angiography; *HbA₁c,* hemoglobin A₁c; *LDL,* low-density lipoprotein cholesterol; *MRA,* magnetic resonance angiography.

KEY DIAGNOSTIC TESTS

- "The resting ABI should be used to establish the lower extremity PAD diagnosis in patients with suspected lower extremity PAD, defined as individuals with 1 or more of the following: exertional leg symptoms, nonhealing wounds, age ≥65 years, or ≥50 years with a history of smoking or diabetes." Also, "The toe-brachial index should be used to establish the lower extremity PAD diagnosis in patients in whom lower extremity PAD is clinically suspected but in whom the ABI test is not reliable due to noncompressible vessels" (Anderson et al., 2013) (SOR: A, ACC/AHA guidelines).
- "Duplex ultrasound of the extremities is useful to diagnose anatomic location and degree of stenosis of PAD. Duplex ultrasound is recommended for routine surveillance after femoral-popliteal or femoral-tibial-pedal bypass with a venous conduit. Minimum surveillance intervals are approximately 3, 6, and 12 months, and then yearly after graft placement" (SOR: A, ACC/AHA guidelines) (Anderson et al., 2013).
- "MRA of the extremities is useful to diagnose anatomic location and degree of stenosis of PAD. MRA of the extremities is useful in selecting patients with lower extremity PAD as candidates for endovascular intervention" (SOR: A, ACC/AHA guidelines) (Anderson et al., 2013).

KEY TREATMENT

- "Patients who are smokers or former smokers should be asked about status of tobacco use at every visit. Patients should be assisted with counseling and developing a plan for quitting that may include pharmacotherapy and/or referral to a smoking cessation program. In the absence of contraindication or other compelling clinical indication, 1 or more of the following pharmacological therapies should be offered: varenicline, bupropion, and nicotine replacement therapy" (Anderson et al., 2013) (SOR: A, ACC/AHA guidelines).
- "Antihypertensive therapy should be administered to hypertensive patients with lower extremity PAD to achieve a goal of less than 140 mm Hg systolic over 90 mm Hg diastolic (individuals without diabetes) or less than 130 mm Hg systolic over 80 mm Hg diastolic (individuals with diabetes and individuals with chronic renal disease) to reduce the risk of MI, stroke, CHF, and cardiovascular death. β-Adrenergic blocking drugs are effective antihypertensive agents and are not contraindicated in patients with PAD" (SOR: A, ACC/AHA guidelines) (Anderson et al., 2013).
- "A program of supervised exercise training is recommended as an initial treatment modality for patients with intermittent claudication. Supervised exercise training should be performed for a minimum of 30 to 45 minutes, in sessions performed at least 3 times per week for a minimum of 12 weeks" (SOR: A, ACC/AHA guidelines) (Anderson et al., 2013).
- "Antiplatelet therapy is indicated to reduce the risk of MI, stroke, and vascular death in individuals with symptomatic atherosclerotic lower extremity PAD, including those with intermittent claudication or CLI, prior lower extremity revascularization (endovascular or surgical), or prior amputation for lower extremity ischemia" (SOR: A, ACC/AHA guidelines) (Anderson et al., 2013).
- Patients should take aspirin 81 to 325 mg/day unless there is a contraindication to aspirin therapy such as active GI bleeding or a history of allergy to aspirin (SOR: A, ACC/AHA guidelines) (Anderson et al., 2013).
- Clopidogrel 75 mg/day can be used as an alternative to aspirin (SOR: A, ACC/AHA guidelines).
- Cilostazol (100 mg orally twice per day) is indicated as an effective therapy to improve symptoms and increase walking distance in patients with lower extremity PAD and IC (SOR: A, ACC/AHA guidelines) (Anderson et al., 2013).
- LDL-C should be lowered to less than 100 mg/dL, preferably to less than 70 mg/dL. A statin should be considered first-line pharmacologic therapy in addition to diet and exercise (SOR: A, ACC/AHA guidelines).
- In patients with CLI and an estimated life expectancy of more than 2 years, bypass surgery, when feasible, may be considered when an autogenous vein conduit is available (SOR: A, AHA/ACC guidelines) (Anderson et al., 2013).
- Patients should be referred for a revascularization procedure when an exercise program and cilostazol therapy fail to adequately alleviate ischemic symptoms (SOR: A, ACC/AHA guidelines).
- All patients with critical limb-threatening ischemia with or without tissue loss should be urgently referred for a revascularization procedure (SOR: A, ACC/AHA guidelines).

Aortic Disease

The aorta is subject to several histopathologies, including atherosclerotic, degenerative, genetic, and vasculitis or inflammatory (Hiratzka et al., 2010). Aneurysms of the aorta can be thoracic, abdominal, or both. Thoracic aortic aneurysms (TAAs) are caused by several factors, including (1) cystic medial degeneration, commonly seen in Marfan syndrome and affecting the root and ascending aorta; (2) genetic, mostly associated with bicuspid aortic valve, Turner syndrome, Ehlers-Danlos syndrome, or familial TAA; (3) atherosclerotic, more frequently seen in the abdominal aorta than the thoracic aorta; (4) inflammatory, as in giant cell aortitis and Takayasu arteritis; and (5) infectious, as in syphilitic aortitis and mycotic aneurysms.

Patients with TAA are generally asymptomatic, with the diagnosis made on a routine chest radiography or CT scan. They may also have aortic valve insufficiency, and the diagnosis becomes evident on an echocardiogram. Large TAAs can have a mass effect and cause dysphagia, cough, and hoarseness. However, they can also present acutely with dissection, intramural hematoma, and rupture. In general, the growth rate of the aneurysm becomes accelerated (0.79 cm/yr) when the size reaches more than 5.0 cm. With the exception of certain inherited disorders, repair of the TAA should be done when the size reaches 5.5 cm or larger or 6.5 cm or larger in high surgical risk patients. A rapid expansion of the TAA size, however (>0.5 cm/yr), severe valvular insufficiency, and the presence of symptoms should warrant earlier repair. Repair of TAA is, however, advised at 4.5 to 5.0 cm in patients with Marfan syndrome (women with Marfan syndrome contemplating pregnancy should have their ascending aortas repaired when they exceed 4 cm), 5.0 to 5.5 cm in patients with bicuspid aortic valve or familial TAA, and 4.4 to 4.6 cm in patients with Loeys-Dietz syndrome. Patients with TAA should be treated with β-blockers as the mainstay of therapy to keep their BP at 110 to 125 mm Hg systolic and heart rate at 50 to 60 beats/min. ARBs are also important in patients with Marfan syndrome (Hiratzka et al., 2010).

Patients with TAA should be followed with an MRA or CTA at the time of diagnosis and then repeated in 6 months. If the size remains stable, then yearly CT or MRA is indicated. In certain genetic disorders such as Loeys-Dietz syndrome, complete imaging of the aorta (ascending, descending, and abdominal) is indicated. Echocardiography should also be performed at least once yearly in patients with TAA. More frequent testing is indicated if the size of the TAA has progressed rapidly (Hiratzka et al., 2010).

Abdominal aortic aneurysm is more prevalent in men. Risk factors include older age, family history of AAA, atherosclerosis, and smoking (Lederle et al., 2000). Predictors of AAA rupture at 3 years of follow-up were female sex, larger initial aneurysm diameter, lower forced expiratory volume in 1 second (FEV_1), current smoking, and higher mean BP (Brown et al., 1999). The USPSTF recommends one-time ultrasound screening of men who have ever smoked and are older than the age of 65 or men older than the age of 60 years with siblings or parents with AAA. Currently, it is recommended that in an average-sized man, a diameter of 5.5 cm or larger is a reasonable target for repair unless preceded by a rapid change in size on follow-up. For women, a threshold of 4.5 to 5.0 cm is appropriate. Monitoring of the aneurysm should be done on a 6-month to yearly basis. Repair can be surgical or endovascular based on several factors, including location and size of the aneurysm, aortic size and tortuosity, surgical risk, and patient's preference.

Acute aortic syndromes are caused by several factors, including a rapidly expanding aortic aneurysm, aortic dissection, intramural hematoma, penetrating atherosclerosis ulcer, or trauma. Aortic dissection is the classic presentation. Predictors of aortic dissection include advanced age, HTN, male gender, history of aortic aneurysm, iatrogenic during angiography or cardiac surgery, pregnancy, or in association with bicuspid valve or Marfan syndrome. This condition is life threatening and is an emergency. Death generally occurs at 1% to 2% per hour. An abrupt onset of severe chest or interscapular tearing or stabbing pain should raise suspicion for aortic dissection, particularly in patients with the described risk factors. CTA can provide an accurate diagnosis of this condition. Aortic dissections involving the ascending aorta or the arch (Stanford type A) are surgical emergencies, but those extending distal to the left subclavian artery (Stanford type B) may be handled medically if no organ compromise, rupture or impending rupture, or intractable pain is present. The mainstay of treatment is β-blockers and IV vasodilators with avoidance of cardiac catheterization and pericardiocentesis for cardiac tamponade. Survivors of acute aortic dissection should be followed closely as outpatients with serial imaging of the aorta (1, 3, and 6 months after discharge and then one or two times per year). BP control and aggressive preventive risk factor modification are strongly indicated.

Peripheral Venous Disease

Venous disease is highly prevalent, with more than 25 million people in the United States being affected (Brand et al., 1988). It is estimated that it costs more than 2 million work days and a cost of $1.4 billion dollars annually to treat. It is estimated that 5% or fewer of patients seek medical attention, the majority of whom have significant venous reflux disease. The incidence of venous reflux disease is higher in women than men irrespective of age. Also, with increasing age, both men and women have a higher incidence of chronic venous insufficiency. Besides age and gender, there are several other risk factors for venous insufficiency, including heredity, obesity, standing occupation, sedentary lifestyle, and prior injury or surgery. The great saphenous vein and its tributaries, the small saphenous vein or perforator veins, are likely to be the culprit in chronic venous insufficiency. These are initially treated with compression stockings, exercise, and weight loss or with nonsurgical ablative methods (radiofrequency or laser). The deep venous system may also have significant reflux, but its treatment is limited to conservative management.

Venous insufficiency may result from overdilation of the veins or actual damage to the venous valve. This leads to an inability of the valves to close properly, leading to blood pooling in the lower legs, venous HTN, edema, pain, itching, heaviness, restless legs, skin hyperpigmentation, and eventually ulcerations. These classic findings are worse as the day progresses and improve in the early hours of the morning when the feet are elevated in bed. Two-thirds of patients also have improvement in symptoms with graded compression stockings, exercise, and weight loss, which are important initial conservative therapies.

A primary care physician needs to obtain a thorough history, including the location and frequency of symptoms; history of deep vein thrombosis or trauma; gynecologic and obstetric history; family history of venous insufficiency or clotting disorder; prior treatment with medications, sclerotherapy, ablation, or surgical stripping; symptoms of itching; involuntary movement of the legs; ulcerations or hyperpigmentation, particularly over the shins or medial aspect of the ankles; change of symptoms with leg elevation or compression stockings; claudication with ambulation; and presence of varicosities. In addition, the legs need to be physically inspected for venous stasis, hyperpigmentation, lower extremity pulses, auscultation over the veins to rule out arteriovenous fistula, varicosities, dermatitis, ulcerations, pitting edema, presence of cords or lipodermatosclerosis, unilateral or bilateral swelling, and CEAP (clinical signs, etiologic classification, anatomic distribution, and pathophysiologic distribution) classification.

The CEAP classification is commonly used to describe the severity of venous disease. The etiologic classification is the most commonly used in an office practice and includes CEAP class 0, no visible or palpable signs of venous disease; CEAP class 1, telangiectasias or reticular veins; CEAP class 2, varicose veins; CEAP class 3, edema; CEAP class 4a and

4b, skin changes, including pigmentation and venous eczema or with lipodermatosclerosis; CEAP class 5, healed venous ulcer; and CEAP class 6, active venous ulcer. Also, photographic documentation of the legs before and after any treatment is advised.

Cardiac Electrophysiology and Arrhythmias

The accurate understanding and interpretation of ECGs, rhythm strips, and unusual cardiac beats is a rewarding practice. Understanding is based not only on recognition of patterns but also on the knowledge of electrical activation and repolarization of individual cells alone and in the aggregate. Anticipation of what should be happening will aid in determining what is happening during any particular beat. Appreciation of the history of electrophysiology and arrhythmology further aids in rhythm management. Through this understanding, accurate interpretation and treatment of arrhythmias in individuals can be made.

Normal cardiac cellular actions may include automaticity, rhythmicity, conductivity, and contractility. Specialized cardiac cells may perform one of these functions better than a prototypical myocyte, thus facilitating organ function. Clinical arrhythmias result from disorders of impulse formation, abnormal impulse conduction, or a combination of these events (Akhtar et al., 1988; Zipes and Jalife, 1990).

The correct action of all cardiac cells is dependent on a normally functioning cell membrane or sarcolemma. Similar to central and peripheral neurons, cardiac cells have bilayer cell membranes composed of phospholipid molecules with specialized channels or pores that function as a semipermeable membrane to a variety of molecules. Sodium (Na^+), potassium (K^+), calcium (Ca^{++}), chloride (Cl^-), and other ions move across the cell membrane in an organized fashion, resulting in depolarization of the cell from a resting electronegative state. Specialized structures along both the long axis and short axis of cardiac cells facilitate the coupling of mechanical and electrical action (Hoyt et al., 1989).

Two specialized electrical cell types with different permeability characteristics for Na^+ and Ca^{++} give rise to specialized action. Slow depolarizing and conducting calcium-dependent cells are more abundantly found in the sinus node and the AV junctional area. Rapidly depolarizing, fast-conducting sodium-dependent cells are more widespread and include atrial and ventricular myocytes and specialized His-Purkinje fibers as well as abnormal cardiac structures such as bypass tracts discussed later in this section. Medications, ischemia, injury, fibrosis, and external stimulation affect these cells differently, allowing for treatment and diagnosis of a variety of arrhythmias.

CARDIAC ANATOMY

The normal heart beat results from a series of electrical and mechanical actions that result in forward output of blood. Alterations in cardiac performance occur from changes in heart rate and contractility in response to variation in autonomic tone and metabolic stress. To carry this out, the heart has developed a specialized conduction system.

Sinus Node Complex

Arising in the right atrium in the superior septal aspect at the junction of the lateral margin of the superior vena cava with the right atrium and the atrial appendage, the sino-atrial (SA) node extends laterally into the crista terminalis (Schlant et al., 1994). The sinus node includes three types of cells: nodal cells, transitional cells, and atrial muscle cells. Impulse formation and rhythmicity in primates are influenced by rich innervation with postganglionic adrenergic and cholinergic nerve terminals (Billman et al., 1989). Impulses leaving the sinus node complex travel through the right and left atrium and converge on the AV node. Controversy still exists as to whether conduction spreads preferentially through specialized internodal and interatrial conduction pathways of the anterior, middle, and posterior internodal pathways or simply through atrial myocytes (Racker, 1989). Regardless, right and left atrial depolarization occurs over 55 to 100 msec, resulting in the surface P wave. Cells residing in the SA node complex are predominantly Ca^{++} dependent and slow conducting and have a higher resting membrane potential than atrial or ventricular myocytes and Purkinje tissue (Sperelakis, 1979).

Atrioventricular Nodal Complex

The AV node lies at the apex of the triangle of Koch. This is formed by the septal leaflet of the tricuspid valve and the tendon of Todaro (Anderson et al., 1988). The AV node is subendocardial and is not visible on gross inspection. The node extends through the A-V groove into the ventricle as the His bundle before branching into the right and left bundle branches of the His-Purkinje system. The AV node contains cells similar to the sinus node P cells. These cells and the associated transitional cells comprise a slowly conducting structure richly innervated with cholinergic and adrenergic fibers. Automaticity and conduction speed is influenced by this innervation. Slow, calcium-dependent cells predominate in the AV node. Conduction time through the AV node is roughly determined from the end of the P wave to the onset of the QRS complex.

Bundle Branch Network and His-Purkinje Tissue

The distal portion of the AV node becomes the His bundle. These cells have fast-conducting sodium channel–dependent cells with more negative resting potentials. Branching off into the right and left bundle branches and finally the endocardial Purkinje network, these fibers transmit impulses 10 times faster than atrial or ventricular myocytes and 50 to 60 times faster than sinus or AV nodal cells (Sperelakis, 1979). Rapid activation of the His-Purkinje network results in global, nearly simultaneous activation of the RV and LV myocytes. Purkinje activation results in a narrow QRS complex (<120 msec) noted on the surface ECG. Abnormalities of the right or left bundle branches result in slower activation of myocardium through cell–cell activation and thus the typical wide bundle branch block QRS on the surface ECG (>120 msec).

Atrial and Ventricular Myocytes

Myocardial cells are specialized cells designed to shorten when activated by a threshold electrical stimulus, thus providing mechanical force to produce contraction. The cell

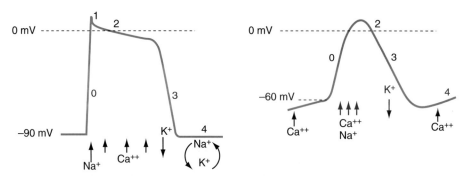

Figure 27-32 Currents and channels involved in generating the resting and action potential: *left,* time course of a stylized action potential of atrial and ventricular cells; *right,* time course of sinoatrial node cells. Above are the various channels and pumps that contribute the currents underlying the electrical events.

membrane is characterized by fast sodium channel activation. Depolarization of the cell results in release of sarcoplasmic calcium and cardiac cell contraction. Conduction velocities are intermediate between SA and AV nodal cells and the Purkinje cells. Cell death, injury resulting in scarring or functional conduction slowing, or changes in cellular automaticity may result in clinical arrhythmias (Zipes, 1992).

THE ACTION POTENTIAL

Considerable consternation on the part of student and physician arises from diagrams of action potentials of cardiac tissue. However, by understanding a few simple concepts on the microscopic or cellular level, arrhythmia evaluation and treatment become easier.

In Figure 27-32, the schematic representation of the transmembrane action potentials of the fast, Na^+ inward current cell and the slow, Ca^{++} inward current cell are shown. In the left panel, *Phase 4* represents the resting transmembrane potential and is −90mV, with the intracellular area being negative. This membrane potential difference is maintained by a sodium/potassium pump using energy to maintain the difference. The membrane is permeable to potassium (K^+) and impermeable to Na^+ at rest. By expending energy, 3 Na^+ ions are pumped out of the cell in exchange for two K^+ ions into the cell. Positive K^+ ions flow across their chemical gradients out of the cell, thus leaving the intracellular space electronegative.

Phase 0 is characterized by the rapid influx of Na^+ ions into the cell, thus depolarizing the cell. Sodium influx is gated. When a sufficiently large depolarization occurs, ion channels are recruited and open, allowing for more influx of ions. Conductance declines as the channel is open and the equilibrium potential for the ion is reached. The channel closes, and Na^+ is again impermeable to influx. *Phase 1* represents a rapid repolarization of the cell through transient K^+ outward currents and β-adrenergic, AMP, and histamine-activated chloride (Cl^-) inward current, restoring the membrane potential toward 0 mV.

Phase 2 or the plateau phase is a long phase that may last several hundred milliseconds. Conductance to all ions falls dramatically. Continued Na^+/K^+ pump activity reduces the membrane potential slightly. An *inward*-rectifying K^+ current further depolarizes the cell, along with continued Ca^{++} influx through the slow inward calcium channels.

Phase 3 represents the final rapid repolarization of the cell membrane. This occurs from inactivation of the slow inward calcium current and from activation of an *outward* K^+ current. The intracellular space becomes more negative, and potassium conductance increases in a regenerative manner.

Phase 4 resumes at the end of phase 3. However, in portions of the heart, a small depolarization current occurs and may result in threshold being reached and depolarization of the cell. This inward-depolarizing current is noted in the SA node, distal AV node, and His-Purkinje fibers. This results in automaticity. The rate of depolarization is greater in the SA node than in other structures and thus results in the SA node as the dominant pacemaker. Adrenergic and cholinergic modulation further results in the SA node as the faster pacemaker, subordinating the automaticity of other pacemaker-like tissues. More frequent stimulation results in shortening of the phase 2 and phase 3 of the action potential, resulting in unchanged or slightly increased conduction velocity.

In the *right panel,* the action potential of the slow inward current type cells is shown. In these cells, calcium and potassium play a greater role in setting the resting membrane potential slightly less negative than in Purkinje or myocytes (phase 4). Phase 0 occurs through activation of slow Ca^{++} current. No phase 1 is noted, and the plateau phase is not as prolonged, owing to the relative importance of the Ca^{++} and K^+ currents dominated by the slow activating and inactivating C^{++} current. More frequent stimulation leads to a decrease in the resting membrane potential, lower peak phase 0 velocity, slower phase 3 repolarization, and ultimately slower overall conduction velocity (Rosen and Schwartz, 1991).

Antiarrhythmic drugs have differential effects on the Na^+, K^+, and Ca^{++} channels or on receptors that mediated the channels. By slowing or enhancing cellular membrane pore activity, one observes changes in either conduction or repolarization characteristics. This may be reflected in changes in the surface ECG as well.

SURFACE ACTION POTENTIAL (ELECTROCARDIOGRAM)

The surface action potential can be thought of as a series of discrete electrical events occurring over time. Figure 27-33 schematically demonstrates cardiac events with the

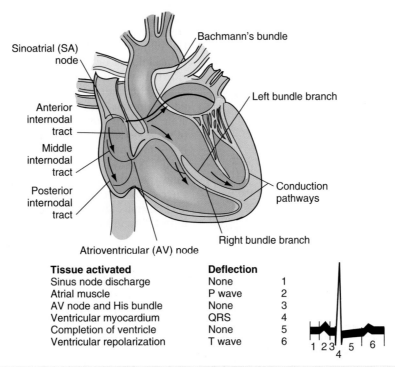

Tissue activated	Deflection	
Sinus node discharge	None	1
Atrial muscle	P wave	2
AV node and His bundle	None	3
Ventricular myocardium	QRS	4
Completion of ventricle	None	5
Ventricular repolarization	T wave	6

Figure 27-33 Schematic diagram of the cardiac chambers and the associated surface electrocardiogram findings.

surface ECG. The P wave begins with spontaneous depolarization of the SA node with propagation throughout the right and left atrium. This is upright in the inferior leads as depolarization occurs from the topmost portion of the atrium and converges on the atrial septum at the AV node. The depolarization of and conduction through the AV node result in no surface activity, resulting in an isoelectric portion beginning at the end of the P wave and continuing to the onset of the QRS. The P-R interval is the total time from SA node activation through the AV node until the beginning of ventricular depolarization. The His-Purkinje network is activated, rapidly depolarizing the large mass of ventricular myocardium. This results in the large QRS complex. The Q-T interval represents myocardial repolarization and may be prolonged in the setting of bundle branch block, drug effect, and genetic disorders causing abnormal ion channel function.

MECHANISMS OF ARRHYTHMIAS

Two main mechanisms for the initiation and perpetuation of arrhythmias have been proposed. Putative mechanisms include disorders of *impulse formation* and disorders of *impulse conduction*. These may occur alone or in combination and result in isolated electrical events and sustained arrhythmias. Alterations in automaticity or triggered activity are two main areas of disordered impulse formation. Clinical examples of abnormal automaticity include inappropriate sinus tachycardia, multifocal atrial tachycardia, sinus pauses, idioventricular rhythm after MI, and ectopy in the setting of HF. Triggered activity, or spontaneous depolarization dependent on prior stimulation, is characterized as early or late after depolarizations. This mechanism may be responsible for arrhythmic events during hypoxia, use of sotalol or the metabolite of procainamide, or in patients with idiopathic and acquired long Q-T syndrome and digitalis toxicity.

Changes in impulse conduction can be clinically divided into *block* with or without *reentry*. Simple block occurs when the propagation of the impulse results in an inadequate depolarization stimulus to the adjacent tissue and the impulse terminates. Clinical examples include SA or AV block or simple bundle branch block. In SA block, normal depolarization of the SA node is inadequate to excite adjacent tissue, resulting in absence of a P wave. In AV block, block may occur within the AV node or as it attempts to depolarize His tissue. This results in a P wave followed by a delayed or absent QRS complex. On the surface ECG, differentiation between block in the AV node or His bundle is only a guess. Bundle branch block or hemiblock is a result of block in a specific branch of the specialized conduction tissue. Activation of tissue beyond the bundle branches must then occur through slower myocyte-to-myocyte activation.

In *block with reentry* (Figure 27-34), unidirectional block within a tissue results in activation of adjacent tissue. Tissue not initially activated then becomes excited by the conducting tissue. Tissue that has had time to recover excitability may then be activated again in a single or perpetual event. Clinical examples may occur within the SA node or AV node, within the atrium such as AFL, and in Purkinje and myocardial tissue as VT. Additional macroreentrant rhythms include atrial reentry and preexcitation with orthodromic and antidromic reciprocating tachycardias.

DIAGNOSIS OF CARDIAC ARRHYTHMIAS

Electrocardiographic Evaluation of Arrhythmias

The basic *single lead* rhythm strip is still used in many offices as a quick verification of ongoing abnormal rhythms. New

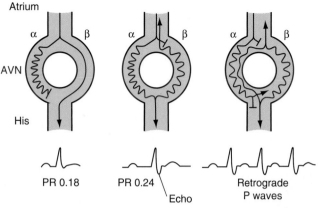

Atrium

AVN

His

PR 0.18   PR 0.24   Retrograde
                   Echo   P waves

Figure 27-34 Mechanism of typical atrioventricular (AV) nodal reentry. The AV node (AVN) is drawn schematically with fast and slow pathways. Differential conduction and refractoriness is noted between the two pathways. The β pathway (fast pathway) has fast conduction and long refractoriness; the α pathway has slower conduction and shorter refractoriness. *Left,* The depolarization wave front from the atrium penetrates both pathways. The β pathway conducts the wave front faster than the slow pathway, and the P-R interval is normal. *Center,* Block occurs in the fast pathway. The slow pathway conducts the wave and depolarizes the ventricle. The β pathway (fast pathway) has time to recover, and conduction proceeds retrograde up the fast pathway and depolarizes the atrial tissue again, resulting in an AV node echo beat. *Right,* Continuation of the reentry can occur. As the fast pathway is activated in the retrograde fashion during an echo beat, the slow pathway, with a shorter refractory period, is able to recover. The excitable tissue can then be activated, and conduction again proceeds back down the slow pathway (α pathway), and the cycle continues.

or used inexpensive equipment can be found through many equipment vendors. This allows for rapid evaluation of symptoms reported during an office visit. Slightly more expensive 12-lead ECG machines provide not only useful information on the ongoing rhythm but may also demonstrate ischemic changes or prior or ongoing injury pattern. Multiple lead analyses helps discern difficult to see P waves during arrhythmia evaluation as well.

Both the single lead and 12-lead ECG are helpful only for ongoing arrhythmia analysis. Obviously, short-lived events or events that occur unpredictably are rarely identified by these simple techniques. Twenty-four-hour ambulatory recording of a single or multiple leads is performed through Holter monitoring. Small patches or electrodes are placed on the skin and are attached to a digital or analog recording device usually worn on the belt. Offline data analysis is performed and relayed to the interpreting provider. Monitoring over 24 to 48 hours allows for increased sensitivity in ambulatory screening. Longer periods of monitoring can be performed using small 30-day recorders. By recording and repeatedly overwriting the last several minutes of a rhythm, individuals with very infrequent events can lock in a symptomatic event and then transmit the information over the phone. This method may also be helpful in monitoring response to pharmacologic therapy such as rate control in AF. However, prolonged electrode contact can result in skin irritation and poor patient acceptance.

Newer, implantable loop monitors became available in the early 1990s. Devices smaller than a disposable lighter are implanted under the skin overlying the chest wall. Lasting 18 to 30 months, these loop recorders have

automatic and activated memory. Evaluation of the recorded events is performed in the clinician's office, remote from the clinical event. Implantation is usually performed by a cardiologist or electrophysiologist when other recording efforts have failed.

Exercise testing may also be useful for clinical events that occur during activity or stress. Elevations in adrenergic state facilitate conduction and repolarization. Unmasking of sinus node, AV node, or His-Purkinje disease resulting in block may occur. Initiation of various supraventricular or even VTs may also occur. Ischemia as a trigger for arrhythmias may also be detected. Exercise testing should be considered in patients with reproducible activity-associated arrhythmias and in patients in whom evaluation suspects long-QT syndrome or manifest preexcitation.

Inpatient evaluation of arrhythmias is seldom needed. However, patients with clinical syncope or the transient loss of postural control thought to be arrhythmic in nature, patients in whom ischemia-induced arrhythmias is a concern, or patients with a clinical history concerning a life-threatening ventricular arrhythmia should be considered for inpatient evaluation. In this setting, an organized testing regimen may be used during continuous ECG monitoring.

A comprehensive discussion of rhythm and 12-lead ECG findings is beyond the scope of this chapter. However, using a standard, stepwise approach to all rhythm strips can be easily learned. Keeping in mind changes in impulse formation and impulse propagation, the correct ECG diagnosis can usually be made. Clinical information such as drug therapy or prior myocardial injury can be equally useful. Similar questions that should be addressed with each rhythm analysis are as follows:

1. What is the origin of the impulse? In essence, determine the P-QRS relationship. Determine if the P wave is the initial event or the secondary event and if it is associated with neighboring depolarizations. If P waves exist, examine the morphology and determine if it is appropriate for the lead reviewed. If the rhythm is irregular, do the irregular beats look the same? These steps will help determine if the rhythm comes from the atrium, AV junction, or ventricle. Further differentiation into irregular atrial events such as AF or multifocal atrial tachycardia can be made. Wide QRS beats may arise from premature ventricular contractions (PVCs), bundle branch block, or preexcitation.
2. What is the basic heart rate? Is the rate appropriate for the origin of the impulse? This will discern tachycardias from bradycardias or normal rates for the rhythm (e.g., sinus arrhythmia).
3. Is the rhythm regular? Is this appropriate? A fixed regular ventricular response in the setting of AF suggests third-degree AV block and may be due to digitalis toxicity if the rate is greater than expected for a junctional escape.
4. Are intervals appropriate and constant? Changes occur in setting of altered origin of impulse, basic heart rate, and with varying degrees of block (e.g., type I second-degree SA or AV block).
5. Are QT segments, ST segments, or T waves helpful? Are Q waves present? This may give clues to ongoing metabolic, ischemic, or drug effects that cause common

arrhythmias. With these few questions in mind, most rhythm strips can be interpreted correctly.

Basic interpretation begins with a rhythm strip of good quality, typically representing lead I, II, or V1. Multiple leads aid in the diagnosis but are not always necessary. Evaluation of heart rate, intervals, and axis is necessary. Regularity of the rhythm; consistency of the P waves, QRS complexes, and T waves; and abnormalities of the ST segment should be characterized. Examples of various rhythms, possible causes, and treatments are presented in the following sections.

PATTERN RECOGNITION OF ARRHYTHMIAS

Atrial Rhythms

Key Point

- Treatment of asymptomatic or minimally symptomatic, non–life-threatening atrial rhythms should be less risky than no treatment at all. The proarrhythmic side effects of drug therapy including VF should be carefully weighed before initiation of drug therapy.

Disorders of sinus rhythm: *Sinus rhythm* is a regular, organized atrial rhythm between 60 and 100 beats/min at rest in healthy individuals. Slower rates as low as 40 to 50 beats/min may be normal in some individuals. Originating in the high right atrium, sinus P waves should be positive in limb leads I and II. *Sinus bradycardia* originates in the sinus node with a P wave indistinguishable from the normal sinus beat but at a rate slower than the established lower limit of 60 beats/min. This is physiologically normal in patients during sleep, in athletic individuals, and as a consequence of many adrenergic-blocking drugs such as β-blockers. Excessive bradycardia may come as a consequence of changes in vagal tone in sleep apnea, during painful stimuli, or with mesenteric stretch. There are typically no significant changes in the P-QRS-T intervals with resting sinus bradycardias. During vagal-mediated sinus slowing, associated prolongation in the P-R interval may give a clue as to the etiology. Typically, no treatment is necessary in this benign condition. If the heart rate slowing is excessive or symptomatic, acute atropine administration, epinephrine, and dopamine may be used acutely. For the long term, pacemaker implantation may be necessary. *Sinus arrhythmia* is the normal variation of heart rate likely caused by changes in volume and vagal tone as a consequence of respiration. Occasional slowing below 60 beats/min at rest is considered acceptable. Patients with high adrenergic tone such as HF often lose normal variations in heart rate and a reduction in the degree of sinus arrhythmia. A *wandering atrial pacemaker* is said to occur if at normal heart rates, there is significant variation in the P-wave morphology and regularity. Associated PR interval and RR intervals are variable because of the different atrial origin and variations in the prematurity of the atrial beat. It is more frequent in young individuals and as a result of changes in vagal tone. The origin of the impulse may arise from within the sinus node complex but at distant sites within the right atrium, giving rise to the changes in P-wave morphology.

A *sinus pause* and the more extreme case of *sinus arrest* are demonstrated as a sudden change in the heart rate, often proceeded by mild slowing in the general sinus rate. A sinus pause is typically due to changes in vagal tone such as gagging, carotid sinus stimulation, or pain and as a consequence of neurocardiogenic activation (Figure 27-35). Very long episodes of no surface atrial activity are considered to have *sinus arrest*. This may occur as a consequence of atrial tissue disease, drug therapy, metabolic derangements, and significant vagal activation. Figure 27-36 demonstrates a long pause noted during neurocardiogenic reflex activation during a tilt-table test in the evaluation of syncope. The pause was approximately 50 seconds and resulted in loss of consciousness. Typically, withdrawal of the offending agent, improvement in cardiac function, and elimination of stimuli causing reflex vagal activation result in improvement in symptoms. In difficult symptomatic

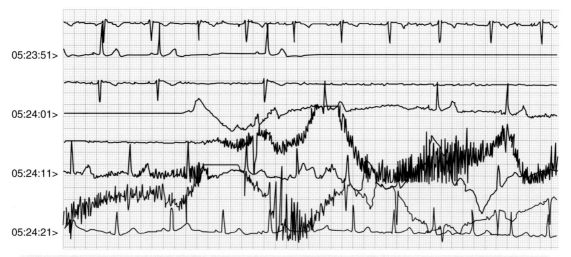

05:23:51>

05:24:01>

05:24:11>

05:24:21>

Figure 27-35 Sinus rhythm is followed by sinus arrest and motion artifact during a seizure. Sinus rhythm then resumes.

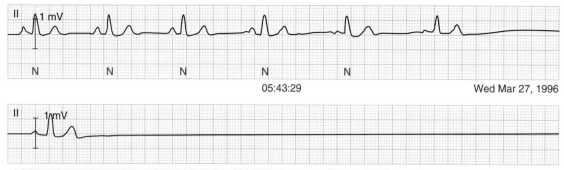

05:43:29   Wed Mar 27, 1996

Figure 27-36 Sinus rhythm slows slightly before sinus arrest occurs for 50 seconds. Return of sinus rhythm is not shown.

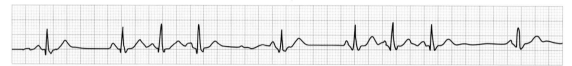

Figure 27-37 Sinus rhythm with type I Wenckebach sinoatrial block. Note shortening of the P-P interval before the dropped P wave and the pause of less than twice the shortest P-P interval. The return cycle length is longer than the cycle length before the pause.

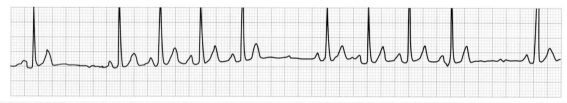

Figure 27-38 Sinus rhythm with type II second-degree sinoatrial block. Note the almost constant P-P interval before loss of P-wave activity. The pause is twice the cycle length of sinus rhythm. The return cycle length is the same as before the pause.

cases and in patients without a reversible cause, pacemakers may be necessary. Demonstration of sinus pauses and sinus arrest as a cause of symptoms of dizziness or syncope may be difficult and require prolonged ambulatory monitoring.

A pause may also occur as a consequence of sinus node disease. In patients with atrial disease, myofibrosis and atrial pressure overload, changes in the automaticity, and rhythmic depolarization of the SA node may be affected. Regular impulses may fail to exit the sinus node complex and depolarize the atrium, resulting in no P wave on the surface ECG and no atrial mechanical contraction. This may occur in regular patterns such as in *type I SA block,* characterized by sequential shortening of the P-P interval and then absence of a P wave. The return cycle length is less than two times the shortest cycle length, and the next cycle is longer than the cycle length just before the dropped P wave (Figure 27-37). *Type II SA block* is characterized by constant P-P intervals followed by a missing P wave. The pause is twice the cycle length of the P-P interval, and the return cycle length is the same as the sinus rate (Figure 27-38).

Premature atrial contractions (PACs) or depolarizations may occur frequently in normal patients. The ECG finding is that of an abrupt early P wave that may or may not be followed by a QRS complex. PACs may occur as isolated events, as couplets, or as sequential events. Most individuals are minimally symptomatic if at all. Benign causes include exogenous stimulants such as tobacco, caffeine, alcohol excess, and sympathomimetic drugs. Digitalis

toxicity should be considered in patients on digitalis treatment. Patients with underlying heart or lung disease or ectopy as a consequence of extrinsic compression on the atrium and adjacent abnormal structures may become symptomatic. Reducing automaticity or triggered activity through antiarrhythmic therapy and treating hypoxia and IHD may reduce the patient's symptoms. In asymptomatic patients, no specific therapy is necessary. β-Blockers and CCBs may reduce ectopy rates and slow or block the ventricular response to the PACs, thus reducing symptoms. Potent antiarrhythmic medications (class Ia, Ic, or III) may occasionally be necessary.

An *ectopic atrial rhythm* is said to occur when the P wave does not have the normal upright morphology in limb leads I, II, and III. Heart rate during the rhythm can be slower than, equal to, or greater than normal sinus rhythm. Ectopic rates greater than 100 beats/min are termed *ectopic atrial tachycardia* (Figures 27-39 and 27-40). The morphology of the ectopic P wave should be consistent, and the P-P intervals should be approximately equal. This helps to distinguish this from sequential PACs. Asymptomatic ectopic atrial rhythms are usually benign and do not require therapy. Patients with incessant, rapid tachycardias may eventually develop rate-related cardiomyopathy. Treatment for or prophylaxis against this type of cardiomyopathy is warranted.

Several additional atrial tachyarrhythmias deserve attention. *Sinus tachycardia* or sinus rhythm at a rate greater than expected for the physiologic state may be seen. Atrial wave morphology is normal. However, sustained increased rates

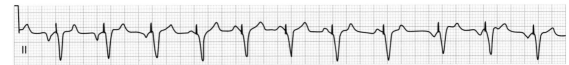

Figure 27-39 An ectopic atrial rhythm at 85 beats/min with negative P waves in lead II is replaced by slower sinus rhythm with upright P waves and then returns at the end of the rhythm strip. A dual-chamber pacemaker senses and tracks both types of P waves and paces the ventricle accordingly.

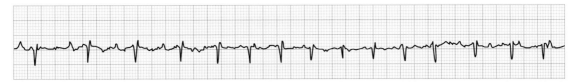

Figure 27-40 Ectopic atrial tachycardia is initiated by a premature atrial complex. Note the P-wave morphology change of the faster ectopic atrial rhythm.

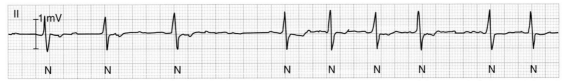

Figure 27-41 The rapid, irregular nature of atrial fibrillation and its chaotic activation of atrial tissue results in no discrete P waves. Conduction through the atrioventricular node is variable, resulting in the irregular ventricular response.

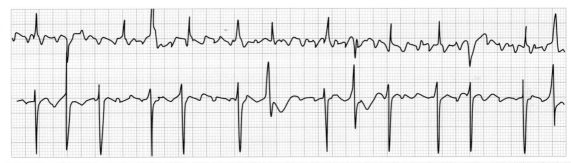

Figure 27-42 Atrial flutter is more organized, resulting in a sawtooth appearance in the limb leads and precordial leads. Atrial rates of almost 300 beats/min are noted, with variations in the ventricular response.

may be related to failure of autonomic regulation, metabolic stress, drug use (prescribed or illicit), or from idiopathic causes. Inappropriate sinus tachycardia syndrome is usually a self-limited problem of the young and may be caused by a variety of factors. Positional orthostatic tachycardia syndrome is a condition of marked increases in heart rate with upright posture, not always associated with a decrease in BP. Volume status is usually normal and differentiates this from simple orthostatic hypotension with reflexive tachycardia. Treatment of these disorders using β-blockers and serotonin antagonists has been helpful in some individuals. Expansion of plasma volume may also be helpful (http://home.att.net/~potsweb/POTS.html).

Multifocal atrial tachycardia is characterized as irregular atrial activity at rates greater than 100 beats/min. There are three or more P waves present as the driving force of the tachycardia. Patients in metabolic stress and with hypoxia are prone to this arrhythmia. Treatment is usually supportive, but verapamil has been shown to help in some. Treatment with digoxin is rarely helpful, and upward titra-

tion may result in toxicity indistinguishable from the original rhythm disorder (Hazard and Burnett, 1987).

The ECG findings of AF are the absence of organized atrial activity with an irregular, usually rapid ventricular response (Figure 27-41). Atria are depolarized from widespread regions of both the left and right atrium and result in chaotic activation at rates exceeding several hundred beats per minute. AF may be asymptomatic or highly symptomatic, ranging from simple palpitations to MI and HF. Recognition of the arrhythmia is the first step in good care. Treatment using an appropriate anticoagulation strategy, ventricular rate control, and consideration of restoration of sinus rhythm is necessary even in asymptomatic patients. Further discussion of AF is provided later in the chapter.

Atrial flutter is also a rapid rhythm of the atrium, usually at a rate near 300 beats/min. The ventricular response may be fixed or variable. Sawtooth flutter waves are usually noted in the inferior limb leads (Figure 27-42). Misidentification of AFL with 2:1 conduction as sinus tachycardia is common and should be considered in all regular

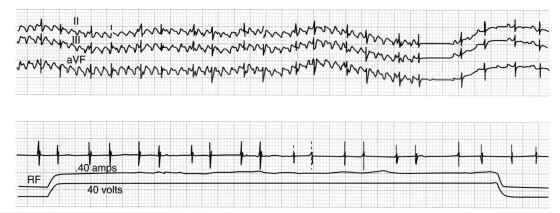

Figure 27-43 Atrial flutter waves noted in leads II, III, and aVF terminate abruptly, and sinus rhythm is restored. An intracardiac ventricular recording and output from a radiofrequency (RF) generator are shown in the lower portion of the diagram. RF application was made at the tricuspid–inferior vena cava isthmus. (From Feld GK, Fleck P, Chen PS, et al. Radiofrequency catheter ablation for the treatment of human type I atrial flutter: identification of a critical zone in the reentrant circuit by endocardial mapping techniques. *Circulation.* 1992;86:1233-1240.)

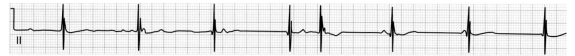

Figure 27-44 Junctional rhythm at a rate greater than the sinus node dominates the rhythm. Conduction through the atrioventricular node occurs with the fifth QRS complex and resets the junctional rhythm. Excessive bradycardia and the associated junctional rhythm may be associated with digoxin toxicity.

tachycardic rhythms. Similar to AF, treatment strategies including anticoagulation with Coumadin should be considered. In contrast to AF, atrial activation is organized and frequently is caused by macroreentry. The wave front ascends the right atrial septum, crosses the roof of the right atrium, and down the lateral wall along the cristae. The wave front then extends between the inferior vena cava and the tricuspid annulus along the isthmus and proceeds to the atrial septum. Targeting the isthmus with linear radiofrequency lesions to effect cure is common (Figure 27-43).

Junctional Rhythms

Similar to PACs, earlier than expected depolarization arising from the AV node complex results in a QRS without a preceding P wave termed a *premature junctional complex* (PJC). Retrograde, inverted P waves may be seen within the early portion of the QRS or following the QRS complex. These are usually benign but may be an early sign of occult cardiac disease. Drugs, adrenergic stimulants, and metabolic stress may be associated with PJCs. In the absence of heart disease or underlying medical condition, these usually asymptomatic beats do not require treatment.

When the AV junction has rhythmic spontaneous depolarization, a *junctional* or *nodal rhythm* occurs (Figure 27-44). The normal pacemaker function of the AV node cells occur at a rate of 35 to 50 beats/min. In sinus node failure, the junctional pacemaker rate may be higher than the sinus rate, resulting in junctional bradycardia. Abnormal reentry within the AV node results in *junctional tachycardia* usually at a rate between 120 and 190 beats/min and is considered a form of supraventricular tachycardia. Differentiation of accelerated junctional tachycardia from more typical supraventricular tachycardias is not possible by surface ECG. Because of simultaneous activation of the

ventricle and retrograde activation of the atrium, junctional rhythms may be more symptomatic than their rate would predict.

DISORDERS OF ATRIOVENTRICULAR NODE CONDUCTION

Key Points

- Atropine may worsen AV block if block occurs at the level of the Purkinje system. Increased sinus rates conducting through the AV node will be blocked because of the refractory His-Purkinje tissue. In contrast, epinephrine may enhance both AV conduction and shorten Purkinje refractoriness, thus resulting in decreased block. Atropine delivery may thus be helpful in distinguishing the level of AV block and determining the urgency of permanent pacing.
- The atrial rate must be faster than the escape rate to confirm complete heart block. A-V dissociation can occur when the escape rate is faster than the atrial rate. This will initially appear to be complete heart block. However, appropriately timed atrial beats may conduct to the ventricle and advance the ventricular cycle, confirming some degree of interaction. Digoxin toxicity and ischemia as well as other drug toxicities may cause accelerated junctional rhythm and should be considered when this rhythm is seen.

First-degree AV block is demonstrated as a P-R interval of greater than 200 msec (Figure 27-45). Persistent AV delay is usually noted, but variations may be seen depending on heart rate. Whereas adrenergic tone shortens the AV delay, drugs such as β–blockers and CCBs may worsen AV conduction, leading to more progressive types of AV block. First-degree AV block is almost always at the level of the AV node. Except for very long AV intervals resulting in atrial contraction while the prior ventricular beat is maintaining AV valve closure, first-degree AV block typically does not require treatment. Advanced age is often associated with this conduction disorder.

Second-degree AV block is separated into type I (Wenkebach); type II, 2 : 1; and high-grade AV block. *Type I second-degree AV block* is characterized by a progressive prolongation of the PR interval followed by failure to conduct and depolarize the ventricle. The PR interval on the return beat will be shorter than the PR just before the block (Figure 27-46). Similar to first-degree AV block, this typically does not require treatment with a pacemaker and does not predict life-threatening complete heart block. In patients with concomitant bundle branch block, one should question if block is actually occurring at the level of the His-Purkinje system. Withdrawal of drugs indicated in AV block is indicated. Dual-chamber pacing in symptomatic patients may be necessary.

Type II second-degree AV block is the abrupt failure of conduction through the AV node and absence of a QRS complex. The PR intervals should be similar before and after block. AV block may occur both at the level of the AV node and His bundle and is indistinguishable without invasive electrophysiology study. Pacing is usually indicated to avoid unpredictable progression to complete heart block. Withdrawal of AV conduction–blocking drugs is indicated. *Two-to-one AV block* can result in very low heart rates and considerable symptoms, including syncope and low-output HF. Loss of ventricular activation every other beat typifies this rhythm. Block at the level of the AV node is suggested by preexistent PR prolongation, but block at the level of the His-Purkinje system cannot be excluded by surface ECG.

High-grade AV block or intermittent complete AV block is similar to type II second-degree AV block. However, greater than one consecutive QRS complex is absent with the block. This degree of AV block is strongly suggestive of significant AV node disease or distal Purkinje disease, and one should strongly consider permanent pacemaker implantation. The one exception may be that of high-grade AV block occurring at night in the setting of sleep apnea.

Third-degree AV block results from failure of atrial impulses from the sinus node to conduct down to the ventricle (Figure 27-47). The finding on a rhythm strip or ECG indicates serious cardiac disease and may be related to significant valvular or coronary disease. An escape rhythm that is narrow suggests that the level of block is above the His–bundle complex and may be more stable. Adrenergic stimulation or atropine may result in an accelerated junctional escape. A slow, wide QRS escape suggests the level is below the His bundle and atropine is unlikely to help. Adrenergic stimulation may help increase the escape rate. Urgent temporary or permanent pacing is indicated. Transcutaneous pacing may be used temporarily but is unreliable and poorly tolerated by the patient.

Ventricular Rhythms

The presence of a wide QRS is usually caused by one of three things: (1) normal AV conduction with bundle branch block aberrancy, (2) presence of preexcitation, or (3) origin of the beat within the ventricle as a PVC or consecutive ventricular activation as seen in VT. A PVC is noted as an early beat, arising before normal atrial activation through the AV node can activate the His–bundle system and depolarize the ventricle. PVCs occur as single beats and couplets but may consecutively appear much like VT. Unifocal PVCs typically are thought of being more benign than multifocal PVCs. The origin of the abnormal beats is usually caused by enhanced automaticity or triggered activity. Cardiac literature has demonstrated higher mortality rates in patients with IHD with decreased EF and increased rates of ventricular ectopy. Suppression of these ectopic beats with class I or III antiarrhythmic medicines, however, has not significantly improved mortality rates (Cardiac Arrhythmia Suppression Trial II Investigators, 1992; Echt et al., 1991).

Ventricular ectopy in patients with normal hearts is not correlated with significant increases in mortality rate.

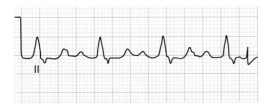

Figure 27-45 Sinus rhythm with first-degree atrioventricular block and bundle branch block.

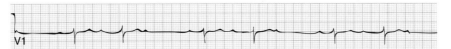

Figure 27-46 Sinus rhythm with type I (Wenckebach) second-degree atrioventricular block. There is prolongation of the P-R interval and then a dropped QRS.

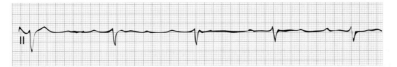

Figure 27-47 Sinus rhythm with third-degree (complete) atrioventricular block. There is complete dissociation of atrial and ventricular activity. The escape rate is less than 30 beats/min, and QRS complex is wide, suggesting a ventricular escape.

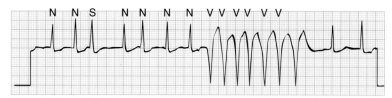

Figure 27-48 Nonsustained monomorphic tachycardia is seen in the setting of underlying atrial fibrillation with increased ventricular response. This terminates spontaneously.

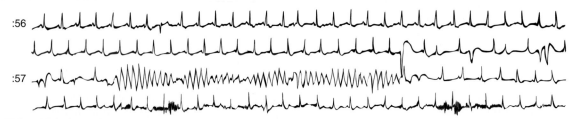

Figure 27-49 Torsades de pointes polymorphic ventricular tachycardia is initiated by sequential premature ventricular contractions (PVCs) that prolong the Q-T interval in a rate-dependent manner. An early PVC landing in the long Q-T interval results in the characteristic twisting about the axis. Spontaneous termination is seen.

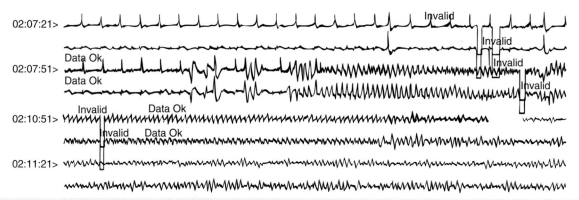

Figure 27-50 Sinus rhythm is noted to degrade initially to a polymorphic ventricular tachycardia and then organizes (not shown in entirety). A premature ventricular contraction during ventricular tachycardia results in ventricular fibrillation, to which the patient ultimately succumbed.

Patients are usually asymptomatic, but in some individuals, even low-frequency ectopy may be quite bothersome. Treatment of these patients with β-blockers often results in symptomatic improvement. In highly symptomatic patients, membrane-active drugs (type I or III) may occasionally be required. Referral to an electrophysiologist should be made if antiarrhythmic medications are used. Some symptomatic patients may also be treated with radiofrequency ablation of the arrhythmic focus.

Ventricular tachycardia is clinically divided into two main categories. In *monomorphic VT*, QRS complexes are nearly identical, and the R-R interval is typically regular. Slight variations at the beginning and end of a run of VT tend to show greater fluctuations in rate. This tends to occur more frequently in scar-related reentry in patients with prior MI and in patients with "normal heart" VT such as RVOT tachycardia and idiopathic LV tachycardia (Figure 27-48). In *polymorphic VT (PMVT)*, the QRS morphology is constantly changing, and the R-R intervals are often inconsistent. Torsades de pointes is a specific clinical PMVT and is characterized by a long QT interval present in the first beat of the tachycardia and a twisting about the axis on a rhythm strip (Figure 27-49). In almost all cases, referral to a cardiologist or electrophysiologist is indicated. Frequently, inpatient evaluation is necessary.

Ventricular fibrillation is a disorganized electrical rhythm of the ventricle and leads to no meaningful ventricular contraction. Without cardiac resuscitation and electrical cardioversion, the individual will die. Figure 27-50 demonstrates a patient hospitalized with an MI. Immediate hospitalization is recommended in patients who have had prior episodes of near syncope or syncope in which VT is suspected because of known underlying ischemic or nonischemic heart disease. Patients suspected of long QT syndrome or VT associated with clinically significant HOCM should be considered for inpatient or invasive evaluation. Patients who are resuscitated from an out-of-hospital VF arrest must be referred to a cardiac specialist for further evaluation and treatment because of the high rate of recurrence (Huikuri et al., 2001). Inpatient evaluation may include invasive coronary angiography or electrophysiology testing.

Paced Rhythms

> ### Key Point
>
> ■ Determination of the site of pacing is important. A bundle branch block pattern on surface ECG contralateral to the site of pacing should occur. Inappropriate LV endocardial lead placement delivered across a patent foramen ovale can be detected before serious consequences of embolic stroke. In addition, appropriate LV epicardial pacing accomplished through lead placement via the coronary sinus can be confirmed through paced right bundle branch block morphology. RV endocardial pacing results in a left bundle branch block pattern on surface ECG.

Temporary or permanent pacemaker implantation is now performed at almost all hospitals in which a cardiologist practices. Activation of myocardium results in a nearly normal P wave but with a notable bundle branch block pattern of ventricular capture on the surface ECG. The ECG recorder may amplify the energy from the pacemaker pulse, resulting in a pacing artifact on the surface 12-lead ECG or rhythm strip to aid in interpretation. Knowledge of the type of pacemaker and the current programming may be necessary for complete analysis. The pacing morphology can be reviewed to confirm consistent and appropriate lead placement. Sensed cardiac events may result in pacemaker inhibition and masking of its presence. Evaluation of unexpected events on the ECG may identify abnormal pacemaker operation, as noted in Figure 27-51. Detailed pacemaker ECG interpretation is beyond the scope of this chapter.

SPECIAL CLINICAL ELECTROCARDIOGRAPHIC SYNDROMES

Sick sinus syndrome is a group of electrocardiographic and clinical findings. Patients often have symptoms of fatigue, palpitations, and heart racing and may have dizzy spells or even syncope. The findings of paroxysmal atrial tachycardia, AF, or AFL results in tachypalpitations and heart racing. Excessive SA node suppression often occurs with drugs used to slow AV conduction or reduce atrial arrhythmias. Figure 27-52 demonstrates typical ECG findings seen in SSS. Pharmacologic treatment to reduce symptoms is often problematic, and permanent pacing is often required. Anticoagulation with Coumadin in patients with documented AF should be considered. Patients without documented AF should be considered for aspirin anticoagulation because of the high frequency of asymptomatic AF in this patient population (Myerburg et al., 1994).

There are at least two types of supraventricular tachycardias that should be routinely considered for referral. Patients with *preexcitation syndrome* (Wolfe-Parkinson-White [WPW] syndrome) or AV reciprocating tachycardia (AVRT) and paroxysmal, symptomatic *AV node reentrant tachycardia* (AVNRT) may benefit from drug therapy or radiofrequency ablation therapy. The ECG signature of WPW is the delta wave. Atrial activation of the ventricle is through the AV node–Purkinje system and is activated through a bundle or bypass tract of muscle inserting along one of the AV valves. The combined activation pattern results in the delta wave. Figures 27-53 and 27-54 demonstrate presence and absence of the delta wave before and after ablation therapy for supraventricular tachycardia associated with the bypass tract. Supraventricular tachycardia results from a macroreentrant circuit in which

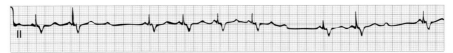

Figure 27-51 Dual-chamber pacing with loss of ventricular output.

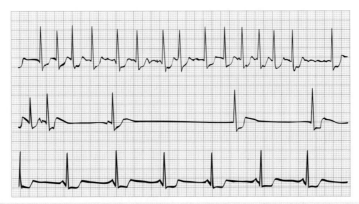

Figure 27-52 Sick sinus syndrome is characterized by rapidly conducted atrial fibrillation, pauses during restoration of sinus rhythm, and excessive bradycardia in normal rhythm.

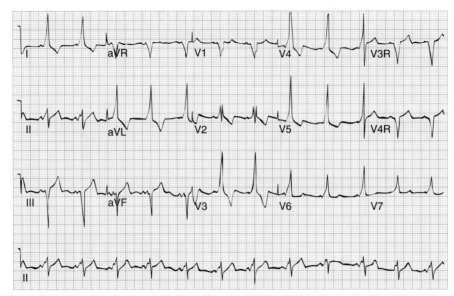

Figure 27-53 Sinus rhythm with obvious delta waves consistent with a right-sided septal or posteroseptal origin. Twelve-lead electrocardiography is performed before radiofrequency ablation.

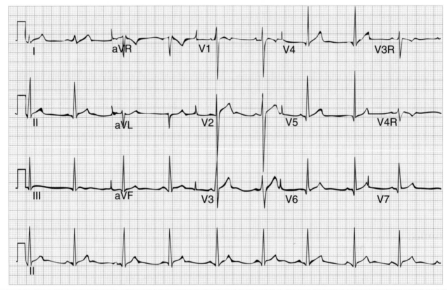

Figure 27-54 Normal electrocardiogram after radiofrequency ablation of the manifest right posteroseptal bypass tract.

conduction proceeds down the AV node into the ventricular myocardium and retrograde up the bypass tract to activate the atrium. The circuit is completed as the AV node is again activated. Tachycardias moving in the opposite direction are identified as wide QRS tachycardias and may be indistinguishable from VT by surface ECG. Adenosine administration during tachycardia may terminate WPW tachycardia but is unlikely to terminate VT. Caution to avoid hypotension or VF during diagnostic atropine administration in nonhypotensive wide complex tachycardia is recommended. Advanced cardiac life support equipment should be available during administration.

In *AVNRT*, sudden rapid onset and offset of narrow complex tachycardia occurs. There is either an inverted P wave immediately after the QRS complex or it may not be visible at all. Termination of the arrhythmia using vagal maneuvers such as carotid sinus massage, Valsalva maneuver, or stimulation with ice cold water may be used clinically. Treatment with AV node–blocking agents can be successful in most patients. Safe, highly effective treatment with invasive electrophysiology study and ablation therapy is common at most larger centers. Figures 27-54 and 27-55 illustrate the mechanism and ECG findings.

Long QT syndrome, a disorder of myocardial repolarization, occurs because of abnormalities in membrane ion channels. Syncope and life-threatening polymorphous VT and VF may result. Autosomal dominant inheritance patterns and variable phenotypic penetrance may be seen. Diagnosis in affected individuals is difficult because the QT interval may be occasionally normal. Provocative maneuvers by a trained specialist may be necessary. Genetic testing for some but not all of the genetic abnormalities are

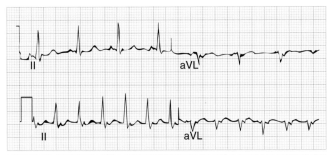

Figure 27-55 Sinus rhythm is noted in the *upper panel*. In the *lower panel,* supraventricular tachycardia consistent with atrioventricular nodal reentrant tachycardia is seen. Retrograde (inverted) P waves immediately after the QRS complex during tachycardia are evident. During the tachycardia at almost 150 beats/min, the normal P-R interval is no longer seen.

available for confirmation. Families with a history of sudden cardiac death or syncope should be evaluated carefully to determine the need for treatment, including β-blockers and implantable defibrillators (Priori et al., 2003).

Atrial fibrillation is the most frequent arrhythmia requiring treatment. In the United States, 2.2 million people have persistent or permanent AF (Feinberg et al., 1997). A basic understanding to the approach of AF can render most patients asymptomatic and dramatically reduce their risk of stroke. The AFFIRM trial represents a landmark study treating all patients with AF with Coumadin. Patients were then randomized to either (1) *control of heart rate* using AV nodal-blocking agents or, if necessary, AV junction ablation and pacemaker therapy or (2) *maintenance of sinus rhythm* using antiarrhythmic drug therapy and repeated direct current cardioversion. Patients were followed for up to 5 years. Patients had similar mortality rates. Patients randomized to rhythm control had more hospitalizations and adverse drug effects mostly related to antiarrhythmic drug therapy. Stroke events were similar but were higher in patients who discontinued Coumadin, regardless of treatment arm (AFFIRM Investigators, 2002).

Based on this study, patients who are candidates for either heart rate control or rhythm control can pursue either treatment strategy with similar efficacy. In patients undergoing restoration of sinus rhythm, the use of direct current cardioversion is safe and effective. Anticoagulation with an INR goal of 2 to 3 in nonvalvular AF is recommended for a minimum of 3 weeks before a cardioversion.

Conscious sedation with short-acting narcotics and IV benzodiazepines allows for synchronized shock delivery in the American Society of Anesthesiologists (ASA) class I and II patients by experienced physicians. In patients adequately anticoagulated with Coumadin, direct current cardioversion can restore sinus rhythm at least transiently in 70% to 90% of patients (Lundrstom and Ryden, 1988; Sodermark et al., 1975; Van Gelder et al., 1991). Maintenance of sinus rhythm at 12 months on antiarrhythmic medications may be as low as 40%, depending on drug selection and the patient population (Van Gelder et al., 1996). Despite this, the practicing physician may elect to gain expertise in conscious sedation and cardioversion when referral electrophysiologists are not readily available and in patients not

requiring or intolerant to drug therapy. Prior recommendations for discontinuation of Coumadin after 6 weeks in sinus rhythm are being scrutinized because of the high stroke rate in patients in the AFFIRM trial who discontinued Coumadin despite being in SR. Caregivers may treat patients long term, even after sinus rhythm is restored or in patients with asymptomatic AF. Because of the high 6-month recurrence rate after cardioversion, many physicians leave patients on anticoagulation for 6 or more months before considering stopping anticoagulation.

Stroke prevention continues to be a primary objective in arrhythmia management. A working knowledge of current anticoagulation guidelines is key to proper management of patients seen in the office and hospital during routine clinical care. For patients with prosthetic mechanical heart valves or with valvular AF (presence of clinically significant MS), the recommendation and use of oral vitamin K antagonists is unchanged. However, changes are ongoing in risk assessment for stroke in patients with paroxysmal, persistent, and permanent nonvalvular AF.

Over the past decade, the $CHADS_2$ score has been used to help objectively quantify a patient's stroke risk in nonvalvular AF. Using the readily available clinical variables of (1) clinical HF, (2) HTN, (3) age 75 years or older, (4) diabetes, and (5) prior stroke or TIA, reasonable prediction of annual stroke risk in the nonanticoagulated patient can be made (Gage et al., 2001). One point is allocated for each of the first four clinical indicators and 2 points for stroke or TIA. Guidelines have recommended no anticoagulation or aspirin only in patients with a $CHADS_2$ score of 0. Warfarin or aspirin is indicated for a $CHADS_2$ score of 1 and warfarin for a score of 2 or greater (Task Force for the Management of Atrial Fibrillation, 2010).

Additional evaluation of stroke rates in individuals with AF has suggested that the $CHADS_2$ scoring system has undervalued age and female gender in the assessment of stroke risk (Karthikeyan and Eikelboom, 2010; Keogh et al., 2011). The CHA_2DS_2-VASc score currently used in Europe and Canada looks at similar risk factors as the $CHADS_2$ scoring system but increases the weight of age and includes female gender if the patient is older than 65 years of age. In addition, CHF is defined as LV systolic dysfunction. Age equal to or greater than 65 years receives 1 point and equal to or greater than 75 years receives an additional point. Female gender (older than 65 years of age) is allocated 1 point and evidence of vascular disease a final point.

The purpose of the CHA_2DS_2-VASc scoring system is to identify very-low-risk patients in whom anticoagulation bleeding risk outweighs stroke reduction benefit, including the use of aspirin. Individuals with CHA_2DS_2-VASc scores of 0 have very low stroke rates, and bleeding risk from either aspirin or full-dose anticoagulation would be excessive. As a consequence, patients with a CHA_2DS_2-VASc score of 0 are currently indicated to be on no anticoagulation for a history of AF (Camm et al., 2012; Oelsen et al., 2011).

In individuals with a CHA_2DS_2-VASc score of 1, oral anticoagulation with adjusted-dose vitamin K antagonist, a direct thrombin inhibitor, or oral factor Xa inhibitor should be considered based on an assessment of the risk of bleeding complications and patient preferences. Individuals with a CHA_2DS_2-VASc score of 2 or greater should be on oral anticoagulation (Camm et al., 2012).

Newer oral anticoagulants have become mainstream in stroke prevention across the globe. As of the publication of this text, three agents have been approved for stroke prevention in patients with nonvalvular AF. Agents fall into one of two classes: the oral direct thrombin inhibitors (dabigatran) and the oral direct factor Xa inhibitors (rivaroxaban, apixaban). These agents, commonly referred to as the novel oral anticoagulants (NOACs), block a specific step in the coagulation cascade in contrast to vitamin K antagonists, which block multiple steps. In addition, these agents have an abrupt onset (within hours) and shorter half-lives (less than 24 hours) compared with warfarin (Camm et al., 2012).

Clinical data from the RE-LY trial, the ROCKET-AF trial, and the ARISTOTLE trial have demonstrated noninferiority or superiority over vitamin K antagonists in stroke prevention and systemic embolism. At currently approved doses, the NOAC are at least noninferior to vitamin K antagonists, and in the case of some of these agents may be superior and associated with decreased bleeding incidence. Importantly, the NOACs are associated with a significant reduction in intracranial hemorrhage (Connolly et al., 2009, 2010; Granger et al., 2011; Patel et al., 2011).

Weighing the risk of anticoagulation against bleeding is a vexing clinical problem in daily practice. Many calculators of bleeding risk have been developed over the past several years. However, the HAS-BLED calculator has grown in popularity (Pisters et al., 2010). Cumulative points are assigned for uncontrolled HTN, abnormal renal or liver function, bleeding tendencies, older age, compounding drug use or abuse, and prior stroke. Individuals with a score greater than or equal to 3 are at high risk of bleeding. A high score does not preclude anticoagulation use, but closer evaluation and follow-up or early discontinuation of anticoagulation may be indicated.

Despite the emergence of risk tools for anticoagulation indication and bleeding probability, predicting the effect of a given anticoagulant on an individual continues to be difficult. Each patient must be clinically evaluated for subtleties in his or her clinical status that improve the safety and efficacy of these potent agents. It is clear, however, that clinicians tend to underanticoagulate patients in current practice. Continued vigilance in evaluating patients for appropriate anticoagulation and the initiation and maintenance of safe dosing in the setting of AF must be maintained to reduce preventable debilitating stroke or systemic embolism.

Syncope is the sudden loss of postural tone and may be due to both cardiac and noncardiac causes. Up to 30% of patients may ultimately have no explanation. A detailed history, including dietary and fluid intake, personal and family history, medication use and timing, and precipitating factors, will aid in the diagnosis. The best single determinant of an etiology is likely the history. Additional testing depends on the presence or absence of structural heart disease. Invasive electrophysiology study in the setting of structural heart disease may identify up to half of patients' causes (Linzer et al., 1997). In the absence of structural heart disease, tilt table testing may identify between 11% and 87% of patients by two reports (Kapoor, 1990, 1992). Referral to an electrophysiologist should be considered in the setting of structural heart disease.

Table 27-26 Classification of Rhythms

Atrial	Sinus rhythm
	Sinus bradycardia
	Sinus pause
	Sinus node exit block (types I and II)
	Sinus arrest
	Sinus tachycardia
	Premature atrial contraction
	Wandering atrial pacemaker
	Ectopic atrial rhythm
	Ectopic atrial tachycardia
	Multifocal atrial tachycardia
	Atrial fibrillation
	Atrial flutter
Junctional rhythms	Premature junctional beat
	Junctional rhythm
	Accelerated junctional tachycardia
	AV nodal reentrant tachycardia
	AV conduction block
	First-degree AV block
	Second-degree AV block
	Type I
	Type II
	2:1
	High grade
	Third-degree AV block (complete AV block)
Ventricular rhythms	Premature ventricular contractions
	Accelerated idioventricular rhythm
	Ventricular tachycardia (monomorphic and polymorphic)
	Ventricular fibrillation
Special rhythms	Preexcitation
	AV reciprocating tachycardia
	Long QT
	Paced rhythms

AV, Atrioventricular.

TREATMENT OF CARDIAC ARRHYTHMIAS

An organized approach to the treatment of cardiac arrhythmias is paramount. Initial steps include identification and verification of the arrhythmia type and an assessment of potential harm to the patient. Table 27-26 outlines various rhythms categorized by their cardiac chamber of origin. As described earlier, inpatient evaluation is recommended in some patients. In patients in whom pharmacologic therapy is recommended, knowledge of the side effects and proarrhythmia potential must be known. Table 27-27 outlines antiarrhythmic agents according to the Vaughan Williams classification system. A newer classification, the Sicilian Gambit, is a system based on channel effects and mechanisms of arrhythmogenesis that, although helpful, is too complex for most individuals to use and has not gained favor in today's era of invasive arrhythmia therapy (Rosen and Schwartz, 1991).

ROLE OF THE CONSULTATIVE CARDIOLOGIST OR ELECTROPHYSIOLOGIST

Evaluation and treatment of patients with arrhythmias is a rewarding practice. Many arrhythmias can be symptomatically improved through use of medications, lifestyle changes, and reassurance. However, meta-analysis of antiarrhythmic drug trials and the CAST studies demonstrate the potential dangers of drug therapy in the treatment of

Table 27-27 Indication, Route of Administration, and Considerations for Use of Common Antiarrhythmic Drugs*

Type of Drug	Typical Indications	Route	Considerations, Contraindications, and Complications	Frequency of General Use
CLASS I				
Class Ia				
Disopyramide (Norpace)	PACs, AF, SVT, PVCs	PO	Useful in normal hearts without ischemia; prolongs QT; atropine effect	Atrial arrhythmias only
Procainamide (Procan, Procanbid)	AF, PAC, PVC, VT	PO, IV	Wider range of use in mild LV dysfunction; lupus side effect; prolongs QT and QRS; best used in normal hearts only; renally excreted with active metabolite (class III)	Atrial arrhythmias; acute suppression of VT after CABG
Quinidine (Quinidex, Quinaglute)	AF, AFL, PACs, PVC, VT	PO, IV	Marked QT prolongation, myasthenia; idiosyncratic blood defects; may enhance AV conduction	Limited use; mostly AF, AFL
Class Ib				
Lidocaine	VT, torsades de pointes	IV	Rapid onset; may cause CNS changes and seizures	Acute VT termination and suppression; being replaced by IV amiodarone
Mexiletine (Mexitil)	PVCs, VT	PO	Significant GI upset; mild proarrhythmia; mild effect; can be used carefully in setting of LV dysfunction	PVC suppression when other agents fail
Phenytoin (Dilantin)	VPB, VT	PO, IV	CNS effects; rash; blood dyscrasias	Rarely used; minimal effect
Tocainide (Tonocard)	VT	PO	CNS effects; blood dyscrasias; GI upset; pneumonitis	Rare use
Class Ic				
Flecainide (Tambocor)	AF, AFL, PACs, EAT, WPW	PO	Well tolerated; may increase conduction of slowed atrial flutter; contraindicated in CHF	Frequently used for AF, AFL
Propafenone (Rythmol)	PACs, EAT, AF, AFL, PVC	PO	Contraindicated in CHF	Frequently used for AF, AFL
CLASS II				
β-Nonselective				
Propanolol	ST, AT, IST, PVCs, VT, AF*	PO, IV	Excess bradycardia; hypotension; CNS effects; negative inotrope; pulmonary bronchospasm	Short acting, rapid onset; increased replacement by longer-acting cardiac selective agents
β-Selective				
Atenolol	ST, AT, IST, PVCs, VT, AF*	PO, IV	Excess bradycardia; hypotension; CNS effects; negative inotrope	Inexpensive, resulting in frequent use
Metoprolol (Lopressor, Toprol)	ST, AT, IST, PVCs, VT, AF*	PO, IV	Excess bradycardia; hypotension; CNS effects; negative inotrope	Frequently used, long-acting preparation with infrequent side effects
Pindolol	ST, AT, IST, PVCs, AF*	PO	Excess bradycardia; hypotension; CNS effects; negative inotrope	Intermediated use
Timolol	ST, AT, IST, PVCs, AF*	PO	Excess bradycardia; hypotension; CNS effects; negative inotrope	Low-frequency use
Esmolol (Brevibloc)	ST, AT, IST, PVCs, AF*	IV	Short acting; excess bradycardia; nonselective at high doses	Low-frequency use because of IV form only
Mixed α and β				
Carvedilol (Coreg)	CHF, PVCs, AF*	PO	Excess bradycardia; hypotension; exacerbation of CHF; fatigue	Infrequent as first choice for arrhythmias but primarily indicated for systolic heart failure
CLASS III				
Ibutilide (Corvert)	AF, AFL	IV	Proarrhythmia frequent, including PVCs, VT, and torsades de pointes; prolongs QT and slows heart rate; requires acute monitoring	Intermediate use has high efficacy in acute AF and AFL but with potential serious acute side effects
Dofetilide (Tikosyn)	PACs, AF, AFL	PO	High efficacy; prolongs QT and QRS; proarrhythmic, including torsades de pointes	Low-frequency use because of inpatient initiation and potential dangerous proarrhythmia; requires training to prescribe; is mortality neutral in CHF and MI patients
Sotalol (Betapace)	ST, AT, IST, PVCs, VT, AF*	PO	Excess bradycardia; prolongs QT with potential torsades de pointes	Moderate-frequency use; reasonably safe in setting of mild LV dysfunction in absence of ischemia

Continued on following page

Table 27-27 Indication, Route of Administration, and Considerations for Use of Common Antiarrhythmic Drugs (Continued)

Type of Drug	Typical Indications	Route	Considerations, Contraindications, and Complications	Frequency of General Use
Amiodarone (Pacerone, Cordarone)	ST, AT, AF, AFL, PVCs, VT, AF*	PO, IV	Class I, II, III, and IV effects; very well tolerated but may produce serious thyroid dysfunction and lethal pulmonary and liver dysfunction; close monitoring for side effects mandatory	High-frequency use owing to very low acute side effect profile and very high efficacy in a variety of arrhythmias; indiscriminate use is discouraged
CLASS IV				
Diltiazem (Cardizem, Cartia)	AF*, PVCs, calcium-dependent VT	PO, IV	Bradycardia; hypotension; exacerbation of systolic heart failure; continuous infusion available	Used frequently for AV node slowing in setting of AF with or without LV dysfunction
Verapamil (Calan, Isoptin)	AF*, PVCs, calcium-dependent VT	PO, IV	Bradycardia; hypotension; exacerbation of systolic heart failure	Used frequently for AV node slowing in setting of AF
CLASS V (OTHER)				
Adenosine (Adenocard)	SVT	IV	Acute onset with very powerful AV node block and to less extent SA block, producing marked bradycardia and transient asystole; temporary pulmonary symptoms	Agent of choice for abrupt termination of most AV node–dependent arrhythmias
Digoxin	AF*	PO, IV	Proarrhythmic, including heart block and enhancing bypass tract conduction; GI side effects	Frequent adjuvant drug for slowing ventricular response in AF
Atropine	SB	IV	Avoid in patients with acute-angle glaucoma	Acute treatment for sinus bradycardia and heart block not caused by Purkinje failure
Magnesium sulphate	Torsades de pointes, PVCs, VT suppression	PO, IV	Caution in renal failure	Frequent adjuvant drug for VT suppression

*Drugs are organized according to the Vaughan Williams classification scheme. Indications represent both approved and nonapproved indications as of the date of publication.
AF, Atrial fibrillation; *AF**, atrioventricular node blockade in atrial fibrillation; *AFL*, atrial flutter; *AT*, atrial tachycardia; *AV, atrioventricular; CABG,* coronary artery bypass graft; *CHF,* systolic congestive heart failure; *CNS*, central nervous system; *GI*, gastrointestinal; *IST*, inappropriate sinus tachycardia; *IV*, intravenous; *LV*, left ventricular; *MI*, myocardial infarction; *PAC;* premature atrial contraction; *PO*, oral; *PVC;* premature ventricular contraction; *SA*, sinoatrial; *SB*, sinus bradycardia; *ST*, sinus tachycardia; *VPB*, ventricular premature beats; *VT*, ventricular tachycardia; *WPW*, Wolfe-Parkinson-White.

cardiac arrhythmias (Echt et al., 1991; Sodermark et al., 1975). In addition, invasive evaluation and treatment of common bothersome or malignant arrhythmias is carried out by cardiac specialists trained in electrophysiology. In addition to drug therapy, an electrophysiologist may offer invasive techniques to treat arrhythmias. Arrhythmia ablation, implantation of pacemakers and defibrillators, and cardiac resynchronization therapy are all techniques to help reduce morbidity and mortality rates.

ELECTROPHYSIOLOGY STUDY AND ABLATION

Patients in whom invasive arrhythmia therapy is recommended are evaluated in special catheterization suites. During an electrophysiology study, several electrodes or wires are inserted through the femoral or jugular vein and advanced to the right atrium, RV, coronary sinus, and the region of the AV node–His-bundle complex. Special pacing sequences and premature beat delivery are used to initiate arrhythmias. The wires may then be moved to different sites within the heart. Application of radiofrequency current through the tip of the catheter electrode results in elimination of the arrhythmia focus. Variations in duration and power of the current are used to alter lesion size. Studies may last less than 1 hour to several hours depending on the

nature of the arrhythmias treated. This essentially painless method replaced the older technique of direct current lesion application, which was poorly controlled, was quite painful, and required general anesthesia to carry out. Radiofrequency ablation is now used as the standard technique is treatment of AV node–dependent arrhythmias, including AVNRT, AV reciprocating tachycardia, and junctional tachycardia. AFL is successfully cured in most cases, and even paroxysmal AF may be suppressed or cured by this technique. Termination of AFL is demonstrated in Figure 27-43. Future refinements of this technique may one day be used to cure countless numbers of patients with bothersome AF.

Alternate energy sources, including microwave, ultrasound, and cryotherapy, are being investigated and used. Radiofrequency, however, remains the energy source in almost all cases for the routine treatment of supraventricular arrhythmias treated with ablation. Treatment of arrhythmias through open-chest procedures was once the only method to cure arrhythmias. Considered high risk in most patients and too invasive for nonlethal arrhythmias in the era of radiofrequency ablation, surgical ablation for AF has enjoyed a resurgence as adjunct therapy during valvular heart surgery with cryotherapy and radiofrequency therapy of pulmonary veins (Todd et al., 2007).

PACEMAKERS AND DEFIBRILLATORS

Significant development in the area of pacing has occurred since transvenous pacemakers were first produced and implanted. Once able to pace only in a single chamber at a preset rate and without the ability to detect underlying rhythms, the pacemakers of today are more sophisticated. A pacemaker is in its simplest form a battery, a pulse generator, and a lead to deliver an impulse. The use of sensing and timing circuits coupled with motion detectors within the pacemaker allow inhibition of pacing when sensed events occur and an increase in paced rate with motion or activity. As technology has advanced, pacemakers are able to pace effectively in the atrium and ventricle, and AV or PR intervals can be adjusted. Telemetry through the skin using proprietary programmers allows adjustment in the physician's office. Miniaturization has now resulted in sophisticated pacemakers in a package not much larger than a half-dollar coin that can pace the heart when necessary, detect rapid rhythms, and attempt to pace terminate the arrhythmia (Figure 27-56; Furman et al., 1993).

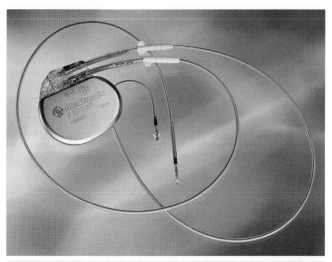

Figure 27-56 Dual-chamber pacemaker with endocardial passive and active fixation leads. (Courtesy Medtronic, Minneapolis, MN.)

Implantable defibrillators with endocardial leads were developed in the early 1990s, allowing for a safer and less invasive procedure. These devices are now able to identify and attempt to terminate ventricular arrhythmias through painless overdrive pacing or using an endocardial shock that can be uncomfortable if the patient is not syncopal (Figures 27-57 and 27-58).

CARDIAC RESYNCHRONIZATION AND DEFIBRILLATOR THERAPY

Patients with refractory clinical CHF have a six- to ninefold increase in sudden cardiac death compared with the general population (AHA, 2002). Despite medical therapy with β-blockers, ACE inhibitors, angiotensin II receptor blockers, diuretics, spironolactone, digoxin, and invasive revascularization strategies, patients continue to have significant morbidity and mortality from systolic CHF. Electrophysiologists for more than a decade have been impacting mortality and morbidity through cardiac pacing resynchronization therapy and defibrillator placement.

The slowing of conduction through the LV in the setting of bundle branch block or significant scarring leads to dyssynchronous lateral and septal contraction. This dyssynchrony results in excess energy expenditure and decreases cardiac performance. Placement of a pacing device capable of pacing in the RV and additionally at the lateral LV has resulted in significant reductions in morbidity and mortality. The addition of a defibrillator further results in reduction of mortality (Abraham et al., 2002; Bristow et al., 2004; Cleland et al., 2005; Young et al., 2003).

Figure 27-59 shows the radiographic appearance of a biventricular system. Pacing in both ventricles demonstrates a shortening of the QRS complex and is associated with improvements in cardiac contractility and over time reduction in LV chamber size, reduction in mitral valve regurgitation, improvements in 6-minute walk test results, quality of life, and NYHA HF classification (Abraham et al., 2002). In Figure 27-60, changes in the QRS morphology are demonstrated depending on the site of electrical

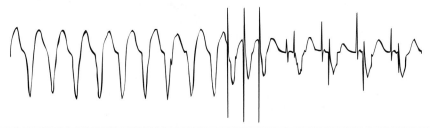

Figure 27-57 Ventricular tachycardia is pace terminated by three rapid ventricular pulses from the implanted pacemaker-defibrillator. Atrioventricular sequential pacing resumes after termination of the ventricular tachycardia.

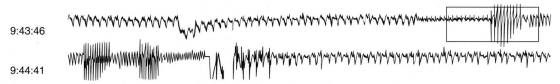

9:43:46

9:44:41

Figure 27-58 Attempt at pace termination of ventricular tachycardia with acceleration of the ventricular tachycardia into ventricular fibrillation. The transient of the endocardial shock is noted, and pacing resumes with organized cardiac activity.

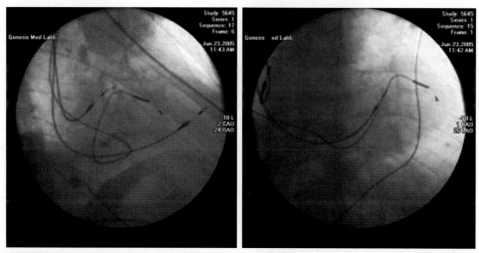

Figure 27-59 Radiographs from a dual-chamber biventricular defibrillator. Right and left anterior oblique views are shown in a patient treated for left ventricular systolic dysfunction and New York Heart Association class III heart failure. Standard leads terminate in the right atrium and the right ventricular septum. A third lead enters the coronary sinus from the right atrium and extends into a branching vein to provide synchronous left and right ventricular activation.

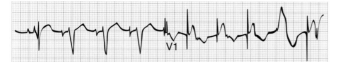

Figure 27-60 Left bundle branch block (BBB) and right BBB are produced from contralateral ventricular pacing. Right ventricular pacing with left BBB morphology is noted on the *left*. Pacing activates one side of the ventricle earlier and therefore results in a BBB pattern of the opposite side of the chamber paced. On the *right*, inappropriate left ventricular endocardial lead placement delivered across a patent foramen ovale was detected before serious consequences of embolic stroke. Epicardial pacing of the left ventricle is also accomplished through lead placement through the coronary sinus.

stimulation. During right and LV activation, the QRS morphology in lead V1 is shown.

Patients with lethal tachycardia events such as VT and VF have been extensively studied. For much of modern electrophysiologic history, the electrophysiologic study was used to induce VT in patients with syncope and structural heart disease, in patients with symptomatic stable VT, and in patients resuscitated from arrhythmic sudden cardiac death. Drugs were then initiated, and repeat testing was performed to test the success of the antiarrhythmic drug. More recent studies have challenged this approach. Drug versus implantable defibrillator therapy trials have demonstrated mortality benefit as secondary prevention of syncopal VT or resuscitated sudden cardiac death with structural heart disease (Antiarrhythmics versus Implantable Defibrillators Investigators, 1997; Connolly et al., 2000; Kuck et al., 2000). Further studies have demonstrated mortality benefit from implantable defibrillators compared with drug therapy in primary prevention trials. Specific groups of patients have demonstrated superiority of device therapy compared with drugs: (1) patients with asymptomatic ventricular ectopy with inducible VT, (2) patients with prior MI and EFs less than 30%, and (3) patients with EFs less than 35% with class II or III NYHA

HF for longer than 3 months (Bardy et al., 2005; Buxton et al., 2000; Moss et al., 1996, 2002). Patients fulfilling these criteria should be referred to an electrophysiologist.

SUMMARY

Treatment of patients with symptoms referable to an arrhythmia is possible for many physicians. Accurate diagnosis of the arrhythmic event may prove difficult, and additional diagnostic tests not readily available to the family physician may need to be used. More conscientious use of antiarrhythmic drugs is necessary as we learn more about the proarrhythmic effects. Implantable device therapy continues to evolve and promises to alter the natural history of many malignant cardiac disease states.

Videos

The following videos are available at www.expertconsult.com.

Video 27-1 Rheumatic Mitral Valve Stenosis

Video 27-2 Mitral Valve Insufficiency

Video 27-3 Normally Functioning Mechanical Mitral Valve Prosthesis

Video 27-4 Right Coronary Artery Occlusion

Video 27-5 Mitral Valve Prolapse

References

The complete reference list is available at www.expertconsult.com.

Web Resources

hypertensiononline.org Slide resource on hypertension management.
www.americanheart.org The American Heart Association's site provides a valuable range of Internet resources on a wide variety of cardiovascular diseases, including statistics on heart disease prevalence.
www.ash-us.org Website and resource center for the American Society of Hypertension.
www.cardiosource.com *Journal of the American College of Cardiology*'s site; outstanding functionality and features; requires subscription.

www.clinicaltrialresults.org Outstanding resource on cardiovascular clinical trials with videos of principal investigators discussing results and slide decks.

www.dashdiet.org Practical instructions on using diet to reduce blood pressure.

www.diabetes.org American Diabetes Association site with information for patients and health professionals.

www.fammed.wisc.edu/integrative/modules/hypertension Summary for clinicians and patients on how to lower blood pressure without medications.

www.lipid.org Website and resource center for the National Lipid Association.

www.lipidsonline.org Slide resource on dyslipidemia management.

www.theheart.org Excellent resource with coverage of all areas of cardiology.

www.vbwg.org Slide resource for management of dyslipidemia, hypertension, insulin resistance, and diabetes mellitus; updated regularly.

Primary care providers can perform many common surgical procedures in an outpatient setting without significant sedation. This chapter provides the foundational competency skills in common procedures, including adequate preparation, appropriate setup, informed consent, good technical skills, and awareness of potential complications. A discussion of the basic surgical skills and setup required, patient consent, and local anesthesia is followed by a review of common office procedures in family medicine, with tips to perform these successfully with minimal complications.

As the U.S. health care system grapples with medical home concepts, family medicine providers must develop proficient skills to carry out common procedures in primary care clinics. The health care system has provided high remuneration for procedural medicine in the past but is evolving to a system driven by outcomes, competency, and the ability to provide cost-effective, competent procedural services in a primary care medical home.

For a brief history of surgery, see eAppendix 28-1 online.

Basic Skills

THE PATIENT HISTORY

The physician must begin with a pertinent comprehensive health history and thorough understanding of the patient and his or her current health condition before undertaking any surgical procedure. Preexisting diagnoses such as diabetes or hemophilia may affect wound healing or bleeding.

Allergies to medication, tape, or preparation agents should be elicited along with any personal or family history of bleeding or thrombosis. Anticoagulant use, including aspirin, clopidogrel, warfarin, nonsteroidal antiinflammatory drugs (NSAIDs), ticlopidine, and dipyridamole, may affect bleeding and hemostasis during any procedure.

Guidelines on perioperative anticoagulation divide these medicines into three categories. There are vitamin K–dependent anticoagulants (VKAs) such as Coumadin, aspirin and NSAIDS, and clopidogrel. Patients taking VKAs who are undergoing minor dental procedures may continue the VKAs and take a dose of vitamin K or stop the VKAs for

2 to 3 days before the minor dental procedure. Patients taking VKAs who are undergoing minor dermatologic procedures are advised to continue vitamin K–dependent anticoagulation, continue aspirin and NSAIDS, and consider stopping clopidogrel if not at high risk for cardiac disease (Douketis et al., 2012).

Aspirin and other antiplatelet medications may be resumed 24 hours after surgery. If a superficial procedure is performed on a high-risk patient, the physician should continue the blood-thinning agent and consider using local anesthesia with epinephrine for vasoconstriction. Local cautery, direct ligation of bleeding vessels, and direct pressure are used as needed for hemostasis.

A change in approach is warranted when a history of delayed healing or keloid (thick scar) formation is elicited. Preventive measures should be undertaken in a patient with a history of a prior vasovagal event or fainting episode during or after a procedure.

KEY TREATMENT

- Patients taking aspirin for secondary prevention of cardiac disease who are having minor dental, dermatologic, or cataract surgery should continue the aspirin *and NOT stop it 7 to 10 days before surgery as previously advised* (SOR: C) (Douketis et al., 2012).
- Warfarin should be stopped 2 to 3 days before the procedure in low-risk patients. High-risk patients may need heparin bridging (SOR: A) (Singer et al., 2008).
- Fish oil and omega-3 fatty acids have not been shown to increase bleeding (SOR: A) (Villani et al., 2013).

SKIN PREPARATION

The skin should be prepared with an appropriate antiseptic solution, starting in the middle of the surgical site and going outward in concentric circles in aseptic fashion. Alcohol, chlorhexidine, povidone-iodine (Betadine), or a combination may be used as an antiseptic cleansing agent (Mangram et al., 1999).

The U.S. Centers for Disease Control and Prevention (CDC) and Healthcare Infection Control Practices Advisory Committee updated guidelines in 2002 on skin preparation related to reducing central line infections. The CDC had issued additional guidelines for the prevention of surgical site infection in 1999. The U.K. National Institute for Health and Clinical Excellence–Surgical Site Infection guidelines from 2008 concurred with the CDC's recommendations. Skin aseptic preparation with chlorhexidine 2% plus 70% isopropyl alcohol was the best at preventing surgical site infections because it achieves greater reductions in skin microflora and has greater residual activity after a single application (Mangram et al., 1999).

Chlorhexidine gluconate is effective even in the presence of blood or serum proteins, but blood and serum proteins may inactivate povidone-iodine. Based on chlorhexidine dilution and duration studies, the best reduction of bacterial load occurred with 4% solution applied at least two minutes before incision. The bacteriocidal effects lasted an hour (Stinner et al., 2011). Isopropyl alcohol 70% is effective immediately, but the antiseptic effect is not sustained. Combinations are superior to isopropyl alcohol or chlorhexidine alone (Adams et al., 2005; Hibbard, 2005).

Many surgical site infections are from endogenous staphylococcal skin flora. An increasing number are also resistant to antibiotics, such as methicillin-resistant *Staphylococcus aureus* (MRSA). Good handwashing and aseptic technique are primary for the prevention of MRSA-related surgical site infections (Siegel et al., 2006). Patients who wash preoperatively with soap and water or chlorhexidine may reduce bacterial skin flora, but this did not reduce the incidence of surgical site infections (Webster and Osborne, 2012). Various guidelines on the prevention of soft tissue surgical site infections found that broad routine MRSA screening is not indicated before surgery (Glick et al., 2013).

KEY TREATMENT

- Chlorhexidine plus alcohol-containing skin preparations were better than povidone-iodine for surgical site antisepsis (Darouiche et al., 2010) (SOR: A).
- Hair should not be removed before surgery unless the hair is at or around the incision site and would interfere with the procedure. If hair removal is required, it should be clipped immediately before surgery, and it should not be shaved (Mangram et al., 1999) (SOR: A).

BITES

Bites represent special risks for laceration repair. Animal bites often involve deep puncture wounds and should be cleaned and irrigated thoroughly. They are generally not closed but are allowed to heal by secondary intention. Facial bites may be primarily closed after wounds are cleansed.

Untreated cat bite infection rates are 18% to 33% (Dire, 1991). Treating cat bites with prophylactic antibiotics significantly reduces infection rates. Dog bites may be more lacerated, and after high-pressure flushing at greater than 7 psi (obtained flushing with a 50-cc syringe and saline), they may be closed primarily in the first 6 hours after the injury. Infection rates for dog bites are less than 20% (Dire, 1992).

Primary suture closure is not generally recommended for nonfacial bite wounds, especially deep punctures, bites to the hand, and clinically infected wounds. Anecdotal data suggest an increased risk of infection after closure of these wounds. Sterile skin closure strips or delayed closure may be appropriate (Singer et al., 2008).

Human bites on the hands and specifically overlying the metacarpophalangeal joints are problematic because of potential damage to underlying tissue, tendons, and joint spaces. Hand injuries may therefore lead to aggressive deep secondary infections. Documentation of sensation, range of motion, and exploration to determine joint or deep space involvement may still miss serious intraarticular bites. Profuse flushing of human hand bites or lacerations, prophylactic antibiotics, and consultation are advised. These wounds may need to be surgically opened under anesthesia to adequately flush them. Seeking care may be delayed, and rates of infection rapidly increase if seen after 24 hours. Late assessment after 24 hours usually involves operative debridement and flushing along with intravenous antibiotics. Bite wounds evaluated, deemed to not involve deep tissues, and flushed within the first 24 hours may be treated conservatively with oral antibiotics; physicians should be aware that there may still be deep penetration, which leads to urgent operative care.

Wounds to both the hands and face need immediate care because infection rates almost double to 29% if not treated within 12 hours. Prophylactic antibiotics should be used with hand and facial bite wounds. Facial wounds may be flushed and closed primarily because of the good blood supply and a risk for poor cosmesis if they are left open (Henry et al., 2007).

KEY TREATMENT

- Antibiotics should be used prophylactically in human bites to the hand (number needed to treat [NNT] = 4) (Medeiros and Saconato, 2001) (SOR: A).
- Prophylaxis with amoxicillin/clavulanate should be considered for all bite wounds that are primarily closed, all puncture wounds, cat bites to the hand and wrist, clenched fist injuries, and crush wounds (Morgan, 2005) (SOR: C).
- Clenched fist human "fight bites" should be radiographed for broken teeth and foreign bodies (Sternberg and Jacob, 2010) (SOR: C).

IMMUNIZATIONS

Tetanus immunization should be updated if indicated with any laceration or open skin injury. If a patient has received three or more primary tetanus immunizations, he or she should receive a booster if the last immunization was more than 10 years ago for a clean wound and if more than 5 years ago with a dirty wound. Patients should receive tetanus immune globulin and begin their tetanus immunization series if they have had fewer than three primary tetanus immunizations in the past. Diphtheria toxoid and pertussis antigens with tetanus toxoid (Tdap) should replace a single dose of Td for adults aged 19 through 64 years who have not received a dose of Tdap previously and require a booster. Tdap may be given as close as 2 years after a Td;

data suggest it is safe even if given within 21 days of Td. Td can be given every 10 years when needed after one Tdap dose is received (CDC, 2010; see Web Resources).

Patients should be offered the hepatitis B immunization series for any human bite or for mucous membrane blood exposure. Patients should be offered and consent to baseline testing for hepatitis B virus (HBV) and C virus (HCV) and human immunodeficiency virus (HIV). Appropriate follow-up based on test results must be arranged (Panlilio et al., 2013). HBIG is indicated if the patient has injuries from a person known to be positive for hepatitis B surface antigen; however, needle stick guidelines suggest that the injured patient receive only a hepatitis B immunization series and not HBIG if the contact person has an unknown or negative carrier status. In the case of a needle stick, HIV prophylaxis with three drugs is recommended if the contact person is known to be HIV positive. If the source patient has an unknown HIV status, postexposure prophylaxis (PEP) generally is not indicated unless there is concern that the source is higher risk, in which case a three-drug PEP is recommended (Clinician Consultation Center, 2014; Panlilio et al., 2005; Schillie et al., 2013; see Web Resources).

PROCEDURE ROOM

A clean procedure room with a table that elevates and an overhead surgical light that can be adjusted and focused gives the provider the best environment to carry out procedures. An adjustable and mobile mayo stand allows the most comfortable access to sterile trays and instruments. Surgical instruments should be stored in sterile packs, ideally set up for specific procedures. Extra equipment may be in individual sterile packs and should be readily available. Sterility expiration dates for all packaged equipment should be checked.

Patients should be made comfortable for the procedure with use of an adjustable bed and pillows as needed. Open, supportive conversation with an empathetic approach encourages relaxation and reassurance before, during, and after the procedure. An assistant is helpful in setup and during the procedure and provides support for the patient during care. In children undergoing a procedure, a family-focused dialog and ongoing conversation are similar to using midazolam in reducing anxiety and speeding recovery (Kain et al., 2007). Prior to starting any procedure, do a "time out" to review a patient procedure check list to make sure everyone agrees on the patient, procedure, and code word to stop the procedure if any team member notes something of concern. This is similar to a pilot's preflight inspection and reduces error (Haynes et al., 2009).

Equipment

The most basic sterile pack for skin procedures contains a needle driver, Adson tissue forceps with teeth, iris or suture scissors, and scalpel handle with blade. The instruments should comfortably fit the provider's hands.

Three primary scalpel blade styles are used in the outpatient setting. A #10 blade has a large, rounded cutting surface and may be used for longer, straight incisions on larger body areas with thicker skin, such as the trunk or limbs. A #15 blade has a smaller, rounded cutting surface to allow more mobility for nonlinear incisions and may be

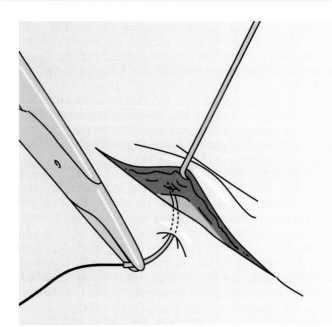

Figure 28-1 The use of forceps or a skin hook to evert the wound edge. This technique allows the operator to see the needle path, thereby ensuring that the proper depth has been reached, and promotes eversion of the skin edges. (From Roberts JR. Methods of wound closure. In Roberts JR, ed. *Roberts & Hedges' clinical procedures in emergency medicine.* 6th ed. Philadelphia: Saunders; 2014.)

used on most skin procedures. A #11 blade has a pointed surface without a curve and is better used for paring superficial lesions, such as warts or calluses, or puncturing skin abscesses. The Adson forceps with teeth has one side with one tooth and the other side with two teeth. Less tissue trauma occurs using the single tooth on the external tissue while everting the skin edges or using a skin hook (Fig. 28-1).

Needle drivers should fit the provider's hand; the ring finger fits in the lower handle hole, and the thumb may fit in the top circle of the handle with the index finger extended along the shaft to stabilize the needle driver. The needle is loaded by locking the needle driver about three quarters of the way up the needle shank, with the needle held perpendicular to the needle driver. Sharps are kept in the same area of the sterile field to reduce needle stick injuries.

Suture

Three basic types of suture exist: natural absorbable, synthetic absorbable, and nonabsorbable. Sutures are sized according to the 1937 U.S. Pharmacopeia classification system. A smaller suture has a higher number of zeroes (e.g., 4-0 is finer than 2-0). The physician should use the smallest suture size that provides adequate initial tensile strength to close the wound and not fail during the healing process. The clinician should use deep subcutaneous sutures to reduce surface tension if the wound is deep and there is high skin surface tension. Ideally, superficial skin sutures gently approximate the skin edges with minimal tension.

Absorbable types of suture include plain gut; chromic gut; and synthetic sutures made of polyglycolic acid, polylactic acid, polydioxanone, and caprolactone. Whereas plain gut suture used externally has a tensile strength lasting 5 to 7 days, chromic gut used internally has a tensile strength lasting 10 to 14 days. The synthetic absorbable

Table 28-1 EMLA Dosing

Age and Weight Requirements	EMLA Cream (maximum total dose, g)	Maximum Application Area (cm²)	Maximum Application Time (hr)
0-3 mo *or* <5 kg	1	10	1
3-12 mo and >5 kg	2	20	4
1-6 yr and >10 kg	1	100	4
7-12 yr and >20 kg	20	200	4

EMLA, Eutectic mixture of lidocaine and prilocaine.
Developed from EMLA drug information. In *Facts and comparisons,* 2010. http://online.factsandcomparisons.com/MonoDisp.aspx?monoID=fandc-hcp1 4927&quick=341644%7c5&search=341644%7c5&isstemmed=true.

types of suture vary in length of tensile strength and rate of absorption. Nonabsorbable suture is made of nylon, special silk, polypropylene, or polyester. These sutures are made in different colors and are inert. Most have long-lasting tensile strength. Nonabsorbable sutures are used externally but can also be used internally for prolonged tissue reinforcement. Nonabsorbable sutures cause less immune response and therefore less scarring. Frequently, they are used superficially when cosmetic outcome is critical.

Traditionally, absorbable suture was only placed below the skin's surface because of its porous structure and concern it would wick bacteria from the skin surface. However, this recommendation is not evidence based. A meta-analysis of two randomized, controlled trials (Jadad scores 3) comparing absorbable versus nonabsorbable sutures in the management of traumatic lacerations and surgical wounds showed no changes in infection rates, scar appearance, patient satisfaction, or dehiscence. In children, the benefit is not requiring suture removal (Al-Abdullah et al., 2007).

Needles

Suture needles are classified by the geometry of their points. Taper needles have a round body that tapers smoothly to a point. Cutting needles are triangular with a sharp cutting edge on the inside curve of the needle; reverse cutting needles have the cutting edge on the outside of the curve. A taper-cut needle is round but ends in a short, triangular cutting point. Some needles are attached permanently to suture and others, called "pop-offs," separate from the suture with a sharp pull. With the wide range of needle types, physicians should be familiar with their own supplies and examine the outsides of packages closely before use. Reverse cutting needles are stronger than conventional cutting needles; both minimize trauma to the skin and so are appropriate for most skin closure.

ANESTHESIA

Topical Anesthesia

An equal mixture of prilocaine 2.5% and lidocaine 2.5%, EMLA (eutectic mixture of lidocaine and prilocaine) cream, may be used as a topical anesthetic. EMLA works best if it is applied to the dermal site at least 1 hour before the procedure and covered with an occlusive dressing. Its use is limited because of the time needed for onset of anesthesia; the increased expense; and the risk of methemoglobinemia in susceptible individuals, such as those with congenital disease; pyruvate kinase–deficient and glucose-6-phosphate dehydrogenase (G6PD)–deficient patients; and those with

rare, acquired forms resulting from medications (e.g., prilocaine, antimalarials, sulfonamides). Patients younger than 3 months of age are vulnerable to developing methemoglobin because the breakdown product, orthotoluidine, can produce methemoglobinemia after systemic doses of prilocaine approximating 8 mg/kg. A rectangle measuring 1.5 × 0.2 inches is about 1 g of EMLA or 25 mg of prilocaine. The maximal area of application is age and weight dependent (Table 28-1).

Other topical anesthetics are used in some circumstances. Ethyl chloride cools the skin superficially and works well for needle punctures. Unfortunately, it is flammable and has a brief action, limiting its usefulness. A 30% lidocaine cream must be applied with an occlusive patch at least 45 minutes before any procedure. Liposomal encapsulation forms of topical tetracaine and lidocaine are as efficacious as EMLA (Eidelman et al., 2005). Lidoderm patches are only at 5% concentration and are not potent enough for topical surgical skin anesthesia (Video 28-1).

Local Anesthesia

For most office procedures, a local injection is a quick and easy way to provide anesthesia by blocking the fast sodium channels and stopping pain fiber neurotransmission. However, an injection of local anesthetic may distort skin edges and adversely affect skin anatomy and alignment. Consider marking incisions and vital points of alignment before infiltrating with a local anesthetic. Anesthetize before flushing the wound in repair of contaminated lacerations. Infiltration of 1% lidocaine does not damage local defenses, promote infection, or exhibit antimicrobial activity that would obscure a culture from a wound (Edlich et al., 2010).

The two groups of local anesthetics are amides and esters. Allergies are more common to the esters. Allergy to an amide is usually caused by the preservative methylparaben. If a patient has an ester allergy, use an amide. No cross-reactivity occurs between classes (Archar and Kundar, 2002) (Table 28-2).

The most common locally injected anesthetic is lidocaine, with or without epinephrine. One percent lidocaine contains 10 mg/mL of lidocaine. Lidocaine dosing should not exceed 4.5 mg/kg without epinephrine (maximum, 300 mg in adults or 30 mL of 1% lidocaine) or 7 mg/kg of lidocaine with epinephrine (maximum, 500 mg in adults or 50 mL of 1% lidocaine with epinephrine) (Tetzlaff, 2000). Others list the recommended safe dose of infiltrated lidocaine as 200 mg or less in an adult, which is 20 mL of 1% lidocaine (Rosenberg et al., 2004). If doing a paracervical or pudendal block, the maximum total dose over 90 minutes is 200 mg of lidocaine or 20 mL of 1% lidocaine total (10 mL

Table 28-2   Local Anesthetic Classifications

Amides	Lidocaine (Xylocaine)
	Bupivacaine (Marcaine)
	Prilocaine (Citanest)
	Etidocaine (Duranest)
	Mepivacaine (Carbocaine)
	Articaine (Septocaine, Zorcaine)
	Ropivacaine (Naropin)
	Dibucaine (Nupercainal)
Esters	Procaine (Novocain)
	Tetracaine (Pontocaine)
	Chloroprocaine (Nesacaine)
	Cocaine
	Benzocaine (Lanacane, Americaine)
	Proparacaine (Alcaine, Ophthetic, Paracaine)

Expanded from Archar S, Kundar S. Principles of office anesthesia. Part I, infiltrative anesthesia. *Am Fam Physician*. 2002;6:91-94.

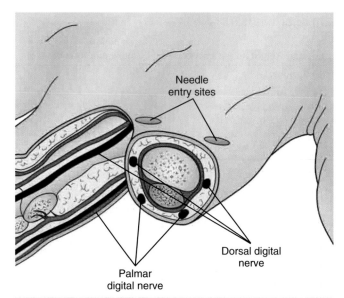

Figure 28-2 Digital nerve block. (From Frank BL. Principles of pain management. In Auerbach PS, ed. *Wilderness medicine*. 6th ed. Philadelphia: Mosby; 2012:420.)

per side). Lidocaine has an elimination half-life of 1.5 to 2.5 hours in most patients, and average infiltrative anesthesia lasts 2 to 6 hours. Bupivacaine has a longer onset and duration of action with an elimination half-life of 2.7 hours in adults and 8 hours in neonates. Data on mixing lidocaine and bupivacaine are limited.

To make the injection more comfortable, the following have been shown to be helpful in some studies: distraction and reassurance, prior application of a topical anesthetic (EMLA or ethyl chloride spray), warming the solution, buffering the solution (1 : 10 dilution with sodium bicarbonate), using a fine-gauge long needle, injecting slowly, using the least amount of solution necessary, infiltrating through the wound edges, injecting from looser subdermal to tighter intradermal skin, and blocking nerves where possible (Quaba et al., 2005).

Some local anesthetics have epinephrine as an additive to help with hemostasis in very vascular locations. The past recommendation was to avoid the use of epinephrine on end-artery areas, including the fingers, ears, nose, lips, penis, and toes. However, a recent review on the use of local anesthesia with epinephrine in a digital block challenges this dogma (Mohan and Cherian, 2007). To be safe, epinephrine should not be used in distal-end vascular beds until the data are more conclusive (Video 28-2).

Local Ring Anesthesia Block

For anesthesia around a superficial skin lesion, a ring block can be placed with good results and reduced tissue distortion. Use a larger needle to draw up the anesthetic and a 25- to 30-gauge needle to infiltrate the tissues. Insert the needle into the subcutaneous skin a few millimeters outside the planned incision line and advance along that circular line around the lesion. Aspirate intermittently for blood to avoid direct instillation of anesthetic into a vein or artery. Infiltrate the local anesthetic as the needle is advanced. Use anesthetized areas to puncture the skin and inject more distal areas as needed around the planned surgical field until the lesion is fully circumscribed.

Digital Block

A digital block can be an effective method for providing anesthesia for fingers and toes. A dorsal or interdigital approach is used to provide anesthesia to the digit. The digital nerves are 3 to 5 mm under the skin at the 2, 4, 8,

and 10 o'clock positions around the digit. Each location can be infiltrated with 1 to 2 cc (mL) of 1% lidocaine without epinephrine. It may take 5 to 30 minutes for distal anesthesia to develop after injection. Occasionally, local anesthesia is needed at the base of the digit circumferentially if achieving complete anesthesia becomes difficult (Fig. 28-2). Patients may continue to feel pressure and motion but should not feel sharp pain when the anesthesia is effective (Video 28-3).

Complications with Local Anesthesia

Recognizing the various side effects and reactions to local anesthesia is critical to prevent serious complications. The most common complication with the use of local infiltrative anesthesia is a vasovagal episode. Lying the patient down in reverse Trendelenburg positioning with both legs elevated can increase blood return to the heart and vagally depressed cardiac output. Atropine can reverse vagal bradycardia but is rarely needed. Recovery occurs spontaneously within minutes, but the queasiness may persist for 30 to 60 minutes.

Inadvertent instillation of an anesthetic into a blood vessel may cause seizures, jitteriness, or palpitations and may be avoided by always aspirating before infiltrating the local anesthetic. If a flash of blood is obtained on aspiration, pull the needle back partially, aspirate again, and instill only if no blood return occurs. Other reactions to local anesthesia are discomfort, bruising, and edema of the injection site. True anaphylaxis to lidocaine is estimated to occur in fewer than 1% of injections (Haugen and Brown, 2007). If anaphylaxis occurs, administer epinephrine 1 : 1000 subcutaneously every 5 minutes as needed and give diphenhydramine (Benadryl), 25 to 50 mg (adult dose) orally, intravenously, or intramuscularly. The adult dose of epinephrine 1 : 1000 is 0.3 to 0.5 mL/kg, and the pediatric dose is 0.01 mL/kg at the same intervals. Emergency response personnel should be immediately notified, and prolonged observation in the emergency department is advised.

Sedation

Some patients may require minimal to mild conscious sedation during a procedure in the outpatient clinic setting. Use of a low-dose benzodiazepine, such as 1 to 2 mg of lorazepam or 0.5 to 1 mg of alprazolam, may be appropriate for light conscious sedation. Sedation may also be accomplished with a dose of an oral opioid such as hydrocodone or oxycodone. These patients should not operate a car or heavy machinery, and another person should provide their transportation. Use of an opioid in combination with a benzodiazepine may cause significant respiratory depression and requires additional constant monitoring of cardiac and oxygenation status, which may not be available in some ambulatory clinical practices.

WOUND IRRIGATION

Wound healing is affected by infection, tension, perfusion, and alignment. Cleaning a wound with tap water or isotonic saline removes debris and bacteria mechanically from the wound and reduces infection rates. One study found no clinically important differences in infection rates between wounds irrigated with tap water or a normal saline solution (Valente et al., 2003).

Many studies recommend 7 psi (lb/in²) or greater for adequate irrigation of dirty wounds and 0.5 psi for clean wounds. Whereas irrigation of the wound with a 35- to 50-mL syringe and a 19-gauge needle produces 7 psi, using a bulb syringe only produces 0.5 psi, which is inadequate to flush and decontaminate a dirty wound. The potential for lateral subcutaneous dissemination with use of high-pressure irrigation can make a clean wound more susceptible to infection, so it should be reserved for contaminated wounds when the benefits are greater than the risk of dissemination. The low-pressure bulb syringe is used for clean lacerations. The pressure is more important in dislodging adherent bacterial and small particles than the amount of solution used. All health care professionals should use a splash protector during irrigation (Edlich et al., 2010).

There is debate on using povidone-iodine (Betadine) to cleanse dirty wounds. In general, avoid Betadine surgical scrubs within the laceration because it can be toxic to tissue. If used, dilute Betadine 1 : 10 with water. Chlorhexidine and hydrogen peroxide may also be toxic to tissue inside a laceration and should be used with care. Poloxamer-188 solutions are safe to use within wounds and are even used on ophthalmologic skin surgeries to cleanse the conjunctiva and by dentists to cleanse oral mucosa.

KEY TREATMENT

- Studies recommend 7 psi or greater for adequate irrigation of dirty wounds (Edlich et al., 2010) (SOR: A).

DEBRIDEMENT

A dirty, uneven wound may benefit from direct, sharp debridement back to clean, viable tissue. Obtaining clean, even skin edges may improve healing, facilitate repair, and reduce scarring. If road grit is present, it must be removed with scrubbing as needed to avoid infection and tattooing.

Generally, unless high-pressure irrigation is unable to remove grit, scrubbing is avoided because it may disrupt clotting along the skin edges. Wounds from high-velocity trauma, deep bites, and soil and fecal contamination are best cleaned in the operating room and allowed to heal open by secondary intention because primary closure is contraindicated (Edlich et al., 2010).

Good anesthesia is critical to appropriate irrigation and debridement. If significant debridement is planned, the physician should document neurologic function in the injured area and distally before infiltration of the anesthetic.

Principles of Healing

Wound healing begins immediately after the initial trauma or cut. Traditional descriptions of wound healing use three distinct but overlapping phases (inflammatory, proliferative, remodeling), but others use four phases to better describe the healing process. Surgical technique and smoking are modifiable risk factors for poor wound healing. Other factors affecting wound healing include anemia, vascularity, diabetes, malnutrition, HIV infection, and cancer.

Trauma to surrounding tissue by the injury and surgical techniques (e.g., too much tension on sutures) may affect healing. Adequate oxygenation and blood flow are critical to good healing. Medications that affect healing include steroids, NSAIDs, and immunosuppressive medications.

STAGES OF HEALING

Exudative or Inflammatory Phase

Immediately after a laceration, fibrin deposits with an influx of platelets, forming a visible clot. The platelets secrete various wound-healing growth factors that activate macrophages and fibroblasts. These growth factors and more than 30 cytokines cause an influx of cellular structures. This phase occurs from 0 to 72 hours (Figure 28-3).

Resorptive Phase

After 24 to 72 hours, the degradation products of fibrin lead to activation of chemotaxis in the resorptive phase. Leukocytes and macrophages migrate into the wound, causing inflammation. The cellular components then begin autolysis and remove injured tissue by a fermentative process. This process creates an effective phagocytosis, a sterilizing defense, and an activation of the immune system.

Proliferative Phase

Between 72 hours and 7 days, fibroblasts migrate into the wound, and vascular proliferation occurs. Granulation tissue formation marks the proliferative phase. Epidermal cells begin to grow at the edges of the wound. A delicate balance of cytokine systems leads to new capillary formation to feed and oxygenate the budding granulation tissue. Extracellular matrices form and act as struts to support the new tissue. The primary clots are broken down by naturally developing fibrinolytic compounds (Figure 28-4).

Regenerative or Remodeling Phase

The remodeling stage is a continuation of the proliferative phase, with ongoing maturation of collagen. The

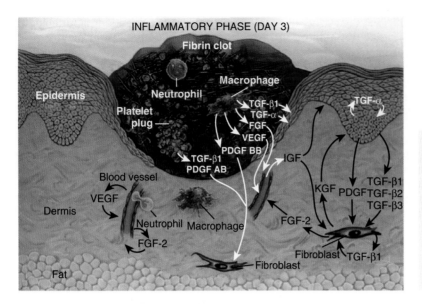

Figure 28-3 A cutaneous wound 3 days after injury. The cells and growth factors necessary to facilitate cell migration into the wound are shown. *FGF,* Fibroblast growth factor; *IGF,* insulin-like growth factor; *KGF,* keratinocyte growth factor; *PDGF,* platelet-derived growth factor; *TGF,* transforming growth factor; *VEGF,* vascular endothelial growth factor. (From Singer AJ, Clark RAF: Mechanisms of disease: cutaneous wound healing. *N Engl J Med.* 1999;341:738, and Leong M, Phillips LG. Wound healing. In Townsend CM, Beauchamp RD, Evers BM, Mattox KL, eds. *Sabiston textbook of surgery: the biological basis of modern surgical practice.* 19th ed. Philadelphia: Saunders; 2012.)

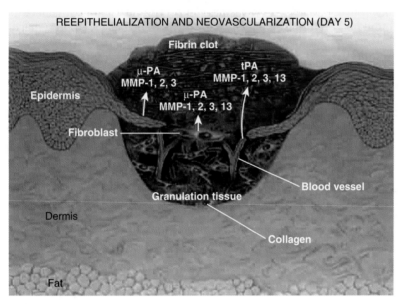

Figure 28-4 Cutaneous wound 5 days after injury. Blood vessels are seen sprouting into the fibrin clot as epidermal cells resurface the wound. Some of the proteinases involved in cell movement at this time point are shown. *MMP-1, -2, -3,* and *-13,* Matrix metalloproteinases 1, 2, 3, and 13 (collagenase 1, gelatinase A, stromelysin 1, and collagenase 3, respectively); *tPA,* tissue plasminogen activator; *uPA,* urokinase-type plasminogen activator. (Adapted from Singer AJ, Clark RAF: Mechanisms of disease: cutaneous wound healing. *N Engl J Med.* 1999;341:738 and Leong M, Phillips LG. Wound healing. In Townsend CM, Beauchamp RD, Evers BM, Mattox KL, eds. *Sabiston textbook of surgery: the biological basis of modern surgical practice.* 19th ed. Philadelphia: Saunders; 2012.)

thickening collagen leads to an increased resistance to shearing and tearing forces. The regenerative phase is characterized by epithelialization and scar formation. This last phase may take up to 1 year. Collagen type III is converted into the mature type I collagen (Figure 28-5). The extracellular matrix and cells within the wound are regulated by cytokines and integrins (transmembrane cell receptors) (Figure 28-6).

KELOIDS

Keloids are fibrous elevated scars that extend outside wound margins. Keloids are unlikely to regress, are likely to recur if excised, and are most likely to occur in patients with darker skin (relative risk, 15-20). Keloids are frequently located over the midline chest, cheeks, and earlobes, and the peak incidence is age 10 to 20 years. Wounds that heal by secondary intention and burn wounds are at high risk for developing keloids. Keloids may be painful as well as

cosmetically unacceptable (Juckett and Hartman-Adams, 2009) (Figure 28-7).

HYPERTROPHIC SCARS

Hypertrophic scars are limited to the wound edges and tend to regress over the first year. The treatment of both keloid and hypertrophic scars is similar, except hypertrophic scars have better outcomes. Genetic expression of various cytokines and inflammatory pathways may affect the myofibrocytes in granulation tissue to continue producing scar tissue, but the exact causes are being investigated. Pressure dressings and colloidal silicone placed on scars after suture removal or on burn scars may reduce the incidence of both keloids and hypertrophic scars, but onion-skin extract (Mederma) alone is not effective (Karagoz et al., 2009). For a review of the prevention and treatment of excessive dermal scarring, review Roseborough et al. (2004).

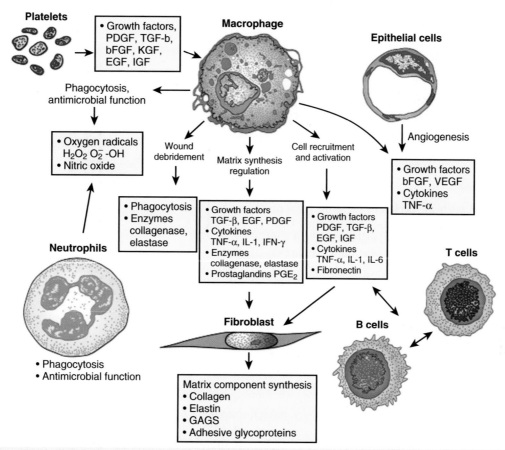

Figure 28-5 Interaction of cellular and humoral factors in wound healing. Note the key role of the macrophage. *bFGF,* Basic fibroblast growth factor; *EGF,* epidermal growth factor; *GAG,* glycosaminoglycan; *H₂O₂,* hydrogen peroxide; *IFN-γ,* interferon-γ; *IGF,* insulin-like growth factor; *IL,* interleukin; *KGF,* keratinocyte growth factor; *O₂-,* superoxide; *PDGF,* platelet-derived growth factor; *PGE₂,* prostaglandin E₂; *TGF-β,* transforming growth factor-β; *TNF-α,* tumor necrosis factor-α; *VEGF,* vascular endothelial growth factor. (Modified from Witte MB, Barbul A. General principles of wound healing. *Surg Clin North Am.* 77:513, 1997 and Leong M, Phillips LG. Wound healing. In Townsend CM, Beauchamp RD, Evers BM, Mattox KL, eds. *Sabiston Textbook of Surgery: The Biological Basis of Modern Surgical Practice.* 19th ed. Philadelphia: Saunders; 2012.)

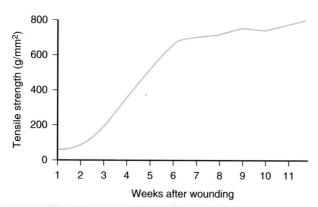

Figure 28-6 Rate of wound healing. Based on the rate of maximum collagen strength; limitation of strenuous activity after 6 weeks of wound healing is not indicated. (From Lawrence WT, Bevin AG, Sheldon GF. Acute wound care. In *Emergency care.* Chicago: Scientific American, American College of Surgeons; 1998 and Chavez MC, Maker VK. Office surgery. In Rakel RE, ed. *Textbook of family medicine.* 7th ed. Philadelphia: Saunders; 2007.)

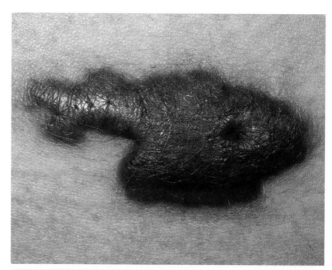

Figure 28-7 Skin keloid. (From Habif TP. *Clinical dermatology.* 5th ed. Philadelphia: Elsevier; 2010:16.)

- Cryotherapy is useful for smaller lesions such as acne scars and keloids (SOR: B).
- Pressure dressings in burns help prevent hypertrophic scars (SOR: B).
- Intralesional corticosteroid injections are first-line primary care therapies for keloids; surgery is a second-line option (SOR: B).

WOUND DRESSINGS

Covering the wound with an occlusive dressing prevents drying and allows the wound to be moist, promoting healing with collagen synthesis and angiogenesis (Field and Kerstein, 1994). Using a topical antibiotic reduces infection only in wound laceration repairs (Dire et al., 1995), not in elective hospital or office surgical procedures (Smack et al., 1996). Studies show no dressing preference for burn wound care (American Burn Association, 2001), but it should be based on wound origin, depth, size, location, exudate, and degree of contamination (Singer et al., 2008). Wounds closed with tissue adhesives provide their own protection and require no additional dressing. Review warning signs of infection with the patient and advise on standard postoperative wound care and timing of suture removal.

NONHEALING WOUNDS

Patients' underlying healing status may be affected by their nutritional status and underlying medical conditions. Healing may be slowed by smoking as well as age. Surgical repairs with too much tension on skin closure increase the chance of tissue necrosis, dehiscence, and reduced healing. In the United States, chronic wounds affect 6.5 million patients. More than $25 billion is spent annually on treatment of chronic wounds (Sen et al., 2009).

Principles of Skin Closure

Closure techniques should minimize skin trauma, result in good skin-edge approximation without undue tension, and result in a cosmetically pleasing appearance (Figure 28-8). The best cosmetic results can be achieved by using the finest suture appropriate for skin thickness and tension. Generally, a 3-0 or 4-0 suture is appropriate on the trunk and scalp, 4-0 or 5-0 on the extremities with finer suture more distal, and 5-0 or 6-0 on the face. Forceps with teeth and skin hooks should be used to reduce crush injury to wound edges. Use the least number of sutures to close the skin with good approximation and without open space deep to the wound. Sutures on the face should be removed on days 3 to 5; wounds not under tension on days 7 to 10; and wounds under tension, on the hands, or over joints on days 10 to 14. If you remove a suture and the wound begins to open, cease removing the other sutures and place a sterile adhesive strip over the area, then ask the patient to return in 2 days.

Sutures are an option along with staples, tissue adhesives, and hair to tie edges together on some scalp wounds.

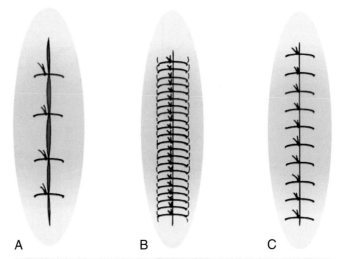

A   B   C

Figure 28-8 Wound repair: skin closure. **A,** Too few stitches used. Note the gaping between sutures. **B,** Too many stitches used. **C,** Correct number of stitches used for a wound under an average amount of tension. (From Lammers RL. Methods of wound closure. In Roberts JR, Hedges JR, eds. *Clinical procedures in emergency medicine.* 5th ed. Philadelphia: Elsevier; 2010.)

Avoid staples in the scalp if computed tomography (CT) or magnetic resonance imaging (MRI) is planned. Expedient cleaning, debridement, and closure with the least trauma to the wound should be the goal.

SKIN TENSION ORIENTATION

Surgeons searching for an ideal guide for elective incisions have developed 36 named guidelines. Karl Langer (1819-1887) studied and drew skin lines of cleavage after noting that round punctures in cadaveric skin produced ellipses. The topographic orientation of these lines coincides with the dominant axis of mechanical tension in the skin. Langer lines were developed by studying skin tension in cadavers with rigor mortis and therefore may not be representative of a living human's skin tension lines. Kraissl noted tension lines in living tissue and developed lines oriented perpendicular to the contraction of the underlying muscles. Later, Borges described *relaxed skin tension lines* (RSTLs), which follow furrows formed when the skin is relaxed and are produced by pinching the skin. These are only guidelines, however, and many factors contribute to the camouflaging of scars, including wrinkles and contour lines. RSTLs are formed by the natural tension on the skin from underlying soft tissue and rigid bony or cartilaginous substructure.

Superior scar revision results occur when making incisions parallel or nearly parallel to RSTLs. The Borges RSTLs and Kraissl lines may be the best guides for elective incisions of the face and body and are often mislabeled "Langer lines." The face can be divided into parallel variations of the four main facial lines: the facial median, nasolabial, facial marginal, and palpebral lines. When performing cosmetically sensitive punch biopsies, stretch the skin 90 degrees perpendicular to the RSTLs so that the resulting ellipse-shaped wound and closure are parallel to the RSTL (Figure 28-9).

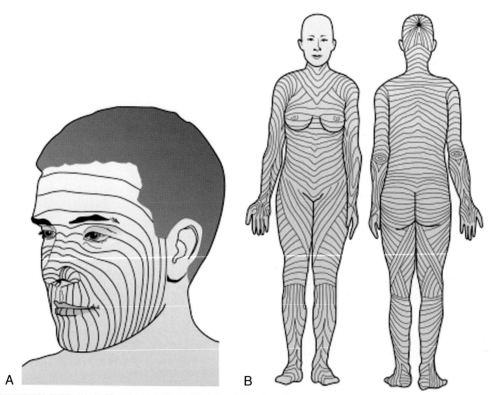

Figure 28-9 A, Facial relaxed skin tension lines (RSTLs). **B,** RSTLs of the entire body. (From Trott A. *Wounds and lacerations: emergency care and closure.* 2nd ed. St. Louis: Mosby; 1997 and Burns JL, Blackwell SJ. Plastic surgery. In Townsend CM, Beauchamp RD, Evers BM, Mattox KL, eds. *Sabiston textbook of surgery: the biological basis of modern surgical practice.* 19th ed. Philadelphia: Saunders; 2012.)

SKIN TENSION ON CLOSURE

Ideally, any wound, excision, or repair should be designed so that the superficial skin edges approximate under minimal tension. The surgeon may undermine surrounding tissue and trim wound edges to improve approximation if it is a clean laceration or elective excision. Debridement or excision of dirty wound edges may remove devitalized tissue, improve alignment, and allow improved closure. Placement of tension-relieving sutures or deep sutures should always be considered to facilitate direct closure of uninfected wounds under tension. If a suture is less than ideal, it is best to remove and replace it.

Wound tips and beveled lacerations are challenging because too much tension may be placed on the narrowest edges and contribute to wound necrosis or breakdown. Ideally, the skin sutures are used to approximate slightly everted superficial edges and not to close deep tissue under high tension. If the wound or excision has a clean approximation under minimal tension, a single-layer repair is preferred. If not, deep interrupted sutures are used to close the underlying space to avoid deep pockets where a hematoma, infection, or abscess could develop (Figure 28-10 and Video 28-4).

TISSUE ADHESIVE

On clean, dry lacerations under low tension, skin adhesives are an appropriate substitute for standard sutures. Adhesives may also work on shallow, irregular, beveled lacerations and are useful on pediatric scalp lacerations.

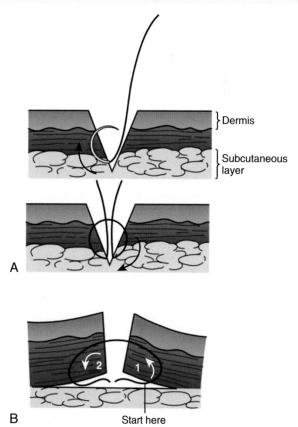

Figure 28-10 Inverted subcutaneous stitches, starting in opposite directions. (From Lammers RL. Methods of wound closure. In Roberts JR, Hedges JR, eds. *Clinical procedures in emergency medicine.* 5th ed. Philadelphia: Elsevier; 2010.)

Since 1998, the medical tissue adhesive 8-carbon 2-octylcyanoacrylate (OCA) has been available in the United States for tissue adhesive closure of wounds. OCA is more durable and flexible than the short-chain butylcyanoacrylates. The longer chain cyanoacrylates create less dehiscence in wounds longer than 8 cm. Avoid adhesive use on moist or hair-bearing areas, mucous membranes, nonhemostatic wounds, over joints or highly mobile tissue, and on bite wounds or dirty lacerations. Consider the adhesives to have about the same strength as 5-0 sutures. If OCAs are used, the patient may shower immediately, but if the butylcyanoacrylates are used, the repaired wound should be kept dry for at least 48 hours. Moisture exposure increases the dehiscence risk (Singer and Dagum, 2008). If the area to repair is under higher tension, deep sutures approximating the skin edges are used before closing with a superficial adhesive (Singer and Thode, 2004).

Tissue adhesive agents form their own bandage, and no additional care is needed. Full tensile strength is achieved after 2.5 minutes. Antibiotic and white petrolatum ointments can dissolve tissue adhesives, so patients should avoid their use (Forsch, 2008).

Dehiscence occurred on 2.5% of wounds closed with tissue adhesives in an animal study compared with 2- and 10-cm laceration repairs with various suture types and stitches. In the 2-cm wounds, results were identical. The 10-cm wounds favored deep suturing even if tissue adhesive was used. The final decision on the method and materials used for wound closure depends on the length and location of the wound as well as the efficiency needed and time of closure (Zeplin et al., 2007 and Video 28-5).

KEY TREATMENT

- Wound closure of superficial lacerations by tissue adhesives is quicker and less painful than conventional suturing, with a similar outcome on appropriate wounds (Aukerman et al., 2005) (SOR: A).

SUTURE PLACEMENT

Interrupted Sutures

Individually placed single sutures are the most common form of wound closure. Although slower to place than a running suture, single sutures have a better cosmetic result and a reduced risk for dehiscence. Slightly everting the skin edges will result in the best wound appearance. Enter the skin 2 to 3 mm from the skin edge with the needle perpendicular to the skin plane and rotate the wrist smoothly. Go an equal distance in depth as the horizontal distance from the wound edge. If unable to obtain an equidistant point on the opposite side of the wound in one step, use an additional pass. Bring the needle out through the laceration, enter at the same level within the laceration, and come out through the skin at a symmetric distance from the wound edge (Figure 28-11 and Video 28-6).

One may reduce the risk for "dog ears" by placing a suture in the middle of a laceration and then another in the middle of the remaining sides until equal tension and alignment approximates the skin edges in a cosmetic and hemostatic fashion. If bleeding persists, ligate or cauterize the

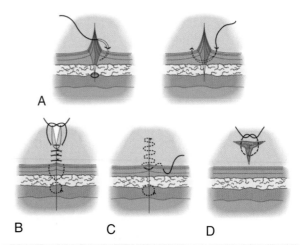

Figure 28-11 Suture technique and methods. **A,** Sutures are placed through the entire thickness of the dermis at right angles to the skin and suture line while everting the wound edge. **B,** Sutures are placed 2 to 3 mm apart and 2 to 3 mm from the wound edge. **C,** The subcuticular stitch prevents crosshatch scarring. **D,** Intradermal sutures help preserve peninsular flaps in this stellate wound. (Modified from Wright CV, Ronaghan JE: Office surgery. In Rakel R, ed. *Textbook of family practice.* 5th ed. Philadelphia: Saunders; 1995.)

vessel before further closure. If suturing a landmark such as vermillion borders on lip edges, consider marking opposing points of the wound before instilling anesthesia and then place an aligning suture at this location first.

Running Sutures

If rapid suture placement is needed and an area is not over a highly mobile joint, the physician can use a running suture. If the suture breaks, however, the entire wound may dehisce. If the running sutures are left too long, "baseball lacing" tracks may remain visible on the skin. In one study (not funded by manufacturers), deeply buried absorbable suture used along with running subcuticular polyglactin 910 (Vicryl) suture left in place resulted in the best results on trunk and extremity scar healing from elective excision of atypical moles (Alam et al., 2006; Halstead, 1889).

Subcuticular Sutures

Halstead first described the subcuticular suturing technique in 1889 as a way to approximate wound edges with the least scarring. A running intradermal, buried subcuticular suture is useful in places where the dermis is shallow and when skin edges are well approximated under minimal tension, such as on the face. Placing subcuticular sutures on the back, chest, and other areas under tension without other supporting deep interrupted sutures may give poor results.

For subcuticular suture placement, use either absorbable or nonabsorbable 4-0 suture and anchor it in the skin on one end external to the wound. Enter the skin and come out in the apex of one end of the wound. Place horizontal zigzagging subcuticular sutures with level symmetric entry and reentry sites on each side of the wound. If using absorbable suture, tie and bury a knot near the end of the wound by tying the knot and then place one more stitch to come out through the skin near the wound; then cut the suture

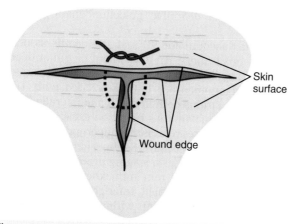

Figure 28-12 View from above stellate laceration, showing closure with half-buried mattress stitches. For some stellate lacerations, it is best to cover them with Steri-Strips and revise the scar later or, if small, excise the laceration and convert it to a linear repair. (From Lammers RL. Methods of wound closure. In Roberts JR, Hedges JR, eds. *Clinical procedures in emergency medicine.* 5th ed. Philadelphia: Elsevier; 2010.)

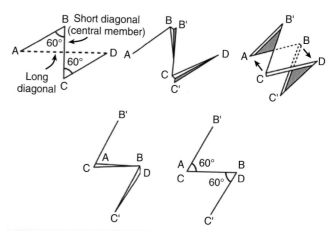

Figure 28-13 Classic equilateral triangle 60-degree Z-plasty. (Modified from Thomas JR, Holt GR. *Facial scars, incisions, revision, and camouflage.* St. Louis: Mosby; 1989 and Thomas JR, Mobley SR. Scar revision and camouflage. In Cummings CW, Flint PW, Haughey BH, et al, eds. *Otolaryngology: head and neck surgery.* 4th ed. Philadelphia: Mosby; 2005.)

flush with the skin while pulling upward on the suture. The knot will be retracted below the skin for later absorption. Alternatively, with either absorbable or nonabsorbable suture, place the last stitch and exit the skin away from the wound and tie off the suture externally. A nonabsorbable suture may be removed after 1 to 3 weeks by cutting one end of suture and gently pulling with countertraction from the other end of the wound (Video 28-7).

Half-Buried Mattress or Tip Sutures

Half-buried mattress sutures can be used on stellate edges and on triangular defects to approximate the skin edges with reduced tension on the tips (Figure 28-12). Tip sutures are similar and used to secure a laceration tip with minimal tension. Tension sutures can reduce blood and oxygen flow to the distal tip and cause ischemia (Video 28-8).

Pulley Sutures

The far-near, near-far pulley sutures are a modification of the vertical mattress suture and may be used as a temporary measure to reduce tension and approximate skin edges to allow placement of interrupted sutures. These sutures are used for longer repairs but should not be left in too long or placed too tightly because cross-hatching scars may occur. For placement, enter with the needle 4 to 6 mm back from the wound edge; come out on the opposite side 2 mm from the wound; and loop back across the wound opening, entering the skin 2 mm from the edge and coming out on the opposite side 4 to 6 mm back from the edge (Wu, 2006).

Modified pulley sutures offer some mechanical advantage in vitro by requiring less force to achieve closure compared with horizontal mattress or single interrupted sutures. These pulley sutures are generally used when a wound is under moderate tension (Austin and Henderson, 2006).

Z-PLASTY

The Z-plasty technique is used to improve the appearance of long scars, correct contractures over joints, and change the orientation of the scar line to align better with RSTLs.

The key is to measure the laceration and then draw a line of the same length as the laceration on each side of the laceration at 60-degree angles for proper alignment on the repair (Figure 28-13).

COMPLICATIONS

Dog-ear formations occur when the two sides of a wound are of unequal length. Tissue may be trimmed before suturing. An ellipse can be cut around the dog ear or an extension laterally at an angle and then repaired (Fig. 28-14). Another technique is called "leashing the dog ear." Tie off the repair near the start of the dog ear. Place a single, interrupted suture by diving through the axis of the wound and out behind the dog ear. When tied down, this suture may flatten a small dog ear (Khachemoune et al., 2005).

Excisions

Incisions should be made perpendicular to the skin with symmetric edges and no angulation. Poor technique may jeopardize healing. In general, the physician should make an elliptical incision with the length three to four times the width. Some limited data suggest less tissue removal and better healing if a round excision is used with adequate margins and subsequent repair of any dog ears. With this technique, though, 59% of the repairs required dog-ear correction (Seo et al., 2008).

If a portion of a pigmented lesion has a worrisome appearance, complete excision is recommended. The American Cancer Society uses the ABCDE mnemonic to recognize lesions of high malignant concern: *A*, asymmetry; *B*, border irregularity; *C*, more than one color; *D*, diameter greater than 6 mm; and *E*, increased elevation or enlargement. If a lesion has one or more of these concerns, an excisional biopsy should be considered. In other lesions, the clinician may consider a shave biopsy or punch biopsy (Videos 28-9 to 28-11).

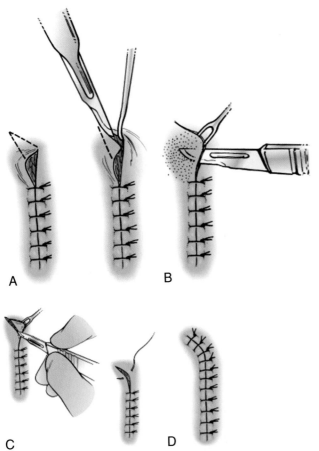

A

B

C

D

Figure 28-14 Dog-ear repair. A dog ear may develop if tension and length vary along both sides of the laceration. **A,** Drawing the wedge to remove to create a "hockey stick" to fix the dog ear. **B,** Undermining the skin. **C,** Removing the wedge of skin. **D,** Repairing the "hockey stick" with both sides having even tension. (Modified from Simon BC. Skin and subcutaneous tissue. In Rosen P, Chan T, Vilke G, et al, eds. *Atlas of emergency procedures.* St. Louis: Mosby; 2001; and Simon B, Hern HG. Soft tissue injuries. In Marx JA, ed. *Rosen's emergency medicine.* 7th ed. Philadelphia: Mosby; 2009.)

ATYPICAL MOLES AND PIGMENTED LESIONS

Elliptic full-thickness excisional biopsies are preferred for any suspicious pigmented mole. Punch biopsies can easily miss positive findings because of fusiform invasion in other portions of the lesion (Chang et al., 2009).

Management of dysplastic nevi with positive margins remains controversial. A National Institutes of Health (NIH) Consensus Conference established margin guidelines for excision of dysplastic nevi (0.2-0.5 cm), but no clear guidelines exist regarding whether an incompletely removed nevus with mild or moderate dysplasia should be reexcised. Dermatopathologists are discordant in identifying dysplasia and differing degrees of atypia, further complicating decision making. Most dermatologists recommend that nevi with severe atypia should be reexcised because they may represent early melanoma or a lesion evolving into melanoma (Goodson et al., 2010).

In 2008, the National Cancer Comprehensive Network published guidelines indicating that a 5-mm excisional margin may be inadequate for lentigo maligna and lentigo maligna melanoma (Bosbous et al., 2009). Despite recurrence rates of 8% to 20% and a growing body of literature suggesting the inadequacy of a 5-mm marginal excision

in these cases, a definitive guideline change has not been made.

Melanomas account for 90% of the deaths associated with cutaneous tumors. An assessment of tumor depth is critical in the diagnosis and prognosis of melanomas. Confirmed melanomas are initially excised with 10- to 20-mm safety margins both in depth and laterally if possible. Unsuspected melanomas found on excisional biopsies should have their bases reexcised for appropriate 1- to 2-cm margins as a second procedure. Sentinel lymph node dissection is routinely offered as a staging procedure in patients with tumors more than 1 mm in thickness, although there is no resultant survival benefit. Interferon-α can be offered as adjuvant therapy to patients with melanoma more than 1.5 mm thick and stage II to III because it increases relapse-free survival.

KEY TREATMENT

- Elliptic full-thickness excisional biopsies are preferred for suspicious pigmented moles (Chang et al., 2009) (SOR: A).
- A 5-mm excisional margin may be inadequate for lentigo maligna and lentigo maligna melanoma (Bosbous et al., 2009) (SOR: A).
- Confirmed melanomas are initially excised with 10- to 20-mm safety margins (SOR: A).

BASAL CELL CANCER

The excision of small basal cell cancers (BCCAs) of less than 20 mm with well-defined borders and a 3-mm peripheral surgical margin will remove the tumor in 85% of cases. A 4- to 5-mm peripheral margin will increase the clearance rate to approximately 95%. Approximately 5% of small, well-defined BCCAs extend more than 4 mm beyond their apparent clinical margins. Morpheic (morpheaform) and large BCCAs require wider surgical margins to maximize the chance of complete histologic removal. On initial removal of morpheic lesions, the rate of complete excision with a 3-mm margin is 66%; 5-mm margin, 82%; and 13- to 15-mm margin, more than 95% (Telfer et al., 2008).

Standard vertical-section processing of excision specimens allows the pathologist to examine only representative areas of the peripheral and deep surgical margins, and at best an estimated 44% of the entire margin can be examined in this manner. Therefore, tumors that appear fully excised occasionally recur (Telfer et al., 2008). If the BCCA is on an area with little extra excisable tissue, consider Mohs microscopic surgery to obtain adequate margins and minimize tissue removal.

If the BCCA lesion is completely excised, the recurrence rate is about 1%. If not completely excised, BCCAs have recurrence rates of 17% to 35% for lateral-margin positivity and 33% for deep-margin positivity. Only one third of positive-margin BCCA lesions recur, so the provider should reexcise the margins but could consider reexcision only if a recurrence develops, with the following exceptions: lesions of long duration, size greater than 2 cm, previous recurrence, and aggressive histologic features (including perineural and perivascular invasion and infiltrative, morpheaform, or micronodular appearance). If marginal positivity is detected in such cases after excision, reexcision and removal of the residual tumor is advised over watchful observance (Ünlü et al., 2009) (Video 28-12).

> **KEY TREATMENT**
>
> - A 4- to 5-mm peripheral margin will increase the cure rate of BCCAs to approximately 95% (Telfer et al., 2008) (SOR: A).
> - Morpheaform and large BCCAs require wider surgical margins (Telfer et al., 2008) (SOR: A).

Cryotherapy

Cryotherapy can be easily mastered for treatment of many skin lesions. Cryotherapy is well tolerated and results in minimal to no scar. It is best used in those with lighter skin and in non–hair-bearing areas because of occasional pigment changes or hair loss with deeper treatments. Liquid nitrogen, the most widely available, cost-effective medical cryogen, boils at −196°C, and temperatures of −25° to −50°C can be achieved in 30 seconds of appropriate skin application. Destruction of benign lesions occurs at −20° to −30°C, and malignant lesions often require temperatures of −40° to −50°C for destruction (Andrews, 2004). Correct use of cryotherapy results in selective cell destruction while sparing the tissue matrix of collagen and fibroelastic tissue and reducing the risk of scar formation. Repeated freeze-thaw applications can increase tissue damage.

INDICATIONS AND CONTRAINDICATIONS

Cryotherapy can be an important treatment option for many lesions commonly encountered in a primary care clinical practice. It can be used in all age groups to treat a number of dermatologic lesions. Even though well tolerated, cryosurgery also has contraindications (Table 28-3). Some body areas or conditions should be approached with prudence because of increased complication risks. BCCAs, particularly in the nasolabial fold or periauricular area, tend to be more extensive than expected and more likely to recur. The vermillion border, periorbital area, and areas overlying cutaneous nerves present confounding variables to safe cryotherapy.

EQUIPMENT AND TECHNIQUE

Liquid nitrogen can be applied with a regular or modified cotton-tipped applicator, cryogen spray device, or cryoprobe, all readily available to providers. The cotton-tipped applicator is the least expensive and can be modified to hold more cryogen or to match the size or shape of the lesion with a cotton ball. Liquid nitrogen can be stored in an insulated device in the office and taken out in small aliquots in a polystyrene cup for individual use with patients.

Handheld cryogen spray devices have significantly improved. Traditional cryotherapy systems provide a reservoir for the liquid nitrogen and an applicator tip to dispense the cryogen. The applicator tip can have a varying aperture for altering cryogen dispersion. Some providers use an otoscopy cone to protect surrounding skin and direct the spray

Table 28-3 Cryotherapy: Indications and Contraindications

Indications	Verruca (warts)
	Condylomata acuminata
	Papular nevi
	Selected basal cell cancer
	Seborrheic keratosis
	Molluscum contagiosum
	Granulation tissue
	Selected squamous cell cancer
	Actinic keratosis
	Acrochordons (skin tags)
	Cervical intraepithelial neoplasia
Contraindications	**ABSOLUTE**
	Prior cryotherapy sensitivity
	Vascular compromise
	Complication nonacceptance
	Steroid therapy
	Melanoma
	Invasive skin cancer
	Need for tissue diagnosis
	Expected poor wound healing
	RELATIVE*
	Hepatitis B and C
	Mononucleosis
	Leukemia
	Lymphoma
	Myeloma
	Systemic lupus
	Nephritic syndrome
	Nephrotic syndrome
	Macroglobulinemia
	Rheumatoid arthritis

*Underlying medical conditions in which medications or the condition itself may slow healing.

onto a small central lesion. The unit is generally held 1 to 2 cm above the lesion and the spray directed at a 90-degree angle and aimed at the lesion center. Newer spray devices use a continuous infrared sensing device to determine the treatment site skin temperature and ensure consistent freeze times. These modifications can improve accuracy and assist in achieving optimum cryotherapy results (Cry-Ac Tracker, http://www.brymill.com).

Before freezing, the depth and diameter of the cryotherapy must be anticipated to minimize injury to surrounding tissues. Mark the skin to ensure adequate treatment in critical cryotherapy sessions. Keratin layers are very resistant to cryotherapy and can be treated for 1 to 2 weeks with topical 40% salicylic acid plaster or mechanically pared away before cryotherapy. Application of salicylic acid alone is equally efficacious to cryotherapy of warts for many patients (Gibbs and Harvey, 2006). A well-hydrated skin lesion can increase cryotherapy success rates.

For superficial benign skin lesions, the cryotherapy applicator should almost cover the lesion and should be applied for 20 to 40 seconds to create an ice ball edge 2 to 3 mm beyond the edge of the lesion. In contrast, deeper or premalignant lesions should be treated with an applicator smaller than the lesion to ensure a depth more equal to the radius of treatment. It should be applied for 40 to 90 seconds to form an ice ball 3 to 4 mm outside the lesion. Superficial malignant lesions also require a smaller applicator but applied for 1 to 3 minutes for an ice ball 5 to 8 mm beyond the lesion. Malignant cells are more resistant to cryotherapy, and destruction requires temperatures at −40° to −50°C. In most cases, the depth of a freeze is similar to the radius of the superficial ice ball formed. The lethal zone for tissue destruction is 2 to 3.5 mm inward from the outer margin of the ice ball (McNabb and Pfenninger, 2010).

COMPLICATIONS

Cryotherapy results in minimal scarring. Vascular or hypertrophic lesions are resistant and sometimes require multiple treatments 2 to 3 weeks apart. Most patients experience pain and burning for 1 to 2 days. During these first days, the skin may be red and sensitive and may form a hemorrhagic bulla followed by sloughing. Infection and pyogenic granuloma formation are rare complications. In deeper cryotherapy, the potential damage to underlying neural structures must be considered (Video 28-13).

KEY TREATMENT

- A significant keratin layer is resistant to cryotherapy (SOR: B).
- The lethal zone for cryogen tissue destruction is 2 to 3.5 mm inward from the outer margin of the ice ball (McNabb and Pfenninger, 2010) (SOR: A).
- Salicylic acid application alone to warts is equally efficacious to cryotherapy (Gibbs and Harvey, 2006) (SOR: A).

Incision and Drainage of Cutaneous Abscesses

A cutaneous abscess is identified by a fluctuance, or compressible softness, in skin surrounded by induration, inflammation, warmth, and tenderness. *Furuncles* are superficial and result from abscess formation in a sweat gland or hair follicle. *Carbuncles* are deeper and extend into the subcutaneous tissue. Offending bacteria include *S. aureus*, streptococci, and occasionally gram-negative rods. These infections can be severe in patients with diabetes or vascular disease. Primary treatment of an abscess is surgical drainage. An area of induration alone with no fluctuance indicates isolated cellulitis and is treated with antibiotics and warm compresses.

When performing an incision and drainage of an abscess, the skin is prepared with a sterilizing and cleansing agent. Local anesthetics do not work well in the acidic environment of an abscess, so a ring or field block can be infiltrated around the periphery of the lesion. Superficial cooling of the surface of the skin with ethyl chloride or liquid nitrogen can also provide brief anesthesia for a stab incision.

A linear incision is made over the area of maximal fluctuance and has been shown to heal in a shorter time than deroofing procedures used in the past (Sørensen et al., 1987). A #11 scalpel blade is inserted with the cutting edge away from the provider in a stabbing motion deep enough to access the abscess but not passing completely through it. The tip is lifted up to create an adequate incision for drainage. The abscess cavity is then probed with a curved hemostat to disrupt any internal loculations. The abscess cavity is packed with ¼- to 1-inch gauze to prevent early superficial wound closure and allow secondary healing. Primary closure is not recommended (Korownyk and Allan, 2007). A bulky sterile dressing can be applied to absorb any drainage and the packing and dressing changed every 1 to 2 days or when soiled. Evidence does not support using oral antibiotics after surgical drainage. Routine swabbing for culture in immunocompetent individuals is not recommended (Korownyk and Allan, 2007). Patients are educated on wound care and return in 2 to 7 days for follow-up (see Video 28-13).

Recurrent skin abscesses should be investigated based on location. Crohn disease, subcutaneous fistulas, and pilonidal cysts can present as recurrent cutaneous abscesses. MRSA should be suspected in recurrence skin infections as well.

KEY TREATMENT

- The primary treatment of an abscess is surgical drainage (SOR: A).
- Incision and drainage of an uncomplicated abscess does not require oral antibiotic treatment (SOR: A).
- Routine culture of abscess drainage in immunocompetent individuals is not recommended (SOR: A).

Lipomas

Lipomas are mature adipose tissue arranged in a nodular formation surrounded by a capsule and commonly located in the subcutaneous tissues. Lipomas can be diagnosed by clinical examination and identification of their unique, well-circumscribed, round, mobile character with a doughy consistency. Although most do not require it, excision may be considered for large tumors, rapidly growing lipomas, and those causing pain. Lipomas can occur in isolation or with other systemic diseases, as a component of genetically inherited disorders or in other connective tissue layers.

A steroid injection or liposuction can be used to treat select lipomas. Steroid injections can be used to treat painful lipomas smaller than 2.5 cm in size and in which pathologic examination is likely unnecessary. An injection of 1 to 3 mL of triamcinolone diluted with 1% lidocaine to a 10 mg/mL concentration can be performed into the center of the lipoma monthly to shrink the tumor to the desired size. Formal liposuction can be done with cannula or 16-gauge syringe under local anesthesia (Salam, 2002). Neither of these procedures is likely to eliminate the lipoma in its entirety, and recurrences are frequent.

Surgical excision of a lipoma removes the neoplasm from the tissue and allows for pathologic examination. Marking the boundaries of the lipoma is helpful for identification of the tumor edges before a local anesthetic field block is placed. The skin is prepared with a povidone-iodine or chlorhexidine solution. Small lipomas can be enucleated with their capsule using blunt dissection through a small incision. Larger lipomas require excision through a linear or elliptic incision. Blunt and, rarely, sharp dissection can be used to free the mass from the surrounding tissues using hemostats or clamps for traction. Hemostasis should be confirmed and cautery or ligature placement used to ensure a dry wound base. The remaining dead space is closed with buried, interrupted, absorbable subcutaneous sutures, and the skin is closed with interrupted sutures or staples depending on location and cosmetic need. A compression dressing should be used for 1 to 2 days to prevent formation of a hematoma, and sutures are removed in 5 to 10 days depending on location. Submit any specimen for pathologic examination. Caution should be used when deciding on removing large lipomas of the low back because they can be larger than the surface appearance suggests. Cases have been reported of an abdominal hernia presenting posteriorly and being mistaken for a lipoma (Video 28-14).

Surgery of the Nail and Digits

INGROWN NAIL (ONYCHOCRYPTOSIS)

The great toe's lateral and distal nail beds are the most common locations for ingrown nails. Poorly fitting shoes, poor nail-trimming techniques, and trauma can result in their formation. Most ingrown nails respond to conservative local treatment of warm soaks and elevation of the distal nail with cotton to allow unobstructed nail growth. If poor toenail trimming is the cause, a shard of nail is usually remaining in the distal lateral nail groove and impaling the skin. It can be simply trimmed and removed for resolution of pain with standard curved or straight iris scissors.

When conservative measures fail, a partial or complete nail excision is performed to remove the portion of offending nail. The toe is cleansed and a digit block placed using 1% lidocaine. A snug tourniquet at the base of the toe can help with hemostasis. A nail elevator is used to separate the section of nail to be removed from the underlying nail bed down to the base of the nail and germinal matrix. The elevator can also remove the cuticle from the nail. Then an iris or bandage scissors can be used to cut the nail longitudinally to the matrix. A straight hemostat is used to grasp the portion of nail to be taken off and the nail is rolled laterally for removal. Hemostasis can be obtained with compression, aluminum chloride solution, or silver nitrate. A bulky tube-gauze dressing can be placed for protection. Recurrent ingrown nails unresponsive to conservative measures can be ablated after nail removal. A phenol solution is applied to a hemostatic germinal nail matrix under the proximal nail fold for 30 to 60 seconds before neutralizing the phenol with rubbing alcohol. (Video 28-15).

NAIL PLATE AVULSION FOR ONYCHOMYCOSIS

Conservative treatment of onychomycosis is the first-line choice for management. A fungal culture of nail clippings can be done to confirm the diagnosis but may take up to 1 month for growth and identification. Oral terbinafine (250 mg/day for 12-16 weeks) produces higher clinical cures than pulse-dosed terbinafine, pulse-dosed itraconazole, or weekly fluconazole (Volk et al., 2013). Even with terbinafine, failure rates can reach 50%. When onychomycosis causes dystrophic nails resulting in pain or toe dysfunction, a complete nail plate avulsion can be performed, with high patient satisfaction (see Ingrown Nail [Onychocryptosis]).

• Oral terbinafine (250 mg/day for 3 months) is the most effective oral treatment for fungally infected toenails (Volk et. al., 2013 (SOR: A).

PARONYCHIA

Whereas an *acute* paronychia is caused by a bacterial infection of the lateral or proximal nail folds after minimal to significant trauma, a *chronic* paronychia results from an inflammatory condition caused by repetitive irritant contact exposure. Acute paronychia without abscess can be treated conservatively with warm soaks, gentle compression, topical steroid creams, and topical or oral antibiotics (Rigopoulos et al., 2008). Chronic paronychias usually respond to removal of the offending agent or treatment of the underlying condition or inflammatory cause, but they sometimes require drainage, oral antibiotics, and antifungals (Franko and Abrams, 2013).

When the local cellulitis of an acute paronychia develops into an abscess, incision and drainage is indicated followed by oral antibiotics to cover both methicillin-sensitive and resistant *S. aureus* and streptococci (Franko and Abrams, 2013). If the fluctuant pocket of the abscess is superficial and underlying the cuticle or nail fold, a 23-gauge needle or #11 blade tip can be used to lift the edge of the fold and allow drainage without local anesthesia. A digital nerve block can be performed if the infection is deeper and requires more extensive drainage or for patient comfort. After anesthetization, an incision into the abscess can be placed parallel to the nail fold with a stab incision using a #11 bladed with subsequent drainage and exploration to break up loculations if warranted. Warm soaks should follow with oral antibiotics for the cellulitis (Figure 28-15).

EVACUATION OF SUBUNGUAL HEMATOMA

Trauma to the nail causing bleeding between the nail plate and nail bed can be excruciatingly painful. Subungual

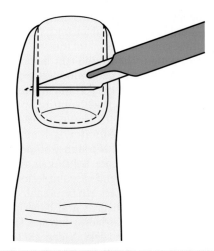

Figure 28-15 Incision and drainage of paronychia. The tip of a #11 scalpel is advanced just under the cuticle and parallel to the nail. The size of the incision should be large enough to include all fluctuant areas and no more. (From Chavez MC, Maker VK. Office surgery. In Rakel RE, ed. *Textbook of family medicine.* 7th ed. Philadelphia: Saunders; 2007.)

hematomas can be drained easily in an office setting by creating a 2-mm hole through the nail and draining the blood using a handheld cautery unit or heated end of a metal paper clip. If trauma was significant or a hematoma involves more than 50% of the nail, the provider should consider an underlying nail bed laceration that may require primary closure after evaluating the digit radiographically. Phalanx tuft fractures can underlie the hematoma after significant trauma (Wang and Johnson, 2001).

Anorectal Disease

Bleeding, pain, discharge, or change in bowel habits can indicate active anorectal disease, and all warrant medical evaluation. The directed complete patient history and anorectal examination lead to a clear diagnosis in most complaints. Inflamed internal hemorrhoids or rectal polyps typically cause painless rectal bleeding because they occur above the dentate line. Painful anal bleeding can result from anal fissures, proctitis, thrombosed external hemorrhoids, or a draining perianal abscess. Palpable chronic masses can indicate an anal skin tag, polyp, or prolapsed rectal mass, and acute masses are usually caused by abscesses or thrombosed hemorrhoids. More than 90% of anorectal complaints can be managed in the primary care physician's office using simple techniques (Pfenninger and Zainea, 2001).

ANOSCOPY

Anoscopy is performed easily in the office to evaluate and treat many anorectal conditions. Scopes can be 7 to 10 cm long and 2 to 3 cm wide and range from a slotted or beveled metal version to a disposable plastic tubular version. The tubular version can be used for diagnosis, and the slotted style allows for ease in treating most anorectal conditions. For a thorough examination, the patient can be placed in a comfortable lateral decubitus position with the hips flexed. The examiner should don nonpermeable protective clothing and eyewear. A digital rectal examination should precede anoscopy to assess for internal pain or mass. The anal tissues should be examined for tags, hemorrhoids, fissures, dermatitis, condylomata, and masses.

During examination, the thumb can be pressed against the internal index finger to determine tenderness, induration, or abscess formation in the perianal tissues in all quadrants. The lubricated anoscope with obturator is introduced fully into the anal canal with gentle, constant pressure. When fully inserted, the obturator is removed and the anorectal mucosa visualized through 360 degrees during gradual withdrawal. Adequate lighting is essential. The Valsalva maneuver may distend vascular lesions for ease in identification. Anal Pap smears can be obtained if warranted for anorectal cancer concerns and biopsies performed using a Kevorkian or Tischler biopsy forceps. Hemostasis is obtained using silver nitrate sticks (Video 28-16).

HEMORRHOIDS

Hemorrhoids are submucosal vascular beds located in the anal and rectal canal that assist with defecation and the sensation of anorectal fullness. These vascular beds can occur in insensate areas above the dentate line as internal hemorrhoids or below the dentate line as external hemorrhoids in exquisitely sensitive areas. Hemorrhoid development may result from genetic factors, aging, or serial local trauma. One study found that 4.4% of the United States. population, or 10 million people, complain of hemorrhoid disease (Reese et al., 2009).

Internal Hemorrhoids

Internal hemorrhoids are classified according to the severity of prolapse. First-degree hemorrhoids do not prolapse, and second-degree disease is characterized by spontaneously reducible prolapse. These can generally be treated with conservative methods. Third-degree hemorrhoids prolapse and require manual reduction, and fourth-degree hemorrhoids have irreducible prolapse. As the prolapse progresses, surgical treatment becomes a more common treatment.

Painless, bright-red rectal bleeding is the primary symptom of internal hemorrhoids. Anoscopy can be used for identification of the site of bleeding acutely. Internal hemorrhoids typically occur in three locations in the anal canal: right anterior, right posterior, and left lateral. A flexible sigmoidoscopy or colonoscopy is performed if the patient's symptoms or history warrants more extensive colonic evaluation or if the site of colorectal bleeding is not easily identified or persists after treatment. Patients older than age 40 years who have hemorrhoidal bleeding may have other colorectal pathology and should have further colorectal evaluation (Chong and Bartolo, 2008).

Dietary management consisting of adequate fluid and fiber intake is the primary noninvasive treatment of symptomatic hemorrhoids (Cataldo et al., 2005). Persistent hemorrhoid symptoms decreased by 53% in those receiving dietary fiber for hemorrhoid care (Alonso-Coello et al., 2005). Conservative therapy can be offered for mild first- and second-degree hemorrhoids, but more advanced disease may require surgical management. Rubber band ligation or hemorrhoid banding is known to be highly effective in outpatient treatment of first-, second-, and some third-degree internal hemorrhoids (Reese et al., 2009). Other options include sclerotherapy, infrared coagulation, radiofrequency coagulation, and cryotherapy (Cataldo et al., 2005).

Prolapsing internal hemorrhoids can be easily treated in the office with rubber band ligation using a McGilvney ligator or similar device. After appropriate consent is obtained, a slotted or beveled anoscope is inserted into the anus. The hemorrhoid is then identified, and with the circular McGilvney ligator in place within the anoscope, the hemorrhoid is grasped with a forceps and drawn into the ligating cylinder. Sensation of the hemorrhoid is assessed to prevent ligation of a high external hemorrhoid. Care is taken not to draw too much tissue into the ligator to avoid denuding the anal canal. When the base of the hemorrhoid is in the ligator, two rubber bands are released from the ligator by one cylinder sliding over the other. The bands cause ischemic necrosis of the hemorrhoid, and the tissue sloughs over days. Bleeding can occur for up to 1 to 2 weeks and is occasionally significant. Patients may feel some rectal fullness, a spasm, or dull ache for a few days after banding.

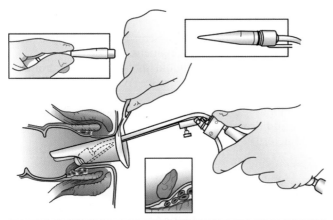

Figure 28-16 Rubber band ligation for an internal hemorrhoid. The band is advanced onto the end of the ligator instrument using a conical attachment *(insets)*. The hemorrhoid is identified at a level proximal to the dentate; this area is tested for sensation before banding. Occluding the suction port of the ligator instrument draws the hemorrhoid into the open end of the ligator, and the instrument is fired. The banded hemorrhoid typically sloughs in 1 week. (Courtesy Mayo Foundation and Nelson H, Cima RR. Anus. In Townsend CM, Beauchamp RD, Evers BM, Mattox KL, eds. *Sabiston textbook of surgery: the biological basis of modern surgical practice.* 19th ed. Philadelphia: Saunders; 2012.)

Rare episodes of pelvic cellulitis have been reported. Only one site should be treated per patient visit (Figure 28-16) (Video 28-17).

Sclerotherapy can be performed on first- and second-degree hemorrhoids using a sclerosant of 5% phenol or saline. The base of the hemorrhoid is injected with 1 to 2 mL of the sclerosant through a syringe while viewed through an anoscope. More late complications can be seen with sclerotherapy than with banding. In a systematic review, sclerotherapy had unknown effectiveness in treating hemorrhoids. Infrared photocoagulation was found to be likely beneficial and as effective as rubber band ligation in the same review. The infrared coagulator light is fired three to five times at the base of the hemorrhoid through an anoscope for 1.5 seconds during one treatment session. Multiple sessions may be required for infrared treatment of first-degree through small third-degree hemorrhoids. Radiofrequency coagulation is performed with a Bicap probe placed at the base of the hemorrhoid above the dentate line and activated four to six times for 2 seconds, forming a white coagulum. Because of prolonged healing after cryotherapy, it is no longer recommended (Reese et al., 2009).

KEY TREATMENT

- Patients older than the age of 40 years who have hemorrhoidal bleeding should have further colorectal evaluation for other pathologic causes. (Chong and Bartolo, 2008) (SOR: B).
- Dietary management of symptomatic hemorrhoids consists of adequate fluid and fiber intake (Alonso-Coello et al., 2005) (SOR: B).
- Rubber band ligation is known to be highly effective outpatient treatment for first-, second-, and some third-degree hemorrhoids (Reese et al., 2009) (SOR: B).

External Hemorrhoids

A nonpainful or painful anal swelling can represent an external hemorrhoid. Hemorrhoids can be differentiated from anal skin tags, condylomata, fissures, and abscesses on anal examination. Symptomatic external hemorrhoids can be excised if conservative treatment fails. The patient is placed in the lateral decubitus position with the hips flexed. The external hemorrhoid or tag is identified and anesthetized at its base with buffered 1% lidocaine with epinephrine. The area is cleansed with povidone-iodine or chlorhexidine. A radially oriented elliptic incision is made around the hemorrhoid or tag and the center removed with the hemorrhoid vein. The resulting defect may need to be cauterized and is frequently left open and allowed to heal. Stool softeners and topical anesthetics may be very beneficial. Because of the vascularity, healing usually occurs in 5 to 10 days (Video 28-18).

Thrombosed External Hemorrhoids. An external hemorrhoid can become thrombosed and be identified by an acute onset of perianal pain and development of a purplish nodule with or without bleeding. Thrombosed hemorrhoids can be managed conservatively with avoidance of constipation, patient analgesia, and ice or sitz baths (Cataldo et al., 2005). Office surgical excision, not incision, of a thrombosed external hemorrhoid results in a lower recurrence rate and earlier resolution of symptoms (Greenspon et al., 2004). Simple incision of the thrombosed hemorrhoid may not remove multiple clots and can result in higher recurrence rate and even extension.

To excise a thrombosed hemorrhoid, the patient is placed in the lateral decubitus position with the buttocks separated for visualization. The surface can be cleansed and anesthesia provided with a local injection of buffered lidocaine or bupivacaine with epinephrine at the base of the hemorrhoid. After anesthetization, an elliptic incision is made in a radial orientation around the hemorrhoid, and all thrombus is removed with excision of the hemorrhoidal vein at its base. Bleeding can be controlled with pressure, Monsel solution, or careful electrocautery. More complex hemorrhoids and those associated with partial rectal prolapse should be referred to a colorectal specialist.

KEY TREATMENT

- Office surgical excision, not incision, of a thrombosed external hemorrhoid results in a lower recurrence rate and earlier resolution of symptoms (Greenspon et al., 2004) (SOR: B).

ANORECTAL ABSCESS

An anorectal abscess can lead to severe pain and disability in patients. Abscesses occur most often in the third or fourth decade of life and in a 3:1 to 2:1 male-to-female ratio (Hebra, 2009). An anorectal abscess develops from an infection originating in the anal glands and crypts at the level of the dentate line and tracking along the lines of least resistance. This tracking results in up to 50% of abscesses being associated with simultaneous fistula development.

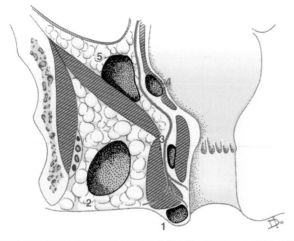

Figure 28-17 Classification of perirectal abscesses: *1,* perianal; *2,* ischiorectal; *3,* intersphincteric; *4,* high intramuscular; and *5,* pelvirectal. (From Hill GJ II, ed. *Outpatient surgery.* 3rd ed. Philadelphia: Saunders; 1988 and Coates WC. Anorectal procedures. In Roberts JR, Hedges JR, eds. *Clinical procedures in emergency medicine.* 5th ed. Philadelphia: Elsevier; 2010.)

Locations of the abscess can vary and may be located in the perianal area (60%), ischiorectal area (20%), intersphincter region (5%), supralevator region (4%), and submucosal location (1%) (Figure 28-17). Abscesses can result from other anorectal infections or pathology such as Crohn disease fistulas, adenocarcinoma, trauma, immunosuppression, and sexually transmitted diseases. A thorough anorectal examination, frequently under anesthesia, is required for complete evaluation. Most abscesses can be localized by physical examination. Deep or large abscesses require a pelvic CT scan to determine the extent of tracking and to plan surgical intervention.

An anorectal abscess should be treated by incision and drainage. The lack of fluctuance should not delay a timely drainage procedure. Antibiotics are an unnecessary addition to routine incision and drainage of uncomplicated perianal abscesses (Whiteford et al., 2005). There is no conclusive evidence that simple drainage is less effective than a sphincter-cutting procedure in the treatment of anorectal abscess (Quah et al., 2006). Antibiotics should be considered only as an adjunct to drainage in patients with immunosuppression, diabetes, prosthetic devices, or significant systemic illness.

Before surgical decompression, an anoscopy should be performed to identify a potential internal draining fistula source at the dentate line. Injecting an agent over or under the mass can provide local anesthesia, although rarely patients may need spinal or general anesthesia. Incision and drainage of superficial abscesses can be accomplished with use of a #11 blade over the area of maximal fluctuance or swelling in a radial orientation. Loculations can be broken by probing with a forceps or gloved finger. A Penrose drain or gauze packing can be placed for continued drainage with appropriate follow-up in 1 to 2 days. Recurrent abscesses can occur when there is an unrecognized and untreated underlying fistula. A fistulotomy must be performed in these cases.

- About 50% of perirectal abscesses are associated with simultaneous fistula development.
- The lack of fluctuance should not delay a timely drainage procedure for perianal abscesses (Whiteford et al., 2005) (SOR: B).
- Antibiotics are an unnecessary addition to routine incision and drainage of uncomplicated perianal abscesses (Whiteford et al., 2005) (SOR: A).

ANAL FISSURE

An anal fissure is a tear in the anal mucosa that can cause severe anal pain and rectal bleeding and results from local stool trauma. Most occur posteriorly in the midline. Other causes or locations should prompt a more complete anorectal evaluation. On examination, the anus is exquisitely tender and may demonstrate internal anal sphincter spasm. Evaluation can occur with gentle spreading of the anus, but some require anoscopy to assess their extent. A radial tear is seen that can be bleeding and very tender.

Most acute anal fissures can be managed conservatively with dietary fiber, prevention of constipation, adequate hydration, and stool softeners. Sitz baths may provide symptomatic improvement. Topical anesthetics such as 5% lidocaine ointment or gel can be used for comfort or before defecation until healing. No surgical treatment is warranted in uncomplicated occurrences. Chronic anal fissures do not resolve after the 3-month acute phase and are generally less tender. Chronic fissures are still associated with significant internal sphincter spasm and may present with a large, protuberant sentinel tag, sometimes confused with a hemorrhoidal tag.

Conservative therapy includes continued constipation prevention. Other therapeutically equal treatment options include topical nitroglycerin ointment, botulinum toxin injections, or calcium channel blockers such as diltiazem or nifedipine for 30 days. However, no conservative medical therapy approximates the efficacy of surgical sphincterotomy for chronic fissures (Nelson, 2006). An open or closed partial lateral internal sphincterotomy appears to be equally efficacious as surgical treatment (Nelson, 2008). An experienced specialist in the technique and anorectal anatomy should perform this procedure.

- No conservative medical therapy approximates the efficacy of surgical sphincterotomy for chronic fissures (Nelson, 2006) (SOR: A).

PILONIDAL CYST AND ABSCESS

Pilonidal disease may manifest itself as a chronically draining sinus or fistula at the base of the spine in the intergluteal crease 5 to 10 cm from the anus. Pilonidal cysts can also become infected and may lead to extensive presacral abscess formation. Multiple hair shafts may be seen within the cyst. Incision and drainage or an elliptic incision under local anesthesia over the sinus track is performed. Drainage is the preferred office management technique and is similar to standard abscess treatment. Packing of the wound should be done, and referral is recommended for excision of the extensive presacral complex. Recurrence is common without excision.

Gynecologic Office Procedures

See also Chapter 25.

PARACERVICAL BLOCK

A paracervical block can be placed before any uterine procedure requiring instrumentation of the cervix or cervical dilation. Contraindications include current desired pregnancy, infection, and bleeding disorders. The local anesthetic used, often 0.5% lidocaine or bupivacaine, is determined by the length of anesthesia required.

The patient is placed in a dorsal lithotomy position, and a vaginal speculum is placed to allow adequate visualization of the cervix. Two 10-mL syringes are drawn up of a 1:1 ratio of 1% lidocaine or bupivacaine and sterile saline. The cervix and vaginal canal are cleansed with chlorhexidine or povidone-iodine. An injection of 1 to 2 mL of this mixture is placed in the anterior cervical lip, where a single-toothed cervical tenaculum is placed. The cervix is lifted upward and deviated laterally to obtain access to the lateral posterior fornix. Eight to 10 mL of this mixture is injected starting in the cervicovaginal reflection at the apex of the posterior fornix at the 4 and 8 o'clock positions and is advanced 2 to 3 cm in depth along the external serosa of the uterus to provide anesthesia to the uterine plexus of nerves near the uterine arteries. Intravascular injection is avoided by aspiration on the syringe plunger before infiltration. Women have less pain during uterine intervention with paracervical block than with placebo injections (SOR: B).

CONTRACEPTIVE DEVICES

Diaphragms

Latex diaphragms have an arcing, coil, or flat spring, and silicone devices have a wide-seal rim and an arcing or coil spring. The arcing spring diaphragm is used most often because it is easier to place in the posterior fornix without an introducer. When fitting a diaphragm, the size can be determined with a simple pelvic examination.

With the patient in a dorsal lithotomy position, the provider inserts the lubricated, gloved index and middle finger straight into the vagina to the posterior fornix. The spot where the inferior pubic arch impacts the index finger is noted. The fingers are withdrawn, and the distance from that point on the index finger to the end of the middle finger is noted; this is about the diameter of diaphragm needed. Diaphragms come in 5-mm increments from 60 to 90 mm, with 75 and 80 mm most common. The diaphragm is then inserted and size confirmed with placement, posteriorly, in the posterior fornix behind the cervix and, anteriorly, behind the pubic arch. Removal of the diaphragm can be accomplished by hooking the anterior rim with a finger and

gently extracting. Women should be given an opportunity to remove and replace the diaphragm to confirm placement in the office before use.

The diaphragm can be placed in the posterior vagina covering the cervix up to 6 hours before intercourse. Generally, women have used 5 mL of spermicide within the diaphragm at insertion, although a Cochrane review failed to prove its contribution to contraceptive effectiveness (Cook et al., 2003). Additional spermicide can be inserted in front of the diaphragm before each act of intercourse without dislodging the diaphragm. The diaphragm is removed at least 6 hours and not more than 24 hours after the last intercourse. An increased risk of urinary tract infections (UTIs) exists with diaphragm use and risk of toxic shock syndrome exists if the diaphragm is left in place for more than 24 hours. The diaphragm size needs to be reestablished after a weight change of 10 to 15 lb, pregnancy, or pelvic surgery. The failure rate for diaphragms is 18% but may be better with perfect use.

Cervical and Vaginal Barrier Methods

Two brands of cervical and vaginal barriers are currently approved and marketed in the United States. Although neither requires specific fitting by a practitioner, both require a prescription for pharmacy or manufacturer dispensation. Whereas FemCap comes in three sizes and is ordered based on pregnancy history, Lea's Shield comes in one size for all women with normal anatomy.

The FemCap is a silicone rubber nonhormonal intravaginal contraceptive (IVC) cervical cap. The smaller rim size (22 mm) is for women who have never been pregnant. The medium size (26 mm) is intended for women who have been pregnant, even for up to as little as 2 weeks with no vaginal delivery. The larger diameter cap (30 mm) is for women who have had a full-term vaginal delivery. When in doubt of prior pregnancy, the 26-mm cap should be used. The patient places the cap over the cervix with up to ¾ tsp of 2% nonoxynol-9 spermicide used around the outside groove at least 15 minutes before sexual arousal. Placement over the cervix is critical and accomplished best while squatting. After it is in place, the cap should be pushed over the cervix for at least 10 seconds to ensure firm placement against the vaginal wall, because it does not fit snug against the cervix. Additional spermicide should be placed with each act of intercourse without removing the cap. Hooking a finger under the removal strap in a squatting position, and withdrawing gently removes the cap. The cap must be removed at least 6 hours but not longer than 48 hours after the last act of intercourse. During a 6-month clinical trial for approval, the FemCap was 86.5% successful in preventing pregnancy (FemCap, 2013). The device is washed and dried thoroughly between uses.

Lea's Shield is a silicone rubber IVC vaginal barrier placed at any time before intercourse. It is inserted with spermicide vaginally to the depth of the cervix, and any trapped air is vented through a one-way valve, creating a tight fit between the vaginal wall and the device. The Shield is removed using the incorporated removal loop with a finger more than 8 hours after the last intercourse. Women had an 8.7% chance of becoming pregnant within 6 months when using the Lea's Shield. The shield is cleaned with warm soapy water and dried for reuse.

- Failure rates for the diaphragm are 18% but may be better with perfect use (Cook et al., 2003) (SOR: A).
- FemCap was 86.5% successful in preventing pregnancy over 6 months of use (FemCap, 2013) (SOR: B).

Intrauterine Devices

Insertion. Long-acting reversible contraception has become increasingly popular in the form of intrauterine devices (IUDs). IUDs are T-shaped devices that are very easy to place in an office setting and have a failure rate less than 1% to 2% per year. They can be used in nulliparous and parous women and have a high continuance rate after 1 year of use (78%-81%). The devices have attached strings at the proximal end for removal in the office, and pregnancy rates return to normal soon afterward. IUDs are contraindicated in women with a current or suspected pregnancy, abnormal uterine cavity, pelvic inflammatory disease or endometritis, known endometrial or cervical malignancy, genital bleeding of unknown etiology, artificial heart valve placement, or allergy to IUD components.

A pregnancy during use of an IUD is more likely to be ectopic, but the overall rate of ectopic pregnancy is less than in sexually active women who use no contraception. Complications of IUD placement include pelvic infection, embedment in the uterine wall, IUD migration or expulsion, and perforation of the uterus. Unlike oral contraceptives, IUDs can be used during lactation and are not contraindicated in women with a history of venous thromboembolic events, those at increased risk of myocardial infarction or stroke, or those who smoke. Perforation rates are 0.6 to 1.6 per 1000 insertions but are higher during the 6 to 8 weeks after delivery, so postpartum placement is delayed until a later visit (McCarthy, 2006).

Before placement of an IUD, the federally mandated patient information included with the IUD should be fully reviewed with the patient and formal written consent obtained after a discussion of risks and benefits. The physician should confirm a pregnancy test result is negative and consider placement during the first 5 to 7 days of her menstrual cycle. A pelvic examination must be performed before insertion to assess the uterine size and location and evaluate for current cervical infection. A prescription dose of an NSAID (e.g., ibuprofen 600-800 mg) should be provided 30 to 60 minutes before placement to help with analgesia. After placement, the patient may continue to use an NSAID for cramping and can expect to have some spotting for a few days. She should be willing to check for the IUD strings monthly to confirm proper retention.

- IUDs have a failure rate less than 1% to 2% per year (SOR: A).
- IUDs can be used during lactation and are not contraindicated in women with a history of venous thromboembolic events, those at increased risk of myocardial infarction or stroke, or those who smoke (SOR: A) (McCarthy, 2006).

Mirena. The Mirena IUD is a levonorgestrel-releasing intrauterine contraceptive system measuring 32 × 32 mm placed for up to 5 years. The 52-mg levonorgestrel-containing IUD releases 20 mcg/day of hormone per day after insertion and decreases to 10 mcg/day after 5 years. Systemic levonorgestrel is minimal at 150 to 200 pg/mL. Variable to no menstrual bleeding is the norm for patients after 3 to 6 months.

The Mirena device is supplied in its own delivery system, aiding with placement. The patient is placed in a dorsal lithotomy position, and a sterile speculum is introduced into the vagina. The cervix and vaginal mucosa is cleansed with a chlorhexidine or povidone-iodine solution. A paracervical block can be placed as described earlier for analgesia. The anterior or posterior cervix is grasped with a single toothed cervical tenaculum for stabilization of the cervix during the procedure. If normal, the uterus should be sounded to depths of 6.5 to 8.5 cm. If the uterus is sounded to a different depth, consider misplacement, cervical stenosis, or uterine perforation. The cervix can be dilated for placement if significant stenosis is present.

Open the Mirena package, release the IUD threads, position the IUD arms, and position the flange at the proper sounded depth. When in the same plane as the inserter system, retract the arms into the inserter by pulling on the strings at the end of the system and pushing forward on the green thumb slider. Lock the strings into the cleft at the end of the inserter. Insert the IUD system gently through the cervix into the uterus but stop 1.5 to 2 cm before the fundus. Pull back on the thumb slider to the designated mark and release the arms outward. Wait for 10 to 15 seconds to allow the arms to fully extend. Hold the slider with the thumb and advance the system fully forward to place the IUD arms against the uterine fundus. Now pull only the slider all the way outward to release the threads at the proximal end of the inserter and then remove the entire inserter system from the cervix, leaving behind the IUD with threads. Cut the two threads to a length of 3 to 5 cm. Remove the tenaculum and observe for any significant bleeding. Monsel solution or pressure can be used for hemostasis. Remove the speculum and give the patient instructions for follow-up visits and postinsertion care (Video 28-19).

Skyla. Skyla is the newest commercially available IUD system in the United States after being approved in 2000 by the U.S. Food and Drug Administration. Skyla is approved for 3 years of use and contains 13.5 mg of levonorgestrel that is released 14 mcg/day at 24 days after insertion and drops to 5 mcg/day in 3 years with an average in vivo release of 6 mcg/day. The dimensions are smaller than the Mirena device at 28 × 30 mm and require a slightly smaller inserter diameter (3.8 mm vs. 4.75 mm). As opposed to other IUD systems, Skyla has been specifically approved for use in nulliparous as well as parous women.

Insertion of Skyla is very similar to the Mirena insertion process above. The primary difference is the internal containment of the strings until insertion is complete. This reduces the variability of string movement during loading and insertion but also prevents reloading of the IUD into the inserter if there is insertion failure. In addition, Skyla has a 99.95% pure silver ring at the top of the vertical stem, making it more visible by ultrasonography. Skyla should be noted on any MRI order because it does require special specific conditions for MRI scanning because of the silver.

Paragard T380A. The Paragard can be placed for up to 10 years in a similar manner as the Mirena IUD. Patients should receive counseling and informed consent for the Paragard IUD, with specific warnings about contraindications in patients with Wilson disease because of the copper content of the Paragard.

Positioning of the patient, placement of the speculum, cleansing of the vagina and cervix, placement of the tenaculum, and uterine sounding are the same as described for Mirena. However, the IUD arms are loaded differently into the Paragard inserter and are folded backward with the distal arm ends inserted into the distal end of the inserter tube to lie next to the IUD shaft. The IUD system is then inserted through the cervix to the uterine fundus. The white inserter plunger is held steady and the outside clear tube retracted 1 to 2 cm to release the arms. The clear tube is then advanced back to the fundus to assist in extending the arms and placing them in the apex of the fundus. The central plunger is then removed before the outside tube to prevent inadvertent removal of the IUD (Figure 28-18). After the inserter is removed, the two threads can be cut to 3 to 5 cm in length and the tenaculum and speculum removed, with hemostasis as needed. The patient is instructed in postplacement care and subsequent monthly cervical thread checks. Warning signs for infection, perforation, and bleeding are given (see Video 28-19).

Removal. Removal of an IUD is quite simple for all devices. An oral NSAID is beneficial to assist with analgesia. The patient is placed in a dorsal lithotomy position, and a speculum is placed in the vagina. The two IUD strings are identified and grasped with a ring forceps. The strings are gently pulled on, and the IUD should easily follow for removal. If the strings are not present, the IUD strings are generally just inside the cervical os. One can use a Cytobrush to retrieve the strings, grasp the strings in the os with a straight hemostat, or consider cervical dilation and use of an IUD hook or extractor for removal. In some women, the IUD may be malpositioned, and ultrasonography or plain abdominal radiography can locate the system for removal. If the IUD is not easily removed or is disconnected from the strings, hysteroscopy-assisted IUD removal may be necessary in rare cases.

Intradermal Contraceptive Device

Implanon is a device 4 cm long and 2 mm wide containing 68 mg of etonogestrel. Nexplanon is the radiopaque version of Implanon. Both are inserted on the inner side of the nondominant upper arm 8 to 10 cm above the medial epicondyle in a subdermal location for up to 3 years of contraception. Insertion should occur during the first 1 to 5 days of a patient's menstrual cycle. The site for insertion is selected, marked, and locally anesthetized. The device is placed using a subdermal insertion trochar. Complications from Implanon insertion are 1% and from removal 1.7%. Irregular bleeding is the most common side effect (11% of patients). The manufacturer requires providers to complete a 3-hour comprehensive training program, which should be completed before device placement (http://www.implanon-usa.com or www.nexplanon-usa.com).

BARTHOLIN GLAND ABSCESS OR CYST

The Bartholin glands are located between the hymen and labia minora bilaterally at the 4 and 8 o'clock positions. Cysts occur when the duct is blocked from trauma or edema, and abscesses occur when retained secretions become infected. Treatment relies on drainage of the cyst or abscess; treatment of any associated cellulitis with oral antibiotics if indicated; and creation of a track that eventually epithelializes, allowing normal gland drainage and reduced recurrence.

For drainage, the patient is placed in the dorsal lithotomy position, and the cyst or abscess is identified by the area of maximal swelling and fluctuance. Topical anesthesia is used on the surface or a local anesthetic injected under the mass for patient comfort. The cyst wall is grasped through the mucosal surface with two clamps 3 to 5 mm apart and a #11 blade used to puncture between the clamps. After drainage, the fluid is cultured and the cyst packed with gauze until healed. To prevent frequent recurrences, a Word catheter can be placed. The latex stemmed catheter with an inflatable balloon is inserted into the incision between the clamps, with care taken to place the balloon in the cyst center. The balloon is then filled with 2 to 3 mL of normal saline and left in place for 4 to 6 weeks to allow epithelialization of the track. The catheter can then be removed. If the incision was done inside the hymen ring, the catheter end can be tucked into the vagina for comfort during the healing process (Video 28-20).

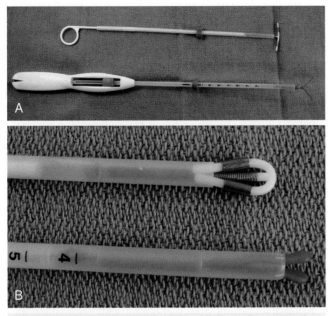

Figure 28-18 A, Paragard T380A is displayed above Mirena. Note that both intrauterine devices (IUDs) have their IUD arms extended. **B,** End of Paragard T380A is displayed above end of Mirena with both IUDs having arms fully retracted in opposite directions and ready for placement.

COLPOSCOPY

Colposcopically directed cervical biopsy and cervical curettage is primarily used to investigate abnormal findings on routine pelvic examination or an abnormal Pap smear. Consensus guidelines for the management of cervical intraepithelial neoplasia have been developed (Massad et al., 2013). Colposcopy requires diligent record keeping and patient communication, with close follow-up pending pathologic results. Colposcopy contraindications are current infection and delivery within the preceding 6 weeks. Pregnancy does not preclude colposcopy, but cervical biopsy or endocervical curettage may cause increased bleeding or miscarriage. A pregnancy test is best performed before a biopsy is contemplated. Patients should receive informed consent and accept their responsibility to follow up based on examination findings.

Colposcopy is performed with a stereoscopic operating microscope with correct focal length. The patient is placed in the dorsal lithotomy position, and the vulva and introitus are inspected for lesions. A speculum is placed in the vagina, with the size selected to maximize visualization of the cervix and minimize patient discomfort. The vaginal canal and cervix are visualized and any lesions of concern noted.

Acetic acid (3%-5%) is applied to the vaginal canal and cervix liberally with a cotton swab. Abnormal areas will display as acetowhite. Higher grade lesions may show punctation, mosaicism, or frank abnormal changes of superficial vessels best seen with a green light filter. Lugol solution, taken up by glycogen in normal mature squamous cells and not by dysplastic, metaplastic, or columnar epithelial tissues, can be applied to improve identification of abnormal tissue. Findings are recorded in a drawing to correlate with biopsy sites and abnormal pathology. Satisfactory examination includes full visualization of the entire transformation zone between squamous and columnar epithelium at the cervical os where most pathology is located. An endocervical speculum can be used to assist in visualization. Planning for lesion treatment options should be done at the time of the colposcopy.

ENDOCERVICAL CURETTAGE

Endocervical sampling is performed frequently with colposcopy and particularly if an ectocervical lesion extends into the cervical canal. Abnormal endocervical lesions can require more extensive evaluation and treatment. Endocervical curettage should precede external cervical biopsies. An endocervical curette is placed into the cervix with the sharp edge against the wall of the canal. The curette is then drawn back and forth against the cervical canal in a 360-degree sampling twice around. The sample removed can be retrieved with an endocervical brush and sent for pathologic assessment separate from any other specimens. Endocervical curettage is contraindicated in pregnant patients (Video 28-21).

CERVICAL BIOPSY

If abnormal areas are identified on the ectocervix, they should be correlated for consistency with the Pap smear results. A biopsy of the abnormal areas identified by the colposcope can be undertaken using a Kevorkian or Tischler biopsy forceps. To aid in visualization and to prevent cross-contamination, biopsies are done on the posterior cervix first followed by the anterior aspect. The fixed end of the biopsy forceps is usually placed into the cervical os, and biopsies are done in a radial orientation to obtain a sampling of the squamocolumnar transition zone where a lesion is identified. Samples should be deep enough to include the epithelial surface and a small amount of underlying stroma.

After biopsies are completed, hemostasis is best achieved with use of a Monsel paste applied with a cotton applicator or silver nitrate stick. The vagina is wiped of remaining debris and the speculum withdrawn. The patient is instructed to use analgesics as needed, to abstain from intercourse and tampon use for 10 to 14 days, and to expect some intermittent spotting. Any excessive bleeding, fever, discharge, or significant pelvic pain should lead to an investigation for the cause. Confirm the preferred method to relay the results and treatment recommendations when the pathologic results return with the patient.

ENDOMETRIAL BIOPSY

An endometrial biopsy can be performed to evaluate abnormal uterine bleeding in women who are premenopausal or postmenopausal in conjunction with ultrasonography. It can also be used to assess for a short luteal phase in infertility and abnormal or atypical glandular cells seen on Pap smear in women older than 40 years of age. Only patients with an endometrial stripe 5 mm or larger need sampling because an endometrial thickness of less than or equal to 4 to 5 mm in patients with postmenopausal bleeding reliably excludes endometrial cancer (American College of Obstetricians and Gynecologists, 2009).

A number of endometrial biopsy devices are available; the disposable flexible plastic aspirator is the easiest to use. This aspirator can be used with most women and even those with mild cervical stenosis. Before biopsy, a pregnancy test should be completed if the patient is of childbearing age and an oral NSAID given. The patient is placed in the dorsal lithotomy position, and uterine size and location are assessed. A speculum is placed to allow full visualization of the cervical os. The vaginal canal and cervix are cleansed with a chlorhexidine or povidone-iodine solution, and a single-toothed tenaculum is placed on the anterior cervix to aid in stabilization. A paracervical block can be placed for patient comfort.

When the preparation is complete, the aspirator is inserted into the cervical os using the tenaculum for countertraction. It is advanced to the fundus, and then the central plunger is retracted to create intrauterine negative pressure for suction of endometrial contents. The aspirator catheter is then withdrawn to the lower uterine segment and advanced again repetitively to the fundus and rotated to sample all aspects of the uterine cavity. Endometrial cells and blood will have entered the aspirator catheter and can be sent for pathologic examination. The tenaculum and speculum are then removed and withdrawn. The patient may experience uterine cramping and bleeding for a few days and should refrain from intercourse until this resolves. Excessive bleeding, fever, or pelvic pain warrants immediate evaluation in the postoperative period. Pathology results are discussed with the patient when available and any treatment arranged. If the sample is insufficient, the patient should be triaged to transvaginal ultrasonography in a low-risk group or full dilation and curettage for any high-risk patients (Brand et al., 2000) (Video 28-22).

- An endometrial biopsy can be performed with ultrasonography to evaluate abnormal uterine bleeding in premenopausal or postmenopausal women.
- Women with spontaneous postmenopausal bleeding and an endometrial thickness greater than 5 mm should be further evaluated with an endometrial biopsy (American College of Obstetricians and Gynecologists, 2009) (SOR: B).
- If the endometrial sample is insufficient, the patient should be triaged to a transvaginal ultrasonography in a low-risk group or dilation and curettage for high-risk patients (Brand et al., 2000) (SOR: B).

CERVICAL POLYP REMOVAL

Cervical polyps are generally benign and asymptomatic and are noted most often during routine gynecologic examinations. Most polyps arise from the endocervical mucosa and occur in perimenopausal women age 30 to 50 years. For polyp removal, the patient is placed in the dorsal lithotomy position, and a speculum is inserted vaginally. A Pap smear should be obtained and the base of the polyp identified to prevent inadvertent removal of a prolapsed endometrial polyp. The polyp is then grasped as close to its base as possible with a ring forceps and twisted. This twisting motion will dislodge the polyp, which should be sent for pathologic assessment. Hemostasis is obtained with Monsel solution or silver nitrate sticks if direct pressure is not sufficient (Video 28-23).

UTERINE ASPIRATION FOR BIOPSY OR MISCARRIAGE MANAGEMENT

Manual vacuum aspiration (MVA) can be used in the office setting for easy sampling of the uterine endometrium using a 4- or 5-mm cannula when a small endometrial biopsy catheter is insufficient (Figure 28-19). The MVA can also be used in the office for removal of retained products of conception after an incomplete or missed miscarriage up to 12 weeks without the added cost of an emergency department visit, surgical suite, and general anesthesia. The MVA device is a handheld plastic aspirator syringe attached to a plastic cannula of varying sizes. The cannula can be flexible or rigid to allow for provider preference. Vacuum aspiration is safe, quick to perform, and less painful than sharp curettage and should be recommended for use in the management of incomplete abortion (Forna and Gulmezoglu, 2001).

Confirmation of a nonviable pregnancy or incomplete abortion is verified with a falling serum β-hCG level, appropriately timed ultrasonography, or clinical findings of uterine bleeding in pregnancy with significant cervical dilation in the first trimester. A blood type and hematocrit are

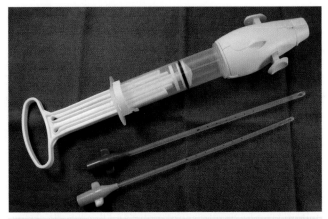

Figure 28-19 The Ipas manual vacuum aspirator (MVA) is displayed with 4-mm and 5-mm cannulas used for miscarriage management in an outpatient setting. Note the thumb buttons that close the barrel entrance to hold negative pressure in the canister when the plunger is retracted. The buttons are then released to transfer the suction pressure to the cannula once in place.

obtained to determine if RhoGAM is necessary or if bleeding has been significant. After informed consent outlining the risks of bleeding, pelvic infection, uterine perforation, Asherman adhesions, and possible need for reaspiration is obtained, the patient may receive a sedative, analgesia, or anesthesia. Most women do well with an oral NSAID for analgesia and a paracervical block for local anesthesia. For comfort, the patient should void before the procedure.

The patient is placed in the dorsal lithotomy position, and uterine size, location, and shape are assessed. Transvaginal or transabdominal ultrasonography can be performed at this time to confirm findings but is not required. A speculum is placed intravaginally, the vagina and cervix are cleansed, and a paracervical block is placed before the procedure. A single-toothed tenaculum is placed on the anterior cervix.

The uterus is sounded to the fundus to determine intracavitary size and position. If not already dilated, the cervical os is successively dilated to a size in millimeters corresponding to the gestational age using Denniston, Pratt, or Hegar dilators. The MVA curette size is generally chosen in millimeters to correspond to the gestational age in weeks as well. Thumb buttons are used to occlude the opening to the MVA barrel, and the plunger is retracted and allowed to snap into place to develop the negative pressure for suction. The cannula is attached to the MVA and placed through the cervix to the uterine fundus. The thumb buttons on each side are released, and the negative suction from the syringe is transferred to the endometrial cavity. The MVA barrel can be rotated and then brought in and out in a piston motion to dislodge the remaining products of conception. These can be observed passing through the cannula and can be evaluated fully by visual or pathologic examination after the procedure. The syringe may need to be emptied and the negative pressure reapplied based on the volume of the uterine contents. A sensation of grittiness is present in the fundus and all four uterine quadrants when the products of conception are completely removed and the cannula makes contact with the myometrium.

On completion, the MVA cannula is removed from the uterus, tenaculum from the cervix, and speculum from the vagina. The patient is observed for 15 to 30 minutes to assess for excessive bleeding, hemodynamic stability, and unusual pain. Intrarectal or intravaginal misoprostol, intracervical or intramuscular methylergonovine, and intramuscular carboprost may be used for excessive bleeding. The patient may be discharged and instructed to refrain from intercourse for 2 weeks or until the bleeding resolves. She should return for excessive bleeding, significant pelvic or abdominal pain, and fever. A form of contraception is provided if the patient desires.

BREAST MASS

In a patient who presents with a breast mass, a careful clinical and family history with focused physical examination, mammography or ultrasonography, and fine-needle aspiration (FNA) of the mass is termed a triple test. Most primary care physicians can perform the triple test that includes (1) careful clinical examination, (2) mammography or ultrasonography, and (3) FNA. A positive triple test (considered positive if any of the three items result in indeterminate, suspicious, or malignant findings) has been found in 99.6% of breast cancers. On the other hand, if the results of all three test components are negative and the patient is deemed low risk by personal or family history, the patient requires no further workup and has a less than 1% risk of cancer (National Breast Cancer Centre, 2006).

BREAST CYST ASPIRATION

When a discrete breast mass is first discovered, a rapid determination can be made with one of two methods. Ultrasonography can be used to identify a cystic or solid mass rapidly with minimal discomfort to the patient. If ultrasonography is not available, an aspiration can be performed to determine if it is a breast cyst.

The patient can be placed in a recumbent position and the skin over the breast cleansed. The mass is stabilized between the thumb and index and middle fingers on the nondominant hand. Anesthesia can be used locally, but most women feel minimal discomfort. A 1.5-inch, 20- to 23-gauge needle is attached to a 10- to 30-mL syringe. The skin is punctured and the end of the needle directed into the mass with continuous suction on the syringe. The fluid of a cyst is aspirated completely before the needle is removed. Fluid should be sent for pathologic evaluation. Straw- to green-colored fluid is usually benign, and bloody brown to red fluid is more suspicious for malignancy. If bloody fluid is obtained in an atraumatic aspirate or if a lump remains, the patient should be referred for a core needle or open biopsy (Video 28-24).

KEY TREATMENT

- Vacuum aspiration is safe, quick to perform, and less painful than sharp curettage and recommended in the management of incomplete abortion (Forna and Gulmezoglu, 2001) (SOR: B).
- The triple test of (1) careful clinical examination, (2) mammography or ultrasonography, and (3) FNA of a breast mass approaches the false-negative rate of surgical breast biopsy and the false-positive rate of frozen section (National Breast Cancer Centre, 2006) (SOR: B).

- If bloody fluid is obtained on an atraumatic breast mass aspirate or if a lump remains after drainage, the patient is referred for surgical consult for core or open biopsy (National Breast Cancer Centre, 2006) (SOR: B).

FINE-NEEDLE ASPIRATION CYTOLOGY OR BIOPSY

Fine-needle aspiration can be performed in the office with minimal equipment for diagnosis of a discrete, solid breast mass. FNA testing results in a sensitivity of 90% and a false-negative rate of 3% to 10% in experienced hands (Valea and Katz, 2007). Contraindications include an overlying skin infection, underlying pulsatile mass, and a history of bleeding disorders.

The patient is properly given informed consent. She is recumbent in position, and the area of puncture is identified, marked, and cleansed. A local injection of 1 to 2 mL of anesthetic is infiltrated into the skin over the mass. The mass is stabilized with the three-finger technique previously mentioned. A 10- to 20-mL syringe with 18- to 22-gauge needle attached is advanced into the mass. Full aspiration suction is performed, and the needle is passed through the mass in different planes three to five times for an adequate sample. The suction is released and the needle removed. The cell sample, frequently only in the needle itself, is placed on a cytology slide and fixed for proper pathologic assessment. FNA provides histologic diagnosis but cannot determine architectural features. FNA should not be used to investigate microcalcifications because FNA cannot distinguish ductal carcinoma in situ from invasive cancer. A core or open biopsy should be performed in these patients for more definitive diagnosis before excision or definitive treatment (see Video 28-24).

Neonatal Circumcision

Circumcision has been used in religious rites for centuries and was used in ancient Egypt as a method for hygiene. Modern data in the United States are conflicting as to the benefits versus risks. By age 5 years, 90% of boys have a spontaneously retractable foreskin. The incidence of phimosis decreases with age and may be treated with a steroid cream. The medical approach to phimosis is initially successful in about 80% of cases, and 1 year later, 60% had no phimosis (Ku and Huen, 2007). Many parents still elect to have their male infants circumcised.

The American Urological Association revised its policy to say that circumcision should be presented for health benefits (Tobian et al., 2010). The American Academy of Pediatrics, American Medical Association, and American College of Obstetrics and Gynecology all consider the procedure elective with minimal benefits (Lannon et al., 1999). The World Health Organization–United Nations program on HIV/AIDS concluded that male circumcision is efficacious in reducing sexual transmission of HIV from women to men. In Africa, circumcision decreased HIV acquisition by 53% to 60%. Herpesvirus type 2 is decreased by 28% to 34% and human papillomavirus prevalence by 32% to 35% in circumcised men. Among female partners of circumcised men in these African studies, the incidence of bacterial vaginosis was reduced by 40% and *Trichomonas vaginalis* by 48%; genital ulcers decreased as well (Tobian et al., 2010).

The incidence of UTI is reduced with circumcision in some populations. If a population has a baseline UTI incidence of 3% or higher and circumcision complication rate less than 2%, circumcision is helpful in reducing UTIs. In normal infants, the risk of UTI is 1% or less; in those with prior UTI, it is 10%; and in those with vesicoureteral reflux, it is 30% (Singh-Grewal, 2005). The main risk is bleeding followed by infection. Actual rates of hemorrhage in medically indicated or ritual hospital-based circumcision range from 0.2% to 3% (Bocquet et al., 2010).

Although numbers may be declining in some U.S. areas, circumcision remains one of the most common procedures performed. A neonatal circumcision is normally performed at 12 to 48 hours old when the infant has stabilized after birth but may be performed up to 4 to 6 weeks of age. Before the procedure, each patient should be examined thoroughly for signs of congenital anomalies of the penis, urethra, or urinary tract. If hypospadias is present, circumcision is stopped or not performed to allow the tissue to be used in a corrective surgical procedure to repair the urethra and glans.

Many locations recommend no oral intake for 1 hour before the procedure to prevent aspiration. Oral sucrose can be used to reduce pain during the procedure (Gatti, 2003). A dorsal penile block or penile ring block is more effective than EMLA cream or sucrose. EMLA cream provides anesthesia but has a risk of methemoglobinemia (Brady-Fryer et al., 2004).

Inspect first to make sure there is no hypospadias or hidden penis. If the penis is normal and parental consent has been obtained, the infant is placed on a circumcision restraint board and the skin prepared. A dorsal block is achieved by injecting 0.4 to 0.5 mL of 1% lidocaine without epinephrine at the base of the penile shaft at both the 10 and 2 o'clock positions and 5 mm distal to the skin reflection onto the pubic area. Inject 1 to 3 mm deep under the Buck fascia after aspirating to ensure you are not in a blood vessel. A ring block can also be done, slightly higher on the penile shaft circumferentially in the subcutaneous tissues, taking care to avoid injury to the urethra or vasculature (Figure 28-20).

When anesthesia is complete, grasp the foreskin distally at 3 and 9 o'clock with two hemostats. All techniques require freeing of adhesions with blunt dissection, usually done with a straight Kelly clamp inserted between the foreskin and glans in a superior direction to avoid the urethra. Open the clamp and sweep laterally. Avoid the highly vascular frenulum. Free the adhesions to the coronal sulcus of the glans. Use a straight hemostat to clamp the free dorsal foreskin, again making sure the tip is held up and away from entering the urethra. Clamp three fourths the length of the foreskin dorsally. Insert iris scissors and carefully cut the foreskin along the crushed line. Peel back the foreskin to reveal the glans. Avoid degloving the shaft and damage to the frenulum.

GOMCO CLAMP

The Gomco is the most common circumcision clamp. Test the clamp's fit with the base before use. Estimate the correct

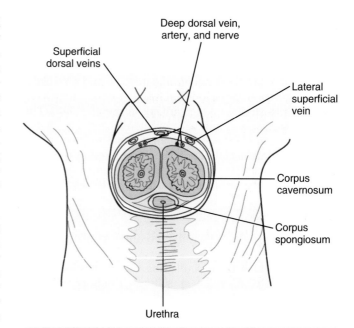

Figure 28-20 Dorsal penile block. The dorsal penile nerve is anesthetized using no more than 1.0 mL total of 1% lidocaine without epinephrine. The anesthetic is administered at the dorsum of the penis approximately 0.5 cm distal to the penile root at the 10 and 2 o'clock positions. (From Pfenninger JL, Fowler G, eds. *Procedures for primary care physicians.* 2nd ed. St. Louis: Mosby; 2003 and Chavez MC, Maker VK. Office surgery. In Rakel RE, ed. *Textbook of family medicine.* 7th ed. Philadelphia: Saunders; 2007.)

size so that the bell covers at least seven-eighths of the glans (1.1, 1.3, and 1.5 sizes available). The glans is then covered with the Gomco bell and the foreskin pulled over it, sometimes with the aid of a clamp or safety pin. The bell and foreskin are then pulled through the hole in the base plate and the foreskin is arranged to ensure even tissue removal. The clamp is then placed on the base plate and the bell stem hooked over the clamp bar. After positioning is confirmed, the clamp is tightened for 5 to 10 minutes and the remaining foreskin removed with a #10 scalpel. If hemostasis is confirmed, the clamp is removed, and the glans is covered regularly with petroleum jelly at each diaper change. Healing should take 4 to 10 days. Complications include bleeding, infection, and trauma to the penis. Bleeding can be controlled with silver nitrate or a simple suture if not resolved with pressure (Video 28-25).

PLASTIBELL

The Plastibell device is a plastic ring on the end of a central removable post. The ring is placed between the glans and foreskin. A tight ligature of moistened suture is placed around the foreskin and tightened into a sulcus on the ring. Foreskin distal to the ring is excised and the handle of the device broken off. The plastic ring stays in place, with the ligature tied tightly around the protective ring, for 5 to 10 days and falls off spontaneously. The appearance of the small amount of necrotic skin may worry parents, and it may be complicated with incomplete or irregular skin edges if the ligature is not tied tightly enough.

MOGAN CLAMP

The Mogan clamp is used in traditional Jewish circumcisions and may cause less pain by being faster. The foreskin is grasped with the nondominant hand and the glans pushed downward. The foreskin is slid into the clamp from anterior to posterior, taking care not to trap the glans. The clamp opens only 3 mm to prevent major glans entrapment. When in place and the glans is confirmed below the plate, the clamp is closed and the distal foreskin removed. The clamp is left in place for a few minutes and then removed, and the foreskin is retracted over the glans.

KEY TREATMENT

- Oral sucrose reduces painful procedures in infants (Gatti, 2003) (SOR: A).
- Dorsal penile block or penile ring blocks are more effective than EMLA cream or sucrose (Brady-Fryer et al., 2004) (SOR: A).
- EMLA cream provides anesthesia but has a risk of methemoglobinemia (Brady-Fryer et al., 2004) (SOR: A)

Musculoskeletal Office Procedures

ASPIRATION OF KNEE JOINT (ARTHROCENTESIS)

The knee is one of the largest and most accessible joints for arthrocentesis or joint injection. Aspiration of joint fluid from the knee is performed to assess for infection, inflammation, crystal deposition, or traumatic complications. Infections may show a significantly high white blood cell infiltrate with visible organisms on Gram stain. Inflammation may show the same without organisms seen. Crystal disease may show urate or calcium pyrophosphate crystals. Trauma may produce a bloody aspirate with tears of a ligament or cartilage and fat lobules with an intraarticular fracture.

Before the aspiration, the patient is consented and placed in a recumbent position with the knee flexed slightly with a rolled towel. The knee is assessed for effusion and the aspiration site marked and cleansed with a sterilizing wash. The knee joint space can be entered with a 22-gauge needle on a syringe on either side but usually from the lateral aspect 1 cm lateral and superior to the patella and directed 45 degrees downward, angling under the patella, with aspiration done during insertion. When the joint space is entered, fluid should enter the syringe rapidly. Milking the lateral and medial recesses of the knee toward the needle tip will remove more fluid. The needle is removed after aspiration, or it is left in place and the syringe changed under sterile conditions for a steroid injection to follow if necessary. Large joints can be injected with 20 to 40 mg of triamcinolone or 6 to 12 mg of betamethasone with 3 to 6 mL of 1% lidocaine for inflammatory conditions unrelated to infections. Procedural risks include septic arthritis, mild injury to the articular cartilage, and hemarthrosis. (Videos 28-26 and 28-28).

SHOULDER INJECTION

The subacromial bursa is another location frequently treated with steroid injection for bursitis or tendonitis. Injections of 10 to 20 mg of triamcinolone with 2 to 4 mL of lidocaine can be performed into the subacromial bursa. The easiest approach to the subacromial space is with the patient seated comfortably and arms resting at the sides. The lateral shoulder is prepared with a sterile solution after palpating landmarks. The acromial process is identified on the lateral shoulder above the humeral head. In the sulcus between the humeral head and the acromial process lies the subacromial bursa. Marking the lateral border of the acromial process can provide some assistance. A 22- to 25-gauge needle on a syringe with the injection is then aimed directly into the sulcus between the bones 1 cm below the acromial process perpendicularly through the deltoid muscle. Ligamentous and muscular structures resist injection, but the bursa should allow free infusion. Relief of pain may be noted in a few minutes if lidocaine is used and confirms the injection was placed appropriately (Video 28-27)

Summary of Additional Online Content

The following content is available at www.expertconsult.com:

eAppendix 28-1 History of Surgery

Videos

The following videos are available at www.expertconsult.com.

Video 28-1 Topical Anesthesia

Video 28-2 Local Anesthesia

Video 28-3 Digital Block

Video 28-4 Inverted Subcuticular Stitches

Video 28-5 Tissue Glue

Video 28-6 Instrument Tie

Video 28-7 Subcuticular Running Stitches

Video 28-8 Mattress Stitches

Video 28-9 Excisional Skin Biopsy

Video 28-10 Punch Biopsy

Video 28-11 Shave Biopsy

Video 28-12 Basal Cell Curettage and Cautery

Video 28-13 Wart Treatment Abscess Incision and Drainage

Video 28-14 Lipoma Removal

Video 28-15 Ingrown Toenail Removal

Video 28-16 Anoscopy

Video 28-17 Internal Hemorrhoid Banding

Video 28-18 External Hemorrhoid Excision

Video 28-19 Intrauterine Device Insertion

Video 28-20 Bartholin Cyst Word Catheter Placement

Video 28-21 Colposcopy

Video 28-22 Endometrial Biopsy

Video 28-23 Cervical Polyp Removal

Video 28-24 Breast Cyst Aspiration

Video 28-25 Neonatal Circumcision

Video 28-26 Knee Aspiration

Video 28-27 Shoulder Injection

Video 28-28 Knee Injection

References

⊕ **The complete reference list is available at www.expertconsult.com.**

Web Resources

emedicine.medscape.com/clinical_procedures Information on additional procedures, including those covered in this chapter.

www.cdc.gov/rabies/exposure/postexposure.html The Centers for Disease Control and Prevention's website has advice on rabies prophylaxis for animal bites.

http://www.cdc.gov/mmwr/PDF/rr/rr5703.pdf Centers for Disease Control and Prevention. Morbidity and Mortality Weekly Report on human rabies prevention 2008.

http://www.cdc.gov/mmwr/pdf/wk/mm6001.pdf Centers for Disease Control and Prevention. 2010 Updated recommendations for use of tetanus toxoid, reduced diphtheria toxoid and acellular pertussis (Tdap) vaccine from the Advisory Committee on Immunization Practices, 2010.

https://www.clinicalkey.com/info/clinicalkey/clinicalkey-for -clinicians/ Clinician search engine resource by Elsevier.

http://www.mdconsult.com/das/patient/view/465780469-2366 MDConsult patient education materials.

www.mpcenter.net Excellent patient education materials.

http://nccc.ucsf.edu/clinician-consultation/post-exposure-prophylaxis -pep/ Clinician Consultation Center for occupational exposures.

www.nejm.org/multimedia/medical-videos Procedural education and videos.

www.npinstitute.com Postgraduate procedural skills training.

www.proceduresconsult.com/medical-procedures Procedural training and videos.

29 *Sports Medicine*

JUSTIN D. ROTHMIER, KIMBERLY G. HARMON, and JOHN W. O'KANE

Sports medicine involves the care of patients with illnesses and injuries related to sports and exercise. Both orthopedic and medical conditions affect a wide spectrum of patients during sports and recreational activities. The field of primary care sports medicine has emerged over the past 30 years as a leader in the comprehensive care of athletes, teams, and exercising individuals. Although sports medicine is often viewed in the context of professional and elite athletes, the principles and practice of sports medicine apply to athletes of all levels and ages.

The role of a sports medicine physician is to promote the health and safety of exercising individuals, prevent injury and illness, optimize function, and minimize disabilities that would preclude sports participation. Sports medicine physicians work closely with a multidisciplinary team of health care providers (specialty physicians and surgeons, athletic trainers, physical therapists, nutritionists, psychologists, and conditioning coaches) to satisfy the complete medical needs of athletes.

Sports medicine includes a rapidly expanding core of knowledge related to medical issues in sports and exercise for which the primary care sports medicine physician is uniquely trained. *Primary care sports medicine* is a subspecialty designation obtained through completion of an accredited sports medicine fellowship and passing the Certificate of Added Qualification examination. Many practicing primary care providers also gain vast experience in sports medicine through office treatment of orthopedic injuries, event coverage, and preparticipation screening evaluations. Musculoskeletal problems account for up to 20% of all primary care office visits (Urwin et al., 1998; Woodwell and Cherry, 2004), and approximately 90% of all sports injuries are treated nonsurgically. Thus, a sound clinical foundation in the evaluation and treatment of musculoskeletal disorders is critical to primary care providers and helps guide appropriate referral to orthopedic and rehabilitative specialists.

This chapter focuses on both the medical aspects of sports medicine and common orthopedic injuries in athletes. Detailed reviews cover the preparticipation physical evaluation (PPE); cardiac disorders in athletes; concussion assessment and management; cervical spine injuries; on-the-field assessment of injured athletes; facial trauma; environmental influences such as exertional heat illness; common infections in athletes; and a systems-based review of dermatologic, pulmonary, hematologic, gastrointestinal (GI), and genitourinary disorders in athletes. Orthopedic areas common in primary care sports medicine are also included, such as athletic low back pain (LBP), muscle strains, tendinopathy, shin pain, stress fractures, and issues unique to pediatric and female athletes. See Chapters 30 and 31 for a comprehensive review of additional musculoskeletal problems relevant to sports medicine and the care of exercising individuals.

Preparticipation Physical Evaluation

Key Points

- The primary objective of the PPE is to detect preexisting medical or musculoskeletal conditions that predispose an athlete to injury, disability, or catastrophic injury.
- Syncope that occurs during exercise is a serious warning sign and warrants a comprehensive cardiology evaluation to rule out an underlying cardiac disorder that predisposes to sudden death.
- Any athlete with a systolic murmur of grade 3/6 in severity, a murmur that gets louder with a Valsalva maneuver or on standing (suspicious for hypertrophic cardiomyopathy), a diastolic murmur, a family history of premature sudden cardiac death, or concerning exertional symptoms should be further evaluated by a cardiovascular specialist.

A PPE, or "sports physical," is frequently required for medical clearance before participation in organized sports.

The *Preparticipation Physical Evaluation* monograph, first introduced in 1992, provides recommendations for the content and format of the evaluation (American Academy of Family Physicians [AAFP] et al., 2010). The fourth edition of the monograph, updated in 2010, is supported by six national medical societies: the AAFP, American Academy of Pediatrics, American College of Sports Medicine, American Medical Society for Sports Medicine, American Orthopaedic Society for Sports Medicine, and American Osteopathic Academy of Sports Medicine. The fourth edition also includes collaboration with the American Heart Association (AHA) regarding the preparticipation cardiovascular evaluation.

The primary objectives of the PPE include the following:

1. Detection of potentially life-threatening or disabling medical or musculoskeletal conditions before athletic clearance
2. Identification of preexisting conditions that may predispose athletes to injury
3. Satisfying legal or administrative requirements

Secondary objectives of the PPE include the following:

1. Promoting the health and safety of athletes in training and competition
2. Serving as an entry point into the health care system for athletes
3. Providing an opportunity for a general health assessment

The recommended frequency of the PPE varies widely according to the requirements of the specific school, organization, or state. AHA first published consensus recommendations for cardiovascular screening in athletes in 1996 and reaffirmed these recommendations in 2007, which have influenced the format and timing of the PPE (Maron et al., 1996b, 2007). A comprehensive PPE is recommended on entry into middle school, high school, and college before participation in competitive sports. For youth and high school athletes, a comprehensive PPE should be repeated every 2 years. For years not requiring a comprehensive PPE, annual updates consisting of a comprehensive history and determination of height, weight, and blood pressure, along with a problem-focused evaluation of new concerns, illnesses, or injuries, should occur on interval years for youth and high school athletes and on all subsequent years for college athletes.

The PPE history focuses on symptoms related to exercise, such as exertional syncope, lightheadedness, chest pain, palpitations, dyspnea, wheezing, and fatigue with less than expected activity (Table 29-1). A past medical history of preexisting cardiac or pulmonary conditions, murmurs, hypertension, coronary artery disease risk factors, asthma, concussions, illicit drug use, prior orthopedic injuries, or other medical conditions that place an athlete at risk of injury should be noted. Specific questions to identify a family history of premature death, cardiovascular disease, and hereditary cardiac disorders (e.g., hypertrophic cardiomyopathy, Marfan syndrome, long QT syndrome) are also recommended.

The PPE examination consists of both medical and musculoskeletal components. The cardiovascular examination

Table 29-1 Preparticipation Physical Evaluation: Cardiovascular History Questions

1. Have you ever passed out or nearly passed out during or after exercise?
2. Have you ever had discomfort, pain, pressure, or tightness in your chest during exercise?
3. Do you get lightheaded or feel more short of breath than expected during exercise?
4. Does your heart ever race or skip beats (irregular beats) during exercise?
5. Has a doctor ever told you that you have a heart problem, high blood pressure, high cholesterol, a heart murmur, a heart infection, Kawasaki disease, or an unexplained seizure disorder?
6. Has a doctor ever ordered a test for your heart (e.g., electrocardiography or echocardiography)?
7. Has any family member or relative died of heart problems or had an unexpected or unexplained sudden death before age 50 years (including drowning, motor vehicle crash, or sudden infant death syndrome)?
8. Has anyone in your family had unexplained fainting, seizures, or near drowning?
9. Does anyone in your family have a heart problem, pacemaker, or implanted defibrillator?
10. Does anyone in your family have hypertrophic cardiomyopathy, Marfan syndrome, arrhythmogenic right ventricular cardiomyopathy, long QT syndrome, short QT syndrome, Brugada syndrome, or catecholaminergic polymorphic ventricular tachycardia?

is a major focus of the medical evaluation and consists of a blood pressure measurement, palpation of the radial and femoral artery pulses, cardiac auscultation with the patient both supine and standing, and recognition of the physical manifestations of Marfan syndrome (Maron et al., 1996b, 2007). Any heart murmur detected should be further assessed during the Valsalva maneuver or while moving the patient from a squatting to a standing position. These maneuvers decrease venous return and may accentuate the murmur of hypertrophic cardiomyopathy, the leading cause of sudden cardiac death in young athletes. However, hypertrophic cardiomyopathy is difficult to detect on examination alone because outflow tract obstruction, which causes the harsh systolic murmur, is present in only about 25% of patients with the disorder (Maron, 1997) (Figure 29-1).

The musculoskeletal assessment serves as a screening evaluation of the spine and upper and lower extremities. Joint range of motion (ROM), strength, and stability should be tested. Several functional tests, such as hopping, squatting, and "duck walking," assess many anatomic areas at once and make the evaluation more efficient. Previous orthopedic injuries can also be evaluated in more detail to detect problems that require further rehabilitation or protective bracing before sports participation.

WARNING SYMPTOMS IN ATHLETES

Warning or "red flag" symptoms that may indicate the presence of an underlying cardiovascular disorder should be recognized and further assessed before medical clearance. Syncope that occurs during but not after exercise is of great concern and warrants a comprehensive cardiology evaluation to rule out the presence of an occult cardiac disorder that may lead to sudden death. Other worrying symptoms include palpitations, chest pain, lightheadedness, and fatigue or dyspnea greater than expected for the level of

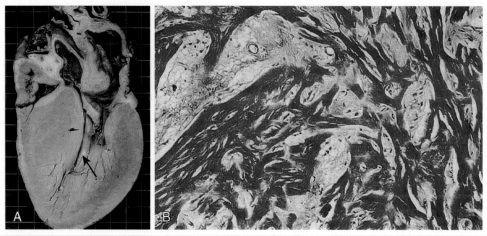

Figure 29-1 Hypertrophic cardiomyopathy. **A,** Gross appearance. **B,** Histologic appearance. Note the myocardial fiber disarray. (From Braunwald E. *Essential atlas of heart diseases.* 3rd ed. Philadelphia: Saunders; 2000.)

activity. Athletes with warning symptoms should be evaluated by an electrocardiogram (ECG), echocardiogram, and exercise stress test and referred to a cardiologist. In addition, systolic murmurs of grade 3/6 in severity, all diastolic murmurs, any murmur that becomes louder with a Valsalva maneuver or on standing (suspicious for hypertrophic cardiomyopathy), and a concerning family history of premature sudden cardiac death or hereditary cardiac disorder should be further evaluated by a cardiovascular specialist.

If a cardiac abnormality is identified, the decision to withhold medical clearance for participation in competitive sports is difficult and should be carefully considered on an individual basis. The American College of Cardiology 36th Bethesda Conference defined eligibility recommendations for athletes with cardiovascular abnormalities (Maron and Zipes, 2005).

LIMITATIONS OF CARDIOVASCULAR SCREENING

Despite efforts to standardize the format and approach to the PPE, several limitations of the screening process still exist. In 2007, only 19% of U.S. states used forms that were considered adequate by AHA, and 35% of states allowed practitioners with limited cardiovascular training to perform the evaluation (Glover et al., 2007). Unfortunately, recommendations to use a comprehensive personal and family questionnaire to guide the PPE are not widely adopted, and recommended screening protocols are often incompletely or inadequately implemented. In addition, the PPE is screening for medical conditions that place an athlete at increased risk of sudden death, and no outcomes-based research has demonstrated that the PPE is effective in preventing sudden death or potentially catastrophic events or for identifying athletes at risk. A complicating feature of the screening process is that athletes who harbor underlying structural heart disease may be asymptomatic until the sudden cardiac arrest. In a review of 134 cases of sudden cardiac death, only 18% of athletes had symptoms of cardiovascular disease in the 3 years before their death, and only 3% were suspected of having a cardiovascular condition after PPE (Maron et al., 1996a).

Limitations in the traditional screening process have led to widespread debate regarding the addition of noninvasive cardiovascular screening techniques, such as ECG, to the PPE. In 2007, the AHA reaffirmed recommendations against universal ECG screening in athletes, citing a low prevalence of disease, poor sensitivity, high false-positive rate, poor cost-effectiveness, and a lack of clinicians to interpret the results (Maron et al., 2007). In contrast, the European Society of Cardiology, the International Olympic Committee, and the governing associations of several U.S. and international professional sports leagues endorse the use of ECG in the screening of athletes (Corrado et al., 2006; Ljungqvist et al., 2009). These recommendations are supported by studies showing that ECG is more sensitive than history and physical examination alone in identifying athletes with underlying cardiovascular disease, including a 77% greater power to detect hypertrophic cardiomyopathy (Corrado et al., 1998).

Corrado and associates reported results from screening 42,386 athletes over 25 years from the national PPE program in Italy. Disqualification on the basis of a screening protocol using history, physical examination, and ECG produced a tenfold reduction in the incidence of sudden cardiac death in young competitive athletes and an 89% reduction of sudden death from cardiomyopathy (Corrado et al., 2005, 2006). Although only 0.2% of athletes were disqualified for potentially lethal cardiovascular conditions, the study reported a 7% false-positive rate and a 2% overall disqualification rate (Corrado et al., 2005). This raised concerns that adopting such a program in the United States would lead to an unacceptable number of disqualifications in athletes with a low risk of sudden death.

Complex issues regarding feasibility, cost-effectiveness, appropriate physician, and healthy system infrastructure remain before large-scale implementation of ECG screening in the United States can be considered. However, some physicians are using ECG during PPE to improve detection of potentially lethal cardiovascular abnormalities. A large-scale study of 32,561 United States high school students performed by cardiologists, administrators, and volunteers who all underwent specialized training and quality review demonstrated an abnormal ECG rate of 2.5% (Marek et al., 2011). When used, ECG interpretation must be based on modern criteria to distinguish abnormal findings from physiologic alterations in athletes to ensure acceptable

Table 29-2 The Seattle Criteria: Abnormal Electrocardiographic Findings in Athletes* (see Table 29-3)

Abnormal ECG Finding	Definition
T-wave inversion	>1 mm in depth in two or more leads: V2-V6, II and aVF or I and aVL (excludes III, aVR, and V1)
ST segment depression	≥0.5 mm in depth in two or more leads
Pathologic Q waves	>3 mm in depth or >40 msec in duration in two or more leads (except III and aVR)
Complete left bundle branch block	QRS ≥120 msec, predominantly negative QRS complex in lead V1 (QS or rS), and upright monophasic R wave in leads I and V6
Intraventricular conduction delay	Any QRS duration ≥140 msec
Left axis deviation	−30 to −90 degrees
Left atrial enlargement	Prolonged P wave duration of >120 msec in leads I or II with negative portion of the P wave ≥1 mm in depth and ≥40 msec in duration in lead V1
Right ventricular hypertrophy pattern	$R\text{-}V_1 + S\text{-}V_5 > 10.5$ mm *and* right-axis deviation >120 degrees
Ventricular preexcitation	PR interval <120 msec with a delta wave (slurred upstroke in the QRS complex) and wide QRS (>120 msec)
Long QT interval[†]	QTc ≥470 msec (male) QTc ≥480 msec (female) QTc ≥500 msec (marked QT prolongation)
Short QT interval[†]	QTc ≤320 msec
Brugada-like ECG pattern	High take-off and downsloping ST segment elevation followed by a negative T wave in ≥2 leads in V1-V3
Profound sinus bradycardia	<30 beats/min or sinus pauses ≥3 sec
Mobitz type II second-degree AV block	Intermittently nonconducted P waves not preceded by PR prolongation and not followed by PR shortening
3-degree AV block	Complete heart block
Atrial tachyarrhythmias	Supraventricular tachycardia, atrial fibrillation, atrial-flutter
Premature ventricular contractions (PVCs)	≥2 PVCs per 10 second tracing
Ventricular arrhythmias	Couplets, triplets, and nonsustained ventricular tachycardia

*These electrocardiographic (ECG) findings are unrelated to regular training or expected physiologic adaptation to exercise, may suggest the presence of pathologic cardiovascular disease, and require further diagnostic evaluation.
[†]The QT interval corrected for heart rate is ideally measured with heart rates of 60 to 90 beats/min. Consider repeating the ECG after mild aerobic activity for borderline or abnormal QTc values with a heart rate less than 50 beats/min.
AV, Atrioventricular.

accuracy and a low false-positive rate (Drezner, 2008). In a study of 2720 competitive athletes and physically active schoolchildren, a U.K. study reported a false-positive rate of 3.7% using history, physical examination, and ECG, with only 1.9% of false-positive results determined by ECG alone (Wilson et al., 2008). Nine athletes (0.3% of those screened) were found to have a cardiovascular condition known to cause sudden cardiac death in young persons, and all athletes were detected by ECG, not by history or physical examination. Physicians interpreting ECGs in athletes should be familiar with common training-related ECG alterations that are normal variants. In contrast, training-unrelated ECG changes suggest the possibility of underlying pathology, require further diagnostic workup, and should be considered abnormal. Current recommendations for ECG interpretation in athletes to distinguish pathologic ECG abnormalities from physiologic ECG alterations have been recently published (Corrado et al., 2009, 2010; Drezner et al., 2013a, 2013b, 2013c). In 2012, a summit of international experts in Sports Cardiology and Sports Medicine convened in Seattle to define contemporary standards in the interpretation of ECGs in athletes. The "Seattle criteria" were developed and subsequently used to develop an online training module for physicians to acquire a common foundation in ECG interpretation in athletes (Tables 29-2 and 29-3). This online training module is available at no cost to any physician worldwide (see Web Resources).

Table 29-3 The Seattle Criteria: Normal Electrocardiographic Findings in Athletes* (see Table 29-2)

1. Sinus bradycardia (≥30 beats/min)
2. Sinus arrhythmia
3. Ectopic atrial rhythm
4. Junctional escape rhythm
5. First-degree AV block (PR interval >200 msec)
6. Mobitz type I (Wenckebach) second-degree AV block
7. Incomplete RBBB
8. Isolated QRS voltage criteria for LVH
   Except: QRS voltage criteria for LVH occurring with any nonvoltage criteria for LVH such as left atrial enlargement, left axis deviation, ST segment depression, T-wave inversion, or pathologic Q waves
9. Early repolarization (ST elevation, J-point elevation, J-waves, or terminal QRS slurring)
10. Convex ("domed") ST segment elevation combined with T-wave inversion in leads V1-V4 in black or African athletes

*These common training-related electrocardiographic alterations are physiological adaptations to regular exercise, considered normal variants in athletes, and do not require further evaluation in asymptomatic athletes.
AV, Atrioventricular; *LVH,* left ventricular hypertrophy; *RBBB,* right bundle branch block.

Cardiac Disorders in Athletes

Key Points

- Bradyarrhythmias caused by increased resting vagal tone are common in athletes and include sinus bradycardia, sinus arrhythmia, first-degree atrioventricular block, and Wenckebach (Mobitz I) second-degree atrioventricular (AV) block.
- Mobitz II second-degree and complete third-degree AV blocks are always pathologic and warrant cardiologic evaluation.
- Supraventricular tachyarrhythmias in athletes are abnormal and require further evaluation and treatment, often with radiofrequency (RF) ablation, before participation in strenuous exercise.
- Ventricular arrhythmias are life-threatening events and usually occur in the presence of structural heart disease or ion channel disorders.
- Hypertrophic cardiomyopathy, coronary artery anomalies, and commotio cordis are the most common causes of sudden cardiac death in young U.S. athletes.

ARRHYTHMIAS

Cardiac arrhythmias in athletes range from benign to life threatening. Bradyarrhythmias are more common in athletes than in the general population because of an increase in resting vagal tone as a response to regular strenuous exercise. Common bradyarrhythmias include sinus bradycardia, sinus arrhythmia, first-degree AV block, and Wenckebach (or Mobitz I) second-degree AV block (Huston et al., 1985; Link et al., 2001). These bradyarrhythmias are usually asymptomatic and should resolve during exercise by the withdrawal of vagal tone and associated catecholamine influx.

Athletes with symptomatic Wenckebach block, such as presyncope or syncope during exertion, require further evaluation by a cardiologist and often placement of a permanent pacemaker and restriction of activities. Higher degrees of heart block, such as Mobitz II second-degree and complete third-degree AV blocks, are always pathologic in any individual, including athletes (Figure 29-2). Mobitz II and complete heart blocks signify marked disease in the His-Purkinje system and are generally accepted as a class I indication for permanent pacemaker placement even in the absence of symptoms (Link et al, 2001).

Tachyarrhythmias in athletes are abnormal and require further evaluation and treatment before participation in strenuous exercise. The treatment of many supraventricular tachyarrhythmias has been greatly advanced by the use

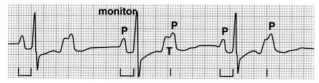

Figure 29-2 Mobitz II second-degree atrioventricular block. Note that every alternate P wave is blocked. (From Goldberger E. *Treatment of cardiac emergencies.* 5th ed. Philadelphia: Saunders; 1990.)

of RF ablation, which might offer an actual cure and obviate the need for lifelong pharmacologic treatment.

The most common tachyarrhythmia in athletes is *atrial fibrillation* (AF). Studies have suggested that AF occurs more frequently in athletes than in the general population (Furlanello et al., 1998; Huston et al., 1985). This might be a consequence of increased vagal tone and bradycardia in athletes, which allows dispersion of atrial repolarization and results in a higher susceptibility to AF. RF ablation is curative in most cases of paroxysmal AF (Link et al., 2001). If pharmacologic treatment is needed, rate control can be accomplished with β-adrenergic blockers or calcium channel blockers, and anticoagulation should be considered with aspirin, warfarin, or possibly the newer factor Xa inhibitors (rivaroxaban, apixaban) and direct thrombin inhibitors (dabigatran), depending on the frequency of AF and other risk factors for thromboembolism. However, any athlete receiving anticoagulation therapy with warfarin should be restricted from sports involving collision or bodily contact.

Atrioventricular nodal reentrant tachycardia (AVNRT) is characterized by abrupt onset and termination of symptoms, a narrow QRS complex, and no evidence of atrial activity on the ECG during the tachycardia. AVNRT caused by an accessory bypass tract, known as Wolff-Parkinson-White (WPW) syndrome, may be evident on the ECG by the characteristic delta wave (slurred upstroke of QRS complex), short PR interval, and prolonged QRS complex (Figure 29-3). Athletes with WPW may be at risk of sudden death and should be strongly considered for RF ablation. RF ablation for both AVNRT and WPW offers cure rates higher than 95% (Link et al., 2001; Manolis et al., 1994).

Atrial flutter is an unusual arrhythmia in trained athletes and typically results from an underlying cardiomyopathy.

Ventricular tachyarrhythmias in athletes are life threatening and usually the result of structural heart disease such as hypertrophic cardiomyopathy, anomalous coronary artery, dilated cardiomyopathy, arrhythmogenic right ventricular dysplasia (ARVD), or atherosclerotic coronary artery disease (CAD). Ventricular arrhythmias and sudden death may also occur in individuals with structurally normal hearts. This may occur from ion channel disorders, such as long QT syndrome, catecholaminergic polymorphic ventricular tachycardia (CPVT), and Brugada syndrome or from commotio cordis. Long QT syndrome is characterized by a prolonged QTc interval, and Brugada syndrome is suggested by an incomplete right bundle branch block and ST segment elevation in the precordial leads. Exercise may provoke ventricular arrhythmias because of high catecholamine levels and make ventricular fibrillation more difficult to terminate. Athletes who experience a resuscitated sudden death should undergo an extensive workup and treatment with an implantable cardioverter-defibrillator (Link et al., 2001).

SUDDEN CARDIAC DEATH

Sudden cardiac death in athletes is a catastrophic event and the leading cause of death in exercising young athletes (Maron et al., 2009). The exact incidence of sudden cardiac deaths per year in the United States is not known. Reported ranges of sudden cardiac death in the United States is

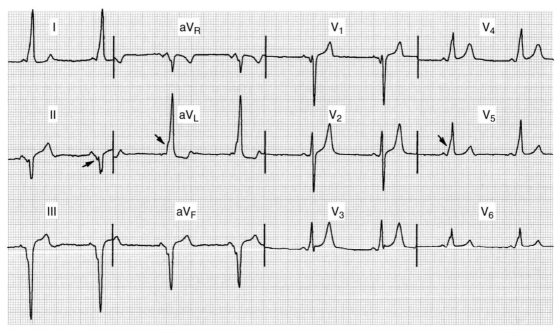

Figure 29-3 Atrioventricular nodal reentrant tachycardia. Notice the characteristic triad of the Wolff-Parkinson-White (WPW) pattern: wide QRS complexes, short PR intervals, and delta waves *(arrows)* that are negative in some leads (e.g., II, III, aV$_R$) and positive in others (aV$_L$ and V$_2$ to V$_6$). The Q waves in leads II, III, and aV$_F$ are the result of abnormal ventricular conduction (negative delta waves) rather than an inferior myocardial infarction. This pattern is consistent with a bypass tract inserting into the posterior wall of the left ventricle. (From Goldberger AL. *Clinical electrocardiography: a simplified approach.* 7th ed. Philadelphia: Saunders; 2006.)

between 0.6 and 13 deaths per 100,000 (Atkins et al., 2009; Drezner et al., 2009; Eckart et al., 2004; Maron et al., 2009). These studies are limited by the lack of a mandatory reporting system for juvenile sudden death and their reliance on electronic databases and media reports to identify cases of sudden death. Thus, current reports likely underestimate the true incidence of sudden cardiac death in athletes.

The cause of sudden cardiac death in young athletes (younger than 35 years of age) is usually a structural cardiac abnormality, with hypertrophic cardiomyopathy and coronary artery anomalies representing 36% and 17% of U.S. cases, respectively (Table 29-4) (Maron et al., 2009). *Commotio cordis,* involving a blunt, nonpenetrating blow to the chest that leads to a ventricular arrhythmia, accounts for approximately 3% of cases. Commotio cordis is most common in younger athletes (mean age, 13 years) with compliant chest walls (Maron et al., 2002). Commotio cordis occurs most often in sports using a firm projectile, such as baseball, softball, hockey, and lacrosse, but can also occur from contact with stationary field equipment, the ground, or another player. In older athletes (older than 35 years of age), atherosclerotic CAD accounts for more than 75% of cases of sudden cardiac death.

AUTOMATED EXTERNAL DEFIBRILLATORS IN ATHLETIC MEDICINE

Limitations of the cardiovascular screening process, the overwhelming desire to protect young athletes from a tragic event, and the success of early defibrillation programs (Caffrey et al., 2002; Page et al., 2000; Valenzuela et al., 2000) using accessible automated external defibrillators (AEDs) have propelled the placement of AEDs into the

Table 29-4 Causes of Sudden Cardiac Death in Young Athletes

Structural	Hypertrophic cardiomyopathy*
	Coronary artery anomalies
	Aortic rupture or Marfan syndrome*
	Dilated cardiomyopathy*
	Myocarditis
	Left ventricular outflow tract obstruction
	Mitral valve prolapse
	Coronary artery (atherosclerotic) disease*
	Arrhythmogenic right ventricular cardiomyopathy*
	Postoperative congenital heart disease
Electrical	Long QT syndrome*
	Wolff-Parkinson-White syndrome
	Brugada syndrome*
	Catecholaminergic polymorphic ventricular tachycardia*
	Short QT syndrome*
	Complete heart block
Other	Drugs and stimulants
	Commotio cordis
	Primary pulmonary hypertension*

*Familial or genetic etiology.

athletic setting (Drezner et al., 2005). Recent research suggests an improved survival rate for young athletes with sudden cardiac arrest if early defibrillation is achieved. A retrospective cohort of 1710 U.S. high schools with onsite AED programs found 14 cases of sudden cardiac arrest in high school student-athletes and a 64% survival rate if early cardiopulmonary resuscitation (CPR) and prompt defibrillation with an AED were provided (Drezner et al., 2009).

Comprehensive emergency response planning is needed to ensure an efficient and structured response to sudden cardiac arrest in the athletic setting. This includes establishing a communication system to activate the emergency medical services system and alert any onsite response team, training of anticipated responders (e.g., coaches) in CPR and AED use, access to an AED, and practice and review of the response plan. High suspicion of sudden cardiac death should be maintained in any collapsed and unresponsive athlete, with application of an AED as soon as possible for rhythm analysis and defibrillation if indicated (Drezner et al., 2007, 2009).

KEY TREATMENT

- High suspicion of sudden cardiac arrest should be maintained in any collapsed and unresponsive athlete, with application of an AED as soon as possible for rhythm analysis and defibrillation if indicated (Drezner et al., 2007, 2009) (SOR: B).

Concussion in Sports

Key Points

- Concussion is defined as a traumatically induced transient disturbance of brain function and involves a complex pathophysiologic process. Concussion is a subset of traumatic brain injury that is generally self-limited (Harmon et al., 2013).
- Animal and human studies support the concept of postconcussive vulnerability, showing that a second blow before the brain has recovered results in worsening metabolic changes (Barkhoudarian et al., 2011; Prins et al., 2010; Shrey et al., 2011).
- Concussion remains a clinical diagnosis ideally made by a health care provider familiar with the athlete and knowledgeable in the recognition and evaluation of concussion (Harmon et al., 2013).
- Initial assessment of concussion should be guided by a symptom checklist, cognitive evaluation, balance tests, and further neurologic physical examination (McCrory et al., 2013).
- Although standardized sideline tests are a useful framework for examination, the sensitivity, specificity, validity, and reliability of these tests among different age groups, cultural groups, and settings is largely undefined. Their practical usefulness with or without an individual baseline test is also largely unknown (Harmon et al., 2013).
- Neuropsychological (NP) tests are an objective measure of brain–behavior relationships and are more sensitive for subtle cognitive impairment than clinical examination (Ellemberg et al., 2009; Van Kampen et al., 2006).
- Most concussions can be managed appropriately without the use of NP testing (Harmon et al., 2013; McCrory et al., 2009).
- A player should never return to play while symptomatic from a concussion.
- When asymptomatic, athletes should follow a stepwise and graded exercise program before return to play (Harmon et al., 2013; McCrory et al., 2009).

In 1966, the Congress of Neurological Surgeons proposed a consensus definition of concussion. Since then, both the definition and our understanding of concussion have been and are continuing to evolve. *Concussion* is defined as a traumatically induced transient disturbance of brain function and involves a complex pathophysiologic process. Concussion is a subset of traumatic brain injury and is generally self-limited (Harmon et al., 2013). There has been increased attention to concussion and brain injury spurred by concern in the NFL and the military. In addition to this concern, there has been increased public awareness, beginning in 2009 with the passage of the Zackery Lystedt Law in Washington State. Nearly every state in the union has passed concussion-related legislation in the past 5 years.

SYMPTOMS AND INCIDENCE

A concussion usually results in the rapid onset of brief neurologic impairment that resolves spontaneously. Symptoms of concussion include loss of consciousness, amnesia, confusion, headache, vision problems, nausea, and balance problems (Table 29-5). A concussion may or may not be associated with a loss of consciousness. More than 90% of concussions are not associated with a loss of consciousness, and unconsciousness is not a marker of the severity of the injury (Lovell et al., 1999). *Amnesia* can include loss of memory of the events before (retrograde amnesia) or after (posttraumatic amnesia) the concussion, or both, and amnesia appears to be the best predictor of severity in athletic concussion (Collins et al., 2003). Conventional imaging studies such as computed tomography (CT) and magnetic resonance imaging (MRI) are normal in concussion. Research protocols show changes related to concussive injury, but no imaging studies are available for clinical use. It is estimated that as many as 3.8 million concussions occur in the United States per year during competitive sports and recreational activities; however, as many as 50% of concussions may go unreported (Centers for Disease Control and Prevention, 1997). In high school football, there are 40,000 concussions per year, with a 3% to 5%

Table 29-5   Signs and Symptoms of Concussion

Disorientation
Confusion
Amnesia
Loss of consciousness
Headache
Dizziness
Balance problems
Poor coordination, gait
Nausea or vomiting
Visual problems (flashing lights)
Hearing problems (tinnitus)
Feeling "foggy" or "dazed"
Inability to focus
Difficulty concentrating
Irritability
Emotional lability
Excessive drowsiness
Delayed verbal or motor response
Vacant, "glassy" stare
Slurred, incoherent speech
Decreased playing performance
Seizure (rare)

incidence (Powell and Barber-Foss, 1999a, 1999b). High-risk sports include contact and collision sports such as football; ice hockey; rugby; wrestling; and to a lesser extent, soccer and basketball. Women appear to be more prone to concussion in some sports (Tierney et al., 2005) for unclear reasons, with further research needed. Younger players also may be more prone to concussion. Concussions in children and younger adolescents appear to have a more prolonged course of recovery (Field et al., 2003; Moser et al. 2005; Zuckerman et al., 2012).

SIDELINE MANAGEMENT

When attending to an athlete with a suspected concussion on the field, attention must first be given to basic first aid. Airway, breathing, and circulation (ABCs) and level of consciousness should be initially assessed followed by an evaluation for potential cervical spine injuries. If loss of consciousness has occurred, the duration of unconsciousness should be determined. A brief loss of consciousness is generally defined as less than 30 to 60 seconds. If a player is unconscious for more than 30 to 60 seconds or still unconscious by the time a medical provider reaches the athlete on the field, most would consider this "prolonged." Patients with concussions involving prolonged loss of consciousness, suspected cervical spine injuries, or gross neurologic impairment should be stabilized and transported to a hospital for further evaluation (see "Catastrophic Cervical Spine Injuries: On-the-Field Assessment" later in this chapter).

After it is determined that the athlete is stable and safe to be moved, further assessment can take place on the sideline. Physical examination should include evaluation of cranial nerves, pupillary dilation and reactivity, balance and coordination, motor strength, and cognitive function (McCrea et al., 1997). Several sideline assessment tools exist to aid medical professionals in the evaluation of an athlete with concussion. The most recent consensus conference on concussion recommended a sideline tool called the Sport Concussion Assessment Tool (SCAT3; http://bjsm.bmj.com/content/47/5/259.full.pdf) (McCrory et al., 2013). This is a modification of earlier versions and consists of several validated measures for concussion. This includes a symptom scale, standard cognitive assessment, and guided physical examination. Such standardized examinations are useful for serial follow-up and if different medical personnel will be evaluating the athlete. It is important to reassess concussed athletes frequently to monitor for resolution of symptoms or signs of deterioration.

RETURN TO PLAY

Return-to-play decisions are driven by the concern of preventing potential complications, primarily second-impact syndrome and permanent neurologic deficit. *Second-impact syndrome* occurs when a player returns to play after a first concussion before the symptoms have completely resolved, and a second, often minor, blow to the head is sustained, which leads to diffuse cerebral swelling, brainstem herniation, and death (Cantu, 1998). The risk for catastrophic injury in athletes returned to play while still symptomatic is of particular concern in children and adolescents.

There is increasing concern that head impact exposure and recurrent concussions contribute to long-term

Table 29-6 Graded Return to Play after Concussion
1. Rest until asymptomatic
2. Light aerobic exercise (stationary cycling, slow jogging)
3. More strenuous aerobic training (running, sprinting)
4. Sport-specific training
5. Noncontact drills
6. Full contact drills
7. Return to competition

neurologic sequelae, including chronic traumatic encephalopathy (CTE). CTE is characterized by the accumulation of tau protein in specific areas of the brain and results in executive dysfunction, memory impairment, depression, and poor impulse control (Baugh et al., 2012). CTE is a diagnosis made only after death with confirmatory histopathology, although imaging techniques are being developed to diagnose it before death. The prevalence of this condition is unknown; however, given the large number of athletes participating in contact or collision sports and the small number of cases described, it is likely that other factors such as genetic predisposition and lifestyle choices play a role in its development.

Current recommendations suggest that management of concussion be based on symptoms and severity. The mildest concussion is one that involves transient symptoms that resolve quickly. More severe concussions involve persistent or prolonged symptoms and cognitive deficits on NP testing. Management of concussion includes both physical and mental rest until all symptoms have cleared followed by a graded and stepwise program of exertion before return to sport (Table 29-6). *Repetitive concussions*, which take longer to return to baseline or that occur with progressively less trauma, are also considered of greater severity (Guskiewicz et al., 2003). Complex or recurrent concussions with persistent cognitive impairment, neurologic findings on examination, or prolonged symptoms may warrant advanced imaging and formal NP testing and should be managed by physicians with specific expertise in sports-related concussion.

Neuropsychological testing in concussion is becoming more common, particularly computerized NP tests. NP tests are a quantitative measure of brain–behavior relationships and are more sensitive to changes secondary to concussion than standard office testing. They can be used both with and without a baseline test. The interpretation of computerized NP testing requires an understanding of the sensitivity, specificity, and reliable change index of the tests used and should be done by someone with training and understanding in this area. These tests should never be used as a sole indicator as readiness to return to play; rather, they should be viewed as one piece of information to be included in the larger clinical picture. Concussions can be properly managed without the use of NP testing. NP testing is sometimes helpful in athletes with prolonged symptoms and those who may not be forthcoming.

Concussion is a common injury in sports. Athletes sustaining a concussion should be medically evaluated by a health care professional with specific training and experience in the management of concussion. No symptomatic athlete should be allowed to return to play, and an athlete should not be allowed to return to play in the same game or practice during which an injury has occurred. When asymptomatic, athletes should follow a graded program before return to play. Referral should be considered in complex or complicated concussions. Further research is needed to provide more information regarding accurate diagnosis, prevention, evidenced-based return-to-play guidelines and long-term sequelae.

KEY TREATMENT

- A player with a concussion who is still symptomatic should be held from practice and competition and should not return to the field of play (SOR: C) (McCrory et al., 2013).
- When asymptomatic, athletes should follow a stepwise and graded exercise program before a return to sport. (SOR: C) (McCrory et al., 2013).

Cervical Spine Injuries

Key Point

- "Stingers" result from a blow to the neck and shoulders with transient unilateral upper extremity pain and paresthesias resolving in minutes.

STRAINS AND SPRAINS

Most sports-related neck injuries are mild and self-limiting. Patients with muscle strains and ligament sprains typically present with minor complaints and no neurologic symptoms. More significant injury should be suspected in the presence of significant cervical muscle spasm, tentative active ROM, severe pain, or abnormal neurologic signs. Evaluation includes active cervical ROM and strength testing of the neck and upper extremities. Manual compression and axial loading to the cervical spine (Spurling maneuver) should not cause pain or radicular symptoms and is helpful in ruling out more significant injury (Magee, 1997). Return to play should be considered when full, pain-free ROM and normal strength of the cervical spine are restored.

STINGERS

Stingers or "burners" are characterized by transient unilateral upper extremity pain and paresthesias resulting from a blow to the neck and shoulders. Stingers are common in American football and have been reported in up to 50% to 65% of college players (Clancy et al., 1977; Sallis et al., 1992). Stingers are peripheral nerve injuries and are considered a transient neurapraxia of the cervical nerve roots, usually involving the upper trunk of the brachial plexus (C5-C6). Stingers typically manifest with dysesthesia (burning pain) that begins in the shoulder and radiates down the arm. They often are associated with transient numbness or weakness, and all symptoms typically resolve in minutes.

Stingers can occur from a tensile or compression overload (Watkins, 1986). In most high school athletes, the mechanism of injury involves a tensile or traction injury when the involved arm and the neck are stretched in opposite directions. This occurs when the neck is forcibly flexed away while the shoulder is depressed. In college and professional athletes, who have a higher likelihood of degenerative changes of the cervical spine, a compression mechanism is more likely. This involves a pinch of the cervical nerve root within the neural foramen as the neck is forcibly extended in a posterolateral direction (Levitz et al., 1997).

Stingers are always unilateral, a distinguishing feature from spinal cord injuries, which involve symptoms in multiple limbs. Athletes are safe to return to play when symptoms have fully resolved and the athlete can demonstrate full cervical ROM and normal neurologic examination results.

Radiography and MRI should be considered in athletes with recurrent stingers to evaluate for cervical degenerative disk disease (Levitz et al., 1997). Rarely, more significant nerve injury involving *axonotmesis* (axon disruption) occurs, causing persistent weakness. Athletes with significant weakness 24 to 48 hours after injury may benefit from treatment with a short burst of oral corticosteroids. If weakness persists, electromyography performed 2 weeks or more after the injury will assess the distribution and degree of injury. Fortunately, most patients with axonotmesis recover within 1 year (Clancy et al., 1977).

CERVICAL CORD NEURAPRAXIA

Cervical cord neurapraxia is characterized by an acute, transient sensory or motor change, or both, to more than one extremity. Symptoms include burning pain, numbness, and tingling with or without paresis or complete paralysis. *Transient quadriplegia* is a type of neurapraxia characterized by temporary paralysis and loss of motor function in all four limbs (Torg et al., 1986). *Burning hands syndrome* is characterized by burning dysesthesias of the hands and associated upper extremity weakness (Maroon, 1977). Episodes of cervical cord neurapraxia usually resolve within 10 to 15 minutes, although gradual resolution may take more than 24 to 48 hours.

Congenital or degenerative narrowing of the anteroposterior (AP) diameter of the cervical spinal canal is an established risk factor for cervical cord neurapraxia (Torg et al., 1997). Athletes with an episode of cord neurapraxia should be held from competition and undergo radiographic evaluation and MRI. Return to play after an episode of cervical cord neurapraxia is a highly controversial area in sports medicine. Several cases of permanent neurologic injury after cervical cord neurapraxia associated with cervical spinal stenosis have been reported (Brigham and Adamson, 2003; Cantu, 1993, 2000). Functional spinal stenosis on advanced imaging in an athlete with a history of cervical cord neurapraxia is an absolute contraindication to return to play in contact and collision sports (Cantu, 2000).

CATASTROPHIC CERVICAL SPINE INJURY

Injury to the spinal cord resulting in temporary or permanent neurologic injury is a rare but potentially catastrophic event during sports competition. Cervical spine trauma is most common in contact and collision sports such as American football, rugby, ice hockey, gymnastics, skiing, wrestling, and diving (Carvell et al., 1983; Cantu and

Mueller, 1999; Tator and Edmonds, 1984; Wu and Lewis, 1985). Cervical spinal cord injuries are the most common catastrophic injury in American football and the second leading cause of death attributable to football. The National Center for Catastrophic Sports Injury Research reported that the incidence of cervical spinal cord injury in American football between 1977 and 2001 was 0.52, 1.55, and 14 per 100,000 participants in high school, college, and professional football, respectively (Cantu and Mueller, 2003). However, the incidence of catastrophic cervical spinal cord injuries in American football between September 1989 and June 2002 was 1.10 and 4.72 per 100,000 participants in high school and college football, respectively (Boden et al., 2006).

Axial loading is the most common mechanism for catastrophic injury to the cervical spine during sports competition (Torg et al., 1979, 1990). Axial loading occurs when a player strikes another player with the top of the head as the point of initial contact ("spear tackling"). In athletes with cervical spinal stenosis, axial loading followed by forced hyperextension or hyperflexion can further narrow the AP diameter of the spinal canal, resulting in compression of the spinal cord and transient or permanent neurologic changes (Eismont et al., 1984; Penning, 1962; Torg et al., 1993).

Recognition of the axial load mechanism as the major cause of catastrophic cervical spine injury in American football resulted in rule changes that banned "spearing," defined as intentionally striking an opponent with the crown of the helmet, as well as other tackling techniques in which the helmet is used as the initial point of contact. In 1976, the incidence of quadriplegia was 2.24 and 10.66 per 100,000 in high school and college athletes, respectively. In 1977, only 1 year after rule changes that banned spear tackling, the incidence decreased to 1.30 and 2.66 per 100,000 in high school and college athletes (Torg et al., 2002). Most recently, the incidence was shown to have decreased even further to 0.50 and 0.82 per 100,000 high school and college athletes (Boden et al., 2006).

On-the-Field Assessment

Medical providers at sporting events must be prepared to assess, stabilize, and transport athletes with suspected cervical spine injuries. Adequate preparation, including the anticipation of required personnel and equipment plus a well designed emergency response plan, are critical to the management of catastrophic neck and spine injuries. In general, any athlete with significant neck or spine pain, diminished level of consciousness, or significant neurologic deficits should be immobilized and prepared for transport.

Guidelines for the prehospital care of spine-injured athletes were established by the Inter-Association Task Force for Appropriate Care of the Spine-Injured Athlete (2001). The initial assessment of an injured athlete begins with a basic assessment of the ABCs and level of consciousness. Unconscious athletes are presumed to have unstable spine injuries until proven otherwise.

The face mask of a protective helmet should be removed as soon as possible regardless of respiratory status (Inter-Association Task Force, 2001). In football, the face mask can be removed with screwdrivers or the loop straps cut with various cutting tools such as pruning shears or a

Trainer's Angel (Knox and Kleiner, 1997). Football helmets and chin straps should be left in place. If the helmet is removed from a downed player wearing shoulder pads, the athlete's head will hyperextend, which may result in secondary injury to the cervical spine. If the athlete is not breathing, an adequate airway can be established by the jaw thrust maneuver, which allows opening the airway while maintaining the cervical spine in a stable position. Rarely, assisted ventilation may be necessary.

If transport is indicated, the athlete should be immobilized to a spine board. A supine athlete can be transferred to a spine board using a six-plus person lift technique, with one person responsible for stabilization of the head and neck (Inter-Association Task Force, 2001). To transfer an athlete who is face down, a logrolling technique is recommended. Transport of a spine-injured athlete should be directed to a trauma center or medical facility with diagnostic and surgical capabilities for spinal injury.

KEY TREATMENT

- Axial loading is the most common mechanism for catastrophic injury to the cervical spine during sports competition (SOR: C) (Torg, 1979, 1990).
- Any athlete with significant neck or spine pain, diminished level of consciousness, or significant neurologic deficits should be immobilized and prepared for transport (SOR: C) (Inter-Association Task Force, 2001).
- Unconscious athletes are presumed to have unstable spine injuries until proven otherwise (SOR: C) (Inter-Association Task Force, 2001).
- The football helmet in a downed player wearing shoulder pads should not be removed to avoid hyperextension of the neck and secondary injury to the cervical spine (SOR: C) (Inter-Association Task Force, 2001).
- Athletes with an episode of cervical cord neurapraxia involving sensory or motor changes (or both) to more than one extremity should be held from competition and undergo radiographic evaluation and MRI to rule out functional spinal stenosis. (SOR: C) (Cantu, 2000; Inter-Association Task Force, 2001).
- In an athlete with a history of cervical cord neurapraxia, functional spinal stenosis on advanced imaging is an absolute contraindication to return to play in contact and collision sports. (SOR: C) (Cantu, 2000; Inter-Association Task Force, 2001).

Environmental Influences

EXERTIONAL HEAT ILLNESS

Key Points

- Hydration sufficient to replace fluid lost in sweat is essential to prevent heat stroke.
- Athletes exercising in the heat who exhibit mental status changes must be immediately removed from competition and cooled.
- Ice-water immersion produces the most rapid decrease in core body temperature.

Heat stroke is the third leading cause of death in high school athletes (Lee-Chiong and Stitt, 1995). Athletes are at the greatest risk during the month of August. High school football poses the greatest risk of heat illness, tenfold that of any other sport (Centers for Disease Control and Prevention, 2010). This is tragic because these deaths are largely avoidable.

An exercising human is an engine operating at about 25% efficiency, resulting in 3 W of heat production for every watt of work, and requires a biologic radiator to avoid overheating. Humans dissipate heat through convection, conduction, radiation, and evaporation, with evaporative sweat loss being the most significant. Higher temperatures limit heat dissipation from convection and conduction, warm sunny days elevate body temperature through radiant heating, and higher humidity decreases evaporative cooling. Thus, the combination of high ambient temperature, radiant heat from the sun, and high humidity works synergistically to create dangerous playing conditions that promote the development of heat illness.

The wet bulb globe temperature (WBGT) index incorporates ambient temperature, relative humidity, and the amount of radiant heat coming from the sun to provide a measure of the risk of overheating. The American College of Sports Medicine Inter-Association Task Force on Exertional Heat Illnesses Consensus Statement (2006) recommends that WBGT readings from 18° to 23°C (64.4°-73.4°F) result in moderate risk, 23° to 28°C (73.4°-82.4°F) in high risk and more than 28°C (82.4°F) in extreme risk. The cumulative effect of successive days of exercise in the heat must also be considered. In a U.S. Marine Corps study, investigators demonstrated that the risk of exertional heat illness was best predicted by considering the current and the previous day's WBGT index (Wallace et al., 2005).

Because evaporative cooling is the primary mechanism for heat dissipation, adequate hydration is essential to keep the biologic radiator functioning. Losses of 2% to 3% of body weight are common with high-intensity exercise in the heat (Galloway, 1999). Below 5% fluid losses, performance and thermoregulation are impaired, and thirst is an inconsistent stimulus to rehydrate, so regular, planned fluid consumption is essential. Fluid recommendations vary, but experts have suggested about 500 mL of fluid intake 2 hours or less before exercise and then about 250 mL every 20 minutes during exercise (Convertino et al., 1996). Because of differences in sweat rate, acclimatization, intensity of exercise, clothing, protective equipment, and environmental factors, individual fluid requirements vary. Thus, recording an athlete's nude weight in the morning and evening is an effective method of determining adequate rehydration. If athletes are losing more than 2% to 3% of their body weight with training, they need to consume more fluids during training. If they cannot regain the lost weight before the next morning's training, they need to consume additional fluids after training and during recovery time. For every kilogram of body weight lost, 1 L of fluid should be consumed. Cooler, flavored fluids are recommended to increase palatability and absorption.

Heat illness is classified as heat edema, heat cramps, heat syncope, heat exhaustion, and heat stroke (Table 29-7) (Binkley et al., 2002; Eichner, 1998). Heat stroke is of the greatest concern, with hallmark features of an elevated core temperature higher than 40.5°C (105°F) and associated mental status changes. Any athlete exhibiting mental status changes and participating in an environment conducive to heat illness requires immediate removal from participation and active cooling. An ice-water tub should be prepared in advance if rapid cooling may be necessary in high-risk events, and an affected athlete should be fully submerged, with only the head above water (Smith, 2005). Other methods of cooling, such as applying ice bags to the neck, axilla, and groin, or using a cold-water spray combined with fanning, can be effective, but the rate of core body temperature loss is slower than in ice-water

Table 29-7   Exertional Heat Illness

	Definition	Management	Prevention
Heat edema	Dependent edema usually occurring before acclimation	Elevation of swollen extremity, rest, cooling Diuretics contraindicated	Gradual acclimation to heat
Heat (exercise-associated) muscle cramps	Painful spasms of single or multiple muscles Likely sodium deficiency and salty sweaters most prone	Rest, stretching, cooling, oral hydration with hypertonic sodium drink IV fluids (normal saline) if oral treatment limited or to expedite recovery	Maintain hydration and increase salt intake Add salt to fluids, especially for those with predisposition based on past history
Heat syncope	Orthostatic dizziness at cessation of exercise, with prolonged standing, or after assuming upright posture	Rest, cooling, place supine with legs elevated, monitor vital signs, and mental status Oral fluid hydration	Adequate hydration and acclimation; if occurs during exercise, requires cardiovascular evaluation
Heat exhaustion	Inability to continue exercise in heat Symptoms: weakness, fainting, dizziness, headache, nausea, vomiting, cramps, dehydration with low urine output Minimal mental status symptoms; core temperature <40°C	Immediate rest, rapid cooling (ice bath), close monitoring of mental status, vital signs (e.g., core temperature) Serum sodium if hyponatremia considered Oral fluid hydration with IV fluids (normal saline) if hypotension present	Adequate acclimation, monitor hydration, adjust training to climate, follow player's weight, and close monitoring for symptoms of heat illness
Heat stroke	Heat exhaustion with core temperature >40°C and mental status alteration or central nervous system collapse	As for heat exhaustion, with hospitalization as soon as possible	As for heat exhaustion, be prepared with ice baths, monitoring equipment, and access to emergency medical services

IV, Intravenous.

immersion. Close monitoring of mental status and vital signs (e.g., core temperature) is indicated, and athletes should be transported to the hospital if they do not exhibit improving mental status with normalization of vital signs. The National Athletic Trainers' Association Exertional Heat Illness Position Statement is an excellent reference regarding proper preparedness for heat illness (Binkley et al., 2002).

EXERTIONAL HYPONATREMIA

Key Points

- Life-threatening hyponatremia develops when excessive hypotonic fluid is consumed, with concomitant sodium sweat loss.
- Exertional hyponatremia most often occurs in women completing endurance races in more than 4 hours who drink copiously throughout the race.
- Symptoms of exertional hyponatremia include mental status changes and peripheral edema without significant elevation in core temperature.

Exertional hyponatremia (serum sodium <130 mmol/L), once considered a rare complication of exercise in the heat, is now recognized as more common and responsible for a number of exercise-related deaths (Almond et al., 2005). Controversy surrounds the exact pathophysiology, but the condition develops in the setting of excessive hypotonic fluid replacement while sodium is progressively lost in sweat (Levine and Thompson, 2005; Noakes, 2002). Typical victims are relatively inexperienced female marathon runners who tend to be light sweaters, finish in more than 4 hours, and drink copiously throughout the race. Nonsteroidal antiinflammatory drugs (NSAIDs) taken before the race may be a contributing factor (Hsieh, 2004). Athletes with a history of exercise-induced hyponatremia do not seem to be predisposed to water overload at rest, although there may be some physiologic mechanism beyond pure water overload that accounts for the condition in some susceptible individuals (Speedy et al., 2001). Symptoms are similar to those of heat exhaustion, including weakness, dizziness, headache, nausea, vomiting, and cramping, but the headache is more prominent and progressively severe, extremity swelling may be noted, and progressive mental status changes occur despite a core temperature lower than 40°C (104°F). Cerebral edema underlies the mental status changes, and pulmonary edema may also occur.

The serum sodium level must be assessed in athletes in whom the diagnosis is suspected to differentiate hyponatremia from heat stroke. Intravenous (IV) fluids, often indicated in heat stroke, can actually worsen hyponatremia if related to excessive hypotonic fluid intake. Prompt hospitalization is indicated for any athlete with mental status changes or persistently altered vital signs after the diagnosis of hyponatremia has been established. Exertional hyponatremic encephalopathy is treated with 3% hypertonic saline boluses (100 mL) (Hew-Butler et al., 2008). Prevention includes following an athlete's weight change with exercise to understand the fluid requirements more precisely, not deviating from established fluid intake on race day to avoid overhydration, incorporating sodium- and electrolyte-containing fluids, and limiting fluid intake to 1 L/hr unless higher fluid requirements have been established (Gardner, 2002).

KEY TREATMENT

- Any athlete exhibiting mental status changes and participating in an environment conducive to heat illness requires immediate removal from participation and active cooling (American College of Sports Medicine, 2006) (SOR: B).
- Patients with exertional hyponatremic encephalopathy are treated with 3% hypertonic saline boluses (100 mL) (Hew-Butler et al., 2008) (SOR: B).

COLD INJURY

Key Points

- Cold-weather exercise requires proper layering of synthetic clothing with a waterproof, breathable outer layer to maintain body temperature, but excessive sweating and environmental dampness should be avoided.
- Hypothermia victims should be sheltered, dried, and warmed, and resuscitation attempts should continue until body temperature is higher than 32°C.

Outdoor sports participation, particularly winter sports, places athletes at risk for cold-induced injury. Two problems commonly encountered are frostbite and hypothermia.

Frostbite most frequently affects the toes, fingers, and exposed skin of the face. As tissue cools, a progressive cell membrane leak results initially in increased extracellular fluid, with progression to extracellular ice crystal formation and then ischemic necrosis. Prevention includes dry layering of clothing that is not constricting; avoidance of skin exposure, especially in windy, cold conditions; and maintaining the core temperature because hypothermic shunting of blood centrally promotes distal extremity freezing. Treatment involves warming, although this is not recommended until the victim has been safely evacuated; warming and then refreezing is more damaging. Antibiotics, tissue debridement, and possibly amputation may be required, depending on the extent of injury. Sallis and Chassay (1999) provide a more in-depth discussion of frostbite and other cold-induced injuries.

Hypothermia is defined as a core temperature at or below 32°C (90°F). Lower ambient temperatures and longer exposure times increase the risk for hypothermia, but *moisture* is the most dangerous variable that must be controlled. Wet clothing results in significant increases in conductive heat loss, which is made worse in the wind. Prevention of hypothermia requires proper clothing for outdoor exercise in the cold. Clothing should be layered so that with increased exertion and endogenous heat production, layers can be removed to avoid excessive sweating. Underlayers should consist of breathable wicking fabrics that move sweat moisture away from the skin. Outer layers should be windproof, waterproof, and breathable. Midlayers, which can be added depending on the temperature and exertion level, should provide loft (synthetic pile or down) to trap air; this provides a temperature gradient between the warm underlayers and cold outer layers similar to the blubber on a marine mammal. Heat loss from the head is significant, so a hat or hood that wicks moisture is necessary, and mittens are warmer than gloves for very cold weather. Dehydration must be avoided because low plasma volume results in peripheral vasoconstriction and increases the risk of frostbite.

Treatment of mild hypothermia involves finding warm shelter away from the wind, removing wet outer layers, and covering with dry blankets. Sharing a sleeping bag with a warm climbing partner can be lifesaving in a desperate situation. In the setting of severe hypothermia, warm IV fluid (40°C), warm humidified oxygen, and warming lamps are indicated, if available. The adage "one is not dead until warm and dead" applies, and ventricular fibrillation or asystole in the settling of hypothermia should be treated with advanced cardiac life support (ACLS) protocols until the patient has a core temperature above 32°C (Sallis and Chassay, 1999; Tom et al., 1994).

ALTITUDE ILLNESS

High-altitude medicine, once the preoccupation of research pulmonologists and physicians practicing at high altitudes and caring for climbers, has become essential for many primary care providers because of increasing numbers of recreational athletes engaging in skiing, hiking, trekking, and other high-altitude pursuits.

Acute mountain sickness (AMS) and its two most significant manifestations, high-altitude pulmonary edema and high-altitude cerebral edema, are complications of travel to higher altitudes with insufficient acclimatization. Symptoms of AMS include headache; sleep difficulty; and GI upset, including loss of appetite, nausea, and vomiting. Symptoms occur a few hours after rapid ascent in 25% of individuals at as low as 8500 feet (Harris et al., 1998), with a higher percentage being affected at higher altitudes. Individuals vary in their susceptibility to AMS, and a high level of physical fitness is not protective. Gradual ascent, allowing acclimatization, prevents symptoms. If symptoms occur, delaying any further ascent with relative rest for 1 to 3 days usually results in improvement. More significant symptoms respond to decreasing altitude. Individuals with a history of AMS are likely to have it recur when they return to a higher altitude. Planning time for acclimatization and avoiding excessive exercise when first arriving at a higher altitude are helpful. Nocturnal periodic breathing probably contributes to worsening hypoxia and subsequent AMS symptoms, so avoiding alcohol and other sedatives is also helpful. Acetazolamide, 125 to 250 mg twice daily, started the day of initial ascent and continuing for 48 hours, has been shown to decrease AMS symptoms and hasten acclimatization, possibly by decreasing nocturnal periodic breathing (Bartsch et al., 2004).

High-altitude cerebral edema (HACE) is defined as a progression of AMS symptoms to include ataxia, mental status changes, lassitude, and eventual coma. HACE is fatal if untreated. Treatment requires immediate descent of at least 2000 feet. Hyperbaric treatment can be lifesaving if immediate descent is not possible; portable hyperbaric chambers are available for mountaineering expeditions. In addition to immediate descent, treatment includes oxygen at 2 to 4 L/min to keep O_2 saturations greater than 90% and dexamethasone, 4 to 8 mg orally followed by 4 mg every 6 hours (Rodway et al., 2003).

High-altitude pulmonary edema (HAPE) is the development of pulmonary edema, dyspnea, and hypoxemia in the setting of AMS. Rapid descent of at least 1000 m is also the primary treatment. The administration of supplemental oxygen, 4 to 6 L/min to maintain O_2 saturations greater than 90%, and nifedipine, 30 mg of sustained-release nifedipine every 12 to 24 hours, is helpful if immediate descent is not possible (Hackett, 2013; Pennardt, 2013).

KEY TREATMENT

- Hypothermia victims should be sheltered, dried, and warmed and resuscitation attempts continued until body temperature is higher than 32°C (90°F) (Sallis and Chassay, 1999; Tom et al., 1994) (SOR: B).
- Pharmacologic prophylaxis can be helpful, but definitive treatment of HAPE or HACE requires descent to lower altitude as rapidly as possible (Pennardt, 2013; Rodway et al., 2003) (SOR: B).

Sports Trauma to the Teeth, Face, and Eyes

Key Points

- Dental trauma is common in many sports and can be largely prevented with a custom-molded mouth guard.
- Avulsed teeth or tooth fragments should be wrapped in saline-soaked gauze, with urgent transport to a dentist and luxated teeth repositioned if possible.
- Facial and nasal injuries requiring immediate referral include those with prolonged loss of consciousness, visual abnormalities suggesting orbital fracture, malocclusion of the teeth suggesting maxillary or mandibular fracture, facial paresthesias suggesting infraorbital nerve injury, open or significantly displaced nasal fractures, and uncontrollable epistaxis.
- Acute auricular hematomas should be fully evacuated to avoid chronic fibrosis and deformity (cauliflower ear).
- Eye trauma is usually preventable using appropriate eye protection.
- Loss of visual acuity, evidence of globe rupture or leaking aqueous humor, limitation or asymmetry of extraocular movements, persisting pupil abnormalities, and evidence of hyphema all require urgent ophthalmologic consultation.

DENTAL TRAUMA

Dental trauma is common, with one third of all dental injuries in the United States occurring with sports activities

(Honsik, 2004). Mouth guards are recommended by the American Dental Association for participation in all collision and contact sports as well as weightlifting, skydiving, skateboarding, gymnastics, racquetball, squash, and skiing. Dental injury is especially common in sports combining collision and a hard ball or puck, such as ice hockey or field hockey. A study of college basketball players found a significant decrease in tooth injuries in participants using custom-fitted mouth guards; however, there was no decrease in oral soft tissue injury or concussion (Labella et al., 2002). Sports physicians and dental professionals agree that although off-the-shelf molded mouthpieces are less expensive and more readily available, they do not protect teeth as effectively as a custom mouthpiece (Honsik, 2004).

Teeth rest in a bony socket, each with a neurovascular root connected to the socket by a periodontal ligament. Above the gum the tooth consists of three layers, dentin, pulp, and superficial enamel. Injuries involve fracture of the tooth or some degree of luxation. *Fractures* range from an enamel chip to those involving the deeper components. *Luxation* can result in a normally positioned loose tooth or a displaced tooth still positioned in the socket. Injury can also result in complete tooth avulsion.

After injury, tooth fragments or avulsed teeth should always be recovered, if possible, and transported to a dentist in saline-soaked gauze. Fractures involving only enamel and dentin can be managed by dental evaluation within 48 hours. Pulp involvement (visible pink or blood in center of the tooth) mandates urgent dental referral, and medical-grade cyanoacrylate (Super Glue) can be placed on the tooth acutely for pain and to prevent infection. Luxation without impaction can be reduced if jaw fracture is not suspected, and return to play with a custom mouth guard can be considered, depending on successful reduction, level of pain, and level of competition. If the tooth is easily repositioned, dental consultation can be delayed 24 hours. Players with impacted luxation or teeth that cannot be repositioned should not return to play, and dental consultation should be sought immediately. Avulsed teeth should be rinsed with sterile saline and replaced, if possible, taking care not to handle or damage the root followed by immediate dental consultation (Honsik, 2004).

FACIAL TRAUMA

Nasal injuries are frequently encountered in sports. The higher the impact velocity, the higher the probability of concomitant injury requiring urgent referral. Situations requiring emergency department (ED) evaluation include associated prolonged loss of consciousness, vision abnormalities suggesting orbital fracture, malocclusion of the teeth suggesting maxillary or mandibular fracture, facial paresthesias suggesting infraorbital nerve injury, open or significantly displaced nasal fractures, and uncontrollable epistaxis. Examination findings prompting early referral include clear rhinorrhea suggesting cribriform plate injury with cerebrospinal fluid leak and impaired extraocular movements, especially unilateral limited upward gaze, which suggests an orbital fracture with inferior oblique, rectus muscle entrapment, or both. Patients with nasal septal hematoma should be referred to an otolaryngologist expeditiously for incision and drainage. If left untreated,

subsequent cartilage degeneration can result in a nasal saddle deformity (Stackhouse, 1998).

If the initial assessment does not mandate immediate referral, subsequent management requires assessing the extent of deformity and controlling epistaxis. In the first few days, swelling can make assessment for bony deformity difficult, but close follow-up is helpful. Any persistent obstruction of the nares or cosmetic abnormality unacceptable to the patient should be referred to an otolaryngologist within 5 days because reduction is best performed within 10 days of injury. Epistaxis is best managed with a topical decongestant such as oxymetazoline nasal 0.05% (Afrin) and compression of the anterior plexus by pinching the nose for 15 minutes. A short nasal tampon soaked with oxymetazoline can be placed into the bleeding nostril to assist with hemostasis and return to play, but anterior packing should only be performed with appropriate visualization to avoid further injury.

Ear trauma in sports can result in auricular hematomas or injury to the tympanic membrane. *Auricular hematomas* mainly occur in wrestling, rugby, and boxing and result in hemorrhage between the perichondrium and the underlying cartilage. Failure to evacuate the hematoma can lead to fibrosis, necrosis, and a chronic deformity known as *cauliflower ear.* An acute auricular hematoma should be drained by needle aspiration under aseptic conditions, and a pressure dressing (using cotton wool soaked in collodion or a silicone splint) carefully applied against the contours of the outer ear and reexamined daily. Occasionally, incision and drainage are required.

Blows across the side of the head can also result in *tympanic membrane rupture,* marked by pain, bleeding, fluid drainage, and impaired hearing. Tympanic membrane ruptures usually heal spontaneously over 4 to 6 weeks. Antibiotic prophylaxis in the first week should be considered, especially if the rupture occurred in a contaminated environment. The ear canal should be kept clean and dry, and a cotton ball coated with petroleum jelly and placed gently into the ear canal can be helpful while showering.

EYE TRAUMA

Ocular injury is common in sports and largely preventable if athletes wear appropriate eye protection. The highest risk sports are those in which intentional injury can occur (e.g., boxing and combative martial arts) and those in which hard projectiles, sticks, or fingers are likely to encounter the eye. High-risk sports include basketball, baseball, softball, cricket, lacrosse, squash, racquetball, fencing, and all varieties of hockey. Squash and racquetball are particularly concerning because of the high likelihood of severe injury. Athletes with preexisting monocular visual impairment must understand the importance of protecting the good eye, and preparticipation visual acuity assessment of binocular and monocular vision is essential. The American Society for Testing and Materials (ASTM) is the primary U.S. organization for certifying eyewear for sports, and experts have provided recommendations for eye protection for different sports (Vinger, 2000).

Common sports-related eye injuries include presence of a foreign body and corneal abrasion. More significant impact results in possible iris injury, posttraumatic iritis, hyphema, or globe perforation or rupture. Athletes presenting with eye pain should be removed from participation and have a thorough eye examination, as follows:

1. Assessment and documentation of visual acuity
2. Inspection for evidence of globe rupture or leaking aqueous humor
3. Assessment of extraocular movements, limitation, or asymmetry suggesting orbital fracture
4. Assessment of pupil reactivity (a dilated, constricted, or sluggish pupil can be transient secondary to iris trauma or may indicate hyphema or globe injury)
5. Inspection of anterior chamber for blood indicating hyphema

Abnormalities identified on this initial examination require consultation with an ophthalmologist. If the examination result is normal, eyelid inversion should be performed, inspecting for a foreign body, with slit-lamp evaluation using fluorescein staining to assess for corneal abrasions. Anesthetic eyedrops may be required to facilitate the examination and for initial pain management but should not be used to allow return to play or for ongoing pain management (Moeller and Rifat, 2003).

Corneal abrasions are treated with antibiotic eyedrops to prevent infection, and topical NSAIDs are given for pain if necessary (Weaver and Terrell, 2003). When they are pain free, with a normal follow-up examination, athletes might return to play. After an ocular injury, an athlete is often more receptive to counseling on protective eyewear.

Infectious Disease

Key Points

- Upper respiratory infections are more common in heavily training athletes, and team physicians must consider both infection control measures and avoiding banned substances when treating high-level athletes.
- Infectious mononucleosis is associated with splenomegaly and a risk of splenic rupture. It requires that athletes avoid heavy exertion and contact sports until the spleen is of normal size, usually within 4 weeks.

Upper respiratory tract infection (URI) is a common complaint in primary care sports medicine. Regular, moderate exercise may decrease the risk for contracting a URI, but acute bouts of heavy exercise, such as running a marathon, and prolonged heavy training increase the risk for URI (Nieman, 2003). Treatment of URI is symptomatic, but health care providers of competitive athletes must consider which substances are banned by the governing body overseeing their sport. Banned substances are subject to change, and physicians must be aware of current regulations. For example, the World Anti-Doping Agency (WADA), responsible for drug regulation for many international sports organizations, bans stimulants and many sympathomimetics. Ephedrine and pseudoephedrine are banned by the WADA above urine concentration thresholds, but

caffeine is not currently banned. The National Collegiate Athletic Association (NCAA) does not ban pseudoephedrine but does ban caffeine above a high urinary threshold. Most governing bodies, such as the World Anti-Doping Agency (WADA) and the NCAA, have websites posting current banned substances (see Web Resources). The WADA also has a smartphone app, which is a convenient resource for both athletes and physicians. These sites should be consulted before prescribing or recommending any medication for athletes subject to drug testing.

Physicians caring for teams must also consider infection control measures. URI, viral gastroenteritis, skin infection, and mononucleosis are of particular concern. Vectors that must be considered include common source spread (enteroviruses), person-to-person spread from sharing secretions (viral, fungal, bacterial skin infection), and airborne droplet spread (picornaviruses). Sharing of water dispensers, bottles, and towels should be eliminated. Handwashing must be encouraged and antibacterial soap or alcohol-based hand sanitizers provided. Shared equipment must be disinfected. Simple infection control measures are often not practiced in the setting of team sports, and educating athletes, coaches, and training staff is the responsibility of the team physician.

MONONUCLEOSIS

Infectious mononucleosis (mono), which is caused by Epstein-Barr virus (EBV) or occasionally by cytomegalovirus (CMV), deserves special mention. Splenomegaly and spleen fragility are often associated with mononucleosis and are a concern for team physicians because of the risk of splenic rupture. The prolonged fatigue accompanying mononucleosis is also especially difficult for athletes trying to return to training as soon as possible.

Epstein-Barr virus is prevalent and shed in saliva. Transmission requires intimate contact with saliva and does not occur via airborne spread, thus mononucleosis's reputation as the "kissing disease." About 50% of the U.S. population seroconverts by age 5 years, with a mild viral syndrome or asymptomatically. If an individual reaches college age (18-22 years) without infection, seroconversion results in a 35% to 50% incidence of mononucleosis. The incubation period is 4 to 6 weeks. Symptoms include 1 week of significant flulike symptoms with anterior and often significant posterior cervical lymphadenopathy and exudative pharyngitis. Splenomegaly occurs in 50% of cases during weeks 2 to 3 of illness and usually resolves by weeks 4 to 6. Splenomegaly is difficult to confirm on examination alone and should be suspected in all athletes with mononucleosis. Significant fatigue is often prevalent, and although most symptoms resolve by 4 weeks, fatigue can last 12 weeks or longer (Rea et al., 2001).

When it is suspected, the diagnosis of mononucleosis should be confirmed because of the risk of splenic rupture and implications for withholding sports participation. The diagnosis can be confirmed by a positive EBV heterophile antibody (Monospot) with 90% sensitivity by 3 weeks. False-negative results are common in the first 2 weeks, with a positive test result in only 40% of those infected during the first week of illness. Therefore, an initially negative Monospot test result in a suspicious case should be repeated

1 week later. An EBV or CMV viral capsid antigen (VCA) immunoglobulin M (IgM) assay can also provide evidence of acute infection, with 90% sensitivity at the onset of symptoms (Cohen, 1998). IgM to VCA usually disappears by 6 weeks, making it a good marker for acute infection, and antibodies to EBV nuclear antigen (EBNA) generally appear after 2 to 4 months of illness and persist for life. Absent IgM in the presence of EBNA is more consistent with prior infection, and acute illness in the presence of both antibodies suggests reactivation (http://www.cdc.gov/epstein-barr/laboratory-testing.html).

Treatment is supportive. Significant tonsillar hypertrophy can be improved with a short course of oral prednisone. There is no clear evidence-based answer for when an athlete with mononucleosis can safely return to sports. The risk of splenic rupture associated with sporting activity occurs almost exclusively in the first 3 weeks of illness (Kinderknecht, 2002). Many authorities recommend restriction from noncontact sports for at least 3 weeks until symptoms have largely resolved and the spleen is not palpable. Returning athletes to contact sports can be considered after 4 weeks of illness, when all symptoms have resolved and splenomegaly is absent (Auwaerter, 2004). The range for normal spleen size varies significantly, and splenic ultrasonography is not necessary in most cases but can be considered before returning an athlete to contact sports. Larger-than-normal ranges for splenic size have been described for taller athletes (Spielmann et al., 2005).

KEY TREATMENT

- For athletes with confirmed mononucleosis, return to sport can be considered after 3 weeks for noncontact sports and after 4 weeks for collision sports after symptoms have largely resolved and the spleen is not palpable (Auwaerter, 2004) (SOR: C).

Sports Dermatology

Key Points

- Fungal, viral, and bacterial skin infections are usually transmitted through person-to-person contact in sports activities.
- Management requires a high index of suspicion, prompt treatment, restriction of participation for contagious athletes, covering lesions when appropriate to allow participation, and appropriate prophylaxis and treatment.
- Skin problems are usually caused by laceration or abrasion, environmental exposure, inflammation, or infection.

FUNGAL INFECTIONS

Tinea (ringworm) is one of the most common fungal infections. Tinea pedis is frequently seen in athletes secondary to group showering, and it can be prevented to some extent by having athletes regularly change socks and use wicking materials in socks to keep their feet dry, drying powders (many of which contain prophylactic topical antifungals), and shower shoes. Treatment with topical antifungals and oral therapy for severe cases are effective.

Fungal infections are spread directly from person to person through contact sports, with the type seen in wrestlers (tinea corporis gladiatorum) being the most problematic. Tinea tonsurans occurs most often, with infection rates in high school wrestlers of 24% to 75% (Adams, 2000; Beller and Gessner, 1994). Infection is caused by contact with an infected opponent and usually occurs on the arms, neck, or head. The lesions often appear initially as annular plaques with raised erythematous borders and may progress without the central clearing often appreciated with ringworm (Adams, 2002). Microscopic evaluation of skin scrapings with potassium hydroxide (KOH) may reveal fungal elements. Topical treatment with azole agents and oral treatment have been studied. A randomized prospective study of topical clotrimazole 1% cream twice daily versus oral fluconazole, 200 mg weekly, showed equal symptomatic improvement after 10 days and a similar 50% lesion reduction at 17 days. However, 50% culture eradication took 11 days with oral treatment and 22 days with topical treatment, leading to the conclusion that weekly fluconazole should be first-line treatment (Kohl et al., 1999). For multiple lesions, a 3-week treatment course with an oral antifungal is recommended.

Return-to-play recommendations after tinea corporis gladiatorum infection vary. The NCAA requires 72 hours of topical therapy for skin lesions and 2 weeks of oral therapy for scalp lesions and stipulates that athletes may participate with an active lesion provided it is covered entirely by an adhesive nonpermeable dressing (NCAA, 2013). The National Federation of State High School Associations does not allow participation with communicable lesions even if they lesions are covered (Landry and Chang, 2004). Prophylaxis using oral itraconazole every other week and oral fluconazole weekly has been shown to be effective (Hazen and Weil, 1997; Kohl et al., 2000), but the potential for exposure and time loss morbidity of an active infection must be weighed against the cost and potential side effects.

VIRAL INFECTIONS

Herpes gladiatorum, caused by herpes simplex virus (HSV), is highly contagious and spread by person-to-person contact, with a predilection for the face, arms, and upper trunk. As the name suggests, herpes gladiatorum is common in wrestling, although epidemics are also reported in other sports, such as rugby (Adams, 2002) (Figure 29-4). Because herpes lacks definitive treatment, it is considered more serious than tinea. Herpes gladiatorum has a prevalence as high as 40% in collegiate wrestlers (Anderson, 1999). Outbreaks generally occur 2 to 5 days after exposure. Lesions typically manifest with prodromal pain or itching followed by clear vesicles on an erythematous base. Primary infections may cause systemic flulike symptoms, and recurrent infections occur in the same dermatome. Often, the vesicles have been traumatized before evaluation, making the rash appear nonspecific, although the prodromal symptoms or history of previous outbreak in the same location suggests herpes. Traditionally, diagnosis was confirmed

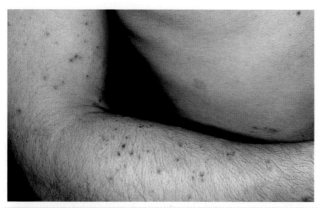

Figure 29-4 Herpes gladiatorum. Lesions may be numerous in wrestlers and involve a wide area of the skin surface. (From Habif T. *Clinical dermatology.* 5th ed. Philadelphia: Elsevier; 2009.)

with Tzanck testing or culture, but the direct fluorescent antibody test or polymerase chain reaction assays provides rapid detection of HSV in specimens with greater sensitivity than traditional methods.

The natural history of a herpes outbreak is to resolve and possibly recur, with the frequency and severity dependent on both host and environmental factors. Treatment with oral antiviral agents can shorten the duration of the outbreak, decrease contagion, and prevent recurrent infection. No one agent has proved superior. The most cost-effective regimen is acyclovir, 400 mg three times daily for 10 days for primary infections and for 5 days for recurrent infections. Treatment is most effective when started at the first sign of infection. Prophylaxis with valacyclovir (500-1000 mg/day) limited herpes gladiatorum recurrence (Anderson, 1999), and acyclovir (400 mg twice daily) has demonstrated effectiveness comparable with valacyclovir, limiting recurrent genital herpes (Reitano et al., 1998) and herpes outbreak among those being treated for cancer (Glenny et al., 2009). Research using antivirals for primary prevention is lacking, but entire teams may be placed on prophylactic doses if a team member or opposing team member has an outbreak. Some team physicians offer prophylactic treatment to the squad before large tournaments or for the entire competitive season.

Return to play after herpes infection is more conservative than with tinea infection. The NCAA requires that wrestlers be free of any systemic symptoms, have no new blisters for 72 hours, have all lesions crusted over, and have taken treatment doses of antiviral medication for 120 hours before competition (NCAA, 2013).

BACTERIAL INFECTIONS

Bacterial infections are common in sports, and treatment is similar for both athletes and nonathletes. Bacterial infections of the skin generally manifest as furuncles, carbuncles, impetigo, cellulitis, or erysipelas. Staphylococcal and streptococcal infections are most common, but community-acquired methicillin-resistant *Staphylococcus aureus* (CA-MRSA), first reported in the late 1990s, has become a significant problem in athletic training facilities (Lindenmighter et al., 1998; Nguyen et al., 2005) and the leading cause of training room skin infection based on a

literature review of published reports from 2005 to 2010 (Collins and O'Connell, 2012).

Sports activities provide a favorable environment for the acquisition and spread of bacterial skin infection. Abrasive surfaces such as artificial turf can harbor bacteria and become a source of infection. Shared equipment, improperly laundered practice gear, person-to-person contact, and inadequate showering facilities without antibacterial soap have all been implicated in the spread of bacterial skin infections in athletes.

Controlling infection in athletes involves prevention; good surveillance; and prompt, appropriate treatment. Shared equipment requires regular cleaning with antibacterial disinfectant. Athletes should shower with antibacterial soap after practice and competition. Abrasions should be addressed expeditiously; scrubbed with antibacterial wash; and covered with sterile dressings, which are changed regularly. Athletes must be instructed to report suspected infections as soon as identified. Topical antibiotics are appropriate for mild infections, with oral or IV antibiotics required for more severe infections. Any significant abscess should have incision and drainage with bacterial culture, including MRSA. Thus far, most CA-MRSA infections in athletes have shown sensitivity to trimethoprim–sulfamethoxazole, with some isolates sensitive to macrolides and quinolones (Arnold and Wojda, 2005). The resistance patterns are susceptible to rapid change, however, making routine culture of these wounds essential. It has been recommended that athletes with recurrent MRSA infections be assessed by nasal culture for colonization with MRSA and treated with topical mupirocin ointment if positive. The role of colonization in infection has been questioned recently, and in a recent study of college athletes, nasal carriage varied through the year and was not associated with infection (Creech et al., 2010).

Pulmonary Problems

Key Points

- Exercise-induced bronchospasm (EIB) is the transient narrowing of the airways in response to exercise.
- Symptoms of EIB include wheezing, coughing, dyspnea, and chest tightness.
- The diagnosis should be confirmed by spirometry testing before and after exercise showing a 10% to 15% reduction in forced expiratory volume in 1 second (FEV_1).

EXERCISE-INDUCED BRONCHOSPASM

Exercise-induced asthma or, more accurately, EIB is a transient narrowing of the airways following vigorous exercise. Ninety percent of known asthmatics and 40% of patients with allergic rhinitis have bronchoconstriction caused or worsened by exercise (Feinstein et al., 1996). In some patients, the only manifestation of airway hyperresponsiveness is EIB, with up to 50% of athletes having EIB in some high-risk sports (Langdeau and Boulet, 2001).

The pathophysiology of EIB involves mucosal drying secondary to large volumes of dry (often cool) air, which causes changes in mucosal pH, osmolarity, and temperature and triggers the release of inflammatory mediators, leading to bronchoconstriction (Hallstrand et al., 2005). This osmotic hypothesis explains the relationship between the intensity and duration of exercise to EIB; the role of inflammation and bronchoconstriction in EIB; and the increased prevalence of EIB in outdoor winter sports, such as cross-country skiing. A refractory period typically follows EIB in which the patient has fewer symptoms on reexercise. This probably occurs because of increased bronchial blood flow after exercise, which enhances water delivery to airway mucosa and makes it more resistant to osmotic changes. The mechanism of EIB in swimmers may be different and related to exposure to direct bronchial irritants, such as chlorine.

Symptoms of EIB include exercise-related wheezing, coughing, dyspnea, and chest tightness. The diagnosis of EIB, however, is difficult, and screening by medical history and physical examination alone is often inaccurate. In a study of 256 adolescent athletes participating in organized sports, 39.5% reported symptoms or a previous diagnosis suggestive of EIB, although only 9.4% were found to have EIB based on an exercise challenge test and serial spirometry (Hallstrand et al., 2002). Thus, any athlete with suspected EIB should be tested with an exercise challenge test, in which pre- and post-exercise spirometry is performed. A decrease in FEV_1 greater than 10% to 15% is indicative of EIB.

Management of EIB involves both nonpharmacologic and pharmacologic methods. Nonpharmacologic treatment includes emphasis on a good warm-up to precipitate the refractory period, exercising in warm and humid environments, and covering the mouth and nose during cold weather. The goal of pharmacologic therapy is for the athlete to be asymptomatic during exercise. First-line pharmacologic treatment involves the use of an inhaled β_2-agonist (e.g., albuterol metered-dose inhaler, 2 puffs) 15 to 30 minutes before exercise. If the athlete is still symptomatic, the addition of a leukotriene modifier (e.g., montelukast, 10 mg) taken at least 1 hour before exercise can provide additional relief (Coreno et al., 2000). Another treatment alternative is an inhaled mast cell stabilizer (e.g., cromolyn) before exercise. Inhaled corticosteroids are not as useful for acute prophylaxis because of their delayed onset of action but can be very useful in patients with chronic persistent asthma and EIB. Any underlying chronic asthma or allergic rhinitis should also be optimally controlled.

PNEUMOTHORAX

Spontaneous and traumatic pneumothorax can occur in the setting of sports. Spontaneous pneumothorax should be suspected in tall, thin male athletes with the acute onset of dyspnea, pleuritic chest pain, and shortness of breath. Traumatic pneumothorax should be considered when an athlete is short of breath after sustaining a blow to the chest, particularly if a rib fracture is suspected (Partridge et al., 1997). The diagnosis is confirmed by chest radiograph, and treatment depends on the amount of lung involved. If the patient is stable and there is less than 15%

to 20% volume loss, this can generally be treated with observation. Return to play after a pneumothorax can usually occur safely in 3 to 4 weeks (Putukian, 2004).

KEY TREATMENT

- Treatment of exercise-induced bronchoconstriction involves an adequate warm-up and use of an inhaled β_2-agonist 15 to 30 minutes before exercise, with the addition of montelukast or cromolyn, if needed (Coreno et al., 2000; Hallstrand et al., 2005) (SOR: B).

Hematologic Problems

Key Points

- Sports anemia is a dilutional anemia caused by the expansion of plasma volume in trained athletes.
- Exertional hemolysis occurs from increased destruction of red blood cells (RBCs), and the diagnosis is confirmed by a low hemoglobin (Hb) or hematocrit (Hct) and low haptoglobin level.
- Low iron stores, even in the absence of anemia, can adversely affect performance in endurance athletes.
- Athletes with sickle cell trait, especially if poorly hydrated, exercising in hot conditions, at a high altitude, or unconditioned, have a higher risk of exertional rhabdomyolysis and sudden death; screening at-risk populations should be considered.

Several hematologic issues are specific to athletes. This section reviews dilutional pseudoanemia or sports anemia, exertional hemolysis, iron-deficiency anemia and low iron stores without anemia, and special considerations regarding athletes who are sickle cell trait positive.

SPORTS ANEMIA

Sports anemia is not representative of true pathology. Rather, it represents an adaptive response to strenuous training and is caused by an expanded plasma volume. The degree of anemia typically correlates with the intensity of training. Plasma volume can expand by 5% to 20%. This adaptive response begins a few days after starting or intensifying training. Moderate exercisers may see a decrease in Hb of 0.5 g/dL, and elite athletes may have an apparent Hb decrease of 1 g/dL. Athletes with low Hb or Hct value and a characteristic history should be checked for iron deficiency. A normal ferritin level, iron level, and total iron-binding capacity confirm the diagnosis of dilutional anemia, or sports anemia, which does not need to be treated (Eichner, 1992; Shaskey and Green, 2000).

EXERTIONAL HEMOLYSIS

Exertional, or "foot strike," hemolysis is another problem often encountered in athletes. Exertional hemolysis was initially described in endurance runners but is also seen in swimmers, rowers, and weightlifters. Hypothesized mechanisms for red RBC destruction include trauma secondary to impact, turbulence in the blood vessel, acidosis, and elevated temperature encountered in working muscles. The diagnosis is made with an elevated mean corpuscular volume and reticulocyte count and a low haptoglobin level. Treatment consists of mitigating impact by having the athlete run in biomechanically correct shoes and on cushioned surfaces and by recommending slow, incremental increases in training (Telford et al., 2003).

IRON-DEFICIENCY ANEMIA

As in the general population, iron-deficiency anemia is common in athletes, especially among female athletes. This is typically caused by low intake of dietary iron, but it can also be caused by exertional GI or genitourinary bleeding or GI bleeding related to NSAID use. Iron requirements of athletes, particularly endurance athletes, may also be higher than for sedentary individuals (Beard and Tobin, 2000). The diagnosis of iron-deficiency anemia is made by a low Hb or Hct level and a low ferritin or iron level. Treatment consists of increasing dietary iron, iron supplementation, and treating the underlying cause if present.

LOW FERRITIN LEVELS IN NONANEMIC ATHLETES

The common belief among coaches and endurance athletes is that a low ferritin level can cause fatigue, poor recovery, and poor performance. The ferritin level generally reflects total body iron, and 82% of female endurance athletes have low ferritin levels (Shaskey and Green, 2000). Many studies have examined whether improvements in performance seen in nonanemic athletes are caused by small increases in Hb level (from a normal to a higher normal Hb level) or by an increase in iron alone (Garza et al., 1997). A review of eight randomized, controlled trials indicates that iron has a positive effect on performance in iron-deficient athletes without anemia, independent of Hb increases (Fogelholm et al., 1992; Friedmann et al., 2001; Hinton et al., 2000; Klingshirn et al., 1992; LaManca and Haymes, 1993; Newhouse et al., 1989; Rowland et al., 1988; Zhu and Haas, 1998).

SICKLE CELL TRAIT AND SUDDEN DEATH

Sickle cell trait occurs in 6% to 8% of the African American population (Kerle and Nishimura, 1996). Among black military recruits, the likelihood of sudden death is 28-fold higher in individuals with sickle cell trait than in those without (Kark et al., 1987) and among college football athletes, those with SCT have a 37-fold increased risk of death (Harmon et al., 2012). Most of these deaths are thought to be associated with *exertional rhabdomyolysis.* This typically occurs when an athlete is poorly hydrated, exercising in hot conditions, at a high altitude, or unconditioned. Athletes with sickle cell trait are generally not restricted from competition; however, consideration should be given to screening high-risk populations, with special precautions taken to ameliorate risk.

Gastrointestinal Problems

Key Points

- Gastroesophageal reflux can be worsened by exercise; treatment with dietary modifications and proton pump inhibitors is usually successful.
- Exercise-induced diarrhea is common in endurance sports; treatment focuses on dietary manipulation before competition and antidiarrheal medications such as loperamide in refractory cases.
- GI bleeding in athletes ranges from microscopic blood loss to ischemic hemorrhagic gastritis or colitis, but pathologic causes of bleeding should be ruled out.

Gastrointestinal problems are common in the general population and in exercising individuals. Although the diagnosis and treatment of many of these issues are similar, exercise may make some issues worse or may present special treatment challenges. See eAppendix 29-1 online for discussions on gastroesophageal reflux, exercise-induced diarrhea, and GI bleeding.

Genitourinary Problems

Hematuria and proteinuria are also common findings in athletes. They may be caused by repetitive mechanical trauma to the bladder or by exercise-related changes in renal physiology. The initial workup is to rule out infection, refrain from exercising for 48 to 72 hours, and retest. If hematuria or proteinuria persists, a full evaluation should be performed (Abarbanel et al., 1990).

Genitourinary problems in male cyclists are particularly common. Pressure from the bicycle saddle can cause compression neuropathies (pudendal nerve), impotence, urethritis, or prostatitis (Leibovitch and Mor, 2005). Pudendal neuropathy manifests with numbness or tingling in the scrotum or penile shaft. Treatment involves relieving pressure by changing the seat type, proper bicycle fitting, and wearing padded shorts.

Low Back Pain

See Chapter 31 and eAppendix 29-2 online.

Spondylolysis

Spondylolysis, a stress fracture of the pars interarticularis, is a common cause of LBP in athletes and is the most common cause of athletic LBP in adolescents (Standaert and Herring, 2000; Standaert et al., 2000) (Figure 29-5). Athletes who participate in sports involving repeated and forceful hyperextension of the spine (e.g., gymnastics, American football) are more likely to develop spondylolysis from the cumulative effect of repetitive loading of the bone imposed by physical activity. Athletes generally have an

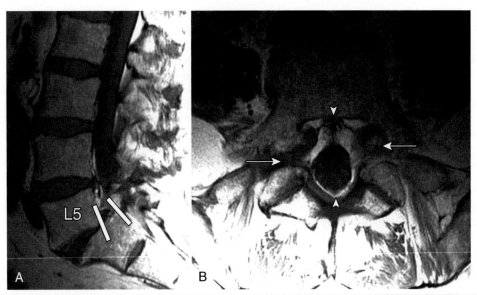

Figure 29-5 Spondylolysis. **A,** Sagittal T1-weighted image. **B,** Axial T1-weighted image. (Used with permission from Czervionke LF, Fenton DS. *Imaging painful spine disorders.* Mayo Foundation for Medical Education and Research Published by Saunders, an imprint of Elsevier Inc, 2011.)

insidious history of increasing focal back pain reproduced by lumbar extension.

Spondylolysis can be identified by plain radiography in approximately 5% of the general population, but the vast majority of these lesions occur without associated symptoms. Identification of spondylolysis on radiographs in an athlete with LBP must be correlated with the clinical presentation and advanced imaging. Single-photon emission CT, high-resolution (thin-slice) CT, and MRI are helpful to determine the metabolic activity of the stress fracture, the acuity of the lesion, and potential for fracture healing and to exclude other spinal pathology that may be present.

Conservative treatment is usually successful in controlling symptoms and restoring function. Treatment requires activity restriction and temporary discontinuation of the aggravating sport or activity. Some patients may require lumbosacral bracing to achieve treatment goals, and only a small percentage of patients require surgical intervention for pain or progressive spondylolisthesis (Standaert and Herring, 2000; Standaert et al., 2000).

Muscle and Tendon Injuries

Key Points

- Eccentric loading produced when the muscle is contracting and lengthening is a common mechanism for muscle and tendon injuries.
- Tendinosis is the predominant pathologic feature in painful overuse tendinopathies.

MECHANISM OF INJURY

Muscle and tendon injuries occur from repetitive microtrauma or a single traumatic event that causes overload to the tensile strength of the myotendinous unit or muscle

fiber itself. *Eccentric loads,* produced when the muscle is contracting and lengthening at the same time, are a common mechanism of injury and can produce higher forces compared with concentric contractions (Stanton and Purdam, 1989). Sports activities with repetitive eccentric demands place the athlete at higher risk of injury. In sprinters, for example, hamstring muscle strains typically occur during the late swing phase of the running cycle as the hamstring muscle contracts while lengthening in an attempt to decelerate the lower leg in preparation for foot strike (Stanton and Purdam, 1989). Achilles tendinopathy and patellar tendinopathy (jumper's knee) also result from repetitive eccentric loading of the tendons during running and jumping.

HISTOPATHOLOGY

Acute muscle injuries go through a predictable cycle of healing and repair. Exercise-induced muscle injury first causes fiber disruption and local microhemorrhage followed by extravasation of inflammatory cells and a phagocytic phase to remove injured tissue and finally a regenerative phase of muscle fiber healing occurs (Armstrong et al., 1991). Limiting overall inflammation decreases pain and minimizes secondary tissue injury caused by hypoxia and inflammatory mediators. However, some amount of inflammation is required in the healing process to remove necrotic muscle fibers and allow scar tissue to bridge the defect (Almekinders and Gilbert, 1986).

In contrast to acute muscle injuries, the pathologic findings in most tendon injuries are consistent with tendinosis, a degenerative condition of the tendon, and not a tendinitis involving inflammation, as was formerly believed (Khan et al., 2000). Healthy tendon contains parallel bundles of tightly packed collagen fibers, with little extracellular matrix (ground substance) and no fibroblasts or myofibroblasts. In contrast, symptomatic tendons contain disorganized collagen fibers, increased mucoid ground substance, prominent capillary proliferation, and increased numbers of fibroblasts and myofibroblasts (Khan et al., 1999). Histopathologic examination is notably devoid of inflammatory cells. Animal models have also suggested that inflammatory cells are absent by 1 week after induced overuse injury (Zamora and Marini, 1988). These findings are present in the most common tendon injuries, including the patella, Achilles, rotator cuff, and extensor carpi radialis brevis tendons, and have important implications in the treatment of tendon disorders (Khan et al., 1999). Use of the term *tendinopathy*, rather than *tendinitis*, is recommended to describe a painful tendon condition.

The generation of pain in chronic tendon injuries appears to involve more than just inflammation. A biochemical hypothesis to explain tendon pain states that biochemical agents are leaked from a degenerated tendon and irritate nociceptors (pain receptors) on adjacent structures (Khan and Cook, 2000). In patellar tendinopathy, higher levels of glycosaminoglycans have been found in the infrapatellar fat pad (Khan et al., 1996), and in patients with partial rotator cuff tears, higher levels of substance P were found in the adjacent subacromial bursa and were significantly associated with pain (Gotoh et al., 1998).

MUSCLE STRAINS

Muscle injuries can be classified as *mild* (grade 1, strain), *moderate* (grade 2, partial tear of myotendinous units), or *severe* (grade 3, complete tear of myotendinous units). Mild injuries are tender and painful with active use but cause minimal strength loss. Moderate injuries demonstrate clear *weakness* with resisted muscle testing and *pain* with passive stretching. Severe injuries cause significant functional and strength deficits and may show ecchymosis and a palpable defect on examination.

In running and sprinting athletes, hamstring muscle strains are the most common muscle injury (Lysholm and Wiklander, 1987; Meeuwisse et al., 2000; Orchard and Seward, 2002). Other common muscle strains include those of the quadriceps (especially the rectus femoris) and the gastrocnemius. The most significant risk factor for a muscle strain is a recent or past history of that same injury, and incomplete rehabilitation may also contribute to recurrent injuries (Ekstrand and Gillquist, 1983; Orchard, 2001). Other risk factors for muscle injury include poor warm-up, muscle fatigue, and muscle imbalance (Agre, 1985; Croisier et al., 2002; Garrett, 1996; Safran et al., 1989).

Initial treatment of an acute muscle strain involves ice application to limit pain and swelling and relative rest to protect the muscle from more significant injury. A short 3- to 5-day course of NSAIDs can help limit overall inflammation and pain in acute muscle injuries. Gentle stretching to restore flexibility should begin when pain allows, and rehabilitation should progress through isometric, concentric, and finally eccentric strengthening exercises before returning to sports-specific activities.

TENDINOPATHY

Tendon injuries can involve acute overuse tendinopathy, chronic tendinosis, partial-thickness tears, or complete rupture of the tendon. The exact role of NSAIDs in the treatment of tendinopathy remains uncertain. NSAIDs are potentially helpful initially after acute tendon injury, when inflammation is most likely to be present. For tendinopathy of longer duration, use of NSAIDs, although an adjunct to pain control, does not contribute to tendon healing. The exact mechanism of action of corticosteroid injections, such as in the treatment of lateral epicondylosis and rotator cuff tendinopathies, is also unclear. Corticosteroid injections bathe the region of tendinosis, alter the chemical composition of the matrix, and may modify nociceptors on nearby structures (Khan and Cook, 2000). NSAIDs and corticosteroids also may have an effect on other biochemical irritants (yet to be defined) that play a role in the generation of tendon pain.

The use of therapeutic methods to stimulate collagen repair is also a major focus in the treatment of tendinopathy. Common strategies to induce collagen remodeling include manual therapies such as deep-friction massage, eccentric conditioning of the tendon, tenotomy (needling a degenerated tendon), and injection of autologous growth factors. Eccentric strengthening programs have shown favorable results for patients with chronic Achilles tendinopathy as well as for athletes with chronic patellar tendinopathy (Alfredson et al., 1998; Purdam et al., 2004). When conservative treatments such as physical therapy fail, treatment options are limited and often lead to either the discontinuation of exercise or surgery. In competitive athletics, chronic tendon injuries can lead to persistent pain, lost time from participation, and suboptimal performance. In occupational injuries, chronic tendon trauma leads to significant cost and morbidity.

With a better understanding of the pathogenesis of tendon injury and healing, newer therapies strive to stimulate the failed healing response in tendinopathies, including percutaneous tenotomy with or without injection of autologous blood or growth factor into the degenerative tendon (Housner et al., 2009; McShane et al., 2006). The most common form of autologous growth factor therapy is platelet-rich plasma (PRP) and is increasingly used to treat tendinosis. Although a relatively novel option for sports-related injuries, PRP has been used in other medical conditions for 2 decades. The use of PRP migrated to orthopedic procedures, in which it has been used effectively to augment bone and soft tissue healing in the operating room, especially in poorly healing fractures and those at high risk for nonunion. Most recently, PRP has been used in the outpatient setting for a variety of sports-related soft tissue injuries, including the treatment of chronic tendinopathies, as well as moderate to severe acute ligament, muscle, and tendon injuries. Autologous growth factor therapy in the treatment of chronic tendinosis can initiate a stalled or failed healing response, leading to a healthier and less symptomatic tendon. There are now many studies, including four randomized controlled studies, that suggest the effectiveness of PRP in tendon healing (de Vos et al., 2010; Filardo et al., 2010; Gaweda et al., 2010; Gosens et al., 2011, 2012; Hechtman et al., 2011; Kon et al., 2009, 2010; Mishra and Pavelko 2006; Peerbooms et al., 2010; Vetrano et al., 2013; Volpi, 2007). In the setting of acute soft tissue injury, it is hypothesized that PRP augments the healing response, leading to faster healing, more rapid recovery, and earlier return to sport or activity. In a series of acute muscle injuries in elite soccer players, PRP therapy was found to significantly shorten the time to return to play (Sánchez et al., 2009).

Although research is still needed to understand the optimal indications and treatment protocols for autologous growth factor therapies, initial findings provide optimism that a new, minimally invasive therapeutic option is available in the management of chronic tendinopathies.

KEY TREATMENT

- Treatment of an acute muscle strain involves ice application to limit pain and swelling; relative rest and protection from more significant injury; gentle stretching to restore flexibility; and progressive rehabilitation through isometric, concentric, and finally eccentric strengthening exercises before returning to sports-specific activities (SOR: C).
- Eccentric strengthening programs can be effective for patients with chronic Achilles or patellar tendinopathy (Alfredson et al., 1998; Purdam et al., 2004) (SOR: B).
- Novel therapies using autologous growth factor injections (platelet-rich plasma) show favorable results in the treatment of chronic tendinopathy (Mishra and Pavelko, 2006; Sánchez et al., 2009) (SOR: C).

Shin Pain

Key Points

- Medial tibial stress syndrome is the most common cause of lower leg pain in running athletes.
- Chronic exertional compartment syndrome is characterized by cramping or burning lower leg pain or numbness, which may radiate to the foot and ankle and resolves within minutes of rest.

MEDIAL TIBIAL STRESS SYNDROME

Exercise-related lower leg pain is an extremely common condition among athletes. The most common presentation is shin pain exacerbated by exercise and diminished with rest. *Shin splints* is a nonspecific term used to describe shin pain in running athletes from almost any cause. *Medial tibial stress syndrome* (MTSS) is the most widely accepted term to describe pain along the medial border of the tibia experienced by running athletes and is considered to be the most common cause of athletic lower leg pain (Kortebein et al., 2000).

The pathogenesis of MTSS is not fully understood. Some support the concept of a traction periostitis along the posteromedial border of the tibia at the origin of the soleus, flexor digitorum longus, and posterior tibialis muscles (Beck and Osternig, 1994; Michael and Holder, 1985). Scintigraphic and biopsy studies, however, have not consistently shown an inflammatory process of the periosteum to support periostitis as the pathogenesis of shin pain. Others suggest that MTSS is caused by a traction fasciitis (involving the crural fascia) or possibly a bony stress reaction and precursor to stress fracture (Batt, 1995). Bone scan and

MRI studies indicate that MTSS is part of a continuum of stress response in bone. Investigation of runners with medial tibial pain demonstrated a spectrum of bone injury, beginning with periosteal edema, progressive marrow edema, and finally frank cortical defects (Fredericson et al., 1995). The mechanism of injury in MTSS probably involves bony overload from the pull of muscle contraction and the impact forces with running.

Athletes with MTSS complain of shin pain that is aggravated with running. Examination reveals tenderness in a broad distribution along the medial border of the tibia, usually spanning the middle and distal thirds of the tibia. In contrast, tibial stress fractures manifest with a focal area of tenderness. Management of MTSS includes rest, activity modification, ice, and antiinflammatory medications. Correction of biomechanical abnormalities is also helpful. Poor hip abductor and external rotator muscle function may contribute to internal femoral rotation and excessive stress on the medial tibia during running. Extreme foot types, both pes planus and pes cavus, may also contribute to impaired shock absorption and force distribution to the tibia and may improve with orthotic devices.

CHRONIC EXERTIONAL COMPARTMENT SYNDROME

Chronic exertional compartment syndrome (CECS) is another cause of athletic lower leg pain. Patients with CECS complain of cramping, burning, or aching lower leg pain with pain or numbness that may radiate to the foot and ankle. The pain is clearly associated with exertion. Pain onset is characteristically at a fixed point in the patient's activity, with progressively increasing pain if the exercise continues and a dramatic reduction in pain within minutes of rest. The pathophysiology of CECS involves elevated intracompartmental pressure, which causes relative ischemia of the involved muscles and pressure on neurovascular structures. The diagnosis of CECS can be confirmed by compartment pressure testing after exercise demonstrating increased intracompartmental pressure correlated with symptom reproduction. Patients with CECS should be questioned about the use of nutritional supplements, such as creatine, that may increase muscle water content and overall muscle mass and contribute to the development of CECS. Surgical treatment by fasciotomy provides good functional improvement and symptomatic cure in a high proportion of cases (Blackman, 2000).

Stress Fractures

Key Points

- Stress fractures typically occur weeks after an abrupt increase in activity level, running distance, or training frequency.
- Navicular stress fractures, anterior tibial stress fractures with a "dreaded black line," and femoral neck stress fractures are high-risk stress fractures for nonunion or progression to a complete fracture and should be referred to an orthopedic specialist.

Stress fractures result from a failure of bone to adapt successfully to repetitive loads encountered during running. Wolff's law of adaptation suggests that a bone responds to external stress by mechanical remodeling. Bone strain may become excessive as a result of increases in load magnitude, rate of loading, or number of loading cycles (Crossley et al., 1999). Advances in imaging techniques and understanding of bone pathophysiology indicate that stress injury to bone occurs on a continuum, ranging from normal bone remodeling to bone strain, to stress reaction, to stress fracture, to frank cortical fracture (Fredericson et al., 1995).

A stress fracture, or *fatigue fracture*, occurs when abnormal stress is applied to normal bone. In contrast, an *insufficiency fracture* occurs when normal or physiologic stress is applied to abnormal bone. Female athletes with premature osteoporosis, as seen in the female athlete triad, may have stress fractures resulting from abnormal stress applied to abnormal bone (Callahan, 2000).

Most stress fractures occur in the lower extremities because of impact forces produced from weight bearing during exercise. Common locations for stress fractures include the metatarsals, navicular, tibia, fibula, femoral shaft, femoral neck, and sacrum. The tibia is the most common site of stress fractures in running and jumping athletes and represents about 50% of all cases (Matheson et al., 1987). Less frequently, stress fractures can occur in the upper extremities, ribs, and clavicle from repetitive activity such as throwing, rowing, or weightlifting.

Lower baseline conditioning and training errors are usually involved in the development of stress fractures. A careful history will often reveal an abrupt increase in activity level, running distance, or training frequency within the 2 or 3 months before symptom onset. Many studies have analyzed bone geometry as a risk factor for stress fracture. In male military recruits and runners, studies have demonstrated that a narrower tibia in combination with a smaller tibial cross-sectional area is a risk factor for tibial stress fractures (Beck et al., 1996; Crossley et al., 1999; Giladi et al., 1987).

Female athletes with a history of eating disorders, oligomenorrhea or amenorrhea, and delayed menarche are more likely to develop stress fractures (Arendt, 2000; Bennell et al., 1995). Inadequate caloric intake relative to energy expenditure, also known as a negative energy balance, has been implicated as the primary cause of menstrual dysfunction in young female athletes and is thought to be responsible in part for bone density changes.

Pain from a stress fracture begins with mild pain during activity that resolves with rest. As the stress fracture progresses, pain increases during activity and continues for hours afterward, usually forcing the athlete to stop exercising. With further progression, pain is present with walking and sometimes at rest. On examination, there is local tenderness at the site of the stress fracture. The hop test (asking the patient to hop on one leg) is a useful functional test for suspected lower extremity stress fractures. If a stress fracture is present, the athlete either is reluctant to hop or will have pain reproduction with hopping. Stress fractures may be seen on radiographs as an area of cortical thickening (periosteal reaction) and may have a linear fracture line visible. Radiographs are positive in only about 50% of cases,

and an advanced imaging study such as MRI or bone scanning is often needed to confirm the diagnosis.

Stress fractures are treated with rest, activity modification, and avoidance of aggravating activities. Ambulation must be pain free to allow for fracture healing. If the athlete cannot achieve pain-free ambulation, a period of non–weight bearing on crutches is indicated. Foot stress fractures may benefit from the use of a rigid walking boot, and tibial stress fractures may benefit from a compressive pneumatic leg brace (Swenson et al., 1997). The time for healing of a stress fracture can vary (range, 4-12 weeks), depending on the site and severity. To maintain overall conditioning, athletes can engage in nonimpact cross-training activities, such as swimming or cycling, assuming that the activity is performed without pain. Athletes with two or more stress fractures should be screened for osteopenia or osteoporosis with a bone density scan. Low bone density requires further investigation to rule out secondary causes of osteoporosis, such as vitamin D deficiency or thyroid abnormalities. Menstrual irregularities, disordered eating, and a negative energy balance in female athletes should also be corrected.

Some stress fractures are at higher risk for nonunion or progression to a complete fracture. High-risk stress fractures include navicular, anterior tibial (diagnosed by the "dreaded black line" on lateral radiograph), and femoral neck stress fractures (Figure 29-6). Athletes with a confirmed or suspected high-risk stress fracture should be made non–weight bearing and referred to a sports medicine or orthopedic specialist.

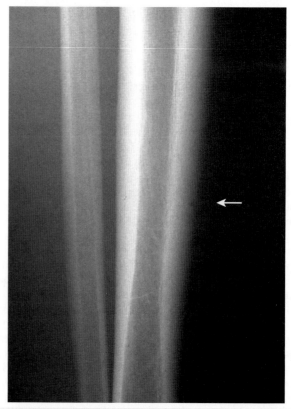

Figure 29-6 Stress fracture. Lateral tibial radiograph shows the "dreaded black line" (*arrow*). Note cortical disruption on the anterior cortex. (From *Delee, Drez's and Miller orthopaedic sports medicine.* 3rd ed. Philadelphia: Elsevier; 2009.)

- Treatment of lower extremity stress fractures include rest, avoidance of aggravating activities, and pain-free ambulation with use of crutches or immobilizing walking boots if needed (SOR: C).

Pediatric Athletes

Key Points

- Children are not "little adults." Sports competition and training must be age appropriate to prevent injury to developing bone and soft tissue and prevent psychological trauma, which could lead to an aversion to physical activity.
- Overuse injuries common in pediatric athletes include articular cartilage injuries (osteochondritis dissecans [OCD]), chronic physeal injuries, and apophysitis.

Pediatric sports injuries are increasing in frequency secondary to increased sports participation, prolonged and overlapping seasons, and children being subjected to adult levels of training and competition prematurely. Although the benefits of exercise and sports participation for children are well recognized, overtraining can have adverse physiologic and psychological consequences. In a review of age-appropriate sports participation from a neurodevelopmental and psychological perspective, Patel and colleagues (2002) suggested that children are not prepared for full competitive participation in complex sports before age 12 years. Children obtain the developmental tools to accomplish complex sports tasks at different ages, and future athletic talent cannot be predicted by childhood performance. Children subjected to age-inappropriate levels of competition or sports-specific skill development are likely to stop participating and create negative associations with sports and exercise, an unfortunate outcome that may affect them adversely for life. Primary care physicians must counsel parents to recognize these issues and not make physical activity and sports participation a negative experience for children.

PHYSEAL AND APOPHYSIAL INJURIES

The adage that "children are not little adults" applies when considering sports injuries. Open physes in long bones and apophyses at tendon attachments to bone provide weak links through which acute and repetitive overuse injury can occur. These growth centers usually close within defined age ranges throughout adolescence, but significant variation among individuals exists. Thus, physeal and apophyseal injury must always be considered when evaluating children or adolescents with musculoskeletal complaints.

Physeal fractures are common and must not be missed because growth arrest can occur if they are not recognized and treated appropriately. The diagnosis of an ankle or knee sprain in a young adolescent with open physes should only be considered after physeal injury has been ruled out. Acute physeal injuries and the Salter-Harris classification system are addressed in greater detail in Chapter 30.

Overuse injuries are increasing in frequency in pediatric athletes, with the most common being articular cartilage injuries (OCD), chronic physeal injury, and apophysitis. OCD involves a focal loss of cartilage and the underlying bone fragment and may be idiopathic or associated with overuse activities. Apophysitis is the pediatric equivalent of tendinopathy in adults. The growth center at the tendon–bone interface is susceptible to injury similar to that sustained by the physes of long bones. Risk factors contributing to the development of pediatric overuse injuries include overtraining; strength and flexibility deficits somewhat inherent in bone and soft tissue development; prior injury with inadequate rehabilitation; faulty technique, often resulting from poor coaching; and excessive pressure from adults to train and perform. The diagnosis is usually straightforward and requires a familiarity with the demands and common overuse injuries of that sport (Lord and Winell, 2004; Thordarson and Shean, 2005). Table 29-8 lists common apophyseal injuries in pediatric athletes.

Table 29-8 Common Apophyseal Injuries in Pediatric Athletes

Eponym/Common Injury	Body Part and Pathophysiology	Common Sports or Activities
Little League shoulder	Proximal humeral epiphysiolysis from repetitive microtrauma	Overhead sports: baseball, softball, tennis, swimming, volleyball
Little League elbow	Medial epicondylar apophysitis from traction to ulnar collateral ligament	Baseball (especially pitchers)
Lateral Little League elbow/ osteochondritis dissecans (OCD)	OCD of capitellum or less likely radial head from repetitive compression-rotation forces	Baseball, gymnastics, overhead throwing and arm weight-bearing sports
Osgood-Schlatter disease	Traction apophysitis of tibial tubercle	Soccer, basketball, running and jumping sports
Sinding-Larsen-Johansson disease	Traction apophysitis to distal patella	Soccer, basketball, running and jumping sports
Sever disease	Calcaneal apophysitis from traction on Achilles insertion	Soccer, basketball, running and jumping sports
Pelvis-ASIS apophysitis	Traction from sartorius origin	Sprinting, kicking, jumping, hurtling
Pelvis-AIIS apophysitis	Traction from rectus femoris origin	Sprinting, kicking, jumping, hurtling
Buttock-ischial apophysitis	Traction from hamstring origin	Sprinting, kicking, jumping, hurtling
Spondylolysis	Stress fracture of vertebral pars interarticularis	Gymnastics, figure skating, football linemen, sports with spine loading in extension

AIIS, Anterior inferior iliac spine; *ASIS,* anterior superior iliac spine.

The treatment of OCD varies according to location, but the offending activity should be stopped immediately and the upper extremity joint immobilized or the lower extremity joint made non–weight bearing. The patient should be referred to an orthopedist for further management, which may involve prolonged rest with radiographic follow-up, reattachment of loose fragments, or removal of fragments with drilling or grafting of joint surfaces.

The treatment for chronic physeal injury or apophysitis consists of initial rest followed by rehabilitation directed at improving flexibility and strength and then a gradual return to activity. Parents and young athletes should be counseled that low-level recurring symptoms can be expected until growth plates have closed but that escalating symptoms should be managed with rest and physician follow-up. The most challenging aspects of treatment are ensuring proper coaching, educating parents regarding appropriate levels of participation and competition for children, and having adults accept reasonable limits for childhood participation in sports.

Special Concerns for Female Athletes

Key Points

- An energy deficit is the primary cause of amenorrhea in athletic women, and treatment should focus on the restoration of a normal energy balance.
- Menstrual dysfunction or hypothalamic–pituitary axis suppression caused by an energy deficit in exercising women is a diagnosis of exclusion, and the workup should include evaluation for medical causes of amenorrhea, including a pregnancy test and determination of prolactin, follicle-stimulating hormone (FSH), luteinizing hormone (LH), thyroid-stimulating hormone (TSH), dehydroepiandrosterone (DHEA), and testosterone levels.
- Bone mineral density is adversely affected by menstrual dysfunction and, although treatment with hormone replacement (e.g., oral contraceptives) should be considered, this does not fully address the mechanisms of bone loss.

Exercise results in many benefits for both male and female athletes. In female athletes, however, exercise coupled with low energy intake can lead to a spectrum of disorders, culminating in the *female athlete triad*, strictly defined as the presence of an eating disorder, amenorrhea, and osteoporosis. It is important to recognize the precursors to the development of the female athlete triad when they may be more amenable to treatment, resulting in less severe long-term sequelae.

The menstrual cycle in the female athlete represents a complex and delicate interplay of hormones. The array of menstrual function seen in athletes ranges from normal ovulatory cycles to luteal-phase defects, to anovulation, to oligomenorrhea, and to amenorrhea. Menstrual dysfunction can exist even in women with normal cycle length, and

various types of cycles are common in an individual athlete (De Souza and Williams, 2004).

Athletic amenorrhea is caused by hypothalamic–pituitary axis suppression and is a diagnosis of exclusion. Other causes of amenorrhea must be ruled out, including pregnancy, hyperthyroidism, hyperprolactinemia, primary deficiency of gonadotropin-releasing hormone, and hyperandrogenic anovulatory syndrome (polycystic ovarian syndrome) (Ahima, 2004). When amenorrhea occurs in the setting of exercise or weight loss and initial hormonal test results are normal, a diagnosis of athletic amenorrhea can be made. Recent research has established that energy deficit is the primary cause of amenorrhea in athletic women (De Souza and Williams, 2004). Strenuous exercise alone in the setting of adequate energy intake does not disrupt the menstrual cycle. An energy deficit results in low concentrations of leptin and in changes in the neuroendocrine axis, including low levels of reproductive hormones, thyroid, and insulin-like growth factor-1 (IGF-1), and an increase in cortisol and growth hormone levels. Similar changes can be seen with psychogenic stress in sedentary women, and stress-induced changes may also contribute to menstrual dysfunction in both normal and underweight female athletes (Ahima, 2004).

The attainment of peak bone mineral density is adversely affected in both the short term and the long term by menstrual dysfunction (Keen and Drinkwater, 1997). The degree of menstrual dysfunction is related to the severity of osteopenia or osteoporosis (Hartard et al., 2004). Initially, the low estrogen state associated with athletic amenorrhea was thought to be solely responsible for bone density problems similar to those seen in postmenopausal women. More recent research has indicated that micronutrient deficiency and low levels of leptin, IGF-1, and other bone trophic factors also contribute to bone mineral deficits (Chan and Mantzoros, 2005).

Treatment of menstrual dysfunction and low bone density has traditionally consisted of hormone replacement therapy, most often with oral contraceptives. Oral contraceptives are not associated with complete bone recovery, most likely because of the multifactorial nature of bone metabolism. Bisphosphonates can increase bone density in adolescents with anorexia but not as effectively as weight restoration (Golden et al., 2005). Bisphosphonates have extremely long half-lives and remain in the skeleton for many years. Because of concern about potential teratogenicity, bisphosphonates should not be used in young women of childbearing age until further studies on their long-term safety.

The primary treatment for athletic amenorrhea should be restoration of a normal energy balance. Disordered eating patterns must be addressed. Anorexia nervosa and bulimia nervosa are common in women, particularly those competing in sports in which there is an emphasis on leanness or appearance, such as gymnastics, figure skating, and cross-country running. Eating disorders are best addressed with an interdisciplinary management team that includes both psychological and nutritional counseling (Otis et al., 1997).

Menstrual dysfunction, although common in female athletes, should prompt evaluation for medical causes and eating disorders. It is never normal or desirable for a female athlete to cease menstrual function, and this should not be seen as a marker of adequate training. Exercise alone should not be blamed for menstrual dysfunction. Treatment should focus on the restoration of energy balance and a safe continuation of activity.

KEY TREATMENT

- The primary treatment for athletic amenorrhea should be restoration of a normal energy balance by addressing disordered eating and training patterns (Otis et al., 1997) (SOR: C).

Summary of Additional Online Content

The following content is available at www.expertconsult.com:

eAppendix 29-1 Gastrointestinal Problems

eAppendix 29-2 Low Back Pain

References

The complete reference list is available at www.expertconsult.com.

Web Resources

bjsm.bmj.com/content/47/5/259.full.pdf Sport Concussion Assessment Tool, 3rd ed. (SCAT3). Tool to assess status following concussion.

http://learning.bmj.com/learning/course-intro/.html?courseId=10042239 BMJ Learning course for ECG interpretation in athletes.

http://www.ncaa.org/sites/default/files/DIII%202014-15%20Banned%20Drugs%20Educational.pdf The National Collegiate Athletic Association's drug-testing program.

list.wada-ama.orgt World Anti-Doping Agency list of prohibited drugs.

30 Common Issues in Orthopedics

JEFFREY A. SILVERSTEIN, JAMES L. MOELLER, and MARK R. HUTCHINSON

Fractures

Key Points

- Always obtain two different radiographic perspectives of a bone or joint when evaluating for fractures.
- Always examine the joint above and below a fracture to look for associated injuries.
- Open fractures are orthopedic emergencies and need to be urgently washed out in the operating room.
- Be particularly alert for growth plate fractures in children.

One of the most common reasons for not identifying a fracture is the failure to examine or radiograph the area or extremity appropriately. When evaluating a patient for a fracture, the primary care physician must be sure to palpate and examine the joint above and below the fracture for potential concomitant injuries. Always obtain orthogonal views from at least two perspectives (e.g., anteroposterior [AP] and lateral). Additional radiographs are necessary only if a fracture is suspected. When communicating about fractures, health care professionals require a similar vocabulary to visualize the description accurately. This is especially true when family physicians and emergency physicians communicate with orthopedic consultants to make treatment decisions. Specific locations of the fracture or fracture fragments are important. They can be proximal or distal, anterior or posterior, medial or lateral. It is also helpful to describe them in relationship (how many centimeters?) to the nearest joint.

Fractures can be oriented in a variety of planes, and certain patterns are associated with a greater risk of instability or complications. Typical fracture orientations are transverse, spiral, oblique, or compression, but they can also be described as buckle, avulsion, stress, or greenstick. Additional features include the specific bone; region within the bone (diaphysis, metaphysis, epiphysis) (Figure 30-1); and whether the fracture is complete or incomplete, open or closed (is bleeding present or bone exposed?), intraarticular or extraarticular, displaced or nondisplaced (if so, how many centimeters?), angulated (if so, pointing in which direction?), shortened (if so, how much?), or comminuted (if so, how many pieces?). In children, physeal involvement is a special concern.

Open fractures are surgical emergencies and require immediate irrigation and debridement, tetanus prophylaxis, and antibiotic coverage. Orthopedists typically refer to the Gustilo-Anderson classification for open fractures, which is based on the size of skin wound, soft tissue damage, and bone comminution (Table 30-1). Even a small puncture wound over a fracture may allow skin flora to infiltrate the fracture site and initiate an infection. Any open fracture warrants an immediate referral to an emergency department (ED) for orthopedic evaluation.

GROWTH PLATE FRACTURES

The physeal plate is a cartilaginous plate present in ends of long bones adjacent to the metaphysis. This is the area that provides longitudinal growth to bones and eventually matures into bone. During growth, the physeal cartilaginous plate is weaker than the surrounding bone and often weaker than the ligaments and tendons that attach nearby, causing it to fracture before other areas. The Salter-Harris classification system describes these injuries (Figure 30-2).

Salter-Harris Type I

The epiphysis is separated from the metaphysis along the physis without an associated fracture through the metaphyseal or epiphyseal bone. The injury goes directly through the cartilaginous physeal plate. These injuries can be displaced or nondisplaced. A nondisplaced Salter-Harris I fracture has a normal-appearing growth plate on radiographs, but patients have pain on palpation directly over the growth plate. Stress radiographs or magnetic resonance imaging (MRI) may be necessary to reveal the injury. Displaced type I injuries are typically easy to reduce because the periosteal attachment remains intact. These injuries have an excellent chance of normal healing with full growth of the injured bone. Despite this, growth delay and growth arrest are complications of growth plate injuries, which should be discussed with the patient and family.

Salter-Harris Type II

The fracture line incompletely extends through the physeal plate and then turns into the metaphysis in an extraarticular fracture pattern. The Salter-Harris II fracture is the most common type of growth plate fracture. The periosteum remains intact on the concave side of the injury, creating a "hinge" and making reduction relatively easy. The prognosis is excellent for future growth when anatomically reduced, with only a minor risk of angular deformity.

Salter-Harris Type III

The fracture line extends incompletely along the physis and then turns through the epiphyseal bone into the joint. Salter-Harris III fractures are intraarticular injuries that imply an increased risk of arthritis, especially if they are not anatomically reduced. Alignment of the joint surface is the

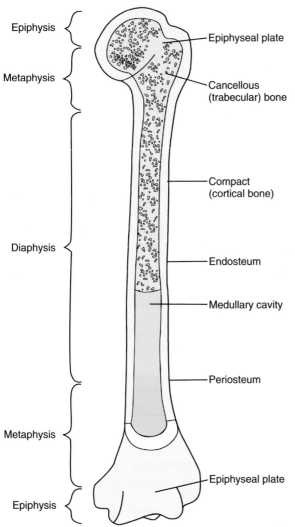

Figure 30-1 Bone regions: the diaphysis, metaphysis, and epiphysis.

Labels: Epiphysis, Metaphysis, Diaphysis, Metaphysis, Epiphysis; Epiphyseal plate, Cancellous (trabecular) bone, Compact (cortical bone), Endosteum, Medullary cavity, Periosteum, Epiphyseal plate

Table 30-1	Gustilo-Anderson Open-Fracture Classification
Type I	▪ Wound is smaller than 1 cm, with minimal soft tissue injury. ▪ Wound bed is clean. ▪ Fracture is usually a simple transverse, short oblique fracture, with minimal comminution.
Type II	▪ Wound is larger than 1 cm, with moderate soft tissue injury. ▪ Fracture is usually a simple transverse, short oblique fracture, with minimal comminution.

Type III	▪ Fracture involves extensive damage to the soft tissues, including muscle, skin, and neurovascular structures.
	▪ Fracture is often accompanied by a high-velocity injury or a severe crushing component.
	▪ Special patterns classified as type III:
	  ▪ Open segmental fracture, regardless of the size of the wound
	  ▪ Gunshot wounds: high-velocity and short-range shotgun injuries
	  ▪ Open fracture with neurovascular injury
	  ▪ Farm injuries, with soil contamination, regardless of size of wound
	  ▪ Traumatic amputations
	  ▪ Open fractures more than 8 hours after injury
	  ▪ Mass casualties (e.g., war, tornado victims)

Subtype IIIA	▪ Adequate soft tissue coverage despite soft tissue laceration or flaps or high-energy trauma, regardless of size of wound; includes segmental fractures or severely comminuted fractures.
Subtype IIIB	▪ Extensive soft tissue lost with periosteal stripping and bony exposure; usually associated with massive contamination.
Subtype IIIC	▪ Fracture with major arterial injury requiring repair for limb salvage.

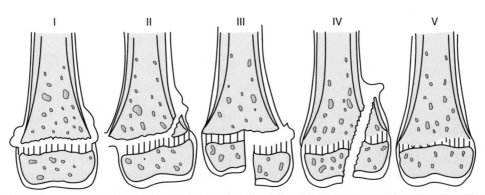

Figure 30-2 Types of growth plate injury (I to V) as classified by Salter and Harris. (From Salter RB, Harris WR. Injuries involving the epiphyseal plate. *J Bone Joint Surg Am.* 1963;45:587.)

top priority, and open reduction is often necessary. The prognosis is good, provided the blood supply to the fracture fragment remains intact.

Salter-Harris Type IV

This intraarticular fracture pattern extends from the epiphysis, across the physeal plate, and through a portion of the metaphysis. Open reduction and internal fixation (ORIF) is usually needed to ensure anatomic alignment of the joint surface and perfect alignment and apposition of the physeal plate. Premature growth arrest and angular deformities can occur with Salter-Harris IV fractures. The prognosis can be good but depends on the ability to restore growth plate.

Salter-Harris Type V

Salter Harris V fractures are crushing injuries in which an axial load compresses the epiphysis into the metaphysis, squeezing the actively growing physis between them. The prognosis for future growth is poor, with a high rate of premature closure of the physis and resultant joint deformity. Fortunately, these are rare injuries.

Shoulder

> ### Key Points
>
> - The diagnosis of joint injuries is usually clinically based and depends on good knowledge of anatomy. Special care should be taken to rule out injury to associated neurovascular structures for all joint injuries.
> - Baseline imaging studies of the shoulder should *always* include a second tangential view of the scapula and glenoid. The best radiographic screening series is an AP view in internal rotation, AP view in external rotation, and axillary view of shoulder. The axillary view is the simplest to assess for joint dislocation.
> - Impingement, rotator cuff injuries, and shoulder instability are best diagnosed with a complete physical examination supported by appropriate imaging studies rather than a single isolated maneuver.
> - Performance, injury prevention, and injury recovery related to the shoulder are optimized when the entire kinetic chain is addressed, including a sound base, core strength, scapular stability, antagonist capsular and muscle stretching, and classic rotator cuff–strengthening program.

The true functional shoulder joint comprises the glenohumeral joint, scapular thoracic joint, acromioclavicular (AC) joint, and sternoclavicular (SC) joint. Problems around the shoulder can be acute or chronic and include pain, weakness, dysfunction, stiffness, and instability. To ensure optimal outcome of treatment, an accurate, anatomic-based diagnosis is necessary. Less targeted treatment regimens tend to be less successful because the specific problem may not be treated. Several evidence-based reviews remain inconclusive regarding specific interventions when a non-specific diagnosis such as "shoulder pain" is targeted.

INJURIES OF CLAVICULAR COMPLEX

> ### Key Points
>
> - Most clavicle fractures can be definitively treated nonsurgically with a sling or a figure-8 dressing if they are minimally displaced or nondisplaced.
> - Grade 1 (tenderness) and grade 2 (tenderness and displacement with intact coracoclavicular [CC] ligaments) AC injuries are managed conservatively with ice, pain control, and a sling for comfort.
> - Anterior shoulder dislocations are more common than posterior shoulder dislocations, but posterior dislocations are more commonly missed.

The diagnosis of clavicle, AC, and SC injuries is straightforward; direct palpation along the clavicular complex should lead to an area of focal pain. Imaging studies should include the entire clavicle and a clear view of the targeted area from at least two planes. All injuries around the shoulder should include examination of the cervical spine and distal neurovascular evaluation. The brachial plexus, subclavian vein, and axillary artery lie immediately beneath the clavicle and can be at risk of injury.

Clavicle fractures account for 5% to 10% of all fractures and can be classified as either displaced or nondisplaced as well as by their specific location (proximal-distal) on the clavicle. Most fractures involve the midshaft (80%); however, distal third (15%) and proximal third (5%) fractures are also possible. Fortunately, most clavicle fractures can be definitively treated nonoperatively with a sling or a figure-8 dressing if they are minimally displaced or nondisplaced. Figure-8 bracing has been linked with skin necrosis over the fracture site, indicating the need for careful observation of skin integrity when used. In most cases, a simple sling for comfort is adequate over the first few weeks followed by progressive range of motion (ROM) activities. More significant displacement (>100%), any tenting of the skin, significant comminution, or excessive shortening (>2 cm) may warrant surgical intervention. Referral to an orthopedic surgeon is recommended. Distal clavicle fractures have a higher rate of nonunion with nonsurgical treatment than midshaft or medial fracture patterns, so careful follow-up is necessary (Khan et al., 2009; McKee et al., 2004).

Acromioclavicular Joint

Acromioclavicular joint injuries are classified by the ligamentous structures involved and the degree of separation of the AC joint (Figure 30-3). A *grade 1* injury involves only a partial injury to the AC ligaments, no displacement occurs, and the CC ligaments are intact. A *grade 2* injury involves the complete injury of the AC ligaments; therefore, mild superior translation of the distal clavicle occurs (<100% translation), and the CC ligaments are intact. Both grade 1 and grade 2 injuries have an excellent prognosis with conservative treatment, which includes local application of ice, reduction of stresses, and a sling for comfort. Most patients have substantial active motion and functional use of the arm within 6 weeks. A *grade 3* involves the complete rupture of both the AC and CC ligaments. The distal end of the clavicle and acromion are now separated by more

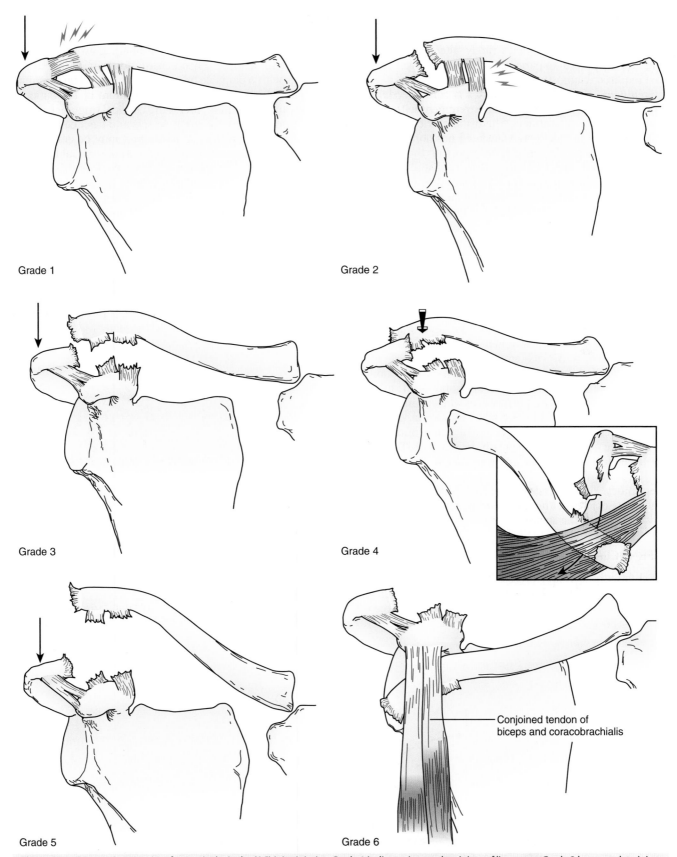

Grade 1

Grade 2

Grade 3

Grade 4

Conjoined tendon of
biceps and coracobrachialis

Grade 5

Grade 6

Figure 30-3 Progressive severity of acromioclavicular (AC) joint injuries. Grade 1 indicates incomplete injury of ligaments. Grade 2 has complete injury of the AC ligaments but intact coracoclavicular (CC) ligaments. Grade 3 injuries have complete injury of both AC and CC ligaments. Grade 4, 5, and 6 injuries are progressively severe, with posterior displacement of clavicle, severe superior displacement of clavicle, and inferior displacement of clavicle beneath the coracoid process.

than a full clavicular width (>100% displacement). Stress radiographic views may magnify this separation even further; however, stress views rarely alter the treatment plan and are painful to patients and thus no longer considered required diagnostic images.

Treatment of grade 3 AC injuries is controversial and ranges from surgical to conservative treatment with a sling. With conservative treatment, the distal clavicle may ultimately heal in a superiorly translated position, leaving a prominent bump over the lateral aspect of the shoulder. However, nonelite athletes can function well and have a full return to activities. Acute repair of grade 3 injuries is suggested for some elite athletes but has not been proved in randomized controlled trials (RCTs) because subtle changes occur at this important point in the kinetic chain. Chronic reconstructions have been suggested in patients who have grade 3 injuries but with residual pain or dysfunction. The more severe injuries of the AC joint have significant posterior, superior, or inferior displacement and require surgical reduction and repair.

A *grade 4* AC separation is a complete injury of both AC and CC ligaments with a posterior subluxation of the distal clavicle relative to the acromion. These are frequently missed on routine AP radiographs but can be easily identified if routine axillary shoulder views are obtained. Fundamental management of bone and joint injuries requires a view from two perspectives. *Grade 5* injuries are basically equivalent to severe grade 3 injuries in which the distal clavicle is riding so high that it either buttonholes through the fascia or tents beneath the skin (300% translation). The fascial injury prevents reduction, and the pressure on the undersurface of the skin risks skin slough or an open injury. Finally, *grade 6* AC injuries are extremely rare and are associated with an inferior dislocation of the distal clavicle beneath the coracoid.

STERNOCLAVICULAR JOINT

Patients with SC injury present with a history of trauma (e.g., landing on lateral aspect of shoulder) or a history of chronic overuse that has led to popping and pain over the medial aspect of the clavicle (Matava et al., 2005). Acute SC joint dislocations can be identified clinically with localized tenderness over the medial clavicular aspect, and gross deformity may be present. More often, however, patients present with a subtle, chronic situation caused by esthetic findings with a palpable or gross asymmetry. The examination should always include an assessment of the patient's airway and circulation, including cervical (jugular) venous distention, because the great vessels and trachea lie immediately posterior to the SC joints and may be compressed or injured (Figure 30-4). Imaging studies should include an AP radiograph of the chest, views of the entire clavicle, and a tangential or serendipity view of the SC joint (Figure 30-5). Because of overlapping shadows, these studies may be difficult to interpret. When suspicious, the best test is computed tomography (CT).

Traumatic SC joint dislocations can be either anterior or posterior. *Anterior dislocations* are generally easily palpated, with the proximal clavicle anteriorly displaced and painful. Anterior injuries may be reduced by placing a rolled towel or beanbag between the shoulder blades and then creating a distraction force along the arm in extension. Anterior dislocations tend to be unstable and to redisplace after

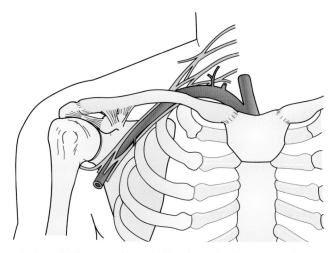

Figure 30-4 Schematic showing the proximity of major neurovascular structures to the sternoclavicular joint.

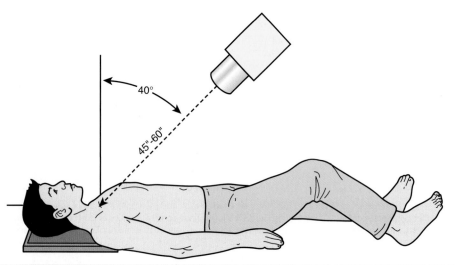

Figure 30-5 Technique in obtaining a tangential radiographic image, the serendipity view, to assess sternoclavicular joint injuries.

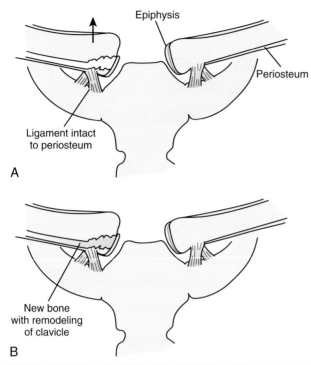

Figure 30-6 Medial clavicle injuries in patients younger than 23 to 25 years are likely physeal injuries and have the potential to remodel. **A,** The initial injury with periosteal sleeve delimitation. **B,** The new callous and bone healing over time.

attempted reduction. Fortunately, anterior injuries usually heal uneventfully, leaving an asymptomatic medial prominence and occasional popping, with minimal effect on the patient's activities of daily living (ADLs). *Posterior dislocations* can be dangerous because of proximity to the great vessels posteriorly. If patients have venous engorgement in the neck and difficulty breathing, closed reduction may be attempted. A towel clip is used at the medial end of the clavicle, pulling anteriorly and creating the reduction. If this is attempted, it is best done in the operating room with a vascular surgeon immediately available in case the proximal clavicle was actually tamponading an injury to the great vessels. This reduction should never be performed on the sideline in the absence of immediate cardiothoracic surgical response unless the patient's life is at risk and there is no other option.

When treating injuries to the proximal clavicle, the age of the patient and normal maturation of the proximal epiphysis are also important considerations. The medial clavicle epiphysis is one of the last to appear, at 19 to 23 years of age, and then the last to fuse, at 23 to 25 years of age. In patients younger than 23 years of age, these injuries are generally physeal injuries and not true dislocations, reducing the need for aggressive treatment (Figure 30-6).

KEY TREATMENT

- Subacromial injection for rotator cuff disease or intraarticular injection for adhesive capsulitis may be effective, although the effect may be minimal and not well maintained (Buchbinder et al., 2003) (SOR: A).
- The use of some physiotherapy interventions is indicated in specific and circumscribed cases of shoulder pain (Green et al., 2003) (SOR: B).

- Little evidence supports the benefit of manual therapy for adhesive capsulitis, shoulder pain, or subacromial impingement syndrome (Ho et al., 2009) (SOR: A).
- The use of acupuncture for shoulder pain can be neither recommended nor refuted (Green et al., 2005) (SOR: A).

SHOULDER IMPINGEMENT AND ROTATOR CUFF DISEASE

Key Points

- Tests to diagnose impingement syndrome include a positive Hawkins test, a painful arc of motion, and weakness with external rotation.
- Tests to diagnose a complete cuff tear include a positive drop-arm test, a painful arc of motion, and weakness to external rotation.
- Incomplete tears of the rotator cuff improve with physical therapy, antiinflammatory medications, or subacromial injection.

By far the two most common diagnostic categories of the shoulder are rotator cuff impingement and shoulder instability. The rotator cuff is a group of four muscles—the supraspinatus, infraspinatus, teres minor, and subscapularis—that originate from the scapular surface, traverse just outside of the glenohumeral capsule, and insert onto the tuberosities of the humerus (Figure 30-7). The rotator cuff initiates motion in the shoulder and stabilizes the humeral head in the glenohumeral joint.

When making the diagnosis of rotator cuff impingement, the clinician should look at the problem as a continuum of progressively more severe pathologies, including subacromial bursitis, AC joint hypertrophy and spurring, rotator cuff tendinosis, partial rotator cuff tears, complete or massive rotator cuff tears, and ultimately, rotator cuff arthropathy (i.e., degenerative disease related to chronic rotator cuff insufficiency) (Almekinders, 2001). Patients generally present with shoulder pain exacerbated by repetitive overhead activities, weakness, and occasionally difficulty sleeping on the shoulder. Physical examination of the shoulder includes provocative maneuvers that exacerbate impingement findings and evaluate the function of each rotator cuff muscle (Tennent et al., 2003a, 2003b). Impingement testing includes straight, forward flexion of the shoulder (Neer sign), abduction and internal rotation of the shoulder (Hawkins sign), and adduction of the shoulder in a 90-degree, forward-flexed position (Figures 30-8 and 30-9). The examiner must be cautious with the latter test because the result may be positive with impingement but also with AC joint hypertrophy alone or with degenerative change of the AC joint.

Isolated testing of the rotator cuff is performed in sequence. To isolate the supraspinatus muscle, the examiner should perform the "empty can" test. This is performed with the arm slightly forward flexed in the plane of the scapula, abducted to 90 degrees, with full internal rotation (i.e., with the thumbs down, or empty can). The examiner should then place resistance on the patient's distal hand in an inferior direction. If this exacerbates pain, it is a positive finding of impingement or rotator cuff tendinopathy. If the

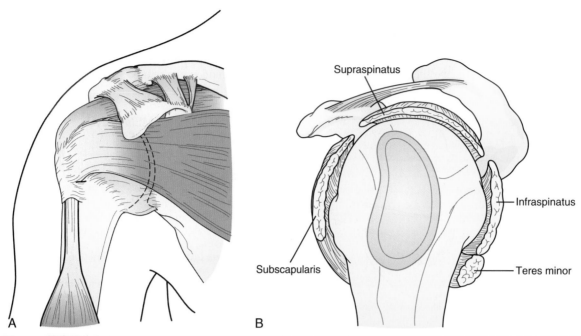

Figure 30-7 Anteroposterior (**A**) and lateral cross-sectional (**B**) schematics of the shoulder demonstrate the relationship of the rotator cuff muscles (supraspinatus, infraspinatus, teres minor, and subscapularis) to the bony structure of the shoulder.

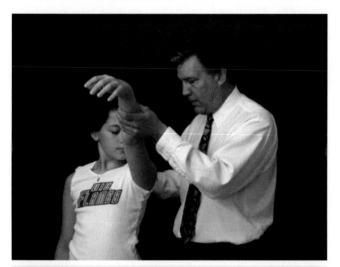

Figure 30-8 The Hawkins test for shoulder impingement is performed by forward elevating the humerus against the fixed scapula. Pain indicates anterior impingement. (Courtesy Mark R. Hutchinson, MD.)

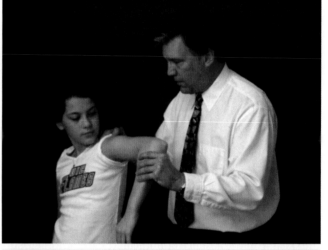

Figure 30-9 The Neer test for shoulder impingement is performed with abduction and internal rotation of the shoulder. Pain indicates lateral impingement. (Courtesy Mark R. Hutchinson, MD.)

patient has a positive "drop arm" sign and is unable to maintain the arm in this position, a complete rotator cuff tear should be suspected. However, this does not confirm a complete rotator cuff tear because the patient may be guarding secondary to pain. Clinically, the examiner can clarify the difference by performing a diagnostic subacromial injection with lidocaine. The injection should significantly diminish pain complaints but not affect the motor function of an intact rotator cuff (Park et al., 2005).

To evaluate the infraspinatus and teres minor muscles, the examiner should evaluate external rotation against resistance. This is best done with the arm at the side, keeping the elbows near the torso, and asking the patient to rotate externally against resistance. Isolating the subscapularis muscle is more difficult. Resisted internal rotation with the

arms at the side will recruit the pectoralis muscles and not isolate the subscapularis. To isolate the subscapularis, two tests have been described. In the *lift-off test*, the patient places the arm behind the back and lifts the hand into further internal rotation against resistance (Figure 30-10). If able to do this, the patient's subscapularis muscle is likely intact. Modification of this test has been described as the "tummy pat" or the "Napoleon" test, in which the patient abducts the elbow, which must be away from the body in the plane of the torso, and is then asked to pat the stomach against resistance (Figure 30-11). Weakness or inability to press against resistance is considered to be a positive test result. After the diagnosis is made clinically, AP and axillary shoulder radiography studies can be obtained to evaluate the extent of injury further or assess for concomitant

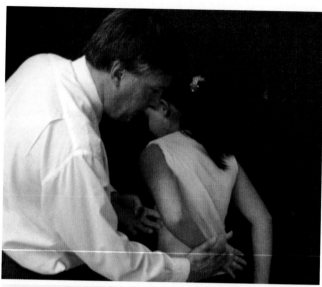

Figure 30-10 The lift-off test is used to assess subscapularis muscle function. Patients are asked to lift their hands off their backs against resistance. Weakness or pain indicates subscapularis pathology. (Courtesy Mark R. Hutchinson, MD.)

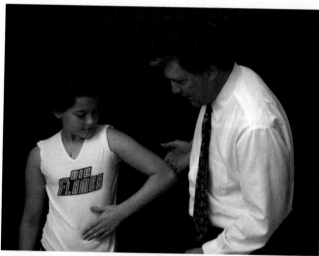

Figure 30-11 The "Napoleon" or "tummy pat" test is a modified lift-off test to evaluate subscapularis function. Patients are asked to maintain their elbow laterally while pressing into their bellies. (Ensure that patients do not drop their arm and use the humerus extensors to mimic subscapularis function.) (Courtesy Mark R. Hutchinson, MD.)

injuries. MRI is not routinely indicated with an intact rotator cuff clinically, and we usually recommend trying a course of physical therapy for 6 to 12 weeks before ordering MRI (Park et al., 2005).

If the patient has symptomatic shoulder pain with overhead motion and cross-body adduction with an intact rotator cuff function on clinical examination and otherwise normal findings on radiographs, a conservative course of physical therapy is indicated for the impingement symptoms. Ninety percent to 95% of patients with incomplete tears of the rotator cuff improve with the course of physical therapy, antiinflammatory medications, or a subacromial injection, although some may require surgery eventually (Matava et al., 2005). Physical therapy should focus on rotator cuff strengthening, ROM, posterior capsular

stretching, and scapular stabilization. If patients fail a 6- to 12-week course of conservative treatment, a corticosteroid injection should be considered before surgery. If a patient is refractory to both corticosteroids and physical therapy, surgical intervention may be indicated. This is a more appropriate time to order MRI because preoperative MR scanning can evaluate the extent of rotator cuff pathology, associated spurring, and degeneration within the shoulder joint. Although not necessary for making the diagnosis, MRI can assist the surgeon at surgery. Platelet-rich plasma injections for partial rotator cuff tears and subacromial bursitis have not been proven in the literature, and only small case reports with short-term follow-up have been reported.

For incomplete rotator cuff tears (<50% of surface), a partial debridement and subacromial decompression using arthroscopy can provide effective, long-term relief of impingement pain. Management of rotator cuff tears greater than 50% or complete with clinical dysfunction is generally surgical. If the tear is identified before chronic retraction and muscle changes, primary arthroscopic or open repair has been effective in reducing pain and improving function. Rehabilitation after rotator cuff repair requires at least 6 weeks of passive ROM only, to protect the repair, followed by a gradual increase to resistance activities for the rotator cuff. Patients usually begin strengthening at 12 weeks. In patients with nonreparable chronic rotator cuff tears or those with advanced rotator arthropathy and degenerative disease, surgical interventions include muscle transfers, soft tissue grafts, hemiarthroplasties, and reverse shoulder hemiarthroplasties.

EVIDENCE-BASED SUMMARY

- In a review of eight clinical trials (>390 patients), no definitive evidence supports or refutes the efficacy of common interventions, including physiotherapy, nonsteroidal antiinflammatory drugs (NSAIDs), corticosteroid injections, or open and arthroscopic surgery, for rotator cuff tears in adults (Ejnisman et al., 2003) (SOR: A).
- Based on limited data from two quality RCTs, no evidence supports the superiority of conservative versus surgical treatment for subacromial impingement syndrome (Dorrestijn et al., 2009) (SOR: B).
- A review of 14 RCTs evaluating rotator cuff surgery showed no long-term pain benefit of surgical decompression versus exercise programs (Coghlan et al., 2009) (SOR: A).

SHOULDER INSTABILITY

Bony anatomy provides minimal stability to the glenohumeral joint; therefore, the primary stability depends on both static and dynamic soft tissue structures. The static soft tissue structures include the fibrocartilaginous labrum, glenohumeral ligaments, and capsule. The labrum attaches to the periphery of the glenoid and serves to deepen the socket, reducing translation out of the socket. The glenohumeral ligaments attach to the labrum, are thickenings in the capsule, and connect to the humeral head. The intrinsic dynamic stabilizers are the rotator cuff and biceps, which help maintain the humeral head in the glenoid socket. The extrinsic dynamic stabilizers include the rhomboid, levator

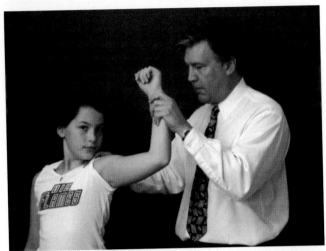

Figure 30-12 The apprehension test is performed with the arm in full abduction and external rotation. A sensation of impending subluxation is a positive finding. (Courtesy Mark R. Hutchinson, MD.)

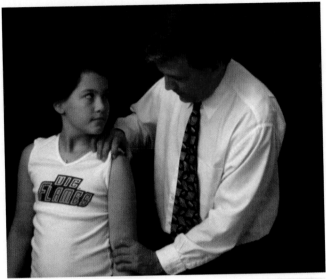

Figure 30-13 The presence or absence of a sulcus sign is evaluated by distracting the arm inferiorly to sublux the humeral head out of the socket. If a sulcus is appreciated as the glenoid is emptied of the humeral head, the clinician should suspect multidirectional instability. (Courtesy Mark R. Hutchinson, MD.)

scapulae, serratus, and trapezius muscles, which position the glenoid beneath the humeral head.

The diagnosis of shoulder instability begins with the patient's history and mechanism of injury, which often include episodes of subluxation, dislocation, or apprehension. Classically, anterior instability is appreciated when the arm is placed in abduction and external rotation (Tennent et al., 2003a, 2003b) (Figure 30-12). *Inferior* instability is appreciated when the patient tries to hold a heavy object and the shoulder subluxes inferiorly. *Posterior* instability is frequently associated with a fall on an outstretched arm or occasionally with weightlifters who lock out their arms in extension while bench pressing. The clinical examination targets these specific pathologies with the classic *apprehension test* for anterior instability, which is performed with the arm in abduction and external rotation and the patient having the sensation of the arm going out of place. In the *relocation test*, the examiner then presses the humeral head back into a reduced position, thus eliminating the sensation of apprehension. Posterior instability is assessed in a supine position with the arm forward flexed 90 degrees with a posteriorly directed force. Inferior instability is assessed by pulling inferiorly on the arm and looking for or feeling the humerus come out the socket and looking for a concavity just below the acromion, called the "sulcus sign" (Figure 30-13).

Some patients may have generalized ligamentous laxity, but laxity itself is not a painful process and is therefore not pathologic. However, some patients with generalized ligamentous laxity do have symptoms of instability and pathology that can be assessed by comparison with the opposite side or looking at the elbows, fingers or thumb, or knees for excessive recurvatum (hyperextension). In general, patients with generalized ligamentous laxity should undergo an extensive course of conservative treatment because of the increased risk of failure associated with most surgical interventions compared with simple unidirectional instability.

The conservative treatment of shoulder instability is targeted at balancing the flexibility, optimizing the motor strength, and optimizing the function of the kinetic chain. The core component is rotator cuff–strengthening exercises

as well as scapular stabilizer exercises. Controversy surrounds the ideal treatment for a first-time shoulder anterior dislocation. In young athletes or military populations, the risk of recurrence and future shoulder problems approaches 90%. Surgical treatment with repair of labral detachments has led to a high rate of return to play and return to performance, with a low risk (<10%) of recurrent instability for a first dislocation. Older nonathletic patients (>40) with first-time dislocations have a reduced risk of recurrent instability (<50%), so surgical treatment is unnecessary. However, if any patient has recurrent instability or pain, surgery to repair the torn capsule or labral lesions is strongly recommended, with good to excellent outcomes occurring 75% to 95% of the time. The Bankart procedure is most often performed and involves direct repair of the torn labrum back to the glenoid from which it was detached (Figure 30-14). Classically, this procedure was performed open, although the current trend is toward arthroscopic assistance.

Posterior instability accounts for only 10% to 15% of isolated instability of the shoulder. The classic treatment for posterior instability is to initiate a course of conservative treatment focused on strengthening the posterior capsular muscles, including the infraspinatus and teres minor. It is important to carefully review a complete series of shoulder images to assess bone anatomy and look for associated glenoid fracture. If a conservative course fails, surgical treatment can again address either capsular laxity or posterior labral injuries.

Multidirectional instability is usually not secondary to a single acute traumatic event. More frequently, the patient will have underlying generalized ligamentous laxity that may or may not be exacerbated by a single traumatic event. These patients are generally loose jointed in all directions and in other joints. Initially, treatment is conservative, although in resistant cases, surgical capsular tightening can be successful in improving symptoms. A thorough

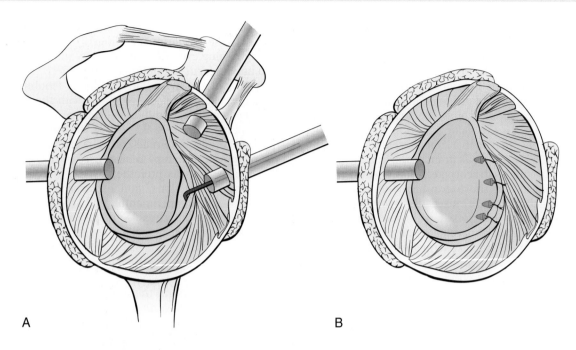

Figure 30-14 A, Detachment of the anterior inferior labrum (a Bankart lesion). **B,** Subsequent suture repair.

history is necessary to rule out psychologic factors (e.g., voluntary dislocation for attention or a party trick). These patients have an extremely high failure rate with surgical intervention.

KEY TREATMENT

- Primary surgical repair is indicated for young athletes engaged in highly demanding physical activities who have sustained their *first* shoulder dislocation (Handoll et al., 2004) (SOR: A).
- Surgical repair of shoulder instability from dislocation results in significantly lower recurrent instability than conservative treatment, especially for younger athletes and those in collision sports (Brophy and Marx, 2009) (SOR: B).
- No significant difference exists between arthroscopic and open techniques in the surgical treatment of recurrent shoulder instability in adults (Pulavarti et al., 2009) (SOR: B).

Elbow

Key Points

- Chronic lateral epicondylopathy (tennis elbow) is a degenerative process of the collagen and not an inflammatory process within the tendon.
- Topical or oral NSAIDs and corticosteroid injections provide short-term relief of lateral epicondylopathy pain but do not treat the underlying tendinopathy.
- Steroids must not be injected into an infectious olecranon bursitis.
- Steroid injections into the medial epicondyle and medial collateral ligament (MCL) can weaken the ligament and increase the risk of rupture.

LATERAL ELBOX TENDINOPATHY

Lateral elbow tendinopathy, commonly called *lateral epicondylitis* or "tennis elbow," is caused by repetitive overuse of the wrist extensor and forearm supinator muscles that originate at the lateral epicondyle of the humerus—more specifically, the extensor carpi radialis brevis tendon. Once thought to result from inflammation, lateral elbow tendinosis is caused by chronic degenerative changes in the collagen fibers themselves (Nirschl, 1992), with minimal inflammation present. Microtears, chronic granulation tissue, and scar tissue formation are often seen in pathologic specimens of surgical cases of tennis elbow. Peritendinous soft tissue inflammation can occur, which may respond to ice and antiinflammatory medications, but these treatments do not address the collagen fiber degeneration.

Patients present because of pain in the lateral aspect of the elbow and less commonly complain of weakness or restricted elbow motion. Pain is made worse by gripping, turning handles, and lifting activities, particularly with the hand in a palm-down position, as in lifting a suitcase, briefcase, or purse. Common positive physical examination findings include tenderness to palpation of the lateral epicondyle of the elbow and over the proximal wrist extensor and forearm supinator muscle tendons just distal to the lateral epicondyle. Pain is intensified with resisted wrist extension and forearm supination. Pain can also limit patient strength. There should be no tenderness directly over the radial head, with normal ligamentous stability and normal neurovascular evaluation. Plain radiographs are not needed to make an accurate diagnosis of lateral epicondylopathy but should be considered in patients with a history of trauma, motion loss, or locking, or those with a prolonged period of pain.

Management focuses on pain control and restoration of normal elbow function. Cryotherapy, ice massage, and NSAIDs or acetaminophen are excellent pain relievers. NSAIDs and corticosteroid injection have been mainstays of treatment, but their use is now questioned because inflammation no longer seems a main factor in the injury process. There seems to be a component of neovascularization, and the tendon is in a chronic state of injury. Corticosteroid injections help quickly reduce the pain of lateral elbow tendinosis related to peripheral peritendinous inflammation but do not alter the long-term outcome (Smidt et al., 2002). Cortisone injection may lead to a short-lived increase in pain in a large percentage of patients (Wang et al., 2003). For recalcitrant cases, treatments such as prolotherapy and extracorporeal shock wave therapy have been studied, but short-term follow-up and isolated reports of effectiveness are mixed (Rabago et al., 2013). Platelet-rich plasma injections for chronic tennis elbow have not been thoroughly evaluated or proven and only small case reports with short term follow-up have been studied.

Counterforce straps can effectively reduce discomfort in some patients (Figure 30-15). The strap is applied just distal to the area of maximal tenderness. The strap may relieve some of the tension exerted on the affected muscle tendon units during activities, thereby reducing pain. However, straps, medications, and injections should not replace therapeutic exercises, which include massage, stretching, and strengthening exercises. The most effective stretch is performed with the elbow extended, forearm fully pronated, and wrist flexed. From this position, gentle traction is applied to the middle and ring fingers toward the olecranon. Strengthening exercises with light weights for wrist extension and forearm supination can be done.

Most patients with lateral elbow tendinopathy will obtain excellent relief of symptoms with the program just described, although minimal evidence exists to support these plans (Bisset et al., 2005). If these measures do not lead to adequate relief, other protocols can be added. Formal physical therapy is often used in recalcitrant cases. Treatments such as prolotherapy, dry needling, platelet-rich plasma injections, and extracorporeal shock wave therapy are still experimental, and studies have not fully proved their effectiveness. Surgical intervention is sometimes needed and has excellent results.

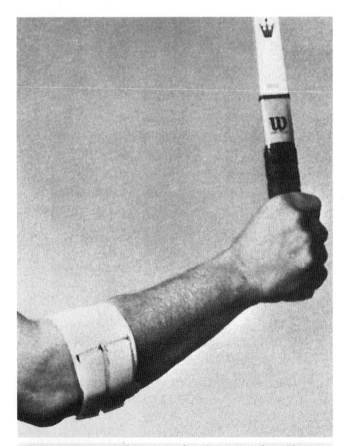

Figure 30-15 Lateral elbow counterforce brace. Note that wide, nonelastic support is curved to fit the conical forearm shape. This does not allow for full muscular expansion, thereby diminishing intrinsic muscular force on the lateral epicondyle. (From Morrey BF, ed. *The elbow and its disorders*. Philadelphia: Saunders; 1985.)

KEY TREATMENT

- No specific physical therapy modality is preferred over another in the treatment of lateral elbow tendinopathy (Smidt et al., 2003) (SOR: A).
- Topical and oral NSAIDs are both effective in providing short-term pain relief from lateral epicondylopathy; topical NSAIDs have fewer adverse effects (Green et al., 2002) (SOR: A).
- Corticosteroid injections are helpful in reducing pain from lateral epicondylopathy but do not alter the long-term outcome (Smidt et al., 2002) (SOR: A).
- Little evidence exists to support the use of therapeutic exercises or braces in the treatment of lateral epicondylopathy (Bisset et al., 2005) (SOR: A).
- Extracorporeal shock wave therapy provides little or no benefit in terms of pain and function in lateral elbow pain (nine placebo-controlled trials, 1006 participants; Buchbinder et al., 2009) (SOR: A).

MEDIAL ELBOW TENDINOPATHY

Medial elbow tendinopathy, commonly called *medial epicondylitis or* "golfer's elbow," is caused by repetitive overuse of the wrist flexor and forearm pronator muscles that originate at the medial epicondyle of the humerus. Patients present because of pain in the medial aspect of the elbow, rarely weakness, and loss of ROM. Pain is worsened by gripping and lifting activities, particularly with the hand in a palm-up position. Common positive findings include tenderness to palpation of the medial epicondyle of the elbow and over the proximal wrist flexor and forearm pronator muscle tendons. Pain is intensified with resisted wrist flexion and forearm pronation (Figure 30-16). Patient discomfort often limits strength. Elbow motion, ligamentous stability, and neurovascular status are typically intact.

As with lateral elbow tendinopathy, plain radiographs are not needed to make an accurate diagnosis of medial elbow tendinopathy but should be considered with a history of trauma, motion loss, locking, or chronic pain. Also similar to lateral epicondylopathy, management of medial epicondylopathy includes ice, medication, prolotherapy or platelet-rich plasma injections, and strapping. Corticosteroid injections are not recommended because of possible ulnar nerve injury and weakening of the MCL. In medial elbow

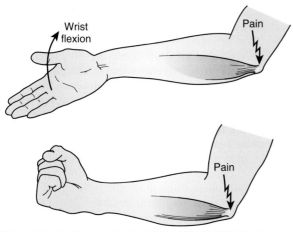

Figure 30-16 Medial epicondylitis may be diagnosed clinically by pain localized to the medial epicondyle during wrist flexion and pronation against resistance. Pain is often elicited after making a tight fist, and grip strength is usually diminished on the affected side. (From Morrey BF, ed. *The elbow and its disorders.* Philadelphia: Saunders; 1985.)

tendinopathy, the most effective stretch is performed with the elbow extended and the wrist and fingers gently pulled into full extension. The forearm can be pronated or supinated. Strengthening focuses on wrist flexion and forearm pronation exercises.

OLECRANON BURSITIS

Olecranon bursitis is a common cause of painless elbow swelling from repetitive friction of the olecranon against a firm surface or traumatic impact. Patients most often present with a painless swelling at the dorsal tip of the elbow, described as "a golf ball" or "goose egg" (Figure 30-17). With trauma-induced swelling, pain and a hematoma may be present. Pain, redness, warmth, and lymphadenopathy may accompany septic bursitis. ROM loss, instability, neurovascular compromise, and strength loss are uncommon. On examination, there is a soft, fluctuant area of swelling directly over the olecranon. Diagnostic studies are generally not necessary to make a diagnosis of olecranon bursitis. However, plain radiographs should be obtained if trauma preceded the bursitis or fracture or dislocation is suspected.

Classic treatment for aseptic bursitis includes compression, ice, and avoidance of impact at the olecranon. NSAIDs may help to reduce swelling. If the fluid collection within the bursa is large or infection is suspected, aspiration of the bursa can be done in the office with a large-bore needle under sterile conditions. The bursa fluid should be clear and straw colored but may be bloody in a traumatic injury. If an infection is not suspected clinically when the fluid is withdrawn, a corticosteroid can be injected. Corticosteroids should never be injected if infection is a possibility. Oral antibiotics can be started if an infection is present. A local incision and drainage may be required in the presence of an infection and abscess. Aspiration does not replace compression wrap, ice, and avoidance of impact. Fluid may reaccumulate but should decrease. Serial aspirations are an option in a recurrent aseptic bursitis, but bursectomy is occasionally needed for definitive treatment.

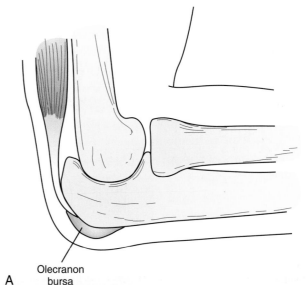

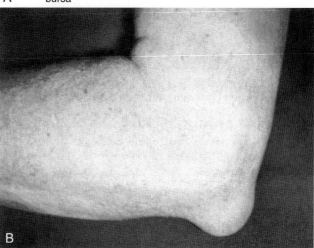

Figure 30-17 A, Relationship of the olecranon bursa to the skin and olecranon. **B,** An enlarged olecranon bursa. (From Singer KM, Butters KP. Olecranon bursitis. In Delee JC, Drez D, eds. *Orthopedic sports medicine: principles and practice.* vol 1. Philadelphia: Saunders; 1994:890, 892.)

Wrist and Hand

Key Points

- Both bracing and cortisone injection may reduce carpal tunnel syndrome (CTS) pain in the short term.
- Surgical treatment of CTS leads to better symptom relief than bracing.
- Immobilization of suspected scaphoid injuries should be instituted while the workup is completed.
- Initial immobilization of any scaphoid fracture should be in a thumb spica cast.
- Proximal pole and displaced scaphoid fractures should be treated by an orthopedic surgeon.

CARPAL TUNNEL SYNDROME

Carpal tunnel syndrome is the most common nerve entrapment syndrome encountered in primary care. CTS is more

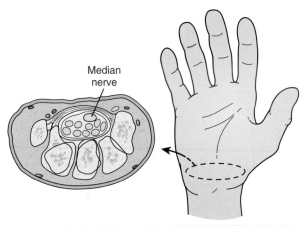

Figure 30-18 Cross-sectional anatomy of the carpal tunnel bounded on three sides by the carpal bones and volarly by the transverse carpal ligament. Nine flexor tendons and the median nerve pass through the tunnel. Anything that causes increased pressure in this canal can produce the symptoms of carpal tunnel syndrome. (From McCue FC, Bruce VF: Hand and wrist. In Delee JC, Drez D, eds. *Orthopedic sports medicine: principles and practice.* vol 1. Philadelphia: Saunders; 1994:997.)

common in women than men and affects about 3% of the adult American population. Of the many possible etiologies, the most common is tenosynovitis of the hand flexors, leading to median nerve compression. CTS can develop during pregnancy as well. Nine flexor tendons course through the carpal tunnel along with the median nerve (Figure 30-18).

Patients typically present because of pain, numbness, paresthesias, and loss of grip strength in the wrist and hand. Symptoms may even radiate into the shoulder region. Symptoms usually involve the radial 3½ digits as supplied by the median nerve and are noted more with repetitive hand motion activities and at night. Physical examination may reveal thenar atrophy and decreased sensation over the radial 3½ digits. These two clinical findings, along with a history of pain in the distribution of the median nerve, are highly suggestive of CTS and correlate to positive nerve conduction study findings (D'Arcy and McGee, 2000).

The Tinel test (sign) at the wrist is performed by tapping over the wrist flexor retinaculum and having increased or reproducible symptoms of pain, numbness, and tingling in the radial 3½ digits. The most sensitive test is the carpal compression test, in which direct compression over the tunnel elicits the symptoms. The Phalen maneuver is performed by having the patient flex the wrists to a 90-degree position, holding the dorsal aspects of the hands back to back. The patient maintains this position up to 1 minute, until symptoms develop.

Diagnostic imaging is not necessary to make a diagnosis of CTS. Electrodiagnostic tests can be used to confirm the diagnosis but are not needed to initiate or direct early treatment in most patients. Although up to 25% are false-negative results in patients with clinical CTS, electrodiagnostic tests should be done before surgery.

Treatment begins with attempts to avoid or at least modify activities known to cause pain for the patient. This may include ergonomic changes in the workplace, such as wrist support pads for computer use. Wrist splinting,

particularly at night, may prove helpful. Nerve gliding exercises are routinely prescribed and can provide relief (Figure 30-19). Oral analgesic and NSAID use may also lead to relief, although studies show these are no more effective than placebo. Corticosteroid injection is a helpful adjunct in many patients and may relieve symptoms better than placebo. A majority of patients will experience good relief of symptoms if these conservative measures are followed. Unfortunately, most of these patients will have a return of symptoms in 1 year (Kanaan and Sawaya, 2001). Surgery is considered in patients who have recurrence of symptoms despite adequate conservative measures, and outcomes are excellent. Both open and endoscopic techniques are available, with equivalent long-term results.

KEY TREATMENT

- Oral analgesics and NSAIDs used to treat symptoms of CTS are no more effective than placebo (Gerritsen et al., 2002) (SOR: A).
- Corticosteroid injection is more effective than placebo in relieving symptoms (short term) (Gerritsen et al., 2002) (SOR: A).
- Bracing for CTS may lead to significant short-term pain reduction (O'Connor et al., 2003) (SOR: A).
- Surgery relieves CTS symptoms significantly better than bracing (Verdugo et al., 2005) (SOR: A).

DEQUERVAIN TENOSYNOVITIS

DeQuervain tenosynovitis is a painful repetitive and overuse condition of the abductor pollicis longus and extensor pollicis brevis along the dorsal radial aspect of the wrist. Patients present because of pain and swelling along the dorsal radial side of the wrist, which is worsened with activities. Physical examination reveals tenderness with palpation, and the classic clinical finding is a positive Finkelstein test result. This is performed by having the patient flex and adduct the thumb to the palm and then close the remaining fingers over the thumb. The examiner then passively takes the patient's wrist into ulnar deviation. Pain along the tendons with this maneuver is considered a positive test result (Finkelstein, 1930). Radiographic tests are not necessary to make an accurate diagnosis.

Treatment begins with avoidance of the inciting activities. Ice may reduce pain and swelling, and analgesic medications are often used as well. Thumb spica splinting is very helpful, allowing the irritated tendons to rest (Winzeler and Rosenstein, 1996). Prolonged splinting may be needed to reduce pain significantly. Corticosteroid injection along the tendon sheath is often used to reduce pain more acutely (Peters-Veluthamaningal et al., 2009a; Wood and Dobyns, 1986). In refractory cases, surgical decompression of the tendons can be performed.

DIGITAL FLEXOR TENOSYNOVITIS

Tenosynovitis of a digital flexor tendon, also called "trigger finger," is quite common. Patients present with the complaint of a finger that "sticks" with motion, primarily flexion, and they must painfully force the finger back into

Starting position 1

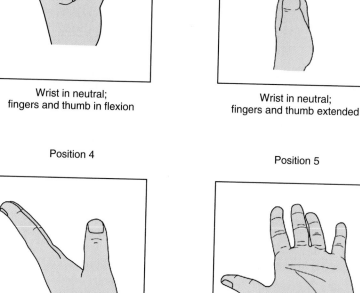

Wrist in neutral;
fingers and thumb in flexion

Position 2

Wrist in neutral;
fingers and thumb extended

Position 3

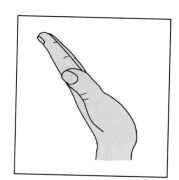

Thumb in neutral;
wrist and fingers extended

Position 4

Wrist, fingers, and thumb extended

Position 5

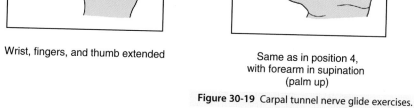

Same as in position 4,
with forearm in supination
(palm up)

Position 6

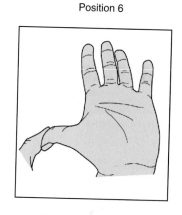

Same as in position 5,
with other hand gently stretching
thumb

Figure 30-19 Carpal tunnel nerve glide exercises.

extension. Usually, a painful palpable nodule on the flexor tendon is present along the distal palmar crease or at the base of the thumb, at the level of the metacarpophalangeal (MCP) joint (Figure 30-20). Motion and activities may be associated with pain. Radiographs and other diagnostic tests are not needed to make an accurate diagnosis.

Treatment options for digital flexor tenosynovitis include antiinflammatory medications, modification of activities, ice, massage, stretching of the flexor tendons, and gentle-grip strength exercises, although these usually provide little relief. Corticosteroid injections are often used to relieve pain and triggering symptoms (Marks and Gunther, 1989; Peters-Veluthamaningal et al., 2009b). Symptoms may return, and repeat injections are considered if the first injection provided reasonable pain relief. However, surgery may be needed in patients with frequent recurrence.

SCAPHOLUNATE SPRAINS

Ligament sprains of the wrist usually result from falls on an outstretched hand. Most are mild and resolve with splinting and symptomatic treatment. However, the clinician must be careful not to miss potentially catastrophic injuries that could compromise a patient's hand and wrist function,

including carpal dislocations, carpal instability (more specifically, scapholunate ligament instability), scaphoid fractures, and displaced intraarticular distal radius fractures. Injury to the scapholunate joint may be missed by physicians who do not consider it in their differential diagnosis of wrist injuries (Figure 30-21).

Patients with scapholunate sprains have pain in the wrist with motion, gripping, and lifting and along the dorsal aspect of the wrist at the scapholunate joint just distal to the Lister tubercle (bump on dorsal aspect of distal radius). Physical examination typically reveals no gross deformities, although dorsal swelling may be noted. The pain may be exacerbated by flexion and extension while palpating directly over the scapholunate joint on the dorsal aspect of the wrist.

Impacts strong enough to cause scapholunate sprain are sufficient to cause fracture. Therefore, plain radiographs should be obtained in all patients with suspected scapholunate sprain to look for associated fracture or avulsion. The series should include a standard AP view, AP with a clenched fist (accentuates scapholunate joint widening), standard lateral view, and posteroanterior (PA) view in ulnar deviation (assesses scaphoid bone for fracture). It is often helpful to obtain a comparison AP view of the

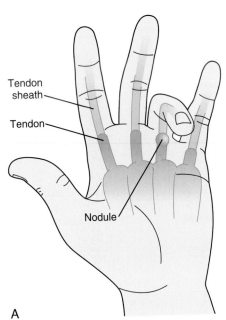

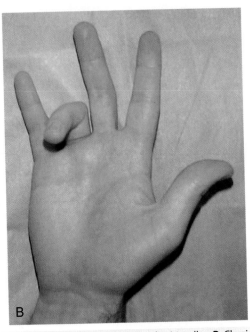

Figure 30-20 Flexor tendon nodule. **A,** Classic trigger finger with a flexor tendon nodule trapped proximal to the A1 pulley. **B,** Classic clinical presentation of a patient with a locked trigger finger.

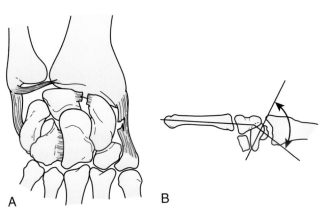

Figure 30-21 A, Disruption of scapholunate and radiocarpal ligaments leads to progressive dissociation between scaphoid and rest of carpal bones. This injury is frequently mistaken for a persistent wrist sprain. **B,** Chronic dissociation of scapholunate joint allows the scaphoid to rotate downward toward the palm. This increases the angle between scaphoid axis and radiolunate–capitate axis. The capitate then slowly migrates toward the radius, and osteoarthritis rapidly develops. (From Connolly JF. *DePalma's the management of fractures and dislocations: an atlas.* 3rd ed. Philadelphia: Saunders; 1981.)

opposite wrist. An increased gap between the scaphoid and lunate bones of 2 to 3 mm on the AP projection (e.g., "Terry Thomas" [United Kingdom] or "David Letterman" [United States] sign because of their gapped-tooth grin) is indicative of scapholunate dissociation (Figure 30-22).

Patients with a "simple" scapholunate sprain require protection and rest with a period of splinting. This can be accomplished with a custom fiberglass or plaster splint or a prefabricated cock-up wrist splint until the patient is asymptomatic. After initial treatment, the patient is weaned from the wrist splint and begins active ROM and hand-strengthening therapy. In patients with scapholunate

dissociation, surgical consultation should be considered early, and referral to a hand specialist is encouraged. Fixation of the joint is often needed to maximize future wrist function (Figure 30-23).

DISTAL RADIUS FRACTURES

Patients with distal radius fractures most often present with wrist pain and deformity immediately after a fall. All patients with wrist pain after a fall should have AP, lateral, and oblique radiographs of the wrist. Deformity may or may not be present, and some patients may complain of paresthesias in the affected extremity. A patient's ability to move the wrist does not rule out a fracture. It is important to palpate the entire extremity to assess any injury above or below the primary injury site for concomitant fractures. If suspected, radiographs should be taken of those areas as well. Neurovascular status should always be evaluated and documented.

Treatment is based on fracture type, patient age, and demand. A nondisplaced or minimally displaced fracture can be initially treated in a splint for 5 to 7 days until swelling subsides and then casted in a short-arm cast. The average healing time is 4 to 8 weeks, and repeat radiographs should be obtained during the healing process at an interval of every 2 to 3 weeks. An extraarticular, angulated fracture is initially treated with closed reduction with block (lidocaine injection into fracture hematoma). If postreduction alignment is adequate, a splint can be placed for 5 to 7 days to maintain the alignment pending casting. Because displacement or angulation of fracture fragments is a high risk even when appropriately splinted or casted, radiographic follow-up is important. Comminuted or displaced intraarticular fractures usually require closed reduction with percutaneous pinning or ORIF to maintain position and articular surface integrity; orthopedic surgery referral is recommended.

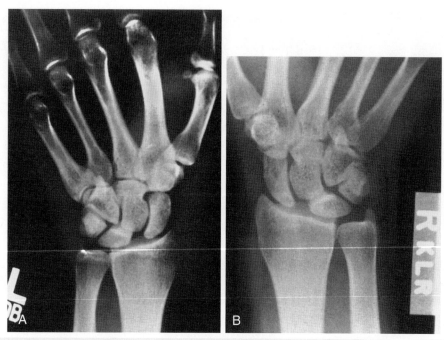

Figure 30-22 A, Posteroanterior radiograph of left wrist in 27-year-old soccer player who fell, landed on his left palm, and complained of pain. Note the abnormal widening of the scapholunate interval. **B,** Comparison view of the uninjured right wrist demonstrates the same scapholunate separation (>3 mm) (the "David Letterman" sign). The patient recovered with only splint support. (From Nicholas J, Hershman E. *The upper extremity in sports medicine.* 2nd ed. St. Louis: Mosby; 1995:456.)

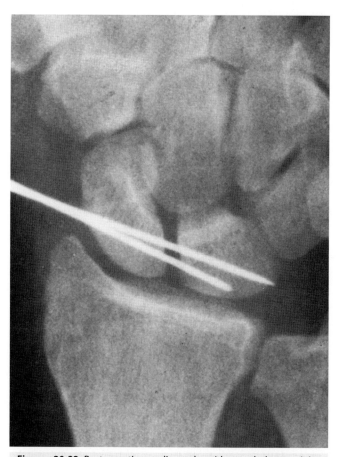

Figure 30-23 Postoperative radiograph with scapholunate joint reduced and two K wires properly positioned to stabilize the joint. (From Nicholas J, Hershman E. *The upper extremity in sports medicine.* 2nd ed. St. Louis: Mosby; 1995:393.)

SCAPHOID FRACTURE

Patients typically present after a fall onto an outstretched hand and complain of pain and swelling in the radial aspect of the wrist, worsened by motion. Gross deformity is not usually seen. The most common physical examination finding is tenderness with palpation over the scaphoid tubercle or in the anatomic snuffbox. Radiographs should be obtained in all patients with suspected scaphoid injury, including AP, lateral, and oblique views, as well as PA ulnar deviation or scaphoid views (Figure 30-24). Importantly, radiographic findings are often negative shortly after immediate injury and may still be negative up to 14 days after the injury; radiographs should be repeated in 2 weeks if suspicion remains high. Because a fracture is suspected, interim splinting or casting is necessary. Other diagnostic tests may be obtained if repeat radiographic results are negative after 2 weeks and the patient is still symptomatic or if definitive diagnosis is needed sooner than the planned 2-week follow-up. These tests may include radionuclide bone scan (usually positive within 2-3 days of injury), CT, or MRI.

Immobilization of a potential scaphoid fracture is initiated if suspicion is high even though radiographic results are initially negative. If fracture is ruled out at follow-up visits, treatment is adjusted accordingly. Nondisplaced scaphoid fractures are treated with cast immobilization. Thumb spica casting is essential, but whether the initial cast needs to be a long- or short-arm variety is controversial. Studies have shown decreased time to union and reduced rates of delayed union and nonunion with a long-arm thumb spica cast (Gellman et al., 1989). However, union rates of up to 95% with short-arm casting have been reported. A combination, with a long-arm cast for the initial 6 weeks followed by short-arm casting from 6 weeks until

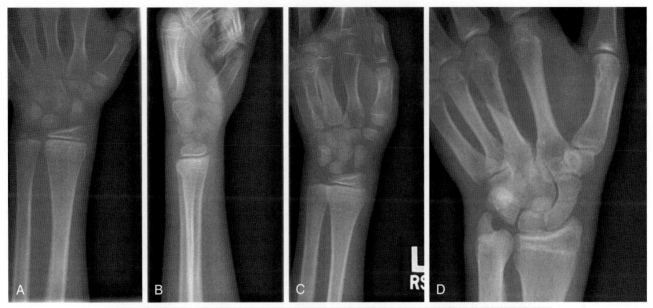

Figure 30-24 Transverse fracture through the waist of the scaphoid. (Courtesy James L. Moeller, MD.)

radiographic healing is present, addresses both of these key issues.

Healing rates and average healing time depend on location of the fracture because the blood supply differs throughout the scaphoid. Nondisplaced distal pole fractures tend to receive a better blood supply and have a healing rate of close to 100%, with average healing time of 10 to 12 weeks. Scaphoid waist fractures have a healing rate of 80% to 90%, with average healing also 10 to 12 weeks. Proximal pole fractures have a healing rate of only 60% to 70%, with average healing time of 12 to 20 weeks. Poor outcomes (i.e., nonunion, malunion) in any scaphoid fracture are more likely to occur if the diagnosis or appropriate treatment is delayed; this is why it is important to initiate treatment based on suspicion of injury with normal radiographs. Displaced fractures (≥1 mm) should be referred to an orthopedic surgeon for consideration of surgical fixation.

EVIDENCE-BASED SUMMARY

- One controlled study showed significant benefit of steroid injections for DeQuervain tenosynovitis. Because of a limited number of patients and limited quality supportive studies, however, definitive recommendations cannot be made (Peters-Veluthamaningal et al., 2009a) (SOR: B).
- Pain and symptoms of people with "trigger finger" may improve with a corticosteroid injection (Peters-Veluthamaningal et al., 2009b) (SOR: A).
- Bone scintigraphy and MRI have equally high sensitivity and high diagnostic value for excluding scaphoid fracture. However, MRI is more specific and better for confirming scaphoid fracture (Yin et al., 2009) (SOR: A). We believe additional studies are needed to assess diagnostic performance of CT.

Hip

Key Points

- Hip osteoarthritis (OA) commonly presents as groin and anterior thigh pain. AP pelvis and lateral hip radiography is recommended for comparison with the other side.
- Greater trochanteric bursitis commonly presents as lateral hip pain that can be reproduced by palpation.
- Avascular necrosis (AVN) of the hip is most commonly associated with prolonged corticosteroid use, alcoholism, and sickle cell disease.
- Hip pain can be referred pain from the lumbar spine.
- Hip fractures are commonly related to osteoporosis, and routine screening should be initiated. Guidelines for screening are updated periodically and based on the United States Preventative Task Force Services Guidelines, http://www.uspreventiveservicestaskforce.org.
- Slipped capital femoral epiphysis (SCFE) is a femoral head growth plate fracture found in adolescent patients. Treatment should be protected weight bearing and urgent referral to an orthopedist for possible surgical intervention.

DEGENERATIVE HIP OSTEOARTHRITIS

An estimated 25% of adults may develop symptomatic hip OA (Murphy, 2010). Degenerative OA of the hip is caused by loss of the hyaline cartilage along the hip joint surfaces. Weight-bearing AP and lateral hip radiographs are strongly recommended to evaluate joint space narrowing and OA extent. MRI is not routinely required and should not be ordered instead of plain radiographs. Radiographic findings include loss of the joint space, presence of osteophytes, subchondral sclerosis, and cysts (Figure 30-25).

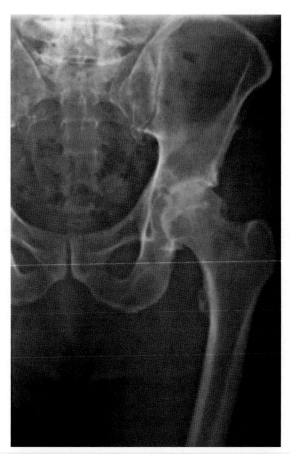

Figure 30-25 Radiograph demonstrating hip arthritis, including joint space narrowing, and superior migration of the femur within the acetabulum. (Reused with permission from Frontera WR, Silver JK, Rizzo TD. *Essentials of physical medicine and rehabilitation.* 2nd ed. Philadelphia: Elsevier; 2008:F48-2.)

Patients with hip OA may complain of groin and anterior thigh pain initially as a deep stiffness or pain when they first get up from a seated position. After a few steps, the pain may subside in the early stages of OA but persist in more severe OA. Additional symptoms include stiffness with walking, difficulty putting on socks and shoes, limping, and difficulty with stair climbing. Physical examination findings often reveal decreased hip ROM (internal rotation and adduction). Logrolling of the hip in a supine position will typically reproduce the symptoms. Additionally, performing the Stinchfield test, resisted supine hip flexion, should reproduce the patient's hip symptoms in the groin and thigh.

Treatment of OA is based on the patient's age, demand, comorbidities, and severity of OA. Conservative treatment for hip arthritis should include a generalized low-impact conditioning program, activity modification to avoid sports or activities that exacerbate the symptoms, weight loss, use of a cane to improve proprioceptive control, use of cushioned shoes, and NSAIDs. Oral supplementation with glucosamine and chondroitin sulfate may also be considered. If these do not provide relief after 4 to 6 weeks, corticosteroid injections can be administered, typically with variable pain relief and duration. Injections may be repeated depending on the patient response. The newest recommendations from the American Academy of Orthopaedic Surgeons (AAOS) do not recommend the routine use of glucosamine

in a routine regimen of approaching patient with OA. Others argue that because they are very low risk, a trial to assess their effectiveness is reasonable. Studies evaluating glucosamine sulfate appear to have better results than those using glucosamine HCl. The dose of glucosamine sulfate is 750 mg twice daily (Sawitzke et al., 2010). Chondroitin is more controversial but may prove helpful in hand OA at a dose of 1200 mg/day (Gabay et al., 2011). In severe OA and resistant cases, a hip replacement can provide excellent pain relief and improve function.

HIP GREATER TROCHANTERIC BURSITIS

Greater trochanteric bursitis is a combination of the inflammation of the bursa surrounding the hip abductor muscles and tendons that attach to the greater trochanteric region of the femur. Typically, this is caused from repetitive overuse or is related to changes in the patient's gait patterns. Evaluate the patient for other musculoskeletal ailments that have changed his or her postures or walking gait (i.e., low back pain, painful ankle, painful knee). The symptoms are typically lateral hip pain with walking and tenderness over the lateral upper part of the femur, which may result in the inability to lie on the affected side.

The diagnosis can be made with a complete history and physical examination and radiography of the hip. Radiography is useful to rule out underlying hip arthritis. MRI is not routinely ordered. The patient will have well-circumscribed area of tenderness over the lateral upper part of the femur. He or she typically has less groin pain, buttock pain, and back pain compared with the lateral areas.

Treatments are based on prevention and correcting body posture and gait patterns, strengthening lower extremity muscles, and increasing flexibility. The primary treatments should start with activity modification, avoiding actions that result in aggravation of the pain; antiinflammatory oral medications; and icing the area. In addition, physical therapy is prescribed for 4 to 6 weeks to work on strengthening and flexibility of the core hip and lumbar spine postural muscles. If these are ineffective, a corticosteroid injection into the inflamed bursal area can be given, which can provide varying amounts of relief. The cortisone shot can be repeated at a minimum of every 3 to 4 months. However, repeated injections of cortisone can weaken and damage the underlying tendons. In rare cases, when the pain does not improve after physical therapy, cortisone shots, and antiinflammatory medication, the inflamed bursa can be removed surgically.

HIP AVASCULAR NECROSIS

Avascular necrosis refers to cellular death of the bone and cartilage due to damage of the blood supply. Most commonly hip femoral head AVN is highly associated with prolonged corticosteroid use, alcoholism, or sickle cell disease (Jacobs, 1978). Specifically, prolonged corticosteroid use for treatment of rheumatologic diseases, asthma, chronic obstructive pulmonary disease, or inflammatory bowel diseases can account for up to 30% of all hip AVN cases (Jacobs, 1978). Alcoholism has been reported to be related to up to 40% of cases of femoral head AVN in several case series (Arlet, 1992; Jacobs, 1978). However, a number of

Table 30-2   Federative Committee on Anatomical Terminology Classification of Avascular Necrosis

	Radiography	MRI	Bone Scan	Clinical Symptoms
Stage 0	Normal	Normal	—	—
Stage I	Normal or minor osteopenia	Edema	Increased uptake	Pain typically in the groin
Stage II	Mixed osteopenia or sclerosis	Geographic defect	Increased uptake	Pain and stiffness
Stage III	Crescent sign and eventual cortical collapse	Same as radiography	+/− Pain and stiffness	Radiation to knee and limp
Stage IV	End stage with evidence of secondary degenerative change	Same as radiography		Pain and limp

MRI, Magnetic resonance imaging.

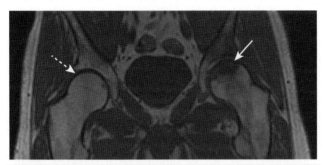

Figure 30-26 Magnetic resonance image of avascular necrosis. A T1-weighted coronal view of both hips demonstrates normal high signal from the fatty marrow in the right femur *(dotted white arrow)* but decreased signal in the left femoral head extending to the subchondral bone of the left hip joint *(solid white arrow).* The joint space is preserved. (Reused with permission from Herring W. *Learning radiology: recognizing the basics.* 2nd ed. Philadelphia: Elsevier; 2011:F21-8.)

Table 30-3   Indications for Bone Mineral Density Testing

Consider bone mineral density testing in the following individuals:
- Women age 65 years and older and men age 70 years and older regardless of clinical risk factors
- Younger postmenopausal women, women in the menopausal transition, and men age 50 to 69 years with clinical risk factors for facture
- Adults who have a fracture after age 50 years
- Adults with a condition (e.g. rheumatoid arthritis) or taking a medication (e.g. glucocorticoids in a daily dose ≥5 mg prednisone or equivalent for ≥3 months) associated with low bone mass or bone loss

From National Osteoporosis Foundation. Having a Bone Density Test. http://nof.org/articles/743.

medical conditions have been associated with AVN, including posttraumatic hip fractures, hemoglobinopathies, hyperuricemia, malignancy, hyperlipidemia, and caisson disease (Arlet, 1992; Jacobs, 1978). AVN often leads to secondary arthritis. Pain is the usual presenting symptoms, most often reported in the groin, radiating to the anterior thigh. Pain is present at rest but worse with weight bearing and hip ROM.

Radiographs of the hip in the AP and lateral plane are recommended. Early stages may not show any changes. Late stages will show cystic and sclerotic changes in the femoral head, subchondral collapse, flattening of the femoral head, and joint space loss. An MRI of the hip without contrast is also recommended in the diagnostic workup to help with the staging. The MRI helps determine the amount or percentage of the femoral head involvement as well as the presence of subchondral collapse, which help determine treatment options (Figure 30-26) (Steinberg, 2001). Hip AVN is a disabling and progressive condition; surgical hip-preserving treatments are successful in the early stages, but more severe cases require a total hip replacement. The key to successful treatment lies in early diagnosis and timely treatments. The FICAT staging system is commonly used to look at the presence or absence of subchondral collapse (Table 30-2). Patients have a more favorable prognosis with hip-preserving procedures such as a core decompression in FICAT stages 1 and 2. After the subchondral bone has collapsed and secondary arthritis has developed, patients typically require a total hip

replacement. The treatment of each patient with hip AVN will depend on the amount and extent of the AVN, presence of subchondral collapse, presence of arthritis, and underlying cause of the AVN.

HIP FRACTURES

Hip fractures in elderly adults pose a significant health care problem worldwide, with a 1-year mortality rate estimated at 30% (Miyamoto, 2008). Hip fractures are most commonly associated from mechanical falls associated with osteoporosis. Osteoporosis is a progressive bone disease characterized by a decrease in bone mass and density, which can lead to an increased risk of fracture. Osteoporosis is defined by the World Health Organization (WHO) as a bone mineral density (BMD) of 2.5 standard deviations or more below the mean peak bone mass (average of young, healthy adults) as measured by dual-energy x-ray absorptiometry (DEXA scan). The National Osteoporosis Foundation (NOF) estimates that more than 10 million people older than age 50 years in the United States have osteoporosis, and another 34 million are at risk for the disease (NOF, 2013). In 2013, the NOF updated its clinical screening guidelines and treatments for patients (NOF, 2013) (Table 30-3).

Treatment focuses on fall prevention and increasing BMD. Modifiable risks factures to prevent falls can focus on balance and gait training through physical therapy and use of an ambulatory aid such as a cane or a walker. In addition, removal of obstacles and loose carpets in the living environment may substantially reduce falls. Proper nutrition and exercise have been shown to increase bone quality.

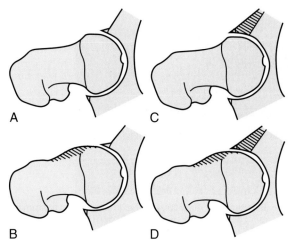

Figure 30-27 Femoral acetabular impingement types. The reduced clearance during joint motion leads to repetitive abutment between the proximal part of the femur and the anterior acetabular rim. **A,** The normal clearance of the hip. **B,** Reduced femoral head and neck offset (cam impingement). **C,** Excessive overcoverage of the femoral head by the acetabulum (pincer impingement). **D,** A combination of reduced head and neck offset and excessive anterior overcoverage (combined impingement). (Reused with permission from Clohisy JC, Beauleé PE, O'Malley A, et al. AOA Symposium: hip disease in the young adult: current concepts of etiology and surgical treatment. *J Bone Joint Surg Am.* 2008;90(suppl A):2267-2281.)

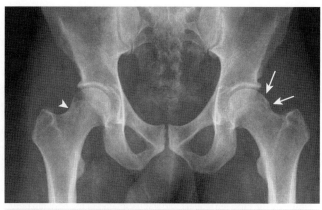

Figure 30-28 Cam-type femoral–acetabular impingement. Frontal radiograph of the pelvis shows osseous prominence *(arrows)* at the anterolateral femoral head–neck junction on the *left* (compare with normal femoral neck concavity on the *right, arrowhead*). (Reused with permission from Miller MD, Sanders TG. *Presentation, imaging and treatment of common musculoskeletal conditions: MRI-arthroscopy correlation.* Philadelphia: Elsevier; 2011:F69-1.)

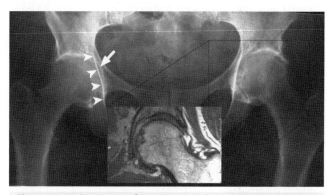

Figure 30-29 Pincer type femoral–acetabular impingement. Frontal radiograph of the pelvis (and coronal magnetic resonance image, *inset*) show a relatively deep acetabular fossa that can lead to overhanging margins and impingement. Note that the medial wall of the acetabulum *(arrow)* extends beyond the margin of the ilioischial line *(arrowheads)*. (Reused with permission from Morrison W. Salvo JP, Busconi B, Wallace R. *Presentation, imaging and treatment of common musculoskeletal conditions.* Philadelphia: Elsevier; 2012:337-344).

Bisphosphonate medications are useful in decreasing the risk of future fractures; this benefit is present when taken for 3 to 5 years, with evidence of little benefit when used for more than 3 to 5 years (Suresh, 2014; Wells, 2008; Whitaker, 2012). With the potential adverse events, it may be appropriate to stop treatment after this time in some.

HIP FEMORAL ACETABULAR IMPINGEMENT

Femoral acetabular impingement (FAI) is a developmental incongruity of the femoral head ball and acetabular socket joint that can cause pain and cartilage damage and lead to secondary hip OA. There are three types of FAI: pincer, cam, and combined impingement (Figures 30-27 to 30-29). Pincer FAI occurs when the acetabulum rim extends too far over the femoral head, providing "overcoverage." The overcoverage of the femoral head from the acetabulum leads to impingement on femoral head and neck bone, with hip flexion, adduction, and internal rotation, which can cause pain. In addition, the hip labrum can be compressed and tear from the abnormal articulation. The hip labrum is a fibrocartilaginous extension of the acetabulum that aids in hip stability. CAM FAI occurs when the femoral head contour is asymmetric or "overgrown" in one area and cannot rotate in the socket freely. Typically, it is the antero-lateral aspect of the femoral head and neck, causing pain with hip flexion, internal rotation, and adduction. The third type of FAI, known as mixed impingement, is a combination of both pincer and CAM FAI.

Femoral acetabular impingement develops from incongruent and asymmetric development of the ball and socket during childhood. It is the deformity of the two bones that leads to FAI, subsequent cartilage damage, and hip pain. Patients with FAI usually have pain in the groin area that

is worse with activities such as twisting at the hip and hip flexion. It can be described as a dull ache or sharp stabbing pain.

Physical examination testing commonly performed involves having the patient lie supine, flexing the hip up to 90 degrees, and internally rotating the hip with combined adduction. This should reproduce the patient's symptoms. FAI can be diagnosed with a radiographic evaluation. The radiographs should include AP and lateral radiographs of the affected hip and possibly the unaffected hip for comparison. CT scans are not routinely ordered. MRI of the hip can be useful and is typically ordered for evaluation of the labrum.

Treatment of FAI varies depending on the severity of FAI, activity level of the patient, age of the patient, and whether secondary OA has developed in the hip joint. Nonsurgical treatment should always be considered first when treating FAI. Nonsurgical treatment will not change the underlying bone incongruity, but FAI symptoms can often be resolved

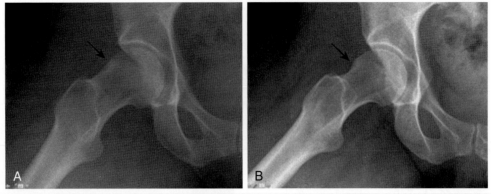

Figure 30-30 Frog-leg lateral radiographic images of the right hip before (**A**) and after (**B**) femoral neck osteoplasty. The *arrow* points to the cam lesion before resection and to the area of bony resection thereafter. (Reused with permission from Chow RM, Kuzma SA, Krych AJ, Levy BA. Arthroscopic femoral neck osteoplasty in the treatment of femoroacetabular impingement. *Arthrosc Tech.* 3(1):e21-5.)

with rest, modifying one's behavior, and a physical therapy or antiinflammatory regimen (or both). An intraarticular hip cortisone injection can also provide relief. Such conservative treatments have been successful in reducing the pain and swelling in the joint. If the pain persists after conservative management, surgery may be recommended. Surgery for FAI varies depending on the severity of the FAI, activity level of the patient, age of the patient, and if secondary OA has developed in the hip joint. Surgery for FAI involves reshaping of the acetabulum and femoral head to remove the impingement. Additional repair of the labrum may be required. Surgery to reshape the femoral head and acetabulum is known as "osteoplasty" and can be done via an open technique or arthroscopically (Figure 30-30). However, if the patient has already developed secondary arthritis because of the FAI, a surgeon may not recommend osteoplasty but rather a total hip replacement. Surgery can successfully reduce symptoms caused by impingement and can prevent future damage to the hip joint. However, sometimes not all of the damage can be completely fixed by surgery, especially if treatment has been put off and the damage is severe and it is possible that more problems may develop in the future (Bedi, 2013).

HIP SLIPPED CAPITAL FEMORAL EPIPHYSIS

SCFE is a fracture through the femoral head growth plate that occurs most commonly in adolescents aged 11 to 15 years. SCFE affects approximately one to 10 per 100,000 children, has a higher prevalence in African American patients, and affects boys twice as often as girls (Kliegman, 2011; Novais et al., 2012). The incidence varies by geographic location, season of the year, and ethnicity. It is strongly linked to obesity, endocrine disorders, trauma, and family history (Kliegman, 2011; Novais et al., 2012). There is a relationship of hypothyroid and short stature specifically with SCFE (Kliegman, 2011; Novais et al., 2012). SCFEs usually cause groin pain on the affected side and can radiate to the knee or thigh. Symptoms include the gradual, progressive onset of hip, thigh, or knee pain with a painful limp. Clinical examination will show obligate external rotation with hip flexion and loss of internal rotation.

Radiographic evaluation should include an AP and frog-leg lateral radiograph of bilateral hips (Figure 30-31).

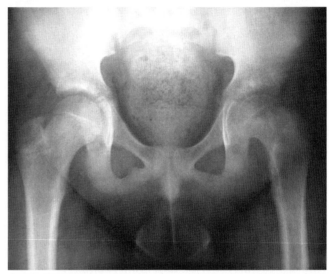

Figure 30-31 Radiographic representation of a slipped capital femoral epiphysis on the left hip. (Reused with permission from Miller MD, Hart J, MacKnight JM. *Essential orthopaedics.* Philadelphia: Elsevier; 2009:F221-1.)

Bilateral involvement occurs in up to 30% of patients. Klein's line is a line drawn along the superior border of the femoral neck and should cross at least a portion of the femoral epiphysis. A slip must be suspected if a straight line drawn up the lateral surface of the femoral neck does not touch the femoral head on the lateral view (Figures 30-32 and 30-33).

Treatment of SCFE is surgical, and the goal is to prevent any additional slipping of the femoral head until the growth plate closes. Surgical treatment will vary depending on the degree of the slip and age of the patient. In mild slips, a single screw can be placed percutaneously across the femoral physis to stabilize the slip in situ and facilitate physeal closure (Figure 30-34). More severe slips with greater deformity may require open reduction and stabilization. Patients should be made non–weight bearing, given crutches, and referred to an orthopedic surgeon urgently. Treatment should be immediate. Early diagnosis of SCFE provides the best chance to achieve the treatment goal of stabilizing the hip.

Knee

Key Points

- In clinical examination of ligament injuries about the knee, the Lachman test is the most sensitive for anterior cruciate ligament (ACL) instability.
- The clinician should maintain a high level of suspicion of associated ligament injuries, especially the lateral collateral ligament (LCL) and posterolateral corner. Acute surgical intervention (within 3 weeks) of LCL and posterolateral corner injuries significantly improves prognosis.

- Viscosupplementation (injection of hyaluronate), corticosteroids injections, therapeutic exercise, and oral supplementation with glucosamine and chondroitin sulfate may all provide some symptomatic relief and functional improvement for generalized knee arthritis. Arthroscopic debridement alone (in the absence of loose bodies, cartilage flaps, and meniscus tears) may not provide relief.
- Vertical, peripheral meniscus tears in the vascular zone of the meniscus of young patients should be treated with meniscus repair whenever possible to avoid focal increased pressures in the articular surface and future risk of degenerative joint disease.
- In older patients with degenerative meniscus pathology and no locking, prevention of arthritic progression may be surgical or nonsurgical. When performed, partial is preferred to complete meniscectomy.

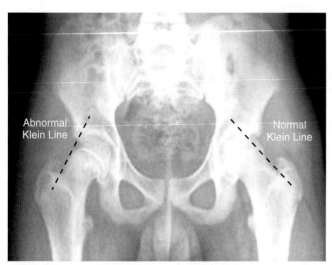

Figure 30-32 Anteroposterior pelvis radiograph demonstrating the Klein line intersecting the epiphysis on the right hip. In the left hip, which shows a slipped capital femoral epiphysis, the Klein line passes just lateral to the epiphysis. (Reused with permission from Aronsson DD, Loder RD, Brerur GJ, Weinstein ST. Slipped capital femoral epiphysis: current concepts. *J Am Acad Orthop Surg*. 2006;14(12):666-679.)

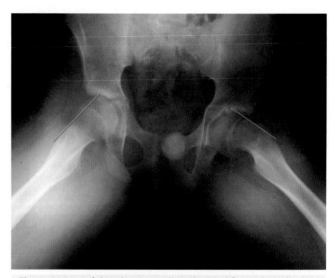

Figure 30-33 Left hip showing a slipped capital femoral epiphysis in the frog-leg lateral, right hip normal position.

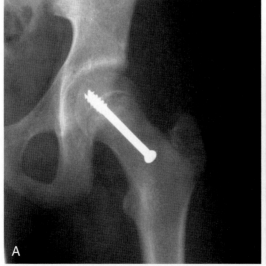
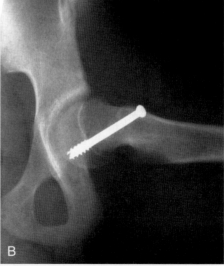

Figure 30-34 Anteroposterior (**A**) and frog-leg lateral (**B**) radiographs of a single in situ pinning of a left slipped capital femoral epiphysis (SCFE). Note that in the image on the left, the relationship between the epiphysis and metaphysis would be considered normal. However, on the lateral view, a large posterior displacement of the epiphysis is seen, thus confirming the SCFE. This emphasizes the necessity of lateral radiographs in making this diagnosis. (Reused with permission from Miller MD, Hart J, MacKnight JM. *Essential orthopaedics*. Philadelphia: Elsevier; 2009:F221-3.)

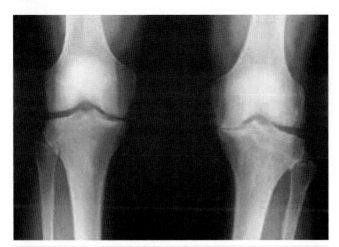

Figure 30-35 Weight-bearing knee radiographs showing osteoarthritis.

DEGENERATIVE OSTEOARTHRITIS

Degenerative OA of the knee is caused by loss of the hyaline cartilage along the knee joint surfaces. This can occur in an isolated compartment or diffusely throughout all three compartments of the knee. OA more often develops in the medial side or medial compartment of the knee, first leading to joint space narrowing and varus, or bowleg, deformity. Loss of articular cartilage and joint space on the lateral aspect of the knee leads to valgus or knock-knee deformity. Weight-bearing (standing flexed-knee PA) radiographs are strongly recommended to evaluate joint space narrowing and OA extent. Lateral and patella sunrise tangential views complete the study (Figure 30-35). MRI is not routinely required and should not be ordered instead of plain radiography. MRI is best reserved for mechanical pathology or preoperative planning. Radiographic findings include loss of the joint space, presence of osteophytes, subchondral sclerosis, and cysts.

Patients with OA typically complain of knee pain and stiffness with walking after prolonged sitting, descending stairs, and early in the morning. Swelling of knees and worse symptoms are typical with weather changes. Physical examination findings often reveal decreased ROM (flexion contractures), knee varus or valgus deformity, joint line tenderness, and crepitus with palpation during ROM.

Treatment of OA is based on the patient's age, demand, comorbidities, and severity of OA. Conservative treatment for knee arthritis should include a generalized conditioning program, weight loss, a knee brace to improve the proprioceptive control, cushioned shoes, and NSAIDs. Oral supplementation with glucosamine and chondroitin sulfate may also be considered. If these do not provide relief after 4 to 6 weeks, corticosteroid or viscosupplement injections can be administered, typically with variable pain relief and duration. Injections may be repeated depending on patient response. The newest recommendations from the AAOS do not recommend the routine use of glucosamine or viscosupplementation in a routine regimen of approaching patients with OA. Others argue that because they are very low risk, a trial to assess their effectiveness is reasonable. In resistant cases, total or partial knee replacement can provide excellent pain relief and improve function. The effect of arthroscopy in patients with degenerative arthritis remains controversial (Hunt et al., 2002; Mosely et al., 2002). However, arthroscopy in the absence of loose bodies, cartilage flaps, or meniscal pathology is unlikely to be unsuccessful (Sihvonen et al., 2013).

EVIDENCE-BASED SUMMARY

- The short-term benefit of intraarticular corticosteroid in treatment of knee OA is well established; however, longer-term benefits have not been confirmed, and the response to viscosupplemental hyaluronic products may have more durability (Bellamy et al., 2005a) (SOR: A).
- Based on a single RCT, bracing for OA may provide additional benefit compared with medical treatment alone (Brouwer et al., 2005) (SOR: B).
- Land-based therapeutic exercise programs reduce pain and improve physical function for patients with OA of the knee (Brosseau et al., 2003; Fransen et al., 2001) (SOR: A).
- Viscosupplementation (injection of hyaluronate) is an effective treatment for OA of the knee, with beneficial effects on pain and function (Bellamy et al., 2005b) (SOR: A).
- Nonglucosamine preparations failed to show benefit, but glucosamine preparations were superior to placebo in the treatment of pain and functional impairment resulting from symptomatic OA (Towhead et al., 2009) (SOR: A).
- Arthroscopic debridement has no benefit for undiscriminated OA with mechanical or inflammatory causes (Laupattarakasem et al., 2009; Sihvonen et al., 2013) (SOR: A).
- In OA patients, exercise results in a modest reduction in pain and a modest improvement in physical function (Fransen and McConnell, 2009) (SOR: B).
- The newest recommendations from the AAOS based on an evidence-based review of the literature do not recommend the inclusion of glucosamine or viscosupplementation in the treatment regimen for OA.

INFECTIONS

Intraarticular joint infections are orthopedic emergencies and require urgent surgical irrigation and debridement as well as long-term antibiotic therapy. The most common source of infection is *Staphylococcus aureus,* which aggressively and quickly destroys cartilage and leaves the patient with permanent OA. Patients with a knee joint infection present with increased pain, swelling, warmth, redness, fever, and decreased ability to ambulate on that leg. Most patients will not want to move their knee at all. The knee should be aspirated and the fluid inspected and sent for laboratory analysis (Gram stain, cell count, culture, crystal evaluation). Crystalline arthropathy such as gout should always be considered because the aspirated fluid often appears cloudy and may mimic a joint infection. C-reactive protein and erythrocyte sedimentation rate should also be obtained. Appropriate antibiotic treatment is initiated based on the offending organism. Although proposed in the medical literature for low-virulent organisms, serial aspiration is discouraged in the orthopedic literature, with surgical irrigation being the preferred treatment.

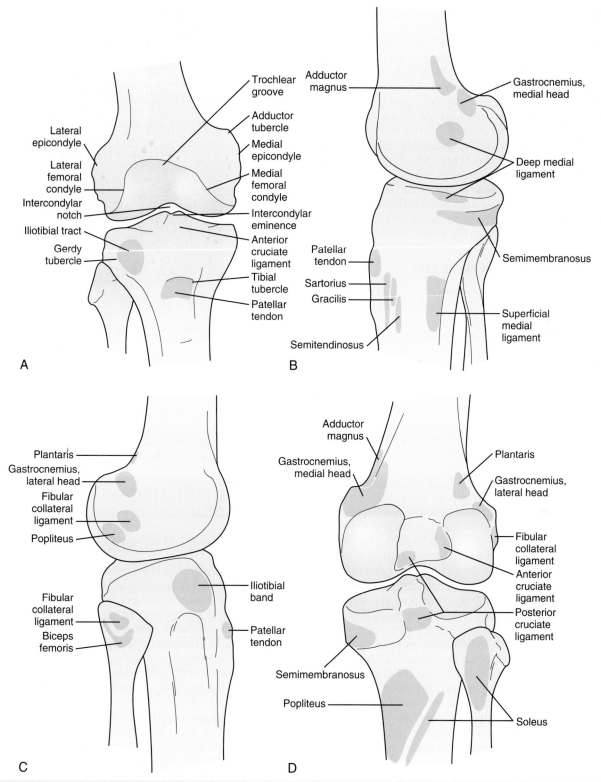

Figure 30-36 Schematic showing anatomic sites of bursae around the knee. **A,** Anterior view. **B,** Medial view. **C,** Lateral view. **D,** Posterior view.

INFLAMMATORY CONDITIONS

Bursae are synovial fluid–filled structures or "cushions" that pad bony prominences as protection against repetitive impact from external forces or snapping anatomic structures, such as ligaments or tendons. Several bursae around the knee can become inflamed; irritated; and rarely, infected, including the prepatellar bursa, infrapatellar bursa, pes anserine bursa, and iliotibial (IT) band bursa (beneath the IT band laterally). Knowing their anatomic location is important so that these bursae can be palpated directly (Figure 30-36).

Treatment of *bursitis* includes compression, ice, protective padding, and avoidance of impact on the bursa. NSAIDs may help to reduce swelling. If the fluid collection is large or an infection is suspected, aspiration of the bursa can be performed in the office with a large-bore needle under sterile conditions. The bursa fluid should be clear and straw colored; it may be bloody in a traumatic injury. If an infection is not suspected clinically after the fluid is withdrawn, a corticosteroid can be injected. Corticosteroids should never be injected if infection is a possibility. Oral antibiotics can be started if an infection is present. Local incision and debridement may be required with infection and abscess. Aspiration does not replace compression wrap, ice, and avoidance of impact. Reaccumulation of fluid may occur, but total volume usually decreases. Serial aspirations are an option in patients with recurrent aseptic bursitis.

EXTENSOR MECHANISM PROBLEMS

The extensor mechanism comprises the quadriceps muscle, quadriceps tendon, patella, and patellar tendon. The differential diagnosis of problems in the extensor mechanism is broad, including muscle or tendon rupture, patellar fracture, patellar tendinopathy, patellofemoral syndrome, patellar instability, Osgood-Schlatter disease, and symptomatic medial plica. Examination of patients with anterior knee pain or extensor mechanism problems should always include a careful evaluation of the lumbar spine and hip to rule out referred pain, as well as assessment of the antagonist hamstring muscles posteriorly. Cores of gluteal weakness as well as hamstring tightness can exacerbate problems of tendinosis, patellofemoral syndrome, and instability.

If the patient presents with focal tenderness over the patellar tendon at the distal pole of the patella, or potentially at the quadriceps insertion onto the patella, the likely diagnosis is tendinopathy. Numerous studies show that chronic repetitive overuse does not actually lead to inflammation of the tendon itself but rather to a central degeneration or tendinosis of the fibers of the tendon (Fithian, 2002). Steroid injections into patellar tendinosis are highly discouraged because they may predispose the tendon to complete failure. Treatment protocols for patellar tendinosis, or "jumper's knee," should include hamstring stretching, quadriceps strengthening with eccentric loading, and occasionally the use of a counterforce brace (Figure 30-37).

Alternative treatments, including deep friction massage, prolotherapy, platelet-rich plasma injections, topical antiinflammatory drugs, ultrasonic waves, and radiofrequency probes, show mixed results. Although no RCTs have yet proved their efficacy, these modalities have had some success. Surgical intervention for debridement of the tendinosis is uncommon but may be necessary to provide long-term relief. In a skeletally immature patient, tenderness at the distal pole of the patella may represent an avulsion apophysitis called Sinding-Larsen-Johansson disease. If a skeletally immature patient has pain at the insertion of the patellar tendon on the tibia, the most likely diagnosis is an apophysitis of the tibial tubercle, or Osgood-Schlatter disease. Both problems are more common during active phases of growth and are generally treated conservatively with rest, flexibility exercises, and a gradual return to activity. Complete failure or rupture of the extensor mechanism

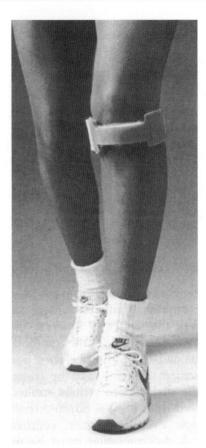

Figure 30-37 A counterforce brace (Cho-Pat strap) can be effective in reducing symptoms of patellar tendinosis (jumper's knee).

at the patellar or quadriceps tendon requires surgical repair (Ilan et al., 2002).

PATELLOFEMORAL SYNDROME

Anterior knee pain has been variously termed patellofemoral syndrome and chondromalacia patellae. When treating anterior knee pain, the physician should identify the specific pathology to initiate targeted treatment. *Chondromalacia patellae*, or degenerative changes on the undersurface of the patella, is more common in young females. Pain complaints related to chondromalacia are exacerbated by sitting for an extended period with a flexed knee, doing deep squats, or going up and down stairs. Each of these activities increases the posteriorly directly forces of the patella, directing increased pressure onto the chondral surfaces.

Treatment of these early arthritic changes is typically rehabilitation. Surgical intervention, such as cartilage scraping and debridement, has not been shown to provide long-term relief or benefit. In rare patients who have associated tight lateral retinacular structures and patellar tilt, surgical release of the lateral retinaculum can provide benefit. Conservative treatment of patellofemoral syndrome includes cushioned shoes, rehabilitation focused on the vastus medialis obliquus muscle, reductive taping techniques, hamstring stretches, and NSAIDs. Correction of the foot alignment with orthotic devices is also a treatment option, but supportive evidence is limited. Seventy percent to 80% of patients will improve with this conservative treatment. Unfortunately, the remaining patients with resistant symptoms can have a frustrating long-term therapeutic course, with a guarded prognosis for any surgical intervention. Ultrasound therapy had no clinically important effect on patients with patellofemoral pain syndrome (Brosseau et al., 2001).

MENISCUS INJURIES

The menisci are fibrocartilaginous structures situated on the tibial plateau both medially and laterally that help disperse the weight-bearing contact forces across the knee joint cartilage surfaces (Figure 30-38). In the presence of a meniscus tear or the complete absence of a meniscus, focal stresses increase. This in turn increases the loading of the hyaline cartilage and early progressive degenerative arthritis (Sherman, 1996). Meniscus tears can occur with axial loading but primarily occur because of twisting, cutting, or rotational forces. In older patients, meniscus tears may simply be a progression of the normal degenerative process. On physical examination, patients have pain over the medial or lateral joint line and may complain of snapping, popping, or catching within the knee (Greis et al., 2002a, 2002b). Varus or valgus loading may exacerbate pain as the meniscus is squeezed between the bony structures. Recurrent effusions may also represent intraarticular pathology. The most common test for meniscus injury is the McMurray test (Figure 30-39). The knee is hyperflexed, stressed with varus

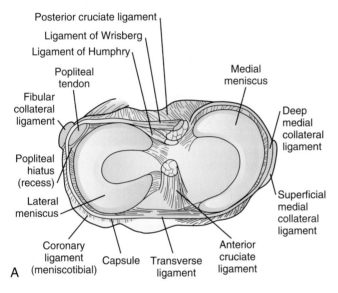

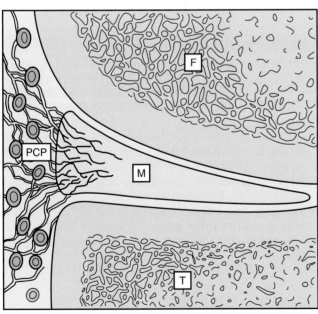

Figure 30-38 Medial and lateral meniscus anatomy as viewed from above (**A**) and via cross-section (**B**). Note the circulation provided to the peripheral third of the meniscus only.

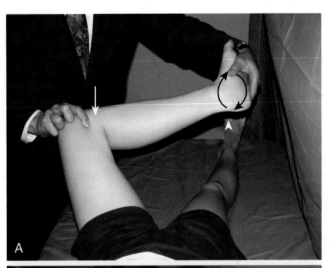

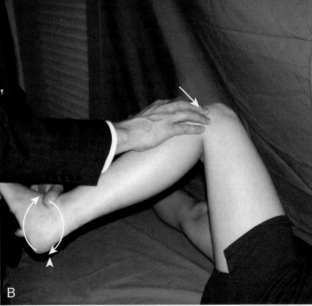

Figure 30-39 Classic examination for meniscal pathology. **A,** The medial McMurray test is performed by palpating along the medial joint line *(thin arrow)* while creating a varus force *(solid triangle)*, ranging the knee through flexion and extension and internally and externally rotating the leg *(yellow arrows)*. A positive finding is noted when the maneuver recreates the symptoms *and* the examiner feels a palpable click. **B,** The lateral McMurray test is done in a similar manner with valgus stress. (Courtesy Mark R. Hutchinson, MD.)

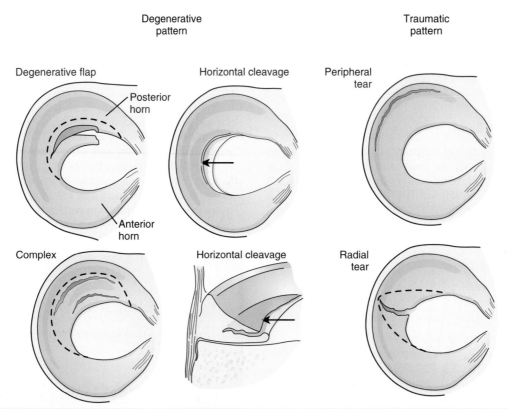

Degenerative pattern   Traumatic pattern

Degenerative flap   Horizontal cleavage   Peripheral tear

Posterior horn

Anterior horn

Complex   Horizontal cleavage   Radial tear

Figure 30-40 Representations of meniscus pathology. Degenerative tears tend to be complex, fibrinous, and horizontal. Acute tears that are vertical in the periphery may be reparable.

or valgus load, and internally and externally rotated as the knee is brought into full extension. More simply, the examiner uses the lower leg and tibia to try to trap the torn meniscus between the tibia and the femur through a full knee ROM. If the examiner feels a snapping or a pop along the joint line and the patient simultaneously complains of pain, the test result is considered positive and highly indicative of a meniscus tear. A single finding may raise suspicion of a tear but does not confirm its presence. Indeed, sensitivity of both findings, the pop and pain, is greater than 90%. MRI can be used to confirm the diagnosis or assist with preoperative planning but should never replace a thorough physical examination.

Definitive treatment of meniscus pathology depends on the actual pattern and location of the meniscus injury on MRI, age of the patient, activity level of the patient, and if coexisting OA is present in the knee. (Greis et al., 2002a, 2002b; Katz et al., 2013; Sherman, 1996; Sihovenon, 2013) (Figure 30-40). Treatment options can be nonsurgical and surgical depending on all of the above factors. Initial treatment may include physical therapy, activity modification, NSAIDs, analgesics, ice, and cortisone injections. If initial conservative treatment fails, then surgery may be indicated. However, surgery may be indicated sooner in younger, more active patients with more substantial meniscus tears. The meniscus can either be reparable or nonreparable depending on the size, location, and patient's age. Because of its essential role in sharing load and preventing the progression of degenerative arthritis, salvageable meniscus tears should always be repaired if possible. After

debridement, patients can bear weight as tolerated and usually return to full activities by about 3 or 4 weeks. With meniscus repair, recovery is extended and requires restricted weight bearing for 3 to 6 weeks, with 2 to 3 months needed before a return to unrestricted activities.

EVIDENCE-BASED SUMMARY

- Definitive treatment of a meniscus tear depends on the actual pattern and location of the meniscus injury on MRI, additional ligament or cartilage injuries, the age of the patient, and the activity level of the patient. If coexisting OA is present in the knee, nonsurgical and surgical options both have a role depending on the aforementioned factors (Greis et al., 2002; Katz et al., 2013; Sherman, 1996; Sihvonen et al., 2013) (SOR: B).
- In a meta-analysis, sensitivity and specificity were 70% and 71% for the McMurray test, 60% and 70% for the Apley test, and 63% and 77% for joint line tenderness, respectively; no single test appears to diagnose a torn tibial meniscus accurately (Hegedus et al., 2007) (SOR: A).

LIGAMENTOUS INJURIES

Four major ligaments keep the knee stable: the ACL, posterior cruciate ligament (PCL), MCL, and LCL. They can be injured in isolation or in combinations related to knee dislocations. Most ligament injuries about the knee are

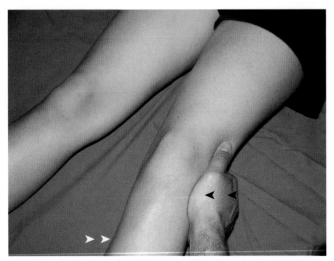

Figure 30-41 Valgus stress is used to assess function of the medial collateral ligament (MCL). To best isolate the MCL, the knee is unlocked to 30 degrees of flexion when stress is applied. If the knee is still unstable in full extension, other structures (posterior cruciate ligament, anterior cruciate ligament, posterior capsule) have been injured. *Black arrowheads* represent a valgus, or medially directed, force, and *white arrowheads* represent a varus, or laterally directed, force. (Courtesy Mark R. Hutchinson, MD.)

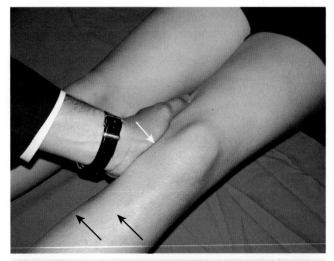

Figure 30-42 Varus stress is used to assess function of the lateral collateral ligament. Varus laxity noted in an acute knee injury should *always* be referred to an orthopedic surgeon; urgent primary repair of injured structures has a better prognosis than delayed reconstruction. *Black arrows* represent a valgus, or medially directed, force, and the *white arrow* represents a varus, or laterally directed, force. (Courtesy Mark R. Hutchinson, MD.)

not urgent. However, the primary care physician must remember (1) always to look out for the potential of a multi-ligament knee injury and the possibility of an arterial injury and (2) always to assess the LCL based on the significantly poorer prognosis if the diagnosis and treatment are delayed beyond 4 to 6 weeks. Early identification and surgical repair of acute LCL injuries improve patient outcomes from 50% to 90%.

Medial Collateral Ligament

The MCL is the most frequently injured ligament of the knee and is often associated with concomitant ligamentous injuries; 95% are associated ACL ruptures. The MCL is the primary knee restraint to valgus loads. The MCL is tested in isolation at 30 degrees of knee flexion with a valgus load (Figure 30-41); at 0 degrees, bony constraints contribute to stability. Valgus laxity at near or full extension implies concurrent injury to the posteromedial capsule or cruciate ligaments. Grade 1 injuries have pathologic laxity, indicated by increased medial joint space widening, of 1 to 4 mm; grade 2, laxity of 5 to 9 mm; and grade 3, more than 10 mm of increased laxity compared to the contralateral side.

Imaging studies should include AP and lateral radiographs looking for associated bone injury or avulsions. MRI may be of benefit in more severe injuries to look for additional associated soft tissue injuries. The initial treatment is nonsurgical for grade 1, 2, and 3 ligament sprains. Protected weight bearing is allowed with crutches and a hinged knee brace until pain resolves medially. Unrestricted ROM is allowed and encouraged. Most patients with MCL injuries do well with conservative treatment. Occasionally, patients with grade 3 injuries who do not respond to nonoperative treatment may require surgery. Timing of return to sports or function is related to severity of injury: grade 1 injuries, usually 1 week; grade 2, 2 to 4 weeks; and grade 3, 4 to 8 weeks.

Lateral Collateral Ligament and Posterolateral Ligament Complex

When evaluating the lateral side of the knee, the physician should evaluate the function of the LCL but also the stability of the knee to posterolateral rotation. The LCL is assessed with the knee unlocked at about 20 to 30 degrees of flexion with varus stress (Figure 30-42). The posterolateral corner is tested by externally rotating the tibia when the knee is flexed at 30 and 90 degrees. If an increased spinout to external rotation is visualized compared with the opposite knee at 30 and 90 degrees, the patient has a posterolateral corner and PCL injury. If the knee spins out only at 30 degrees compared with the opposite side, an isolated posterolateral corner injury is present (Figure 30-43). Imaging usually includes AP and lateral radiographs and MRI. Perhaps the simplest rule for primary care physicians is that any patient with acute varus instability (injury of LCL) should be referred to an orthopedic surgeon as soon as possible.

Treatment is based on the severity of the injury. Nonsurgical treatment with protected weight bearing and protected ROM early for a few weeks is recommended for isolated grade 1 or 2 LCL; grade 1 is an opening of the lateral joint line less than 5 mm, and grade 2 is an opening of 6 to 10 mm. Progressive ROM and functional rehabilitation are initiated. Return to sports can be expected in 6 to 8 weeks. Surgical indications are recommended for isolated grade 3 LCL injuries (>10 mm gapping) and any rotator instability of the posterolateral corner. Acute surgery has more favorable outcomes, and early referral to an orthopedic surgeon is recommended.

Posterior Cruciate Ligament

The PCL is the primary restraint to posterior tibial translation in the knee. The most sensitive test for the PCL is the posterior drawer, which is a posterior-directed force on the

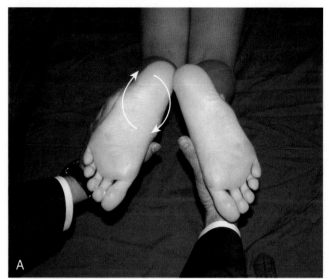

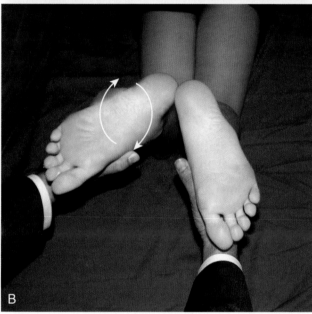

Figure 30-43 The dial test is used to assess the posterior cruciate ligament (PCL) and posterolateral corner and is best done with patient prone and knees together. **A,** A normal examination result should reveal symmetry with forced external rotation. **B,** If increased external rotation is identified with knee flexed 30 degrees, an injury to the posterolateral corner is identified. If asymmetry persists as knee is flexed to 90 degrees, the PCL is likely also involved. (Courtesy Mark R. Hutchinson, MD.)

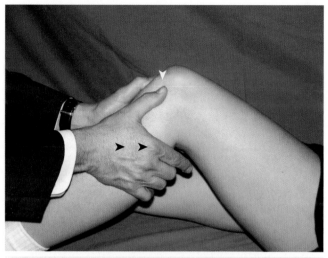

Figure 30-44 The posterior drawer test is the most sensitive test for evaluating posterior cruciate ligament function. Place the thumbs on the femoral condyles, feeling the tibial offset at the level of the joint line *(black arrow).* Then create a posteriorly directed force *(white arrows)* and reassess the tibial step-off. (Courtesy Mark R. Hutchinson, MD.)

Typically, grades I, II, and III are treated nonsurgically with bracing and functional rehabilitation to focus on quadriceps strengthening. PCL ruptures, unlike ACL ruptures, tend to heal, and often a grade III will heal as a grade II and a grade II as a grade I, with appropriate bracing and protection. Mild PCL laxity is usually not symptomatic for patients. If the knee becomes unstable over time, reconstruction can be performed with exactly the same technique that would have been used if performed acutely.

Anterior Cruciate Ligament

The ACL is perhaps the most famous of knee ligaments because of its notoriety in twisting and cutting sports. The common presentation of an ACL injury is an athlete landing in a twisting and cutting sport, feeling a pop, and having an acute hemarthrosis within 24 hours. The most sensitive test for ACL rupture is a Lachman test, which is basically an anterior translation of the tibia on the femur with the knee flexed 20 to 30 degrees (Figure 30-45). The anterior drawer test is also used but is less sensitive (Figure 30-46). The most specific test is the "pivot shift."

The initial treatment of ACL injury focuses on rehabilitation to regain ROM and strengthen the knee. Surgical indications are based on the patient's function as well as future demands (Beynnon et al., 2005). For young athletes who want to play a twisting or cutting sport more than two or three times per week, ACL reconstruction is strongly recommended. The key reason for that indication is the absolute requirement to avoid the current instability or pivoting. Recurrent wobbling or pivoting of the knee leads to an increase in stress along the meniscus, meniscal failure, meniscal degeneration, hyaline cartilage degeneration, and degenerative changes in the knee. If the athlete is willing to give up his or her sport, with no complaints of instability performing ADLs, surgical ACL reconstruction is not always necessary.

knee with the knee flexed to about 90 degrees (Figure 30-44). The PCL is usually injured secondary to a posteriorly directed force on the tibia, from a fall, or potentially from a dashboard injury during a motor vehicle crash. Grading of the PCL injury is based on the posterior drawer test and the relationship of the proximal tibia to the femoral condyles. In grade I PCL injuries, the tibial plateau is slightly anterior to the femoral condyles; in grade II, the plateau and condyles sit flush at the same level; and in grade III, the tibia is posterior to the level. Treatment of a PCL injury is guided by injury severity and associated ligamentous injuries (Cosgarea and Jay, 2001; Wind and Bergfield, 2004).

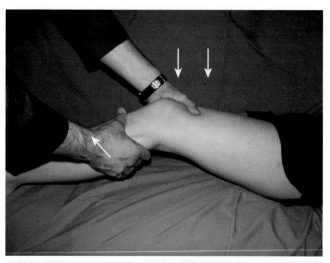

Figure 30-45 The Lachman test is the most sensitive approach to assess anterior cruciate ligament function. The femur is stabilized *(white arrows)* with the knee flexed about 15 to 20 degrees and the tibia drawn anteriorly *(white arrow)*. Comparison with the opposite side and assessment of a ropelike end point are key.

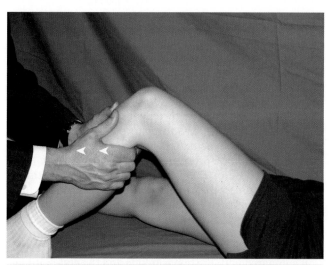

Figure 30-46 The anterior drawer test is less sensitive for isolating anterior cruciate ligament injuries but may assist in diagnosing associated pathology. The knee is flexed 90 degrees, and the tibia is drawn anteriorly. The *white arrowheads* represent an anteriorly directed force as the examiner pulls the tibia anteriorly with respect to the femur. (Courtesy Mark R. Hutchinson, MD.)

Skeletally immature athletes pose a unique challenge because of their open growth plates. Treatment options include delay of definitive surgical reconstruction until maturity, extraarticular reconstruction, and reconstruction with soft tissue across the physis (Bates et al., 2004). Most studies have shown that children are not fully cooperative with programs that have them reduce activities until skeletal maturity. This leads to recurrent episodes of instability with associated meniscal and cartilage damage. Based on this, there has been a strong trend to surgically stabilize these young athletes to reduce the risk of arthrosis at a young age.

EVIDENCE-BASED SUMMARY

- No RCTs have compared surgical and nonsurgical outcomes in reduction of future osteoarthritic change for PCL injuries (Peccin et al., 1995) (SOR: A).
- Based on two clinical trials in the 1980s and insufficient RCTs, no conclusions can be drawn about conservative versus surgical treatment of ACL ruptures in adults (Linko et al., 2005).
- Surgical stabilization should be considered for skeletally immature patients with ACL injuries because they carry a high risk of recurrent instability and subsequent injury and damage to the meniscus (Bates et al., 2004) (SOR: B).

Ankle and Foot

Key Points

- Radiographs for foot and ankle imaging should be weight bearing if a fracture does not preclude it.
- Radiographs are not necessary in all cases of suspected ankle sprain.
- Early mobilization with an external supportive device usually leads to a quicker recovery from ankle sprain, although it may not affect the long-term outcome.
- Although corticosteroid injections can provide short-term relief of plantar fasciitis pain, no single intervention appears superior to another.
- Fractures through the watershed area of blood supply in the proximal fifth metatarsal (Jones fracture) have a high risk of nonunion or malunion.

The foot and ankle are complex structures that provide the foundation to gait and the upright musculoskeletal structure. They are intimately related to a person's ability to ambulate, run, jump, and traverse unstable and variable terrain. Optimal foot and ankle function implies a higher level of function for ADLs. Thorough examination and imaging should consider a broad differential diagnosis of common problems, including ligament sprains, stress fractures, fractures and avulsions, chronic tendinopathies, and tendon ruptures. A more expansive differential diagnosis includes nerve entrapment, circulatory dysfunction, and systemic disease, as well as congenital and developmental problems. All radiographic imaging of the foot and ankle for pain should be weight-bearing views, in the absence of suspicion of a fracture, to allow a more accurate clinical picture because the patient usually experiences pain when weight bearing and not at rest (Stiell et al., 1992, 1993).

ANKLE SPRAINS

Sprains are injuries to the ligamentous structures of the ankle. About 85% of ankle sprains involve the lateral ligaments; medial and syndesmosis sprains make up the remaining 15%. The diagnosis is based primarily on the history and physical examination, although radiographs are often helpful. Advanced diagnostic testing is not usually

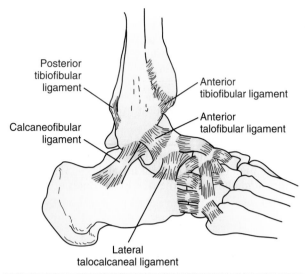

Figure 30-47 Anatomy of lateral ankle ligaments. (From Nicholas J, Hershman E. *The lower extremity and spine in sports medicine.* Vol 1, 2nd ed. St. Louis: Mosby; 1995:424.)

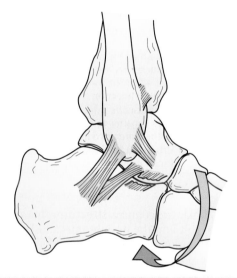

Figure 30-48 Forceful inversion of the hindfoot with a plantarflexed ankle, possibly tearing the anterior talofibular and interosseous talocalcaneal ligaments. (From Meyer JM, Garcia J, Hoffmeyer P, et al. The subtalar sprain: a roentgenographic study. *Clin Orthop.* 1988;226:169-173.)

necessary. The family physician must be aware of the many potential pitfalls in the diagnosis of ankle sprains as well.

Lateral Ankle Sprains

The anterior talofibular ligament (ATFL), calcaneofibular ligament (CFL), and posterior talofibular ligament (PTFL) are the three ligaments of the lateral ankle (Figure 30-47). The ATFL primarily restricts anterior motion of the talus within the ankle mortise, the CFL restricts inversion, and the PTFL restricts posterior translation. The most common mechanism of lateral ankle sprain is an *inversion* ankle injury. Inversion events with the ankle in a plantarflexed position often lead to ATFL injury (Figure 30-48); inversion events with the ankle in a dorsiflexed position more often lead to CFL injury (Figure 30-49). Patients present because of ankle pain that may be associated with swelling,

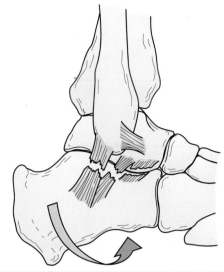

Figure 30-49 Forceful inversion of the hindfoot with a dorsiflexed ankle, possibly tearing the calcaneofibular, cervical, and interosseous talocalcaneal ligaments. The *curved pink area* describes a rotational inversion force as the calcaneus/hindfoot is rotated beneath the ankle mortis, causing tension and failure of the lateral ligamentous structures. (From Meyer JM, Garcia J, Hoffmeyer P, et al. The subtalar sprain: a roentgenographic study. *Clin Orthop.* 1988;226:169-173.)

bruising, decreased motion, and increased pain with weight bearing if they are able.

Examination begins with observing the patient's gait; a limp is often noted. Gross observation of the foot and ankle often reveals lateral edema and ecchymosis. Active motion may be severely restricted. Neurovascular structures are usually normal. Along with palpation of the ATFL, CFL, and PTFL, important structures to palpate on the lateral aspect of the ankle include the fibula (entire length), peroneal tendons, lateral process of the talus, neck of the talus, cuboid, and base of the fifth metatarsal. Stress testing is performed to assess the integrity of ligamentous structures. The anterior drawer test translates the talus within the mortise and assesses the ATFL, performed with the ankle in slight plantarflexion to place the ATFL under tension while decreasing CFL tension. Both the amount of excursion compared with the opposite side and the end-point feel to the test are important determinants in the evaluation. The CFL is tested by the talar tilt. The ankle is placed in a neutral position, putting tension on the CFL and decreasing tension on the ATFL. The talus is then inverted within the mortise while the examiner assesses excursion and end-point feel. Again, these findings are compared with the opposite side to determine the severity of injury.

In the United States, patients presenting for ankle injury often undergo radiographic evaluation, but the utility of routine radiographs to evaluate ankle injuries is under debate. Well-designed studies from Canada have shown that many patients with ankle injuries can be managed safely without routine radiographs. Indications for lateral ankle radiograph include age younger than 18 or older than 55 years; inability to bear weight for four consecutive steps, either immediately after injury or in the examination room; and pain over the posterior portion of the distal 6 cm or at the tip of the fibula (Stiell et al., 1992, 1993). If pain is noted in the proximal or midshaft fibula, tibia and fibula radiographs should be obtained, and pain over the base of the fifth metatarsal indicates the need for foot radiographs.

Various scales are available to grade ankle injuries, and inter- and intraexaminer variability is high. The most common scale is mild (grade 1), moderate (grade 2), and severe (grade 3). However, grading does not significantly affect treatment, complication rates, or long-term outcomes. Grading may have a predictive role in duration of recovery.

Treatment of lateral ankle sprains has changed drastically over the past 25 years. Complete immobilization and rest were once thought to be important initial components of treatment. Currently, early mobilization with an external support device and rehabilitation are common therapies. Early immobilization may lead to greater stability and patient compliance, and the risk for early reinjury is low. In the early mobilization and rehabilitation plan, recovery tends to occur slightly more quickly (based on full return to work), and early discomfort may be decreased (Eiff et al., 1994; Karlsson et al., 1996). With immobilization, the ankle joint can become stiff and lead to muscle atrophy. This may require a prolonged postimmobilization program focused on regaining motion and strength. Long-term outcomes of early mobilization and immobilization treatment plans are not significantly different.

Basic stages of treatment include early external support and, depending on severity, limited weight bearing, pain control, reducing swelling with ice and elevation, and maintaining motion. After the initial acute injury subsides, weaning from supportive devices such as crutches, walking boots, or casts should be done and formal rehabilitation initiated. Rehabilitation should focus on motion, strength, and proprioception activities. The final phase of rehabilitation is reintroduction of sport-specific tasks and return to sports. Participation in a prevention-based training program with a focus on balance and proprioception reduces the incidence of ankle sprain without increasing the incidence of other injuries (Bahr et al., 1997). Bracing the ankle on return to sports may reduce the risk of recurrent injury. Whether bracing reduces the risk of an initial sprain is under debate (Sitler et al., 1994; Surve et al., 1994).

When treating skeletally immature patients, it is important to remember that physeal plate fractures through the distal fibula result from the same mechanism as an ankle sprain. If the physical examination reveals tenderness along the distal fibular growth plate, a growth plate fracture must be considered even if the radiographic results are negative. In this case, a short period of immobilization followed by repeat imaging in 2 weeks is appropriate.

Medial Ankle Sprains

The main ligament on the medial side of the ankle is the deltoid ligament (Figure 30-50). Deltoid injuries are typically caused by an eversion mechanism. Medial ankle examination is similar to that of the lateral ankle. Observation of gait usually reveals a limp, and gross observation of the ankle often reveals medial edema but no other deformity. Active motion may be severely restricted, and neurovascular status should be normal. Careful palpation of bony, tendinous, and ligamentous structures of the medial ankle include the deltoid ligament, medial malleolus, medial process of the talus, neck of the talus, medial cuneiform,

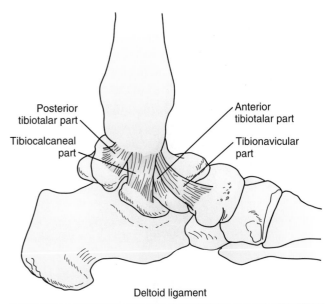

Figure 30-50 Anatomy of medial ankle ligaments. (From Nicholas J, Hershman E. *The lower extremity and spine in sports medicine.* Vol 1, 2nd ed. St. Louis: Mosby; 1995:424.)

cuboid, navicular, and medial ankle tendons (posterior tibialis, flexor digitorum longus, and flexor hallucis longus).

Stress testing of the deltoid ligament is performed by an eversion stress test, usually performed with the ankle in neutral position. The amount of excursion compared with the opposite side and the end-point feel determine the severity of the injury. Deltoid function should be carefully assessed with eversion stressing the ankle in eversion as well as translation stressing from side to side. Mortis widening indicates an injury of the syndesmosis. Any offset increases the stresses on the articular cartilage and increases the risk of arthritis. Obtaining radiographs in the patient with medial ankle injury is decided on a case-by-case basis but should be done more readily than for the typical lateral ankle sprain. Treatment plans are similar to those for lateral ankle sprains. It is widely believed that medial sprains take longer to heal than their lateral counterparts.

Syndesmosis Ankle Sprains (High Ankle Sprains)

The ankle *syndesmosis* is the area of the distal tibia–fibula joint. The five soft tissue structures in the syndesmosis region include the anterior tibiofibular, posterior tibiofibular, transverse tibiofibular, and interosseous ligaments and the interosseous membrane; of these, the anterior tibiofibular ligament is most often injured. Syndesmosis sprains account for 1% to 18% of ankle sprains, with a higher incidence in high-level athletes. Syndesmosis sprains are generally thought to take longer to heal than lateral or medial sprains (Hopkinson et al., 1990), and persistent ankle pain and persistent dysfunction are more common (Gerber et al., 1998); syndesmosis injuries are often associated with fractures. The mechanism of injury is different than for the more common lateral and medial sprains; syndesmosis sprains are most often caused by forceful external rotation and hyperdorsiflexion injuries.

Physical examination often reveals an antalgic gait limp and anterolateral ankle swelling over the anterior

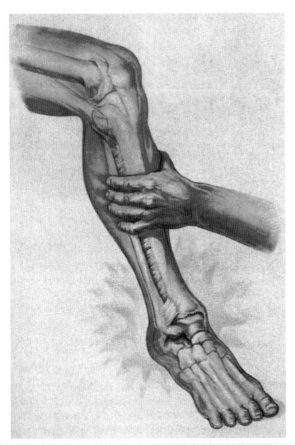

Figure 30-51 The squeeze test. (From Hopkinson WJ, St. Pierre P, Ryan IB, et al. Syndesmosis sprains of the ankle. *Foot Ankle Int.* 1990;10:325-330. Copyright American Orthopedic Foot and Ankle Society, 1990.)

tibiofibular ligament just proximal to the joint line. Ecchymosis is often a delayed finding and is usually noted proximal to the ankle joint in contrast to that noted in lateral and medial sprains, which is often below the ankle and occasionally throughout the foot. Careful palpation reveals tenderness directly over the anterior tibiofibular ligament. Syndesmosis injuries may be present along with medial ankle injury, so tenderness over the deltoid ligament may be noted as well. Be sure to palpate the proximal fibula because extreme forced external rotation may lead to a Maisonneuve fracture (proximal fibular fracture). Strength testing is often limited by pain, and neurovascular status remains intact.

Special stress tests to evaluate the syndesmosis include the squeeze, external rotation, and dorsiflexion–compression tests. The squeeze test is performed by compressing the fibula and tibia above the midpoint of the calf (Hopkinson et al., 1990) (Figure 30-51). The test result is positive if compression causes pain in the region of the syndesmosis ligament. The external rotation test is performed with the knee at 90-degree flexion and the ankle in neutral position. An external rotation force is applied to the foot while the remainder of the leg is stabilized. Pain in the anterior tibiofibular region is a positive test result. The external rotation test is thought to be the most reliable of the common clinical tests used to diagnose syndesmosis sprains.

Because of the risk of concurrent fracture with syndesmosis sprains, radiographs should be obtained. Plain radiographs are adequate to assess for frank *diastasis* (widening between fibula and tibia). Stress radiographs may be necessary to discover latent diastasis. The three major radiographic considerations are the (1) *tibiofibular clear space*, the distance between the medial border of fibula and the lateral border of the posterior tibia, measured 1 cm above tibial plafond; (2) *tibiofibular overlap*, the maximum amount of overlap of the distal fibula and anterior tibial tubercle; and (3) *medial clear space*, the distance between medial malleolus and the medial border of the talus, measured 1 cm below the tibial plafond (Figure 30-52).

Additional testing such as CT can be helpful early in the workup to look for occult fracture and later to assess for heterotopic ossification, a common complication of syndesmosis sprains. MRI is sometimes used and has a high sensitivity and specificity for detecting anterior and posterior tibiofibular ligament injuries (Oae et al., 2003).

The initial treatment begins with protection of the joint, relative rest, ice, compression, and elevation. Various modalities to reduce swelling and inflammation can be used. Rehabilitation includes ROM exercises, strengthening and balance exercises, and proprioception training. Activities can be advanced when pain is reduced, and rehabilitation exercises can be performed pain free. Return to full activities can be entertained when the patient has full motion, full strength, no tenderness on examination, and no functionally limiting pain.

Minimal diastasis can be treated nonoperatively if reduction can be achieved. Therapy includes immobilization with non–weight bearing followed by progressive weight bearing beginning at about 4 weeks and full weight bearing by 2 months. Surgery is needed if reduction cannot be achieved or if diastasis recurs despite immobilization. Frank diastasis is treated surgically.

A common adverse outcome of syndesmosis sprain is heterotopic ossification. Plain radiographs are adequate to make the diagnosis in patients with persistent pain (Figure 30-53). Affecting 25% to 90% of patients, heterotopic ossification may or may not be symptomatic. Ossification may cause pain without causing frank synostosis. The discomfort comes from an inflammatory response in early stages and then from pressure on adjacent bones. Fracture of the ossification is also a potential cause of pain. Frank synostosis can occur. Pain typically results from restricted tibiofibular motion, particularly during full ankle dorsiflexion. Conservative treatment may reduce the pain, but surgical excision may be required (Hopkinson et al., 1990; Taylor et al., 1992).

ACHILLES TENDINOPATHY

Achilles tendinopathy is a common problem, especially in running and jumping athletes. The Achilles tendon consists of the distal ends of the gastrocnemius and soleus muscles and attaches broadly across the posterior aspect of the calcaneus. Contraction of the Achilles results in plantarflexion of the ankle. Activities that cause eccentric loading of the tendon may result in tendonitis. Achilles tendonitis is considered an overuse injury.

Patients present with pain in the posterior aspect of the distal lower leg or heel. Pain is worsened with push-off activities, such as walking up hills or stairs, running, and

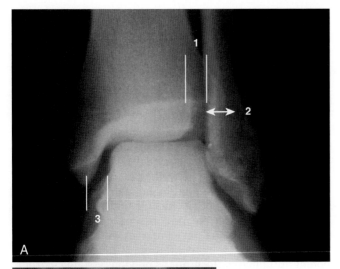

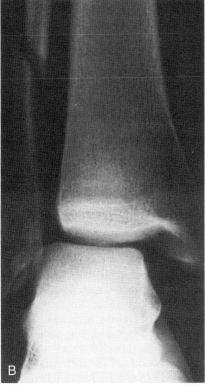

Figure 30-52 A, Normal anteroposterior radiograph of the ankle revealing (1) a normal tibiofibular clear space, (2) normal tibiofibular overlap, and (3) normal medial clear space. Significant mortise widening is noted with widening of all three of these parameters. Note the distal fibula fracture. This injury is best treated with internal fixation of the fracture and stabilization of the ankle mortise with a syndesmosis screw. **B,** A football eversion injury shows widening medial mortise with associated deltoid tear, widening distal tibiofibular syndesmosis, a high fibular fracture, and a small posterior malleolus fracture (not seen here). (Part A courtesy James L. Moeller, MD; part B from Nicholas J, Hershman E. *The lower extremity and spine in sports medicine.* Vol 1, 2nd ed. St. Louis: Mosby; 1995:465.)

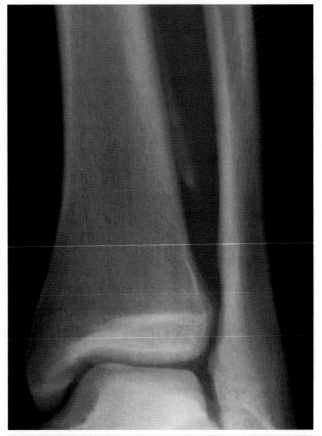

Figure 30-53 Heterotopic ossification noted after a syndesmosis ankle sprain. (Courtesy James L. Moeller, MD.)

jumping. Examination reveals tenderness to palpation of the distal portion of the tendon. A palpable area of swelling and firmness may be noted as well as "wet crepitus" from fluid in the peritenon. Strength may be limited because of discomfort. This can be assessed by direct manual testing or by having the patient perform repeated single-foot toe-raise exercises.

Assessment of the integrity of the Achilles tendon is essential and best done by the Thompson test. Asking the patient simply to plantarflex the ankle actively is not sufficient because there are several secondary plantarflexors. The patient should lie prone on the examination table with the knee flexed to 90 degrees and the ankle in neutral position. Squeeze the midgastrocnemius area and observe for passive ankle plantarflexion. If the Achilles is intact, the ankle will plantarflex (negative test result). If the Achilles is torn, the ankle will remain in a neutral position (positive test result).

Radiographs generally are not necessary to make an accurate diagnosis of Achilles tendinopathy or to initiate treatment. Radiographs are considered in chronic cases, primarily to rule out calcific tendinopathy and Haglund deformity (a bump on the back of the calcaneus near the Achilles insertion). Ultrasonography and MRI are not routinely needed early on but may be used to assess for partial tears, as well as assess the vascular integrity of the injured area. Ultrasonography and MRI changes in the tendon can persist even after functional recovery (Khan et al., 2003).

Treatment of Achilles tendinopathy is similar to that for other forms of tendinopathy and includes ice treatment, relative rest, NSAIDs, stretching and strengthening programs, and proprioception exercises. An exercise program focused on eccentric training has been described and renders promising results in many cases (Alfredson et al., 1998). Most experts agree that corticosteroid injection should not be considered because of the risk of tendon rupture. For recalcitrant cases, treatments such as prolotherapy and extracorporeal shock wave therapy have been studied, but short-term follow-up and isolated reports of effectiveness are mixed. Platelet-rich plasma injections for chronic Achilles tendinopathy have no benefit over saline injections. Surgical debridement is reserved for chronic cases and involves debridement of the diseased tendon and may require tendon transfers for grafting.

ACHILLES TENDON RUPTURE

Tears of the Achilles tendon are most often encountered in men 40 to 60 years old. The most common mechanism of injury is sudden, forceful eccentric loading of the tendon. This can occur from a sudden forceful push-off from a single foot or landing on a single foot. Patients present because of a sudden onset pain in the posterior heel and decreased push-off strength. Patients often describe a feeling of being kicked or hit in the heel, often hearing or feeling a pop at the time of injury. Examination may reveal a palpable gap in the tendon, usually distally. The Thompson test result is positive, with no ankle plantarflexion when the examiner squeezes the calf. Imaging studies are not typically needed to make an accurate diagnosis of Achilles tendon rupture.

Both surgical and nonsurgical treatment options exist (McComis et al., 1997; Weber et al., 2003). Patient selection and including the patient in the decision-making process are important. Generally, younger patients who desire or require greater posttreatment push-off power are likely to be good surgical candidates, and older patients or patients who require less push-off power are nonsurgical candidates. The nonoperative risk of repeat rupture is as high as 10% versus up to 2% with surgery. Skin necrosis of the surgical wound occurs in 5% to 10% of patients.

Conservative treatment entails a period of immobilization accomplished through casting or brace use, usually for 8 to 10 weeks; early weight bearing is controversial. After immobilization, progressive rehabilitation to regain motion, strength, and proprioception is initiated. Surgery is associated with improved push-off power and a reduced rate of repeat rupture and generally allows for the best functional recovery (Wong et al., 2002).

PLANTAR FASCIITIS

Plantar fasciitis is the most common cause of plantar heel pain in active individuals. The plantar fascia is a fibrous band of tissue that originates at the medial calcaneal tubercle, fans out across the plantar aspect of the foot, and then splits before inserting into the plantar aspects of the proximal phalanges. Plantar fasciitis is an overuse injury often seen in people who stand for prolonged periods, as well as in runners and regular exercisers. Many believe plantar fasciitis is an inflammatory condition, but it is more likely caused by chronic changes and microtears of the fascia.

The most common clinical presentation is plantar heel pain. Pain has often been present for several months before presentation. The pain can be described as sharp and stabbing and tends to be worst in the morning, on arising from prolonged sitting, and after standing for prolonged periods. Other symptoms, such as bruising, swelling, weakness, numbness, and tingling, are uncommon. The primary finding on physical examination reveals tenderness over the origin of the plantar fascia.

Treatment protocols are variable, and it may take several months for the patient to feel significant pain relief. Most treatment plans include plantar fascia stretching, ice or ice massage, heel cushioning, and analgesic medication. NSAIDs are often used but are helpful most likely because of their analgesic, not antiinflammatory, effects. Other common treatment options include night splints, physical therapy, orthotic devices, and cortisone injection. Cortisone injection reduces pain from plantar fasciitis, but the mechanism is unclear (Hunt and Sevier, 2004). Cortisone is a potent antiinflammatory, but as previously stated, chronic plantar fasciitis is probably not an inflammatory problem. Risks with cortisone injection include plantar fascia rupture and necrosis of the plantar fat pad, the natural heel cushion. These adverse outcomes should be reviewed with patients before injection.

New modalities for the treatment of plantar fasciitis are under investigation. Extracorporeal shock wave therapy has shown mixed results (Rompe et al., 2002, 2003). Prolotherapy and autologous blood injection involve injecting substances into the area of pathology. Dry needling is also being studied. None of these options has proved to be consistently helpful. Surgical intervention is sometimes needed in recalcitrant cases.

METATARSAL FRACTURES

Nondisplaced fractures of the midshaft and distal portions of the metatarsals are treated with immobilization. Short-leg casting and immobilizer boots can lead to adequate healing in 6 to 8 weeks in most cases. Postoperative shoe use without formal immobilization can also lead to adequate healing of metatarsal fractures, although the risk of adverse outcome is higher. Displaced, angulated, and rotated fractures may require operative fixation.

Fractures of the proximal portion of the metatarsal (first through fourth metatarsals) should be approached with great care. Nondisplaced fractures may be associated with injury to the intermetatarsal ligaments, leading to widening of these joints; surgical consultation is recommended in these cases. If there is no apparent injury to the tarsometatarsal (Lisfranc) joint, cast immobilization typically leads to adequate fracture healing.

Fractures of the base of the fifth metatarsal deserve special discussion. A watershed area of blood flow in the proximal portion of the fifth metatarsal puts it at particular risk for malunion and nonunion. Avulsion fractures off the most proximal portion of the bone have an opportunity to heal with conservative management. Fractures that occur in the watershed area, so-called Jones fractures, have a high chance for malunion and nonunion that should be discussed with the patient. Jones fractures occur in the proximal third of the metatarsal and do not involve the tarsometatarsal joint. Screw fixation of Jones fractures often leads to more acceptable outcomes.

- Early mobilization with an external support device after ankle sprain leads to better short-term outcomes (reduction of pain and return to work and sport activities) compared with early immobilization; long-term outcomes are similar (Eiff et al., 1994; Karlsson et al., 1996; Kerkhoffs et al., 2004) (SOR: A).
- Use of an external ankle brace after ankle sprain reduces the risk of recurrent sprain. Evidence also supports balance and proprioception training for reducing risk of recurrent sprain (Bahr et al., 1997; Surve et al., 1994) (SOR: B).
- An eccentric training program is effective in treating chronic Achilles tendinopathy (Alfredson et al., 1998) (SOR: B).
- Surgery for acute Achilles tendon ruptures reduces the risk of repeat rupture compared with nonsurgical treatment but produces a significantly higher risk of other complications, including wound infection (Khan et al., 2004) (SOR: A).
- Corticosteroid injection can reduce plantar fasciitis pain in the short term (Hunt and Sevier, 2004) (SOR: B).
- For acute Jones fractures in recreationally active patients, early intramedullary screw fixation results in lower failure rates and shorter times to both clinical union and return to sports than non–weight-bearing short-leg casting (Vu et al., 2006) (SOR: B).

References

The complete reference list is available at www.expertconsult.com.

Web Resources

Shoulder

emedicine.medscape.com/article/1260953-overview Clavicle fractures.
emedicine.medscape.com/article/92974-overview Shoulder impingement syndrome.
orthoinfo.aaos.org/topic.cfm?topic=A00032 Shoulder impingement.
orthoinfo.aaos.org/topic.cfm?topic=a00033 Shoulder separation.
orthoinfo.aaos.org/topic.cfm?topic=A00072 Clavicle fracture.
orthoinfo.aaos.org/topic.cfm?topic=A00406 Rotator cuff tear.
orthoinfo.aaos.org/topic.cfm?topic=A00529 Shoulder instability.
www.emedicinehealth.com/rotator_cuff_injury/article_em.htm Rotator cuff injury.
www.eorthopod.com/node/10838 Acromioclavicular sprain.
www.eorthopod.com/node/10847 Sternoclavicular sprain.
www.shoulderdoc.co.uk/article.asp?section=497 Review of the shoulder examination with specific instructions on the physical examination.

Elbow

emedicine.medscape.com/article/1231903-overview Lateral epicondylitis surgery.
emedicine.medscape.com/article/327860-overview Physical medicine and rehabilitation for epicondylitis.
orthoinfo.aaos.org/topic.cfm?topic=A00068 Lateral tendinopathy.
www.mayoclinic.com/health/golfers-elbow/DS00713 Medial tendinopathy.

Wrist and Hand

orthoinfo.aaos.org/topic.cfm?topic=A00012 Scaphoid fracture of the wrist.
orthoinfo.aaos.org/topic.cfm?topic=a00412 Distal radius fracture.
www.handuniversity.com/topics.asp?Topic_ID=30 Scaphoid fracture.
www.handuniversity.com/topics.asp?Topic_ID=45 DeQuervain tenosynovitis.
www.mayoclinic.com/health/carpal-tunnel-syndrome/DS00326 Carpal tunnel syndrome.
www.mayoclinic.com/health/de-quervains-tenosynovitis/DS00692 DeQuervain tenosynovitis.
www.mayoclinic.com/health/trigger-finger/DS00155 Trigger finger.

Knee

orthoinfo.aaos.org/topic.cfm?topic=A00197 Joint infection.
orthoinfo.aaos.org/topic.cfm?topic=A00212 Degenerative osteoarthritis.
orthoinfo.aaos.org/topic.cfm?topic=A00297 Ligament injury.
orthoinfo.aaos.org/topic.cfm?topic=a00358 Meniscus tear.
www.mayoclinic.com/health/patellar-tendinitis/DS00625 Patellar tendinitis.
www.webmd.com/a-to-z-guides/anterior-cruciate-ligament-acl-injuries-topic-overview Anterior cruciate ligament injuries.
www.webmd.com/a-to-z-guides/patellofemoral-pain-syndrome-topic-overview Patellofemoral pain.

Ankle and Foot

emedicine.medscape.com/article/399372-overview Metatarsal fracture.
orthoinfo.aaos.org/topic.cfm?topic=a00150 Ankle sprain.
www.emedicinehealth.com/achilles_tendon_rupture/article_em.htm Achilles tendon rupture.
www.emedicinehealth.com/ankle_sprain/article_em.htm Ankle sprain.
www.mayoclinic.com/health/achilles-tendinitis/DS00737 Achilles tendinitis.
www.mayoclinic.com/health/achilles-tendon-rupture/DS00160 Achilles tendon rupture.
www.mayoclinic.com/health/plantar-fasciitis/DS00508 Plantar fasciitis.

31 *Neck and Back Pain*

RUSSELL LEMMON and JIM LEONARD

Introduction

Neck and lower back pain are common, often frustrating, presenting complaints for primary care physicians. Up to 85% of patients have low back pain at some point in their lives, and it is the fifth most common reason for visiting a physician (Manusov, 2012). Neck pain has an estimated prevalence of 30% to 50% (Manchikanti, 2009). The cost of spinal pain to the United States alone is enormous, accounting for $89 billion in 2005 (Martin et al., 2008). Furthermore, chronic low back pain is the leading cause of opioid prescriptions for noncancer pain (Chou et al., 2009).

Spinal pain is a frustrating problem for clinicians and patients. Factors associated with pain include mood, coping skills, relationship problems, and sleep disorders. Physicians identify chronic pain as a factor contributing to a patient being labeled "difficult" (Edgoose, 2012). Patients turn to complementary therapies for pain more than any other diagnosis, often because of dissatisfaction with their treatment choices (National Institutes of Health, National Center of Complementary and Alternative Medicine, 2004). In addition, the overall societal burden of these conditions is increasing because of unnecessary imaging, unjustified procedures, and the effects of increasing opioid prescribing.

Family physicians are ideally suited to manage the complex problem of spinal pain. They have an understanding of the patient's psychosocial milieu, comorbidities, and functional status. However, many family physicians do not feel equipped to effectively diagnose and treat spinal pain. Multiple guidelines do exist addressing these areas, but they are often not used in routine clinical care (Manusov, 2012).

This section can serve as a framework to the diagnostic and therapeutic challenge of spinal pain. With improved understanding of these conditions, we can better partner with patients, helping them become active in their care and improve their quality of life.

HISTORY

The initial assessment is focused on questions that elucidate the history of the presenting pain condition, including location, quality, severity, duration, timing, context, modifying factors, and associated signs and symptoms. Of particular importance in the initial history are the acuity of pain and a description of any inciting trauma. Further questioning has several goals: identifying an underlying etiology when possible, identifying urgent medical or surgical issues, and assessing psychosocial barriers to successful treatment (Table 31-1).

Emergent conditions are rare but essential considerations in the evaluation of spinal pain. Emergencies such as cauda equina syndrome and spinal infections are examples of conditions that must be identified as quickly as possible. Physicians can efficiently evaluate for these conditions by considering "red flag" symptoms (Table 31-2).

It is also important to consider and assess the psychosocial aspects of pain. Clinicians should ask about the impact of the pain on daily activities, any recent life stressors, and any history of psychiatric disorders.

PHYSICAL EXAMINATION

The physical evaluation of neck and lower back pain begins with inspection of the spine and assessment of motion. Inspection is focused on alignment of major bony landmarks and assessment of the normal spinal curves. The skin should be directly assessed because dermatologic conditions such as herpes zoster can be a cause of neck or back pain. Both the cervical and lumbar spine normally have a lordotic curve. Absence of this can indicate underlying muscular pathology. Range of motion (ROM) should be tested in flexion, extension, side bending, and rotation. Specific muscle testing can also be useful, such as testing hamstring and psoas muscle motion.

The examination should include palpation of bony landmarks and soft tissue structures related to the area of pain. Checking for costovertebral angle tenderness can help rule out renal involvement. A neurologic examination is of particular importance in assessing for more urgent concerns. This should include assessment of gait, strength, sensation, and reflexes. This information can then be correlated with history findings of radicular pain, subjective weakness, or numbness. Finally, special tests can be done to further clarify the differential diagnosis. Several special tests for spinal pain may be appropriate (Table 31-3). They are of limited utility when taken in isolation, so they should always be considered in the context of the entire evaluation. Finally, it may be necessary to evaluate the adjacent joint structures, most commonly the temporomandibular joint,

Table 31-1 Top 10 Questions to Assess Spinal Pain

1. Is this the first episode or a recurrence?
2. Was there any inciting trauma?
3. What increases and decreases your pain?
4. What is your pain pattern over a 24-hour period?
5. Can you diagram the pain pathway?
6. Is there any focal weakness or numbness?
7. Are there any new bowel or bladder symptoms?
8. What previous treatments have been used? Did they help?
9. Did you have any joint problems or sports injuries in childhood?
10. How is this pain affecting your daily life?

Table 31-2 Historical Red Flags

Fever, weight loss, nausea	History of IV drug use
Saddle anesthesia	History of cancer
Recent trauma	History of immune suppression
Bowel or bladder incontinence or retention	History of chronic steroid use
Recent UTIs	History of tuberculosis

IV, Intravenous; *UTI,* urinary tract infection.

Table 31-3 Physical Exam Testing of the Spine

Test	Description	Purpose
GENERAL		
Inspection, including posture Gait assessment Range of motion Neurologic testing Palpation Adjacent joint testing		
SPECIAL TESTS		
Spurling test	The neck is passively extended and then side bent toward the symptomatic side. A compressive force is then applied through the top of the patient's head.	Tests for cervical radiculopathy. A positive test result is an increase in pain and radicular symptoms. This test has a low sensitivity but a high specificity (Rubinstein et al., 2007).
Cervical distraction test	The patient is supine. The examiner has one hand on the chin and another on the occiput. The head is then gently lifted and cervical traction applied.	Tests for cervical radiculopathy. A positive test result is an improvement in pain and radicular symptoms. This test has a low sensitivity but a high specificity (Rubinstein et al., 2007).
Upper limb tension test	The patient is supine. The examiner uses one hand to compress the scapula. The other hand places the patient's shoulder in flexion and abduction and then extends the elbow, wrist, and fingers. The neck is side bent toward the contralateral side.	Tests for cervical radiculopathy. A positive test result is an increase in pain and radicular symptoms. This test has a sensitivity of more than 90% but a low specificity (Rubinstein et al., 2007).
Straight-leg raise	The patient is supine with the legs straight. The leg on the symptomatic side is lifted with the knee in extension.	Tests for lumbar disc herniation. A positive test result is pain between 30 and 70 degrees in the low back or leg. Sensitivity has been published at 91% and specificity at 26% (Deville et al., 2000).
Standing flexion test	The patient is standing with the examiner behind the patient. The examiner places the thumbs on the base of the sacrum and asks the patient to forward flex.	A positive test result is one thumb tracking asymmetrically higher on one side; this indicates iliosacral dysfunction. Thoracic and lumbar ROM can also be assessed from this position.
Psoas muscle test	The patient is prone. The knee is flexed to 90 degrees and then lifted off the table to assess ROM.	Tightness in one or both psoas muscles can contribute to low back pain through attachments on the lumbar spine. Asymmetry in ROM or reproducing low back pain symptoms may indicate psoas involvement in the underlying etiology.
Piriformis test	The patient lies on his or her side. The lower leg is flexed at the hip and knee for stability. The upper leg is straightened off the table. The examiner stabilizes at the pelvis and then pushes down on the upper leg.	Tests for piriformis muscle involvement. A positive test result is pain in the buttocks. If pain radiates down the leg, the test is suggestive of sciatic nerve impingement at the piriformis.

ROM, Range of motion.

shoulder joint, or hip joint, to assess for nonspinal sources of pain.

IMAGING

A history and physical examination are adequate for making a diagnosis and determining a treatment plan for the vast majority of patients with neck or low back pain. The potential benefits of imaging in spinal pain are to advance the diagnosis, exclude urgent medical and surgical pathology, or guide evidence-based treatment. In most cases, imaging does not add useful information or value. Despite this, use of magnetic resonance imaging (MRI) in lower back pain increased by 307% from 1994 to 2005 with no evidence of improved outcomes (Maus, 2010).

In acute neck pain, the presence or absence of trauma guides the decision-making process for imaging. Acute neck trauma is a special consideration because of the concern for catastrophic spinal injury. The National Emergency X-Radiography Utilization Study (NEXUS) criteria provide a clinical guideline to aid in selecting patients for imaging. If a patient meets the criteria listed in Table 31-4, no acute imaging is required (Hoffman et al., 1998). For patients in acute neck pain without trauma or neurologic findings, imaging is not indicated. Chronic neck pain warrants radiographic imaging according to consensus guidelines, but its usefulness remains controversial (Daffner, 2010). If initial radiographic results are normal and there are no neurologic findings, then no further imaging is required. If neurologic findings are present on examination or there is history of significant whiplash injury, MRI is indicated to evaluate further.

Early imaging in acute back pain has not been shown to improve either short- or long-term outcomes and is not recommended by several clinical guidelines (Davis et al., 2009; Maus, 2010). This has been shown to be costly and can be harmful, and findings do not correlate to clinical course (Maus, 2010). Avoiding the use of imaging in the early evaluation of low back pain has been identified as one of the top five ways to improve value in primary care (Good Stewardship Working Group, 2011). Without red flag symptoms or concerning neurologic findings, imaging before 6 weeks of symptoms is discouraged.

Even after the acute period, patients should undergo imaging only if it may reasonably guide treatment decisions. Several limitations are associated with the use of radiographic and MRI testing that can lead to increased risks to patients. A major problem is the poor correlation between anatomic abnormalities and the underlying source of pain. For example, even if a patient has a known disc abnormality on imaging, there is no standard to identfiy the disc as the source of the patient's symptoms. Also, MRI findings of degenerative changes in facet joints are not predictive of a patient benefiting from a facet joint injection (Maus, 2010). The same is true of degenerative changes in the sacroiliac joints. This makes interpreting studies difficult and may overestimate the importance of imaging studies when trying to correlate information to the patient presentation. Potential harms of advanced imaging include unnecessary subsequent procedures and "labeling" a patient with a condition, such as degenerative disc disease, that may ultimately have no bearing on the course of his or her clinical symptoms. If the decision is made to proceed with imaging in low back pain, radiographs are recommended initially (Figure 31-1). If there is a specific neurologic concern or the patient is considering interventional treatments, an MRI may help guide treatment.

Cervical Sprains and Whiplash Syndromes

Table 31-4 The NEXUS Low-Risk Criteria

Cervical spine imaging is recommended in acute trauma unless all of the following criteria exist:

No posterior midline tenderness

A normal level of alertness

No focal neurologic deficits

No evidence of intoxication

No distracting injuries (other injuries that are large enough as to possibly distract from cervical injury)

NEXUS, National Emergency X-Radiography Utilization Study.
From Hoffman JR, Wolfson AB, Todd K, Mower WR. Selective cervical spine radiography in blunt trauma: methodology of the National Emergency X-Radiography Utilization Study (NEXUS). *Ann Emerg Med.* 1998;32: 461-469.

> ### Key Points
>
> - It is important to rule out fracture, joint instability, and neurologic deficit early in the evaluation process
> - Long-term comprehensive treatment should include patient education, lifestyle modifications, and use of psychological interventions to aid in pain coping mechanisms.

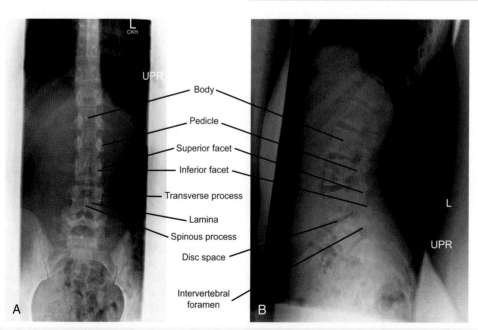

Figure 31-1 Standing lumbar anteroposterior (**A**) and lateral (**B**) radiographs. Note the important labeled bony and soft tissue structures of the vertebrae.

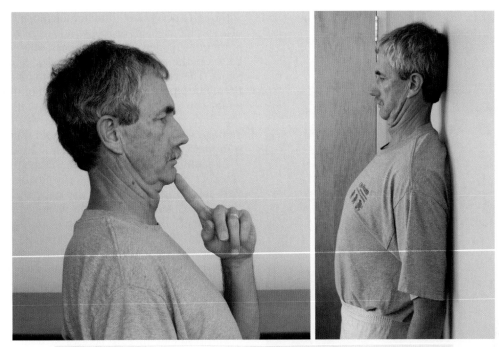

Figure 31-2 Neck retraction used to correct head protraction and to self-mobilize facets.

Whiplash is a term coined by Crowe in 1928. Before that, the term *railway spine* was used to describe these types of injuries (Otte, 2001). The mechanism of injury is due to a combination of forces, including flexion-extension, dynamic loading, shear, and others (Nordin et al., 2008). Abnormal neck postures or axial rotation at the time of the collision increases the risk of structural injury. Pain generators include facets, dorsal root ganglia, discs, ligaments, muscles, vertebral artery, psychosocial factors, and generalized hyperalgesia (Nordin et al., 2008). Fractures, ligamentous instability, significant disc herniation, and degenerative changes such as osteophytes can be identified on imaging studies. Subtle microscopic injuries to facets, nerves, muscles, and bone are not seen on these studies, relegating patients with these types of injuries to the subjective pain category (Curatolo et al., 2011).

CLINICAL FEATURES

Symptoms vary but frequently include neck pain and stiffness, dizziness, headache, radiating pain, numbness, and weakness in the upper extremities and may include cognitive impairment (Walton et al., 2013). It is important to document the onset of symptoms in relation to the time of injury and the presence or absence of preexisting symptoms before the injury. Of note, evidence indicates that factors related to the collision itself, such as amount of vehicle damage, are not reliably predictive of the degree of pain and injury to the individual (Walton et al., 2013).

Evaluation includes review of posture, gait, ROM of the spine and extremities, and neurologic tests (including cranial nerves and cognitive function when indicated). In addition, special tests such as the Spurling test, manual cervical traction, and palpation are done to assess the cervical spine. The Spurling test is done by slightly extending the cervical spine and bending the neck toward the painful side. Pressure is then applied through the top of the head (axial loading). A positive test result is increased pain and radicular symptoms, suggestive of a cervical radiculopathy. The maneuver is thought to be specific but not sensitive for cervical radiculopathy (Tong et al., 2002). With any area of injury, the proximal and distal joints should be evaluated. For a cervical injury, this includes the temporal–mandibular joint above and the scapula and glenohumeral joint below (Hol, 2008). In the acute setting, imaging should be done based on the NEXUS criteria (see Table 31-4).

TREATMENT

With acute injuries, emphasis is initially placed on pain control, mechanisms to decrease inflammation, and passive modalities. As the patient tolerates more activity, emphasis should shift to more active approaches such as aerobic and joint-specific exercise (Figures 31-2 and 31-3), and sport-specific activity. Cervical collars and supportive devices should be reserved for short-term use only when no instability is present (Hurwitz et al., 2008).

Risk factors for poor recovery include female gender, a low level of education, higher baseline scores for neck pain intensity and somatization, and lower baseline scores for work-related activities. Of these, neck pain intensity and work disability are the most consistent predictors (Hendriks, 2005; Walton et al., 2013). Most rigorous studies suggest that half of those with whiplash-associated disorders report neck symptoms 1 year after their injury (Carroll et al., 2008).

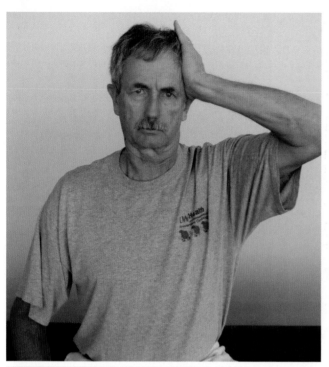

Figure 31-3 Isometric cervical strengthening. This is done in four quadrants as part of a general cervical strengthening program.

Cervical and Lumbar Disc Syndromes

Key Points

- Disc herniations are usually the result of a long-standing degenerative process.
- A careful neurologic examination is mandatory to determine the clinical level of involvement.

Although a cervical or lumbar radiculopathy can be a result of a specific incident or injury, it is usually a manifestation of an ongoing degenerative process. There is a fine balance between the vertebrae–disc complex and the two facet joints. The combination of muscle imbalances, coordination issues, postural abnormalities, and disc degeneration alters the center of axis of motion of this three-joint complex. Dysfunctional movement can result in tissue damage, such as fraying of the annulus fibrosis, and microtrauma to the facet joints and their fluid-filled capsules.

In addition, Wolff's law states that bone responds to the stressors placed on it by hypertrophying, an example of form following function. As the spine seeks a more stable state, facet and ligamentum flavum hypertrophy may result in a central, lateral recess or foraminal stenosis (Kirkaldy-Willis, 1988; Wolff, 1986). In the cervical spine, the uncus is a unique structure that is a site of osteophyte formation (Figure 31-4). A combination of disc herniation, uncovertebral hypertrophy (disc–osteophyte complex), and facet hypertrophy may result in stenosis of the foramen, lateral recess, or central canal (White and Panjabi, 1990) (Figure 31-5).

The result of these processes in either the cervical or lumbar spine is an unstable joint that eventually may result in disc herniation caused by joint laxity (Kirkaldy-Willis, 1988). Describing disc herniation as the end result of a multifactorial, chronic process rather than an isolated event is helpful in counseling patients and planning effective treatments.

CLINICAL FEATURES

A pain diagram and a through history and physical are key to defining a radicular pattern. Other structures such as facet joints, myofascial trigger points, or the sacroiliac joint may have a radiating pain that mimics a compressed nerve root pattern (Kellgren, 1939). In the lumbar spine, disc

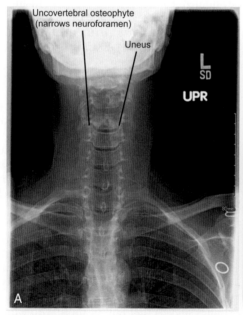
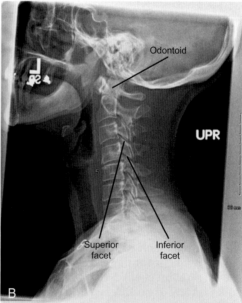

Figure 31-4 Cervical anteroposterior (**A**) and lateral (**B**) radiographs. Note the uncus and upward pointing lateral projection of the vertebral body. Osteophytes are prone to develop here (note right C4-C5 level), and frequently project into the neural foramen, impinging the exiting nerve root.

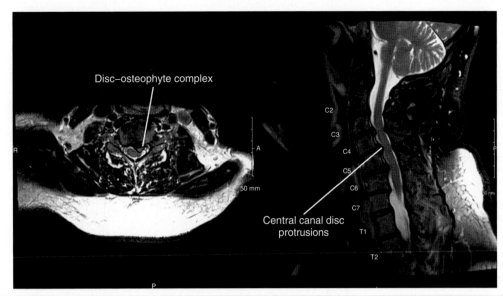

Figure 31-5 Cervical MRI axial and sagittal views. Note the disc–osteophyte complex to the left of center at C4 to C5 that impinges on both the spinal cord and the exiting nerve root.

Table 31-5 Common Radiculopathies

Level of Disc Herniation	Nerve Root Involved	Muscle to Be Tested	Area of Sensory Loss	Reflex
C5-C6	C6	Bicep	Lateral forearm	Biceps
C6-C7	C7	Triceps	Index finger	Triceps
L3-L4	L4	Tibialis anterior	Medial calf	Patellar
L4-L5	L5	Extensor hallucis longus	Lateral calf	None
L5-S1	S1	Gastrosoleus	Lateral foot	Achilles
Cauda equina syndrome	S2-S3-S4	External anal sphincter	Perirectal	None

herniations most frequently increase pain with sitting (Nachemson, 1981; White and Panjabi, 1990).

Lumbar herniations are more frequently noted to be central or in the paramedian position in the spinal canal. This results in the compression of the nerve root exiting at the next lower level (e.g., an L4-L5 herniation compressing the L5 nerve root) (Table 31-5 and Figure 31-6). The exception is when there is a far lateral herniation into the neuroforamen (e.g., an L4-L5 foraminal protrusion compressing the exiting L4 nerve root).

In the cervical spine, disc herniations usually compress the nerve root at the same level (e.g., a C5-C6 herniation compressing the C6 nerve root) (Figure 31-7). The amount of compression of the nerve root varies according to the degree of disc herniation (i.e., protrusion, extrusion, sequestered fragment).

Although the extent of the herniation can be visualized on MRI, the process is dynamic and subject to pressure and positional influences. Therefore, the clinical picture takes precedent over the imaging studies. Thorough neurologic examinations are required to define any deficit that exists, including any potential cauda equina involvement.

TREATMENT

Although treatment guidelines are available, evidence-based rules are not well defined. The absolute indication for surgery is loss of bowel or bladder control or progressive neurologic involvement. Relative indications for surgery include static motor loss or intractable pain that causes debilitating functional loss. Other potential indications include neoplasm, infection, congenital conditions, or deformity (Cole and Herring, 2003).

Conservative approaches are multiple. The major categories of these are listed in Table 31-6. After an initial short period of rest, aerobic exercise should be one major component of the program. Recommendations for spine-specific exercises vary, but family physicians should feel comfortable initiating a few commonly effective exercises. In the cervical spine, these include neck retraction and isometric strengthening (see Figures 31-2 and 31-3). In the lumbar spine, rehabilitation can include the supine knee-to-chest and prone extension initially (Figures 31-8 and 31-9). As the patient progresses, strengthening exercises such as the four-point balance exercise and lateral plank are good options (Figures 31-10 and 31-11). Other specific exercises can be included based on individual needs, often with the help of a physical therapist.

Although passive modalities and medications may be included, these should not be a mainstay of treatment. Active modalities as described earlier and activity modification based on sound ergonomic principles should be emphasized. With lumbar radiculopathy, limiting prolonged sitting is frequently required. With cervical radiculopathy, limiting

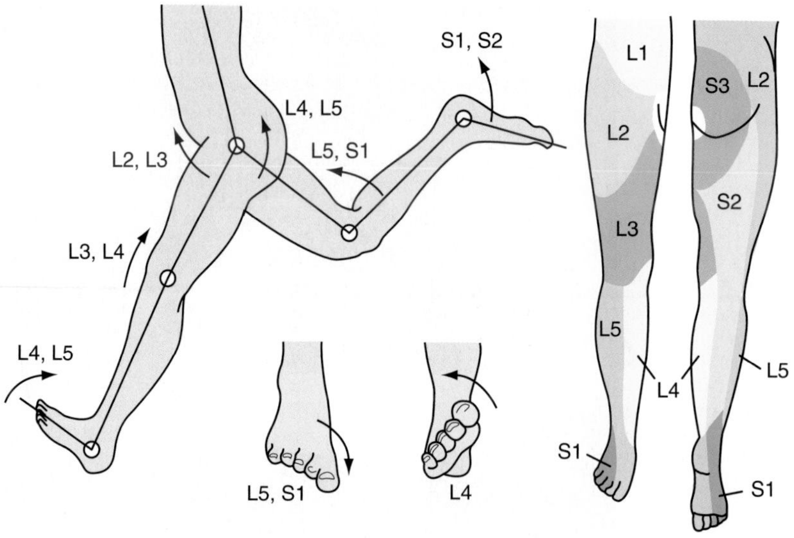

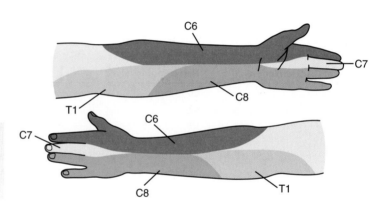

Figure 31-6 Root (segmental) distribution. Note that motion in each joint is controlled by four nerve roots running in sequence: hip—flexion, L2 and L3 and extension, L4 and L5; knee—extension (and knee jerk), L3 and L4 and flexion, L5 and S1; ankle—dorsiflexion, L4 and L5 and plantarflexion (and ankle jerk), S1 and S2. (Inversion involves L4 and eversion L5 and S1.) A useful mnemonic for the low limb dermatomes is that "we kneel on L3, stand on S1, and sit on S3." (Redrawn from McRae R, Kinninman AWG. *Orthopedics and trauma.* New York: Churchill Livingstone; 1997:26.)

Figure 31-7 Volar and dorsal dermatome patterns of the forearm and hand. Pain and paresthesias may radiate into these areas when the affected nerve root is compressed. Note that extremity symptoms as a result of disc disease are almost always unilateral. (Redrawn from Mercier R. *Practical orthopedics.* 5th ed. St. Louis: Mosby; 2000:29.)

Table 31-6   Types of Modalities Used to Treat Neck and Back Pain

Thermal	Mechanical	Electrical	Injections
Moist heat	Spinal traction	Electrical stimulation	Nerve blocks
Cold packs	Massage	TENS unit	Trigger points
Ice massages	Myofascial treatment	Nerve stimulators	Spinal injections
Contrast baths	Joint mobilization	Spinal cord stimulators	Botox injections
Infrared heat lamps	Manipulation	Iontophoresis	Joint injections
Diathermy	Compression garments	Interferential current	Prolotherapy
Ultrasonography			
Laser			
Hydrotherapy	**Bracing**	**Medications**	**Psychological**
Whirlpool	Soft or rigid braces	Analgesic	Counseling
Warm water pool	Joint immobilizers	Antiinflammatories	Biofeedback
Swimming pool	Orthotics	Neuromodulators	Cognitive based
Contrast baths	Shoe lift	Antispasmodic	Group sessions
		Antidepressant	
		Topical	
		Intrathecal	
Surgery	**Exercise**	**Integrative**	**Forensic**
Spinal decompression	Aerobic	Medication	Case closure
Fusion	Joint specific	Nutrition	Disability evaluation
Disc replacement	Stretching and strengthening	Yoga, Pilates, and Tai Chi	
Arthroscopy	Coordination	Weight loss	
Discectomy	Sport and activity specific	Acupuncture	

TENS, Transcutaneous electrical nerve stimulation.

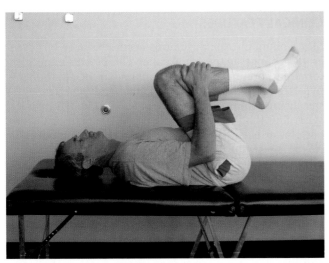

Figure 31-8 Supine bilateral knee-to-chest maneuvers used to improve flexion ability. Also, flexion maneuvers increase the antero-posterior dimensions of spinal canal and neuroforamen, which may decompress pain-sensitive structures.

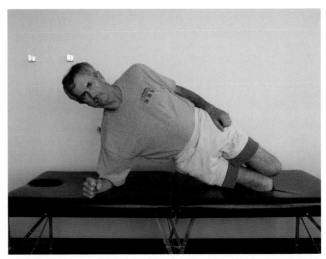

Figure 31-11 Lateral plank used to improve the strength of the quadratus lumborum, a lateral stabilizer of the spine.

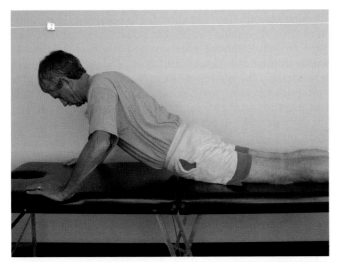

Figure 31-9 Prone extension exercise used with radiculopathies in an attempt to centralize the radiating pain to the lumbar spine and work it out from there.

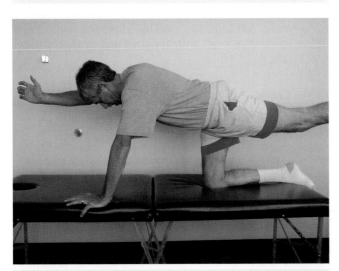

Figure 31-10 Four-point balance exercise used to improve postural strength and coordination.

static postures such as prolonged computer use or limiting overhead and repetitive upper extremity work can avoid further exacerbation of a painful disorder (Figure 31-12).

Considerations regarding return to play and return to work follow parallel guidelines. The general exertion categories to consider with return to work are listed in Table 31-7. Return to play criteria include the following general principles: resolution of any neurologic deficit, full ROM, and little or no pain, and the athlete is able to perform adequately in practice. In addition, the athlete should have the proper protective equipment, have the confidence to play, and should not be at significant risk of injury by participating (Cole and Herring, 2003).

Spinal Stenosis

Key Points

- Spinal stenosis is a multifactorial process that is most commonly an end result of the degenerative cascade.
- Spinal stenosis most often presents as neurogenic claudication in older adults.
- Clinical findings need to be confirmed with imaging to make a definitive diagnosis, but imaging will not change management in mild symptoms.

Spinal stenosis is a clinical syndrome of buttock or lower extremity pain associated with diminished space available for neural and vascular structures within the spinal canal (Doorly et al., 2010). An understanding of spinal stenosis is important in primary care because it is a common cause of pain, disability, and back surgery in the elderly population. It is also a common source of confusion among clinicians because *spinal stenosis* is both a clinical and radiologic term that must be correlated to determine its clinical significance.

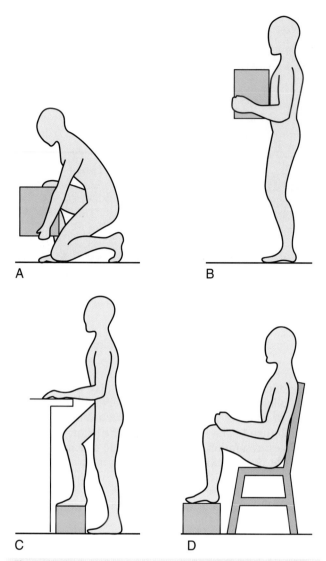

Figure 31-12 General postural instructions. **A,** Bend the knees and hips and keep the back straight when lifting. **B,** Hold objects close to the body when carrying. **C,** Place one foot on a stool when standing. **D,** Keep the knees higher than the hips when sitting and keep the back straight when standing by tucking in the abdomen and tightening the buttocks to decrease swayback. In addition, patients should avoid high-heeled shoes and sleeping on the abdomen, activities that increase lordosis. (Redrawn from Mercier L. *Practical orthopedics.* 5th ed. St. Louis: Mosby; 2000:125.)

Table 31-7   Components of a Return to Work Form

	Occasional Lift Limit (lb)	Frequent Lift Limit (lb)
Sedentary	10	5
Light	20	10
Light to medium	35	20
Medium	50	25
Heavy	75	30-40

Also comment on:
- Number of hours per day and days per week
- Sitting, standing, walking, and driving times
- Ability to do overhead work
- Ability to use the feet and hands for repetitive activity

CLINICAL FEATURES

Most commonly, spinal stenosis occurs because of degenerative changes in the spinal canal. This process is multifactorial and originates from a combination of disc bulging, hypertrophy of arthritic facet joints, and hypertrophy of the ligamentum flavum (Suri et al., 2010). The clinical syndrome that results is variable, but patients can have both lower back pain and lower extremity symptoms. The classic presentation is that of neurogenic claudication in older adults. The lower extremity pain and weakness can be unilateral or bilateral, worsens with walking, and is relieved with sitting (Backstrom et al., 2011). It is a slow, progressive disorder and typically does not present until after age 60 years. Additional findings in the history suggestive of the diagnosis are improvement of symptoms with flexion and worsening with extension. This correlates with the common scenario of symptoms improving when leaning on a shopping cart in the supermarket. Overall, improvement in symptoms with forward bending and absence of pain while seated are the most useful historical findings suggestive of spinal stenosis (Suri et al., 2010). Physical examination tests are not as reliable as symptoms in making the diagnosis, but the presence of a wide-based gait and an abnormal Romberg test result make lumbar spinal stenosis more likely (Suri et al., 2010). The Romberg test is part of the neurologic examination that tests balance and proprioception by having a patient stand with the feet together and the eyes closed. In a positive test result, the patient will not be able to maintain balance with the eyes closed.

An important consideration in the differential diagnosis is evaluating for peripheral vascular disease (PVD). The presentation of neurogenic claudication could certainly be confused with vascular claudication. Differing characteristics include postural changes, which should improve pain in spinal stenosis but not PVD. Also, the discomfort of vascular claudication may be more consistently reproducible with ambulation than neurogenic claudication in terms of walking time and distance (Suri et al., 2010). If concern for vascular disease persists, ankle-brachial index (ABI) studies should be obtained. The ABI compares blood pressures from the ankle and arm both at rest and after exercise. A decreased ABI indicates that blood pressures are lower in the ankle compared with the arm and is suggestive of underlying PVD.

DIAGNOSIS

A history and examination are usually enough to make a presumptive diagnosis of spinal stenosis. To confirm the diagnosis, an MRI is the imaging test of choice (Kreiner et al., 2013). It is not necessary to initially obtain imaging in most cases. For patients with mild or moderate symptoms, imaging will not change the initial management. Furthermore, it is important to recognize that isolated radiographic findings of spinal stenosis without appropriate symptoms do not make the diagnosis of the clinical syndrome of lumbar spinal stenosis. Clinical symptoms that correlate with the radiologic findings must be present to make the diagnosis. Clinicians should be aware of the tendency to use the term *stenosis* in a more general sense to avoid confusion when evaluating or discussing patients (Suri et al., 2010).

TREATMENT

The treatment approach is based on symptom severity. The overall treatment goals are to relieve pain and improve function. Importantly, the symptoms, not radiologic findings, should direct the treatment approach. On the other hand, classification of stenosis as mild, moderate, or severe is based on radiologic measurements. Radiographically, an anteroposterior (AP) diameter of less than 10 mm in the spinal canal is considered severe stenosis. Although there are objective measures to determine the severity of spinal canal narrowing, the degree of severity has not been shown to correlate to any clinical measure. Specifically, there is poor correlation between MRI assessment of stenosis and walking distance, degree of disability, patient-reported pain, and physician clinical impression (North American Spine Society, 2011). In the absence of reliable objective evidence, physicians must clinically assess the severity of the clinical symptoms in the context of comorbid conditions to determine the most appropriate treatment approach.

Treatment options are generally divided into conservative and surgical approaches. In patients with mild to moderate symptoms, conservative care is effective 70% of the time at 6 months, decreasing to 57% at 4 years (North American Spine Society, 2011). In patients with severe symptoms, conservative care is effective approximately 33% of the time, in contrast to 80% effectiveness of surgical decompression (North American Spine Society, 2011). Conservative care options include physical therapy, analgesic medications, lumbosacral braces, manual therapy, and weight loss. Choosing among the nonsurgical options is challenging because treatments have been poorly investigated in clinical trials (Doorly et al., 2010). Although there is currently no standard of care for conservative treatments, current guidelines state that physical therapy and exercise may be effective in improving outcomes as part of a comprehensive treatment strategy (Kreiner et al., 2013). Regarding pharmacologic treatments, recommendations have been adapted from other more general pain recommendations and have limited evidence when specifically applied to spinal stenosis (Doorly et al., 2010). As with other causes of spinal pain, acetaminophen and nonsteroidal antiinflammatory drugs (NSAIDs) are typical first-line pharmacologic agents despite the lack of data specific to spinal stenosis. There is insufficient evidence to support other agents such as skeletal muscle relaxants or calcitonin (North American Spine Society, 2011). Gabapentin warrants specific mention in this discussion because its use is common given the neurogenic origin of symptoms. However, the evidence supporting its use in spinal stenosis is limited to one study of 55 patients with several limitations (North American Spine Society, 2011).

Interventional treatments include epidural steroid injections and spinal surgery. Current recommendations support the use of epidural injections for short term relief of neurogenic claudication symptoms, but evidence is not as strong for long-term benefit (North American Spine Society, 2011). Spinal decompression surgery is recommended for patients with moderate to severe radicular symptoms, especially when not benefiting from conservative care. Patients with primarily axial back pain as opposed to radicular pain do not typically get as much benefit from surgery. Of note, patients older than 75 years of age undergoing decompression surgery have outcomes similar to younger patients and should be considered for debilitating symptoms (Doorly et al., 2010).

KEY TREATMENT

- Patients with mild to moderate symptoms should be offered conservative treatment options, including analgesia, physical therapy, lumbar braces, and weight loss (Kreiner et al., 2013). (SOR: C).
- Patients with severe symptoms should be considered for surgical evaluation. This recommendation includes patients older than the age of 75 years because outcomes are similar to those in younger patients (North American Spine Society, 2011) (SOR: B).

Spondylolisthesis

Key Points

- Spondylolisthesis is defined as a forward slippage of one vertebral body relative to the one below.
- The most common underlying causes are a bilateral pars interarticularis defect in the younger population and degenerative changes in older adults.

BACKGROUND

Spondylolisthesis is a condition commonly seen by family physicians in both the pediatric and adult population. It is also an important condition to consider relative to the previous section on spinal stenosis because spondylolisthesis can be a cause of spinal stenosis. First, it is important to define terms used in discussing this topic. Spondylo*lysis* is a defect of the pars interarticularis of a lumbar vertebra. Spondylo*listhesis* is the forward slippage of a vertebral body relative to the one below. There are five underlying causes of spondylolisthesis (Table 31-8). Types I and II are more common in the pediatric population, and type III is more commonly seen in older adults. This discussion focuses on the two most common types, which are types II and III.

In spondylolisthesis caused by pars defects, it is generally agreed that genetic predisposition plays a role, but

Table 31-8 Types of Spondylolisthesis

Type	Description
I	Congenital abnormality
II	Defect of the pars interarticularis
III	Degenerative
IV	Traumatic
V	Pathologic

otherwise the exact etiology is unclear. The overall incidence is quite high, with quoted rates of 6% by age 14 years. Clinical significance varies significantly based on the individual, but a slippage greater than 25% tends to correlate with the presence of pain (Tallarico et al., 2008).

Degenerative spondylolisthesis is a major cause of spinal stenosis. It is thought to be a multifactorial problem similar to other causes of spinal stenosis, stemming from arthritis of facet joints, ligamentous laxity, and poor muscular stabilization (Kalichman and Hunter, 2008). Degenerative spondylolisthesis occurs mostly at L4 to L5, as opposed to spondylolysis, which occurs at L5 to S1 in approximately 90% of cases (Tallarico et al., 2008).

DIAGNOSIS

The most common complaint is low back pain. This can be exacerbated by activities that stress extension of the spine such as gymnastics or football. In degenerative cases presentation is similar to that of spinal stenosis.

Anteroposterior and lateral plain radiographs are the standard views taken. Oblique views can be added if a pars interarticularis defect is suspected. MRI can be considered for those with persistent symptoms or concerning findings on a neurologic examination. An MRI or bone scan may be useful if there is a need to determine the acuity of a pars fracture. Grading of spondylolisthesis can be done in two ways but is most commonly expressed as a percentage of the AP diameter of the top of the lower vertebrae. Of note, there is some subjectivity in this assessment, so caution is advised when assessing for progression (Kalichman and Hunter, 2008). Low-grade slips are defined as less than 50%, and high-grade slips are greater than 50% (Tallarico et al., 2008).

TREATMENT

The prognosis is excellent in patients with spondylolisthesis caused by a pars defect. Treatment recommendations are variable in this group but depend on age, acuity of the pars defect, level of activity, and degree of impairment. Treatment is based on relative rest from sports with progressive rehabilitation as symptoms decrease. Lumbosacral bracing can be used, especially in the setting of acute pars fractures in younger patients (Tallarico et al., 2008). Bracing is less often done in adult patients but can be used if there are significant symptoms. Surgical treatment is generally reserved for those who have failed conservative care for 6 months. One notable exception is in skeletally immature patients with high-grade vertebral slippage. It is often recommended that these patients undergo fusion because of the risk of further slippage (Tallarico et al., 2008). Return to activity in spondylolysis and spondylolisthesis caused by pars defects is based on improvement of symptoms rather than radiologic improvement. Follow-up is based on age. Whereas patients who are skeletally immature may benefit from serial imaging every 6 months to monitor for progression, those who are near skeletal maturity do not require routine follow-up (Tallarico et al., 2008).

Degenerative spondylolisthesis also has a favorable prognosis, but this often depends on the degree of neurologic symptoms present because of spinal stenosis. Having neurologic symptoms at baseline is predictive of a poorer prognosis when treated non-surgically (Kalichman and Hunter, 2008). Nonoperative treatment of degenerative spondylolisthesis is similar to that for spinal stenosis and includes progressive aerobic exercise, weight reduction, and analgesic medications. Specific physical therapy modalities that can be of benefit include lumbar bracing, strengthening of back flexor and extensor muscle groups, and back stabilization training (Kalichman and Hunter, 2008). Surgical indications are persistent pain or neurologic deficit that affects quality of life, resistant to conservative care, progressive neurologic deficit, or bowel and bladder symptoms. Of note, progression of slippage does not correlate well to clinical symptoms and is typically not used to guide treatment as much as the clinical presentation (Kalichman and Hunter, 2008).

Vertebral Compression Fractures

> ### Key Points
>
> - Vertebral compression fractures (VCFs) are often identified incidentally and are most commonly asymptomatic.
> - They are most commonly caused by osteoporosis but can also be caused by underlying systemic pathology.
> - Plain radiographs are the test of choice when a compression fracture is suspected.

Vertebral compression fractures are a common cause of pain and disability, especially in the elderly population. Family physicians play an important role not only in the treatment of recognized fractures but also in prevention of future fractures.

A useful concept when considering the pathophysiology of VCF is the three-column spine theory proposed by Francis Denis in 1983 (Denis, 1983). This concept separates the spine into anterior, middle, and posterior columns by conceptually dividing the vertebral body in half. The anterior column comprises the anterior longitudinal ligament and the anterior half of the vertebral body. The middle column consists of the posterior half of the vertebral body and the posterior longitudinal ligament. The posterior column consists of the pedicles, the facet joints, and the supraspinous ligaments. This concept is significant when assessing the stability of a spinal fracture. If two of the three columns are involved, then the fracture is more likely to be unstable. Most compression fractures are stable because they involve a wedge deformity of the anterior column alone. The middle column remains intact to prevent compression of neural elements (Denis, 1983).

CLINICAL FEATURES

The presentation of VCF is highly variable: most are asymptomatic and identified incidentally (Patel and Shah, 2011). It is estimated that just one third of vertebral fractures are symptomatic (Longo et al., 2012). When they do cause symptoms, there may be a history of minor trauma preceding the pain, but the event may be as minor as a cough or sneeze. The physical examination may reveal decreased ROM typical of many etiologies of back pain and localized vertebral tenderness but otherwise is not usually helpful in making the diagnosis. An increased kyphosis may also be present, caused by several factors associated with aging. These include a decline in bone mass; weakness of vertebral end plates; and reduction in axial muscle strength, mostly with spinal extension (Sinaki, 2012). These changes can occur with or without vertebral fractures and thus are not helpful in making a diagnosis. The neurologic examination should be normal in an uncomplicated vertebral fracture.

The most common site for fractures is at the thoracolumbar junction. Fractures superior to T7 and those occurring in patients without osteoporosis should prompt further workup to look for potential underlying systemic disease (Patel and Shah, 2011). Possible etiologies include malignancy, hyperparathyroidism, osteomalacia, and tuberculosis.

DIAGNOSIS

As noted, a vertebral fracture should be considered a potential source of back pain in individuals with risk factors for osteoporosis, a prior diagnosis of osteoporosis, or red flags for systemic disease predisposing the patient to vertebral fractures. Given that most patients present without significant trauma, it is appropriate to obtain imaging to make the diagnosis when concern for vertebral fracture exists. If there is concern for a cause other than osteoporosis, a laboratory workup is also appropriate. This can include a complete blood count, erythrocyte sedimentation rate, C-reactive protein, serum calcium, parathyroid hormone, and a vitamin D level. In addition, tuberculosis screening may be indicated.

Plain radiographs are appropriate initial tests when VCF is suspected (Alexandru and So, 2012). Radiographic characteristics of compression fractures include anterior wedging of one or more vertebrae with vertebral collapse, demineralization, and vertebral end-plate irregularity (Patel and Shah, 2011). VCF is defined by a decrease in vertebral height by 20% or at least 4 mm compared with baseline (Longo et al., 2012). Imaging findings that indicate an unstable fracture include loss of greater than 50% of vertebral body height and multiple adjacent compression fractures or failure of two of the three columns. MRI or computed tomograph is appropriate if there is a neurologic abnormality on examination or if there is suspicion for a malignancy-associated vertebral fracture. A bone scan may also be useful if there is concern for malignancy (Longo et al., 2012).

TREATMENT

The overall goals of management include pain control and prevention of further fractures and disability. Treatment options include both conservative measures and interventional methods. Management of acute compression fractures is still controversial, but recent research suggests that an initial trial of conservative treatment is likely most appropriate (Kallmes and Comstock, 2012; Longo et al.,

2012). Common conservative therapies include analgesic medications, bed rest, back braces, and physical therapy.

As with most causes of pain, nonopioid analgesic medications should be used initially. Risks associated with opioids that are especially relevant to the osteoporotic population include falls and constipation. Nasal calcitonin can be used as an adjunct to analgesic medications. It may take up to 2 weeks for optimal pain control but has nearly no side effects or drug interactions (Silverman and Azria, 2002). Physical therapy–based approaches center around rehabilitation of the back extensors (Figure 31-9). This has a role even in the management of acute fractures because isometric exercises of the extensor muscle groups can decrease pain (Sinaki, 2012). For pain that persists beyond 6 weeks despite conservative care, consideration can be given to interventional treatment. Balloon kyphoplasty and vertebroplasty are options for refractory symptoms, but the indications of these procedures are currently not clear. Some studies have shown quicker pain relief with both procedures compared with conservative care, but others have found no improvement in pain and functional measures at 6 months (Anselmetti et al., 2013). Surgical intervention is normally reserved for unstable fractures.

In addition to acute management of vertebral fractures, it is essential for family physicians to address underlying osteoporosis to prevent future fractures. A comprehensive approach to osteoporosis includes regular exercise, adequate calcium and vitamin D intake, smoking cessation, and bisphosphonate medications. Exercise should be considered a standard part of osteoporosis management to improve axial stability. Spinal extensor exercises can decrease the risk of future vertebral fractures even without an increase in bone mass (Sinaki, 2012). In addition, back extensor strength has been correlated to better quality of life in patients with osteoporosis (Sinaki, 2012).

KEY TREATMENT

- Conservative treatments are the appropriate initial approach for the majority of compression fractures and include rest, physical therapy, analgesic medications, and back braces (Kallmes and Comstock, 2012) (SOR: C).
- Nasal calcitonin can be used as a safe adjunctive treatment for pain associated with compression fractures (Silverman and Azria, 2002) (SOR: C).
- Treatment of compression fractures should include a comprehensive treatment of underlying osteoporosis (Wells et al., 2008) (SOR: A).

Myofascial Pain

Myofascial pain is considered a regional pain syndrome caused by myofascial trigger points. Trigger points are discrete, focal, hyperirritable spots located in a taut band of skeletal muscle (Travell and Simons, 1992). The spots are painful on compression and can produce referred pain (Travell and Simons, 1992). Frequently, this is a diagnosis of exclusion, and other pathology, including bone abnormalities, nerve deficits, and inflammatory disorders, should be investigated. Comorbidities should be considered, including but not limited to depression, anxiety, and central sensitization from a previous or coexisting injury (Travell and Simons, 1992).

Treatment is focused on eliminating factors perpetuating muscular overuse, physical modalities, judicious use of analgesic medicines, and encouraging activity (Alvarez and Rockwell, 2002). Acetaminophen and NSAIDs are good medication choices for periodic use. Symptomatic trigger points can be treated with several modalities such as manual therapies, dry needling, or trigger point injections (Alvarez and Rockwell, 2002). In addition, more integrative approaches should address lifestyle issues such as sleep disturbance, mood disorders, dietary intake, and stress reduction. As with any musculoskeletal disorder, emphasis should be placed on aerobic and specific exercises along with biomechanical approaches to limit exacerbations. This is especially important with chronic pain conditions, defined as pain that lasts more than 3 to 6 months. The ill effects of long-term immobilization and lack of exercise with resultant deconditioning can result in a state that is worse than the original myofascial pain problem.

Chronic Low Back Pain

> ### Key Points
>
> - There are multiple potential pain generators in chronic low back pain, contributing to the difficulty of making a specific diagnosis.
> - Chronic back pain is often grouped into mechanical back pain, radicular pain, and pathologic back pain.
> - Evaluating for common red flag symptoms helps clinicians efficiently rule out urgent conditions.
> - Imaging modalities are not indicated before 6 weeks of back pain symptoms unless red flag symptoms are present.

Chronic low back pain is a very common and costly problem, as well as a source of frustration for both patients and providers. Back pain is by nature a complex problem because of the multiple potential sources of pain, and this complexity is magnified when pain becomes chronic. Having an understanding of this complexity can help guide therapies and provide better patient counseling. Primary care clinicians need to have an approach to caring for patients with chronic back pain. This section expands on the physiologic basis for low back pain, discusses a diagnostic and therapeutic approach, and discusses thoughts on how to uses office visits to improve patient care and provider satisfaction.

PHYSIOLOGY

Acute pain is based on nociceptive receptors peripherally at an anatomic site. There are multiple potential pain generators, including the discs, facet joints, sacroiliac joints, ligaments, muscles, and fascia (Salzberg, 2012). In chronic low back pain, there is often increased motion, decreased cushioning, abnormal bone formation, and weakening of

muscles and ligaments, all of which can cause pain to innervated structures. Pain processing occurs in the spinal cord at the dorsal root ganglia and dorsal horn and in the brain at the limbic system, thalamus, and cerebral cortex (Salzberg, 2012).

Chronic pain results in changes to the nervous system such as neuron hyperexcitability, changes in gene expression, and signal amplification to the thalamus. In addition, emotional and psychological changes that take place also color the pain experience (Salzberg, 2012). Taken together, these changes can result in continued pain signals even when there is no further tissue damage. This knowledge is useful clinically because pharmacologic and physical treatments can be focused at different target sites. Possible targets include the peripheral site of pain, the spinal cord, or sites of pain modulation in the brain. In addition, it is important to address the psychological and emotional components because they directly impact pain perception.

DIAGNOSTIC APPROACH

The diagnostic approach to low back pain differs from many other symptoms in that an exact diagnosis is not the end result of most evaluations. Only 15% of patients have a specific identifiable cause of back pain (Manusov, 2012). This has led to multiple classifications systems in attempt to find efficient ways to identify immediate red flag concerns and categorize others with the goal of initiating treatment. There is no evidence that one classification system should be used over another (Manusov, 2012). A commonly used approach is one that was recommended in 2007 by a joint statement from the American College of Physicians and the American Pain Society. It uses the following three categories: nonspecific back pain, radicular pain, and red flag–associated symptoms (see Table 31-2). This and other guidelines have the approach of ruling out tumor, infection, organic causes, and surgical emergencies first and then proceeding with management of mechanical-type back pain.

Early imaging is not indicated unless red flags are present. Advanced imaging, most commonly MRI, may be considered when more invasive treatments are likely but does have downsides. MRI may lead to more surgery without improving outcomes and the "labeling" of a condition that may not in fact fully explain symptoms (Vanwye, 2010).

TREATMENT APPROACH IN PRIMARY CARE

After establishing a working diagnosis of nonspecific or mechanical back pain, developing a therapeutic approach remains challenging. There is a long list of potential therapies from which to choose (see Table 31-6), and symptomatic improvement often does not happen quickly. Physicians need to be comfortable following patients with back pain over the long term, assisting patients with necessary changes, monitoring progress, and dealing with setbacks.

A good place to start is determining the treatment goals. In chronic pain of any type, "curing the pain" is often not a reasonable goal. Consider both patient and provider goals in this process and attempt to agree upon using these goals to judge outcomes because this may improve the therapeutic alliance (Yelland and Schluter, 2006). If a patient is having difficulty with this process, a question to shed light

Table 31-9 Stages of Change

Precontemplation	Not seeing a problem behavior or considering change
Contemplation	Acknowledging a problem but not yet acting to make changes
Preparation	Taking the steps to get ready for change
Action	Making the change
Maintenance	Maintaining the behavior change

From Prochaska JO, DiClemente CC: Stages and processes of self-change of smoking: toward an integrative model of change, *J Consult Clin Psychol* 1983;51:390-395.

Table 31-10 Follow-up Visits for Patients Taking Opioid Medications: Monitoring the Five As

Analgesia
Activities of daily living: physical function, mood, sleep
Aerobic exercise
Adverse effects
Aberrant behaviors

Modified from Sehgal N, Manchikanti L, Smith HS. Prescription opioid abuse in chronic pain: a review of opioid abuse predictors and strategies to curb opioid abuse. *Pain Physician.* 2012;15:ES67-E92.

on patient values can be, "What do you want your health for?" This may help reframe the discussion, focusing appropriate treatment and outcome goals on what truly matters to the patient.

It may also be helpful at this point to determine how willing a patient is to change any potentially destructive lifestyle habits. Central to the treatment approach is helping the patient become more active and functional, and this often requires changes to existing lifestyle habits, such as increasing physical activity and losing weight. A tool that can be helpful in this assessment is the stages of change model (Table 31-9). This model can help clinicians individualize counseling approaches depending on the patient's readiness to make necessary lifestyle changes.

After establishing some baseline goals, consider patient preferences in treatment options. A patient-centered approach has become the standard of care and is included in guidelines on management of back pain (National Institute of Health and Clinical Excellence [NICE], 2009). The United Kingdom's NICE established evidence-based guidelines for treatment of chronic back pain in 2009. The recommended treatment approach is to offer information about self-care in addition to a therapeutic course of physical therapy, manual therapy, or acupuncture. These modalities were judged to have evidence of both clinical and cost effectiveness (NICE, 2009).

The self-care information should include instruction on how to remain active. This likely reduces pain and disability while lowering the number of visits and cost (Vanwye, 2010). Recommendations should include both rehabilitation exercises specific to the spine and aerobic exercise recommendations. Rehabilitation exercises should progress from passive to more active therapies as the pain moves from acute to more chronic or as the patient progresses and regains function. Aerobic exercise directly impacts a person's functional status in addition to improving mood and possibly pain perception. Several guidelines may be considered when making aerobic recommendations to patients. One is from the American College of Sports Medicine, which recommends 150 minutes of moderate-intensity exercise per week (Haskell et al., 2007). For patients who are not at this level of exercise, this goal can become part of the treatment plan.

Medication options for nonspecific back pain start with acetaminophen as a first-line recommendation. NSAIDs and weak opioids (such as codeine) are second-line choices. NSAIDs should be cautiously used in elderly patients because of an increased risk of heart disease and renal

failure (American Geriatrics Society 2012 Beers Criteria Update Expert Panel, 2012). For insufficient pain relief, consider a tricyclic antidepressant (NICE, 2009). Muscle relaxant medications may be useful for the short term but have not been shown helpful in chronic management of low back pain. Anticonvulsant medications such as gabapentin may be indicated for neuropathic pain but do not have evidence of effectiveness in more general musculoskeletal pain (Turk et al., 2011).

Starting opioid medications is a common source of tension for primary care physicians. In general, opioids can be considered as a backup plan when other modalities and medications have failed to give adequate pain relief and pain is still having an impact on function. Risks of opioids include nausea, constipation, sedation, hyperalgesia, misuse, and addiction. Opioids have been shown to improve pain but have not been shown to improve function more than other analgesics (Turk et al., 2011). Because of this lack of functional improvement and several risks associated with its use, the chronic use of opioids remains controversial. It is best to use opioids with defined functional goals in mind, which again should be made mutually with patients. When considering opioid therapies, several tools are available to clinicians to help determine the future risk of medication abuse. Among the most popular are the diagnosis, intractability, risk, and efficacy (DIRE) and the screener and opioid assessment for patients with pain (SOAPP) screening tools. The SOAPP may be more accurate in predicting risk of abuse. If the decision is made to start opioid medications, this can be viewed as a "trial of therapy." If functional goals are not being achieved, side effects are limiting, or there is evidence of aberrant use, the trial of therapy should be stopped (Table 31-10).

Goals of office visits include monitoring ongoing treatments, monitoring medications for side effects, and helping the patient stay engaged as an active participant in his or her care. One tool that can be useful in this process is the SMART goals (Table 31-11). Helping patients develop attainable goals can assist in behavior changes that are part of their treatment plans and allow for focused discussion in subsequent office visits.

For patients who are worsening or not progressing in terms of function, the first step is reevaluating the diagnosis and making sure no new red flag symptoms are present. Then consideration should be given to a change in therapy, additional workup, or specialist consultation. Reasons for consultation include complex cases with questions about the diagnosis, questions regarding appropriate

Table 31-11 SMART Goals (Using the Example of Wanting to Increase Exercise)

Specific	Walk 15 minutes every day before breakfast (avoid generic goals such as "exercise more")
Measurable	On a kitchen calendar, track time spent walking for the next month
Attainable	"I currently am able to walk 15 minutes but do so sporadically. Physically, I am able to do this, and it is realistic to wake up 15 minutes earlier."
Relevant	"Increasing exercise is a vital part of my pain treatment plan."
Time sensitive	"I will find my tennis shoes today and start walking tomorrow."

management after a failed treatment course, or when a specific diagnostic or therapeutic procedure is indicated. In addition, consider a psychology referral if a patient has completed one treatment course and still has significant disability or high levels of psychological stress (NICE, 2009).

KEY TREATMENT

- An initial treatment approach should include information on self-care in addition to a course of physical therapy, manual therapy, or acupuncture (Haskell et al., 2008) (SOR: A).

- Self-care information should include instructions on how to best remain active (Haskell et al., 2008) (SOR: A).
- Acetaminophen is the first-line medication choice with NSAIDs and weak opioids being second line. Consider a tricyclic antidepressant for patients with persistent or refractory pain (Haskell et al., 2008) (SOR: A).
- Opioid medications have been shown to improve pain but have not been shown to improve functional measures more than other analgesics (Turk et al., 2011) (SOR: C).

References

The complete reference list is available at www.expertconsult.com.

Web Resources

theacpa.org American Chronic Pain Association. Patient site with multiple resources, including a chronic pain diary.

www.americanbacksoc.org American Back Society. Nonprofit organization offering information for health care professionals on all aspects of spinal pain care.

www.familydoctor.org American Academy of Family Physicians (AAFP) Patient Information. Consumer health information on a variety of disorders, provided by the AAFP.

www.fammed.wisc.edu/integrative/modules/low-back-pain University of Wisconsin Integrative Medicine patient handouts. Information for clinicians and patient handouts on integrative and comprehensive management of chronic low back pain.

www.painedu.org/soapp.asp SOAPP opioid risk assessment tool.

32 Rheumatology and Musculoskeletal Problems

DOUGLAS COMEAU and DEANNA COREY

Arthritis is the most common health complaint in the United States and a common reason for office visits to family physicians despite the numerous over-the-counter treatments for joint pain and other musculoskeletal problems. In a Centers for Disease Control and Prevention (CDC) National Ambulatory Medical Care Survey, 49 million American adults reported physician-diagnosed arthritis, 21 million of whom reported chronic joint symptoms (Hootman and Helmick, 2006). The 30-year projection rate of patients age 65 and older will increase from 21.4 million to 41.4 million. These statistics lead to 75,000 hospitalizations and 36 million outpatient visits annually.

The term *arthritis* actually applies to more than 180 different disorders, all with pain in or around one or more joints, some with an inflammatory component. Although patients and physicians refer to this collection of diseases as arthritis or "rheumatism," family physicians must attempt to identify the disease process more precisely because of the many treatments available. Musculoskeletal symptoms might be harbingers of other, serious diseases affecting other organs. Patients should know their prognosis, whether their symptoms will most likely be self-limited, chronic, or progressive.

Rheumatic diseases greatly impact the U.S. health care system and society. Approximately 1% of the U.S. gross national product is spent each year on rheumatic diseases alone. Work absences, lost wages, and long-term disability also impact the quality of life of patient and family. Family physicians must be knowledgeable about new treatment options in the evaluation, assessment, and treatment of these conditions.

Evaluation of Joint and Other Musculoskeletal Symptoms

Precise anatomic localization of pain is the first task of the physician caring for a patient presenting with joint pain while also evaluating stiffness, redness, warmth, or swelling in the absence of trauma. It is important to distinguish pain that is truly articular from *periarticular* pain. Causes of *localized* periarticular pain include bursitis, tendonitis, and

carpal tunnel syndrome; fibromyalgia, polymyalgia rheumatica (PMR), and polymyositis all can cause *diffuse* periarticular pain.

The number of involved joints and presence or absence of symmetry are criteria for further diagnosis of articular pain (Figures 32-1 and 32-2). Monoarticular (one joint) or *oligoarticular* (several joints) arthritides can be caused by conditions such as *osteoarthritis* (OA), gout, pseudogout, or septic arthritis. Asymmetric polyarthritis occurs in ankylosing spondylitis (AS), psoriatic arthritis, Reiter disease, and spondyloarthropathies. *Symmetric* arthritis, meaning that the same joint is affected on the contralateral side but not necessarily to the same degree, is characteristic of *rheumatoid arthritis* (RA), *systemic lupus erythematosus* (SLE), Sjögren syndrome (SS), polymyositis, and scleroderma. Fibromyalgia, reflex sympathetic dystrophy, and predominantly psychological factors must be considered when pain is diffuse, not relatable to specific anatomic structures, or described in vague terms.

Other differentiating criteria include the correlation with activity or rest and the character of the pain. Mechanical causes tend to be more directly related to the joint's activity than inflammatory conditions. Whereas neuropathies tend to cause burning or prickling sensations, arthritides often cause an aching pain. The presence of joint stiffness after a period of inactivity might also aid in diagnosis; whereas RA is characterized by morning stiffness lasting 30 to 60 minutes or longer, OA-related morning stiffness lasts a shorter period, typically less than 30 minutes, but stiffness might also occur during the day. In neurologic conditions such as Parkinson disease, stiffness might be relatively constant. Vascular pain, such as intermittent claudication, is felt with activity, relieved quickly by rest, and described as a "deep, aching" sensation.

Constitutional symptoms such as fatigue, weakness, malaise, and weight changes are common chief complaints heard in a primary care office practice and often associated symptoms of specific rheumatic diseases. The patient's functional ability, occupational history, and activities requiring repetitive joint movement, as well as the ergonomics of such activities, should also be considered routinely in initial and serial evaluations. How are the symptoms affecting the patient's ability to perform self-care

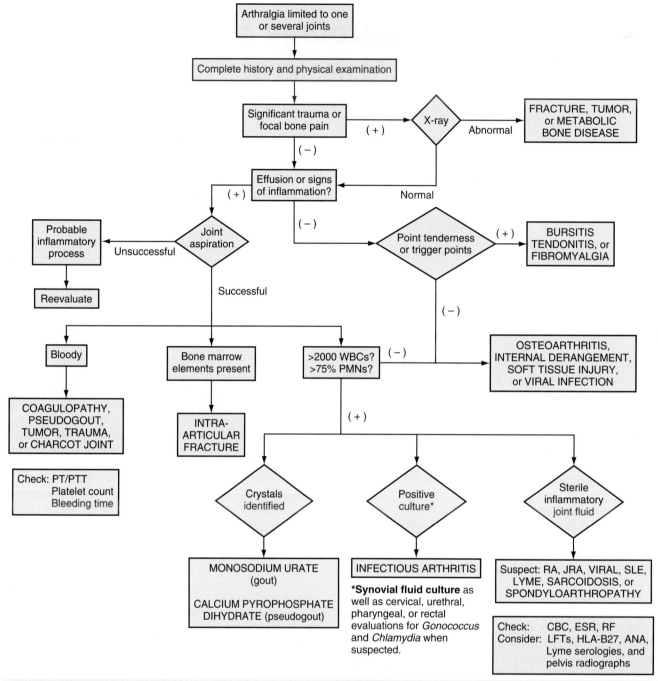

Figure 32-1 Evaluation of monoarticular or pauciarticular symptoms. *ANA*, Antinuclear antibody; *CBC*, complete blood cell count; *ESR*, erythrocyte sedimentation rate; *JRA*, juvenile rheumatoid arthritis; *LFT*, liver function test; *PMN*, polymorphonuclear (leukocyte) neutrophil; *PT*, prothrombin time; *PTT*, partial thromboplastin time; *RA*, rheumatoid arthritis; *RF*, rheumatoid factor; *SLE*, systemic lupus erythematosus; *WBCs*, white blood cells. (From American College of Rheumatology Ad Hoc Committee on Clinical Guidelines. Guidelines for the initial evaluation of the adult patient with acute musculoskeletal symptoms. *Arthritis Rheum.* 1996;39:1.)

activities of daily living (ADLs) such as bathing, dressing, and eating? Is the patient able to do instrumental activities of daily living (IADLs) such as buying groceries, cooking, using the telephone, and opening jars? Rheumatic disease can have a devastating effect on quality of life for both the patient and the family, with serious psychosocial and economic consequences. Therefore, the physician should address effects on occupational, recreational, and sexual activities in the context of family and other support systems.

PHYSICAL EXAMINATION

A thorough physical examination should be performed on all patients presenting with joint pain, including examination of asymptomatic joints and other organ systems that might be involved. Joints should be examined for swelling, tenderness, deformity, instability, and limitation of motion. Comparisons with the patient's contralateral side can be made in all these parameters, as well as with the physician's

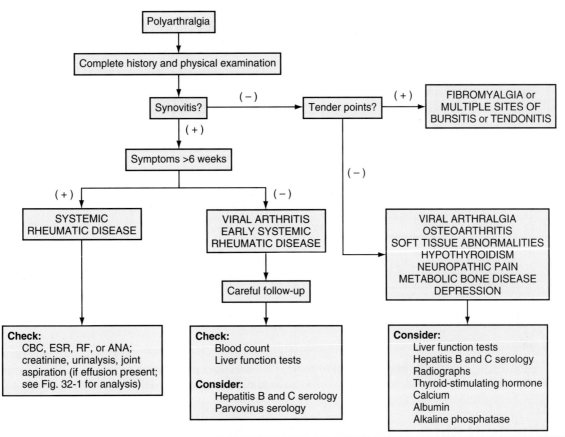

Figure 32-2 Evaluation of polyarticular symptoms. *ANA,* Antinuclear antibody; *CBC,* complete blood cell count; *ESR,* erythrocyte sedimentation rate; *RF,* rheumatoid factor. (From American College of Rheumatology Ad Hoc Committee on Clinical Guidelines: Guidelines for the initial evaluation of the adult patient with acute musculoskeletal symptoms. *Arthritis Rheum.* 1996;39:1.)

joints as a control. Instability can be tested by moving adjacent bones in the direction opposite to normal movement and observing for greater-than-normal motion. Serial grip strength measurements can be made by asking the patient to squeeze a blood pressure (BP) cuff inflated to 20 mm Hg and recording the maximal grip force in millimeters of mercury. Signs of systemic disease include fever; weight loss; oral or nasal ulcerations; liver, spleen, or lymph node enlargement; neurologic abnormalities; rashes; subcutaneous nodules; eye iritis; conjunctivitis or scleritis; and pericardial or pulmonary rubs. Because of circadian changes in patients with RA, serial comparisons of the physical examination are more accurate if the time of day is also recorded. Using skeleton diagrams of joint involvement facilitates the recording of a comprehensive joint examination (Figure 32-3).

Myalgias can be caused by localized trauma or overuse, systemic infection, metabolic disorder, or primary muscle disease. Multiple tender sites in an otherwise healthy patient suggest fibromyalgia. An elevated creatine kinase (CK) level with proximal weakness may be caused by an inflammatory myopathy such as polymyositis or dermatomyositis.

Rheumatic and other musculoskeletal problems are properly diagnosed by careful history and physical examination rather than by just ordering many laboratory tests, the results of which might actually confuse the diagnosis. Laboratory tests and radiologic imaging help confirm a

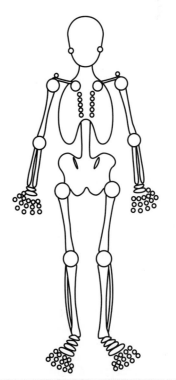

Figure 32-3 Skeleton diagram for recording joint examination findings. (From Polley HF, Hunder GG. *Rheumatologic interviewing and physical examination of the joints.* 2nd ed. Philadelphia: Saunders; 1978.)

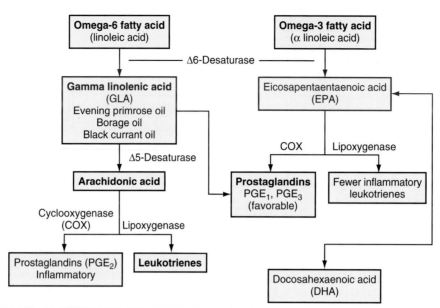

Figure 32-4 Influence of omega-6 fatty acids and omega-3 fatty acids on inflammation. (From Rakel R. *Integrative medicine*. Philadelphia: Saunders-Elsevier; 2007.)

presumptive clinical diagnosis made from a careful history and physical examination.

Pathogenesis of Rheumatic and Other Musculoskeletal Diseases

As with most disease, research into the causes of rheumatologic and musculoskeletal diseases shows that the cause of each disease is actually multifactorial. Further identification of these factors will help the family physician and rheumatologist modify the course of disease and eventually perhaps even prevent them.

Genetic factors have been identified for several arthritides. The presence of the human leukocyte antigen (HLA) system's HLA-DR4 antigen is associated with an increased incidence and severity of RA. The HLA-B27 antigen is found in a higher percentage in patients with AS and other spondyloarthropathies than in the general population. Other factors are apparently involved, however, because its presence or absence neither guarantees nor excludes development of arthritis. Testing for these antigens is not routinely performed. A National Institutes of Health (NIH) study found that genetic factors contributed 39% to 65% of OA variance. About 80% of patients with chondrodysplasias were found to have a type II collagen gene mutation likely linking these findings to OA (Prockop, 1998).

Inborn errors of metabolism are well known to cause diseases such as gout, in which uric acid is overproduced or underexcreted by the kidneys. Poorly controlled metabolic diseases such as diabetes or hemochromatosis might lead to arthropathies. Mechanical or traumatic factors cause OA in soccer players but not in long-distance runners, indicating that the type and direction of joint stress might be more important than the stress itself. Obesity is also an identified factor in OA of the knee, possibly because of metabolic influences as well as mechanical forces (Eaton, 2004).

Infectious agents such as parvovirus B19, human immunodeficiency virus (HIV), *Neisseria gonorrhoeae*, *Borrelia burgdorferi* (Lyme disease), and streptococci (rheumatic fever) are all well-known causes of arthritides. Some speculate that dietary factors might contribute to autoimmune syndromes, and fasting or a vegan diet (or both) can lead to improvement in RA (Kjeldsen-Kragh et al., 1991; McDougall et al., 2002; Smedslund et al., 2010). More specifically, a gluten-free vegan diet can induce changes that are atheroprotective and antiinflammatory in patients with RA (Elkan et al., 2008). The imbalance of omega-6 and omega-3 fatty acids in the standard American diet (a ratio of 30:1, as opposed to the ratio of 1:2 that is thought to have been present in Paleolithic diets) is also postulated to contribute to a more inflammatory state. Whereas omega-6 fatty acids are preferentially converted to more inflammatory prostaglandins such as arachidonic acid, omega-3 fatty acids can be converted into eicosapentaenoic acid (EPA) and docosahexaenoic acid (DHA), which contribute to antiinflammatory series-3 prostaglandin production (Figure 32-4). Omega-3 fatty acids are useful in RA, showing a decrease in use of nonsteroidal antiinflammatory drugs (NSAIDs) and decreased levels of pain (Oh, 2005).

Other medical systems, such as traditional Chinese medicine, may have completely different explanations for the changes seen in rheumatologic conditions. Although a conventional practitioner may not be aware of these, it is helpful to know about complementary modalities that may be beneficial (e.g., acupuncture helping patients with OA and fibromyalgia). See Chapter 12, Integrative Medicine.

Laboratory Studies

A complete blood cell count (CBC) with differential, urinalysis, and renal and liver function tests (LFTs) should be performed if asymptomatic rheumatic disease is suspected. Importantly, the frequency of abnormal laboratory results increases with increasing age in the normal population, even in the absence of disease, including common tests such as erythrocyte sedimentation rate (ESR), uric acid, antinuclear antibodies (ANAs), and rheumatoid factor (RF). Thus, arthritis panels can confuse the situation and should not be performed routinely. For example, only 80% of patients with RA have a positive RF. RF is a serum auto-antibody against immunoglobulin G (IgG). Up to 4% of the healthy population has a positive RF, which is also frequently positive in patients with *chronic obstructive pulmonary disease*, viral hepatitis, and sarcoidosis and can also be positive in malignancy and primary biliary cirrhosis and other autoimmune diseases. The higher the RF titer, however, the more likely it is caused by RA. ANA test results are positive in 95% of patients with lupus, and the test is often used to screen for SLE, but the result is also positive in 5% of the normal population. Drug use, age, and other factors might also cause a positive ANA test result. ANA titer also does not correlate exactly with changes in disease activity, so it should not be ordered in the absence of systemic symptoms. A patient with a positive ANA without clinical features is unlikely to have SLE. However, higher titers of ANA make it more likely that the result is related to lupus or another rheumatologic disorder.

Laboratory studies can be helpful in monitoring disease activity and drug toxicity as well as in establishing a diagnosis. CBC can detect anemia secondary to the chronic disease of RA or from NSAID-induced gastrointestinal (GI) blood loss. Patients with SLE can have hemolytic anemia, thrombocytopenia, or lymphopenia. Urinalysis can detect renal disease secondary to SLE, NSAIDs, or disease-modifying antirheumatic drugs (DMARDs) being used to treat RA. An elevated uric acid level can suggest gout. Acute-phase reactants such as ESR and C-reactive protein (CRP) can be useful to monitor disease activity but are nonspecific; they can also be negative in the presence of active disease. Patients with temporal arteritis and PMR almost always have a greatly elevated ESR. As a rule of thumb, for men, the upper limit of the normal ESR is age divided by 2; for women, it is age plus 10 divided by 2.

With weakness or muscle pain, CK level should be measured and arthralgias with abnormal liver enzyme levels followed up with hepatitis viral serologies.

Other tests, such as HLA-B27, antineutrophil cytoplasmic antibody, Lyme or parvovirus serologies, myositis-specific antibodies (anti–Jo-1), and antiphospholipid antibodies, are useful only when the clinical suspicion is high for spondyloarthropathies, Wegener granulomatosis, Lyme or parvovirus infection, inflammatory myositis, or antiphospholipid antibody syndrome, respectively (American College of Rheumatology [ACR], 1996).

SYNOVIAL FLUID ANALYSIS

Synovial fluid analysis can be helpful in evaluating a febrile patient with an acute joint to rule out septic arthritis or acute monoarthritis. Synovial fluid should be analyzed for white blood cell (WBC) count differential, cultured, and tested with polarized light microscopy for crystals. Purulent synovial fluid with greater than 90% polymorphonuclear leukocytes (PMNs), low viscosity, and turbid clarity can be caused by infection or crystal arthropathy

Table 32-1 Interpretation of Synovial Fluid Cell Count

Leukocyte Count (WBCs/mm³)	Interpretation
<200	Normal synovial fluid
<2000	Noninflammatory fluid
>2000	Inflammatory fluid
2000-20,000	Mild inflammation (e.g., SLE)
20,000-50,000	Moderate inflammation (e.g., RA, reactive arthritis)
50,000	Severe inflammation (e.g., sepsis, gout)
>100,000	Sepsis, until proved otherwise

RA, Rheumatoid arthritis; *SLE*, systemic lupus erythematosus; *WBC*, white blood cell.
From Towheed TE, Hochberg MC. Acute monoarthritis: a practical approach to assessment and treatment. *Am Fam Physician* 1996;54:2239.

(gout or pseudogout). Urate crystals are needle-shaped and negatively birefringent; calcium pyrophosphate dihydrate crystals are rhomboidal and weakly positively birefringent. Noninflammatory fluids generally have a clear appearance, normal viscosity, fewer than 2000 WBCs/mm³, and less than 75% PMNs (Table 32-1).

Synovial fluid analysis should always be performed on freshly obtained fluid. A simple bedside test is to attempt to read newsprint through the synovial fluid; newsprint can be read through noninflammatory fluid (Figure 32-5). Traditional tests on synovial fluid that are of limited or no value include measurement of glucose, lactate, and protein levels; subjective determination of viscosity; mucin clot test (examining the friability of the precipitate formed by mixing synovial fluid with dilute acetic acid); and immunologic tests. When looking for crystals and infection, direct examination, Gram stain, culture, and WBC count with differential are the only tests worth performing on synovial fluid. Inflammatory synovial fluid must be considered secondary to infection until proved otherwise by culture. The presence of crystals in the joint does not exclude the possibility of joint infection.

Synovial biopsy can facilitate a diagnosis in some settings. Arthroscopy has greatly simplified the acquisition of synovial tissue. This might be helpful in the diagnosis of granulomatous disease or infiltrative processes such as lymphoma, metastatic disease, or amyloidosis (Klippel, 2001).

IMAGING STUDIES

Plain radiographs are still the most common imaging studies done for evaluation and management of rheumatic diseases. Techniques such as magnetic resonance imaging (MRI) and radionuclide scintigraphy (bone scan) are being used more often, but they are costly and often unnecessary. Many arthritides have characteristic radiographic findings, but these techniques are not indicated for most patients with acute and new symptoms of SLE, gout, mechanical lower back pain, or RA because radiographs are usually normal early in the course of the disease. Normal radiographs also do not rule out OA. In established RA, the physician might see periarticular osteoporosis, soft tissue

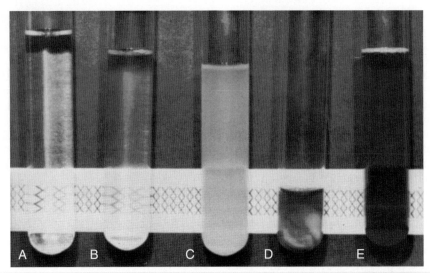

Figure 32-5 Synovial effusions. **A,** Normal or edema fluid is clear, pale yellow, or colorless. Print is easily read through the tube. **B,** Fluid from noninflammatory joint disease is yellow and clear. **C,** An inflammatory effusion is cloudy and yellow. Print may be blurred or completely obliterated, depending on the number of leukocytes. The effusion is translucent. **D,** A purulent effusion from septic arthritis contains a dense clump that does not even allow light through the many leukocytes. **E,** Hemorrhagic fluid is red. The supernatant may be darker yellow-brown (xanthochromic). A traumatic tap is less uniform and often has blood streaks. (From Schumacher HR. Synovial fluid analysis and synovial biopsy. In Kelley WN, Harris ED, Ruddy S, et al, eds. *Textbook of rheumatology.* 5th ed, vol 1. Philadelphia: Saunders; 1997:609-625.)

swelling, and marginal erosions. Gouty erosions cause characteristic overhanging edges because of reparative changes. (See later in this chapter.)

The severity of radiographic changes in association with severe symptoms can help guide the aggressiveness of treatment. Overreliance on radiographs, however, can lead to undertreatment or overtreatment of disease. Treatment of RA with a DMARD should usually be initiated long before severe radiographic abnormalities are present. The near-ubiquitous presence of osteophytes on the lumbar vertebrae should not be used to justify aggressive surgical treatment for low back pain; on the other hand, many patients with chronic lower back pain have normal lumbar radiographs. Radiographs for acute joint symptoms might be helpful to rule out fractures, metastases, or infection, especially in older patients. If symptoms persist for more than 10 days, the physician should consider repeat radiography, looking for callus formation.

Besides rotator cuff injuries, MRI studies are particularly useful for possible cruciate ligament, complete lateral collateral ligament, and meniscal tears in the knee for potential surgical candidates. Although expensive, MRI shows soft tissue destruction long before plain radiographs. Bone scans also are costly and are nonspecific but demonstrate RA changes before radiographs.

FUNCTIONAL ASSESSMENT

A functional assessment screen is a practical tool for the family physician and takes only minutes (see eTable 32-1 online). Focusing on disease impact on the patient as well as on the patient's joints can be an important contribution by the family physician. Functional assessment helps the primary care physician determine the role of other team physicians (rheumatologist, orthopedic surgeon, physical therapist, occupational therapist, mental health professional). Assessment of function can also lead to a discussion of disease impact on the family and help them deal with this chronic, possibly progressive condition.

Arthrocentesis

Arthrocentesis is most helpful in diagnosing crystal-induced and septic arthritis. Synovial fluid analysis can also be helpful in ruling out the coexistence of two or more types of arthritis in a single patient and even in a single joint. RA might coexist with a septic joint, secondary OA, hemarthrosis, or calcium pyrophosphate dihydrate (CPPD) disease. Hemarthrosis and bacterial infections usually occur in joints already damaged by arthritis. Arthrocentesis is a simple office procedure that can rule out bacterial infection in an acutely inflamed joint. Untreated or delayed treatment of infectious arthritis can cause rapid joint destruction, necessitating prompt diagnosis. A second line of treatment for RA should generally not be started until crystal arthropathy first has been ruled out. A physician is much more likely to harm a patient by not obtaining synovial fluid analysis when needed to make an accurate diagnosis. This is more common than the relatively rare occurrence of iatrogenic infection (particularly if proper sterile technique is used) or hemarthrosis (usually seen in patients with coagulopathies). The iatrogenic infection rate is generally estimated at one in 10,000, much less common than missed diagnosis of a septic joint. Anticoagulation therapy is not an absolute contraindication in the setting of acute arthritis.

The preferred route of entry for arthrocentesis traverses the shortest distance through tissue and avoids major vessels, tendons, and nerves. The knee, ankle, wrist, and elbow are the easiest joints to aspirate, and aspiration can be performed with only a moderate amount of trauma. Other joints normally require more extensive experience. Sterile technique normally does not require draping, but the same needle should not be used to aspirate the joint and to transfer the aspirated fluid to collection bottles.

The knee is the easiest joint to aspirate, best done with a medial or lateral approach at the superior third of the patella between it and the femur. Ankle arthrocentesis entry is midline, equidistant from the medial and lateral malleoli. A lateral entry between the olecranon process and the lateral epicondyle is best for the elbow. The shoulder can be approached posteriorly below the posterolateral aspect of the acromion process or anteriorly just lateral to the coracoid process.

A local anesthetic can be used but might distort landmarks; ethyl chloride spray immediately before needle insertion is usually sufficient. An 18-gauge needle is used for the knee and a 20-gauge needle for other joints; only 1 to 5 mL of synovial fluid is needed for diagnostic purposes. Fluid aspiration by itself is often therapeutic because it reduces articular pressure. Cartilage puncture should be avoided, if possible, by inserting the needle only as deeply as needed to obtain fluid, obtaining as much fluid as possible without risking unnecessary trauma by trying to aspirate every last drop, and avoiding side-to-side needle movement.

Therapeutic Corticosteroid Injection. Arthrocentesis can also be a therapeutic technique to deliver local corticosteroid to a joint that has not responded to systemic therapy and after infection has been excluded. Synovial fluid is first aspirated to ensure proper positioning in the joint space followed by 1 to 2 mL of corticosteroid to large joints (knees, hips, shoulders); 0.5 to 1 mL to wrists, elbows, and ankles; and 0.25 to 0.5 mL to small joints and soft tissue sites. A 1:2 dilution with lidocaine can be used to provide instant relief, although many believe lidocaine adds to the risk of infection (e.g., requiring a more complex procedure, changing needles) with limited benefit and therefore do not use it. After injection, the joint should be moved through its passive range of motion (ROM) followed by at least 24 hours of rest. Steroid injections should be limited to no more than three to four times per joint per year because of concerns about possible cartilage and ligamentous damage from repeated injections.

Nonsteroidal Antiinflammatory Drugs. The NSAIDs are among the most frequently prescribed drugs and are used by family physicians for almost all rheumatic and musculoskeletal pain conditions. By suppressing the synthesis of prostaglandins, NSAIDs reduce inflammation and therefore pain but do not prevent tissue injury or joint damage. Cyclooxygenase-2 (COX-2) inhibitors are used for rheumatologic and musculoskeletal pain because of decreased GI side effects. The Vioxx Gastrointestintal Outcomes Research (VIGOR) (Bombardier et al., 2000) and Celecoxib Long-term Arthritis Safety (CLASS) (Silverstein et al., 2000) studies for rofecoxib and celecoxib, respectively, showed that the decreased GI effects outweighed any cardiovascular risk. The Adenomatous Polyp Prevention on Vioxx (APPROVe) study linked rofecoxib (Vioxx) to an increased risk of cardiovascular disease (Bresalier et al., 2005). The Alzheimer's Disease Anti-Inflammatory Prevention Trial (ADAPT) study compared celecoxib (Celebrex) and naproxen (Naprosyn, Aleve) in Alzheimer disease prevention and was stopped secondary to a 50% increase in cardiovascular events in subjects not taking placebo (NIH, 2004). Overall, COX-2 inhibitors have produced minimal decrease in GI bleeding and thus should be used cautiously for rheumatologic and musculoskeletal pain because the cardiovascular risk outweighs the GI benefit. Currently, celecoxib has a "black box" warning; rofecoxib was removed from the market.

Patients respond to different classes of NSAIDs for unknown reasons, and no NSAID appears superior to others in efficacy. Treatment is largely empiric. Most clinicians start with a low dose and titrate upward if needed. An adequate trial of an NSAID requires that the patient take a maximum dose for 3 weeks before changing to a different NSAID, although many patients will expect a change in medication before this. It is usually best to switch to an NSAID from a different class. There is no benefit to combining nonsalicylate NSAIDs. All COX-1 NSAIDs can cause dyspepsia and GI toxicity, interfere with platelet function, and prolong bleeding times. Other common side effects include renal toxicity; hypertension; and central nervous system (CNS) symptoms such as drowsiness, dizziness, and confusion. A 2004 Cochrane review of NSAIDs for lower back pain concluded that the various types of NSAIDs (e.g., COX-2 inhibitors) are equally effective, and selection of an NSAID for OA should be based on relative safety and patient acceptability.

Combining NSAIDs with misoprostol (Cytotec), 100 to 200 mg four times daily with meals, or omeprazole (Prilosec), 20 mg/day (Hawkey et al., 1998) has been shown to decrease the incidence of gastric and duodenal ulcers. But combining with proton pump inhibitors (PPIs) for prolonged periods of time can interfere with absorption of other nutrients, including B vitamins, iron, magnesium, and calcium, which can lead to neuropathy, anemia, arrhythmia, and fracture (Wilhelm et al., 2013). A meta-analysis of 112 randomized controlled trials (RCTs) found no evidence supporting the effectiveness of H_2 receptor antagonists, while the risk of symptomatic ulcers was significantly reduced by PPIs, misoprostol, and COX-2 inhibitors (Koch et al., 1996). Omeprazole and other PPIs are better tolerated than misoprostol and famotidine (Hawkey et al., 1998). The physician should monitor for decreased renal function, interaction with antihypertensives, and transaminase (alanine aminotransferase [ALT], aspartate transaminase [AST]) elevations when starting NSAID therapy or increasing dosage or when the patient's condition changes.

A common issue for the family physician is whether a patient prescribed aspirin for cardiac prophylaxis needs to stop the aspirin when prescribed a traditional NSAID. Patients taking both do not appear to be at significantly increased risk of GI toxicity. However, the aspirin might not yield any additional cardioprotective benefit because these patients already benefit from the traditional nonselective NSAID antiplatelet effect. If taking both aspirin and NSAID, it is best to take the aspirin at least 4 hours before the NSAID for its full protective effect.

ARTHRITIS OF SYSTEMIC DISEASE

Arthritis can be a component of many systemic diseases, including metabolic disorders; infections; malignancies; and various endocrine, hematologic, and GI diseases. Parvovirus B19 is responsible for erythema infectiosum and can also cause polyarthritis, especially in the hands, knees, and ankles. HIV infection sometimes causes symmetric polyarthritis, spondylitis, or acute oligoarthritis. Hepatitis B and *C* can cause acute symmetric polyarthritis in large and small joints. Inflammation in a few large joints and back pain are among the earliest symptoms of infective endocarditis in about 25% of patients with this disorder (Totemchokchyakarn and Ball, 1996).

Lyme arthritis caused by *B. burgdorferi* can cause migratory monoarthritis or oligoarthritis in the knees or shoulders weeks to months after the rash of erythema chronicum migrans has developed. Poorly controlled *diabetes* (affecting foot, ankle, and knee), *hyperthyroidism* (affecting fingers and toes), *hypothyroidism* (causing noninflammatory effusions in knees, wrists, and hands), and *parathyroid disease* (causing chondrocalcinosis) are all endocrine disorders that can cause arthritis.

Metabolic disorders can cause degenerative arthritis. *Hemochromatosis* (caused by iron deposition) typically affects the second and third metacarpophalangeal (MCP) joints, wrists, knees, hips, and shoulders. *Wilson disease* (caused by copper deposition) can cause premature OA in wrists and knees. Sickle cell disease can be complicated by knee arthritis; arthritis is also often seen in patients with hemophilia and leukemia. Arthritis is associated with inflammatory bowel disease (IBD) and primary biliary cirrhosis. Reactive carcinoma synovitis can be the presenting symptom of an underlying malignancy, particularly of the breast or the prostate.

REFERRAL TO THE RHEUMATOLOGIST

As for all types of disease conditions, referral to the subspecialist largely depends on the family physician's knowledge, interest level, and logistical ability to provide state-of-the-art care to a given patient for a given disease entity at a given time in the disease course. Patients with specific conditions, such as suspected septic arthritis, acute myelopathy or mononeuritis multiplex, suspected acute tendon or muscle rupture, or acute internal derangement, should probably be referred. In addition, referral should be considered for patients without a specific diagnosis after 6 weeks; those with difficulty in symptom control, systemic symptoms in pregnancy, or severe symptoms; patients requiring steroid, immunosuppressive, or other drugs unfamiliar to the primary care physician; and those with end-stage joint disease. The often nonspecific nature and psychosocial impact of rheumatic symptoms require continued active involvement of the family physician in the patient's care, regardless of referral.

Rheumatic Diseases

OSTEOARTHRITIS

> ### Key Points
>
> - OA affects 20% of the U.S. population; 44% of OA patients are not active.
> - Primary and secondary OA must be differentiated.
> - NSAIDs, not COX-2 inhibitors, are still the pharmacologic treatment of choice for OA.

Osteoarthritis, also known as "degenerative joint disease," is the most common form of arthritis and causes more work disability in the United States (17%) than any other disease. Arthritis affects 20% of the U.S. population, about half of whom primarily have OA. In 2005, it was estimated that 27 million Americans had OA (Lawrence et al., 2008). Long thought to result from "wear and tear," OA is now known to have genetic, traumatic, metabolic, and developmental causes, which complicate prevention and treatment. OA is found radiographically in almost all 75-year-old patients, most of whom are asymptomatic. OA occurs about equally in men and women ages 45 to 55 years, but after 55 years is more common in women (CDC, 2005). Most patients with OA are not seriously affected and are asymptomatic. Others, however, require joint replacement surgery because of its severity.

Although OA is considered a noninflammatory type of arthritis affecting primarily the cartilage, it actually involves active biochemical disease processes as well as mechanical forces that affect the entire synovial joint. An OA variant affecting primarily the hands runs in families and is inflammatory. Women are more prone to this inflammatory variant of OA of the hands that causes Heberden nodes (in distal interphalangeal [DIP] joints) and Bouchard nodes (in proximal interphalangeal [PIP] joints). The articular cartilage may not even be involved, with the disease process centered more on subchondral bone turnover (Peterson et al., 1998). Quadriceps muscle weakness might precede the onset of knee OA, indicating the importance of biomechanical factors (Slemenda et al., 1997).

Osteoarthritis can be separated into primary (idiopathic), hereditary (resulting from collagen gene defects), and secondary. Secondary OA results from previous cartilage damage. Occupations causing repetitive joint trauma predispose a patient to OA. Episodic trauma, congenital anatomic abnormalities (slipped capital femoral epiphyses, congenital hip dysplasias), neuropathies, and endocrine-metabolic causes (obesity, hemochromatosis, Wilson disease, CPPD disease, Paget disease, acromegaly) all might lead to OA. Inflammatory arthritides such as RA, infections, or gout damage cartilage and are often followed by the development of OA.

Occupational kneelers (e.g., shipyard workers, miners, carpet or floor layers) have a significantly higher incidence of knee OA than control groups of clerical workers (Maetzel et al., 1997). However, repetitive sports activities such as long-distance running are unlikely to cause OA in the absence of joint injury or antecedent joint abnormality (Panush and Lane, 1994). More than 44% of patients with diagnosed OA are inactive (Gordon et al., 1998). Low-impact activity in normal joints is not associated with OA, but high-intensity and high-impact activity resulting in injury is associated with OA. Mechanical risk factors might affect the initiation more than the progression of OA. Most mild OA does not progress to severe joint damage. Mild OA might be a different disease than severe OA, which depends on processes other than early OA.

Clinical Findings

Most OA is asymptomatic, an incidental finding on radiographs performed for other reasons. No treatment or further evaluation is indicated for asymptomatic OA. Early symptomatic OA is characterized by local pain of gradual onset exacerbated by using the involved joint. Pain typically worsens as the day progresses and is relieved by rest. There is less than 30 minutes of localized morning stiffness and no constitutional or systemic symptoms, and the gel phenomenon (stiffness after periods of rest and inactivity) resolves within several minutes of activity. Damp, cool, rainy weather often exacerbates symptoms because of changes in intraarticular pressure associated with changes in barometric pressure. Patients with OA of the knees might complain of buckling or instability, especially when descending stairs. OA of the hip can manifest as pain radiating from the groin and down the anterior thigh. OA of the neck might be felt in the neck, back, or upper extremities, causing pain, weakness, or numbness. As OA progresses, pain can become continuous, including at night.

Primary OA can be divided into three classifications: generalized OA, large-joint OA, and erosive OA. *Generalized* OA involves five or more joints, most often the DIP joints of the hand (Herberden nodes), the PIP joints of the hand (Bouchard nodes), the first carpometacarpal joint, the first MTP joint of the feet, and the knee, hip, and spine. There is a significant familial component. *Large-joint* OA of the knees and hips might occur as part of generalized OA or alone. OA of the knees often occurs in the medial and patellofemoral compartments. OA of the hips can be characterized in two subsets, central and superior poles. Central or medial involvement of the hip joint space occurs in the setting of generalized OA, is usually bilateral, and is seen in women more than men. Most hip OA is superior pole, usually unilateral, seen more in men, and occurs without other joint involvement. As many as 40% to 90% of cases of adult hip OA might arise from subtle developmental abnormalities of the hip, including acetabular dysplasia, developmental (formerly "congenital") hip dislocation, Legg-Calvé-Perthes disease, and slipped capital femoral epiphysis (Brandt and Slemenda, 2004).

A rare form of primary OA known as *erosive OA* involves the hand's PIP and DIP joints equally, with significant inflammation. Other joints are often not involved, although 15% of erosive OA cases might subsequently evolve into seropositive RA (Kujala et al., 1995).

Physical Findings

Physical findings of OA typically include joint swelling, tenderness, crepitus, and enlargements at joint margins, causing deformity. The location of pain should be precisely localized as to whether it is truly articular or periarticular; if pain is located in the joint, an inflammatory or infectious cause should be ruled out first. Patients might have reduced ROM or, in severe cases, joint instability, resulting in excess motion or locking because of loose cartilage fragments. Warmth and soft tissue swelling because of joint effusion might be present, but a markedly swollen, hot, erythematous joint suggests a septic or microcrystalline disease rather than OA.

Laboratory Studies

Clinical study criteria for OA classification are helpful as a means to standardize the diagnosis (see eTables 32-2 and 32-3 online). Although the diagnosis of OA can almost always be made by history and physical examination,

Table 32-2 Criteria for Classification of Idiopathic Osteoarthritis of the Knee

Clinical and Laboratory	Clinical and Radiographic	Clinical*
Knee pain *plus* at least five of nine: Age >50 yr Stiffness <30 min Crepitus Bony tenderness Bony enlargement No palpable warmth ESR <40 mm/hr RF <1:40 SFOA	Knee pain *plus* at least one of three: Age >50 yr Stiffness <30 min Crepitus *plus* Osteophytes	Knee pain *plus* at least three of six: Age >50 yr Stiffness <30 min Crepitus Bony tenderness Bony enlargement No palpable warmth
92% sensitive	91% sensitive	95% sensitive
75% specific	86% specific	69% specific

ESR, Erythrocyte sedimentation rate (Westergren); *RF*, rheumatoid factor; *SFOA*, synovial fluid signs of OA (clear, viscous, or white blood cell count <2000/mm³).
*Alternative for the clinical category would be four of six, which is 84% sensitive and 89% specific.
From Altman R, Asch E, Bloch G, et al. Development of criteria for the classification and reporting of osteoarthritis: classification of osteoarthritis of the knee. *Arthritis Rheum.* 1986;29:1039-1049, with permission of the American College of Rheumatology.

definitive diagnosis can be helped by synovial fluid analysis; radiography; and normal ESR, ANA, and RF during symptomatic periods. Synovial fluid analysis of large-joint effusions can be used to exclude other processes. Joint effusions in OA typically show leukocyte counts lower than 1000 WBCs/mm³, predominantly lymphocytes (Table 32-2). Serum tests might be misleading because ESR rises with age, and 20% of healthy older adults have positive RF levels. A greatly elevated ESR suggests a process other than OA. Although many have been identified, biochemical markers of OA are not generally useful to practicing clinicians at this time.

Imaging Studies

Radiographs are generally the first-line confirmation of the presence of OA. Treatment should not be based solely on radiographic abnormalities, however, given the frequency of asymptomatic joints demonstrating radiographic OA changes. OA changes include osteophyte formation, asymmetric joint space narrowing (defined as <3 mm on a weight-bearing knee), and subchondral bone sclerosis (Figures 32-6 and 32-7). Later in the disease process, subchondral cysts with sclerotic walls might develop. Periarticular osteoporosis and marginal erosions suggest RA or some other inflammatory arthritis rather than OA. Patients with OA involving atypical joints (MCP joints, wrists, elbows, shoulders, or ankles) should be evaluated for an underlying disorder such as CPPD or hemochromatosis.

Treatment

Treatment of OA includes pharmacologic therapy, nonpharmacologic therapy, and surgery. Before initiating treatment, a definitive diagnosis of OA must be made by careful history and physical examination. No currently available treatment has been shown to alter the natural history of the disease. Therefore, the goal of management of OA is primarily to relieve pain, stiffness, and swelling. The physician seeks to reduce limitation of motion and disability without causing iatrogenic side effects. Patients and their families must also be educated about the disease and their treatment options (Table 32-3).

Nonpharmacologic therapy includes rest during pain episodes, exercise, weight control, avoidance of trauma, patient and family education, and assistive devices. The patient's ability to perform both self-care ADLs and IADLs requiring higher functioning (e.g., shopping, driving, writing) should be assessed. Physical and occupational therapists can provide great benefit by offering an exercise program and assistive devices to maintain independence and minimize symptoms (Fransen et al., 2001). Patients benefit from the use of canes, walkers, bathtub and toilet wall bars, and dressing sticks for socks and from the other methods of joint protection and symptom relief, such as heat massage. Rest is important for patients with acute pain. Otherwise, helpful exercise programs include swimming, other aerobic conditioning, and walking (van Baar et al., 1999). Weight control and weight reduction have also been shown to improve symptoms (Messier et al., 2004).

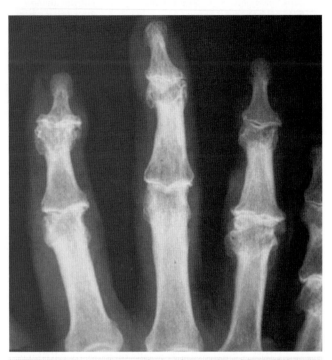

Figure 32-6 Osteoarthritis in the hand. (From Resnick D, Yu JS, Sartoris D. Imaging. In Kelley WN Harris ED, Ruddy S, et al, eds. *Textbook of rheumatology*. 5th ed, vol 1. Philadelphia: Saunders; 1997:626-686.)

Table 32-3 Options in the Management of Patients with Osteoarthritis

Nonpharmacologic therapy	Patient education and self-management programs
	Social support through telephone contact
	Physical and occupational therapy
	ROM and strengthening exercises
	Aerobic conditioning
	Weight loss
	Assistive devices for ambulation and activities of daily living
Pharmacologic therapy	Oral nonopioid analgesics (e.g., acetaminophen)
	Topical analgesics (e.g., capsaicin cream)
	NSAIDs
	Intraarticular steroid injections
	Opioid analgesics
Surgical therapy	Closed tidal joint lavage
	Arthroscopic debridement and joint lavage
	Osteotomy
	Total joint arthroplasty

NSAID, Nonsteroidal antiinflammatory drug; *ROM,* range of motion.

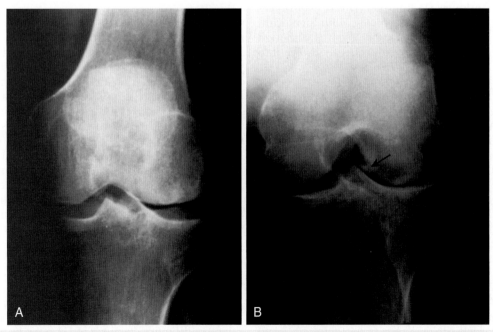

Figure 32-7 Osteoarthritis in the knee. **A,** Anteroposterior (AP) radiograph of knee showing asymmetric joint narrowing. **B,** AP radiograph showing osteophyte formation in knee (*arrow*). (From Resnick D, Yu JS, Sartoris D. Imaging. In Kelley WN Harris ED, Ruddy S, et al, eds. *Textbook of rheumatology*. 5th ed, vol 1. Philadelphia: Saunders; 1997:626-686.)

First-line pharmacologic therapies for symptom control include acetaminophen, up to 1000 mg four times daily in the absence of liver disease, and traditional NSAIDs, beginning with ibuprofen. Because few RCTs studied differences in efficacy of NSAIDs, the initial choice is empiric. Therefore, relative safety, patient adherence, and cost should determine selection. Risk factors for upper GI bleeding with NSAIDS include age older than 65 years, history of peptic ulcer disease or upper GI bleeding, concurrent use of oral corticosteroids and anticoagulants, and possibly smoking and alcohol consumption. Evidence suggests that NSAIDs are superior to acetaminophen for improving knee and hip pain from OA. No significant difference in overall safety was found, although patients taking NSAIDs were more likely to experience an adverse GI event (Towhead et al., 2006). Particular care must be taken with use among geriatric patients because several studies have shown increased hospital admissions caused by NSAID-related complications in this population (Liantonio and Simmons, 2013). Capsaicin (Zostrix) topical cream four times daily, formerly a first-line agent, now has been shown to have minimal benefit, especially when considering side effects that impair compliance (Mason et al., 2004). Combination therapy (NSAIDs with analgesics) may also be helpful. The addition of tramadol (Ultram, 200 mg/day) in patients responding to 1000 mg/day of naproxen has been shown to allow a significant reduction (by half) in the naproxen dose needed without compromising pain relief (Schnitzer et al., 1999).

Currently, NSAIDs plus a PPI such as omeprazole remain the treatment of choice for prevention of NSAID-induced gastric ulcers. Opioid analgesics and limited intraarticular corticosteroid injections (up to 4 injections per joint per year) are the remaining traditional choices. Opiates should generally be avoided for long-term use but might be helpful for acute exacerbations.

Intraarticular glucocorticoids are often used and are particularly useful in patients with contraindications or continued pain despite NSAIDs. This modality is postulated to work by decreasing cartilage catabolism and osteophyte formation. A meta-analysis found that patients receiving intraarticular steroid injections for OA of the knee were twice as likely to have short-term improvement as control participants (Arroll et al., 2004). Data on injection of the hip and knee joint show the most promise, but efficacy at other sites is less certain. Aseptic technique should be used to prevent iatrogenic complications of infection. Patients should be counseled on postinjection complications such as bleeding, infection, skin hypopigmentation, fat necrosis, and steroid flare.

Because OA is a common incurable disease that causes pain, many other treatments, including dietary supplements and other alternative therapies, have been tried for centuries. Balanced hormone therapy, copper bracelets, bee venom, vitamins, herbs, homeopathic remedies, and certain types of foods are promoted as effective treatments or cures for OA. Family physicians should be aware of proven and unproven remedies used by their patients. One therapy shown to be efficacious is glucosamine sulfate.

Glucosamine and chondroitin sulfates both stimulate the production of proteoglycan in cartilage and inhibit its breakdown. Over-the-counter formulations vary in the amount of glucosamine (made from crab shells) and chondroitin (processed from cow cartilage). Research has shown that patients have moderately benefited from glucosamine and chondroitin supplements over 3 years with less knee joint space narrowing on radiography, significant reduction of symptoms, and no adverse effects (Richy et al., 2003; Sherman et al., 2012). The major studies of glucosamine used two different formulations of the supplement, which yielded different results: the sulfate and HCl formulations. A 2005 Cochrane review found that whereas the glucosamine HCL preparation failed to show benefit in pain and function, the glucosamine sulfate preparation showed that glucosamine was superior to placebo in the treatment of pain and functional impairment resulting from symptomatic OA. Studies for chondroitin are less convincing, with no consistent improvement in pain or functional status (Ebell, 2006) except for possibly hand OA (Erickson and Messer, 2013; Reginster, 2012), although a more recent study comparing glucosamine sulfate to HCL found no difference between the two formulations (Provenza et al., 2014). The safest daily intake is 1500 mg/day of glucosamine sulfate and 1200 mg/day of chondroitin. Most capsules containing both minerals are also formulated with manganese, theorized to assist in proteoglycan metabolism but not studied (Richy et al., 2003).

A meta-analysis of 11 studies found that S-adenosylmethionine (SAMe) was as effective as NSAIDs at reducing pain and functional limitations, with a somewhat better adverse effect profile (Soeken et al., 2002). This is a stimulating supplement and should not be used at bedtime due to potential insomnia.

A Cochrane review of herbal therapies for OA found two studies demonstrating that avocado–soybean unsaponifiables showed beneficial effects on function, pain, intake of NSAIDs, and global evaluation (Little et al., 2000). Another beneficial intervention is transcutaneous electrical nerve stimulation (TENS) for OA of the knee; electrical stimulation has been shown to improve knee OA moderately by 25% and cervical OA by 12% (Osiri et al., 2004).

Studies comparing acupuncture with a sham control found greater improvement in those receiving the actual treatment (Berman et al., 2004; Ezzo et al., 2001; Vas et al., 2004). A meta-analysis found that acupuncture was more effective than placebo in pain reduction in peripheral OA (Kwon et al., 2006). Two studies found that therapeutic touch, an energy modality, showed benefit in OA (Gordon et al., 1998). Although previously cited as beneficial for OA secondary to antioxidants, the literature reports an increased risk of cardiovascular disease with vitamins C and E (Alkhenizan and Palda, 2003).

Other, less traditional therapies have received much media attention but have not shown effectiveness. Cycles of three or more weekly intra-articular injections of hyaluronic acid (viscous substance in synovial fluid that lubricates and protects joints) have been used, with partial success (Abramowicz, 1998a). Hyaluronate sodium (Hyalgan) and hylan G-F 20 (Synvisc) are approved by the Food and Drug Administration (FDA) for OA of the knee. Onset of pain relief can take several weeks and can last for 6 months or longer. Meta-analyses of hyaluronic acid have shown minimal effectiveness versus placebo. The cost-to-benefit ratio favors therapies other than joint injection (Lo et al., 2003).

- Treatment of OA begins with nonpharmacologic modalities, including weight loss (Messier et al., 2004), physical therapy (Fransen et al., 2001), exercise (van Baar et al., 1999), and orthotics if needed (SOR: A).
- Acetaminophen and NSAIDs are both first-line pharmacotherapy for pain associated with OA, although NSAIDs appear to be more effective (Towhead et al., 2006) (SOR: A).
- Intraarticular glucocorticoids show short-term improvement in pain associated with OA of the hip and knee (Arroll et al., 2004) (SOR: B).
- Treatments such as Synvisc (Lo et al., 2003), glucosamine (Richy et al., 2003), and acupuncture (Kwon et al., 2006) are often used for OA relief before surgical measures (SOR: B).

RHEUMATOID ARTHRITIS

Key Points

- RA affects women 3 : 1 more than men, with 70% having an insidious onset.
- Symmetric synovitis with morning stiffness longer than 1 hour is the hallmark of RA.
- Constitutional symptoms are common in patients with RA.

Rheumatoid arthritis is a chronic inflammatory systemic disease in which cellular and autoimmune mechanisms result in destruction of tissues, primarily the synovium. A genetic predisposition appears to be important, but a specific inciting infectious agent or other cause has still not been found. RA manifestations vary from very mild, self-limited disease to multiorgan destruction and early death. Increasing knowledge of the modulating factors in disease progression is transforming the treatment of RA. Without treatment, the normally fluctuating disease course results in progressive joint destruction. Patients with active, polyarticular, RF-positive RA have more than a 70% chance of developing joint damage or erosion within 2 years (Fuchs et al., 1989). Because RA is relatively uncommon compared with OA and is now treated quite differently, the family physician must be able to make the correct diagnosis and initiate disease-modifying therapy early, before joint destruction.

Epidemiology

Rheumatoid arthritis affects women more frequently than men (≈3 : 1 ratio) and occurs in all age groups but has a peak incidence between 20 and 50 years. The prevalence is 1% to 2% of adults, ranging from 0.3% of the population younger than age 35 years to about 10% of those older than age 65 years. There is a higher concordance of RA in monozygotic twins than in dizygotic twins because of gender differences and differences in major histocompatibility complex (MHC) class II gene products (HLA-DR). Combinations of different genes most likely predispose patients to the disease. The HLA-DR antigen appears to be

triggered by many stimuli. After this inciting event, the synovial lining cells and subsynovial vessels proliferate, forming a pannus. Leukocytes invade, followed by a further inflammatory cascade involving proteases and cytokines. RF produces autoantibodies to IgG Fc fragment, influenced by HLA-DR polymorphism and associated with more severe, extraarticular disease. Again, RF is not specific to RA and can be detected in normal persons.

Diagnosis

Rheumatoid arthritis is a clinical diagnosis made by careful history and physical examination. Laboratory testing can be confirmatory but is also misleading if not interpreted in context. Radiographic evidence of erosions appears only several months to 1 year after disease onset. The ACR published useful criteria in 1987 for the diagnosis of RA (Table 32-4). Symptoms must be present for at least 6 weeks for the initial diagnosis.

Symmetric synovitis is the hallmark of RA and can be suggested by joint aspiration of synovial fluid, yielding more than 2000 WBCs/mm³ without crystal or by radiographic evidence of erosions. Because the cause of synovitis cannot be differentiated clinically, extraarticular manifestations can help distinguish RA from other inflammatory conditions.

Table 32-4 American College of Rheumatology Revised Criteria for Classification of Rheumatoid Arthritis (Traditional Format)

Criterion*	Definition
1. Morning stiffness	Morning stiffness in and around the joints lasting at least 1 hour before maximal improvement
2. Arthritis of three or more joint areas	At least three joint areas with simultaneous soft tissue swelling or fluid (not bony overgrowth alone) observed by physician. The 14 possible joint areas are right or left PIP, MCP, wrist, elbow, knee, ankle, and MTP joints.
3. Arthritis of hand joints	At least one joint area swollen as above in a wrist, MCP, or PIP joint
4. Symmetric arthritis	Simultaneous involvement of the same joint areas on both sides of the body; bilateral involvement of PIP, MCP, or MTP joints is acceptable without absolute symmetry.
5. Rheumatoid nodules	Subcutaneous nodules over bony prominences or extensor surfaces or juxtaarticular nodules regions, observed by physician
6. Serum rheumatoid factor	Demonstration of abnormal amounts of serum RF by any method that has been positive in fewer than 5% of normal control participants
7. Radiologic changes	Radiologic changes typical of RA on posteroanterior hand and wrist radiographs, which must include erosions or unequivocal bony decalcification localized to, or most marked adjacent to, the involved joints (osteoarthritis changes alone do not qualify)

*Four or more criteria are needed for the diagnosis of rheumatoid arthritis (RA). Criteria 1 through 4 must be present for 6 weeks or longer. The presence of criteria is not conclusive evidence for the diagnosis of RA. The absence of criteria is not conclusively negative.
MCP, Metacarpophalangeal; MTP, metatarsophalangeal; PIP, proximal interphalangeal; RF, rheumatoid factor.
From Arnett FC. Revised criteria for the classification of rheumatoid arthritis. *Bull Rheum Dis.* 1989;38:1. Used with permission.

History

Approximately 70% of patients with RA experience an insidious onset over weeks to months, 10% have an acute abrupt onset, and 20% have an intermediate onset, with increasing symptoms for days to weeks. Morning stiffness occurring for more than 1 hour is suggestive of RA. Morning stiffness results from joint immobilization during sleep and is not related to the time of day. As opposed to patients with OA, patients with RA have constitutional symptoms such as fatigue, malaise, weight loss, low-grade fever, and anemia. Small joints in the hands and feet (PIP, MCP) are typically involved first, with larger joints involved later. The joints themselves might be warm to the touch but are usually not erythematous. A pannus of inflamed synovium palpable as a rubbery mass of tissue strongly suggests RA.

The presentation of exacerbations of chronic rheumatoid synovitis might differ from those of early acute synovitis. Chronic inflammation causing fibrosis decreases synovial vascularity, reducing the amount of swelling from previous episodes. Although the frank swelling of burned-out RA appears less severe, the amount of pain, morning stiffness, constitutional symptoms (fatigue, malaise), and joint destruction on radiography shows this physical finding to be misleading. These episodes in patients with chronic, long-term RA should therefore not be considered improvement over more visible, earlier episodes of synovitis.

Less common presentations of RA include acute onset (which has the best prognosis) and palindromic RA, which is characterized by brief episodes of swelling of a large joint such as a knee, wrist, or ankle. Palindromic RA can therefore be easily misdiagnosed as gout.

Approximately 20% of patients with RA have intermittent symptoms. The rest have progressive disease of varying severity from slow to rapid progressive. In addition to morning stiffness, synovitis, and structural damage, RA exhibits classic manifestations in specific joints. Whereas cervical spine involvement is common, thoracic and lumbar spine involvement is rare. Early symptoms are neck stiffness and decreased motion, which can lead to neurologic complications from C1 to C2 instability resulting from tenosynovitis of the transverse ligament of the first cervical vertebra (C1, which stabilizes odontoid process of C2), as well as disease of the apophyseal joints.

Neck pain without neurologic features tends to be self-limited and usually improves, but neck pain and neurologic symptoms often do not correlate well. A neurologic examination, even in the absence of neck pain, is therefore prudent in patients with RA. Radiographs of the cervical spine in flexion and extension might be needed to detect C1 to C2 involvement, which necessitates caution during surgical procedures requiring intubation.

Physical Examination

Upper Extremity. Shoulder RA usually manifests as decreased ROM. Elbow RA is more accessible than shoulder RA for physical examination and joint aspiration. Elbow involvement can manifest with elbow pain and swelling; ulnar compression syndrome (paresthesia and weakness of fourth and fifth digits) can develop from the synovitis. The wrists are affected in most RA patients, in contrast to OA patients; carpal tunnel syndrome is seen frequently. RA usually involves the MCP and PIP joints rather than the DIP joints. Classic late changes such as swan neck and boutonnière deformities and ulnar deviation of the MCP joints caused by ligamentous laxity might occur. The swan neck deformity is characterized by flexion of the DIP and MCP joints and hyperextension of the PIP joint, probably resulting from shortening of the interosseous muscles and tendons and shortening of the dorsal tendon sheath. The boutonnière deformity results from avulsion of the extensor hood of the PIP because of chronic inflammation. This causes the PIP to pop up in flexion while the DIP stays in hyperextension.

Lower Extremity. Hip involvement in RA might be difficult to detect on physical examination and might manifest as only a small decrease in ROM. If pain develops, it can be felt in the buttock, lower back, groin, thigh, or medial aspect of the knee. RA of the knee is usually easily apparent on examination. A *Baker cyst* (posterior herniation of the joint capsule to the popliteal area) might occur and can be diagnosed by ultrasound. Rupture of a Baker cyst into the posterior leg might mimic thrombophlebitis. RA might involve the MTP, talonavicular, and ankle joints, causing gait problems. The tarsal tunnel containing the posterior tibial nerve can be compressed by synovitis, causing burning paresthesias on the sole of the foot made worse by weight bearing.

Joint Deformities. The synovitis of RA has many effects on cartilage, bone, muscles, tendons, and ligaments. Cartilage and bone erode, and muscles and tendons shorten in response to chronic inflammation. Ligaments are weakened by collagenases released by inflamed synovium and pannus. Upper extremity joints (shoulder, wrist, elbow) are prone to more severe deformities, as previously noted, than knees and ankles because splinting (avoiding joint motion to minimize pain) is easier in these lower extremity joints. The decreased use of these joints leads to more destruction by tendon shortening and contraction of the articular capsule.

Extraarticular Manifestations. Systemic constitutional symptoms such as fatigue, malaise, anorexia, weight loss, and fever occur in addition to joint inflammation and destruction in RA. Significant inflammation of almost all organ systems occurs. Patients have an increased incidence of renal, cardiac, pulmonary, and neurologic disorders; serious infections; and hematologic malignancies such as non-Hodgkin lymphoma. Subcutaneous rheumatoid nodules occur frequently in RA patients, usually in areas subject to pressure such as the elbows and sacrum. Their onset can be abrupt or gradual, and they might also resolve spontaneously. Biopsies are sometimes required to differentiate these from a gouty tophus or xanthoma. Rheumatoid nodules can also occur throughout the body, including (rarely) organs such as the lungs and heart.

Pulmonary involvement can include pleural effusions, interstitial fibrosis, solitary or multiple nodular lung disease, and pleurisy. Asymptomatic pericarditis diagnosed by echocardiography during RA exacerbations is relatively common but rarely results in cardiac-related sequelae. Nodules can occur rarely in the myocardium, heart valves, and aorta. Renal and GI complications are generally secondary to the treatment of RA rather than arising from the disease itself.

Eye dryness from keratoconjunctivitis sicca, episcleritis, or scleritis is associated with RA. Hematologic complications of RA include a hypochromic microcytic anemia with a low serum ferritin level and low or normal iron-binding capacity. Because many RA patients are taking NSAIDs, it can be difficult to distinguish anemia associated with their RA from NSAID-induced GI blood loss. *Felty syndrome* (RA, splenomegaly, leukopenia, leg ulcers, lymphadenopathy, thrombocytopenia, HLA-DR4 haplotype) is most common in patients with severe, nodule-forming RA.

Laboratory Studies

Arthritis panels should not be routinely performed and might only confuse the diagnosis. RF, ESR, uric acid level, ANA, and radiographic abnormalities all increase with age in the general population, even in the absence of disease. Therefore, laboratory studies should be reviewed as confirmatory of the clinical diagnosis made by careful history and physical examination.

Rheumatoid factor, ANA, and ESR are normally the most helpful tests to diagnose RA. RF is present in 80% to 90% of patients with RA. Therefore, 10% to 20% of patients with RA never have a positive RF. Also, up to 4% of normal young persons have low levels of RF. Moreover, RF titers are not helpful in following disease progression; when a patient is discovered to have a positive RF, repeating the test is of no value. Repeating a RF 6 to 12 months later for patients with initially negative RF results may be useful when RA is still being strongly considered. RF can be increased in other diseases, mainly chronic infections (Lyme disease, subacute bacterial endocarditis, tuberculosis, syphilis), viral infections (infectious mononucleosis, cytomegalovirus, influenza), parasitic infections, and other chronic inflammatory diseases such as sarcoidosis, pulmonary interstitial disease, and noninfectious hepatitis.

Anti-cyclic citrullinated peptide (anti-CCP) antibody is another laboratory test useful in the diagnosis of RA when the diagnosis is in question or the RF result is negative. Anti-CCP is more specific than RF for RA with 95% specificity and 69% sensitivity. Positive anti-CCP serology has also been linked with more severe radiologic progression of joint erosions from RA (Nishimura et al., 2007). Anti-CCP results can also be positive in patients with active tuberculosis or other autoimmune diseases.

Other serum tests include ANA titers, complement, ESR, and CBC. Abnormal ANA titers indicate SLE, SS, and scleroderma, but up to 30% of RA patients also have abnormal ANAs. Complements (CH50, C3, and C4) are decreased in SLE but are normal or increased in RA. The ESR, a nonspecific marker of inflammation, might help differentiate RA from other noninflammatory diseases. CRP, an acute-phase reactant, is also nonspecific but increases more rapidly than the ESR in early inflammation. A CBC showing a mild normochromic, normocytic anemia and a normal WBC count suggests RA. Thrombocytosis might also mimic disease activity as another acute-phase reactant, and eosinophilia might be seen.

Synovial fluid analysis in RA shows a yellow-white and turbid but sterile fluid without crystals. WBC counts of synovial fluid in RA are typically 10,000 to 20,000 cells/mm^3 but are at least higher than 2000/mm^3, with more than 75% PMNs. Synovial CH50 is lower than serum

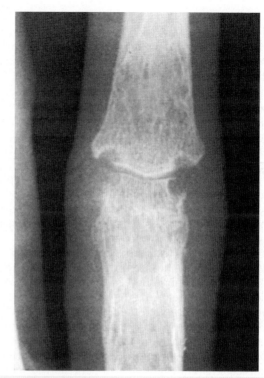

Figure 32-8 Rheumatoid arthritis marginal erosions and joint space narrowing. (From Resnick D, Yu JS, Sartoris D. Imaging. In Kelley WN Harris ED, Ruddy S, et al, eds. *Textbook of rheumatology.* 5th ed, vol 1. Philadelphia: Saunders; 1997:626-686.)

levels, and the serum and synovial glucose difference is usually higher than 30 mg/dL.

Imaging Studies

Radiography is indicated early when infection or fracture must be ruled out, the patient has a history of malignancy, the physical examination fails to localize the source of pain, or pain persists despite conservative treatment. Early RA might show only soft tissue swelling. Advanced destruction on radiographs should not be required to initiate disease-modifying therapy if a diagnosis of RA is strongly suspected clinically. In late-stage disease, radiographs might show marginal bony erosions, periarticular osteoporosis, and joint space narrowing, especially in the hands and feet (Figures 32-8 and 32-9).

Course

Almost 90% of joints ultimately affected in a given patient are involved during the first year of the disease, allowing the family physician to alert the patient with chronic RA about which joints will ultimately be affected (Anderson, 2004). The rate of spontaneous remission is extremely low, usually occurring within 2 years of disease onset. The presence of RF, nodules, extraarticular manifestations, and HLA-DR4 haplotype is associated with a more severe course. Mortality rates for patients with severe RA are higher secondary to infections; cardiovascular, pulmonary, and renal disease; GI bleeding; and excess malignancy. The strongest predictors of survival appear to be extraarticular manifestations of the disease and comorbidities (Gabriel et al., 2003).

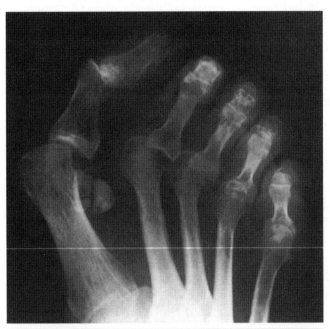

Figure 32-9 Classic forefoot deformities of rheumatoid arthritis. (From Resnick D, Niwayama G. *Diagnosis of bone and joint disorders.* Philadelphia: Saunders; 1988.)

Treatment

Initiation of early aggressive treatment of RA is essential to achieve the best prognosis in an individual patient. An integrated approach using up-to-date pharmacotherapy, patient education, physical and occupational therapy, and surgery is optimal. The family physician's role in early diagnosis of RA and subsequent initiation of DMARDs gives patients the best chance for minimizing joint destruction. The early aggressive treatment of RA begins with initial sign and symptom onset through the first 1 to 2 years of the disease. Considering symptomatology such as the patient's overall function, fatigue, inflammation and erosion of joints, and extraarticular symptoms can lead to an early diagnosis.

Although long used as the mainstay of pharmacologic therapy, NSAIDs provide only symptomatic relief without improving the prognosis. Therefore, almost all patients should start taking a DMARD as soon as the diagnosis of RA has been made (Figure 32-10). Many DMARDs are no more toxic than high-dose NSAIDs. Treatment options include DMARDs (hydroxychloroquine, sulfasalazine, and methotrexate) and minocycline. After 1 to 2 years of this therapy, the disease will have progressed to established RA. For moderate signs and symptoms, single and combination therapy is applicable, with options such as methotrexate, anti-TNF (tumor necrosis factor), anti–K-1, leflunomide, azathioprine, gold, cyclosporine, and other medications for mild RA (Osiri et al., 2003; Wells et al., 2000). The disease progresses to severe RA if the treatment options for established RA have failed. Therapy such as cyclophosphamide (Cytoxan), a different DMARD selection, pulse steroids, and Prosorba Column (protein A) could then be considered. Along with prescribing the DMARD, the family physician must educate the patient and family about the importance of DMARD compliance. Physical and occupational therapy are important for joint protection during exacerbations, as

is exercise to improve function and ROM. Early consultation with a rheumatologist is generally recommended.

Disease-Modifying Antirheumatic Drugs. Although traditional first-line therapy has included aspirin and NSAIDs, DMARDs are now used more frequently in early RA (Table 32-5). Because of the potential for toxicity, it is important to differentiate RA from other causes of synovitis as well as from OA. The 2008 ACR recommendations identified four adverse prognostic factors that would encourage use of DMARDs: functional limitation, extraarticular disease, RF positivity or presence of anti-CCP antibodies, and bony erosions documented on radiographs. Hydroxychloroquine appears to be the least toxic of the DMARDs followed (in order) by sulfasalazine (Azulfidine), methotrexate (Rheumatrex), intramuscular (IM) gold sodium thiomalate (Myochrysine), and aurothioglucose (Solganal). Hydroxychloroquine is dosed at 200 mg orally once or twice daily; however, patients need ophthalmologic follow-up in 6 months (Carmichael et al., 2002; Wassenberg and Rau, 2003). Hydroxychloroquine is generally only used for patients with milder RA symptoms. Significant improvement was seen in patients with mild RA taking hydroxychloroquine compared with those taking placebo (Davis et al., 1991).

Sulfasalazine is given at 2 to 3 g/day in two divided doses (Suarez-Almazor et al., 2000a). Before prescribing sulfasalazine, a sulfa drug, the physician must be aware of potential allergy and check CBC and LFTs weekly for 1 month and then every 4 to 6 weeks. Using sulfasalazine as the sole DMARD for treatment should be limited to patients lacking the poor prognostic factors noted earlier or those with contraindications to methotrexate. A meta-analysis of 15 trials showed that sulfasalazine was effective for treatment of RA (Weinblatt et al., 1999b). Oral gold, or auranofin (Ridaura), is not as effective as IM preparations and should be used only for early mild RA or in combination with other DMARDs (Suarez-Almazor et al., 2000c). Gold is given as 3 mg twice daily, and a CBC must be done every 4 to 6 weeks. Diarrhea is a frequent side effect. The onset of action of most DMARDs is at least several months, so adequate pain control with analgesics should be given and the patient counseled about realistic expectations.

Methotrexate. Many rheumatologists consider methotrexate to be the DMARD of first choice; it is the most frequently used DMARD in the United States. Methotrexate inhibits folic acid synthesis and is the primary choice for moderate to severe RA, showing significant short-term benefit but adverse effects on abrupt withdrawal (Ortiz et al., 2000; Suarez-Almazor et al., 2000a). Folic acid (1 mg/day) reduces methotrexate-induced mouth sores without decreasing the drug's efficacy. Patients cannot drink alcohol and must have LFTs every 4 to 6 weeks. Increasing the dose up to 25 mg/week and using the subcutaneous or IM route might enhance efficacy. Liver biopsies are no longer recommended during therapy unless abnormal alanine transaminase (ALT) or albumin levels persist (Kremer et al., 1994). Methotrexate toxicities include hepatotoxicity, bone marrow suppression, rare development of B-cell non-Hodgkin lymphoma, subcutaneous nodules (treated with colchicine), opportunistic infections,

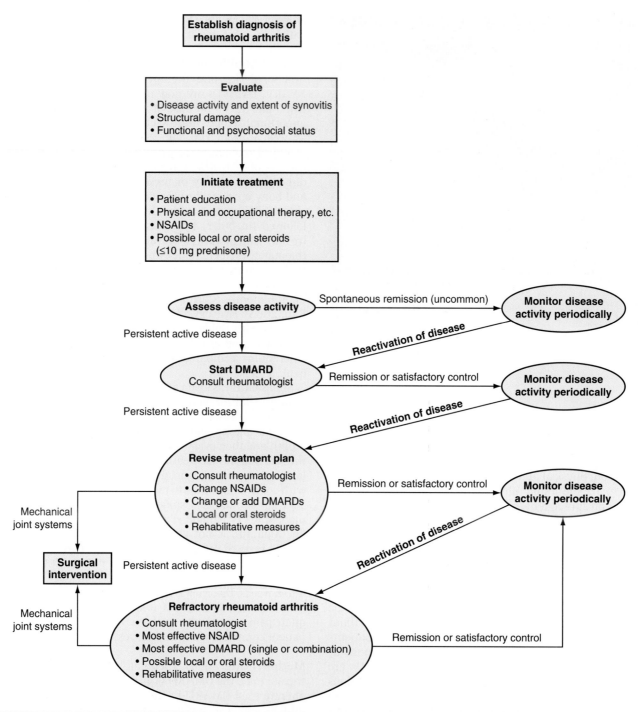

Figure 32-10 Algorithm for management of rheumatoid arthritis. *DMARD*, Disease-modifying antirheumatic drug; *NSAID*, nonsteroidal antiinflammatory drug. (From American College of Rheumatology Ad Hoc Committee on Clinical Guidelines. Guidelines for the initial evaluation of the adult patient with acute musculoskeletal symptoms. *Arthritis Rheum*. 1996;39:1.)

and hypersensitivity pneumonitis (treated with corticosteroids). It can be difficult to withdraw methotrexate after it has been started without causing a disease flare.

Other Disease-Modifying Antirheumatic Drugs. Azathioprine (Imuran) is used for moderate and severe RA as a second- or third-line drug after methotrexate, sulfasalazine, gold, and hydroxychloroquine have been tried. It suppresses bone marrow and can lead to infection. After the initial DMARD therapy, azathioprine can be tried for a 2- to 6-week course. No evidence has demonstrated increased

effectiveness over other DMARDs (Suarez-Almazor et al., 2000d).

Cyclosporine (Sandimmune, Neoral) is used in combination with methotrexate and is given as a 2.5-mg/kg dose to prevent hypertension and renal disease. It has shown modest efficacy in short-term treatment with progressive RA (Wells et al., 2000). D-Penicillamine (Depen, Cuprimine) has unpredictable toxicity, making it a less attractive choice. The alkylating agents cyclophosphamide and chlorambucil, as well as cyclosporine, are effective but are reserved for refractory severe cases because of their toxicities. All

Table 32-5 Selected Disease-Modifying Antirheumatic Drugs

Class/Drug (Brand)	Recommended Dosage	Toxic Effects	Recommended Monitoring
GOLD COMPOUNDS			
Gold sodium thiomalate (Myochrysine)	IM: 10 mg followed by 25 mg 1 wk later; then 25-50 mg weekly until there is toxicity, major clinical improvement, or cumulative dose of 1 g; if effective, interval between doses is increased	Pruritus, dermatitis (frequent in one third of patients), stomatitis, nephrotoxicity, blood dyscrasias, "nitritoid" reaction: flushing, weakness, nausea, dizziness 30 min after injection	CBC, platelet count before every other injection U/A before each dose
Auranofin (Ridaura)	PO: 3 mg BID or 6 mg QD; may increase to 3 mg TID after 6 mo	Loose stools, diarrhea (≤50%), dermatitis	Baseline CBC, platelet count, U/A, renal, liver function at onset; then CBC with platelet count, U/A at 9 mo
ANTIMALARIALS			
Hydroxychloroquine (Plaquenil)	PO: 400-600 mg QD for 4-12 wk; then 200-400 mg QD	Retinopathy, dermatitis, muscle weakness, hypoactive DTRs, CNS	Ophthalmologic examination every 3 mo (visual acuity, slit-lamp funduscopic, visual field tests); neuromuscular examination
Penicillamine (Cuprimine)	PO: 125-250 mg QD; then increasing doses by 125-250 mg at monthly intervals to a maximum of 750-1000 mg	Pruritus, rash, or mouth ulcers; bone marrow depression; proteinuria; hematuria; hypogeusia myasthenia; myositis; GI distress; pulmonary toxicity; teratogenic	CBC every 2 wk until dose stable; then every month U/A weekly until dose stable; then every 9 mo hCG as needed
Methotrexate (Rheumatrex)	PO: 7.5-20 mg weekly	Pulmonary toxicity, ulcerative stomatitis, leukopenia, thrombocytopenia, GI distress, malaise, fatigue, chills, fever, CNS, elevated LFTs or liver disease, lymphoma, infection	CBC with platelet count LFTs weekly for 6 wk; then monthly U/A periodically hCG as needed
Azathioprine (Imuran)	PO: 50-100 mg QD, increase at 4-wk intervals by 0.5 mg/kg/day, up to 2.5 mg/kg/day	Leukopenia, thrombocytopenia, GI, neoplastic if previous therapy with alkylating agents	CBC with platelet count, weekly for 1 mo, twice monthly for 2 mo, then monthly hCG as needed
Sulfasalazine (Azulfidine)	PO: 500 mg/day; then increase, up to 3 g daily	GI, skin rash, pruritus, blood dyscrasias, oligospermia	CBC, U/A every 2 wk for 3 mo; then monthly for 9 mo; then every 6 mo
ALKYLATING AGENTS			
Cyclophosphamide (Cytoxan)	PO: 50-100 mg/day, up to 2.5 mg/kg/day	Leukopenia, thrombocytopenia, hematuria, GI, alopecia, rash, bladder cancer, non-Hodgkin lymphoma, infection	CBC with platelet count, regularly hCG as needed
Chlorambucil (Leukeran)	PO: 0.1-0.2 mg/kg/day	Bone marrow suppression, GI, CNS, infection	CBC with platelet count every wk WBC count 3-4 days after each CBC during first 3-6 wk at therapy hCG as needed
Cyclosporine (Sandimmune)	PO: 2.5-5 mg/kg/day	Nephrotoxicity, tremor, hirsutism, hypertension, gum hyperplasia	Renal function, liver function
PYRIMIDINE SYNTHESIS INHIBITOR			
Leflunomide (Arava)	Loading dose: 100 mg/day for 3 days Maintenance therapy: 20 mg/day; if not tolerated, 10 mg/day	Hepatotoxicity, carcinogenesis Immunosuppression, long half-life	LFTs every month, drug levels after discontinuation (after 1-mo therapy, remains in blood for 2 yr without cholestyramine)
TUMOR NECROSIS FACTOR INHIBITORS			
Etanercept (Enbrel)	2-5 mg SC twice weekly or 50 mg SC weekly	Sepsis, opportunistic infections, congestive heart failure, injection site pain	PPD, CBC, ALT at baseline monthly until dose is stable; then every 2-3 mo
Infliximab (Remicade)	5 mg/kg IV on weeks 0, 2, 6; then biweekly	Sepsis, opportunistic infections, reactivation of hepatitis B and TB, pancytopenia	PPD, CBC, ALT at baseline monthly until dose is stable; then every 2-3 mo
Adalimumab (Humira)	40 mg SC every 2 wk	Sepsis, opportunistic infections, reactivation of TB	PPD, CBC, ALT at baseline monthly until dose is stable; then every 2-3 mo
EXTRACORPOREAL*			
Staphylococcal protein A immunoadsorption	IV weekly for 12 wk	Hypotension (especially with ACE inhibitor), injection site infection, anemia, flulike symptoms, joint pain	CBC routinely

*Use only in patients whose disease is refractory to disease-modifying antirheumatic drugs (DMARDs).
ACE, Angiotensin-converting enzyme; *ALT,* alanine transaminase; *BID,* twice daily; *CBC,* complete blood count; *CNS,* central nervous system; *DTR,* deep tendon reflex; *GI,* gastrointestinal; *hCG,* human chorionic gonadotropin; *IM,* intramuscular; *IV,* intravenous; *LFT,* liver function test; *PO,* oral; *PPD,* purified protein derivative; *QD,* once daily; *SC,* subcutaneously; *TB,* tuberculosis; *TID,* three times daily; *U/A,* urinalysis; *WBC,* white blood cell.

second-line drugs are teratogenic, so a family physician must help the patient establish an effective means of birth control. The risk of toxic effects is an important factor in choice of these agents, and selection is generally best handled in consultation with the rheumatologist.

Leflunomide (Arava) inhibits pyrimidine synthesis, is given orally, and is considered a possible alternative to methotrexate for decreasing erosion and controlling inflammation, but it provides no apparent benefit over methotrexate and is expensive. Leflunomide has been shown not only to reduce symptoms but also to slow disease progression. The routine dosage is 100 mg/day for 3 days followed by a maintenance dosage of 10 to 20 mg/day. LFTs must be ordered, and as with methotrexate, leflunomide is better for short-term therapy (Suarez-Almazor et al., 2000a). Research continues into combining DMARDs to lower drug resistance. DMARD combination therapy in early RA has shown minimal benefit (Mottonen et al., 1999).

Anticytokine Therapy. Cytokines such as interleukin-1 (IL-1), TNF-α, granulocyte-macrophage colony-stimulating factor, IL-6, and chemoattractant cytokines (known as chemokines) are derived from macrophages and fibroblasts and appear to be the most important cytokines involved in RA treatment (Kavanaugh, 2006). TNF-α is produced by synovial macrophages and causes many destructive inflammatory actions in the rheumatoid joint. Synovial macrophages proliferate; synoviocytes (fibroblast-like cells lining the joint) produce prostaglandins and cytokines, continuing the inflammatory process. Administering monoclonal antibodies such as infliximab (Remicade) to bind TNF-α and block its activity and giving TNF-α receptors such as etanercept (Enbrel) are two approaches to decrease TNF activity. Patients with a suboptimal response to methotrexate at 25 mg/wk (maximum dose) are the best candidates for etanercept or infliximab. Before starting any anticytokine therapy, CBC and tuberculin test (purified protein derivative [PPD]) are required.

Etanercept, a recombinant p75 TNF-α receptor–Fc fusion protein, is given subcutaneously once to twice weekly. It decreases binding of TNF-α to cellular receptors and avoids downstream inflammation. It is well tolerated and is indicated for use alone or with methotrexate for methotrexate-refractory disease (Blumenauer et al., 2003; Weinblatt et al., 1999a). The most common side effect is injection site erythema, which must be carefully watched in RA patients with diabetes mellitus. Etanercept has significantly reduced disease activity in a dose-related manner over 6 months, with no laboratory abnormalities noted (Moreland et al., 1999).

Infliximab, an anti–TNF-α monoclonal antibody, is given intravenously for refractory disease every 4 to 8 weeks. It is 75% human and 25% mouse antibody to TNF-α. The primary mechanism is halting joint space narrowing, with subsequent decreased erosion. It is FDA approved only in combination with methotrexate. Again, caution is warranted in patients with diabetes for skin ulcers. If the patient has a positive PPD, isoniazid and vitamin B6 therapy must be given for 9 months with the treatment. Fewer appropriate trials exist for infliximab than etanercept; however, the benefit in refractory disease has been demonstrated (Blumenauer et al., 2002).

Adalimumab (Humira), 40 mg subcutaneously every other week, has a greater therapeutic potential when used with methotrexate (OnMedica, 2005). It is a full human anti–TNF-α. Fewer studies exist on its long-term efficacy, but short-term studies show a greater effect than infliximab or etanercept. Risk factors with this regimen include skin infection, malignancy, and demyelination.

Nonsteroidal Antiinflammatory Drugs. The NSAIDs improve inflammation and pain but do not alter disease progression. Therefore, most patients with RA should take a DMARD. NSAIDs are used for analgesia and to help control symptoms. DMARDs generally have a slow onset of action, necessitating use of other agents to help keep the patient comfortable while awaiting onset of the DMARD's action. NSAID-associated GI bleeding is a widespread problem; one in three RA patients will be hospitalized or will die from a GI bleed at some point. Selection of NSAID is largely empiric (Table 32-6). The least toxic NSAIDs are coated or buffered aspirin, salsalate (Disalcid, Mono-Gesic, Salflex), ibuprofen (Advil, Motrin, Nuprin, Rufen), and naproxen sodium (Aleve). The most toxic are indomethacin (Indocin), tolmetin sodium (Tolectin), meclofenamate sodium (Meclomen), and ketoprofen (Orudis, Oruvail). High-toxicity NSAIDs provide no more clinical benefit than lower-toxicity drugs (Fries et al., 1991).

Patients receiving long-term nonselective NSAIDs should be monitored several times annually for hematocrit abnormalities and should undergo stool guaiac testing and have renal and liver function evaluated. There is no benefit to combining different NSAIDs.

Aspirin and Salicylates. High-dose aspirin (900-1050 mg four times daily) is as effective as much more expensive NSAIDs but is often less well tolerated and less convenient to take.

Glucocorticoids. Glucocorticoid articular injections are often used for temporary localized suppression of RA but are not recommended for use more than three times per joint per year. Common drugs for injection (used with lidocaine to minimize patient discomfort) include hydrocortisone, triamcinolone (Kenalog, Aristocort), methylprednisolone (Depo-Medrol), dexamethasone (Decadron-LA), and betamethasone (Celestone Soluspan), in ascending order of duration of action.

Systemic corticosteroids are used primarily as bridge therapy for several months when initiating DMARDs and awaiting their onset. Prednisone might be especially useful for constitutional symptoms such as fatigue and malaise. Low-dose prednisone (<7.5 mg/day) in a single morning dose might particularly be useful in older adult patients when other drugs have more potential for toxicity.

Surgery

Surgery is useful in RA patients with more severe disease who, despite optimal medical treatment, develop joint erosions and severe destruction resulting in pain and limitation of function. Surgical procedures range from carpal tunnel release to synovectomy, joint fusion, and arthroplasty. About 90% of older adult patients with severe incapacitating rheumatoid joint disease can expect

Table 32-6 Selected NSAIDs Used in Rheumatoid Arthritis and Osteoarthritis

Class/Drug (Brand)	Usual Dosage Range for Arthritis
I. ARYLCARBOXYLIC ACIDS	
A. Salicylic Acids	
1. Acetylated	
Aspirin, extended release	1600 mg BID
Aspirin, enteric coated	1000 mg QID
2. Nonacetylated	
Diflunisal (Dolobid)	250-500 mg BID; maximum, 1500 mg/day
Choline-magnesium salicylate	3 g/day in 1-3 doses
Salsalate (Disalcid, Salflex)	3-4 g/day in 2-3 doses
B. Anthranilic Acid	
1. Meclofenamate Sodium	200-400 mg/day in 3-4 doses
II. ARYLALKANOIC ACIDS	
A. Arylacetic Acid	
1. Diclofenac (Voltaren)	150-225 mg/day in 3-4 divided doses
2. Naproxen (Naprosyn)	250-500 mg BID-TID
3. Naproxen sodium (Anaprox)	275-550 mg BID
B. Arylpropionic Acids	
1. Ibuprofen (Advil, Motrin)	300-800 mg/TID-QID
2. Ketoprofen (Oruvail)	100-200 mg/day
3. Fenoprofen (Nalfon)	300-600 mg TID-QID
C. Oxazolepropionic Acid	
1. Oxaprozin (Daypro)	600-1800 mg/day in 1-2 doses
D. Heteroarylacetic Acid	600-1800 mg/day in 3-4 doses
1. Tolmetin	
E. Indoleacetic and Indeneacetic Acids	
1. Indomethacin (Indocin, Indocin SR)	25-50 mg TID-QID 75 mg QD-BID
2. Sulindac (Clinoril)	150-200 mg BID
F. Pyranocarboxylic Acid	
1. Etodolac (Lodine)	300-500 mg BID
III. ENOLIC ACIDS—OXICAM	
A. Piroxicam (Feldene)	20 mg/day
IV. NONACIDIC AGENT	
A. Nabumetone (Relafen)	1000-2000 mg divided QD-BID
B. Meloxicam (Mobic)	7.5-15 mg QD
V. CYCLOOXYGENASE (COX-2) INHIBITOR	
A. Celecoxib (Celebrex)	100-200 mg BID

BID, Twice daily; *NSAID,* nonsteroidal antiinflammatory drug; *QD,* once daily; *QID;* four times daily; *TID,* three times daily.

excellent pain relief and increased ROM after total hip or knee replacement (Harris and Sledge, 1990).

Other Therapies

Antimicrobial Therapy. On the basis of the theory that persistent mycoplasma infection might cause RA, tetracyclines such as minocycline (Minocin) have been used by some physicians for years. Minocycline, 100 mg orally twice daily, has shown modest efficacy but can lead to dizziness and dosing sensitivity in early RA (O'Dell et al., 2001). A small study showed that use of minocycline (100 mg twice daily) in early RA (first 3 months after diagnosis) resulted in more frequent remissions, and the need for DMARD therapy was reduced after follow-up for 4 years (O'Dell et al., 1999). These antibiotics result in mild improvement in RA patients, and other actions may include inhibition of collagenase activity, direct antiinflammatory effect, and interference with leukocyte function.

Mind–Body Therapy. Stress management, cognitive-behavioral pain management techniques, relaxation training, biofeedback, and family-oriented behavior therapy have all been shown to improve daily functioning, pain reports, and disease activity in RA patients (Parker et al., 1995). A small RCT showed a 28% decrease in mean disease severity at 4 months using writing therapy (Smyth et al., 1999). Another study showed that 20% of the disability of RA was related to psychosocial factors (Escalante and del Rincon, 1999). Educating patients about methods to cope with their disease can significantly improve quality of life. Interventions shown to improve outcomes include tai chi (Han et al., 2004) and journaling (Smyth et al., 1999). A meta-analysis of psychological interventions (e.g., biofeedback, relaxation, cognitive-behavioral therapy) found significant effects on pain, disability, functional status, and coping, although these might be more effective for patients with RA of shorter duration (Astin et al., 2002).

Nutrition. Nutritional changes are hypothesized to decrease RA signs and symptoms. A Cochrane review of herbs found that γ-linolenic acid (GLA) resulted in some improvement in clinical outcomes (Little and Parsons, 2000; Zurier et al., 1996), consistent with other findings on essential fatty acids. Fish oil, high in omega-3 fatty acids, significantly improved the number of tender joints and morning stiffness (Fortin et al., 1995; Volker et al., 2000); the recommended dose would be 3 g/day, and symptom relief might not be evident until 12 weeks of use. Changes in the total diet have been studied as well. Fasting has anecdotal evidence for inducing remission of symptoms. A 7- to 10-day fast followed by a gluten-free vegan diet was found to sustain improvements (Kjeldsen-Kragh et al., 1991; McDougall et al., 2002). Proceeding immediately to a vegan gluten-free diet resulted in RA symptom improvement (Hafstrom et al., 2001). Symptoms were exacerbated with challenges of foods that patients had reacted to on skin-prick test (Karatay et al., 2004). Therefore, a trial of such a diet or an elimination diet would be reasonable options (Table 32-7). In general, a plant-based Mediterranean diet appears to be a healthy option for patients with RA (Sales et al., 2009).

Monitoring Arthritic Activity

Because RA is a chronic disease with significant psychosocial impact, the continuity that the family physician provides is crucial. The frequency of visits depends on disease activity, need for drug toxicity monitoring, and psychosocial functioning of the patient (see eTable 32-4 online). Periodic ESR and CRP levels, radiography, and functional status

Table 32-7   Elimination Diet: Patient Handout

Special diets called *elimination diets* are sometimes used to discover whether food allergies or sensitivities are related to symptoms you might be having. The goal of an elimination diet is to identify problem foods. The diet is temporary and must be followed very carefully so that a permanent diet to help you feel better can be planned. The steps in an elimination diet follow:

1. Decide which foods might be causing problems.	This step involves describing your diet for your doctor and sharing your ideas about what foods might be causing problems. Sometimes food allergy tests are used to help with the decision.
2. Avoid the foods completely for 2 to 4 weeks.	This is the actual elimination step. This step involves the greatest restrictions in your diet. • The foods need to be avoided completely for symptoms to be noticeable when the foods are added back. • Foods should be avoided both in their whole form and as ingredients in food. • Keeping track of how you feel during this step is important. It is useful to keep a written record. You may feel worse before you feel better, but that should last only 1 or 2 days. If you feel worse for longer, please call your doctor.
3. Add the foods back one at a time.	This is called the *challenge step*. It allows you to learn which foods, if any, are causing symptoms. • Decide with your doctor which food to add back first. • Keep track of how you feel throughout this step with a written record. • On the day a food is added, eat that food twice. For the next 2 days, do not eat that food again but continue to follow the elimination diet. You can have a reaction up to 3 days after a food is eaten. • Add a new food every 3 days because you can have a reaction up to 3 days after the challenge food is eaten. • If the food does not cause a reaction, that food "passes" and can be added back to your diet when the entire process is over. Do not eat the foods you have added back, even if they "passed," until you have tested all the foods. • After following the elimination diet carefully, you and your doctor will have a better picture of which foods, if any, are causing your problems. Remember that problems with foods can be intermittent, and it is sometimes difficult to tell exactly whether foods are a problem.

From Rakel D. *Integrative medicine.* Philadelphia: Saunders; 2002.

assessment are important in addition to serial joint examination. A team approach using the expertise of a rheumatologist and physical and occupational therapists is generally indicated. Patients' ability to perform their jobs must be considered, and using modified work profiles or absences may be necessary. Osteoporosis resulting from RA should be monitored and prevented. The patient should also be monitored for infection, pulmonary disease, renal disease, or GI bleeding, taking a general health maintenance approach to this systemic disease.

KEY TREATMENT

- NSAIDS are the preferred treatment for pain in RA (SOR: C).
- Treatment of RA with DMARDs should be started as soon as possible (SOR: C).

- Methotrexate has substantial benefit in the treatment of RA and is generally the first-line DMARD (Suarez-Almazor et al., 2000a) (SOR: A).
- Sulfasalazine has proven benefits on RA disease activity (Weinblatt et al., 1999b) (SOR: A). However, it should be used as the sole therapy only in patients with minor symptoms and no poor prognostic signs of RA.
- Hydroxychloroquine has been shown to be effective in the treatment of RA (Davis et al., 1991). However, it is generally used with another DMARD or methotrexate in refractory cases when initial treatment fails (SOR: B).
- Biologic agents such as etanercept and infliximab reduce RA disease activity and are important treatment options in patients with moderate to severe RA who have failed treatment with methotrexate or combination therapy (Blumenauer et al., 2003; Weinblatt et al., 1999a) (SOR: A).

CRYSTAL ARTHROPATHIES

Gout and pseudogout are conditions caused by deposition of crystals of urate and calcium pyrophosphate dihydrate, respectively, with a resulting inflammatory response. These conditions can be distinguished from each other and from other causes of an acutely swollen joint or joints by synovial fluid examination, looking for crystals using polarized light microscopy.

Gout

Key Points

- Hyperuricemia is present (usually >8 mg/dL) in patients with gout.
- Gout affects more men than women.
- Negative birefringent crystals are seen on fluid analysis in gout.

Gout primarily affects middle-aged men (40-60 years) and postmenopausal women. It typically manifests as an acutely painful monoarticular arthritis, possibly becoming chronic after years of progressively more severe and frequent episodes, interspersed with variable symptom-free periods. *Hyperuricemia* is a marker for gout, but each can exist without the other. Asymptomatic hyperuricemia is not a disease. The risk of gout, however, is proportional to the degree and duration of hyperuricemia. Multiple genetic and environmental factors affect uric acid concentration. Uric acid is derived from ingestion of a diet rich in purines (e.g., typical American diet), as well as from endogenous production of purines. Inborn errors of metabolism, either reduced excretion (90% of patients) or increased production (10%) of uric acid, cause primary hyperuricemia. Secondary hyperuricemia results from diseases or drug therapies that raise uric acid levels.

In addition to attempting to prevent acute flares, the family physician's goal in treating patients predisposed to gout is to minimize the risk of developing other sequelae. These include interstitial nephropathy with renal function impairment; accumulation of urate crystal deposits in joints, soft tissue, cartilage, and bone, called *tophi;* and uric acid calculi in the genitourinary (GU) tract.

Clinical Presentation. The first MTP joint (great toe) is involved in 50% of initial acute gouty attacks (podagra) and is eventually affected in 75% to 90% of patients with gout. This joint sustains more microtrauma and is relatively cool compared with the rest of the body. The heel, ankle, knee, midtarsal joints, and olecranon bursa can all be initially involved but are so less frequently than the first MTP joint. Gout severity ranges from vague aches and pains to severe pain, swelling, redness, and exquisite tenderness. Acute attacks resolve within several days to weeks, even in untreated gout.

In contrast to the typical middle-aged male presentation, gout in women and in older adult patients tends to be polyarticular. Because gout in these patient subgroups tends to involve more than one joint, it can often be misdiagnosed as RA (tophi are mistaken for rheumatoid nodules) or septic joint cellulitis, especially if low-grade fever, leukocytosis, redness, or desquamation is present. Synovial fluid analysis is necessary for definitive diagnosis.

Synovial Fluid Examination. A presumptive diagnosis of gout can be made by clinical signs and symptoms, a negative joint culture, response to NSAIDs or colchicine, and hyperuricemia. However, definitive diagnosis can be made only by finding needle-shaped, negatively birefringent urate crystals on synovial fluid examination or in tophi.

Clinical Stages of Primary Gout. Hyperuricemia is defined as two standard deviations above the individual laboratory's mean based on gender, usually 8 mg/dL in men and 7 mg/dL in women. Hyperuricemia is present in 5% of men, only 5% to 10% of whom develop acute gout. It normally takes at least 20 years of hyperuricemia before a patient has a first episode of gouty arthritis. Lowering the serum uric acid level does not decrease the risk of gouty nephropathy; chronic renal disease is almost always caused by concurrent diseases such as diabetes or hypertension. Because of expense and potential drug toxicity, treatment of asymptomatic hyperuricemia is generally not recommended.

The two most important factors in the development of acute gouty arthritis are obesity and alcohol (Choi et al., 2005). Ethanol metabolism blocks renal excretion of uric acid, leading to gouty attacks. Studies have shown a 2.5-fold increase in the risk of gout in men who drink 2 or more beers per day. This risk was similar but slightly lower in men who drank the same amount of distilled alcohols. In contrast, drinking two 4-oz glasses of wine or more per day was not associated with an increased risk of gout (Choi at al., 2004). Other factors include rapid decrease or increase in serum urate level (thus a possible attack at start of allopurinol treatment), emotional stress, infection, and surgery. Dietary excesses of purine-rich foods (e.g., sweetbreads, sardines, anchovies, kidney, liver) have traditionally been mentioned but are in reality rarely responsible for acute gouty attacks. Diuretics, both hydrochlorothiazide and loop, have been associated with increased serum uric acid. Risks, benefits, and cost must be evaluated before deciding to change or stop these medications for hypertension.

After an initial gouty attack, more than half of patients will have a recurrent attack. The timing is highly variable, however, and the recurrent attack can be weeks or years later. As time passes, gouty attacks tend to become more frequent, more severe, and less responsive to therapy and to involve more joints. Between acute attacks, urate crystals can still be aspirated from asymptomatic joints, demonstrating that this so-called intercritical or interval gout represents a progression of disease. Chronic tophaceous gout occurs at least 10 years into the disease and is now seen infrequently because of more aggressive treatment of gout and hyperuricemia. Tophi can occur anywhere but tend to occur in the helix of the ear, on the proximal ulnar surface of the forearm, on the olecranon, on the Achilles tendon, on the prepatellar bursa, or near active joints. Tophi are not seen on plain radiographs unless they are calcified. The classic radiographic finding of chronic gout is sharply marginated erosions proximal to the joint space, with an overlying rim of cortical bone (Figure 32-11).

Secondary gout is caused by drugs or disease processes affecting uric acid metabolism or excretion. Myeloproliferative and lymphoproliferative diseases, hemolytic anemia, multiple myeloma, and other malignancies result in overproduction. Renal disease, diuretics, salicylates, alcohol, nicotinic acid, and chronic lead intoxication (saturnine gout) all cause underexcretion. Chemotherapy for

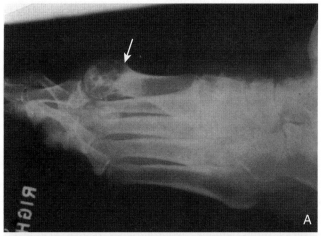

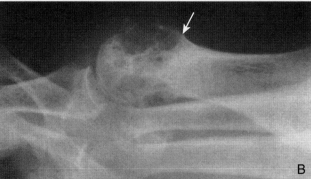

Figure 32-11 Advanced gout in the feet. **A,** Calcified tophi (*arrow*) of gout seen on a radiograph. **B,** Osteophyte formation in knee (*arrow*). (From Visual Aids, Subcommittee of the Professional Education Committee of the Arthritis Foundation. *Clinical slide collection on the rheumatic diseases.* New York: Arthritis Foundation; 1972:82.)

hematologic or myeloproliferative disorders can result in gouty nephropathy unless adequate hydration and possibly allopurinol prophylaxis are initiated before therapy.

Treatment of Gouty Arthritis. The NSAIDs are generally used first because of their efficacy and relative lack of toxicity. Indomethacin (Indocin) has been used for years for gouty arthritis attacks, but any NSAID can probably be used with similar efficacy as long as an initial maximal dose is given. After 2 days of therapy at the maximal dose, the NSAID can be tapered over the next several weeks.

Colchicine decreases inflammation associated with lactic acid production and phagocytosis of urate; it terminates most gouty attacks within 6 to 12 hours but is limited by GI side effects (nausea, vomiting, abdominal cramps, diarrhea). Two 0.5- or 0.6-mg tablets are taken initially and then 1 tablet every hour until clinical response has been achieved, GI side effects cause discontinuation, or a total of 6 mg has been given (Cox, 2004). Colchicine at 0.5 to 1 mg every 6 hours intravenously, up to 4 mg total, can also be given for a single attack, but the parenteral route is associated with increased bone marrow suppression, renal and hepatic toxicity, and myopathy. No additional colchicine should be given for at least 1 week if the patient is given the full 4-mg total dose.

When NSAIDs and colchicine are ineffective or contraindicated, corticosteroids might be used. Treatment options include oral corticosteroids using prednisone, 0.5 mg/kg, followed by tapering the dose by 5 mg/day. An intraarticular injection can be given using triamcinolone hexacetonide (Aristospan), triamcinolone acetonide, or methylprednisolone (Medrol); typical doses are 10 to 40 mg in large joints and 5 to 20 mg in small joints. Intraarticular injection is preferred for monoarticular episodes. Finally, adrenocorticotropic hormone, 40 to 80 mg intravenously or intramuscularly every 8 to 12 hours, has been successful when all other therapies fail, but it is quite expensive.

Prophylaxis of Recurrent Gout. Asymptomatic hyperuricemia need not be treated, but after one episode of acute gouty arthritis or acute nephrolithiasis, patients should be offered the option of prophylaxis. Some choose not to take a daily drug, particularly if their gouty attacks are not severe or are infrequent. For patients with recurrent gouty attacks, renal damage, nephrolithiasis, or uric acid levels higher than 12 mg/dL or those undergoing cancer chemotherapy, uric acid–lowering therapy should be initiated. Prophylaxis may be discontinued when uric acid levels are brought down to normal levels for 2 months. Patients should be instructed to avoid alcohol, aspirin, diuretics, prolonged fasting, and high-purine foods. Several days before initiating uric acid–lowering therapy, it is prudent to start colchicine, 0.5 mg twice daily, to avoid precipitating an acute attack. This therapy can continue for up to 6 months after the desired uric acid levels have been obtained.

Allopurinol (Zyloprim) is a xanthine oxidase inhibitor that decreases uric acid production but also produces a more soluble metabolite. Allopurinol is therefore effective regardless of the cause of the hyperuricemia. Allopurinol therapy should never be initiated until an acute attack has subsided. Allopurinol is started at 100 mg/day with food and then increased at weekly intervals by 100 mg/day

until the serum uric acid level is lower than 6 mg/dL. The usual effective dose is 200 to 300 mg/day, although some patients require up to 600 mg/day (Perez-Ruiz et al., 1998). Patients should ensure adequate fluid intake to produce more than 2 L of urine output daily. The dose needs to be adjusted for decreased creatinine clearance. If an acute attack occurs when the patient is taking allopurinol, the dose should be maintained and the attack treated as usual (NSAIDs, colchicine, corticosteroids). Allopurinol can cause rash, liver transaminase level elevations, and renal toxicity if used with thiazide diuretics. It might also potentiate the effect of anticoagulants and cause a rash if used with amoxicillin.

The uricosuric drugs probenecid and sulfinpyrazone (Anturane) block renal tubular reabsorption of uric acid. Probenecid is started at 250 mg twice daily for 1 week; increased to 500 mg twice daily; and then increased by 500 mg/week, up to 3 g/day, until the urate level is normal. Sulfinpyrazone is started at 100 mg twice daily, increasing to 400 mg twice daily. These drugs should also never be started during an acute attack but should be maintained if the patient is already taking them. Urate stone formation risk can be minimized by a high fluid intake and alkalinization of the urine. A 24-hour urine sample for determination of creatinine clearance and uric acid level should be obtained before starting these drugs, because the glomerular filtration rate must be higher than 50 mL/min and uric acid excretion less than 800 mg/24 hr.

KEY TREATMENT

- Patients with gout who are overweight should be instructed on weight loss (Choi et al., 2005) (SOR: B).
- Patients with gout should limit their intake of beer and distilled alcohol (Choi et al., 2005) (SOR: B).
- Colchicine is an effective treatment for acute gout but should be used as second-line therapy when NSAIDs or corticosteroids are ineffective (SOR: C).
- Allopurinol should be started for prophylaxis in patients with frequent severe attacks, nephrolithiasis, or gouty tophi (Perez-Ruiz et al., 1998) (SOR: B).
- Antihyperuricemic therapy should be titrated to a dose that results in a serum urate level less than 6 mg/dL (slowly, <0.6 mg/dL/mo) (SOR: C).
- Before starting allopurinol, colchicine prophylaxis can be used for up to 6 months after desired uric acid level is reached to prevent acute attacks (SOR: C).

Pseudogout

Key Points

- The knees are the most common sources of pain in pseudogout (CPDD).
- Genetic factors are present in calcium pyrophosphate deposition disease (CPDD).
- Positive birefringent crystals are seen on fluid analysis in CPPD disease.
- Radiographic appearance of CPDD is punctate or linear densities in cartilage.

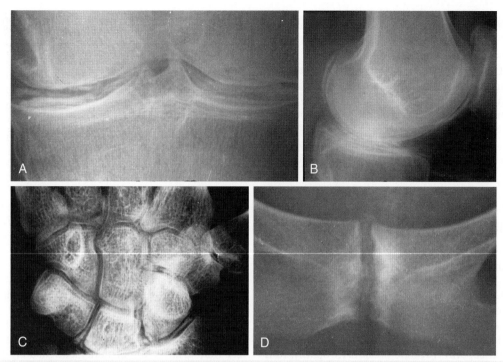

Figure 32-12 Chondrocalcinosis in calcium pyrophosphate deposition disease. **A,** Anteroposterior (AP) radiograph of the knee. **B,** Lateral radiograph of the knee. **C,** AP radiograph of the wrist. **D,** Radiograph of the pelvis. (From Reginato AJ, Reginato AM. Diseases associated with deposition of calcium pyrophosphate or hydroxyapatite. In Kelley WN Harris ED, Ruddy S, et al, eds. *Textbook of rheumatology.* 5th ed, vol 2. Philadelphia: Saunders; 1997:1352-1367.)

Calcium pyrophosphate deposition disease is known as pseudogout because of the acute goutlike attacks that CPPD crystals can cause. *Chondrocalcinosis* refers to radiographically detectable densities in cartilage and joint inflammation caused by these calcium-containing crystals. Calcium pyrophosphate (CP) crystals can be deposited not only on articular cartilage but also in ligaments, tendons, soft tissues, and synovium.

This arthritis is caused by genetic factors (autosomal dominant inheritance pattern) secondary to trauma and various metabolic diseases or is sporadic or idiopathic. CPDD is most often associated with aging, and about 4% of the adult U.S. population has articular CP crystal deposits at death (Agudelo and Wise, 2000). CPPD disease can be associated with hyperparathyroidism, hypothyroidism, hypomagnesemia, hypophosphatemia, hemochromatosis, and amyloidosis. Therefore, newly diagnosed CPDD should be followed up with serum measurements of calcium, magnesium, phosphorus, thyroid-stimulating hormone, ferritin, transferrin, serum iron, and alkaline phosphatase (ALP) levels.

The most common site is the knee, although the first MTP joint is also often affected, resulting in difficulty differentiating CPDD from gout. Any joint can be affected, however. Synovial fluid examination for rhomboid or rod-shaped, weakly positively birefringent crystals is diagnostic. Analysis needs to be done promptly after aspiration because identification of crystals diminishes over time. The crystals are also smaller and more difficult to detect, so careful preparation of the slide to avoid false-positive results must be taken. Pseudogout can also cause pseudo-RA. CPDD can be misdiagnosed as RA because of its often multiple joint involvement with symmetric distribution, morning stiffness, and elevated ESR and because 10% of CPDD patients have positive RF test results. CPDD might also be confused with OA because of its knee and hip involvement, but it also often affects the wrists, MCP joints, elbows, and shoulders. An acute attack of CPDD can cause low-grade fever, leukocytosis (12,000-15,000/mm^3), and elevated ESR. The typical radiographic appearance of CPDD is punctate or linear densities in cartilage (chondrocalcinosis) (Figure 32-12). Definitive diagnosis relies on either the typical radiographic signs or synovial fluid confirmation.

Treatment of acute pseudogout consists of removal of the crystals through joint aspiration, use of NSAIDs or colchicine during the acute inflammatory period; intraarticular joint injection with a glucocorticoid when possible; and a limited period of joint immobilization. No solid data support removal of crystals and prevention of crystal deposition, which are done only for diagnostic purposes and pain relief. If only one or two joints are involved, intraarticular injections may give the most symptomatic relief; if more joints are involved, an NSAID or colchicine is a better option. Because of severe pain associated with acute events, limited weight bearing may be needed for a short period while symptoms improve.

For patients with recurrent episodes of pseudogout, prophylaxis with colchicine, 0.6 mg twice daily, should be considered. In 10 patients with recurrent attacks, colchicine was associated with a marked decrease in the number of episodes (10) in 1 year compared with the previous year (32 episodes) (Alvarellos and Spilberg, 1986).

- Aspiration of the knee joint is done for symptomatic relief and diagnosis of pseudogout (CPDD) (SOR: C).
- A patient with CPDD receives intraarticular injection of glucocorticoid if septic joint has been ruled out and fewer than two joints are involved (SOR: C).
- An NSAID or colchicine is prescribed for acute pain of pseudogout (SOR: C).
- For recurrent pseudogout attacks, colchicine can be used for prophylaxis to decrease number of episodes (Alvarellos and Spilberg, 1986) (SOR: B).

SPONDYLOARTHROPATHIES

The spondyloarthropathies are a group of multisystem inflammatory disorders that affect predominantly the spine but also other joints and extraarticular tissues. Most are linked to the HLA-B27 gene, but HLA-B27 by itself does not explain the development of these diseases; the pathogenesis of these conditions is still unknown. They include AS, reactive arthritis (Reiter syndrome), psoriatic arthropathy, enteropathic arthropathy, juvenile-onset arthropathy, and undifferentiated spondyloarthropathy. Both genetic and environmental factors probably contribute to the onset and progression of these diseases. Most people with HLA-B27 do not develop these diseases, and these diseases occur in the absence of HLA-B27.

Ankylosing Spondylitis

Key Points

- Back pain and progressive stiffness are primary symptoms of this chronic inflammatory disease of axial skeleton.
- The male predominance for AS is 5:1.
- Clinical history, physical examination, and radiologic findings are key to the diagnosis of AS.

Primary or uncomplicated AS is a systemic inflammatory disorder predominantly affecting the sacroiliac joints and the spine. Patients with secondary AS have IBD, psoriasis, or Reiter syndrome in addition to their arthropathy. Hip and shoulder joints may also be involved in AS. Inflammation occurs at the intervertebral disk's annulus fibrosis–vertebral bone margin. This area is replaced by fibrocartilage and then ossified. Progression of this process results in the classic vertebral fusion known as *bamboo spine;* this ankylosis is a very late finding. Inflammation also occurs at the sites of ligament and tendon attachments (enthesitis) in the spine and pelvis, which become ossified.

Ankylosing spondylitis usually affects men (male:female ratio, 5:1) in their 20s and 30s. It often manifests as vague, somewhat diffuse low back pain, felt generally in the buttocks or sacroiliac area but often in the lumbar area. Pain becomes more persistent and bilateral. Back stiffness after inactivity, such as on awakening, becomes more predominant and is relieved by activity or a hot shower. AS can also disturb sleep, leading to complaints of fatigue, and can be associated with systemic symptoms such as malaise, low-grade fever, and weight loss. Symptoms can be subtle, but AS should be considered if back stiffness or discomfort persists, is relieved by exercise, and occurs in a man younger than 40 years. In juvenile-onset AS, hip and shoulder symptoms might predominate first, but in adult AS, the back is usually the first affected area. Disease progression is highly variable and can be mild and self-limited or can cause disability.

The two most common techniques to detect AS are palpation of the sacroiliac joints and assessment for spinal mobility. Decreased mobility early on is usually caused by pain and muscle spasm rather than by ankylosis. Flexion, hyperextension, axial rotation, and forward flexion should be assessed. Over time, the spine becomes increasingly stiff at an unpredictable rate, and stiffness might or might not eventually involve the entire spine.

Other extraarticular manifestations of AS include acute uveitis (iritis), aortitis, and neurologic complications resulting from cervical spine fractures from even minor trauma. Diaphragmatic breathing and limited chest excursion can be seen as a result of costovertebral involvement. The earliest radiographic abnormality can usually be seen in the sacroiliac joints, with sacroiliitis progressing to bony erosions and sclerosis (Figures 32-13 and 32-14). These changes might also be seen at the sites of ligamentous attachments to bones. Bone scans, computed tomography (CT), and MRI should be used only if plain radiography does not confirm clinical suspicion of AS.

Seventy percent to 80% of AS patients report substantial relief of their symptoms with NSAIDs, the mainstay of AS therapy (Song et al., 2008). Continuous NSAID use may decrease radiographic progression of the disease (Ward, 2005). However, the benefits must be weighed against the risks associated with prolonged NSAID use. Corticosteroids have not been shown to be helpful. Physical therapy focusing on strengthening of back extensor muscles might improve functional status and, at the very least, help maintain an erect position if spinal ossification occurs (Dagfinrud et al., 2004). Patients should be encouraged to walk erect and to keep the spine erect as much as possible, sleep on a firm mattress with the spine extended, and swim for exercise. Splints and braces do not help.

A home exercise program is better than no intervention for AS patients, and supervised group exercise is better than home exercise. Combined inpatient spa treatment and exercise (group physical exercises, walking, correction therapy, hydrotherapy, sports, sauna) followed by supervised outpatient weekly group physiotherapy is better than weekly physiotherapy alone (Dagfinrud et al., 2004).

Second-line drug therapies include etanercept, sulfasalazine, and methotrexate, as well as topical or oral steroids for associated uveitis, in consultation with an ophthalmologist. Second-line drugs, however, have shown no clear effect on the progression of decreased spinal mobility (Dagfinrud et al., 2004). A meta-analysis indicated that all three of the anti-TNF agents were similar in efficacy for patients with AS and that 80% of patients responded to treatment, with improved global, pain, and functional assessment and reduced inflammation, based on morning stiffness (MacLeod et al., 2007). Sulfasalazine in general is only used for

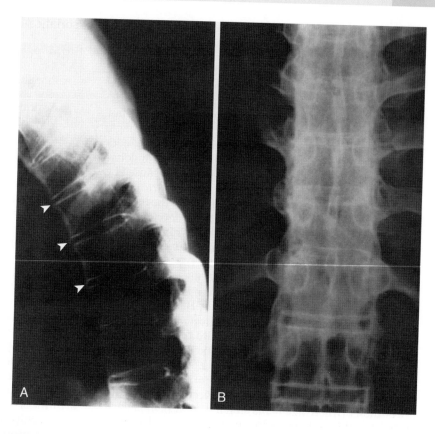

Figure 32-13 Ankylosing spondylitis. **A,** Bone erosion of dorsal aspect of thoracic spine. **B,** Classic appearance of bamboo spine. (From Resnick D, Yu JS, Sartoris D: Imaging. In Kelley WN Harris ED, Ruddy S, et al, eds. *Textbook of rheumatology.* 5th ed, vol 1. Philadelphia: Saunders; 1997:626-686.)

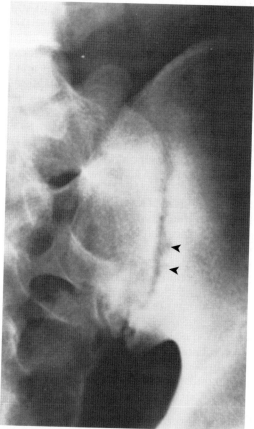

Figure 32-14 Ankylosing spondylitis. *Arrowheads* indicate sacroiliitis progressing to bony erosions and sclerosis. (From Resnick D, Yu JS, Sartoris D. Imaging. In Kelley WN Harris ED, Ruddy S, et al, eds. *Textbook of rheumatology.* 5th ed, vol 1. Philadelphia: Saunders; 1997:626-686.)

peripheral AS. Methotrexate, sulfasalazine, and leflunomide are ineffective for axial disease of AS.

KEY TREATMENT

- NSAIDs are the recommended initial therapy for AS (Song et al., 2008) (SOR: A).
- Patients with AS should initiate an exercise program (Dagfinrud et al., 2004) (SOR: B).
- Systemic glucocorticoids are not recommended for AS therapy (SOR: C).
- For AS patients with axial disease who do not respond to NSAIDs, anti-TNF therapy is recommended (MacLeod et al., 2007) (SOR: A).

Reactive Arthritis (Reiter Syndrome)

Key Points

- Signs and symptoms of reactive arthritis develop within 1 month after a GU or GI infection.
- Chlamydia infection or common enteric bacterial infections are the primary cause of Reiter syndrome.
- Only one third of patients with reactive arthritis will present with the classic triad of urethritis, conjunctivitis, and arthritis.

Reactive arthritis, or Reiter syndrome, is characterized by asymmetric oligoarticular arthritis with other extraarticular manifestations within 1 month of GU or GI tract (and possibly pulmonary) infection. The arthritis often occurs after the urethritis, uveitis, or gastroenteritis has resolved.

The classic triad of nongonococcal urethritis, conjunctivitis, and arthritis is fully present clinically in only one third of patients.

Reactive arthritis occurs secondary to *Chlamydia trachomatis* and possibly *Ureaplasma urealyticum* urethritis. Urethritis is sometimes asymptomatic or, in male patients, might manifest not with a mucopurulent discharge but rather with gross hematuria secondary to a hemorrhagic cystitis. *Neisseria gonorrhoeae* infection does not cause reactive arthritis, but a septic joint, including that from gonococcal infection, must be ruled out. GI infections caused by *Shigella, Salmonella, Campylobacter, Klebsiella, Clostridium,* or *Yersinia* spp. can all lead to reactive arthritis. By the time the gastroenteritis has resolved and arthritis has developed, the inciting bacterial agent cannot be cultured from the stool. Pulmonary infections with *Chlamydia pneumoniae* might also cause the disease (Braun et al., 1994). Conjunctivitis occurs at the same time or several days after the arthritis, if it occurs at all. The relationship between Reiter syndrome and HIV infection is most likely caused by HIV's association with *Chlamydia* and enteric bacterial infections rather than by HIV itself. Two thirds of patients with reactive arthritis are HLA-B27 positive, indicating genetic factors as well as infectious causes.

Reactive arthritis usually affects several joints, most often in the lower extremity (knees, ankles, feet). Common sites are entheses (where ligaments attach to bones), in particular the Achilles tendon attachment, which causes heel pain. Extraarticular manifestations of reactive arthritis include oral ulcers, aortitis, keratoderma blennorrhagicum (a papulosquamous skin rash occurring most commonly on the palms and soles), and balanitis circinata.

Reactive arthritis usually resolves within 1 year. Although there is no cure, the underlying illness should be treated. When *Chlamydia* is suspected, patients might be given doxycycline or an analogue for up to 3 months, but the optimal duration of therapy is unknown (Mandell et al., 2010). Antibiotics might limit recurrences as well as shorten the course after an episode of urethritis; however, antibiotic use after enteric infections has not been shown to affect the course of reactive arthritis. Reactive arthritis is treated with NSAIDs or intraarticular corticosteroid injections acutely and subsequently with sulfasalazine, 1 g two or three times daily, or methotrexate, 7.5 to 25 mg weekly. No specific studies using anti-TNF therapy have been done, but antidotal research indicates it may be helpful. Long-term disability is uncommon but is usually caused by chronic foot or heel pain or vision problems.

KEY TREATMENT

- NSAIDs are the mainstay of treatment for symptomatic reactive arthritis but do not alter or shorten its course (SOR: C).
- Intraarticular injections can be helpful and are not contraindicated in Reiter syndrome (SOR: C).
- When there is unsatisfactory response to NSAIDs or steroid injections, a trial of sulfasalazine is suggested for patients with reactive arthritis (SOR: C).
- For patients with contraindications or intolerance to sulfasalazine, a trial of etanercept can be attempted (SOR: C).

Psoriatic Arthritis

Key Points

- Psoriatic arthritis affects 5% to 7% of patients with psoriasis.
- Arthritis can occur before or after psoriatic lesions.
- Obtaining family history for psoriasis is important in those without current diagnosis and active psoriatic lesions.

Psoriatic arthritis is seen in approximately 5% to 7% of psoriasis patients, but it might affect up to 40% of hospitalized patients with extensive psoriatic lesions (Cuellar et al., 1994). The associated inflammatory peripheral arthritis might be monoarticular, asymmetric oligoarticular, or symmetric polyarticular, resembling RA. RF is usually absent. Psoriatic arthritis is associated with multiple HLA genes; environmental factors such as infections and physical trauma likely are also involved.

Psoriatic skin lesions predate arthritis in 70% of patients, occur with arthritis in 15%, and follow arthritis in 15%. Family history of psoriasis is therefore important for diagnosis in patients with an arthritis similar to psoriatic but without a known history. Psoriatic arthritis often manifests initially as an asymmetric monoarticular or oligoarticular arthritis of a large joint, such as a knee, evolving into asymmetric polyarticular arthritis. The distribution of involvement of psoriatic arthritis might resemble RA but involves the DIP joints more often, as well as causing enthesitis. Psoriatic arthritis might also cause spondylitis, sacroiliitis, chest wall pain from enthesitis, arthritis mutilans (destruction of phalanges and metacarpals, causing telescoping of fingers), conjunctivitis, and Achilles tendon and plantar fascia involvement. Radiographic abnormalities include marginal erosions at DIP and PIP joints, with new bone formation.

In addition to treating the psoriatic skin lesions, the arthritis is treated first with NSAIDs followed by DMARDs for widespread disease and corticosteroid injections if only one or two joints are involved (Cuellar et al., 1994). A Cochrane analysis showed that high-dose methotrexate and sulfasalazine have efficacy in psoriatic arthritis (Jones et al., 2000). Azathioprine, etretinate, low-dose methotrexate, and colchicines all had some effectiveness versus placebo, but more studies are necessary. Anti-TNF medications are also used if patients continue to have symptoms despite DMARD treatment or if axial disease is present and NSAIDs have not worked. A meta-analysis of RCTs showed that anti-TNF drugs are effective against psoriatic arthritis (Saad et al., 2008). When contemplating a local steroid joint injection, the physician should keep in mind that bacterial colonization of psoriatic skin lesions with streptococcus or staphylococcus is common. Injecting through skin lesions should therefore be avoided.

KEY TREATMENT

- NSAIDs are the first line of treatment for psoriatic arthritis (Cuellar et al., 1994) (SOR: B).
- Methotrexate and sulfasalazine have proven efficacy in the treatment of psoriatic arthritis (Jones et al., 2000)

(SOR: B) used as second-line agents if inadequate response to NSAIDs.
- Patients with axial disease or who have peripheral disease without improvement to DMARD treatments are candidates for anti-TNF medications, which have proven efficacy (Saad et al., 2008) (SOR: A).

Enteropathic Arthropathy

There seems to be a connection between the gut and spondyloarthropathies. Of patients with IBD (ulcerative colitis and Crohn disease), 10% to 20% have a peripheral arthritis different from other defined arthritides. Migratory arthralgias, especially of the knees, ankles, and feet, often coincide with periods of GI disease flares. Other joints, including the spine and sacroiliac joints, might be involved but are seemingly less coincident with bowel exacerbations. HLA-B27 is found in 50% of patients with IBD-associated spondylitis but is not found in a higher percentage than in the general population for this type of spondylitis. RF and ANA are negative. NSAIDs are normally used but must be taken with caution given the patient's underlying GI disease. As noted earlier, dietary factors might increase the patient's baseline inflammatory state, so a trial of dietary manipulation or the addition of omega-3 fatty acids is reasonable.

INFECTIOUS ARTHRITIS

Septic Arthritis

> **Key Points**
> - The knees are the most common sources of infectious arthritic pain.
> - Septic arthritis is a surgical emergency.
> - *Staphylococcus aureus* and *Neisseria gonorrhoeae* are the two most common causes.

Acute bacterial arthritis is one of the few rheumatologic emergencies. Failure by the primary care physician to diagnose this entity and to initiate prompt antibiotic therapy results in significant morbidity (functional disability, joint destruction) and at least 5% mortality. Even in patients with known rheumatologic disease, a bacterial infection may cause an acutely inflamed joint. The three mechanisms of a septic joint are (1) hematogenous spread from a distant location, such as a urinary tract infection (UTI) or pneumonia; (2) contiguous spread from a wound infection, abscess, or osteomyelitis; and (3) direct introduction of bacteria through trauma, surgery, or arthrocentesis. Concern about the third mechanism should not prevent the family physician from ruling out bacterial infection by performing synovial fluid analysis in an inflamed joint if the diagnosis is unclear. As for lumbar puncture, if the physician thinks it should, arthrocentesis probably should be done.

From 80% to 90% of acute bacterial articular infections are monoarticular. In adults with nongonococcal bacterial arthritis, the most common sites are the knee (50%), hip (20%), shoulders (8%), ankles (7%), wrists (7%), elbow (6%), other (5%), and more than one joint (usually two; 12%) (Brusch, 2005). In children, the most common sites

are the knee (40%), hip (28%), ankle (14%), shoulder (4%), wrist (3%), elbow (11%), other (3%), and more than one joint (7%) (Baker and Schumacher, 1993). About 20% of patients are afebrile. Septic joints are normally painful, swollen, red, and warm. Diabetes mellitus, malignancy, chronic liver disease, and other rheumatic diseases (e.g., RA, SLE) increase the risk of a septic joint and probably its severity. Other risk factors for a septic joint include advanced age, intravenous (IV) drug abuse, HIV infection, and having a prosthetic joint. Almost half of adults with septic arthritis are older than 60 years, and the condition usually affects an arthritic hip, knee, or shoulder. Septic arthritis in older adults causes a fever in only 10% of patients and a marked leukocytosis in only one third, although ESR elevation is usually marked. Joint and blood culture results are usually positive.

Most polyarticular disease is seen in immunosuppressed patients or those with underlying rheumatic disease. The causative organism is usually *Staphylococcus aureus*. The mortality rate in patients with polyarticular septic joints approaches 40% (Youssef and York, 1994).

Most cases of septic arthritis are secondary to hematogenous spread of infection. In drug abusers, the causative organism is usually *S. aureus* or gram-negative organisms and affects predominantly the joints of the axial skeleton (hip, shoulder, vertebrae, symphysis pubis, costochondral, sternoclavicular, sacroiliac). Iatrogenic septic arthritis is usually caused by *S. aureus, Staphylococcus epidermidis*, and gram-negative organisms. This complication might be difficult to recognize because the joint is already symptomatic (which prompted the arthroscopy or arthrocentesis) before infection. Bacterial infection after arthroscopy is 0.04% to 4% and after arthrocentesis is 0.01%. Septic arthritis complicating RA is polyarticular in 50% of patients, usually caused by *S. aureus*, and arises from pulmonary or UTIs, infected rheumatoid nodules, or foot infections. Prosthetic infections are from direct inoculation or hematogenous spread; the prosthesis often must be removed.

Septic arthritis in children normally involves the lower extremities (knee, hip, and ankle). An infant or child with a septic joint often presents with not moving the infected joint and being generally irritable. Septic arthritis can complicate otitis media, an umbilical catheter, meningitis, or osteomyelitis. *S. aureus* and group B streptococci are the most common organisms in infants and children, except ages 6 months to 2 years, when *Haemophilus influenzae* and *Kingella kingae* organisms predominate. *H. influenzae* septic arthritis is seen especially in partially immunized children.

The most common form of acute bacterial arthritis is disseminated gonococcal infection, which causes a migratory polyarthritis and tenosynovitis, affecting predominantly the small joints of the hands, wrists, elbow, ankles, and knees. Papules and vesicles are often apparent on the trunk and extremities, including the palms and soles. Patients usually do not have symptoms of urethritis, cervicitis, or pharyngitis. If gonococcal arthritis is suspected, empiric treatment should be initiated immediately while culture results are pending. *Neisseria meningitidis* can cause a similar arthritis and rash syndrome after an illness, ranging from a mild upper respiratory infection to frank meningitis. In contrast to gonococcal infections, the meningococcus might cause oral mucosal lesions as well as skin lesions.

Acute gonococcal arthritis can be confirmed by Gram stain in only 25% of patients and by culture in 50%; nongonococcal bacterial arthritis can be confirmed in 50% and 90% of patients, respectively. It is therefore important to make a clinical diagnosis rather than rely solely on laboratory studies. Fever is often absent or of low grade. Blood cultures are also positive only approximately half the time but might be positive when synovial fluid cultures fail to identify an organism. Synovial fluid analysis usually shows WBC count over 50,000/mm³, with more than 90% PMNs. Crystals can coexist with bacterial infections, and their presence should not rule out bacterial infection. Plain radiography might detect an osteomyelitis and should be done as a baseline study because destruction can be seen on radiographs 10 to 14 days later. Air in the joint suggests an anaerobic infection, which accounts for 1% of septic joints.

The duration of appropriate IV antibiotic treatment depends on the presumptive or culture-identified causative organism. Initial therapy depends on the Gram stain result from synovial fluid. If gram-positive cocci are seen, IV vancomycin should be started empirically. If gram-negative bacilli are seen, a third-generation IV cephalosporin should be initiated. If the Gram stain result is negative, IV vancomycin should be considered. When sensitivity data return, antibiotic therapy can be narrowed appropriately. The duration varies, but often the patient will receive 2 weeks of IV therapy followed by 2 weeks of oral therapy. Intraarticular antibiotic injections are unnecessary. A joint might need repeated needle aspirations or tidal lavage with arthroscopy to sterilize the joint space (Klippel, 2001).

KEY TREATMENT

- Empiric treatment of infectious arthritis with appropriate IV antibiotics is based on Gram stain results; joint and blood culture sensitivities narrow the antibiotic regimen (SOR: C).
- Joints may need drainage in patients with septic arthritis (SOR: C).

Viral Arthritis

See eAppendix 32-1 online.

Lyme Arthritis

Key Points

- *B. burgdorferi* is the most common source of Lyme disease.
- Lyme titer is diagnostic but might have a high false-negative ratio.
- False-positive titers can be caused by RA or lupus.
- About 80% of Lyme disease patients have classic erythema migrans (EM) rash.

Lyme disease is caused by the *Ixodes* tick-borne spirochete *B. burgdorferi* and was first described in 1975 after an apparent outbreak of juvenile RA in Lyme, Connecticut. The characteristic target rash of EM develops within 1 month (mean 1 week) of a tick bite and can be complicated by CNS disease (meningitis, neuritis), cardiac disease (atrioventricular conduction blocks), and arthritis. It occurs most often in northeastern states (New York, Connecticut, Massachusetts, New Jersey, Rhode Island, Pennsylvania) and upper Midwestern states (Wisconsin, Minnesota). As with other rheumatologic diseases, Lyme disease is a clinical diagnosis, with laboratory tests used only to clarify the diagnosis.

Although most patients with Lyme disease do not recall an actual tick bite, most (80%) manifest the EM rash, which might be confluent or have central clearing or darkening. This rash may enlarge quickly and may be accompanied by arthralgia, myalgia, fatigue, fever, and chills. Weeks to months after the EM rash, neurologic involvement can occur. A facial nerve palsy is common, although most facial nerve palsies are not caused by Lyme disease, even in endemic areas. As with neurologic signs, carditis might be the first presenting symptom, often manifesting as a first-, second-, or third-degree atrioventricular block or bundle branch block. Cardiac symptoms normally do not occur for 1 to 2 months after onset of symptoms.

Arthritis can occur in approximately half of untreated patients with Lyme disease but is rare in treated patients. Rheumatic symptoms occurring late in the clinical course include polyarthralgias, a migratory polyarthritis, or an oligoarticular arthritis with few systemic symptoms. In untreated patients developing an arthritis, some develop a chronic arthritis resistant to antibiotics.

Laboratory Studies

The current recommended approach is a two-tier strategy using a sensitive enzyme-linked immunosorbent assay (ELISA) and, if the result is positive, Western blot. ELISA is associated with a high false-positive rate, so all positive results must be confirmed with a positive Western blot. Western blot can test for both immunoglobulin M (IgM) and IgG antibodies to *B. burgdorferi*. IgM antibodies typically appear within 1 to 2 weeks and IgG in 2 to 6 weeks after onset of EM rash. Only one third of patients with a single lesion of EM are seropositive at diagnosis (Verdon and Sigal, 1997). The presence of EM is itself enough to make the clinical diagnosis, and testing is not required. Negative serology in a suspected case should be followed by acute- and convalescent-phase samples (2-4 weeks after initial sample). False-positive ELISA test results can occur in RA, juvenile rheumatoid arthritis (JRA), SLE, and infectious mononucleosis. Serologic testing after treatment is not helpful because seroreactivity persists long after successful treatment.

Treatment

Treatment of early Lyme disease in adults includes doxycycline, 100 mg twice daily, or amoxicillin, 500 mg three times daily, for 21 days. Amoxicillin is first-line therapy in children younger than 8 years old; cefuroxime axetil or erythromycin is used in cases of doxycycline or amoxicillin allergy (Worsmer et al., 2006). Oral therapy is as effective as IV therapy for patients with either early Lyme disease or Lyme arthritis and is less costly (Eckman et al., 1997). Concern about the risk of late neurologic sequelae should not lead to more aggressive treatment with IV antibiotics for these patients (Wormser et al., 2000). Early treatment prevents recurrent arthritis as well as neurologic and cardiac sequelae. IV therapy with ceftriaxone (Rocephin), cefotaxime (Claforan), or penicillin G is used for early disseminated and late Lyme disease. IV antibiotic therapy is preferable for patients with neurologic symptoms, with the possible exception of those with facial palsy alone (Steere, 1989). Most patients are symptomatically better with 20 days of treatment. Continued symptomatology in patients with treated infection does not respond to further antibiotics (Klippel, 2001). Antibiotic treatment failures can occur but are rare and usually associated with poor absorption. Antibiotic resistance to typically used agents has not been shown.

For preventive measures against Lyme disease, see eAppendix 32-2 online.

KEY TREATMENT

- Adults and children 8 years and older should be treated with oral doxycycline for 21 days for early Lyme disease (Worsmer et al., 2006) (SOR: A).
- Pregnant women and children younger than 8 years should be treated with oral amoxicillin or cefuroxime (SOR: C).
- Patients with neurologic (excluding isolated facial nerve palsy) or cardiac manifestation are treated with IV antibiotic therapy for Lyme disease (Wormser et al., 2000) (SOR: B).

Other Infectious Arthritides

Although mycobacteria, parasites, and fungi rarely cause arthritis, the incidence has increased with increasing numbers of HIV/AIDS and other immunosuppressed patients. *Mycobacterium tuberculosis* arthritis occurs by hematogenous spread from the lung and is diagnosed by synovial fluid culture. The classic tuberculosis infection involves the spine and is known as Pott disease. Thoracic vertebrae are most often involved, but a monoarticular arthritis can also occur in large, weight-bearing joints. Mild arthritides might also be caused by *Giardia lamblia* infection, histoplasmosis, cryptococcosis, blastomycosis, sporotrichosis, coccidioidomycosis, actinomycetes, and atypical mycobacteria.

RHEUMATIC FEVER

Key Points

- Rheumatic fever is seen 2 to 4 weeks after β-hemolytic streptococcal pharyngitis.
- Antibiotic treatment for streptococcal infection can help prevent development of rheumatic fever.
- The Jones criteria and ASO titers are helpful in diagnosis of rheumatic fever.

Rheumatic fever is a systemic inflammatory process initiated by group A β-hemolytic streptococcal pharyngitis. Often, younger children in particular do not recall

Table 32-8 Revised Jones Criteria for Diagnosis of Acute Rheumatic Fever*

Major manifestations	Carditis
	Polyarthritis
	Chorea
	Erythema marginatum
	Subcutaneous nodules
Minor manifestations	*Clinical:*
	Arthralgia, fever
	Laboratory:
	Elevated acute-phase reactants (ESR, CRP)
	Prolonged PR interval

Plus:
Supporting evidence of antecedent group A streptococcal infection
Positive throat culture or rapid streptococcal antigen test
Elevated or rising streptococcal antibody titer

*If supported by evidence of preceding group A streptococcal infection, the presence of two major manifestations or of one major and two minor manifestations indicates a high probability of acute rheumatic fever.
CRP, C-reactive protein; *ESR,* erythrocyte sedimentation rate.
From Gibofsky A, Zabriskie JB. Rheumatic fever. In Klippel JH, ed. *Primer on the rheumatic diseases.* 12th ed. Atlanta: Arthritis Foundation; 2001:282.

antecedent pharyngitis, which usually occurs 2 to 4 weeks before symptom onset. Rheumatic fever appears to be linked only to pharyngitis; group A streptococcal (GAS) impetigo does not seem to be associated with rheumatic fever. Rheumatic fever most often affects children 4 to 9 years of age, and the onset is usually characterized by an acute febrile illness that can cause large-joint migratory arthritis, CNS involvement (Sydenham chorea), characteristic rash, and carditis with inflammation of heart valves and subsequent damage. Antibiotic treatment of GAS pharyngitis greatly reduces the development of rheumatic fever. The 1992 revised Jones criteria are useful in the diagnosis of acute rheumatic fever (Table 32-8).

Rheumatic fever–related arthritis is often preceded by arthralgias out of proportion to frank swelling, lasting approximately 1 week. Arthralgias usually migrate to lower extremity joints and then to the upper extremities. Children experience this arthritis less frequently than adolescents and adults. The arthritis then resolves spontaneously. Carditis involving the valves, particularly the mitral valve, is the most severe sequela. Rheumatic heart disease is the most common serious sequela and usually occurs 10 to 20 years after the original attack. Patients might also have erythema marginatum, a rash with open or closed ring lesions with sharp outer edges or macular rings with pale centers, or both. The rash spreads centrifugally from the trunk to the extremities with lesions that come and go.

The antistreptolysin O (ASO) titer is the most useful laboratory test because pharyngeal culture results are often negative by the time rheumatic fever develops. The ASO titer rises 4 to 5 weeks after the onset of GAS pharyngitis or 2 to 3 weeks after development of rheumatic fever. Because only 80% of patients with rheumatic fever develop an increase in ASO titer, clinically suspicious rheumatic fever with a negative ASO titer should be followed up by testing for antistreptococcal antibody, such as anti-DNase, anti-DNase B, and antihyaluronidase antibody tests.

Aspirin is the drug of choice for acute rheumatic fever and usually results in a dramatic response. The usual dosage is 80 to 100 mg/kg/day for children and 4 to 8 g/day for adults. Penicillin should also be given for a 10-day course whether or not pharyngitis is present, and family members and other close contacts should be cultured and treated if necessary. IM penicillin is more effective than oral penicillin in clinical trials. No benefit has been shown from IV immune globulin (IVIG) or corticosteroids for rheumatic fever, but studies continue (Manyemba and Mightosi, 2004).

Patients who have had documented rheumatic fever and who develop subsequent GAS pharyngitis are at high risk for a recurrent rheumatic episode and thus at increased risk for worsening rheumatic heart disease. For this reason, prevention of recurrent episodes requires continuous antimicrobial prophylaxis (Gerber et al., 2009). Before prophylaxis initiation, a full treatment course for GAS pharyngitis should be completed. In the United States, typical prophylactic therapy is with long-acting IM benzathine penicillin G every 4 weeks until early adulthood ($\approx$18 years of age).

KEY TREATMENT

- Patients with acute GAS pharyngitis should receive antibiotic therapy to help prevent the complication of acute rheumatic fever (Denny et al., 1950) (SOR: B).
- Patients with acute rheumatic fever should receive appropriate antibiotic therapy to eradicate the GAS infection, regardless of whether pharyngitis is present at diagnosis (SOR: C).
- Use of aspirin is the treatment of choice for the acute symptoms of acute rheumatic fever (SOR: C).
- Prevention of recurrent acute rheumatic fever requires prophylactic treatment for GAS pharyngitis with antibiotics (Gerber et al., 2009) (SOR: A).

SYSTEMIC LUPUS ERYTHEMATOSUS

Key Points

- The 5-year survival rate of SLE patients is 90%.
- The female : male ratio is 2 : 1 before and 4 : 1 after puberty.
- Four of 11 criteria are needed for SLE diagnosis.

Systemic lupus erythematosus is a generalized autoimmune disease of unknown cause characterized by the production of antibodies to numerous antigens. The most common antibodies found in SLE are those directed against the cell nucleus (ANAs). These antibodies bind DNA, RNA, nuclear proteins, and protein–DNA or protein–RNA complexes. Antibodies to double-stranded DNA and an RNA–protein complex called Sm are found almost exclusively in SLE. Immune complex deposition results in inflammation and vasculitis, causing multiorgan pathology.

Systemic LE is most common in women of reproductive age (15-40 years), and the female : male ratio is approximately 2:1 before puberty and 4:1 after puberty. However, SLE can be seen in all ages, including infants and older adults; in these two subpopulations, the female : male ratio is only 2:1. SLE affects approximately one in 1000 to 2500

in the general population, but the disease incidence in African American and Latino women is much higher (up to one in 250 in African American women ages 18-65 years). The 5-year survival rate after diagnosis is 90%.

Systemic LE also shows a strong familial tendency. An association with MHC genes *DR2, DR3, DR4,* and *DR5* has been found. As with other rheumatologic diseases, SLE appears to result from a genetic abnormality that can be triggered by environmental factors. Some of these hypothesized factors include infections, stress (neuroendocrine changes), exposure to sunlight, diet, and toxins, including drugs. In addition to autoantibody production, SLE involves immune cell (B, T, monocyte) abnormalities. Because of the wide variety of presentations, the ACR created a classification system to standardize the diagnosis of SLE (Table 32-9). To confirm a diagnosis of SLE, patients must have at least 4 of 11 criteria present either serially or simultaneously.

Clinical Features

Constitutional symptoms found in patients with SLE include fatigue, malaise, fever, and weight loss. The family physician therefore has an important role to play in the diagnosis of this multisystem disease, which must be differentiated from infections such as HIV (which often is false positive in SLE) and subacute bacterial endocarditis; other connective tissue diseases such as vasculitis, RA, and mixed connective tissue disease; and malignancies such as lymphomas. SLE is characterized by specific organ system abnormalities. The disease most often affects the skin, joints, kidneys, CNS, GI tract, and lungs, with a spectrum of disease severity and an unpredictable course. SLE is truly systemic; other asymptomatic organ involvement must be searched for during active periods of disease, regardless of the presenting sign or symptom.

Mucocutaneous Manifestations. More than 90% of SLE patients eventually have a mucocutaneous manifestation. The classic malar butterfly rash gave lupus its name because it was thought to resemble the bite of a wolf. This rash is present in only one third of patients; when it occurs, it is often after sunlight exposure. One third to two thirds of SLE patients are extremely photosensitive. Sun exposure not only can cause a maculopapular, erythematous rash but also can induce a flare of systemic symptoms. Other lesions can occur, such as bullae or generalized erythema.

Subacute cutaneous lupus erythematosus (SCLE) occurs in sun-exposed areas of the skin, particularly on the upper torso, in two forms—annular or papulosquamous lesions. The former variant might be confused with erythema annulare and the latter with psoriasis or lichen planus. About 70% of patients with photosensitivity have anti-Ro antibodies (Boumpas et al., 1995). SCLE lesions do not result in scarring. Discoid lupus lesions are raised plaques that often occur in the absence of any other systemic manifestations, most often on the face, neck, scalp, and external ears. Unlike SCLE lesions, these erythematous plaques with heavy scales can cause scarring, with a hypopigmented, atrophic central area. Other mucocutaneous manifestations of SLE include alopecia, which resolves when the acute SLE exacerbation ends, unless the alopecia is secondary to discoid scarring. Oral, nasal, and vaginal ulcerations as well as palpable purpura also occur.

Table 32-9 Criteria for Classification of Systemic Lupus Erythematosus*

1. Malar rash	Fixed erythema, flat or raised, over the malar eminences, tending to spare the nasolabial folds
2. Discoid rash	Erythematous raised patches with adherent keratotic scaling and follicular plugging; atrophic scarring may occur in older lesions
3. Photosensitivity	Skin rash as a result of unusual reaction to sunlight, by patient history or physician observation
4. Oral ulcers	Oral or nasopharyngeal ulceration, usually painless, observed by a physician
5. Arthritis	Nonerosive arthritis involving two or more peripheral joints, characterized by tenderness, swelling, or effusion
6. Serositis	a. Pleuritis—convincing history of pleuritic pain or rub heard by a physician or evidence of pleural effusion *or* b. Pericarditis—documented by electrocardiogram or rub or evidence of pericardial effusion
7. Renal disorder	a. Persistent proteinuria higher than 0.5 g/day or higher than 3+ if quantitation not performed *or* b. Cellular casts: may be red cell, hemoglobin, granular, tubular, or mixed
8. Neurologic disorder	a. Seizures—in the absence of offending drugs or known metabolic derangements (e.g., uremia, ketoacidosis, electrolyte imbalance) *or* b. Psychosis: in the absence of offending drugs or known metabolic derangements (e.g., uremia, ketoacidosis, electrolyte imbalance)
9. Hematologic disorder	a. Hemolytic anemia—with reticulocytosis *or* b. Leukopenia—less than 4000/mm^3 total on two or more occasions *or* c. Lymphopenia—less than 1500/mm^3 on two or more occasions *or* d. Thrombocytopenia—less than 100,000/mm^3 in the absence of offending drugs
10. Immunologic disorder	a. Positive lupus erythematosus cell preparation *or* b. Anti-DNA: antibody to native DNA in abnormal titer *or* c. Anti-Sm: presence of antibody to Sm nuclear antigen *or* d. False-positive serologic test for syphilis known to be positive for at least 6 months and confirmed by *Treponema pallidum* immobilization or fluorescent treponemal antibody absorption test
11. Antinuclear antibody	An abnormal titer of antinuclear antibody by immunofluorescence or an equivalent assay at any point in time and in the absence of drugs known to be associated with "drug-induced lupus" syndrome

*The proposed classification is based on 11 criteria. For the purpose of identifying patients in clinical studies, a person is said to have systemic lupus erythematosus if any 4 or more of the 11 criteria are present, serially or simultaneously, during any interval of observation.
From Tan EM, Cohen AS, Fries JF, et al. The 1982 revised criteria for the classification of systemic lupus erythematosus (SLE). *Arthritis Rheum.* 1982;25:1271-1277, with permission of the American College of Rheumatology.

Latent lupus refers to the condition of those patients who do not meet the ACR criteria for diagnosis of SLE but have many features consistent with lupus. This form is mild and is treated symptomatically. Many of these patients never develop classic SLE; there are no identifiable prognostic indicators of propensity for progression to frank lupus.

Drug-induced lupus occurs when a patient taking a drug develops clinical and serologically consistent lupus, which then resolves (clinically and then serologically) on discontinuation of the drug. Drugs known or suspected to cause lupus include *antituberculous* drugs (e.g., isoniazid, streptomycin), *antibiotics* (e.g., penicillin, tetracycline, sulfa, griseofulvin), *anticonvulsants* (e.g., phenytoin [Dilantin], ethosuximide [Zarontin], carbamazepine [Tegretol]), *phenothiazines* (e.g., perphenazine [Trilafon], promethazine [Phenergan], thioridazine [Mellaril]), and *antihypertensives* (e.g., hydralazine, methyldopa, reserpine), as well as oral contraceptives, lithium, propylthiouracil, and procainamide. Symptoms are usually mild and do not involve the CNS or kidneys.

Musculoskeletal Manifestations. Arthralgias and arthritis are the most common initial symptoms of SLE. The typical pattern is symmetric involvement of the hands, wrists, or knees, either migratory or persisting in an involved joint. There may be subcutaneous nodules similar to those of RA, but SLE usually does not cause RA-like erosions. Subluxations causing swan neck deformities and other deformities in the hands are known as *Jaccoud arthropathy*, which is characterized by deformity without erosion of bone and cartilage. Patients with SLE sometimes experience myalgias but usually not to the degree seen in dermatomyositis.

Musculoskeletal complications of SLE also include osteoporosis and avascular necrosis of bone (osteonecrosis), especially in corticosteroid-treated children with SLE. In one study, 65% of premenopausal women with SLE had abnormal bone mineral density (Petri, 1995). Screening for osteoporosis, even in premenopausal women, and treatment, if indicated, are therefore prudent measures, as is minimizing the use of corticosteroids. Late SLE can cause osteonecrosis, particularly of the hip, independent of active SLE episodes. Major risk factors for osteonecrosis include a prednisone dosage higher than 20 mg/day for 1 month or longer and the presence of Raynaud disease or vasculitis. Avascular necrosis of the hip is diagnosed early by MRI.

Renal Disease. Called *lupus nephritis*, SLE-induced renal disease is typically asymptomatic until relatively late. More than 50% of all patients and 75% of African American patients with SLE have renal involvement. Immune complex deposition along the glomerular basement membrane leads to the nephrotic syndrome or renal failure, which can be the presenting sign. An elevated serum creatinine level can be found, as well as proteinuria, hematuria, pyuria, and casts in the absence of infection. Definitively diagnosed by renal biopsy, lupus nephritis constitutes a spectrum of severity from mild to more severe that involves mesangial, focal proliferative, diffuse proliferative, and advanced sclerosing forms of glomerulonephritis (Petri, 1998). Patients with SLE should have an annual urinalysis and renal function test to rule out proteinuria. An elevated creatinine level

(>2 mg/dL) is the best predictor of prognosis. Patients with SLE have had successful renal transplants, although lupus nephritis can recur.

Neuropsychiatric Disease. Neuropsychiatric symptoms are common when SLE is active but can occur in isolation. Manifestations include headache, generalized seizures (20% of SLE patients), stroke, cranial and peripheral neuropathies, psychosis, severe depression (40%), cognitive abnormalities, and organic brain syndrome. Cranial neuropathies may manifest as visual defects, tinnitus, vertigo, nystagmus, ptosis, or facial palsies. A migraine-type headache is common and can be intractable. *Neuropsychiatric lupus* is a diagnosis of exclusion after other causes of the patient's symptoms have been ruled out. Electroencephalographic findings are often abnormal but nonspecific. MRI of the head can show diffuse, small focal areas of increased signal density on the cerebral white matter and cortical gray matter that clear with corticosteroid treatment. Cerebrospinal fluid (CSF) studies are important to rule out infectious causes. Even in long-term mild disease, neurocognitive abnormalities affecting memory or causing speech abnormalities often persist. Antiribosomal P antibody presence correlates with cognitive impairment in SLE (Hirohata and Nakanishi, 2001).

Cardiovascular Manifestations. Patients with SLE have an increased risk of premature atherosclerosis from the disease itself as well as from its treatment; up to 40% of SLE patients have been found to have this complication in screening studies. Corticosteroids increase cardiac risk factors such as weight, BP, cholesterol, and homocysteine levels, which the family physician must keep in mind. Primary coronary disease prevention monitoring and patient education plans for the SLE patient are important because the mortality rate from myocardial infarction is approximately 10 times that in an age- and gender-matched population (Klippel, 2001). Myocarditis and endocarditis are rare, but pericarditis can occur in up to 45% of patients with SLE (25% in most series). Symptoms might be mild or severe, but constrictive pericarditis and cardiac tamponade are rare.

Thrombosis is a major cause of morbidity and mortality in lupus patients. Between 30% and 50% of SLE patients make antiphospholipid autoantibodies to the phospholipid part of the normal cell membrane, although most people with these antibodies do not have lupus. Types of antiphospholipid antibodies include anticardiolipin antibody, β2-GP-I antibody and lupus anticoagulant. Lupus anticoagulant antibodies might result in prolonged partial thromboplastin time (PTT) and prothrombin time (PT) but paradoxically result in an increased risk of thrombotic events for these patients. This might be caused by an antibody-induced vasculopathy. Anticardiolipin and β2-GP-I antibodies can be detected using ELISA, but there is no direct testing for the lupus anticoagulant. If the lupus anticoagulant is clinically suspected but activated PTT is normal, more sensitive coagulation tests should be done, including kaolin clotting time (KCT), modified Russell viper venom time (RVVT), and platelet neutralization procedure (PNP) (Petri, 1994).

Antiphospholipid antibody syndrome is defined as the presence of lupus anticoagulant, β2-GP-I antibody or anticardiolipin antibody with one of these four entities: arterial thrombosis, venous thrombosis, recurrent first-trimester or one late (second- or third-trimester) spontaneous abortion, or thrombocytopenia. This acquired autoimmune hypercoagulability is more common in patients with SLE than in the general population.

The incidence of spontaneous abortion, intrauterine death, and prematurity is also increased in women with SLE alone. Studies differ, but currently pregnancy is not thought to exacerbate SLE, as formerly thought. It is recommended that women be flare-free for 6 months and do not have serious comorbidities such as renal disease before deciding to become pregnant. Fertility is not affected by SLE. Women with either recurrent first-trimester or late pregnancy loss can reduce their risk of pregnancy loss with heparin and low-dose aspirin therapy.

Other Manifestations. Serositis that causes pericarditis, pleurisy, and peritonitis is common in SLE. Bilateral pleural effusions are usually small and are seen most often in drug-induced lupus patients and in older adult patients. Pleurisy is clinically more common than pericarditis, which rarely becomes severe enough to be constrictive.

Systemic LE can cause multiple GI symptoms such as nausea, vomiting, anorexia, and abdominal pain, often as a result of peritoneal inflammation. Mesenteric vasculitis can cause lower abdominal pain and rectal bleeding. Hepatomegaly with increases in liver enzyme levels and pancreatitis with amylase level elevations can occur with SLE. In addition to hepatomegaly, splenomegaly and lymphadenopathy can occur with lupus exacerbations.

Lung involvement can include pulmonary hemorrhage, pulmonary hypertension, and pneumonitis. *Lupus pneumonitis* often manifests as a diffuse interstitial disease. *Shrinking lung syndrome*, seen in late SLE, is a restrictive condition with decreased lung volumes resulting from abnormal musculoskeletal respiratory function.

Laboratory Abnormalities

There are no specific tests for lupus. The lupus erythematosus cell, formed when complexes of nuclei and antibodies are phagocytosed by PMNs, is highly specific but of low sensitivity. ANA, anti–double-stranded DNA, and antiphospholipid antibody are all markers for SLE, but antibody test results are misleading if not considered in the clinical context. From 2% to 5% of patients with SLE are ANA negative, but 5% of the normal population and up to 20% of healthy young women are ANA positive (Fritzler et al., 1985). Antibodies to an RNA–protein complex called Sm (anti-Smith antibody) and to double-stranded DNA (dsDNA) are almost unique for SLE, both being 95% specific. Whereas ESR is normally increased, CRP is normal (Linares et al., 1986).

Autoantibodies in SLE include ANA and anticytoplasmic antibodies (including lipoproteins), antibodies against blood cells, antibodies against various organs and structures (e.g., gastric mucosa, neurons, muscle sarcolemma, thyroglobulin), and antibodies against collagen. Different antibodies against different parts of the cell nucleus appear as the four patterns of ANA staining. These include membranous antibodies against single-stranded DNA, speckled antibodies against extractable ribonucleoproteins, dsDNA antibodies against native dsDNA, nucleolar antibodies against nucleolar antigens and sometimes associated with scleroderma, and homogeneous antibodies against deoxyribonucleoproteins.

In active SLE, serum complement (C3, C4, and often CH50) levels are depressed. ESR is often elevated during active disease but is not a precise indicator of disease activity. DNA autoantibodies also do not correlate well with periods of active disease. A normochromic normocytic anemia, leukopenia (2500-4000 WBCs/mm^3), and thrombocytopenia are common because of bone marrow suppression or the autoimmune process, although other causes must be ruled out first. SLE can manifest as immune thrombocytic purpura years before the patient develops other symptoms of lupus.

The confirming tests for lupus (e.g., ANA, anti-DNA titers) are generally not helpful in follow-up. Monitoring for disease or treatment sequelae often involves serial CBC; renal function testing (creatinine); urinalysis; C3 and C4; and laboratory tests monitoring specific drug toxicities, including homocysteine and cholesterol levels for patients taking corticosteroids.

Treatment

The major goal of treatment is to treat the active disease without causing iatrogenic long-term complications and to be supportive of the patient and family. The family physician has a vital role in educating patients with SLE about signs and symptoms of disease flares. Continued monitoring, even when the disease appears inactive, is also important. General advice includes avoiding sun exposure or using potent sunscreens, early evaluation of unexplained fevers, annual influenza vaccine, adequate rest and exercise, and weight control. Other specific information tailored to the patient's needs is also important, such as SLE and its effect on pregnancy.

Vigilance for severe infections, particularly when corticosteroids are being used, should be continual. Proper monitoring for drug toxicities must include ophthalmologic examination with antimalarials and monitoring for corticosteroid-induced side effects. Treatment approaches for SLE emphasize using a drug combination to minimize corticosteroid use. Corticosteroids increase cardiovascular risk factors, including weight, BP, and cholesterol and homocysteine levels. Too-rapid steroid tapering should also be avoided. Immunosuppressive drugs are also being used more often, requiring careful monitoring.

The NSAIDs are still the drugs of choice for musculoskeletal manifestations, especially mild symptoms. The potential renal and GI toxicity of these drugs being used for a disease that in itself causes renal and GI damage must be kept in mind and monitored. Gastroduodenal cytoprotective therapy should be strongly considered for patients taking NSAIDs.

For minor polyarthritic disease activity, prednisone at 0.5 mg/kg/day in a single dose can be given, but many recommend other agents if the daily maintenance prednisone dose is 10 mg or more. Antimalarials such as hydroxychloroquine (Plaquenil) are often used for lupus arthritis but require ophthalmologic monitoring every 6 to 12 months. For severe arthritis or flare-ups, prednisone at 1.0 mg/kg/day; intraarticular injection with triamcinolone

hexacetonide; or IV methylprednisolone sodium succinate (Solu-Medrol), 1000 mg over 90 minutes daily for 3 days, can be used, followed by oral prednisone. Methotrexate, 7.5 mg orally once weekly, along with folic acid supplementation or azathioprine, can also be used to minimize prednisone dosage, although methotrexate cannot be used during pregnancy.

Cutaneous lupus is treated with sunscreen and sun avoidance, topical or intralesional corticosteroids, topical cryotherapy with liquid nitrogen (less often), and antimalarials. The most common antimalarials are hydroxychloroquine, chloroquine (Aralen), and quinacrine. For patients who cannot take antimalarials, dapsone and retinoids such as etretinate (Tegison) or isotretinoin (Accutane) might be used with appropriate precautions. Fluocinonide cream has greater effect than hydrocortisone for discoid lupus (Jessop et al., 2001). Dapsone should not be used in patients with glucose-6-phosphate dehydrogenase (G6PD) deficiency, and retinoids should be avoided in pregnant patients. Severe cutaneous lupus can be treated with high-dose corticosteroids, but if the daily dose of prednisone exceeds 10 mg, methotrexate or azathioprine should be considered. Finally, thalidomide is effective for discoid lupus, but its use is limited by concerns about neuropathy and teratogenicity.

Lupus nephritis, once diagnosed by renal biopsy, can be treated with high-dose corticosteroids alone or with steroid-sparing drugs such as methotrexate or azathioprine. Cyclophosphamide for rapidly progressive or severe nephritis is effective but has substantial toxicities and is generally best left for the rheumatologist to prescribe. Toxicity can be minimized somewhat with prehydration and a mesna (Mesnex) injection, a cyclophosphamide metabolite binder, to avoid hemorrhagic cystitis. Later development of hematologic malignancies (rare) and premature ovarian failure (common) can result from cyclophosphamide use. If cyclophosphamide is indicated in a young woman, her family physician should raise options such as egg harvesting to preserve fertility.

Patients with SLE and antiphospholipid antibody syndrome who consequently have venous or arterial thrombosis can be treated with warfarin (Coumadin) to keep the international normalized ratio between 2 and 3. Although somewhat controversial, therapy should continue for at least 3 to 6 months, and often, lifelong anticoagulation is recommended based on high risk for subsequent events. Severe hemolytic anemia responds to IV methylprednisolone. Leukopenia rarely requires treatment. Severe thrombocytopenia with platelet counts below 50,000/mm^3 can be treated with methylprednisolone, danazol (Danocrine), immunosuppressive drugs, and possibly splenectomy.

Arthritis, serositis, and constitutional signs usually respond to 0.5 mg/kg/day of prednisone; nephritis and CNS disease usually require doses of 1 mg/kg/day. Patients who do not respond to high-dose steroids after 7 weeks should be considered for immunosuppressive drugs.

Rarely, plasma exchange is necessary for severe thrombotic thrombocytopenic purpura and pulmonary hemorrhage. Plasmapheresis has not shown long-term benefit for lupus nephritis. End-stage lupus nephropathy is treated with dialysis or kidney transplantation. Other experimental therapies for SLE include immunotherapy with anti-CD4, anti–TNF-α, and interferon-α.

Treatment of SLE has been successful in decreasing morbidity and mortality in what used to be considered a universally progressive, terminal disease. More than 90% of treated patients survive at least 15 years. SLE evolves over time with new manifestations and sometimes vague symptomatology arising unpredictably. Therefore, good communication in an ongoing physician–patient relationship and teamwork between the family physician and the rheumatologist are necessary for optimal care.

KEY TREATMENT

- Cutaneous lupus should initially be treated with topical corticosteroids (Jessop et al., 2001) (SOR: B) and avoidance of precipitating factors such as sun exposure (SOR: C).
- Patients with persistent cutaneous lesions should be considered for treatment with antimalarials such a hydroxychloroquine (SOR: C).
- NSAIDs are the initial treatment for SLE-associated myositis, serositis, and arthritis. Refractory cases can be treated with 0.5 to 1 mg/kg/day of prednisone (SOR: C).

SJÖGREN SYNDROME

Sjögren syndrome is an autoimmune disorder caused most likely by T cell–mediated exocrine gland destruction characterized by dry eyes (keratoconjunctivitis sicca) and dry mouth (xerostomia). Patients with secondary SS have these symptoms in association with other autoimmune diseases such as RA, SLE, polymyositis, systemic sclerosis, or biliary cirrhosis.

A diagnosis of definite SS requires a minor salivary gland biopsy; a probable SS diagnosis can be based on demonstrating decreased salivary function. Exclusions to the diagnosis based on the San Diego Criteria include patients with HIV, primary fibromyalgia, sarcoidosis, preexisting lymphoma, keratitis sicca, hepatitis B or C, or salivary gland enlargement (Table 32-10). Objective evidence of ocular dryness can be obtained by the Schirmer II test, which involves stimulating the nasolacrimal reflex by inserting a cotton swab into the nostril; the increase in tear flow is then measured for both eyes (Tsubota, 1991). Rose bengal staining of the corneal or conjunctiva epithelial layer is another objective test. Serologic evidence of SS includes an elevated RF (>1:320), elevated ANA (>1:320), or presence of anti–SS-A (Ro) or anti–SS-B (La) antibodies.

Salivary secretions can be quantified by asking the patient to suck on a sugarless piece of candy for 3 minutes and then expectorate. If there is very little or no expectorant, a probable diagnosis of SS can be made; a follow-up minor salivary gland biopsy is definitively diagnostic. Patients not fitting these objective criteria can be reassured that their dry eyes or mouth are most likely not caused by an autoimmune disorder. Other manifestations of SS include constitutional symptoms such as fatigue, dry skin, vaginal dryness, upper respiratory tract dryness, and difficulty swallowing (caused by decreased saliva). SS is not the only entity that can cause enlarged lacrimal and salivary glands and glandular dysfunction. SS needs to be differentiated from infiltrative processes (lymphoma, sarcoidosis, fatty

Table 32-10 San Diego Criteria for Sjögren Syndrome

I. Primary Sjögren syndrome*	A. Symptoms and objective signs of ocular dryness 1. Schirmer test <8 mm wetting per 5 minutes *and* 2. Positive rose bengal staining of cornea or conjunctiva to demonstrate keratoconjunctivitis sicca B. Symptoms and objective signs of dry mouth 1. Decreased parotid flow rate using a Lashley cup or other method *and* 2. Abnormal findings from biopsy of minor salivary gland (focus score of ≥1 based on average of four evaluable lobules) C. Serologic evidence of a systemic autoimmunity 1. Elevated rheumatoid factor >1:320 *or* 2. Elevated antinuclear antibody <1:320 *or* 3. Presence of anti–SS-A(Ro) or anti–SS-B(La) antibodies
II. Secondary Sjögren syndrome	Characteristic signs and symptoms of Sjögren syndrome (described above) plus clinical features sufficient to allow a diagnosis of rheumatoid arthritis, SLE, polymyositis, scleroderma, or biliary cirrhosis
III. Exclusions	Sarcoidosis, preexisting lymphoma; HIV infection; hepatitis virus B or C infection; primary fibromyalgia; and other known causes of autonomic neuropathy, keratitis sicca, or salivary gland enlargement

*Definite Sjögren syndrome requires objective evidence of dryness of eyes and mouth and autoimmunity, including a characteristic minor salivary gland biopsy (criteria IA, IB, and IC). Probable Sjögren syndrome does not require a minor salivary gland biopsy but can be diagnosed by demonstrating decreased salivary function (criteria IA, IB-1, and IC).
SLE, Systemic lupus erythematosus.
From Fox RI, Saito I. Criteria for diagnosis of Sjögren syndrome. *Rheum Dis Clin North Am.* 1994;20:391.

infiltrates, hemochromatosis), infectious diseases (blepharitis, HIV, hepatitis B and C, tuberculosis, syphilis), neuropathic dysfunction of the glands caused by multiple sclerosis or Bell palsy, autonomic neuropathy, and drug side effects.

Treatment of keratoconjunctivitis sicca consists of the use of artificial tears while monitoring for blepharitis caused by preservatives used in these preparations. Punctal plugs can be used to increase eye moisture, with either collagen plugs that dissolve after 2 days or silicone plugs, which are more durable but can be removed if excessive tearing occurs. If this is helpful, permanent punctal occlusion surgery might be considered. Humidifiers may also be helpful. Cyclosporine ophthalmic preparations are FDA approved for treatment of keratoconjunctivitis sicca, with objective and subjective improvement in dry eyes (Sall et al., 2000).

Dry mouth can be relieved by sugarless mints or gum. Frequent sips of water are also helpful. Those with continued symptoms may be candidates to try artificial saliva solutions (Salivart, Mouth Kote). Meticulous dental care should be encouraged because caries can occur more frequently with reduced salivary flow. Secretagogues such as pilocarpine or cevimeline can be used, but adverse effects such as flushing, increased perspiration, and increased bowel or bladder motility might outweigh their benefits. Topical antifungal troches are useful for low-grade oral infections.

Systemic treatment of SS is similar to that of SLE. NSAIDs and antimalarials, in particular, are useful for concomitant arthralgias and other systemic symptoms, but corticosteroids and immunosuppressants might be needed for refractory severe systemic disease.

- Simple treatments such as the use of humidifiers, artificial tears, sugarless gums, and frequent sips of water are adequate in most patients with keratoconjunctivitis sicca and xerostomia of SS (SOR: C).

VASCULITIC SYNDROMES

Vasculitis refers to a broad spectrum of conditions involving inflammation of blood vessels. Although many classification schemes have focused on the size of the vessels involved, this might not be very useful clinically because of the significant amount of overlap between these disorders. Many vasculitides characteristically affect certain age groups for unknown reasons: Kawasaki disease in children, temporal arteritis in elderly adults, and Henoch-Schönlein purpura with a bimodal distribution. Most vasculitic syndromes are of unknown cause. Pathologic findings are usually not diagnostic for a specific syndrome; the diagnosis is still made primarily on clinical grounds. Most vasculitides tend to cause sporadic involvement of vessels with skip lesions. That is, they involve only part of the vessel wall for only part of the segmental length of the vessel and do not occur uniformly in other vessels of the same size.

Giant Cell Arteritis

Also known as *temporal arteritis,* giant cell arteritis (GCA) usually occurs in patients older than 50 years. It is most common in Caucasians, particularly in people of northern European ancestry. Giant multinucleated cells are found in vessel walls, most frequently in the temporal arteries but sometimes in the vertebral or carotid arteries. The disease usually begins gradually, with constitutional symptoms, such as fatigue, malaise, fever, weight loss, and PMR (a separate entity characterized by proximal muscle pain and stiffness, elevated ESR, and constitutional symptoms), occurring for weeks or even months. Specific symptoms then develop, such as jaw claudication (masticatory muscle discomfort with chewing); new-type or new-onset headache; scalp tenderness, particularly overlying the temporal arteries; diplopia; and visual loss secondary to retinal ischemia. Patients might also have loss of taste or hearing. About 30% of patients have neurologic symptoms such as peripheral neuropathies and transient ischemic attacks. About 10% of patients have respiratory tract symptoms such as a sore throat, cough, and hoarseness.

On physical examination, the temporal arteries might be tender, thickened, and erythematous. New carotid artery bruits should also raise suspicion. The aortic arch or its branches might be involved, manifested by reduced BP in one or both arms or arm claudication. Temporal artery biopsies confirm the diagnosis before initiating treatment, although the skip lesion nature of involvement means that a negative temporal artery biopsy does not rule out the diagnosis. The ESR tends to be high in GCA, usually 80 to 100 mm/hr, although in one small study, 25% of all patients

with GCA on temporal artery biopsy had a normal ESR (Weyand et al., 2000). ALP and AST levels are mildly elevated in one third of patients. Serum IL-6 levels parallel inflammatory activity, and CRP may also be used to follow inflammation. The family physician should consider the diagnosis of GCA for any patient older than 50 years presenting with new-onset or new-type headache, elevated ESR, abrupt loss of vision, PMR, and prolonged fever.

The treatment for temporal arteritis or clinically suspected temporal arteritis with a negative biopsy result is prednisone, 40 to 60 mg/day for 2 to 4 weeks. One should not wait for the biopsy results if clinical suspicion is high; treatment should start immediately. If symptoms and laboratory values suggest that the disease is under control, the dose is decreased 10 mg every 2 weeks for 1 month and then by 10% of the daily dose every 2 weeks (serum ESR and CRP levels are measured before decreasing the dose). Full courses often last 9 to 12 months. Prednisone often eliminates symptoms within 12 to 48 hours. GCA is usually self-limited, up to 2 years, at which time prednisone can be discontinued in most patients, although some still require small doses of corticosteroids for years to control symptoms. Because thoracic aortic aneurysms and renal artery stenosis are relatively common sequelae, the patient should be evaluated for these.

- Prednisone is the treatment of choice in temporal arteritis (SOR: C).

Polymyalgia Rheumatica

As with GCA, PMR usually occurs in Caucasians older than 50 years, especially those of northern European ancestry. Constitutional symptoms such as fever, fatigue, malaise, and weight loss occur early on followed by neck and proximal upper extremity muscle aches. PMR is sometimes misdiagnosed as a frozen shoulder because of this. PMR later involves the lower extremity proximal muscles of the hips and thighs. Morning stiffness of large joints can make it difficult for the patient to perform ADLs, such as getting out of bed or combing the hair. The only typical physical finding is muscle tenderness but without other objective signs. A transient mild synovitis of the knees, wrists, and sternoclavicular joints might occur. The diagnosis is made clinically by noting the combination of proximal extremity and truncal muscle pain and stiffness, increased ESR, and response to steroids.

Both PMR and GCA (temporal arteritis) are often seen together. PMR can precede, appear simultaneously with, or follow the onset of GCA symptoms. These two conditions might represent different manifestations of the same pathologic process. The best treatment for PMR is corticosteroids, with the dose determined by patient characteristics as well as by whether GCA is present. The typical dose is 15 to 30 mg/day of prednisolone; the daily dose is reduced by 5 mg/week until the dose is 15 mg/day, at which point the dosage is decreased by 2.5 mg/month.

Treatment can be stopped after 6 to 12 months if the ESR remains normal and the patient remains asymptomatic at a daily dose of 2.5 mg. Serial ESRs should be performed every 2 to 3 weeks, although following the patient's symptoms closely is more important than simply following laboratory values. For recurrences, 15 mg of prednisolone is restarted and gradually tapered. NSAIDs might help relieve symptoms but do not protect against vasculitis.

KEY TREATMENT

- Prednisone is the treatment of choice in PMR (SOR: C).

Other Vasculitic Conditions

See eAppendix 32-3 online for discussions on:

- Takayasu arteritis
- Polyarteritis nodosa
- Churg-Strauss syndrome
- Wegener granulomatosis
- Cryoglobulinemia
- Hypersensitivity vasculitis
- Behçet disease

Inflammatory Myopathies

This heterogeneous group of diseases causes inflammation of skeletal muscle, increases in levels of enzymes derived from muscle, and proximal muscle weakness or myopathy. The two most common myopathies are dermatomyositis and polymyositis. Inflammatory myopathies are classified by patient age at onset or by coexisting diseases, such as myositis associated with neoplasia or myositis associated with collagen vascular diseases (e.g., systemic scleroderma, SLE, SS). They have a bimodal distribution and are seen most often between age 10 to 15 and 45 to 60 years. Myositis is most common after age 50 years. The cause of inflammatory myopathies is unknown, but evidence suggests a genetic predisposition (associated with certain HLA markers) combined with an environmental insult, such as viruses, thereby initiating an autoimmune process.

Patients usually experience progressive, symmetric, proximal muscle weakness with fatigue, malaise, and morning stiffness. Muscles often affected are those of the shoulder, neck, and pelvic girdle. Pulmonary (interstitial pneumonitis or fibrosis), cardiac (cardiomyopathy, congestive heart failure, arrhythmias), pharyngeal (dysphagia), and musculoskeletal (myalgias, arthralgias) symptoms might occur, although most patients do not experience synovitis. CK as well as ALT, AST, and lactate dehydrogenase (LDH) levels might be elevated, although ESR is elevated only half the time. Muscle biopsy can also be helpful in diagnosis. *Dermatomyositis* is characterized by all of these manifestations plus a scaly, erythematous, or violaceous rash on the face and neck, upper back (shawl sign), and upper anterior chest and neck (V sign). Other signs include dystrophic cuticles, mechanic's hands (darkened or dirty-appearing horizontal lines across palmar aspect of fingers), and Gottron's papules seen on dorsal aspects of the PIP, DIP, or MCP joints, elbows, patellae, and medial malleoli (Olsen and Wortmann, 2004). Disease in patients with skin changes but without muscle inflammation is termed *amyopathic dermatomyositis.*

Inflammatory myopathies can result from malignancies. Screening for malignancies common for the patient's gender and age should be undertaken, but further exploration is not indicated. However, ovarian cancer appears to be associated with dermatomyositis, so the family physician should consider evaluation for this.

Before treatment, a thorough motor neurologic examination is done, with muscle enzyme levels (CK, aldolase, ALT, AST, LDH) and cancer screening tests appropriate for patient age and gender. Prednisone, 1 mg/kg/day for up to several months, is the drug of choice; the earlier it is started in the disease process, the more effective it normally is. If prednisone is not sufficient, methotrexate, azathioprine, or another immunosuppressant is added.

Systemic Sclerosis

Key Points

- CREST syndrome and diffuse cutaneous systemic sclerosis are the primary manifestations of systemic sclerosis.
- The female : male predominance is 8 : 1 for sclerosis.
- The major ACR criterion for systemic sclerosis is skin thickening proximal to the MCP and MTP joints.

"Scleroderma," or hardening of the skin, is now recognized to be a disorder involving almost every organ system in the body and is therefore more appropriately referred to as *systemic sclerosis.* Systemic sclerosis is characterized by a progressive fibrosis of the skin, blood vessels, lungs, kidneys, heart, and GI tract. The degree of skin involvement (diffuse or limited) is useful for prognosis. *Diffuse cutaneous systemic sclerosis* (DCSS) involves almost the entire body, including the trunk, face, neck, and extremities. Cardiopulmonary disease is the leading cause of death in DCSS. Limited cutaneous systemic sclerosis has a more benign course and involves the face, neck, and distal extremities below the knee and elbow. CREST syndrome (calcinosis, Raynaud phenomenon, esophageal dysmotility, sclerodactyly, and telangiectasias) is one of the limited forms of systemic sclerosis, characterized by cutaneous thickening of the distal limbs only. Skin biopsy showing subcutaneous fibrosis is helpful if the diagnosis is in doubt.

Systemic sclerosis affects women up to eight times more often than men; the peak incidence is in the 40s and 50s. There is no significant familial connection, but systemic sclerosis patients typically have a family history of autoimmune disease. Many chemicals and toxins have been implicated, most clearly silica exposure in coal miners.

The major ACR classification criterion for systemic sclerosis is skin thickening proximal to the MCP or MTP joints. The three minor ACR criteria are involvement distal to the MCP joints (sclerodactyly), fingertip-pitting scars or loss of subcutaneous tissue, and chronic pulmonary interstitial changes. Patients with the major criterion or two of the three minor criteria are considered to have systemic sclerosis; however, many patients with clear-cut systemic sclerosis do not meet these criteria because their disease might be early or undifferentiated or in an overlap category with other connective tissue diseases. Ninety-five percent of patients have a positive ANA test result, most often nucleolar staining. Various serologic tests, including anti-RNA polymerase, anticentromere antibody, and antifibrillarin, can provide prognostic information.

The vast majority (>90%) of patients with systemic sclerosis have *Raynaud phenomenon,* which is the initial complaint in most patients, although some might complain first of puffy hands and fingers and of arthralgias. Patients with Raynaud phenomenon experience cold hands and feet, usually triggered by cold temperature or emotional stress. Vasospasm of the digital arteries and arterioles causes skin pallor followed by cyanosis. With rewarming, the digits have a hyperemic or red color, thus completing this white, blue, and red phenomenon.

Scleroderma's skin changes result from inflammation and subsequent collagen deposition. The skin feels (and is) thickened, with decreased flexibility. As the skin becomes more fibrotic and thickened, it becomes very dry, causing pruritus. Late-stage skin changes include atrophy. Arthralgias and myalgias progress to muscle atrophy and weakness.

Patients with scleroderma can develop two different pulmonary diseases: pulmonary hypertension and pulmonary fibrosis. Pulmonary hypertension (which can occur independently of fibrosis) is associated with a poor prognosis. GI symptoms include dysphagia with heartburn, dry mucosal membranes, esophageal reflux, and dysmotility. Cardiac manifestations are usually late and caused by coronary vasospasm, myocardial fibrosis, and pericardial effusions.

Scleroderma renal crisis is characterized by accelerated hypertension, rapidly progressive renal failure, or both (Steen, 1994). Depression is present in more than 50% of patients with systemic sclerosis and is often amenable to antidepressants. Thyroid fibrosis might lead to hypothyroidism; sicca syndrome can be treated with artificial tears and good dental care.

Treatment. Treatment for systemic sclerosis is difficult. Penicillamine, immunosuppressive drugs, and other agents have been used to treat scleroderma, but none has yielded dramatic results. Localized sclerosis can soften with ultraviolet-A (UVA) light therapy, with dramatic improvement in symptoms seen in two small non-RCTs (Kreuter et al., 2004; Stege et al., 1997). Other options include high-dose topical corticosteroids and methotrexate. Treatments for calcinosis, including probenecid, colchicine, and warfarin, have not shown improvement. A five-patient study showed that the calcium channel blocker (CCB) diltiazem caused significant regression in calcinosis and clinical improvement (Palmieri et al., 1995); more studies are needed. Raynaud phenomenon is treated by cold avoidance for the entire body (not only hands), tobacco avoidance, and biofeedback or other stress reduction techniques; pharmacologic therapy includes CCBs, topical nitroglycerin, and prazosin (Pope et al., 2000). A meta-analysis concluded that CCBs are efficacious for reduction in frequency and severity of attacks (Thompson et al., 2005). Skin care consists of avoiding excessive bathing and using moisturizers.

The NSAIDs are used first for musculoskeletal symptoms of systemic sclerosis, but low-dose corticosteroids or narcotic analgesics might be needed. No studies have been performed, but in general, acid-reducing medications such as PPIs or H_2 blockers are used to prevent the development of possible esophageal strictures, given the high rates of esophageal dysmotility in the systemic sclerosis. Delayed small intestinal tract transit time may lead to bacterial overgrowth, causing GI symptoms; antibiotics might be effective. Angiotensin-converting enzyme inhibitors are useful in the treatment of renal crisis manifested by hypertension and renal failure.

For scleroderma-like disorders, see eAppendix 32-4 online.

KEY TREATMENT

- Systemic sclerosis is difficult to treat. UVA therapy is the most effective treatment for localized skin sclerosis (Kreuter et al., 2004; Stege et al., 1997) (SOR: B).
- Pharmacologic therapy with calcium channel blockers is effective at decreasing the frequency and severity of Raynaud's phenomenon (Thompson et al., 2005) (SOR: B).

Diffuse Fasciitis with Eosinophilia

See eAppendix 32-5 online.

FIBROMYALGIA SYNDROME

> ### Key Points
>
> - Fibromyalgia syndrome (FMS) accounts for 20% of visits to rheumatologists.
> - The diagnosis is confirmed by 3 months of widespread pain with associated fatigue, cognitive dysfunction, and unrestful sleep.
> - The female : male predominance is 9 : 1 for FMS.

Fibromyalgia syndrome is one of the most common rheumatic diseases, affecting up to 20% of patients seen in rheumatology practices (Keefe and Caldwell, 1997). The diagnosis of FM was modified in 2010 from counting trigger points to the evaluation of widespread pain persisting for 3 months. Pain is considered widespread when it affects all four quadrants of the body, meaning it must be felt on both the left and right sides of the body as well as above and below the waist. The traditional areas of discomfort can be seen in Figure 32-15. The widespread pain along with associated symptoms, including fatigue, awaking unrefreshed, and difficulty with cognition, help make the diagnosis (Wolfe et al., 2010).

The diagnostic criteria require a subjective assessment by the clinician. The most important ingredient is widespread pain for three months. To solidify the diagnosis, then ask, "Are you having problems with fatigue? Waking up tired? Thinking or remembering things?" Then the clinician should follow up with more detailed inquiries about other somatic conditions such as irritable bowel syndrome, headache, dry mouth, or bladder spasms. Three months of pain accompanied by these other symptoms suggest the diagnosis.

Psychological factors and comorbid conditions might aggravate symptoms. FMS is more common than RA and causes a comparable degree of disability and loss of family income. About 90% of FMS patients are women, and there

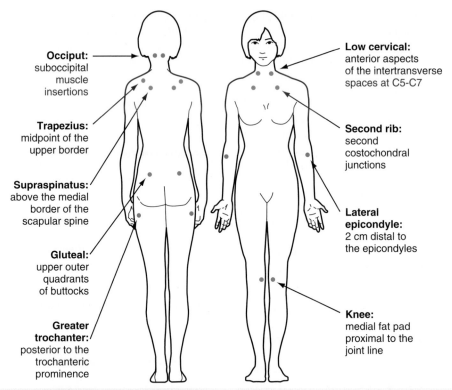

Occiput: suboccipital muscle insertions

Trapezius: midpoint of the upper border

Supraspinatus: above the medial border of the scapular spine

Gluteal: upper outer quadrants of buttocks

Greater trochanter: posterior to the trochanteric prominence

Low cervical: anterior aspects of the intertransverse spaces at C5-C7

Second rib: second costochondral junctions

Lateral epicondyle: 2 cm distal to the epicondyles

Knee: medial fat pad proximal to the joint line

Figure 32-15 Location of the specific tender points in fibromyalgia. (From Freundlich B, Leventhal L. Diffuse pain syndromes. In Klippel JH, ed. *Primer on the rheumatic diseases.* 11th ed. Atlanta: Arthritis Foundation; 1997:123-127.)

is evidence of familial aggregation. Fibromyalgia might also be present in patients with autoimmune disorders such as SLE, RA, and AS, and should be suspected when symptoms are unresponsive to antiinflammatory therapies.

Fibromyalgia syndrome is probably caused by central pain mechanism dysfunction, possibly in neurotransmitters. Several studies have found that FMS patients have up to three times higher levels of substance P in CSF than normal control participants (Russell et al., 1994). FMS can be initially triggered by trauma or peripheral inflammatory arthritis, but peripheral, ongoing inflammation is not present in this syndrome. Important secondary factors contributing to the patient's pain include nonrestorative sleep, muscle deconditioning secondary to pain, and psychological factors. Pain is most common in the neck, back, shoulders, pelvic girdle areas, and hands. Paresthesias in the extremities are also common, as are tension-type headaches, irritable bowel syndrome, primary dysmenorrhea, chronic fatigue syndrome, restless legs syndrome, temporomandibular joint (TMJ) dysfunction, and regional fibromyalgia (myofascial pain syndrome). Although some patients with FMS have depression, most do not. Physical examination reveals tenderness with moderate pressure in the traditional defined points seen in Figure 32-15. Care must be taken on examination not to palpate too softly or too firmly. The proper amount of palpation pressure is about the amount of pressure required to blanch the nail of the examining finger when it is pressed against the patient's forehead (Yunus, 1996).

No laboratory tests are available to diagnose FMS. CBC results; tests for ESR, muscle enzyme, electrolyte, and ANA levels; and radiography are all normal in the absence of comorbid disease. Sleep electroencephalograms are often

abnormal and should be considered if a history of particular sleep disturbances is suspected (see eTable 32-5 online). Because FMS is often seen in association with other rheumatic diseases, the diagnosis is often missed because FMS symptoms might be mistaken for the comorbid disease. Conversely, patients presenting with FMS should be evaluated for an underlying condition.

The cause of fibromyalgia is unknown. Muscle biopsies reveal no apparent abnormalities. There is great overlap with chronic fatigue syndrome, but there is no evidence that an infection such as chronic Epstein-Barr virus (EBV) is associated with fibromyalgia. About 80% of fibromyalgia patients have sleep disturbances, particularly disrupted non–rapid eye movement (non-REM) sleep (stages 3 and 4, which is deep, restorative sleep). Non-REM sleep deprivation studies have reproduced the signs and symptoms of FMS, which make the sleep disturbance possibly an integral part on the pathogenesis and continuation of fibromyalgia. Patients with RA and other rheumatic diseases have disrupted sleep with nocturnal awakening and arousals to a lighter stage of sleep throughout the night. Sleep studies reveal that patients often cannot recall these episodes on awakening the next day but do feel fatigued or describe themselves as light sleepers.

Treatment

It is important to educate patients with FMS and to reassure them that FMS is a common disease, that it is not psychiatric, and that there are treatments available.

Tricyclic antidepressants (TCAs), selective serotonin reuptake inhibitors (SSRIs), and serotonin-norepinephrine reuptake inhibitors (SNRIs) help relieve pain associated with fibromyalgia. A meta-analysis (18 RCTs with a variety of antidepressants) concluded there was strong evidence of efficacy for antidepressants for relief of pain, fatigue, mood, sleep disturbance, and health-related quality of life (Hauser et al., 2009). The effect size for pain reduction was large for TCAs and small for the SSRIs and SNRIs, although newer studies of SNRIs were not included. Studies of the SNRIs milnacipran (Savella) and duloxetine (Cymbalta) have shown significant reductions in pain, and both have been FDA approved for the treatment of fibromyalgia. Amitriptyline doses are typically 25 to 50 mg at night, much lower than the doses used for the treatment of depression. The addition of amitriptyline to SSRIs or SNRIs showed a trend toward improvement versus medication alone, but results were not statistically significant (Goldenberg et al., 1996).

Cyclobenzaprine has a chemical structure similar to TCAs, and various dosing regimens have been studied in the treatment of fibromyalgia. A meta-analysis found that pain was significantly decreased in patients receiving cyclobenzaprine over placebo at 4 weeks but not statistically significant at 8 or 12 weeks. Overall, patients treated with cyclobenzaprine were three times more likely to report subjective improvement, and five patients would need to be treated for one patient to experience symptom improvement (Tofferi et al., 2004).

Pregabalin (Lyrica), a second-generation anticonvulsant, was the first medication to be FDA approved for the treatment of fibromyalgia. As with gabapentin, pregabalin has effects on cellular calcium channels and may exert its analgesic effects by blocking various neurotransmitters. Multiple large studies have shown its efficacy for the treatment of pain, fatigue, and improvement in sleep (Mease et al., 2008). Gabapentin has not been FDA approved for this use but is efficacious for reducing pain in fibromyalgia (Arnold et al., 2007).

The NSAIDs and corticosteroids are usually not helpful because no evidence indicates FMS is an inflammatory disease, and NSAIDs are no better than placebo in the treatment of pain. Combination analgesic therapy with acetaminophen and tramadol was found to decrease pain significantly in these patients (Bennett et al., 2003). However, the long-term use of tramadol needs to be carefully considered, and this approach is best used after other therapies (e.g., antidepressants) have failed.

At least two thirds of FMS patients use some type of complementary method, such as herbal supplements or acupuncture. A meta-analysis of acupuncture suggested benefit, but study quality was generally poor (Berman et al., 1999). Local anesthesia injected into tender points can sometimes relieve pain, and topical capsaicin (Zostrix) cream has helped some patients. Treatment of underlying depression is also important.

Daily exercise programs, particularly aerobic exercise, and physical therapy might also help FMS patients; it is important that exercise regimens begin at a low intensity and build up slowly. A review of controlled trials for aerobic exercise for fibromyalgia found beneficial effects in overall global function, physical function, and possibly in reduction of pain and tender points (Busch et al., 2008).

Cognitive-behavioral treatment (CBT) is promising for FMS patients, although there have been few controlled studies. There might be even more benefit if CBT is combined with physical exercise. Patients are often resistant to starting exercise programs such as walking or bicycling because they fear exacerbation of pain. CBT programs can overcome negative self-statements that prevent the initiation of exercise or limit the amount of exercise that can be done. An emphatic ongoing relationship with a caring physician is particularly important treatment for patients with FMS. Although musculoskeletal rehabilitation has no effect by itself, physical therapy can help subacute low back pain and other comorbidities. Subacute aerobic exercise is also effective in decreasing symptoms but might need to begin at very low levels (Busch et al., 2002; Busch et al., 2008).

KEY TREATMENT

- Aerobic exercise programs have positive effects for overall global function, physical function, and pain (Busch et al., 2008) (SOR: A).
- Antidepressant therapy is effective for fibromyalgia patients; TCAs show the greatest improvements (Hauser et al., 2009) (SOR: A).
- Pregabalin improves pain, fatigue, and sleep in patients with fibromyalgia (Arnold et al., 2007; Mease et al., 2008) (SOR: A).
- Acetaminophen and tramadol significantly reduce pain associated with fibromyalgia (Bennett et al., 2003) (SOR: B), but prolonged use of tramadol should be considered only after inadequate response to antidepressant therapy (SOR: C).

TEMPOROMANDIBULAR JOINT SYNDROME

See eAppendix 32-6 online.

Rheumatic Disease in Children

JUVENILE RHEUMATOID ARTHRITIS

Juvenile rheumatoid arthritis, formerly known as Still disease, is a heterogeneous group of diseases clinically distinct from adult RA. Although much less common than RA, JRA is four times more common than sickle cell anemia or cystic fibrosis and 10 times more common than other pediatric diseases, such as hemophilia, muscular dystrophy, acute lymphocytic leukemia, and chronic renal failure (Gortmaker, 1984). Fortunately, most children with JRA have long remissions without loss of function or significant residual deformity.

There are no specific laboratory tests to diagnose JRA. Other causes for arthritis must be excluded, including reactive arthritis from extraarticular infection, septic arthritis, neoplastic disorders, endocrine disorders (thyroid disease, type 1 diabetes mellitus), degenerative or mechanical disorders, and idiopathic pediatric joint pain. The diagnosis of JRA requires true arthritis (signs of inflammation rather than simply arthralgias) persisting for more than 6 weeks, with onset at or before age 16 years.

The three major subtypes of JRA are pauciarticular (40%-50%), polyarticular (30%), and systemic (5%-10%), all with different clinical presentations and courses; their differentiation determines treatment. *Pauciarticular* JRA involves four or fewer joints, usually large joints asymmetrically. Early-onset pauciarticular JRA affects mostly girls younger than 4 years and has a 30% risk of chronic iridocyclitis and a 10% risk of ocular damage. Late-onset pauciarticular JRA affects mostly boys older than 8 years, many of whom later develop spondyloarthropathies; 10% develop iridocyclitis. Slit-lamp ophthalmic examinations are recommended. *Polyarticular* JRA is defined as arthritis in five or more joints; patients are RF positive or negative. RF-positive patients usually are girls age 8 years or older, have symmetric small-joint arthritis, and have a worse functional prognosis than RF-negative patients. *Systemic-onset* JRA is characterized by high intermittent fevers (>38.8° C; 102° F), rash, hepatosplenomegaly, lymphadenopathy, arthralgias, pericarditis, pleuritis, and growth delay. Anemia, leukocytosis, and thrombocytosis are common laboratory findings. Extraarticular symptoms are usually mild and self-limited. Boys and girls are equally affected. The severity of the arthritis is a harbinger of prognosis.

The NSAIDs are the first-line treatment for JRA, but patience is necessary because clinical improvement might not be seen for up to 1 month. Approximately two thirds of patients need another agent in addition to NSAIDs; methotrexate is often used, particularly for systemic and polyarticular JRA. Corticosteroids are used orally for severe, life-threatening, systemic JRA and intraarticularly for pauciarticular JRA. Eye inflammation is best treated by an ophthalmologist.

Juvenile RA is an excellent example of a disease that significantly affects the entire family. JRA can actually have a greater negative psychological impact on siblings than on the patient (White and Shear, 1992). Most children with JRA require extensive physical as well as psychological support. Encourage families to receive support from social programs and JRA advocacy and support groups. The consulting rheumatologist and physical and occupational therapists are vital, but patients and families also benefit greatly from a continuous, supportive relationship with the family physician. Physical and occupational therapy are important because children often stop using painful joints, adding to disability.

SPONDYLOARTHROPATHIES

Four spondyloarthropathies are seen in children: juvenile AS, psoriatic arthritis, Reiter syndrome (reactive arthritis), and IBD-associated arthritis. Definitive diagnoses of these conditions are often delayed. Patients with JAS must have their lumbar spine motion monitored. Plain radiographs often do not show the changes characteristic of adult AS. NSAIDs are used for treatment. Significant arthritis can be seen in 7% to 20% of IBD patients.

SYSTEMIC LUPUS ERYTHEMATOUS IN CHILDHOOD

Systemic lupus erythematosus primarily affects adolescent girls, many of whom do not have the typical malar rash. The small joints of the hands or feet and the kidneys are typically affected; the patient should be monitored for proteinuria and hematuria. Because of steroid side effects, immunosuppressant drugs are often used for severe cases.

HENOCH-SCHÖNLEIN PURPURA

Henoch-Schönlein purpura is a small-vessel vasculitis seen mostly in children. Immune complexes are deposited, causing petechiae, nephropathy, or renal disease (40%) and GI bleeding. The purpura is usually in dependent areas such as the buttocks and lower extremities. Affected children often present with abdominal pain after an upper respiratory infection. Symptoms typically resolve spontaneously without treatment within 2 weeks, but serious GI and renal involvement can occur, requiring steroids. NSAIDs might be helpful for arthralgias.

KAWASAKI SYNDROME

Kawasaki syndrome (KS), also known as Kawasaki's disease, is the leading cause of acquired heart disease in children. Prolonged high fever (up to 40° C [104° F]), with an urticaria-like rash and injection of mucous membranes, including a strawberry tongue, is followed by erythema of the palms and soles and desquamation of the fingertips. Most patients have cervical lymphadenopathy. A myocarditis is present in more than 50% of patients and is manifested by a tachycardia. Many other symptoms might also occur, such as respiratory, neurologic, and GI symptoms (Table 32-11). Because KS symptoms resolve spontaneously, cardiac manifestations might not be diagnosed. A coronary arteritis and even aneurysms might develop, with significant morbidity and mortality. Laboratory studies are not helpful. Serial electrocardiograms are recommended at diagnosis, 2 to 3 weeks into the illness, and 1 month after that.

Although KS's seasonal variation (winter and spring) and epidemics suggest an infectious cause, none has yet been identified. IV fluids, aspirin, and IVIG have been used most frequently for KS. Antibiotics are of no use unless there is a concomitant bacterial infection. Steroids might actually increase the incidence of aneurysms and should be avoided, if possible.

Table 32-11 Diagnostic Guidelines for Kawasaki Syndrome*

Fever lasting >5 days *plus* four of the following five criteria:

1. Polymorphous rash
2. Bilateral conjunctival infection
3. One or more of the following mucous membrane changes:
   • Diffuse infection of oral and pharyngeal mucosa
   • Erythema or fissuring of the lips
   • Strawberry tongue
4. Acute, nonpurulent cervical lymphadenopathy (one lymph node must be >1.5 cm)
5. One or more of the following extremity changes:
   • Erythema of palms, soles, or both
   • Indurative edema of hands, feet, or both
   • Membranous desquamation of the fingertips

Other illnesses with similar clinical signs must be excluded.

*Based on the Centers for Disease Control and Prevention case definition. From Freundlich B, Leventhal L. Diffuse pain syndromes. In Klippel JH, ed. *Primer on the rheumatic diseases.* 12th ed. Atlanta: Arthritis Foundation; 2001:409.

NONARTICULAR RHEUMATISM

Any pain and stiffness without true inflammation in the joint and with normal laboratory results in children is termed *nonarticular rheumatism,* or "growing pains." These usually occur at night, last several hours, and often resolve spontaneously or are helped by massage or analgesics. Pain is sometimes felt behind the knees. No further evaluation is indicated unless pain occurs during the day. Overuse or hypermobile joints are two possible explanations; nonarticular rheumatism does not normally cause any reduction in activity.

Rheumatology Information on the Internet

A great deal of information on rheumatic diseases for both physicians and patients can be found on the Internet. This can be a valuable tool for family physicians in this era of active research and new treatment modalities in rheumatology. Patients might receive online support from numerous advocacy and support groups for these conditions, although the Internet can also be a source of misinformation, with charlatans touting arthritis cures. Websites of the ACR, Arthritis Foundation, and Medline Plus are particularly good sources of information (see Web Resources).

Summary of Additional Online Content

The following content is available at www.expertconsult.com.

eTable 32-1 Functional Assessment Screen

eTable 32-2 Classification Criteria for Osteoarthritis of the Hand, Traditional Format

eTable 32-3 Classification Criteria for Osteoarthritis of the Hip, Traditional Format

eTable 32-4 Monitoring Rheumatoid Arthritis Activity

eAppendix 32-1, Viral Arthritis

eAppendix 32-2, Prevention of Lyme Disease

eAppendix 32-3, Other Vasculitic Conditions

eAppendix 32-4 Scleroderma-Like Disorders

eAppendix 32-5 Diffuse Fasciitis with Eosinophilia

eTable 32-5 Conditions Associated with Sleep Disturbance and Fibromyalgia

eAppendix 32-6 Temporomandibular Joint Syndrome

References

The complete reference list is available at www.expertconsult.com.

Web Resources

General Reference

www.arthritis.org Arthritis Foundation. Excellent site, primarily for patients.

www.curearthritis.org Arthritis National Research Foundation. Information on financial support for research.

www.nih.gov/niams National Institute of Arthritis and Musculoskeletal and Skin Diseases (NIAMS) and National Institutes of Health (NIH), which conducts research in these areas.

www.nlm.nih.gov/medlineplus/arthritis.html Medline Plus.

www.rheumatology.org American College of Rheumatology. Internet resources, academic and government sites, foundations, and associations.

Disease-Specific Sites

http://www.rheumatology.org/practice/clinical/classification/fibromyalgia/fibro_2010.asp The American College of Rheumatology 2010 Fibromyalgia Diagnostic Criteria.

www.aarda.org American Autoimmune Related Diseases Association. Patient education.

www.aldf.com American Lyme Disease Foundation.

www.lupus.org Lupus Foundation. Patient advocacy, patient information, and local chapters.

www.myositis.org Myositis Association of America. Polymyositis, dermatomyositis.

www.rheumatology.org/Practice/Clinical/Patients/Diseases_And_Conditions/Fibromyalgia/ American College of Rheumatology. Fibromyalgia.

www.risg.org Reiter's Information and Support Group. Patient education.

www.sjogrens.org Sjögren's Syndrome Foundation.

www.spondylitis.org Spondylitis Association of America. Patient education on ankylosing spondylosis, psoriatic arthritis, and other types of spondylitis.

33 *Dermatology*

RICHARD P. USATINE and JENNIFER KREJCI-MANWARING

Principles of Diagnosis

Dermatologic diagnoses often begin with *pattern recognition.* Experts can look at most lesions and make an immediate and accurate diagnosis through pattern recognition. The basic terms used to describe lesion morphology and patterns provide the vocabulary to describe what is seen. The physician then combines keen observation of the lesions (including type and distribution) with a careful history to create an informed differential diagnosis. If the diagnosis is still not known, the physician can consult a dermatology atlas (online or print), textbook, or expert to complete the diagnosis. In some cases, further testing (scraping, culture, biopsy) may be needed.

INITIAL EVALUATION

Although medical school teaches students to perform the history before doing the physical examination, this is not the most efficient way to approach the diagnosis of a skin condition. When the patient has a skin complaint, immediately look at the skin while asking your questions. Look carefully at the lesions and determine the lesion morphology. Table 33-1 provides definitions for the terms used to describe primary and secondary morphology. A magnifying glass and good lighting help to distinguish the morphology of many skin conditions. Next, touch the lesions, with gloves when appropriate. For some lesions, such as actinic keratosis (AK) with scaling or the sandpaper rash of scarlet fever, lightly feeling the skin provides much information. For deeper lesions, such as nodules and cysts, deep palpation is needed. Observe the distribution of the lesions. Try to determine if the primary lesions are arranged in groups, rings, lines, or merely scattered over the skin.

Determine which parts of the skin are affected and which are spared. Be sure to look at the remainder of the skin, nails, hair, and mucous membranes. Patients often show only one small area and appear reluctant to expose the rest of their skin, especially their feet. With many skin conditions, it is essential to look beyond the most affected area because other areas may provide important clues (e.g., nail pitting when considering psoriasis). Patients may have lesions on their back or feet that they have not observed. For example, a patient may have a papular eruption on the hands or arms that represents an autosensitization reaction *(id reaction)* to a fungal infection on the feet; not looking for the fungus on the feet will lead to a missed diagnosis (Figures 33-1 and 33-2). Some skin diseases have manifestations in the mouth; finding white patches on the buccal mucosa may lead to the correct diagnosis of lichen planus (Figure 33-3).

When the physician starts to look at the skin, the patient history will be more focused, directed toward finding the correct diagnosis. The following information assists in making a dermatologic diagnosis and planning treatment:

- Onset and duration of skin lesions: continuous or intermittent?
- Pattern of eruption: Where did it start? How has it changed?
- Any known precipitants, such as exposure to medication (prescription, over the counter [OTC]), foods, plants, sun, topical agents, chemicals (occupation, hobbies)?
- Skin symptoms: itching, pain, paresthesia
- Systemic symptoms: fever, chills, night sweats, fatigue, weakness, weight loss
- Underlying illnesses: diabetes, thyroid disease, human immunodeficiency virus (HIV)
- Family history: acne, atopic dermatitis (AD), psoriasis, skin cancers, dysplastic nevi

The most important in-office examinations of the skin are the following:

Microscopy. To diagnose a fungal infection, scrape some of the scale onto a microscope slide, add 10% potassium hydroxide (KOH) (best with dimethyl sulfoxide [DMSO] and fungal stain), and look for the hyphae of dermatophytes or the pseudohyphae of *Candida* or *Pityrosporum* species.

Wood's light examination. This is helpful in diagnosing tinea capitis and erythrasma. Tinea capitis caused by *Microsporum* spp. produces green fluorescence, but *Trichophyton* spp. do not fluoresce. Erythrasma has a coral-red fluorescence. A Wood's lamp also helps distinguish lesions of vitiligo in patients with fair skin.

Table 33-1 Primary and Secondary Skin Lesions

Lesions	Description
PRIMARY (BASIC) LESIONS	
Macule	Circumscribed flat discoloration (≤5 mm)
Patch	Flat nonpalpable discoloration (>5 mm)
Papule	Elevated solid lesion (≤5 mm)
Plaque	Elevated solid lesion (>5 mm) (often a confluence of papules)
Nodule	Palpable solid (round) lesion, deeper than a papule
Wheal (hive)	Pink edematous plaque (round or flat), topped and transient
Pustule	Elevated collection of pus
Vesicle	Circumscribed elevated collection of fluid (≤5 mm in diameter)
Bulla	Circumscribed elevated collection of fluid (>5 mm in diameter)
SECONDARY (SEQUENTIAL) LESIONS	
Scale (desquamation)	Excess dead epidermal cells
Crusts	Collection of dried serum, blood, or pus
Erosion	Superficial loss of epidermis
Ulcer	Focal loss of epidermis and dermis
Fissure	Linear loss of epidermis and dermis
Atrophy	Depression in skin from thinning of epidermis or dermis
Excoriation	Erosion caused by scratching
Lichenification	Thickened epidermis with prominent skin lines

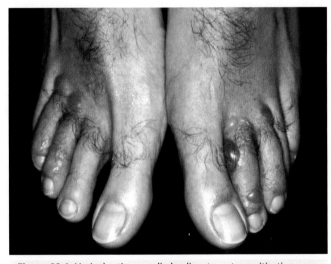

Figure 33-1 Vesicular tinea pedis leading to autosensitization reaction. (© Richard P. Usatine.)

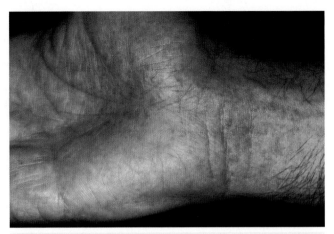

Figure 33-2 Autosensitization reaction secondary to vesicular tinea pedis (id reaction). (© Richard P. Usatine.)

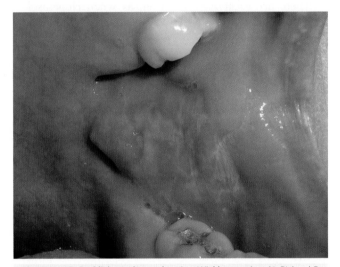

Figure 33-3 Oral lichen planus showing Wickham striae. (© Richard P. Usatine.)

Surgical biopsy. The biopsy can be used as a diagnostic and treatment tool. Having a reasonable differential diagnosis will help the physician choose shave, punch, or elliptic biopsy. Similarly, when submitting your specimen to pathology, always include background information and the differential to aid the pathologist.

General Management

TOPICAL CORTICOSTEROIDS

The choice of a topical steroid involves maximizing benefit and minimizing adverse effects. Many skin conditions benefit greatly from topical steroids. However, local adverse effects of topical steroids are common with regular use over weeks to months. The most common adverse effect of topical steroids is skin *atrophy*, in which the epidermis becomes thin and the superficial capillaries dilate. Epidermal atrophy can be accompanied by hypopigmentation and telangiectasias. If atrophy involves the dermis, striae may occur. Although the epidermal atrophy may be reversible in months, striae are irreversible. When steroids are continuously applied to the face, perioral dermatitis acne or rosacea-like eruptions can occur.

Systemic adverse effects are rare and occur when large amounts of topical steroids are absorbed systemically. The risk of such absorption increases with stronger steroids, thinner skin, younger patients, longer duration of therapy, and the use of occlusion in therapy. Prescribing the minimum strength needed for the shortest duration required helps prevent adverse effects. In choosing the best topical steroid, consider the following factors:

1. **Skin disorder.** As the severity of the disorder increases, the need for higher-potency steroids increases. Also,

Table 33-2 Potency of Topical Corticosteroids

Potency	Generic Drugs	Brand Names
"Superpotent" (class 1)	Clobetasol, betamethasone dipropionate, halobetasol, fluocinonide	Clobex, Diprolene, Olux, Psorcon, Temovate, Ultravate, Vanos
High potency (classes 2 and 3)	Betamethasone dipropionate, mometasone, halcinonide, fluocinonide, desoximetasone, triamcinolone 0.1%, fluticasone, amcinonide	Diprolene, Elocon, Halog, Lidex, Psorcon, Topicort, Aristocort, Cutivate, Cyclocort
Midpotency (classes 4 and 5)	Prednicarbate, mometasone, betamethasone valerate, hydrocortisone probutate, fluocinolone, desoximetasone, hydrocortisone valerate, triamcinolone 0.025%	Dermatop, Elocon, Luxiq, Pandel, Synalar, Topicort, Westcort, Cordran, Cutivate, Locoid
Low potency (classes 6 and 7)	Alclometasone, desonide, fluocinolone, hydrocortisone	Aclovate, DesOwen, Synalar, Hytone, Desonate

thicker lesions (e.g., psoriatic plaques, lichen planus) need higher-potency steroids.

2. **Site.** Use only the weakest-potency steroids on the face, genitals, and intertriginous areas, where skin is thin or moist and skin atrophy and striae occur most rapidly. There are exceptions, however, as when clobetasol is needed to treat certain vulvar disorders such as lichen sclerosis. The skin on the palms and soles is so thick that the most potent steroids are often needed.

3. **Age.** Avoid the use of high-potency topical steroids in infants and children because they have greater surface area per body mass than adults and have greater risk and consequences of systemic absorption.

4. **Steroid potency** (strength and concentration). There are more than 50 types and brands of steroids; family physicians should know at least one steroid from each of four basic strengths (Table 33-2). Generic agents can be used from all the potency groups to save on costs.

5. **Vehicle.** The vehicle is the substance in which the steroid is dispersed. The most common vehicles are ointments, creams, gels, solutions, lotions, and foams. The choice of vehicle is determined by the characteristics of the lesion (dry or moist), the site involved, and patient preference. Furthermore, the vehicle affects the potency of the steroid because it determines the rate at which the steroid is absorbed through the skin.

Most skin preparations can be applied twice a day, conveniently in the morning and evening. Try to estimate and prescribe an appropriate amount; many topical products are supplied in 15-g, 30-g, 60-g, and 80-g sizes; 80 g is about the size of a tube of toothpaste. Based on common practice, it is accepted that 2 g of cream is required to cover the face or one hand, 3 g for an arm, 4 g for a leg, and 12 to 30 g for an entire body. Therefore, if you calculate that out to 1 month's worth of medication, you would need a 30- to 60-g tube for the face but up to 900 g or almost 2 lb for the whole body. To avoid adverse effects of steroid overuse, do not prescribe large quantities for small lesions and specify the duration of use. On the other end of the spectrum, prescribing only 15 g of steroid for a large area of involvement will be frustrating to the patient when the steroid is depleted before completing the prescribed treatment. Generic triamcinolone comes in 1-lb tubs (454 g), which is extremely helpful for patients with inflammatory conditions covering much of the body. It is therefore important to specify the quantity you want on the prescription; otherwise, the pharmacist may choose whatever size is in stock.

The duration of therapy is usually the time required for resolution of symptoms or lesions. To avoid adverse effects, the highest potency steroids should not be used for longer than 2 to 4 weeks continuously. However, these can be used intermittently for chronic conditions such as psoriasis in a pulse-therapy mode (e.g., apply every weekend, with steroid-sparing medication on weekdays). For conditions with dry skin, liberal use of emollients between steroid applications can minimize steroid exposure while maximizing the benefits of therapy.

MANAGEMENT OF PRURITIS

Often, patients present because of the pruritus associated with a skin condition rather than the skin condition itself. Itching associated with visible lesions often responds to relatively nonspecific antipruritic treatments. If the itching is generalized, patients may obtain temporary relief from cool or tepid baths with the addition of colloidal oatmeal (Aveeno). Soap should be avoided. Oral antihistamines can be given every 6 to 8 hours, especially at bedtime to promote sleep. Diphenhydramine (Benadryl) and hydroxyzine (Atarax, Vistaril) are first-generation antihistamines that are relatively safe and effective, although caution should be used in older adult patients. Second-generation antihistamines are similarly effective for reducing pruritus in the daytime and are less sedating for some patients. These include fexofenadine (Allegra), loratadine (Claritin), desloratadine (Clarinex), cetirizine (Zyrtec), and levocetirizine (Xyzal). Usually, second-generation antihistamines are given once daily.

Skin Problems Beginning in Childhood

ATOPIC DERMATITIS (ECZEMA)

Key Points

- AD is a common inherited childhood disorder that may occur with other atopic conditions such as allergic rhinitis and asthma.
- Topical steroids and emollients are the mainstays of treatment for AD.
- Topical and systemic antibiotics are used for AD secondarily infected with bacteria.

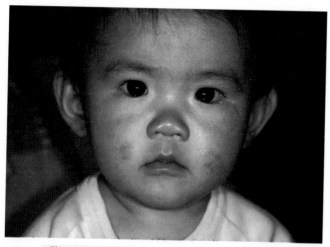

Figure 33-4 Atopic dermatitis. (© Richard P. Usatine.)

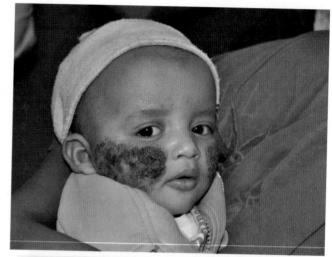

Figure 33-6 Impetiginized atopic dermatitis. (© Richard P. Usatine.)

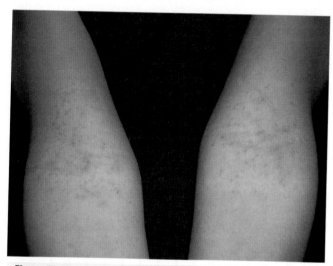

Figure 33-5 Atopic dermatitis in the antecubital fossa. (© Richard P. Usatine.)

age. When required for rare severe cases, oral corticosteroids can be used.

Always look for signs of bacterial superinfection, such as weeping of fluid and crusts (Figure 33-6). Superinfection with *Staphylococcus aureus* may lead to worsening of AD because the bacteria functions as a super antigen. *S. aureus* superinfections are usually sensitive to methicillin, so oral cephalexin is frequently a good choice for treatment. Bleach baths are helpful to cut down on colonization. (Add ¼-½ cup regular bleach per full tub of lukewarm water and soak for 5 to 10 minutes before washing off the bleach water.) Apply emollients or topical medications (or both) immediately after the bath.

KEY TREATMENT

- Topical steroids and emollients are the mainstay of treatment for AD (Hanifin et al., 2004) (SOR: A).
- Topical and systemic antibiotics are used for AD with secondary bacterial infection; weeping fluid and crusting during an exacerbation should prompt consideration of antibiotic use (Hanifin et al., 2004) (SOR: A).
- Topical calcineurin inhibitors (immunomodulators such as pimecrolimus and tacrolimus) reduce the rash severity and symptoms of AD in children and adults (Hanifin et al., 2004) (SOR: A).
- Dietary restriction is useful only for infants with proven egg and cow's milk protein allergies (Hanifin et al., 2004; Lifschitz & Szajewska, 2014) (SOR: B).
- The value of antihistamines in AD is controversial; if used, the sedating agents are most effective and can be given at night (Hanifin et al., 2004) (SOR: B).

Atopic dermatitis is a potentially debilitating condition that can compromise quality of life. Its most frequent symptom is pruritus. Pruritus leads to scratching, resulting in secondary skin changes such as excoriation, crusting, and lichenification. Consequently, AD has been referred to as "the itch that rashes."

Atopic dermatitis is a common problem affecting up to 15% of all children. In most cases, AD occurs before 5 years of age, frequently on the face or extensor surfaces in the first year of life (Figure 33-4). As children grow, the antecubital and popliteal fossae (flexural surfaces) are often involved (Figure 33-5). The disease may occur intermittently between periods of complete remission. By adulthood, the incidence becomes less than 1%. Treatment should be directed at limiting itching, repairing the skin, and decreasing inflammation. Lubricants and topical corticosteroids are the mainstays of therapy. Topical pimecrolimus and tacrolimus are considered steroid-sparing agents and are effective for short-term use or in cases unresponsive to topical corticosteroids. These agents are only approved for second-line treatment in patients older than 2 years of

PITYRIASIS ALBA

Pityriasis alba is a common hypopigmented dermatitis that may affect nearly one third of school-age children in the United States. The condition is more common in patients with a history of AD. Patients present with numerous hypopigmented macules ranging from 1 to 4 cm in size on the face, neck, and shoulders (Figure 33-7). The macules

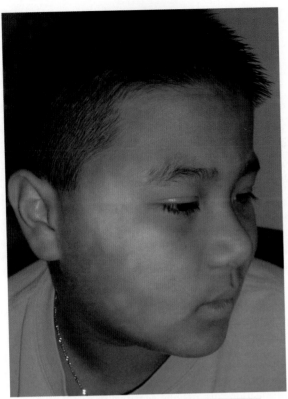

Figure 33-7 Pityriasis alba. (© Richard P. Usatine.)

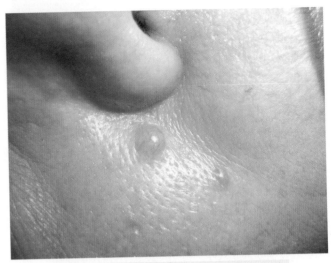

Figure 33-8 Intradermal nevi. (© Richard P. Usatine.)

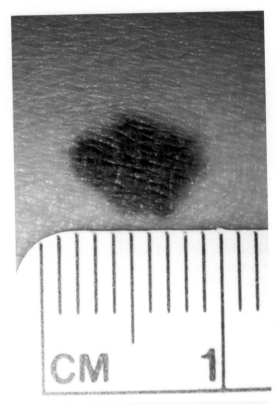

Figure 33-9 Compound nevus. (© Richard P. Usatine.)

are poorly defined and may have fine scales. Occasionally, erythema and pruritus occur before the lesions. Sun exposure can cause more contrast of the lesions as the surrounding normal skin tans. Generally, pityriasis alba is self-limited and asymptomatic, so therapy is typically unnecessary. Lesions usually fade by adulthood. Topical steroids, emollients, and phototherapy have limited efficacy. Hydrocortisone 1% cream or ointment may provide some benefit, and if used for no more than 2 weeks, the patients should be relatively safe from adverse effects.

KERATOSIS PILARIS

Keratosis pilaris is very common and presents as tiny (<1 mm) keratotic follicular papules found on extensor arms and thighs and occasionally the cheeks. The numerous papules give the skin a rough feeling. Often there is a ring of erythema around the follicle. The incidence of keratosis pilaris is increased in patients with AD. Treatment consists of emollients combined with keratolytic agents; common preparations are 5% or 12% ammonium lactate (AmLactin, Laclotion, Lac-Hydrin) and urea-based creams or lotions. Microdermabrasion has also been used to treat keratosis pilaris. Patient education should stress that keratosis pilaris is genetic and cannot be cured. Any smoothing with topical or mechanical agents is temporary and will return if the treatment is stopped.

MELANOCYTIC NEVI

Nevi (moles) are benign lesions composed of collections of nevus cells of neuroectodermal origin. They appear in childhood, tend to increase in number throughout the adult years, and then resolve with age. *Pigmented* nevi can be flat, raised, or pedunculated and have impressive variations in size, color, and surface characteristics. Histologically, *junctional* nevi are located in the epidermis, *intradermal* nevi in the dermis, and *compound* nevi in the epidermis and dermis. Junctional nevi are flat and pigmented, intradermal nevi are raised and skin colored, and compound nevi are raised and pigmented (Figures 33-8 and 33-9).

Unless they become suspicious for melanoma, nevi need not be removed except for cosmetic reasons or because of chronic irritation based on their location. Nevi should be examined frequently, however, for changes in color, shape, or size. These changes may herald the onset of a melanoma

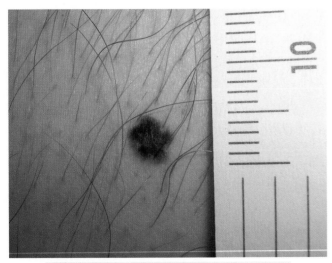

Figure 33-10 Dysplastic nevus. (© Richard P. Usatine.)

in a previously benign nevus and warrant excision with pathologic evaluation of the tissue.

Nevi that are present at birth and are visible shortly thereafter are considered *congenital* nevi. Although these nevi may have a slightly higher risk of developing melanoma than acquired nevi, it is not cost effective or sensible to recommend the removal of all congenital nevi. It is even controversial with regard to removal of large, "bathing suit" nevi, which have the highest risk of melanoma. Children born with these nevi are at risk for developing melanoma in the central nervous system (CNS) as well as subcutaneous melanoma, which is not visible as a color or surface change and requires palpation to detect it on routine skin examination.

Dysplastic nevi (atypical moles) are markers for an increased risk of melanoma. These nevi have more atypical features but are not at high risk of converting to melanoma (Figure 33-10). Therefore, removing dysplastic nevi does not provide a survival benefit for patients. The presence of five or more dysplastic nevi should alert the patient and physician to this higher risk of melanoma, and therefore regular skin examinations should be performed along with sun protection and avoidance.

INFANTILE HEMANGIOMA

A hemangioma is an extremely common type of benign tumor that occurs most frequently in infants and children. It is composed of newly formed blood vessels that result from malformation of angioblastic tissue during fetal life. The two main types are capillary (superficial) and cavernous (deep) hemangiomas (Figures 33-11 and 33-12).

Hemangiomas undergo a growth phase before resolving spontaneously. Although some regression begins by the end of the first year of life, many hemangiomas do not completely resolve until the child is 10 to 12 years old, and some may leave permanent textural or color changes. Although typically benign, rapidly proliferating hemangiomas can ulcerate. Those on the face may obscure vision and can cause blindness. Those on the anterior neck can compress the upper respiratory track during proliferation and can be life threatening. Hemangiomas of the genital region are

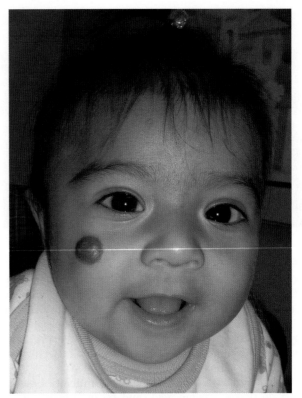

Figure 33-11 Strawberry hemangioma. (© Richard P. Usatine.)

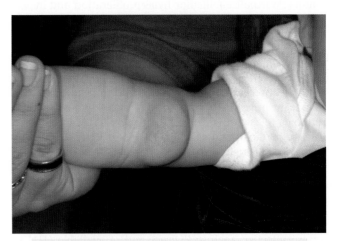

Figure 33-12 Cavernous hemangioma. (© Richard P. Usatine.)

also problematic and may indicate other internal malformations. Persistent or obstructive hemangiomas have been successfully treated with propranolol, lasers, excision, systemic corticosteroids, interferon, imiquimod, and cryosurgery.

ACNE VULGARIS

Acne is a disorder of the pilosebaceous follicles on the face, chest, and back. Follicular obstruction leads to comedones, and inflammation results in papules, pustules, and nodules. The four most important steps in acne pathogenesis are (1) sebum overproduction related to androgenic hormones and genetics, (2) abnormal desquamation of follicular epithelium (keratin plugging), (3) *Propionibacterium acnes*

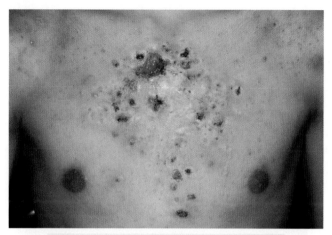

Figure 33-13 Acne fulminans. (© Richard P. Usatine.)

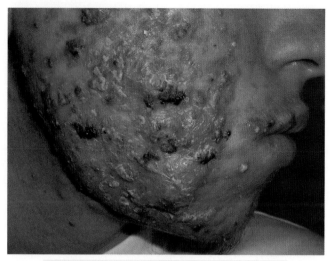

Figure 33-14 Acne conglobata (© Richard P. Usatine.)

proliferation, and (4) neutrophil chemotaxis, which leads to inflammation. These steps are stimulated by androgens, and strong genetic factors determine a person's likelihood of developing acne. Although common, acne can cause physical pain, psychosocial suffering, and scarring. Acne may be associated with fever, arthritis, and other systemic symptoms in acne fulminans (Figure 33-13).

Topical treatments include retinoids, antibiotics, benzoyl peroxide (BPO), azelaic acid, and α- or β-hydroxyl acid products. Topical retinoids are comedolytic and antiinflammatory; normalize follicular hyperproliferation and hyperkeratinization; and reduce the numbers of microcomedones, comedones, and inflammatory lesions. The most frequently prescribed topical retinoids include tretinoin (Retin-A), adapalene (Differin), and tazarotene (Tazorac). Topical retinoids frequently cause skin irritation, peeling, and redness. Mild cleansers and noncomedogenic moisturizers can reduce the inflammation, as does less frequent dosing of the retinoids (every other day or twice weekly). Glycolic acid (α-hydroxy acid) and salicylic acid (β-hydroxy acid) come in various products, are used in chemical peels, and are also effective for hyperkeratinization.

Topical antibiotics are effective against *P. acnes* and act as antiinflammatories. Erythromycin and clindamycin are frequently used once or twice daily. Topical dapsone (Aczone) was approved in 2008 for acne treatment. Benzoyl peroxide is also effective against *P. acnes* and is available OTC in various preparations. Combination products with antibiotics, retinoids, or BPO are convenient methods of delivering synergistic medications in one preparation. If two separate products are to be used instead of a combination product, it is best that they are applied at different times to avoid one product inactivating the other.

Oral medications used in acne treatment include antibiotics, hormone therapies, and isotretinoin. Isotretinoin is a known teratogen and should not be used in women of childbearing age unless avoidance of pregnancy is ensured. Contraception counseling is mandatory, and two negative pregnancy test results are required before initiation of therapy. The baseline laboratory examination should also include determination of cholesterol, fasting triglycerides, transaminase levels, blood urea nitrogen (BUN) or creatinine, and a complete blood count (CBC). Pregnancy tests must be repeated monthly for women of childbearing

potential. Other laboratory examinations should be repeated routinely during treatment.

- Topical benzoyl peroxide (gel, cream, lotion, wash) has an antimicrobial effect in acne treatment. Higher percentage products (10%) cause more irritation and are not more effective (Agency for Healthcare Research and Quality [AHRQ], 2001) (SOR: A).
- Topical antibiotics such as clindamycin and erythromycin are beneficial treatments (AHRQ, 2001) (SOR: A).
- Combination products with antibiotics and BPO deliver synergistic medications in one preparation (AHRQ, 2001) (SOR: B).
- Topical retinoids (tretinoin, adapalene, tazarotene) are excellent to treat all types of acne and the primary treatment in comedonal acne (AHRQ, 2001) (SOR: A).
- Azelaic acid is useful to treat postinflammatory hyperpigmentation and acne (AHRQ, 2001) (SOR: B).
- Oral antibiotics with proven benefit in acne include tetracycline, doxycycline, minocycline, and erythromycin and are particularly useful for inflammatory acne and trunk acne (AHRQ, 2001; Strauss et al., 2007) (SOR: A).
- Isotretinoin is the most powerful treatment for cystic and scarring acne that has not responded to other therapies (Figure 33-14) (Strauss et al., 2007) (SOR: A).
- Prolonged use of tetracycline antibiotics, particularly doxycycline, may be associated with an increased risk of inflammatory bowel disease, particularly Crohn disease (Margolis et al., 2010) (SOR:B).

VIRAL EXANTHEMS

Viral causes of rashes include varicella, rubeola, rubella, roseola, and erythema infectiosum (fifth disease). Treatment is aimed at symptoms using acetaminophen or ibuprofen for fever and diphenhydramine for pruritus.

Varicella

Varicella is now much less common because of universal varicella vaccination of children. Occasionally, a family

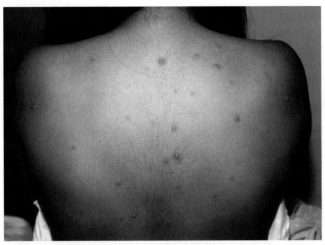

Figure 33-15 Chickenpox. (© Richard P. Usatine.)

physician sees a case of breakthrough chickenpox in a vaccinated child. Unvaccinated adults may also present with varicella. Patients with varicella have fever and general malaise as a mild prodrome lasting 1 to 2 days before the rash appears. The rash typically begins on the face, scalp, or trunk and then spreads to the extremities. The lesions appear as erythematous macules and progress to papules with an edematous base. The papules quickly evolve into vesicles, appearing as "dewdrop on a rose petal" (Figure 33-15). The vesicles evolve into pustules, which become umbilicated and subsequently crust over in the ensuing 8 to 12 hours. A defining characteristic of varicella is that lesions may be present in all stages simultaneously.

In children, the most common varicella complication is secondary bacterial infection of excoriated lesions. Other complications include cerebellar ataxia, encephalitis, meningitis, transverse myelitis, and rarely Reye syndrome. Varicella pneumonia and encephalitis can be serious complications in adults. Because of the risk of Reye syndrome, aspirin use should be avoided in patients with varicella. Acyclovir is recommended for adolescents, adults, and children with varicella who are taking steroids or otherwise immunocompromised.

Measles (Rubeola) and Rubella

Rubeola presents as maculopapular (morbilliform) eruption. It starts on the face and spreads centrifugally. It is associated with cough, coryza, conjunctivitis, fever, and Koplik spots (red-white-blue macules in mouth). As with varicella, rubeola is now uncommon because of vaccinations.

The exanthem of rubeola (measles) begins around the fourth febrile day, with discrete lesions that become confluent as they spread from the hairline downward, sparing the palms and soles. The exanthem typically lasts 4 to 6 days. The lesions fade gradually in order of appearance, leaving a residual yellow-tan coloration or faint desquamation. Rubeola is also distinguished by the presence of Koplik spots in the oral mucosa. These are usually small white or bluish macules with a ring of erythema on the buccal mucosa.

Rubella is similar to rubeola and is caused by a togavirus. It causes less severe symptoms, and its exanthem characteristically has a duration of 2 to 3 days. Rubella is associated with tender cervical lymphadenopathy, most notably in the posterior cervical and occipital areas. Another unique feature is Forchheimer spots, which are pinpoint red macules and petechiae over the soft palate and the uvula.

Hand, Foot, and Mouth Disease

This common childhood illness usually occurs in the summer or early fall and presents as flat-topped vesicles on hands, feet, and mouth, especially on the palms and soles. Every case may not involve all three sites. Hand, foot, and mouth disease is most often caused by coxsackievirus A16.

However, a number of atypical hand-foot-and-mouth disease cases are now being reported with an expanded range of cutaneous findings that are associated with coxsackievirus A6 infection (Lott et al., 2013). In a recent series, two adults and three children with atypical hand, foot, and mouth disease were identified. Four of five patients exhibited widespread cutaneous lesions, and systemic symptoms prompted four of five patients to seek emergency care. In two patients with a history of AD, accentuation in areas of dermatitis was noted. Infection with CV-A6 was confirmed in all patients (Lott et al., 2013).

Erythema Infectiosum (Fifth Disease)

Erythema infectiosum is caused by human parvovirus B19 and primarily affects children 3 to 12 years old. The prodrome may consist of fever, anorexia, sore throat, and abdominal pain. After the fever resolves, the classic erythematous facial rash ("slapped cheek") appears. The exanthem progresses to a diffuse, reticular or "lacy" pattern on the extensor extremities that may wax and wane for several weeks.

Roseola Infantum (Sixth Disease, Exanthem Subitum)

Roseola infantum, or exanthem subitum, is caused by human herpesvirus 6. This disease occurs in children younger than 3 years. As in fifth disease, the rash of sixth disease appears after the resolution of several days of high fever. The diffuse morbilliform eruption often spares the face and is of short duration, typically fading within 3 days.

Inflammatory Dermatologic Diseases

SEBORRHEA

Seborrheic dermatitis is a chronic inflammatory disorder affecting areas of the head (scalp, face) and body where sebaceous glands are prominent. The inflammation is thought to be caused by *Malassezia (Pityrosporum)* spp. All age groups may be affected, and seborrhea can be chronic or intermittent. On the scalp, seborrhea can range from mild dandruff to thick, adherent plaques. Seborrhea on the face and body appears as erythema with greasy or waxy scales. On the face, two common locations are around the eyebrows and nose and around the beard and mustache in men (Figures 33-16 and 33-17). When on the body, it is found on the chest and groin.

Treatments are aimed at the inflammation and the *Malassezia* overgrowth and include shampoos containing

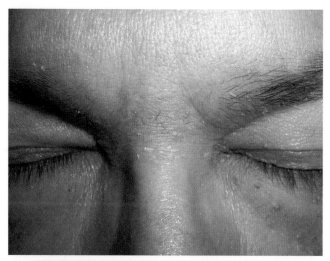

Figure 33-16 Seborrheic dermatitis. (© Richard P. Usatine.)

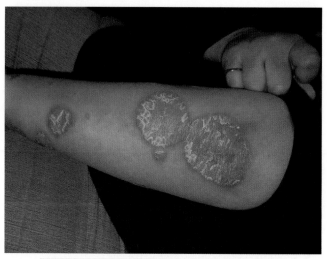

Figure 33-18 Psoriatic plaques. (© Richard P. Usatine.)

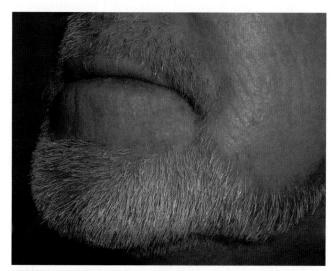

Figure 33-17 Seborrheic dermatitis around beard and mustache. (© Richard P. Usatine.)

selenium sulfide, ketoconazole, or pyrithione zinc. Topical antifungal lotions and corticosteroid preparations are also effective. Low-potency corticosteroids used intermittently are safe and effective. In infants, seborrheic dermatitis might only involve the scalp (cradle cap) or can be seen in other areas of skin folds such as the diaper area. If not treated prophylactically, seborrheic dermatitis has a tendency to recur.

KEY TREATMENT

- Shampoos containing ketoconazole, selenium sulfide, or zinc pyrithione are effective for moderate to severe seborrhea capitis (Danby et al., 1993; Pierard-Franchimont, 2002) (SOR: A).
- Ketoconazole 2% cream, gel, or emulsion is safe and effective for facial seborrheic dermatitis (Chosidow et al., 2003; Pierard et al., 1991) (SOR: B).
- Oral terbinafine, 250 mg daily for 4 weeks, is effective for moderate to severe seborrhea (Scaparro, 2001; Vena et al., 2005) (SOR: A).

- Hydrocortisone 1% cream or lotion can be used twice daily on face, scalp, or other affected area (Firooz et al., 2006) SOR: B).
- Desonide 0.05% lotion is safe and effective for short-term treatment of seborrheic dermatitis of the face (Freeman, 2002) (SOR: B).
- For moderate to severe seborrhea on the scalp, 0.05% fluocinonide solution once daily is affordably priced and beneficial (SOR: C).

PSORIASIS

Psoriasis is a common skin disorder that most often appears as inflamed plaques covered with a thickened, silvery-white scale. Psoriasis is divided into the following nine categories, although a patient can have more than one type at the same time:

1. *Plaque* psoriasis accounts for 80% to 90% of patients with psoriasis (Figure 33-18).
2. *Scalp* psoriasis causes plaques on the scalp (Figure 33-19).
3. *Guttate* psoriasis appears as small, round plaques that resemble water drops (Figure 33-20).
4. *Inverse* psoriasis causes lesions in the intertriginous areas (skin folds) of the axilla, groin, inframammary, inguinal and intergluteal regions. Inverse psoriasis may not exhibit classic scaly plaques, and the erythema, scaling, or maceration in these areas is often mistaken for fungal infection (Figure 33-21).
5. *Palmar-plantar* psoriasis occurs on the plantar aspects of the hands and feet (palms and soles) (Figure 33-22).
6. *Erythrodermic* psoriasis is widespread erythema and scales.
7. *Pustular* psoriasis can be localized or generalized. In the generalized form, superficial pustules may appear and coalesce to form lakes of pus that dry and desquamate in sheets (Figure 33-23).
8. *Nail* psoriasis causes the nails to develop pits, onycholysis, "oil spots," or onychauxis (nail thickening).

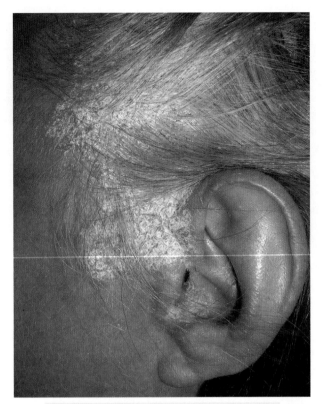

Figure 33-19 Scalp psoriasis. (© Richard P. Usatine.)

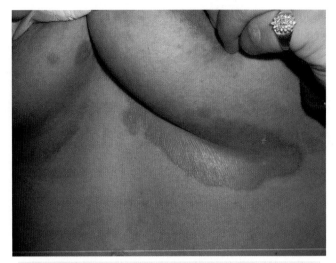

Figure 33-21 Inverse psoriasis under breasts. (© Richard P. Usatine.)

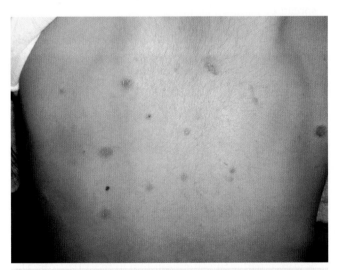

Figure 33-20 Guttate psoriasis after streptococcal throat infection in child. (© Richard P. Usatine.)

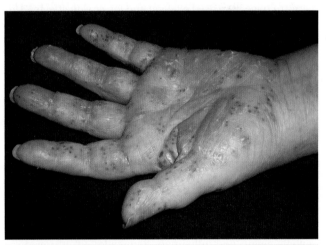

Figure 33-22 Palmoplantar psoriasis as a form of localized pustular psoriasis. (© Richard P. Usatine.)

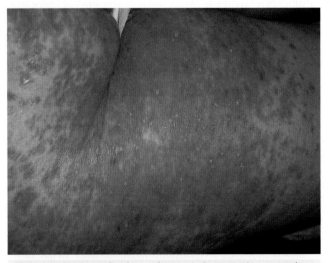

Figure 33-23 Generalized pustular psoriasis presenting as erythroderma. (© Richard P. Usatine.)

9. *Psoriatic* arthritis commonly affects the joints of the hands, feet, and knees but can involve other joints as well.

One percent to 2% of the U.S. population has plaque psoriasis. Genetic factors are involved: when both parents are affected by psoriasis, the rate of psoriasis may be as high as 50%; with one parent affected, the rate is approximately 16%. Psoriasis can appear at any age, but the two peak age ranges are 16 to 22 years and 57 to 60 years. Guttate psoriasis often occurs after streptococcal pharyngitis or another upper respiratory infection. Pustular psoriasis may be provoked by the withdrawal of systemic steroids in a patient already diagnosed with psoriasis.

The most common areas involved include the elbows, knees, extremities, trunk, scalp, face, ears, hands, feet, genitalia, intertriginous areas, and the nails. In most cases, diagnosis of psoriasis is based on the clinical appearance. The differential diagnosis list is long, but a KOH (potassium hydroxide) preparation or skin biopsy may be needed. A biopsy may also be helpful to establish the diagnosis in less common types of psoriasis (pustular, palmar-plantar, inverse). Psoriasis should not be treated with oral or systemic steroids; this can precipitate a life-threatening case of generalized pustular psoriasis.

A meta-analysis showed that 68% to 89% of patients treated with clobetasol (ultrahigh-potency steroid) had clear improvement or complete healing (Nast et al., 2007). Comparable efficacy was shown for topical calcipotriene (vitamin D analog) and tazarotene (retinoid), with a slight increase in adverse effects for tazarotene (Afifi et al., 2005). Combination topical steroids and calcipotriene or tazarotene is the most promising current topical treatment and seems to have increased efficacy and fewer side effects (Afifi et al., 2005; Nast et al., 2007). Clinical trials suggest that tacrolimus (0.1%) ointment twice daily produces a good response in a majority of patients with facial and intertriginous (inverse) psoriasis (Brune et al., 2007; Lebwohl et al., 2004; Martin et al., 2006). Methotrexate as a weekly oral dose of 5 to 15 mg can be very effective for widespread psoriasis not responding to topical treatments (Saporito and Menter, 2004). Acitretin (Soriatane) is a potent systemic retinoid used for psoriasis that is widespread or palmar-plantar and not responding to topical treatments (Pearce et al., 2006)

Etanercept (Enbrel) is a subcutaneous biologic agent that is especially valuable in patients with psoriatic arthritis, as well as those with moderate to severe cutaneous psoriasis (Nast et al., 2007). Adalimumab (Humira), a subcutaneous biologic agent, and infliximab (Remicade), an intravenous (IV) biologic agent, are effective for patients with psoriatic arthritis as well as those with moderate to severe cutaneous psoriasis (Bansback et al., 2009). Ustekinumab (Stelara), the most recently approved subcutaneous biologic agent, significantly reduced signs and symptoms of psoriatic arthritis and diminished skin lesions compared with placebo (Gottlieb et al., 2009).

KEY TREATMENT

- Potent topical steroid ointments are a good choice for first-line therapy of psoriasis (Afifi et al., 2005) (SOR: A).
- Clobetasol successfully treated 68% to 89% of patients with psoriasis (Nast et al., 2007) (SOR: A).
- Topical calcipotriene and tazarotene show comparable efficacy as clobetasol for psoriasis (Afifi et al., 2005) (SOR: A).
- Topical steroids and calcipotriene or tazarotene show increased efficacy in psoriasis and fewer side effects (Afifi et al., 2005; Nast et al., 2007) (SOR: A).
- Tacrolimus (0.1% ointment twice a day) helps most patients with facial and inverse psoriasis (Brune et al., 2007; Lebwohl et al., 2004; Martin et al., 2006) (SOR: B).

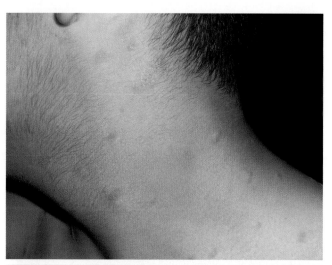

Figure 33-24 Pityriasis rosea with herald patch on neck. (© Richard P. Usatine.)

- Narrow-band ultraviolet B (UVB) is safer and more effective than broadband UVB for psoriasis (Ibbotson et al., 2004) (SOR: A)
- Methotrexate (5-15 mg/wk) is effective for widespread psoriasis not responding to topical treatments (Saporito and Menter, 2004) (SOR: A). It is also beneficial for psoriatic arthritis.
- Acitretin (Soriatane) is used for unresponsive widespread or palmar-plantar psoriasis (Pearce et al., 2006) (SOR: A).
- Etanercept (Enbrel) and other biologic agents are especially valuable in patients with psoriatic arthritis or cutaneous psoriasis (Ash et al., 2012) (Nast et al., 2007) (SOR: A).

PITYRIASIS ROSEA

Pityriasis rosea is a common acute eruption usually affecting children and young adults; the cause is unknown. It is characterized by the formation of an initial herald patch (Figure 33-24) followed by the development of a diffuse papulosquamous rash. Pityriasis rosea is difficult to identify until the appearance of characteristic, smaller, secondary lesions that follow Langer lines in a "Christmas tree" pattern (Figure 33-25). The rash of pityriasis rosea typically lasts 5 to 8 weeks, with complete resolution in most patients. The rash is usually asymptomatic, but treatment for pruritus may be needed and can include calamine lotion, topical steroids, and oral antihistamines. Systemic steroids are generally not recommended.

Ultraviolet (UV) radiation and erythromycin have been used with varying results. Because no bacterial cause has been associated with the disease, the likely effect of erythromycin is a result of its antiinflammatory properties. Postinflammatory hyperpigmentation may occur with UVB radiation therapy, so some experts recommend against its use. High-dose acyclovir (800 mg four times a day) may help shorten disease, especially if instituted early in the disease course, but studies are limited.

Patients should be reassured about the self-limited nature of pityriasis rosea. Persistence of the rash or pruritus beyond 12 weeks should prompt reconsideration of the

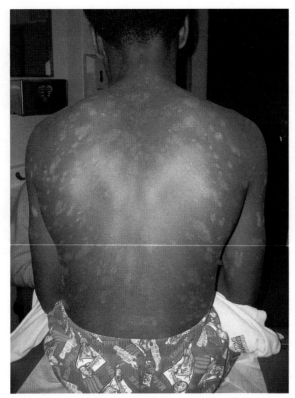

Figure 33-25 Pityriasis rosea with "Christmas tree" pattern on back (© Richard P. Usatine and E.J. Mayeaux, Jr. *The Color Atlas of Family Medicine.*)

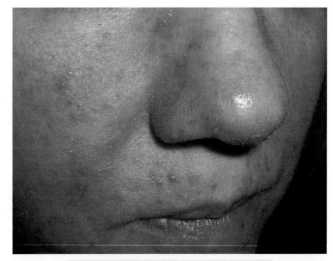

Figure 33-26 Rosacea. (© Richard P. Usatine.)

original diagnosis, such as secondary syphilis and consideration of laboratory work or biopsy to confirm the diagnosis, and questioning the patient again about use of medications that may cause a rash similar to that of pityriasis rosea.

ROSACEA

Rosacea, sometimes called "acne rosacea," is an inflammatory disease with unknown etiology. Various facial manifestations occur, and symptoms differ from patient to patient. The four types of rosacea are erythematotelangiectatic, papulopustular, phymatous, and ocular. Patients may have overlapping features of more than one type. The predominant manifesting complaints of *erythematotelangiectatic* rosacea are intermittent central facial flushing and erythema. Many patients complain of a stinging or burning pain associated with flushing episodes. Common triggers include exposure to the sun, cold weather, sudden emotion (including laughter or embarrassment), hot beverages, spicy foods, and alcohol consumption.

Papulopustular rosacea presents with acnelike papules and sterile pustules and can occur alone or in combination with the erythema and telangiectasias (Figure 33-26). Intermittent or chronic facial edema may also occur in all forms. Some patients develop *rhinophyma,* a coarse hypertrophy of the connective tissue and sebaceous glands of the nose. This can be extremely disfiguring and even cause nasal airway obstruction. Approximately one third of patients with rosacea develop ocular symptoms, including eyes that are itchy, burning, or dry; a gritty or foreign body sensation; and erythema, swelling, or hordeolum of the eyelid. The ocular changes can become chronic. Corneal

neovascularization and keratitis can occur, leading to corneal scarring and perforation. Episcleritis and iritis have also been reported to occur in patients with rosacea.

First-line treatment is avoidance of triggering or exacerbating factors. Although patients have different trigger(s), almost all patients benefit from strict sun avoidance and protection. Acne-like lesions respond well to long-term topical treatment using metronidazole, azelaic acid, erythromycin, and clindamycin. Oral tetracyclines used in antimicrobial (high) doses or antiinflammatory (low) doses are helpful for moderate to severe rosacea. Topical retinoid therapy may also be effective, but irritation can limit its tolerability. Laser treatment is an option for progressive telangiectasia, erythema, or rhinophyma. Ocular symptoms generally require oral tetracyclines. Consultation may be required for the management of rhinophyma, ocular complications, or severe disease.

KEY TREATMENT

- Best evidence supports the topical use of metronidazole (0.75% or 1%) and azelaic acid (15% or 20%) for rosacea (van Zuuren et al., 2011) (SOR: A).
- If the skin lesions are more extensive, oral antibiotics, such as doxycycline, are recommended for rosacea (van Zuuren et al., 2011) (SOR: C).
- Both antiinflammatory (low-dose) doxycycline (40-mg delayed-release Oracea) and 100-mg doxycycline are equally effective once-daily treatments for moderate to severe rosacea; a higher dosage (100 mg) is associated with a higher incidence of adverse effects (mostly gastrointestinal [GI] symptoms) (Del Rosso et al., 2008) (SOR: B).
- Pulsed-dye laser and intense pulse light result in significant reduction in erythema, telangiectasia, and patient-reported associated symptoms (Neuhaus et al., 2009) (SOR: B).
- Ocular rosacea may be treated with oral doxycycline. (Bartholomew et al., 1982; Seal et al., 1995) Cyclosporin 0.05% ophthalmic emulsion is an option for topical treatment of ocular rosacea (van Zuuren et al., 2011) (SOR: C).

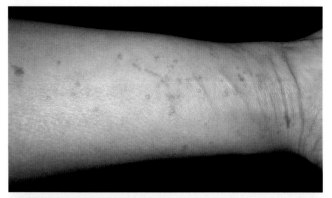

Figure 33-27 Lichen planus with linear papules. (© Richard P. Usatine.)

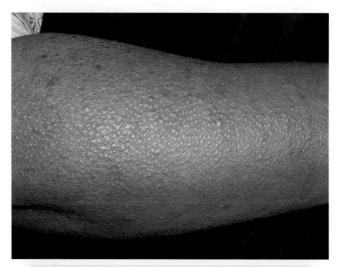

Figure 33-29 Lichen simplex chronicus. (© Richard P. Usatine.)

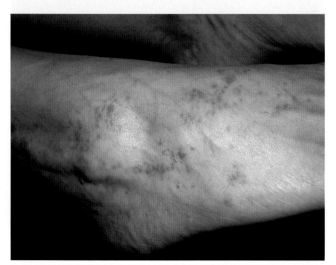

Figure 33-28 Lichen planus on the lateral ankle. (© Richard P. Usatine.)

LICHEN PLANUS

Lichen planus is a papular pruritic skin eruption characterized by its violaceous color and polygonal shape. Most frequently, flat-topped papules and plaques are found on the flexor surfaces of the upper extremities, on the genitalia, around the ankles, and on the mucous membranes (Figures 33-27 and 33-28). Skin lesions can be intensely pruritic. Lichen planus is most commonly associated with hepatitis C infection and the association is strongest for the oral form of lichen planus.

Patients with lichen planus are usually between 30 and 60 years old, although the disorder may occur at any age. Men and women are equally affected, and there is no racial predisposition. The cutaneous form spontaneously resolves within 6 months in about half of patients, and most forms resolve within 18 months. Mucous membrane lesions may become chronic and persist for years. Most cases can be treated symptomatically with mid- to high-potency topical steroids and oral antihistamines. Topical steroids can be used in the mouth in various vehicles, including gel, ointment, or oral paste. Many drugs cause lichenoid reactions, so a review of the medication history may find a precipitating medication that needs to be stopped. More severe cases or those involving the mucous membranes can be treated with systemic steroids, oral acitretin, or UV light.

- Treatment of lichen planus starts with high-potency topical steroids twice daily to the affected areas (Usatine & Tinitigan, 2011) (SOR: C).
- Intralesional triamcinolone (3 mg/mL) is considered for hypertrophic or mucous membrane lichen planus lesions (Usatine & Tinitigan, 2011) (SOR: C).
- Systemic treatment with oral steroids or acitretin can be considered for severe cases of lichen planus that involve mucous membranes (Zakrzewska et al., 2005) (SOR: B).

LICHEN SIMPLEX CHRONICUS

Lichen simplex chronicus (LSC) is a secondary condition that results from repeated mechanical trauma to the skin, usually through rubbing and scratching, which causes lichenification (thickening of epidermis). Skin appears leathery, violaceous to hyperpigmented, and scaly (Figure 33-29). Involved areas are within the patient's easy reach, such as the arms, legs, posterior neck, upper back, buttocks, and scrotum. The cycle of pruritus, which is alleviated by scratching, perpetuates the condition. Pruritus is usually worse during periods of inactivity, usually at bedtime and during the night. Stress also may provoke pruritus, which is relieved by rubbing and scratching and often becomes an unconscious behavior.

Treatment of LSC is aimed at treating existing lesions, reducing pruritus, providing insight into the itch–scratch cycle, and eliciting behavioral changes, Topical steroids decrease inflammation and pruritus and help "thin down" the hyperkeratosis. Because lesions are by nature chronic, long-term treatment should be stressed. Occlusion can be used to increase potency and enhance delivery of the topical steroid and also provides a barrier to scratching. Flurandrenolide tape (Cordran) is very effective and can be cut to fit each lesion of LSC. Anxiolytics and antihistamines such as diphenhydramine and hydroxyzine may be considered as adjunct treatments. Behavior modification is also useful. In severe, debilitating cases, oral doxepin and clonazepam may be considered. For secondary infections, a topical or oral antibiotic is appropriate.

CONTACT DERMATITIS

Key Points

- Contact dermatitis is classified as irritant (ICD) or allergic (ACD).
- Clinical findings of ICD and ACD can be identical, and both entities can be present simultaneously.
- Nickel is the most common cause of ACD.
- Avoidance of irritating substances or environments and allergens is key to therapy. Dry-skin care and topical corticosteroids are also helpful.
- Referral for patch testing can help identify the causative agent in ACD.

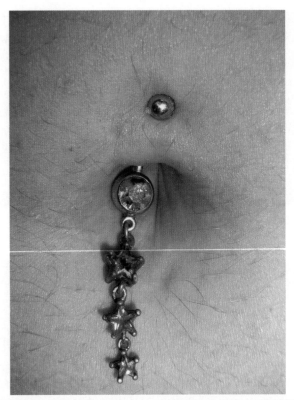

Figure 33-30 Contact dermatitis to nickel jewelry in the umbilicus. (© Richard P. Usatine.)

Contact dermatitis may be classified by cause into two subgroups, ICD and ACD. ICD occurs when the skin is exposed to an environment or substance in a sufficient frequency, quantity, or duration that it overcomes the barrier function of the skin. Therefore, given adequate exposure, anyone may experience ICD. ACD is a delayed-type hypersensitivity (type 4) reaction to a topical agent and requires initial contact with a substance causing a T helper cell type 2 (Th2)–mediated immune response in a predisposed individual. Only with repeated exposure do the primed T cells cause the clinical response of dermatitis.

Findings of contact dermatitis can include erythema, vesicles, bullae, exudation, crusting, blisters, swelling, and scaling. Common areas affected are the hands, neck, eyelids, face, genitalia, and legs. ICD and ACD can look identical and can present on similar body areas. Both may be intensely pruritic, further complicating the diagnosis. In addition, ACD and ICD can be present simultaneously, as with health care workers allergic to latex who wash their hands repeatedly throughout the day. A careful history and patch testing are often the key to diagnosis.

Each year, millions of patients develop an allergic rash after contact with poison ivy, poison sumac, or poison oak, and contrary to popular belief, the fluid within these vesicles does not cause poison ivy "to spread." Nickel is the most common nonplant cause of ACD and is historically more common in women because of costume jewelry and ear piercing (Figure 33-30). With the increased popularity of jewelry and body piercing, the prevalence is rising in men.

The top 15 most frequently positive allergens are nickel sulfate (19.5%), Myroxylon Pereira (11.0%), neomycin (10.1%), fragrance mix I (9.4%), quaternium-15 (8.6%), cobalt chloride (8.4%), bacitracin (7.9%), formaldehyde (7.7%), methyldibromoglutaronitrile/phenoxyethanol (5.5%), p-phenylenediamine (5.3%), propolis (4.9%), carba mix (4.5%), potassium dichromate (4.1%), fragrance mix II (3.6%), and methylchloroisothiazolinone/methylisothiazolinone (3.6%) (Fransway et al., 2013).

In the workplace, ACD is very common. For skin conditions, 90% of workers' compensation claims result from contact dermatitis. Common offenders in specific occupations are rubber or latex in health care workers, hair and clothing dyes in hairdressers, chromates in cement workers, and the Rhus family (poison ivy, oak, and sumac) in agricultural workers. ICD most often develops in response to excessive exposure to soaps, cleansers, hand sanitizers, and water exposure. Therefore, the primary treatment is avoidance of these irritating substances, application of a barrier ointment such as petrolatum, and protective equipment such as gloves.

For ACD caused by plants, the skin and clothes should be thoroughly washed with soap and water as soon as possible to minimize exposure to the antigen. Cool, wet soaks for 10 to 15 minutes may be soothing. Superpotent topical steroids, such as clobetasol propionate or betamethasone dipropionate applied twice daily for 1 to 2 weeks, are effective for treating small areas of moderate ACD. Systemic steroids are reserved for severe episodes and should be continued for at least 2 weeks to prevent rebound dermatitis. In otherwise healthy persons, a tapering dose of prednisone is not required for short courses of systemic therapy. Severe pruritus may respond to antihistamines such as hydroxyzine, diphenhydramine, or a nonsedating H_2 blocker such as loratadine, cetirizine, or fexofenadine.

If ACD is suspected based on history, consultation for patch testing with a dermatologist can be customized to the patient's occupation or hobbies. After the offending agent is identified, avoidance is crucial. When the offending agent is occupational, a change in jobs may be required. Alternative protective equipment can be sufficient in other cases, such as substituting nitrile gloves for latex. Generalized dry-skin care, topical steroids, or immunomodulators (pimecrolimus, tacrolimus) can help prevent recurrence and treat flares.

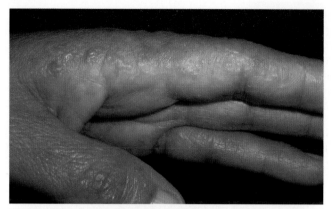

Figure 33-31 Dyshidrotic eczema with tapioca vesicles (pompholyx). (© Richard P. Usatine.)

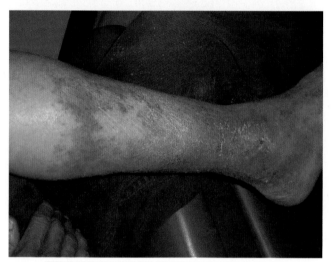

Figure 33-32 Stasis dermatitis. (© Richard P. Usatine.)

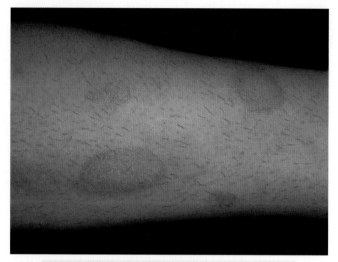

Figure 33-33 Nummular eczema. (© Richard P. Usatine.)

DYSHIDROTIC ECZEMA (POMPHOLYX)

Dyshidrotic eczema is a form of dermatitis characterized by a pruritic vesicular eruption on the fingers, palms, and soles (Figure 33-31). Patients may be affected at any age, with women affected twice as often as men. The condition may be acute, intermittent, or chronic. Eruptions occur with varying severity and can be mild or debilitating. Before the formation of vesicles, patients describe itching or burning of the hands and feet. Small vesicles appear along the lateral aspects of the fingers or feet, palms, and soles. Lesions may persist for weeks and may be accompanied by erythema of the palms and soles.

Treatment of dyshidrotic eczema includes high-potency topical steroids and cold compresses for symptomatic relief of the burning sensation. Greasy emollients are helpful to moisturize, protect, and prevent fissures. If fissures do occur, cyanoacrylate ("superglue") can be used to seal small cracks in the skin and decrease pain. Short courses of oral steroids may be used for acute flares.

STASIS DERMATITIS

Stasis dermatitis occurs on the lower extremities in patients with chronic venous insufficiency (Figure 33-32). Impaired function of the venous valves permits backflow of the blood from the deep venous system to the superficial system, causing increased venous hydrostatic pressure and increased permeability of dermal capillaries. The condition typically affects middle-aged and older-adult patients, except for patients with acquired venous insufficiency resulting from surgery, trauma, or thrombosis.

Stasis dermatitis can range from mild to severe. In all stages, reddish brown discoloration is caused by staining from hemosiderin that has leaked out of red blood cells in the overtaxed dermal capillaries. Pedal edema and scaling are also present in various degrees, and one leg can be more affected than the other. ACD is often superimposed on stasis dermatitis and can mislead the physician into suspecting cellulitis because of a sudden reddening, weeping, or induration of the area. Because of the impaired skin barrier and frequent use of OTC products and "home remedies," neomycin, lanolin, iodine, fragrances, and preservatives are common triggers for ACD in these patients.

Long-term treatment focuses first on reducing pedal edema with compression therapy after assessing the integrity of the arterial circulation to prevent claudication or ischemic necrosis. Compression stockings are best applied early in the morning before the patient rises from bed, when leg edema is at a minimum. For the pruritus and dermatitis, stasis dermatitis is treated in the same manner as other forms of acute eczematous dermatitis. Dry skin care with mild cleansers (Dove, Cetaphil) and bland emollients (petrolatum, Aquaphor, or Absorbase) should be used liberally. Medium-potency topical corticosteroids (e.g., triamcinolone 0.1% ointment) should be used twice daily when inflammation and pruritus are present. If infection is suspected, mupirocin should be used preferentially over other topical antibiotics to avoid ACD to bacitracin or neomycin. For severe cases with exuberant purulent drainage and induration, oral antibiotics with activity against *Staphylococcus* and *Streptococcus* should be used.

NUMMULAR DERMATITIS (NUMMULAR ECZEMA)

Nummular dermatitis consists of well-demarcated, coin-shaped lesions of eczema, typically on the extremities and less often the trunk in adults (Figure 33-33). Nummular

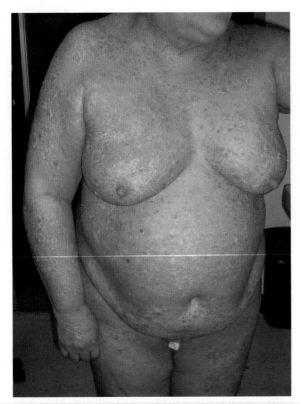

Figure 33-34 Erythroderma secondary to pustular psoriasis. (© Richard P. Usatine.)

dermatitis tends to worsen in dry, cold weather. Lesions may be mildly to severely pruritic and as a result become excoriated or even lichenified with scratching. Nummular dermatitis can be confused with plaques of psoriasis or tinea corporis, but skin scrapings will not reveal hyphae on KOH preparation. Also, lesions lack the typical central sparing of tinea corporis. If necessary, a biopsy can help differentiate nummular eczema from psoriasis.

As with all eczematous dermatitis, general dry skin care is recommended with mild cleansers and bland emollients. An intermediate to potent topical steroid may be applied two to four times daily to the affected areas. When lesions improve, a lower potency steroid or immunomodulator (tacrolimus, pimecrolimus) should be used to minimize skin atrophy. Pruritus may be treated with an antihistamine if needed.

GENERALIZED EXFOLIATIVE DERMATITIS

Exfoliative dermatitis, also known as *erythroderma*, is an uncommon but serious skin disorder defined as erythema and scale covering over 90% of the body surface area (Figure 33-34). The four most common causes of erythroderma are psoriasis, AD, cutaneous T-cell lymphoma (CTCL), and drug reactions. More than 60 drugs (more often allopurinol, β-lactam antibiotics, antiseizure medications, and sulfa drugs) have been implicated in cases of exfoliative dermatitis. More than half of patients will have a known underlying skin disease, but in up to 25%, an etiology may never be determined and is termed *idiopathic* erythroderma. The majority of patients are adults older than age 40 years.

The long-term prognosis is good in patients with drug-induced exfoliative dermatitis. The course tends to be remitting and relapsing in idiopathic cases. The prognosis of patients with associated malignancy usually depends on the outcome of the malignancy. A skin biopsy can help establish the diagnosis when the underlying skin disease is not known. The approach to treatment should include discontinuation of potentially causative medications and a search for any underlying malignancy. Initial evaluation and treatment usually require hospitalization for fluid and electrolyte replacement, temperature modulation, and prevention and treatment of secondary infection.

ERYTHEMA NODOSUM

Erythema nodosum is an acute inflammatory process involving the fatty tissue layer underlying the skin (panniculitis). The condition is more frequently seen in women, and although it is often idiopathic, many cases are associated with streptococcal infections of the upper respiratory tract, drugs such as estrogens or oral contraceptives, sarcoidosis, and inflammatory bowel disease. Other, less frequent bacterial causes include tuberculosis, brucellosis, mycoplasma, and chlamydia. Fungal infections such as blastomycosis and histoplasmosis may also cause erythema nodosum. Rare causes are Behçet disease, acute myelogenous leukemia, and Hodgkin disease.

Patients present with tender red nodules, most frequently on the pretibial area or lower legs. The nodules may become fluctuant but do not suppurate or ulcerate. New lesions may continue to appear for several weeks. Additional symptoms may include fever, malaise, and arthralgia. Treatment is aimed at determining any underlying cause. Infectious processes should be evaluated and treated appropriately. Discontinuation of any possible offending agents is also advised. Bed rest, leg elevation, and nonsteroidal antiinflammatory drugs (NSAIDSs) are the mainstays of therapy. Spontaneous resolution occurs within 4 to 6 weeks in most patients, but residual leg pain and ankle edema can persist for weeks.

GRANULOMA ANNULARE

Granuloma annulare is a benign, self-limited dermatosis characterized by a raised annular distribution (Figure 33-35). The condition may be localized, generalized, perforating, or subcutaneous. Except for subcutaneous granuloma annulare, the subtypes have similar appearances, but each follows a distinct clinical course. *Subcutaneous* granuloma annulare appears differently, with deep dermal or subcutaneous nodules. Patients with *localized* granuloma annulare present with groups of 1- to 2-mm papules in an annular arrangement over the distal extremities, ranging in color from skin tone to erythematous. Lesions most frequently appear on the dorsal surfaces of the hands and feet, fingers, and extensor aspects of the arms and legs. In *generalized* granuloma annulare, patients have a few to thousands of papules and rings that involve many body regions. The rings tend to be distributed symmetrically. Patients with *perforating* granuloma annulare present with up to hundreds of grouped 1- to 4-mm papules that may evolve into pustular lesions that drain and umbilicate, leaving atrophic

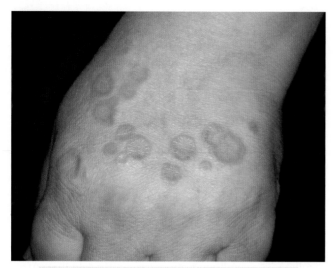

Figure 33-35 Granuloma annulare. (© Richard P. Usatine.)

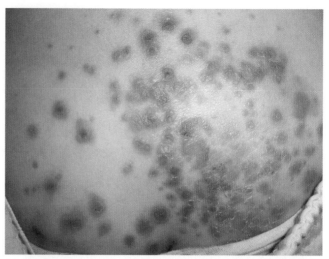

Figure 33-36 Impetigo on the back and buttocks of a child showing honey crusts. (© Richard P. Usatine.)

scars. These lesions tend to appear on the extensor surfaces of extremities and the dorsa of the hands and fingers. Granuloma annulare may resolve spontaneously but can take several years. When patients request treatment, steroid injections are most effective.

Infectious Skin Diseases

BACTERIAL INFECTIONS

Key Points

- Most bacterial skin infections are caused by *Streptococcus pyogenes* or *S. aureus.*
- Impetigo is the most superficial bacterial skin infection and often appears with honey-crusted lesions.
- Erysipelas is a superficial bacterial skin infection that extends into the cutaneous lymphatics, most often on the face or lower leg.
- Cellulitis is a deeper skin infection that requires oral antibiotics active against *S. pyogenes* and *S. aureus.*
- Abscesses often require incision and drainage to resolve completely.
- Community-acquired methicillin-resistant *S. aureus* is a common cause of abscesses and other bacterial skin infections.

Impetigo

Impetigo is a bacterial infection of the epidermis caused by *S. aureus* and group A β-hemolytic streptococci (GABHS). Both organisms may be present at the same time in the affected site. Community-acquired methicillin-resistant *S. aureus* (CA-MRSA) may cause impetigo. Various types of dermatitis can become secondarily infected with bacteria, and the skin is then called "impetiginized." About 30% of people are colonized in the anterior nares by *S. aureus.* Impetigo is highly infectious, and the bacteria are readily transmitted from one person to another through direct contact, entering through broken skin created by

cutaneous diseases, burns, surgery, trauma, radiation therapy, and insect bites.

Impetigo is a common condition that occurs in all age groups and in both genders equally. The incidence in those younger than 6 years is higher than in adults. The peak incidence occurs during the summer and fall. Most patients recover without complications. Individuals with impetigo from streptococcal infections can develop glomerulonephritis as a rare complication. Impetigo is usually diagnosed clinically based on its characteristic appearance of honey crusts and superficial erosions (Figure 33-36). Exudate from beneath the skin crust should be obtained for culture and sensitivity testing if a community outbreak has occurred, MRSA is suspected, or poststreptococcal glomerulonephritis is present.

Mupirocin ointment is the treatment of choice for small areas of impetigo and is as effective as oral antibiotics, including cases caused by MRSA and GABHS. Mupirocin three times daily for 5 days each month is also recommended intranasally for patients found to be chronic nasal carriers. Oral antibiotics are used in patients with extensive impetigo or with refractory infection. A cephalosporin, semisynthetic penicillin, or β-lactam–β-lactamase inhibitor is recommended. If bacterial cultures reveal MRSA, trimethoprim–sulfamethoxazole, doxycycline (older than age 10 years), or clindamycin are appropriate. Gentle debridement of crusts using antibacterial soap and a washcloth is also recommended. Patients should be encouraged to use careful handwashing to prevent further spread of infection.

Erysipelas (St. Anthony's Fire)

Erysipelas is a superficial bacterial skin infection that extends into the cutaneous lymphatics. Usually, this infection is caused by *S. pyogenes* infection and occurs on the face or lower leg. Bacterial inoculation into an area of damaged skin is the initial event in developing erysipelas, although patients may not recall the precipitating event. The source of the bacteria is often from the host's nasopharynx. A history of recent streptococcal pharyngitis is reported in up to one third of patients.

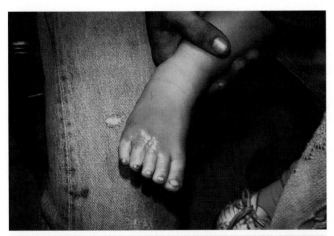

Figure 33-37 Cellulitis on the foot of a child after a break in the skin. (© Richard P. Usatine.)

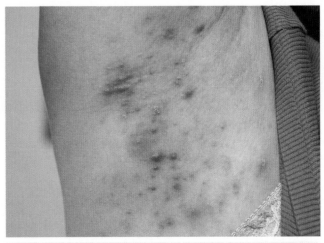

Figure 33-38 Folliculitis secondary to methicillin-resistant *Staphylococcus aureus* (MRSA). (Courtesy of Alisha N. Plotner, MD, and Robert T. Brodell, MD, with permission from *J Fam Pract* 2008; 57(4):253-255.)

The most common complaints during the acute infection are pain, fever, chills, and swelling of the skin. Infants, young children, and older adult patients are the groups most often affected, with a peak incidence at age 60 to 80 years. Erysipelas may become a red, indurated, tense, and shiny plaque with sharply demarcated margins. Local inflammatory signs, such as warmth, edema, and tenderness, are universal. Lymphatic involvement is manifested by a peau d'orange look to the skin, with sharp borders and regional lymphadenopathy. More severe infections may include numerous vesicles or bullae, petechiae, and even skin necrosis. Streptococci cause erysipelas in as many as 80% of cases, with two thirds of those caused by group A and 25% by group G streptococci. *S. aureus* has been implicated in cases of recurrent erysipelas secondary to lymphedema. Atypical forms have been caused by *Streptococcus pneumoniae*, *Klebsiella pneumoniae*, *Yersinia enterocolitica*, and *Moraxella* spp. and should be considered in cases refractory to standard antibiotic therapy.

In cases involving the extremities, elevation and rest of the affected limb are recommended to reduce local swelling and inflammation. Oral or intramuscular penicillin for 10 to 14 days is sufficient for many cases of erysipelas. A macrolide such as erythromycin or azithromycin may be used if the patient is allergic to penicillin. Hospitalization for close monitoring and IV antibiotics are recommended for severe cases and for infants, older adults, and immunocompromised patients. Facial erysipelas should be treated empirically with a penicillinase-resistant antibiotic such as dicloxacillin to cover for possible *S. aureus*. Predisposing skin lesions, such as tinea pedis and stasis ulcers, should be treated aggressively to prevent superinfection.

Cellulitis

Cellulitis is an acute infection of the skin and soft tissues, usually developing after a break in the skin. The condition is characterized by localized pain, swelling, tenderness, erythema, and warmth (Figure 33-37). The vast majority of cases are caused by *S. pyogenes* or *S. aureus*. Other causes include *Vibrio vulnificus* and *Pseudomonas* spp. Cellulitis is generally localized and nonrecurrent when treated appropriately. Death is extremely rare but may occur when the condition is neglected or caused by a highly virulent

organism. Patients typically present with a red, hot, swollen, and tender area of skin. Unlike erysipelas, the borders are neither elevated nor sharply demarcated. Lymphangitis and local lymphadenopathy may be present. Fever is common, and patients with severe cases may develop hypotension. Those with mild cellulitis may be treated as outpatients. Oral antibiotics are usually effective for treatment of cellulitis in immunocompetent hosts. Severe cases or patients with comorbid conditions (e.g., cardiac, renal, or hepatic failure, immunosuppression) should be initially treated with IV antibiotics in the hospital setting. Elevation of affected limbs improves resolution of swelling.

Folliculitis

Folliculitis is caused by infection or irritation of individual hair follicles. Patients with folliculitis present with pustules at the bases of hairs, particularly on the scalp, back, legs, buttocks, and arms (Figure 33-38). Folliculitis occurs more often in obese, immunocompromised, or diabetic patients. *S. aureus* is the most common pathogen. A form of folliculitis caused by *Pseudomonas* spp., "hot tub folliculitis," occurs when patients use poorly maintained hot tubs. The condition may be self-limited, requiring only the use of antibacterial soap, or may persist and require topical or systemic antibiotic therapy. If a pseudomonal infection is suspected and lesions persist for more than 5 days without treatment, an oral fluoroquinolone (e.g., ciprofloxacin) should be considered. The hot tub must also be drained and cleaned.

Abscesses: Furuncles and Carbuncles

Furuncles, or "boils," are small abscesses in the skin. Patients present with a painful, often fluctuant swelling in areas of friction such as the axilla, inframammary, buttocks, and inner thigh. A *carbuncle* is a collection of furuncles and usually occurs on the back of the neck in middle-aged and older men. Antibiotic therapy should be considered if the furuncle is not yet fluctuant, there is evidence of surrounding cellulitis or lymphadenitis, or the lesion is on the face. Carbuncles have many interconnecting sinuses and tend to recur despite drainage and antibiotics. Surgical

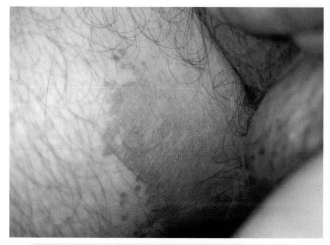

Figure 33-39 Erythrasma in the groin. (© Richard P. Usatine.)

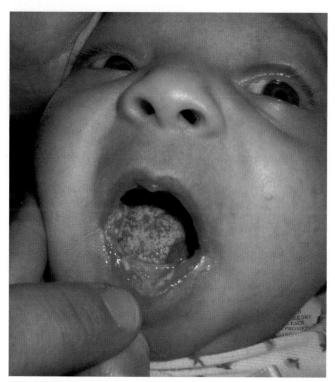

Figure 33-40 Thrush caused by Candida albicans. (© Richard P. Usatine.)

drainage and resection of the lesions are often necessary. Many abscesses are now caused by MRSA, and if fluctuant, the first-line treatment is incision and drainage.

Erythrasma

Erythrasma is a superficial skin infection caused by *Corynebacterium* spp., a normal inhabitant of the skin. The infection typically occurs in intertriginous spaces, especially in obese, hyperhidrotic, or diabetic patients (Figure 33-39). Moderate itching and discomfort may occur, and the infected skin is often reddish brown and may be slightly raised, with some central clearing. The lesions are largely confluent but may have poorly defined borders. Because of the production of porphyrins by the infecting corynebacteria, Wood's light demonstrates the lesions as a coral red. However, if the patient has recently washed the affected area, the coral-red fluorescence may be absent. Erythrasma is often confused with a fungal infection. Erythrasma may be treated with topical erythromycin or clindamycin. Oral antibiotics are only needed in very extensive involvement.

FUNGAL INFECTIONS

Key Points

- Tinea capitis should be treated with oral antifungal agents.
- Tinea infections may be transmitted from person to person by animals (pets, livestock) and through fomites.
- OTC topical antifungals are often effective for tinea pedis.
- Tinea versicolor is caused by infection with *Malassezia* spp. and can be treated by topical antidandruff shampoos or oral antifungals (ketoconazole, fluconazole).

Dermatophytosis (Tinea)

Mucocutaneous fungal infections are caused by dermatophytes (*Microsporum*, *Epidermophyton*, and *Trichophyton* spp.) and yeasts. About 40 species in the three dermatophyte genera can cause tinea pedis and manus, tinea capitis,

tinea corporis, tinea cruris, and onychomycosis. Yeasts of *Candida* spp. can cause diaper dermatitis, balanitis, vulvovaginitis, and thrush (Figure 33-40). The yeastlike organism of *Malassezia (Pityrosporum)* spp. causes tinea versicolor and contributes to seborrhea. Although tinea versicolor has the name *tinea* in it, it is not a true dermatophyte.

The most important test for a suspected fungal infection is the KOH prep. Scrape the leading edge of the lesion onto a slide using the side of a #15 scalpel or another slide. Use the coverslip to push the scale into the center of the slide. Add 2 drops of KOH (with or without fungal stain) to the slide and place a coverslip on top. Examine with microscope starting with 10× magnification and low light to look for the cells and hyphae. The fungal stain helps the hyphae to stand out among the epithelial cells. Look for groups of cells that appear to have fungal elements within them; do not be fooled by cell borders that look linear and branching. Switch to 40× magnification to confirm any areas that appear to have fungal elements by looking for true fungal morphology. The fungal stains bring out these characteristics, including cell walls, nuclei, and arthroconidia (Figure 33-41). KOH test characteristics without fungal stain are sensitivity, 77% to 88%, and specificity, 62% to 95% (Thomas, 2003).

Tinea Corporis

Tinea corporis is a superficial dermatophyte infection of the cornified layers of skin on the trunk and extremities. Lesions are typically annular with central clearing and a scaling border and may be pruritic (Figure 33-42). Infection may be transmitted from person to person, by animals such as household pets or farm animals, and through fomites. Because the cornified layer of skin is involved, topical

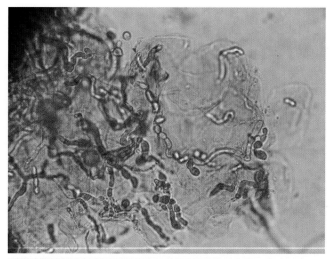

Figure 33-41 *Trichophyton rubrum* seen after potassium hydroxide (KOH) preparation using fungal stain. (© Richard P. Usatine.)

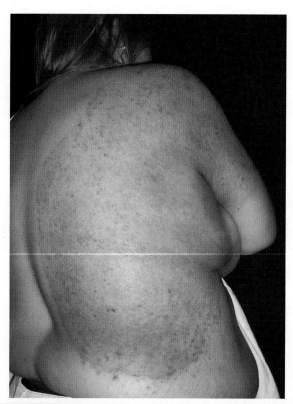

Figure 33-43 Tinea corporis covering half the body. (© Richard P. Usatine.)

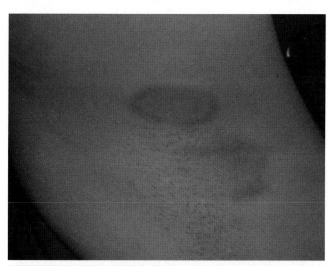

Figure 33-42 Tinea corporis showing concentric circles. (© Richard P. Usatine.)

- All topical antifungal agents (not nystatin) may be effective, but evidence supports the greater effectiveness of the allylamines (e.g., terbinafine) over the less expensive azoles (e.g., clotrimazole) for tinea pedis and corporis (Crawford et al., 2000) (SOR: A).
- Terbinafine 1% cream or solution once daily for 7 days is highly effective for tinea corporis or cruris (Budimulja et al., 2001) (SOR: B).
- Oral terbinafine, 250 mg once daily, showed higher cure rates for tinea corporis and cruris than griseofulvin (Voravutinon, 1993) (SOR: B).

Tinea Pedis

Tinea pedis, or "athlete's foot," is most often caused by *Trichophyton rubrum*. Typically, patients describe pruritic scaly soles, often with painful fissures between the toes. The most characteristic type of infection is interdigital (Figure 33-44). Erythema, maceration, and fissuring occur between the toes and are accompanied by intense pruritus. Patients may also have chronic hyperkeratotic tinea pedis, characterized by plantar erythema and hyperkeratosis (dry-looking scaly feet) that may be completely asymptomatic or mildly pruritic. This is described as a moccasin distribution (Figure 33-45). Inflammatory tinea pedis causes painful vesicles on the foot (see Figure 33-1).

Tinea pedis is more common in men than in women and rarely occurs in children. Infection can occur through contact with infected scales on bath or pool floors, so wearing protective footwear in shared areas may help

therapy is usually sufficient for localized cases. A topical antifungal should be applied to the lesion and proximal surrounding skin twice daily for a minimum of 2 weeks. Various agents have demonstrated effectiveness, including the azoles (miconazole, clotrimazole, ketoconazole, itraconazole) and the allylamines (naftifine, terbinafine). Terbinafine 1% cream (available OTC as Lamisil AF) produced a mycologic cure of 84.2%, versus 23.3% with placebo (Budimulja et al., 2001). In another study, patients with mycologically diagnosed tinea corporis and tinea cruris were randomly allocated to receive either 250 mg of oral terbinafine once daily or 500 mg of griseofulvin once daily for 2 weeks. The cure rates were higher for terbinafine at 6 weeks (Voravutinon, 1993). Patients should be instructed to avoid direct contact with others and avoid sharing towels and clothing to prevent spread of the infection. Oral antifungal agents should be considered for first-line therapy for tinea corporis covering large areas of the body (Figure 33-43).

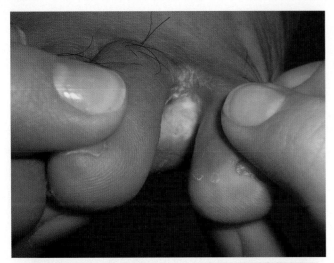

Figure 33-44 Tinea pedis between the toes. (© Richard P. Usatine.)

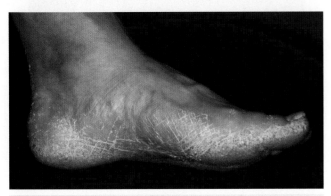

Figure 33-45 Tinea pedis in a moccasin distribution. (© Richard P. Usatine.)

decrease the likelihood of infection. Occlusive footwear promotes infection by creating warm, humid, macerating environments; therefore, patients should try to minimize foot moisture by limiting the use of occlusive footwear and frequently changing socks.

The treatment of tinea pedis involves application of an antifungal cream to the web spaces and other infected areas. Topical antifungal agents containing allylamines (naftifine, terbinafine, butenafine) or azoles (clotrimazole, miconazole, econazole) all work to treat tinea pedis. Allylamines cure slightly more infections than azoles but are more expensive. No differences in efficacy were found between individual allylamines or individual azoles (Crawford et al., 2000) Infrequently, systemic therapy is used for refractory infections. Twice-daily application of the allylamine terbinafine has resulted in a higher and more rapid cure rate than twice-daily application of the imidazole clotrimazole (Lotrimin AF).

KEY TREATMENT

- With topical antifungals to treat tinea pedis, allylamines cure slightly more infections than azoles but are more expensive (Crawford et al., 2000) (SOR: A).

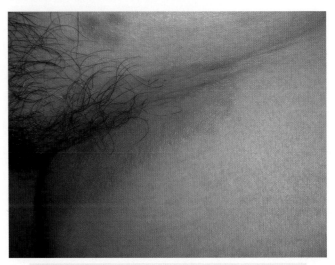

Figure 33-46 Tinea cruris in a woman. (© Richard P. Usatine.)

- Consider oral antifungals such as terbinafine, 250 mg daily for 2 weeks, when tinea pedis is severe or does not respond to topical agents (Bell-Syer et al., 2004) (SOR: B).
- Oral itraconazole is equal to oral terbinafine in patient outcomes. Itraconazole can be prescribed as two 100-mg tablets daily for 1 week (Bell-Syer et al., 2004; Thomas, 2003) (SOR: B).

Tinea Cruris

Tinea cruris, commonly called "jock itch," is a dermatophyte infection of the groin. This dermatophytosis is more common in men than women and is frequently associated with tinea pedis. Tinea cruris occurs when ambient temperature and humidity are high. Occlusion from wet or tight-fitting clothing provides an optimal environment for infection. Tinea cruris involves the proximal medial thighs and may extend to the buttocks and lower abdomen (Figure 33-46). The scrotum tends to be spared. Patients with this dermatophytosis frequently complain of burning and pruritus. Care should be taken to evaluate the feet as a source of infection.

Treatment is identical to tinea pedis with topical antifungals. Oral antifungal therapy is needed if the tinea cruris has spread beyond the groin (Figure 33-47). Inverse psoriasis may be mistaken for tinea cruris but will not respond to antifungal treatment (Figure 33-48). The fungicidal allylamines naftifine and terbinafine and the allylamine derivative butenafine are more costly topical tinea treatments but allow for a shorter duration of treatment compared with fungistatic azoles (clotrimazole, econazole, ketoconazole, oxiconazole, miconazole, sulconazole) (Nadalo et al., 2006).

KEY TREATMENT

- Tinea cruris may be treated with a topical allylamine or a topical azole (Nadalo et al., 2006) (SOR: B).
- Fluconazole, 150 mg once weekly for 2 to 4 weeks, appears effective against tinea cruris (Nozickova et al., 1998) (SOR: B).

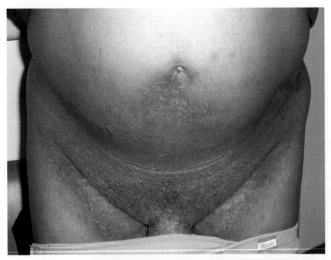

Figure 33-47 Tinea cruris that has spread up to umbilicus. (© Richard P. Usatine.)

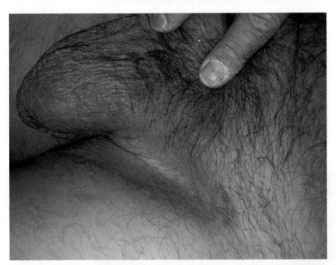

Figure 33-48 Inverse psoriasis that resembles tinea cruris. Note nail pitting of psoriasis. (© Richard P. Usatine.)

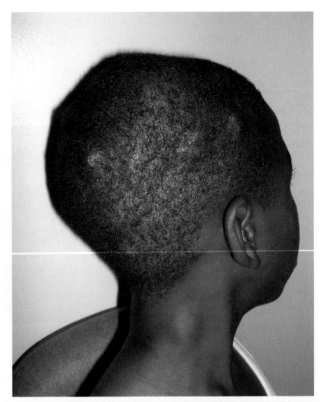

Figure 33-49 Tinea capitis with prominent cervical lymphadenopathy. (© Richard P. Usatine.)

Oral griseofulvin daily for 6 to 8 weeks is a proven treatment for tinea capitis, even if it requires a somewhat longer course than the other antifungal agents (Fleece et al., 2004). It is available in a liquid form for children. Alternatively, 4 weeks of oral terbinafine daily is as effective as 8 weeks of griseofulvin, but at week 12, the efficacy of griseofulvin decreased to 44%, but the efficacy of terbinafine was 76% (Caceres-Rios et al., 2000). Oral fluconazole is another option because it is available in liquid form and appears to be effective and safe, but fewer clinical trials have been done (Foster et al., 2005).

KEY TREATMENT

- Give oral griseofulvin daily for 6 to 8 weeks to treat tinea capitis (Fleece et al., 2004) (SOR: B).
- Consider 4 weeks of oral terbinafine daily (Caceres-Rios et al., 2000) (SOR: B).
- Consider oral fluconazole (available as liquid) as an option to treat tinea capitis (Foster et al., 2005) (SOR: B).

Onychomycosis

Onychomycosis is a fungal infection that affects the toenails or fingernails. It may involve any component of the nail unit, including the nail matrix, nail bed, or nail plate. Onychomycosis may be unsightly but is often asymptomatic. In the worst cases, it causes enough discomfort and disfigurement to produce physical and occupational limitations. Use of topical agents should be limited to cases involving less than half the distal nail plate and patients unable

Tinea Capitis

Tinea capitis, the most common dermatophytosis in children, is an infection of the scalp and hair follicle. Transmission is fostered by poor hygiene and overcrowding and can occur through contaminated hats, brushes, and pillowcases. After being shed, affected hairs can harbor viable organisms for more than 1 year. Tinea capitis is characterized by irregular or well-demarcated alopecia and scaling (Figure 33-49). Cervical and occipital lymphadenopathy may be prominent. When hairs fracture a few millimeters from the scalp, "black dot" alopecia is produced. Tinea scalp infection also may result in a cell-mediated immune response termed a *kerion*, which is a boggy, sterile, inflammatory scalp mass (Figure 33-50). A kerion does not require antibiotics or incision and drainage. If a kerion does not respond to oral antifungals alone, an oral steroid may be added for a short course.

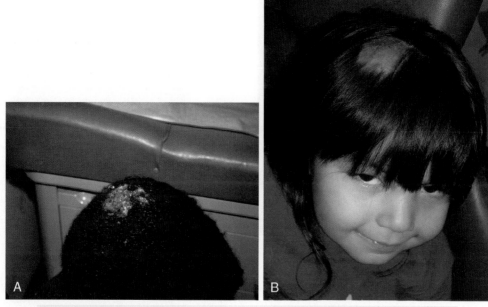

Figure 33-50 Kerions secondary to tinea capitis inflammation (**A** and **B**). (© Richard P. Usatine.)

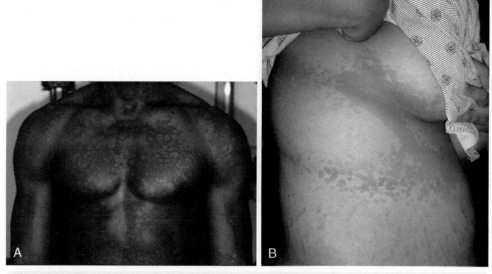

Figure 33-51 Tinea versicolor with hypopigmentation (**A**) and hyperpigmentation (**B**). (© Richard P. Usatine.)

to tolerate systemic treatment. Agents include ciclopirox 8% (Penlac), azoles, and allylamines. Topical treatments are poorly effective because of inadequate nail plate penetration. Oral antifungal agents such as terbinafine and itraconazole have replaced older therapies in the treatment of onychomycosis. Oral antifungals offer shorter treatment regimens, higher cure rates, and fewer adverse effects.

KEY TREATMENT

• Terbinafine is more effective than griseofulvin, and terbinafine and itraconazole are more effective than no treatment (Cochrane review; Bell-Syer et al., 2004) (SOR: A).

• Two clinical trials of nail infections found no evidence of benefit for topical treatments (did not include ciclopirox) compared with placebo (Cochrane review; Crawford et al., 2000) (SOR: A).

Tinea Versicolor

Versicolor means varied colors and tinea versicolor presents with hypopigmented, pink, or brown macules and patches with fine scale (Figure 33-51). Tinea versicolor is also called *pityriasis versicolor* as pityriasis stems from a Greek word meaning "bran," indicating flaking or scaly skin. Tinea versicolor is found on the back, chest, abdomen, and upper arms, often in a capelike distribution. Tinea versicolor is caused by *Malassezia furfur (Pityrosporum)*, a lipophilic

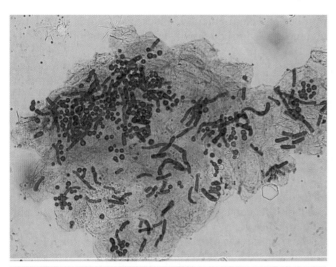

Figure 33-52 "Spaghetti and meatballs" pattern of tinea versicolor on microscopy (blue fungal stain, 40×). (© Richard P. Usatine.)

yeast that can be normal human cutaneous flora. *Pityrosporum* is also associated with seborrhea, and thus antidandruff shampoos are effective in treating this tinea. *Pityrosporum* spp. thrive on sebum and moisture and tend to grow on the skin in areas where sebaceous follicles secrete sebum. Topical and oral treatments are effective, but tinea versicolor tends to recur, especially during the warmer months. The diagnosis can usually be made with the clinical examination, and if there is any doubt, a KOH prep can be examined for the typical "spaghetti and meatballs" pattern (Figure 33-52). The spaghetti or "ziti" is the short mycelial form, and the meatballs are the round yeast of *Pityrosporum ovale*.

Patients may apply selenium sulfide 2.5% lotion or shampoo to the involved areas daily for 1 week. A double-blind study found that selenium sulfide (2.5%) lotion applied daily for 10 minutes for 7 consecutive days was effective in the treatment of tinea versicolor (Sanchez and Torres, 1984). A single oral dose of 400 mg of oral fluconazole or ketoconazole can also be used to treat tinea versicolor. Fluconazole provided the best clinical as well as mycologic cure rate, with no relapse during 12 months of follow-up (Bhogal et al., 2001). Oral itraconazole, 200 mg twice daily for 1 day a month, has been shown to be safe and effective as a prophylactic treatment for tinea versicolor (Faergemann et al., 2002).

KEY TREATMENT

- Selenium sulfide 2.5% lotion (or shampoo) daily for 1 week is effective treatment of tinea versicolor (Sanchez and Torres, 1984) (SOR: B).
- Ketoconazole 2% shampoo (Nizoral) may be applied daily for 3 days to treat tinea versicolor (Lange et al., 1998) (SOR: B).
- Oral fluconazole or ketoconazole (400 mg) also treats tinea versicolor (Bhogal et al., 2001) (SOR: B).
- Oral itraconazole (200 mg twice a day, 1 day a month) is effective prophylactic treatment for tinea versicolor (Faergemann et al., 2002) (SOR: B).

VIRAL INFECTIONS

Key Points

- Herpes simplex virus type 1 (HSV-1) is the most common cause of oral herpes infection (80%). HSV-2 is the primary pathogen in genital herpes (70%-90%). Both can cause oral or genital lesions.
- HSV-1 and HSV-2 are characterized by a primary infection, latent periods, asymptomatic shedding, and reactivation.
- Approximately 10% to 20% of the U.S. population develop zoster, but rates are likely to decrease with varicella-zoster virus (VZV) vaccine for children.
- Corneal involvement should be suspected when herpes zoster involves the tip of the nose and is an ophthalmologic emergency because it can lead to blindness.
- For herpes zoster, antiviral therapy (acyclovir, valacyclovir, famciclovir) should be started within 3 days of onset of symptoms to reduce disease severity and incidence of postherpetic neuralgia.
- Human papillomavirus (HPV) types 6 and 11 are associated with condylomata acuminata (genital warts); HPV types 16 and 18 are associated with carcinoma. The quadrivalent HPV vaccine (Gardasil) is active against HPV types 6, 11, 16, and 18 and is approved for both genders ages 9 to 26 years. The bivalent vaccine (Cervarix) is active against HPV types 16 and 18 and is approved only for girls and women ages 9 to 25 years.
- Molluscum contagiosum is a common, self-limited viral infection most often affecting children. It is considered sexually transmitted in adults.
- Lesions of molluscum usually resolve spontaneously over months to years; with or without treatment, lesions can leave pitted scars.

Herpes Simplex

Herpes simplex virus types 1 and 2 are very common pathogens that cause orolabial and genital blisters and erosions. Seroprevalence of HSV-1 is estimated at 80% to 90% worldwide and is the most common cause of oral herpes infection (80%). HSV-2 is the primary pathogen in genital herpes (70%-90%) and is one of the most common sexually transmitted infections (STIs). Approximately 50 million Americans have genital herpes, and an estimated 1 million new cases occur each year.

Herpes simplex infection can be characterized by an initial infection, episodes of latency, asymptomatic viral shedding, and recurrent activation. Spread of HSV-1 is primarily through direct contact with contaminated saliva or other secretions. Symptoms of primary orolabial herpes usually occur 3 to 7 days after exposure and include a prodrome of fever, sore throat, and lymphadenopathy. Localized pain, tingling, tenderness, or burning can occur before the eruption of the vesicles, which are usually grouped on a background of erythema and edema (Figure 33-53). The lesions coalesce, ulcerate, and heal within 2 to 3 weeks.

Herpes simplex type 2 is usually transmitted through genital contact and must involve mucous membranes or open or damaged skin. Primary HSV-2 occurs up to 3 weeks after exposure to the virus and has more severe clinical

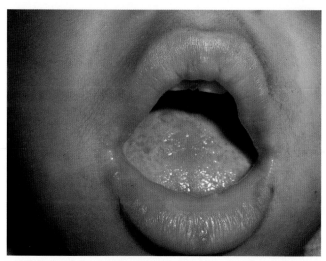

Figure 33-53 Oral herpes gingivostomatitis as primary infection in 2-year-old child. (© Richard P. Usatine.)

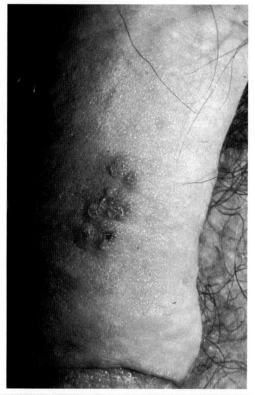

Figure 33-54 Herpes simplex type 2 recurrence on the penis with a cluster of vesicles. (Courtesy Jack Rezneck, Sr., and *The Color Atlas of Family Medicine*.)

manifestations. Systemic symptoms include fever, malaise, edema, inguinal lymphadenopathy, dysuria, and vaginal or penile discharge. These are more common in women. In men, painful vesicles and erosions usually occur on the penis but can also appear on the buttocks or perineum (Figure 33-54). In women, lesions occur primarily on the labia but may also appear on the cervix, buttocks, or perineum. Symptoms of the primary episode typically last 2 to 3 weeks. Risk factors for genital herpes include age 15 to 30 years (the ages of greatest sexually activity), increased

number of sexual partners, black or Hispanic race, lower income levels and education, female gender, homosexuality, and HIV.

In both serotypes, HSV may be latent for months to years after the primary infection. During latency, the virus resides in the sensory nerve root ganglia. Recurrent outbreaks are often preceded by a prodrome of pain, itching, tingling, burning, or paresthesias and are usually less severe than the primary outbreak.

The diagnosis of herpes simplex is conveniently done with a direct fluorescent antibody (DFA) test, and results may be obtained within hours. A viral culture can be performed, but results take 2 to 5 days. Serologic testing is also available that can establish serostatus, but this is not helpful for acute disease.

The treatment of HSV depends on whether the infection is a first episode or a recurrence. Many different dosing schedules are available with oral antivirals, including acyclovir (Zovirax), valacyclovir (Valtrex), and famciclovir (Famvir). Suppressive therapy may be considered in patients with recurrent genital herpes. Women who are pregnant or contemplating pregnancy should receive information regarding neonatal transmission and possible cesarean delivery if active lesions are present at the onset of labor. The risk of transmission is highest for women with a primary infection during the third trimester of pregnancy. Neonatal herpes infection can cause long-term CNS morbidity, such as mental retardation, chorioretinitis, seizures, and even death.

Herpes Zoster (Shingles)

Zoster is caused by the reactivation of the VZV (human herpesvirus 3 [HHV-3], chickenpox). After the primary infection, VZV lies dormant in the dorsal root ganglia. The time between the onset of primary chickenpox and reactivation can be any time, but usually is decades later. Approximately 10% to 20% of the U.S. population eventually develop one or more cases of zoster in their lifetime. The incidence is much higher in immunocompromised patients and older adults. These rates are likely to decrease over time now that a VZV vaccine is given as part of the routine immunization schedule in children.

Patients typically experience pain and paresthesias followed by the appearance of small groups of vesicles on an erythematous base in a dermatomal distribution (Figure 33-55). The rash rarely crosses the midline of the body and is usually confined to a single dermatome. The eruption may be accompanied by a fever, headache, and malaise. Lesions usually resolve in 2 to 3 weeks. Pain can be severe and may persist long after skin lesions heal in a condition known as *postherpetic neuralgia*. Corneal involvement should be suspected when lesions appear on the tip of the nose or in the distribution of cranial nerve V1 (ophthalmic branch of trigeminal nerve) and should prompt an emergency ophthalmology consultation because this can cause permanent blindness (Figure 33-56).

Antiviral therapy such as acyclovir, valacyclovir, and famciclovir should be started within the first 3 days of onset of symptoms to reduce the severity and duration of symptoms and skin lesions. Early treatment may also reduce the incidence and severity of postherpetic neuralgia. However, benefits can be seen even if started up to 7 days after onset

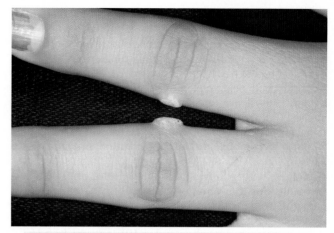

Figure 33-57 Kissing warts on the fingers. (© Richard P. Usatine.)

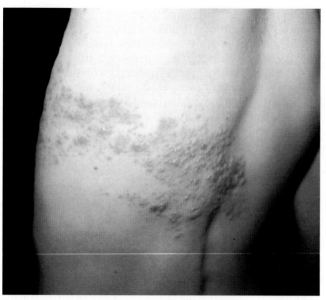

Figure 33-55 Herpes zoster in a dermatomal pattern. (© Richard P. Usatine.)

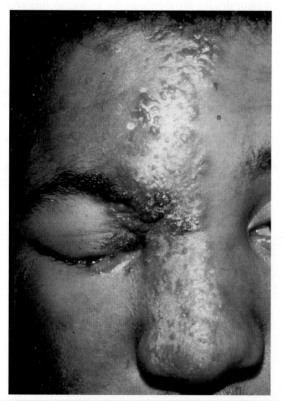

Figure 33-56 Herpes zoster on the face with herpes ophthalmicus. (© Richard P. Usatine.)

of symptoms. Analgesics such as acetaminophen and even narcotics are sometimes required to control the pain caused by zoster. Cool compresses may also help soothe during the acute phase. Postherpetic neuralgia occurs in up to 40% of adult patients older than age 60 years but in less than 10% of patients younger than 60 years. In 2006, the Food and Drug Administration (FDA) approved a live, attenuated vaccine (Zostavax) for adults older than 60 years who are

immunocompetent and have not already had zoster. The vaccine decreased the burden of illness by 61% and decreased the incidence of postherpetic neuralgia by 67% in large clinical trials (Oxman et al., 2005).

Verruca (Warts)

Warts are common growths of skin and mucosa caused by the HPV. Currently, more than 100 types of HPV have been identified. Specific HPV types often correlate to the lesion location, morphology, or oncogenic potential. Although most are benign, warts can be disfiguring or can cause significant psychological distress, and some cause cancer.

Verruca vulgaris (common warts) are dome-shaped keratotic papules that usually develop on the dorsal hands, fingers, or other sites on the extremities (Figure 33-57). *Palmoplantar* warts are on the palms or soles and are surrounded by hyperkeratotic callus-like skin. These can be painful when occurring on weight-bearing surfaces. Multiple plantar warts may combine to become a large mosaic wart. Both common warts and palmoplantar warts have characteristic punctuate black dots, mistakenly leading to the common term "seed warts," but these black dots actually represent thrombosed capillaries. *Filiform* warts have fingerlike projections and often appear on the face. *Verruca plana* (flat warts) are smooth, small (1-4 mm) flesh-colored papules, often occurring on the face or legs and often spread by scratching or shaving (Figure 33-58). Although inconspicuous at first, flat warts propagate rapidly, often into the hundreds.

Condylomata acuminata (genital warts) occur on the external genitalia, perineum, perianal, or adjacent intertriginous regions but can also be found on the oral mucosa. These lesions are generally considered sexually transmitted, but it is usually impossible to determine when the inoculation occurred. The lesions begin as small papules, which often become whitish with maceration and take on a cauliflower-like appearance as they grow (Figure 33-59). Condylomata are associated with cervical carcinoma and penile cancer. Among the many subtypes of HPV, types 6 and 11 are most often associated with condylomata, but types 16 and 18 are most often associated with the development of carcinoma.

There is no standard treatment for warts. Most warts spontaneously regress over many months to years. Local treatments include cryotherapy, salicylic acid, imiquimod, podophyllin, 5-fluorouracil (5-FU), cantharidin, and duct tape. For physician-applied treatments such as cryotherapy or podophyllotoxin, patients should be seen every 3 to 4 weeks for repeat treatment as needed. For home treatments with salicylic acid, podofilox (Condylox), or imiquimod (Aldara), most are applied daily, and patients should be advised that treatment can take months of extreme persistence for resolution. Office and home treatment modalities can also be combined to hasten resolution, but studies are lacking.

Women with condylomata should have annual Papanicolaou tests to evaluate for cervical neoplasia. For both men and women, it is advisable to refrain from sexual activity while genital lesions are present, to prevent transmission. In 2006, the FDA approved an HPV vaccine (Gardasil),

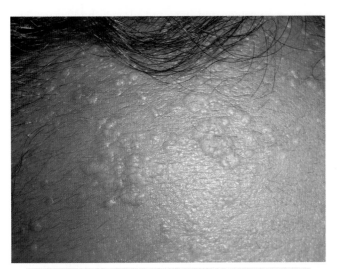

Figure 33-58 Flat warts on the forehead. (© Richard P. Usatine.)

recommended for girls and women age 11 to 26 years regardless of abnormal Pap history, positive HPV status, or genital warts. It is active against HPV types 6, 11, 16, and 18. In clinical trials, Gardasil decreased the incidence of cervical intraepithelial neoplasia, cervical cancer, and anogenital warts by 90% (Villa et al., 2006). Since it was first released, the indications have now been expanded to include both genders ages 9 to 26 years.

Molluscum Contagiosum

Molluscum contagiosum is a common, self-limited viral infection seen most frequently in children and can occur anywhere on the body, most often on the trunk, face, and extremities. In adults, mollusca are considered sexually transmitted and occur in the genital region or lower abdomen. Infection occurs through direct skin-to-skin contact or indirect contact with fomites. The typical molluscum lesion is a pink to flesh-colored, firm, smooth, dome-shaped papule with central umbilication (Figure 33-60). A white material can sometimes be visualized in the umbilication and can be easily expressed. This caseous material is teeming with viral particles. Lesions are usually 2 to 5 mm in diameter and number less than 30 but can number in the hundreds. Particularly in immunocompromised patients, the infection may be much more extensive, may fail to resolve spontaneously, and may be resistant to treatment. Over months to years, lesions of molluscum normally resolve spontaneously.

Some patients or parents desire treatment, and cryotherapy, cantharidin, trichloroacetic acid, tretinoin (Retin-A), or imiquimod may be effective. Cantharidin is most easily given to young children because its application is painless. Cryotherapy is another good option, but many young children will not willingly submit to this therapy, which is painful. Often it is best to reassure parents that molluscum is not harmful and will eventually resolve, although with or without treatment, lesions can leave pitted scars.

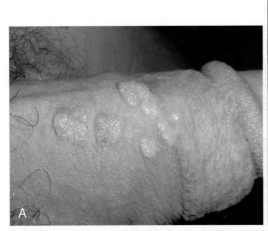

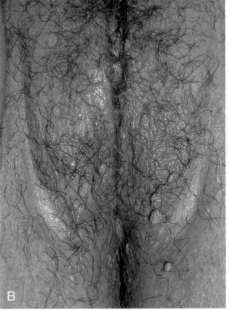

Figure 33-59 A, Condyloma acuminata on penis. **B,** Condyloma acuminata on the vulva. (© Richard P. Usatine.)

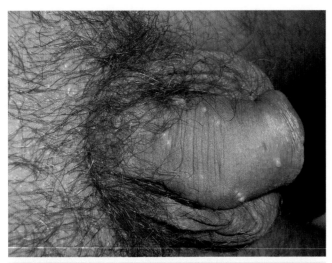

Figure 33-60 Molluscum contagiosum on the penis as a sexually transmitted disease. (© Richard P. Usatine.)

Infestations

Key Points

- Scabies is a pruritic rash involving interdigital spaces, wrists, ankles, waist, groin, and axillae.
- The three types of human lice infest the scalp hair, the body, or the pubic hair.

SCABIES

Scabies is caused by the mite *Sarcoptes scabiei,* an obligate human parasite. Patients present with a pruritic rash that is often worse in the night. Skin findings include papules, nodules, burrows, and vesiculopustules (Figure 33-61). The distribution includes the interdigital spaces, wrists, ankles, waist, groin, and axillae. Pruritic nodules around the axillae, umbilicus, or on the penis and scrotum are highly suggestive of scabies. In children, the head can also be involved. Look for burrows because these are pathognomonic of scabies and will be the best site to find mites.

For the most part, scabies is a clinical diagnosis based on the typical rash and the history. It is often helpful if other family members have pruritus and a similar rash. In cases in which the diagnosis is in question or there appears to be multiple recurrences, the scraping is worthwhile to confirm the clinical impression. A dermatoscope or magnifying lens can be used to look for the small arrowhead-appearing mite at the end of a burrow. Scraping of active lesions can yield the identification of mites, eggs, or feces under the microscope (KOH or mineral oil can be used on the slide) (Figure 33-62).

Crusted (Norwegian) scabies is a highly contagious form with a propensity for older adults and immunocompromised or physically debilitated patients (Figure 33-63). Widespread, crusted lesions appear with thick, hyperkeratotic scales over the elbows, knees, palms, and soles. Infections may occur with thousands of mites at a time and can be especially problematic in nursing homes or assisted-living environments. Ivermectin is an oral treatment for

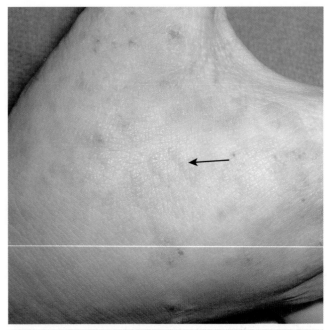

Figure 33-61 Scabies with a visible burrow *(arrow).* (© Richard P. Usatine.)

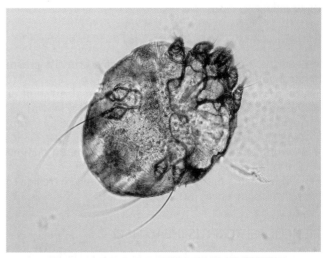

Figure 33-62 Scabies mite (40×). (© Richard P. Usatine.)

resistant or crusted scabies with demonstrated safety and efficacy. Most studies used a single dose of ivermectin at 200 µg/kg (Strong and Johnstone, 2007).

Permethrin cream is applied from the neck down (including the head when involved) and rinsed off 8 to 14 hours later. Usually this is done overnight. Repeating the treatment in 1 to 2 weeks increases the cure rate. Unfortunately, scabies resistance to permethrin is increasing. Antihistamines and midpotency steroid creams can be used for symptomatic relief of itching. It is important to note that pruritus may persist for weeks or months after successful treatment because the dead mites and eggs still have antigenic qualities that may cause persistent inflammation. Environmental decontamination is a standard component of all therapies. Clothing, bed linens, and towels should be machine-washed in hot water. Clothing or other items (e.g., stuffed animals) that cannot be washed may be

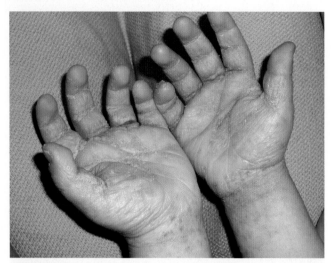

Figure 33-63 Crusted scabies on the hands of a 2-year-old child. (© Richard P. Usatine.)

dry cleaned, heated in hot dryer for 15 minutes, or stored in sealed bags for 1 month. All household or family members living in the infested home should be treated. Failure to treat all involved individuals often results in recurrences within the family.

KEY TREATMENT

- Begin treatment of scabies with permethrin 5% cream (Strong and Johnstone, 2007) (SOR: A).
- Oral ivermectin (200 μg/kg) is used to treat resistant or crusted scabies. (Strong and Johnstone, 2007) (SOR: A).
- Antihistamines and steroid creams can be used for symptomatic relief of itching (SOR: C).
- Environmental decontamination is a standard component of all scabies therapy (SOR: C).
- All those living in the infested home should be treated to prevent recurrences (SOR: C).

PEDICULOSIS CAPITIS (HEAD LICE)

Lice are obligate human parasites transmitted by person-to-person contact. Infestations are increasing in frequency because of the development of resistance to current treatments. The infestation is usually detected because of intense itching and the presence of eggs or nits adherent to the hair shaft (Figure 33-64). After the nit is attached to the hair shaft, the head louse develops over 3 to 4 days. Within 12 days of hatching, the nymph becomes a sexually mature adult capable of reproducing. After a single fertilization, each female lays up to 10 eggs a day during her 30-day life span. Typically, infestation occurs over a 2-week period, resulting in an allergic reaction to the louse saliva, causing the pruritus. Without frequent blood meals from the host, lice survive only 15 to 20 hours.

Detection of a single live louse is sufficient for diagnosis of infestation. Nits should be examined for viable embryo, which will show some movement under magnification. Because of the route of transmission, outbreaks are often seen in daycare centers, classrooms, and homeless shelters.

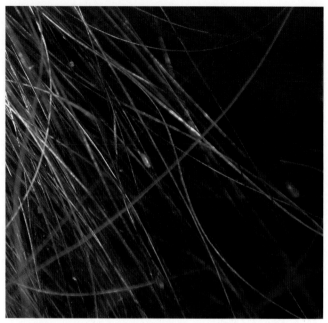

Figure 33-64 Pearly nits of head lice. (© Richard P. Usatine.)

Effective eradication of pediculosis often requires two treatments given 7 to 10 days apart. Several OTC preparations are available, including 4% piperonyl butoxide with 0.33% pyrethrins (RID, Pronto, A-200) and permethrin (Nix). Malathion is available by prescription for treatment of resistant strains but should not be used in infants or children younger than 6 years. Instructions for use must be followed carefully, including treatment of all household contacts. Removal of all nits is not necessary after eradication but can be done with a fine-toothed comb if desired. Schools often require no visible nits before permitting children to return to classes. Use of a 50% vinegar and water rinse after shampooing may help reduce adherence of nits to the hair shaft.

Bedding and clothing should be washed in the hottest water possible or dry cleaned. Combs, barrettes, and hair ornaments may be soaked in hot water for 10 minutes. Items that cannot be otherwise cleaned, such as stuffed animals and decorative pillows, can be sealed in plastic bags for 2 weeks.

KEY TREATMENT

- Pediculicides effective in the treatment of head lice include 1% permethrin cream rinse, pyrethrins with piperonyl butoxide shampoo, and malathion cream; no evidence shows one is better than another (Cochrane review; Dodd, 2006) (SOR: A).

PEDICULOSIS CORPORIS (BODY LICE)

Body lice are most frequently seen in patients who live in environments that prevent regular changing of clothing and bedding, such as homeless people. Diagnosis should be suspected in patients with generalized itching and excoriations and poor hygiene. Body lice are more likely to be found in the seams of clothing than on the patient (Figure 33-65).

Initial treatment of body lice entails washing the entire body surface and wearing clean clothing. In severe infestations, topical use of permethrin, pyrethrin, or malathion may be indicated. Again, clothing and bedding should be washed in hot water or dry cleaned. As an alternative to topical treatment, ivermectin may be given orally.

PHTHIRUS PUBIS (PUBIC LICE, CRAB LICE)

Pubic lice are sexually transmitted and may be transmitted through clothing and towels. Treatment is the same as for head lice and should include any sexual contacts. Additionally, the presence of pubic lice should prompt consideration of other STIs.

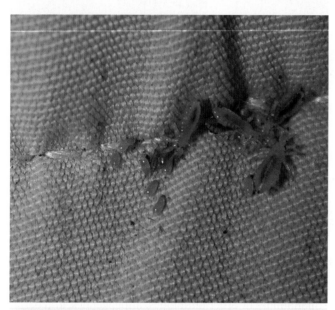

Figure 33-65 Body lice on the seams of clothing. (© Richard P. Usatine.)

Hypersensitivity Reactions and Other Eruptions

Key Points

- Morbilliform drug reactions occur 1 to 2 weeks after initial exposure but occur much quicker (1-3 days) on repeat exposure.
- Urticaria can be acute or chronic and is triggered by drugs, infections, arthropods, autoimmune disease, food, and even emotional stress.
- The mainstay of therapy for urticaria is avoidance of known triggers and antihistamines.
- Oral corticosteroids for urticaria should be limited to short-term therapy of severe episodes.
- Erythema multiforme (EM) is a reaction pattern secondary to a variety of etiologic agents and characterized by distinctive target lesions.
- Half of EM cases are caused by HSV; drugs and other infections are also common causes.
- Stevens-Johnson syndrome (SJS) and toxic epidermal necrolysis (TEN) typically occur 7 to 21 days after starting NSAIDS, antibiotics, or antiepileptics.

"MORBILLIFORM" (MACULOPAPULAR, EXANTHEM-LIKE) REACTION

Morbilliform eruption is by far the most common type of drug eruption, reported in response to almost every drug. Small pink to red papules and macules usually start on the face or upper chest and can extend to limbs, resembling measles (Figure 33-66). The rash may be relatively asymptomatic or extremely pruritic. The typical course begins 7 to 14 days after drug initiation if the first exposure. On reexposure to the same medicine, the eruption will occur much more quickly, within 1 to 3 days. A maculopapular

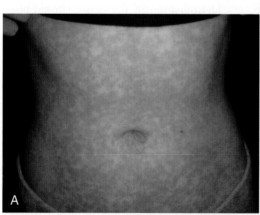
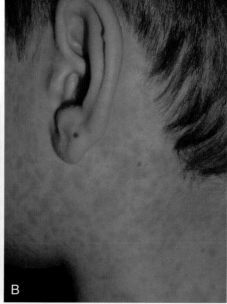

Figure 33-66 A, Amoxicillin drug eruption in a young woman with mononucleosis. **B,** Amoxicillin rash in a child with otitis media. (© Richard P. Usatine.)

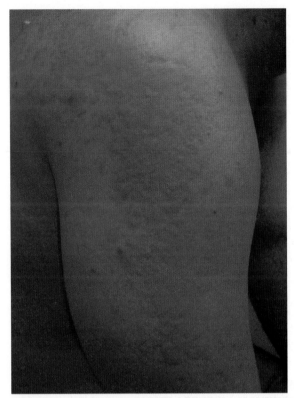

Figure 33-67 Urticarial drug eruption secondary to trimethoprim–sulfamethoxazole therapy. (© Richard P. Usatine.)

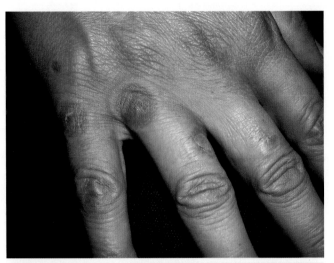

Figure 33-68 Erythema multiforme secondary to recurrent genital herpes simplex. (© Richard P. Usatine.)

reaction is not generally life threatening and does not proceed to anaphylaxis; therefore, when no alternative drug is available, the offending agent can be continued. The eruption can be treated symptomatically with antihistamines and midpotency topical corticosteroids.

URTICARIA

Urticaria, commonly known as "hives," can be acute or chronic, and the numerous triggers include drugs, food, infections, arthropods, autoimmune disease, and stress. The wheals consist of circumscribed areas of raised erythematous plaques that are often annular and very pruritic (Figure 33-67). These wheals can occur on any skin area and are transient and migratory. The acute form of urticaria lasts less than 4 to 6 weeks, and the chronic form lasts more than 6 weeks. When there is an obvious new drug causing the eruption, the causation is easy to determine.

For patients taking multiple medications who have no evidence of infection or illness, the diagnosis can be very difficult. Skin prick testing or radioallergosorbent assay testing (RAST), typically done through an allergy specialist, may help determine the cause but may be elusive. Patients with chronic urticaria unresponsive to antihistamines require an extensive workup. In more than 50% of cases of chronic urticaria, no etiology is found, and it is considered idiopathic or chronic "autoimmune" urticaria.

The mainstay of therapy for urticaria is avoidance of known triggering agents and antihistamines. Classic antihistamines are effective (diphenhydramine, hydroxyzine, doxepin), but sedation limits their use to primarily nighttime dosing. Second- and third-generation antihistamines

are helpful for daytime use, and dose escalation up to four times the normal daily dose may be necessary (cetirizine, loratadine, fexofenadine, desloratadine, levocetirizine). Oral corticosteroids are useful but should be limited to short-term therapy of severe acute urticaria. H_2-receptor antagonists (cimetidine, ranitidine, famotidine) and leukotriene antagonists are sometimes helpful as adjunctive therapy.

ERYTHEMA MULTIFORME

Erythema multiforme is a reaction pattern secondary to a variety of etiologic agents characterized by distinctive target lesions. About 50% of cases of EM are caused by infections, most often HSV and *Mycoplasma pneumoniae* (Figure 33-68). The other 50% are caused by drugs, most often NSAIDs, sulfonamides or other antibiotics, antiepileptics, and barbiturates. A small number of cases are due to foods and other allergens, immunologic or connective tissue disease, malignancy, and hormones.

Lesions begin as dull-red macules or urticarial plaques on the palms, soles, or extensor surfaces of the extremities and tend to expand in size. A small papule, vesicle, or bulla develops in the center with concentric rings forming around the blister. The center of the lesion becomes dusky or violaceous from necrosis of the epidermis. Most EM cases spontaneously subside within 3 weeks without sequelae.

Identification of the cause should be made, if possible. Patient should be queried for prescription and OTC medications and history of HSV. A thorough examination should be performed, looking for oral or genital ulcers with Tzanck prep or DFA test for HSV. Cultures of the skin, nose, throat, and conjunctiva are indicated to evaluate for infections and treated appropriately.

STEVENS-JOHNSON SYNDROME AND TOXIC EPIDERMAL NECROLYSIS

Both SJS and TEN are rare, severe, life-threatening reactions that are almost always drug related. The most common offending medications are NSAIDS, antibiotics, and antiseizure medications. SJS or TEN typically occurs 7 to 21 days after the start of the medication.

Stevens-Johnson syndrome often presents with a prodrome of fever, painful swallowing, stinging eyes, and *painful* skin. Two or more mucosal surfaces eventually become involved (conjunctiva, oral mucosa, genitalia) with vesicles, bullae, erosions, or hemorrhagic crusts. Skin lesions usually begin as dusky purpuric macules that progress to bullae or erosions on the trunk and spread centrifugally. *Targetoid lesions,* similar to EM, may also be present. By definition, less than 10% body surface area (BSA) is involved in SJS. A similar presentation occurs in TEN, but the bullae and erosions involve greater than 30% BSA. Also, the skin that initially appears normal may easily slide off with gentle tangential pressure (the Nikolsky sign), leaving more denuded skin. When skin and mucosal involvement is 10% to 30% BSA, it is considered a SJS–TEN overlap.

Both SJS and TEN can be fatal; the mortality rate is 1% to 5% for SJS and 25% to 35% for TEN, but it may be even higher in elderly patients or those with comorbidities. Above all, removal of the offending agent is paramount. Most patients are treated in a burn unit because the skin is necrotic and no longer functioning as a barrier. Care is supportive and aimed at regulation of fluids, electrolytes, protein, temperature, and prevention of infection. Neither systemic steroids nor intravenous immune globulin demonstrate consistent clinical efficacy in clinical studies, which are limited because of the rarity of SJS and TEN.

Skin Signs of Systemic Disease

LUPUS ERYTHEMATOSUS

Key Points

- Lupus erythematosus (LE) is an autoimmune disease of connective tissue that may be limited to the skin (cutaneous lupus), or the skin findings may indicate systemic disease.
- All LE variants are photosensitive, and primary treatment should include education in sun protection and avoidance.

Lupus erythematosus is an autoimmune disease of connective tissue that has frequent dermatologic manifestations. LE may be limited to the skin, or the skin findings may indicate systemic disease. For dermatologic purposes, there are three main variants:

1. *Acute cutaneous* (ACLE): exemplified by the malar rash, usually associated with systemic disease and positive antinuclear antibodies (Figure 33-69)
2. *Subacute cutaneous* (SCLE): characteristic photosensitive papulosquamous annular lesions of the trunk and arms, associated with anti-Ro antibodies (70%); up to 25% will have systemic involvement (Figure 33-70)
3. *Discoid* (DLE): inflammation involves deeper adnexal structures, with predilection for head and neck; results in scarring; fewer than 10% have systemic involvement (Figure 33-71)

Acute cutaneous LE presents as the classic "butterfly rash" and tends to follow sun exposure. Erythema and

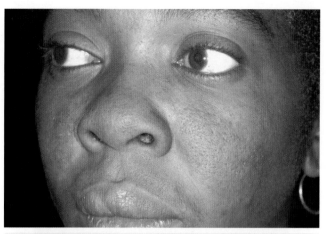

Figure 33-69 Systemic lupus erythematosus and with malar rash. (© Richard P. Usatine.)

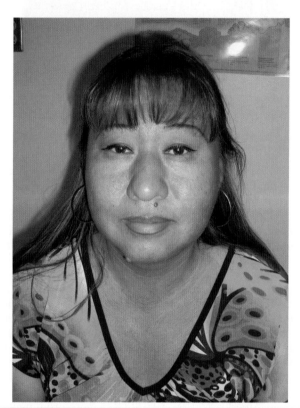

Figure 33-70 Subacute cutaneous lupus erythematosus in sun-exposed areas. (© Richard P. Usatine.)

edema may be mild to severe. The presence of *poikiloderma* (patches of hypopigmentation, hyperpigmentation, telangiectasias, and epidermal atrophy) may help to differentiate the malar rash of lupus from other skin diseases of the midface, such as rosacea or seborrheic dermatitis, which are not poikilodermatous. There is sparing of the nasolabial folds and the skin under the nose and upper lip, areas that are shaded from the sun.

Lesions of SCLE are very photosensitive and appear as annular, scaly, erythematous patches or papulosquamous rings with central clearing. These usually affect the lateral face (instead of central face), upper chest, arms, and shoulders, areas that are sun exposed. Discoid lesions are

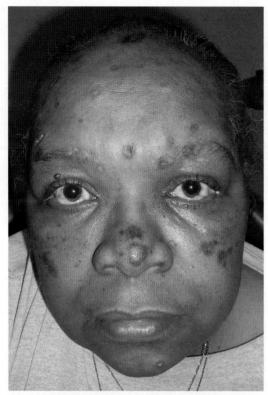

Figure 33-71 Discoid lupus with hyperpigmentation atrophy and scarring. (© Richard P. Usatine.)

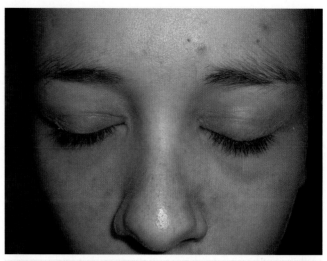

Figure 33-72 Heliotrope rash of dermatomyositis. (© Richard P. Usatine.)

somewhat photosensitive but also found on nonexposed skin and mucosal surfaces. Most often these present on the ears, face, and neck and appear as scaly, brightly erythematous to violaceous plaques. Because of the deeper involvement of inflammation, as DLE lesions resolve, they often leave behind hyper- or hypopigmentation, even depigmentation. Severe scarring, alopecia, and disfigurement may also occur. ACLE, or systemic lupus erythematosus (SLE), is more common in women, especially of childbearing age (female : male ratio, 6-10 : 1), suggesting a hormonal factor in susceptibility. The female : male ratio for patients with only cutaneous forms of lupus is much lower (3-4 : 1 for SCLE; 2 : 1 for DLE). The prevalence of ACLE and SLE is also fourfold higher in African American women than white American women, and DLE is slightly more common in African Americans. However, SCLE is more prominent in whites (80%).

Occasionally, drugs can induce ACLE or SCLE. Whereas procainamide, hydralazine, isoniazid, quinidine, and phenytoin are most frequently reported for ACLE, hydrochlorothiazide, calcium channel blockers (diltiazem), angiotensin-converting enzyme inhibitors, terbinafine, NSAIDs, griseofulvin, and tumor necrosis factor antagonists are most frequently reported for SCLE. Drug-induced ACLE usually fades after the drug is discontinued but may take many months. Drug-induced SCLE may or may not clear with cessation of the drug.

For skin lesions of lupus, sun protection and sun avoidance are crucial because all types are photosensitive. Although discoid lesions are not as photosensitive as the other variants, some patients with ACLE, SLE, or SCLE can even be triggered by indoor light. Topical corticosteroids and calcineurin inhibitors (pimecrolimus, tacrolimus) are the mainstay in treatment of skin lesions. If oral medications are required to control skin disease, antimalarials (most often hydroxychloroquine) are first-line therapy.

DERMATOMYOSITIS

Key Points

- Dermatomyositis is an autoimmune disease of unclear etiology but sometimes triggered by malignancy, drugs, or infection.
- High-dose corticosteroids with a slow taper over 2 to 4 years are the primary treatment, and muscle disease usually responds more rapidly than skin disease.

Dermatomyositis is presumably an autoimmune disease that is triggered by an outside factor. Antinuclear antibodies or anticytoplasmic antibodies (antisynthetase) are found in up to 95% of patients. Clinically, dermatomyositis is characterized by a symmetric proximal inflammatory myopathy and distinct skin lesions. Proximal muscle weakness may precede the skin findings, may follow them, or may be absent ("dermatomyositis sine myositis"). Classic cutaneous lesions include the *heliotrope rash*, pink to lilac, poikilodermatous or edematous patches of the periocular skin (Figure 33-72). The *shawl sign* consists of poikiloderma of the upper chest, shoulders, and upper back. Gottron papules are erythematous, scaly or lichenified papules or plaques over the knuckles. Similar plaques may be seen on the elbows, mimicking psoriasis. Other common cutaneous findings are periungual telangiectasias (visible dilated capillary loops) and ragged cuticles (cuticular dystrophy).

Although the etiology of dermatomyositis is unknown, triggers may include malignancy, drugs, and infection. In adults with dermatomyositis, studies report a wide range of association with internal malignancy (10%-50%). Common malignancies include genitourinary, ovarian, colon, breast, lung, pancreatic, and lymphoma. The same association is not found in juvenile cases of dermatomyositis. Therefore, any adult with a new diagnosis of dermatomyositis should be screened with a chest, abdominal, and pelvic computed tomography with close surveillance for 2 to 3 years.

Double-blind, placebo-controlled trials are lacking for this rare disease, but the mainstay of treatment for dermatomyositis is high-dose corticosteroids with slow taper over 2 to 4 years. Other immunosuppressants used include methotrexate, azathioprine, cyclophosphamide, and cyclosporine. In general, the myopathy responds more rapidly and easily than the skin lesions, and severe pruritus can persist long after muscle disease is controlled. For skin lesions, sun protections, topical corticosteroids, or antimalarials may help.

SARCOIDOSIS

Sarcoidosis is a systemic granulomatous disease of unknown etiology that most often involves the lungs (90%). The skin is involved in about one third of patients with systemic sarcoidosis. In the United States, women and African Americans are more frequently affected. As with syphilis, sarcoidosis is considered a "great imitator" because it has widely variable presentations and may involve almost any organ system.

Classic skin lesions of sarcoidosis are red-brown, nonscaly papules and plaques appearing on the face, especially around the nose or mouth (Figure 33-73). The color can vary significantly from yellow to red to brown, and lesions also occur on the trunk or extremities and tend to be symmetric. Lesions on the alar rim of the nose, also known as *lupus pernio*, are highly associated with granulomatous infiltration of the upper airway. Patients with cutaneous sarcoidosis should have a complete evaluation for systemic disease, including history and physical examination, renal and hepatic function testing, chest radiography, pulmonary function tests, electrocardiography, and ophthalmologic evaluation.

Lesions of cutaneous sarcoidosis are difficult to treat and tend to recur. The most effective therapy is intralesional injection of corticosteroids repeated at 2- to 4-week intervals. Topical corticosteroids are often ineffective because they do not penetrate the skin lesions adequately. Systemic corticosteroids are effective in treating lesions that are widespread or impairing function. In especially difficult cases, agents such as hydroxychloroquine or methotrexate may be used.

Benign Growths

Key Points

- The most important reason to be able to recognize benign skin growths is to differentiate them from skin cancers.
- Seborrheic keratoses (SKs), epidermal cysts, and dermatofibromas can be surgically excised if they are suspicious for cancer or causing symptoms.
- Pyogenic granulomas bleed easily and should be excised and sent for pathology to rule out amelanotic melanoma.
- SKs and dermatofibromas have characteristic patterns with dermoscopy that can help guide the need for a biopsy.

SEBORRHEIC KERATOSIS

Seborrheic keratoses are hyperkeratotic lesions of the epidermis that often appear to be stuck on the surface of the skin (Figure 33-74). SKs usually have a discrete border and vary in color from pink or tan to brown, gray, or even black. Most lesions have a rough surface and usually range from 2 mm to 3 cm in diameter but can be larger. SK may start as a hyperpigmented macule and progress to the characteristic plaque. The trunk is the most common site, but the lesions can be found on the extremities, face, and scalp.

The incidence of SK increases with age in men and women. *Stucco keratoses,* a variant of SK, are many skin-colored or white, dry scaly lesions often seen on the arms and legs. *Dermatosis papulosa nigra* is another type of SK consisting of many small, brown or black papules on the faces of patients with highly pigmented skin.

Differentiating between SK and melanomas can be a challenge, especially in patients with numerous lesions. Both have varying dark colors, the potential for large size, and irregularity. SKs have a rough surface, and the keratin can have horn cysts or look cerebriform. The best way to differentiate a SK from a melanoma is with a dermatoscope. This special magnifying light can distinguish specific characteristics of the keratosis with higher specificity than with the naked eye. These characteristics are comedo-like openings and milia-like cysts (see Figure 33-74).

Some patients want their SKs treated for cosmetic reasons or to decrease irritation from abrasion on clothing.

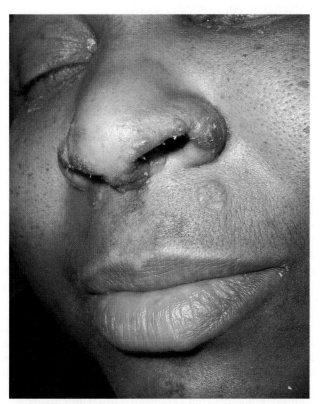

Figure 33-73 Cutaneous sarcoidosis. (© Richard P. Usatine.)

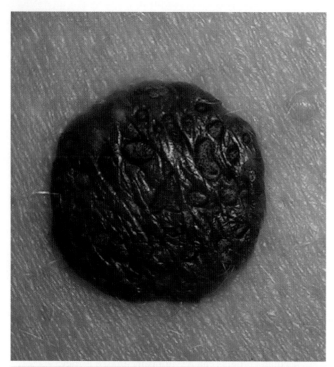

Figure 33-74 Seborrheic keratosis with horn cysts (comedo-like openings). (© Richard P. Usatine.)

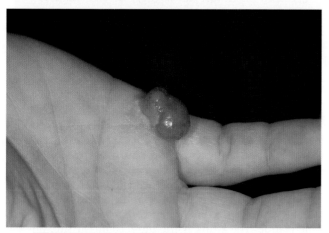

Figure 33-75 Pyogenic granuloma. (© Richard P. Usatine.)

Cryosurgery, curettage, and shave excision are the most frequently used methods of removal. Cryotherapy with liquid nitrogen is effective for most SKs, except for extremely thick lesions. Repeat treatments may be necessary. Curettage can be performed with or without electrocautery after administration of local anesthesia. Excisional biopsy should be used to remove lesions suspicious for melanoma.

PYOGENIC GRANULOMA

Pyogenic granulomas (lobulated capillary hemangiomas) are benign vascular lesions that occur most often in young adults and children (Figure 33-75). These rapidly growing hemangiomas may start at sites of trauma. Treatment is surgical removal. Pyogenic granulomas do not have malignant potential, but it is important to send the tissue for pathology to rule out an amelanotic melanoma. Lesions

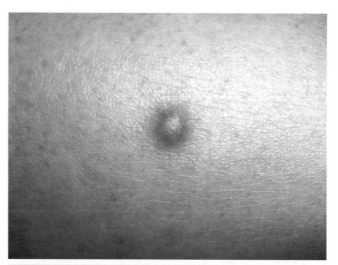

Figure 33-76 Dermatofibroma on the leg with a hyperpigmented halo. (© Richard P. Usatine.)

most commonly occur on areas of trauma or friction such as the fingers, head, neck, and extremities and on mucous membranes. Pyogenic granulomas frequently occur on the gingiva during pregnancy and regress spontaneously after childbirth. Patients usually are acutely concerned that the lesion has grown quickly and bleeds easily with little or no trauma.

Removal can be accomplished with shave excision and then curettage and electrodesiccation of the base to reduce chances of recurrence. Alternatively, the whole lesion can be cut out down to subcutaneous fat. Pyogenic granulomas will recur if any residual tissue remains after excision.

EPIDERMAL INCLUSION CYSTS

Epidermal inclusion cysts, also known as *sebaceous cysts,* are filled with keratin and lined with stratified squamous epithelium. Epidermal cysts usually occur on the back, face, and chest and open to the skin through a small, central punctum or keratin-filled plug. The cysts may remain small for years or may grow rapidly. Rupture of the cyst wall into the dermis initiates an inflammatory response.

Acutely inflamed, fluctuant cysts should be incised and drained. However, unless the cyst wall is removed or destroyed, there is a high risk of cyst recurrence. Alternately, the cyst may be removed intact by excision and blunt dissection. Complete drainage is enhanced with gauze packing, which is changed frequently during wound healing. The use of antibiotics is unnecessary unless a concurrent cellulitis exists. If a patient requests removal of an epidermal cyst before an acute inflammatory event, the cyst wall can be more easily shelled out, minimizing the risk of recurrence.

DERMATOFIBROMA

Dermatofibromas (benign fibrous histiocytomas) are most likely fibrous reactions to minor trauma, insect bites, viral infections, ruptured cysts, or folliculitis. The nodules can be found anywhere on the body but most often appear on the legs and arms. Dermatofibromas are firm, raised papules, plaques, or nodules that vary from 3 to 10 mm in diameter (Figure 33-76). Dermatofibromas have a central fibrous

it is important to limit removal of unaffected skin. It is also useful for poorly defined or recurrent head and neck BD (Cox et al., 2007). Excision should be an effective treatment with low recurrence rates, but the limited evidence cannot address specific lesion sites (Cox et al., 2007).

The overall risk of progression of BD to invasive cancer is about 3% to 5%. However, the risk is greater for patients with oral and genital lesions (≈10%), as well as those with a history of arsenic exposure or lesions located in a chronic scar or ulcer.

KEY TREATMENT

- Curettage and electrodesiccation may be superior to cryotherapy in treating BD, especially for lesions on the lower leg (Ahmed et al., 2000) (SOR: A).
- Use of 5-FU is more practical than surgery for large BD lesions, especially at potentially poor healing sites (Cox et al., 2007) (SOR: B).
- Imiquimod effectively clears BD lesions in most patients (Patel et al., 2006) (SOR: B).
- Mohs surgery is recommended for BD at the digits or penis and is useful for poorly defined or recurrent head and neck BD (Cox et al., 2007) (SOR: B).

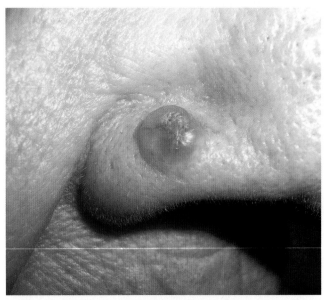

Figure 33-80 Nodular basal cell carcinoma on nasal ala. (© Richard P. Usatine.)

BASAL CELL CARCINOMA

Basal cell carcinoma is the most common human malignancy. In the United States, BCC affects almost 3 million people per year, and this estimate is likely low because no national registry exists for nonmelanoma skin cancers. BCC typically appears in areas of sun-exposed skin, is usually slow growing, and rarely metastasizes. The prognosis is excellent with proper therapy, but BCC can cause significant local destruction and disfigurement if neglected. The estimated lifetime risk in whites is approximately one in five, but it increases to one in three in those older than age 65 years living in southern latitudes. The incidence is extremely low in those with highly pigmented skin. Organ transplant recipients have a five to 10 times greater risk of BCC.

Patients often present with a nonhealing sore on the face, ears, scalp, neck, or upper trunk. The most common type of BCC is *nodular*, which is usually a pink papule or nodule, with a central depression or ulceration and pearly, rolled borders with overlying telangiectasias (Figure 33-80). *Superficial* BCC is the second most common type (Figure 33-81). *Sclerosing* (morpheaform, infiltrating) BCC is the least common (Figure 33-82). It is not unusual to see pigment in a nodular BCC (Figure 33-83). A shave biopsy is usually adequate to confirm the diagnosis.

Superficial BCC can be treated with ED&C or topically with 5-FU or imiquimod. Imiquimod 5% cream once daily five times weekly for 6 weeks for superficial BBC produced an initial clearance rate of 90%, with 80% of subjects clinically clear at 2 years (Gollnick et al., 2005). In another study, superficial BCC lesions on the trunk or limbs were treated with 5-FU cream twice daily for up to 12 weeks. The histologic cure rate was 90%, and the mean time to clinical cure was 10.5 weeks. 5-FU was generally well tolerated, with a good cosmetic outcome; most patients

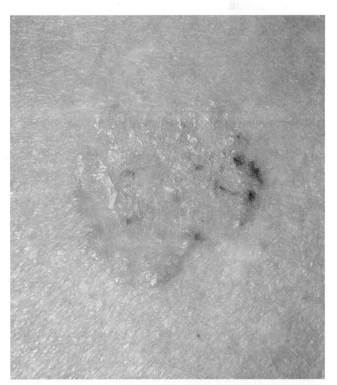

Figure 33-81 Superficial basal cell carcinoma on back. (© Richard P. Usatine.)

had no pain or scarring and only mild erythema (Gross et al., 2007).

Nodular BCC can be excised with 3- to 5-mm margins or treated with ED&C, depending on location and patient comorbidities and preference. Cryotherapy is another option but is infrequently performed because of poor wound healing. Tumors that are more aggressive by histologic pattern (morpheaform, micronodular, or infiltrating) or

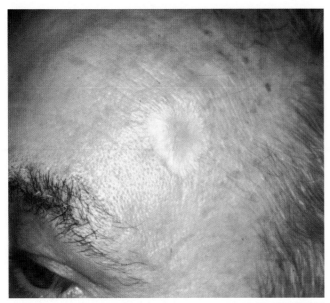

Figure 33-82 Sclerosing basal cell carcinoma. (© Richard P. Usatine and the Skin Cancer Foundation.)

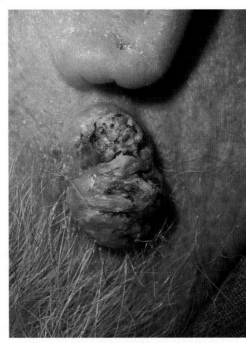

Figure 33-84 Squamous cell carcinoma under ear. (© Richard P. Usatine.)

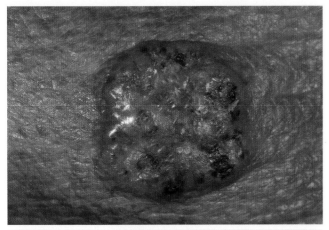

Figure 33-83 Pigmented nodular basal cell carcinoma. (© Richard P. Usatine.)

those occurring near vital or cosmetically sensitive structures are best treated with MMS. This tissue-sparing method also allows for examination of almost 100% of the tissue margins. MMS is the removal of tumor by scalpel in sequential layers, in which each tissue sample is frozen, stained, and microscopically examined. This is repeated until all the margins are clear. MMS is the treatment of choice for BCCs greater than 2 cm, with poorly defined margins, aggressive histology, involving areas of cosmetic or functional importance (mouth, ears, nose, eyelids), or recurrent lesions (Thissen et al., 1999).

Patients diagnosed with BCC have an approximately 30% higher risk than the general population of being diagnosed with another BCC unrelated to the previous lesion. Because BCC can recur, patients should have frequent full-body skin examinations at least twice yearly for the first 2 years and then yearly if no new lesions occur. As with all sun-related malignancies and precancerous lesions, patients must be instructed on sun protection and sun avoidance.

KEY TREATMENT

- Mohs surgery (three studies; $n = 2660$) is the "gold standard" but is not needed for all BCCs. The recurrence rate was 0.8 to 1.1. Systematic review also showed the following (Thissen et al., 1999) (SOR: A):
  - Surgical excision (three studies; $n = 1303$): the recurrence rate was 2 to 8. The mean cumulative 5-year rate was 5.3. Recommended margins are 4 to 5 mm.
  - Curettage and desiccation (six studies; $n = 4212$): the recurrence rate was 4.3 to 18.1. The cumulative 5-year rate was 5.7 to 18.8. Three cycles of curettage and desiccation can produce higher cure rates then one cycle.
  - Cryosurgery (4 studies; $n = 796$): the recurrence rate was 3.0 to 4.3. The cumulative 5-year rate (3 studies) was 0 to 16.5.
- Superficial BCC is effectively treated with imiquimod 5% cream (Gollnick et al., 2005) or 5-FU cream (Gross et al., 2007) (SOR: B).

SQUAMOUS CELL CARCINOMA

Cutaneous SCC is the second most common form of skin cancer, also arising primarily on sun-exposed skin of middle-aged and older adults. Most SCCs arise from sun-induced precancerous lesions (AKs). As in BD, there is a higher risk of SCC in patients with radiation dermatitis (x-ray damage), leukoplakia or erythroplakia (in oral or

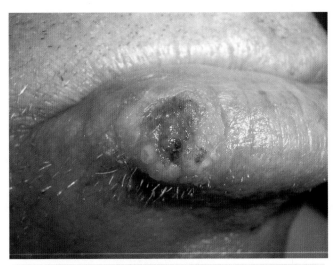

Figure 33-85 Squamous cell carcinoma on lip. (© Richard P. Usatine.)

Table 33-3 Mnemonic for Signs and Symptoms of Melanoma

ABCDE	Description
Asymmetry	Half the mole does not match the other half
Border irregularity	Edges of mole are ragged, blurred, or notched
Color	Color over mole is not homogeneous; may be varying shades of tan, brown, or black; patches of red, blue, or white in some cases
Diameter	Mole is >6 mm
Evolution	Previously stable mole that is changing (evolving) in color, size, or other signs or symptoms

genital mucosa), burn scars, and chronic skin ulcers. It is important to note that organ transplant recipients have a 40 to 250 times greater risk of developing SCC, purportedly from interaction of HPV and immunosuppression.

Lesions are typically pink to flesh-colored papules or nodules, often with crusting or ulceration (Figure 33-84). They may also be keratotic or may develop a cutaneous horn. The most common locations include the face, scalp, lips, ears, neck, dorsal arms and hands, and genitalia (Figure 33-85). Although many SCCs are asymptomatic, symptoms such as bleeding, pain, and tenderness may be noted. SCC has an overall *metastasis* rate of 2% to 3%, but it is highly variable based on location, size, depth, invasion, and immunosuppression; rates can be as high as 30% to 40%. High-risk areas for metastasis include the ear, lip, genitalia, and areas of chronic inflammation (burns, scars, ulcers). A biopsy is required for diagnosis, which can be done with the shave or punch technique. Treatment of superficial SCC is covered under BD.

Many SCCs can be excised with 4- to 5-mm margins. Smaller lesions may be amenable to ED&C. Several series report excellent cure rates with ED&C, and experience suggests that small (<1 cm), well-differentiated, primary slow-growing tumors arising on sun-exposed sites can be removed by experienced physicians with curettage (Motley et al., 2003). As with BCC, tumors of SCC that are large, invasive, recurrent or near vital or cosmetically sensitive structures are best treated with Mohs surgery. Surgical resection with 4-mm margins should be adequate for well-defined low-risk tumors less than 2 cm in diameter. Such margins are expected to remove the primary tumor mass completely in 95% of cases. MMS should therefore be considered as first-line treatment of high-risk SCC, particularly at sites where wide surgical margins may be difficult to achieve without functional impairment (Motley et al., 2003). In a prospective, multicenter case series of 1263 patients with SCC who underwent MMS, recurrence after MMS was diagnosed in 15 of the 381 patients (3.9%) who completed the 5-year follow-up: 2.6% in patients with primary SCC, and 5.9% in patients with previously recurrent SCC (Leibovitch et al., 2005).

KEY TREATMENT

- Surgical resection with 4-mm margins should remove small cell carcinoma (low risk, <2 cm) completely in 95% of patients (Motley et al., 2003) (SOR: A).
- MMS is considered first-line treatment of high-risk SCC (Motley et al., 2003) (SOR: B).

MELANOMA

Melanoma is the most lethal of the cutaneous malignancies, causing more than 77% of skin cancer deaths. In the United States, more than 68,000 new cases of invasive melanoma and almost 57,000 new cases of melanoma in situ were diagnosed in 2010. Melanoma arises from the pigment-producing cells (melanocytes) located predominantly in the skin, but it also found in the eyes, ears, GI tract, leptomeninges, and oral and genital mucous membranes. Early detection and treatment of melanoma are the best means of reducing mortality.

The development of melanoma is not completely understood and is not as directly linked to chronic sun exposure as is BCC or SCC. Risk factors include a fair complexion, red or blond hair, inability to tan or predisposition to burn, freckles, excessive childhood sun exposure, more than three blistering childhood sunburns, an increased number of moles (nevi) or dysplastic nevi, a family history of melanoma, a personal history of melanoma, immunosuppression, and older age.

One third of melanomas arise in a preexisting nevus. A changing or newly acquired nevus in a person older than age 20 years is the most common warning sign for melanoma. An increase in size, change in color, asymmetry of borders, and variegated pigmentation are signs that warrant a biopsy. The mnemonic ABCDE (asymmetry, border irregularity, color, diameter, evolving) is helpful to assess lesions that may be melanocytic (Table 33-3). Symptoms such as bleeding, itching, ulceration, and pain in a pigmented lesion are less common but also warrant further evaluation.

The subtypes of melanoma include superficial spreading melanoma (60%-70%), nodular melanoma (15%-30%), lentigo malignant melanoma (5%-15%), and acral lentiginous melanoma (5%-10%). These are essentially histologic subtypes but do tend to favor certain areas or populations. Superficial spreading, the most common type, usually

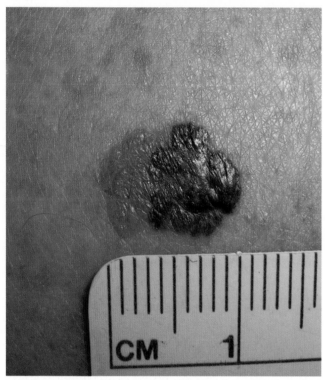

Figure 33-86 Superficial spreading melanoma on back. (© Richard P. Usatine.)

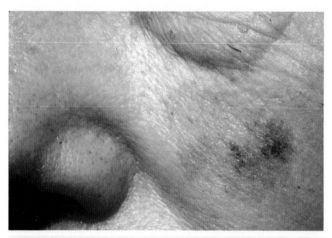

Figure 33-87 Lentigo maligna melanoma on the face. (© The Skin Cancer Foundation.)

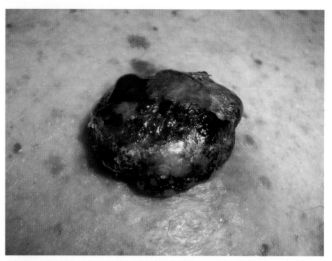

Figure 33-88 Nodular melanoma with 22-mm Breslow depth. (© Richard P. Usatine.)

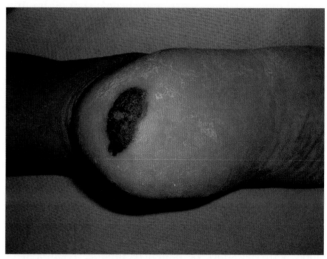

Figure 33-89 Acral lentiginous melanoma on heel of African American woman. (© Richard P. Usatine.)

occurs on the trunk or legs (Figure 33-86). Lentigo maligna melanoma is a superficial variant and usually found on the face in elderly persons (Figure 33-87). Nodular melanomas often have a solid-black color, and their thickness predicts a worse prognosis (Figure 33-88). Acral lentiginous melanoma is most often found on the great toe or thumb and is the most common type to occur in African Americans (Figure 33-89).

Excisional biopsy, including 1 to 2 mm of normal skin surrounding the pigmented lesion, is optimal to provide accurate diagnosis and histologic staging. Referral for biopsy may be appropriate based on the location and size of the lesion. "Scoop shave" biopsies can be performed as long as the depth of the specimen obtained is greater than 1 to 2 mm. This is important because the depth of tumor invasion (Breslow depth) is the most important prognostic indicator and used in staging. Melanomas are also staged based on the presence of ulceration (histologically), lymph node involvement, and location of metastasis. Diagnosing melanoma early is critical to a good prognosis. Most thin tumors (Breslow depth <1 mm) have a greater than 90% 10-year survival rate.

Treatment for melanoma is primarily surgical and depends on the depth of the tumor. Lesions with Breslow thicknesses less than 1 mm can be excised with 1-cm margins. Lesions with Breslow thicknesses of 1 mm or greater should be referred for sentinel lymph node biopsy to provide accurate staging. There is limited adjuvant therapy for melanoma that has spread to the lymph nodes other than interferon-α. However, two new medications have been approved for metastatic melanoma. Ipilimumab (Yervoy) is a CTLA-4 inhibitor (found on T-cells) and dosed intravenously every 3 weeks for a total of four doses. Vemurafenib (Zelboraf) is a kinase inhibitor for BRAF-positive patients only and is dosed 1 tablet twice daily (Culos et al., 2013; Heakal et al., 2011). Ipilimumab is slow to take effect, and only about one in four patients respond, but responses can be very long lasting. Vemurafenib, on the other hand, usually demonstrates a fast antitumor response, but it does not last and is often followed by treatment resistance. Vemurafenib can only be used for patients who have the *BRAF* mutation, which accounts for just half of all patients with metastatic melanoma. Patients who do not have the mutation should not take vemurafenib because data show that it could accelerate their disease (Heakal et al., 2011).

For 2 to 3 years after any diagnosis of melanoma, patients should be seen every 3 to 6 months because most metastases occur in the first few years. If no new tumors are found, annual full-body skin examinations should be performed for life because of the higher risk of subsequent primary melanomas. Strict sun protection and sun avoidance should also be followed.

KEY TREATMENT

- World Health Organization recommendations for excision margins are 5 mm for melanoma in situ lesions, 1 cm for lesions less than 1 mm, and 2 cm for melanomas 2 to 4 mm in thickness (Lens et al., 2002) (SOR: A).
- Sentinel lymph node biopsies are recommended for melanomas 1 mm or greater in depth for staging purposes but do not improve survival (Tanis et al., 2008) (SOR: B).
- Interferon-α may offer some benefit in recurrence-free and overall survival of melanoma patients (Garbe and Eigentler, 2007) (SOR: B).
- Ipilimumab (Yervoy) is a new biologic agent that may extend survival in cases of metastatic melanoma and can be used in any patient (Culos et al., 2013) (SOR B).
- Vemurafenib (Zelboraf) is an oral therapy for metastatic melanoma but is only effective for cases that are BRAF positive.

References

The complete reference list is available at www.expertconsult.com.

Web Resources

dermatlas.org DermAtlas. A large international atlas of dermatology from Johns Hopkins University.

dermis.net DermIS (Derm Information Systems). A large dermatology information service containing adult and pediatric dermatology atlases; founded at the University of Erlangen.

www.dermatlas.net Interactive Dermatology Atlas. Contains more than 1500 photographs, a sophisticated search tool, quiz mode, and more than 60 interactive cases developed by Dr. Richard Usatine.

www.dermnet.com Dermnet skin disease atlas with more than 23,000 images of skin diseases.

www.skinsight.com/Skinsight (Logical Images). Contains free information for patients and professionals. Although promoting the VisualDx product, the site has good information and images.

34 *Diabetes Mellitus*

JEFF UNGER and RUSSELL WHITE

Introduction

Diabetes mellitus is a heterogeneous group of disorders with distinct genetic, etiologic, immunologic, and pathophysiologic mechanisms that result in glucose intolerance and hyperglycemia. Patients with diabetes develop insulin deficiency, impaired peripheral insulin action, or both. Chronic exposure to hyperglycemia, glycemic variability, and resultant oxidative stress in genetically prone individuals can result in both acute (diabetic ketoacidosis [DKA] and hypoglycemia) and long-term (micro- and macrovascular) complications.

Diabetes is currently classified into four major types on the basis of etiology and clinical presentation:

1. **Type 1 diabetes (T1DM):** characterized by a gradual loss of insulin-producing pancreatic β-cells secondary to autoimmune destruction
2. **Type 2 diabetes (T2DM):** genetically predisposed individuals develop a chronic progressive disease characterized by insulin resistance and subsequent β-cell failure
3. **Gestational diabetes mellitus (GDM):** defined as hyperglycemia with onset or first recognition during pregnancy
4. **Other specific types,** including monogenetic forms of diabetes (i.e., neonatal diabetes and maturity onset diabetes of the young), diabetes attributable to diseases of the exocrine pancreas (i.e., cystic fibrosis), other endocrinopathies, and drug-induced diabetes (e.g., steroids) (American Diabetes Association [ADA], 2011a)

The prevalence of diabetes is increasing throughout the Western world. The World Health Organization estimates that more than 347 million people worldwide currently have diabetes, and 90% of all cased involve T2DM (ADA, 2011a; World Health Organization, 2013). This number is projected to grow to 439 million individuals worldwide (7.7% of the population) by 2030 (Shaw et al., 2010).

HISTORICAL OVERVIEW

In 1920, diabetes was a terminal disease with a life expectancy of 6 to 12 months (Bliss, 1982). Its treatment consisted of restricting caloric intake to less than 500 calories per day. Individuals who breached that nutrition threshold in an attempt to appease their hunger would develop DKA and die within hours to days. Life for patients with diabetes in the early 1900s was, in a word, miserable. Patients suffered from malnutrition, cataracts, blindness, gangrene, impotence, and immune-resistant infections (e.g., pneumonia, tuberculosis, boils, and carbuncles). Surgeons recognized the futility of operating on gangrenous, rotting legs; patients were equally likely to die from surgical complications as from the underlying infection. Women who were able to conceive were unable to carry their macrosomic babies to term. The "sickish sweet smell of rotten apples" breeched the halls of hospital wards as dehydrated patients with DKA lay hopelessly waiting to die (Bliss, 1982). All too often, death from diabetes would be considered a blessing by those who long suffered the consequences of chronic hyperglycemia.

The first human injection of insulin (derived from extracts obtained from dog pancreases) was given to a 14-year-old patient named Leonard Thompson in Toronto, Canada, on January 11, 1922. Weighing only 64 lb on admission, this "hopeless charity case" who was near death from DKA received a 7.5-cc injection of "thick black muck" in each hip (Bliss, 1982). The dose was calculated by Dr. Frederick Banting, who discovered insulin, and his medical student Charles Best based on their work with pancreatectomized dogs. Thompson nearly died from boils and sepsis because the "iletin" extract was impure and unsterile. Yet, to the amazement of all in attendance, his blood glucose level declined from 420 mg/dL to 330 mg/dL. Shortly after the pancreatic extract was purified, Thompson received additional injections. He was eventually discharged from the hospital and later died at 27 years of age secondary to complications from pneumonia.

In October 1922, another patient, Elsie Needham, became the first individual to ever have DKA reversed with the use of insulin. Although insulin was in short supply, physicians such as Eliot Joslin used the drug successfully to treat patients who were starving or dying of acute diabetes complications. Although the insulin extract had an immediate effect on reducing mortality, Joslin professed that lifestyle intervention remained the foundation of care for all individuals with diabetes.

Thus, less than a century ago, the discovery of insulin saved the lives of millions of people with diabetes while changing the process through which medicine is studied and practiced to this day. In short order, drug purification methods were developed and perfected. The field of endocrinology was born. Other hormones were discovered and purified. Pharmaceutical companies began to fund clinical trials, allowing clinicians and scientists the opportunity to evaluate the safety and efficacy of new compounds.

Before 1920, clinicians relied on their own marketing skills to sell their homemade snake oil products from horse-drawn buggies. Various folkloric remedies, which rarely worked, were available to anyone and promoted to "cure whatever ails you." People were becoming skeptical about the practice of medicine, as well as about those who claimed to be experts at curing diseases such as diabetes, tuberculosis, senility, and sexually transmitted diseases. Doctors had not yet gained the public's trust in them as healers. After all, what could these men actually heal?

After the discovery of insulin was solidified, Banting refused to take the traditional approach of proclaiming his findings to the news media. Instead, he took the then-unprecedented route of publishing his data in a reputable medical journal (Banting and Best, 1922). People slowly began to trust physicians, not merely as quasi-mystical healers but as practitioners who could identify and cure disease through scientific discovery. Importantly, however, as Eliot Joslin noted in 1923, "Insulin is not a cure for diabetes" (Bliss, 1982).

By 1945, the lifespan of patients with diabetes had increased by nearly 45 years. Starvation and DKA gave way to long-term micro- and macrovascular complications as the primary causes of death in patients with diabetes. In 1955, sulfonylureas became the first oral medications developed and marketed for the treatment of diabetes. However, testing urine for the presence of sugar was still used as a crude means by which therapeutic decisions could be rationalized. The Ames glucometer, introduced in 1970, provided patients with the first tool for performing self-monitoring of blood glucose (SMBG), which has since become an important component of diabetes management. Metformin was approved by the U.S. Food and Drug Administration (FDA) in 1995. In 2010, more than 48 million prescriptions for generic metformin were filled in the United States alone (IMS Institute for Healthcare Informatics, 2011).

In 1993, the Diabetes Control and Complications Trial (DCCT) demonstrated that intensive glycemic control (i.e., keeping blood glucose levels as close as possible to the normal range) reduces the incidence and progression of microvascular complications (e.g., retinopathy, nephropathy, and neuropathy) in T1DM (DCCT Research Group, 1993). Whether the same held true in T2DM remained uncertain until 1998, when the U.K. Prospective Diabetes Study (UKPDS) established that intensively lowering blood glucose levels reduces microvascular complications in T2DM as well (UKPDS Study Group, 1998). However, these and other landmark long-term, randomized controlled trials (RCTs) have consistently demonstrated that individuals whose diabetes is intensively managed have a higher risk of hypoglycemia; weight gain; and, in some cases, all-cause mortality than their peers who are treated to a more relaxed or conventional glycemic target (Action to Control Cardiovascular Risk in Diabetes [ACCORD] Study Group, 2008, The Action in Diabetes and Vascular Disease: Preterax and Diamicron Modified Release Controlled Evaluation

[ADVANCE] Collaborative Group, 2008, DCCT Research Group, 1993; Duckworth et al., 2009; UKPDS Study Group, 1998).

Based on the findings of the DCCT and UKPDS, the ADA recommends an A1C target of 6.5% to 7% for most healthy patients in the United States (ADA, 2013b). However, rather than focusing on a specific glycemic target, care should be customized based on factors such as the patient's age, disease duration, hypoglycemia risk, presence or absence of significant comorbidities, expected longevity, and capability for and attitudes regarding diabetes self-management (Ismail-Beigi et al., 2011). Metabolic targets for lipids and blood pressure should also be customized. Following a healthy lifestyle, including a healthy eating plan, adequate physical activity, modest weight reduction (8-10 lb), and smoking cessation, is crucial for reducing the risk of long-term complications. Finally, SMBG should be incorporated into every patient's daily routine as a means of identifying glycemic variability, predicting hypoglycemia, and evaluating immediate responses to therapeutic interventions.

The recent guideline modifications regarding individualizing metabolic targets notwithstanding, American medicine is achieving a historic level of success in treating this chronic progressive illness. Ninety percent of all patients with diabetes are managed in the primary care setting (Unger, 2012c). Some critics argue that practitioners are failing to treat patients successfully to their metabolic targets; apparently, these naysayers do not understand the importance of positive trending. Recently published data from the National Health and Nutrition Examination Survey (NHANES) suggested that, in 2010, 18.8% of all patients with diabetes successfully achieved an A1C of less than 7%, a blood pressure less than 130/80 mm Hg, and a low-density lipoprotein (LDL) cholesterol level less than 100 mg/dL compared with only 1.7% of surveyed individuals with diabetes from 1988 to 1994 (Stark Casagrande, et al., 2013).

American medicine is changing. Our treatments for diabetes, hypertension, and hyperlipidemia have improved. These improvements in the management of diabetes and related disorders may be attributed in large part to the primary care providers who care for the increasingly high numbers of patients exposed to prolonged glycemic burden, as well as to patients' desire to become more active participants in their own diabetes care. The renewed emphasis on individualized, patient-centered diabetes care may further expand our success in this area in the near future.

Prediabetes: A Treatable Precursor of Type 2 Diabetes

Diabetes affects 25.8 million Americans (18.8 million have been diagnosed with diabetes, and an estimated 7 million remain undiagnosed). Based on NHANES data obtained between 2005 and 2008, 35% of U.S. adults 20 years of age or older and 50% of individuals 65 years of age and older meet the diagnostic criteria for prediabetes. In 2010, 79 million Americans were estimated to have prediabetes. In 2011, an estimated 280 million people were estimated to have *prediabetes* worldwide (ADA, 2011b). By 2030, the

Table 34-1   Diagnosing Prediabetes and Diabetes

Parameter	Euglycemia	Prediabetes	Diabetes
Fasting glucose (mg/dL)	<100	100-125 (impaired fasting glucose)	>126
2-hour postprandial glucose (mg/dL)	<140	140-199 (impaired glucose tolerance)	>200
A1C (%)	<5.7	5.7-6.4	>6.5

Data from American Diabetes Association. Diagnosis and classification of diabetes mellitus. *Diabetes Care.* 36(suppl 1):S67-S74, 2013.

International Diabetes Federation predicts that this number will increase to 400 million as westernization and obesity push into Asia, Africa, and South America (Unger and Moriarty, 2008).

The costs of caring for patients with diabetes will continue to rise. Annual health care costs in the United States for a person without diabetes are $5615. Diabetes inflicts a 2.3-fold increase in annual costs of care, raising this figure to $12,195. In 2012, diabetes cost $245 billion in health care expenditures, an increase of 41% since 2007. Astonishingly, diabetes care now accounts for nearly 30% of the total Medicare budget. Thus, screening and implementing preventive strategies for prediabetes warrant political, medical, and bioethical consideration (ADA, 2013a).

Diabetes is a chronic, progressive disorder that, over the course of time, exposes patients to a prolonged, excessive glycemic burden, which activates pathways favoring oxidative stress and endothelial cell dysfunction. Complication pathways are propagated, resulting in micro- and macrovascular disease. Given the physical, emotional, and financial consequences associated with diabetes, screening high-risk patients could identify those with an intermediate form of dysglycemia who are likely to progress to clinical diabetes. The diagnostic criteria for prediabetes and diabetes are shown in Table 34-1.

Between 6% and 10% of patients with impaired glucose tolerance (IGT) progress to clinical diabetes each year, but up to 65% of individuals with both impaired fasting glucose (IFG) and IGT progress to clinical diabetes annually (Garber et al., 2008). Progression rates of IFG or IGT to diabetes vary according to degrees of initial hyperglycemia, racial and ethnic backgrounds, and environmental influences. The higher the glucose values, the greater the risk of progression to diabetes and diabetes complications. Primary care physicians are trained not only in managing patients within effective chronic disease-state models but also in identifying patients who are likely to develop diseases such as hypertension, diabetes, obesity, and cancer. High-risk individuals, after they have been identified (Table 34-2), should be screened for prediabetes and diabetes.

A1C has also been shown in prospective studies to predict progression to clinical diabetes. Zhang et al. (2010) noted that whereas individuals with a screening A1C at baseline of between 5.5% and 6% had a 5-year progression rate of 9% to 25%, those with an A1C of 6% to 6.5% progressed over 5 years at a rate of 25% to 50%.

Diagnostic tests for prediabetes and diabetes should be repeated to rule out laboratory error unless the diagnosis is unequivocal. A screened symptomatic patient with an A1C of 7.9% and a random blood glucose of 265 mg/dL can simply be treated for diabetes. However, a patient with a screening A1C of 6.2% with a euglycemic 2-hour

Table 34-2   Screening Patients at High Risk for Developing Prediabetes

Patients at Risk for Developing Prediabetes	Patients to Target for Prediabetes Screening
History of PCOS	Family history positive for diabetes
History of GDM	History of cardiovascular disease
Children of parents with T2DM	Obesity
Patients with abdominal obesity	Sedentary lifestyle
	Nonwhite ancestry
	Previous history of IGT or IFG
	History of hypertension
	History of elevated triglycerides, low HDL cholesterol, or both
	History of GDM
	History of PCOS
	Delivery of a baby weighing >9 lb
	Patients with schizophrenia or bipolar disorder

GDM, Gestational diabetes mellitus; *HDL,* high-density lipoprotein; *IFG,* impaired fasting glucose; *IGT,* impaired glucose tolerance; *PCOS,* polycystic ovary syndrome; *T2DM,* type 2 diabetes mellitus.
Data from Garber AJ, Handelsman Y, Einhorn D, et al. Diagnosis and management of prediabetes in the continuum of hyperglycemia: when do the risk of diabetes begin? A consensus statement from the American College of Endocrinology and the American Association of Clinical Endocrinologists. *Endocr Pract.* 14:933-945, 2008.

post–glucose challenge value should be rescreened. Preferably, the same test should be repeated for confirmation. If the initial A1C is 6.4% with a secondary measurement performed 2 months later of 6.3%, the diagnosis of prediabetes is confirmed. One can also make the diagnosis of prediabetes if the results of two different tests such as the A1C and the 2-hour post–glucose challenge are higher than diagnostic thresholds.

A1C can be useful as a screening tool for patients who present to the emergency department for management of an acute illness. An A1C greater than 5.7% performed in the acute-care setting has a sensitivity of 54.8% and a specificity of 71.3% for detecting prediabetes. An A1C of 6% has a sensitivity of 76.9% and a specificity of 87.3% for diagnosing diabetes in the acute-care setting (Silverman et al., 2011).

To prevent progression to clinical diabetes, the ADA recommends moderate exercise, weight loss (7%-10% of baseline weight in obese individuals), consideration of metformin (in patients with a body mass index [BMI] >35 kg/m^2; age younger than 60 years; or, in women, a history of GDM) (ADA, 2013b). Modifiable cardiovascular disease (CVD) risk factors must also be addressed, including smoking cessation, targeting blood pressure to less than 140/90 mm Hg, and targeting LDL cholesterol to less than 100 mg/dL. A recent study suggested that a single period of moderate exercise expending 350 kcal of energy can improve insulin sensitivity for obese patients into the following day (Newsom et al., 2013). In the Nurses' Health Study, whereas each 2-hour increment spent watching television daily was associated with a 14% increased risk of developing T2DM, a similar increment spent standing or walking was associated with a 12% risk reduction (Hu et al., 2011).

The relationship among environmental factors, the increased risk of obesity, and a reduction in desire to increase physical activity is well established. Unfortunately, the acute medical models fail to address meaningful and effective strategies that may prevent or reverse the diabetes epidemic. Proactive public health initiatives designed to educate parents and children about the importance of healthy lifestyle choices may be our best hope for minimizing the nuclear burden of the looming health care costs associated with chronic hyperglycemia.

Zhang et al. (2003) suggested that screening obese patients for prediabetes is cost effective. Screening studies cost less than $200 per case. Patients who screen positive for prediabetes can initiate low-cost lifestyle interventions and metformin, if necessary. These noninvasive therapies will result in a savings of greater than $8000 per quality-adjusted life year gained for screened individuals.

Weight reduction and physical activity can improve insulin-mediated glucose disposal, reduce postprandial hyperglycemia, delay pancreatic β-cell death, and slow the progression of glucose intolerance to clinical T2DM.

The Diabetes Prevention Program (DPP) was the most comprehensive clinical trial to date evaluating the importance of lifestyle modification as a deterrent to diabetes in high-risk patients (Knowler et al., 2002). A total of 3234 overweight subjects with prediabetes were randomized to one of three cohorts. The intensive lifestyle intervention (ILI) group received intensive instruction in diet, physical activity, and behavioral modification. The patients assigned to this group were counseled to reduce their fat and calorie consumption and to exercise for 150 minutes per week and were targeted to lose 7% of their baseline weight. Subjects in the ILI group reduced their risk of progression to diabetes by 58% over 4 years. The second group used metformin, 850 mg twice daily, and received information regarding lifestyle intervention but no intensive counseling. Their risk of progression to clinical diabetes was reduced by 31%. The control group was given a placebo in place of metformin and attended classes related to lifestyle intervention. About 5% of the lifestyle intervention group developed diabetes each year during the study period compared with 11% of those in the placebo group. A follow-up to the DPP showed that preservation of β-cell function and delay of progression to diabetes in high-risk individuals can persist for at least 10 years with lifestyle intervention or metformin (DPP Research Group, 2009).

The FDA has not approved any pharmacotherapeutic agents for the treatment of prediabetes. However, several therapies have proven to be effective at delaying or preventing the progression of prediabetes to diabetes. Compared with placebo, acarbose has been shown to reduce progression of prediabetes to T2DM by 25% over a 3.3-year period regardless of age, sex, or BMI (Chiasson et al., 2003).

Pioglitazone reduced the risk of conversion to diabetes in patients with isolated IGT or with combined IFG and IGT in both men and women, as well as in all age and weight groups compared with placebo (DeFronzo et al., 2011). Unfortunately, the mean weight gain in pioglitazone-treated patients was 3.6 kg. Thus, one might argue that pioglitazone may be a strong candidate as a pharmacologic intervention for prediabetes. However, use of pioglitazone in this patient population will likely result in weight gain.

The ORIGIN Trial (Outcome Reduction with Initial Glargine Intervention) was a 6-year RCT designed to assess the effects of treatment with insulin glargine compared with standard care on cardiovascular outcomes in more than 12,500 subjects worldwide. Study participants had either prediabetes or early T2DM, as well as a high cardiovascular risk profile. A total of 6264 patients were randomized to receive glargine titrated to achieve fasting normoglycemia. Glargine achieved the targeted long-term glycemic control (median fasting glucose of 93.6 mg/dL and A1C of 6.2%) over 6.2 years without increasing the overall incidence of cancer or heart disease. In addition, glargine delayed the progression from prediabetes to T2DM by 28%. However, patients randomized to the glargine group experienced nearly three times the frequency of hypoglycemia events compared with those in the standard cohort and gained on average 3.5 lb over the course of the study (Gerstein et al., 2012).

Recommended treatment strategies for managing prediabetes vary depending on the particular published guidelines consulted and are summarized in Table 34-3.

In summary, patients who are at high risk for diabetes should be screened for prediabetes and clinical diabetes using a fasting blood glucose, 2-hour post-glucose challenge, or A1C test (assuming patients are not pregnant). Unless a patient has symptoms strongly suggestive of diabetes (e.g., thirst, weight loss, blurred vision, paresthesias, and fatigue) in association with significantly abnormal screening laboratory values, a diagnosis of abnormal glucose tolerance should be confirmed with repeat testing.

For individuals who are diagnosed with prediabetes (IFG or IGT), adoption of healthy lifestyle choices with the goal of restoring normal glucose regulation becomes the key to preventing disease progression to T2DM. Every 1 kg of weight lost is associated with a 16% reduction in the risk of progression to diabetes. Physical activity improves peripheral insulin resistance and enhances weight loss.

Patients also should be instructed to monitor their blood glucose levels. One common recommendation is to perform 7-point SMBG (before and after each meal and at bedtime) for 3 successive days before each clinic appointment. This will allow the clinician to gauge changes in fasting and postabsorptive glucose values that require attentive intervention.

The American Association of Clinical Endocrinologists (AACE) recommends initiating off-label use of metformin in patients likely to progress to clinical diabetes whose A1C level is greater than 6.0% (Garber et al., 2008). The pharmacologic goal of prediabetes management should be directed toward pancreatic β-cell preservation. Patients who have prediabetes have lost 80% of their β-cell function and are considered to be maximally insulin resistant (Gastaldelli et al., 2004).

Ambitious screening of high-risk patients and encouragement of healthy lifestyle principles by primary care

Table 34-3   Management and Prevention of Type 2 Diabetes Mellitus in High-Risk Individuals

Published Guidelines	Clinical Recommendations for the Management of Prediabetes
American Diabetes Association	Refer to effective ongoing support program targeting a weight loss of 7% from baseline At least 150 min/wk of moderate physical activity such as walking Consider metformin if A1C increases above the threshold of 6% despite lifestyle intervention Monitor annually for progression to clinical diabetes
American Association of Clinical Endocrinologists	Lifestyle intervention strategies, including weight reduction of 5% to 10% from baseline with long-term maintenance Moderate-intensity exercise program for 30 to 60 min/day at least 5 days/wk Dietary recommendations: lower sodium intake, avoidance of excessive alcohol, caloric restriction, increased fiber intake, possible limitation on carbohydrate intake Initiation of metformin or acarbose for "low-risk" patients or pioglitazone for "high-risk" patients or for those in whom lower-risk therapies have not succeeded Incretin therapies may also prove effective in β-cell preservation No targeted A1C is recommended Use statins to achieve an LDL cholesterol level <100 mg/dL, non-HDL cholesterol <130 mg/dL, and/or apolipoprotein B ≤90 mg/dL) Target blood pressure of <130/80 mm Hg Antiplatelet therapy (low-dose aspirin) for all patients with prediabetes for whom there is no identified excess risk for GI, intracranial, or other hemorrhagic condition

GI, Gastrointestinal; *HDL,* high-density lipoprotein; *LDL,* low-density lipoprotein.
Adapted with permission from Unger J. *Diabetes management in primary care.* 2nd ed. Philadelphia: Lippincott, Williams and Wilkins; 2012.

physicians will reduce the number of individuals who ultimately progress to clinical diabetes and suffer the consequences of a chronic hyperglycemia burden.

Type 2 Diabetes Mellitus

PATHOGENESIS

The Genome-Wide Association study has detected 18 polymorphisms (genetic variations) that may increase a person's likelihood of developing T2DM (Hamman, 1992). Over time and under the influence of environmental triggers, the activation of these alleles distorts the homeostatic control of normal glycemia (Unger, 2012d). Several of the recently described activators of prediabetes and T2DM pathogenesis that may be of particular interest to family physicians are discussed in Table 34-4. Other environmental triggers include low levels of vitamin D; obesity; high-fat diets; lack of physical activity; concurrent illnesses; and use of certain prescription medications, which may induce treatment-emergent diabetes.

Genetically susceptible individuals may possess polymorphisms (alterations in the normal DNA sequencing that form a typical allele) that favor reduction in satiety, increased appetite, reduced energy expenditure, and increased intraabdominal fat accumulation. These individuals will become obese, which will induce physiological stress and overproduction of insulin by their pancreatic β cells. Over time, genetic coding will begin the process of programmed β-cell death (apoptosis). The San Antonio Metabolism Study demonstrated that patients with prediabetes who have 2-hour postprandial glucose levels of 140 to 180 mg/dL have effectively lost 80% of their β-cell function and are maximally insulin resistant. Additionally, 18% of patients with prediabetes are already diagnosed with diabetic retinopathy (Gastaldelli et al., 2004). Thus, the dreaded long-term microvascular (i.e., retinopathy, neuropathy, and nephropathy) and macrovascular (i.e., coronary heart disease, peripheral vascular disease, and stroke) complications are already in the progressive stages long before these patients progress to T2DM.

MAINTENANCE OF NORMAL GLUCOSE HOMEOSTASIS AND DIABETES PATHOGENESIS

Glucose homeostasis is rigidly maintained within the range of 85 to 140 mg/dL via the interaction of multiple hormones (i.e., insulin, glucagon, amylin, leptin, resistin, glucagon-like peptide 1 [GLP-1], glucose-dependent insulinotropic polypeptide [GIP], adiponectin, growth hormone, cortisol, and somatastatin). Insulin modulates the metabolism of fat and protein while regulating intracellular transport of glucose. Insulin also regulates hepatic glucose production and peripheral glucose uptake and disposal by skeletal muscles and limits lipolysis. The body stores approximately 450 g of glucose, which is used as an energy source for the brain, skeletal muscles, and cellular metabolism. The brain requires 125 g of glucose daily. Another 125 g of glucose is used by the rest of the body. Daily intake of 180 g of dietary glucose and 70 g of glucose from gluconeogenesis (via the kidneys and liver) replenishes the body's glucose stores (Unger, 2012a).

A decrement in plasma glucose of as little as 20 mg/dL (i.e., from 90 to 70 mg/dL) will suppress β-cell insulin release while triggering the release of counterregulatory hormones (i.e., glucagon, catecholamines, cortisol, and growth hormone) (Gerich, 1988). Likewise, a 10-mg/dL increase in plasma glucose will stimulate insulin secretion and mitigate glucagon release by the pancreatic α cells (Shrayyef and Gerich, 2010).

Postabsorptive endogenous glucose release is maintained by hepatic glycogenolysis (the breakdown of glycogen, accounting for 50% of the total basal glucose) and hepatic gluconeogenesis (the formation of glucose from noncarbohydrate molecules such as amino acids and lactic acidosis, accounting for 30% of the body's basal glucose). Renal gluconeogenesis provides an additional 20% of the body's total endogenous energy stores. This "basal glucose" prevents hypoglycemia while supplying sufficient energy

Table 34-4 Environmental Activators of Type 2 Diabetes Mellitus

Environmental Activator	Suspected Mechanism Leading to Induction of Type 2 Diabetes Mellitus
Advanced age	Aging-related alterations of DNA methylation can affect cell signaling and gene transcription. This may upregulate a state of chronic inflammation in older individuals.
Late-morning rising and large caloric intake at dinner (late chronotype)	Late bedtimes and late-morning rising are associated with skipping breakfast and shifting more calories consumed to later in the day. This increases the risk of obesity and diabetes.
Sleep disorders (e.g., obstructive sleep apnea, defective REM sleep, shift work–related, insomnia, and restless leg syndrome)	Circadian misalignment affects sleep architecture as well as glucose–insulin metabolism, substrate oxidation, homeostasis model assessment of insulin resistance index, leptin concentrations, and hypothalamic–pituitary–adrenal axis activity. Depression is common in people with sleep disorders and can also increase diabetes risk.
Mental illness	Patients with major depression, bipolar disorder, or schizophrenia tend to smoke, be physically inactive and overweight, and have increased levels of C-reactive protein (favoring an inflammatory state). Low levels of tissue plasminogen activator in patients with schizophrenia may affect signaling within dopamine neurotransmitters, affecting insulin resistance and promoting diabetes.
Exposure to second-hand smoke	Women exposed to second-hand smoke from at least one parent have been found to have an 18% higher rate of diabetes than nonexposed women. Smoking causes adipocyte hypertrophy, insulin resistance, leptin resistance, and chronic pancreatic inflammation.
History of physical or sexual abuse	Results of the Nurses' Health Study II indicate the following associations: Physical abuse: ■ Moderate: 26% higher diabetes risk in adults ■ Severe: 54% higher diabetes risk in adults Forced sexual activity before adulthood: ■ 1 occasion: 34% higher diabetes risk in adults ■ >1 occasion: 69% higher diabetes risk in adults
Chemical exposure	In patients with a genetic predisposition to the development of diabetes, 10 chemicals have been determined to activate alleles that, in turn, favor the onset of β-cell apoptosis. Chemicals that have the greatest propensity toward β-cell destruction include arsenic, dioxin (a contaminant chemical in Agent Orange), hexachlorobenzene (a banned fungal chemical for agriculture), and perfluorooctanoic acid (a chemical found in Teflon, which is known to be toxic in animals and is found in the blood of 98% of the U.S. population).
Early menarche	Menarche occurring between the ages of 8 and 11 years may increase T2DM risk by up to 70%. Early menarche is associated with obesity and insulin resistance.

REM, Rapid eye movement; *T2DM,* type 2 diabetes mellitus.
References: Audouze et al., 2013; Elks et al., 2013; Gonnissen et al., 2013; Hoirisch-Clapauch and Nardi, 2013; Johansson et al., 2013; Lajous M et al., 2013; López-Otín et al., 2013; Pouwer et al., 2013; Reutrakul et al., 2013; and Rich-Edwards et al., 2010.

sources for the brain in the fasting state (Gerich et al., 2001). As noted earlier, ingested carbohydrates provide an exogenous source of glucose for the body's energy needs.

Intracellular transport of glucose occurs within skeletal muscles and adipose tissue as endogenous insulin binds to membrane-bound receptors. Glucose transporter type 4 (GLUT4) actively transports glucose intracellularly for storage as glycogen or in adipose tissue as fat.

The gastrointestinal (GI) tract participates in glucose homeostasis by permitting glucose entry to the body during digestion. Approximately 60% of the insulin response to an oral glucose load is prompted by the potentiating effect of two gut-derived incretin hormones. GLP-1, secreted by L cells, helps regulate the rate of glucose appearance by inhibiting glucagon secretion and hepatic glucose production, regulating gastric emptying, and reducing food intake by postulated centrally mediated mechanisms. GIP is secreted by the K cells of the proximal duodenum in response to glucose stimulation enhanced by fat and promotes triglyceride storage in adipose cells.

The levels of both GLP-1 and GIP increase within minutes of eating, probably as a result of a combination of endocrine and neural signals that stimulate incretin release before digested food comes into contact with the L cells of the small bowel and colon. Plasma levels of GLP-1 are low (5-10 pmol/L) in the fasting state and increase rapidly after eating, reaching 15 to 50 pmol/L. Circulating levels of both

GLP-1 and GIP decrease rapidly because of enzymatic inactivation via dipeptidyl peptidase-4 (DPP-4) and renal clearance. Approximately two thirds of the insulin response to an oral glucose load results from the potentiating effect of gut-derived incretin hormones.

The pancreas regulates glucose homeostasis by secreting insulin from centrally positioned β cells and glucagon from α cells located on the periphery of the pancreatic islet. Insulin is secreted in response to high plasma glucose levels and GLP-1 stimulation after nutrient intake.

Insulin is normally secreted into the portal circulation in two phases. In the fasting state, basal insulin is secreted at the approximate rate of 1 unit/hr to minimize hepatic glucose production (Kruszynska et al., 1987). Basal insulin also limits lipolysis and excess flux of free fatty acids (FFAs) to the liver, which can result in a state of postabsorptive insulin resistance. The circulating glucose levels are maintained at a level that allows for the extraction of this energy source by obligate glucose consumers such as the central nervous system. Basal insulinopenia (in T1DM) stimulates hormone-sensitive lipase and FFA release from fat stores, which, in turn, triggers hepatic production and release of ketone bodies, leading to ketogenesis and DKA.

The second-phase postprandial glucose peak occurs between 1 and 2 hours after a meal, with a mean peak time of 75 minutes (Slama et al., 2006). Eating prompts a five- to 10-fold increase in prandial insulin release from pancreatic β cells in euglycemic individuals. The meal-stimulated insulin response is triggered by a rise in plasma glucose and FFA concentrations, as well as neuroendocrine-augmented release of incretin hormones GIP and GLP-1. At basal insulin levels of 5 to 10 microunits/mL, hepatic glucose production and lipolysis (FFA release) are suppressed, which effectively counteracts the hyperglycemic effects of glucagon. Proximal uptake of glucose within skeletal muscles is not effective. As postabsorptive insulin levels exceed 40 to 50 microunits/mL, hepatic glucose suppression becomes optimally suppressed (Shrayyef and Gerich, 2010). This postabsorptive state may last between 4 and 6 hours and is dependent on the food content of each meal. High-fat meals such as pizza prolong the postabsorbtive state (Sheard et al., 2004).

The liver performs two different functions, depending on the level of circulating insulin. In the presence of low levels of insulin (≤25 mU/mL; e.g., in the fasting state), glucose is derived from glycogenolysis and gluconeogenesis to maintain euglycemia (Consoli, 1987). As circulating insulin levels rise, glucose is stored in the liver as glycogen and released into the plasma in response to hypoglycemia. After an overnight fast, the liver of a euglycemic individual produces glucose at a rate of approximately 2 mg/kg/min. Interestingly, in T2DM, despite a threefold increase in circulating plasma insulin levels, the liver will secrete an additional 25 to 30 g of glucose nightly into the plasma. Thus, the primary defect in T2DM appears to be related to peripheral glucose disposal caused by defective skeletal muscle transport rather than excessive hepatic glucose production (Unger, 2012A).

Amylin is a peptide hormone that is co-secreted from pancreatic β cells with insulin and is thus deficient in patients with diabetes. Amylin inhibits glucagon secretion, delays gastric emptying, and acts to increase satiety. Amylin also suppresses postprandial triglyceride concentrations and is known to reduce markers of oxidative stress and endothelial cell dysfunction (Unger, 2008b).

Although FFAs are the primary fuel for most organs, glucose is the obligate energy source of the brain under most physiological conditions. Glucose transport across the blood–brain barrier is more efficient than FFA absorption. During a prolonged fast, FFAs and ketone bodies supply the brain with its metabolic requirements (Shrayyef and Gerich, 2010). Lipolysis increases plasma levels of FFAs, which augment insulin resistance at multiple levels. The rise in FFAs impairs both the first- and second-phase insulin response in genetically predisposed individuals (DeFronzo, 2009). This portends to glucotoxicity occurring with each meal. Chronic exposure to elevated plasma glucose favors β-cell apoptosis (cell death). Hepatic glucose production is also accelerated by a rise in FFAs. Additionally, FFAs competitively bind to insulin receptors on myocytes, after which the GLUT4 transport mechanism is blocked from carrying glucose as an energy source from plasma into cells (DeFronzo, 2009).

Intracellular signaling occurs between the β and α cells such that glucose levels are tightly regulated, minimizing the likelihood of postprandial hypoglycemia. In the presence of decreasing plasma glucose levels, the α cells will signal the β cells to cease insulin production and secretion as glucagon levels rise. The secretion of glucagon results in

Table 34-5   Regulators of Normal Glucose Homeostasis

Regulating Component	Glucose Production	Glucose Disposal	Lipolysis
Insulin	↓	↑	↓
Glucagon	↑	—	—
Epinephrine	↑	↓	↑
Cortisol	↑	↓	↑
Growth hormone	↑	↓	↑
FFAs	↑	↓	—
Amylin	—	↓	—*

*Free fatty acids (FFAs) may stimulate release of insulin and amylin.

hepatic gluconeogenesis and a return to euglycemia. As β cell function and mass deteriorates, the neurologic pathways of communication between the α and β cells are disrupted, resulting in excess glucagon production. Clinically, patients experience elevations in fasting and postabsorptive glucose levels.

The role of the kidneys in maintaining normoglycemia through the filtration and reabsorption of glucose and gluconeogenesis is well established. Each day, 180 L of plasma filters through the kidneys, translating into a filtration load of approximately 180 g of glucose. Ninety percent of renal glucose reabsorption occurs within the proximal glomeruli tubules, where sodium–glucose co-transporter 2 (SGLT2) is present. Ten percent of circulating glucose is reabsorbed in the distal tubules via sodium–glucose co-transporter 1 (SGLT1). SGLT1 is also expressed in the gut and is responsible for absorption of both dietary glucose and galactose. The glucose transport mechanism becomes saturated when plasma glucose levels exceed 180 to 190 mmol/L. Beyond the point of transporter saturation, any additional glucose is detected as glycosuria (DeFronzo et al., 2012). The key hormonal and metabolic regulators of normal glucose homeostasis are shown in Table 34-5.

Insulin acts as a growth factor in the brain and supports neuronal repair, dendritic sprouting and synaptogenesis, and protection from oxidative stress. The increased risk of Alzheimer disease, Parkinson disease, and stroke in people with T2DM suggests that shared mechanisms or pathways of cell death, possibly related to insulin dysregulation, may underlie all of these disorders. Although the disease anatomy varies with each disorder, a wide range of genetic and environmental factors triggers activation of similar biochemical pathways in all of them, suggesting a complex network of biochemical events that feed into a final common path toward cellular dysfunction and death (Rasool et al., 2013).

Patients with T2DM exhibit multiple abnormalities in glucose homeostasis, including impaired first- and second-phase insulin secretion; inappropriately timed and excessive glucagon secretion; increased hepatic glucose production despite elevations in endogenous plasma insulin levels; reduced peripheral uptake of glucose within skeletal muscle cells; loss of central neural protection promoting alterations in satiety and weight gain; an overexpression of SGLT2 within the renal proximal tubules, subsequently increasing plasma reabsorption of glucose and promoting insulin resistance; amplified lipolysis, resulting in β cell apoptosis; and loss of the meal-triggered insulin response, which may

Table 34-6 Summary of Pathological Deficits Associated with Type 2 Diabetes Mellitus

Target Organ/Tissue	Physiological Defects	Glycemic Effects
Pancreatic β cells	Loss of first-phase insulin secretion Delayed second-phase insulin secretion Loss of amylin secretion	Glucose toxicity results in β-cell apoptosis.
Pancreatic α cells	α-Cell hypertrophy Loss of α- and β-cell signaling results in loss of appropriate and timely counterregulation; patients are more likely to develop hypoglycemia awareness autonomic failure over time. Exaggerated, paradoxical, and untimely secretion of glucagon during both the fasting and postprandial states	Hyperglucagonemia results in glucose toxicity, β-cell destruction, and excessive hepatic glucose production. Patients experience an increase in fasting and postprandial glucose levels; this increases their A1C. Insulin resistance is exacerbated.
Hepatocytes	Excessive hepatic glucose production despite initial elevations in circulating plasma insulin levels The liver excretes >25 g/day of extra glucose into the plasma	Increases insulin resistance Increases gluconeogenesis and glycogenolysis
Myocytes	Impaired uptake and intracellular utilization of glucose	Increases peripheral insulin resistance Increases fasting and postabsorptive glucose levels Marked deficiency in peripheral glucose utilization is the most significant defect observed in insulin resistance.
Gut	Reduction in secretion of GLP-1 and GIP by the intestines in response to oral glucose stimulation When GLP-1 is secreted, ≈80% of the gut hormone is immediately deactivated by DPP-4; reduced levels of GLP-1 result in proportionally lower amounts of GLP-1 being expressed at pancreatic β-cell receptors. GLP-1 resistance at target tissue site Amylin levels are reduced within pancreatic islets; amylin and insulin are co-secreted in a glucose-dependent manner.	Alters gastric emptying Causes weight gain Increases fasting and postprandial glucose levels Reduces sense of satiety Causes loss of neuroprotection against Alzheimer disease and Parkinson disease Reduction in amylin accelerates gastric emptying and impairs satiety. The overall effect is a rise in postprandial glucose values.
Adipose tissue	Increased lipolysis in response to a reduction in circulating endogenous insulin	β-cell destruction Increases FFAs Increases hepatic glucose production because the liver is unable to store glycogen Impairs GLUT4 transport of glucose into muscle, exacerbating peripheral insulin resistance
Brain	Loss of neuroprotection	Increases appetite Favors obesity Increases oxidative stress Insulin resistance appears to be associated with Alzheimer disease and Parkinson disease.
Kidneys	Increased expression of SGLT2 in the proximal glomerular tubules Daily renal filtered glucose threshold increases from 180 to 240 g/day.	90% of filtered glucose is absorbed via SGLT2 in the proximal tubules, and 10% is absorbed by SGLT1 in the distal tubules. SGLT1 is also expressed in the gut, where daily dietary glucose absorption of 180 g occurs. If the renal glucose threshold of the SGLT2 transport mechanism is surpassed, glycosuria occurs. In T2DM, the threshold is increased from 180 to 240 g/day, which results in an increased renal absorption of glucose regardless of the patient's state of chronic hyperglycemia. Excessive reabsorption of glucose from the kidneys exacerbates insulin resistance.

DPP-4, Dipeptidyl peptidase-4; *FFA*, free fatty acid; *GIP*, glucose-dependent insulinotropic polypeptide; *GLP-1*, glucagon-like peptide 1; *GLUT4*, glucose transporter type 4; *SGLT2*, sodium–glucose co-transporter 2; *T2DM*, type 2 diabetes mellitus.
Data from DeFronzo RA. From the triumvirate to the ominous octet: a new paradigm for the treatment of type 2 diabetes mellitus. *Diabetes*. 58:773-795, 2009.

maintain weight and euglycemia for years. Table 34-6 summarizes the common pathogenic pathways related to T2DM.

The pathogenesis of T2DM is multifactorial. Genetically or environmentally challenged individuals begin the transformation from euglycemia to clinically apparent T2DM as their skeletal muscles and hepatocytes exhibit early evidence of insulin resistance. Initially, pancreatic β cells attempt to compensate for IGT by overproducing insulin. Obesity plays a major role in the progression of prediabetes to T2DM. Compared with lean individuals, overweight euglycemic subjects appear to require a longer time to achieve satiety, and the magnitude of their appetite suppression also reduced (Matsuda, 1999). Thus, obesity tends to

become self-promoting. As meal portions increase, so does the secretion of GLP-1, resulting in β-cell hypertrophy.

Few individuals can maintain hypersecretion of insulin for a prolonged period of time. Patients who have primary relatives with T2DM will lose their acute, first-phase insulin response to a glucose stimulus and experience a delay in the initiation of their second-phase response. IGT will now become apparent as patients progress into a state of prediabetes. Over time, other metabolic defects appear, which tend to aggravate the existing state of hyperglycemia. As endogenous insulin levels decline, lipolysis is accelerated because insulin action normally stabilizes fat cells. Lipolysis further aggravates the first-phase insulin response, promotes

Table 34-7   Factors Promoting Patients' Adherence to Their Diabetes Management Regimen

Higher socioeconomic status and level of education
Resolution of comorbid mental illness symptomatology
Spousal, familial, and communal support
Satisfaction with doctor–patient relationship
Availability of and support from a diabetes health care team
Appointment reminder cards, reminder phone calls regarding upcoming appointments, minimal clinic waiting room delays, and emphasis on the positive aspects of patient's diabetes self-management efforts rather than on patient's failures or oversights
Simplified treatment regimens
Particular aspect of the regimen; patient adherence to medication regimens surpasses their adherence to lifestyle or behavioral recommendations
Co-management of "complex" patients with a mental health professional

Reprinted with permission from Unger J. *Diabetes management in primary care.* 2nd ed. Philadelphia: Lippincott, Williams and Wilkins; 2012.

Table 34-8   Medical Nutrition Therapy Recommendations for Patients with Diabetes

Patients with diabetes should receive customized MNT recommendations from a registered dietitian who is familiar with the components of diabetes nutritional interventions.
Portion control and healthy food choices are suitable options for patients with literacy and numeracy concerns. Older adults may also benefit from this simplified approach to meal planning.
Reducing food intake and increasing energy expenditure is recommended to promote weight loss in obese adult patients with T2DM.
Modest weight loss may result in improvement in glycemia, blood pressure, and lipids, especially when initiated soon after patients are diagnosed with diabetes. Intensive lifestyle education and management is recommended for newly diagnosed patients with diabetes.
The optimal mix of macronutrients (i.e., carbohydrates, fats, and proteins) in the daily diet should be individualized.
Patients' personal preferences regarding foods and metabolic goals should be considered when discussing eating patterns and meal planning.
Substituting low–glycemic index foods for higher–glycemic index foods may modestly improve glycemic control.
People with diabetes should consume fiber and whole grains in a manner similar to what is recommended to the general public.
People with diabetes should minimize their consumption of sugar-containing beverages.

MNT, Medical nutrition therapy; *T2DM,* type 2 diabetes mellitus.
Data from Evert AB, Boucher JL, Cypress M, et al. Nutrition therapy recommendations for the management of adults with diabetes. *Diabetes Care.* 36:3821-3842, 2013.

glycogen breakdown by hepatocytes, and prevents the peripheral uptake of glucose by skeletal muscle cells.

The complex pathogenesis of diabetes underscores the importance of combining rational polypharmacy designed to target specific metabolic defects with ILIs when managing patients with T2DM.

LIFESTYLE INTERVENTIONS FOR TYPE 2 DIABETES MELLITUS

Lifestyle interventions focusing on both diet and physical activity are clearly beneficial for patients with diabetes. Reducing caloric intake to 1100 kcal/day has been shown to decrease fasting blood glucose levels in obese patients with T2DM and in those with normal glucose tolerance in as few as 4 days (Markovic et al., 1998).

Behavior changes are almost always necessary for patients to adopt and maintain a healthy lifestyle, reduce their long-term risks, and perform daily self-care tasks essential to attaining adequate glycemic control. By some estimates, fewer than 50% of patients with diabetes adhere to recommended lifestyle and behavioral guidelines (Peyrot et al., 2005). Furthermore, adherence is a multidimensional concept in that some patients may comply with their medication regimens while ignoring dietary or physical activity recommendations. Others, who say they "feel just fine," may try to exercise for 2 to 3 hours per day in an attempt to avoid starting medications that are needed to manage their hyperglycemia, hypertension, and hyperlipidemia. In addition, a study of NHANES data collected from patients with T2DM found that 29% of insulin-treated patients, 65% of those taking oral medications, and 80% of those whose diabetes was managed by diet and exercise alone either never performed SMBG—a key component of diabetes self-management—or did so less than once a month (Harris, 2001). Factors that promote patient adherence to their diabetes management regimen are listed in noted in Table 34-7.

New ADA nutrition guidelines published in 2013 focus on overall nutrition and patient preferences rather than any particular dietary prescription (Evert et al., 2013). The "diabetic diet" has been officially replaced with concepts such as "healthful eating patterns" and "individualized eating plans." Clinicians should emphasize personal characteristics and preferences (e.g., patients' tradition, culture, religion, health beliefs, health goals, and financial circumstances) when providing nutrition counseling. In addition, clinicians should refer newly diagnosed patients with diabetes to a registered dietitian to ensure that they receive timely and appropriate medical nutrition therapy (MNT). Highlights of the ADA nutrition recommendations are listed in Table 34-8.

The Look AHEAD study was a 4-year RCT comparing ILI with standard diabetes education and support in 4503 adult patients with T2DM and BMIs of 25 kg/m^2 or greater. The study sought to determine the frequency of remission from T2DM to prediabetes or normoglycemia between the two groups of subjects. Partial or complete remission of diabetes was defined as transition from meeting the criteria for a diagnosis of diabetes to having prediabetic or nondiabetic levels of glycemia (fasting plasma glucose <126 mg/dL and A1C <6.5% with no antihyperglycemic medication). Partial or complete remission was observed in 11.5% (95% confidence interval, 10.1%-12.8%) of the ILI group at 4 years compared with 1.5% to 2.7% of the conventionally managed individuals (P <0.001), thus supporting the importance of early lifestyle intervention after patients are diagnosed with diabetes (Gregg et al., 2012).

Intensive lifestyle intervention also has been considered as a means by which cardiovascular risk may be reduced. Although the Look AHEAD study successfully improved T2DM remission rates when ILI was initiated soon after diagnosis, weight loss and exercise did not translate into a reduction in cardiovascular risk. Weight loss was greater in the intervention group than in the control cohort throughout the study (8.6% vs. 0.7% at 1 year and 6.0% vs. 3.5%

at study end after 9.6 years). The ILI group also demonstrated greater reductions in A1C and greater initial improvements in fitness and cardiovascular risk factors. However, cardiovascular end points occurred in 403 patients in the intervention group and in 418 patients in the control group ($P = 0.51$). Thus, ILI focusing on weight loss did not appear to reduce the rate of cardiovascular events in overweight or obese adults with T2DM (Look AHEAD Research Group, 2013).

Obesity prevalence rates began to increase sharply 30 years ago, and obesity has since emerged as a global public health hazard. Thirty-five percent of the U.S. adult population is obese (BMI ≥30 kg/m²), and another 35% is classified as overweight (BMI, 25-29.9 kg/m²) (Flegal et al., 2012). Obesity is associated with disorders such as metabolic syndrome, prediabetes, T2DM, and CVD. Indeed, 80% of patients with T2DM are overweight or obese (National Diabetes Information Clearinghouse, 2013). The third report of the U.S. National Cholesterol Education Program (NCEP) Expert Panel on Detection, Evaluation, and Treatment of High Blood Cholesterol in Adults classified T2DM as a coronary heart disease risk equivalent (NCEP Expert Panel, 2002). This classification was based in part on the observation that people with T2DM and no prior myocardial infarction (MI) (mean age, 58 years) were at the same risk as people without diabetes who had a prior MI (mean age, 56 years) for MI (20% and 19%, respectively) and coronary mortality (15% and 16%, respectively) (Haffner et al., 1998).

Therapy for obesity includes lifestyle modification, pharmacologic interventions, and bariatric surgery. The presence and severity of obesity-related complications should be assessed before initiating therapy for overweight patients. Complications related to insulin resistance include hypertension, hyperlipidemia, treatment-resistant diabetes, obstructive sleep apnea, proteinuria, and fatty liver disease. Patients also may have complications related to mechanical or functional disorders, including gastroesophageal reflux, stress incontinence, immobility, and joint pain.

Weight loss medications (i.e., phentermine/topiramate ER, lorcaserin) should be considered for overweight or obese patients with T2DM who fail to achieve moderate weight loss (i.e., ≈10% of their baseline weight) through lifestyle modification (Garvey, 2013). Weight loss drugs can also be used in conjunction with certain oral agents for diabetes (e.g., metformin, SGLT2 inhibitors, and GLP-1 receptor agonists), which are discussed in greater detail in the Long-Term Complications of Diabetes section of this chapter. Patients who fail to improve their metabolic profiles while using FDA-approved weight loss agents may be candidates for bariatric surgery (also known as "metabolic surgery").

Bariatric surgery consists of several well-defined procedures. Restrictive surgeries such as laparoscopic adjustable gastric banding (LAGB) and vertical banded gastroplasty (VBG) reduce the volume of the stomach by 85% to decrease food intake and induce early satiety. VBG is also known as sleeve gastrectomy. LAGB is considered a minimally invasive intervention through which a restrictive band is placed around the upper stomach to partition a small proximal pouch. Initially, these bands were designed for open surgical placement and were not adjustable. However, further refinement has now enabled surgeons to place the adjustable

Table 34-9 Preoperative Factors Positively Predicting Diabetes Resolution after Bariatric Surgery in Severely Obese Patients with Type 2 Diabetes Mellitus

Baseline A1C of 6.5% to 7.9% (77% remission rate vs. 50% remission rate for those having a baseline A1C >10%)
Duration of diabetes of ≤5.5 years
Baseline C-peptide >3 ng/mL (suggestive of severe insulin resistance)
Baseline BMI >45 kg/m²
Significantly elevated basal and 2-hour postprandial insulin levels

BMI, Body mass index.
Data from Schernthaner G, Brix JM, Kopp HP, et al. Cure of type 2 diabetes by metabolic surgery? A critical analysis of the evidence in 2010. *Diabetes Care.* 34(suppl 2):S355-S360, 2011.

Table 34-10 Benefits of Bariatric Surgery in Severely Obese Patients with Type 2 Diabetes Mellitus

Average 1.72 life-years gained in patients with a history of diabetes for <5 years before surgery
Patients with a BMI of 30-34 kg/m₂ have the most cost-effective outcomes over time
Cost-effectiveness ratio of $7,000 to $12,000 per quality-adjusted life year gained
Cost savings greatest in patients 65 to 74 years of age who have had diabetes for <5 years
Bariatric surgery resulted in a remission rate of ≈40% to 80% (After bariatric surgery, the likelihood of diabetes relapse is 8% annually.)
Systolic blood pressure reduced 11.25% during the first 2 years followed by an additional 1.4% reduction until year 10; no further improvement in blood pressure observed thereafter
Total cholesterol reduced 16.1% during the first 2 years followed by a 1.2% reduction each year thereafter until year 10
HDL cholesterol improves 10% during the first 2 years and then decreases by 0.05% through year 10

BMI, Body mass index; *HDL*, high-density lipoprotein.
Data from Hoerger TJ, Zhang P, Segel JE, et al. Cost-effectiveness of metabolic surgery for severely obese adults with diabetes. *Diabetes Care.* 33:1933-1939, 2010.

appliance laparoscopically. Malabsorptive procedures such as biliopancreatic diversion (BPD) shorten the small intestine to decrease nutrient absorption. Combined procedures such as the roux-en-Y gastric bypass (RYGB) incorporate both restrictive and malabsorptive elements. RYGB surgery is considered the gold-standard treatment for severe obesity. Both BPD and RYGB alter the secretion of gut hormones that affect satiety. Factors that predict the resolution of T2DM after bariatric surgery are listed in Table 34-9. Table 34-10 lists the benefits of bariatric surgery for patients with T2DM.

Patients who are considering bariatric surgery should be counseled about the risks and benefits of the different types of available procedures. Specific contraindications to bariatric surgery are few and include mental or cognitive impairment that limits patients' ability to understand the procedure and thus precludes informed consent. Very severe coexisting medical conditions such as unstable coronary artery disease or advanced liver disease with portal hypertension may, in some instances, render the risks of surgery unacceptably high. On average, bariatric surgery is associated with a mortality risk in the range of 0.3%. Significant or major complications occur in just over 4% of patients (Flum et al., 2009).

Physical activity and weight loss lower the risk of developing T2DM by 58% in high-risk individuals (American College of Sports Medicine and ADA, 2010). Physical activity decreases peripheral insulin resistance by improving glucose uptake by skeletal muscle cells. During muscle activity, glucose is transported into myocytes and used to replenish muscle glycogen stores. Glycogen is metabolized during exercise in a process known as glycogenolysis. Moderate exercise consisting of the use of 350 kcal of energy will result in improvement of peripheral insulin sensitivity over the course of 24 hours (Newsom et al., 2013). In T2DM, GLUT4 is impaired at rest but enhanced by the muscle contractions that occur during physical activity. Thus, insulin resistance at the periphery improves with exercise (Wang Y et al., 2009) Recommendations for T2DM physical activity prescribing are shown in Table 34-11.

Self-monitoring of blood glucose allows patients to evaluate their individual responses to lifestyle and pharmacologic interventions and to assess whether they are achieving their short-term glycemic targets. SBGM can also be used to detect extreme changes in blood glucose levels, including hypoglycemia, hyperglycemia, and DKA. Patients who successfully use SBGM can learn to adjust insulin doses, alter activity levels, and better understand the correlation between food intake and pharmacologic therapy.

Structured glucose testing is useful for recognizing specific problematic glycemic patterns such as hypoglycemia, fasting hyperglycemia, and postprandial hyperglycemia. Identifying the most likely cause of these patterns can assist patients in altering behaviors or changing medications or dosages to improve overall glycemic control (Polonsky et al., 2009). Structured testing can be performed before and after meals to determine the effect of food intake on glycemic excursions. Patients who perform SMBG before and after exercise will learn how insulin resistance at peripheral muscle sites appears to improve with mild to moderate activity performed 5 days per week. In addition, by testing pre- and postprandial blood glucose at breakfast for 2 or 3 days before initiating exercise, they can better determine at what time of day exercise will have the greatest glucose-lowering effect. When a patient begins an exercise program, this paired testing pattern is simply repeated, and exercise-related reductions in blood glucose can be identified. The same SMBG testing pattern can be repeated for each meal but should be individualized based on patients' eating, working, exercise, and sleeping habits.

The difference between premeal and 2-hour postprandial blood glucose levels is known as the Δ (or delta, a math symbol indicating the difference between two values). A physiological response to a meal should result in a positive Δ value of 0 to 50 mg/dL. For example, an insulin-requiring patient with T2DM checks his blood glucose before lunch and notes the blood glucose level as 100 mg/dL. He anticipates that he will require 8 units of rapid-acting insulin to cover the carbohydrates consumed for that meal. Two hours after eating, his postmeal glucose is 134, and his Δ is +34. This means that he administered the correct amount of insulin for that meal. The interpretation of Δ values resulting from structured SMBG around meals is explained in more detail in Table 34-12. Note that any negative Δ values 2 hours postprandially would indicate that the patient is at risk for developing postabsorptive hypoglycemia. Thus,

Table 34-11 Summary of Physical Activity Recommendations for Patients with Type 2 Diabetes Mellitus

- Perform at least 150 minutes of moderately intense physical activity (50%-70% of maximum heart rate) over at least 3 days/wk with no more than 2 consecutive days void of exercise.
- Indications for exercise stress testing:
  - Age >40 years with or without cardiovascular risk factors in addition to diabetes
  - Age >30 years plus:
    - T1DM or T2DM of a disease duration >10 years
    - Hypertension
    - Current cigarette smoker
    - Dyslipidemia
    - Proliferative or preproliferative retinopathy
    - Chronic kidney disease, including microalbuminuria
  - Known history of stroke, coronary artery disease, or peripheral vascular disease
  - Autonomic neuropathy
  - End-stage renal disease
- Unless contraindicated, patients should be encouraged to participate in resistance training (2 to 4 sets of 8 to 10 repetitions each) twice weekly.
  - Adults should train each major muscle group 2 or 3 days/wk using a variety of exercises and equipment.
  - Very light or light intensity is best for older people or previously sedentary adults starting exercise.
  - Two to four sets of each exercise will help adults improve strength and power.
  - For each exercise, 8 to 12 repetitions will improve strength and power, 10 to 15 repetitions will improve strength in middle-aged and older people starting exercise, and 15 to 20 repetitions will improve muscular endurance.
  - Adults should wait at least 48 hours between resistance training sessions.
  - Contraindications for resistance training include poor left ventricular function, unstable angina, proliferative diabetic retinopathy, cardiac autonomic neuropathy, a history of exercise-induced ventricular dysthymias, vertigo, and vestibular dysfunction.
- Monitor blood glucose before and after exercise. Proactively treat for hypoglycemia:
  - If pre-exercise blood glucose level is <100 mg/dL, patients using secretagogues or insulin should consume 15 g of carbohydrates before initiating physical activity.
  - Consuming 5 to 30 g of carbohydrates may be necessary to minimize hypoglycemia risk during intense or prolonged physical activity lasting more than 30 minutes.
- Patients requiring supervised cardiovascular rehabilitation programs include:
  - Those with cardiac autonomic neuropathy, coronary artery disease, peripheral vascular disease, stroke, proliferative retinopathy, macular edema, autonomic neuropathy (loss of sweating capacity), or peripheral neuropathy (increased risk of falls and foot ulcerations)

T1DM, Type 1 diabetes mellitus; *T2DM,* type 2 diabetes mellitus.
American College of Sports Medicine and American Diabetes Association, 2010; Bjarnason-Wehrens et al., 2004; Garber CE et al, 2011.

patients with negative Δ values should continue monitoring their blood glucose 3 and 4 hours after the meal to ensure that they do not experience a rapid decline in blood glucose.

In summary, lifestyle intervention provides the foundation of care for all patients with diabetes. Patients at high risk for developing diabetes should be encouraged to increase their physical activity and to adopt a healthier meal plan in an attempt to reduce both their weight and their cardiometabolic risk. ILI appears to have a greater effect on inducing diabetes remission if it is initiated soon after patients

Table 34-12   Interpretation of Structured Self-Monitoring of Blood Glucose Δ Values*

Δ (mg/dL)	Interpretation	Intervention
0-50	Correct insulin was given for amount of carbohydrates consumed Correct lag time procedure was followed	None
51-100	Insulin-to-carbohydrate undercalculation Incorrect lag time Possible snacking between end of meal and 2-hour test	Increase prandial insulin dose by 1 to 2 units next time this type of food is eaten Make sure to inject insulin at least 15 minutes before meals
100-200	Patient possibly had elevated blood glucose before the meal and did not take a correction dose of insulin Insulin-to-carbohydrate mismatch Insulin may have been omitted Possible error in SMBG technique	Teach patient how to use a premeal insulin sensitivity factor (see discussion of physiological insulin replacement) If a patient omitted insulin, the Δ value illustrates the effect of this decision If postmeal Δ is consistently elevated, increase prescribed baseline insulin dose by 1 unit/day until Δ is 0-50 or 2-hour postprandial glucose is <140 mg/dL Educate patient on proper SMBG technique; touching fruit, cake, or ice cream after a meal may leave sugar deposits on the fingertips and result in falsely high SMBG results
Any negative value (e.g., −25)	Miscalculation of insulin-to-carbohydrate ratio; too much insulin bolused for amount of carbohydrates eaten; patient is likely to become hypoglycemic in the next 1 to 2 hours	Educate patient regarding insulin absorption principles: 1 hour after administering bolus, 90% of rapid-acting insulin analog remains in depot; 2 hours after bolusing, 60% of insulin remains in depot. Thus, if 10 units of insulin are given at 8:00 AM, 6 units remain to be absorbed at 10:00 AM. A premeal glucose value of 120 mg/dL and a 2-hour postprandial value of 90 mg/dL yield a Δ of −30 mg/dL. The patient still has 6 units remaining to be absorbed and is likely to become hypoglycemic. Appropriate surveillance and intervention should be initiated.

*The Δ value is calculated by determining the difference between the premeal and 2-hour postprandial glucose values. A physiological rise in 2-hour postprandial glucose levels from baseline in euglycemic individuals is ≤50 mg/dL.
SMBG, Self-monitoring of blood glucose.
Adapted with permission from Unger J. *Diabetes management in primary care.* 2nd ed. Philadelphia: Lippincott, Williams and Wilkins; 2012.

are diagnosed with impaired glycemic control. Patients should be referred to a registered dietitian soon after being diagnosed to receive their customized MNT and meal program.

The ADA and the American College of Sports Medicine encourage the prescribing of cardiovascular and resistance training for nearly all patients with diabetes. Before initiating any form of intensive physical activity, patients with a disease duration of longer than 10 years should undergo a stress test. Patients with advanced disease should exercise in a supervised environment.

Obese or overweight patients with T2DM may be considered candidates for antiobesity pharmacotherapeutic interventions, especially if they are at high risk for CVD. Patients who are unable to modify their weight should be referred to a bariatric surgeon.

The use of structured SMBG will allow patients to determine patterns of glycemic control in relation to the use of their medications, meals, and exercise habits. In addition, structured SMBG may be useful in predicting the onset of hypoglycemia.

MEDICAL MANAGEMENT OF PATIENTS WITH TYPE 2 DIABETES MELLITUS

The goals of therapeutic intervention in patients with T2DM are to (1) encourage the adoption of healthy lifestyle choices (i.e., cease alcohol, nicotine, and substance abuse; follow a healthful eating plan; and increase physical activity); (2) encourage modest weight reduction (5%-10% from baseline); and 3) introduce safe, effective, and rational pharmacologic interventions in a timely manner that will allow patients to achieve their customized metabolic targets.

Primary care physicians are actively involved in screening, diagnosing, and managing patients with diabetes; 90% of all patients with diabetes are managed in the primary care setting. Diabetes is a multifactorial disease state that is chronic and progressive. As such, its management requires frequent reassessment and adjustment.

ENCOURAGING PATIENT SELF-CARE

Clinicians should be viewed as "coaches" who direct diabetes care, although patients are ultimately responsible for carrying out the complex daily self-management regimen. Unlike with other chronic diseases such as cancer, patients with diabetes are required to make multiple decisions each day that may affect their glycemic control. Glucose levels may vary based on physical activity, sleep duration, timing and dosing of antihyperglycemic therapies, food consumption, macronutrient intake, renal and hepatic status, concomitant prescribed medications, recent history of hypoglycemia, and accuracy of SMBG technique. Therefore, patients must take an active role to achieve their metabolic targets and successfully manage their diabetes.

Diabetes self-management can become all-encompassing and distressful. Patients with diabetes have to make choices and decisions throughout each day in hopes of keeping their blood glucose levels within the physiological range of 90 to 130 mg/dL. Patients should never be blamed for failing to achieve their fasting blood glucose, postprandial glucose, or A1C targets. Instead, clinicians must work with patients to provide the tools they need to become successful at diabetes self-management.

When euglycemic individuals eat, their glucose levels are maintained within a narrow range (85-126 mg/dL). This occurs because the normally functioning pancreas is provided with neuroendocrine signals, allowing its α and β cells to coordinate the perfect level of insulin secretion to cover the carbohydrates consumed in each meal. Patients with diabetes have multiple physiological deficits. Over time, their β-cell function deteriorates to the point at which insulin must be used to maintain adequate control of plasma glucose levels. When insulinopenic patients eat, exogenous insulin must be given based on a dose calculation they determine before each meal. Dose determinations are not always simple, and by no means are they always correct. Patients have to substitute their brain for their pancreas to control their glycemia and self-manage their disease. Therefore, criticism of patients with diabetes should be tempered at all times, and patients should be encouraged to attain the best level of glycemic control of which they capable.

INDIVIDUALIZED METABOLIC TARGETS

Randomized controlled trials such as the DCCT in patients with T1DM (DCCT Research Group, 1993) and the UKPDS (U.K. Prospective Diabetes Study Group, 1998) and Kumamoto Study (Ohkubo et al., 1995) in those with T2DM established glycemic therapeutic goals that minimize the risk of long-term complications. Neither the DCCT nor the UKPDS was successful at maintaining A1C levels below 7% in their intensively treated cohorts.

More recently, published RCTs have attempted to intensify patients' glycemic control to a target A1C below 6.5% using a variety of interventions. The primary objective of the ACCORD study (ACCORD Study Group, 2008) was to decrease CVD in high-risk patients. More than 10,000 patients either with or at risk for developing CVD were randomized either to an intensive intervention targeting an A1C level of less than 6.0% or to an intervention with a more conservative A1C target of less than 7.9%. The intensively treated cohort demonstrated a 22% higher rate of cardiovascular mortality than the more conservatively managed patients. Based on ACCORD data, the ADA now recommends that clinicians consider patients' disease duration, severity of comorbidities, hypoglycemia history, and life expectancy when setting individualized metabolic targets. Patients deemed to be at high risk should have an A1C target of 7.5% to 8%, but most healthy patients should be treated to an A1C target of 6.5% or less to 7% (ADA, 2013b; Ismail-Beigi et al., 2011).

Some have speculated that the excess mortality rate in ACCORD may have been related to hypoglycemia. Interestingly, however, severe hypoglycemia was associated with an increased risk of death in the more conservative treatment cohort more so than in the intensively managed cohort (Bonds et al., 2012). Additionally, severe hypoglycemia events were more prevalent in patients having a higher baseline A1C; those with A1C levels closer to the 7% target had more frequent, but less severe, hypoglycemia episodes. Hypoglycemia results in the release of counterregulatory hormones, including cortisol, norepinephrine, and epinephrine. Hypoglycemia may also increase the risk of QTc prolongation (Beom et al., 2013). Patients who experience QTc prolongation during an episode of severe hypoglycemia would be subject to potentially fatal arrhythmias (i.e.,

torsades de pointes ventricular tachycardia) induced by the release of catecholamines (Figure 34-1).

Could repeated episodes of hypoglycemia be protective against sudden death, as observed in ACCORD patients who were closer to the prescribed A1C target? A single episode of hypoglycemia will result in defective counterregulation and a blunted adrenergic response to future events. Additionally, patients who become hypoglycemic lose their ability to recognize the symptoms of low blood glucose. Thus, hypoglycemia awareness autonomic failure (also called "hypoglycemia unawareness") may result in a form of hypoglycemia preconditioning that protects against the development of a fatal arrhythmia.

Patients with suboptimal glycemic control who are ambitiously treated to a fasting glucose or A1C level based on politically motivated incentive payment programs may be at risk for developing fatal arrhythmias. Clinicians must consider all aspects of patients' medical, behavioral, and social history before determining their optimal individualized glycemic targets.

Metrics other than A1C are also important to evaluate to identify and mitigate each patient's long-term risk for complications. Hirsch and Brownlee have suggested that A1C and duration of diabetes (glycemic exposure) accounted for only 11% of the total risk in the retinopathy cohort of T1DM patients in the DCCT (Hirsch and Brownlee, 2010). The remaining 89% of a patient's likelihood for developing microvascular complications may be derived from genetics, environmental factors, poorly controlled lipids, and hypertension. Although targeting glycemic control patients is a noble goal, clinicians must never forget the complex metabolic nature of T2DM. Normalization of lipids, blood pressure, and renal function cannot be overshadowed by the struggle to become a "glycemic perfectionist."

The ADA and AACE have each published statements providing a framework for initiating and titrating pharmacologic therapies for patients with T2DM in the primary care setting (ADA, 2013b; Garber et al., 2013) A summary of the highlights for the AACE comprehensive diabetes management algorithm is offered in Table 34-13. Both the ADA and AACE statements include recommended metabolic treatment targets, which are summarized in Table 34-14. Clinicians should remember that managing patients with diabetes entails customizing targets for blood pressure, weight, and lipids, in addition to glycemia.

The American Academy of Family Physicians has yet to publish any guidelines on diabetes management. Patients are unique entities with individual concerns, fears, and abilities to address their given disease state. Primary care physicians must never lose sight of the importance of directing individualized care toward what is safe and efficacious for each patient.

PHARMACOLOGIC MANAGEMENT OF TYPE 2 DIABETES MELLITUS

After pharmacotherapy is initiated, patients must become even more active participants in their diabetes self-management. Performing SMBG, adhering to MNT and physical activity recommendations, and undergoing professional surveillance to determine whether metabolic targets

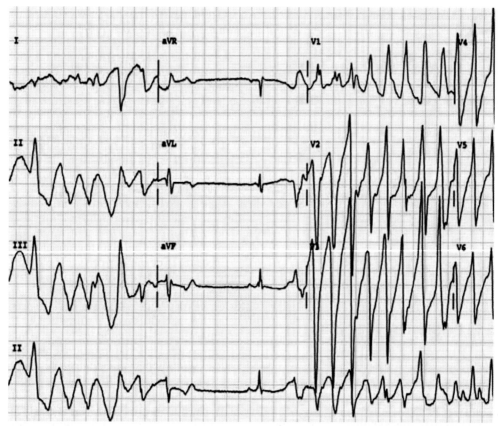

Figure 34-1 Torsades de pointes is a distinctive form of polymorphic ventricular tachycardia characterized by a gradual change in the amplitude and twisting of the QRS complexes around the isoelectric line. Torsades de pointes is associated with a prolonged QTc interval, which may be congenital or acquired. The arrhythmia usually terminates spontaneously but may reoccur and degenerate into a fatal form of ventricular fibrillation.

Table 34-13   Summary of the American Association of Clinical Endocrinologists 2013 Treatment Algorithm for Diabetes

- Lifestyle intervention remains the foundation of diabetes care across all A1C levels.
- If a patient's A1C is ≥9%, initiate and titrate basal insulin.
- Patients with an A1C <7.5% may be treated with monotherapy, as follows:
  - Metformin is considered first-line therapy.
  - Second-line therapies include GLP-1 receptor agonists, DPP-4 inhibitors, and α-glucosidase inhibitors.
  - If A1C is >6.5% after 3 months of therapy, add a second agent.
- Consider dual or triple combination therapy in patients with A1C levels ≥7.5% and ≤9%, as follows:
  - GLP-1 receptor agonists and DPP-4 inhibitors are the preferred agents.
  - Basal insulin may also be used.
  - SGLT2 inhibitors are acceptable drugs for combination therapy (ADA guidelines do not mention SGLT2 inhibitors).
  - If A1C is not at goal after 3 months, add a third agent.
- For patients who are symptomatic with an A1C of 8.5%, initiate basal insulin.
- Practical strategies to consider when customizing pharmacologic intervention include:
  - Prescribe medications that are less likely to result in hypoglycemia.
  - Medications that minimize weight gain should be preferred.
  - A1C testing should be repeated every 3 months until patients achieve their individualized goals.
  - Lifestyle intervention should be emphasized at each visit.
  - Smoking is unacceptable; encourage patients to stop nicotine use. Patients may be referred to 800-QUIT-NOW for free smoking cessation assistance.
  - Combination therapy using agents with complementary mechanisms of action is often required to help patients to achieve their prescribed glycemic targets.
  - When using insulin, DPP-4 inhibitors, SGLT2 inhibitors, metformin, GLP-1 receptor agonists, and bromocriptine may be continued. Sulfonylureas and thiazolidinediones should be discontinued because of increased risks of weight gain and hypoglycemia.
- Cost is important, but safety trumps cost.

ADA, American Diabetes Association; *DPP-4,* Dipeptidyl peptidase-4; *GLP-1,* glucagon-like peptide 1; *SGLT2,* sodium–glucose co-transporter 2.
Adapted from Garber AJ, Abrahamson MJ, Barzilay JI, et al. American Association of Clinical Endocrinologists' comprehensive diabetes management algorithm 2013 consensus statement: executive summary. *Endocr Pract.* 19:536-557, 2013.

Table 34-14 Metabolic Treatment Targets for Most Patients with Diabetes

Metabolic Target	AACE Guidelines	ADA Guidelines
A1C (%)	≤6.5	≤7.0
Fasting or premeal blood glucose (mg/dL)	<110	70-130
2-hour postprandial blood glucose (mg/dL)	<140	<180
Blood pressure (mm Hg)	<130/80	<140/80
LDL cholesterol (mg/dL)	<100 (<70 for high-risk patients with CVD)	<100
HDL cholesterol (mg/dL)	>40 for men; >50 for women	>50
Triglycerides (mg/dL)	<150	<150

AACE, American Association of Clinical Endocrinologists; *ADA,* American Diabetes Association; *CVD,* cardiovascular disease; *HDL,* high-density lipoprotein; *LDL,* low-density lipoprotein.
Adapted from Garber AJ, Abrahamson MJ, Barzilay JI, et al. American Association of Clinical Endocrinologists' comprehensive diabetes management algorithm 2013 consensus statement: executive summary. *Endocr Pract.* 19:536-557, 2013; American Diabetes Association. Standards of medical care in diabetes—2013. *Diabetes Care.* 36(suppl 1):S11-S66, 2013.

are being achieved are all necessary to lessen the impact of diabetes-related complications.

Patients should be aware of the potential risks and clinical benefits of the different types of oral agents. Some medications may increase weight or induce hypoglycemia; others must be held before undergoing certain diagnostic procedures. The continued use of oral agents during acute inpatient care may be detrimental. Insulin is the preferred drug for patients with diabetes who are admitted to the hospital for acute illness. Insulin also may be necessary in certain situations that complicate T2DM management, including concomitant use of corticosteroids, surgery, restricted oral nutrient intake, and pregnancy. Table 34-15 lists the noninsulin medications currently approved for patients with T2DM, as well as their mechanisms of action and safety concerns. Information on dosing adjustments required for incretin agents based on renal status is provided in Table 34-16.

In summary, clinicians should individualize metabolic targets for patients with diabetes. Lifestyle intervention remains the foundation of care for all patients with diabetes. Patients whose glycemic control deteriorates over time should be ambitiously managed initially with metformin or a combination of medications designed to address their particular pathophysiological defects. Treatment-naive patients will likely have some remaining β-cell function at the time of diagnosis and should respond to oral agents or incretins. Over time, β-cell function and mass will deteriorate, necessitating the use of insulin to control fasting and postprandial glucose excursions. Pharmacotherapy agents that have a low risk for potentiating hypoglycemia and weight gain should be preferred. Specific agents should be selected based on their likely effectiveness in reducing blood glucose levels to patients' individualized target range while taking into consideration patients' unique characteristics and preferences.

INSULIN INITIATION FOR PATIENTS WITH TYPE 2 DIABETES MELLITUS

Insulin is the most powerful tool in the diabetes pharmacologic armamentarium. Timely initiation of exogenous insulin appears to reduce insulin resistance and induce β-cell rest and does not increase cardiovascular or cancer risk over time (Gerstein et al., 2012). Thus, insulin initiation should be considered for symptomatic patients who have an A1C higher than 8.5% or for any patients who have an A1C higher than 9.0%. Basal insulin is simple to initiate and may be used safely in combination with several oral agents and with GLP-1 receptor agonists.

Type 2 diabetes mellitus is a progressive disease. Therefore, its effective treatment requires early initiation of appropriate therapies, frequent monitoring, and reassessment to make certain that therapeutic goals are attained.

Exposure to chronic hyperglycemia can cause micro- and macrovascular complications, many of which may already be apparent at the time of diabetes diagnosis. Multiple defective metabolic pathways work to overcome the body's defensive mechanisms, resulting in loss of β-cell function and mass. Ultimately, genetically prone individuals whose β cells become exposed to a progressively antagonistic metabolic environment will demonstrate apoptosis. As endogenous insulin levels are unable to prevent lipolysis, plasma FFA concentrations increase, further promoting apoptosis. FFAs also impair the body's first-phase insulin response and amplify hepatic glucose production. FFAs potentiate peripheral insulin resistance by blocking the ability of GLUT4 to transport glucose from the plasma into the myocytes. Patients exposed to chronic hyperglycemia may or may not experience symptoms similar to those with poorly controlled T1DM (i.e., fatigue, thirst, weight loss, hunger, frequent urination, and dry skin secondary to dehydration).

Intensified and individualized therapy targeting glycemic control is crucial for reducing the incidence of microvascular complications in patients with T2DM. Evidence supports efforts that appear to induce "metabolic memory," a theoretical protective mechanism through which early reversal and avoidance of hyperglycemia appear likely to minimize the risk of developing long-term complications (DCCT/EDIC Research Group, 2005). The fact that early initiation of intensive insulin therapy reduces insulin resistance and appears to induce β-cell rest suggests that such a regimen should be initiated sooner rather than later in treatment-naive patients with T2DM (Weng et al., 2008).

Recent RCTs have demonstrated that insulin interventions can be readily initiated and successfully titrated in the primary care setting (Gerstein et al., 2006; Meneghini et al., 2007) Additionally, with few exceptions, "needle phobia" often is less of an issue for patients than for clinicians. Most patients are willing to intensify their diabetes management according to the best guidance provided by their physicians. Clinicians are encouraged to develop several basal and prandial insulin protocols (perhaps using insulin pens or even disposable insulin patch pump devices) that can be introduced easily to patients (Figure 34-2).

Before initiating an insulin regimen, clinicians must consider patients' eating, sleeping, and exercise patterns and their ability to carry out diabetes self-management tasks. Perhaps most important, patients will need education

Table 34-15   Food and Drug Administration–Approved Noninsulin Pharmacologic Agents for Type 2 Diabetes Mellitus Treatment

Agents (Trade Name[s])	Mode of Action	Safety Concerns, Within-Class Distinctions, and Other Important Considerations
SULFONYLUREAS		
Glyburide (Micronase, Diabeta) Glipizide (Glucotrol) Glipizide-GITS (Glucotrol XL) Glyburide, micronized (Glynase) Glimepiride (Amaryl)	Insulin secretagogue	Increase the risk of hypoglycemia, especially in elderly adults and those with renal insufficiency or weight gain Meta-analysis suggests that sulfonylureas may increase stroke risk (Monami et al., 2013b) Short effective durability of drug except in patients with monogenetic T2DM (i.e., maturity-onset diabetes of the young) Glimepiride lowers fasting and postprandial glucose and has the best safety profile; avoid glyburide in elderly patients and those with CVD
BIGUANIDES		
Metformin (Glucophage) Metformin XL (Fortamet) Metformin XR (Glucophage XR, Glumetza) Metformin oral suspension	Decrease hepatic glucose production and glucose absorption from the GI tract and increase peripheral utilization of glucose	Must take with food to avoid gastritis and GI side effects Caution required for use in elderly patients and those with an estimated GFR rate <45 mL/min Withhold before contrast studies are performed; metformin may be restarted after serum creatinine is repeated and determined to be within a safe targeted range ≤10% of patients may be intolerant to side effect profile May reduce cancer risk in some patients with diabetes May improve fertility in patients with PCOS Some diabetologists prefer a dosing protocol involving rapid titration from 500 mg/day extended release with food to 2 g/day over 2 weeks
α-GLUCOSIDASE INHIBITORS		
Acarbose (Precose) Miglitol (Glyset)	Slow gut absorption of carbohydrates by inhibiting α-glucosidase enzymes	Contraindicated in inflammatory bowel disease, malabsorption syndromes, and partial bowel obstructions May induce hypoglycemia when used in combination therapy; oral glucose (dextrose), whose absorption is not inhibited by α-glucosidase inhibitors, should be used instead of sucrose (cane sugar) for hypoglycemia treatment; hypoglycemia will also respond to glucagon injection Glycemic efficacy of acarbose has been noted to be equal to that of metformin in treatment naive Chinese patients (Yang et al., 2014)
THIAZOLIDINEDIONE		
Pioglitazone (Actos)	Enhances tissue sensitivity to insulin in skeletal muscles by activating intracellular peroxisome proliferator-activated receptors	May cause resumption of ovulation in anovulatory premenopausal women Cases average weight gain of 0.9-2.6 kg Contraindicated in any patient with advanced heart failure (NYHA class III or class IV) or a history of bladder cancer Liver function testing required at baseline and every 2 months for the first year and then periodically thereafter Increases fracture risk in women
GLITINIDES		
Repaglinide (Prandin) Nateglinide (Starlix)	Rapid-acting insulin secretagogue with short (1- to 2-hour) duration of action; same mechanism of action as sulfonylureas but with a different binding site to pancreatic β cells	More effective than metformin, sulfonylureas, and thiazolidinediones at lowering postprandial blood glucose Less risk of hypoglycemia than sulfonylureas because of more rapid kinetics Must be taken 15 minutes before meals Approximately 1 month of therapy is required before fasting blood glucose decreases May either be weight neutral or result in slight weight increase
D2-DOPAMINE AGONIST		
Bromocriptine (Cycoset)	Resets dopaminergic and sympathetic tone within the central nervous system	Reduces glucose, triglycerides, and insulin resistance in patients with T2DM Can be used with all other oral agents and insulin Should be taken daily within 2 hours of rising Consider for use in patients who are shift workers; improving dopaminergic and sympathetic tone within the SCN may reduce insulin resistance; shift workers have disruption in their SCN pacemaker
BILE ACID SEQUESTRANT		
Colesevelam (Welchol)	Uncertain mode of action; may affect secretion of GLP-1	Not indicated as monotherapy in T2DM; may be used with metformin or metformin + sulfonylurea May be considered for off-label use in patients with prediabetes to reduce LDL cholesterol to <100 mg/dL and preserve β-cell function May be considered for use in T2DM patients who have elevated LDL cholesterol

Continued on following page

Table 34-15   Food and Drug Administration–Approved Noninsulin Pharmacologic Agents for Type 2 Diabetes Mellitus Treatment (Continued)

Agents (Trade Name[s])	Mode of Action	Safety Concerns, Within-Class Distinctions, and Other Important Considerations
DPP-4 INHIBITORS		
Sitagliptin (Januvia) Sitagliptin + metformin/sitagliptin + metformin, extended release (Janumet/Janumet XR) Saxagliptin (Onglyza) Saxagliptin + metformin, extended release (Kombiglyze XR) Linagliptin (Tradjenta) Linagliptin + metformin (Jentadueto) Alogliptin (Nesina) Alogliptin + metformin (Kazano) Alogliptin + pioglitazone (Oseni)	Block the action of DPP-4 enzymes, resulting in a two- to threefold increase in plasma levels of endogenous GLP-1	Most common side effects are rash and rhinitis Doses of all DPP-4 inhibitors, with the exception of linagliptin, must be adjusted based on renal status (see Table 34-15) As a class, DPP-4 inhibitors do not appear to increase the risk of CAD, HF, or hospitalizations for CHF; they also do not mitigate cardiovascular risk (Monami et al., 2013a) Oseni is contraindicated in patients with established NYHA class III or class IV HF and is not recommended in patients with symptomatic HF
GLP-1 RECEPTOR AGONISTS		
Exenatide (Byetta) Liraglutide (Victoza) Exenatide QW (Bydureon)	Enhance nutrient-stimulated insulin secretion via activation of GLP-1 receptors on β cells; inhibit glucagon secretion; delay gastric emptying; reduce appetite	Associated with weight loss Favorable effect on cardiovascular biomarkers Low rates of hypoglycemia Favor preservation of β-cell function GLP-1 infusion studies demonstrate favorable effects on endothelial cell function in humans Direct link to acute pancreatitis has not been demonstrated Contraindicated in patients with personal or family history of medullary thyroid carcinoma or MEN II (medullary thyroid cancer + pheochromocytoma) Most common adverse effect is nausea, which can be avoided if patients do not eat beyond the point of satiety When used with insulin secretagogue or insulin, reduce dose of secretagogue or insulin to minimize the likelihood of inducing hypoglycemia Exenatide is injected twice daily within 1 hr of eating; liraglutide is injected once daily without regard to meals; exenatide QW is injected once weekly Contraindicated in patients with a history of pancreatitis. Pancreatitis has been observed in patients taking GLP-1 receptor agonists or DPP-4 inhibitors. However, no direct signal has been noted that would implicate the incretin class as inducers of pancreatitis or pancreatic cancer in patients with diabetes Discontinue use in patients suspected of having pancreatitis Exenatide QW may cause injection nodules
SYNTHETIC AMYLIN ANALOG		
Pramlintide (Symlin)	Exogenous replacement of amylin, which is deficit in proportion with insulin deficiency in diabetes	Adjunct treatment in patients with T1DM or T2DM who use mealtime insulin therapy and have not achieved desired glucose control despite optimal insulin therapy May be used with or without sulfonylurea or metformin in T2DM Injected before meals Adverse effects include nausea and severe hypoglycemia Should be used only in patients who do not have hypoglycemia awareness autonomic failure (i.e., hypoglycemia unawareness) Can result in weight loss and satiety Challenging to titrate
SGLT2 INHIBITOR		
Canagliflozin (Invokana)	Reduces the renal threshold of glucose absorption from 180 g/day to approximately 70 g/day by blocking the SGLT2 co-transporter in the distal tubules of the glomeruli. Because glucose is not absorbed in the plasma, insulin resistance improves in a glucose-dependent manner, and patients experience a reduction in fasting and postprandial glucose levels, A1C, weight, and BP.	Side effects include increased frequency of urination, glycosuria, UTIs, mycotic infections, and diarrhea. Elderly patients should be carefully observed for treatment-induced orthostatic hypotension. Contraindicated in patients with renal insufficiency and a GFR <45 mL/min/1.73 m² Canagliflozin dose should be 100 mg/day taken in the morning if the estimated GFR is 45-60 mL/min/1.73 m²; can be titrated to 300 mg if the GFR is >60 mL/min/1.73 m² Co-administration with nonselective inducers of UGT enzymes (Rifampin, phenytoin, phenobarbital, ritonavir) will decrease the efficacy of canagliflozin

Table 34-15 Food and Drug Administration–Approved Noninsulin Pharmacologic Agents for Type 2 Diabetes Mellitus Treatment (Continued)

Agents (Trade Name[s])	Mode of Action	Safety Concerns, Within-Class Distinctions, and Other Important Considerations
Dapagliflozin (Farxiga)	Starting dose is 5 mg daily. Can increase to 10 mg daily for patients requiring additional glycemic control	Should not be initiated in patients with an eGFR <60 mL/min/1.73 m²
	As with other agents in this class, SGLT2 inhibitors interfere with 1,5-anhydroglucitol assays	Results in approximately 70 g of glucose excretion in urine weekly
Empagliflozin (Jardiance)	Doses are 10 and 25 mg daily	Do not initiate in patients with eGFR <45 mL/min/1.73 m² and discontinue if eGFR is persistently <45 mL/min/1.73 m²

BP, Blood pressure; *CAD*, coronary artery disease; *CHF*, congestive heart failure; *CVD*, cardiovascular disease; *DPP-4*, Dipeptidyl peptidase-4; *GFR*, glomerular filtration rate; *GI*, gastrointestinal; *GLP*, glucagon-like peptide; *HF*, heart failure; *LDL*, low-density lipoprotein; *MEN*, multiple endocrine neoplasia; *NYHA*, New York Heart Association; *PCOS*, polycystic ovary syndrome; *SCN*, suprachiasmic nucleus; *T2DM*, type 2 diabetes mellitus; *UTI*, urinary tract infection.
Boehringer Ingelheim Pharmaceuticals and Eli Lilly: Jardiance product information. http://bidocs.boehringer-ingelheim.com/BIWebAccess/ViewServlet.ser?docBase=renetnt&folderPath=/Prescribing+Information/PIs/Jardiance/jardiance.pdf. Assessed November 2014; Bristol-Myers Squibb and AstraZeneca Pharmaceuticals: Farxiga product information. http://www.azpicentral.com/farxiga/pi_farxiga.pdf. Accessed November 2014; Janssen Pharmaceuticals: Invokana product information. http://www.invokanahcp.com/prescribing-information.pdf. Accessed November 2014; Monami M, Genovese S, Mannucci E. Cardiovascular safety of sulfonylureas: a meta-analysis of randomized clinical trials. *Diabetes Obes Metab.* 15:938-953, 2013; Yang W, Liu J, Shan Z, et al. Acarbose compared with metformin as initial therapy in patients with newly diagnosed type 2 diabetes: an open-label, non-inferiority randomised trial. *Lancet Diabetes Endocrinol.* 2013; doi: 10.1016/S2213-8587(13)70021-4; Monami M, Ahren B, Dicembrini I, et al. Dipeptidyl peptidase-4 inhibitors and cardiovascular risk: a meta-analysis of randomized clinical trials. *Diabetes Obes Metab.* 15:112-120, 2013.

Table 34-16 Dosing Adjustments Required for Incretin Agents Based on Renal Status

Drug	Mild Renal Insufficiency*	Severe Renal Insufficiency or Disease Requiring Dialysis†
DPP-4 INHIBITORS		
Linagliptin	No adjustment required	No adjustment required
Saxagliptin	No adjustment required	Reduce to 2.5 mg/day
Sitagliptin	50 mg/day	25 mg/day
Alogliptin	≥30 to ≤60 mL/min use 12.5 mg/day	6.25 mg/day
GLP-1 RECEPTOR AGONISTS		
Exenatide	Use with caution	Contraindicated
Exenatide QW	Use with caution	Contraindicated
Liraglutide	Use with caution	Use with caution

*Creatinine clearance ≥50 mL/min; serum creatinine ≤1.7 mg/dL in men and <1.5 mg/dL in women.
†Creatinine clearance <30 mL/min; serum creatinine >3.0 in men and >2.5 in women.
DPP-4, Dipeptidyl peptidase-4; *GLP-1*, glucagon-like peptide 1.
References: Amylin Pharmaceuticals, 2013; Boehringer Ingelheim, 2011; Bristol-Myers Squibb, 2011, 2013; Monami et al., 2014; Merck, 2011; Novo Nordisk, 2013; Takeda, 2013.

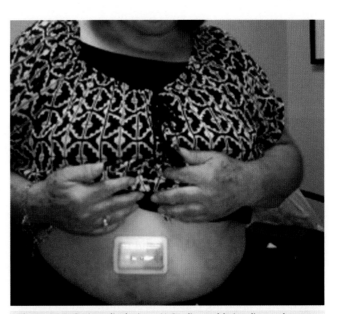

Figure 34-2 Patient displaying a V-Go disposable insulin patch pump (Valeritas, Bridgewater, NJ). Designed for use in patients with type 2 diabetes mellitus and available in three sizes (V-Go 20, V-Go 30, and V-Go 40), these devices deliver rapid-acting lispro or aspart insulin at a single specific basal rate of 0.83, 1.25, or 1.67 units/hr. An additional 36 units of prandial (bolus) insulin may be delivered by the patient before meals or for correction dose if glucose levels are elevated. Patients must remove and replace the pump after 24 hours. The advantages of the pump include improvement in A1C, adherence to mealtime bolus insulin prescribing, no visual association with needle therapy, and a reduction in total daily Insulin dose (Rosenfeld and Grunberger, 2013). Most patients can learn to use the V-Go system in 5 to 10 minutes.

about how to prevent, predict, and effectively manage hypoglycemia.

Optimal insulin replacement regimens replicate physiological insulin secretion in the fasting and postabsorptive states. Euglycemic individuals produce sufficient insulin to maintain plasma glucose levels in the range of 85 to 140 mg/dL. Exogenous basal insulin replacement is prescribed to reduce the magnitude of excessive hepatic glucose production in the fasting state. The two available basal insulin analogs are glargine and detemir. Both are characterized by a relatively flat time-action profile with an onset of action within 1 to 4 hours. A double-blind, randomized, crossover, investigator-initiated study of once-daily dosing demonstrated that the pharmacokinetics (i.e., absorption, metabolism, distribution, and excretion) and pharmacodynamics (i.e., variability of absorption from injection site, time to peak effect, and duration of action) of these insulin analogs were equivalent (King, 2009).

Table 34-17 Simple Basal Insulin Protocols That May Be Effectively and Efficiently Initiated in the Primary Care Setting

Protocol	Initial Dose of Basal Insulin	Titration Schedule	Comments	Reference(s)
Canadian INSIGHT Trial	10 units at 9:00 PM	Increase dose by 1 unit at 9:00 PM daily until fasting glucose is ≤110 mg/dL.	Very simple titration schedule. Can also increase dose by 5 units every Monday instead of adjusting daily	Gerstein et al., 2006.
PREDICTIVE 303 Protocol TITRATE Protocol	10 units at 9:00 PM	Perform SMBG every morning and base insulin dose on 3-day average of glucose values. The target fasting glucose is 80-110 mg/dL. Adjust 9:00 PM dose based on the average fasting glucose level over 3 days as follows: <80 mg/dL = −3 units 80-110 mg/dL = no adjustment >110 mg/dL = +3 units	Treatment goals can be modified. TITRATE study targets were set at 70-90 mg/dL. PREDICTIVE 303 Protocol should be considered perpetual; patients should not stop adjusting doses unless instructed by their clinicians.	Meneghini et al., 2007; Blonde et al., 2009
Insulin-Resistant Weight Protocol	0.4 units/kg of body weight at 9:00 PM	For patients who are obese, treatment-naive, and have symptomatic hyperglycemia who require a more rapid method of insulin initiation and titration; can increase the dose by 5 units each Monday up to a maximum of 60 units. After a patient has reached the 60-unit dose of basal insulin, add prandial insulin targeting a specific meal ("basal-plus" regimen) or reduce the basal dose by 20% and initiate either exenatide or liraglutide.	Can use in combination with a GLP-1 receptor agonist, SGLT2 inhibitor, DPP-4 inhibitor, or prandial insulin. Continue metformin unless patient is metformin intolerant.	Unger, 2011

DPP-4, Dipeptidyl peptidase-4; *GLP-1,* glucagon-like peptide 1; *SMBG,* self-monitoring of blood glucose; *T2DM,* type 2 diabetes mellitus.

Approximately 60% of patients with T2DM are able to achieve an A1C of 7% or less using basal insulin replacement in combination with oral agents or a GLP-1 receptor agonist. Patients who are still unable to achieve their target fasting, postprandial, or A1C goals should be transitioned to a basal-plus (basal insulin plus one prandial injection at the largest meal) or basal-bolus (basal insulin plus prandial injections for all meals) insulin regimen that provides long-acting insulin for basal needs and rapid-acting insulin (i.e., lispro, aspart, or glulisine) to minimize the peak rise in glucose levels after carbohydrate ingestion.

Table 34-17 lists several practical regimens that may be used to initiate patients on basal insulin. Successful initiation of basal insulin requires patients to understand their individualized glycemic targets and to know how to safely achieve these objectives. In clinical trials, patients who are provided with a specific algorithm are almost always able to safely and effectively lower their A1C to their prescribed target. Thus, allowing patients to self-titrate should be the rule rather than the exception.

Table 34-18 lists the appropriate time to consider adding prandial insulin to one's basal regimen. Physiological insulin regimens should be individualized and titrated based on the factors shown in Table 34-19. Rapid-acting insulin analogs exhibit a peak onset of pharmacodynamics (blood glucose–lowering capacity) 60 minutes after injection. Peak carbohydrate absorption after a meal occurs 75 to 90 minutes after eating. Thus, to synchronize the peak activity of insulin with the expected risk in postprandial glucose, the analog should be injected 15 minutes before meals unless premeal blood glucose is less than 80 mg/dL (Unger, 2011). The delay between the time of injection and the start of the meal is known as the "lag time." Patients who inject just before eating may experience postprandial hypoglycemia within 1 hour of starting the meal only to develop postprandial hyperglycemia 2 to 3 hours later.

Table 34-18 Practical Considerations for Initiating Prandial Insulin

Consider adding prandial insulin:

- For patients who have not attained the recommended A1C of ≤7% despite successful basal insulin dose titration and the achievement of fasting glucose levels of <100 mg/dL (An alternative to starting prandial insulin is to add an incretin-based therapy to basal insulin, which will reduce postprandial and fasting glucose levels; however, exenatide QW is not approved for use with insulin.)
- When basal insulin dose titration has resulted in repeated episodes of nocturnal hypoglycemia
- When the basal insulin dose has exceeded 60 units/day
- For patients who have not met their A1C goal within 1 year of initiating basal insulin
- If the "BeAM factor" is >55 mg/dL
  - BeAM factor: the difference between bedtime and morning ("AM") blood glucose levels
  - Patients titrating basal insulin to a fasting glucose target of ≤100 mg/dL who have a BeAM factor >55 mg/dL are less likely to achieve an A1C ≤7% without experiencing nocturnal hypoglycemia; therefore, these patients should initiate prandial insulin
  - A BeAM factor >55 mg/dL is associated with an increased risk of nocturnal hypoglycemia, but not overall hypoglycemia

Holman RR, Farmer AJ, Davies MJ, et al. Three-year efficacy of complex insulin regimens in type 2 diabetes. *N Engl J Med.* 361:1736-1747, 2009; Zisman A, Aleksandra V, Zhou R. The BeAM factor: an easy-to-determine, objective, clinical indicator for when to add prandial insulin vs. continued basal insulin titration. Presented at the American Diabetes Association 71st Scientific Sessions (Abstract 1121-P), San Diego, CA, June 2011.

For a basal-plus regimen (basal insulin plus one prandial dose per day), identifying the meal to target for intervention might be simplified with the use of structured SMBG, as described in the Type 1 Diabetes Mellitus section of this chapter. SMBG should be performed before and 2 hours after each meal for 3 days. The meal with the highest Δ (difference between premeal and 2-hour postprandial

Table 34-19 Factors to Be Considered When Prescribing Physiological Insulin Replacement Therapy

Factor	Comment
Meal consumption	Does patient skip meals?
	Are meals consumed on a scheduled basis?
	What are the approximate sizes and carbohydrate contents of meals?
	Has patient received meal planning education from a registered dietitian or certified diabetes educator?
	Does patient have an eating disorder?
Work schedule	Does patient work irregular shifts?
	Does an irregular work schedule affect sleep?
	Does patient frequently travel?
	Does travel schedule require flexible meal and insulin injection scheduling?
Adherence history	Does patient have a history of omitting insulin doses?
	Is patient willing to perform frequent SMBG?
	Does patient understand how to properly perform SMBG and interpret glucose values, patterns, and averages?
Physical activity	Does patient exercise?
	What type of exercise does patient do?
	What time of day does exercise occur?
	Does exercise time vary?
	Is patient a professional athlete?
	Is patient planning to initiate an exercise program for the first time?
	What are patient's glucose targets before, during, and after exercise?
	Does patient know how to predict and treat hypoglycemia?
Hypoglycemia history	Does patient have a history of hypoglycemia unawareness?
	Does patient live alone?
	Does patient know how to predict and treat hypoglycemia?
	Are there comorbidities (e.g., heart disease, chronic kidney disease, seizures, hypoglycemia unawareness) that could preclude patient from being intensively managed and thereby increasing their risk of hypoglycemia?
	Does patient have access to and wear a CGM device?
	Does patient know to perform SMBG before driving?
	What is patient's target A1C?
Comorbidities of concern	Coronary artery disease or cardiac arrhythmias
	Preconception planning or pregnancy
	Cancer
	End-stage renal disease
	Mental illness
	Diabetic neuropathy
	Diabetic retinopathy
	Advanced age
Learning skill deficiencies	Does patient have deficient reading, writing, or math (numeracy) skills?
	Is there a language barrier that may affect patient's ability to learn how to administer and self-titrate insulin?

CGM, Continuous glucose monitoring; *SMBG,* self-monitoring of blood glucose.
Adapted with permission from Unger J. *Diabetes management in primary care.* 2nd ed. Philadelphia: Lippincott, Williams and Wilkins, 2012.

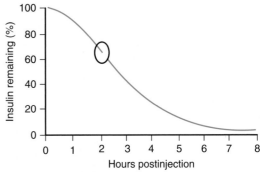

Figure 34-3 Insulin disappearance curve. This graph demonstrates the amount of insulin remaining in the subcutaneous depot over time after a subcutaneous injection (insulin on board). After 2 hours *(circle),* 64% of the original dose remains in the depot waiting to act. Thus, if 10 units of insulin are given at 10:00 AM, 6 units remain as active drug at noon. The glucose-lowering effects of rapid-acting analogs persist for up to 6 hours after a subcutaneous injection. If a patient gives a correction dose of insulin before the insulin from the previous injection is completely absorbed (a practice known as "insulin stacking"), hypoglycemia is likely to occur. For example, if the blood glucose level is 200 mg/dL at noon and the patient injects an additional 6 units for lunchtime, the subcutaneous depot has now been increased to 12 units. Patients should always calculate insulin on board from the previous injection before injecting supplemental insulin. Insulin stacking is a major cause of hypoglycemia and can easily be avoided. (Adapted with permission from Unger J. *Diabetes management in primary care.* 2nd ed. Philadelphia: Lippincott, Williams and Wilkins; 2012.)

glucose levels) becomes the initial point of intercession. The goal is to achieve a physiological Δ (0-50 mg/dL) for the meal. For example, if the pre-breakfast glucose is 100 mg/dL and the 2-hour postprandial glucose after breakfast is 142 mg/dL, the breakfast Δ = 142 − 100, or 42 mg/dL. Patients with A1C levels above 12% may require immediate initiation of a basal-bolus regimen to reduce postprandial hyperglycemia after all meals.

Structured SMBG also allows patients to identify impending hypoglycemia. Any negative Δ (difference between premeal and 2-hour postprandial glucose resulting in a negative value) would predict a high risk of impending hypoglycemia. For example, if a patient has a premeal glucose level of 187 mg/dL and a 2-hour postprandial glucose level of 100 mg/dL after taking 10 units of insulin, one could predict impending hypoglycemia based on the Δ of −87 mg/dL. If the patient received two 10 units of insulin 2 hours before eating, he or she would be at risk for impending hypoglycemia (Figure 34-3). Calculating Δ values from structured SMBG can also help patients adjust their baseline doses of prandial insulin based on glycemic patterns that become apparent over several days. Table 34-12 lists the causes of low and elevated Δ values.

After a basal-plus or basal-bolus insulin regimen is initiated, a repeat A1C should be obtained to determine if the patient is beginning to trend toward the prescribed glycemic target. Insulin therapy may be intensified based on the patient's A1C level and structured SMBG results.

The initial dose of any prandial rapid-acting insulin can be approximated as 0.1 unit/kg of body weight per meal. Thus, a 100-kg person would require 10 units of rapid-acting insulin, which would be injected 15 minutes before eating. If the 2-hour postprandial glucose is 0 to 50 mg/dL, the correct amount of insulin was given to cover the

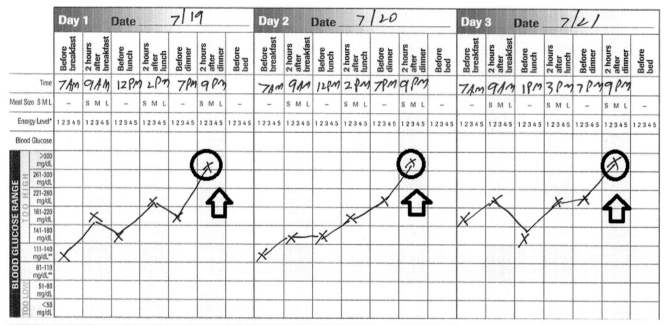

Figure 34-4 Insulin initiation and intensification for patients with advanced type 2 diabetes mellitus (T2DM). *Although any meal may be targeted for rapid-acting insulin intensification, structured self-monitoring of blood glucose should be performed before and 2 hours after each meal for 3 days before a scheduled office visit. The meal that shows the greatest 2-hour postprandial glucose increase (the greatest Δ value) should be targeted for intensification. Note: "Advanced T2DM" refers to patients who have had diabetes for more than 5 years, those whose A1C is greater than 9%, and those who are no longer able to control their glucose with triple combination drug therapy. In this example using the Accu-Check 360 blood glucose analysis system, the patient and his physician were able to determine that the greatest rise in prandial glucose values occurred consistently with dinner. Therefore, basal-plus insulin therapy was initiated, targeting the postprandial excursions at dinner.

carbohydrate content of that meal. However, if the 2-hour postprandial glucose level is consistently above 50 mg/dL, the patient can adjust the mealtime dose of insulin by 1 unit/day until the Δ target is achieved. Figure 34-4 summarizes a popular approach to initiating basal-bolus therapy in the primary care setting. The keys to successful initiation of insulin are summarized in Table 34-20.

PREMIXED INSULIN FORMULATIONS

Premixed preparations combine rapid-acting (prandial) and long-duration (basal) insulins in a single vial or pen injector. Using these fixed-dose insulins can reduce dosing errors that may occur when patients attempt to mix neutral protamine Hagedorn (NPH) and regular insulin in the same syringe. Such formulations are also helpful in other situations. For example, when combining NPH with a rapid-acting analog, the injection must be made immediately to avoid alteration in the glucose-lowering effects of the analog. Patients with visual impairments may have a family member preload their rapid- and intermediate-acting insulin into syringes for use later in the day. However, this may result in absorption variability and hypoglycemia. By contrast, using premixed insulin preparations is simple, user friendly, and more physiological than NPH-plus-regular-insulin injections.

The human premixed insulins (Humulin 50/50, Humulin 70/30, and Novolin 70/30) combine regular and NPH insulin in a single dose. Thirty units of 50/50 insulin would consist of 15 units of regular plus 15 units of NPH. The 70/30 preparations consist of 70% NPH and 30% regular

insulin. When used, these insulins must be injected at least 30 minutes before a meal.

Analog premixed insulins (lispro mix 75/25, lispro mix 50/50, and biaspart mix 70/30), unlike human mixed insulins, consist of a set percentage of rapid-acting insulin (either lispro or aspart) plus the rapid-acting insulin combined with protamine, which delays the absorption of that insulin component. By prolonging the duration of action of a percentage of the aspart or lispro within the mixed formulation, protamine improves the glucodynamic effect of the insulin. Patients using a mixed insulin would receive the benefits of a basal and a bolus insulin in a single injection. Thus, a 20-unit dose of lispro 75/25 would contain 5 units of lispro plus 15 units of lispro plus protamine. The analog premixed insulins should be injected 15 minutes before eating to minimize postprandial glycemic excursions.

Although less expensive than the analog premixed formulations, human premixed insulins are less effective at minimizing postprandial glycemic excursions. Using premixed analogs can result in hypoglycemia; however, the incidence of severe hypoglycemia appears to be slightly higher for individuals using human premixed formulations (2%-14% of patients) versus those using premixed analogs (2%-8% of patients).

Premixed insulin analogs might be useful for patients who have a baseline A1C between 8.5% and 10%. Other candidates who might be successful users of premixed analogs include those who eat three meals daily and adhere to a regular schedule for work and physical activity. Another advantage of premixed analogs is that patients receive two insulins for a single insurance copayment.

Table 34-20 Keys to Successful Insulin Initiation in Patients with Type 2 Diabetes Mellitus

Suggest that insulin will help patients achieve their individualized fasting, postprandial, and A1C targets in a timely, safe, and efficient manner.

Provide each patient with a written, individualized treatment plan for insulin intensification.

Use insulin pens or disposable pumps rather than syringes and vials; this may improve dosing accuracy and adherence.

Teach patients how to proactively identify impending hypoglycemia using structured SMBG.

Patients should always be allowed to titrate their basal and prandial insulin doses with prescribed guidance and tutorials from their clinician.

Use insulin analogs; regular human insulin increases the risk of hypoglycemia.

Explain the differences between "basal" and "bolus" insulin to patients to minimize dosing errors.

When adding a GLP-1 receptor agonist to basal insulin, consider reducing the dose of the basal insulin by 20%.

Patients with renal insufficiency should reduce their insulin doses by 10% and monitor their glucose levels carefully because insulin is secreted in the urine. Renal insufficiency may increase circulating insulin levels and increase the risk for hypoglycemia.

To reduce weight gain when insulin is initiated, consider discontinuing any thiazolidinedione, sulfonylurea, or glitinides. Agents that may be continued safely after initiating insulin include metformin, bromocriptine, SGLT2 inhibitors, α-glucosidase inhibitors, DPP-4 inhibitors, and GLP-1 receptor agonists.

Some patients may be able to discontinue insulin if their doses are relatively low (<20 units/day), and they attain an A1C <7.5%. Thus, initiating insulin does not always mean that the patient will be on insulin forever.

Patients must be instructed about how to inject insulin properly. Also, be sure to discuss the proper timing of basal and prandial insulin administration with each patient.

Patients who are shift workers should consider using an insulin pump (continuous subcutaneous insulin infusion) to improve their glucose levels.

Patients with high A1C levels (>10%) do not feel well after eating. This is because their postprandial glucose levels go from bad to worse. After initiating insulin, their symptoms of fatigue and sluggishness should improve dramatically, motivating them to intensify their insulin therapy, if necessary.

DPP-4, Dipeptidyl peptidase-4; *GLP-1,* glucagon-like peptide 1; *SGLT2,* sodium–glucose co-transporter 2; *SMBG,* self-monitoring of blood glucose.

The initiation and titration of premixed insulins has proven successful in allowing patients to achieve their glycemic targets. In a 48-week, multicenter, open-label trial, patients with T2DM and who were not achieving targets on oral agents with or without once-daily basal insulin were placed on premixed biaspart (70/30) in three phases. In phase 1, patients initiated treatment with the premixed formulation once before supper. The dosing frequency was increased to twice daily in phase 2 and to three times daily in phase 3 at 16 and 32 weeks, respectively, if patients did not achieve an A1C of less than 6.5%. Patients reached the end of their participation in the study when they achieved an A1C of 6.5% or less or at 48 weeks, whichever came first. At the end of the trial, 77% of patients had achieved A1C levels of less than 7.0%, and 60% of patients attained an A1C level of 6.5% or less through dosing once, twice, or three times with premixed biaspart (Garber et al., 2006).

Whether treatment-naive patients should begin treatment with basal insulin or a premixed insulin analog was the primary study question of the Initiating insulin therapy in type 2 diabetes: a comparison of biphasic and basal insulin analogs [INITIATE] trial (Raskin et al., 2004). A total of 233 patients with poorly controlled diabetes on oral agents who had a baseline A1C greater than 8% were randomized to take either insulin glargine or premixed biaspart (70/30) for 28 weeks. At the conclusion of the study, 66% of patients taking premixed biaspart reached the recommended ADA target A1C of less than 7% compared with 40% of those taking glargine. As expected, postprandial glycemic excursions for the biaspart group were approximately 25% lower than for patients using glargine. Minor hypoglycemia occurred more commonly in patients taking the premixed insulin, but no episodes of severe hypoglycemia were recorded during the trial.

Treatment of patients with T2DM should no longer be protocol driven. The ACCORD trial demonstrated that intensive therapy can be used successfully to reduce A1C to less than 6.5% in patients with T2DM. Unfortunately, the all-cause mortality rate in ACCORD was 22% in intensively managed patients (ACCORD Study Group, 2008). Not all patients are at risk if ambitiously treated, however. In fact, the patients who were able to lower their A1C to below 6.5% within 4 months of randomization did not demonstrate in increase in all-cause mortality. Those who were unable to achieve their targeted goal by intensification appeared to have elevated postprandial glucose levels that were more refractory to treatment. These individuals also had longer disease durations and were at higher risk of experiencing fatal arrhythmias caused by severe hypoglycemia (Riddle et al., 2010).

Thus, metabolic targets for diabetes must be individualized based on the patient's age, disease duration, number and severity of comorbidities, history of hypoglycemia awareness autonomic failure, ability to participate in self-diabetes management, and life expectancy. Most newly diagnosed patients with diabetes should attempt to lower their A1C to 6.5% or less. Pharmacotherapy choices should be selected based on their ability to correct and reverse the metabolic defects associated with T2DM and insulin resistance. Simply attempting to target a given glycemic parameter is no longer a safe or acceptable practice when managing patients with either T1DM or T2DM.

Type 1 Diabetes Mellitus

Type 1 diabetes mellitus accounts for 5% to 10% of all individuals diagnosed with diabetes and results from a cellular-mediated autoimmune destruction of the pancreatic β cells. Markers of immune destruction of β cells include islet cell autoantibodies (ICAs), autoantibodies to insulin (IAAs), autoantibodies to glutamic acid decarboxylase (GAD65), antibodies to an insulinoma-associated antigen-2 (ICA512), and autoantibodies to the tyrosine phosphatases (IA-2 and IA-2β) (ADA, 2012). One or more of the autoantibodies are present in 85% to 90% of individuals who initially experience fasting hyperglycemia.

The rate of β-cell destruction in T1DM varies. Whereas infants and children tend to demonstrate rapid β-cell death, adults typically present with a lengthy prodromal phase leading to latent autoimmune diabetes of adulthood (LADA)

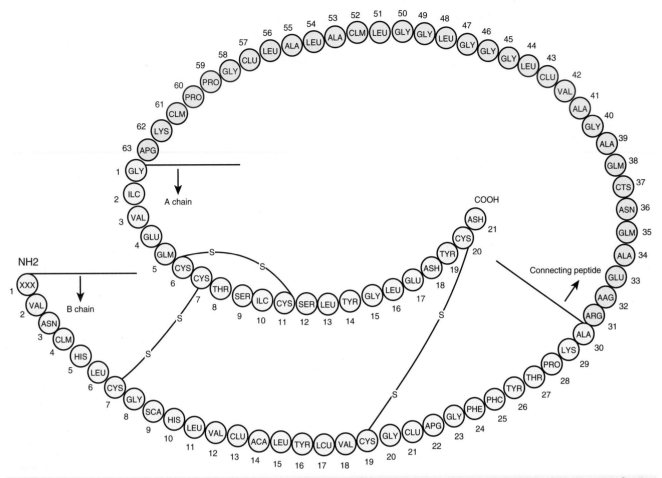

Figure 34-5 Structure of human insulin. The precursor of insulin, proinsulin, is produced within the endoplasmic reticulum of the pancreatic β cells. Proinsulin is then transported to the Golgi apparatus and packaged into secretory vesicles. The C-peptide chain is released from the center of the proinsulin sequence while the two disulfide bonds remain intact. One C-peptide molecule is formed with each insulin molecule. Therefore, C-peptide levels can serve as an accurate measure of endogenous insulin production. C-peptide levels in euglycemic individuals range from 0.5 to 2.0 ng/mL. Patients with type 1 diabetes mellitus are deficient in C-peptide. (Adapted with permission from Unger J. *Diabetes management in primary care.* 2nd ed. Philadelphia: Lippincott, Williams and Wilkins; 2012.)

(Unger, 2008a). Some children and adolescents may present with DKA as the first manifestation of the disease. Others have modest fasting hyperglycemia that can rapidly change to severe hyperglycemia or DKA in the presence of infection or other stress. Adults may retain residual β-cell function (remaining C-peptide positive; Figure 34-5) that is sufficient to prevent DKA for many years. Residual β-cell function detected 3 to 6 years after the onset of T1DM has also been associated with a lower risk of hypoglycemia, reduced exogenous insulin requirement, and improved glycemic control (Sorensen et al., 2013).

Patients with near-complete insulin deficiency who remain antibody negative are classified as having "type 1B diabetes" (Notkins and Lernmark, 2001). Most patients with type 1B diabetes are of African or Asian ancestry.

Patients with T1DM are prone to other autoimmune disorders such as autoimmune thyroid disease (15%-30%), celiac disease (4%-9%), and Addison disease (0.5%) (Unger, 2012e). Assays for thyroid peroxidase autoantibodies (for autoimmune thyroid disease), tissue transglutaminase autoantibodies (for celiac disease), and 21-hydroxylase autoantibodies (for Addison disease) may be used to screen asymptomatic patients to identify those at high risk for clinical progression to these conditions. Thirty-three percent of patients with T1DM screen positive for at least one additional organ-specific autoantibody when initially diagnosed with diabetes, and 19% have evidence of clinical disease. Given the high preponderance of these antibodies at the onset of T1DM, screening for coexisting autoimmune disorders appears to be warranted (Triolo et al., 2011).

To date, no intervention has been developed that can unequivocally prevent the development of T1DM or arrest the progression of immune system destruction of β cells after diagnosis. Although some promising studies in the area of diabetes prevention and reversal have given the field much encouragement, most of these efforts are unfolding at large academic or research-focused medical centers. Nonetheless, family physicians play a vital role in working with patients who are at high risk for developing T1DM. In families with established T1DM, all first-degree relatives, including the parents of the patient (if they are younger than 45 years of age), are at increased risk for T1DM and should be counseled about this risk. Identical twins are at the greatest risk. Second- and third-degree relatives of patients with T1DM are also at heightened risk if they are younger than 21 years of age.

Table 34-21   Features of Type 1 Diabetes Mellitus, Type 2 Diabetes Mellitus, and Latent Autoimmune Diabetes of Adulthood

Condition	DKA	Cardiovascular Complications	Microvascular Complications*	Pathophysiology	Autoantibodies	Insulin Requirements
T1DM	Develops rapidly unless patient receives insulin therapy	Increased risk of cardiovascular morbidity and mortality related to stroke, acute coronary event, or coronary revascularization; high incidence of cardiovascular complications compared with euglycemic people, especially in women	Increased risk	Autoimmune destruction of pancreatic β cells	Patients typically test positive for ≥2 autoantibodies	Insulin required at diagnosis
LADA	Absent at diagnosis but may develop with severe insulinopenia	Risk is two to four times higher than in euglycemic people	Increased risk	Latent autoimmune destruction of pancreatic β cells	Glutamic acid decarboxylase autoantibodies most common; islet cell antibodies less common Patients typically test positive for only one autoantibody	Insulin therapy is ultimately necessary; may be considered if autoantibodies are identified
T2DM	Usually absent	Risk is two to four times higher than in euglycemic people	Increased risk	Peripheral insulin resistance; reduced pancreatic β-cell mass and function; reduced insulin	Usually absent	Usually needed late in the disease course when the remaining β-cell mass and function can no longer support acceptable glycemic control with oral agents or incretin mimetics

*Retinopathy, nephropathy, and neuropathy
LADA, Latent autoimmune diabetes of adulthood; *T1DM,* type 1 diabetes mellitus; *T2DM,* type 2 diabetes mellitus.
Unger J. Diagnosing and managing latent autoimmune diabetes in adults. *Pract Diabetol.* 21:32-37, 2008.

After being apprised of their diabetes risk, such individuals should be made aware of T1DM screening and intervention studies such as the National Institutes of Health's T1DM TrialNet (http://www.diabetestrialnet.org). The advantages of screening for T1DM risk through such research-oriented programs include state-of-the-art antibody determinations in specialized research laboratories, a superb follow-up and support network of T1DM specialists, protection of laboratory data from insurance carriers, and the opportunity to participate in further clinical research studies aimed at diabetes prevention. Participating in a research study incurs no cost to patients or their insurance companies.

Early vitamin D supplementation may protect against T1DM progression, although the exact mechanism is uncertain. Vitamin D is a potent modulator of the immune system and is involved in regulating cell proliferation and differentiation (Zella and DeLuca, 2003). A meta-analysis of data from five observational studies recently indicated that children supplemented with vitamin D had a 29% reduction in T1DM risk compared with their unsupplemented peers (Zipitis and Akobeng, 2008).

LATENT AUTOIMMUNE DIABETES IN ADULTS

Latent autoimmune diabetes in adults is a slowly progressive form of autoimmune diabetes characterized by older age at diagnosis, the presence of pancreatic autoantibodies, and the lack of an absolute insulin requirement at diagnosis. Although patients with LADA present with more preserved β-cell function than those with classic T1DM, they tend to have a rapid and progressive loss of β-cell function necessitating intensive insulin intervention. Approximately 10% of all patients diagnosed with T2DM actually have LADA (Isomaa et al., 1999). Table 34-21 compares the characteristics of T1DM, T2DM, and LADA.

Although the exact pathogenesis of LADA is unclear, the underlying immune-mediated destruction of β cells in patients with this form of the disease leads to insulin dependency more rapidly than in patients with T2DM. Protective alleles appear to delay absolute exogenous insulin dependency in people with LADA compared with those with T1DM.

Suspicion of LADA should be heightened in patients with coexisting autoimmune disorders such as hypothyroidism, who are not excessively overweight, and who have deteriorating glycemic control despite intensification of oral therapies and the use of incretin mimetics. Physicians may consider GAD65 testing to determine whether LADA is present.

Because of the ambiguous pathophysiology and clinical characteristics of LADA, no specific guidelines have been established for its treatment. Nevertheless, theoretical advantages of intensive insulin therapy exist. Eighteen years after the DCCT, a follow-up study showed that early control of diabetes over 6.5 years seems to provide continued protection against micro- and macrovascular complications (DCCT Research Group, 1993; DCCT/EDIC Research Group, 2005). This result occurred despite the fact that patients in the DCCT who received intensive treatment had deteriorating A1C levels over time, but those in the conventional treatment group showed improvement upon completion of this landmark study. Early stabilization of glycemic control in patients with T1DM is postulated to establish "metabolic memory," which theoretically protects against long-term complications.

PATHOGENESIS OF TYPE 1 DIABETES MELLITUS

Type 1 diabetes mellitus occurs in individuals in whom genetic susceptibility outweighs genetic protection. Distinctive environmental triggers play a supporting role in provoking a cellular-mediated autoimmune process directed to one or more β-cell proteins (autoantigens). As islet cell destruction occurs, autoantibodies are delivered into the pancreatic lymph nodes, where destructive T-effector cells are produced and outnumber the stabilizing T-regulatory cells. Initially, the decline in β-cell function and loss of β-cell mass present clinically as loss of first-phase insulin response to an intravenous glucose challenge. Over time, patients progress through stages of "dysglycemia" (glucose values >200 mg/dL at 30, 60, or 90 minutes during an oral glucose tolerance test). Ultimately, the clinical syndrome of T1DM becomes evident when the majority of β-cell function has been lost and most β cells have been destroyed. At this juncture, frank hyperglycemia supervenes. To date, no intervention has been developed that can unequivocally prevent the development of T1DM or arrest the progression of immune system destruction of β cells after diagnosis, although some promising studies have given the field much encouragement (Unger, 2012e).

OUTPATIENT MANAGEMENT OF ADULTS WITH TYPE 1 DIABETES MELLITUS

The ultimate goal of insulin replacement therapy is to mimic the normal insulin response to hyperglycemia in both the fasting and postprandial states. Physiological insulin replacement regimens include the use of basal-bolus insulin preparations administered in a multiple daily injection (MDI) regimen or through continuous subcutaneous insulin infusion (CSII; insulin pump therapy). Nonphysiologic regimens include NPH insulin with or without a rapid-acting insulin, premixed insulin analogs, or analog basal insulin therapy alone given once or twice daily. Such regimens fail to mimic the normal glucose-stimulated insulin response of pancreatic β cells. Physiological insulin

therapies require individualization and titration based on the factors shown in Table 34-19.

Insulin Analog Formulations

Basal Insulin Analogs. The two available basal analogs include glargine and detemir. Glargine provides glycemic control that is at least comparable with NPH in adults, adolescents, and children. However, the risks of mild and severe episodes of hypoglycemia are significantly reduced with glargine compared with NPH use in adults. Combining glargine with a rapid-acting insulin analog as part of an MDI regimen provides benefits over the use of NPH plus regular human insulin (Garg et al., 2011).

The absence of clear peaks in the time-action profiles of glargine and detemir contributes to the lower risk of hypoglycemia with these analogs compared with NPH. In addition, the analogs demonstrate less variability in absorption compared with NPH, suggesting that the analog formulations have a more predictable glucose-lowering effect than NPH in T1DM (Heise et al., 2004).

Rapid-Acting Insulin Analogs. Rapid-acting insulin analogs begin to exhibit their glucose-lowering effects within 10 to 15 minutes after an injection compared with the 30- to 60-minute onset of action of regular human insulin. The three available rapid-acting insulin analogs are lispro, aspart, and glulisine. Aspart and glulisine have also been approved for injection immediately after a meal. Postprandial administration can be useful for patients who forget to take their insulin before eating. Pediatric and elderly patients whose food consumption and mealtimes are unpredictable may also bolus after eating.

Table 34-22 lists the pharmacologic characteristics of commercially available insulin preparations, as well as an investigational long-acting basal insulin (degludec), which is now in phase 3 clinical trials.

INITIATING AND INTENSIFYING PHYSIOLOGICAL INSULIN THERAPY IN PATIENTS WITH TYPE 1 DIABETES MELLITUS

Findings from large RCTS clearly demonstrate that early and aggressive management of glycemia significantly decreases the development and progression of both micro- and macrovascular complications of diabetes (DCCT Research Group, 1993; DCCT/EDCIC Research Group, 2005). Unfortunately, intensification of therapy and improved glycemic control are often associated with an increased frequency of severe hypoglycemia (DCCT Research Group, 1993). Thus, the rate-limiting step to diabetes intensification remains fear on the part of patients or providers of inducing iatrogenic hypoglycemia. Patients must receive education about how to avoid, recognize, and treat hypoglycemia. If necessary, clinicians should consider the use of a continuous glucose monitoring (CGM) devices, which have alarms to help patients avoid hypoglycemia. Table 34-23 lists self-management goals for patients who are prescribed basal-bolus insulin therapy.

Patients with T1DM must make many therapeutic decisions, most often without physician guidance, on a daily basis. Amazingly, most patients become quite adept at adjusting their insulin doses according to their specific and

Table 34-22 Pharmacologic Characteristics of Commercially Available Insulin Preparations

Insulin Preparations	Onset of Action	Peak Action (hr)	Duration of Action (hr)
HUMAN INSULINS			
Prandial			
Regular	30-60 min	2-4	6-8
Intermediate Acting			
NPH	1-4 hours	6-10	10-16
Premixed			
70/30 (70% NPH, 30% regular)	0.5-1.0 hr	First peak 2-3 hr; second peak several hours later	10-16
50/50 (50% NPH, 50% regular)	0.5-1.0 hr	First peak 2-3 hours; second peak several hours later	10-16
INSULIN ANALOGS			
Basal			
Glargine	1-4 hr	No pronounced peak	24 (terminal half-life = 12.5 hr)
Detemir	1-4 hr	No pronounced peak	20-24
Degludec*	—	No peak	>24 hr (terminal half-life = 25 hr)
IDegAsp* (degludec + aspart)	10 min[†]	No peak	>24 hr (equal to degludec)
PRANDIAL			
Lispro/aspart/glulisine	5-15 min	1-2	3-4
Premixed			
Lispro mix 75/25 (75% protamine lispro/25% lispro)	15 min	0.5-1.2	10-16
BiAsp 70/30 (70% protamine aspart/30% aspart)	15 min	0.5-1.2	10-16
Lispro mix 50/50	15 min	0.5-1.2	10-16

*These insulins are in phase 3b clinical trials and have been submitted for review to the Food and Drug Administration.
[†]Degludec has a flat profile under steady-state conditions. There is no peak. Therefore, "time to peak action" and onset of action become irrelevant. Steady state for degludec is achieved on the third day of treatment. The effect of the previous injection will cover the time between injection and onset of action of the subsequent injection. The duration of action is dose dependent. Higher doses increase the duration of action for any insulin. The terminal half-life of insulin degludec is 25 hours compared with 12.5 hours for insulin glargine. There are no published data regarding the duration of action of insulin degludec. However, the end of action (end of action is defined as blood glucose levels >150 mg/dL) was not reached by 42 hours after the conclusion of glucose clamping for subjects receiving either 0.6 or 0.8 units/kg. The duration of action of IDegAsp is determined by the degludec component. The onset of action of IDegAsp is based on the aspart component. BiAsp has an onset of action of 10 minutes and a duration of action of 1 to 3 hours.
NPH, Neutral protamine Hagedorn.
References: Aventis, 2003; Garg and Ulrich, 2006; Heise et al., 2011; Hirsch, 2005; Lepore et al., 2000; Nosek et al., 2011; Novo Nordisk, 2005.

Table 34-23 Self-Management Goals for Patients Using Basal-Bolus Insulin Therapy

Prescribe a protocol that will allow patients to successfully and safely achieve the ADA's fasting blood glucose target of 90-130 mg/dL.
Target 2-hour postprandial blood glucose levels <180 mg/dL.
Minimize the rise in postprandial blood glucose levels from premeal baseline levels of ≤50 mg/dL.
Minimize the risk of developing hypoglycemia by instructing patients about appropriate pattern glucose testing and means by which hypoglycemia may be predicted and treated proactively.
Allow patients to self-titrate their basal and prandial insulin doses based on specified treatment targets (fasting and postprandial glucose excursions).
Encourage use of certified diabetes educators and registered dietitians to assist patients in learning and appropriately incorporating their treatment regimens into their active lifestyles.
Individualize insulin regimens to include considerations for exercise, travel, and sleep.
Recognize and effectively manage patients with mental illness and eating disorders.
Individualize treatment based on cultural, religious, and personal preferences.
Periodically review injection and SMBG technique to ensure that these basic skills are being performed properly.

ADA, American Diabetes Association; *SMBG,* self-monitoring of blood glucose.

immediate metabolic requirements. On occasion, patients may bolus inappropriate doses of insulin. In such cases, clinicians should never rebuke patients for missing their fasting or postprandial glucose targets. After all, they are doing the best they can with the insulin dosing resources provided by their health care providers.

The following steps may be used to safely and effectively initiate and titrate basal-bolus insulin for insulin-requiring patients (Unger, 2007):

Step 1. Determine the total daily dose (TDD) of insulin. The TDD is equal to the weight in kg × 0.7. For example, a 70-kg patient would require a total of $70 \times 0.7 = 49$ units of insulin daily.

Step 2. Determine the starting dose of basal insulin analog (glargine or detemir) and rapid-acting insulin (aspart, lispro, or glulisine).

$$\text{Basal insulin dose}/24 \text{ hours} = 50\% \text{ of TDD}$$

$$\text{Bolus insulin dose}/24 \text{ hours} = 50\% \text{ of TDD}$$

Basal insulin minimizes the effects of hepatic glucose production, thus keeping blood glucose levels regulated in the fasting state. The basal insulin requirement is equal to 50% of the TDD. Thus, a patient requiring 50 units/day of insulin would require approximately 25 units of basal insulin. The remaining 50% would be dedicated to bolus insulin.

These percentages may vary from patient to patient. Some individuals may require a 40/60 split favoring bolus insulin. Basal insulin should be injected at a consistent time each day or night because its maximum duration of action is 24 hours. After it is initiated, the basal insulin can be titrated by increasing the dose by 1 unit/day until fasting blood glucose is less than 100 mg/dL (Harris et al., 2008).

Step 3. Establish a prandial dosing regimen.

A. Determine baseline prandial insulin dosage:

Dose of prandial insulin = 0.1 units/kg/meal (e.g., a 70-kg patient would require 70 × 0.1 units = 7 units of rapid-acting insulin per meal)

B. Establish the lag time for insulin injection:
Insulin should be injected 15 minutes before a meal unless the blood glucose level before eating is less than 80 mg/dL, in which case insulin should be injected at the onset of the meal.

C. Allow the patient to adjust the insulin dose based on the size of the meal (Table 34-24). For example, a patient with a baseline prescribed prandial insulin dose of 7 units plans to eat a Thanksgiving-sized feast. The dose of insulin would be 7 + 3 = 10 units injected 15 minutes before eating. The baseline prandial insulin dose can be further adjusted based on structured glucose testing (Table 34-25).

D. Adjust the patient's initial baseline dose of insulin periodically based on the results of structured SMBG.

Step 4: Fine tune basal-bolus doses of insulin based on structured SMBG.

- Perform SMBG before eating and 2 hours after each meal.
- If 2-hour postprandial glucose is consistently more than 50 mg/dL above baseline for a given meal, increase insulin dose by 1 to 2 units. The target 2-hour postprandial Δ is 0 to 50 mg/dL (see Table 34-12).
- Any negative Δ (e.g., −25 mg/dL from baseline) predicts hypoglycemia. Blood glucose levels must be rechecked in 1 hour to monitor for hypoglycemia.
- A pattern of negative Δ values for a given meal suggests a mismatch between insulin dosing and carbohydrate intake for that meal. Reduce insulin dose by 1 to 2 units.

Table 34-25 shows examples of how structured glucose testing may be used to fine tune prandial insulin regimens.

Step 5: Establish an insulin sensitivity factor to determine correction doses for premeal hyperglycemia.

- Correction doses may be used to correct an elevated blood glucose value before eating.
- Patients can safely correct if their premeal glucose level is greater than 180 mg/dL.
- Postcorrection blood glucose target should always be 150 mg/dL (to avoid overshooting that conservative goal and inducing hypoglycemia).
- Insulin sensitivity factor is the number of mg/dL that 1 unit of insulin is expected to lower blood glucose and is based on the "rule of 1800."

1800/TDD = Expected drop in blood glucose from 1 unit of insulin. Example: If TDD is 70 units, the insulin sensitivity factor would be:

$$1800/70 = 25.7 \text{ (Round off to 25.)}$$

Thus, if the premeal blood glucose is 200 mg/dL and the target blood glucose is 150 mg/dL, the patient would give

Table 34-24   Prandial Dose Adjustments of Rapid-Acting Insulin

Meal Size	Prandial Insulin Dose Adjustment
Standard meal	No change
Very large meal with dessert	+3 units from baseline dose
Large meal without dessert	+1 to 2 units from baseline dose
Smaller than usual meal	−1 to 2 units from baseline dose

Table 34-25   Example of Structured Self-Monitoring of Blood Glucose for Patients with Type 1 Diabetes Mellitus

Date	Pre-Lunch Glucose (mg/dL)	2-Hour Post-Lunch Glucose (mg/dL)	Δ (Difference between Baseline Glucose and 2-Hour Postmeal Glucose)	Reasons for Δ Being <0 (a "Negative Δ") (Could Indicate Impending Hypoglycemia; List Actions Taken for Hypoglycemia)	Reasons for Δ Being >50 mg/dL (List Corrective Actions)
2/13	125	225	+100	—	Bolus given at meal time rather than 15 minute before eating Mismatch of insulin to carbohydrate (ate dessert); will give 2 units for dessert next time
2/14	110	154	44 (at target)	—	—
2/15	227	117	−110	Overcorrected on premeal insulin dose; became hypoglycemic 3 hours after eating but consumed 15 g of carbohydrate	
2/16	153	169	+16	Perfect	No need for adjustments for this type of food
3/17	125	200	+75	Stopped daily afternoon workouts; caring for ailing mother-in-law	Advised to increase baseline lunchtime prandial insulin dose by 2 units
3/18	100	190	+90		
3/19	135	235	+100		

a correction dose of 2 units (to correct for 50 mg/dL above target) in addition to the baseline prandial insulin dose at that particular meal. A patient who normally boluses 7 units before eating and has a 200 mg/dL premeal glucose value would add 2 units to the prandial dose for a total bolus dose of 7 + 2 = 9 units before eating.

- Patients who plan to eat a large meal may adjust their mealtime dose further according to the options mentioned in Table 34-24.
- SMBG should be performed 2 hours after eating to ensure that the correction dose did not cause glucose levels to trend toward hypoglycemia as a result of overcorrection.

Multiple daily injections should be initiated and maintained with the use of insulin pens rather than syringes and vials. Insulin pens allow for accuracy, portability, flexibility, and ease of use. Insulin pens typically do not need refrigeration, which may provide for additional patient adherence to therapy over vial-and-syringe insulin delivery. Patients must be familiar with the nuances of using each type of pen delivery device. Most important, errors in insulin delivery can be avoided if patients make certain that they are giving the appropriate formulation of insulin for basal or prandial coverage.

Patients whose A1C levels rise despite being provided adequate dosing protocols for a basal-bolus regimen may be nonadherent to their prescribed insulin regimen. One study found that 64% of T1DM patients were incorrectly assessing their prandial insulin requirements (Ahola et al., 2010). Barriers to insulin intensification in T1DM include fear of hypoglycemia, weight gain, inconvenient dosing protocols, and confusion about appropriate dosing of mealtime insulin (Cavan et al., 2012). Table 34-26 lists the advantages of insulin pens over syringes and vials (Asamoah, 2008).

Table 34-26 Advantages of Insulin Pen Delivery Systems versus Syringes and Vials

Clinicians can teach pen use to patients in <3 min on average. There is no need to inconvenience patients by having them learn the technique of insulin injection offsite.

Use of 30- or 31-gauge short needles with pens has significantly reduced the needle phobia that patients have about taking injections. Also, needles are less painful when they do not have to be inserted through the rubber stopper of a vial, which destroys the fine tip needle coating and thus increases injection pain.

Pens are easier then vials and syringes to carry in a pocket or purse.

Pen devices have been shown to be more accurate than syringes for delivering insulin doses ≤5 units, so they may benefit children and adolescents, who usually require smaller doses (Gnanalingham et al, 1998).

Older patients with diabetes who have comorbidities or disabilities (e.g., visual impairments, tremors, or impaired motor skills) that may exacerbate the difficulties of self-injection and increase the risk of dosing errors often find that pen devices can help to overcome such limitations.

Numerous patient surveys have demonstrated that patients prefer pens over vials and syringes (Asamoah, 2008).

Gnanalingham MG, Newland P, Smith CP. An evaluation of NovoPen, BD-Pen, and syringe devices at small doses of insulin [Abstract P118]. Presented at the British Diabetes Association's Medical and Scientific Section Spring Meeting in Edinburgh, Scotland, March 25-27, 1998; Asamoah E. Insulin pen: the "iPod" for insulin delivery: why pen wins over syringe. *J Diabetes Sci Technol.* 2:292-296, 2008.

INSULIN PUMP THERAPY AND CONTINUOUS GLUCOSE SENSORS

Continuous subcutaneous insulin infusion, also known as insulin pump therapy, allows patients with diabetes to achieve improved glycemic control while using less daily insulin, reducing the likelihood of weight gain and hypoglycemia, and limiting diurnal glycemic variability compared with insulin delivery via vials and syringes or insulin pen devices (Weissberg-Benchell et al., 2003). Because of the lifestyle flexibility that insulin pump users enjoy, quality-of-life assessment scores consistently favor CSII over MDI regimens. Switching from an MDI regimen to CSII will limit the number of short-term complications such as hypoglycemia and DKA, as well as reduce the risk for long-term microvascular complications (Weissberg-Benchell et al., 2003).

Although CSII is certainly the most sophisticated and precise insulin-delivery method currently available, patients who initiate pump therapy must be solidly committed to diabetes self-management. SMBG must be performed six to eight times daily unless patients use concomitant CGM devices. Patients must understand insulin pharmacokinetics, become adept at appropriate dosing and timing of prandial insulin, and be knowledgeable about exercise physiology. Pumps are machines that may fail, malfunction, or even be lost. Therefore, pump users must be trained to fall back to an emergency protocol such as pen or syringe insulin delivery to allow them to control hyperglycemia and minimize the risk of DKA if their pump malfunctions.

Fortunately, the vast majority of insulin pump users are skilled diabetes self-managers who often put clinicians to shame with their disease state knowledge. Because pump users are both challenging and intelligent members of the diabetes community, primary care physicians should learn the basics of pump therapy. Clinicians who feel comfortable intensively managing patients with MDI regimens are also capable of initiating and titrating insulin pump regimens (Unger, 2012b).

Ideally, insulin replacement should mimic the normal glucose and endogenous insulin response to the fasting and prandial states. However, prandial injection therapy, whether given by a syringe or a pen device, cannot provide an exact physiological dose to replicate first- and second-phase insulin secretion. A pen- or syringe-delivered dose of insulin mimics only first-phase (acute) insulin secretion. The bolus dose may not be sufficient to cover a delayed rise in glucose that may occur if the consumed meal is high in fat. Thus, patients may experience an insulin-to-carbohydrate mismatch, resulting in early postabsorptive hypoglycemia followed by an increase in plasma glucose as the rapid-acting insulin analog absorption is mitigated. To address this problem, insulin pumps allow patients to provide a bolus of insulin in percentages over time. For example, 20% of the insulin dose may be bolused immediately, and the remainder can be released as an "extended bolus" over several hours.

A similar problem exists regarding basal insulin delivered via pen or syringe. Giving one dose via pen or syringe assumes that basal insulin requirements will not change during the 24-hour period after the dose is given. However, patients who exercise will have reduced basal insulin requirements. Before patients arise in the morning, their

Table 34-27   Candidates for Continuous Subcutaneous Insulin Infusion Therapy

CSII should be considered for patients who:
- Have frequent hypoglycemia or hypoglycemia unawareness
- Fail to reach goal A1C with MDI insulin regimen
- Exercise regularly
- Experience the dawn phenomenon, which cannot be controlled with a single daily injection of basal insulin
- Travel frequently or are employed in shift work
- Are pregnant or planning for pregnancy
- Are children or adolescents
- Have gastroparesis
- Have a history of frequent DKA
- Experience severe insulin resistance (requiring >250 units of insulin daily)
- Would prefer to use an insulin pump rather than following an MDI regimen
- Are undergoing chemotherapy; glycemic variability may increase cancer-related mortality
- Have multiple micro- and macrovascular complications; hypoglycemia increases mortality in these patients
- Have ESRD
- Are athletes at any level of competition

CSII, Continuous subcutaneous insulin infusion; *DKA,* diabetic ketoacidosis; *ESRD,* end-stage renal failure; *MDI,* multiple daily injection.

basal insulin requirements increase in response to physiological insulin resistance caused by increased production of cortisol and growth hormone (a circumstance known as the "dawn phenomenon"). In the afternoon hours, insulin requirements are typically lower than during the morning and evening hours. Unfortunately, after a pen or syringe injection of basal insulin is given, the drug's influence on basal insulin levels cannot be altered; one cannot turn up or turn down the level of basal insulin injected the evening before in response to exercise or varying degrees of insulin resistance occurring in the 24-hour period after the injection. Insulin pumps address this issue by allowing patients to program multiple basal insulin delivery rates to match their individualized sleep patterns, physical activity, menstrual schedule, medications, and travel plans. (Such a feature is ideal for steroid-dependent patients who experience postprandial hyperglycemia and normal fasting glucose values.)

Thus, CSII allows patients with T1DM or insulin-requiring T2DM to enjoy a flexible lifestyle while avoiding hypoglycemia. By programming changes to both basal and bolus insulin delivery rates, pump users adjust their regimen to closely simulate normal endogenous β-cell insulin secretion.

Insulin pumps have been available since the 1980s, and more than 400,000 pump devices are sold annually worldwide (Unger, 2012b). Table 34-27 lists some of the indications for considering CSII in insulin-requiring patients with diabetes.

Patients may also integrate their CSII regimen with CGM. CGM systems operate by measuring glucose levels in interstitial fluid. The devices consist of three components: a disposable sensor that measures glucose levels, a transmitter that is attached to the sensor, and a receiver that displays and stores glucose information. The information stored in the receiver is then converted into estimated mean values of glucose standardized to capillary blood glucose levels

measured during calibration. Using an applicator or self-insertion device, patients insert a thin plastic sensor just under the skin of the abdomen or upper arm. These devices can display real-time glucose values and trends, and some can help patients avoid hyper- and hypoglycemia by sounding an alarm or vibrating when glucose levels rise above or fall below preprogrammed upper and lower thresholds. The receiver can store information for later use, and long-term data can be downloaded to a computer. Real-time trend graphs can be downloaded to a computer or displayed on the pump screen, which can be useful in identifying glycemic trends in response to physical activity, meals, insulin doses, menstruation, illness, or other factors.

The Medtronic MiniMed 530G system integrates CGM with CSII in one device that uses sensor-augmented pump technology. The CGM communicates with the pump and will automatically suspend insulin delivery when glucose values reach a pre-programmed low threshold.

EXERCISE AND TYPE 1 DIABETES MELLITUS MANAGEMENT

During the transition from rest to exercise, skeletal muscles shift from using predominantly FFAs released from adipose tissue to a mixture of muscle triglycerides, muscle glycogen, and glucose derived from glycogenolysis. During the initial stages of moderate exercise, muscle glycogen is the primary energy source. However, as exercise becomes more prolonged, glycogen stores become depleted, requiring the body to rely on circulating FFAs and plasma glucose as fuel sources. During heavy exercise (30-60 minutes at 80% of maximal oxygen uptake), peripheral glucose utilization may be as high as 1 to 1.5 g/min (Wasserman et al., 2002). This source of energy must be continuously replaced at an equal rate to prevent the onset of exercise-induced hypoglycemia.

In euglycemic individuals, plasma glucose levels are sustained during exercise because pancreatic insulin secretion decreases while levels of glucagon, growth hormone, cortisol, and catecholamines increase. Patients with T1DM lack the ability to regulate both endogenous insulin secretion and counterregulatory hormones in response to exercise, making maintenance of physiological fuel regulation nearly impossible. Thus, patients must adjust their carbohydrate consumption and insulin doses, as well as their exercise intensity, mode, and duration, to minimize the risk of hypoglycemia and exercise-induced DKA.

Intensive management of T1DM increases the risk of exercise-induced hypoglycemia. Exercise acutely increases peripheral glucose utilization within skeletal muscles, thus making circulating exogenous insulin "turbo-charged."

Patients with poorly controlled T1DM are at risk for exercise-emergent DKA (Riddell and Perkins, 2006). Prolonged exercise triggers hepatic glucose production. Insulinopenic patients with a baseline plasma glucose level greater than 240 mg/dL experience a rise in plasma glucose levels as exercise intensifies. Low circulating insulin levels cannot suppress hepatic glucose production during exercise. Dehydration combined with an exercise-induced increase in catecholamines will likely hasten the onset of DKA in these individuals (Marliss and Vranik, 2002). Table 34-28 lists suggested practical guidelines to minimize blood

Table 34-28 Suggestions for Minimizing Blood Glucose Excursions before, during, and after Exercise for Patients with Type 1 Diabetes Mellitus

Time Period	Recommendations
Before exercise	Determine the timing, mode (aerobic vs. resistance training), and intensity of exercise to be performed.
	Perform SMBG before exercising.
	A safe target blood glucose before moderate exercise is 120-180 mg/dL.
	If blood glucose is <120 mg/dL, consume 15 g of carbohydrates to provide an energy source during exercise.
	Do not exercise if blood glucose is ≥250 mg/dL and ketosis is present or if glucose is ≥300 mg/dL and no ketones are present.
	If activity is moderate or strenuous, lasts <90 min, and begins within 90 min of a meal, a reduction in prandial doses of lispro, aspart, or glulisine is warranted.
	Insulin doses may need to be increased and monitored more frequently during periods of prolonged resistance training or when training occurs in a warm environment.
	Consume 250 mL of fluids 20 min before exercise to maintain hydration.
During exercise	Monitor blood glucose level every 30 min.
	Continue fluid intake of 250 mL every 20 min during vigorous exercise.
	If blood glucose drops to <100 mg/dL during periods of moderate or intense exercise, consume 15 g of carbohydrates every 20-30 min.
	Consider using a CGM device, which will indicate the directional trend in blood glucose during exercise.
After exercise	Perform SMBG overnight if exercise is atypical.
	Consider consuming additional slow-acting carbohydrates to protect against exercise-induced nocturnal hypoglycemia.
	Patients with hypoglycemia awareness should wear a CGM device, which will alert them to impending nocturnal hypoglycemia.

CGM, Continuous glucose monitoring; *SMBG*, self-monitoring of blood glucose.

glucose excursions before, during, and after exercise for patients with T1DM.

Each year, 13,000 Americans are diagnosed with T1DM. Early intervention using an MDI or CSII insulin regimen is likely to minimize patients' long-term risks of micro- and macrovascular complications. Modern insulin formulations and delivery systems allow more patients to achieve their target glycemic and metabolic goals. T1DM is no longer an acute disease with a "death sentence" of 6 months as it was before the discovery of insulin. As our understanding of T1DM pathogenesis expands and our treatment armamentarium becomes more accessible, patients with diabetes are now able to life full and productive lives.

As clinicians, we must give our patients credit for making multiple decisions each day that will ultimately determine their ability to physiologically control glucose levels against incredible odds. We should never chastise our patients or imply that they are "noncompliant" because their glucose levels are poorly controlled. As family doctors, our role is to coordinate care for our patients and to make sure all patients are treated toward success rather than failure. T1DM is a challenging chronic disease. No specialty is better equipped to manage all aspects of diabetes than family medicine.

Long-Term Complications of Diabetes

Prolonged exposure to hyperglycemia, glycemic variability, genetic predisposition, oxidative stress, obesity, environmental factors, duration of disease, and timing of intensive management initiation are important determinants in the development of long-term diabetes-related complications. Microvascular disease resulting in small vessel injury can lead to disorders affecting the peripheral, sensory, and autonomic nerves; kidneys; and eyes. Macrovascular complications damage large vessels, resulting in coronary artery disease, MI, angina, peripheral arterial disease, and stroke. The link between glycemic burden and induction of disease-specific complication pathways has been established to involve four independent biochemical abnormalities: increased polyol pathway flux, increased formation of advanced glycation end products, activation of protein kinase C, and increased hexosamine pathway flux. These seemingly unrelated pathways have an underlying common denominator, which is an increase in oxidative stress caused by the overproduction of superoxide by the mitochondrial electron transport chain (Figure 34-6). Hyperglycemia, whether acute (postprandial) or chronic, has tissue-damaging effects on cell types such as capillary endothelial cells of the retina, mesangial cells in the renal glomerulus, and peripheral neurons. Cells that can effectively assimilate glucose as an energy source before transporting nonessential glucose out of the cell are less prone to complications. Cells such as neurons and nephrons, which are inefficient interstitial transporters of glucose, undergo oxidative stress, which induces endothelial dysfunction, vascular inflammation, and activation of pathways that trigger complications. Other cells, such as those in the GI tract, are more efficient at transporting excessive glucose out of the cell, thereby minimizing the risk of oxidative stress.

Vascular endothelial cells form physical and biological barriers between vessel walls and circulating blood cells, with the endothelium playing an important role in the maintenance of vascular homeostasis. Central to this role is the endothelial production of nitric oxide (NO), which is synthesized by the constitutively expressed endothelial isoform of NO synthase. Vascular diseases, including hypertension, diabetes, and atherosclerosis, are characterized by impaired endothelium-derived NO bioactivity that may contribute to clinical cardiovascular events. Endothelial cells exposed to oxidative stress generate high levels of reactive oxygen species via their mitochondrial electron-transport chain. Susceptible cells activate biochemical pathways

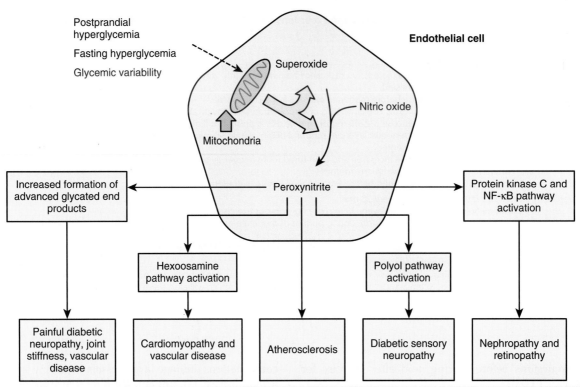

Figure 34-6 Downstream effects of oxidative stress–induced diabetes complication pathways. Postprandial and fasting hyperglycemia, as well as glycemic variability, result in the production of superoxide within the mitochondria of endothelial cells. Nitric oxide regulates vascular tone and minimizes adhesion molecule penetration of the vascular walls. When superoxide interacts with peroxynitrate, the endothelial cell's mitochondrial electron transport system becomes impaired, resulting in endothelial dysfunction. Transcription of endothelial- derived cytokines induce pathways known to activate microvascular complications. Peroxynitrate also favors lipid oxidation leading to atherosclerosis and macrovascular disease. Activation of the protein kinase C and nuclear factor κB pathways favors induction of nephropathy and retinopathy. Neuropathic induction is activated through the polyol pathway. Excessive advanced glycation results in painful diabetic neuropathy. *NF-κB*, Nuclear factor-κB. (Adapted with permission from Unger J. *Diabetes management in primary care.* 2nd ed. Philadelphia: Lippincott, Williams and Wilkins; 2012.)

likely to progress to long-term micro- and macrovascular complications unless metabolic stability is restored.

Brownlee (2001) determined that patients with both acute and chronic hyperglycemia live in a constant state of oxidative stress favoring end-stage complications. Exposure to blood glucose levels greater than 180 mg/dL results in prolonged endothelial cell dysfunction and vascular inflammation that persist for 7 days even after the acute episode of hyperglycemia is reversed. Clinically, patients who record a fasting blood glucose level greater than 180 mg/dL have likely been exposed to oxidative stress that has persisted throughout their resting hours. Failure to recognize and correct the chronic hyperglycemic state will place patients at risk for all-cause mortality and long-term complications.

Tables 34-29 and 34-30 list practical pointers related to each of the major long-term micro- and macrovascular complications observed in patients with diabetes. Table 34-31 summarizes the ADA's recommendations for use of angiotensin-converting enzyme inhibitors and angiotensin receptor blockers in patients with diabetic nephropathy.

Primary care physicians should play a proactive role in screening patients for micro- and macrovascular complications. All patients with diabetes should be provided with written, individualized glycemic targets for fasting glucose,

postprandial glucose, and A1C. Glycemic targets should be determined based on patients' duration of disease, presence or absence of significant comorbidities (especially macrovascular disorders), ability to safely and effectively perform SMBG, history of hypoglycemia unawareness, and psychosocial support mechanisms. Patients with renal insufficiency are at risk for treatment-emergent hypoglycemia and should have their prescription and herbal medications reviewed at each visit. Patients with chronic liver disease should discontinue use of sulfonylureas and consider lowering insulin doses. Chronic liver disease appears to increase β-cell sensitivity to sulfonylureas and reduce hepatic clearance of insulin, both of which can lead to a higher risk of hypoglycemia.

Undoubtedly, diabetes is a very complex disorder that requires a comprehensive treatment plan for most patients. Primary care physicians should not hesitate to communicate with consulting physicians who are co-managing their diabetes patients. Primary care physicians need to develop better means for monitoring their patients for compliance related to their specialty care visits. In addition, clinicians must communicate their concerns about patients' poor metabolic control to co-managing specialists to ensure that patients receive timely and appropriate screening and management of their long-term complications.

Table 34-29   Diabetes-Related Microvascular Complications: Practical Pointers

Complication	Statistics of Interest	Clinical Presentation	Treatment Strategies	Prevention or Reversal
Neuropathy	50% of patients with clinical neuropathy may be asymptomatic Affects 25%-30% of all patients with diabetes Cardiac autonomic neuropathy associated with a threefold increased risk of mortality	Pain derived from small nerve fibers may be sharp, burning, and lancinating Patients describe pain as "bee stings through socks" or "walking on hot coals" Pain typically worse at rest and improves with activity Negatively affects sleep, quality of life, and balance; may lead to anxiety and depressive symptoms Autonomic symptoms include loss of sweating on forehead and feet; abdominal distention; nocturnal diarrhea and constipation; erectile dysfunction and vaginal dryness; orthostatic hypotension; cardiac autonomic dysfunction; and hypoglycemia awareness autonomic dysfunction	FDA-approved drugs include duloxetine and pregabalin Avoid tricyclic antidepressants in patients >65 years of age because of adverse side effects For refractory pain, consider gabapentin + methadone	Smoking cessation Weight reduction Improvement in triglycerides Consider use of vitamin D_3, 4000 IU, and magnesium oxide, 250 mg, at bedtime For autonomic dysfunction, glycemic variability must be minimized and A1C should be brought as closely and safely as possible to the range of 7%-7.5%
Nephropathy	30% of patients with T1DM and 10%-40% of patients with T2DM will eventually develop ESRD Diabetes accounts for 38% of all ESRD in the United States The mean A1C of patients initiating treatment for ESRD is 7.6%, suggesting that risk factors such as genetics, BP, smoking, obesity, and hyperlipidemia may be influential in determining both disease progression and outcomes Diabetes-related ESRD declined in all age groups by 3.9% per year from 1996 to 2006 as physicians became more aware of the importance of intensive metabolic management of glucose, BP, and hyperlipidemia The highest mortality rates are observed with macroalbuminuria (albumin-to-creatinine ratio >300 mg/g) and a GFR <60 mL/min/1.73 m²	CKD is defined as having an estimated GFR <60 mL/min/1.73 m² over 6 months CKD stages are based on the estimated GFR (mL/min/1.73 m²) as follows: ■ Normal: >90 ■ Stage 1: >90 with kidney damage ■ Stage 2: 60-89 with kidney damage ■ Stage 3: 30-59 ■ Stage 3A: 45-59 ■ Stage 3B: 30-44 ■ Stage 4: 15-29 ■ Stage 5: <15	Discontinue nicotine and alcohol Screen high-risk patients for sleep apnea, vitamin D deficiency, and secondary hyperparathyroidism DCCT: intensively managing T1DM reduces the incidence of microalbuminuria by 39% ADVANCE: 21% reduction in the risk of new or worsening nephropathy noted in patients as systolic BP was reduced to 110 mm Hg ACE inhibitors and ARBs decrease the risk of progression to macroalbuminuria by as much as 60%-70% A moderately low-protein diet (0.9 g /kg/day) used in patients with T1DM and progressive diabetic nephropathy reduced the risk of ESRD and death by 76% without affecting the decline in GFR Drugs that require dosage adjustments in patients with nephropathy include metformin, sulfonylureas, α-glucosidase inhibitors, glitinides, and insulin. The incretin-based therapies exenatide, sitagliptin, saxagliptin, and alogliptin require dosage reductions in people with a creatinine clearance of <50 mL/min; liraglutide and linagliptin require no adjustments. SGLT2 inhibitors are ineffective at estimated GFR <45 mL/min/1.73 m² Screen and treat patients for anemia to reduce the risk of heart failure and CKD progression; maintain hemoglobin levels ≥12 g/dL Use aspirin to prevent CVD; higher doses are needed because patients with CKD are aspirin resistant Lowering LDL cholesterol to <100 mg/dL may minimize CVD risk but not CKD progression	Yearly measurements of creatinine, urinary albumin excretion, and potassium

Continued on following page

Table 34-29   Diabetes-Related Microvascular Complications: Practical Pointers (Continued)

Complication	Statistics of Interest	Clinical Presentation	Treatment Strategies	Prevention or Reversal
Retinopathy	Prevalence of diabetic macular edema in the United States is 28% Only 63% of diabetes patients have had screening eye examinations	"Mild" refers to the presence of microaneurysms only. "Moderate" NPDR is defined as the presence of microaneurysms and either hard exudates or blot hemorrhages caused by the deposition of lipoproteins and the exudation of red blood cells from retinal microaneurysms. "Severe" NPDR is characterized by a large number of retinal hemorrhages or the presence of cotton-wool exudates (microinfarcts within the nerve fiber layer of the retina) and the development of intraretinal microvascular abnormalities (collateral vessels) in the resulting ischemic areas of the retina. PDR is associated with the development of abnormal new retinal blood vessels that may bleed into the vitreous cavity and become fibrotic; the resulting traction on the macula leads to visual loss. Diabetic macular edema results in thickening of the retina and decreased central visual activity.	Minimize glycemic variability DCCT: intensive diabetes management reduced risk of proliferative retinopathy by 47% UKPDS: intensive BP control resulted in a 47% risk reduction in vision loss for patients treated to a target of <150/85 mm Hg vs. those treated to 180/95 mm Hg	Screen T1DM patients 3–5 years after initial diagnosis; repeat annually if no retinopathy observed Screen T2DM patients at time of diagnosis; repeat annually if no retinopathy observed Screen before conception and during the first trimester of pregnancy; reevaluate every 1 to 3 months if retinopathy is present Optical coherence tomography can demonstrate intraretinal edema affecting the macula Digital retinal photography allows for rapid acquisition of high-quality retinal images without requiring pupillary dilatation; these cameras can be used by primary care physicians with interpretation by trained ophthalmologists

ACE, Angiotensin-converting enzyme; *ADVANCE,* The Action in Diabetes and Vascular Disease: Preterax and Diamicron Modified Release Controlled Evaluation trial; *ARB,* angiotensin receptor blocker; *BP,* blood pressure; *CKD,* chronic kidney disease; *CVD,* cardiovascular disease; *DCCT,* Diabetes Control and Complications Trial; *ESRD,* end-stage renal disease; *GFR,* glomerular filtration rate; *FDA,* Food and Drug Administration; *LDL,* low-density lipoprotein; *NPDR,* nonproliferative diabetic retinopathy; *PDR,* proliferative retinopathy; *T2DM,* type 2 diabetes mellitus; *T1DM,* type 1 diabetes mellitus; *T2DM,* type 2 diabetes mellitus; *UKPDS,* U.K. Prospective Diabetes Study.

Tarantola RM, Maturi RK, Kushal S, et al. Screening, prevention, and ambitious management of diabetic macular edema in patients with type 1 diabetes. *Curr Diab Rep.* 13:679-686, 2013; Unger J. *Diabetes management in primary care.* 2nd ed. Philadelphia: Lippincott, Williams and Wilkins; 2012.

Table 34-30   Diabetes-Related Macrovascular Complications: Practical Pointers

Complication	Statistics of Interest	Clinical Presentation	Treatment Strategies	Prevention or Reversal
Coronary heart disease, stroke, and peripheral arterial disease	The mortality rate at the time of acute MI is essentially doubled in patients with diabetes compared with those without diabetes. For MI survivors, follow-up mortality in patients with diabetes is essentially doubled compared with those without diabetes. 80% of diabetes-related deaths are attributable to coronary heart disease, stroke, and peripheral arterial disease.	Chest pain, shortness of breath, anxiety (in women), orthostatic hypotension, loss of beat-to-beat variability, abnormalities in QT interval (QT prolongation), depression, erectile dysfunction, low testosterone levels in men, fatigue, peripheral edema, congestive heart failure, and sudden death For peripheral arterial disease: ■ Some patients are asymptomatic ■ Pain with ambulation; subsides with rest ■ Hair loss ■ Brittle nails ■ Dry, scaly, atrophic skin ■ Dependent rubor ■ Pallor with leg elevation after 1 minute at 60 degrees (normal color should return in 10-15 seconds; >40 seconds indicates severe ischemia) ■ Ischemic tissue ulceration (punched-out, painful, with little bleeding), gangrene ■ Absent or diminished femoral or pedal pulses ■ Arterial bruits	Low-dose aspirin Lower LDL cholesterol to <100 mg/dL Lower BP to <130/80 mm Hg Target A1C to lowest and safest level using rational pharmacology to minimize risk of hypoglycemia, especially in patients with T2DM and preexisting coronary artery disease	Screen for and manage risk factors related to unhealthy lifestyle choices: inactivity, obesity, smoking, alcohol, and inactivity. Reduce and slow progression of microalbuminuria and CKD. Recommendations for ABI screening to detect peripheral arterial disease in patients with diabetes: ■ A resting ABI should be used to established diagnosis of peripheral arterial disease in high-risk patients. ■ Index is calculated as the ratio of systolic BP at the ankle to that at the arm. ■ High-risk patients include those with exertional claudication, nonhealing wounds, and age ≥65 years or age ≥50 years with a history of smoking or diabetes. ■ Normal values defined as 1.00 to 1.40; borderline 0.91 to 0.99. ■ Abnormal values are ≤0.90.

ABI, Ankle-brachial index; *CKD,* chronic kidney disease; *MI,* myocardial infarction; *LDL,* low-density lipoprotein; *T2DM,* type 2 diabetes mellitus.
Rooke TW, Hirsch AT, Misra S, et al. 2011 ACCF/AHA focused update of the guideline for the management of patients with peripheral artery disease (updating the 2005 guideline): a report of the American College of Cardiology Foundation/American Heart Association Task Force on Practice Guidelines. *Circulation.* 124:2020-2045, 2011; Fowler MJ. Complications of diabetes. *Clinical Diabetes.* 29:116-122, 2011; Unger J. *Diabetes management in primary care.* 2nd ed. Philadelphia: Lippincott, Williams and Wilkins; 2012

Table 34-31   Treatment for Diabetic Nephropathy

Category	Recommended Treatment
T1DM or T2DM with micro- or macroalbuminuria	ACE inhibitors or ARBs
T1DM with hypertension and albuminuria	ACE inhibitors delay progression of nephropathy
T2DM with hypertension and microalbuminuria	ACE inhibitors or ARBs delay the progression to macroalbuminuria
T2DM with hypertension, macroalbuminuria, and renal insufficiency (serum creatinine >1.5 mg/dL)	ARBs delay the progression of nephropathy
T1DM or T2DM with microalbuminuria and normal BP	ACE inhibitors or ARBs

ACE, Angiotensin-converting enzyme; *ARB,* angiotensin receptor blocker; *BP,* blood pressure; *T1DM,* type 1 diabetes mellitus; *T2DM,* type 2 diabetes mellitus.
References: American Diabetes Association. Clinical practice recommendations, 2011. *Diabetes Care.* 34(suppl 1):S33, 2011; Gross JL, de Azevedo MJ, Silveiro SP, et al. Diabetic nephropathy: diagnosis, prevention and treatment. *Diabetes Care.* 28:164-176, 2005.

Table 34-32   Five Key Behaviors to Help Patients Become Successful Diabetes Self-Managers

1. Know your metabolic targets (A1C, BP, and lipids).
2. Know how to achieve your metabolic targets.
   a. Increase physical activity.
   b. Consume a healthy diet.
   c. Perform SMBG in a timely manner.
3. Stop smoking and alcohol use.
4. Take your prescribed medications.
5. Be certain your health care providers understand how to successfully and intensively manage diabetes.

BP, Blood pressure; *SMBG,* self-monitoring of blood glucose.

Five Things Patients Must Do to Become Successful Diabetes Self-Managers

A diagnosis of diabetes presents numerous challenges for patients, their families, and the clinicians who direct their care. At times, the burden of having diabetes may seem overwhelming. Unfortunately, diabetes is a chronic disease requiring daily adjustments in care and, in most cases, adoption of intensive lifestyle alterations. Rather than increase their concern about the future risk of long-term complications, newly diagnosed patients with diabetes should be reassured that their lives can be long, productive, and healthy if they adopt the five specific behaviors listed in Table 34-32. Of primary importance is reassuring patients that the number 1 complication of *well-controlled* diabetes is ... nothing!

Acknowledgment

The authors thank Debbie Kendall of Kendall Editorial in Richmond, Virginia, for her assistance in the editing and preparation of this chapter.

Videos

 The following video is available at www.expertconsult.com:

Video 34-1 Demonstration of the Use of Selected Equipment Used in the Management of Diabetes

References

The complete reference list is available at www.expertconsult.com.

Web Resources

www.cdc.gov/diabetes/ Centers for Disease Control and Prevention. National Diabetes Fact Sheet provides general information and national estimates on diabetes in the United States.

www.endotext.org/ Endotext. Up-to-date, comprehensive source of information on all topics in clinical endocrinology.

www.who.int/diabetes/facts/en/ World Health Organization. Diabetes program fact sheet.

35 Endocrinology

GEORGE A. WILSON and MAE SHEIKH-ALI

Key Points

- The hypothalamic–pituitary axis (HPA) orchestrates the hormonal secretions of the other endocrine glands.
- The pituitary is composed of the adenohypophysis, or anterior lobe, and the neurohypophysis, or posterior lobe.
- The hormonal secretions of the anterior pituitary are regulated by a number of hypothalamic-releasing hormones and inhibitory molecules.
- The posterior lobe of the pituitary is where nerve endings, originating in the paraventricular and supraoptic nuclei, project as the supraopticohypophyseal tract.

Hypothalamic–Pituitary Axis

The hypothalamus affects several nonendocrine functions, including appetite, sleep, body temperature, and activity of the autonomic nervous system. In addition, the hypothalamus modulates the pituitary hormone secretions. The other half of the HPA, the pituitary gland, is often referred to as the "master gland" in recognition of its role in orchestrating the hormonal secretions of the other endocrine glands (Mooradian and Korenman, 2007; Mooradian and Morley, 1988).

The pituitary gland is located in the anterior fossa, in the sella turcica, in close proximity to the optic chiasm. The pituitary is composed of the adenohypophysis, or anterior lobe, and the neurohypophysis, or posterior lobe, and is connected to the hypothalamus by the pituitary stalk.

See Table 35-1 for a listing of hormones from each lobe of the pituitary.

Control of pituitary hormones is a complex process involving the hypothalamus, both lobes of the pituitary, and hormones endogenously produced by the various organs of the endocrine system.

Hormones secreted from the anterior pituitary lobe are regulated by a number of hypothalamic-releasing hormones and inhibitory molecules. These factors reach the pituitary through the portal circulation and, upon interaction with specific receptors, either stimulate or inhibit the secretion of the anterior pituitary hormones.

The main releasing hormones produced in the hypothalamus include thyrotropin-releasing hormone (TRH), gonadotropin-releasing hormone (GnRH), corticotropin-releasing hormone (CRH), and growth hormone–releasing hormone (GHRH). There are two major inhibitory factors: dopamine, which principally inhibits prolactin release, and somatostatin, a potent inhibitor of growth hormone (GH) and, to a lesser extent, thyrotropin or thyroid-stimulating hormone (TSH).

A number of other factors have been identified and shown to have important regulatory effects on anterior pituitary function. The kisspeptin hormones are a family of peptides encoded by the *KiSS-1* gene and are thought to play a critical role in reproduction. Kisspeptin receptors stimulate GnRH release and activation of the mammalian reproductive axis. Mutations in kisspeptin receptor GPR-54 cause idiopathic hypogonadotropic hypogonadism (HH) characterized by delayed or absent puberty (Jayasena and Dhillo, 2009).

There is a short-loop regulatory system within the HPA, which, via the portal circulation, allows pituitary hormones to flow in a retrograde direction back to the hypothalamus to feedback on their own releasing hormones. In addition, there is a long-loop negative feedback on the pituitary, mediated by hormones secreted by endocrine glands in the periphery (Mooradian and Korenman, 2007; Mooradian and Morley, 1988). It is the interplay between the effects of the hypothalamic-releasing hormones, the short-loop regulatory system and the long-loop negative feedback that controls pituitary hormonal secretions. For example, a rise in plasma thyroid hormone level feeds back and suppresses pituitary TSH and hypothalamic TRH secretion.

As we achieve better understanding of the intricacies of these processes and feedback controls, new therapeutic modalities are postulated. Secretion of GH is regulated by two hypothalamic hormones, GHRH and somatostatin. New data suggest that γ-aminobutyric acid (GABA) may also play a role in GH secretion. Although research in this area is relatively new, it does suggest a possible alternative approach to growth retardation caused by insufficient GH secretion or gigantism caused by GH excess (Powers, 2012).

The posterior pituitary lobe is essentially an extension of the hypothalamus, where the nerve endings, originating in the paraventricular and supraoptic nuclei, project as the supraopticohypophyseal tract. The posterior pituitary

Table 35-1 Pituitary Hormones

Hormones of the adenohypophysis or anterior pituitary lobe	Thyroid-stimulating hormone (TSH or thyrotropin) Follicle-stimulating hormone (FSH) Luteinizing hormone (LH) Prolactin (PRL) Growth hormone (GH or somatotropin) Adrenocorticotropic hormone (ACTH) α-Melanocyte-stimulating hormone (α-MSH)
Hormones of the neurohypophysis (pars nervosa) or posterior pituitary lobe	Antidiuretic hormone (ADH or vasopressin) Oxytocin

hormones are directly controlled by neural impulses and are released into the inferior hypophyseal veins and then into the systemic circulation (Mooradian and Morley, 1988).

Approach to Pituitary Disease

Key Points

- Pituitary disease may manifest with pituitary hormone excess or deficiency or symptoms of mass expansion, including headaches and visual disturbances.
- Pituitary adenoma is the most common cause of pituitary dysfunction in adults.
- HPA function should be assessed whenever a mass is discovered in the sella turcica.
- Evaluation of pituitary function (deficiency or excess) involves imaging and serum measurements of prolactin, GH, insulin-like growth factor type 1 (IGF-1), free thyroxine (FT_4), TSH, adrenocorticotropic hormone (ACTH), cortisol, luteinizing hormone (LH), follicle-stimulating hormone (FSH), testosterone (in men), and estradiol (in women). Twenty-four-hour urinary free cortisol and dexamethasone suppression tests (DSTs) are used for evaluating cortisol excess.

The most common cause of pituitary disease is the development of benign tumors (adenomas). These tumors can cause symptoms because of excessive production of hormones such as prolactin, GH, or ACTH or can cause pituitary hormone insufficiency secondary to tissue destruction. The pituitary hormones that can be lost early from gradual destruction of pituitary tissue include GH and GnRH followed by TSH and ACTH (Mooradian and Korenman, 2007; Mooradian and Morley, 1988). However, occasionally, the autoimmune destruction of the pituitary can be cell specific and cause selective pituitary hormone deficiency.

Pituitary tumors can expand into surrounding tissue such as the optic chiasm and hypothalamus and cause visual field defects and symptoms of hypothalamic disease, respectively. Early manifestations of optic chiasm impingement can be subtle and include seeing images that float apart or seeing half of a face higher than the other half (the Picasso effect or hemifield slide phenomenon). These symptoms emerge when the patient is tired or anxious and are the result of failure to fuse the images from both eyes because of the lack of nasal fields (Mooradian and Morley, 1988). Expansion of tumors into the hypothalamus can cause disturbances in sleep, appetite, temperature regulation, sweating, water balance, and memory (Mooradian and Morley, 1988).

In children, pituitary adenomas are less common, and hypothalamic pituitary dysfunction is usually the result of hypothalamic tumors, notably craniopharyngiomas.

When microadenoma (<10 mm) is discovered incidentally, the initial evaluation should seek hormone hypersecretion by measuring levels of serum prolactin, IGF-1, TSH, and FT_4, as well as 24-hour urine free-cortisol or a 1-mg overnight DST (Mooradian and Korenman, 2007; Mooradian and Morley, 1988). More extensive workup is required for pituitary masses larger than 10 mm (macroadenoma) regardless of symptoms.

The overall workup and management of pituitary disease should include identifying and treating hormonal deficiency or excess as well as diagnosing and managing mass effects of the tumors.

HYPOPITUITARISM

Key Points

- Hypopituitarism refers to total or partial deficiency of one or more pituitary hormones.
- Hypopituitarism could be the result of a genetic cause; a deficiency in hypothalamic releasing factor; or, more commonly, the result of pituitary tissue destruction secondary to mass expansion, infiltrative process, autoimmune or infectious disease, vascular accidents, radiation injury, or trauma.
- Pituitary apoplexy may result in life-threatening hypocortisolism.
- Lymphocytic hypophysitis is a rare autoimmune disease of the pituitary occurring in women during late pregnancy or in the postpartum period. This disease may mimic pituitary tumor but does not require resection.
- Kallmann syndrome is characterized by an isolated defect in GnRH secretion.
- Approximately 10% of patients with empty sella syndrome have clinically apparent hypopituitarism, and some may have pituitary adenomas.
- Systemic disease, including end-stage liver disease or chronic renal failure, is associated with variable degrees of hypopituitarism without significant histopathologic changes in the pituitary.

Hypopituitarism refers to total or partial deficiency of one or more pituitary hormones resulting in end-organ changes or reduced hormonal secretion of target endocrine glands (Toogood and Stewart, 2008). The deficiencies could be the result of primary disease of the pituitary or secondary to failure of hypothalamic hormone synthesis or transport. There are no good estimates of the incidence of hypopituitarism because the disease is often subclinical.

Causes

Hypopituitarism could be the result of a genetic cause; a deficiency in hypothalamic releasing factor; or, more commonly, the result of pituitary tissue destruction secondary to mass expansion, infiltrative process, autoimmune or infectious disease, vascular accidents, radiation injury, or trauma (Toogood and Stewart, 2008). Sometimes the etiology of hypopituitarism cannot be identified and is considered idiopathic. Most of these cases are sporadic, although there are well described familial causes of hypopituitarism.

The most common cause of hypopituitarism in the adult population is *intrasellar pituitary tumors*. Occasionally, hypopituitarism is resolved with surgical or medical treatment of the pituitary mass. Parasellar masses that cause hypopituitarism include craniopharyngiomas, meningiomas, optic nerve gliomas, teratomas, germinomas, chordomas, metastatic cancer, and lymphomas.

The second most common cause of hypopituitarism in adults is *postpartum pituitary necrosis* (Sheehan syndrome). The portal system of the anterior pituitary vascular supply, increased oxygen demand of an enlarged pituitary gland during pregnancy, excessive blood loss, and possibly increased intravascular coagulation converge to cause ischemic injury of the pituitary. Other ischemic causes of pituitary necrosis can occur in systemic vascular diseases such as diabetes mellitus, temporal arteritis, and sickle cell disease. These diseases can also result in hemorrhagic infarction *(apoplexy)* of the pituitary with acute onset of severe headache, visual impairment, altered mental status, and hypopituitarism. The sudden decline in ACTH, and thus hypocortisolism, may be the most life-threatening consequence of hypopituitarism, requiring emergency treatment with corticosteroids. Although pituitary adenomas are the most common cause of pituitary apoplexy, often it may be related to complications of diabetes, radiotherapy, or open heart surgery (Toogood and Stewart, 2008).

Rarely, infectious diseases can lead to hypopituitarism. Examples include meningitis, intracranial abscess, septic shock, fungal infections of the central nervous system (CNS), tuberculosis (TB), malaria, and syphilis.

Infiltrative diseases of the pituitary, and more commonly of the hypothalamus, can cause hypopituitarism. Sarcoidosis can present with hypopituitarism along with polydipsia and polyuria. Histiocytosis X may present as a suprasellar tumor. Lipid storage diseases and hemochromatosis can cause hypopituitarism often with hypogonadotropin deficiency.

Lymphocytic hypophysitis is a rare autoimmune disease of the pituitary occurring in women during late pregnancy or in the postpartum period. Lymphocytes and plasma cells infiltrate the pituitary gland, which results in the destruction of anterior pituitary cells (Toogood and Stewart, 2008). Lymphocytic hypophysitis cannot be distinguished from tumor except by biopsy. The diagnosis is suspected in women who develop hypopituitarism during or immediately after pregnancy in the absence of a history of hemorrhage during delivery or previous history of infertility or menstrual disorders.

Mutations in the *PROP-1* gene are the most common causes of congenital hypopituitarism and present as deficiencies of GH, prolactin, TSH, LH, and FSH. Older adults with *PROP-1* gene mutations may manifest with ACTH deficiency (Wu et al., 1998). Mutations of genes that code for specific anterior pituitary hormones have also been described, the most common of which is isolated genetic deficiencies of GH, which manifests with short stature and begins in infancy or childhood. *Kallmann syndrome* is characterized by an isolated defect in GnRH secretion. Young men develop a eunuchoid appearance and testosterone deficiency, and women manifest with amenorrhea or oligomenorrhea. The syndrome may also be associated with hyposmia or anosmia (Oliveira et al., 2001). Iatrogenic causes of hypopituitarism include surgical ablation and radiotherapy. Hypothalamic and pituitary deficiency may occur after several years, with GH and gonadotropin deficiencies the most common. Prolactin level may be mildly elevated.

Approximately 10% of patients with *empty sella syndrome* have clinically apparent hypopituitarism and some may have pituitary adenomas (Mooradian and Morley, 1988). The empty sella syndrome occurs when a defect in the sellar diaphragm allows the subarachnoid space to herniate into the pituitary fossa. It is a relatively common disorder found in 5% to 8% of autopsies. Systemic disease, including endstage liver disease or chronic renal failure, is associated with variable degrees of hypopituitarism without significant histopathologic changes in the pituitary (Mooradian, 2001; Nowak and Mooradian, 2007).

Clinical Manifestations

Key Points

- Progressive loss of hormones occurs in pituitary injury with loss of GH and gonadotropin followed by TSH and ACTH deficiency.
- ACTH deficiency results in cortisol deficiency, leading to hypotension, shock, and cardiovascular collapse.
- TSH deficiency results in signs and symptoms of hypothyroidism.
- Gonadotropin deficiency results in signs and symptoms of hypogonadism.
- GH deficiency causes short stature in children and may be asymptomatic in adults.

The clinical manifestations of hypopituitarism are highly variable and depend on the age and sex of the patient as well as on the etiology of the pituitary disease (Toogood and Stewart, 2008). Patients can be completely asymptomatic for many years or present with dramatic symptoms of nausea, vomiting, headache, and vascular collapse. The latter is more common in pituitary apoplexy when the sudden withdrawal of ACTH and ensuing adrenal insufficiency cause hemodynamic instability. It is believed that at least 75% of the glandular tissue must be destroyed before an individual becomes clinically symptomatic. If the etiology is a space-occupying lesion, such as an expanding adenoma or carotid aneurysm, the clinical manifestations will include headache and visual field defects, which are classically bitemporal hemianopsia (loss of peripheral vision). Other subtle changes in vision include changes in color perception, patchy scotomas, and difficulty in passing a thread through the eye of a needle (Mooradian and Morley, 1988).

Failure to lactate may be the first clinical sign of Sheehan syndrome. Lethargy, anorexia, weight loss, failure to resume normal menstrual periods, and loss of pubic hair may also be present later in the postpartum period. On the other hand, symptoms and signs of pituitary infarction may be subtle and not recognized for years.

Patients with *panhypopituitarism* (Simmonds syndrome) are usually pale and lethargic; have dry skin and low blood pressure (BP); and, rarely, may look cachectic (Mooradian and Morley, 1988; Toogood and Stewart, 2008). These patients have lost all the anterior pituitary hormones, and the clinical manifestations are the result of a mixture of hypogonadism, hypothyroidism, adrenal insufficiency, and GH deficiency. The clinical manifestations depend on whether the deficiency is partial or complete. Individual signs and symptoms are reflections of the biologic actions of various hormones secreted by the pituitary.

Growth hormone deficiency manifests as growth retardation in children. The body proportion and primary teeth are normal, but secondary tooth eruption is delayed. In up to 10% of children with GH deficiency, symptomatic hypoglycemia may occur. In adults, GH deficiency may be asymptomatic. Subtle changes may occur in insulin sensitivity, manifested by reduced insulin requirements in patients with diabetes, decreased muscle and bone mass with increased adiposity, delayed wound healing, and fasting hypoglycemia, and may contribute to anemia of hypopituitarism. Additional adverse effects associated with GH deficiency in adults include an increase in low-density lipoprotein (LDL) and a decrease in high-density lipoprotein (HDL) cholesterol, decreased cardiovascular function, increased risk of cardiovascular events, and a diminished sense of well-being. Life expectancy is reduced in these patients compared with age-matched control participants (Svensson et al., 2004).

Gonadotropin deficiency results in HH or secondary hypogonadism (Toogood and Stewart, 2008). In prepubertal children, HH manifests as failure to achieve pubertal changes along with a lack of a pubertal growth spurt. Girls have primary amenorrhea and lack breast development and widening of the pelvis. In boys, the testicular size remains small; the scrotal skin does not thicken; and penile growth, muscle development, and hoarseness of voice do not appear. In adults, HH presents as infertility, loss of libido, decreased facial hair, and muscle mass in men and amenorrhea, decreased breast size, and atrophic vaginal mucosa in women. If left untreated, men and women with hypogonadism develop osteoporosis. A deficiency in TSH causes secondary hypothyroidism unless the patient has concomitant Graves disease or an autonomously functioning thyroid nodule. The classical clinical manifestations of hypothyroidism include lethargy, easy fatigability, dry skin, cold intolerance, constipation, fine silky hair, slow mentation, and slow relaxation phase of deep tendon reflexes. Other features include anemia and hyponatremia secondary to increased antidiuretic hormone (ADH) secretion. In general, these symptoms are less severe in patients with TSH deficiency compared with patients with primary thyroid failure, and other findings, such as hypercholesterolemia, hypercarotenemia, myxedema, and effusions in body cavities, may occur less frequently (Toogood and Stewart, 2008).

A deficiency in ACTH results in deficiency of cortisol secretion and is referred to as *secondary adrenal insufficiency*. The clinical features resemble primary adrenal disease such as Addison disease. In both entities, anorexia, lethargy, nausea, vomiting, abdominal pain, postural hypotension, and vascular collapse may occur. Whereas hyponatremia is more common in ACTH deficiency, hyperkalemia is seen only in primary adrenal insufficiency and loss of aldosterone secretion, primarily regulated by the renin–angiotensin system (RAS) and serum potassium and sodium concentrations. Hyperpigmentation of the skin and vitiligo are features of primary adrenal insufficiency, and patients with ACTH deficiency have difficulty tanning upon exposure to sunlight. Mild ACTH deficiency may be asymptomatic and go undiagnosed for a long time.

Diagnosis

> ### Key Points
>
> - If one pituitary hormone insufficiency is documented, the other pituitary hormones should be tested.
> - An 8 AM plasma cortisol level below 3 µg/dL strongly suggests hypocortisolism. A level 18 µg/dL or greater excludes ACTH deficiency.
> - Serum FT$_4$ must be used with serum TSH concentration in assessing thyroid function.
> - A normal or subnormal LH level in menopausal or amenorrheic women, in the presence of a low estradiol level, indicates secondary hypogonadism (in men, a low testosterone level).
> - The diagnosis of GH deficiency requires provocative testing.

Because the presenting complaints of hypopituitarism can be subtle, clinicians need a high index of suspicion to arrive at the correct diagnosis (Toogood and Stewart, 2008). If the clinical manifestations fit hypogonadism, hypothyroidism, or adrenal insufficiency, those hormonal tests should be ordered to confirm the diagnosis. After one pituitary hormone insufficiency is documented, every attempt should be made to test the status of the other pituitary hormones as well. The underlying etiology of the disease should be determined by computed tomography (CT) or magnetic resonance imagining (MRI) of the hypothalamic–pituitary area. Occasionally, angiography is needed when carotid artery aneurysm is suspected or to define the blood supply of the tumor. Formal ophthalmologic examination, with visual field evaluation, should be ordered if the patient is symptomatic or harbors a pituitary mass lesion.

Pituitary hormone secretion is episodic, and in general, dynamic testing is more valuable than single baseline hormone measurements. For practical reasons, however, screening can be done with pituitary hormone and target hormone measurements simultaneously. For evaluating suspected hypopituitarism, tests include thyroid function, LH, serum testosterone in men and estradiol in women, IGF-1 (because GH has a short half-life in blood), prolactin, and morning cortisol. Provocative testing for GH and ACTH reserves may be required as well. Patients with known pituitary disease and deficiencies of ACTH, TSH, or gonadotropins have a 95% chance of subnormal provocative stimulus for GH. Also, patients with known pituitary disease and a serum IGF-1 concentration lower than normal can be presumed to have GH deficiency (Gharib et al., 2003). Provocative tests for GH are either physiologic (sleep or exercise) or pharmacologic, such as insulin-induced hypoglycemia, GHRH with arginine test, and levodopa with arginine test (Biller et al., 2002; Gharib et al., 2003). GH deficiency is diagnosed when GH does not rise above 5 ng/mL in response to two or more stimuli.

A plasma cortisol level below 3 μg/dL at 8 AM on two occasions in a patient with a disorder known to cause hypopituitarism strongly suggests hypocortisolism, and in the presence of normal or low serum ACTH concentration, it establishes the diagnosis of secondary adrenal insufficiency. Conversely, a cortisol level of 18 μg/dL or greater virtually excludes the diagnosis of ACTH deficiency.

To evaluate ACTH reserve, an insulin hypoglycemia test (0.1-0.15 U/kg IV) should be done. A normal cortisol response to adequate hypoglycemic stimulus (blood glucose <50 mg/dL) is either an incremental level of 6 to 10 μg/dL or an absolute level greater than 20 μg/dL. The test allows for concomitant evaluation of GH reserve; however, it is contraindicated in elderly adults and those with coronary artery disease (CAD) or epilepsy (Nowak and Mooradian, 2007).

An alternative is the metyrapone test, 750 mg orally every 4 hours for 6 doses, which assesses the sensitivity of the pituitary to negative inhibition of cortisol. Metyrapone blocks 11β-hydroxylase, an enzyme that catalyzes the final step in cortisol biosynthesis, which inhibits cortisol production. The decrease in cortisol secretion after metyrapone is given should result in a compensatory increase in the ACTH level. The level of the precursor steroid 11-deoxycortisol should also increase. A normal response is an increase in serum 11-deoxycortisol level greater than 10 μg/dL, when serum cortisol level is reduced to less than 8 μg/dL, indicating adequate suppression of glucocorticoid synthesis. In the more convenient overnight test, metyrapone 30 mg/kg orally, is administered at midnight. An increase in the 8 AM serum 11-deoxycortisol level to greater than 7 μg/dL is found in healthy persons. If symptomatic postural hypotension occurs after metyrapone administration, hydrocortisone should be administered exogenously.

Cosyntropin (synthetic ACTH), 250 μg administered intramuscularly or intravenously should result in an increase in the serum cortisol level to 18 μg/dL or greater at 60 minutes in normal subjects. The test may not reliably determine the ACTH reserve, especially in those with recent ACTH deficiency and in patients whose adrenal glands may not be atrophied enough. There is some controversy whether the 1-μg cosyntropin stimulation test (intravenous [IV] only) may be more sensitive for the diagnosis of subtle secondary adrenal insufficiency.

Thyrotropin (TSH) deficiency is diagnosed when low baseline FT$_4$ and low or normal TSH is documented on more than one measurement. Gonadotropin deficiency in men is tested with measurements of baseline LH, FSH, and total testosterone. Serum samples are drawn between 8 AM and 10 AM, and low concentrations should be confirmed with a second serum sample. The 8 AM to 10 AM serum testosterone concentration generally should be 300 to 1000 ng/dL.

A low testosterone value (< 200 ng/dL) with low or normal LH is indicative of HH (Mooradian and Korenman, 2006). For serum total testosterone levels between 200 and 400 ng/dL, free testosterone level should also be ordered (Mooradian and Korenman, 2006).

The presence of amenorrhea in premenopausal women, along with a low estrogen level (<30 pg/mL), establishes the diagnosis of HH. In menopausal women, the absence of elevated FSH and LH is sufficient for the diagnosis.

Elevated serum prolactin levels in a hypogonadal individual suggest a pituitary adenoma. Prolactin deficiency often indicates severe intrinsic pituitary disease and is uncommon without concomitant deficiencies of other anterior pituitary hormones.

Conditions known to mimic hypopituitarism should be excluded when evaluating patients, including anorexia nervosa, protein-calorie malnutrition, systemic illness, chronic renal failure, and liver cirrhosis.

Treatment

> **Key Points**
>
> - Hydrocortisone is given to ACTH-deficient adults at 20 to 30 mg/day and increased twofold to threefold during times of illness and other stresses.
> - Serum IGF-1 concentration and growth rate in children are used for monitoring the effectiveness of GH replacement.

The treatment of hypopituitarism depends on the etiology and the particular hormonal deficiency (Mooradian and Morley, 1988; Toogood and Stewart, 2008). Surgical and medical interventions may be necessary for treatment of pituitary masses, infiltrative diseases, and carotid aneurysms.

Growth hormone deficiency is treated with recombinant human GH (somatotropin) preparations (Gharib et al., 2003). The recommended GH dose in children with GH deficiency is 0.04 mg/kg/day. In adults, recombinant human GH is administered subcutaneously at 0.001 to 0.008 mg/kg/day. The usual starting dose is 0.1 to 0.3 mg/day for a 70-kg man with a typical maintenance dose of 0.3 to 0.6 mg/day (Gharib et al., 2003). In general, women require higher doses than men because estrogen increases GH resistance. Serum IGF-1 concentration should be monitored to maintain it at the midnormal range. Side effects that should be monitored include edema, carpal tunnel syndrome, arrhythmias, paresthesias, and glucose intolerance.

Growth hormone can also be used in other causes of growth retardations such as chronic renal disease, Turner syndrome, and Prader Willi syndrome . Mortality caused by hypopituitarism is a significant issue; however, this may not translate when GH is used alone. For a pediatric patient who has one of these other nonpituitary causes of growth retardation, this might be a clinically appropriate option to consider. Early referral to a pediatric endocrinologist bears consideration (Sherlock and Stewart, 2013).

Treatment of secondary hypogonadism depends on the gender of the individual and whether fertility is desired.

Estradiol and progesterone replacement is the treatment of choice for secondary hypogonadism in premenopausal women who have intact uteri and do not desire fertility. These hormones can be given cyclically or daily in fixed-dose combinations. In individuals who have undergone hysterectomy, estrogen replacement alone is sufficient to maintain vulvar and vaginal lubrication, relieve symptoms of vasomotor instability, and reduce bone loss.

HYPERFUNCTIONING PITUITARY ADENOMAS

Key Points

- Pituitary adenomas may present with visual impairment, headache, or hormonal abnormalities.
- Prolactinomas are the most common type of functioning pituitary adenoma. These adenomas manifest with galactorrhea and hypogonadism.
- Nonpathologic causes of hyperprolactinemia are sought, and primary hypothyroidism is excluded.
- MRI is the imaging modality of choice for the anatomic evaluation of the hypothalamus and pituitary gland.
- Prolactin level greater than 150 ng/mL and pituitary adenoma not identified on imaging studies suggest macroprolactinemia.
- A dopamine agonist (bromocriptine or cabergoline) is the first-line treatment of prolactinomas.

Pituitary adenomas can arise from any cell type and can be either functioning or nonfunctioning. The precise pathogenesis of these adenomas is not known, but mutations found in several genes can play a role in the development of many adenomas.

With prolactinomas the most common type, other functioning pituitary adenomas include gonadotropic, thyrotropic, somatotropic, and corticotropic adenomas.

Hyperprolactinemia and Prolactinomas

Diagnosis. Prolactin is a polypeptide secreted from the lactotrophs of the anterior pituitary (Leung and Pacaud, 2004; Mancini et al., 2008). Its main function is the development of breast tissue in preparation for milk production and the maintenance of lactation during the postpartum period. Unlike the other pituitary hormones, the regulation of prolactin release is predominantly under inhibitory control. Whereas dopamine is the principal inhibitor, prolactin stimulators, such as TRH and estrogen, have minor roles.

Hypersecretion of prolactin may be physiologic or pathologic in origin (Leung and Pacaud, 2004; Mancini et al., 2008). Physiologic stimulators include exercise, pain, breast stimulation, sexual intercourse, general anesthesia, and pregnancy. Pathologic causes of hyperprolactinemia include prolactinomas, decreased dopaminergic inhibition of prolactin secretion through pharmacologic agents, and decreased clearance of prolactin.

Early manifestation of prolactin hypersecretion is galactorrhea and menstrual irregularities, notably amenorrhea in women and erectile dysfunction or loss of libido in men. Rarely, galactorrhea with gynecomastia can occur in men.

These patients are at risk of developing osteoporosis secondary to hypogonadism as well as a result of the direct inhibitory effect of prolactin on bone formation. Galactorrhea is rarely found in postmenopausal women with hyperprolactinemia and mass effect of prolactinomas, such as headache or visual disturbance, cause the principal presenting symptoms (Mancini et al., 2008). Similarly, the diagnosis of prolactinomas in men is often delayed because the clinical signs and symptoms of hyperprolactinemia are less obvious.

Clinical evaluation of patients suspected to have prolactinomas should include a thorough evaluation of medication history and the presence of comorbidities. Many drugs are known to cause hyperprolactinemia, including phenothiazines, haloperidol, metoclopramide, H2 antagonists, imipramines, selective serotonin reuptake inhibitors (SSRIs), calcium channel blockers, and hormones (Leung and Pacaud, 2004; Mancini et al., 2008). The physical examination may reveal galactorrhea and visual field defects. Women may have mild hirsutism, and men may have decreased facial hair growth.

Laboratory tests include serum prolactin and thyroid function. Primary hypothyroidism is associated with hyperprolactinemia secondary to elevated levels of TRH that induces prolactin secretion. Laboratory testing should also seek systemic illnesses, such as liver or renal failure. MRI is the imaging modality of choice for the anatomic evaluation of the hypothalamus and pituitary gland. Complete pituitary hormone evaluation should be performed when an adenomatous mass is noted in the region of the pituitary.

Features to distinguish hyperprolactinemia associated with pituitary tumors include (1) prolactin levels greater than 150 ng/mL, (2) loss of normal sleep-associated increases in prolactin levels, and (3) failure of prolactin levels to rise in response to exogenous TRH. None of these tests are absolute, and the diagnosis of prolactinoma depends on radiologic studies.

Clinicians should be aware of two prolactin assay-related conditions that may cause diagnostic confusion. In *macroprolactinemia,* large-molecular-weight prolactin aggregates with globulins, which are then recorded in the assay as elevated levels of prolactin in the absence of any physiologic or pathologic cause of hyperprolactinemia (Mancini et al., 2008). This condition is suspected when the patient is found to have very high prolactin level without galactorrhea or any tumor demonstrated on pituitary MRI. The second area of confusion occurs when very high concentrations of serum prolactin overwhelm the assay reagents such that the measurements underestimate the true concentration of prolactin. This is referred to as the "hook" effect.

The gold standard for differentiating hyperprolactinemia from macroprolactinemia is via gel filtration chromatography (GFC). But if available, a simple, inexpensive, and suitable alternative to GFC that should be considered is polyethylene glycol (PEG) precipitation. Because macroprolactinemia is a benign condition, early laboratory testing, such as PEG, which can definitively determine the presence of macroprolactin molecules, eliminating the need for further hormonal or imaging investigation or surgery (Kasum et al., 2012).

Treatment. The treatment of hyperprolactinemia depends on the etiology, presence or absence of mass effects, (e.g., visual changes), presence of bothersome galactorrhea or associated pituitary hormone deficiencies, and whether fertility is desired (Leung and Pacaud, 2004; Mancini et al., 2008). If possible, drugs known to cause prolactin elevation should be discontinued, and the serum prolactin concentration should be measured again. Persistent hyperprolactinemia requires imaging of the pituitary and hypothalamus.

Treatment of prolactinomas includes dopamine agonists as first-line therapy. In select subgroups, surgical excision is recommended, usually through the transsphenoidal approach. In rare cases, with large residual tumor mass postsurgery, nonresponsive to medical therapy, radiation therapy may be offered. Associated hormone deficiency should also be targeted. Often, as the prolactin levels are normalized, symptoms of hypogonadism can be reversed.

Bromocriptine and cabergoline are U.S. Food and Drug Administration (FDA)–approved dopamine agonists for treatment of hyperprolactinemia. Cabergoline has greater tolerability than bromocriptine and is more effective in achieving normalization of prolactin levels in 90% of individuals with prolactinomas. Because of long-standing experience, however, bromocriptine is the preferred agent in women who wish to become pregnant. Bromocriptine should be discontinued after pregnancy has been confirmed even though the risk of teratogenicity is small. Pregnant women with prolactinomas should be warned to report any visual disturbances or headaches because up to 10% of microprolactinomas and 30% of macroprolactinomas increase in size sufficient to cause symptoms. During pregnancy, prolactin levels should be monitored periodically, but interpretation of the results may be difficult. Pregnant women with macroadenomas should receive similar advice and have serial visual field testing. Pergolide is an alternative to bromocriptine and cabergoline, but it is not FDA-approved for this use. Caution should be exercised with all of these ergot derivatives because of rare case reports of valvular heart damage in patients taking the drug at very high doses for prolonged periods.

The dosage of dopamine agonist may be reduced when prolactin levels have been normalized for 1 year and tumor size has been significantly reduced. Medication withdrawal may be considered after 2 years in those with normal prolactin levels and an MRI scan showing no tumor or tumor reduction more than 50% and more than 5 mm from the optic chiasm with no invasion of the cavernous sinus. Withdrawal of therapeutic drug may lead to recurrent prolactin hypersecretion and adenoma growth, although in some patients, microadenomas have resolved after a few years of treatment. MRI of the pituitary and serum prolactin levels should be monitored closely thereafter.

Indications for transsphenoidal surgery in patients with prolactinomas include medical treatment failure or medication intolerance, very large tumors threatening visual pathways, or hemorrhagic infarcts (apoplexy). Approximately 30% of macroadenomas can be successfully removed surgically.

ACROMEGALY AND GIGANTISM

See eAppendix 35-1 online.

CUSHING DISEASE

Key Points

- Cushing syndrome is categorized into ACTH-dependent and ACTH-independent cases. Pituitary ACTH-dependent Cushing syndrome is Cushing disease.
- The diagnosis is established when the clinical findings of Cushing syndrome are associated with laboratory documentation of excess cortisol production.
- Measurement of 24-hour urinary free cortisol excretion is a good screening tool.
- Comparison of serum ACTH concentration with serum cortisol level can help determine the cause of hypercortisolism.
- Treatment of Cushing syndrome is directed at the cause of hypercortisolism. The treatment of choice for Cushing disease is selective transsphenoidal resection.

Hypercortisolemia, (also hypercortisolism, hyperadrenocorticism) caused by either exogenous administration of cortisol or other synthetic glucocorticoids or endogenous overproduction of cortisol leads to a constellation of clinical and biochemical findings referred to as Cushing syndrome (Arnaldi et al., 2003; Biller et al., 2008; Findling and Raff, 2005). The multiple causes include pituitary adenomas, excess production of CRH leading to hyperplasia of corticotropes in the pituitary, ectopic production of ACTH and CRH, and adrenal cortical adenomas and carcinomas. The term *Cushing disease* specifically refers to pituitary-dependent cortisol hypersecretion (Biller et al., 2008).

Whereas pituitary, ACTH-dependent Cushing disease accounts for at least 70% of endogenous cases, the most common cause of ACTH-independent Cushing syndrome is prolonged glucocorticoid therapy.

Patients who have undergone bilateral adrenalectomy for hypothalamic pituitary–dependent Cushing syndrome may develop pituitary tumors associated with marked skin pigmentation. This condition is referred to as *Nelson syndrome.* The skin hyperpigmentation occurs because of excess production of melanocyte-stimulating hormone (MSH), which is a product of the gene that also encodes ACTH and β-endorphin.

Diagnosis

A high index of suspicion is required to make the diagnosis of Cushing syndrome as manifestations of the disease are insidious and develop over months (Arnaldi et al., 2003; Findling and Raff, 2005). The clinical features include weight gain with centralized obesity distributed in the face, neck, trunk, and abdomen with facial rounding and plethora. The thinning of the skin and loss of subcutaneous tissue results in easy bruising and emergence of violaceous abdominal striae (Arnaldi et al., 2003; Findling and Raff, 2005).

In cases of ectopic ACTH-dependent Cushing syndrome, extreme elevations of ACTH levels cause rapid hyperpigmentation and are more likely to demonstrate features of mineralocorticoid excess, such as hypokalemia and metabolic alkalosis (Findling and Raff, 2005).

Gonadal dysfunction is associated with decreased testosterone levels in men; in women, it is associated with decreased serum estradiol levels and menstrual disorders, notably amenorrhea. Virilization and androgen excess are more common in cases of Cushing syndrome caused by adrenal carcinomas. Glucocorticoid excess also interferes with calcium and bone metabolism and leads to osteoporosis. Catabolic effects of excess glucocorticoid on muscles cause proximal muscle weakness. Glucose intolerance is found in 30% to 60% of those with hypercortisolism.

Other complications of hypercortisolism include risk of opportunistic infections, including *Pneumocystis jiroveci* (formerly *carinii*) pneumonia, and hypercoagulable state with thromboembolic events secondary to increased plasma concentration of several clotting factors and neuropsychiatric changes (Arnaldi et al., 2003; Findling and Raff, 2005).

Establishing the Cause

The diagnosis is established when the clinical findings of Cushing disease are associated with laboratory documentation of excess cortisol production, loss of diurnal variation of plasma cortisol level, and more than 50% suppression of plasma and urine cortisol after the administration of 2 mg of dexamethasone every 6 hours (high-dose DST). Measurement of 24-hour urinary free cortisol excretion is a good screening tool (Arnaldi et al., 2003; Findling and Raff, 2005). Late night salivary cortisol is another good screening tool (Nieman et al., 2008). Alternatively, impaired suppression of cortisol, after an overnight 1-mg DST, can be used as a screening tool in nonobese individuals. A plasma ACTH concentration less than 5 pg/mL and a serum cortisol concentration greater than 15 μg/dL suggest an ACTH-independent cause. Plasma ACTH concentration greater than 15 pg/mL in a patient with hypercortisolism suggests ACTH-dependent hypercortisolism (Arnaldi et al., 2003; Findling and Raff, 2005).

Suppression of urinary cortisol excretion after administration of high-dose dexamethasone is consistent with the diagnosis of Cushing disease, but urinary cortisol excretion in cases of ectopic ACTH syndrome is usually not suppressible. When the high-dose DST fails to differentiate an ectopic source from a pituitary source of ACTH and radiographic imaging is not conclusive, further CRH testing and petrosal sinus sampling of ACTH are indicated to localize the tumor to the pituitary.

The vast majority of patients with ACTH-dependent Cushing syndrome have a pituitary adenoma as the cause. The few who have an ectopic source of ACTH must be identified with high-resolution CT scanning of the chest, abdomen, and pelvis.

Treatment

The treatment of choice for Cushing disease is selective transsphenoidal resection of the pituitary adenoma. The cure rate for this procedure, at experienced centers, is 70% to 80% for microadenomas. In some patients, total hypophysectomy is considered when the disease recurs after transsphenoidal resection. Many postsurgical patients require low-dose cortisol replacement for up to 12 months until their endogenous adrenal function recovers.

Bilateral adrenalectomy with or without pituitary irradiation is offered to patients who have recurrence of hypercortisolemia or have severe disease. For those who are poor surgical candidates, adjunctive medical therapy is offered and includes metyrapone (a blocker of 11-β-hydroxylase), mitotane, and cyproheptadine. These treatment options have variable efficacy (Biller et al., 2008; Nieman et al., 2008).

CRANIOPHARYNGIOMAS, THYROTROPIN-SECRETING PITUITARY ADENOMAS, GONADOTROPIC ADENOMAS, AND OTHER ADENOMAS

See eAppendix 35-2 online.

POSTERIOR PITUITARY DISORDERS

Arginine vasopressin (AVP) and oxytocin are the principal hormones secreted from the posterior pituitary (Mooradian and Korenman, 2007; Mooradian and Morley, 1988). The two major stimuli of oxytocin secretion are suckling during lactation and dilation of the cervix during labor. Oxytocin is not essential for initiation of labor but can be used pharmacologically to initiate labor or to control postpartum hemorrhage and uterine atony. Rarely, it has been used to induce milk ejection. The physiologic role of this hormone in males is not known (Mooradian and Morley, 1988).

Arginine vasopressin differs from oxytocin by only one amino acid. AVP is found in all mammals except pigs and related species in which lysine vasopressin replaces AVP. In humans and many mammals, AVP and oxytocin are associated with two neurophysins (Mooradian and Morley, 1988). The exact roles of the latter are not known except that they are carrier proteins involved in storage and transport of posterior pituitary hormones.

Antidiuretic hormone is synthesized in the hypothalamus and migrates down into the posterior lobe of the pituitary to be stored and later secreted. Some ADH is secreted directly into the cerebrospinal fluid (CSF) rather than the posterior pituitary. Thus, pathologic lesions affecting the hypothalamus below the median eminence may preserve some functional ADH that migrates from the CSF into the systemic circulation.

The half-life of AVP in circulation is only 20 minutes because of its susceptibility to peptidases. Loss of the terminal amino group in position 1 makes this peptide resistant to degradation; substitution of the *levo* analogue of arginine for dextro-arginine in position 8 reduces presser effect without altering its antidiuretic properties (Mooradian and Morley, 1988). The resultant peptide deamino-8-D-arginine vasopressin (DDAVP; desmopressin) is currently the treatment of choice for central diabetes insipidus (DI).

The biologic effects of AVP are initiated at two receptors referred to as V1 and V2. The V1 receptors are located in the vascular system, and their stimulation results in vasoconstriction. V2 receptors are located in the kidneys, and stimulation of these receptors results in free water reabsorption (Korbonits and Carlsen, 2009).

Plasma osmolality, blood volume, and BP are the most important physiologic stimuli of AVP secretion. Other factors that modulate AVP secretion include pain, stress, nausea, hypoglycemia, hypercapnia, angiotensin II, atrial natriuretic hormone, and a host of drugs. Many stimuli of AVP release also promote thirst. Thirst is less sensitive for AVP release than these other stimuli and therefore thirst is a second-line defense against dehydration.

Central Diabetes Insipidus

Key Points

- DI is characterized by excessive dilute urine with thirst and polydipsia and results from decreased ADH secretion.
- The differential diagnosis of hypotonic polyuria includes neurogenic DI (vasopressin sensitive), nephrogenic DI (vasopressin resistant), and primary polydipsia.
- The water restriction test assists in the diagnosis.
- DDAVP is the primary treatment for central DI.

Clinical Features. The disease is characterized by the production of excessive dilute urine with secondary thirst and polydipsia. *Polyuria* is defined as 3 L/day or greater in adults and 2 L/day or greater in children. Central DI can be familial or sporadic and can be caused by head trauma, neurosurgery, neoplasms, granulomas, infections, inflammation, chemical toxins, vascular disorders, congenital malformations, and genetic causes. Other causes include hypoxic encephalopathy; infiltrative disorders, notably *histiocytosis X* (Hand-Schuller-Christian disease); anorexia nervosa; acute fatty liver of pregnancy; and Wolfram syndrome (central DI, diabetes mellitus, optic atrophy, and deafness) (Reddy and Mooradian, 2009). An autoimmune process is probably the cause of idiopathic DI and accounts for 30% to 50% of cases of central DI (De Bellis et al., 1999).

Thickening or enlargement of the posterior pituitary seen on MRI may represent lymphocytic infiltration and inflammation. Classically, DI after head trauma or neurosurgical procedures goes through three phases. Polyuria appears in the first 1 to 2 days after surgery followed by a period of oliguria for 3 to 4 days, which culminates in a polyuric phase. These phases are a reflection of the early paralysis of vasopressin-producing cells followed by neuronal degeneration and massive release of vasopressin with subsequent permanent loss of vasopressin production.

Vasopressin-resistant DI is usually a familial disorder, although sporadic causes are recognized in chronic medullary kidney disease associated with sickle cell disease, multiple myeloma, amyloidosis, Sjögren syndrome, and renal medullary cystic disease. In addition, prolonged primary polydipsia can wash out the normal medullary concentration gradient and may mimic vasopressin-resistant nephrogenic DI.

Diagnosis. Although a variety of diseases may present as polyuria and polydipsia, thorough history and routine laboratory evaluation can narrow the differential diagnosis of hypotonic polyuria to three possibilities: neurogenic DI (vasopressin sensitive), nephrogenic DI (vasopressin resistant), or primary polydipsia (Mooradian and Morley, 1988).

Serum sodium concentrations less than 137 mEq/L and polyuria are usually manifestations of primary polydipsia. For patients with serum sodium concentrations less than 143 mEq/L, a water deprivation test should be carried out after an overnight fast, with hourly measurement of body weight, urine volume, and osmolality. In severe cases, the dehydration test can be started at 6 AM. When the urine osmolality remains constant during three consecutive measurements or if the patient loses more than 5% total body weight, then plasma osmolality, vasopressin, and sodium concentrations should be determined, and aqueous vasopressin (0.1 unit/kg subcutaneously) or 10 µg of nasal desmopressin should be administered and the response evaluated. An increase in urine osmolality of 150 mOsm/kg above baseline will exclude nephrogenic DI.

In central DI, administration of 10 µg of nasal desmopressin will result in increases in urine osmolality of as much as 800%. The response to desmopressin in partial central DI may result in urine osmolality increases of 15% to 50%.

Patients with nephrogenic DI continue to have urine osmolality levels that remain below isosmotic. Patients with primary polydipsia respond to the water deprivation test with urine concentrating to 500 mOsmol/kg, or higher. In comparison, urine osmolality in normal subjects undergoing the water deprivation test will increase to 800 mOsmol/kg or higher. Administration of exogenous vasopressin produces no further concentration in cases of primary polydipsia.

When the water suppression test yields equivocal results, the serum AVP concentration at baseline and following the water restriction test should be measured. However, the results of these tests may still be misleading because primary polydipsia results in submaximal secretion of AVP, mimicking the pattern of AVP secretion in partial central DI.

Treatment. The treatment of choice for central DI is DDAVP. DDAVP can be administered intravenously, subcutaneously, nasally, or orally. An initial nasal inhalation of 5 µg at bedtime is given. The dose is increased by 5-µg increments until nocturia has been resolved. After nocturia is successfully treated, a morning dose is given. The total daily dosage of nasally administered desmopressin is 5 to 20 µg /day (Loh and Verbalis, 2008). Desmopressin given by mouth should be given on an empty stomach. Absorption can be reduced by up to 50% when desmopressin is taken with food. A 0.1-mg tablet is equivalent to 2.5 to 5.0 µg of nasal inhalation spray (Loh and Verbalis, 2008).

Patients with partial DI will benefit from oral agents that potentiate AVP action or stimulate the release of AVP. These agents include chlorpropamide, carbamazepine, or clofibrate. In such cases, desmopressin requirements may be lower than available preparations can provide. Patients with nephrogenic DI benefit from thiazide diuretics or indomethacin.

Patients with DI should wear a medical ID bracelet. When the ability to drink fluids is impaired, IV hydration will be required to avoid dehydration and hypernatremia.

Syndrome of Inappropriate Antidiuretic Hormone Secretion

Key Points

- Laboratory evaluation of plasma osmolality, urine osmolality, and urine sodium concentration assist in determining the cause of hyponatremia.
- Water restriction and salt replacement are the most important treatment modalities in hyponatremia. The underlying cause should be identified and treated when possible.
- Vasopressin antagonists are currently indicated for the treatment of euvolemic and hypervolemic hyponatremia.

The syndrome of inappropriate antidiuretic hormone secretion (SIADH) is associated with plasma ADH concentrations that are inappropriately high for the plasma osmolality. Laboratory and clinical features of SIADH include (1) euvolemic hyponatremia; (2) decreased measured plasma osmolality (< 275 mOsm/kg); (3) urine osmolality greater than 100 mOsm/kg; (4) urine sodium usually greater than 40 mEq/L; (5) normal acid–base and potassium balance; (6) blood urea nitrogen (BUN) less than 10 mg/dL; (7) hypouricemia less than 4 mg/dL; (8) normal thyroid and adrenal function; and (9) absence of advanced cardiac, renal, or liver disease (Reddy and Mooradian, 2009).

Conditions or factors associated with SIADH include CNS trauma and infections, tumors, drugs, major surgery, pulmonary disease (e.g., TB), hormone administration, human immunodeficiency virus (HIV) infection, hereditary SIADH, idiopathic causes, and cerebral salt wasting. In some cases, it is difficult to differentiate SIADH from mild to moderate depletional hyponatremia (Reddy and Mooradian, 2009) (Table 35-2).

The response of urinary and plasma sodium concentration to an infusion of 1 to 2 L of 0.9% (isotonic) saline may help in the differential diagnosis. In a patient with SIADH who is at equilibrium, the administered saline will be excreted; therefore, there will be an increase in urinary sodium while plasma sodium concentration will either not change or decrease slightly. If the patient has depletional hyponatremia from renal losses, sodium from the administered saline is retained, and the excess water is excreted. Urinary sodium decreases, and plasma sodium concentration increases (Reddy and Mooradian, 2009).

A *reset osmostat* may be suspected when mild hyponatremia persists despite changes in fluid and salt intake. A reset osmostat may be confirmed by having the patient receive a fluid bolus of 10 to 15 mL/kg. Normal patients, or those with a reset osmostat, should excrete 80% of this bolus in 4 hours, which does not occur with SIADH (Reddy and Mooradian, 2009).

Cerebral salt wasting induces SIADH-like symptoms. Salt wasting followed by volume depletion occurs in some cases of cerebral disease. This leads to a secondary rise in ADH levels. The mechanism underlying cerebral salt wasting is unclear (Reddy and Mooradian, 2009).

Treatment. Management of SIADH should begin with water restriction and treatment or elimination of the underlying etiology. In all patients with hyponatremia, free water intake from all sources should be restricted to less than 1 to 1.5 L/d. In patients with mild symptoms, the rate of urinary solute excretion, which is the main determinant of urine output, can be increased by a high-salt, high-protein diet or supplementation with urea (30-60 g/day) or salt tablets (200 mEq/day) (Reddy and Mooradian, 2009). However, salt therapy is generally contraindicated in patients with hypertension and edema because it leads to exacerbation of both conditions. In addition, water restriction is contraindicated in patients with subarachnoid hemorrhage with hypovolemia, in whom water restriction may result in hypotension, creating a risk for cerebral infarction. This risk is more pronounced if the patient has cerebral salt wasting, which must be treated first with isotonic or hypertonic saline solution until adequate volume status has been demonstrated.

In general, plasma sodium concentration should be corrected at a rate of 1 mEq/L/hr until the reversal of neurologic symptoms (Reddy and Mooradian, 2009). Then the correction rate is reduced to 0.5 mEq/L/hr until the plasma sodium has reached a level of 120 to 125 mEq/L. This approach effectively prevents the devastating neurologic consequences of acute hyponatremia and is associated with reduced risk of osmotic demyelination of pontine and extrapontine neurons.

The most specific treatment for SIADH is to block the V2 receptors in the kidney that mediate the diuretic effect of ADH. Vasopressin antagonists are currently indicated for the treatment of euvolemic and hypervolemic hyponatremia (Loh and Verbalis, 2008; Reddy and Mooradian, 2009).

For hospitalized patients, conivaptan is given as an IV loading dose of 20 mg delivered over 30 minutes and then as 20 mg continuously over 24 hours. Subsequent infusions may be administered every 1 to 3 days at 20 to 40 mg/day by continuous infusion (Reddy and Mooradian, 2009). More recently, an orally active vasopressin receptor antagonist, tolvaptan, became available. Rapid correction of hyponatremia has been reported in patients receiving these agents; therefore, frequent checks of plasma sodium are needed.

Chronic SIADH can occur in patients with ectopic ADH-producing tumors and in patients in whom antipsychotic drugs cannot be discontinued. If water restriction and salt tablet therapy are ineffective, the following drug therapy could be attempted: (1) administration of loop diuretic along with salt tablets, (2) demeclocycline, (3) lithium carbonate, and (4) orally active vasopressin antagonists such as tolvaptan. (Cost and increased liver enzymes limit tolvaptan's utility. In addition, tolvaptan should not be used for longer than 30 days and should not be used in patients with liver disease.) Demeclocycline is nephrotoxic in patients with cirrhosis and is contraindicated in children because of interference with bone development and teeth discoloration. (It also has a cost consideration.) Lithium carbonate may induce interstitial nephritis and renal failure; therefore, lithium should be considered for use only in patients in whom demeclocycline is contraindicated (Reddy and Mooradian, 2009).

Table 35-2   Select Causes of Syndrome of Inappropriate Antidiuretic Hormone Secretion

Nonosmotic stimuli	Nausea, pain, stress Human immunodeficiency virus (HIV) Acute psychosis Surgery Pregnancy (physiologic) Hypokalemia Congestive heart failure exacerbation
CNS lesions	Tumors (neuroblastoma) Cerebrovascular accident (stroke) Meningitis, encephalitis Abscess Guillain-Barré syndrome Hydrocephalus Pituitary stalk lesion Delirium tremens Demyelinating disease Acute porphyria
Malignancies	Lymphoma, leukemia, Hodgkin disease Carcinoma of the uterus Ureteral, prostate, and bladder carcinoma Carcinoma of the duodenum and pancreas Ectopic production of vasopressin by tumors (small cell lung carcinoma, carcinoids) Cancers of the head and neck and nasopharynx Renal cell carcinoma Osteosarcoma
Increased intrathoracic pressure	Mediastinal tumors (thymoma, sarcoma) Positive-pressure ventilation Infections (pneumonia, TB, aspergillosis, lung abscess) Bronchogenic carcinoma, mesothelioma Bronchiectasis, empyema COPD Pneumothorax
DRUG INDUCED	
Antipsychotics	Phenothiazines Haloperidol
Antidepressants	SSRIs, TCAs, MAOIs Bupropion
Anticonvulsants	Carbamazepine, oxcarbazepine Sodium valproate
Analgesics and recreational drugs	Morphine (high doses) Tramadol MDMA ("ecstasy")
Nonsteroidal antiinflammatory drugs	Colchicine, venlafaxine Duloxetine (Cymbalta)
Cardiac drugs	Thiazides, clonidine ACE inhibitors, aldosterone antagonists Amiloride, loop diuretics Methyldopa, amlodipine Amiodarone, lorcainide Propafenone, theophylline, terlipressin Unfractionated heparin (aldosterone antagonist)
Antidiabetic drugs	Chlorpropamide Tolbutamide, glipizide
Lipid-lowering agent	Clofibrate
Antineoplastic agents	Cyclophosphamide Vincristine, vinblastine Cisplatin, hydroxyurea Melphalan
Immunosuppressives	Tacrolimus, methotrexate Interferon-α and -γ, levamisole Monoclonal antibodies
Antibiotics	Azithromycin, ciprofloxacin Trimethoprim–sulfamethoxazole Cefoperazone–sulbactam, rifabutin

ACE, Angiotensin-converting enzyme; *CNS,* central nervous system; *COPD,* chronic obstructive pulmonary disease; ; *MAOI,* monoamine oxidase inhibitor; *MDMA,* 3,4-methylenedioxymethamphetamine; *SSRI,* selective serotonin reuptake inhibitor; *TB,* tuberculosis; *TCA,* tricyclic antidepressant.

Modified from Reddy P, Mooradian AD. Diagnosis and management of hyponatremia in hospitalized patients. *Int J Clin Pract.* 2009;63:1494-1508.

- Hydrocortisone is given to ACTH-deficient adults at 20 to 30 mg/day, increased twofold to threefold during times of illness and other stresses (Toogood and Stewart, 2008) (SOR: A).
- The goal of thyroid replacement should be to achieve a normal serum free thyroxin concentration and clinical euthyroidism (Oiknine and Mooradian, 2006) (SOR: A)
- A dopamine agonist is first-line treatment of prolactinomas (Mancini et al., 2008) (SOR: A).
- Transsphenoidal surgery to remove the pituitary adenoma is usually the treatment of choice in individuals with acromegaly (Melmed et al., 2009) (SOR: A).
- Octreotide (Sandostatin) is often effective in normalizing GH and IGF-1 levels. Pegvisomant is a GH receptor antagonist also approved for the treatment of acromegaly (Melmed et al., 2009) (SOR: A).
- Treatment of Cushing syndrome should be directed at the cause of hypercortisolism. The treatment of choice for Cushing disease is selective transsphenoidal resection (Biller et al., 2008) (SOR: A).
- Desmopressin is the primary treatment for central DI (Loh and Verbalis, 2008; Reddy and Mooradian, 2009) (SOR: A).
- Water restriction and salt replacement are the most important treatment modalities in hyponatremia. The underlying cause should be identified and treated when possible (Reddy and Mooradian, 2009) (SOR: A).
- Vasopressin antagonists are currently indicated for the treatment of euvolemic and hypervolemic hyponatremia (Loh and Verbalis, 2008; Reddy and Mooradian, 2009) (SOR: A).

Pineal Gland

The pineal gland, in general, is rarely thought of and especially not as part of the endocrine system, which is not surprising because there are rare (if any) diseases directly attributed to the pineal gland. The one area where there does seem to be consensus is the role the pineal gland appears to play in our orientation to day and night. It is also widely accepted that this is probably a teleologic holdover from more primitive parts of the human brain. There appears to be an interrelationship between some of our neurohormones, sleep, and what is generally referred to as the circadian rhythm (or sleep cycle). Sleep appears to have a significant effect on some hormones (GH) but little effect on others (MSH). One area where this occurs, of which most physicians are aware, is the normal cortisol surge that occurs in early morning and that seems to be absent or dulled when sleep deprived.

The deleterious effect of sleep deprivation is well known, anecdotally, in long-haul truckers and airline transport pilots. Over the past 15+ years, there have been significant changes in work hours for medical and surgical residents in an effort to eliminate, or at least ameliorate, sleep deprivation–induced iatrogenic errors. The negative physiologic effects of sleep deprivation have long been documented. Animal studies have definitively shown that when sleep deprived long enough (total sleep deprivation), the animal dies (Rechtschaffen et al., 1989). New data suggests that during sleep, the brain clears "toxins," specifically β-amyloid, which is associated with Alzheimer disease (Spira et al., 2013; Xie et al., 2013).

Thyroid Disorders

Thyroid disorders can be categorized into processes that affect function (physiology) as well as structure (anatomy). The etiology of some of these are extraglandular, including metastatic neoplasia, pituitary disorders, dietary issues, autoimmune diseases, infections, and genetic or familial diseases (multiple endocrine neoplasia [MEN] IIA and familial medullary thyroid carcinoma [FMTC]). Other causes are intrinsic to the thyroid and include cysts, nodules, goiter, and primary neoplasia.

Irrespective of the disease process, all thyroid diseases exist in one of three functional states: euthyroid, hyperthyroid, or hypothyroid, each defined by the level of total bound and free circulating thyroid hormone. The presence of any one of these states in an individual can be transient, static, or progressing. Laboratory abnormalities of circulating thyroid hormone, at any point in time, do not prove disease and do not depend on the etiology of thyroid dysfunction. All three states may exist at different times during the course of an illness, and each state can exist with or without disease or clinical findings. In addition, the various thyroid structures can reflect disease independent of endocrinologic function.

Accurate assessment of thyroid function, with determination of presence or absence of disease, requires data in addition to levels of circulating thyroid hormones. These data include serum free thyroid hormone levels; thyrotropin (TSH) levels; and in some cases, antithyroid antibody titers. This battery of tests provides diagnosis in the majority of common thyroid disorders. When imaging studies and fine-needle aspiration are added, 90% to 95% of patients with thyroid disease who present in the primary care setting can be diagnosed and appropriately managed (Figure 35-1).

Thyroid disorders affect 60 to 80/1000 adults worldwide and up to 8.9% of the adult U.S. population (Bagchi et al., 1990; Vanderpump et al., 1995). Because most thyroid disorders have an insidious onset or closely mimic other. more common disorders, they are easily missed and, although rarely fatal, can cause significant morbidity. Early recognition is critical to minimizing that morbidity. With the exception of conditions such as simple goiter or visible nodule, patients who ultimately are diagnosed with thyroid disease rarely present to family physicians with complaints suggesting thyroid disorder.

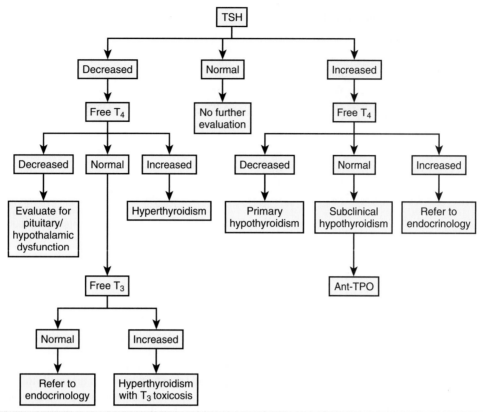

Figure 35-1 Algorithm for the diagnosis of thyroid dysfunction, beginning with an abnormal serum thyrotropin level. *anti-TPO,* Anti-thyroid antibodies; T_3, triiodothyronine; T_4, thyroxine; *TSH,* thyroid-stimulating hormone.

ANATOMY AND PHYSIOLOGY

Key Points

- Thyroxine (T_4) is the major product of the thyroid gland.
- Triiodothyronine (T_3) is the active hormone at the cellular level.
- The majority of circulating T_3 is formed in the peripheral circulation by deiodination of T_4.
- T_4 serves as a reservoir (prohormone) for T_3.
- Serum thyrotropin (sTSH) is required in all evaluations of dementia and depression.

Histologically, the thyroid gland consists of five primary elements: follicular cells, colloid, interstitial tissue, "C" cells, and lymphoid cells. The most prominent element is the follicular cell, which produces colloid. The thyroid follicle is the functional unit of the gland and the site where colloid is stored. It is within the follicle where thyroid hormone (thyroxine or T_4) synthesis occurs. The remaining cellular elements are "C" cells, which are few in number, and lymphoid cells. The few "C" cells are located in the intrafollicular space and produce calcitonin. Lymphoid cells are found scattered throughout the gland stroma in small, isolated clusters.

Circulating Thyroid Hormones

Biosynthesis of thyroid hormone is unique among endocrine glands because final assembly occurs extracellularly in the follicular lumen. The source of thyroid hormones (T_4 and triiodothyronine [T_3]) is *thyroglobulin* (Tg), an iodoprotein, produced by the follicular cells. Thyroglobulin is the major portion of intraluminal colloid and is the most important protein of the thyroid gland (Kopp, 2005). Thyroglobulin provides a matrix for the synthesis of thyroid hormones and a vehicle for subsequent storage. Stored thyroglobulin is oxidized by thyroid peroxidase (TPO), adding an iodine molecule to tyrosine to form monoiodotyrosine (MIT) and diiodotyrosine (DIT). MIT and DIT are then assembled into the final products, tetraiodothyronine (T_4) and triiodothyronine (T_3), which are stored in the follicular colloid for future use. When stimulated by serum thyrotropin (sTSH), thyroglobulin within the colloidal space is internalized by thyroid cells and enzymatically degraded to release T_4 and T_3 into the peripheral circulation. Approximately one third to half of T_4 released into the peripheral circulation is deiodinated to form T_3.

In the peripheral circulation, T_4 and T_3 are bound to thyroid-binding globulin (TBG). Thyroxine is bound to TBG in concentrations 10 to 20 times greater than T_3, and neither bound T_4 nor bound T_3 is directly available to tissues. Only unbound or "free" portions of T_4 and T_3 are metabolically available at the cellular level. The free portion of T_4 represents 0.02% to 0.05% of total serum T_4, and the free portion of T_3 represents 0.1% to 0.3% of total serum T_3 (Benvenga, 2005; Meier and Burger, 2005; Toft and Beckett, 2005). Most T_3 (>99.5%) is bound to TBG, but T_3 is not as tightly bound as T_4, allowing easier release into the free-state.

Table 35-3 Laboratory Tests for Evaluation of Thyroid Function

	Screening	Hyper	Hypo	Graves	CAT	Nodule	Thyroiditis	Other
TSH	Yes	Yes	Yes	Yes	Yes	Yes	Yes	No
T_4	No	No	No	No	No	No	No	No
T_3	No	Yes	No	Yes	No	No	No	No
FT_4	No	Yes	Yes	Yes	No	Yes	Yes	No
FT_3	No	No	No	No	No	No	No	No
Thyroglobulin	No	No	No	No	No	No	No	Yes
TSH-RS Abs	No	Yes	No	Yes	No	No	No	No
TPO Abs	No	No	No	No	Yes	No	No	No
Tg Abs	No	No	No	No	±	No	No	No
Thyroid microsomal Abs	No	No	No	No	No	No	Yes	±

CAT, Chronic autoimmune thyroiditis; *FT₃,* free triiodothyronine; *FT₄,* free thyroxine; *T₃,* triiodothyronine; *T₄,* thyroxine; *Tg Abs,* thyroglobulin antibodies; *TPO Abs,* thyroid antiperoxidase antibodies; *TSH,* thyroid-stimulating hormone (thyrotropin); *TSH-RS Abs,* TSH receptor-stimulator antibodies.

Thyroid hormones exert their effect by binding to thyroid receptors (TRs) within cells. At the cellular level, T_3 is roughly twice as biologically active as T_4. This is, in part, because T_3 binds more strongly to TR than T_4 does, thus, it easily displaces T_4 from binding sites (Yen, 2005). T_3 is the biologically active form of thyroid hormone. Thyroxine's role in this process appears to be that of a prohormone, providing a readily accessible reservoir for conversion to T_3. What other purpose(s) or role(s) T_4 plays is unknown (Bianco and Larsen, 2005).

Thyroid hormones (T_4 and T_3) regulate growth, development, and metabolism by affecting oxygen consumption and protein, carbohydrate, and vitamin metabolism. Around puberty, the effect on growth and development begin to wane, and in adults, thyroid hormones essentially affect only metabolism (Yen, 2005).

Normal thyroid function, in terms of circulating levels of T_4, T_3, FT_4, and free T_3 (FT_3) and the thyrotropin feedback system, appears to remain stable throughout life. Without intrinsic disease of the hypothalamic–pituitary–thyroid axis, age does not appear to have an adverse effect on the function of the thyroid gland or its component parts in terms of serum concentration of T_4 and T_3 (Hassani and Hershman, 2006; Oiknine and Mooradian, 2006). Although changes in measurable levels of total serum T_4 and T_3 do occur as a result of changes in transport protein concentrations, FT_4 and FT_3 levels remain mostly constant (Hassani and Hershman, 2006).

LABORATORY TESTING

Tests for thyroid disorders include laboratory studies, imaging, and biopsy. Before imaging or biopsy is undertaken, it is important to determine the functional state of the thyroid gland even when the initial presentation is a thyroid mass or thyromegaly. This is accomplished via laboratory testing of a peripheral blood sample. These simple and readily available tests provide direction for further workup. Initial laboratory tests, regardless of presenting complaint or finding, include sTSH and FT_4. The results of these initial studies help determine the functional state of the gland (hyperthyroid, euthyroid, or hypothyroid) and

thus suggest which additional tests are required (Garber et al., 2012) (Table 35-3).

Second-tier laboratory tests include thyroid antibodies and FT_3 if T_3 toxicosis is suspected. As noted previously, aging and comorbidities that affect circulating levels of thyroid transport protein can result in T_4 levels that appear to be abnormally low, suggesting a hypothyroid state. However, FT_4 and FT_3 will be normal, as will sTSH. Thyroid antibodies are useful in evaluating several disease states, primarily Graves disease and chronic autoimmune thyroiditis (CAT or Hashimoto thyroiditis). In Graves disease, the primary antibody culprit is TSH receptor-stimulator antibody (TSH-RS Abs). In CAT, the primary antibodies are thyroid anti-peroxidase antibodies (TPO Abs) and thyroglobulin antibodies (Tg Abs). Patients with hypothyroidism occasionally exhibit TSH receptor-blocker antibodies (TSH-RB Abs), but the role this plays in the disease course is unclear. Thyroid microsomal antibodies (TPO Abs, Tg Abs) are occasionally seen in the self-limited processes of postpartum thyroiditis and silent thyroiditis. Figure 35-1 provides an algorithm for diagnosing thyroid dysfunction.

Imaging

Thyroid ultrasonography is the first-line study a primary care physician should obtain for a palpable thyroid mass. The goal is to determine whether the mass is cystic, solid, or mixed. It is also used as a presumptive screen for malignancy in the hands of an experienced radiologist because malignant thyroid nodules have unique ultrasonographic characteristics. If the patient is hyperthyroid, with suppressed sTSH, ultrasonography is done in conjunction with radioisotope scan.

Nuclear imaging uses iodine 123 (^{123}I) to evaluate gland activity. Patients with normal gland function show homogeneity throughout the gland, with the exception of areas where cysts or nonfunctioning nodules are located. Patients with autonomously functioning nodules or multinodular goiter show uptake of ^{123}I in nodular areas, with the remainder of the gland, under the control of sTSH, being hypoactive or inactive.

CT and MRI are not useful in diagnosis and treatment of nonmalignant diseases of the thyroid and thus are not recommended as initial studies. For biopsy-proven malignancy, CT and MRI can be useful preoperatively to define the area of involvement and for postoperative follow-up. CT and MRI should be reserved for the surgeon and oncologist.

Biopsy

Ultrasound-guided fine-needle aspiration (FNA) biopsy is a well-defined procedure for evaluating thyroid masses. It is safe and virtually painless in the hands of an experienced interventional radiologist, endocrinologist, or pathologist. When a definitive diagnosis cannot be made and there is concern for possible malignancy, surgical referral is required. This usually results in a lobectomy or subtotal thyroidectomy.

HYPERTHYROIDISM

Key Points

- Hyperthyroidism is diagnosed with a suppressed sTSH and increased FT_4.
- Graves disease is caused by an abnormal response to circulating antithyroid antibodies.
- Serum TSH in Graves disease is usually less than 0.01 mIU/L and may be unmeasurable. TSH-RS Abs are often present.
- Diagnosis of Graves disease in a patient without goiter and ophthalmic abnormality should be suspect.

Hyperthyroidism is a biochemical process represented by an increase in thyroid hormone biosynthesis and secretion (Bahn et al., 2011; Toft, 2001). The diagnosis of hyperthyroidism is based on sTSH level less than 0.1 mIU/L and elevated FT_4 and FT_3 and is often associated with symptoms consistent with a hypermetabolic state (Table 35-4). Determining the exact etiology requires further testing, including laboratory studies and imaging (Table 35-5).

Table 35-4 Symptoms Consistent with a Hypermetabolic State

Tachycardia, wide pulse pressure
Systolic hypertension
Fever, tremor
Warm moist skin
Anxiety, hyperactivity
Diarrhea, weight loss

Modified from Braverman LE, Utiger RD. Introduction to thyrotoxicosis. In Braverman LE, Utiger RD, eds. *The thyroid: a fundamental and clinical text.* 9th ed. Philadelphia: Lippincott, Williams & Wilkins; 2005.

Table 35-5 Common Causes of Hyperthyroidism

Autonomous functioning (toxic) nodule
Toxic multinodular goiter (TMNG, Plummer disease)
Factitious disorder (Munchausen disease)
Iatrogenic disease
TSH receptor-stimulator antibody production (Graves disease)
Acute thyroiditis
TSH-producing pituitary tumor (adenoma)

TMNG, Toxic multinodular goiter; *TSH,* thyroid-stimulating hormone (thyrotropin).

Graves Disease

Graves disease is the most common cause of hyperthyroidism and results from the development of TSH-RS Abs. These antibodies attach to TSH receptors in the thyroid gland and "mimic" the action of TSH, stimulating production and release of T_4. Because of excess circulating T_4, the pituitary feedback loop for TSH production is suppressed, resulting in sTSH levels significantly below 0.01 mIU/L. Serum TSH levels greater than 0.05 mIU/L, although not impossible with Graves disease, should make the diagnosis suspect.

Graves disease can present at the family physician's office as thyrotoxicosis or thyroid storm but more often presents with hypermetabolic symptoms or goiter. How it is treated initially is determined by the patient's age, comorbidities, and acuity of symptoms. The primary symptomatic treatment is directed toward the cardiovascular responses of tachycardia, systolic hypertension, and volume depletion. Concurrent with this is the administration of antithyroid medication (propylthiouracil [PTU] or methimazole [MMI]). After the patient's symptoms have been controlled and there is evidence the hyperthyroid state is resolving, planning for long-term treatment can ensue.

Three courses of action can be followed for long-term treatment of patients with Graves disease. The goal is to maintain a euthyroid state. This can be accomplished with continued use of antithyroid medication, adjusting the dose to maintain sTSH in a normal range. A second option is ablation of the thyroid gland using ^{131}I or total thyroidectomy (Bahn et al., 2011). Either is appropriate, and in either case, the patient must take some medication on a permanent basis. As a third option, an occasional patient will undergo spontaneous remission, so a trial of antithyroid medication for 6 months to 1 year may be worthwhile. When this approach is tried, it requires close follow-up in case the patient rebounds. The majority of patients with Graves disease elect radioactive ablation and long-term treatment with thyroxine replacement.

Intervention to treat the symptoms of hyperthyroidism begins with a β-adrenergic receptor blocker as a temporizing agent to control sympathetically mediated symptoms. Specific therapy is deferred pending confirmation of the cause. For Graves disease, autonomously functioning nodule, or toxic multinodular goiter (TMNG), specific intervention includes PTU or MMI to control thyroxine synthesis and, with PTU, to reduce conversion of T_4 to T_3 in the peripheral circulation. Cases of serious liver injury have been associated with PTU use; thus, some experts suggest that MMI be used in every patient who chooses antithyroid medications as treatment for Graves disease with the exception of the women in the first trimester of pregnancy, in whom PTU is preferred (Bahn et al., 2011). After the patient is converted to a euthyroid state, specific treatment, based on cause, can be instituted.

With treatment of Graves disease, the goiter, which is found in more than 90% of these patients, may shrink. However, large goiters often require surgery for a satisfactory cosmetic appearance.

Thyroxine-Producing Nodules

Autonomously functioning thyroid nodules are found occasionally during workup for a hypermetabolic state or palpation of a thyroid mass. Autonomous nodules have a much higher incidence of occurring in iodine deficient areas, accounting for approximately 60% of cases of thyrotoxicosis.

Autonomous functioning nodules and TMNG (Plummer disease) produce values for sTSH and FT_4 similar to those found in Graves disease, although sTSH is generally not less than 0.05 mIU/L. In both cases, one would expect the TSH-RS Abs to be negative or, at most, at an extremely low titer. Evaluation includes radioisotope scan with ^{123}I, which will demonstrate the nodule(s). These tumors are rarely malignant, and treatment is surgical after appropriate thyroid suppression. Long-term results are excellent, with no expectation of recurrence.

For patients with TMNG, and those with autonomous nodules who cannot tolerate surgery, ^{131}I ablation can be used. The ^{131}I is picked up by the most active portion(s) of the gland, so residual normally functioning thyroid gland often remains. However, iatrogenic hypothyroidism is always possible. After ^{131}I treatment of an autonomous nodule or TMNG, sTSH levels are required to determine if the gland can provide sufficient T_4 to meet physiologic requirements.

Other Causes of a Hyperthyroid State

Two often overlooked causes of a hyperthyroid state are fictitious and iatrogenic hyperthyroidism caused by excess exogenous T_4. In each case, patients have suppressed sTSH but generally only in the low normal range. From a laboratory perspective, these entities mimic painless, sporadic thyroiditis, with elevated T_4, low sTSH, and negative thyroid antibodies. If one measures FT_4 and FT_3, the relative ratio ($FT_4 : FT_3$) will be altered from what is normal. To identify fictitious thyrotoxicosis, it may be necessary to obtain an ^{123}I uptake study, which will demonstrate a minimally active thyroid gland. With Graves disease, autonomous functioning nodule, or TMNG, there is marked glandular activity. Elevated sTSH and elevated FT_4 levels are consistent with central hyperthyroidism or thyroid hormone resistance syndrome, and an evaluation of the pituitary for a TSH-producing tumor is required.

Thyrotoxicosis

Thyrotoxicosis is a physiologic process manifesting as hypermetabolism and hyperactivity that is caused by high serum concentrations of T_4, T_3, or both (Braverman and Utiger, 2005). It is not necessarily caused by excess hormone production and therefore may not represent a true hyperthyroid state. Although in the majority of patients the cause of thyrotoxicosis is excess T_4, in 2% to 4% of patients, it is due to elevated T_3 levels, with concomitant upper limit of normal T_4 levels (Meier and Burger, 2005).

Thyrotoxicosis is more common in female patients and in persons of northern European extraction and is rare in blacks. Spontaneous thyrotoxicosis is most often caused by Graves disease, accounting for 60% to 90% of all cases, followed by silent, or postpartum, thyroiditis caused by the sudden spike of circulating T_4, although it is transient and usually not clinically significant. Other less common, but not rare, causes of thyrotoxicosis include TMNG, autonomous functioning adenoma, and ingestion of exogenous thyroid hormone. Acute onset of thyrotoxicosis is almost always caused by thyroiditis. Thyrotoxicosis associated with Graves disease has a more insidious course, evolving over a more protracted period. If a patient is thyrotoxic and the thyroid gland is not palpable, consider painless thyroiditis, unsuspected Graves disease, or exogenous thyroxine. A thyrotoxic patient with a goiter or ophthalmopathy has Graves disease until proven otherwise. Treatment of hypermetabolic symptoms should not be delayed pending further testing or referral.

Symptoms of hyperthyroidism in younger individuals are usually the result of sympathoadrenal activity, but elderly patients have an age-related desensitization of β-adrenergic receptors, which probably accounts for a blunting of some symptoms usually associated with hyperthyroidism (Hassani and Hershman, 2006; Oiknine and Mooradian, 2006; Trivalle et al., 1996).

In older individuals with altered sympathetic and parasympathetic function, symptoms of thyrotoxicosis tend to include cardiovascular dysfunction, dyspnea, weight loss, and proximal muscle weakness. Cardiovascular symptoms in elderly adults usually consist of resting tachycardia, wide pulse pressure, exercise intolerance, and dyspnea on exertion. Atrial fibrillation is uncommon but occurs more often in older individuals (5%-15%) (Franklyn and Gammage, 2005).

Other cardiovascular effects that affect both young and old individuals are decreased peripheral resistance, decreased cardiac filling times, increased blood volume, and fluid retention. Individuals with preexisting CAD may have ischemic congestive heart failure (CHF) as a result of their hypermetabolic state, but this generally improves with appropriate antithyroid therapy. Atrial flutter, paroxysmal supraventricular tachycardia, premature ventricular beats, and ventricular fibrillation are rare complications of thyrotoxicosis and may represent unsuspected CAD.

Signs and symptoms of CHF are common in both young and old individuals with thyrotoxicosis (Trivalle et al., 1996). Because of decreased effective circulating arterial volume, aldosterone secretion increases, with a concomitant increase in sodium retention that results in dependent edema. After the thyrotoxicosis is effectively treated, all CHF symptoms quickly resolve. When periorbital edema is present, a diagnosis of Graves disease should be considered, and TSH-RS Abs titers should be checked.

Apathetic thyrotoxicosis is an uncommon presentation but represents the most common mental disorder associated with excess thyroid hormone production and release. Symptoms include apathy, lethargy, pseudodementia, weight loss, and depressed mood. It usually occurs in older patients without symptoms of tachycardia, hyperphagia, sweating, warm skin, or goiter (Wagle et al., 1998). This syndrome is easily confused with depression or dementia and, unless specifically sought, is easy to miss. A screening sTSH should be included in every depression or dementia workup.

The treatment of thyrotoxicosis is straightforward with three objectives; ameliorate acute symptoms, suppress synthesis and secretion of thyroid hormones, and treat the primary cause to prevent recurrence (Bahn et al., 2011). Acute symptoms respond readily to β-adrenergic receptor blocking agents, which should be continued until FT_4 levels have returned to the normal range. Calcium channel blockers can be used in patients who cannot tolerate β-blockers. Inhibition of synthesis of thyroid hormones is achieved with PTU or MMI. Adjunct therapies include fluid resuscitation with D5 or D10 normal saline and administration of steroids. Fever generally responds satisfactorily to acetaminophen. The high fevers associated with thyroid storm may require cooling blankets. Nonsteroidal drugs and salicylates should be avoided in the acute phase because of competition for thyroid hormone binding sites on transport proteins. This can cause release of bound thyroid hormone into the peripheral circulation. With aggressive therapy, acute symptoms of thyrotoxicosis should improve within 12 to 24 hours. After acute symptoms are controlled, treatment of the primary cause can be considered. This could include watchful waiting in the case of thyroiditis, surgery for an autonomously functioning adenoma, or ^{131}I in Graves disease.

Thyroid Storm

> **Key Points**
>
> - Unrecognized thyroid storm has a mortality rate as high as 75%.
> - Thyroid storm is usually the result of another disorder that unmasks a preexisting, but unidentified, hyperthyroid state.
> - Thyroid storm is a clinical diagnosis, not defined by levels of TSH, T_4, or T_3.
> - Suspicion of thyroid storm is a medical emergency with close monitoring in the intensive care unit and appropriate consultation by an endocrinologist.

Thyroid storm is a severe variant of thyrotoxicosis in which the metabolic state is sufficiently increased such that organ system failure can occur. It represents a rare complication of thyrotoxicosis and has a mortality rate as high as 75%, depending on how quickly it is recognized and treated (Tiegens and Leinung, 1995; Trzepacz et al., 1989; Wartofsky, 2005).

The diagnosis of thyroid storm is based on clinical findings, not measured levels of circulating T_4 or sTSH. Thyroid storm is often precipitated by infection, with associated symptoms that mask a thyrotoxic state. Clinical findings in thyroid storm include hyperpyrexia (>102° F), tachycardia out of proportion to temperature, gastrointestinal (GI) dysfunction (nausea, vomiting, diarrhea, jaundice), and CNS dysfunction (marked hyperirritability, anxiety, confusion, apathy, coma) (Wartofsky, 2005). There is usually pronounced decompensation of one or more organ systems. Any patient presenting with goiter, fever, and marked tachycardia should be considered to be in thyroid storm and treated accordingly. Admission to the medical intensive care unit and consultation with an endocrinologist are appropriate.

Treatment of thyroid storm includes β-blockers, antithyroid drugs, corticosteroid therapy, antipyretics, aggressive fluid replacement, and identification and treatment of any precipitating process. For patients with severe symptoms, Lugol solution or supersaturated potassium iodide will help inhibit release of T_4 into the peripheral circulation.

Table 35-6   Causes of Hypothyroidism

Insufficient intake of dietary iodine (uncommon in the United States)
Autoimmune disease (primarily Hashimoto thyroiditis)
Surgery (thyroid surgery)
Radiation exposure (head and neck)
Viral infection
Central disease (primary pituitary failure)

If either is used, it should only be given after loading doses of antithyroid drugs, to block iodine-induced synthesis of T_4. Lithium also has an antithyroid effect and can be used in severe cases of thyroid storm. Severe thyrotoxic symptoms, unresponsive to all of these regimens, may respond to sodium ipodate at 500 mg/day.

HYPOTHYROIDISM

Hypothyroidism is a hypometabolic state resulting from levels of circulating thyroid hormone insufficient to meet body requirements. Serum TSH will be greater than 10 mIU/L and can be significantly increased (>25 mIU/L) in protracted cases. Primary causes are listed in Table 35-6.

Chronic Autoimmune Thyroiditis (Hashimoto Thyroiditis)

> **Key Points**
>
> - Hashimoto thyroiditis is an autoimmune disorder that results in fibrosis of the thyroid gland.
> - Hashimoto thyroiditis is the most common cause of hypothyroidism in the United States.
> - Diagnosis of Hashimoto thyroiditis is based on an elevated sTSH, low normal to low FT_4, and TPO Abs.

The most common cause of hypothyroidism worldwide is inadequate dietary intake of iodine. Because of the addition of iodine to table salt, however, this is a rare cause in the United States. In the United States and the rest of the developed world, the most common cause of hypothyroidism is CAT (Hashimoto disease). CAT is caused by the development of antithyroid antibodies that attack the thyroidal struma, causing progressive fibrosis. TPO Abs and Tg abs appear to be responsible, with TPO Abs considered the primary cause (Dayan and Daniels, 1996). Diagnosis is based on elevated sTSH, a low normal or low FT_4, and the presence of TPO Abs (Garber et al., 2012).

Hashimoto thyroiditis occurs most often in women, with a female-to-male ratio of 10-14:1. CAT is usually diagnosed in the fifth decade of life and is progressive (Vanderpump, 2005). As it progresses, more functioning thyroid gland becomes fibrotic, and less indigenous T_4 is produced. After diagnosis, replacement doses of T_4 should be used. In adults, the average replacement dose of L-thyroxine is 1.6 μg/kg/day. Serum TSH is followed annually to ensure adequate control.

Other Forms of Hypothyroidism

Central hypothyroidism is caused by pituitary failure and is rare. The diagnosis is suggested with low to nonexistent sTSH levels in a patient without symptoms of hypermetabolism (thyrotoxicosis) and with low circulating FT_4. Generally, when presented with these data, further evaluation to determine the etiology of the hypothyroidism is not necessary. However, the patient should be evaluated for pituitary failure if this has not already been done (see Approach to Pituitary Diseases).

Depending on the degree of injury, thyroiditis (postpartum, sporadic, or subacute) can result in a transient hypothyroid state, with eventual recovery. Subacute thyroiditis is more likely to undergo this process with insufficient T_4 production for 3 to 6 months. Treatment is usually unnecessary, but low-dose thyroxine replacement can be used on a temporary basis for patients who become symptomatic.

Other causes of hypothyroidism include dietary iodine deficiency, surgery, ^{131}I radiation therapy, and nonthyroid head and neck cancer treatment.

Hypothyroidism is typically treated with L-thyroxine replacement alone. However, some believe that patients occasionally have T_4-resistant disease and recommend mixed T_4–T_3 replacement. Although true T_4 resistance is controversial, if a patient receiving replacement T_4 has sTSH in the therapeutic range but continues to complain of hypothyroid symptoms, combination T_4–T_3 can be tried to alleviate symptoms. But it is prudent to ensure that the sTSH is maintained above 1.0 mIU/L to guard against unintended consequences of iatrogenic hyperthyroidism (Gencer et al., 2013; Taylor et al., 2013).

Initial dose of L-thyroxine will depend on the patient's age, duration of hypothyroid state, and comorbidities. In a young healthy adult, treatment with L-thyroxine may start with full replacement dosing. For someone older than 50 to 60 years without evidence of CAD, an L-thyroxine dose of 0.05 mg (50 µg) daily is recommended, with increases weekly of 0.025 mg to 0.05 mg, depending on clinical response (Garber et al., 2012). If the patient becomes tachycardic, is tremulous, or sweats, the time interval should be extended between increases in dosage to every 2 to 3 weeks. After the patient is stabilized on 0.1 to 0.125 mg of L-thyroxine daily, further increases are made based on sTSH response. Serum TSH only needs to be checked every 4 to 6 weeks. More frequent testing does not allow a sufficient interval for developing homeostasis and can result in overdosing. When the patient is on a steady dose, further treatment is adjusted so that sTSH remains at 0.5 to 4.5 mIU/L (mean, 2.5 mIU/L). Doses of L-thyroxine resulting in sTSH less than 0.1 mIU/L indicate iatrogenic hyperthyroidism and should be avoided (Gencer et al., 2013).

Thyroiditis

Forms of thyroiditis include tender thyroiditis such as subacute granulomatous thyroiditis (probable viral etiology), infectious thyroiditis (probable bacteria etiology), radiation thyroiditis, and palpation- or trauma-induced thyroiditis. Nontender thyroiditis includes silent thyroiditis, postpartum thyroiditis, drug-induced thyroiditis, fibrous thyroiditis, and CAT (Hashimoto thyroiditis) (Bahn et al., 2011; Farwell, 2005; Lazarus, 2005).

The mechanism of injury to the thyroid gland is disruption of thyroid architecture caused by lymphocytic infiltration, resulting in leakage of colloid-stored thyroxine into the peripheral circulation. This nonphysiologically triggered leakage of stored T_4 causes a spike in peripheral circulating T_4 and transient hypermetabolic symptoms. Early testing in the disease can demonstrate an elevated FT_4 level, although not necessarily outside the normal range. Depending on the duration of the destructive process and degree of injury, sTSH may be normal, low normal, or low. If the cause of this variability is not appreciated, it could lead to the erroneous initial diagnosis of Graves disease (increased FT_4 and low sTSH). With protracted acute thyroiditis, however, sTSH is not as low as in Graves disease, and TSH-RS Abs titers are low to absent. In addition, patients with acute thyroiditis lack Graves disease optic findings and goiter.

As a general rule, acute thyroiditis is a short-lived process, with T_4 stores being rapidly depleted. This represents a case of thyrotoxicosis (increased circulating T_4) but not hyperthyroidism (increased production of T_4). Follow-up testing over the next few weeks demonstrates progressively lower T_4 levels, which eventually return to normal. As T_4 levels return to normal, the acute hypermetabolic symptoms begin to decline. The duration of T_4 elevation determines how low the sTSH will go and how quickly it will return to normal.

Treatment of Hypothyroid Disease

Synthetic levothyroxine (L-thyroxine) is the drug of choice for the treatment of TSH-deficient hypothyroidism (Oiknine and Mooradian, 2006). A typical replacement dose in adults is approximately 1.6 µg/kg/day. The daily requirements should be individually determined based on clinical and biochemical evaluations. The FT_4 level should be in the middle to upper third of normal range. Attention to other, coexistent diseases is required when replacing thyroid hormone (Garber et al., 2012). Thyroid replacement increases the clearance of cortisol and will uncover a subclinical adrenal insufficiency. This must be considered when replacing thyroxine in a patient with secondary hypothyroidism. The ACTH status should be assessed and, if deficient or the status is uncertain, glucocorticoid replacement is indicated before thyroid hormone is replaced.

Subclinical Thyroid Disease

> ### Key Points
>
> - Subclinical thyroid disease is based on a TSH level that is above the normal reference range in an asymptomatic patient with normal FT_4.
> - The American Thyroid Association (ATA) and the American Association of Clinical Endocrinologists (AACE) recommend that screening for hypothyroidism should be considered in all adults over the age of 60 years.
> - The decision to treat subclinical hypothyroidism when serum TSH is less than 10 mIU/L should be individualized
> - The ATA and AACE suggest treatment of subclinical hypothyroidism (sTSH <10 mIU/L in patients positive for TPO Abs or a history of atherosclerotic vascular disease or symptoms consistent with hypothyroidism).

Discussion about subclinical thyroid disease has focused on whether it is a real clinical entity. Subclinical thyroid diseases are defined as (1) subclinical hyperthyroidism (or subclinical thyrotoxicosis) with sTSH less than 0.1mIU/L and normal circulating FT_4 and FT_3 or (2) subclinical hypothyroidism with sTSH greater than 4.5 mIU/L but less than 10.0 mIU/L with normal circulating FT_4. Both entities assume a patient who is asymptomatic or has minimal signs and symptoms.

The primary questions concerning subclinical thyroid disease are whether early intervention is beneficial and whether patients should be screened. The only disease state that has been directly related to subclinical thyroid disease is overt hypothyroidism. Individuals with subclinical hypothyroidism have a higher incidence of progression to overt hypothyroidism than the general population. Annually, 3% to 5% of patients identified with subclinical hypothyroidism progress to overt hypothyroidism with sTSH levels greater than 10.0 mIU/L (Toft and Beckett, 2005). The majority of these represent early CAT. For patients with subclinical hypothyroidism, a TPO Ab measurement should be considered.

Currently, no consensus exists among national organizations as to whether these individuals should start therapy during this phase of their disease. Treating those with symptoms seems appropriate, but there is no evidence to support the premise that early treatment alters the disease course or associated comorbidities (hyperlipidemia, hypertension, CAD).

Studies have demonstrated a two to three times higher incidence of atrial fibrillation in patients with subclinical hyperthyroidism compared with individuals with normal sTSH levels (Ross, 2005a, 2005b). The Framingham data suggest that some individuals with subclinical hyperthyroidism are at increased risk for paroxysmal atrial fibrillation (Oiknine and Mooradian, 2006). In addition, good evidence indicates that osteoporosis is associated with overt hyperthyroidism. New evidence suggests that osteoporosis is also associated with subclinical hyperthyroidism (Gencer et al., 2013).

Although data supporting adverse consequences of subclinical hyperthyroidism continue to accumulate, there still are no outcomes data to show a decrease in mortality or morbidity from early intervention. The AACE, however, does recommend treatment of subclinical hyperthyroidism caused by nodular thyroid disease (AACE, 2002).

New guidelines from the ATA and AACE, published in 2012, have moved from their previous position of not recommending treatment of subclinical hypothyroidism to suggesting that treatment be considered for individuals with a sTSH between 4.5 and 10 mIU/L who are positive for TPO Abs or have a history of atherosclerotic vascular disease and anyone with symptoms suggestive of hypothyroidism (Garber et al., 2012).

A review of the literature on how variation of thyroid function tests affect cardiovascular, bone, metabolic, pregnancy, neurologic, and psychologic outcomes, suggests there may be a correlation between these and thyroid test variability (i.e., "normal" range) (Taylor et al., 2013). Evidence synthesis shows that higher sTSH and lower T_4 levels are associated with more cardiovascular risk factors and cardiovascular events and worse metabolic parameters

and pregnancy outcomes. Furthermore, it shows that lower sTSH and higher T_4 levels are associated with reduced bone mineral density (BMD) and increased fracture risk. High-quality data are lacking for neurologic and psychological outcomes. The conclusion suggests that even with thyroid function data within currently accepted normal range (0.1-4.5 mIU/L), there is an association with adverse health outcomes (Taylor et al., 2013). Data from the Thyroid Studies Collaboration support these findings. Specifically, subclinical hypothyroidism is associated with an increased risk of coronary heart disease (CHD) events, increased CHD mortality, and heart failure (HF). Subclinical hyperthyroidism is associated with an overall risk of total mortality, CHD mortality, HF, and atrial fibrillation. Atrial fibrillation is particularly increased in individuals whose sTSH is suppressed below 0.1 mIU/L (Gencer et al., 2013; Rodondi et al., 2005).

By extrapolation from the results of these data, it is reasonable to assume that treatment of subclinical thyroid disease could be beneficial, but definitive outcomes data are lacking. However, it is clear that careful control and follow-up of treatment of overt thyroid disease is essential.

ANATOMIC DISEASES

Anatomic diseases of the thyroid gland include a number of primary and secondary disorders (Table 35-7). The list includes goiter, nodules, primary neoplasia, metastatic neoplasia (rare), and familial disorders.

Goiter

Goiter is the most common anatomic disease, and the major cause of goiter worldwide is iodine deficiency. When simple goiter occurs in areas of adequate iodine intake, there appears to be a strong genetic component to the disease. In the United States, goiter found independent of Graves disease is usually associated with CAT as the disease progresses to a hypothyroid state. Goiter is the result of both hypertrophy and hyperplasia of the thyroid gland. In the case of iodine deficiency, this is caused by excess thyrotropin production, leading to glandular growth and colloid production.

In Graves disease, stimulation of the thyroid by TSH-RS Abs causes excess production of T_4 and T_3, in turn resulting in uncontrolled production of colloid to store the excess production of thyroid hormone. In fact, goiter is the most common clinical finding in Graves disease after thyrotoxicosis, occurring in nearly 100% of patients (Chiovato et al., 2001).

Goiter is one of the five hallmarks of Graves disease. Goiter associated with hypothyroidism often improves after euthyroid doses of thyroxine have been achieved, although

Table 35-7	Anatomic Diseases of Thyroid
Goiter	Simple, toxic, iodine deficiency
Nodule	Adenoma, incidental, toxic
Cyst	Simple, complex
Malignancy	Primary: papillary or follicular, medullary, lymphoma
	Metastatic: lymphoma, breast, pulmonary, other
	Familial: multiple endocrine neoplasia type IIA

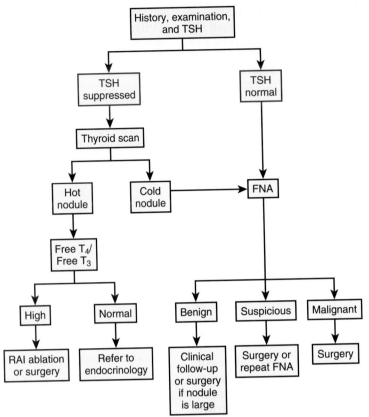

Figure 35-2 Algorithm for the clinical evaluation of thyroid nodule. *FNA,* Fine-needle aspiration; *RAI,* radioactive iodine; *T₃,* triiodothyronine; *T₄,* thyroxine; *TSH,* thyroid-stimulating hormone.

it may take 6 months to 1 year. If the goiter does not involute with thyroxine replacement, excision may be required. Besides goiter, the other four hallmarks of Graves disease are thyrotoxicosis, ophthalmopathy, local myxedema, and acropachy (clubbing of fingers and toes).

Nodules and Cysts

Thyroid nodules come in a variety of sizes and types. The incidence of malignancy in nodules smaller than 1.0 cm in size, which typically are found incidental to some non–thyroid-related diagnostic procedure (e.g., head and neck ultrasonography), is less than 0.5%. Current recommendations for evaluation of these "incidentalomas" include TSH and FT₄ levels and careful palpation of the thyroid gland (Ross, 2005a) and adjacent cervical nodes (Cooper et al., 2009) (Figure 35-2).

If results of tests and palpation are normal or negative, annual follow-up with palpation by the physician is recommended. As long as growth remains minimal and there were no ultrasonographic hallmarks of malignancy on the initial scan, these nodules can be monitored clinically.

The exception to annual follow-up in nodules smaller than 1.0 cm is when a solitary nodule occurs before 14 years of age because these have a greater than 50% incidence of malignancy. Other reasons to obtain FNA of a nodule smaller than 1.0 cm include high-risk history (nodules >5 mm) or presence of cervical adenopathy (all nodules regardless of size) (Cooper et al., 2009).

A nodule that is palpable on examination or 1.0 cm or larger on ultrasonography requires further evaluation. If the sTSH is within normal range and a local endocrinologist experienced in FNA is available, referral without imaging is appropriate. However, if ultrasonography is performed and it shows a purely cystic lesion, FNA is not necessary. As long as the cyst remains small or is asymptomatic, no intervention is required. However, if the cyst increases in size or becomes symptomatic, it can be drained via FNA.

If the patient with a palpable nodule has a suppressed sTSH, this would suggest a nodule that is functioning autonomously. Before any intervention (surgical or FNA), a radioisotope ^{123}I scan is indicated. If the lesion is "hot," suppression is the course of action before FNA or surgery is performed. If "cold," it could represent a cystic, mixed, or solid mass, thus requiring further evaluation by FNA (first choice) or surgical exploration.

Benign nodules do not require therapeutic intervention unless the nodule's size is causing symptoms (tracheal compression or pain). These generally do not respond to suppression; thus, surgical excision is the treatment of choice.

Malignancy

Malignancy of the thyroid, both primary and secondary, is rare, accounting for fewer than 2% of all cancers, and generally, tumors are not aggressive. *Papillary carcinoma* is the most common, accounting for approximately 80% of primary thyroid malignancies. Follicular carcinoma, which arises from the same cell type as papillary carcinoma, accounts for about 5% of thyroid neoplasia. Undifferentiated and anaplastic carcinoma makes up fewer than 10% of all thyroid malignancies, and medullary carcinoma of the thyroid about 5% of thyroid malignancies (Baloch and Livolsi, 2005).

The most common cancers that metastasize to the thyroid are breast, lung, and kidney. Primary lymphoid cancer occurs in the thyroid, but its incidence is unknown because it cannot be distinguished from lymphoma that originates elsewhere in the body. Treatment of thyroid cancers is generally surgical with ^{131}I therapy with subtotal thyroidectomy. As with cancers elsewhere in the body, primary treatment will depend on tissue diagnosis and clinical evaluation. New imaging techniques are being used to evaluate patients who are thyroglobulin positive but whole-body iodine scan negative for differentiated thyroid cancer. This imaging technique uses [18]fluorine-labeled fluorodeoxyglucose positron emission tomography/computed tomography (^{18}F FDG PET/CT), and ATA guidelines from 2009 recommend this screening in select patients with any one of five main indicators. Presently, this level of nuclear scan may only be available in larger metropolitan areas and academic medical centers (Cooper et al., 2009; Palaniswamy and Subramanyam, 2013).

Two familial thyroid malignancies include MEN IIA and FMTC. MEN IIA is an autosomal dominant disorder that can cause "C"-cell hyperplasia and hyperparathyroidism. The diagnosis is often serendipitously found during evaluation for hypercalcemia or renal calculi.

LONG-TERM FOLLOW-UP OF THYROID DISORDERS

For patients receiving long-term thyroid therapy for hypothyroidism, monitoring is done via sTSH unless there is hypothalamic-pituitary disease. It takes 4 weeks after initiating treatment (or changing dose) before clinically significant change occurs in sTSH level. In most patients, checking sTSH once every 4 weeks is sufficient until steady state is reached. After the patient is stabilized, sTSH can be checked at 6 months and then annually unless the patient develops new symptoms (Garber et al., 2012).

Patients determined to have benign nodules after adequate evaluation are followed annually with careful palpation of the thyroid gland. Unless there is a size change or new symptoms, no additional testing is required. Ultrasound imaging of the thyroid is not recommended for follow-up of nodules smaller than 1.0 cm. Repeat ultrasonography is required in patients with an enlarging nodule, evidence of a new thyroid mass, or who complain of pain or pressure. Unless the patient is experiencing symptoms of hyper- or hypothyroid, repeat testing of sTSH or FT$_4$ is not indicated (Cooper et al., 2009).

SICK EUTHYROID SYNDROME (THYROID HORMONE ADAPTATION SYNDROME)

Thyroid function can appear suppressed during severe illness and may not represent abnormal thyroid function. Serious illness has been shown to affect laboratory tests of thyroid function (sTSH, T$_4$, thyroglobulin), but there is no clear evidence that this reflects a disease state (Chopra, 1997). Because these changes appear to have no direct adverse effect on the patient's overall clinical state, this condition is labeled "sick euthyroid syndrome." In broad terms,

sick euthyroid syndrome is more of academic interest than clinical. Administration of T$_4$ to a seriously ill individual does not improve the outcome for most patients, but evidence suggests that high doses of T$_3$ after cardiac surgery may be beneficial (Wiersinga, 2005).

The physician should remember the rare patient whose thyroid disease is uncovered by serious illness. If a seriously ill patient is not responding as expected, (e.g., difficulty in weaning from ventilator support), checking thyroid function may be appropriate, although any interpretation of results should be reviewed by a clinician experienced in interpreting thyroid tests in seriously ill patients before intervention (Garber et al., 2012).

DRUGS AFFECTING THYROID FUNCTION AND TESTING

Key Points

- Therapeutic drugs have a variety of effects on thyroid function, including delayed or suppressed synthesis.
- Therapeutic drugs may block the effect of thyroid hormone at the cellular level.
- Phenothiazines, dopamine, phenytoin, and glucocorticoids block release of TSH from the pituitary.
- Amiodarone can cause both hyperthyroidism and hypothyroidism. Approximately 20% of patients can develop hypothyroidism from fibrosis of the gland.

Many common drugs can affect thyroid function, bioavailability of thyroid hormone, and laboratory testing. Drugs that affect thyroid function fall into several categories: some inhibit synthesis of T$_4$, some block secretion of T$_4$, some block TSH release, some affect extrathyroidal conversion of T$_4$ to T$_3$, and some influence thyroxine at the tissue or cellular level (Table 35-8). PTU and MMI inhibit thyroid hormone synthesis by interfering with thyroid peroxidase. PTU has the added advantage of inhibiting extrathyroidal conversion of T$_4$ to T$_3$. Neither PTU nor MMI inhibits T$_4$ release (secretion) from the thyroid gland. Amiodarone, lithium, and cytokines can affect synthesis and secretion. In the absence of iodine, amiodarone can precipitate both hyperthyroid and hypothyroid events. In the United States, where dietary iodine is plentiful, patients taking amiodarone tend to develop hypothyroidism from fibrosis of the

Table 35-8 Drugs That Affect Thyroid Function at the Glandular Level

Drug	Inhibits T$_4$ Synthesis	Blocks T$_4$ Secretion	Blocks TSH Release
Iodine	Yes	—	—
Propylthiouracil	Yes	—	—
Methimazole	Yes	—	—
Antipsychotic	—	—	Yes
Amiodarone	Yes	Yes	—
Lithium	Yes	Yes	—
Phenytoin	—	—	Yes
Dopamine	—	—	Yes
Glucocorticoid	—	—	Yes
Cytokines	Yes	Yes	—

T$_4$ Thyroxine; *TSH,* thyroid-stimulating hormone (thyrotropin).

Table 35-9 Drugs and Oral Agents That Affect Thyroid Function at the Peripheral Level

Drug	Compete for Protein Binding	Inhibit Deiodination of T_4 to T_3	Inhibit Action at Tissue Level	Inhibit Uptake of T_3 at Tissue Level	Affect Thyroid Hormone Clearance Time	Inhibit GI Absorption	Adverse Effect on Lab Tests
Phenytoin	—	—	—	—	Yes	—	—
Phenobarbital	—	—	—	—	Yes	—	—
Carbamazepine	—	—	—	—	Yes	—	—
Rifampin	—	—	—	—	Yes	—	Yes
Salicylates	Yes	—	—	—	—	—	Yes
NSAID	Yes	—	—	—	—	—	Yes
Furosemide	Yes	—	—	—	—	—	Yes
Heparin	Yes	—	—	—	—	—	Yes
Enoxaparin	Yes	—	—	—	—	—	—
Sucralfate	—	—	—	—	—	Yes	—
Ca carbonate	—	—	—	—	—	Yes	—
Al hydroxide	—	—	—	—	—	Yes	—
Soy	—	—	—	—	—	Yes	—
Ferrous sulfate	—	—	—	—	—	Yes	—
PTU	—	—	Yes	—	—	—	Yes
Dexamethasone	—	Yes	—	—	—	—	Yes
β-Blocker	—	Yes	Yes	—	—	—	Yes
Benzodiazepine	—	—	—	Yes	—	—	—
CCB	—	—	—	Yes	—	—	—
Amiodarone	—	Yes	—	—	—	—	—
Contrast agent	—	Yes	—	—	—	—	—

Al, aluminum; *Ca,* calcium; *CCB,* Calcium channel blocker; *GI,* gastrointestinal; *NSAID,* nonsteroidal antiinflammatory drug; *PTU,* propylthiouracil; *T₃,* triiodothyronine; *T₄,* thyroxine.

thyroid gland. The incidence is approximately 20% (Harjai and Licata, 1997; Roti and Vagenakis, 2005). Patients taking these drugs, especially amiodarone, should be screened regularly with sTSH for developing thyroid dysfunction. Dopamine, glucocorticoids, and phenytoin have been shown to inhibit release of TSH from the anterior pituitary. Salicylates and other NSAIDs, furosemide, heparin, and enoxaparin compete for binding sites on thyroid hormone transport proteins. Use of these drugs in acute thyroid disease can potentially exacerbate thyrotoxic symptoms by releasing thyroid hormone into the peripheral circulation. Serum TSH and FT_4 should be monitored in regular users of these medications (Table 35-9).

Phenytoin, phenobarbital, carbamazepine, and rifampin stimulate hepatic enzymatic activity, thus shortening thyroid hormone clearance times and increasing conversion of T_4 to T_3. Serum TSH levels should be monitored routinely, until stable, when these medications are added or deleted from a patient's regimen. Sucralfate, cholestyramine, calcium carbonate, aluminum hydroxide, soluble fiber, soy products, and ferrous sulfate inhibit absorption of exogenous L-thyroxine from the gut. Oral L-thyroxine should be taken on an empty stomach.

β-Blockers exert their effect on thyroid hormones at the cellular level, and benzodiazepines block uptake of T_3 at the cellular level (Hedley et al., 1989; Tiegens and Leinung, 1995; Wartofsky, 2005). Calcium channel blocking agents inhibit uptake of thyroid hormone by hepatic and muscle cells (Table 35-9).

THYROID DISEASE IN PREGNANCY

Pregnancy can exacerbate an already existing thyroid disorder, thus requiring extra vigilance on the part of the family physician. Careful monitoring and proactive clinical intervention are key. The majority of women with hypothyroidism, who are euthyroid on stable doses of thyroid replacement, require increased doses of thyroxine replacement during their pregnancy. In pregnancy, the normal range for sTSH is trimester specific. If trimester-specific sTSH ranges are not available at the local laboratory, the recommended upper levels for normal are 2.5 mIU/L for the first trimester, 3.0 mIU/L for the second trimester, and 3.5 mIU/L for the third (Garber et al., 2012). Being aware of this need and being prepared to make dosage adjustments in a timely manner are important. Consulting an endocrinologist to help with the care of these patients is advised (Shankar et al., 2001).

Silent or postpartum thyroiditis during pregnancy is essentially a benign, short-term disease and requires only symptomatic treatment. Occasional checks of sTSH and FT_4 levels are justified to monitor recovery. For the rare pregnant patient who requires suppression of T_4 synthesis, judicious use of antithyroid drugs (PTU and MMI) is generally considered to be safe. There is some concern that MMI may cross the placental barrier more readily than PTU, but this has not proven to be of concern in a clinical setting. It is important, however, to remember that prolonged suppression of the thyroid or suppression late in pregnancy can result in a transient depression of neonatal thyroid function and may induce goiters in the neonate. PTU and MMI can be found in breast milk. This has not proven to be of concern as long as the dose is kept low. PTU (maximum, 150 mg/day) and MMI (maximum, 20 mg/day) caused no problems with a nursing child (Glinoer, 2005). Both PTU and MMI are category D pregnancy risk, and the American Academy of Pediatrics reports no sign or symptom in infants or adverse effects on lactation and supports use of these drugs during breastfeeding. In the United States, PTU has generally been the antithyroid drug of choice in pregnant and nursing women; however, recent reports concerning hepatotoxicity from PTU have limited use of PTU to the preferred agent during the first trimester of pregnancy, and MMI is first-line therapy during the second and third trimesters of pregnancy and nursing.

SCREENING FOR THYROID DISEASE

Screening for asymptomatic thyroid disease is controversial, but screening in specific populations may be beneficial (American Academy of Family Physicians [AAFP], 2009; Bahn et al., 2011; Garber et al., 2012; Helfand, 2004; Ladenson et al., 2000). Women older than the age of 50 years have the highest incidence of spontaneous hypothyroidism compared with all males and mixed younger populations, approaching 5% per year. Thus, screening has a good chance of finding disease early. However, the evidence supporting benefit from early intervention is not strong and probably does not justify the cost. However, the ATA and AACE changed their guidelines in 2012 to say that screening for hypothyroidism should be considered in adults older than 60 years old (Garber et al., 2012). Patients who present with paroxysmal atrial fibrillation should be routinely screened for hyperthyroidism, although the incidence of positive findings is low.

One area where screening is advantageous is patients with newly diagnosed dementia. This is especially true if the clinical course is atypical or accelerated. Both hypothyroidism (myxedema) and hyperthyroidism (apathetic thyrotoxicosis) can present with dementia-like symptoms and, in these patients, timely intervention can completely reverse the signs and symptoms of dementia or depression caused by thyroid dysfunction.

If screening is undertaken, the test of choice is a sTSH. When coupled with FT_4, the vast majority of clinically significant hyperthyroidism and hypothyroidism can be diagnosed. If symptoms are present or there are overt signs of disease, the initial testing should include sTSH, FT_4, and FT_3. Thyroid panels providing T_4, T_3, T_7, FT_4 index, and T_3 uptake are no longer advocated.

KEY TREATMENT

- Thyrotoxicosis is treated initially with β-blockers and antithyroid medication to control symptoms and stop synthesis and release of thyroid hormone into the peripheral circulation (Bahn et al., 2011; Oiknine et al., 2006; Trivalle et al., 1996) (SOR: A).
- Hypothyroid (TSH >10 mIU/L) replacement T_4 dose is approximately 1.6 μg/kg/day (Oiknine et al., 2006) (SOR: A).

- With the exception of thyroid antibody–positive subclinical hypothyroidism with TSH less than 10 mIU/L, prophylactic treatment has not been shown to have a positive effect on lipids or CAD risk (Bahn et al., 2011; Garber et al., 2012; Helfand, 2004; Ladenson et al., 2000) (SOR: A).
- Treatment of subclinical hyperthyroidism should be considered when TSH is less than 0.1 mU/L in all patients older than 65 years and in patients younger than 65 years with any of the following comorbidities: heart disease, osteoporosis, menopause, or hyperthyroid symptoms (ATA and AACE, 2011) (SOR: B).

Adrenal Glands

PHYSIOLOGY

The adrenal glands are located at the superomedial aspects of the kidneys. The glands consist of two endocrine tissues of different embryologic origins: the primarily steroid-producing adrenocortical tissue in the cortex and the catecholamine-producing chromaffin cells in the medulla. The adrenal cortex consists of three zones that vary in both their morphologic features and the hormones they produce. The outer, *zona glomerulosa*, is the unique source of the mineralocorticoid aldosterone. The intermediate, *zona fasciculate*, and the inner, *zona reticularis*, produce the glucocorticoids cortisol and corticosterone and the androgens dehydroepiandrosterone (DHEA) and DHEA sulfate (DHEA-S). The chromaffin cells in the adrenal medulla mainly secrete the catecholamines epinephrine and norepinephrine (Table 35-10) (Williams and Dluhy, 2008).

Mineralocorticoids are major regulators of extracellular fluid volume and potassium metabolism. Volume is regulated through a direct effect on the collecting duct of the kidney, where aldosterone causes an increase in sodium retention and in potassium excretion. The release of aldosterone is regulated by the RAS, plasma potassium levels, and ACTH. The RAS maintains the circulating blood volume by regulating aldosterone secretion. Aldosterone-induced sodium retention occurs in volume deficiency states, but aldosterone-dependent sodium retention is reduced when volume is ample. An increase in plasma potassium or a decrease in plasma sodium stimulates aldosterone release. ACTH stimulates mineralocorticoid output, but this effect on aldosterone secretion is transient.

Table 35-10   Adrenal Gland Anatomy and Steroids

Cortex	Zona glomerulosa
	Aldosterone
	Zona fasciculata
	Zona reticularis
	Glucocorticoids
	Cortisol
	Corticosterone
	Dehydroepiandrosterone (DHEA)
	DHEA sulfate (DHEA-S)
Medulla	Epinephrine
	Norepinephrine
	Dopamine

The release of *cortisol*, the main glucocorticoid in humans, is pulsatile and directly stimulated by ACTH or its precursors, such as pro-opiomelanocortin. The release of ACTH from the anterior pituitary is regulated by corticotrophin-releasing hormone (CRH), which is produced by the hypothalamus. High cortisol levels inhibit the biosynthesis and secretion of CRH and ACTH through a negative feedback mechanism. Cortisol release follows a circadian rhythm with its highest level in the morning and is sensitive to light, sleep, stress, and disease. The glucocorticoid effects are multisystemic. They stimulate proteolysis and gluconeogenesis, inhibit muscle protein synthesis, and increase fatty acid mobilization. Gluconeogenesis results in an increase in blood glucose concentrations. At high levels, glucocorticoids are catabolic and result in loss of lean body mass. Glucocorticoids modulate the immune response through their antiinflammatory effects and modulate perception and emotion in the CNS.

The production of the adrenal androgens is controlled by ACTH, not by gonadotropins. Among the adrenal androgens, DHEA is the most abundant circulating hormone in the body and is readily conjugated to its sulfate ester DHEA-S. The adrenal androgens are converted into androstenedione and subsequently into potent androgens (testosterone) or estrogens (estradiol) in the peripheral tissues. Adrenal secretion of DHEA and DHEA-S increases in children around 6 to 8 years of age and peaks between the ages of 20 to 30 years. However, the production of DHEA-S by the adrenal glands is reduced by 70% to 95% during the aging process; by age 70 years, serum DHEA-S levels are approximately 20% of their peak values and continue to decrease with age. Adrenal androgens have minimal effects in men, whose sexual characteristics are predominantly determined by gonadal steroids (testosterone). In women, adrenal-derived testosterone is important in maintaining pubic and axillary hair. Adrenal androgen hypersecretion in men causes no clinical signs but in women manifests with signs of hirsutism and masculinization.

The adrenal medulla secretes epinephrine, norepinephrine, and dopamine. Most catecholamine output in the adrenal vein is epinephrine; norepinephrine also enters the circulation from noradrenergic nerve endings. In emergency situations, the secretion of adrenal catecholamines is increased to prepare the individual for stress ("fight or flight" response). Hypoglycemia and certain drugs are also potent stimuli to catecholamine secretion.

DISORDERS OF CORTICAL HYPOFUNCTION

Primary Adrenal Insufficiency

Key Points

- Primary adrenal insufficiency is defined as the failure of the adrenal cortex to produce glucocorticoids and mineralocorticoids.
- The most frequent cause of primary adrenal insufficiency is autoimmune. In the developing world, however, TB remains the most common cause.
- Symptoms are usually insidious and include fatigue, orthostatic hypotension, weight loss, and hyperpigmentation.

- Acute adrenal insufficiency should be considered in critically ill patients with unexplained hypotension.
- A baseline cortisol and ACTH level followed by an ACTH stimulation test can establish diagnosis.
- Detection of adrenal cortex antibodies or 21-hydroxylase autoantibodies supports the diagnosis of autoimmune adrenalitis. Abdominal CT may be helpful if other causes are suspected.

Primary adrenal insufficiency (AI) is defined as the failure of the adrenal cortex to produce adequate amounts of glucocorticoids and mineralocorticoids (Arlt and Allolio, 2003; Salvatori, 2005). Primary AI can result from processes that damage the adrenal glands or from drugs (e.g., ketoconazole, etomidate) that block the synthesis of cortisol. All causes of primary AI involve the adrenal cortex as a whole and result in a deficiency of cortisol and aldosterone (plus adrenal androgen), although the severity of the deficiencies may vary. An exception is the *syndrome of isolated glucocorticoid deficiency*. The reported prevalence of primary AI (Addison disease) in developed countries is 39 to 60 persons per 1 million population. In adult patients, the mean age at diagnosis is 40 years (range, 17-72 years).

The most frequent cause of primary AI in developed countries is *autoimmune adrenalitis*. However, in the developing world, TB remains the most common cause of adrenal failure. Autoimmune adrenalitis is sometimes accompanied by other autoimmune endocrine deficiencies (autoimmune polyglandular syndromes [APS]). The adult form (type II, Schmidt syndrome) of polyglandular syndrome consists mainly of AI, autoimmune thyroid disease, and insulin-dependent (type 1) diabetes mellitus. Several infectious processes associated with acquired immunodeficiency syndrome (AIDS) such as cytomegalovirus (CMV), *Mycobacterium tuberculosis*, *Cryptococcus neoformans*, *Mycobacterium avium intracellulare*, *Histoplasma capsulatum*, and Kaposi sarcoma may damage the adrenal gland and lead to insufficiency. In young males, adrenoleukodystrophy (or the less severe adrenomyeloneuropathy), an X-linked recessive disorder of metabolism of long-chain fatty acids, can cause spastic paralysis and adrenal insufficiency. AI can precede neurologic symptoms and should prompt the clinician to perform a careful neurologic examination in young males with primary AI. Other causes are listed in Table 35-11.

Chronic (Primary) Adrenal Insufficiency. Most of the symptoms are nonspecific and occur insidiously. Chronic AI manifestations include weakness, chronic fatigue, anorexia, unintentional weight loss, listlessness, joint pain, and orthostatic hypotension. Some patients may initially present with GI symptoms (abdominal pain, nausea, vomiting, diarrhea), but others may present with symptoms that can be attributed to depression or anorexia nervosa. In contrast to secondary AI, primary AI is often associated with lack of aldosterone as well as cortisol. Thus, signs of mineralocorticoid deficiency (salt craving, postural hypotension, electrolyte abnormalities) are usually indicative of primary AI. The most specific sign of primary AI is hyperpigmentation of the skin and mucosal surfaces, which results from the melanocyte-stimulating activity of β-lipotropin that derives from the same precursor as ACTH.

Table 35-11 Causes of Primary Adrenal Insufficiency

Autoimmune	Isolated adrenal insufficiency (Addison disease)
	Polyglandular autoimmune syndrome types I and II
Infectious	Tuberculosis
	Fungal
	Histoplasmosis
	Paracoccidioidomycosis
	HIV/AIDS
	Cytomegalovirus
	Syphilis
	African trypanosomiasis
Vascular	Bilateral adrenal hemorrhage
	Sepsis (Waterhouse-Friderichsen syndrome)
	Coagulopathy
	Thrombosis, embolism
	Infarction
Infiltrative	Metastatic carcinoma (most often lung, breast, stomach, or colon)
	Lymphoma
	Sarcoidosis
	Amyloidosis
	Hemochromatosis
Congenital	Congenital adrenal hyperplasia
	21α-Hydroxylase deficiency
	11β-Hydroxylase deficiency
	3β-ol-Dehydrogenase deficiency
	20,22-Desmolase deficiency
	Familial adrenocorticotropic hormone resistance syndromes
	Familial glucocorticoid deficiency
	Adrenoleukodystrophy
	Adrenomyeloneuropathy
	Adrenal hypoplasia
Iatrogenic	Bilateral adrenalectomy
	Anticoagulation therapy
	Drugs
	Adrenolytic: mitotane, aminoglutethimide, metyrapone, trilostane
	Other: ketoconazole, rifampin, etomidate, phenytoin, barbiturates, megestrol acetate

Patients with autoimmune adrenalitis present with vitiligo, Hashimoto thyroiditis (70% in APS II), type I diabetes, and pernicious anemia. Thinning or loss of pubic and axillary hair may occur in women as a result of lack of androgen production by the adrenal cortex. Both systolic and diastolic BP are usually reduced (systolic BP <110 mm Hg).

Acute (Primary) Adrenal Insufficiency. In critically ill patients, it is crucial to consider the possibility of adrenal insufficiency. AI should be suspected in the presence of unexplained catecholamine-resistant hypotension, especially if the patient has pallor, hyperpigmentation, vitiligo, scanty axillary and pubic hair, hyponatremia, or hyperkalemia. Furthermore, AI caused by adrenal hemorrhage and adrenal vein thrombosis should be considered in a severely ill patient with abdominal pain or rigidity, vomiting, confusion, and arterial hypotension. In acutely ill patients, a plasma cortisol level greater than 25 μg/dL rules out adrenal insufficiency, but a level in the normal range does not. Further testing may be required.

Laboratory Evaluation. Patients with adrenal insufficiency present with hyponatremia (frequent), hyperkalemia, acidosis, mild elevation of plasma creatinine concentrations, hypoglycemia, hypercalcemia (rare), mild normocytic anemia, lymphocytosis, and mild eosinophilia. In addition, hormone levels are useful in diagnosis. A random measurement of serum cortisol level is usually inadequate to assess adrenal function caused by the pulsatile and diurnal variation of cortisol secretion. However, a morning cortisol level (measured between 8 and 9 AM) of 3μg/dL or less indicates primary AI and obviates the need for further tests. A level of 19 μg/dL or greater rules AI out. Patients with levels between 3 and 19 μg/dL need further testing. If primary AI is suspected, basal ACTH and cortisol levels should be measured followed by a short ACTH stimulation test. For testing, synthetic ACTH (cosyntropin) is given intravenously or intramuscularly at 250 μg, and the serum cortisol level is measured 60 minutes after injection. A normal response to this test (cortisol ≥20 μg/dL) excludes primary AI. In patients with severe secondary AI, plasma cortisol increases little or not at all after the administration of cosyntropin because of adrenocortical atrophy.

Detection of adrenal cortex antibodies or 21-hydroxylase autoantibodies supports the diagnosis of autoimmune adrenalitis. Antibodies against other endocrine glands are common in patients with autoimmune AI, and evaluation might be warranted. However, the incidence of antiadrenal antibodies in serum from patients with normal adrenal function who have other autoimmune endocrine diseases is low (2%), with the exception of those with hypoparathyroidism (16%). Abdominal CT scan may be helpful if infection, hemorrhage, infiltration, or neoplastic disease is suspected.

Treatment. In chronic AI, any underlying cause, such as infection or malignancy, should be treated. Glucocorticoid replacement is usually required for symptomatic patients and is given in two or three daily doses with half to two thirds of the daily dose given in the morning to mimic the physiologic daily pattern of cortisol secretion. Hydrocortisone (15-25 mg) or cortisone acetate (25-37.5 mg) is preferred because of its mineralocorticoid action and shorter biological half-life, which prevents unfavorably high nighttime glucocorticoid activity. The goal is to use the smallest dose that relieves the patient's symptoms to prevent side effects from steroid use, such as weight gain and osteoporosis. Because a reliable marker of glucocorticoid action is lacking, clinical judgment and careful assessment of clinical signs and symptoms guide treatment.

In patients with primary AI, mineralocorticoid replacement is necessary and is attained by fludrocortisone, in a single daily dose of 0.05 to 0.2 mg, as a substitute for aldosterone. The dose can be adjusted based on measurements of BP, serum sodium and potassium, and renin activity (aiming at concentrations within the middle or upper normal range). All patients should carry a card or wear a bracelet or necklace with information on current treatment and recommendations in emergency situations. Patients should be advised to double or triple the dose of hydrocortisone temporarily when they have a febrile illness or injury. In addition, they should be given ampoules of glucocorticoid for self-injection or glucocorticoid suppositories to be used in case of vomiting.

Patients with ACTH deficiency should be treated with glucocorticoids, preferably hydrocortisone (i.e., the glucocorticoid that the adrenals produce). Hydrocortisone replacement, usually 10 to 12 mg/m^2, should be given orally as 20 to 30 mg/day divided into two doses with two thirds of the daily dose given in the morning and one third given in the early afternoon or evening (Coursin and Wood, 2002; Toogood and Stewart, 2008). Alternatively, prednisone is given at a total daily dosage of 5 to 7.5 mg/day in one to two doses. Clinical evaluation is the primary modality to assess the adequacy of cortisol replacement. It is important to increase the dose of hydrocortisone two- to threefold in time of illness and other stresses. All patients should carry medical alert tags or cards to identify the need for high-dose glucocorticoids in an emergency. Those with secondary adrenal insufficiency usually do not require mineralocorticoid replacement because ACTH is not essential for aldosterone secretion.

Secondary and Tertiary Adrenal Insufficiency

> **Key Points**
>
> - Secondary adrenal insufficiency results from ACTH deficiency and is often seen in panhypopituitarism or after chronic glucocorticoid excess.
> - Lack of production of CRH from the hypothalamus results in tertiary adrenal insufficiency.
> - In secondary adrenal insufficiency, mineralocorticoid production is maintained by the RAS. Thus, hyperkalemia is absent, but hyponatremia may occur as a result of loss of glucocorticoid effect on free-water clearance.
> - Low ACTH and cortisol levels suggest secondary or tertiary adrenal insufficiency.

Secondary adrenal insufficiency is defined as a deficiency of ACTH. Isolated ACTH deficiency is rare and may be congenital or caused by lymphocytic hypophysitis. Secondary AI more commonly occurs in the setting of panhypopituitarism from underlying causes such as pituitary or metastatic tumors, craniopharyngioma, infections (TB, histoplasmosis), infiltrative disease (sarcoidosis), head trauma, or postpartum pituitary necrosis (Sheehan syndrome). Chronic glucocorticoid excess, either exogenous (glucocorticoid treatment for >4 weeks) or endogenous (Cushing syndrome), causes secondary AI by prolonged suppression of the production of CRH. Tertiary adrenal insufficiency results from the lack of CRH production from the hypothalamus.

Clinical Presentation. Signs and symptoms are similar with those of primary AI, but electrolyte and fluid abnormalities or hypotensive symptoms are absent because the mineralocorticoid production is still maintained by the RAS. Hyperpigmentation is not seen. Menstrual dysfunction, headache and visual symptoms, hypothyroidism, and DI may be present as a result of panhypopituitarism (see Approach to Pituitary Diseases).

Laboratory Evaluation. Plasma cortisol and ACTH levels should be checked initially. Low ACTH (<5 pg/mL) and cortisol levels suggest secondary or tertiary adrenal insufficiency, and pituitary CT or MRI is indicated. The cosyntropin stimulation test may be helpful in identifying adrenal insufficiency. With an abnormal result, ACTH level may determine primary (high ACTH) versus secondary (normal or low ACTH) disease. However, in secondary AI, the ACTH stimulation test might not be abnormal because sufficient ACTH might be present to prevent adrenal gland atrophy. In these patients, CRH stimulation test can assess ACTH response. Secondary AI shows little or no increase in the ACTH or cortisol level throughout the test but in tertiary AI, the ACTH increases in an exaggerated fashion and remains elevated longer. The insulin tolerance test and the metyrapone test are also available but less commonly used to assess the integrity of the HPA axis by its response to hypoglycemia or inhibited cortisol synthesis, respectively.

Treatment. As described in primary AI, treatment of underlying disorders and glucocorticoid replacement are necessary in secondary and tertiary AI; however, mineralocorticoid replacement is not.

Isolated Aldosterone Deficiency

See eAppendix 35-3 online.

DISORDERS OF CORTICAL HYPERFUNCTION: HYPERCORTISOLISM

Cushing Syndrome

> **Key Points**
>
> - Cushing syndrome results from chronic exposure to excessive levels of glucocorticoids.
> - Cushing syndrome may be ACTH dependent (pituitary or ectopic tumors) or ACTH independent (adrenal or exogenous glucocorticoids).
> - Reddish purple striae, plethora, proximal muscle weakness, easy bruising, and unexplained osteoporosis are discriminatory symptoms.
> - CT or MRI of the adrenal glands may differentiate among the various types of ACTH-independent Cushing syndrome.

Cushing syndrome is a group of signs and symptoms that result from prolonged and inappropriately high exposure of tissue to glucocorticoids (Nieman et al., 2008). Excess cortisol production is the hallmark of endogenous Cushing syndrome and may result from excess ACTH secretion from the pituitary (Cushing disease) or from ectopic tumors secreting ACTH or CRH. ACTH-independent adrenal production of cortisol is caused by adrenocortical tumors or hyperplasias. However, the most common cause of Cushing syndrome is *iatrogenic* from exogenous glucocorticoid administration. Certain psychiatric disorders (anxiety, depression), poorly controlled diabetes, and alcoholism can be associated with mild hypercortisolism and may produce results suggestive of Cushing syndrome.

Clinical Presentation. Although Cushing syndrome might be easy to diagnose when full blown, the diagnosis can be challenging in mild cases. The spectrum of clinical presentation is broad. Some discriminatory symptoms include reddish purple striae, plethora, proximal muscle weakness, bruising without any obvious trauma, and unexplained osteoporosis. More often, patients present with features caused by cortisol excess such as obesity, depression, diabetes, hypertension, or menstrual irregularity. A dorsocervical fat pad (buffalo hump), facial and supraclavicular fullness, thin skin, peripheral edema, hirsutism or female balding, and poor skin healing are typically seen in Cushing syndrome. Children usually have slow growth, abnormal genital virilization, short stature, and pseudoprecocious or delayed puberty.

Laboratory Evaluation. Before the diagnosis of Cushing syndrome is considered, exogenous intake of glucocorticoids should be excluded. According to the 2008 Endocrine Society Clinical Practice Guidelines (Nieman et al., 2008), tests to be considered for diagnosis include urine free cortisol (UFC); a late-night salivary cortisol, 1-mg overnight DST; or the longer, low-dose DST (2mg/d for 48 h). UFC and salivary cortisol should be obtained at least twice. The diagnosis of Cushing syndrome is made if two test results are unequivocally abnormal. The diagnostic accuracy of other tests previously used, such as random cortisol levels, is too low to recommend them for testing (Figure 35-3).

The UFC provides an integrated assessment of cortisol secretion over 24 hours and measures the cortisol not bound to cortisol-binding globulin (CBG). Unlike serum cortisol, which measures both free and CBG-bound cortisol, UFC is not affected by conditions and medications that alter CBG. A 24-hour urine cortisol secretion or an overnight urine sample (10 PM to 8 AM) can be ordered in conjunction with urine creatinine to assure accuracy of the results. UFC reflects renal filtration, and values are significantly lower in patients with moderate to severe renal impairment. A patient can be assumed to have Cushing syndrome if basal urinary cortisol secretion is more than three times the upper limit of normal and one other test is abnormal. However, UFC may be normal in mild cases of Cushing syndrome, in which case salivary cortisol may be more useful.

Late-night salivary cortisol is usually measured at bedtime or between 11 PM and midnight because the loss of circadian rhythm, with absence of a late-night cortisol nadir, is a consistent biochemical abnormality in those with Cushing syndrome. The active free cortisol in the blood is in equilibrium with cortisol in the saliva, and the concentration of salivary cortisol does not appear to be affected by the rate of saliva production. Overall, in adults, the accuracy of the test is similar to that of UFC.

Various protocols have been used for the DST, but most commonly 1 mg of dexamethasone is given between 11 PM and midnight, and cortisol is measured between 8 AM and 9 AM the following morning. In patients with endogenous Cushing syndrome, a low dose of dexamethasone fails to suppress ACTH and cortisol secretion. A normal response is a serum cortisol of 5 µg/dL or less. To enhance DST sensitivity, experts have advocated requiring a lower cutoff for suppression of the serum cortisol to 1.8 µg/dL or less to achieve sensitivity rates greater than 95%.

Some endocrinologists prefer to use the 48-hour 2-mg/day, low-dose DST (LDDST) as an initial test because of its improved specificity compared with the 1-mg test. The LDDST may be helpful in conditions with overactivation of

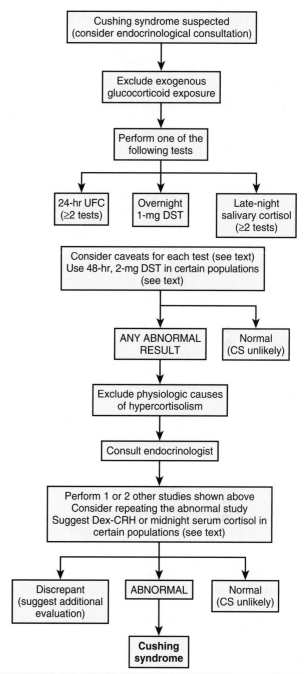

Figure 35-3 Clinical approach to a patient with suspected Cushing syndrome. *CS,* Cushing syndrome; *Dex-CRH,* dexamethasone/corticotropin-releasing hormone test; *DST,* dexamethasone suppression test; *UFC,* urine free cortisol. (Courtesy The Endocrine Society.)

the HPA axis but without true Cushing syndrome, such as in certain psychiatric disorders, obesity, and alcoholism. Dexamethasone is given in doses of 0.5 mg every 6 hours for 48 hours, beginning at 9 AM on day 1. Serum cortisol is measured at 9 AM on the second day 6 hours after the last dose of dexamethasone (Funder et al., 2008).

New studies have shown a link between baseline levels of ACTH and major depressive disorder. One study published in the *Journal of Affective Disorders* in 2013 using a combined dexamethasone suppression–CRH stimulation test found higher baseline levels of ACTH in patients with major depressive disorder compared with control participants (Sher et al., 2013). These results implied decreased feedback control of ACTH by circulating cortisol levels. The correlation between these finding is not known but may represent a new area for diagnosing and treating major depression. Additional testing is recommended for patients with initial abnormal or discordant results, such as the dexamethasone–CRH stimulation test or the midnight serum cortisol test. The dexamethasone–CRH stimulation test has been developed to improve the sensitivity of the LDDST. The administration of dexamethasone at a dose of 2 mg/day over 48 hours is followed by administration of CRH (1 µg/kg IV) 2 hours after the last dose of dexamethasone. Cortisol is measured 15 minutes later. ACTH and cortisol should increase after administration of CRH in patients with Cushing disease.

After hypersecretion of cortisol is confirmed, the next step is to determine whether the Cushing syndrome is ACTH dependent or independent. This is accomplished through measurement of the late-afternoon ACTH level when it is normally low. Cushing syndrome is ACTH *dependent* if plasma ACTH is greater than 10 pg/mL and ACTH *independent* if ACTH level is less than 5 pg/mL. For an intermediate ACTH level, further testing with the CRH stimulation test is performed. A rise in cortisol by 20% or in ACTH of at least 50% over baseline after administration of CRH is considered evidence for an ACTH-dependent lesion. In these patients, high-dose dexamethasone suppression test (HDDST), combined with cranial MRI studies, may help in localizing the site of ACTH overproduction. HDDST (2 mg of dexamethasone every 6 hours for 2 days) provides close to 100% specificity if the criterion used is suppression of urinary free cortisol by more than 90% and can differentiate Cushing disease from ectopic ACTH production. If the workup results are still equivocal or suggestive of ectopic ACTH production, inferior petrosal sampling is performed, obtaining ACTH samples from the periphery and petrosal sinuses simultaneously. A ratio of petrosal sinus to peripheral ACTH of 2 to 1 is diagnostic of a pituitary source and can be further used to localize the side of ACTH production from the pituitary gland. For patients with ACTH-independent lesions, abdominal CT or MRI may localize the site of the lesion.

Treatment. The treatment of Cushing syndrome depends on the cause. For endogenous disease, surgical resection of the causative tumor is indicated. The treatment of choice for Cushing disease is transsphenoidal hypophysectomy. Other treatment modalities include various forms of radiation therapy and pharmacologic inhibition of ACTH secretion.

Patients with adrenal adenomas are treated with unilateral adrenalectomy and have an excellent prognosis. These patients require glucocorticoid therapy both during and after surgery until the residual adrenal gland recovers. For patients with biopsy-proven adrenal carcinoma that is not amenable to surgery, mitotane is the treatment of choice. For ectopic ACTH syndrome, ideal treatment is the excision of identified benign tumors. However, for ectopic tumors that are unidentified or unresectable, medications that block steroidogenesis, such as ketoconazole, metyrapone, or aminoglutethimide, may be useful.

Aldosteronism

Key Points

- In primary aldosteronism (PA), secretion of aldosterone is inappropriately high and, when it is the result of an adrenal adenoma, it is relatively autonomous from renin–angiotensin secretion.
- Secondary aldosteronism is generally related to hypertension, and the aldosterone secretion is driven by high plasma renin.
- Patients present with hypokalemia and hypertension that may be resistant to treatment (Conn syndrome).
- The ratio of plasma aldosterone to renin is the most reliable test for screening for PA.
- A ratio of plasma aldosterone to renin of 20 or greater and a plasma aldosterone higher than 15 ng/dL support the diagnosis of primary hyperaldosteronism.

Background. Primary aldosteronism was first described by Jerome Conn in 1955 as a syndrome (Conn syndrome) characterized by hypertension and hypokalemia caused by an adrenal aldosterone-producing adenoma (APA). The secretion of aldosterone from the adrenal *zona glomerulosa* is regulated mainly by the RAS and by potassium anions. PA is now recognized to be the most common form of secondary hypertension. In PA, the secretion of aldosterone is inappropriately high, relatively autonomous from the RAS, and nonsuppressible by volume expansion or sodium loading. In secondary aldosteronism associated with hypertension, the aldosterone secretion is driven by high plasma renin and is suppressed by volume expansion.

Primary aldosteronism is commonly caused by an APA (35% of cases); unilateral or bilateral idiopathic adrenal hyperplasia (IHA) (2% and 60% of cases, respectively); an adrenal carcinoma (rare); or in rare cases, familial hyperaldosteronism (FH), either type I (glucocorticoid-remediable aldosteronism [GRA]) or type II (familial occurrence of APA, IHA, or both). There are two types of aldosteronomas: a corticotrophin-responsive (and renin-unresponsive) type and a renin-responsive type. PA had been previously described in fewer than 1% of patients with hypertension. However, recent studies estimate the prevalence of PA is 5% to 13% among hypertensive patients.

Clinical Presentation. Few symptoms are specific to the syndrome. Patients present with moderate to severe hypertension that may be resistant to usual pharmacologic treatments. Hypokalemia is usually present, and the serum sodium concentration tends to be high-normal or slightly above the upper limit of normal. Patients with marked hypokalemia may have muscle weakness and cramping, headaches, palpitations, polydipsia, polyuria, or nocturia (Funder et al., 2008). However, hypokalemia might be absent; thus, any patient with hypertension could be a candidate for this disorder. Patients with PA may be at higher risk than other patients with hypertension for target organ damage of the heart and kidney. A significantly higher rate of cardiovascular events (i.e., stroke, atrial fibrillation, and myocardial infarction [MI]) has been noted in patients with APA or IHA compared with patients matched for age, gender, and hypertension. Patients with APA have more severe hypertension, more frequent hypokalemia, and

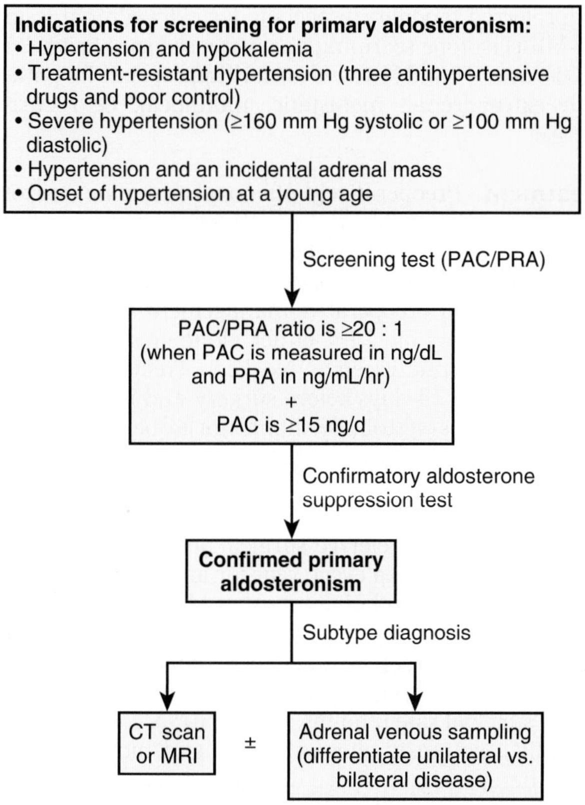

Indications for screening for primary aldosteronism:
- Hypertension and hypokalemia
- Treatment-resistant hypertension (three antihypertensive drugs and poor control)
- Severe hypertension (≥160 mm Hg systolic or ≥100 mm Hg diastolic)
- Hypertension and an incidental adrenal mass
- Onset of hypertension at a young age

↓ Screening test (PAC/PRA)

PAC/PRA ratio is ≥20 : 1 (when PAC is measured in ng/dL and PRA in ng/mL/hr) + PAC is ≥15 ng/d

↓ Confirmatory aldosterone suppression test

Confirmed primary aldosteronism

↓ Subtype diagnosis

CT scan or MRI ± Adrenal venous sampling (differentiate unilateral vs. bilateral disease)

Figure 35-4 Indications for screening for primary aldosteronism and flow chart for clinical assessment. *CT,* computed tomography; *MRI,* magnetic resonance imaging; *PAC,* plasma aldosterone concentration; *PRA,* plasma renin activity.

higher plasma and urinary levels of aldosterone and are younger (<50 years) than those with IHA.

Hypokalemia, when present, strongly suggests associated mineralocorticoid excess. However, most patients with PA have baseline blood levels of potassium in the normal range. Therefore, hypokalemia should not be the criterion used to make the diagnosis of PA. Screening for PA should be considered in patients with hypertension and hypokalemia, treatment-resistant hypertension (three antihypertensive drugs and poor control), severe hypertension (≥160 mm Hg systolic or ≥100 mm Hg diastolic), hypertension and an incidental adrenal mass, and onset of hypertension at a young age (Figure 35-4). When an evaluation for secondary hypertension is performed, the diagnosis of PA should also be considered. In patients with suspected PA, the screening can be accomplished by measuring a morning ambulatory paired random plasma aldosterone concentration (PAC) and plasma renin activity or concentration (PRA or PRC). This test can be performed while the patient is taking antihypertensive medications (except for spironolactone, eplerenone, and high-dose amiloride) and without posture stimulation. The aldosterone-to-renin ratio (ARR) is currently the most reliable available means of screening for PA. A test result is considered positive when the PAC/PRA ratio is 20:1 or greater (when PAC is measured in nanograms per deciliter and PRA in nanograms per deciliter per hour) and the PAC is higher than 15 ng/dL. All positive results should be followed by a confirmatory aldosterone suppression test to verify autonomous aldosterone production before treatment is initiated.

If the diagnosis of PA is confirmed, lateralization of the source of the excessive aldosterone secretion is critical to guide further management. All patients with PA should undergo an adrenal CT scan as the initial study in subtype testing and to exclude large masses that may represent adrenocortical carcinoma. MRI has no advantage over CT in subtype evaluation of PA. In patients with PA, adrenal venous sampling is the reference standard test to differentiate unilateral from bilateral disease. This is important because unilateral adrenalectomy in patients with APA or primary adrenal hyperplasia results in normalization of hypokalemia and improvement of hypertension in all patients and cure of hypertension in 30% to 60%. Glucocorticoid-remediable aldosteronism is an autosomal dominant disease and may be diagnosed by genetic testing.

Treatment. The treatment approach depends on the cause of PA. Unilateral laparoscopic adrenalectomy is an excellent treatment option for patients with APA or unilateral hyperplasia. BP control improves in almost 100% of these patients postoperatively, and the average long-term cure rates of hypertension after unilateral adrenalectomy for APA range from 30% to 72%. A potassium supplement or a mineralocorticoid receptor antagonist (or both) should be given preoperatively to correct the hypokalemia but should be discontinued postoperatively.

Medical management is recommended for patients with APA who do not undergo surgery and for those with IHA or GRA. Spironolactone has been the drug of choice for PA and is titrated to achieve BP control and normokalemia without the aid of oral potassium supplement. Eplerenone is a competitive and selective aldosterone receptor antagonist and may be used as an alternative agent. Compared with spironolactone, eplerenone has less antiandrogenic and progestational actions but is more expensive. In patients who are intolerant to aldosterone receptor antagonists, amiloride may be an alternative treatment that can reduce BP and normalize potassium levels, but it does not protect against the negative effects of aldosterone excess. Patients with IHA may be resistant to drug therapy caused by hypervolemia and may require a second antihypertensive agent such as a thiazide diuretic in combination with the aldosterone receptor antagonist.

DISORDERS OF HYPERFUNCTION: ADRENAL MEDULLA

Pheochromocytoma

Key Points

- Pheochromocytomas are catecholamine-secreting neuroendocrine tumors that originate in the adrenal medulla (80% to 85% of cases) or in any sympathetic ganglion (paragangliomas).
- Hypertension, tachycardia, pallor, palpitations, diaphoresis, and anxiety are common.
- Paroxysmal hypertension often occurs, even in normotensive persons, and may be severe and result in hypertensive emergencies.
- Plasma and urine catecholamines and metanephrines are measured to diagnose pheochromocytoma.
- CT, MRI, and iodine-123-meta-iodo-benzyl-guanidine (^{123}I-MIBG) may be helpful for tumor localization.

Pheochromocytomas are catecholamine-secreting neuroendocrine tumors arising from chromaffin cells of neural crest origin (Lenders et al., 2005). About 80% to 85% of pheochromocytomas originate in the adrenal medulla, and 15% to 20% are extraadrenal (paragangliomas). Pheochromocytomas are rare tumors with an incidence of one to two per 100,000 adults per year. Sporadic forms of pheochromocytoma are usually diagnosed in individuals age 40 to 50 years, but hereditary forms are diagnosed earlier, most often before age 40 years. The traditional "rule of 10" for pheochromocytomas (10% bilateral, 10% extraadrenal, 10% familial, 10% malignant) is now challenged by advances in diagnosis and genetics. Hereditary pheochromocytomas occur in MEN II, von Hippel-Lindau syndrome, neurofibromatosis type 1, and familial paragangliomas. Pheochromocytoma is rare in children but, when found, is often extraadrenal, multifocal, and associated with hereditary syndromes.

Clinical Presentation. Paroxysmal signs and symptoms due to the episodic secretion of catecholamines provide clues to the diagnosis of pheochromocytoma. The presentation can vary greatly, and therefore the pheochromocytoma is often referred to as the "great mimic." Anesthesia and tumor manipulation are the most well-known stimuli to elicit a catecholaminergic crisis. Hypertension, tachycardia, pallor, palpitations, diaphoresis, headache, and feelings of panic or anxiety are common. The hypertension is often paroxysmal and may occur in patients with hypertension or in normotensive persons. The hypertensive episodes can be severe, resulting in hypertensive emergencies. Persons with paragangliomas may have normal BP or hypotension. Orthostatic hypotension (a result of hypovolemia), fever, nausea, flushing, leukocytosis, and polycythemia are less common findings. Metabolic abnormalities may be present and include hyperglycemia, lactic acidosis, and weight loss.

Laboratory Evaluation. All patients with suspected pheochromocytoma should undergo biochemical testing. Traditional tests include measurements of urinary and plasma catecholamines, urinary metanephrines (normetanephrine and metanephrine), and urinary vanillylmandelic acid. Measurement of plasma-fractionated metanephrines (normetanephrine and metanephrine) is a newer test. Plasma and urine metanephrine measurements are the most sensitive tests for diagnosis but do not always indicate a pheochromocytoma. Many physiological stimuli (i.e., stress), drugs (e.g., phenoxybenzamine, tricyclic antidepressants), and clinical conditions (i.e., hyperthyroidism, heart failure, stroke) may cause an increase in circulating catecholamines and metabolites and lead to false-positive test results. The use of clonidine or glucagon to suppress catecholamine release from the sympathoadrenal system provides a dynamic pharmacologic test to distinguish increased catecholamine release caused by sympathetic activation from increased release caused by a pheochromocytoma.

If there is biochemical evidence for pheochromocytoma, tumor localization by CT scan of the entire abdomen (and pelvis), with and without contrast, should be performed. MRI with gadolinium has similar diagnostic sensitivity (90%-100%) and specificity (70%-80%) and is usually the preferred modality, especially for extraadrenal lesions. ^{123}I-MIBG isotope scanning has increased specificity (95%-100%) over CT and MRI and is more appropriate for patients with extraadrenal, metastatic, multifocal, or recurrent disease.

Treatment. Preoperatively, phenoxybenzamine, prazosin, doxazosin, or urapidil can be used for the blockade of the a-adrenoceptors. Phenoxybenzamine is often preferred because it blocks α-adrenoceptors noncompetitively. Alternative drugs for preoperative management are labetalol or calcium channel blockers, either alone or in combination with α-adrenergic receptor blockers. Treatment must be initiated 10 to 14 days before surgery and is titrated until mild orthostasis (systolic BP should not fall below 90 mm Hg in standing position) is present. Blockade of β-adrenoceptors should never be initiated before blockade of α-adrenoceptors. Laparoscopic removal of intra- and extraadrenal pheochromocytomas is the preferred surgical approach. All patients should be followed up every year for at least 10 years after surgery. BP and catecholamines should be monitored indefinitely in patients with extraadrenal or familial pheochromocytoma to detect possible recurrence. For malignant disease, radical surgical removal is recommended, but the 5-year survival rate remains poor (~50%). Treatment with ^{131}I-MIBG, cytotoxic chemotherapy, and molecularly targeted therapies have shown disappointing results.

MIXED DISORDER: CONGENITAL ADRENAL HYPERPLASIA

See eAppendix 35-4 online.

KEY TREATMENT

- In primary adrenal insufficiency, long-term glucocorticoid and mineralocorticoid replacement is necessary. The baseline steroid dose should be increased two- to threefold during periods of febrile illness or injury (Arlt and Allolio, 2003; Salvatori, 2005) (SOR: A).
- Therapeutic intervention for secondary and tertiary adrenal insufficiency requires treatment of underlying disorders. Glucocorticoid replacement is necessary (Arlt and Allolio, 2003) (SOR: A).
- Oral fludrocortisone (0.05-0.15 mg/day) is the treatment of choice for aldosterone deficiency. In hyporeninemic hypoaldosteronism, furosemide with reduced salt intake can ameliorate acidosis and hyperkalemia (Arlt and Allolio, 2003) (SOR: A).
- Surgical resection is usually the treatment of choice for Cushing disease and ACTH-independent Cushing syndrome (Nieman et al., 2008) (SOR: A).
- Treatment of aldosteronism is directed at the underlying cause. Aldosterone antagonists such as spironolactone are effective therapy (Funder et al., 2008) (SOR: A).
- Laparoscopic removal of intra- and extraadrenal pheochromocytomas after α-adrenoceptor blockade is the preferred treatment (Lenders et al., 2005 (SOR: A).
- Treatment of congenital adrenal hyperplasia with glucocorticoids may result in amelioration of symptoms (New, 2004, 2010) (SOR: A).

Ovarian and Testicular Disorders

Sexual development in both males and females is driven by the HPA. The normal process is the result of pulsatile release of GnRH from the hypothalamus, which stimulates the pituitary to release FSH and LH (GHRH and GH also play a role). Release of FSH and LH activates the ovaries and testes to produce estrogen and testosterone and is responsible for stimulation of gametogenesis. This process is assisted by conversion of adrenal androgens from the adrenal cortex into androstenedione and subsequently into potent androgens (testosterone) or estrogens (estradiol) in the peripheral tissues (see Adrenal Glands section). Errors can occur along this complex pathway, resulting in early sexual development (precocity), delayed sexual development (delayed menarche), errors of translation (male feminization syndrome), early loss of reproductive function (premature menopause), and inappropriate response to stimuli (polycystic ovary syndrome [PCOS])

NORMAL SEXUAL DEVELOPMENT

Sexual differentiation in humans is controlled by genetics (presence of Y chromosome determines development of testis and absence determines the development of ovary with additional X chromosome), environment (e.g., nutrition), and hormones (MacLaughlin and Donahoe, 2004). Congenital conditions associated with aberrations of chromosomal, gonadal, or anatomic sex development are called "disorders of sex development" (Houk et al., 2006).

In the postgonadal phase, hormones control external genitalia differentiation and secondary sexual development. Puberty refers to a physiological transition phase (>4 years long) between childhood and adulthood during which there is pubertal growth spurt and development of secondary sexual characteristics. Puberty is preceded by adrenarche (6-7 years in girls and 7-8 years in boys), marked by increasing amounts of adrenal androgens (DHEA, DHEA-S, and androstenedione). The growth spurt (a striking increase in growth velocity during puberty) is a complex hormonal phenomenon in which GH, thyroid hormones, and sex steroids play major roles. Gonadarche (the secretion of gonadal sex steroids) follows adrenarche and is initiated by activation of the GnRH pulse generator in the hypothalamus. These GnRH pulses result in increased gonadotropin secretion and subsequent production of sex hormones by the gonads.

Sexual maturation in females starts with breast development (thelarche) at a mean age of 11 years followed by pubic hair development and menses (menarche). In males, it starts with scrotal corrugation and testicular enlargement at a mean age of 11.5 years followed by growth of the penis and pubic hair.

In males, release of LH stimulates testicular Leydig cells to produce testosterone. FSH, in conjunction with testosterone, stimulates spermatogenesis. In females, FSH stimulates development of primary ovarian follicles and increases production of estrogen from ovarian granulosa cells. LH in females stimulates ovarian theca cells to produce androgens and the corpus luteum to synthesize progesterone. LH induces ovulation through the midcycle surge.

Estradiol production in males increases the bone age, BMD, and the rate of epiphyseal fusion. In females, it stimulates the development of the breasts, labia, vagina, and uterus and proliferation of endometrium. In addition, estradiol enhances development of and increase in the ducts of the breast and body fat. Whereas estrogen in low levels enhances linear growth, high levels increase the rate of fusion of epiphyses. Testosterone is responsible for the increase in muscle mass, sebaceous glands, and voice changes seen in pubertal males, and it is a linear growth accelerator. In females, testosterone accelerates linear growth and stimulates pubic and axillary hair development. Progesterone in females is responsible for development of a secretory endometrium and plays a role in breast development. Lineal growth and pubic hair development in both males and females is caused by androgens from the adrenal gland.

Figures 35-5 and 35-6 show normal pubertal developmental stages of Marshall and Tanner.

ABNORMAL PUBERTY

Key Points

- Evaluation should begin if signs of puberty develop in girls younger than 8 years or in boys younger than 9 years.
- Diagnoses of true puberty and pseudopuberty should be differentiated.
- Evaluation includes a comprehensive history and physical examination, growth chart, and wrist radiograph.
- If true puberty is suspected, consider cranial CT or MRI to rule out CNS lesions.

Evaluation of suspected abnormal puberty begins with obtaining a detailed history, including growth and development (timing of physical and developmental milestones), medical conditions, dietary history, social history, ethnicity, and family history. Physical examination should be thorough, including current weight, and a complete examination, with focused examination for development of secondary sexual characteristics and genitalia. A detailed growth chart from birth to the present day should be obtained. A radiograph of the left wrist is needed to estimate bone age (Blondell et al., 1999).

Precocious Puberty

Precocious puberty (premature onset of puberty) may be defined as the appearance of secondary sexual maturation at an early age. The age of onset of puberty before the age of 8 years in girls and before the age of 9 years in boys is considered precocious puberty. The Lawson Wilkins Pediatric Endocrine Society guidelines recommend that breast development or pubic hair in white girls before age 7 years and in black girls before age 6 years should be evaluated for precocious puberty. Boys of all races should be evaluated for precocious puberty with signs of secondary sexual development at 9 years of age or younger (Kaplowitz and Oberfield, 1999). These guidelines are under some debate as setting perhaps too early an age for defining

Tanner stage	Breasts*	Standard	Pubic hair*	Standard	Growth	Other
1	Prepubertal, elevation of papilla only	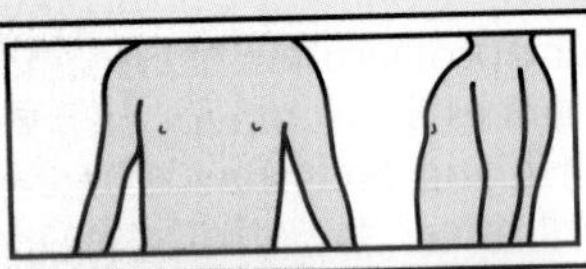	Prepubertal, villus hair only	—	Basal; about 5.0 to 6.0 cm (2.0 to 2.4 in) per year	Adrenarche Ovarian growth
2	Breast buds appear under enlarged areaolae (11.2 years)	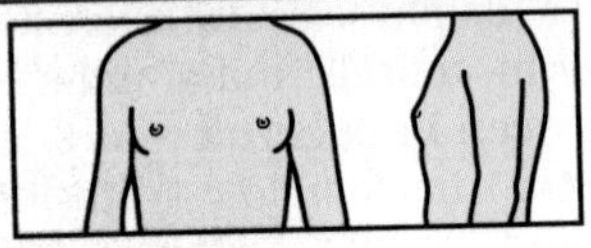	Sparse growth of slightly pigmented hair along the labia (11.9 years)	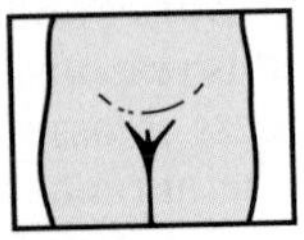	Accelerated: about 7.0 to 8.0 cm (2.8 to 3.2 in) per year	Clitoral enlargement Labia pigmentation Uterus enlargement
3	Breast tissue beyond areola without contour separation (12.4 years)	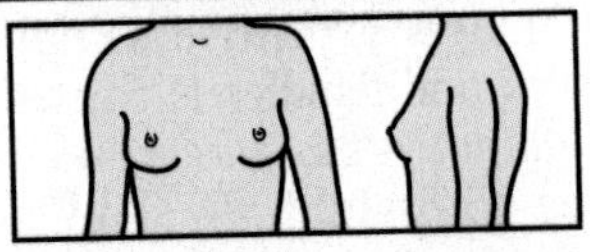	Hair is coarser, curled, and pigmented; spreads across the pubes (12.7 years)	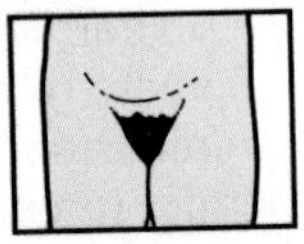	Peak velocity: about 8.0 cm (3.2 in) per year (12.5 years)	Axillary hair (13.1 years) Acne (13.2 years)
4	Projection of areola and papilla forms a secondary mound (13.1 years)	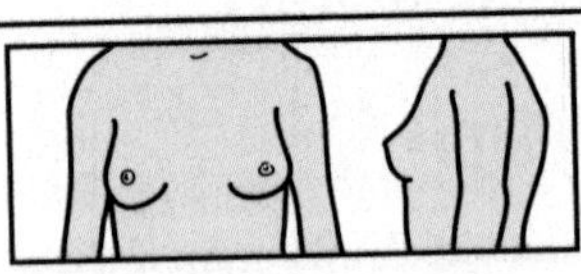	Adult-type hair but no spread to medial thigh (13.4 years)	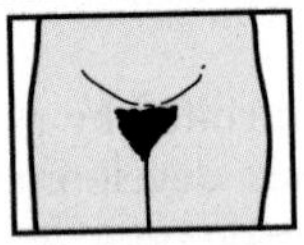	Deceleration: <7.0 cm (2.8 in) per year	Menarch (13.3 years) Regular menses (13.9 years)
5	Adult breast contour with projection of papilla only (14.5 years)	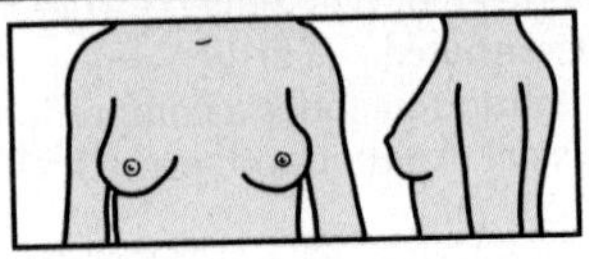	Adult-type hair with spread to medial thigh but not up linea alba (14.6 years)	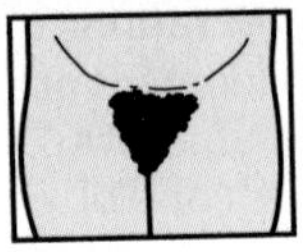	Cessation at about 16 years	Adult genitalia

*The Tanner stages of puberty in girls are based on breast size and shape and pubic hair distribution. Mean age of milestone attainment is shown in parentheses for the reference population of Marshall and Tanner. Actual age at milestone attainment may vary among individuals and among different study populations.

Figure 35-5 Pubertal milestones for girls. (From Blondell RD, Foster MB, Dave KC. Disorders of puberty. *Am Fam Physician*. 1999;60:209, 223.)

precocity. Some child endocrinologists believe that defining precocity as only children with sexual development younger than 7 years will lead to missing some conditions that may respond to early intervention; they prefer the formerly used age of younger than 8 years old in girls to trigger investigation (Carel and Léger, 2008; Midyett et al., 2003; Traggiai and Stanhope, 2003). Children with developmental disabilities have a higher incidence of precocity (Siddiqui et al., 1999). However, the majority of children (>75%) investigated for precocious puberty have benign diagnoses that are considered to be normal variations and do not require any treatment (Kaplowitz, 2004).

Precocious puberty is classified as *central* (GnRH dependent) or *peripheral* (non-GnRH dependent). The peripheral group includes autonomous gonadal activation, gonadal tumors with production of sex steroids, adrenal disorders, and exposure to exogenous agents with properties of sex steroids. Precocious puberty may be differentiated into *progressive* (one stage to next in 3-6 months) or *nonprogressive* (no progression of pubertal signs over time). Other terminology is based on the pubertal signs in relation to the individual's gender. *Isosexual* refers to precocity in the same gender (e.g., feminization of a female). *Heterosexual* (or contrasexual) would be precocious puberty resulting in virilization of a female.

Benign variants of precocious pubertal development (incomplete precocious puberty or variations in pubertal development) include nonprogressive precocious puberty, isolated precocious thelarche, isolated precocious pubarche, isolated menarche, and adolescent (male) gynecomastia. *Isolated thelarche* (unilateral or bilateral breast development) without progression of other signs of puberty generally resolves spontaneously, especially in girls younger than 2 years and requires no treatment. *Isolated precocious pubarche* (pubic hair development) as a result of early adrenarche is usually self-limited. Evaluation beyond a complete history, physical examination, and bone age determination would include an ACTH stimulation test to rule out late-onset congenital adrenal hyperplasia. *Gynecomastia* in adolescent males is common and presents more of a social than a

Tanner stage	Standard	Genitalia*	Pubic hair*	Growth	Other
1	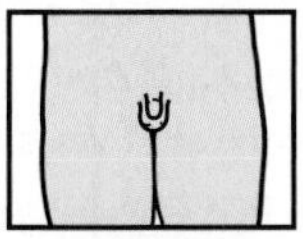	Prepubertal testes: <2.5 cm (1.0 in)	Prepubertal, villus hair only	Basal: about 5.0 to 6.0 cm (2.0 to 2.4 in) per year	Adrenarche
2	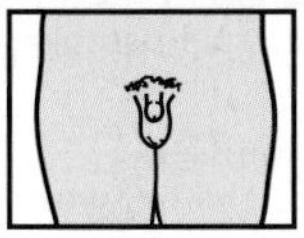	Thinning and reddening of scrotum (11.9 years) Testes: 2.5 to 3.2 cm (1.0 to 1.28 in)	Sparse growth of slightly pigmented hair at base of penis (12.3 years)	Basal: about 5.0 to 6.0 cm (2.0 to 2.4 in) per year	Decrease in total body fat
3	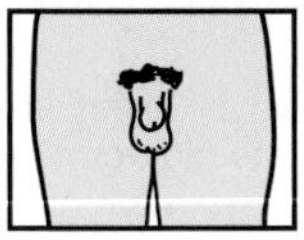	Growth of penis, especially length (13.2 years) Testes: 3.3 to 4.0 cm (1.32 to 1.6 in)	Thicker, curlier hair spreads to the mons pubis (13.9 years)	Accelerated: about 7.0 to 8.0 cm (2.8 to 3.2 in) per year	Gynecomastia (13.2 years) Voice breaks (13.5 years) Muscle mass increases
4	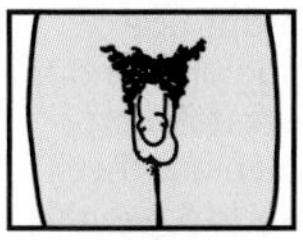	Growth of penis and glands, darkening of scrotum (14.3 years) Testes: 4.1 to 4.5 cm (1.64 to 1.8 in)	Adult-type hair but no spread to medial thigh (14.7 years)	Peak velocity: about 10.0 cm (4.0 in) per year (13.8 years)	Axillary hair (14.0 years) Voice change (14.1 years) Acne (14.3 years)
5	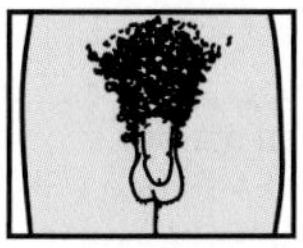	Adult genitalia (15.1 years) Testes: >4.5 cm (1.8 in)	Adult-type hair with spread to medial thigh but not up linea alba (15.3 years)	Deceleration and cessation (about 17 years)	Facial hair (14.9 years) Muscle mass continues to increase after stage 5

*The Tanner stages of puberty in boys are based on the development of the genitalia and pubic hair distribution. Mean age of milestone attainment is shown in parentheses for the reference population of Marshall and Tanner. Actual age at milestone attainment may vary among individuals and among different study populations.

Figure 35-6 Pubertal milestones for boys. (From Blondell RD, Foster MB, Dave KC. Disorders of puberty. *Am Fam Physician*. 1999;60:209, 223.)

physical problem. Careful explanation and reassurance for the child and parent that this is a self-limited condition is the best approach.

Accidental precocity occasionally results from unusual dietary habits or inappropriate use of medications (estrogen creams). A careful review for these, early in the evaluation, is helpful.

Central (GnRH-Dependent) Precocious Puberty. Central (or true) precocious puberty is caused by early activation of hypothalamic GnRH secretion. Most patients have no identifiable cause, and the precocity is labeled as "idiopathic." Initial evaluation begins with history, examination, growth chart, and wrist radiographs. Morning testosterone levels are useful in boys, and GnRH-agonist stimulation tests are helpful in females to identify a central etiology. A wide variety of CNS lesions are known to cause central isosexual precocity, so cranial CT or MRI is indicated to rule out these pathologies. An underlying CNS disorder is not unusual in boys presenting with precocious puberty. Treatment is focused on managing the underlying cause. GnRH analogues that reversibly inhibit gonadotropin secretion can be used to prevent secondary sexual development and early epiphyseal fusion that occurs in children who are

very young at the onset of puberty, especially when it progresses rapidly (Carel et al., 2004). The optimal age to discontinue therapy is 11 years. When therapy is discontinued, puberty commences normally. There is a slowly progressive form of central isosexual precocity in which no height is lost. These patients may be considered for a nontherapeutic approach with careful observation (Palmert et al., 1999) (Table 35-12).

In many studies, the most common causes of precocity are benign and need no treatment. Detailed evaluation with hormonal studies and imaging may be reserved for patients with severe symptoms and signs (Kaplowitz, 2004, 2005; de Vries and Phillip, 2005).

KEY TREATMENT

- Common causes of precocity are benign and require no treatment. Careful nontherapeutic observation may be considered (Carel et al., 2004) (SOR: A).
- Treatment of precocity with GnRH analogues, which reversibly inhibit gonadotropin secretion, can be used to prevent secondary sexual development and early epiphyseal fusion (Carel et al., 2004) (SOR: A).

Table 35-12   Precocious Puberty: Types, Causes, and Treatment

Etiology	Symptoms	Tests and Treatment
CENTRAL PRECOCITY*		
Idiopathic	Development of secondary sexual characteristics	GnRH analogues Discontinue at 11 years
CNS lesions (including congenital defects): hamartomas, tumors, infection, trauma, radiation, after androgen exposure, craniopharyngioma, others	History of trauma Medical history Headache, visual changes possible	FSH, LH, prolactin, sex steroids, TSH MRI of brain Treatment per pathology
Primary hypothyroidism	Signs of hypothyroidism without increase in growth velocity	Thyroid profile Treatment with thyroxine
INCOMPLETE ISOSEXUAL PRECOCITY		
Females: Isolated precocious thelarche	Breast enlargement without other secondary sexual changes	Most cases are benign
Females: Isolated precocious adrenarche	Pubic hair development, adult odor, acne	DHEA may be increased Adrenal steroid hormones and sex hormones: normal ACTH stimulation test to exclude CAH Usually benign; no treatment needed
Females: Isolated precocious menarche	Menarche precedes breast development or appearance of pubic hair	Normal bone age Ultrasonography: normal pelvis with prepubertal uterus Usually benign; check for abuse and ovarian and genital pathology
Females: Estrogen-secreting tumors of ovary or adrenal glands Ovarian cysts	Abdominal symptoms Signs of precocious puberty	CT or MRI in addition to hormonal tests Treat as per pathology
Females and males: McCune-Albright syndrome	Autonomous hyperfunction of gonads; rapid development of precocity Café au lait spots, fibrous dysplasia	Ultrasonography or CT of abdomen: large ovarian masses LFTs, DHEA sulfate, TSH, phosphate, cortisol
Males: Gonadotropin-secreting tumors; excessive androgen production Testicular or adrenal tumors Virilizing CAH Premature Leydig and germinal cell maturation	Excessive virilization Enlargement of testis (unilateral)	CT or MRI of abdomen Ultrasonography Hormonal tests Treat per pathology Surgery may be indicated
Males and females: Iatrogenic	History of using sex steroids and related products	Stop causative agent
CONTRASEXUAL PRECOCITY (ISOLATED VIRILIZATION)		
Isolated Precocious Adrenarche		
Females: Virilizing CAH, androgen-secreting ovarian or adrenal neoplasm, Cushing syndrome, glucocorticoid resistance, arrhenoblastoma	Prepubertal masculinization	Tests for CAH Cortisol Testosterone MRI of abdomen and pelvis Treat per pathology
Males: Estrogen-secreting tumor, chorionepithelioma; increased extraglandular aromatization of adrenal steroids causing increased extraglandular estrogen production and unusual CAH variations	Prepubertal feminization in boys is rare	Tests for CAH Cortisol and estrogen levels Testosterone MRI of abdomen and pelvis Treat per pathology
Iatrogenic	History of using sex steroids and related products	Stop causative agent
Nonprogressive precocious puberty	Stabilization of precocity Normal bone age	Normal bone age Ultrasonography: normal pelvis with prepubertal uterus

*True precocious puberty: gonadotropin dependent.
ACTH, Adrenocorticotropic hormone; *CAH,* congenital adrenal hyperplasia; *CNS,* central nervous system; *CT,* computed tomography; *DHEA,* dehydroepiandrosterone; *FSH,* follicle-stimulating hormone; *GnRH,* gonadotropin-releasing hormone; *LFT,* liver function test; *LH,* luteinizing hormone; *MRI,* magnetic resonance imaging; *TSH,* thyroid-stimulating hormone.
Modified from Carel JC, Léger J. Precocious puberty. *N Engl J Med.* 2008;358(22):2366-2377.

DELAYED PUBERTY

Key Points

- Lack of thelarche (breast development) by the age of 12 years in girls or lack of testicular enlargement by the age of 14 years in boys indicates delayed puberty.

- Whereas constitutional delay is characterized by delayed but spontaneous onset of puberty, organic delay is caused by gonadal, pituitary, or central dysfunction.

Delayed puberty in girls is defined as lack of thelarche by age 12 years or duration between thelarche and menarche longer than 5 years (age 17 years). In boys, delayed puberty is defined as no testicular enlargement by age 14 years with more than 5 years between initial and complete development of the genitalia (age 19 years). Delayed puberty in both males and females is classified as *constitutional* (idiopathic) or *organic* (gonadal, pituitary, or central cause). A retrospective study of 232 male and female patients with delayed puberty revealed that the majority (53%) had constitutional delay of growth and maturation, with much higher incidence in males (63%) compared with females (30%). The remaining 47% of the total 232 patients had mixed etiologies; 19% had functional HH, 12% had permanent HH, 13% had permanent hypergonadotropic hypogonadism, and there was no clear etiology for the remaining 3% (Sedlmeyer and Palmert, 2002).

Constitutional delay is characterized by physiologic delay but subsequent spontaneous onset of puberty, and it is a diagnosis of exclusion. The cause is a delay in GnRH pulse generation, with low levels of gonadotropins. Height and weight in these children tend to be below the fifth percentile, but most catch up during adolescence, reaching normal adult height and weight. Family history may reveal similar delays of puberty in one or both parents, which can be reassuring for the child and parent. Values for FSH, LH, DHEA-S, prolactin, testosterone, and estradiol levels will be consistent with prepubertal values until onset of puberty and normal sexual maturation.

The two common causes of delayed puberty from organic etiologies are pituitary dysfunction and HH. Panhypopituitarism in children may present as delayed puberty, but it would occur in conjunction with growth failure, secondary hypothyroidism, and adrenal insufficiency. Differentiation of organic forms of delay from constitutional delay may be difficult to establish in certain patients, requiring a series of observations and testing (no single study or imaging technique will differentiate these). HH presents with low levels of FSH and LH as a result of defective GnRH pulsation. Causes include anorexia nervosa, excessive weight loss, extreme exercise (cross country runners), tumors, head trauma, infiltrative processes, infection, and radiation. *Hypergonadotropic* hypogonadism is usually caused by gonadal failure and presents with high levels of gonadotropins and low levels of sex steroids (Table 35-13).

Evaluation of delayed puberty, as with all evaluations for abnormal sexual development, begins with a detailed history focusing on growth patterns, presence of any secondary sexual development, diet, exercise habits, congenital abnormalities, neurologic symptoms, and family history. Physical examination includes a thorough search for early signs of sexual maturation using Tanner staging. Measurement of arm span in relation to height is helpful in growth assessment. Arm span that exceeds height more than 5 cm is consistent with adult configuration. When this is present in children, it may mean delayed epiphyseal closure caused by hypogonadism. Wrist radiography is useful to determine bone age. Initial laboratory screening should include complete blood cell count, erythrocyte sedimentation rate, and liver function tests. Serum FSH, LH, estradiol, and testosterone levels can distinguish between primary and secondary hypogonadism. In primary hypogonadism (ovarian and testicular failure), serum gonadotropin levels are elevated. In patients with constitutional delay

Table 35-13 Causes of Hypogonadotropic Hypogonadism

CONGENITAL	
Isolated gonadotropin deficiency	Idiopathic HH
	Kallmann syndrome
	Non–X-linked
	Partial HH (fertile eunuch syndrome)
Associated with CNS disorders	Prader-Willi syndrome
	Laurence-Moon-Biedl syndrome
	Möbius syndrome
	Lowe syndrome
	Noonan syndrome
	LEOPARD syndrome
	X-linked ichthyosis
	Genetic defects
	GnRH receptor gene mutations
	FGFR1
	GPR54
	Adrenal hypoplasia, congenital
	Multiple pituitary hormone deficiency
ACQUIRED	
Organic lesions	Tumors
	Craniopharyngiomas
	Pituitary adenomas (e.g., prolactinoma, nonfunctioning tumor)
	Meningioma
	Pituitary apoplexy
	Infiltrative disorders
	Sarcoidosis, hemochromatosis
	Histiocytosis X
	Head trauma
	Leydig cell tumors, choriocarcinoma
	CNS radiation therapy
Systemic disorders affecting HPT axis	Critical illness, including burns
	Extreme exercise
	Malnutrition (anorexia nervosa)
	Morbid obesity
	Anabolic steroid abuse
	Glucocorticoid excess (endogenous: Cushing syndrome; exogenous)
	Narcotics

CNS, Central nervous system; *GnRH,* gonadotropin-releasing hormone; *HH,* hypogonadotropic hypogonadism; *HPT,* hypothalamic–pituitary–testicular; *LEOPARD,* lentigines, electrocardiographic defects, optic hypertelorism, pulmonary stenosis, abnormalities of genitalia, retarded growth, deafness.
From Allan CA, McLachlan RI. Androgen deficiency disorders. In DeGroot LJ, Jameson, JL, eds. *Endocrinology.* 5th ed, vol 3. Philadelphia: Saunders; 2006.

of puberty and congenital GnRH deficiency, serum gonadotropin levels are low. Prolactin, TSH, adrenal androgens, and karyotype (to rule out Turner, Klinefelter, and Noonan syndromes) should be evaluated if the clinical presentation warrants.

Therapy for delayed puberty is targeted at the underlying disorder, if identified. If the cause is unknown, observation with reassurance and psychosocial support and reevaluation after 4 to 6 months is an option. Hormonal therapy with estrogen (girls older than 12 years) or testosterone (boys older than 14 years) is an option. Short-term use of exogenous hormones does not appear to have long-term sequelae, except for the potential effect on skeletal maturation, which might result in failure to achieve potential adult height. In females taking estrogen replacement therapy, progestins should be added to the regimen after breakthrough bleeding occurs or after 1 year of therapy.

PROBLEMS OF THE TESTICLE AND OTHER MALE ENDOCRINE ISSUES

Male Hypogonadism

Male hypogonadism is defined as "inadequate gonadal function" manifested by deficiency in gametogenesis or secretion of gonadal hormones. Primary hypogonadism is caused by dysfunction in the testes from either chromosomal or acquired disorders (Table 35-13). Secondary hypogonadism is caused by an abnormality of the HPA. Males may present with infertility, decreased testicular size, changes in libido, impotency, gynecomastia, delayed puberty, or a combination of these (Swerdloff and Wang, 2004).

Diagnosis. The clinical diagnosis begins with history, including information about sexual developmental milestones, current symptoms, ambiguous genitalia at birth, cryptorchidism, behavioral abnormalities, anosmia, surgeries, sexually transmitted diseases (STDs), and medications. The history should include the presence of acute and chronic medical conditions and neurologic symptoms. The physical examination is directed toward sexual characteristics, body habitus, gynecomastia, and signs of hypogonadism. The testes should be measured for length and width with an orchidometer. Consistency of the testes should be noted and a scrotal examination done for the presence of varicocele. A nonpalpable prostate may imply testosterone deficiency. A low morning (8-10 AM) serum testosterone level is suggestive of hypogonadism. Serum LH and FSH levels are elevated in primary hypogonadism and normal to low in secondary hypogonadism. Semen analysis assesses the capability of spermatogenesis. An increase in sex hormone–binding globulin (SHBG) may imply hyperthyroidism, severe androgen deficiency, liver disease, or estrogen excess. A low level of SHBG may indicate hypothyroidism, PCOS, obesity, or acromegaly. The prolactin level should be measured to identify a prolactinoma followed by CT or MRI if the level is elevated. Other studies, such as BMD; pituitary imaging; genetic studies; and, in some cases, testicular biopsy may be indicated.

Two congenital conditions causing hypogonadism are Klinefelter syndrome and Kallmann syndrome. Klinefelter syndrome is the most common genetic cause of male infertility caused by hypogonadism. It is caused by a chromosomal aberration, most often 47,XXY. Phenotypic males can present with small, firm testicles; infertility; tall height; long legs; gynecomastia; and varying symptoms of androgen deficiency and undervirilization. Kallmann syndrome is an inherited disorder (see Approach to Pituitary Diseases [Hypopituitarism]). The most common form is isolated gonadotropin deficiency caused by defective GnRH secretion from the hypothalamus. Patients with Kallmann syndrome usually come to medical attention because of delayed puberty or incomplete sexual development. Anosmia or hyposmia is present in 80% of patients and establishes the diagnosis of Kallmann syndrome in those with isolated gonadotropin deficiency.

Requests to measure serum testosterone have become common in primary care. The increased interest in this disorder has been brought about by a number of things. First, and perhaps most important, is access to information. For example, if one enters "male hypogonadism" in Google, there are more than 300,000 results. It is common now for a patient to present with a list of symptoms and Internet data supporting his belief that he has a problem. In addition, there are now a wide variety of pharmacologic options available, including testosterone injections, topical gels, and oral medications. Added to this is the plethora of over-the-counter preparations on the market which are touted to increase testosterone. In addition, there are growing numbers of articles in the scientific literature (albeit perhaps not totally objective) supporting hypogonadism as a disorder causing significant morbidity that requires therapeutic intervention (Dandona and Rosenberg, 2010).

Laboratory Evaluation. To start the discussion of laboratory evaluation, it is important to understand that a low serum testosterone level does not, by itself, provide a diagnosis of hypogonadism. Whether or not a low level represents a pathologic condition or is merely a laboratory phenomenon is not clear cut. An article published in the *American Family Physician* (2006) provides a very good review of this topic, and one of its main points is that in the absence of specific symptoms or physical findings, there is no clearly agreed upon normal testosterone level for defining hypogonadism (Margo and Winn, 2006). Generally accepted normal values for total serum testosterone are 300 to 1000 ng/dL, but when hypogonadism becomes a real physiologic condition is unclear. The level most often used for defining hypogonadism is 200 ng/dL, which is the level set by the AACE in its 2002 guidelines (update). But data clearly defining this level as a pathologic state are lacking (AACE, 2002).

When a low serum total testosterone level is obtained, it is necessary to verify that this does represent a pathologic condition before any consideration of therapeutic intervention can be entertained. Specific testing to evaluate a low testosterone level includes a repeat total serum testosterone and FSH. Some experts recommend that the serum testosterone be checked in the early morning (8-10 AM). Although this does improve reproducibility, it must be remembered that pituitary gonadotrophs are released in surges so limiting collection of serum testosterone to a specific time of day is not a guarantee that the results represent actual 24-hour circulating levels.

If the second testosterone level is low and the FSH level is normal or elevated, a free testosterone level is obtained (reference range, 9-30 ng/dL). If the free serum testosterone level is low, then there is good evidence to support a diagnosis of primary hypogonadism. To further document this assumption, LH and prolactin levels are obtained (see Approach to Pituitary Diseases [Clinical Manifestations]). These tests are sufficient to determine if the testosterone level is truly low and whether it is due to testicular failure (primary) or failure somewhere along the HPA (secondary). Further workup, if any, is determined by these results.

Screening. There are clear instances in which hypogonadism is a defined entity (i.e., secondary to pituitary failure, congenital hypogonadism, premature aging of the testes, testicular cancer, intraabdominal cryptorchidism). In these patients, screening of testosterone is warranted. But in the primary care setting, the large majority of patients interested in testing their serum testosterone level are concerned about decreased libido, strength, and stamina; loss of muscle mass (sarcopenia); increasing truncal obesity; frailty; and overall lethargy in the absence of specific common diseases and etiologies.

Data in support of screening for hypogonadism are lacking. At the present time, there are insufficient data to determine if male hypogonadism is increasing in the population or is only a phenomenon of more access to laboratory testing. So, when is it appropriate to screen for hypogonadism? One is male infertility. Screening testosterone is part of an infertility workup given appropriate history or physical findings. The American Urologic Association's (AUA's) position on endocrine testing in evaluating male infertility is discussed in its publication *The Optimal Evaluation of the Infertile Male: AUA Best Practice Statement* (Jarow et al., 2010). The AUA recommends endocrine testing when there is an abnormal semen analysis, with impaired sexual function, or with other clinical findings suggestive of endocrinopathy.

Other reasons to screen for low testosterone include clearly identified physical signs of decreased testosterone such as lack of facial hair, sparse or lacking pubic hair, atrophic testes, or clinical evidence of pituitary dysfunction. After these, however, screening for hypogonadism is not recommended. As occurs with other conditions in which screening provides a very low yield ("n" to diagnose), screening for low testosterone is not justified.

Testosterone Replacement Therapy (Risk versus Benefit)

When presented with a below published normal total serum testosterone, especially when definitive physical findings are absent, it is essential to try and provide a precise cause before therapeutic intervention is initiated. Once a diagnosis of hypogonadism is confirmed and categorized as either primary or secondary, then consideration for hormone replacement can begin. But, before moving on to treatment, it is necessary to discuss risk versus benefit. This is especially true when the patient is elderly and/or has other disease processes that could be aggravated by testosterone therapy.

Recent data published in the *Journal of the American Medical Association* (November 2013) report on the incidence of mortality, MI, and stroke in men with low total serum testosterone levels (<300 ng/dL) who receive replacement therapy ($n = 1223$). When those treated with testosterone replacement were compared with those who did not receive exogenous testosterone ($n = 7486$), there was a statistically significant difference in outcomes for the two groups. The group receiving replacement therapy had a 25.7% higher event (death, MI, stroke) level compared with an event level of 19.9% in the untreated group (an absolute risk difference of 5.8%) (Vigen et al., 2013).

A meta-analysis by a group from University of Hong Kong had results similar to those above, although their analysis of risk was reported as odds ratio (OR) instead of relative or absolute risk. In their review of 27 trials, testosterone therapy increased risk of cardiovascular events to an OR of 1.54 (with OR of 0.0 being no difference). There was, however, an unexpected finding in their analysis. The OR for each individual study varied depending on funding source for the study. Whereas studies funded by pharmaceutical industry had an OR of 0.89, studies funded by other entities (nonpharmaceutical) had an OR of 2.06. The conclusion was that "Appropriately prescribed testosterone is undoubtedly beneficial. However, caution needs to be exercised to ensure that the associated health benefits of testosterone therapy outweigh the potential increased risk of cardiovascular-related events, particularly in older men when cardiovascular disease is common" (Xu et al., 2013).

Treatment. Once a definitive diagnosis of hypogonadism is made, referral to an endocrinologist for management is certainly appropriate. However, if the cause is definitely primary hypogonadism, and the risk to benefit analysis has been completed, initiation of treatment and ongoing management can be done by the primary care physician.

In some cases, such as Klinefelter and Kallmann syndromes, hormone replacement is aimed at specific end points. In Klinefelter syndrome, treatment is directed to preventing the sequelae of androgen deficiency. For Kallmann syndrome, treatment is directed at virilization by the administration of testosterone. In both of these, the primary care physician may want to refer to an endocrinologist, at least for initiation of therapy. This may also be the best choice for secondary hypogonadism when restoration of fertility is the goal. In these cases, gonadotropin replacement or human chorionic gonadotropin therapy is required. If the defect is in the hypothalamus, GnRH is the treatment of choice.

In primary hypogonadism, testosterone replacement is the treatment of choice. Many preparations are now available for testosterone replacement (Mooradian and Korenman, 2006). The currently used injectable testosterone esters, such as testosterone enanthate or testosterone cypionate, act similarly. The usual replacement dose is 200 mg intramuscularly every 2 weeks. In older men, it may be prudent to start at 50 to 75 mg weekly. Testosterone undecanoate is available as an oral preparation that does not have hepatotoxicity; however, because of its short half-life, it must be taken three times daily. Transdermal preparations can be given as patches or gels. Some androgen skin patches are associated with a high incidence of skin reactions. The commercially available transdermal gel preparations (Androgel 1% or 1.62%, Testim 1%, Fortesta 2%, and Axiron 2%) are applied over the trunk of the body daily (Mooradian and Korenman, 2006). Subcutaneous pellets, sublingual preparations, and buccal preparations of testosterone are also available for replacement therapy (Mooradian and Korenman, 2006).

Side effects of testosterone replacement should be monitored carefully. Digital rectal examinations, hematocrit (Hct), and prostate-specific antigen (PSA) should be measured at 3, 6, and 12 months of follow-up and then annually or semiannually (preferable). Bone density measurements should be obtained at baseline and, if low, at 2-year intervals to monitor improvement. In addition to monitoring clinical response, serum testosterone levels should be measured with the goal of achieving a midnormal range midway between injections of testosterone enanthate or cypionate, at 3 to 10 hours after application of a testosterone patch, or at any time after application of a testosterone gel.

Absolute contraindications to testosterone therapy currently are history of prostate or breast cancer, Hct of 55%

or greater, elevated PSA level that has not been completely investigated by a qualified urologist, or sensitivity to ingredients of the testosterone preparation (Mooradian and Korenman, 2006). There are currently no data to suggest testosterone replacement aggravates subclinical prostatic cancer.

Relative contraindications include obstructive sleep apnea, CHF, obstructive symptoms of prostatic hyperplasia, and Hct of 52% or greater. Patients with hyperlipidemia, atherosclerotic vascular disease, diabetes, and morbid obesity should be treated with caution and careful follow-up.

Cryptorchidism

See eAppendix 35-5 online.

Male Infertility

Infertility is defined as failure to achieve pregnancy after 1 year of unprotected intercourse. A specific cause can be identified in approximately 80% of couples, one third of which are female factors alone, one third male factors alone, and one third a combination of both. Unexplained infertility, in which no specific cause can be identified, occurs in approximately 20% of infertile couples. The initial step in evaluation of the male is a thorough medical history, focusing on general health, erectile function, STD history, medications, surgical history, previous successful pregnancy, contraception use, drug or alcohol use, and family history of genetic diseases. The first, and often only, test needed in evaluating male factors is semen analysis. If two consecutive analyses indicate oligospermia or azoospermia, ordering blood tests for testosterone, LH, FSH, and prolactin levels is warranted. *Varicocele* is the most common cause of male infertility (Griffin and Wilson, 2003) (Table 35-14).

Management consists of treating the underlying infection with appropriate antibiotics, varicocelectomy, appropriate counseling about environmental factors, and referral to an infertility specialist for more extensive therapy (Frey and Patel, 2004).

Table 35-14 Common Diagnoses in Men Evaluated for Infertility

Diagnostic Category	Incidence (%)
Idiopathic infertility	50-60
Primary testicular failure (chromosomal disorders, including Klinefelter syndrome, Y chromosome microdeletions, undescended testis, irradiation, orchitis, drugs)	10-20
Genital tract obstruction (congenital absence of vas, vasectomy, epididymal obstruction)	5
Coital disorders	<1
Hypogonadotropic hypogonadism (pituitary adenomas, panhypopituitarism, idiopathic hypogonadotropic hypogonadism, hyperprolactinemia)	3-4
Varicocele	15-35
Other (sperm autoimmunity, drugs, toxins, systemic illness)	5

From Griffin JE, Wilson JD. Disorders of the testes and the male reproductive tract. In Larsen PR, Kronenberg HM, Melmed S, Polonsky KS, eds. *Williams' textbook of endocrinology.* 10th ed. Philadelphia: Saunders; 2003.

Gynecomastia

> ### Key Point
>
> ■ Although breast cancer is an uncommon cause of breast enlargement in men, this diagnosis must be ruled out because the prognosis is worse for men diagnosed with breast cancer than for women.

Gynecomastia refers to a benign enlargement of the male breast resulting from proliferation of breast glandular tissue. When the male breast is enlarged from adipose tissue, it is called *lipomastia* or *pseudogynecomastia* and is not caused by proliferation of breast tissue. Gynecomastia can be unilateral, bilateral, or asymmetric. Any palpable breast tissue in men is abnormal except for three physiologic situations: transient gynecomastia of the newborn (caused by maternal or placental estrogens), pubertal gynecomastia (observed in 40%-70% of adolescent boys, resolving by 18 years of age), and gynecomastia that occasionally occurs in older adult men (resulting from changes in estrogen and androgen metabolism). Gynecomastia can also be iatrogenic, caused by use of some medications. Gynecomastia is occasionally seen in male adolescents from marijuana use (Mayo Clinic Health Information, 2014).

Gynecomastia occurs as concentric, palpable glandular tissue beneath the areola that is not fixed to underlying structures. The prevalence is highest in men 50 to 80 years old and generally presents as bilateral. The cause of pathologic gynecomastia is a relative or absolute increase in circulating estrogen compared with androgen. Careful history (including drugs, legal and illegal) and physical examination can usually rule out Klinefelter syndrome, androgen insensitivity syndrome, and testicular tumors (Griffin and Wilson, 2003) (Table 35-15).

Breast cancer is rare in men, but it does occur, and generally the prognosis is much worse for men than for women diagnosed with breast cancer. Typically, breast cancer presents as a painless, central breast lump that may advance to pain, bloody discharge, and skin ulceration. Although there may be some benefit to obtaining breast ultrasonography or mammography, definitive diagnosis must be confirmed by biopsy (Wise et al., 2005).

Treatment of nonphysiologic gynecomastia involves removal of the offending drug or correction of the underlying condition, either of which usually results in regression of the glandular breast tissue. If the gynecomastia persists, a trial of antiestrogen therapy may be considered. Gynecomastia present for more than 1 year will undergo fibrosis and usually not respond to medications. Surgical correction is required for alleviation of symptoms.

PROBLEMS OF THE OVARY AND OTHER FEMALE ENDOCRINE ISSUES

Menopause and Hormone Replacement Therapy

Normal menopause is defined as the cessation of menstruation for 12 months after the age of 40 years without other known (physiological or pathological) causes of amenorrhea (Table 35-16). Perimenopause refers to an indefinite period before, during, and after cessation of menstruation.

Table 35-15   Causes of Pathologic Gynecomastia

ESTRADIOL EXCESS

Estradiol Secretion

Adrenal tumors
Sporadic testicular tumors (sex cord, Sertoli, germ, Leydig cells)
Testicular tumors associated with familial syndromes (Peutz-Jeghers, Carney complex)

Exogenous Estrogens or Estrogenic Substances

Drug therapy with estrogens
Estrogen creams and lotions
Embalming fluid exposure
Delousing powder
Hair oil
Marijuana
Estrogen analogues: digitoxin

ELEVATED ESTROGEN PRECURSORS: AROMATIZABLE ANDROGENS

Human chorionic gonadotropin (hCG) excess (eutopic or ectopic)

Exogenous Hormones

Testosterone enanthate
Testosterone propionate
Anabolic steroids
hCG administration

TESTOSTERONE DEFICIENCY

Anorchia
Hypogonadotropic syndromes
Drugs or exogenous substances
Ketoconazole
Heroin
Methadone
Alcohol

ESTRADIOL/TESTOSTERONE IMBALANCE

Hypergonadotropic syndromes
Hypogonadotropic hypogonadism syndromes
Primary gonadal diseases
Drugs

REGULATORY HORMONE EXCESS

Hyperthyroidism
Acromegaly
Prolactin Excess
Hypothyroidism
Pituitary tumor

Drug therapy with:

Catecholamine antagonists or depleters
Domperidone
Haloperidol
Methyldopa
Metoclopramide
Phenothiazines
Reserpine
Sulpiride
Tricyclic antidepressants
Administration of growth hormone
Cushing syndrome

OTHER CAUSES

Local Trauma

Hip spica cast
Chest injury
Herpes zoster of chest wall
Post thoracotomy
Spinal cord injury
Primary breast tumor

Uncertain Causes

Other Chronic Illnesses

Renal failure
Pulmonary tuberculosis
HIV
Diabetes mellitus
Leprosy
Refeeding gynecomastia
Persistent pubertal macromastia
Idiopathic

Drugs Associated with Gynecomastia with Uncertain Mechanisms:

Cytotoxic Drug-Induced Hypogonadism from:

Busulfan
Nitrosourea
Vincristine
Combination chemotherapy
Steroid synthesis inhibitory drugs

Androgen Resistance

Complete testicular feminization
Partial: Reifenstein, Lubs, Rosewater, and Dreyfus syndromes

Androgen Antagonistic Drugs

Bicalutamide
Cimetidine
Cyproterone acetate
Flutamide
Spironolactone

Blockers of 5α-Reductase

Finasteride

Tumor Related

hCG-producing tumors (e.g., testis, lung, gastrointestinal tract)
Hypogonadotropic syndromes
Isolated gonadotropin deficiency, particularly fertile eunuch syndrome
Panhypopituitarism
Systemic illnesses
Renal disease
Severe liver disease
Amiodarone
Amphetamines
Auranofin
β-Blockers
Calcium channel blockers
Captopril
Cyclosporin
Diazepam
Diethylpropion
Enalapril
Ethionamide
Etretinate
Griseofulvin
Heparin
Indinavir
Isoniazid
Methotrexate
Metronidazole
Narcotic analgesics
Nitrates
Omeprazole
Penicillamine
Phenytoin
Quinidine
Sulindac
Theophylline
Thiacetazone
Vitamin E

From Santen RJ. Gynecomastia. In DeGroot LJ, Jameson, JL, eds. *Endocrinology*. 5th ed, vol 3. Philadelphia: Saunders; 2006.

Table 35-16 Menopausal Symptoms* and Treatment

Symptoms	Pre (%)	Peri (%)	Post (%)	Treatment
Vasomotor symptoms	14-51	35-50	30-80	ET/EPT (SOR: A)
Vaginal dryness and painful intercourse	4-22	7-39	17-30	ET/EPT Vaginal ET preferred (SOR: A)
Mood symptoms	8-37	11-21	8-38	ET may be beneficial (SOR: A)
Urinary symptoms	10-36	17-39	15-36	Vaginal estrogens (SOR: B)
Sleep disturbances	16-42	39-47	35-60	Sleep hygiene; other agents

*Incidence of *premenopausal*, *perimenopausal*, and *post*menopausal symptoms.
ET, Estrogen therapy; *EPT*, cyclic combined estrogen-progestogen therapy; *SOR*, strength of recommendation.
Modified from NIH State of the Science Conference on Management of Menopausal-Related Symptoms. Bethesda, Maryland, 2005.
  http://consensus.nih.gov/2005/menopausestatement.htm.

The term *climacteric* refers to the period of time after the cessation of reproductive function. Premature menopause, sometimes referred to as premature ovarian failure, is the same syndrome but occurring before age 40 years and is often thought to be the result of an autoimmune process. Premature menopause can also be the result of surgical removal of the ovaries or chemotherapy. When amenorrhea is associated with a negative pregnancy test result, elevated levels of FSH (≥35 mIU/mL) and low estradiol levels (≤35 pg/mL), it is primary ovarian failure until proven otherwise. Fluctuations in the level of various hormones (FSH, LH, estrogen, progestin) are common during the perimenopausal period. A single reading of these hormones during this period may be unreliable for a definitive diagnosis of menopause. The combination of clinical presentation plus laboratory test results in these circumstances is useful.

Menstrual Patterns and Symptom Overview

Decreasing levels of estrogens and androgens are responsible for most menopausal symptoms. Typical hormonal changes include increases in FSH and LH with a significant reduction in estradiol (E2), a moderate reduction in estrone (E1) and androstenedione, a mild reduction in testosterone, and changes in cortisol levels that are insignificant. Not all women experience symptoms associated with hormone deprivation. Obese women may experience no or relatively few symptoms of hormone deficiency and are at reduced risk of osteoporosis, but they are at increased risk for cancer (e.g., uterine cancer) and cardiovascular disease (CVD).

The most common symptoms of menopause are hot flashes (vasomotor symptom complex with sudden sensations of intense heat, sweating, and flushing, typically lasting 5 to 10 minutes, and night sweats), sleep and mood disturbances, decreased libido, and vaginal dryness. Hot flashes tend to be most intense in duration, severity, and frequency in younger women and during the first year of menopause, generally tapering thereafter. A small percentage of women have hot flashes on a lifelong basis.

Treatment of Hormonally Mediated Symptoms

Key Points

- Hormone replacement therapy (HRT) may be appropriate for the relief of severe vasomotor symptoms in selected postmenopausal women.
- HRT has previously been used for broad segments of the population. Currently, individualized therapy, predominantly nonhormonal, is advised.

- HRT increases the risks of breast cancer, CVD and stroke, deep vein thrombosis (DVT), and cognitive decline (much of this is contrary to previous findings).
- If HRT is used, the lowest dose for the shortest duration should be administered.
- HRT has been shown to improve bone density and osteoporosis and decrease colon cancer risk.

Beliefs about HRT for menopausal women have shifted substantially in recent years because of randomized clinical studies, including the landmark Women's Health Initiative (WHI) study (Anderson et al., 2004). These studies showed that hormonal therapy, particularly with combined conjugated estrogen and medroxyprogesterone regimens, not only increases the risk for developing breast cancer and thromboembolic disease but also increases the risk of cardiovascular events (Anderson et al., 2004; Hulley et al., 1998; Nelson et al., 2002; Rossouw et al., 2002; Tomson et al., 2005).

Side effects of HRT are related to the age of the patient, her baseline disease risk strata, age at time of menopause, time interval since menopause, duration and dosage of estrogen administered, and emerging medical conditions during treatment. WHI also showed hormone therapy initiated less than 10 years since menopause had a lower incidence of CHD compared with that initiated 10 years after menopause. Although the absolute risk for any individual woman for severe complications was low, the cumulative risk over large populations has led to substantial changes in prescribing patterns and recommendations for postmenopausal therapy (Anderson et al., 2004).

Recent analysis has raised the question of whether unopposed estrogen may actually be safer than combined estrogen and progesterone even in women who still have their uteruses (Rossouw et al., 2002). Prescribing progesterone to prevent endometrial cancer may be incorrect in that an increased incidence of breast cancer and other risks from adding progesterone might actually outweigh the benefit of preventing uterine cancer—the incidence of breast cancer is actually substantially higher than that of uterine cancer. The WHI estrogen-only therapy arm for hysterectomized women (average follow-up, 6.8 years) revealed reduced breast cancer (0.77 [0.59-1.01]; 95% confidence interval [CI]) and hip fracture (0.61 [0.41-0.91]), but there was a small increase in total CVD (1.12 [1.01-1.24]) and an absolute increase in strokes (12 in 10,000 person-years) with six fewer fractures per 10,000 person-years. Conjugated equine estrogen is not recommended for chronic

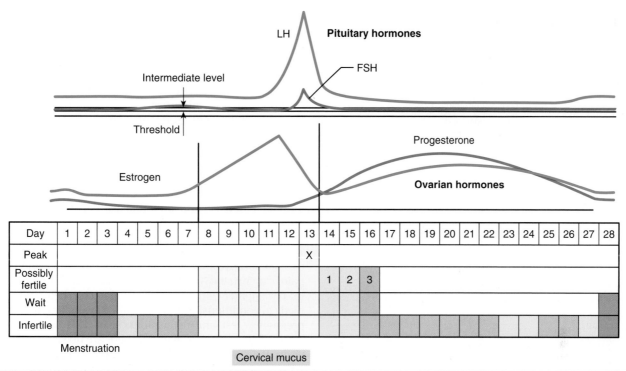

Figure 35-7 Female reproductive physiology. *FSH,* Follicle-stimulating hormone; *LH,* luteinizing hormone. From Brown, JB: Hormones of a woman's reproductive cycle [Epub, www.pearsoncustom.com].

disease prevention in post-menopausal women (Anderson et al., 2004).

Transdermal preparations of progesterone-only creams have helped relieve hot flashes (Leonetti et al., 1999). Their risks are poorly defined but may include an increased risk of breast cancer because many postmenopausal breast cancers are positive for estrogen and progesterone receptors.

Hormone therapy with estrogen-containing regimens is the most effective treatment for vasomotor symptoms. However, the U.S. Preventive Service Task Force (USPSTF) recommendations (2005) warn against the routine use of unopposed estrogen or combined estrogen and progestin for the prevention of chronic conditions in postmenopausal women (USPSTF, 2005). The use of SSRIs, clonidine, and gabapentin is recommended. Although studies are smaller and efficacy appears to be lower, the associated risks, particularly of serious complications, are lower.

Depressed Libido in Women

See eAppendix 35-6 online.

Amenorrhea

> #### Key Points
>
> - Amenorrhea is categorized as primary or secondary; however, this distinction may be misleading in certain patients.
> - Primary amenorrhea can be caused by obstruction of the outflow tract; androgen insensitivity; gonadal dysgenesis; hyperprolactinemia; and dysfunction of the hypothalamus, pituitary, or thyroid.
> - Pregnancy is the most common cause of secondary amenorrhea.

Primary Amenorrhea. Menses is a normal, physiologic function in a sexually mature female. Amenorrhea is the absence of menses in a sexually mature woman. Amenorrhea is divided into two large categories, primary and secondary, depending on whether the female has ever had menarche, with attendant menstrual flow. *Primary* amenorrhea is defined as failure of menarche by age 16 years in a female with apparently normal sexual development or in a female age 14 years who does not demonstrate evidence of developing secondary sexual characteristics. *Secondary* amenorrhea is failure of menstruation after normal menses are established with the caveat that at least 3 months have passed with apparently normal menses or 9 months have passed in a woman with oligomenorrhea.

Menstruation is a very complex process, with many interacting and codependent processes that must occur in specific chronologic order (Figure 35-7). Dysfunction of any organ or system involved with these processes has the potential to disrupt the menstrual cycle and cause amenorrhea. The organs and systems that are involved in the menstrual cycle are the CNS (influenced by environment, stress), hypothalamus (through GnRH), anterior pituitary (FSH, LH), thyroid gland, adrenals, ovary (estrogen, progesterone), and uterus. Secondary amenorrhea is more common than primary amenorrhea, with the most common cause being pregnancy. The distinction between etiologies of primary and secondary amenorrhea may be misleading, as in the case of a woman with PCOS who presents with primary amenorrhea or a woman with partial gonadal dysgenesis who has rudimentary ovarian development and may initially ovulate, thus presenting with secondary amenorrhea (Table 35-17; see Figure 35-8).

The more common causes of primary amenorrhea fall into congenital or anatomical abnormalities. Congenital

Table 35-17   Causes of Amenorrhea*

Hyperprolactinemia	Prolactin-secreting tumor Centrally acting medications, including dopamine antagonists
Pituitary disease	Non–prolactin-secreting pituitary tumor Generalized pituitary insufficiency, including previous pituitary surgery
Hypothalamic amenorrhea	Nutrition/exercise disorders Idiopathic hypogonadotropic hypogonadism

*Resulting from disorders of the hypothalamus and pituitary.
From Illingworth P. Amenorrhea, anovulation, and dysfunctional uterine bleeding. In DeGroot LJ, Jameson, JL, eds. *Endocrinology.* 5th ed, vol 3. Philadelphia: Saunders; 2006.

Table 35-18   Causes of Primary Ovarian Failure

Iatrogenic	Surgery Chemotherapy Radiotherapy
Environmental	Smoking Viral infections
Autoimmune	Association with other autoimmune disease
Abnormal karyotypes	46,XY 45,XO
Genetic disorders with normal karyotype	Fragile X permutations Galactosemia Carbohydrate-deficient glycoprotein syndrome type 1 Inhibin α-gene mutations Follicle-stimulating hormone receptor gene mutations

From Peter Illingworth. Amenorrhea, anovulation, and dysfunctional uterine bleeding. In DeGroot LJ, Jameson, JL, eds. *Endocrinology.* 5th ed, vol 3. Philadelphia: Saunders; 2006.

absence of the uterus and vagina, known as müllerian agenesis or Mayer-Rokitansky-Küster-Hauser (MRKH) syndrome, is a significant cause of amenorrhea. Other congenital causes of primary amenorrhea include chromosomal abnormalities, prenatal adrenal hyperplasia, and female virilization syndrome. An anatomic cause of primary amenorrhea, usually discovered at time of menarche, is imperforate hymen.

To evaluate a patient with primary amenorrhea, after a thorough clinical history, the physical examination must focus on development of hormonally mediated secondary sexual characteristics (breast development, pubic or axillary hair). Although rare as a cause of primary amenorrhea, pregnancy occasionally does occur before a woman's first menstrual period, therefore, it should always be excluded before any testing or imagining is initiated.

Laboratory testing includes FSH, LH, TSH, and prolactin. If FSH is normal or reduced, this may mean the patient has chronic anovulation, functional hypothalamic amenorrhea, or PCOS. Increased FSH with breast development is likely secondary to ovarian failure. Increased FSH without secondary sexual characteristics may be caused by congenital agenesis of the ovaries. In a patient without a uterus, serum testosterone level and karyotype should be determined. In the presence of a uterus and normal secondary sexual characteristics, serum TSH levels should be evaluated (Sybert and McCauley, 2004) (Table 35-18).

Secondary Amenorrhea. Pregnancy is the most common cause of secondary amenorrhea and must always be ruled out at the initial clinical visit. Structural changes may cause amenorrhea, such as adhesions after instrumentation (Asherman syndrome) or infection in the form of TB or endometritis. Patients with PCOS present with irregular or absent menses, hirsutism, acne, subfertility secondary to a hyperandrogenic state, or a combination. Adrenal or ovarian tumors, hyperthecosis, and late-onset or mild congenital adrenal hyperplasia may also result in secondary amenorrhea and hyperandrogenism. Hypergonadotropic hypogonadism (premature ovarian failure), HH, thyroid disease, menopause, extreme exercise, anorexia nervosa, bulimia, and hyperprolactinemia are all potential causes of secondary amenorrhea.

A thorough history and physical examination will provide the diagnosis, with laboratory studies and imaging serving as collaborative evidence. Particular attention should be paid to menstrual history, diet, exercise, medications, pubertal development, hirsutism, acne, galactorrhea, and other medical conditions. Initial laboratory evaluation includes a pregnancy test and determination of TSH and prolactin levels. If these are normal and there are no signs of hyperandrogenism (e.g., hirsutism, acne, voice change), proceed with progesterone challenge by using medroxyprogesterone (Provera) 10 to 20 mg/day for 5 to 10 days. In the presence of a uterus, the progesterone withdrawal test will induce withdrawal bleeding within 10 days in a woman with adequate estrogen production. If there is no withdrawal bleed, consider repeating the test with progesterone in oil (100-200 mg intramuscular) or with norethindrone or micronized progesterone. If these test results are also negative, a 21-day course of conjugated estrogen (1.25 mg/day) or a cycle of combined oral contraceptives (OCs) should provide adequate stimulation of the endometrium to support a withdrawal bleed. If all of these fail to result in menstrual flow, additional tests may be ordered, beginning with FSH, and if there are clinical signs of hyperandrogenism, a check for DHEA-S and testosterone levels. Elevated FSH level indicates ovarian failure (including gonadal dysgenesis and secondary ovarian failure or menopause); normal or low values indicate HH or uterine abnormality (Asherman syndrome). Proceed with a workup for PCOS (discussed later), late-onset congenital adrenal hyperplasia, or Cushing syndrome if there are features consistent with these illnesses. Features of hyperandrogenemia or substantially increased serum testosterone levels should prompt appropriate studies to rule out a neoplastic source of androgen. Figure 35-8 is a diagnostic algorithm for evaluating a patient with primary or secondary amenorrhea.

Management of amenorrhea depends on establishing a diagnosis, specific treatment directed to the underlying cause, restoration of ovulatory cycles, and treating infertility if desired. Also, appropriate treatment must be provided for hypoestrogenemia and hyperandrogenemia, both medical and surgical.

Female Infertility

Infertility is defined as failure of conception after 1 year of unprotected intercourse. From 15% to 20% of all couples are infertile. In women, fertility peaks between ages 20 and 24 years. After this, there is progressive decline in fertility

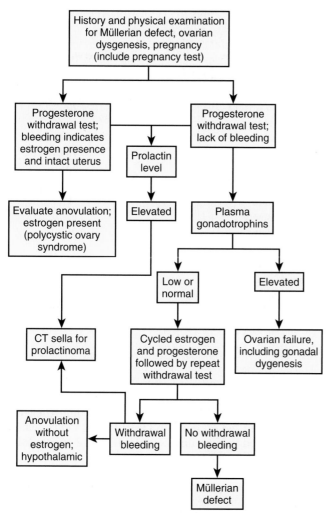

Figure 35-8 Diagnostic algorithm for evaluating a patient with primary and secondary amenorrhea. *CT*, Computed tomography. (Modified from Carr BR. Disorders of the ovaries and female reproductive tract. In Wilson JD, Foster DW, eds. *Williams' textbook of endocrinology.* 8th ed. Philadelphia: Saunders; 1992.)

Table 35-19 Tests for Evaluating Female Infertility

Female Infertility	Common Tests
Ovulatory factors	Basal body temperature or urinary LH test (ovulatory predictor test); serum progesterone (during luteal phase); transvaginal ultrasound; TSH, FSH, prolactin, and androgens
Cervical factors	Cervical mucus evaluation; postcoital test (not sensitive)
Uterine factors	Ultrasonography, hysterosalpingography, hysteroscopy, sonohysterography (for submucosal myomas and endometrial polyps), MRI
Tubal factors	Hysterosalpingography; laparoscopy and chromotubation; fluoroscopic or hysteroscopic tubal cannulation
Peritoneal factors	Ultrasonography, laparoscopy

FSH, Follicle-stimulating hormone; *LH,* luteinizing hormone; *MRI,* magnetic resonance imaging; *TSH,* thyroid-stimulating hormone.
Modified from Brassard M, AinMelk Y, Baillargeon JP. Basic infertility including polycystic ovary syndrome. *Med Clin North Am.* 2008;92: 1163-1192.

Treatment should be directed toward the underlying cause. Ovulatory dysfunction is treated based on the underlying cause: bromocriptine for prolactinoma, metformin or clomiphene citrate for PCOS, human menopausal gonadotropin for HH, clomiphene citrate plus glucocorticoids for adrenal hyperplasia with elevated levels of androgens, and antibiotics for infection. The family physician should strongly consider early referral to a reproductive specialist if the patient or couple has complex medical histories or advanced reproductive age.

Women who have secondary infertility (pituitary) wishing to restore fertility should be referred to specialized centers for pharmacologic induction of ovulation with exogenous pulsatile GnRH and exogenous FSH and LH treatment. GnRH can be used to restore fertility when hypothalamic disease and tertiary hypogonadism are present. Women older than the age of 50 years with secondary hypogonadism should be treated as menopausal, taking into consideration the risk-to-benefit ratio of estrogen replacement therapy in this age group.

Assessment of fallopian tube patency is accomplished by hysterosalpingography (first choice) or laparoscopy (if history strongly suggests prior tubal damage). Postcoital tests, endometrial biopsies, and basal body temperature records are no longer recommended as routine studies in the initial evaluation (Mancini et al., 2008; Practice Committee of the American Society of Reproductive Medicine, 2004) (Table 35-19).

Galactorrhea and Hirsutism

See eAppendix 35-7 online.

Polycystic Ovary Syndrome

Polycystic ovary syndrome is the clinical condition seen most commonly with androgen excess. Women with PCOS present with complaints of abnormal menses, infertility, hirsutism, acne, and obesity, all of which are related to excess androgen. PCOS is the single most common endocrine abnormality of women of reproductive age and affects

until about age 32 years followed by a steep decline after 40 years. Causes of infertility in couples tend to be one third male factors, one third female factors, and one third combination. Female causes of infertility include ovarian dysfunction (40%), tubal factors (20%), cervical factors (infection, stenosis), uterine factors (infection, fibroids), and other (endometriosis, adhesions). The course of investigation for infertility should be based on a couple's wishes for fertility, their age, the duration of infertility, and unique features in the history and physical examination.

After congenital and other nonhormonal causes are excluded, ovulation should be verified by urinary ovulation prediction kits that detect the LH surge, determination of the midluteal phase serum progesterone level (7 days before anticipated menses), or both. Daily rectal temperature measurements to establish ovulation are no longer recommended. Women older than the age of 35 years should have a serum FSH level checked on day 3 of the menstrual cycle. A value higher than 12 IU/L is associated with poor ovarian response, and referral to a reproductive endocrinologist should be considered.

Table 35-20   Causes of Androgen Excess in Women

Adrenal hyperandrogenism	■ Premature adrenarche ■ Functional adrenal hyperandrogenism ■ Congenital adrenal hyperplasia ■ Cushing syndrome ■ Hyperprolactinemia and acromegaly ■ Abnormal cortisol action or metabolism ■ Adrenal neoplasms
Gonadal hyperandrogenism	■ Ovarian hyperandrogenism 　■ Functional ovarian hyperandrogenism or polycystic ovary syndrome 　■ Adrenal virilizing disorders and rest tumors 　■ Ovarian steroidogenic blocks 　■ Syndromes of extreme insulin resistance 　■ Ovarian neoplasms ■ True hermaphroditism ■ Pregnancy-related hyperandrogenism
Peripheral androgen overproduction	■ Obesity ■ Idiopathic

From Ehrmann DA, Barnes RB, Rosenfeld RL. Hyperandrogenism, hirsutism, and the polycystic ovary syndrome. In DeGroot LJ, Jameson, JL, eds. *Endocrinology*. 5th ed, vol 3. Philadelphia: Saunders; 2006.

Table 35-21   Signs and Symptoms in Relation to Presence of Polycystic Ovary Syndrome (PCOS)

Symptoms and Signs	Patients with PCOS (%)
Hirsutism and unwanted hair growth	78.4
Alopecia	36.5
Hyperandrogenemia	70
Persistent acne	20-40
Normal androgen levels	20-40
Overt menstrual dysfunction	75-85
Oligomenorrhea	79.11
Polycystic ovaries	75-90
LH-to-FSH ratio	40
Insulin resistance	50-70
Type 2 diabetes	26.7
Dyslipidemia	70
Oligoanovulation	40
Obesity	50
Hyperprolactinemia	<1

FSH, Follicle-stimulating hormone; *LH*, luteinizing hormone.
Modified from Azziz R, Carmina E, Dewailly D, et al. Task Force on the phenotype of the polycystic ovary syndrome of the Androgen Excess and PCOS Society. The Androgen Excess and PCOS Society criteria for the polycystic ovary syndrome: the complete task force report. *Fertil Steril*. 2009;91:456-488.

6% to 8% of women worldwide (Azziz et al., 2009). The definition of PCOS is constantly being revised. The latest Task Force on the Phenotype of the Polycystic Ovary Syndrome from the Androgen Excess and PCOS Society (AE-PCOS Society) defines PCOS by the presence of hyperandrogenism (clinical or biochemical), ovarian dysfunction (oligo-anovulation or polycystic ovaries), and the exclusion of related disorders (Azziz et al., 2009) (Table 35-20).

The typical presentation of PCOS includes hirsutism, menstrual dysfunction, obesity, insulin resistance, acanthosis nigricans, decreased fertility, and polycystic appearance to the ovaries. The onset of symptoms is usually around the time of menarche, but it may occur after puberty as a result of weight gain or other environmental factors. The differential diagnosis includes idiopathic hirsutism, ovarian hyperthecosis, ovarian tumor, adrenal tumor, nonclassic adrenal hyperplasia, Cushing syndrome, glucocorticoid resistance, and androgen-producing neoplasms.

A patient with PCOS is at higher risk for infertility, dysfunctional bleeding, obesity, endometrial hyperplasia, endometrial carcinoma, type 2 diabetes mellitus, dyslipidemia, hypertension, obstructive sleep apnea, and possibly CVD with a familial tendency (increased risk for mother and daughter) (Azziz et al., 2009; Ehrmann, 2005) (Table 35-21).

The diagnosis of PCOS is made with evidence of hyperandrogenism (clinical or biochemical), presence of ovarian dysfunction (clinical or anatomic), and excluding other conditions producing hyperandrogenism and ovarian dysfunction. Initial laboratory testing should include the determination of serum free testosterone, androstenedione, DHEA-S, and 17-hydroxyprogesterone. Other studies include prolactin, TSH, fasting glucose and insulin, and serum lipid profile. Obtaining circulating levels of LH and FSH does not contribute significantly to the diagnosis of PCOS, so these laboratory tests are not indicated with initial evaluation. Pelvic or transvaginal ultrasonography should be performed to identify the ovaries and determine their size and shape and the presence of cysts; typical PCOS ovaries have increased volume and contain 10 to 12 subcapsular follicular cysts 2 to 9 mm in diameter.

Treatment of hirsutism and acne in PCOS focuses on decreasing androgen levels, production, and effects. Metformin is used extensively to reduce insulin resistance and hyperinsulinemia related to hormonal changes and ovulation (Nestler, 2008). To decrease the risk of endometrial hyperplasia and carcinoma, cyclic progestin or a combination OC should be considered to inhibit endometrial proliferation.

In the long-term management of PCOS, steps should be taken to reduce CV complications, diabetes, obesity, and psychosocial morbidities (Figure 35-9). Screening for glucose intolerance with a 75-g 2-hour FTT and determination of serum lipid levels (total cholesterol, LDL, HDL, triglycerides) should be carried out. Lifestyle management changes include weight loss, exercise, and use of metformin and thiazolidinediones for those individuals with abnormal GTT results. In addition, clinicians should consider cardiovascular risk reduction, psychosocial issues, management of subfertility and hirsutism, and other lifetime management with insulin sensitizers and protection of the endometrium with hormonal manipulations (Figure 35-9).

KEY TREATMENT

• Patients with PCOS require cardiovascular risk reduction, psychosocial counseling, management of subfertility and hirsutism, and possible insulin sensitizers and protection of endometrium with hormonal manipulations (Azziz et al., 2009; Ehrmann, 2005; Nestler, 2008) (SOR: A).

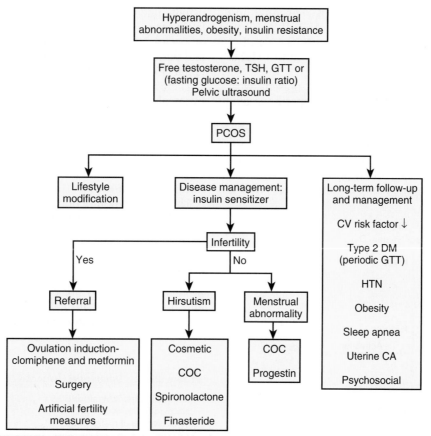

Figure 35-9 Therapeutic algorithm for management of polycystic ovary syndrome. *CA,* cancer; *COC,* combined oral contraceptives; *CV,* cardiovascular; *DM,* diabetes mellitus; *GTT,* glucose tolerance test; *HTN,* hypertension; *PCOS,* polycystic ovary syndrome; *TSH,* thyroid-stimulating hormone. (Modified from Samraj GPN, Kuritzky L. Polycystic ovary syndrome: comprehensive management in primary care. *Comp Ther.* 2002;28:208-221q.)

Disturbances in Calcium and Phosphate

Calcium homeostasis is a delicate balance among a number of organ systems and functions. These include the kidneys, thyroid, parathyroid, bone, adrenal glands, GI tract, nutrition, infectious disease, and medication. Malfunction in any of these modalities can result in hypercalcemia or hypocalcemia with the potential for serious morbidity and mortality. Total body calcium is balanced between plasma and the bony skeleton in a state of dynamic equilibrium. Approximately 1% of total calcium is in circulation, and the remaining 99% is stored in bone. In plasma, circulating calcium is approximately 40% protein (albumin) bound, 45% exists in an ionized state (Ca^{++}), and roughly 15% is found as various salts (calcium citrate, calcium lactate, calcium phosphate, and calcium sulfate). Bony calcium exists in an active state with constant deposition and resorption under the influence of parathyroid hormone (PTH, parathormone), calcitonin, osteoclastic and osteoblastic activity, and neoplastic disease.

The primary factor driving increases in circulating calcium is PTH, which increases bone resorption and converts vitamin D_3 (cholecalciferol) into 1,25-dihydroxy-cholecalciferol, the active form of vitamin D_3. Cholecalciferol is primarily formed in the skin from solar irradiation, and some evidence suggests that ultraviolet radiation exposure

of tanning beds can raise vitamin D levels. However, the latter is not recommended as an appropriate source of vitamin D_3 (Tangpricha et al., 2004). Dietary sources of vitamin D_3 are also important and can be obtained from fortified milk, fruit juices, fish oil, and other sources. The active form of vitamin D_3 is required to facilitate calcium absorption from the gut. Calcium homeostasis is further maintained by circulating levels of ionized calcium and calcitonin's negative effect on osteoclastic bone resorption (Guyton and Hall, 2006) (Figure 35-10).

Normal levels of total circulating calcium, with normal albumin levels, range between 8.5 and 10.5 mg/dL ($\approx$2.4 mmol/L). Ionized levels, which are not albumin dependent, will range between 1.17 and 1.33 mmol/L ($\approx$4.7 mg/dL) (Bringhurst and Leder, 2006).

HYPERCALCEMIA

Causes of hypercalcemia are generally divided into two types: primary and secondary. Primary causes are due to excessive parathormone secretion, and secondary causes include disease processes that directly affect bone metabolism and calcium excretion. The most common cause of primary hyperparathyroidism (PHPT) is a solitary parathyroid adenoma, accounting for approximately 80% of cases. Multiple adenomas are found in 2% to 4% of cases. The second most common cause of PHPT (15%) is parathyroid hyperplasia of multiple (usually $\geq$4) parathyroid glands.

The etiologies for these include a mix of congenital and familial diseases such as MEN-I and MEN-IIA. Fewer than 1% of cases of PHPT are caused by primary parathyroid malignancy (Silverberg and Bilezikian, 2006) (Table 35-22).

Primary hyperparathyroidism does not present with classic symptoms. Symptoms may be as nonspecific as generalized weakness in the proximal muscles, fatigue, headache, weight loss, and constipation all the way to being as profound as renal failure, hypovolemic shock, and death (usually in patients with malignancy but sometimes previously undiagnosed). Patients rarely present with signs and symptoms immediately suggesting hypercalcemia. PHPT is usually uncovered through routine, nonspecific screening laboratory tests; during evaluation for nephrolithiasis; or, occasionally in a patient with accelerated osteoporosis and pathologic fracture (Silverberg and Bilezikian, 2006) (Table 35-23).

There is a classic "quadrad" of symptoms associated with hypercalcemia that, although seen in many disease processes, may be helpful in a patient with hypercalcemia, irrespective of etiology. The mnemonic is "bones, stones, moans, and abdominal groans," representing the four symptoms of the classic quadrad, which are bone pain, renal calculi, psychiatric disorder, and nausea and vomiting (Silverberg and Bilezikian, 2006).

The primary dysfunction in PHPT is an excess of circulating PHT. However, with bony metastases, PHT levels will be appropriately suppressed in the presence of elevated serum calcium levels because of osteolytic metastases. When the cause of hypercalcemia is malignancy, the patient usually has a history; an exception is unsuspected multiple myeloma, which may present with chronic low back pain and an elevated serum calcium level. Calcium levels in malignancy are typically higher (>14 mg/dL) than those

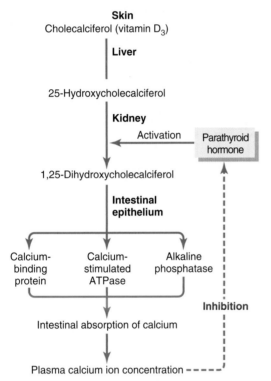

Figure 35-10 Pathway for conversion of vitamin D_3 into its active form (1,25-dihydroxycholecalciferol) and the role vitamin D plays in control of plasma calcium concentration. (From Hall JE. Parathyroid hormone, calcitonin, calcium and phosphate metabolism, vitamin D, bone, and teeth. In Guyton AC, Hall JE, eds. *Textbook of medical physiology.* 12th ed. Philadelphia: Saunders; 2011.)

Table 35-22   Differential Diagnosis of Hypercalcemia

Primary hyperparathyroidism
Parathyroid carcinoma
Hypercalcemia of malignancy
Nonparathyroid endocrine causes
Thyrotoxicosis
Pheochromocytoma
Addison disease
Islet cell tumors
Drug-related hypercalcemia
Vitamin D
Vitamin A
Thiazide diuretics
Lithium
Estrogen and antiestrogens
Familial hypocalciuric hypercalcemia
Miscellaneous
Immobilization
Milk-alkali syndrome
Parenteral nutrition

From Silverberg SJ, Bilezikian JP. Primary hyperparathyroidism. In DeGroot LJ, Jameson, JL, eds. *Endocrinology.* 5th ed, vol 2. Philadelphia: Saunders; 2006.

Table 35-23   Biochemical Profile in Primary Hyperparathyroidism

	Patients (mean ±SEM)	Reference Range
Serum calcium	10.7 ± mg/dL	8.2-10.2 mg/dL
Serum phosphorus	2.8 ± 0.1 mg/dL	2.5-4.5 mg/dL
Total alkaline phosphatase	114 ± 5 IU/L	<100 IU/L
Serum magnesium	2.0 ± 0.1 mg/dL	1.8-2.4 mg/dL
PTH (IRMA)	119 ± 7 pg/mL	10-65 pg/mL
25(OH) vitamin D	19 ± 1 ng/mL	9-52 ng/mL
1,25(OH)$_2$ vitamin D	54 ± 2 pg/mL	15-60 pg/mL
Urinary calcium	240 ± 11 mg/g creatinine	
Urine DPD	17.6 ± nmol/L/mmol/L creatinine	<14.6 nmol/L/mmol/L creatinine
Urine PYD	46.8 ± 2.7 nmol/L/mmol/L creatinine	<51.8 nmol/L/mmol/L creatinine

DPD, Deoxypyridinoline; *IRMA,* immunoradiometric assay; *PTH,* parathyroid hormone; *PYD,* pyridinoline.
From Silverberg SJ, Bilezikian JP. Primary hyperparathyroidism. In DeGroot LJ, Jameson, JL, eds. *Endocrinology.* 5th ed, vol 3. Philadelphia: Saunders; 2006.

found with parathyroid adenomas (<13 mg/dL), although this is not always the case.

Thiazide diuretics, lithium, and calcium carbonate are common medications seen in primary care that, if not properly monitored and prescribed, can result in hypercalcemia. It is also important to inquire about nonprescription medications (OTC) because excess vitamin D (intoxication) can be a cause. If a patient is taking any of these substances, the patient is asymptomatic, and the serum calcium level is less than 14 mg/dL, the approach is to discontinue the medication and repeat the calcium level in 1 week. If the serum calcium is stable or declining, continue to monitor it until it returns to normal. Occasionally, adrenal insufficiency and hyperthyroidism are uncovered in the evaluation of a patient with an elevated serum calcium level.

Patients who have symptoms consistent with hypercalcemia or serum calcium levels in excess of 13.5 mg/dL may require more aggressive treatment. These patients will almost always be volume depleted as a result of hypercalciuria with resultant polyuria. Treatment is aimed initially at aggressive rehydration. Isotonic saline, at the rate of 2 to 4 L/day until the calcium level returns to normal, is appropriate. Furosemide (loop diuretic) can be used in conjunction with fluid replacement in older patients and those with renal or cardiac disorders to prevent fluid overload. Careful fluid management must be maintained to prevent inadvertent fluid overload or depletion. Other treatments include IV bisphosphonate, calcitonin, and gallium nitrate or plicamycin (Tables 35-24 and 35-25).

Parathyroidectomy is indicated in symptomatic patients and is considered to be the first and generally the only option to cure PHPT. In addition, surgical treatment is recommended for asymptomatic patients who meet any of the following conditions: serum calcium more than 1 mg/dL or more above the upper limit of normal,

Table 35-24 Summary of the Most Generally Useful Medical Therapies for Hypercalcemia

Treatment	Onset of Action	Duration of Action	Advantages	Disadvantages
Rehydration	Hours	During treatment	Rapid action Rehydration invariably needed	None
Forced saline diuresis (with or without loop diuretics)	Hours	During treatment	Rapid action	Modest calcium-lowering effect Potential for volume overload Electrolyte disturbance Transient efficacy Inconvenient for patients
Calcitonin	Hours	1-2 days	Rapid action	Modest calcium-lowering effect Tachyphylaxis develops in a few days
BISPHOSPHONATES				
Etidronate	1-3 days	5-7 days	First-generation bisphosphonate Well tolerated	3-day infusion protocol Less effective than other bisphosphonates
Pamidronate	1-2 days	Weeks to months	Second-generation bisphosphonate Normalizes calcium levels in many patients	Fever Occasional hypocalcemia, hypophosphatemia, and hypomagnesemia
Zoledronate	1-2 days	Weeks to months	Third-generation bisphosphonate More potent than second-generation bisphosphonates Normalizes calcium levels in 90% of patients Can be given in 30 min	Fever Hypophosphatemia Hypocalcemia Renal toxicity occasional

From Finkelstein JS, Potts JT. Medical management of hypercalcemia. In DeGroot LJ, Jameson, JL, eds. *Endocrinology.* 5th ed, vol 2. Philadelphia: Saunders; 2006.

Table 35-25 Summary of Therapies for Hypercalcemia Useful in Special Circumstances

Treatment	Onset of Action	Duration of Action	Advantages	Disadvantages
Gallium nitrate	5 days	7-10 days	May normalize calcium in patients resistant to bisphosphonates	Must be infused continuously over 5 days Occasional nephrotoxicity or hypophosphatemia
Glucocorticoids	Days	Days to weeks	Oral administration	Effective in granulomatous disorders and certain types of malignancies, especially hematologic
Dialysis	Hours	During use and for 24-48 hr afterward	Rapid onset of action Useful in patients with renal failure and heart failure Useful to treat life-threatening hypercalcemia	Complex procedure Reserved for extreme or special circumstances
Oral phosphate	24 hr	During use	Minimal toxicity if serum phosphate low Oral administration	Modest calcium-lowering effect Diarrhea

From Finkelstein JS, Potts JT. Medical management of hypercalcemia. In DeGroot LJ, Jameson, JL, eds. *Endocrinology.* 5th ed, vol 2. Philadelphia: Saunders; 2006.

creatinine clearance less than 60 mL/min, osteoporosis, and age younger than 50 years (Bilezikian et al., 2009; Silverberg and Bilezikian, 2006).

For patients who have failed surgery and those who do not meet surgical criteria, medical treatment includes calcimimetics (cinacalcet), moderate calcium intake, estrogen replacement (when applicable), bisphosphonates, and selective estrogen receptor modulators (SERMs) (Bilezikian et al., 2009; Silverberg and Bilezikian, 2006).

For a patient with PHPT not caused by malignancy, determining if there is one adenoma or multiple functioning adenomas and the location(s) is important in minimizing both the duration and extent of surgery. It is possible to determine preoperatively which parathyroid gland(s) may be the source of the PTH using technetium-labeled (Tc-99m) sestamibi nuclear scan. If the latter did not provide definitive results, then ultrasonography, CT, or MRI may be used to localize the adenoma (Silverberg and Bilezikian, 2006).

HYPOCALCEMIA

Hypocalcemia has a number of primary and secondary causes. Primary causes are due to some defect in PTH availability, including (1) a lack of production (surgical removal of the parathyroid gland or hypoparathyroidism due to autoimmune disease), (2) impaired secretion (with profound hypomagnesemia), and (3) end-organ resistance. With the first two, there is a deficit in circulating PTH, but with the third, the PTH is elevated, in contrast to a low serum calcium level and hypophosphatemia. An example of end-organ resistance is Albright syndrome. Secondary causes include severe vitamin D deficiency, "hungry bone syndrome" with chondrosarcoma, and HIV/AIDS (Table 35-26).

Signs and symptoms of hypocalcemia are generally lacking in the outpatient setting. The primary clinical findings are caused by neuromuscular irritability. If hypocalcemia is suspected, two physical tests can be performed, which may help to make the diagnosis, although negative responses do not rule out hypocalcemia: the Chvostek sign (tapping the facial nerve across the cheek with contraction of the facial muscle) and Trousseau sign (carpal spasm via a BP cuff). Deep tendon reflexes may be hyperactive, and the patient may appear anxious, confused, demented, or psychotic. The signs and symptoms of hypocalcemia are related to the level of ionized calcium rather than total calcium, as well as the rapidity of decline (Levine, 2006). Alkalosis, either primary or compensatory, can cause a shift in ionized calcium to a bound state, thus exacerbating a borderline hypocalcemia situation.

Cardiac changes caused by hypocalcemia include prolongation of the QT interval, resulting in life-threatening dysrhythmia and cardiac dysfunction. Generalized seizures are also possible. The cardiac dysfunction is generally reversible with normalization of the ionized calcium levels. In acute and severe cases, IV calcium is the treatment of choice. Concurrent management of hyperphosphatemia, alkalosis, and hypomagnesemia is required. Long-term management is with oral calcium and vitamin D. Although use of thiazide diuretics is contraindicated in patients with hypercalcemia, they can be used with hypocalcemia and may, in

Table 35-26   Causes of Functional Hypoparathyroidism

A. Surgery
B. Toxic agents
  1. High-dose radiation (rarely)
  2. Asparaginase
  3. Ethiofos
C. Infiltrative processes
  1. Iron deposition
  2. Copper deposition
  3. Tumor or granuloma
D. Defective secretion of PTH
  1. Magnesium deficiency
  2. Magnesium excess
  3. Activating mutation of calcium-sensing receptor gene (MIM 145980)
  4. Antibodies that activate the calcium-sensing receptor
  5. Burn injury and upregulation of calcium-sensing receptor
  6. Alcohol
  7. Maternal hypercalcemia
  8. Neonatal hypocalcemia
E. Autoimmune destruction of parathyroid glands
  1. Autoimmune hypoparathyroidism
  2. Autoimmune polyglandular syndrome, type 1 (APECED, MIM 240300)
F. Idiopathic hypoparathyroidism
  1. Autosomal recessive (MIM 241400)
  2. X-linked (MIM 307700)
G. Embryologic defects in parathyroid gland development
  1. DiGeorge syndrome (del 22q or TBX1 mutation); DGS1; MIM 188400
  2. DiGeorge syndrome (del 10p) DGS2; MIM 601362
  3. Velocardiofacial syndrome (del 22q); MIM 192430
    a. Kenny-Caffey and Sanjad-Sakati syndromes (TBCE, MIM 244460)
H. Defective synthesis of parathyroid hormone (MIM 168450)
  1. Autosomal dominant mutation in prepro-PTH gene
  2. Autosomal recessive mutation in prepro-PTH gene
I. Metabolic defects and mitochondrial neuromyopathies
  1. Kearn-Sayre syndrome
  2. Person syndrome
  3. tRNA *leu* mutations
J. Resistance to PTH
  1. Pseudohypoparathyroidism type 1a (MIM 103580)
  2. Pseudohypoparathyroidism type 1b
  3. Pseudohypoparathyroidism type 1c
  4. Pseudohypoparathyroidism type 2

APECED, Autoimmune polyendocrinopathy-candidiasis-ectodermal dystrophy; *DGS,* DiGeorge syndrome; *MIM,* designator that represents an autoimmune gene mutation; *prepro-PTH,* preproparathyroid hormone; *PTH,* parathyroid hormone; *TBCE,* tubulin folding cofactor E.
From Levine MA. Hypoparathyroidism and pseudohypoparathyroidism. In DeGroot LJ, Jameson, JL, eds. *Endocrinology.* 5th ed, vol 2. Philadelphia: Saunders; 2006.

fact, have somewhat of a beneficial effect. On the other hand, loop diuretics must be used very cautiously because they increase renal excretion of calcium and may exacerbate the problem.

Pseudohypoparathyroidism is a rare phenomenon representative of several congenital, endocrinologic disorders in which tissue resistance to PTH is present. The classic form of this disorder is *Albright hereditary osteodystrophy* (AHO). Patients with AHO have short stature, mental retardation, brachydactyly, and PTH resistance (elevated PTH levels). Another form of AHO, called pseudopseudohypoparathyroidism, does not have PTH dysfunction. Although the clinical course for these diseases may be variable and, in some cases, is protracted, AHO usually is associated with a shortened life expectancy. Treatment is primarily supportive (Levine, 2006).

HYPERPHOSPHATEMIA

The most common cause of hyperphosphatemia, and most familiar to primary care physicians, is impaired renal function. It is also a characteristic of all forms of hypoparathyroidism from the loss of inhibitory effect of PTH on phosphate reabsorption at the proximal renal tubule (Kolon et al., 2004). High-phosphate formula provided to infants can result in hypocalcemia and tetany (Table 35-27).

HYPOPHOSPHATEMIA

Dietary causes of hypophosphatemia are virtually nonexistent, although excessive use of oral phosphate binders (aluminum and magnesium hydroxide antacids) can result in binding of phosphate in the intestine, thus preventing absorption. Generally, when use of oral antacids is excluded, the most common cause of hypophosphatemia is elevated levels of serum calcium caused by increased PTH or malignancy (Silverberg and Bilezikian, 2006). Hypophosphatemia, in association with hypocalcemia, is usually attributable to renal wasting or seen in severe illness. One form of infant hypophosphatemic rickets is transmitted as an autosomal dominant trait (Table 35-28).

Table 35-27 Causes of Hyperphosphatemia

Impaired renal phosphate excretion	Renal insufficiency Tumoral calcinosis Hypoparathyroidism, pseudohypoparathyroidism Acromegaly Etidronate Heparin
Increased extracellular phosphate	Rapid administration of phosphate (IV, oral, rectal) Rapid cellular catabolism or lysis Catabolic states Tissue injury Hyperthermia Crush injuries Fulminant hepatitis Cellular lysis Hemolytic anemia Rhabdomyolysis Cytotoxic therapy Transcellular shifts of phosphate Metabolic acidosis Respiratory acidosis

IV, Intravenous.
From Bringhurst FR, Leder BZ. Regulation of calcium and phosphate homeostasis. In DeGroot LJ, Jameson, JL, eds. *Endocrinology.* 5th ed, vol 2. Philadelphia: Saunders; 2006.

Table 35-28 Causes of Hypophosphatemia

IMPAIRED INTESTINAL PHOSPHATE REABSORPTION

Selective binding of dietary phosphate
  Aluminum-containing antacids

IMPAIRED RENAL TUBULAR PHOSPHATE REABSORPTION

Renal tubular disorders

Fanconi syndrome(s), other renal tubular disorders
Cystinosis
Wilson disease
Inactivating NA/P12 mutations
Dent disease
Hypophosphatemia in idiopathic hypercalciuria

Elevated PTH or PTHrP

Primary hyperparathyroidism
PTHrP-dependent hypercalcemia (malignancy)
Secondary hyperparathyroidism
  Vitamin D deficiency resistance
  Calcium starvation or malabsorption
  Bartter syndrome
  Autosomal recessive renal hypomagnesemia or hypercalciuria

Humoral phosphate-wasting syndromes

X-linked hypophosphatemic rickets
Autosomal dominant hypophosphatemic rickets
Tumor-induced osteomalacia
McCune-Albright syndrome

Other systemic disorders

Glucosuria
Hyperaldosteronism
Magnesium or potassium depletion
Amyloidosis
Renal transplantation
Rewarming, induced hyperthermia

Drugs and toxins

Ethanol
Ifosfamide
Acetazolamide
Cisplatin
Toluene
Heavy metals
Glucocorticoids
Rapamycin
Estrogens
Foscarnet
Suramin
Pamidronate

ACCELERATED PHOSPHATE REDISTRIBUTION INTO CELLS OR BONE

Acute intracellular shifts

Insulin therapy (for hyperglycemia, diabetic ketoacidosis)
IV glucose, fructose, glycerol (in NPO patients)
Catecholamines (epinephrine, albuterol, terbutaline, dopamine)
Acute respiratory alkalosis (salicylate intoxication, acute gout)
Gram-negative sepsis, toxic shock syndrome, thyrotoxic periodic paralysis
Recovery from acidosis, starvation, hypothermia

Rapid formation of new cells

Leukemic blast crisis
Bone marrow, stem cell therapy
Erythropoietin, GM-CSF therapy
Treatment of pernicious anemia
Status post–partial hepatectomy

Accelerated net bone formation

Postparathyroidectomy
Treatment of vitamin D deficiency
Early phase of bisphosphonate therapy
Osteoblastic metastases

GM-CSF, Granulocyte-macrophage-colony-stimulating factor; *IV,* intravenous; *NPO,* nothing by mouth; *PTH,* parathyroid hormone; *PTHrP,* parathyroid hormone-related protein.
Bringhurst FR, Leder BZ. Regulation of calcium and phosphate homeostasis. In DeGroot LJ, Jameson, JL, eds. *Endocrinology.* 5th ed, vol 2. Philadelphia: Saunders; 2006.

OSTEOPOROSIS AND OSTEOMALACIA

See eAppendix 35-8 online.

Summary of Additional Online Content

 The following content is available at www.expertconsult.com:

eAppendix 35-1 Acromegaly and Gigantism

eAppendix 35-2 Craniopharyngiomas, Thyrotropin-Secreting Pituitary Adenomas, Gonadotropic Adenomas, and Other Adenomas

eAppendix 35-3 Isolated Aldosterone Deficiency

eAppendix 35-4 Mixed Disorder: Congenital Adrenal Hyperplasia

eAppendix 35-5 Cryptorchidism

eAppendix 35-6 Depressed Libido in Women

eAppendix 35-7 Galactorrhea and Hirsutism

eAppendix 35-8 Osteoporosis and Osteomalacia

References

The complete reference list is available at www.expertconsult.com.

Web Resources

www.aace.com/pub/guidelines American Association of Clinical Endocrinologists.

www.aafp.org/online/en/home/clinical.html The American Academy of Family Physicians maintains a website that can be accessed by members (more selection) and nonmembers with information on recommendations for clinical screening and treatment.

www.acponline.org/clinical_information/guidelines The American College of Physicians maintains this website for general information as well as specific information on disease screening.

www.endo-society.org/guidelines Direct access to current and past treatment guidelines for most endocrine-related diseases.

www.hormone.org/Resources/Patient_Guides Ready resource for current recommendations for physicians and the public for endocrine disorders.

www.jama.ama-assn.org Reference site sponsored by the American Medical Association with access to current and past *JAMA* publications, by author, subject, and so on.

www.ncbi.nlm.nih.gov/sites/entrez PubMed is a general reference source that provides search access based on subject, author, journal, and so on.

36 *Obesity*

ELIZABETH BOHAM, P. MICHAEL STONE, and RUTH DEBUSK

Overview

Key Points

- The prevalence of obesity is a global concern.
- Obesity leads to increased health risks.
- Obesity is associated with increased economic burden on a nation's health care system.

The prevalence of obesity is a growing health concern globally (Swinburn et al., 2011). For the United States, data reported from the ongoing National Health and Nutrition Examination Survey (NHANES) suggest that more than one third of adult men and women age 20 years or older (35.7%, 78 million) and almost one fifth of young people age 2 to 19 years (17.9%, 12.5 million) are obese (Ogden et al., 2012, 2013). Overall, older adults (≥60 years), particularly older women, are more likely to be obese than younger adults. Among young people, a greater proportion of boys was found to be obese compared with girls (Ogden et al., 2012).

The high prevalence of obesity is of concern from several perspectives. Being obese increases the risk for developing chronic disorders such as heart disease, stroke, hypertension, type 2 diabetes, and some cancers, which in turn impairs an individual's quality of life. The economic burden to the United States of having a large percentage of the population with obesity can be measured in direct and indirect costs. The direct costs for obesity-related services such as inpatient and outpatient care, medical tests, and drug therapy have been reported to be $190 billion per year, with a per capita medical spending of $2741 higher (in 2005 dollars) for obese individuals than for those who are not obese (Cawley and Meyerhoefer, 2012). Indirect costs caused by workplace absenteeism, lost economic productivity, and higher insurance premiums are more difficult to estimate but are widely considered to be of equal concern (Dall et al., 2009).

A 2012 report projects that, over the next two decades, the prevalence of obesity in the United States will increase by 33% and 130% for severe obesity (Finkelstein et al., 2012). Just holding obesity prevalence at the 2010 level is estimated to save $549.5 billion in obesity-related direct medical costs alone. Family medicine physicians are well positioned to assist patients in attaining and maintaining a desirable weight. However, effective strategies and tools are needed. This chapter explores the approaches to caring for patients with excess weight and proposes a functional medicine approach to healthy weight management.

Defining Obesity

Key Points

- Obesity is derived differently for adults and children.
- In adults, obesity is defined as a body mass index (BMI) of 30.0 kg/m² or greater.
- Adult obesity is further categorized as class I, BMI of 30.0 to 34.9; class II, BMI of 35.0 to 39.9; and class III, BMI of 40.0 or greater.
- In children, obesity is defined as weight exceeding the 95th percentile on standard growth charts.

The BMI is derived from height and weight and expressed in kg/m². BMI is a convenient measurement used worldwide. For adults, BMI is age independent and the same for both sexes. In the United States, adults with a BMI of 18.9 to 24.9 are considered to be of normal weight. Overweight is a BMI of 25.0 or greater but less than 30.0, and obesity is defined as a BMI of 30.0 or greater. The World Health Organization (WHO) subdivides obesity into three classes according to BMI: 30.0 to 34.9 for class I, 35.0 to 39.9 for class II, and 40.0 or greater for class III, often referred to as extreme obesity (WHO Global Database, 2013) (Table 36-1).

In contrast to adults, weight for children varies with height but also age and sex. Growth charts issued in 2000 by the Centers for Disease Control and Prevention (CDC) for U.S. children provide sex- and age-specific reference values and allow determination of a BMI percentile (CDC, 2000; Kuczmarski et al., 2002). Obesity is defined as a BMI percentile at or greater than the 95th percentile on the sex-appropriate growth chart, and overweight is between the 85th and 95th percentiles (Krebs et al., 2007; Ogden and Flegal, 2010). Additional approaches to assessing the composition of the body mass of overweight and obese patients are discussed in the Assessment section.

Table 36-1   Classification and Types of Obesity

Class	BMI
I	30.0-34.9
II	35.0-39.9
III	≥40.0

Source: World Health Organization. http://apps.who.int/bmi/
index.jsp?introPage=intro_3.html.

Determinants of Obesity

Key Points

- A number of factors have been found to affect weight regulation, including genes and their epigenetic modifications; maternal weight during pregnancy; metabolic imbalances; and environmental factors, including food intake, movement and physical activity, sleep, psychosocial stress, toxin exposure, and microbiome composition.
- These factors can provide leverage points for successful weight regulation.

Many factors contribute to a person's susceptibility to becoming overweight or obese (Barabas, 2007; NHLBNA, 2000). Overconsumption of calories and insufficient physical activity are two common contributors to weight gain, but several additional factors appear to be at play as well, including the quantity and quality of calories consumed; genetics and epigenetics; mother's weight gain during pregnancy; inadequate amount and quality of sleep; a wide variety of psychosocial stressors; exposure to environmental toxins; and the composition of the various body cavities in which microbiota exist, such as the intestinal, vaginal, respiratory, and oral cavities. Increasingly, no one component appears to be solely responsible for obesity. Rather, interactions among our genome, epigenome, and environment throughout our lifespan mutually influence weight regulation.

GENES AND THEIR EPIGENETIC MODULATION

There is general confusion as to contribution of genes in terms of developing obesity. A certain percentage is often assigned to the contribution of genes. This percentage reflects the balance between the relative contribution of genes and environment in the risk of someone becoming overweight or obese. It appears that the susceptibility for becoming obese is a continuum ranging from highly likely to highly unlikely, depending on one's particular genome (set of genes). Each of us has our individual genetic susceptibility with respect to becoming obese. There are genes that, when mutated, provide a high risk for developing obesity, even under environmental conditions that promote normal weight. These genes would contribute to the 100% (high risk) end of the spectrum. Fortunately, the prevalence of these genes appears to be rare, so only a minority of people have such a high risk for obesity. The vast majority of us appear to have a number of mutations (genetic variations) whose contributions are not strong enough in

themselves to lead readily to obesity, but when these variants interact with particular environmental factors, the chance for weight gain increases. In this case, genetics would fall at the low-risk end of the spectrum, and the influence of the environment would fall towards the high end. It's the extent of interaction among various genes and environmental factors that appears to determine our susceptibility to gain and maintain excess weight.

Severe early-onset obesity results from a strong genetic influence on weight regulation and is typically accompanied by hyperphagia. In this case, single gene mutations (monogenic obesity) have been identified that, when present, tend to result in obesity that manifests in childhood. Although the genetic influence is much stronger than the environmental influence, excessive consumption of calories and insufficient physical activity can further exacerbate the situation. Examples of genes that have been identified as conferring a high risk for early-onset obesity include leptin (*LEP*) and the leptin receptor (*LEPR*) (Dubern and Clement, 2012), proopiomelanocortin (*POMC*) (Raffin-Sanson et al., 2003), and melanocortin-4 receptor (*MC4R*) (Panaro and Cone, 2013). These genes are collectively referred to as the leptin–POMC–melanocortin axis, a major hypothalamic circuit controlling energy homeostasis and food intake.

More recently, a number of gene variants have been described that, in the presence of an obesegenic environment, can promote overweight and obesity. These variants may influence any of the key components that factor into weight regulation, such as appetite control, energy metabolism, or physical activity, and interact with environmental factors such as dietary fats or carbohydrates. Examples of such variants include those that promote an increased absorption of dietary fat (e.g., *FABP2*); those involved with increased storage of fat in adipocytes (e.g., *ADRB2*, *ADRB3*); those that regulate transcription of key genes (e.g., *PPARG2*, *TCF7L2*); those that uncouple energy metabolism (e.g., the *UCP* gene family); and genes such as *FTO*, which is the most common weight-associated variant but whose function is not yet understood. Numerous other variants are being investigated for their role in weight regulation, including variants of genes involved with circadian rhythm (*CLOCK*, *REV-ERB-ALPHA*), which affect feeding behavior and weight regulation (Garaulet et al., 2013a, 2013b). Abete and colleagues (2012) provide a current review of the spectrum of genetic mutations associated with weight management.

Several of these variants form the basis of the weight management genetic tests that are presently on the market. However, these variants represent only a fraction of the many genes that are involved in the myriad of underlying biochemical mechanisms that can lead to obesity. As research continues to explore the numerous genes involved in all aspects of excessive weight, many more gene variants that influence weight management are expected to be identified.

Learn more about epigenetic regulation in eAppendix 36-1 online.

METABOLIC IMBALANCES

The adipocyte does more than store fat for future energy needs. It is a major endocrine organ that has a profound impact on the metabolism of other tissues, the regulation of appetite, insulin sensitivity, immunologic responses, and the risk of vascular disease (Ali et al., 2013). Adipocytes secrete multiple inflammatory cytokines such as interleukin-6 and tumor necrosis factor α, which can lead to increased systemic chronic inflammation. Weight gain furthers inflammation in the body, and when inflammation is present, losing weight is more difficult. Visceral adipose tissue is particularly active metabolically. Insulin resistance, present in the cardiometabolic syndrome (characterized by elevated waist circumference, low high-density lipoprotein cholesterol, elevated triglycerides, elevated blood pressure, and elevated blood sugar), is strongly associated with visceral adiposity. When insulin levels are high, as is the case in insulin resistance, the body is more likely to store calories. Weight gain in the abdominal area is associated with elevated insulin levels and inflammation. The elevated insulin levels can increase hunger levels and make it more difficult for a patient to lose weight. The interconnectivity of these metabolic factors promotes a vicious cycle that can make achieving a healthy weight difficult.

Other hormones influence weight and need to be considered when evaluating patients for weight gain and obesity. Hypothyroidism can result in weight gain. Other signs and symptoms of hypothyroidism include hair loss and hair thinning, cold intolerance, constipation, depression, arthralgias, elevated low-density lipoprotein cholesterol, dry skin, fatigue, memory impairment, menorrhagia, myalgias, and weakness (Gaitonde et al., 2012). Weight gain also influences hormone levels in the body. Estrogen can be produced in the adipocyte through the action of the enzyme aromatase. As an individual's percentage of body fat increases, dehydroepiandrosterone (DHEA) and testosterone are converted into estrogen by aromatase in adipose tissue. For men, this conversion can result in a lower testosterone level. This hormonal change has been associated with estrogen-related cancers, such as breast cancer, prostate cancer, and endometrial cancer (Williams, 2010).

MATERNAL WEIGHT DURING PREGNANCY

Maternal prenatal weight and weight gain during pregnancy have been associated with weight issues for the infant during childhood. A mother's prepregnancy weight and weight gain during pregnancy may also influence her children's weight. In a meta-analysis in which 45 studies met the researchers' selection criteria, Yu and coworkers (2013) found that children of mothers who were overweight or obese before pregnancy had a significantly increased risk of being overweight or obese during childhood. In a meta-analysis of 12 studies, Tie and colleagues (2014) found a significant association between excessive gestational weight gain and childhood overweight and obesity. Similarly, children of mothers who had gestational diabetes during pregnancy were found to have an increased risk of being overweight or obese later in life (Nehring et al., 2013). Undernutrition during pregnancy has also been associated with an increased risk of weight gain in children born to these mothers (Cunha et al., 2013). These reports suggest that maternal nutrition during pregnancy may be an important factor in weight management of offspring. Other contributing factors that should also be considered include

features of infant feeding, the overall nutritional sufficiency during childhood, and how health promoting the eating patterns are within the home.

ENVIRONMENTAL FACTORS

Food Intake

Over the past 40 years, the tendency in the U.S. population has been to consume more calories than needed. Per capita consumption of calories increased from 2200 kcal in 1970 to 2680 kcal in 1997 (Putnam, 2000). Increased portion sizes, the energy density of today's commonly eaten foods, and the trend in consuming meals outside the home where food portions tend to exceed standard serving sizes all contribute to the increase in calorie consumption. Satiety helps determine food intake and is partially determined by the volume and weight of the food consumed. Foods that are high in calorie content for a given volume, such as highly processed, low-fiber foods, can lead to excessive calorie intake.

It is important to recognize that the reasons a person gains or loses weight are not always simple. In a laboratory setting, 3500 calories equals 1 lb, and so it has been assumed that if a person consumes 3500 fewer calories than his or her body requires, they will lose 1 lb. In the office setting, this calculation does not always hold, and it is important to recognize and accept this when working with patients. Why does someone overeat? Many factors contribute to overeating, including stress, boredom, nutritional insufficiencies, emotional lability, access to food, and the changing of our diet to one that is highly processed. In a randomized, blinded crossover design study by Lennerz and colleagues (2013), overweight or obese young men age 18 to 35 years ate test meals that differed only in glycemic index (GI). The high-GI meal contained rapidly digested carbohydrate; the low-GI meal contained slowly digested carbohydrate (see Glycemic Index and Glycemic Load).

Plasma glucose, serum insulin, and hunger were monitored after each test meal and compared between those who ate the high-GI meal and those who ate the low-GI meal. After the low-GI meal, plasma glucose initially rose and by 1 hour had dropped to a relatively steady plateau over the next 3 hours. In those who ate the high-GI meal, plasma glucose initially surged and then dropped steeply over the next 3 hours to a level lower than seen with the low-GI meal. A similar pattern was seen with serum insulin levels. At the 4-hour mark, subjects who had eaten the high-GI meal reported greater hunger, and brain imaging showed intense activation of the nucleus accumbens, the brain region considered "ground zero" for conventional addiction (e.g., involving drug abuse or gambling). Remarkably, every subject who ate the high-GI meal responded in exactly the same way on the brain scans, producing extremely strong confidence in the results ($P < 0.001$).

This study showed that highly processed carbohydrate foods can cause food cravings in susceptible individuals, providing qualified support for the notion of "food addiction." The findings suggest that limiting consumption of highly processed carbohydrates, such as white bread, white rice, white potato products, and products with concentrated sugar, could help weight gain–prone individuals avoid overeating.

Glycemic Index and Glycemic Load

- Two values are commonly used to describe how rapidly a food or meal is digested. The GI value of a food is measured by the rise in blood glucose after consumption of 50 g of that food. This is then compared with the rise in blood glucose after consumption of 50 g of sugar. Carbohydrates that break down quickly have high GI values. Carbohydrates that break down slowly have low GI values.
- The glycemic load describes the rise in blood glucose after an edible portion of that food is consumed along with other foods. For example, carrots may have a high GI, but because it is very difficult to consume 50 g of carbohydrate from carrots, they have a low glycemic load.
- Examples of foods with high GIs include candy, soda, and fruit juice. Broccoli is an example of a food with a low GI. A meal with a high glycemic load would be pancakes with syrup and orange juice; fish with ½ cup of brown rice and 2 cups of mixed greens would be a meal with a low glycemic load.

Movement and Physical Activity

In a recent review, Denham et al. (2013) summarized the ability of physical activity to influence epigenetic modifications of histones or DNA in the brain, skeletal muscle, and peripheral blood. Aerobic exercise over many weeks was the primary variable studied that led to activity-induced benefits. Several of the studies found benefits with 30 minutes of daily moderate activity.

Yoga also appears to be an effective type of movement activity for improving weight, mental well-being, and health in general. In a narrative review of yoga intervention clinical trials, Rioux and Ritenbaugh (2013) reported that overall therapeutic yoga programs were effective in reducing body weight and improving body composition. A community-based 12-week yoga and Pilates program was found to be helpful for weight loss in postpartum women (Ko et al., 2013). In a small 8-week randomized controlled trial of 20 obese adolescent Korean boys, yoga was found to significantly decrease body weight, BMI, body fat mass, and percentage of body fat and to significantly increase fat-free mass and basal metabolic rate (Seo et al., 2012). Although the trends appear positive in terms of yoga's health benefits, larger controlled trials are needed to explore the full potential of yoga for health promotion.

Sleep

There is an association between too little or too much sleep and overweight and obesity. In a survey of more than 54,000 U.S. adults age 45 years or older, sleeping too little (≤6 hours) and sleeping too much (≥10 hours) were significantly associated with obesity (Liu et al., 2013). Throughout the life cycle, a short sleep duration is independently associated with weight gain (Gillman and Ludwig, 2013; Patel and Hu, 2008). When sleep duration and BMI were followed for 7.5 years in more than 83,000 U.S. adults age 51 years or older, researchers found an inverse relationship between the length of sleeping and BMI (Xiao et al., 2013). Sleep deprivation is associated with elevated ghrelin, elevated cortisol, elevated insulin, decreased leptin, and increased hunger (Patel and Hu, 2008). These hormonal changes are associated with weight gain and can result in less than expected weight loss in patients who are sleep deprived, even when they are restricting their caloric intake (Nedeltcheva et al., 2010). In a longitudinal study of adolescents, sleep duration and BMI were followed at 6-month intervals between age 14 and 18 (Mitchell et al., 2013). Shorter sleep duration was associated with greater BMI. Mesarwi and colleagues (2013) found a correlation between short duration of sleep, obesity, and type 2 diabetes and recommended assessing sleep quantity and quality during patient visits.

We must assess our patients' sleep when addressing weight gain and obesity. In addition, we must be alert to signs of obstructive sleep apnea (OSA) because this process is proinflammatory. Patients with OSA have higher inflammatory markers than BMI-matched individuals without OSA (Steiropoulos et al., 2010). Insulin resistance, type 2 diabetes, obesity, and weight gain are frequently associated with sleep apnea, which can result from weight gain and can also cause weight gain through the increase in inflammation and changes in metabolism that result from inadequate sleep (Alam et al., 2007). Signs and symptoms of sleep apnea include elevated blood pressure, difficulty in controlling blood pressure, fatigue, hypersomnolence, retrognathia, snoring, mood changes, and attention issues. When a child is gaining weight, it is important to screen for sleep apnea by asking the parents about snoring and examining the tonsils and adenoids for enlargement.

PSYCHOSOCIAL STRESS

In addition to the negative influences of physiological stress from poor nutrition, insufficient appropriate activity, and inadequate sleep, psychosocial stress can also contribute to excess weight. Psychosocial stress can arise from a wide variety of environmental stressors, such as change in routine, difficult decisions, depression, chronic health issues, lack of access to health care, economic challenges, a dysfunctional home environment, an unsafe neighborhood, inadequate social support, abusive relationships, illiteracy, job dissatisfaction, poor adjustment to life-cycle transitions such as retirement, and legal problems.

This type of stress is often associated with weight gain, elevated BMI, and poor food choices. The amount of weight someone gains when exposed to stress depends on the intensity of the stress, the duration of the stress, and the type of food available for consumption during stressful times (Block et al., 2009). Increased cortisol levels can lead to weight gain around the abdominal region (central adiposity). It is important to screen for emotional stress with patients, identify how this stress may be negatively impacting their weight, and help them incorporate stress reduction programs to achieve their weight loss goals. Even when we are unable to control the existence of stressors, controlling our response to stress can positively influence our weight and our overall health.

Similarly, cultivating supportive relationships with oneself and with friends and family is particularly helpful when undergoing behavioral change, which is often necessary with weight loss. Persons of the same sex have a greater influence on each other than those of the opposite sex (Christakis and Fowler, 2007). Our social networks can be a positive influence as well. People who exercise together are more likely to exercise. If you tell a friend, colleague or spouse that you are making a change in your lifestyle, you are more likely to maintain those changes.

TOXIN EXPOSURE

One environmental toxin in particular, the family of endocrine-disrupting chemicals (EDCs), is being investigated for its contribution to the high prevalence of obesity. Examples of EDCs include polychlorinated bisphenyls (PCBs), diethylstilbestrol (DES), bisphenol A, and persistent organic pollutants (POPs) such as tributyltin (TBT). This group of chemicals can interfere with the normal functioning of the endocrine system, which can affect development, reproduction, insulin production and utilization, and metabolic rate. Recent reviews of the literature suggest that exposure to EDCs during development is associated with excessive weight later in life and that these chemicals should be given serious consideration as potential contributors to obesity (Engel and Wolff, 2013; Newbold 2010; Tang-Péronard et al., 2011). Furthermore, these toxins have also been associated with insulin resistance and its associated obesity. An examination of selected POPs in the NHANES 1999 to 2002 data showed that elevated BMI and waist circumference were associated with POPs levels (Elobeid et al., 2010). BPA has also been linked to increased insulin levels and weight gain (Nadal et al., 2009).

MICROBIOME COMPOSITION

The microorganisms that inhabit the body cavities, such as the mouth, vagina, and respiratory and gastrointestinal tracts, appear to play an active role in our overall health. The gastrointestinal tract has been the subject of considerable interest in this regard. Multiple studies have suggested an association between our intestinal microbiota and weight. Fecal microbial cultures from healthy donors transplanted into recipients with metabolic syndrome were found to ameliorate the insulin resistance phenotype (Vrieze et al., 2012). High numbers of Bifidobacteria and low numbers of *Staphylococcus aureus* in the digestive tract in infancy may provide protection against the development of weight gain and obesity later in life. Bifidobacteria typify the gut microbiota composition of a healthy breastfed infant. Breastfeeding is associated with a 13% to 22% reduced likelihood of being overweight or obese in childhood (Kalliomäki et al., 2008).

However, just how the microbiota influence obesity remains unclear. What is clear so far is that the microbes are readily transmissible between individuals, after being transmitted can alter the outcome (obese vs. lean), and diet can further influence the outcome. The quality of the food we eat, as well as the influence our food has on our microbiota, have implications for the level of inflammation in our body and subsequent weight gain (Badman et al., 2005). Again, we see that all calories are not created equal.

See eAppendix 36-2 online to learn more about current research on how the microbiome can influence weight.

Assessment

Key Points

- Many of the environmental factors that lead to excess weight are lifestyle related.
- The patient's readiness to change is an important predictor of successful weight management.
- A thorough patient history provides important clues to the root cause of obesity.
- The patient assessment is conducted through a nutrition-oriented lens.
- Assessing percent body fat and its distribution helps inform the therapeutic intervention.
- Beyond nutrition, multiple modifiable lifestyle factors are also assessed.

Many of the environmental factors that lead to excess weight are lifestyle related. Typically, these factors are modifiable through an individual's actions, which provides the physician and patient with multiple leverage points in developing a personalized plan that can lead to successful weight management. The components of a thorough assessment are described in this section. Each of the chapter authors uses a nutrition-oriented approach to enhancing the standard patient health assessment, and key aspects are described here. Poetic license is taken with the term "nutrition" because it not only encompasses valuable clues as to nutritional status but also other lifestyle factors such as physical activity, sleep, thoughts and emotions, and relationships and system of meaning that can contribute to the root cause of overweight and obesity. Assessing your patient's readiness to change will help you decide where best to begin the journey toward attaining and maintaining a desirable weight.

READINESS TO CHANGE

The majority of the determinants of overweight and obesity are related to choices that can be modified. However, unless patients are ready to change their habits, successful weight management is not likely. Therefore, it is helpful to assess a patient's readiness to change. One particularly successful approach has been the transtheoretical or stages of change model pioneered by psychologist James Prochaska and colleagues (1992). This model describes the stages that a person passes through while changing a behavior: precontemplation, contemplation, preparation, action, and maintenance. Unless patients are ready to take action, they frequently are not able to sustain behavioral change. Validated questionnaires are available to help you determine the patient's stage (University of Rhode Island Change Assessment Scale, 2013). You can also get a quick feel for patient readiness with the question: "On a scale of 1 to 10, with 1 being not ready and 10 being very ready, how would you rate your readiness to change?"

In addition to using an open-ended questioning approach, motivational interviewing is particularly helpful when working with patients with chronic disorders in whom behavioral change is a key factor (Miller and Rollnick,

Table 36-2   Antecedents, Triggers, and Perpetuators in Obesity

Antecedents (genetics)	*Ob* gene (chromosome 7) FTO (fat mass and obesity-associated gene) is located on chromosome 16 and is associated with being overweight or obese (Fawcett et al., 2010; Frayling et al., 2007) A defect in the melanocortin-4 receptor is the most common single gene mutation associated with severe obesity in 5% of the population (Chambers et al., 2008) Brain-derived neurotrophic factor (BDNF) gene has been shown to cause spontaneous mendelian obesity in humans (Fisler et al., 2013) Fatty acid binding protein gene (*FABP2*) is associated with fat absorption Peroxisome proliferator receptor-γ gene (PPAR-γ) plays a key role in the formation of fat cells Adrenergic β_2-receptor gene (*ADRB2*) mobilizes fat cells for energy Adrenergic β_3-receptor gene (*ADRB3*) regulates the breakdown of fat from tissues in response to exercise Glutamate decarboxylase 2 gene (*GAD2*) is released from pancreatic and brain cells coding for GABA neurotransmitter, which regulates food intake
Triggers	Food insecurity; supplemental nutrition programs with high–glycemic index foods (Leung et al., 2012; Ludwig et al., 2012; Nickols-Richardson et al., 2005); high fructose intake; infection (chronic, bacterial, viral, or parasitic); sources of injury and chronic inflammation; endocrine imbalance, adrenal insufficiency, thyroid hypofunction (consider autoimmune, radiation induced, chemical induced, or medication induced) (Hochberg et al., 2010; Thaler et al., 2013); food sensitivity or genetic overlap (celiac, food, and environmental hypersensitivity); environmental toxicity (bisphenol A; Dolinoy et al., 2007); and even cell phone use alters glucose metabolism in the brain, disrupting appetite-related chronobiology (Fragopoulou et al., 2012; Kohlstadt, 2013; Volkow et al., 2011)
Perpetuators	Altered sleep (disrupted chronobiology: shift work, jet lag) (Kohlstadt, 2013; Stempfer et al., 1989) and sleep apnea Minimal exercise (Jakicic et al., 2011; Sausse, 2013; Vincent et al., 2012; Warburton et al., 2006) Persistent stress (psychologic, physical, relationship, socioeconomic, environmental) Nutrition (high glycemic index [Ruottinen et al., 2008; Fava et al., 2013], poor vegetable or fruit intake)

GABA, γ-Aminobutyric acid.

2002). Motivational interviewing focuses on identifying, examining, and resolving the ambivalence that a patient feels about behavioral change. Key web resources are listed at the end of this chapter.

PATIENT HISTORY

A careful history helps identify common antecedents, triggers, and perpetuators of obesity (Table 36-2). Multiple factors can lead to overweight and obesity, and each patient will have his or her own path leading to excess weight. Determining some of the contributing factors will help you identify an intervention that is most likely to be successful for that patient. When gathering your patient's history, ask open-ended questions that will help identify the factors that may have predisposed them towards obesity: Was he or she overweight as a child? Did he or she gain weight all of a sudden or slowly over many years? Is there a family history of overweight or obesity? Is his or her activity level low because of pain or injury, inflammation, or fatigue? A slow, steady weight gain of 2 to 5 lb per year is typical for many adults who are not exercising adequately or eating too many calories. Alternatively, if your patient gained weight quickly, it is important to rule out thyroid disorders, hormonal changes, stress, family trauma, infection, and inflammation. A variety of clues such as these can come out during the information-gathering phase of the assessment if you ask open-ended questions and listen carefully (i.e., be "present" to the patient during this process).

During the patient history, evaluate the timeline of the weight gain. When did the weight gain begin? When did it markedly increase? Through the identification of environmental triggers as well as epigenetic and metabolic drivers for the obesogenic environment, therapeutic interventions can be developed. These environmental pressures, from the prenatal period through adulthood, are associated with weight gain and obesity (Table 36-3).

Obese patients frequently have comorbidities that often require therapeutic medications. These therapeutic drug regimens for diabetes, depression, hypertension, seizures, and HIV disease can trigger weight gain and worsen obesity (Table 36-4). Additionally, many of the most commonly prescribed medications can alter nutritional biochemistry and the obesogenic environment by multiple mechanisms (Table 36-5).

THE ABCDs OF NUTRITION EVALUATION

The ABCDs of nutrition evaluation of the obese patient include anthropometrics, biochemical markers, clinical indicators, and diet and lifestyle evaluation (Institute for Functional Medicine, 2010). Anthropometrics and vital signs include the height; weight; BMI; waist circumference; hip circumference; waist-to-hip ratio or waist-to-height ratio; percent body fat (fat mass); percent fat-free mass (lean body mass); extracellular water content; intracellular water content; blood pressure; respiratory rate; temperature; pulse; and for patients with diabetes, microfilament testing of the feet to test for feeling sensation. Biochemical markers typically include the comprehensive metabolic panel that includes a fasting lipid panel, thyroid panel or at least thyroid-stimulating hormone, 25-hydroxy vitamin D, high-sensitivity C-reactive protein, hemoglobin A_{1c}, complete blood count, urinalysis, and other laboratory analyses as needed (e.g., fasting insulin). The physical examination is a standard comprehensive examination with the assessment of additional clinical indicators as seen through a nutrition lens, such as including an examination of the mouth; evaluation of the nails, skin, and hair; and peripheral sensation using monofilament, 128 Hz tuning fork, and a reflex hammer.

The ABCDs of the nutrition-oriented evaluation of the obese patient should be completed and will help clarify the role of lifestyle in the root causes of the underlying chronic condition (Jones et al., 2010; Minich et al., 2013).

Table 36-3 Environmental Influences on Obesity

Environmental Influences	Behavior, Condition, or Exposure	Associated Impact
Prenatal	Maternal smoking Higher maternal BMI at conception Maternal diabetes	Increase odds of adult obesity by 50% by age 33 Increase body weight of child Increase overweight as a child and adult
Breastfeeding	Primarily breast fed (vs. formula)	Less likely to be obese as a child Each additional month of breastfeeding can result in a 4% decrease in risk of obesity
Viruses (e.g., adenovirus-36 antibody)	Increased glucose uptake, decreased leptin secretion	Associated with increased body weight in twin studies
Toxins (e.g., endocrine-disrupting chemicals)	Bisphenol A, organotins, phytoestrogen exposure during development	Higher serum toxin levels can lead to greater obesity in children
Smoking cessation	People who discontinue smoking	Increased odds ratio of obesity by at least twofold
Sleep deprivation	Associated with increased food intake, decreased physical activity, and decreased body temperature with fatigue	Consistently associated with development of obesity in children and young adults
Movement	Increased leisure time Declining work activity Declining walking, biking, etc. as a means of transportation Declining activity at home Increased electronic interface (computers, games, TV time) High risk of inactivity	A low level of physical activity decreases total energy expenditure and unless matched by a decrease in energy intake can lead to weight gain

BMI, Body mass index.
Adapted from Polsky S, Catenacci VA, Wyatt HR, Hill JO. Obesity: epidemiology, etiology and prevention. In Ross AC, Caballero B, Cousins RJ, et al, eds. *Modern nutrition in health and disease.* 11th ed. Baltimore: Wolters Kluwer/Lippincott Williams and Wilkins; 2014:771-785.

Table 36-4 Concomitant Pharmacology That Promotes Weight Gain and Influences Body Weight

Steroid hormones	Glucocorticoids, estrogens, progestins, testosterone, tamoxifen
Diabetes therapies	Some insulins, sulfonylureas, thiazolidinediones; metformin, glucagon-like peptide agonists, sodium glucose cotransporter 2 inhibitors
Certain antiretroviral protease inhibitors	Lipodystrophy during treatment with protease inhibitors, lipohypertrophy after successful suppression of viral load
Certain β-adrenergic blockers	Propranolol
Certain antihistamines	Diphenhydramine
Certain antidepressants	Tricyclic antidepressants, MAO inhibitors, some SSRIs (paroxetine), antiserotonin agents (pizotifen)
Certain antiseizure medications	Valproate, gabapentin, carbamazepine
Certain antipsychotropic drugs	Clonazepine, olanzapine, risperidone, thioridazine

MAO, Monoamine oxidase; SSRI, selective serotonin reuptake inhibitor.
Anuurad et al., 2010; Polsky et al., 2014; Seger, 2013.

Table 36-5 Many Commonly Used Medications Promote Weight Gain

Rank in Prescriptions Written (Million)	Medication	Mechanism
2 (94.1)	Simvastatin	Reduces exercise tolerance, promotes insulin resistance, depletes CoQ10
5 (57.2)	Amlodipine besylate	Increases appetite centrally in some patients
6 (53.4)	Omeprazole	Contributes to vitamin B_{12} deficiency and diet indiscretion
9 (48.3)	Metformin	Lowers absorption of vitamin B_{12}
10 (47.8)	Hydrochlorothiazide	Increases appetite, reduces cardiac response to exercise
By Sales (Billions)	**Medication**	**Mechanism**
1 (7.2)	Lipitor	Reduces exercise tolerance, promotes insulin resistance, depletes CoQ10 within muscle cells in genetically susceptible patients
2 (6.3)	Nexium	May contribute to vitamin B_{12} deficiency, fatigue, altered methylation, diet indiscretion
4 (4.7)	Advair Discus	Potentially protects against weight gain by reducing need for corticosteroids
5 (4.6)	Abilify	Increases appetite centrally
6 (4.4)	Seroquel	Increases appetite centrally
8 (3.8)	Crestor	Reduces exercise tolerance, promotes insulin resistance, depletes CoQ10
9 (3.5)	Actose	Associated with weight gain

CoQ10, Coenzyme Q10.
Adapted from Kohlstadt I. Obesity-primary care approaches to weight reduction. In Kohlstadt I, ed. *Advancing medicine with food and nutrients.* 2nd ed. Boca Raton, FL: CRC Press; 2013: 349-372 and Report of the IMS Institute for Healthcare Informatics. The use of medicines in the United States: review of 2010. Parsippany, NJ: IMS Health; 2011. http://www.imshealth.com/imshealth/Global/Content/IMS%20Institute/Documents/IHII_UseOfMed_report%20.pdf.

Table 36-6   Anthropometric Evaluation

Quantitative direct measurements	**COMMONLY USED**
	Weight, height (length)
	Waist circumference (<35 in women; <40 in men)
	Hip circumference
	Skinfold thickness measurements (three sites)
	Reactance/resistance (BIA)
Calculations	BMI (normal, 18.5-24.9; overweight, >25; obese, >30)
	Waist-to-hip ratio (<0.8 in women; <0.9 in men)
	Waist-to-height ratio (<0.5)
	Deurenberg Equation (BMI, Age, Gender)
	% Body fat = (1.2 × BMI) + (0.23 × Age [yr]) − (10.8 × G) − 5.4
	G = 1 for male; G = 0 for female
	Bioelectrical imepdance analysis
	Fat mass, fat-free mass, extracellular water, intracellular water, phase angle, BMR (weight, height, and activity dependent)
Quantitative testing	**LESS COMMONLY USED**
	BOD POD
	Quantitative magnetic resonance
	Underwater weighing
	Deuterium dilution

BIA, Bioelectrical impedance analysis; *BMI,* body mass index; *BMR,* basal metabolic rate; *BOD POD,* whole-body air displacement plethysmography (Deurenberg et al., 2003; Srikanthan et al., 2009; Wang et al., 2010).

Anthropometrics

Assessing anthropometrics is the first step in the nutritional evaluation of the patient. Starting with birth, the weight and height are determined and then routinely checked throughout the lifespan. The use of these basic measurements and associated ratios that can be calculated, such as waist-to-hip ratio, are commonly used in clinics. The initial stratification is by BMI calculation from height and weight (underweight, <18.5; normal, 18.5-24.9; overweight, 25-29.9; obese, >30), waist circumference (women, <35 in; men, <40), and waist-to-hip ratio (women, <0.8; men, <0.9) or waist-to-height ratio (<0.5 ideal). BMI is the primary parameter used to categorize weight for height (Weight/Height/Height × 703) and, in fact, has recently been mandated to be included in all patient charts. The BMI is bimodal. There is increased risk of mortality and morbidity when BMI is below 18.5 and above 24.9. The risk of inflammatory disease, including cardiovascular disease, occurs at both ends of the bimodal curve.

Body mass index is a quick and easy screening tool to use in the office setting but is imperfect. For muscular individuals, the BMI overestimates risk. For patients with too little lean muscle mass (sarcopenia), the BMI underestimates risk. Table 36-6 lists the many ways to assess body composition. A comparison of the various assessment methods is provided by Saltzman et al. (2013).

A more informative assessment of adiposity as well as risk for disease than BMI is body fat percentage. Table 36-7 lists the fat percentage in healthy individuals. Although underwater (hydrostatic) weighing and dual-energy X-ray absorptiometry (DXA) scan are considered the preferred methods for measuring percent body fat, these methods are not readily available in most clinics. Each method has its own confounders and advantages (Carroll et al., 2008;

Table 36-7   Classification by Percentage Body Fat

Classification	Female (%)	Male (%)
Essential fat	10-13	2-5
Athletes	14-20	6-13
Fitness	21-24	14-17
Acceptable	25-31	18-24
Obesity	>32	>25

Adapted from ACE Pro. Percent body fat calculator: skinfold method. http://www.acefitness.org/acefit/healthy_living_tools_content.aspx?id=2.

Kushner and Blatner, 2005; Wang et al., 2010). Bioelectrical impedance analysis (BIA) has emerged as a more convenient technique for in-office measurements of body fat and fat-free mass, of particular interest in detecting malnutrition. The inclusion of BIA in the NHANES with comparison with the more traditional multisite skinfold measurements has validated the use of this tool. BIA is best used as a tool for tracking a patient's progress from one time point to another rather than as a precise measurement of any one component of body composition. Many practitioners use sequential BIA analysis to follow the progression of treatment, which allows for determining that the weight loss is the desired fat mass and not muscle mass loss or excessive water loss.

Additional anthropometric measurements, waist and hip circumference, and the calculated waist-to-hip ratio help to further stratify obesity by location of fat accumulation (Figure 36-1). If a man's waist circumference is greater than 40 inches (102 cm) and a woman's abdominal circumference is greater than 35 inches (>89 cm), then they are considered obese. The presence of android obesity (visceral adiposity) with a waist-to-hip ratio of greater than 0.8 in women and greater than 0.9 in men portends of a more inflammatory metabolism and is characterized by the apple shape. The gynoid obesity (increased BMI, increased body fat percentage) hallmark is subcutaneous obesity with a waist-to-hip ratio of less than 0.8 for women and less than 0.9 for men and a characteristic pear-shaped body type. Android obesity (increased BMI, increased percentage of body fat with an elevated waist-to-hip ratio) correlates with adiposopathy and with metabolic disease (insulin resistance, metabolic syndrome). Those with android obesity have an increased visceral adipose tissue percentage. The waist measurement accuracy depends on the use of the same landmarks. Some suggest the waist at the top of the iliac crest (Anderson and Hensrud, 2011); others use the waist as the midpoint between the bottom of the 10th rib and the superior iliac crest at the midaxillary line.

Figure 36-2 provides a case example in which the combined used of multiple anthropometric measures, including BIA, is helpful in following treatment progression.

After the pattern of fat distribution has been determined (android or gynoid distribution), the necessary biochemical indicators are ordered to help determine drivers of the obesity-promoting condition (Table 36-8). This approach helps improve the metrics for health risk analysis (Ahima and Lazer, 2013).

The pattern of morbidity in an obese patient is influenced by whether the patient has the sequel of adiposopathy (dysmetabolic syndrome), which is associated with elevated

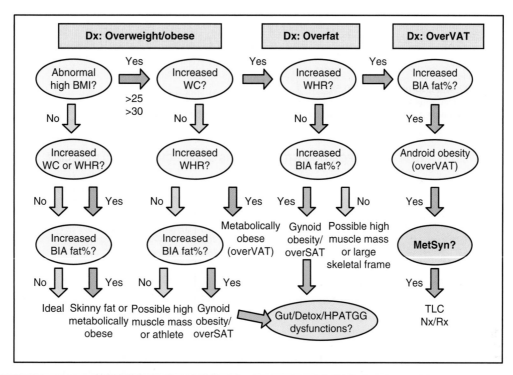

Abnormal BMI	Increased Waist Circumference	Increased Waist-to-Hip Ratio	Increased % Body Fat	Obese/Fat Distribution	Workup
No	No	No	No	No	Ideal normal health monitoring
No	No	No	Yes	Skinny fat—sarcopenic adiposity	Metabolically obese inflammatory workup; workup for causes of sarcopenia or sarcobesity (Parr et al., 2013)
Yes	No	No	No	No	High-muscle athlete; normal health monitoring
Yes	No	Yes	Yes	Yes: android obesity, visceral adiposity	Inflammatory workup; root causes of inflammation associated with weight gain and adiposopathy (e.g., infection, glucose dysregulation, toxins)
Yes	No	No	Yes	Yes: gynoid obesity, subcutaneous fat adiposity	Gastrointestinal, biotransformation, HPATGG dysfunction, toxicity, and endocrine evaluations
Yes	Yes	No	No	No: large frame; high muscle mass	No intervention; normal health monitoring
Yes	Yes	No	Yes	Yes: gynoid obesity subcutaneous fat adiposity	Gastrointestinal, biotransformation, HPATGG dysfunction, toxicity, and endocrine evaluations
Yes	Yes	Yes	Yes	Yes: android obesity, visceral adiposity	Therapeutic lifestyle change, nutritional and inflammatory workup, root causes of inflammation associated with weight gain and adiposopathy (e.g., infection, glucose dysregulation, toxins)

Figure 36-1 Assessing body composition by body mass index (BMI), waist circumference, waist-to-hip ratio, and percent fat mass. *BIA,* Bioelectrical impedance analysis; *fat %,* bioelectrical impedance analysis fat percentage; *HPATGG,* hypothalamic–pituitary–adrenal–thyroid–gonadal–gastrointestinal axis; *METSyn,* metabolic syndrome; *overSAT,* high percentage of subcutaneous adipose tissue; *overVAT,* high percentage of visceral adipose tissue; *TLC Nx/Rx,* therapeutic lifestyle change and intervention, nutritional and pharmacologic treatment; *WC,* waist circumference; *WHR,* waist-to-hip ratio. (From Saxena S: Cardiovascular advanced practice module, *Institute for Functional Medicine,* 2012, Federal Way, WA, and Stone PM: Functional nutrition–head to toe. Toolkit, *Institute for Functional Medicine,* 2013, Federal Way, WA.)

Case Study:
Anthropometrics: height, 72 in; weight, 202 lb
BMI: 27.4
Waist circumference: 39 in
Hip circumference: 38 in
Waist-to-hip ratio: 10.02; **waist-to-height ratio:** 0.54
BIA: fat mass, 28.1%; **fat-free mass:** 71.9%
Assessment: android body type, increased abdominal visceral body fat, grade 1 obesity
Treatment: low glycemic impact diet

WEIGHT AND BODY COMPOSITION WITH 4 MONTHS OF DIET CHANGE AND EXERCISE

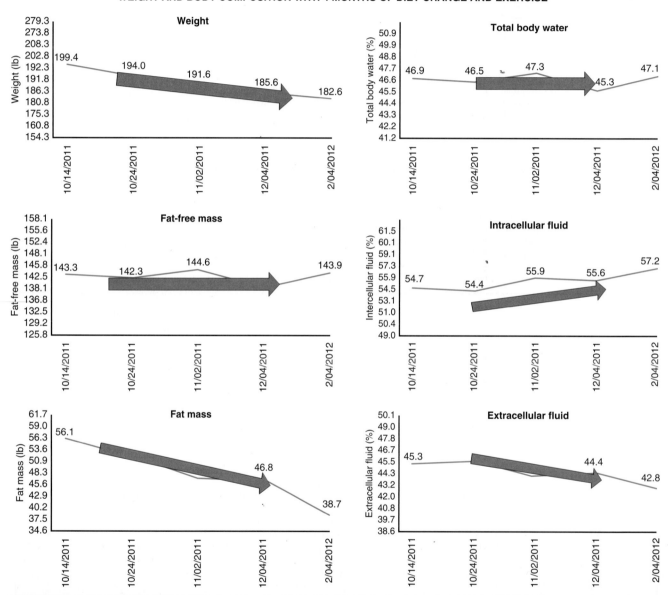

Case Study:
Anthropometrics: height, 72 in; weight, 182.3 lb
BMI: 24.7
Waist circumference: 33 in
Hip circumference: 37.5 in
Waist-to-hip ratio: 0.88; **waist-to-height ratio:** 0.45
BIA: fat mass, 20.9%; **fat-free mass:** 78.1%

Figure 36-2 Case Study: Case example using sequential bioelectrical impedance analysis (BIA) to follow treatment progression. The patient was a 56-year-old man with hyperlipidemia and erectile dysfunction taking prevastatin and Viagra. BIA was used over the 4-month period of increased exercise, food choice, and quantity intervention to follow anthropometric changes in weight, fat-free mass, and fat mass to confirm that the weight loss was composed of fat mass loss and not loss of muscle mass or total body water. The shift in extracellular fluid to intracellular fluid is considered a healthy sign.

Table 36-8 Physical Examination Findings in the Obese with Associated Comorbidities

System	Condition
Body composition	Monitoring fat and muscle mass with weight, waist circumference, waist-to-hip ratio, BIA, and resting metabolic rate; DEXA assesses bone densitometry and body composition (Heber et al., 1996; Kohlstadt, 2013) Age of onset in adolescence: increased BMI (23-25) strongly associated with obesity in adulthood Age 25-40 yr: increases in BMI associated with worse profile biomarkers later in adulthood
Hydration	Dry mucous membranes, pedal edema, poor skin turgor, dry mouth generally indicative of intracellular dehydration; need corroboration with urine specific gravity Poor hydration is associated with less favorable BIA and alters accuracy of skinfold measurements (Kohlstadt et al., 2013)
Oral cavity	Xerostomia, periodontal disease, tooth decay, amalgam fillings, and odor may indicate barriers to weight reduction, inducing dehydration unfavorable microbiota, inadequate mastication, undermethylation, and insulin resistance (Kohlstadt, 2013)
Neck circumference	Predictor of OSA and severity which is obesogenic (men, >17 in [43 cm]; women, >16 in [41 cm]) (Pinto et al., 2011)
Cardiovascular	Hypertension, CAD, essential hypertension, LVH, CHF, cor pulmonale, obesity-associated cardiomyopathy, accelerated atherosclerosis, pulmonary hypertension of obesity, thromboembolic pulmonary emboli Peripheral vasculature: venous varicosities, thrombophlebitis, lower extremity venous and or lymphatic edema, lower limb circulatory stasis
Pulmonary	Predisposition to respiratory infections, increased bronchial asthma, obesity hypoventilation syndrome (Pickwickian syndrome), dyspnea, OSA, hypoventilation syndrome, Pickwickian syndrome, asthma
Neurologic	Cranial nerve I: olfactory nerve function loss is associated with altered food choices, including oversalting and oversweetening of food (Hirsch and Whitman, 2013; Kohlstadt, 2013) Intracranial hypertension caused by increased abdominal pressure, sleep apnea, and so on Stroke, nerve entrapment (meralgia paresthetica, carpal tunnel syndrome)
Gastrointestinal	Gallbladder disease (cholecystitis, cholelithiasis), NASH, fatty liver infiltration, reflux esophagitis, hernias
Genitourinary	Urinary stress incontinence, nephrotic syndrome, focal glomerulosclerosis, erectile dysfunction
Reproductive	Obstetric and perinatal complications: pregnancy-induced hypertension, increased risk of gestational diabetes, shoulder dystocia, fetal macrosomia, pelvic dystocia Women: anovulation, early puberty, infertility, hyperandrogenism, polycystic ovaries Men: hypogonadotropic hypogonadism
Musculoskeletal	Musculoskeletal: general: abdominal hernias, ventral and inguinal, immobility Musculoskeletal and orthopedic: osteoarthritis of major joints, coxa vera, slipped capital femoral epiphysis, Blount disease, Legg-Calvé-Perthes disease, chronic lumbago Pain with moderate pressure over adult patients' shin bones or ribs: associated with osteomalacia; vitamin D deficiency, which perpetuates insulin resistance; can lower mood and limits physical activity, increasing fall risk (Brady et al., 2013; Holick, 2006; Kimmons et al., 2006; Wicherts et al., 2007)
Integument	Intertrigo (bacterial or fungal), acanthosis nigracans, hirsutism, increased risk of cellulitis and carbuncles, skin tags (epiliths) secondary to insulin resistance, stasis dermatitis, ulcerations, stria distensae (skin stretch mark), stasis pigmentation, venous stasis ulcers
Metabolic and endocrine	Type 2 diabetes mellitus, prediabetes, metabolic syndrome, dyslipidemia
Psychologic	Social stigmatization and depression
Malignant	Associations with endometrial, prostate, colon, breast, gallbladder, and lung cancer
Lifestyle	Sleep duration <5 hr to >8 hr associated with increased visceral and subcutaneous body fat with decreased leptin hormone and increased ghrelin hormone levels
Obesity in women	Being overweight contributes to menstrual disorders, infertility, miscarriage, poor pregnancy outcome, impaired fetal well-being, and type 2 diabetes; changes in sensitivity to insulin may occur Pregnant women who are obese are more at risk for pregnancy-induced hypertension and preeclampsia (Escott-Stump, 2012)
Age of onset	History of rapid weight gain in infancy, childhood, or early puberty, and excessive weight gain in pregnancy increase the risk for obesity (Johnson et al., 2006) Total energy expenditure and physical activity level declines progressively in both overweight and normal weight men and women, falling ≈150 kcal/decade; the thermic effect of food does not change (Roberts and Dallal, 2005)
Obesity in elderly adults	Increasing prevalence along with related macro and micronutrient deficiencies (Flood and Carr, 2004)

BIA, Bioelectrical impedance analysis; *BMI,* body mass index; *CAD,* Coronary artery disease; *CHF,* congestive heart failure; *DEXA,* dual-energy x-ray absorptiometry; *LVH,* left ventricular hypertrophy; *NASH,* nonalcoholic steatohepatitis; *OSA,* obstructive sleep apnea.
Hamby and Griffing, 2013; Kushner and Roth, 2003.

blood sugar, elevated blood pressure, and dyslipidemia. Fat mass disease is associated with stress on the weight-bearing joints, immobility, tissue compression (sleep apnea, gastrointestinal reflux, high blood pressure), and tissue sheer forces (intertrigo) (Allende-Vigo 2010; Bays et al., 2005, 2008; Bays, 2009, 2012; Seger et al., 2013).

Bioelectrical impedance analysis provides additional information on fat-free mass (lean body and muscle mass), extracellular water, and intracellular water. Being able to monitor whether body fat, rather than lean muscle mass, is being lost is a particularly valuable contribution of BIA testing. There is often a lower than predicted metabolic rate observed in extremely obese individuals (Livingston and Kohlstadt, 2005). This is because muscle caloric burn rate per pound per day is 6 calories for muscle and 2 calories for fat. The coincident loss of muscle and replacement weight fat leads to a 66% decrease in resting burn rate per pound of tissue (Kohlstadt, 2013).

In morbidly and super obese individuals, there is a shift in percentage of body water, and body fat percentage increases. Whereas an adult with a healthy weight is 60% to 65% body water, someone who is extremely obese tends to have a total body water of 35% to 45%. This shift places the obese at an increased vulnerability for volume depletion (dehydration), which is a common problem in obese individuals (Batmanghelidj and Kohlstadt, 2006; Kohlstadt, 2013; Livingston and Kohlstadt, 2005).

Biochemical Indicators

The distribution of fat, percent body fat, and associated muscle mass help the clinician determine which laboratory and biochemical indicators would be most revealing and helpful for determining interventions (see Figure 36-1 and Table 36-9). Using this sorting of fat distribution determined by BMI, waist circumference, waist-to-hip ratio, and bioimpedance analysis, the laboratory tests considered extend beyond the evaluation of simply thyroid function. See Table 36-9 for further clarity on how body fat percent and distribution inform the intervention.

Clinical Indicators

The clinical indicators (see Table 36-8) uncovered during the physical examination of the obese patient help identify comorbidities and physical examination features unique to the patient with android or gynoid obesity caused by adiposopathy or fat mass disease (see Table 36-9). The pathology of cardiovascular, pulmonary, rheumatologic, neurologic, and endocrinologic comorbid disease drives the obesogenic metabolic environment within the patient. The physical examination is a key component to the nutritional evaluation of the obese patient.

Diet and Lifestyle Evaluation

At a minimum, include a food diary in your patient information packet and, preferably, a broader diet and lifestyle assessment to assess your patient's risk of becoming overweight or obese. The diet and lifestyle evaluation should include a diet record from the patient that ranges from 1 to 7 days in length. The diet is evaluated for adequacy of protein; essential fats; and complex carbohydrates, including fiber. The overabundance of any major nutrient or the imbalance of saturated or transaturated fats, simple carbohydrates, or incomplete protein is identified. Also assess whether your patient has adequate intake of water and a wide variety of colorful vegetables and fruits, which are rich in phytonutrients. Assuring that these aspects of the diet are adequate will increase the likelihood of sufficiency of minerals and vitamins.

The diet and lifestyle assessment helps uncover and improve understanding of the obesogenic drivers. During the gathering of the patient history, the antecedents, triggers, and perpetuators combine with the anthropometrics, biochemical indicators, and clinical findings to direct the development of an intervention and its treatment plan.

If possible, make the information packet available so the patient can complete it in advance. You can create a simple 7-day diet and lifestyle assessment form by listing the days of the week across the top and down the left side listing food intake (breakfast, snack, lunch, snack, dinner, optional snack), water intake (cups or ounces), physical activity (time, type), sleep (quality), emotional stress (thoughts and emotions), and one thing patients did for themselves each day that brought them joy. If, however, you use only a food and activity log, include room to note activity for each day of the week and at least 3 days of food intake that includes two weekdays and one weekend or nonwork day because people tend to eat differently when their schedules are more flexible. Have patients indicate the type of activity and length as well as which foods and beverages and how much was consumed.

Below are recommendations for ways to assess each of the key modifiable lifestyle factors that contribute to disease.

Food Diary. Key information you can obtain from the food diary includes whether the patient eats breakfast, snacks at night, or drinks an excessive amount of sugar-sweetened beverages. Skipping breakfast has been associated with increased calories eaten later in the day and with weight gain. Nighttime snacking is a common pattern that you want to fully assess and help curtail. How much soda, juice drinks, 100% fruit juice, or sweetened caffeinated beverages are drunk most days? Drinking your calories through high soda or juice intake is associated with obesity. An easy recommendation that you can make during many office visits is to have your patients stop drinking all sugar-sweetened beverages. It is important to ask about all sugar-sweetened beverages, including soda, sports drinks, juice drinks, and coffee and tea (Han and Powell, 2013) (see Figure 36-1). Table 36-9 reviews key diagnostic nutritional tests that can be considered in weight loss therapy. The calories from these beverages can add up quickly and should not be included on a daily basis.

A food diary can also help determine the quality of the carbohydrates eaten, which may come from foods with a high GI or from sugar-sweetened beverages. There is compelling evidence that carbohydrate quality has important influences on obesity as well as on comorbidities associated with obesity, such as cardiovascular disease, metabolic syndrome, and type 2 diabetes. Dietary fiber is an important determinant of satiety and weight gain and helps protect against hyperlipidemia and hyperglycemia. Vegetables and fruits are excellent sources of fiber and phytonutrients and help protect against cardiovascular disease, diabetes, and cancer. Assess the record for high-GI carbohydrates (see Glycemic Index and Glycemic Load earlier in the chapter). It is common for patients to replace saturated fat with high-GI carbohydrates, which may increase the risk of developing type 2 diabetes and cardiovascular disease. As noted earlier, soft drink consumption is a proven cause of weight gain, which may relate to the lack of satiation provided by these drinks. In large amounts, the fructose contained in these drinks leads to greater adverse metabolic changes than equivalent amounts of glucose (Slyper, 2013).

Another aspect of food intake that can lead to excess weight (not necessarily excess body fat) is the presence of food sensitivities, as measured by elevated IgG antibodies

Table 36-9 Nutritional Diagnostic Tests to Guide Weight Loss Reduction

Testing	Interpretation	Mechanism	Treatment	Relevance to Weight Loss
Albumin (serum)	Low level suggests protein malnutrition	Inadequate intake, malabsorption	Dietary protein, supplemental amino acids, digestive enzymes	Maintain lean body mass, avoid sarcopenia (Kohlstadt, 2008)
C-reactive protein (CRP)	High-sensitivity CRP should be <10 mg/L	Inflammation from various sources, including food allergies, infection, autoimmune issues, and weight reduction	Supplemental fiber, alkaline diet, avoidance of food allergens, multiple vitamin, supplemental curcumin 2-4 g/d	Inflammation exacerbates sarcopenia
Carnitine	Deficiency if low plasma carnitine or elevated urinary adipic, suberic, and ethylmalonic acids	Impaired absorption; decreased synthesis, associated with Fe deficiency, high demand during fat metabolism	L-acetyl carnitine 2 g/day	Fat metabolism increases demand for carnitine; carnitine drop is associated with fatigue in pregnancy; carnitine is needed to transport free fatty acids into the mitochondria
Carotenes	α-Carotene, 9-101 mcg/L β-Carotene, 42-373 mcg/L, lutein, 50-250 mcg/L, zeaxanthin, 8-80 mcg/L	Nutrient deficiencies (i.e., Zn) and medications can interfere with synthesis	Green leafy vegetables; cooking with spices, phytonutrient-rich supplements	Obesity is a risk factor for reduced fat-soluble nutrients
Coenzyme Q10 (CoQ10)	Low serum CoQ10 signifies depletion of tissue CoQ10; high levels of pyruvate, succinate, fumarate, and malate in the urine suggest insufficient CoQ10 to meet energy needs	Nutrient deficiencies and medications can interfere with synthesis	Supplemental CoQ10 up to 300 mg/day	Fat metabolism increases demand for CoQ10
Fatty acid profile	RBC fatty acid profiles can identify omega-3, omega-6, trans, very long chain, and saturated fatty acids	Skewed dietary intake; inappropriate supplement use; reduced delta 6 desaturase enzyme activity; fat malabsorption	Balance mono- and polyunsaturated fatty acids with diet and supplements	Guides strategic use of dietary and supplemental fatty acids for weight reduction; fatty acid imbalances may stem from prior medical or surgical treatment for obesity
Homocysteine	Elevation signifies deficiency in vitamin B_{12}, folate, vitamin B_6, or interactive insufficiencies of riboflavin, niacin, and thiamine	Impaired absorption and inadequate intake of the B vitamins (B_1, B_2, B_3, B_6, B_{12}, folate)	Supplementation of methyl folate, folacin, and vitamin B_{12} can improve methylation	Maintain energy metabolism and harvest of calories through intermediary metabolism of carbohydrates and proteins
Iron studies	Low ferritin and percent saturation ≤15 suggest iron-deficient erythropoiesis even when HCT is normal; elevation suggests hemochromatosis	Deficiency from impaired absorption; inadequate intake excess from primary hemochromatosis, a nutrient–gene interaction	Treat deficiency with supplemental minerals, dietary iron, and cooking with an iron skillet with citrus; hemochromatosis is managed medically and by minimizing dietary iron intake	Deficiency tends to coexist with other mineral deficiencies, exacerbated by some diets; iron, zinc, and chromium alter food preferences; hemochromatosis contributes to the inflammatory component of obesity
Magnesium	RBC magnesium below laboratory-specified range	Impaired absorption, inadequate dietary intake, competitive absorption with calcium	Increase fruit and vegetable intake; supplement calcium and magnesium in a ratio of 2:1	Optimizing magnesium supports hydration, fat metabolism, and extracellular–intracellular fluid flux
Triglycerides	Fasting values >100 mg/dL or even 75 mg/dL suggest impaired fat metabolism	Steatosis, increased oxidative stress, consumption of synthetic fats, and refined carbohydrates	Diet low in refined carbohydrates and no trans or highly processed fats; liver support; supplemental L carnitine 2 g/d	Elevated triglycerides represent a treatable impairment in fat metabolism; also may indicate increased intestinal production of lipids from simple carbohydrates

Continued on following page

Table 36-9   Nutritional Diagnostic Tests to Guide Weight Loss Reduction (Continued)

Testing	Interpretation	Mechanism	Treatment	Relevance to Weight Loss
Vitamin D	25-OH vitamin D: 30-50 ng/mL throughout the year <10 ng/mL deficient, <30 ng/mL insufficient, <36 ng/mL associated with insulin resistance, <50 ng/mL associated with double the solid cancer incidence; when associated with a high normal or high 1,25–DHCC, associated with underlying infection	Low vitamin D associated with decreased innate immunity function, increased insulin resistance; impaired absorption is associated with certain medications, sunblock use, or inadequate outdoor sunlight exposure Obesity increases the demand for preactivated vitamin D	Food rich in vitamin D; augment digestive enzymes if postsurgical or pancreatic insufficiency; consider supplementation as needed to address deficiency states Dietary sources include cold water fish, dairy (if supplemented), mushrooms (ergocalciferol)	Obesity is associated with lower serum levels of vitamin D and plays a role in the mechanism of hyperparathyroidism and bone loss in obesity; low vitamin D levels are associated with increased musculoskeletal pain, increased fall risk, and increased insulin resistance Optimizing vitamin D may facilitate weight loss
Vitamin B$_{12}$	Serum concentration <540 mg/mL and elevated urine methyl malonate, homocysteine, and mean cell volume suggest deficiency	Impaired absorption partly from drug interactions; reduced intake from some diets Impaired absorption caused by age-related decrease	Oral, sublingual, or IM supplementation	Maintain energy metabolism
Uric acid	Serum uric acid >5.9 mg/dL needs further evaluation	If increased TG, LDL, homocysteine, platelets >385,000 consider atherosclerotic disease	Quercetin and folic acid inhibit xanthine oxidase	Consider low-purine diet; address oxidative stress; look for confounders (fructose intake >100 g/day) associated with metabolic syndrome; chronic inflammation promotes weight gain via insulin resistance
Hemoglobin A$_{1c}$	<5.4, good; 5.5-6.0, increased oxidative stress, age; >6.0, insulin resistance; and >6.5, diabetes	Low–glycemic index diet change; consider adequacy of protein intake; evaluate root causes	Consider adequacy of vitamin D; evaluate and treat root pathology, oral hypoglycemia, and insulin if necessary Low–glycemic index foods; reduce simple sugars; increase exercise	Elevated HgA$_{1c}$ as an advanced glycosylation endproduct is a marker of prolonged oxidative stress and can decrease as BMI drops into normal range if diabetes is under control Hypertriglyceridemia artificially raises HgA$_{1c}$ readings (Xavier and Carmichael, 2013)
Thyroid-stimulating hormone	>2 mIU/L requires further evaluation	Lowered metabolic rate and marked decrease in exercise tolerance	Consider appropriate treatments for diminished thyroid function; nutritional evaluation of zinc, iodine, selenium, and protein adequacy should be considered	Maintain optimal metabolic rate; reduce myalgias, fatigue, and gastrointestinal symptoms
Urinalysis	Specific gravity >1.025 suggests inadequate hydration; the presence of protein may require additional evaluation	Medical barriers to adequate hydration may be present; urinary protein losses can suggest chronic kidney disease	Address medical barriers to hydration; diet may need to be modified if chronic kidney disease	Hydration facilitates weight reduction; urine protein loss may require modifying the patient's diet

1,25-DHCC, 1,25-Dihydroxycholecalciferol; *BMI,* body mass index; *HCT,* hematocrit. *IM,* intramuscular; *LDL,* low-density lipoprotein; *RBC,* red blood cell; *TG,* triglyceride.
Adapted from Escott-Stump, 2012; Kohlstadt, 2013; Lysen et al., 2012; Xavier and Carmichael, 2013; Cunningham et al., 2005.

against foods. Elevated levels of food sensitivities have been associated with obesity in children. Obese children have been found to have higher serum C-reactive protein values, more IgG food sensitivities, and higher carotid intimal thickness on ultrasonography (Wilders-Truschnig et al., 2008). Could it be that the inflammation resulting from the immune response is a trigger or perpetuator in the development of obesity? A food diary and careful questioning of the patient can detect gastrointestinal dysfunction. Sometimes the patient can associate symptoms such as bloating, gas, cramping, or increased motility to particular foods, but often the effects of food sensitivities are delayed and appear 24 to 48 hours after ingesting the problem food. In the authors' opinion, there is no one test that provides unequivocal identification of foods that cause delayed hypersensitivity, but many practitioners have found IgG4 testing, mediator release testing, and the antigen leukocyte cellular antibody test helpful in identifying problem foods. Often an elimination diet is the best test to determine if food sensitivities or allergies are present.

As discussed earlier, modifiable lifestyle factors, including sleep and relaxation, exercise and movement, and stress and relationships, need to be assessed as well to determine the causes of the individual patient's weight gain.

Intervention

How best to counsel a patient about long-term weight management is as individual as each patient. Many patients are uncomfortable discussing their weight. They may be ashamed of their size if they believe that it reflects weak self-control. Often speaking with patients about the role of a healthy weight in overall health as simply another valuable component of a multipronged approach to being healthy in the same way that not smoking, regular seatbelt use, and washing hands regularly help protect one's health can be nonthreatening. Asking patients whether they would like to discuss weight management also helps to establish a nonjudgmental environment in which patients will feel comfortable voicing their concerns. Ask patients what has worked for them in the past. Help patients identify their strengths and discuss ways to build on these strengths from a weight management perspective. Alexander and colleagues (2011) have proposed the 5A's of obesity treatment as a recommended framework for approaching weight management with overweight and obese patients (Table 36-10).

LIFESTYLE THERAPY

Interventions for overweight and obese patients are tailored to each patient's needs and include lifestyle therapy, either alone or in combination with pharmacotherapy, and when appropriate, bariatric surgery. Lifestyle therapy, including behavioral change, is the cornerstone of evidence-based weight control. Using a slow, steady approach, as many of the modifiable lifestyle factors as possible are addressed so that patients come to adopt health-promoting habits and eliminate health-detracting ones. This process can be challenging for patients and, ideally, the physician and patient will work together as partners in this endeavor. The physician or other team members supply the guidance, tools, and encouragement, and the patient supplies the long-term commitment to achieving a healthy weight. Health care practitioner support and peer group support are powerful modalities for effecting behavioral change.

The most successful treatments for obesity incorporate nutrition professionals in the care and counseling of the patient. The diet and lifestyle evaluations are most frequently completed by a nutrition professional, lifestyle educator, or counselor involved in the team approach to helping the obese patient successfully intervene in his or her condition. When the physician partners with the nutritionist and other treatment team members, the patient is more successful in addressing the multifactorial aspects of obesity (Table 36-11).

DIET

A health-promoting diet is an integral part of weight management. Numerous diets are available; the challenge is to select one that meets the individual nutritional needs and food preferences of each patient. In general, the food plan should include adequate quantity (i.e., sufficient calories) and quality, which includes macronutrients (protein, fats, and carbohydrates) and micronutrients (minerals, vitamins, and phytonutrients). Basic principles of a health-promoting diet include consuming sufficient calories to support a healthy weight; eating a variety of foods to maximize nutritional value; meeting macronutrient needs with food selections of high nutritional value; consuming at least one and preferably two servings of each of the six categories of richly colored foods each day (6-10 total servings/day); and drinking adequate amounts of clean, filtered water. Protein content should range from 10% to 25% of calories, fats 30%, and carbohydrates 40% to 55%. A diet high in fiber and low in sodium is commonly recommended as part of a health-promoting eating plan. For starters, however, virtually all of these details can be rolled into the following simple guidelines: become familiar with serving size so as not to overeat; select whole foods rather than processed foods; choose plant foods over animal foods as often as possible; and drink clean, filtered water (measured in ounces) equal to approximately half your desirable weight (in pounds).

For patients who meet criteria for dysmetabolic syndrome or android obesity, a low glycemic impact diet has been show to result in more weight loss (Pittas et al., 2005) and improvement in blood sugar, insulin, and lipids. In this population, limitation of refined carbohydrates is especially important.

CALCULATING IDEAL WEIGHT

We caution against using the life insurance tables of weight for height. These values are observational and reflect what

---

Table 36-10   The 5 A's of Obesity Treatment

Ask	Ask for permission to discuss body weight and explore readiness for change.
Assess	Assess body mass index, waist circumference, and obesity stage; explore drivers and complications of excess weight.
Advise	Advise the patient about the health risks of obesity, the benefits of modest weight loss, the need for a long-term strategy, and treatment options.
Agree	Agree on realistic weight-loss expectations, targets, behavioral changes, and specific details of the treatment plan.
Arrange or assist	Assist in identifying and addressing barriers, provide resources, assist in finding and consulting with appropriate providers, and arrange regular follow-up.

Adapted from Alexander SC, Cox ME, Boling et al. Do the five A's work when physicians counsel about weight loss? *Fam Med.* 2011;43:179-184.

Table 36-11 Interventions

Dietary	Moderately energy-deficit diets Low-calorie diets Very-low-calorie diets Low-carbohydrate, high-protein diets Low-fat, low-energy-dense diets Low–glycemic index diets Balanced-deficit/portion-control diets Meal replacement diets	Requires a nutrition professional partnering with the patient and medical provider
Physical activity	Moderate intensity: 30 min 5 days a wk Vigorous activity: 30 min 3 days a wk (>6 MET) >200 min a wk (moderate exercise) 90 to 150 min a wk (vigorous activity) Resistance training	Often requires partnering for accountability and persistent change
Behavior therapy	Readiness to change Setting goals Reliable support system Building in maintenance Making gradual changes Keeping records Making it enjoyable Being flexible	Often requires counselors, lifestyle educators, awareness and desire to change health trajectory
Pharmacologic	Orlistat Phentermine–topiramate ER Lorcaserin	Requires monitoring from informed physician
Surgical	LAGB Vertical sleeve gastrectomy Roux-en-Y gastric bypass Distal-roux-en-Y gastric bypass Duodenal switch with biliopancreatic diversion Jejunoileal bypass	Requires surgical and bariatric specialty BMI >40 kg/m² BMI 35-40 kg/m² with significant obesity-related comorbidities such as hypertension or type 2 diabetes Unsuccessful attempt at weight loss by nonoperative means Clearance by dietitian and mental health professional No contraindications for surgery

BMI, Body mass index; *LAGB,* laparoscopic adjustable gastric band; *MET,* metabolic equivalent.
Adapted from Cheskin and Poddar, 2014.

the people surveyed actually weighed rather than derived through research studies of what desirable weight for height would be. Typically, these tables overestimate desirable weight. Instead, use the Hamwi formula, which is a quick method that has been in use clinically since it was introduced in 1964 by the American Diabetes Association (Hamwi, 1964). It is a handy way to get an estimate of desirable weight during a brief office visit. For women, assign 100 lb to the first 60 in and 5 lb for each additional inch of height (for those under 60 inches, subtract 2.5 lb for each inch under 60 in). This calculation will yield an approximate ideal weight. Adjust this weight to a desirable weight by discussing with the patient what she believes has been a comfortable weight for her in the past, her goal weight (which may be much lower than her comfortable weight), and your clinical judgment. If she is 64 in and 200 lb and wants to get down to 140 lb, talk with her about the advisability of losing 1 to 2 lb per week for a healthy approach and to increase the success for long-term maintenance of weight lost and then stage the weight loss using 1 to 2 lb per week weight loss. Perhaps discuss a first goal of losing 20 lb and be sure she understands that will take approximately 3 months. To estimate desirable weight for men, use 106 lb for the first 60 inches and 6 lb for each additional inch. These are estimates for medium frames and can be adjusted ±10% to accommodate small or large frames as needed.

CALCULATING CALORIES

To calculate an appropriate calorie level, the Mifflin–St. Jeor modification of the Harris-Benedict equation (Mifflin et al., 1990) is commonly used because it takes into account age, sex, and activity level (including metabolic needs resulting from medical conditions). It does, however, underestimate calories needed for muscular individuals and overestimates calories for obese individuals. For office visit purposes of arriving at a reasonably good estimate of calorie levels, use the rule of thumb of 10 calories per pound of desirable weight as being the least amount of calories to recommend to keep metabolism humming along. A range of 12 to 13 calories per pound is appropriate for active women and 13 to 15 calories per pound for an active man. This approach guards against recommending calorie levels below 1200 for women and below 1500 for men. Again, the nutrition professional will make any needed adjustments and develop a longer-term plan.

Address weight and healthy eating at each office visit, even if only briefly. Success with weight management is associated with the patient making behavioral changes in small steps. For most physicians, the goals will be to point the patient in the right direction; provide basic guidelines of healthy eating (and physical activity); and refer the patient to a nutrition professional who can personalize the diet to the patient's weight loss needs, comorbid conditions, food preferences, economic status, family requirements

Table 36-12 Centers for Disease Control and Prevention's Physical Activity Guidelines for Americans

Age	Duration and Frequency (Total Time Includes All Three Types of Activity)	Weekly Time (Includes All Three Types of Activities)		
		Aerobic Activity*	Muscle-Strengthening Activities*	Bone-Strengthening Activities*
Children, 6-17 yr	60 min at least 3 days per wk	Moderate or vigorous	Push-ups, gymnastics	Jumping rope, running
Adults, 18-64 yr	Regular activity throughout the week rather than as a single session	150 min per wk of moderate activity, 75 min of vigorous activity, or an equivalent mix of moderate and vigorous activity	2 or more days per week	Not specifically addressed
Older adults, ≥65 yr	Regular activity throughout the week rather than as a single session	150 min per wk of moderate activity, 75 min of vigorous activity, or an equivalent mix of moderate and vigorous activity	2 or more days per week	Not specifically addressed

*Examples of *moderate activities* include brisk walking, water aerobics, riding a bike on level ground or with few hills, playing doubles tennis, pushing a lawn mower, and dancing. Examples of *vigorous activities* include running, swimming laps, riding a bike fast or on hills, playing singles tennis, and playing basketball. *Muscle-strengthening activities* work all major muscle groups (legs, hips, back, abdomen, chest, shoulders, and arms). Examples include lifting weights (machines or hand weights), working with resistance bands, exercises that use your body for resistance (sit-ups, push-ups, pull-ups, gymnastics), heavy gardening (digging, shoveling), climbing wall, and yoga. Bone-strengthening activities include hopping, skipping, jumping, running, jumping rope, tennis, basketball, and gymnastics

From Centers for Disease Control and Prevention. http://www.cdc.gov/physicalactivity/everyone/guidelines/children.html.

(e.g., whether there are children, elders, or other family members with specific health requirements in the home), and overall lifestyle. It is common today for patients not to be skilled in planning, shopping for, and preparing healthy meals. Many need education concerning basic nutrition and the role of food in health. The nutrition professional will be able to address each of these issues and help the patient plan meals appropriate to his or her needs.

If you have reason to believe the patient has food sensitivities, an elimination diet is an inexpensive way to help identify which foods are problematic for the patient. This type of food plan typically eliminates the most common food sensitivities (e.g., dairy, gluten, nuts, citrus, seafood, beef) and environmental toxins for a 21-day period. Each eliminated food category is then added back systematically and the patient's response noted. After suspect foods have been identified, these foods can be removed from the diet or rotated so they are infrequently eaten. If symptoms persist with a food or food grouping, these foods are eliminated for a longer period (e.g., 6-9 months), and reintroduction is again tested and recorded by the patient. If no symptoms are noted, these foods are added back to the diet. If symptoms are noted, the foods are eliminated and may need to be avoided indefinitely.

MOVEMENT AND PHYSICAL ACTIVITY

Physical activity is a key component of a healthy lifestyle for reasons ranging from stress reduction to decreased risk of cardiovascular disease. It is also an important component of preventing and treating overweight and obesity. Movement should be a normal part of life, from a formal exercise program to becoming more physically active in daily routines. Exercise itself burns calories but also promotes the development of lean muscle mass that in turn can increase the amount of calories used even when we are at rest. In general, the goal should be 30 minutes of moderately vigorous physical activity most days of the week. To promote weight loss, a goal of 60 minutes per day may be more appropriate and, to maintain weight loss, up to 90 minutes a day may be necessary. A popular program

promoting physical activity encourages people to walk 10,000 steps each day or at least an initial increase of 2000 steps over baseline. A pedometer is a great way for patients to track their progress. The National Weight Control Registry, which was started in 1993, is the longest ongoing study of individuals who have lost at least 30 lb and have kept it off for a minimum of 1 year. Registry participants who have been successful at weight loss maintenance report exercising at least 1 hour per day every day (Phelan et al., 2007).

Physical activity has three key components: aerobic activity, muscle strengthening (resistance) activity, and bone-strengthening activity. Table 36-12 shows guidelines from the CDC for duration and frequency for physical activity and recommendations for the types of activities to engage in while physically active.

In addition to traditional aerobic and resistance exercise, many people are turning to yoga as a way to strengthen muscles and bones and to combat stress, improve feelings of self-worth, and develop a sense of community with others. See previous discussion on yoga under the heading Environmental Factors.

SLEEP

As discussed earlier, too little sleep, too much sleep, and poor-quality sleep in adults and children have been associated with weight gain, overweight, and obesity (Liu et al., 2013; Mesarwi et al., 2013; Xiao et al., 2013).

The amount of sleep needed varies with the individual. Recommendations for the amount of sleep needed per day are typically given by age and are intended to be guidelines only. The National Sleep Foundation's recommendations for sleep durations across the lifespan are shown in Table 36-13.

Many patients are counseled to lose weight to help their sleep-disordered breathing. Although this approach can be helpful, it is important to remember that for some patients, sleep apnea is the cause or at least a contributing factor for their weight gain. As a result, these patients will have a difficult time losing weight if they have untreated sleep apnea.

Table 36-13   National Sleep Foundation Recommendations for Sleep Durations across the Lifespan

Age	Duration (hr/day)	Schedule
Infants, 1-2 mo	10.5-18	As needed (irregular schedule)
Infants, 3-11 mo	9-12	Naps of 0.5-2 hours
Toddlers, 1-3 yr	12-14	Nap of 1-3 hours
Preschoolers, 3-5 yr	11-12	Nap up to 5 years
School-age children, 5-10 yr	10-11	Nighttime
Teens, 10-17 yr	8.5-9.25	Nighttime
Adults, ≥18 yr	7-9	Nighttime

Adapted from information provided by the National Sleep Foundation. http://www.sleepfoundation.org.

A referral to a sleep specialist is often necessary to help patients reach their goals.

Additionally, the discussion of good sleep hygiene should be included in the office visit. Remind patients to stop work and turn off their computers, phones, and TV an hour before bedtime and keep to a similar schedule to go to bed and to get up. Yoga is being examined as a beneficial modality to improve sleep quality (Afonso et al., 2012; Innes and Selfe, 2012; Taibi and Vitiello, 2011). Add in relaxation exercises such as breathing, yoga, or a calming bath before bedtime to help quiet the mind and body and assist with the transition to sleep.

PSYCHOSOCIAL STRESS

Many patients would benefit from assistance with identifying their stressors, reducing the intensity and number of stressors experienced, learning skills for coping with stressful situations, and changing their maladaptive perceptions. As with improving nutrition, the behavioral changes needed require a slow, steady approach to changing long-term perceptions and behaviors. Most patients are likely to be more successful making these changes for the long term if they are able to work with a behavioral medicine professional, either individually or in a group setting. If you do not have such a professional available to your practice, either as a member of the health care team or on contract, there may be hospital- or community-based programs that host stress management programs. These programs can be quite effective when the patient is at the action stage of the readiness to change continuum.

Mindfulness programs are showing promise for long-term weight management as well as stress reduction. A mindful approach to each of the modifiable lifestyle factors can help overweight and obese patients identify the root cause of their excess weight and develop effective strategies for building resiliency in multiple areas of their lives. The mindfulness approach to behavior change originated in 1985 at the University of Massachusetts Medical Center under the guidance of Jon Kabat-Zinn. Mindfulness means paying attention in a particular way: on purpose, in the present moment, and nonjudgmentally. Mindfulness has been used successfully for therapeutic applications for more than 30 years. Among the better researched mindfulness programs are mindfulness-based stress reduction (MBSR)

(Kabat-Zinn et al., 1985), mindfulness-based cognitive therapy (MBCT) developed by Segal and colleagues (Bieling et al., 2012), and mindfulness-based eating (MB-EAT) (Kristeller and Wolever, 2011).

In a recent overview, Kabat-Zinn and colleagues discuss the current state of MBSR and the neuroscience underlying mindfulness (Paulson et al., 2013). The MBSR program was adapted by Zindel Segal, Mark Williams, and John Teasdale to develop a MBCT program that focuses on thoughts and emotions, particularly in reference to recurring depression and unhappiness. The approach has been incorporated into the clinical guidelines established by the American Psychiatric Association (2000). Although rooted in the Buddhist philosophy, mindfulness programs have been carefully developed as secular programs designed to be acceptable to everyone, regardless of religious orientation.

As with many emerging modalities, mindfulness-based programs originally lacked strong scientific documentation for their efficacy. However, more recently, the studies have used rigorous scientific methodology and integrated the latest in understanding the neuroscience principles that underlie mindfulness. In a review of the current status of mindfulness programs, Marchand (2012) reviewed the studies conducted to date and concluded that the research was of very high quality and published in journals with very high impact factors. Mindfulness approaches singled out as particularly efficacious included conditions commonly seen in primary care, such as depression, anxiety, and pain.

More recently, the field of positive psychology has emerged, founded by Martin Seligman at the University of Pennsylvania (Seligman and Csikszentmihalyi, 2000). This approach came from the realization that the field of psychology focused primarily on what was wrong, identifying and repairing damage to human functioning within a disease model, rather than on what made individuals and communities thrive and flourish. Seligman and his colleagues have worked to turn this orientation around and created a strong movement within academia and clinical practice. Clinicians are particularly subject to focusing on what's wrong as patients tend to come to them when they have a problem. Rather than asking, "What are your concerns?" try asking, "What's going well for you today (or in your life)?" Simple changes such as this one change the tenor of the physician–patient interaction. Focus on what works. Similarly, identify positive psychology-based programs in your community that can assist patients in becoming more positive in spite of their medical challenges.

The physician should also encourage patients to rethink their relationships with themselves and others. Are they comfortable with themselves? Are they able to tap into and trust their own inner wisdom? Do they feel worthy and able to set aside time each day to do one thing that brings them joy? Do they have a strong social support network? If not, what is one thing they could do today that would begin to strengthen existing relationships or develop a new one? Again, mindfulness practice can help significantly in developing relationships with oneself and others. You can find helpful resources at Dr. Seligman's website (http://www.pursuit-of-happiness.org) and the Wholebeing Institute (http://www.wholebeinginstitute.com).

ENVIRONMENTAL TOXIN EXPOSURE

As discussed previously, the environment presents numerous toxins that can enter our bodies through the food we eat, the water we drink, and the air we breathe. Toxins are potential triggers for harmful effects within the body. Help patients identify the sources of potential toxins and ways to eliminate them. In parallel, consider ways to lower the level of toxins that already exists within the patient. Here, nutrition is key. The detoxification and biotransformation process that occurs in the gut and the liver is dependent on nutrients as cofactors for the various reactions. If you are able to assess whether the patient has one or more genetic variants in the phase I cytochrome P450s (*CYP* genes) or phase II glutathione-S-transferase (*GST*) or N-acetyltransferase (*NAT*) genes, use nutrition therapy to compensate for any genetic limitations that in turn affect activity of the key biotransformation enzymes coded for by these gene variants. Use the cruciferous (cabbage family) vegetables to upregulate other GST genes that are unimpaired. Examples of appropriate foods are broccoli, Brussels sprouts, cabbage, greens (e.g., beet, collard, kale, mustard, turnip), and horseradish root.

MICROBIOME

Although it is not yet clear whether the intestinal microbiome plays a significant role in the risk of becoming overweight or obese, it is becoming clear that the human microbiome does contribute to our overall health status. Clues that an overweight or obese patient's microbiome may be unbalanced include gastrointestinal distress, such as gas, bloating, cramping, or motility issues, and a strong history of antibiotic use. Promoting a healthy microbiome through attention to sufficiency of both prebiotics and probiotics would seem to be prudent. Microorganisms enter the digestive tract primarily through the food we eat. Whether the overall microbial composition is pathogenic or beneficial depends in large part on the types of foods eaten. Consuming fermented foods that contain live active cultures is one approach. Examples of such foods include various dairy foods (yogurts, kefir) and nondairy foods (fermented soy, kim chi, natto, miso, sauerkraut, tempeh, and various pickled vegetables). How much of a food containing live active cultures will be needed depends on the patient's beginning microbiome, but a serving a day can be helpful for maintaining a healthy microbial community in the gut. When it is clear that the patient needs to eliminate pathogenic organisms and recolonize the gut with beneficial ones, it is typically more efficient to use a concentrated form of live active cultures, called a "probiotic," available in dietary supplement form. A probiotic will provide a higher titer of microorganisms and appears to colonize the gut more quickly than most food sources. Probiotics come in liquid and capsule forms and may or may not need to be refrigerated, depending on the brand selected. Also depending on the brand, products can be obtained that are dairy free and do not contain ingredients such as wheat, gluten, soy, egg, peanuts, tree nuts, fish, crustacean shellfish, colors, artificial sweeteners, artificial flavors, or preservatives for patients with food sensitivities. A probiotic should contain titers in the billions of organisms per serving. All of this information can be found on the Dietary Supplement Facts panel on the product. These live organisms thrive on soluble fiber, which is often referred to as a "prebiotic." One or more prebiotic ingredients may be included in the probiotic, but they can also be obtained through a health-promoting diet that includes daily servings of foods such as fruit, vegetables, legumes, and grains.

Caution your patients that they may initially experience some gas and bloating as the microbial population expands within the digestive tract but that the situation will usually fade away within 1 week or so. Allow approximately 1 month for a healthy microbiome to become established and then cut back on the therapy. Daily use of live active cultures of probiotics can be continued because this practice appears to have no known adverse effects. Alternatively, patients may wish to reseed their guts periodically or after antibiotic use with the same protocol they used initially to support the ongoing health of their gut microbiome.

INTERVENING WITH OUR PEDIATRIC POPULATION

Of increasing concern is the growing excessive weight in children. Research shows that children who are obese or overweight rate their well-being as similar to that of children with cancer. Helping our families with prevention of weight gain is of utmost importance. The American Heart Association recently analyzed NHANES data and discovered that fewer than 50% of our adolescents exhibited more than five of seven ideal cardiovascular markers. Markers analyzed included blood pressure, blood sugar, cholesterol, level of physical activity, weight, use of tobacco, and health of their diet (Shay et al., 2013). Poor diet and lack of physical activity in adolescents increases their risk of obesity throughout their lives. Prevention is key, and a family physician is the ideal person to help our children get set up for a healthy life. A good resource for families is *Ending the Food Fight* by David Ludwig, MD, PhD. It is important that we encourage parents to act as good role models and that the family become active together.

In an infant, breastfeeding should be encouraged up to the age of 1 year. Restriction or elimination of sweetened beverages such as soft drinks and sports drinks can greatly reduce caloric consumption in children. The American Academy of Pediatrics (AAP) recommends that even 100% fruit juices be limited to 4 to 6 oz daily for children age 1 to 6 years.

For children age 2 to 5 years, whether they are overweight or obese, the goal is weight maintenance and not weight loss. They will have improvement in their BMI as they grow taller. For overweight children between the ages of 6 and 11 years old, the goal is also weight maintenance. If they meet the criteria for obesity, the goal is 1 lb of weight loss every 2 weeks. For overweight or obese children between the ages of 12 and 18, up to 2 lb of weight loss per month is an acceptable goal (Rao, 2008). It is important to focus on long-term behavioral patterns and lifestyle change with a slow, steady weight loss that can be maintained. Healthy lifestyle modification should be the goal. Overly restrictive diets have the potential of interfering with growth rate, bone mineralization, and menstruation. For a child with a BMI above the 95th percentile (obesity), a more structured and aggressive approach may be appropriate. Many children and families benefit from working with nutrition professionals. It is very important that the whole family is involved in the lifestyle change to prevent the overweight child from feeling uncomfortable. When the whole family focuses on eating more vegetables and incorporating 60 minutes of exercise every day, it is more likely that the child will be successful. Small, specific, measurable goals will make everyone more successful.

Also encourage parents to make meal time be family time, a time when the family gathers to eat together without distractions, such as television or electronic devices. This practice can help to improve the nutritional status of parents and children alike, encourages interpersonal connections among family members, and provides space for each member to share his or her successes and concerns. Establishing a positive environment is essential for many reasons, including optimal digestion as well as providing a safe space for children to express their concerns and feel heard. Avoiding squabbles over the child's food choices is essential to preserving the positive environment sought. Table 36-14 provides meal time guidelines for parents and children that can promote harmony along with good nutrition.

Prevention is key and can be implemented in every primary care office. Encourage your families to remember the 5-2-1-0 rule recommended by the AAP as part of the White House Obesity Initiative:

- Five servings of fruits and vegetables per day
- Two hours or less of screen time per day
- One hour of physical activity per day
- Zero sweetened beverages per day

The AAP provides prescription forms for the 5-2-1-0 program for use in the clinic (http://www.aap.org/en-us/professional-resources/practice-support/Patient-Management/Pages/Healthy-Active-Living-Prescriptions.aspx).

Table 36-14   A Suggested Division of Responsibility at Meal Time

3 Ps for parents	1. Plan healthy meals and snacks. Have healthy food options in the home. 2. Prepare and serve meals. 3. Provide support so your child can make healthy choices.
3 Cs for the children	1. Choose to eat or not. The child chooses whether to eat the healthy meal the parent has prepared and does not have the option to eat other foods not served. 2. Choose what to eat from what is served. It is healthier for the child to choose, and often the child will take a smaller portion than the parent would serve. 3. Choose how much to eat. The child eats until full. The parent should not instruct the child to clean the plate or restrict the quantity of food.

Adapted from Dunlop A, Blount B. Childhood obesity: management. FP Audio 405 (AAFP). Feb 2013.

Weight loss targets depend on many factors, such as the age of the patient and his or her health status. Even small amounts of weight loss can have a profound impact on a patient's health. In multiple studies, 5% to 10% of weight loss has been associated with a reversal of metabolic syndrome, type 2 diabetes, heart disease, and cancer (Liebermeister, 2003). This is important when counseling patients to make changes. When obesity is approached nonjudgmentally from the perspective of health risk, patients may be more accepting of the need to change and more willing to partner with the physician in addressing the problem. A patient does not need to lose weight to reach a normal BMI in order to achieve the health benefits. It also may not be possible for some patients to achieve a normal BMI. That does not mean that they cannot be successful. Have many markers to follow your patient outside of weight, including waist circumference, fasting blood glucose, blood pressure, fasting insulin and triglyceride levels as well as their energy level and how clothes fit for them. If we just focus on weight, patients may feel that they failed if the scale does not decrease enough, when in fact they may have made substantial changes in biomarkers and health risk. What we eat and how active we are is often more important than the amount we weigh. Include more markers to follow so you can motivate your patients with their improvements. Readiness to change should be addressed, and addressing barriers to success is key in weight loss and maintenance. Barriers may include emotional factors (stress, depression) or time constraints that limit exercise or proper food preparation. A support system can be helpful for someone attempting weight loss, including friends, a spouse, or an organized program put together by a local nutritionist.

WHEN LIFESTYLE THERAPY IS NOT SUFFICIENT

Treatment interventions of adult patients with overweight or obesity as a disease are multifactorial depending on the underlying causes and the timeline of weight excess onset. Patients are weighed every day in clinic, and certain weight markers should trigger nutrition and lifestyle counseling and intervention (Table 36-15). For the best results, the interventions should include many aspects of personal lifestyle: nutrition, physical activity, behavior therapy, pharmacotherapy, and, in certain cases, bariatric surgery. The pharmacologic and bariatric treatments for obesity are discussed here.

Pharmacotherapy

Adding weight loss medication to lifestyle counseling increases average weight loss (Carvajal et al., 2013; Garvey et al., 2012), but they have been approved for only short-term use. Until the mid 1990s, diet, physical activity, and behavior modifications were the key components of a weight loss program, but the pharmacotherapy option was added as the understanding of the metabolic risks of disease that occurred when the BMI was greater than 27 (Seagle et al., 2013). Many medications have appeared on the market and have been subsequently withdrawn because of side effects. Three classes of medications continue to be available in the United States approved by the U.S. Food and Drug Administration: (1) decreasing fat digestion and absorption (e.g., Orlistat, a gastric and pancreatic lipase

Table 36-15   Nutritional Biomarkers to Check before Bariatric Surgery, 6 Months after Surgery, then Annually

Nutrient	Biomarker	Primary Symptoms/Signs
Thiamin (vitamin B$_1$)	Serum thiamin	Ophthalmoplegia, nystagmus, ataxia, rapid vision loss, Wernicke encephalopathy, peripheral neuropathy with proximal weakness
Folate	RBC folate, homocysteine	Megaloblastic anemia, glossitis
Vitamin B$_{12}$	Serum vitamin B$_{12}$, methylmalonic acid	Megaloblastic anemia, neuropathy, memory loss, vision loss, darkening of the skin, decreased vibratory and position sense
Iron	Serum ferritin, TIBC, CBC	Microcytic anemia, fatigue, pallor, koilonychias, glossitis
Vitamin D	25-OH vitamin D, calcium, phosphorus, parathyroid hormone	Decreased bone density, secondary hyperparathyroidism, tender anterior tibia, increased inflammation, periodontal disease
Protein	Serum albumin, plasma amino acids	Edema, excessive alopecia, poor wound healing, sarcopenia, neurotransmitter inadequacy, poor biotransformation
Vitamin A	Plasma retinol	Reduced night vision, hyperkeratosis pilaris, poor immune function
Vitamin E	Plasma α-tocopherol	Neuropathy, ataxia
Vitamin K	PT, serum uncarboxylated osteocalcin	Bleeding tendency, easy bruising, osteoporosis

CBC, Complete blood count; *PT,* prothrombin time; *TIBC,* total iron-binding capacity.
Adapted from Xanthakos SA. Nutritional deficiencies in obesity and after bariatric surgery. *Pediatr Clin North Am* 2009;56:1105-1121 and Stone PM. Physical signs indicative or suggestive of undernutrition. In Jones DS, ed. *Textbook of functional medicine.* Gig Harbor, WA: Institute for Functional Medicine; 2005:786-788.

inhibitor for long-term use and available over the counter), (2) norepinephrine reuptake inhibitor as an appetite suppressant (e.g., phentermine), and (3) 5-hydroxytryptamine agonist (e.g., Lorcaserin, also used as a centrally acting appetite suppressant).

Orlistat works by inhibiting lipases in the gastrointestinal tract, which partially blocks fat absorption. It is approved for up to 2 years of continuous use and has been shown to improve weight loss and lipids, lower blood pressure, and enhance glucose metabolism. In a combined lifestyle intervention study involving Orlistat, the study treatment for 4 years delayed development of type 2 diabetes in obese subjects by 37% (Nicolai et al., 2012).

Phentermine as a norepinephrine reuptake inhibitor is a schedule 4 medication. It is has been approved for use for up to 12 weeks since its release in 1959. A continuous off-label use pattern in bariatric medicine has validation in the international literature (Nicolai et al., 2012). The side effect precautions include dry mouth, palpitations, hypertension, constipation, and insomnia.

Phentermine HCl–topiramate extended release is also a schedule 4 medication. It is a combination shorter- and longer-acting medication that combines a shorter-acting sympathomimetic amine and a longer-acting neurostabilizer approved as monotherapy for seizure disorders and migraine headache prevention. Phentermine is metabolized by the liver and excreted by the kidney; topiramate is excreted by the kidney (Garvey et al., 2012; Seger et al., 2013). This combination has been associated with up to a 10% weight loss in phase 3 trials (Garvey et al., 2012).

Lorcaserin is a 5-hydroxytryptamine 2c receptor agonist weight management agent that is a schedule 4 medication used twice a day. Serotonin (5-HT) has been implicated as a critical factor in the short-term (meal-bymeal) regulation of food intake. Its safety profile with coadministration with other serotonergic, antidopaminergic agents has not been established. The drug has multiple multisystem potential side effects (Seger et al., 2013) and should not be used in pregnancy. When combined with a 600-kcal decrease in food intake, lorcaserin twice a day was associated with a 10% weight loss in 20% of patients compared with 7% in the placebo group in phase 3 trials (Redman and Ravussin, 2010).

Indications for consideration of pharmacotherapy include obesity with a BMI greater than 30; overweight patients (BMI >27) with presence of obesity complications, including type 2 diabetes, hypertension, and dyslipidemia; and no improvement in a 12-week program of therapeutic lifestyle change, including consultation and routine evaluation with a behavioral therapist, nutritionist, and exercise program specialist. When used as an isolated therapy, pharmacotherapy to reduce obesity is not cost effective (Veerman et al., 2011).

Surgery

Indications. Bariatric surgery for patients with BMIs of greater than 40 or patients with BMIs greater than 35 with multiple comorbid conditions is now endorsed by different groups (Buchwald et al., 2004; Buchwald 2005). Over the past 2 decades, the prevalence of severe obesity (BMI >40 kg/m^2) has increased from 1 in 200 to 1 in 50 Americans. A new category of the extremely obese (BMI >50) was developed by the CDC to better inform the spectrum of disease and varies in frequency from state, gender, and ethnic background (Kushner and Herrington, 2013). Nearly 6% of adult Americans are severely obese, with the highest prevalence (nearly 14%) in adult African American women. Weight loss surgery has been found to be effective in carefully selected patients and has been reviewed elsewhere (Anderson and Hensrud, 2011; Medical Advisory Secretariat, 2009).

Evaluation for a patient with a BMI greater than 30 and one or more adverse health conditions caused by excessive fat or a BMI greater than 40 with or without adverse health conditions caused by fat mass disease or excessive body fat are the basic considerations now outlined for bariatric surgery (Seger et al., 2013). A thorough medical evaluation, including a bariatric surgery specialty consultation, with cardiology, pulmonary, gastroenterology, nutrition, and mental health evaluations, should be completed (Mechanick et al., 2013). Surgery alters the morbidity of obese patients with diabetes by varying mechanisms

(Cummings et al., 2004). There has been a recent meta-analysis review noting that after bariatric surgery, there was 76.8% complete resolution of type 2 diabetes in the 1846 patients evaluated (Medical Advisory Secretariat, 2009). The patients with gastric banding had a 47.9% resolution of their diabetes; gastroplasty, 71%; gastric bypass, 83.7%; and biliopancreatic diversion or duodenal switch, 98.9% (mean change in HbA$_{1c}$ was −2.7%; Medical Advisory Secretariat, 2009).

Techniques and Procedures

PREOPERATIVE. The guidelines for weight loss surgery suggest that patients who cannot comprehend the nature of the surgical interventions and the lifelong measures required to maintain an acceptable level of health should be excluded from surgery (Consensus Development Conference Panel, 1991). Often the patient must show documentation of a 6 to 18 month supervised diet program before insurance authorization for the bariatric procedure (Brethauer, 2011). Exclusion criteria usually include previous weight reduction surgery; previous gastric operations, including gastric or duodenal ulcer, in the past 6 months; active malignancy in the past 5 years; myocardial infarction in the past 6 months; bulimic eating pattern; abuse of alcohol or drugs; psychological problems resulting in poor cooperation; regular use of cortisone or nonsteroidal anti-inflammatory drugs; and other severe illness, including certain autoimmune conditions (Sjostrom et al., 2004).

TYPES OF PROCEDURES. The types of bariatric procedures are illustrated in Figure 36-3. The procedures create one of three post–bariatric surgical states: malabsorptive (Figure 36-3, A to C), restrictive (Figure 36-3, D and E), or a combined malabsorptive and restrictive state (Figure 36-3, F

and G). The malabsorptive conditions are more effective at weight loss, but they have a higher morbidity complication rate. The goal of the restrictive procedures is to limit food intake capacity and to slow the rate of stomach emptying. These include the laparoscopic adjustable gastric banding (LAGB) versus the vertical banded gastroplasty. Because of the ease of procedures and the lack of effectiveness of the vertical banding in trials, gastric banding is common and routinely completed. The adjustable gastric band involves the placement of the banded sleeve that can band a reservoir around the upper quarter of the upper stomach. Gastric banding is followed by the gastric sleeve and finally the roux-en-Y gastric bypass (RYGB) procedure for the lowest cost effectiveness (Seger et al., 2013).

The laparoscopic adjustable gastric band is a silicone ring placed around the proximal portion of the stomach and inflated to create a small proximal gastric pouch and a narrowed opening between the proximal and distal stomach with the gastric pouch holding approximately 30 cc (DeLegge et al., 2013; Shikora et al., 2007). This has been advocated for obese adolescents and those with a lower obese BMI (DeLegge et al., 2013). The lap band procedure is less complicated and is the most often performed in the United States. Weight loss occurs more slowly. Most patients can expect to lose 30% to 50% of their excess weight over 3 to 5 years, with an average of 47% (Buchwald et al., 2004; DeLegge et al., 2013). Laparoscopic adjustable banding is generally an outpatient procedure (Seger et al., 2013). The recovery is usually 1 week, and the contraindications include being a poor surgical candidate because of nutritional status or having severe comorbidities, severe psychiatric disorder, intolerance to general anesthesia, pregnancy, untreated esophagitis, or drug or alcohol

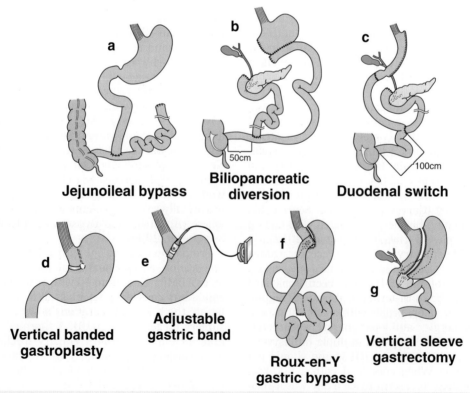

Figure 36-3 Malabsorptive, restrictive, or combined restrictive, and malabsorptive bariatric procedures. (Reprinted with permission from Xanthakos SA. Bariatric surgery for extreme adolescent obesity: indications, outcome and physiologic effects on the gut-brain axis. *Pathophysiology*. 2008;15:135.)

addiction. The acute complications include the band being too tight with gastrointestinal obstruction symptoms, leakage of gastric contents into the abdomen, hemorrhage, gastrointestinal bleeding, infection, cardiac dysrhythmias, atelectasis and pneumonia, deep vein thrombosis (DVT), and occasional death. The chronic complications can include weight regain with no weight loss, band slippage erosion, ulceration, port infection, disconnection, and displacement. The patients may develop esophageal dilation, and there are rarer nutrient deficiencies that can occur if persistent vomiting is marked and there is a sustained decrease in nutritional intake. Depression may also develop.

The sleeve gastrectomy involves surgically reducing the stomach to about 25% of its original size with the surgical removal of a large portion of the stomach along the greater curvature, resulting in a narrower sleeve or tube like structure. The vertical sleeve gastrectomy removes 85% of the stomach, leaving a narrow, tubular, banana-shaped portion of the stomach (stomach capacity, 50-150 cc), and is sometimes advocated for those with a very high BMI (>55 kg/m^2). The detached section of the stomach is primarily responsible for production of ghrelin, and weight loss is further enhanced by the lower levels of this hormone that result after the surgery (Frezza, 2007). In general, the hospital stay is 1 to 2 days, with recovery in 1 to 2 weeks. The contraindications are similar to those for the LAP-BAND with the additional contraindications of Barrett esophagus, severe gastroparesis, achalasia, previous gastrectomy, and gastric bypass surgery. The acute complications are similar with addition of pulmonary emboli, rhabdomyolysis, or dehydration. Long-term complications may include marginal ulcers, dumping syndrome with reactive hypoglycemia, and small bowel obstruction caused by internal hernias or adhesions. Additional documented complications include luminal stenosis, anastomotic staple line leak, fistula formation, gallstones, calcium deficiency, secondary hyperparathyroidism, iron deficiency, protein malnutrition, and nutritional and mineral deficiencies (including vitamins A, C, D, E, K, B, and B$_{12}$, folate, zinc, magnesium, and thiamin). Anemia related to mineral and nutrition deficiencies, metabolic acidosis, bacterial overgrowth, and kidney stones (oxalates) may also develop. Increased frequency of neuropathies, osteoporosis, and depression is seen in this post-surgical population without ongoing assessment and appropriate interventions (Seger et al., 2013; Xanthakos, 2009).

The purely malabsorptive procedures such as the biliopancreatic diversion with or without the duodenal switch (stomach capacity, 50-150 cc) are not commonly performed because of the significant nutritional complications that develop after the procedure, including significant protein, essential fat, vitamin, and mineral deficiencies (DeLegge et al., 2013). The RYGB, the combined malabsorptive and restrictive procedure, usually leaves a gastric pouch of 20 to 30 cc. The patient generally has a hospitalization of 2 to 4 days, with a recovery 2 to 4 weeks or longer. The contraindications are poor surgical candidate, severe psychotic disorder, intolerance to general anesthesia, pregnancy, drug or alcohol addiction, untreated esophagitis, and unwillingness or inability for appropriate long-term follow-up. The acute complications include gastrointestinal obstruction, hemorrhage, gastrointestinal bleeding, anastomotic leaks, infection, cardiac dysrhythmia, atelectasis

and pneumonia, DVT, pulmonary emboli, rhabdomyolysis, dehydration, and death. Chronic complications can include weight regain, marginal ulcers, esophageal dilation, dumping syndrome with reactive hypoglycemia, small bowel obstruction caused by internal hernias or adhesions, anastomotic stenosis, gallstones, calcium deficiency, secondary hyperparathyroidism, iron deficiency, protein malnutrition, other nutritional mineral deficiencies, anemia, metabolic acidosis, bacterial overgrowth, kidney stones (oxalates), neuropathies resulting from nutritional deficiencies, osteoporosis (often caused by calcium deficiency and chronically elevated parathyroid hormone levels), and depression (Seger et al., 2013). The efficacy of the more aggressive surgeries is partially tied to the gastrointestinal endocrine system effects, which are significant. Gut hormones (glucagon-like peptide 1, peptide YY, leptin, and ghrelin) are not affected by restrictive operations such as LAGB and therefore do not contribute to weight loss. The adiposity hormones (leptin and insulin) are elevated in obese individuals and decrease with weight loss. It is suggested that RYGB surgery restores leptin sensitivity (DeLegge et al., 2013). Ghrelin is a known appetite stimulant produced by the stomach and duodenum and increases before eating and decreases afterward (DeLegge et al., 2013). It stimulates mealtime hunger associated with initiation of a meal. Successful weight loss surgery is not associated with lowering of the ghrelin levels.

Dumping Syndrome. Dumping syndrome following RYGB or other gastric surgeries that bypass the pylorus or interfere with gastric innervation is common. Up to 70% of RYGB patients report dumping in the postoperative period (DeLegge et al., 2013), but a minority will have an ongoing problem. It is categorized into early or late dumping syndrome. The early dumping syndrome is handled with low-volume, high-protein, carbohydrate-controlled mini meals (DeLegge et al., 2013) and the addition of soluble fiber from guar gum, glucomannan, or pectins to delay gastric emptying and alter the transit time in the bowel (DeLegge et al., 2013). A host of medications have been used to help alleviate the issue. Octreotide has been used to improve the symptoms of dumping syndrome (Ukleja, 2006)

A successful outcome from bariatric surgery is the loss of 50% of excess weight. A meta-analysis of 22,000 patients demonstrating outcomes reported a weight loss of 61.6% for RYGB and 47% for LAGB. Weight regain occurs in 30% to 50% of the patients, with significant weight regain of 15% to 30% (DeLegge et al., 2013; Hsu et al., 1998; Magro et al., 2008). There is significant success with the correctly selected patient in undergoing a significant body composition change and reductions in type 2 diabetes, hypertension, and dyslipidemia (Table 36-16). The morbidity and mortality from the procedures are markedly affected by the discernment and preoperative screening of the potential surgical patient (Table 36-17). The advantages and disadvantages of the different procedures have been reviewed elsewhere (Anderson and Hensrud, 2011; DeLegge et al., 2013; Medical Advisory Secretariat, 2009; Xanthakos, 2009).

Postprocedure Treatment and Monitoring

There is no doubt that the success of continued weight loss after bariatric surgery requires multiple team members,

Table 36-16 Summary of Findings on Excess Weight Loss and Resolution of Comorbid Conditions

Procedure	Excess Weight Loss (%)*	Resolution of Comorbid Conditions (Range %)†
MALABSORPTIVE		
Roux-en-Y gastric bypass	60-90	Diabetes mellitus: 74-99 Hypertension: 67-93 Dyslipidemia: 73-99
RESTRICTIVE		
Adjustable gastric banding	42-60	Diabetes mellitus: 29-92 Hypertension: 29-40 Dyslipidemia: 24
Vertical banded gastroplasty	58-67	Diabetes mellitus: 100 Hypertension: 50-60 Dyslipidemia: 14-72

*Percentage of excess weight loss = (Weight loss/Excess weight) × 100 (where Excess weight = Total preoperative weight – Ideal weight)
†Defined as the stopping of medication taken for comorbid condition.
From Medical Advisory Secretariat. Bariatric surgery: an evidence-based analysis. *Ont Health Technol Assess Ser.* 2005; 5(1).

Table 36-17 Mortality and Adverse Effects from Bariatric Surgery

Procedure	Mortality Range (%)	Adverse Effects Range (%)
MALABSORPTIVE		
Roux-en-Y gastric bypass	0.1-4.1	0.1-70
RESTRICTIVE		
Adjustable gastric banding	0-0.9	1.1-18
Vertical banded gastroplasty	0-0.8	1.0-30.4

Medical Advisory Secretariat. Bariatric surgery: an evidence-based analysis. *Ont Health Technol Assess Ser.* 2005;5(1).

including the patient with the will for prolonged lifestyle and nutrition habit change; the nutrition professional for continued counseling and education about diet and nutritional interventions; often input from a counselor involved in behavior change; the primary care physician, who continues to be alert to monitor nutrition and disease-associated laboratory and physical examination findings suggestive of under- or malnutrition; and the surgeon, who is involved in any procedural issues associated with the ongoing monitoring and adjustment of the postsurgical patient. Nutrition-directed biomarker tracking needs to be completed before bariatric surgery, at 6 months, and annually after bariatric surgery (see Table 36-15). It is noted that the increased use of malabsorptive and restrictive bariatric surgical procedures has increased the incidence of nutrition deficiency signs and symptoms in the treated obese population (Kumar, 2010; Xanthakos, 2009). Depending on the procedure location in the patient, the full range of nutritional mineral, vitamin, and major nutrient deficiencies can develop over time. The routine and consistent application of the ABCDs of nutrition assessment of obese and postoperative obese patients will aid in their healthful recovery.

Summary

Overweight and obesity and their reduction in quality of life and increase in economic burden are global concerns. Family medicine physicians can make a valuable contribution to decreasing the prevalence of weight-related diseases by addressing weight issues at each office visit. Through the evaluation of the basis for the patient's overweight or obesity and the patient's readiness to change, the physician can identify appropriate ways to move patients in a positive direction along their journey to achieving and maintaining a healthy weight. A number of environmental factors contribute to why a patient is overweight or obese, and a number of modalities are available. It is critical that patients not be overwhelmed with the magnitude of the journey ahead. Help them to take one step at a time. For example, have patients identify one modifiable lifestyle factor each day and ask, "What can I do for myself today that would move me in the direction of the goals I set in partnership with my physician?" Alternatively, if addressing each of the modifiable lifestyle factors is overwhelming, have patients focus on just one domain and select a different one tomorrow. Help them to think in terms of small steps. For example, have them think about making just a small change: eating 5% less today than they typically eat, increasing their physical activity by 5% today, increasing their sleep time by 5% tonight, keeping a gratitude journal for 30 days, or making a commitment to phoning a friend today or attending their church social hour this week to strengthen relationships.

Summary of Additional Online Content

The following content is available at www.expertconsult.com:

eAppendix 36-1 Epigenetic Regulation

eAppendix 36-2 Current Research on How the Microbiome Can Influence Weight

References

The complete reference list is available at www.expertconsult.com.

Web Resources

www.calculator.net/calorie-calculator.html Calorie calculator based on Mifflin-St. Jeor modification of the Harris-Benedict equation.

www.cellinteractive.com/ucla/physcian_ed/interview_alg.html UCLA Center for Human Nutrition helpful algorithm for motivational interviewing.

www.heartmath.org/free-services/solutions-for-stress/gps-for-the-soul.html GPS for the Soul measures your heart rate and heart rate variability. This is helpful to assess the parasympathetic nervous system, calm the body, and make better lifestyle choices.

www.loseit.com Lose It application. A great app that helps patients track their calories and activity against a goal.

www.motivationalinterviewing.org Clinical resources for motivational interviewing.

www.myfitnesspal.com MyFitnessPal is a free website that allows for calorie tracking along with a food diary. It helps individuals track their progress and lifestyle habits toward achieving and maintaining their ideal weight.

www.nhlbi.nih.gov/guidelines/obesity/BMI/bmicalc.htm Standard body mass index calculator.

37 Nutrition and Family Medicine

MARGARET THOMPSON and MARY BARTH NOEL

Overview

The goal of improving the health of the U.S. population through approaches such as physical activity and nutrition has come to the forefront of public and medical attention. The efforts of public health and other health care professionals in promoting nutrition's potential to improve health are beginning to result in constructive action, but the majority of the public still reports being confused by what a healthy diet is. The public health approach to improving diet through education is part of the focus on preventing chronic diseases in an aging population, and clinical medicine should join in this effort. Additionally, the clinical medicine approach to nutrition may implement nutritional therapies as part of disease management. For these approaches to work for the public, a unified approach between public health and clinical medicine for improving the nutritional health of the public is necessary. This chapter discusses both approaches.

CURRENT DIETARY GUIDANCE

The latest version of the public health dietary program was introduced in 2013. This is in connection with the MyPlate food system (www.MyPlate.gov).

The new ChooseMyPlate.gov incorporates food choices and other ways to customize the food plan, as well as key concepts, into a visual image (see Web Resources). Although there is general agreement, many argue that the recommendations are vague and that food amounts and groupings are inappropriate. The major omission in this version of the dietary system has been *physical activity*, which the last version (MyPyramid.gov) had and seems to be critical in the considerations of diet and the balancing of energy needs with intake. The overarching concepts of the 2010 Dietary Guidelines (www.dietaryguidelines.gov) explain the educational framework for the MyPlate, as follows:

- Maintain calorie balance over time to achieve and sustain a healthy weight.
- Focus on consuming nutrient-dense foods and beverages.

There are more than 23 key recommendations in the latest 2010 Dietary Guidelines (which will be revised in 2015) for the general population and six additional key recommendations for specific populations. The Dietary Guidelines that are emphasized in this version of the public guidance are as follows:

- Build a healthy plate.
- Cut back on foods high in solid fats, added sugars, and salt.
- Eat the right amount of calories for you.
- Be physically active your way.

Along with providing the 10 tips to help the public and professionals who educate the public, the goal is to improve the nutritional quality of the American diet to prevent the leading chronic diseases of obesity, heart disease, and type 2 diabetes. The 10 tips that go along with ChooseMyPlate are as follows:

1. Balance calories.
2. Enjoy your food but eat less.
3. Avoid oversized portions.
4. Foods to eat more often include vegetables, fruits, whole grains, and low-fat milk and dairy products.
5. Make half your plate fruits and vegetables.
6. Switch to fat-free or low-fat (1%) milk.
7. Make half your grains whole grains.
8. Foods to eat less often include foods high in solid fats, added sugars, and salt.
9. Compare sodium in foods.
10. Drink water instead of sugary drinks.

There are additional recommendations for women capable of becoming pregnant, women who are pregnant or breastfeeding, infants and children, and individuals ages 50 years and older.

The specifics of the ChooseMyPlate are many, and the latest dietary guidelines might be as confusing as previous guidelines. The American plans are a combination of food- and nutrient-based recommendations, the latter of which are often difficult to explain to and are not well understood by the public. Both the professional community and the general public recognize the important role of proper nutrition in maintaining health, but neither always heeds current evidence. Physical activity also needs to be part of any discussion about nutrition. This chapter highlights the current evidence for supporting nutritional approaches to common medical and health concerns. Recent research emphasizes that the whole-food diet (rather than specific nutrients or supplements) seems to be most important to influencing positively the prevention and treatment of chronic diseases.

Nutrition Assessment

A nutrition assessment is the process of determining an individual's nutritional status or whether adequate amounts of required nutrients are available to and absorbed by the body. Every patient in a family medicine practice deserves some level of nutrition assessment. This assessment can be a brief screen when the patient is relatively healthy or more in-depth if the patient appears to have nutritional inadequacy or risk factors for malnutrition. The depth of the assessment is based on the patient and the presenting situation. Those who may require a more in-depth evaluation include patients who are grossly overweight or underweight, patients with a chronic or severe acute illness, growing infants and children, patients in poverty or otherwise unable to obtain a variety of foods, most frail older adults, and patients who maintain nontraditional diets such as recent immigrants or fad dieters (American Dietetic Association, 2012).

HISTORY

Patients with chronic illness deserve a more thorough history assessment, as do patients with symptoms or signs potentially related to poor nutrition (Table 37-1). Physicians should review gastrointestinal (GI) symptoms and elicit information about supplemental vitamins and other nutritional products, alcohol and illicit drugs, appetite suppressants or stimulants, glucocorticoids, and laxatives. In at-risk patients and those with clinical evidence of poor nutrition, clinicians should consider the presence of conditions that may increase nutritional requirements. Physicians should also investigate the patient's ability to obtain, ingest, digest, metabolize, and absorb nutrients; consider whether a treatment or medication will require modification of the diet; and use information obtained in the history to plan for that change.

Conditions That May Increase Nutritional Requirements

Any condition that increases the metabolic rate of the patient is likely to increase nutritional requirements (Table 37-2).

Ability to Obtain Food. Patients in poverty and who cannot or do not receive financial assistance are at risk for poor nutrition because of an inability to obtain enough food or a variety of foods. Those who lack transportation or have other shopping access issues, such as language barriers or distance from a store, may also not be able to acquire sufficient food. Patients who rely on others to provide food, prepare food, or both may have inadequate dietary intake. Many patients, because of poor mobility and declining health, gradually lose the ability to perform activities of daily living, such as shopping, cooking, and cleaning, so the

history should contain specific questions directed at these activities. Individuals with substance abuse problems or poor mental health may lack the initiative or ability to acquire healthy foods.

Ability to Ingest Nutrients. Various conditions may contribute to a patient's inability or lack of desire to eat (see Table 37-2).

Digestion. A number of processes can affect the normal digestive process. Any factor that interferes with the secretion of acid or enzymes into the stomach or small intestine may impair digestion. For example, patients with partial gastrectomy or even vagotomy for peptic ulcer disease may have maldigestion and nutritional deficiencies. Similarly, patients with chronic pancreatitis or on chronic acid-suppressing medicines may lack acid and certain digestive enzymes and thus cannot absorb all nutrients.

Absorption. Patients may demonstrate poor absorption of nutrients for a variety of reasons, including loss of absorptive surface area in the intestinal tract from surgery; Crohn disease; infectious processes; or other inflammatory conditions, such as celiac disease. It is important to be aware of hidden sources of gluten in a variety of foods (National Digestive Diseases Information Clearinghouse, 2008) (Table 37-3). Incomplete digestion and processing of fats, carbohydrates, proteins, and vitamins can also lead to decreased absorption of those nutrients. Table 37-4 lists various nutrients and their sites of metabolism and absorption.

Metabolism and Excretion. Many chronic diseases result in poor metabolism of foods, which leads to poor availability of calories and other nutrients. Additionally, any condition that results in excessive losses of nutrients through the intestinal tract or kidneys may also result in malnutrition. Certain foods, such as nonabsorbable fat substitutes, cause excessive loss of fat-soluble vitamins, with steatorrhea caused by the fat not being absorbed (Table 37-5).

Dietary History

It is important to obtain information about the patient's usual and recent diet as part of the history. The dietary history refers to a patient's usual pattern of food intake and any factors that may influence food choices and availability. Screening questions include number of daily meals and examples of food consumed. A more thorough evaluation delves into cultural or religious food practices, personal preferences, and use of a table or picture of the food groups as a tool to help patients identify food groups from which they may be consuming too few or too many servings.

A specific part of the dietary history is a *nutrient intake analysis*. This history relies on a food diary kept by the patient for a specific period, usually 3 to 7 days, including times, food and beverages consumed, and activity. Clinicians also use *dietary recall* as a method to assess nutrient intake. With this tool, patients report foods and beverages consumed over the past 24 to 48 hours. This retrospective analysis has less validity than the prospective food diary because people typically are unable to remember the details

Text continued on page 898

Table 37-1 Summary of Major Nutrients

Nutrient	Major Dietary Sources	Major Functions	Signs of Deficiency	Usual Causes of Deficiency	Effects of Excess	Normal Laboratory Value
Protein (supplies 4 kcal/g)	Fish, chicken, beef, other animals; lentils, seeds, legumes, dried beans; dairy products; eggs; nuts	Building materials (AAs) for growth, maintenance, repair of all cells; regulates fluid balance between blood and cells; provides energy; essential AAs are threonine, tryptophan, histidine, lysine, leucine, isoleucine, methionine, valine, and phenylalanine	Kwashiorkor (protein malnutrition); decreased immune response; edema; stunted growth and development; poor musculature; marasmus (protein-energy malnutrition)	Poor intake of protein, especially high-quality protein; too few calories so that protein is used for energy; malabsorption; genetic diseases of protein, AAs (e.g., PKU)	Reduced calcium retention; weight gain; obesity	Albumin, 3.5-5.0 g/dL; BUN, 9-20 mg/dL; creatinine, 0.3-1.3 mg/dL; prealbumin, 10-40 mg/dL; total protein, 6.0-8.0 g/dL
Carbohydrates (CHO) (supply 4 kcal/g)	Cereal grains, dried peas and beans, bread, pasta, vegetables, fruits, dairy products, sugar, jellies, other sweets	Provide energy for body processes and physical activity; aid in use of fat and spare protein; provide energy; many vitamins and most fibers are CHO	Growth retardation; weight loss	Poor intake; malabsorption; genetic diseases of CHO (e.g., glycogen storage disease)	Weight gain; obesity; increased blood triglyceride levels	None
Fat (supplies 9 kcal/g)	Saturated fats: meats, dairy fats (e.g., ice cream, sour cream, butter); bacon, sausages. Unsaturated fats: avocado, oils (e.g., corn, safflower, vegetable). Monounsaturated fats: olive oil, canola oil	Supplies concentrated source of energy; carries fat-soluble vitamins; supplies essential fatty acids (e.g., linoleic, linolenic, arachidonic acids); membrane structures; transport processes of cells	Flaky, scaly skin; poor growth; hair loss; impaired wound healing and immune functioning	Poor intake; malabsorption; extreme diets or supplementary feedings for long periods (e.g., IV lines, TPN without fats)	Increased blood cholesterol or triglyceride levels; weight gain; obesity	Total cholesterol, <200 to >140 mg/dL; HDL >45 mg/dL; LDL <100-130 mg/dL
Water	Water, beverages, fruits; almost all foods contain some water	Provides substrate for most of body's reactions; helps move materials to and waste from cells; helps control body temperature; lubricates joints in body	Dehydration; death	Poor intake; medications; diarrhea; vomiting; high temperatures	Excess retention of fluid related to imbalance of minerals; overconsumption is rare but can result in death	Dehydration: increased albumin, BUN. Fluid overload: decreased albumin, BUN
VITAMINS						
Water-Soluble Vitamins						
Vitamin B₁ (thiamin)	Lean pork, wheat germ, whole or fortified cereals, legumes, bread products	Assists in use of CHO and fat for energy; promotes growth, appetite, and muscle tone; promotes normal functioning of nervous system; coenzyme in metabolism of CHO branched-chain AAs	Beriberi; changes in nerves; excessive water retention; loss of appetite; depression; muscle tenderness; high-output cardiac failure; polyneuritis	Poor intake; malabsorption; hemodialysis	None reported	Thiamine pyrophosphate (TPP); stimulation >20% (index >0.2% indicates deficiency)

Continued on following page

Table 37-1   Summary of Major Nutrients (Continued)

Nutrient	Major Dietary Sources	Major Functions	Signs of Deficiency	Usual Causes of Deficiency	Effects of Excess	Normal Laboratory Value
Vitamin B₂ (riboflavin)	Dairy products, liver and other organ meats, meat, fish, dark green vegetables, fortified grain products	Functions as part of energy release; essential for growth; part of flavin coenzymes required in cellular oxidation	Cheilosis; photophobia; angular stomatitis; magenta tongue; glossitis; seborrhea; corneal vascularization	Poor intake; malabsorption	None reported	FAD; stimulation >40% (index >1.4% indicates deficiency)
Vitamin B₆ comprises six compounds: pyridoxal, pyridoxine, pyridoxamine, and three 5′-phosphates: pyridoxal (PLP), pyridoxine (PNP), and pyridoxamine (PMP)	Liver, pork, poultry, whole or fortified grain products, bananas, legumes, lentils, fortified soy-based meat substitutes, nuts	Cofactor for many enzymes in metabolism of protein and AAs; functions in hemoglobin synthesis	Anemia; irritability; convulsions (in infants); skin lesions; smooth red tongue (glossitis); peripheral neuropathies; impaired all-mediated immunity	Poor intake; malabsorption; aging (increased need); medications	Sensory neuropathy marked by changes in gait and peripheral sensation	—
Vitamin B₁₂* (cobalamin)	Liver, beef, poultry, fish, eggs, brewer's yeast (not present in plant foods) Oral initial dose: 1000-2000 µg per 1-2 weeks Maintenance: 1000 µg daily for life IM initial dose: 100-1000 µg daily or every other day for 1-2 weeks Maintenance: 100-1000 µg every 1-3 months	Maintenance of nervous tissue and blood formation; nucleic acid synthesis; recycling of tetrahydrofolate	Megaloblastic anemia (pernicious anemia); permanent damage to nervous system; peripheral neuropathy; weight loss; glossitis	Deficiency of hydrochloric acid in stomach (as occurs with aging); strict vegetarians; high intakes of folate can mask deficiency of vitamin B₁₂	None reported	Schilling test: 8% of radioactivity per 24-hour urine†
Vitamin C (ascorbic acid)	Citrus fruits and juices, tomatoes, potatoes, cabbage, broccoli, strawberries, spinach	Cofactor for reactions requiring reduced copper or iron metalloenzymes; protective antioxidant	Scurvy; easy bruising; slow wound healing; degeneration of skin, teeth, gums, blood vessels	Smokers have increased need; poor intake	GI disturbances; kidney stones; excess iron absorption	Plasma or leukocyte vitamin C measured by chromatography; plasma vitamin C, 0.50-1.40 mg/dL (30-80 µmol/L)
Folate (folic acid, folacin, pteroylpoly-glutamates)	Dark-green leafy vegetables, whole grains, legumes, nuts, organ meats, orange juice, fortified cereal products	Assists in red blood cell maturation; cofactor for synthesis of purine and pyrimidine; coenzyme in metabolism of nucleic acids and AAs	Megaloblastic anemia; general weakness; depression; polyneuropathy; GI upsets; poor growth; maternal deficiency linked to neural tube defects in fetus (400 µg/day recommended prepregnancy)	Poor intake; malabsorption	Masks deficiency of vitamin B₁₂	Red blood cell folate, 4-20 ng/mL
Niacin (includes nicotinic acid amide, nicotinic acid, nicotinamide)	Liver, meat, bran or fortified cereal products, fish, poultry, whole or fortified grains, peanuts, tuna	Part of coenzymes for oxidation-reduction reactions; active in release of energy and biosynthesis of fatty acids	Pellagra; pigmented dermatitis; dementia; diarrhea; inflammation of mucous membranes; weakness; tremors	Poor intake; malabsorption; consumption of processed grains that have niacin removed; hemodialysis	Flushing, burning, tingling around face, neck, hands; liver damage; GI distress	—

Nutrient	Major Dietary Sources	Major Functions	Signs of Deficiency	Usual Causes of Deficiency	Effects of Excess	Normal Laboratory Value
Pantothenic acid	Liver, egg yolks, meat, mushrooms, whole grains, brewer's yeast, broccoli, skim milk, sweet potatoes, avocados	Component of coenzyme A; functions in release of energy from CHO, protein, and fat; coenzyme in fatty acid metabolism	Fatigue; malaise; insomnia; burning paresthesias; depression; weakness (rare)	Poor intake; malabsorption; incomplete PEN or TPN formulas	Unknown	—
Biotin	Nuts, soy, eggs, nonfat milk, sweet potatoes	Coenzyme for carboxylation reactions; plays a role in CHO and fat metabolism; coenzyme in synthesis of fat, glycogen, and AAs	Dermatitis; neuritis; appetite loss; nausea; glossitis; insomnia; thin hair; depression; hypercholesterolemia (few known cases)	Incomplete PEN or TPN formulas	Unknown	—
Fat-Soluble Vitamins						
Vitamin A (includes provitamin A such as retinols, carotenoids)	Liver, dairy products, fish; turkey (carotene), carrots, dark-green leafy vegetables, sweet potatoes, cantaloupe, apricots, broccoli, tomatoes	Maintenance of skin and mucous membranes; component in visual process; particular adaptation to darkness; immune function	Night blindness; xerophthalmia; keratomalacia; Bitot spots; follicular hyperkeratosis; reduced immunity; poor growth	Poor intake; malabsorption with steatorrhea; liver disease	Loss of appetite; headache; vomiting; blurred vision with eventual eye damage; liver toxicity; teratogen in fetal growth	Serum retinol and retinol ester vitamin A, 30-80 µg/dL (1.0-2.8 µmol/L)
Vitamin D (calciferol) uptake; glucocorticoid	Fortified dairy products,‡ fish, eggs; sunlight (15 min/day for 3-4 days/wk)	Mineralization of bones and teeth; intestinal regulation of calcium and phosphorus	Rickets (children); osteomalacia (adults); costochondral beading; muscle weakness and twitching; low serum calcium	Poor sunlight exposure; poor intake; with aging, poor uptake glucocorticoid therapy may need additional vitamin D	Poor growth; weight loss; poor appetite; calcium deposits in soft tissues	25-hydroxy-vitamin D test, costochondral
Vitamin E (also called α-tocopherol)	Nuts, fats, polyunsaturated vegetable oils, margarine, seeds, whole grains	Antioxidant; prevents peroxidation of polyunsaturated lipids; free radical scavenger	Hemolytic anemia of newborn; increased fragility of red blood cells; nerve and muscle disturbances in severe malabsorption	Lipid malabsorption	Interferes with vitamin K (risk of bleeding, especially in trauma); hemorrhagic toxicity; monitor patients taking anticoagulants and vitamin E supplements	Serum tocopherol measured by chromatography, 0.5-1.8 mg/dL (12-42 µmol/L)
Vitamin K	Dark-green leafy vegetables, liver, vegetable oils, margarines, cabbage family	Synthesis of prothrombin and clotting factors II, VII, IX, and X	Bleeding (especially in newborns); ecchymosis; epistaxis; prolonged clotting time	Bacteria destroyed in gut that produce vitamin K; liver disease; lipid malabsorption	Unknown; monitor patients taking anticoagulants with vitamin K intake	PT to assess vitamin K indirectly
MINERALS						
Calcium	Dairy products, fish with small bones, dark-green leafy vegetables (mustard greens, kale), corn tortillas, calcium-set tofu	Structure of bones and teeth; nerve transmission; muscle contraction; essential role in blood clotting	Stunted growth; bone loss; rickets; osteomalacia; osteoporosis; tetany; possibly hypertension	Poor intake; poor consumption of vitamin D; poor sunlight exposure; lack of physical activity; high phosphorus intake	Decreased absorption of other minerals; kidney stones; hypercalcemia; milk-alkali syndrome; renal insufficiency	8.5-10.5 g/dL

Continued on following page

Table 37-1 Summary of Major Nutrients (Continued)

Nutrient	Major Dietary Sources	Major Functions	Signs of Deficiency	Usual Causes of Deficiency	Effects of Excess	Normal Laboratory Value
Chloride	Table salt, seafood, meat	Acid–base balance; constituent of gastric juice; major anion of ECF	Rare; mental apathy, muscle cramps, usually seen with sodium depletion	Rare in United States (has occurred in babies whose formula did not have chloride)	None reported	96–106 mEq/L
Chromium	Fish, cheese, meat, poultry, whole-grain cereals, beer	Insulin cofactor; glucose and energy metabolism	Insulin resistance; glucose intolerance	Unknown	None reported	—
Cobalt	Organ and muscle meats, dairy products	Constituent of vitamin B$_{12}$	Only as vitamin B$_{12}$ deficiency; pernicious anemia	Those associated with vitamin B$_{12}$	None reported	—
Copper	Liver, shellfish, nuts, whole grains, cereals, legumes, cocoa products	Absorption and use of iron; enzyme cofactor; in myelin nerve sheath	Anemia; kinky hair; neutropenia; disturbance of bone formation	Usually genetic	Wilson disease (genetic); iron-deficiency anemia; chronic renal failure	—
Fluoride	Fluoridated drinking water, fluoridated dental products, seafood	Structure of bone and teeth enamel; reduces dental caries	Dental caries	Nonfluoridated water or dental products	Mottled teeth; enamel and skeletal fluorosis	—
Iodine	Iodized salt, seafood, saltwater fish	Constituent of thyroid hormone	Goiter; cretinism	Lack of iodine in food or in soil where food is grown	Rare; goiter may be caused by excess iodine; elevated TSH	—
Iron	Liver, lean meats, legumes, egg yolk, fortified cereals and breads	Constituent of hemoglobin; involved in oxygen and electron transport	Microcytic hypochromic anemia; fatigue; decreased immune response	Poor intake; blood loss	Liver and pancreas damage; large dose at one time: shock, death; GI distress	Serum iron, 50–150 μg/dL
Magnesium	Bran cereals, nuts, legumes, green leafy vegetables, meat	Part of protein synthesis; helps muscles contract and helps nerve impulse transmission	Rare; behavioral disturbances, tremor, spasms, neuromuscular irritability	Rare	Rare; diarrhea; fatigue; nervous system disturbances (usually from pharmacologic agents, not food sources)	1.5–2.5 mEq/L
Manganese	Nuts, legumes, whole-grain cereals	Involved in formation of bone and enzymes in AAs, cholesterol, and CHO metabolism	Rare; dermatitis; weight loss	Rare	Rare; inhaled manganese linked to CNS disorders, neurotoxicity	—

Nutrient	Major Dietary Sources	Major Functions	Signs of Deficiency	Usual Causes of Deficiency	Effects of Excess	Normal Laboratory Value
Molybdenum	Whole-grain cereals, legumes, nuts	Oxidation-reduction reactions; enzyme helps in catabolism of sulfur AAs; metabolism of purine, pyrimidines	None	None	Unknown	—
Phosphorus	Dairy products, eggs, meat, whole-grain cereals, soda	Structure of bone and teeth; component of phospholipids; helps regulate acid–base balance; energy metabolism	Rare; demineralization of bone; weakness; poor growth; paresthesias of hands and feet	Rare in United States	May cause deficiency of calcium, skeletal porosity; interference with calcium absorption	2.5–4.5 mg/dL
Potassium	Fruits (particularly bananas, citrus juices), dairy products, potatoes, vegetables	Major component of intracellular fluid; regulates acid–base and water balance; maintains heart and nerve function	Muscle weakness; rapid, irregular heart rate; paralysis; death	Medications (e.g., diuretics), especially with poor intake	Electrolyte imbalance; muscle weakness; disturbed heart function; death	3.5–5.0 mEq/dL
Selenium	Organ meat, seafood, plants from selenium-containing soil	Antioxidant; constituent of glutathione oxidase	Rare; cardiac myopathy; muscle tenderness	Rare	Rare; hair and nail brittleness and loss	—
Sodium	Table salt, processed foods, in most foods except fruits	Maintains water balance; influences muscle contraction and nerve irritability	Rare; muscle cramps; reduced appetite	Rare; restricted diet with excessive medication	In some people, retention of fluids and hypertension	135–145 mEq/dL
Sulfur	Protein foods (e.g., meat, dairy, legumes)	Constituent of coenzyme A, AAs, hair, cartilage	No dietary deficiency with adequate protein	Rare	Rare	—
Zinc	Meat, seafood, dark meat of poultry, whole grains, legumes	Component of enzymes and proteins; involved in regulation of gene expression	Growth failure; impaired wound healing; taste changes; decreased immune response	Poor consumption of protein foods; phytate consumption inhibits absorption	Fever, nausea, vomiting, diarrhea; reduction in copper	115 ± 12 ng/dL

*Dosages from Lederle FA. Oral cobalamin for pernicious anemia: medicine's best kept secret? *JAMA*. 1991;265:94-95.
†From Mahan LK, Escott-Stump S. *Krause's Food and Nutrition Therapy*. 11th ed. Philadelphia: Saunders; 2003:1208-1219.
‡Not all dairy products are fortified.

AA, Amino acid; *BUN*, blood urea nitrogen; *CNS*, central nervous system; *ECF*, extracellular fluid; *FAD*, flavin adenine dinucleotide *GI*, gastrointestinal; *HDL*, high-density lipoprotein; *IM*, intramuscular; *IV*, intravenous; *LDL*, low-density lipoprotein; *PEN*, peripheral enteral nutrition; *PKU*, phenylketonuria; *PT*, prothrombin time; *TPN*, total parenteral nutrition; *TSH*, thyroid-stimulating hormone.
Modified from Noel T. Nutrition and obesity. In Paulman PM, Susman J, Harrison J, et al, eds. *Family medicine clerkship guide*. St. Louis: Mosby-Elsevier; 2005.

Table 37-2 Select Conditions That Increase Nutrient Requirements

Pregnancy
Lactation
Healing wounds, including skin ulcers
Surgery
Trauma
Burns
Chronic lung disease
Cancer
AIDS
Infection
Inflammatory diseases
Hyperthyroidism

Table 37-3 Celiac Disease: Grains with and without Gluten

Grains or Flours Allowed		Grains or Flours with Gluten: Not Allowed
Rice	Millet	Wheat (e.g., durum, semolina, kamut, spelt)
Soy	Buckwheat	
Potato	Arrowroot	Rye
Tapioca	Amaranth	Barley
Beans	Tef	Triticale
Garfava	Wild grass seeds (Montina)	Oats (most likely because of contamination)
Sorghum		
Quinoa	Nut flours	

Table 37-4 Nutrients and Sites of Metabolism and Absorption

Nutrient	Site of Absorption
MACRONUTRIENTS	
Amino acids	Throughout small intestine (more rapid proximally)
Sugars	Throughout small intestine
FATS	
Fatty acids	Throughout small intestine (mostly proximal)
Bile acids	Ileum
Short-chain fatty acids	Colon
MINERALS	
Calcium	Duodenum, jejunum
Iron	Duodenum
Magnesium	Small intestine
VITAMINS	
Folic acid	Proximal small intestine
Vitamin B_{12}	Ileum
Fat-soluble vitamins (A, D, E, K)	Small intestine

Table 37-5 Conditions Affecting Metabolism and Excretion

Type of Impairment	Possible Contributing Condition
Impaired dietary intake	AIDS
	Anorexia nervosa
	Cancer
	Depression
	Dental problems
	Hyperemesis gravidarum
	Poverty
	Stroke
	Substance abuse
Maldigestion	Cholestasis
	Enzyme deficiencies
	Intestinal bacterial stasis
	Pancreatitis or insufficiency
	Radiation enteritis
	Short bowel syndrome
Malabsorption	AIDS
	Celiac disease
	Intestinal lymphoma
	Radiation enteritis
Impaired metabolism	AIDS
	Cancer
	Chronic disease (liver, kidney)
	Corticosteroid use
Increased excretion of nutrients	Diarrhea (zinc, magnesium)
	Glucosuria
	Inflammatory bowel disease
	Protein-losing enteropathy
	GI bleeding (iron)
Increased requirements	Burns
	Trauma
	Surgery
	Chronic infection
	Inflammation
	Chronic lung disease
	Hyperthyroidism
	Sepsis

AIDS, Acquired immunodeficiency syndrome; *GI,* gastrointestinal.
Modified from Newton JM, Halsted CH. Clinical and functional assessment of adults. In Shils ME, Olson JA, Shike M, Ross AC, eds. *Modern nutrition in health and disease.* 9th ed. St. Louis: Lippincott-Williams & Wilkins; 1999.

of their past eating habits accurately (Hammond, 2004). There are currently several smartphone applications and software programs that allow patients to track their own food intake. A recent study evaluated the content of several of these apps to determine which best aligned with weight loss theory, including providing motivation, diet tracking, healthy cooking, wise grocery shopping choices, and weight and body mass index (BMI) tracking. Lose It by FitNow, Inc. best fulfills those criteria (Azar et al., 2013). Another useful app is the eTools app from Weight Watchers, which allows members to track meals online or through the app, as well as document activity, find ideas for healthy recipes,

and read tips on how to choose healthy options while eating out. A recent study demonstrated that individuals enrolled in Weight Watchers with access to the eTools mobile app and online system as well as the support meetings were more successful with weight loss than individuals enrolled in a self-help system (Johnston et al., 2013). Both Lose It and eTools include bar code scanner capability, which allows automatic logging of nutritional information on packaged foods.

HealthyOut is an app and website that was developed for New York City and is now available as a resource listing different restaurant food options throughout the country. HealthyOut allows the user to select a type of dietary pattern (healthy, low carbohydrate, vegan, and many others) and find nearby restaurants offering appropriate foods. The application gives ideas for what to order at a particular restaurant, as well as nutritional information (see Web Resources).

Although these apps and websites facilitate the process, studies have shown that patients continue to struggle to accurately determine portion size when reporting (Nelson et al., 1994).

PHYSICAL EXAMINATION

> ### Key Points
>
> - Significant weight loss—5% in 1 month, 7.5% in 3 months, or 10% in 6 months, from usual weight—indicates the need for further evaluation to determine the cause.
> - Although BMI is a validated independent measure of body fat, it may not accurately reflect body composition in certain subsets of individuals, such as trained athletes and elderly adults.

Table 37-6 Weight Categories According to Body Mass Index (BMI)

Category	BMI (kg/m^2)
Underweight	<18.5
Normal	18.5-24.9
Overweight	25-29.9
Obese	≥30

From National Heart, Lung, and Blood Institute (NHLBI). Clinical guidelines on the identification, evaluation, and treatment of overweight and obesity in adults, BMI calculator. http://www.nhlbisupport.com/bmi/bmicalc.htm.

A systematic physical examination is important in evaluating nutritional status. General inspection may immediately reveal obvious overweight or underweight. Anthropometry, or physical measurements of an individual that are compared with reference standards, plays a role as well. These parameters include height, weight, skinfold thickness, head circumference (especially in infants and children), and waist and hip circumferences. These measurements are most helpful when taken at several intervals over time.

Height and Weight

It is useful to measure height and weight to assess nutrition. Patients tend to overestimate their height and underestimate their weight. In considering weight alone in adults, the *usual body weight* is a more useful parameter than ideal body weight obtained from published tables. In children, body weight is more useful than height in estimating body fat and provides information about recent nutrient intake (Hammond, 2004). Changes in weight over time from the usual body weight may reflect a change in nutritional status. However, it is important to remember that acutely, weight loss or gain may signify a change in fluid status rather than in nutritional well-being. In an obese individual or older adult, loss of lean body mass indicating malnutrition may be masked by the presence of excess body fat.

Significant weight loss is defined as a 5% loss in 1 month, a 7.5% loss in 3 months, or a 10% loss in 6 months. A severe weight loss is defined as any loss higher than those percentages in the same interval. The following method is also used to assess nutritional status as a function of weight loss (Hammond, 2004):

- Weight within 85% to 90% of usual body weight—*mild* malnutrition
- Weight within 75% to 84% of usual body weight—*moderate* malnutrition
- Weight less than 74% of usual body weight—*severe* malnutrition

Both height and weight are needed to calculate BMI, which is highly correlated with independent measures of body fat in adults (Balcombe et al., 2001; Keys et al., 1972). The formula for calculating BMI is Weight (kg)/[Height (m)]^2. Table 37-6 lists parameters for overweight, obesity, and underweight according to the BMI (see Web Resources for a BMI calculator).

It is important to note the limitations of the BMI as a nutritional assessment tool. It may overestimate body fat in trained athletes, and it may underestimate body fat in older patients and in those who have lost lean body mass because of nutritional deficiency. Studies show that body composition is probably more predictive than BMI of chronic diseases such as metabolic syndrome (Gomez-Ambrosi et al., 2012). Additionally, there is fairly strong evidence that individuals who are overweight by National Heart, Lung and Blood Institute (NHLBI) guidelines (BMI, 25 to <30 kg/m^2) actually have lower age-related all-cause mortality than individuals at normal BMI (18.5 to <25 kg/m^2) (Flegal et al., 2012; Flegal et al., 2013; Ogden et al., 2012).

Body Composition

Assessment of body composition reveals the relative amount of body fat and lean body mass. One common method for assessing subcutaneous fat is the measurement of *skinfold thickness*. Several areas of the body have demonstrated good correlation with body fat, including the triceps, biceps, subscapular tissue, and tissue above the iliac crest. Measurements are taken with calipers and compared with standardized tables to determine the percentage of body fat. This type of assessment can be limited by the accuracy of the measuring technique. Changes in skinfold thickness take place over 3 to 4 weeks, so this measurement is not a useful gauge for determining acute changes in nutritional status.

Circumference measurements are useful in assessing nutritional status. The waist circumference correlates with abdominal fat content. Increased waist circumference has been associated with cardiovascular disease risk factors (Dalton et al., 2003). The correct method for waist circumference is to measure the distance around the smallest area below the rib cage and above the umbilicus. Waist measurements of more than 40 inches in men and 35 inches in women are independent risk factors for disease (NHLBI, 2005). The waist circumference has less predictive value in patients shorter than 5 feet tall and in those with BMI greater than 35.

General Physical Examination

Certain findings on physical examination may alert the physician to the potential for malnutrition. Many of the physical signs of nutritional deficiency are age dependent. General findings include loss of subcutaneous fat (orbital or in triceps area), temporal wasting, decreased muscle mass in general, proximal muscle weakness, reduced grip strength, and certain skin changes (e.g., scaling, poor wound healing, bruising). Tissues in the body that undergo rapid cell turnover, such as mucous membranes, skin, and hair, may be the first to show signs of nutritional insufficiency (see Table 37-1). In children, decelerating linear growth, lethargy, and fat depletion may signal malnutrition.

Macronutrient deficiencies present with specific signs, depending on the nutrient. For example, dietary fat deficiency, which may be seen with disordered eating, may be evidenced through flaky skin, hair loss, or poor wound healing. A deficiency of protein (kwashiorkor) that is severe will present with a protuberant abdomen, hair loss, loss of skin pigmentation, and growth retardation (Hoffer, 2012).

Overall, most vitamin deficiencies are uncommon in the United States, but some signs should alert physicians to evaluate for those nutritional deficits or malabsorption. For example, several B vitamin deficiencies may result in glossitis, or a smooth tongue appearance. A niacin deficiency (seen in individuals with alcoholism or malabsorption) may cause diarrhea, inflamed mucous membranes, and skin ulcerations. Thiamine deficiency (most commonly seen in those with alcoholism) may present with peripheral neuropathy, gait disturbance, and nystagmus. Iron deficiency from nutritional or non-nutritional causes may present with koilonychias (spooning of the nails).

LABORATORY EVALUATION

Key Points

- Albumin and transferrin can be artificially low when C-reactive protein (CRP) level (inflammation) is high. Prealbumin is a more accurate marker of nutritional status with systemic inflammation.

Physiologic changes related to adequacy of nutrition occur slowly; the first signs of a change in nutritional status usually appear at the cellular level. These changes may be detected by a variety of laboratory tests. Single laboratory tests may have value in screening for nutritional problems, but a series of values is important for assessing ongoing nutritional problems and treatment.

What to Order to Assess Malnutrition

No general laboratory studies will diagnose malnutrition. Laboratory investigation should be directed toward specific nutrients that the physician suspects may be missing from a patient's diet, for which the patient may be at risk based on disease or because of history or physical examination findings that suggest a nutritional deficiency (see Table 37-1).

Unexplained weight loss with no other specific symptoms is often associated with inflammation, and inflammatory markers such as CRP and erythrocyte sedimentation rate may be elevated. Table 37-7 lists common laboratory evaluations for frequently encountered micronutrient deficiencies.

Measuring Visceral Protein: Albumin. The protein contained in visceral organs constitutes about 10% of total body protein, and the protein in plasma and extravascular body fluids makes up about 3% of total protein. *Albumin*

Table 37-7 Laboratory Tests for Nutritional Deficiencies

Nutrient Deficiency	Laboratory Evaluation
Vitamin A	Serum retinol
Vitamin D	25(OH)D
Vitamin E	Not usually assayed for diagnosis
Vitamin K	PT, INR
Vitamin B$_{12}$	MMA, tHcy
Folate	MMA, tHcy
Vitamin B$_2$ (riboflavin)	Serum EGRAC
Vitamin B$_1$ (thiamine)	Erythrocyte thiamine diphosphate level
Iron	CBC, serum ferritin, total iron binding capacity
Zinc	Serum or plasma zinc level (not good assessment of zinc stores)

CBC, Complete blood count; *ECGRAC*, erythrocyte glutathione reductase activity coefficient; *INR*, international normalized ratio; *MMA*, methylmalonic acid; *PT*, prothrombin time; *tHcy*, total homocysteine; *25(OH)D*, 25-hydroxy-vitamin D.

is a plasma protein produced by the liver that can be used as an indicator of visceral protein balance. The measurement of serum albumin reflects changes in the protein status over time because albumin has a serum half-life of 2 to 3 weeks.

Using serum albumin as a marker for protein nutrition status has limitations. Albumin is a negative acute-phase reactant and tends to decrease in concentration under conditions of inflammation. Because of its long half-life, this change may be misleading. In protein-calorie starvation, albumin levels tend to decrease, but in total-calorie deprivation, albumin levels may remain more stable (Hammond, 2004). Finally, there is a large extravascular albumin pool, which tends to equilibrate by entering the vascular system when plasma concentration of albumin decreases.

Transferrin. Transferrin is another plasma protein that reflects overall protein balance. Similar to albumin, transferrin is a negative acute-phase reactant, but because of its shorter half-life (8 days), it may be somewhat more accurate than albumin as a tool for assessing nutritional status. Transferrin has limitations, however, in that its concentration is related to the patient's overall iron status. Also, as with albumin, serum concentration of transferrin does not change rapidly with changes in protein-calorie intake.

Other Plasma Proteins. Several other plasma proteins have been proposed as good markers for protein energy status. The level of transthyretin (TTY), also known as *prealbumin*, has been shown to correlate with visceral protein status, but it is an acute-phase reactant and is also affected by zinc concentrations. It has a half-life of 2 to 3 days. Retinol-binding protein (RBP) has a short serum half-life (12 hours) and correlates with protein energy status in some patients with malnutrition, but it also is a negative acute-phase reactant and has limitations for the assessment of nutritional status.

It is possible to circumvent the problems raised by inflammation in interpreting the plasma levels of the proteins mentioned. CRP level provides an indication of the amount of inflammation present at a given time. Some clinicians may ascribe more usefulness to levels of albumin, transferrin, TTY, and RBP when the CRP level is low.

Urinary Creatinine and Creatinine-to-Height Ratio

The urinary creatinine level reflects the amount of ongoing muscle metabolism. The amount of creatinine excreted in the urine is proportional to the muscle mass of an individual. Using a mathematical formula, it is possible to derive an expected amount of creatinine excretion over 24 hours based on a person's height. This formula is limited in the case of a tall, thin subject or short, muscular subject. The amount of urinary creatinine also varies depending on the diet; diets high in meat will result in increased urinary creatinine excretion.

Vitamin and Mineral Assays

In general, protein-calorie malnutrition is associated with low levels of vitamin A, zinc, and magnesium. Fat-soluble vitamins may be deficient in conditions of malabsorption of fat. Folic acid and iron are not well absorbed in celiac disease.

Hematologic Tests

Changes in red blood cell production may result from insufficient levels of iron, vitamin B_1, folic acid, and other vitamins. It is important to note that determining the complete blood count (CBC) is important in assessing nutritional status. Patients with poor nutritional status may also demonstrate weak immune status. T cell–mediated responses are more severely affected by nutritional inadequacy than B-cell functions, such as immunoglobulin function. Evaluating the total lymphocyte count can be helpful in assessing T cells. Using skin testing for anergy is one method of testing T-cell immune competence.

Nutrition in the Life Cycle

Key Points

- Recommendations regarding vitamin D and calcium supplements for prevention of osteoporosis continue to evolve, but the United States Preventive Services Task Force (USPSTF) currently recommends against routine supplementation in healthy men and premenopausal women.
- The USPSTF finds insufficient evidence to determine the benefits and harms of daily supplementation with more than 400 IU of vitamin D_3 and more than 1000 mg of calcium for primary prevention of fractures in healthy men and postmenopausal women.

PREGNANCY AND LACTATION

Pregnancy has long been recognized as a time of increased nutritional needs. Recommendations vary, but one constant remains: with adequate caloric intake comes a greater likelihood of ingesting adequate nutrients. Weight checks are a standard part of all prenatal visits. In recent years, concern has focused on the woman's health status after the pregnancy. As Table 37-8 demonstrates, in older pregnant

Table 37-8 Pregnancy Outcomes Linked to Weight Gain

Increased Risk of LBW Infant	Best Outcomes		Increased Risk of Gestational Diabetes*
Biologically immature or too thin (BMI <18.5 kg/m²)	BMI 18.5-24.9 kg/m²	BMI 25-29.9 kg/m²	BMI ≥30 kg/m² or older than 35 years
RECOMMENDED WEIGHT GAIN			
≈28-40 pounds (1.1 lb/wk)	25-30 lb (0.7 lb/wk) Not nursing: 0.8 lb/wk Nursing: 0.9 lb/wk Twins: 1.4 lb/wk	15-25 lb	11-20 lb

*Increased risk of low-birth-weight (LBW) infant or infant too large.
BMI, Body mass index.
Data from Institutes of Medicine. *Report on weight gain during pregnancy: reexamining the guidelines*. Washington, DC: Institutes of Medicine; 2009.

women or biologically immature women (those who become pregnant within 5 years of starting to menstruate), the caloric intake and weight gain are specific to the particular health needs of the woman during as well as after the pregnancy. The usual weight retained with each pregnancy by women in the United States is 10 lb (McGanity et al., 1999). This retained weight may have a significant influence on future chronic disease development for women.

It is now known that the nutritional needs for pregnancy begin before conception. The state of nutrition 60 to 90 days before conception influences pregnancy outcomes. The major nutrient changes from conception through the first trimester are increases in folic acid, iron, and calories. The overall nutritional needs throughout the pregnancy are as follows:

1. Adequate calories for development of the fetus, placenta, and lactation after delivery (with adequate calories increasing the opportunity for adequate nutrients)
2. Adequate protein
3. Adequate iron
4. Adequate folic acid, vitamin C (especially critical if the woman is a smoker because there is a much higher need in smokers), and vitamin B_{12}
5. Adequate calcium and iodine

Community-based programs such as Women, Infants, and Children (WIC) can be resources for helping women in need. It has been demonstrated that infants of women who participate in these programs have higher birth weights than those who were not in the programs and who are in the same social, economic, or other problematic circumstances.

Although not well understood yet, there seems to be some evidence indicating that what occurs nutritionally before pregnancy and during pregnancy for the mother may affect the potential for chronic diseases later in the life of the child. Such diseases as hypertension and diabetes may have their start in the embryonic stage of life (Roseboom et al., 2006, 2011).

Many of the nutritional issues in *lactation* are influenced by the nutritional status of the pregnant woman. The nutritional stores of the postpartum woman are an important source of supplies for her and the infant. Certain nutrients are stable regardless of the maternal diet. Studies of lactation have found that after about 6 months of breast-feeding, maternal weight decreases by about 10 lb without any changes in the composition or production of breast milk (Barbosa et al., 1997). This may be important when considering that the average weight retained with each pregnancy is about 10 lb.

INFANCY AND CHILDHOOD

An excellent summary of the nutrients and development needs for food in this age group is available in Figure 37-1. This figure provides guidance about major nutrient needs and how the infant and child can meet these needs. These evidence-based guidelines were developed by a panel of pediatricians, nutritionists, and the U.S Department of Agriculture (USDA) after comprehensive review of the literature.

It is important to help parents understand that the introduction of new foods takes time. Researchers have found that it takes at least eight different attempts of introducing a new food before a child will show true acceptance or rejection (Birch et al., 1991; Satter, 2000). Parents must understand that their role is to provide a healthy range and variety of foods in a pleasant eating environment, and the child's role is to consume the food in the amounts that he or she needs and wants. This foundation of good food habits will carry through to the adolescent stage, in which independence and finding ways of expressing this independence are achieved not only in social functioning but also in food and health habits.

ADOLESCENCE

Adolescents gain independence by taking a greater role in food choices and amounts eaten. It is frustrating for parents who worked to establish standards to see the young person seek independence even with foods consumed. This is a stage in life that demands high caloric intake because growth needs are second only to those in infancy—more kilocalories per kilogram are required than in any other life stage. This high caloric consumption is favorable to nutritional status because with high calories comes the increased likelihood of taking in more nutrients. Parents must remain hopeful that good health habits will guide the teenager. There may be concern over peer pressure leading to "strange" or different food habits, such as disordered eating, sports nutrition, and vegetarian diets, which many teens attempt. Such exploration is often a natural part of expressing independence. These food patterns can be healthy, such as improving food habits with vegetarianism or sports nutrition. The family physician needs to determine when the teen's exploration could become harmful. Nutrition assessment is appropriate in this life stage in regard to determining whether a nutritional problem is present.

ADULTHOOD

The study of adult nutrition tends to focus on prevention and treatment of chronic diseases. There is new interest in

optimizing nutrition during this stage to enhance older adults' quality of life. Many individuals attempt to use foods and nutritional products as a type of alternative medicine. Some of these developments, such as increased ingestion of supplemental antioxidant vitamins, plant-based estrogens, and other functional foods, have not had the desired outcomes (i.e., longer life, enhanced functional status). The *Dietary Reference Intakes* (National Academy of Sciences, 2005) has addressed the concept of enhanced nutrient intakes through supplements and other products by introducing a new category called *tolerable upper intake levels* (see Terminology). Many values in this category of nutrient levels are still under investigation.

Osteoporosis ("Holes in Bones")

With the possibility of a 20% bone mass loss in the 5 to 7 years after menopause, the best treatment for osteoporosis (reduction in amount of bone mass) is the prevention of bone loss. The following three steps are recognized as most helpful for women (80% of osteoporosis population). It is important to realize that all foods that have calcium (e.g., cheeses) do not necessarily have vitamin D unless they are fortified (see Table 37-1).

1. Balanced diet rich in calcium and vitamin D (see Table 37-1)
2. Weight-bearing exercise, such as walking
3. Healthy lifestyle, with no smoking or excessive alcohol intake

Peak bone development occurs throughout adolescence, with smaller bone gain during the 20s, and thus less calcium is needed at this age. Bone loss starts with menopause for women, which increases the need for calcium and vitamin D to prevent bone loss. High dietary intake of calcium does not seem to present any risk; previous concern about kidney stone formation with increased calcium intake appears to be unfounded (Curhan et al., 1997). Side effects of high amounts of calcium supplement intake include constipation and dyspepsia. There is evidence that high supplemental calcium intake is associated with cardiovascular disease (Xiao et al., 2013).

Calcium supplementation with more than 2000 mg/day of vitamin D may lead to soft tissue calcification. Currently, the USPSTF recommends *against* supplementation with 400 IU or less of vitamin D_3 and 1000 mg of calcium or less per day for primary prevention of fractures in post-menopausal women (level D recommendation). The USPSTF finds insufficient evidence to determine the benefits and harms of greater amounts of supplementation in post-menopausal women or any supplementation in premenopausal healthy women (USPSTF, 2013).

Osteomalacia ("Soft Bones")

Adult-onset osteomalacia (adult form of rickets) is being studied more and seems to be identified more frequently. This is of concern in northern climates with low sunlight and in climates where intense sun blocks are used because of low levels of vitamin D.

Cancer Prevention Through Nutrition

Caloric Restriction. In animal studies, caloric restriction has shown promise in increasing the life span of the animals

Development stage	Newborn	Head up	Supported sitter	Independent sitter	Crawler	Beginning to walk	Independent toddler
Physical skills	• Needs head support	• More skillful head control with support emerging	• Sits with help or support • On tummy, pushes up on arms with straight elbows	• Sits independently • Can pick up and hold small object in hand • Leans toward food or spoon	• Learns to crawl • May pull self to stand	• Pulls self to stand • Stands alone • Takes early steps	• Walks well alone • Runs
Eating skills	• Baby establishes a suck-swallow-breathe pattern during breastfeeding or bottle feeding	• Breastfeeds or bottle feeds • Tongue moves forward and back to suck	• May push food out of mouth with tongue, which gradually decreases with age • Moves pureed food forward and backward in mouth with tongue to swallow • Recognizes spoon and holds mouth open as spoon approaches	• Learns to keep thick purees in mouth • Pulls head downward and presses upper lip to draw food from spoon • Tries to rake foods toward self into fist • Can transfer food from one hand to the other • Can drink from a cup held by feeder	• Learns to move tongue from side to side to transfer food around mouth and push food to the side of the mouth so food can be mashed • Begins to use jaw and tongue to mash food • Plays with spoon at mealtime, may bring it to mouth but does not use it for self-feeding yet • Can feed self finger foods • Holds cup independently • Holds small foods between thumb and first finger	• Feeds self easily with fingers • Can drink from a straw • Can hold cup with two hands and take swallows • More skillful at chewing • Dips spoon in food rather than scooping • Demands to spoon-feed self • Bites through a variety of textures	• Chews and swallows firmer foods skillfully • Learns to use a fork for spearing • Uses spoon with less spilling • Can hold cup in one hand and set it down skillfully
Baby's hunger and fullness cues	• Cries or fusses to show hunger • Gazes at caregiver, opens mouth during feeding indicating desire to continue • Spits out nipple or falls asleep when full • Stops sucking when full	• Cries or fusses to show hunger • Smiles, gazes at caregiver, or coos during feeding to indicate desire to continue • Spits out nipple or falls asleep when full • Stops sucking when full	• Moves head forward to reach spoon when hungry • May swipe the food toward the mouth when hungry • Turns head away from spoon when full • May be distracted or notice surroundings more when full	• Reaches for spoon or food when hungry • Points to food when hungry • Slows down in eating when full • Clenches mouth shut or pushes food away when full	• Reaches for food when hungry • Points to food when hungry • Shows excitement when food is presented when hungry • Pushes food away when full • Slows down in eating when full	• Expresses desire for specific foods with words or sounds • Shakes head to say "no more" when full	• Combines phrases with gestures, such as "want that" and pointing • Can lead parent to refrigerator and point to a desired food or drink • Uses words like "all done" and "get down" • Plays with food or throws food when full
Appropriate foods and textures	• Breastmilk or infant formula	• Breastmilk or infant formula	• Breastmilk or infant formula • Infant cereals • Thin pureed baby foods	• Breastmilk or infant formula • Infant cereals • Thin pureed baby foods • Thicker pureed baby foods • Soft mashed foods without lumps • 100% juice	• Breastmilk or infant formula • 100% juice • Infant cereals • Pureed foods • Ground or soft mashed foods with tiny soft noticeable lumps • Foods with soft texture • Crunchy foods that dissolve (such as baby biscuits or crackers) • Increase variety of flavors offered	• Breastmilk, infant formula, or whole milk • 100% juice • Coarsely chopped foods, including foods with noticeable pieces • Foods with soft to moderate texture • Toddler foods • Bite-sized pieces of foods • Bites through a variety of textures	• Whole milk • 100% juice • Coarsely chopped foods • Toddler foods • Bite-sized pieces of foods • Becomes efficient at eating foods of varying textures and taking controlled bites of soft solids, hard solids, or crunchy foods by 2 years

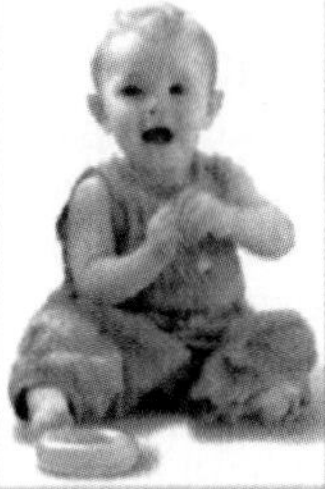

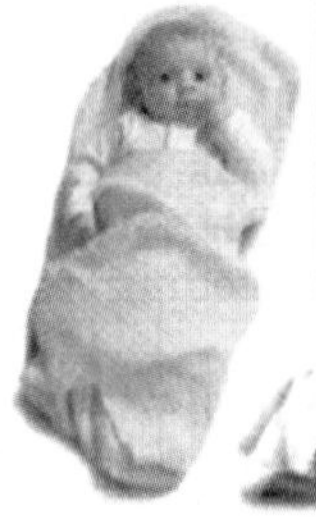

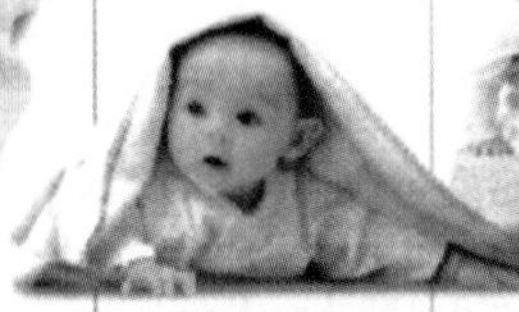

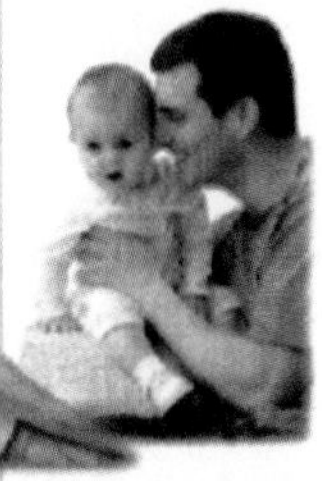

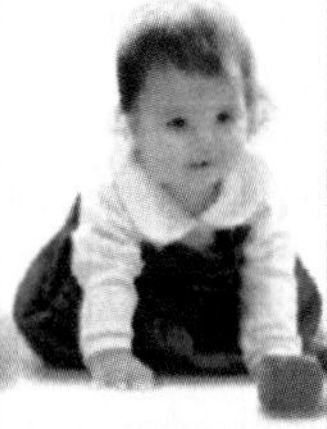

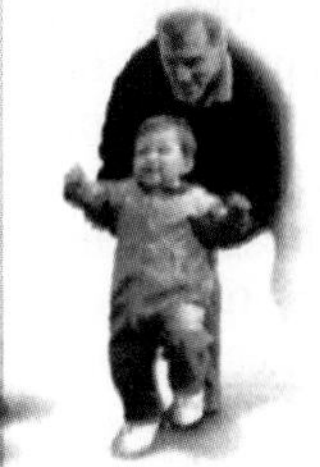

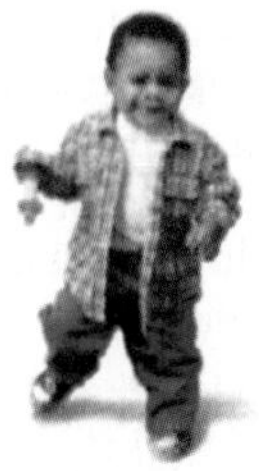

© 2003 Gerber Products Company

Figure 37-1 Summary of physical and eating skills, hunger and fullness cues, and appropriate food textures for infants and children. (From Butte N, Cobb K, Dwyer J, et al. The Start Healthy feeding guidelines for infants and toddlers. *J Am Diet Assoc.* 2004;104:455-467.)

studied, but human studies have not been as encouraging. This may be an extremely difficult area to investigate because there is no clear understanding of where in the human life span caloric restriction would be the most beneficial. In humans, the balance between starvation and overnutrition seems to be more difficult to determine. People with a BMI less than 18 kg/m² seem to have a higher mortality rate, but those who are obese (BMI >30) also probably do less well. Currently, there is insufficient evidence to recommend caloric restriction as a means of treatment or prevention of cancer, although evidence does suggest that a high BMI (>30) may be a cancer-promoting factor. Physical activity to balance the energy intake is probably the best preventive measure against cancer at this time.

Vitamin Supplementation. Epidemiologic studies note that populations who consume diets high in vitamins and minerals have a lower incidence of cancer. Three studies, the Alpha-Tocopherol Beta-Carotene Cancer Prevention Study Group (1994), β-Carotene and Retinol Efficacy Trial (CARET; Omenn et al., 1996), and Physicians' Health Study (Hennekens et al., 1996), investigated smokers and asbestos workers to see whether provitamin A and beta-carotene supplementation would decrease the incidence of cancer. Those who received supplementation developed cancers earlier than those who did not, and the studies were suspended. The USPSTF currently recommends against supplementation with beta-carotene, either alone or in combination with other supplements, for the prevention of cardiovascular disease and cancer (USPSTF, 2003). It is important to understand that current research on the importance of these nutrients is furthering the understanding that the individual nutrients have a food basis of enhancement of health. The disease–mortality response curves are U-shaped for many nutrients (i.e., there is an increased risk of adverse outcomes if the nutrient is ingested in either too low or too high amounts) (Alexander et al., 2013; Ohlhorst et al., 2013).

Therefore, the dietary elements that seem to be the most favorable, according to epidemiologic studies, are as follows:

- *More* fruits, vegetables, whole-grain products, and calcium-containing foods
- *Less* saturated fats, particularly those found in red meats

Aging

The only difference in the nutritional needs of older adults was long thought to be the decrease in caloric needs, about a 2% to 5% decrease with each decade of life. The smaller decrease in caloric need (2%) is for those who exercise and the higher decrease (5%) is for those who do not exercise. A decrease in caloric need is complicated by the well-established phenomenon that weight gain tapers as humans age. Peak weights for men are at around 55 years, with weight loss after that age (slowly because rapid weight loss has significant risks in the older adult) (Sperrin et al., 2013). Peak weights for women are at around 65 years with decreases after that age. Rapid weight loss can identify critical problems; one of the first signs of dementia is often unintended weight loss. Additional changes in nutrient needs occur mainly because of the physiologic changes of aging (Table 37-9). The Tufts University USDA Human

Table 37-9   Different Nutrient Needs in Aging

Decreased Need	Calories Vitamin A
Increased Need	Fluid needs Protein (slightly increased) Vitamin D Calcium Vitamin B₁₂ Vitamin B₆ (pyridoxine)

Nutrition Center on Aging has developed a food pyramid based on the different nutrient needs that are critical to older adults (Russell et al., 1999). A part of aging is muscle loss, and fat stores increase. Current research supports the need for adequate (not excessive) calorie intake for protein sparing, as well as adequate protein intake (0.9-1.0 g/kg body weight) and muscle-retaining exercise to retain or lessen loss of muscle mass with aging. Diet with protein alone, or exercise alone, does not seem to retain muscle as well as the combination of exercise and protein intake.

Because psychosocial components are so important in determining nutritional status in older adults, reliable nutrition assessment includes consideration of these elements for evaluation (Figure 37-2). Functional status and mental status influence nutrition and well-being. Undernutrition in older individuals is defined by the type of body tissue loss. *Wasting* is an unintentional weight loss caused by insufficient intake of calories. *Cachexia* is loss of fat-free body mass (from muscle, bone, organs) caused by catabolism (e.g., in cancer or heart failure) and results in a change of body composition accompanied by an ongoing inflammatory process. *Sarcopenia* is the loss of skeletal muscle mass and is a common condition in aging adults. The causes of sarcopenia are multifactorial, including a decline in physical activity, changes in anabolic hormone levels, and chronic inflammation (Hoffer, 2012).

Dietary Patterns in Prevention and Management of Major Diseases

Key Points

- The Mediterranean diet has been shown to be more effective than a low-fat diet in primary prevention of cardiovascular events in patients at high risk (SOR: A).
- Consuming a Mediterranean diet is associated with a decrease in all-cause mortality as well as a reduced risk for cardiovascular disease, neurodegenerative disease, and cancer (SOR: B).
- The DASH (Dietary Approaches to Stopping Hypertension) diet significantly reduces systolic (>11 mm Hg) and diastolic (>5 mm Hg) blood pressure (BP) in persons with stage I hypertension (Appel et al., 1997; Svetkey et al., 1999) (SOR: A).
- Patients following the DASH diet may have a lower risk of developing stroke and myocardial infarction and may have a lower risk of cardiovascular mortality (SOR: B).
- A low-carbohydrate diet (high protein and fat) is as effective as low-fat diets in weight loss and may be associated with a better lipid profile.

NESTLÉ NUTRITION SERVICES

Mini Nutritional Assessment
MNA®

Updated Version

| Last name: | First name: | Sex: | Date: |

| Age: | Weight, kg: | Height, cm: | I.D. Number: |

Complete the screen by filling in the boxes with the appropriate numbers.
Add the numbers for the screen. If score is 11 or less, continue with the assessment to gain a Malnutrition Indicator Score.

Screening

A Has food intake declined over the past 3 months
due to loss of appetite, digestive problems,
chewing or swallowing difficulties?
0 = severe loss of appetite
1 = moderate loss of appetite
2 = no loss of appetite ☐

B Weight loss during last months
0 = weight loss greater than 3 kg (6.6 lbs)
1 = does not know
2 = weight loss between 1 and 3 kg (2.2 and 6.6 lbs)
3 = no weight loss ☐

C Mobility
0 = bed or chair bound
1 = able to get out of bed/chair but does not go out
2 = goes out ☐

D Has suffered psychological stress or acute
disease in the past 3 months
0 = yes   2 = no ☐

E Neuropsychological problems
0 = severe dementia or depression
1 = mild dementia
2 = no psychological problems ☐

F Body Mass Index (BMI) (weight in kg)/(height in m)^2
0 = BMI less than 19
1 = BMI 19 to less than 21
2 = BMI 21 to less than 23
3 = BMI 23 or greater ☐

Screening score (subtotal max. 14 points) ☐ ☐

12 points or greater   Normal – not at risk –
no need to complete assessment

11 points or below   Possible malnutrition –
continue assessment

Assessment

G Lives independently (not in a nursing home or hospital)
0 = no   1 = yes ☐

H Takes more than 3 prescription drugs per day
0 = yes   1 = no ☐

I Pressure sores or skin ulcers
0 = yes   1 = no ☐

J How many full meals does the patient eat daily?
0 = 1 meal
1 = 2 meals
2 = 3 meals ☐

K Selected consumption markers for protein intake
• At least one serving of dairy products
(milk, cheese, yogurt) per day?   yes ☐   no ☐
• Two or more serving of legumes
or eggs per week?   yes ☐   no ☐
• Meat, fish or poultry every day   yes ☐   no ☐
0.0 = if 0 or 1 yes
0.5 = if 2 yes
1.0 = if 3 yes ☐.☐

L Consumes two or more servings
of fruits or vegetables per day?
0 = no   1 = yes ☐

M How much fluid (water, juice, coffee, tea, milk…)
is consumed per day?
0.0 = less than 3 cups
0.5 = 3 to 5 cups
1.0 = more than 5 cups ☐.☐

N Mode of feeding
0 = unable to eat without assistance
1 = self-fed with some difficulty
2 = self-fed without any problem ☐

O Self view of nutritional status
0 = view self as being malnourished
1 = is uncertain of nutritional state
2 = views self as having no nutritional problem ☐

P In comparison with other people of the same age,
how do they consider their health status?
0.0 = not as good
0.5 = does not know
1.0 = as good
2.0 = better ☐.☐

Q Mid-arm circumference (MAC) in cm
0.0 = MAC less than 21
0.5 = MAC 21 to 22
1.0 = MAC 22 or greater ☐.☐

R Calf circumference (CC) in cm
0 = CC less than 31   1 = CC 31 or greater ☐

Assessment (max. 16 points) ☐ ☐.☐

Screening score ☐ ☐

Total Assessment (max. 30 points) ☐ ☐.☐

Malnutrition Indicator Score

17 to 23.5 points   at risk of malnutrition ☐

Less than 17 points   malnourished ☐

06.98 USA

® Société des Produits Nestlé S.A., Vevey, Switzerland, Trademark Owners

Figure 37-2 The mini nutritional assessment (MNA). (From Vellas B, Garry PJ, Guigoz V, eds. *Mini nutritional assessment [MNA]: research and practice in the elderly.* vol 1. Nestlé Nutrition Workshop Series. Basel, Switzerland: Karger; 1999:158.)

- Diet as a whole should be considered in the balanced food intake (with energy expenditure and basal metabolic rate) for determining needs of patients with diabetes. Diet should be individualized to the patient's unique needs (American Diabetes Association [ADA], 2008) (SOR: A).
- Lifestyle changes (increased activity, weight loss, smoking cessation, decreased saturated fat and increased fiber intake, moderation in alcohol intake) are the only treatments shown to affect all components of the metabolic syndrome and should be implemented in all patients (Finnish Medical Society, 2007) (SOR: A).

MEDITERRANEAN DIET

The Mediterranean diet is used extensively as a regional diet in southern Europe, northern African, and the Middle Eastern countries. Although it has many cultural variations, such as the types of seasonings, use of different starches (rice to pasta to couscous), and use or non-use of alcohol, most of the research and popular use of the term Mediterranean diet relates to the diet commonly found in southern Italy, Sicily, and Corsica during the late 1950s to 1960s. It is not currently what is practiced in these regions to the extent it was during the research of Ancel Keyes, who first described its effects on prevention of many of the chronic diseases common to Western countries. Currently, research has shown positive effects on the prevention and to a lesser extent treatment of diseases such as cardiovascular, diabetes, Parkinson disease, dementia, and cancer.

The foods commonly used in the Mediterranean diet are as follows:

- Eating primarily plant-based foods, such as fruits and vegetables, whole grains, legumes, and nuts as the basis of the diet
- Replacing butter with healthy fats, such as olive oil
- Eating fish and poultry at least twice a week
- Drinking red wine in moderation (optional)
- Including regular exercise and physical activity
- Limiting red meat and sweets to no more than a few times a month

Several Mediterranean Diet Pyramid schematics may be helpful in directing patients toward this type of eating pattern. In most representations of the Mediterranean diet, exercise is considered an important component to the diet to maintain energy balance. This is critical to the health outcomes with the diet (see Web Resources).

The Mediterranean diet has been shown to reduce cardiovascular events compared with a traditional low-fat diet in patients at high risk for disease (Estruch et al., 2013). Several observational studies have strongly suggested a decrease in all-cause mortality and in morbidity. These studies include evidence of reduction in cardiovascular disease, neurodegenerative disease, and cancer (Sofi et al., 2010). Another study has shown that when patients with cardiovascular risk factors and at risk for developing type 2 diabetes followed the Mediterranean diet, the risk of developing type 2 diabetes actually decreased (Salas-Salvado et al., 2011). In fact, the Mediterranean diet can be very effective in helping patients with diabetes maintain appropriate blood glucose control. Specific studies have demonstrated that following a Mediterranean diet may decrease the risk for developing cancer (Cottet et al., 2005; Couto et al., 2011). There is also evidence that patients who adhere to the Mediterranean diet have a decreased risk of developing dementia, especially when the diet is combined with physical activity (Scarmeas et al., 2009). The risks of following a Mediterranean diet are few and include deficiencies in calories (because of the filling nature of high-fiber foods).

Dietary Approaches to Stopping Hypertension Diet

A combination diet known as DASH is low in saturated fat, high in fruits and vegetables (8-10 servings, or 4-5 cups/day), and high in low-fat dairy products, with physical activity and some salt restriction. DASH resulted in significant reductions in systolic (>11 mm Hg) and diastolic (>5 mm Hg) BP in persons with stage I hypertension (Appel et al., 1997; Svetkey et al., 1999). With the addition of sodium restriction (<2 g daily), further BP reductions have been observed (He and MacGregor, 2004; National Institutes of Health [NIH], 2006). A recent meta-analysis confirmed the finding that low-sodium diets result in lowered BP but also found that sodium-restricted diets were associated with an increase in plasma levels of renin, aldosterone, cholesterol, and triglycerides compared with a non–sodium-restricted diet (Graudal et al., 2011). The DASH diet, or a similar combination, with modest sodium restriction should be considered as first-line treatment for prehypertension and early stage I hypertension. There is some evidence that patients following the DASH diet have lower risk of stroke, cardiovascular mortality, and myocardial infarction (Fung et al., 2008).

The foods commonly used in the DASH diet are as follows (serving range is because of different calorie consumption—lower number of servings for lower caloric intake and higher number for higher caloric consumption):

- Whole grains: 6 to 11 servings per day (1 serving = 1 slice bread; 1 oz dry cereal; $\frac{1}{2}$ cup cooked rice, pasta or cereal)
- Vegetables: 3 to 6 servings/day (1 serving = $\frac{1}{2}$ cup cut up raw or cooked; 1 cup leafy green)
- Fruits: 4 to 6 servings/day (1 serving = 1 medium piece; $\frac{1}{2}$ cup juice or cut up)
- Low-fat dairy: 2 to 3 servings/day (1 serving = 1 cup yogurt, milk; $1\frac{1}{2}$ oz cheeses)
- Lean meats: 3 to 6 servings (1 serving = 1 oz meat or 1 egg for a total of 3 to 6 oz/day)
- Nuts and legumes: 1 serving per day to 3 servings per week (1 serving = 1/3 cup nuts; 2 Tbsp peanut butter; $\frac{1}{2}$ cup legumes)
- Fats and oils: 2 to 3 servings per day (1 serving = 1 tsp oils or soft margarine; 2 Tbsp salad dressings)
- Sweets: 0 to no more than 2 per day (1 serving = 1 Tbsp sugar or jam or jelly; $\frac{1}{2}$ cup gelatin or sorbet; 1 cup lemonade)

There are many similarities between the Mediterranean and DASH diets, such as the high use of whole grains, vegetables, fruits, nuts, and legumes and the limited use of red meats and sweets. The DASH plan does include the consumption of more dairy products than does the Mediterranean diet. The DASH diet does not explicitly include fish or olive oil as the Mediterranean plan does. Whether these are significant differences is yet to be determined.

Low-Carbohydrate Diets (Higher in Fat and Protein)

The low-carbohydrate diet plan—for example, the Atkins Diet (and variations) or the South Beach Diet—has few similarities to either the DASH diet or the Mediterranean diet. It prescribes much more protein than either of the previously discussed dietary patterns. The South Beach Plan is not as high in saturated fat because the protein source is mainly fish. Research actually shows that low-carbohydrate diets may have a more favorable effect on serum lipids than do low-fat diets (Foster et al., 2010; Shai et al., 2008). Some evidence indicates that recommending an increase in some types of dietary fat, such as olive oil and fish oil, may be helpful in managing diabetes (Shai et al., 2008). There are a few hypotheses as to why low-carbohydrate diets confer less cardiovascular risk than low-fat diets. One idea is that low-fat diets are high-carbohydrate diets, which often means that individuals substitute refined carbohydrates for fat. This type of carbohydrate consumption contributes to the risk of type 2 diabetes and hence cardiovascular disease. A second hypothesis is that energy balance is more important than the specific macronutrient in the diet (Schwingshackl & Hoffman, 2013). This means that whether the diet is high in fat, protein, or carbohydrate, the important issue is that the patient maintains energy balance by not consuming more calories than are expended each day. Energy balance is more important to chronic disease prevention than is consumption of a high- or low-macronutrient content diet (Sacks et al., 2009).

Risks of the low carbohydrate diets include potential deficiencies in the B vitamins, vitamin C, and possibly fat-soluble vitamins D and K, depending on the sources of fat and protein in the diet.

Vegetarian Diets

For a variety of reasons, many people follow a vegetarian dietary pattern. These dietary patterns may or may not include animal products such as milk (lactovegetarians), cheese, or eggs (lacto-ovo vegetarians). Strict vegans consume no animal products at all. Children and adolescents are at a particular risk for micronutrient deficiencies when adhering to vegetarian dietary practices. For example, adolescents may consume too little zinc, iron, and vitamin C and are also at risk for having low vitamin B_{12} levels. Individuals who completely exclude animal and fish food sources from their diets may be at risk for deficiencies of essential fatty acids and vitamin D, although there are some mushroom sources as well as sunlight for vitamin D. Family physicians should ask about specifics of dietary intake in patients who claim to be vegetarian to ensure that adequate levels of calcium, micronutrients, and an adequate mix of plant proteins are being consumed. Additionally, adolescents and young adults who follow a restrictive vegetarian diet may have a higher prevalence of unhealthy dieting behaviors and disordered eating (American Dietetic Association, 2009).

When properly incorporated, vegetarian diets have been shown to be effective in lowering total cholesterol and low-density lipoprotein cholesterol in patients with hyperlipidemia (American Dietetic Association, 2009). Vegetarian diets can also be effective for weight loss.

Nutrition Decisions in the Hospitalized Patient

Key Points

- The Joint Commission requires a nutritional screen be completed on each patient within 24 hours of admission (SOR: C).
- If nutrition screening and assessment indicate that a patient is at risk for malnutrition or malnourishment, then nutrition support intervention is indicated (SOR: B).

Patients who are hospitalized require appropriate nutritional support to heal wounds and recover from illness. Up to 40% of hospitalized patients have some degree of malnutrition (Coates et al., 1993). Clinical studies have shown that length of stay and hospital costs are higher in patients at risk for poor nutrition than patients who are not at risk (Chima et al., 1997). The Joint Commission (formerly Joint Commission on Accreditation of Healthcare Organizations, JCAHO) requires a nutritional screen to be completed on each patient within 24 hours of admission, although evidence to support this practice is not of top quality (Mueller et al., 2011). The Malnutrition Screening Tool (MST) and the Short Nutritional Assessment Questionnaire (SNAQ) have both been shown to have specificities and sensitivities of greater than 70% (Neelemaat et al., 2011) and are considered "quick and easy" screening tools, as is the Mini Nutritional Assessment (see Figure 37-2). When a screen indicates that a patient is at nutritional risk, the patient should undergo a complete nutrition assessment. The rationale for this is that malnourished patients tend to have longer hospital stays and more complications as well as potentially higher mortality rates. Often, patients with chronic illness are nutritionally depleted before hospitalization, and trauma and surgery increase nutritional demands significantly. Patients, particularly older adults, may rapidly fall behind in caloric and nutrient intake.

SUBJECTIVE GLOBAL ASSESSMENT

A useful instrument for the more detailed assessment of nutritional status in hospitalized patients is the subjective global assessment (SGA) (Brugler et al., 2005). The SGA incorporates five features of the history and four components of the physical examination findings, enabling the physician to make a rapid determination of a patient's nutritional status (Figure 37-3). The history components are weight loss, food intake, presence of significant GI symptoms, functional status or energy level, and metabolic demand of the underlying disease state. The physical components are depletion of subcutaneous fat, muscle wasting in the quadriceps and deltoid muscles, edema, and ascites. Each component is evaluated as category A (patient well nourished), B (mildly malnourished), or C (severely malnourished).

Weight loss is one of the most important components of the assessment. Generally, if the patient loses at least 5% of

SUBJECTIVE GLOBAL ASSESSMENT SCORING SHEET

Patient name: _____   Patient ID: _____   Date: _____

Part 1: Medical history

SGA Score

	A	B	C

1. Weight change

    A. Overall change in past 6 months: _____ kgs.

    B. Percent change: _____ Gain < 5% loss
                         _____ 5–10% loss
                         _____ > 10% loss

    C. Change in past 2 weeks: _____ Increase
                             _____ No change
                             _____ Decrease

2. Dietary intake

    A. Overall change: _____ No change
                     _____ Change

    B. Duration: _____ Weeks

    C. Type of change:
        _____ Suboptimal solid diet   _____ Full liquid diet
        _____ Hypocaloric liquid   _____ Starvation

3. Gastrointestinal symptoms (persisting for >2 weeks)
    ____ None   ____ Nausea   ____ Vomiting ____ Diarrhea ____ Anorexia

4. Functional impairment (nutritionally related)

    A. Overall impairment: _____ None
                                 _____ Moderate
                                 _____ Severe

    B. Change in past 2 weeks: _____ Improved
                                 _____ No change
                                 _____ Regressed

Part 2: Physical examination

SGA Score

	Normal	Mild	Moderate	Severe
5. Evidence of: Loss of subcutaneous fat				
Muscle wasting				
Edema				
Ascites (hemo only)				

Part 3: SGA rating (check one)

    A. ☐ Well-nourished   B. ☐ Mildly-moderately malnourished   C. ☐ Severely malnourished

Figure 37-3 The subjective global assessment (SGA). (From Kalantar-Zadeh K, Kleiner M, Dunne E, et al. Total iron-binding capacity-estimated transferring correlates with nutritional subjective global assessment in hemodialysis patients. *Am J Kidney Dis.* 1998;31:263-272; and Brugler L, Stankovic AK, Schlefer M, Bernstein L. A simplified nutrition screen for hospitalized patients using readily available laboratory and patient information. *Nutrition.* 2005;21:650-658.)

body weight over 2 weeks, the ranking in that category is B; a 10% loss puts the patient in category C.

After completing the assessment, the clinician makes a global judgment about the overall status. This is not a numeric assessment but rather is based on the clinician's sense of the overall nutritional picture, mainly through evidence of weight loss, poor intake, muscle wasting, and loss of subcutaneous fat. This instrument has been validated with trained clinicians (Baker et al., 1982a, 1982b; Detsky et al., 1984) but not with untrained physicians.

Other assessment tools have been proposed and may eventually be validated (Brugler et al., 2005). Most of these take into account the same key factors: risk for malnutrition based on preexisting conditions, oral intake, need to heal wounds, and biochemical or hematologic parameters (e.g., serum albumin level and total lymphocyte count). The family physician can find most of these data readily and obtain a reasonable assessment of nutritional status. If nutrition screening and assessment suggest that a patient is at risk for malnutrition or malnourishment, then nutrition support intervention is indicated.

DETERIORATION OF NUTRITIONAL STATUS AND NEED FOR SUPPORT

Caloric Requirements

Even previously healthy patients may lose nutritional ground rapidly when they are hospitalized. Surgery and the stress of disease increase caloric requirements. The amount of these increases can be calculated using one of a number

Table 37-10   Estimated Caloric Need*

Weight Goal	Level of Activity or Severity of Illness		
	Low kcal/kg	Moderate kcal/kg	High kcal/kg
Lose weight	15	20	25
Maintain weight	20	25	30
Gain weight	25	30	35

*Examples: A 165-lb woman (height 5 ft, 2 in; BMI, 30.2) needs to lose weight but does not want to do any physical activity (low activity, lose weight); 165 lb = 75 kg, 75 × 15 = 1125 kcal estimated. A 200-lb man (height 6 ft, 4 in; BMI, 24.3) is hospitalized with sepsis and needs to maintain his weight (moderate activity, maintain weight); 200 lb = 91 kg, 91 × 25 = 2275 kcal estimated.
BMI, Body mass index.

Table 37-11   Determining Total Daily Needs

- To determine total daily calorie needs, multiply the BMR by the appropriate activity factor:
  - Sedentary (little or no exercise; mild stress): BMR × 1.2
  - Light activity (light exercise, sports 1-3 days/wk; moderate stress): BMR × 1.4
  - Moderately active (moderate exercise, sports 3-5 days/wk; severe stress): BMR × 1.6
  - Very active (hard exercise, sports 6-7 days/wk): BMR × 1.725
  - Extra active (very hard exercise, sports + physical job or cross-training): BMR × 1.9
- To determine the BMR or BEE, use the online calculator (http://www.calculator.org/bmr.html).
- Whenever possible, nutritional supplementation should be through the enteral route rather than parenteral.

BEE, Basal energy expenditure; BMR, basal metabolic rate.

of predictive equations for determining *resting metabolic rate* (RMR) in kilocalories per day (kcal/day), which is the largest component of overall calorie expenditure. One frequently used model is the *Harris-Benedict equation* (1919), as follows:

For men: $\text{RMR} = 66.47 + (13.75 \times \text{Weight [kg]}) + (5.0 \times \text{Height [cm]}) - (6.75 \times \text{Age [yr]})$

For women: $\text{RMR} = 665.09 + (9.56 \times \text{Weight [kg]}) + (1.84 \times \text{Height [cm]}) - (4.67 \times \text{Age [yr]})$

Frankenfield and colleagues (2005) compared validation studies on several equations and found that the *Mifflin–St. Jeor equation* performed best in terms of predicting RMR compared with calorimetry. Although all the equations are less accurate for obese subjects, the following Mifflin–St. Jeor equation is least affected by obesity.

For men: $\text{RMR} = (9.99 \times \text{Weight [kg]}) + (6.25 \times \text{Height [cm]}) - (4.92 \times \text{Age [yr]}) + 5$

For women: $\text{RMR} = (9.99 \times \text{Weight [kg]}) + (6.25 \times \text{Height [cm]}) - (4.92 \times \text{Age [yr]}) - 161$

In critically ill patients (on ventilators), the Penn State 2003 equation or the Penn State 2010 equation for obese patients is most appropriate (Academy of Nutrition and Dietetics, 2012). (See Web Resources for RMR/BMR and resting energy/basal energy expenditure calculators.) Many online and handheld device BMR and RMR calculators are available (Table 37-10).

These predictive equations do have weaknesses. They have not been validated in all subsets of the population, such as elderly adults and nonwhite ethnic groups. Chronic illness can affect the relationship between RMR and body size, with loss of lean body mass in chronic illness.

These equations predict the *resting* metabolic rate, and caloric requirements increase beyond this figure, based on the patient's illness and other metabolic demands. The *resting energy expenditure* (REE) is 1.2 to 1.3 multiplied by the RMR. This figure is further altered by the level of stress. An example is to multiply REE by 1.1 by the number of degrees (Celsius) above normal in a patient with fever. Other multiples are 1.2 for mild stress, 1.4 for moderate stress, and 1.6 for severe stress. It is important to remember that all these calculations only *estimate* caloric requirements

and should be considered as a starting point in nutrition repletion rather than the goal (Table 37-11).

Macronutrient Requirements

Hospitalized patients, and especially surgery and trauma patients, often develop *protein-calorie malnutrition*. It is important that patients in the hospital receive adequate calories to meet energy needs and adequate protein to maintain cellular integrity. Caloric requirement can be estimated by a formula, as noted earlier. Protein should make up 1.5 to 2 g/kg/day of that caloric requirement. Specific amino acids (e.g., glutamine, arginine) may be especially important in catabolic states (e.g., cancer, burns). These amino acids are therefore called *conditionally essential* amino acids. Carbohydrates make up about 70% of the remaining total caloric requirement and lipids about 30%.

When to Start Nutritional Supplementation

There is a general trend to delay nutritional supplementation in hospitalized patients in the belief that oral intake will improve imminently, but this may exacerbate the existing malnutrition. The decision to initiate supplemental feeding (over what the patient willingly consumes at meals) must be individualized according to the patient's overall health and likely clinical outcome.

Calorie counts can be obtained for patients receiving oral nutrition. If the patient is falling short on caloric or protein intake, oral supplements are appropriate, given one to three times daily. The commercially available, canned oral supplements provide about 250 kcal and 9 g of protein per can.

For a variety of reasons, hospitalized patients are often unable to consume the calories and protein required to maintain nutrition. At some point, a patient may require enteral or parenteral nutrition. The American Society for Enteral and Parenteral Nutrition has published evidence-based guidelines for assessment and management of supplemental nutrition in patients with various disease states and surgical procedures (available through the National Guideline Clearinghouse, http://www.guideline.gov). Depending on the disease state, these guidelines recommend that hospitalized patients begin *specialized nutrition support* (SNS) (enteral or parenteral feeding) when it is anticipated that patients will not otherwise be able to meet their nutritional needs for 7 to 10 days and within 24 to 48 hours of admission to an intensive care unit as long as enteral nutrition is not contraindicated (Academy of Nutrition and Dietetics, 2012).

Enteral Nutrition

Most experts agree that when SNS is required, enteral feeding is the most appropriate method as long as the GI tract is competent (ADA, 2006; SOR: A). This is partly because enteral feeding can supply complex nutrients such as fiber and intact proteins that parenteral nutrition cannot supply. Also, evidence indicates that enteral feeding has beneficial effects on the GI mucosa. Some cells lining the GI tract rely on luminal nutrients to flourish, and enteral feeding maintains the absorptive capacity of the epithelial cells. Enteral feeding also stimulates the immune function of the gut. Enteral feeding is usually safer and less expensive than parenteral feeding.

Delivery Methods. Nasogastric feeding is the least invasive form of enteral feeding and is appropriate when there is no gastric outlet obstruction, delayed gastric emptying, or elevated risk for aspiration. If a patient does not tolerate gastric feeding, has one of the previous contraindications, or requires prolonged nutritional supplementation, as is often the case with head and neck cancers, a *postpyloric feeding method* such as duodenal or jejunal tube placement is appropriate. Jejunal tubes are preferred to duodenal tubes because the latter still pose a reasonably high risk for aspiration.

FORMULAS. One type of tube-feeding formula is blenderized food, which can be any type of food that can be successfully liquefied. There are also nutritionally complete commercial formulas that are sterile, easy to use, and appropriate for patients with normal digestive and absorptive function. Elemental formulas contain predigested, chemically formulated nutrients in low-molecular-weight form and may be useful in patients with stressed GI tracts that cannot digest and absorb nutrients in a more complex form. Specialized modular formulas are available for specific disease states, such as a formula appropriate for a patient with chronic kidney or lung disease.

Complications. Clinicians should be aware of the potential complications of enteral feeding, such as aspiration (especially with gastric feeding), gut perforation, and functional problems (e.g., gastric distention, nausea, vomiting, diarrhea). Current guidelines recommend that unless contraindicated, the head of the bed should be elevated 30 to 40 degrees for a patient receiving enteral nutrition (Academy of Nutrition and Dietetics, 2012). Serum electrolyte and glucose level abnormalities are common in patients receiving enteral nutrition, and monitoring of these parameters is important.

Parenteral Nutrition

Most hospitals now use multidisciplinary teams to help plan and implement parenteral nutrition when it is deemed appropriate. *Peripheral parenteral nutrition* (PPN), using a peripheral vein, is appropriate for short-term administration of nutrients (7-10 days) when the GI tract is not functional. *Total parenteral nutrition* (TPN) is administered through a more central vein and is used longer term (>10 days). TPN may be used to administer higher concentrations of glucose and protein than PPN, as well as for infusion of lipids.

Complications. The complications of PPN and TPN include phlebitis and other local reactions to infusion, maintenance of venous access, infection, air embolism, and refeeding syndrome. The *refeeding syndrome* is more common with TPN and may result in sudden death, more often affecting severely malnourished patients as they transition suddenly from deriving energy from stored fat to obtaining energy from infused glucose. This can cause a sudden depletion of phosphate stores, resulting in cardiac dysfunction. Patients who have lost more than 30% of their body weight should undergo gradual repletion of nutrients, with a slow increase in the rate of TPN over several days.

Future in Nutrition

MICROBIOME: GUT BACTERIA AND NUTRITION

Recent research on the synergistic relationship between the hundreds of bacteria that live symbiotically with each human has taken on new understandings with the NIH Human Microbiome Project (The NIH HMP Working Group, 2009). The understanding that different bacteria may have different effects on diseases, such as obesity, antibiotic resistance, and other conditions, has led to revision in how diseases are treated. In the past, we have seen such a paradigm shift with ulcers going from a disease related to stress (and bland diets) to a disease of bacterial origin, resulting in the appropriate change in focus of the treatment. The microbiome of an individual changes with age and diet, and there is ongoing research into how diet and disease influence and are influenced by the individual's microbiotic makeup.

CONSUMER TECHNOLOGY AND NUTRITION

With the wide availability of smartphones and just-in-time information, there has also been a proliferation of applications designed to help with health and fitness, including weight loss. The appropriate research to determine the effectiveness of these applications to affect sound nutrition is just beginning. A recent study has determined that of the more than 10,000 weight loss and fitness applications, none is very strong at incorporating theory-based behavior change concepts. Food tracking has been shown to be effective for people attempting to lose weight, and many tracking applications are available. However, these apps are currently weak at providing motivation (other than positive reinforcement) or helping dieters identify eating triggers (Azar et al., 2013).

In addition to consumer-based technology, there is currently a great deal of research underway to look for better ways for professionals (nurses, physicians, dieticians) to assess nutrition in vulnerable groups. The use of digital photography and electronic databases has the potential to enhance customization of diets for community-dwelling patients by more accurately documenting intake and micronutrient content.

Terminology

The following list of definitions is taken from *Dietary Reference Intakes* (National Academy of Sciences, 2004).

- *Recommended daily allowance* (RDA): Average daily nutrient intake level sufficient to meet the nutrient requirements of nearly all those (97%-98%) in a life stage and gender group. It is intended to be used for assessing the diets of healthy subjects, not for assessing or planning diets for groups.
- *Estimated energy requirement* (EER): Dietary energy intake that is predicted to allow for a level of physical activity consistent with normal health and development and for the deposition of tissues at a rate consistent with growth
- *Acceptable macronutrient distribution range* (AMDR): Range of macronutrient intakes for a particular energy source associated with reduced risk of chronic disease while providing adequate intakes of essential nutrients
- *Tolerable upper intake levels* (TULs): Highest average daily nutrient intake likely to pose no risks of adverse health effects to almost all those in a life stage and gender group
- *Adequate intake* (AI): Recommended average daily nutrient level based on observed or experimentally determined estimates of average nutrient intakes by a group of healthy subjects. It is used when an RDA cannot be determined and may be used to plan and evaluate diets of individual subjects or groups.
- *Estimated average requirement* (EAR): Nutrient intake value estimated to meet the requirement defined by a specific indicator of adequacy in 50% of those in a life stage and gender group, expressed as a daily value over time (for most nutrients, at least 1 week). It includes an adjustment for bioavailability, is intended to be used as one factor in assessing the adequacy of intake of groups or individual subjects, and should not be used as an intake goal for just one person.

Conclusion

Nutrition is a foundation for human health. In the future, as more is understood about genetics, nutritional needs will become more tailored to individual diverse needs. In the review of a person's nutritional status, the clinician should consider food and supplements, as well as how these balance with exercise, diseases, and other environmental factors (e.g., smoking). Overweight, normal-weight, and underweight people are not necessarily well nourished, and weight may not be an indicator of healthy eating. *Biologic balance* involves energy balance (between what is needed or eaten and what is used) and nutrient balance; too few nutrients can cause malnutrition and even chronic diseases, and too many nutrients may be toxic or may even cause chronic disease.

References

The complete reference list is available at www.expertconsult.com.

Web Resources

diabetes.niddk.nih.gov/dm/pubs/eating_ez/ National Institutes of Health. Information on diabetes and diet for the public.

mayoclinic.com/health/weight-loss/NU00595 Mayo Clinic Healthy Weight Pyramid Tool.

ndb.nal.usda.gov/ U.S. Department of Agriculture National Nutrient Database for Standard Reference. Lists the nutrient content of foods.

www.aafp.org/afp/20000301/1409.html American Association of Family Physicians. A "stages of change" approach for helping patients change their behavior.

www.calculator.org/bmr.html For calculating basal metabolic rate for adults.

www.cdc.gov/healthyweight/assessing/bmi/index.html Body Mass Index calculator from the Centers for Disease Control and Prevention.

www.ChooseMyPlate.gov Current food guidance.

www.diabetes.org The American Diabetes Association.

www.dietaryguidelines.gov Dietary Guidelines for Americans.

www.eatright.org The Academy of Nutrition and Dietetics (formerly the American Dietetic Association) public information site.

www.healthfinder.gov/prevention Health Topics A to Z.

www.healthyout.com/ Site for researching restaurants for particular dietary patterns and nutritional needs.

www.heart.org/HEARTORG/Getting-Healthy/NutritionCenter/ Mediterranean_Diet_UCM_306004_Article.jsp Information on the Mediterranean diet from the American Heart Association.

www.iom.edu/Global/Topics/Food-Nutrition.aspx Institute of Medicine reference on topics related to food and nutrition.

www.mayoclinic.com/health/healthy-diet/NU00190 Different healthy food pyramids from the Mayo Clinic (Asian diet, Latin American diet, Mediterranean diet, MyPlate, vegetarian diet).

http://www.nhlbi.nih.gov/health/health-topics/topics/dash/ The DASH diet.

www.nlm.nih.gov/medlineplus National Library of Medicine, National Institutes of Health (MedlinePlus). Reliable health information on nutrition, diet, and dietary supplements.

www.nutrition.gov Portal for all government websites on nutrition information. Available through the U.S. Department of Agriculture, National Agricultural Library.

www-users.med.cornell.edu/~spon/picu/calc/beecalc.htm Basal energy expenditure (Harris-Benedict equation) calculator from Weill Medical College, Cornell University.

38 *Gastroenterology*

JOEL J. HEIDELBAUGH and SCOTT KELLEY

He who does not mind his belly will hardly mind anything else.

—SAMUEL JOHNSON (1763)

Thought depends absolutely on the stomach, but in spite of that, those who have the best stomachs are not the best thinkers.

—VOLTAIRE (1770)

Epidemiology and Social Impact of Gastrointestinal Disease

Although diseases of other organ systems (e.g., cardiovascular disease) may appear to be more dramatic illnesses with higher rates of morbidity and mortality, the overall impact of gastrointestinal (GI) disorders is often underestimated from both a biopsychosocial and a resource standpoint. Typically, diseases of the GI tract are misdiagnosed, mistreated, misunderstood, or missed altogether, ultimately leading to substantial psychological morbidity and tremendous direct and indirect expense. Digestive diseases cost an estimated $91 billion annually in U.S. health care costs, lost days from work, and premature deaths. More than 70 million Americans are diagnosed each year with disorders of the digestive tract, including gastroesophageal reflux disease (GERD), peptic ulcer disease (PUD), inflammatory bowel disease (IBD), GI cancers, motility disorders, hepatitis, cirrhosis, and foodborne illness (Foundation for Digestive Health and Nutrition, 2009).

This chapter serves as an overview of common GI diseases and disorders encountered in family medicine practices, encompassing both adult and pediatric populations. The most recent evidence-based diagnostic and therapeutic guidelines and reviews are highlighted, and radiographs, endoscopy photos, and video segments are integrated when applicable.

APPROACH TO THE PATIENT WITH GASTROINTESTINAL COMPLAINTS

Psychosocial Factors of Gastrointestinal Disease

Locke's review in *Sleisenger and Fordtran's Gastrointestinal and Liver Disease* (8th edition) provides an excellent framework of the biopsychosocial approach to the patient with GI complaints. In caring for patients with both acute and chronic GI disorders, family physicians should obtain a patient-centered, nondirected history using open-ended questions that enable patients to tell the history in their words. Medical and social histories should be integrated so that symptomatic complaints are described in the context of the psychosocial events surrounding the presenting illness, including the setting of symptom onset and exacerbation. Throughout the encounter, the provider's questions should communicate a sincere willingness to address both biologic and psychologic aspects of the illness. Evaluation and treatment of GI symptoms depend on a strong physician–patient therapeutic relationship, allowing the family physician to elicit, evaluate, and communicate the role of potential psychosocial factors in the disease state. Patient reassurance, acknowledgment of patient adaptations to chronic illness, reinforcement of healthy behaviors, and the consideration of psychopharmacologic medication are paramount (Locke, 2006).

The failure to find a specific structural etiology for a patient's GI symptoms is usually the rule rather than the exception in the ambulatory care setting. Because functional GI disorders may represent an "illness without an evident disease," some providers do not regard these as legitimate, especially within the biopsychosocial model of disease. This phenomenon often leads physicians (and patients to coerce physicians) to pursue unnecessary, costly, and invasive diagnostic tests to find the etiology of a patient's symptoms rather than focusing directly on symptom management and potential psychological comorbidities. Family physicians must establish clear boundaries with their patients to prevent unnecessary workups and, when indicated, should consider a referral to a mental health professional skilled in the care of patients with functional GI conditions to assist in symptom management (Locke, 2006).

THE ABDOMINAL EXAMINATION

For descriptive purposes of location, the abdomen has been divided into four quadrants, constructed by an imaginary vertical line from the tip of the xyphoid process to the pubic symphysis and an imaginary horizontal line bridging the anterior superior iliac crests referred to as the right upper (RUQ), right lower (RLQ), left upper (LUQ), and left lower (LLQ) quadrants (Bickley, 2008). The abdomen can be further divided into the epigastric, umbilical, hypogastric or suprapubic, and right and left flank regions. Knowledge of anatomic structures that lie in each of these quadrants and regions is imperative for the clinician to form an accurate differential diagnosis in relation to a patient's presenting symptoms (Table 38-1).

Clinicians should remember that a comprehensive physical examination, not just abdominal, should be performed in patients presenting with digestive complaints. The clinician should ensure patient comfort and modesty because the abdominal examination (and pelvic, if indicated) may cause significant pain, anxiety, and embarrassment to the patient. Infants, young children, and pregnant women may require additional care during the abdominal examination. A thorough explanation of examination techniques and findings is necessary to minimize patient anxiety.

The anorectal examination is an important component of the abdominal examination that may often be omitted. Although uncomfortable and embarrassing to the patient, it should not be neglected and should be approached with a calm, gentle attitude on the part of the clinician. The examiner should comment on both external and internal components of the anorectal examination, specifically anal sphincter tone; presence or absence of hemorrhoids, fissures, fistulas, or masses; prostatic abnormality in male patients; and consistency of the stool. Anoscopy should be considered as an adjunct to the anorectal examination when indicated, allowing for direct visualization of the internal anorectal canal. In female patients, the pelvic examination may provide additional information in the diagnosis of abdominal symptoms because it is often challenging to differentiate between GI and genitourinary complaints.

Common Pediatric Gastrointestinal Disorders

INFANTILE REGURGITATION

In an infant with recurrent vomiting, a thorough history and physical examination are often sufficient to establish a diagnosis of uncomplicated GERD, labeling the infant as "the happy spitter." Diagnostic evaluation is indicated if there are signs of poor weight gain, GI obstruction, excessive crying and irritability, disturbed sleep, or feeding or respiratory problems suggesting suspected asthma or recurrent pneumonia. In an infant with uncomplicated GERD, parental education, reassurance, and anticipatory guidance are recommended; no specific intervention is

necessary because the process is usually self-limited. Thickened formula and a trial of a hypoallergenic formula are the best treatment options. A trial of time-limited acid-suppression therapy, usually with histamine-2 receptor antagonists (H_2RAs), is useful in determining if GERD is causing vomiting and regurgitation. If symptoms worsen or do not improve by 18 to 24 months of age, reevaluation for complications of GERD is recommended, including an upper GI series (barium swallow study) and consultation with a pediatric gastroenterologist. In otherwise normal children who have recurrent vomiting or regurgitation after age 2 years, management options include an upper GI series, upper endoscopy with biopsy, and anti-secretory therapy (National Digestive Diseases Information Clearinghouse, 2006).

DIARRHEA AND DEHYDRATION

Diarrhea is exceedingly common in pediatric and adult populations worldwide. Dehydration and electrolyte (e.g., sodium, potassium, bicarbonate) losses associated with severe diarrhea account for significant morbidity and may lead to mortality in cases of acute gastroenteritis, especially in countries with poor access to adequate health care. Rotavirus infection is the most common cause of diarrhea in U.S. infants and children, especially in winter months and temperate climates; Norwalk-like virus is the most common agent in adults (King et al., 2003).

A thorough history should be the first step in evaluating a patient who presents with a significant diarrheal illness, including the following (Guerrant et al., 2001):

- When and how the illness began (abrupt or gradual onset and duration of symptoms)
- Stool characteristics (watery, bloody, mucous, purulent, greasy)
- Frequency of bowel movements and relative quantity of stool produced
- Presence of dysenteric symptoms (fever, tenesmus, blood or pus in stool)
- Symptoms of volume depletion (increased thirst, tachycardia, orthostasis, decreased urine output, lethargy, decreased skin turgor, decreased tear production)
- Associated symptoms and their frequency and intensity (nausea, vomiting, abdominal pain, cramps, headache, myalgias, altered sensorium)

In addition, all patients should be asked about potential epidemiologic risk factors for diarrheal diseases, including the following:

- Travel to an underdeveloped area
- Daycare center attendance or employment
- Consumption of unsafe foods (e.g., raw meats, eggs, or shellfish; unpasteurized milk or juices) or swimming in or drinking untreated fresh surface water from a lake or stream
- Visiting a farm or petting zoo or having contact with reptiles or with pets with diarrhea
- Knowledge of other ill persons (e.g., in a dormitory, office, or social function)
- Recent or regular medications (e.g., antibiotics, antacids, antimotility agents)

Table 38-1   Differential Diagnosis for Abdominal Pain Based on Location

Left upper quadrant	*Cardiac:* angina pectoris, myocardial infarction *Dermatologic:* herpes zoster *Gastric:* peptic ulcer disease, gastritis, pyloric stenosis, hiatal hernia *Intestinal:* high fecal impaction, perforated colon, diverticulitis *Pancreatic:* pancreatitis, neoplasm, stone in pancreatic duct or ampulla *Pulmonary:* pneumonia, empyema, pulmonary infarction *Renal:* calculi, pyelonephritis, neoplasm *Splenic:* splenomegaly, rupture, abscess, splenic infarction Trauma *Vascular:* dissecting or ruptured aortic aneurysm
Right upper quadrant	*Biliary:* calculi, infection, inflammation, neoplasm *Cardiac:* myocardial ischemia or infarction (particularly involving the inferior wall), pericarditis *Dermatologic:* herpes zoster Fitz-Hugh-Curtis syndrome (perihepatitis) *Gastric:* peptic ulcer disease, pyloric stenosis, neoplasm, alcoholic gastritis, hiatal hernia *Hepatic:* hepatitis, abscess, hepatic congestion, neoplasm, trauma *Pancreatic:* pancreatitis, neoplasm, stone in pancreatic duct or ampulla *Pulmonary:* pneumonia, pulmonary infarction, right-sided pleurisy *Renal:* calculi, infection, inflammation, neoplasm, rupture of kidney *Intestinal:* retrocecal appendicitis, intestinal obstruction, high fecal impaction, diverticulitis Trauma
Left lower quadrant	*Intestinal:* diverticulitis, intestinal obstruction, perforated ulcer, inflammatory bowel disease, perforated descending colon, inguinal hernia, neoplasm, appendicitis Psoas abscess *Renal:* renal or ureteral calculi, pyelonephritis, neoplasm *Reproductive:* ectopic pregnancy, ovarian cyst, torsion of ovarian cyst, salpingitis, tuboovarian abscess, mittelschmerz, endometriosis, seminal vesiculitis Trauma *Vascular:* dissecting, ruptured, or leaking aortic aneurysm
Right lower quadrant	Cholecystitis *Intestinal:* acute appendicitis, regional enteritis, incarcerated hernia, cecal diverticulitis, intestinal obstruction, perforated ulcer, perforated cecum, Meckel diverticulitis Psoas abscess *Reproductive:* ectopic pregnancy, ovarian cyst, torsion of ovarian cyst, salpingitis, tuboovarian abscess, mittelschmerz, endometriosis, seminal vesiculitis *Renal:* renal or ureteral calculi, pyelonephritis, neoplasm Trauma *Vascular:* dissecting, ruptured, or leaking aortic aneurysm
Other regions	**EPIGASTRIC** *Biliary:* cholecystitis, cholangitis *Cardiac:* angina, myocardial infarction, pericarditis *Duodenal:* peptic ulcer disease, duodenitis *Gastric:* peptic ulcer disease, gastric outlet obstruction, gastric ulcer *Hepatitic:* hepatitis, abscess *Intestinal:* high small bowel obstruction, early appendicitis Pancreatitis *Pulmonary:* pneumonia, pleurisy, pneumothorax Subphrenic abscess *Vascular:* dissecting, ruptured, or leaking aortic aneurysm, mesenteric ischemia **PERIUMBILICAL** *Intestinal:* small bowel obstruction or gangrene, early appendicitis *Vascular:* mesenteric thrombosis, dissecting, ruptured, or leaking aortic aneurysm **SUPRAPUBIC** *Genitourinary:* cystitis, rupture of urinary bladder *Intestinal:* colonic obstruction or gangrene, diverticulitis, appendicitis *Reproductive:* ectopic pregnancy, mittelschmerz, torsion of ovarian cyst, pelvic inflammatory disease, salpingitis, endometriosis, rupture of endometrioma
Diffuse	*Genitourinary:* urinary tract infection, pelvic inflammatory disease *Intestinal:* diverticulitis, early appendicitis, gastroenteritis, inflammatory bowel disease, intestinal obstruction, irritable bowel syndrome, mesenteric adenitis, insufficiency, or infarction *Metabolic:* toxins, lead poisoning, uremia, drug overdose, diabetic ketoacidosis, heavy metal poisoning Pancreatitis Peritonitis Pneumonia (rare) Sickle cell crisis Trauma *Other:* acute intermittent porphyria, tabes dorsalis, periarteritis nodosa, Henoch-Schönlein purpura, adrenal insufficiency *Vascular:* aortic aneurysm

Table 38-2 Common Pathogens and Recommended Therapy for Acute Diarrhea

Pathogen	Therapy (Adult Doses)
Campylobacter jejuni	Azithromycin, 500 mg QD for 3 days, or ciprofloxacin,* 500 mg BID for 7 days
Clostridium difficile	Metronidazole, 500 mg TID or 250 mg QID for 10-14 days, or vancomycin, 125 mg QID for 10-14 days
Entamoeba histolytica	Metronidazole, 500-750 mg TID for 10 days, or tinidazole, 2 g QD for 3 days, followed by paromomycin, 500 mg PO TID for 7 days, or iodoquinol, 650 mg TID for 20 days
Escherichia coli 0157:H7	No treatment with antimicrobials or antimotility drugs
E. coli (toxigenic)	Azithromycin, 1 g in 1 dose, or rifaximin, 200 mg TID for 3 days, or levofloxacin,* 500 mg for 1 dose
Giardia lamblia	Tinidazole, 2 g in 1 dose, or nitazoxanide, 500 mg BID for 3 days, or metronidazole, 500-750 mg TID for 5 days
Salmonella spp. (nontyphi)[†]	Ciprofloxacin, 500 mg BID for 5-7 days, or azithromycin, 1 g for 1 day, then 500 mg QD for 6 days
Shigella spp.	Ciprofloxacin, 500 mg BID for 5-7 days, or levofloxacin, 500 mg QD for 3 days, or TMP-SMX-DS, 1 tablet BID for 3 days, or azithromycin, 500 mg for 1 dose, then 250 mg QD for 4 days
Staphylococcus aureus (food poisoning)	No treatment with antimicrobials or antimotility drugs
Vibrio cholerae	Ciprofloxacin, 1 g in 1 dose, plus aggressive fluid hydration
Vibrio parahaemolyticus	No treatment with antimicrobials or antimotility drugs
Yersinia enterocolitica	No treatment unless severe; if severe: Doxycycline, 100 mg IV BID, and tobramycin or gentamicin, 5 mg/kg/day QD, or TMP-SMX and fluoroquinolones as alternatives

*Avoid fluoroquinolones in pediatric patients and pregnant women.
[†]Antimicrobial therapy not indicated in asymptomatic patients or those with mild illness. Treatment is advised in patients younger than 1 year old or older than 50 years old, if immunocompromised, or if patient has a vascular graft or prosthetic joints.
BID, Twice daily; DS, double strength; IV, intravenous; PO, oral; QD, once daily; QID, four times daily; TID, three times daily; TMP-SMX, trimethoprim–sulfamethoxazole.
Modified from Gilbert DN, Moellering RC, Eliopoulos GM, et al. The Sanford guide to antimicrobial therapy. 39th ed. Sperryville, VA: Antimicrobial Therapy, 2009.

- Underlying medical conditions predisposing to infectious diarrhea (AIDS, immunosuppressive medications, prior gastrectomy, extremes of age)
- Receptive anal intercourse or oral-anal sexual contact
- Occupation as a food handler or caregiver

In the majority of patients with acute gastroenteritis, the "gold standard" stool cultures and ova and parasite testing are seldom required because the disease is most often viral in etiology and self-limited. In more severe cases with dehydration, metabolic derangement, longer duration, bloody stools (dysentery) and mucus in the stool, or known or suspected transmission of a pathogen, these tests are often required to identify the pathogen and to direct appropriate antimicrobial therapy (Table 38-2). Viral cultures are rarely performed and are unnecessary except in rare cases and immunocompromised patients. Although fecal leukocytes and lactoferrin often suggest an inflammatory etiology of diarrhea, there is no consensus regarding the routine use of these tests in the initial testing of patients with either community-acquired or nosocomial diarrhea. Hospitalized patients with diarrhea, especially those with abdominal pain, should be tested for Clostridium difficile toxin (Surawicz et al., 2013). Therapy with metronidazole remains the choice for mild to moderate disease but may not be adequate for patients with severe or complicated disease. Oral vancomycin is significantly more expensive and may select for colonization with vancomycin-resistant enterococci but may be required when a patient has had multiple bouts of C. difficile–associated diarrhea treated with metronidazole.

Nonpathogenic causes of diarrhea should be considered when a viral etiology is unlikely and a diagnostic evaluation has not identified a pathogen. The differential diagnosis includes irritable bowel syndrome (IBS), inflammatory or ischemic bowel disease, laxative abuse, partial bowel obstruction, rectosigmoid abscess, Whipple disease, pernicious anemia, diabetes mellitus, malabsorption syndromes (e.g., celiac disease), small bowel diverticulosis, and scleroderma in primarily adult patients, and an appropriate workup should be considered.

KEY TREATMENT

- Oral metronidazole is the first-line therapy for treatment of C. difficile–associated diarrhea; oral vancomycin is reserved for resistant cases (Surawicz et al., 2013) (SOR: A).
- In cases of traveler's diarrhea, (e.g., enterotoxigenic Escherichia coli, Shigella spp., Salmonella spp., or Campylobacter spp.), prompt treatment with a fluoroquinolone or, in children, trimethoprim–sulfamethoxazole (TMP-SMX) has been shown to reduce the duration of the illness from 3 to 5 days to less than 1 to 2 days (Guerrant et al., 2001) (SOR: A).

APPENDICITIS

A diagnosis of appendicitis should be considered in any pediatric patient presenting with acute abdominal pain. Acute appendicitis often presents with a constellation of signs and symptoms, including fever, anorexia, nausea, vomiting, tenesmus, migratory RLQ abdominal pain, abdominal tenderness and guarding, and signs of peritoneal irritation. Classically, hours after onset, the pain migrates to the McBurney point, defined as the point two thirds the distance from the umbilicus along a straight line toward the anterosuperior iliac spine of the pelvis. The

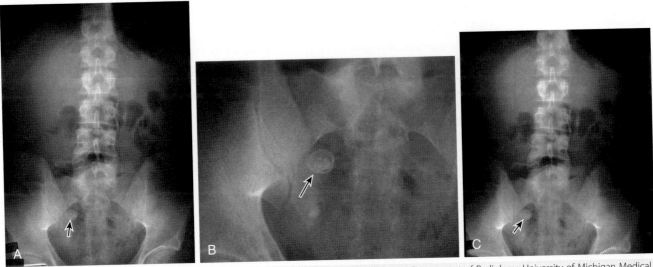

Figure 38-1 Appendicolith (**A** to **C**). (Courtesy Dr. Perry Pernicano, Clinical Assistant Professor, Department of Radiology, University of Michigan Medical School, Ann Arbor, MI.)

Rovsing sign (referred tenderness from LLQ to RLQ during palpation), *psoas sign* (pain elicited by extending hip posteriorly with patient lying prone), and *obturator sign* (pain elicited by abducting right hip with patient lying supine) are often conducted but are of little diagnostic value. No sign or combination of signs has accurately predicted acute appendicitis in children (Cincinnati Children's Hospital Medical Center, 2002).

Although none has proved adequately predictive of acute appendicitis in the pediatric population, laboratory studies are typically performed in the emergency department because other diagnoses may need to be excluded. A series of studies discovered an elevated white blood cell (WBC) count in 87% to 92% of patients with acute appendicitis, although 8% to 13% of patients with appendicitis had normal WBC counts (Cincinnati Children's Hospital Medical Center, 2002). The abdominal examination is particularly unreliable in women of reproductive age, so pelvic examination, urinalysis, and urine pregnancy test represent a reasonable clinical strategy to exclude genitourinary pathology.

Diagnostic imaging is not routinely recommended in patients with a high or a low probability of appendicitis because it can alter management strategies and has not proved cost effective; imaging is most helpful when the clinical assessment is equivocal. Controversy exists over the superiority of ultrasonography versus computed tomography (CT) in accurately diagnosing appendicitis, and both tests have a positive predictive value approaching 100%. Although ultrasonography may be advantageous in thin patients, CT is preferred in the evaluation of a more obese child (Halter et al., 2004). Typical radiographic findings in the evaluation of acute appendicitis include appendicoliths (Figure 38-1), dilation of the appendix with adjacent hazy fat (Figure 38-2), and periappendiceal abscesses (Figure 38-3). If the abdominal CT does not show evidence of acute appendicitis, the patient may either be admitted for observation or discharged at the discretion of the examiner and parents, with instructions for follow-up if symptoms worsen. Expert opinion states that if there is high suspicion

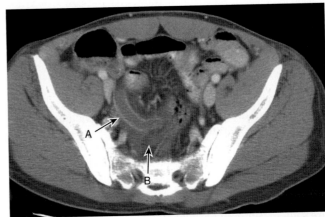

Figure 38-2 Appendicitis. Dilated thickened appendix (**A**), with adjacent hazy fat (**B**). (Courtesy Dr. Perry Pernicano.)

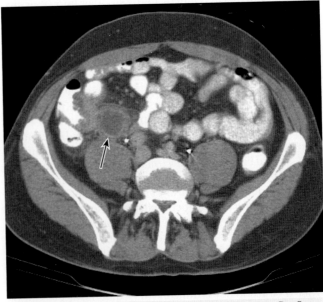

Figure 38-3 Periappendiceal abscess *(arrow)*. (Courtesy Dr. Perry Pernicano.)

of appendicitis on the basis of history, physical examination, and laboratory studies, the patient should go directly to the operating room for an exploratory laparotomy to evaluate the appendix, without an imaging study.

Common Adult Gastrointestinal Disorders

ESOPHAGUS

Barrett Esophagus and Esophageal Adenocarcinoma

Barrett esophagus (BE) is a premalignant condition related to chronic GERD. The hallmark is a change in the mucosal lining of the distal esophagus from the normal squamous epithelium to columnar-appearing mucosa resembling that of the stomach and small intestines, referred to as *intestinal metaplasia* (Figure 38-4). The estimated risk of progression to adenocarcinoma of the esophagus with BE is approximately 0.5% per year, but without BE, the risk is 0.07%, prompting development of clinical practice guidelines for surveillance endoscopy. The risk of development of BE increases linearly with age; if a patient has GERD symptoms for fewer than 20 years with an age of onset of symptoms between 30 and 49 years of age, the odds ratio for development of BE is 6.93 (Thrift et al., 2013).

Adenocarcinoma of the esophagus has had the fastest rising incidence of any cancer in the United States and Western Europe over the past 2 decades. Family and other primary care physicians who see the vast majority of patients with GERD in its nonerosive and more complicated forms are charged with the task of suspecting and appropriately referring patients with BE for esophagogastroduodenoscopy (EGD). Although risk factors for BE and adenocarcinoma are not evidence based, there is suggestive evidence that male gender, white race, older age, dysplasia,

smoking, and obesity place patients at a higher risk (Wang and Sampliner, 2008). Current evidence-based guidelines exist for the assessment and surveillance of patients with BE, yet routine screening will not be cost effective unless criteria can be identified to select patients at high risk. Recommendations from the American College of Gastroenterology (ACG) state that screening EGD for BE should be considered in select patients with chronic, longstanding GERD. After a negative screening examination result, further screening endoscopy is not indicated. For patients with established BE of any length and with no dysplasia, after two consecutive examinations within 1 year, an acceptable interval for additional surveillance is every 3 years. Surveillance in patients with low-grade dysplasia is recommended, although the optimal interval and biopsy protocol have not been established. A follow-up EGD at 6 months should be performed, and if low-grade dysplasia is confirmed, surveillance at 12 months and yearly thereafter as long as dysplasia persists is advised (Wang and Sampliner, 2008).

STOMACH AND DUODENUM

Dyspepsia

Dyspepsia ("bad digestion") accounts for approximately 5% of all visits to family practitioners and is the most common reason for referral to a gastroenterologist in the United States, accounting for 20% to 40% of consultations (Jones and Lacy, 2004). The term *dyspepsia* refers to episodic or recurrent pain or discomfort arising from the proximal GI tract related to meals and is associated with heartburn, reflux, regurgitation, indigestion, bloating, early satiety, and weight loss. The lack of a standardized definition affects accurate prevalence data, given the challenge of clearly defining dyspepsia as either *functional* or *nonulcer dyspepsia* (NUD) (~60% of cases) or that caused by structural or biochemical disease (40%) (Dickerson and King, 2004). Regardless of cause, dyspepsia has a profoundly negative impact on patients' health-related quality of life (HRQOL) and results in significant economic burden.

Nonulcer dyspepsia is defined in patients who have undergone either formal radiographic or endoscopic evaluation and who do not have an organic lesion (e.g., ulcer, tumor) to explain their symptoms. Potential etiologies for NUD include gastric acid hypersecretion, gastroduodenal dysmotility, visceral hypersensitivity, emotional stress, and psychological factors. As with other functional GI disorders, the potential for underlying psychosocial and lifestyle factors must be addressed. There is no current recommendation on the role of prokinetics, cytoprotectives, or antidepressants in the management of functional dyspepsia; similarly, no clear evidence supports specific diet and lifestyle modifications or psychosocial interventions.

Peptic Ulcer Disease

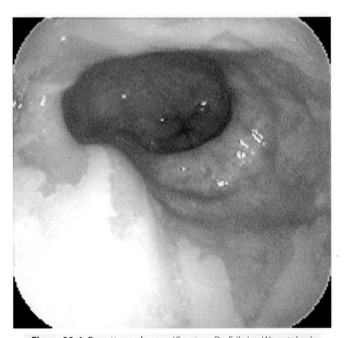

Figure 38-4 Barrett esophagus. (Courtesy Dr. Erik-Jan Wamsteker.)

> ### Key Points
>
> ■ A noninvasive *Helicobacter pylori* "test and treat" strategy is as effective as endoscopy in the initial management of patients younger than age 45 with uncomplicated dyspepsia.

- Eradication of *H. pylori* infection in patients with a duodenal or gastric ulcer reduces symptom recurrence.
- Ulcer prophylaxis with an H₂RA or proton pump inhibitor (PPI) should be considered in patients at high risk for nonsteroidal antiinflammatory drug (NSAID)–associated PUD, including those with a history of PUD, elderly patients, and patients taking corticosteroids or anticoagulants.

Peptic ulcer disease is the most common cause of *upper gastrointestinal bleeding* (UGIB) and a leading cause of dyspepsia (Table 38-3), with a cumulative lifetime prevalence of 8% to 14% (Figure 38-5). Although up to 70% of patients with gastric and duodenal ulcers are 25 to 64 years old, the peak prevalence of complicated ulcer disease requiring hospitalization is age 65 to 74 years (Saad and Scheiman, 2004).

Numerous options exist for the management of uninvestigated dyspepsia in primary care (Figure 38-6). Given the high cost and often limited access to endoscopy testing, not all patients with uninvestigated dyspepsia should undergo an invasive investigation of their symptoms. The presence of "alarm symptoms" for PUD raises concern for a gastric malignancy. The American Gastroenterological Association (AGA, 2005) endorses prompt endoscopic evaluation in any patient older than age 45 years with new-onset dyspepsia.

The most common complications of PUD include UGIB, perforation, penetration, and gastric outlet obstruction. An upper GI hemorrhage can occur in up to 15% of patients with PUD and is most common in patients older than 60 years, with mortality rate as high as 10%. Perforation occurs in approximately 7% of patients with PUD, again classically in elderly patients receiving long-term NSAIDs. Perforation can be confirmed on plain abdominal radiography; barium contrast studies and upper endoscopy are contraindicated with suspected perforation, and urgent surgical consultation is mandatory. The mortality rate may be as high as 30% to 50% in patients with perforation, particularly in elderly and debilitated patients. Penetration occurs when the ulcer crater erodes through and into adjacent organs, including the small bowel, pancreas, liver, and biliary tree. Often subtle, it typically presents as acute pancreatitis. Gastric outlet obstruction occurs in 1% to 3% of PUD patients, resulting from acute inflammation or mechanical obstruction caused by scarring at the gastroduodenal junction (Saad and Scheiman, 2004).

Approaches to confirm a diagnosis of PUD include double-contrast barium esophagography (upper GI series) and upper endoscopy. Although the upper GI series has accuracy of 80% to 90%, upper endoscopy is the preferred diagnostic modality, with multiple studies showing consistent diagnostic superiority in identifying gastric and duodenal ulcers. Despite a higher procedural cost and a slightly increased risk in procedure-related complications (bleeding, perforation, oversedation), upper endoscopy should be the initial diagnostic study performed in suspected PUD. Most important, upper endoscopy provides the distinct advantage of permitting biopsies and brushings to identify underlying pathology.

Fecal–oral infection with the bacterium *H. pylori* is a major risk factor for the development of PUD. Its prevalence and association with PUD is higher in populations who have a lower standard of living than in the United States, especially in Africa and Central America, although this may be declining. Approximately 90% of patients worldwide with duodenal ulcers are infected with the *H. pylori* pathogen, but 30% to 40% of U.S. ulcer patients are infected (Chey and Wong, 2007). The strongest evidence to support the role of *H. pylori* as an etiology of PUD is the elimination of ulcer recurrence when the infection has been successfully eradicated.

The evidence-based standard of care dictates that patients with dyspepsia and no alarm symptoms should be tested for *H. pylori* infection and then given eradication therapy if the

Table 38-3	Causes of Dyspepsia
Common*	GERD (with and without esophagitis)
	Functional (nonulcer dyspepsia)
	Peptic ulcer disease
Less common†	Alcohol consumption
	Biliary colic
	Celiac sprue
	GI malignancy
	Gastroparesis
	Infection (viral, bacterial, spirochetal, parasitic)
	Inflammatory and infiltrative processes (esophagus, stomach, small bowel)
	Intestinal ischemia
	Lactose intolerance
	Medications (primarily aspirin and NSAIDs)
	Pancreatitis
	Pregnancy
	Other systemic and metabolic disorders

*In order of relative frequency.
†Alphabetical order.
GERD, Gastroesophageal reflux disease; *GI,* gastrointestinal; *NSAID,* nonsteroidal ant-inflammatory drug.
Modified from Saad R, Scheiman JM. Diagnosis and management of peptic ulcer disease. *Clin Fam Pract* 2004;6:569-587.

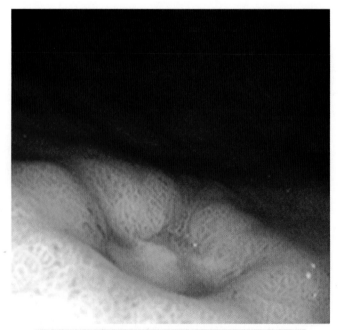

Figure 38-5 Gastric ulcer. (Courtesy Dr. Erik-Jan Wamsteker.)

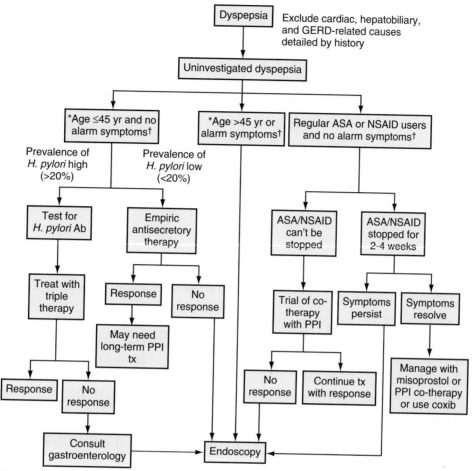

Figure 38-6 Evaluation of uninvestigated dyspepsia. *Age cutoff is controversial. Risk of pathology increases slightly with age but older age (50-55 years) cutoff is used in many guidelines. †Alarm symptoms include rectal bleeding or melena, weight loss, anorexia, early satiety, persistent vomiting, and anemia. The presence of an abdominal mass, lymphadenopathy, dysphagia, odynophagia, family history of upper gastrointestinal cancer, personal history of peptic ulcer, prior gastric surgery, or malignancy should eliminate consideration of noninvasive approaches. *ASA*, Acetylsalicylic acid; *GERD*, gastroesophageal reflux disease; *NSAID*, nonsteroidal antiinflammatory drug; *PPI*, proton pump inhibitor; *tx*, treatment. (Modified from Saad R, Scheiman JM. Diagnosis and management of peptic ulcer disease. *Clin Fam Pract* 2004;6:569-587.)

result is positive ("test and treat") (Chey and Wong, 2007). *H. pylori*–positive or *H. pylori*–negative patients who do not undergo endoscopy initially should do so if their symptoms persist. The effectiveness of this approach depends on the prevalence of *H. pylori* infection in patients with ulcers in the community; as in some geographic areas, the prevalence may be too low to make this approach effective.

Nonendoscopic testing for *H. pylori* includes a quantitative assay for serum immunoglobulin G (IgG) antibodies, the radiolabeled urea breath test, and the stool antigen test. The median sensitivity and specificity for serologic IgG tests are 92% and 83%, respectively (Scottish Intercollegiate Guidelines Network, 2003). Some patients may have persistently positive IgG antibodies for months to years after eradication therapy, yielding a false-positive result during that period if retested. In comparative studies, urea breath tests are more accurate than serologic tests. The stool antigen test is recommended as the preferred initial noninvasive diagnostic test. The urea breath test is the recommended standard to determine if *H. pylori* has been successfully eradicated (Chey and Wong, 2007).

Several medication regimens have been developed for the treatment of confirmed *H. pylori* infection based on

data from randomized controlled trials (RCTs), meta-analyses, and systematic reviews (Table 38-4). The best evidence-based recommendation for *H. pylori* eradication is for 14-day triple therapy with the use of a PPI, clarithromycin, and either amoxicillin or metronidazole, yielding eradication rates from 70% to 85%. The most common salvage regimen in patients with persistent *H. pylori* is bismuth quadruple therapy. Recent data suggest that 10-day therapy with a PPI, levofloxacin, and amoxicillin is more effective and better tolerated than bismuth quadruple therapy for persistent *H. pylori* infection (Chey and Wong, 2007).

Another major etiology of PUD is the increasing and widespread use of both NSAIDs and aspirin. The use and overuse of these medications is the most common cause of PUD in *H. pylori*–negative patients, and up to 60% of unexplained cases of PUD are attributed to unrecognized NSAID use. In a meta-analysis of observational studies of GI bleeding risk from various NSAIDs, a fourfold increased risk associated with NSAID-use persisted throughout therapy and fell to baseline within 2 months of discontinuation of the drug (Hernandez-Diaz and Rodriguez, 2000). Although both *H. pylori* and aspirin and NSAIDs are involved in the

Table 38-4   First-Line Regimens for *Helicobacter pylori* Eradication

Regimen	Duration (days)	Eradication Rates (%)	Comments
Standard-dose PPI BID (esomeprazole, QD); clarithromycin, 500 mg, *or* amoxicillin, 1000 mg	10-14	70-85	Consider in non–penicillin-allergic patients who have not previously received a macrolide
Standard-dose PPI BID; clarithromycin, 500 mg, *or* metronidazole, 500 mg	10-14	70-85	Consider in penicillin-allergic patients who have not previously received a macrolide or are unable to tolerate bismuth quadruple therapy
Bismuth subsalicylate, 525 mg QID; metronidazole, 250 mg QID; tetracycline, 500 mg QID; ranitidine, 150 mg BID; *or* standard-dose PPI QD-BID	10-14	75-90	Consider in penicillin-allergic patients
PPI + amoxicillin, 1 g BID, followed by: PPI + clarithromycin, 500 mg; tinidazole, 500 mg BID	5 5	>90	Requires validation in North America

BID, Twice daily; *PPI,* proton pump inhibitor; *QD,* once daily; *QID,* four times daily.
Modified from Chey WD, Wong BC. American College of Gastroenterology guideline on the management of *Helicobacter pylori* infection. *Am J Gastroenterol* 2007;102:1808-1825.

Table 38-5   Etiology of Peptic Ulcer Disease

Major causes	*Helicobacter pylori* infection NSAIDs Aspirin
Minor causes	Duodenal obstruction from annular pancreas Use of topically injurious drugs (potassium chloride, nitrogen-containing bisphosphonates) Immunosuppressants (e.g., mycophenolate) *Helicobacter heilmannii* infection Mucosal infection (herpes simplex 1, CMV, tuberculosis, syphilis) Systemic processes (systemic mastocytosis, Crohn disease, lymphoma, carcinomas) Radiation involving duodenum Use of cocaine or "crack" cocaine Zollinger-Ellison syndrome

CMV, Cytomegalovirus; *NSAID,* nonsteroidal anti-inflammatory drug.
From Heidelbaugh JJ. Peptic ulcer disease. In Rakel RE, ed. *Essential family medicine.* 3rd ed. Philadelphia: Saunders; 2006.

overwhelming majority of PUD cases, other factors contribute to the remaining 1% to 5% (Table 38-5).

Independent risk factors that augment the impact of *H. pylori* and NSAID-related PUD risk and may promote ulcer complications include advancing age; history of PUD or complicated ulcer disease with perforation, penetration, or gastric outlet obstruction; use of multiple NSAIDs (including concomitant use of low-dose aspirin and an NSAID); and concurrent warfarin or corticosteroid use. Evidence suggests that smoking may increase the risk of PUD and ulcer complications by impairing gastric mucosal healing. Alcohol use may increase the risk of ulcer complications in NSAID users, but its overall effect in patients without concomitant liver disease has not been clearly defined. Currently, no solid evidence implicates dietary factors in the development of PUD.

Use of NSAIDs and aspirin is frequently associated with symptoms of dyspepsia even in the absence of PUD. Empiric antisecretory therapy with PPIs is an attractive strategy that involves subjecting to upper endoscopy only patients who fail to respond to a 4-week course of pharmacotherapy. The rationale for this approach is that most patients with dyspepsia do not have *H. pylori* infection or PUD (most typically have GERD), and their response to antisecretory therapy eliminates the need for further expensive and invasive diagnostic testing (Saad and Scheiman, 2004).

> **KEY TREATMENT**
>
> • The most efficacious therapy for *H. pylori* eradication consists of 14-day triple therapy with a PPI, clarithromycin, and amoxicillin or metronidazole, yielding eradication rates of 70% to 85% (Chey and Wong, 2007) (SOR: A).

Gastroesophageal Reflux Disease

> **Key Points**
>
> ■ The PPIs provide the most rapid symptomatic relief and healing of esophagitis in the highest percentage of patients.
> ■ Although less effective than PPIs, H₂RAs given in divided doses may be effective in some patients with less severe symptoms of GERD; continuous therapy to control symptoms and prevent complications is appropriate.
> ■ Chronic acid suppression has been associated with malabsorption of iron, magnesium, vitamin B_{12}, and calcium; small bowel bacterial overgrowth; increased risk of hip fracture; *C. difficile* colitis; and community-acquired pneumonia.

A complex, chronic, and relapsing condition, GERD carries a risk of significant morbidity and resultant complications. Population-based studies revealed that 40% of U.S. adults experience heartburn at least once a month; age- and gender-adjusted prevalence of weekly heartburn or acid regurgitation approaches 20% (*Heartburn Across America,* 1998; Locke et al., 1997). Most patients with GERD self-treat with over-the-counter medications and do not seek medical attention for their symptoms.

Most patients with GERD evaluated in primary care practices have *nonerosive reflux disease* (NERD), although some progress to *erosive esophagitis* (Figure 38-7) and even fewer to more severe disease resulting in esophageal strictures, BE, and adenocarcinoma of the esophagus (Katz et al.,

2013). Patients with NERD are prone to develop atypical or extraesophageal manifestations of disease (Table 38-6). Because of a small risk of disease progression, however, they generally do not require long-term surveillance despite persistent reflux symptoms. Symptom relapse rates in patients with NERD are similar to those in patients with erosive esophagitis, and although many require continuous pharmacotherapy to control their symptoms, almost all continue to exhibit no definable erosive esophagitis on upper endoscopy (Fass, 2002).

Upper endoscopy is considered the gold standard in assessing esophageal complications of GERD (e.g., erosive esophagitis, BE) but lacks an appreciable sensitivity and specificity for identifying pathologic reflux (DeVault & Castell, 2005). Double-contrast barium radiography has limited usefulness in making an accurate diagnosis of GERD but may be useful in defining the presence of anatomic abnormalities, such as pyloric stenosis, malrotation, and annular pancreas in vomiting infants, as well as hiatal hernia and esophageal strictures in children and adults.

The goals of GERD treatment are to relieve symptoms, heal erosive esophagitis if present, manage and prevent complications, and avoid recurrence and progression of disease using acid-suppressive medications. Clinicians should recommend lifestyle and dietary modifications before consideration of pharmacotherapy, including limitation and avoidance of caffeine, smoking, alcohol, chocolate, carbonated beverages, and citrus and spicy foods, as well as weight reduction and exercise (Katz et al., 2013). Lifestyle modifications should be recommended as adjunctive therapy in all patients with GERD (Table 38-7). Evidence is lacking to support the use of nonpharmacologic measures as the sole initial or long-term therapy for GERD, but expert opinion considers these to be of some potential benefit and no proven harm, although they are not sufficiently effective in treatment.

Initial empiric pharmacotherapy should consist of either an H2RA or a PPI without the need for immediate diagnostic testing in the vast majority of cases. Expert opinion supports either step-up or step-down therapy for the initial treatment of patients with GERD (Inadomi, 2002). In patients who incompletely respond to H2RAs, PPIs taken once daily 30 minutes before the first meal of the day are preferred over continuing H2RA therapy because of greater efficacy and faster symptom control with PPIs. An inadequate response to a 4- or 8-week trial of standard-dose PPI may indicate the need for longer treatment, more severe disease, or an incorrect diagnosis (Figure 38-8). Additional benefit may be obtained by extending treatment for another 4 to 8 weeks with the same or a double dose of PPI (Medical Advisory Panel for the Pharmacy Benefits Management Strategic Healthcare Group, 2003).

Diagnostic testing is recommended in patients with GERD who have an inadequate response to PPI therapy, need continuous chronic therapy to control frequent GERD symptoms, have chronic symptoms (>5 years) and are at risk for BE, have atypical or extraesophageal manifestations suggesting complicated disease, or have alarm symptoms suggesting cancer (Table 38-8).

The basic tenets of antireflux surgery include reduction of the hiatal hernia, repair of the diaphragmatic hiatus, strengthening of the gastroesophageal junction–posterior

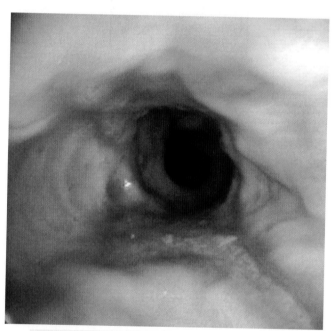

Figure 38-7 Esophagitis. (Courtesy Dr. Erik-Jan Wamsteker.)

Table 38-6 Atypical or Extraesophageal Manifestations of Gastroesophageal Reflux Disease

Aspiration
Asthma
Chronic cough
Dental enamel loss
Globus sensation
Noncardiac chest pain
Recurrent laryngitis
Recurrent sore throat
Subglottic stenosis

Modified from Heidelbaugh JJ, Nostrant TT. Medical and surgical management of gastroesophageal reflux disease. *Clin Fam Pract* 2004;6:547-568.

Table 38-7 Suggested Lifestyle Modifications in the Management of Gastroesophageal Reflux Disease

Avoid acidic foods (citrus and tomato-based products), alcohol, caffeinated beverages, chocolate, onions, garlic, salt, and peppermint.
Avoid large meals.
Avoid medications that may potentiate GERD symptoms (calcium channel blockers, β-agonists, α-agonists, theophylline, nitrates, sedatives).
Avoid recumbency 3 to 4 hours after meals.
Avoid tight clothing around the waist.
Decrease dietary intake of fat.
Elevate the head of the bed 4 to 8 inches (10-20 cm).
Lose weight.
Stop smoking.

GERD, Gastroesophageal reflux disease.
Modified from DeVault KR, Castell DO. Updated guidelines for the diagnosis and treatment of gastroesophageal reflux disease. The Practice Parameters Committee of the American College of Gastroenterology. *Am J Gastroenterol* 1999;94:1434-1442 and Nilsson M, Johnsen R, Ye W, et al. Lifestyle related risk factors in the aetiology of gastro-oesophageal reflux. *Gut* 2004;53:1730-1735.

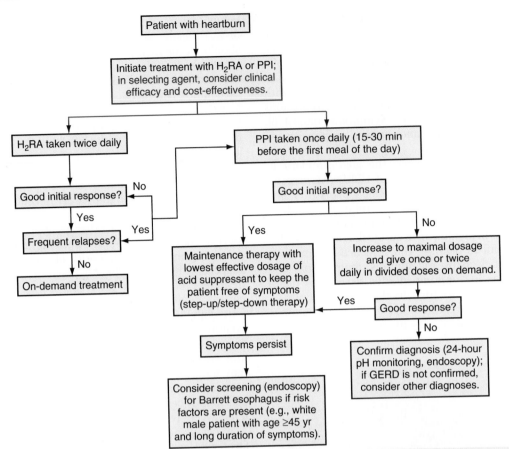

Figure 38-8 Algorithm for the diagnosis and treatment of gastroesophageal reflux disease. *H₂RA*, histamine-2 receptor antagonist; *PPI*, proton pump inhibitor. (Modified from Heidelbaugh JJ, Nostrant TT. Medical and surgical management of gastroesophageal reflux disease. *Clin Fam Pract* 2004;6:547-568.)

Table 38-8   Alarm Symptoms of Gastroesophageal Reflux Disease Suggesting Complicated Disease

Black or bloody stools
Choking
Chronic coughing
Dysphagia
Early satiety
Hematemesis
Hoarseness
Iron deficiency anemia
Odynophagia
Weight loss

Modified from Heidelbaugh JJ, Nostrant TT. Medical and surgical management of gastroesophageal reflux disease. *Clin Fam Pract* 2004;6:547-568.

diaphragm attachment, and strengthening of the antireflux barrier by adding a gastric wrap around the gastroesophageal junction (Nissen or Toupet fundoplication). In controlled studies comparing antireflux surgery with H₂RAs and PPIs, surgery has shown marginal superiority as measured by heartburn relief, esophagitis healing, and improved quality of life in patients with erosive esophagitis. Long-term follow-up trials found that more than half of patients resumed taking antireflux medications 3 to 5 years after surgery, most likely as a result of poor patient selection and surgical breakdown (Heidelbaugh and Nostrant, 2004).

KEY TREATMENT

- Lifestyle modifications, including weight management, elevation of the head of the bed, and improving nutrition with eliminating triggering foods should be recommended to patients with GERD (Katz et al., 2013) (SOR: B).
- Acid suppression with PPIs is the mainstay of pharmaceutical therapy for esophagitis (Katz et al., 2013) (SOR: A).

Upper Gastrointestinal Bleeding

Key Points

- Comorbid risk factors for GI bleeding severity, including advanced age, shock, congestive heart failure, ischemic heart disease, and stigmata of recent hemorrhage, accurately predict the likelihood of death or rebleeding.
- UGIB is confirmed by upper endoscopy, permitting direct visualization of the cause and location of the bleeding and allowing an attempt at immediate hemostasis.

Significant UGIB is defined as bleeding that results in hemodynamic instability and a decrease in the hemoglobin and hematocrit. Although most patients with UGIB resolve

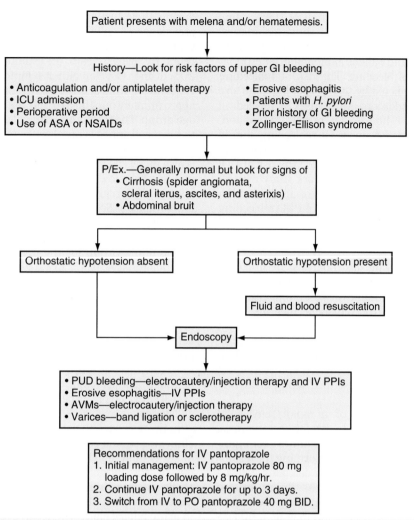

Figure 38-9 Algorithm for the evaluation of acute upper gastrointestinal (GI) bleeding. *ASA*, acetylsalicylic acid; *AVM*, arteriovenous malformation; *BID*, twice daily; *ICU*, intensive care unit; *IV*, intravenous; *NSAID*, nonsteroidal antiinflammatory drug; *PO*, oral; *PPI*, proton pump inhibitor; *PUD*, peptic ulcer disease. (Modified from Oh DS, Pisegna JR. Management of upper gastrointestinal bleeding. *Clin Fam Pract* 2004;6:631-645.)

spontaneously, those with an acute UGIB requiring hemostasis often present with a recent history of hematemesis (vomiting fresh blood) or "coffee ground" emesis (black, partially digested blood). UGIB has an incidence of 40 to 150 episodes per 100,000 persons annually in the United States, with mortality of 6% to 10% (Oh and Pisegna, 2004). Table 38-9 lists the most common causes of UGIB.

It is important to characterize patients with risk factors for the development of UGIB to identify potential preventive measures, including aspirin or NSAID use and anticoagulation or antiplatelet therapy. *H. pylori* infection, erosive esophagitis, history of UGIB, perioperative period, intensive care unit (ICU) admission, and Zollinger-Ellison syndrome are also significant risk factors for UGIB. Figure 38-9 outlines an algorithm for the diagnosis and management of acute UGIB. Hemodynamically unstable patients should be admitted to the ICU, have a large-bore intravenous (IV) and nasogastric tube placed, and should not be fed orally.

Confirmation of UGIB is by upper endoscopy, permitting direct visualization of the cause and location of the bleeding and an attempt at immediate hemostasis. During the diagnostic evaluation, the endoscopist can treat the source

Table 38-9 Common Causes of Upper Gastrointestinal Bleeding

AVMs
Bleeding from the nose or pharynx
Dieulafoy lesion (ruptured mucosal artery)
Erosive esophagitis (severe)
Esophageal rupture (Boerhaave syndrome)
Helicobacter pylori infection
Hemobilia
Hemoptysis
Mallory-Weiss tears (esophagogastric mucosal tears)
Neoplasm (carcinoma, lymphoma, leiomyoma, leiomyosarcoma, polyps)
NSAIDs
Ulcers (gastric, duodenal)
Vascular-enteric fistulas, usually from aortic aneurysm or graft
Varices (esophageal, gastric, duodenal)

AVM, Arteriovenous malformation; *NSAID*, nonsteroidal antiinflammatory drug.
Modified from Oh DS, Pisegna JR. Pharmacologic treatment of upper gastrointestinal bleeding. *Curr Treat Options Gastroenterol* 2003;6:157-162.

of UGIB by using electrocautery, injection of 0.9% saline or 100% ethanol, or a combination of these techniques. Alternative methods include laser photoablation, band ligation, and sclerotherapy and balloon tamponade for esophageal and gastric variceal bleeding. The risk of rebleeding after therapy can be predicted by the morphology and size of the ulcer at upper endoscopy. Most cases of rebleeding occur within the first 72 hours after hospital admission; patients at increased risk for upper GI rebleeding should have ICU monitoring during their admission (Oh and Pisegna, 2004). The use of PPIs in reducing the risk of UGI rebleeding was demonstrated in a landmark study with IV omeprazole, showing the clinical efficacy of acid reduction therapy in preventing the complications of PUD rebleeding (Lau et al., 2000).

Gastroparesis

Clinical symptoms suggesting gastroparesis, or impaired and delayed gastric emptying, include nausea, vomiting, and postprandial abdominal fullness. Most often, gastroparesis is related to poorly controlled diabetes mellitus, autonomic neuropathies, postsurgical conditions (e.g., vagotomy, Billroth pyloroplasty), and anorexia nervosa. Vomiting needs to be differentiated from regurgitation, rumination, and even bulimia; the duration, frequency, and severity of symptoms together should be described along with any associated symptoms.

Gastric-emptying scintigraphy of a radiolabeled solid meal is the most accepted method to test for gastroparesis. Conventionally, the test is performed for 2 hours after ingestion of a radiolabeled meal; however, performing the test for up to 4 hours may increase the yield in detecting delayed gastric emptying in symptomatic patients. Breath testing can be used to measure gastric emptying using the nonradioactive isotope carbon 13 ($_{13}$C) (Parkman et al., 2004).

Primary treatment of gastroparesis includes dietary manipulation and administration of antiemetic and prokinetic agents. Dietary recommendations include eating more frequent and smaller meals and replacing solid food with liquids, such as soups. Foods consumed should be low in both fat and fiber content. Common antiemetic agents include prochlorperazine, trimethobenzamide, and promethazine. Currently used prokinetic agents include metoclopramide and erythromycin, administered orally or intravenously. Domperidone, a dopamine (D_2) receptor antagonist, is not approved in the United States for treatment of gastroparesis but is available in Canada, Mexico, and Europe (Parkman et al., 2004). Endoscopic injection of botulinum toxin into the pyloric sphincter can aid in relaxing pyloric sphincter resistance, allowing more food to empty from the stomach. No placebo-controlled trials have yet been reported for this therapy, and long-term control of gastroparesis should not be expected from using botulinum toxin.

Gallbladder

CHOLELITHIASIS AND CHOLECYSTITIS

Gallstones are exceedingly common among women and men of all ages, affecting approximately 20% of Americans

during their lifetimes. Population-based studies reveal a prevalence of gallbladder disease in women age 20 to 55 years of 5% to 20%, increasing to 25% to 30% after age 50 years. By age 75 years, an estimated 35% of women and 20% of men develop either symptomatic or asymptomatic gallstones (Attili et al., 1995). The prevalence for men is approximately one third to half that for women in any given age group. The traditional clinical picture of a patient likely to have gallstones is an obese woman older than 40 years of age (the four Fs: female, "fat," 40, and fertile). Prevalence is also increased in patients with cystic fibrosis with pancreatic insufficiency, diabetes mellitus, or family a history of biliary colic; pregnancy; rapid weight loss; Native American Pima Indian or Scandinavian descent; patients taking estrogens, progestins, or ceftriaxone; and those requiring total parenteral nutrition.

The Rome Group for the Epidemiology and Prevention of Cholelithiasis (GREPCO, 1984) found that the overall cumulative probability of developing biliary colic in those with gallstones over time was 11.9% at 2 years, 16.5% at 4 years, and 25.8% at 10 years, with a cumulative probability of 3% of developing complications at 10 years. The incidence of the development of biliary complications as the presenting complaint of gallstone disease is rare, ranging from 0% to 5.5%. Based on these data, evidence from well-designed cohort and case-control studies summarized by GREPCO favors expectant treatment of asymptomatic gallstones.

In the approach to patients with symptomatic gallstones, clinicians should effectively rule out other potential causes of RUQ and epigastric abdominal pain, distinguishing biliary from nonbiliary etiologies as the primary source of disease (see Table 38-2). A gallstone blocking the cystic duct or common bile duct (CBD; *choledocholithiasis*) results in acute biliary colic, which can evolve into acute suppurative cholecystitis or cholangitis. The onset of pain from biliary colic is rarely related to meals or the type of food consumed, contrary to popular opinion. Many patients with postprandial abdominal pain believe that they have gallbladder disease, but many of them actually have dyspepsia or GERD. One meta-analysis found that heartburn, flatulence, regurgitation, and fatty food intolerance were not associated with gallstones but that epigastric pain, nausea, and vomiting were associated with a higher odds ratio of having gallstones (Kragg et al., 1995).

In cases of acute cholecystitis, laboratory tests frequently lack adequate predictive value in making an accurate diagnosis. A complete blood count (CBC) usually reveals a moderate leukocytosis, often with a "bandemia" in cases of ascending cholangitis. Serum amylase and lipase values are usually normal but may be elevated if there is associated pancreatitis. Serum alkaline phosphatase (ALP), liver transaminases, and bilirubin levels are rarely elevated except when CBD stones are causing obstruction. Patients with choledocholithiasis often present similar to those with cholelithiasis, although they may also have obstructive jaundice, cholangitis, and pancreatitis.

The evaluation of gallstones using abdominal ultrasonography is currently the best screening modality, with sensitivity and specificity above 90%. When calculi, gallbladder wall thickening, and gallbladder sludge are found, the diagnosis of acute cholecystitis is almost certain, yet the

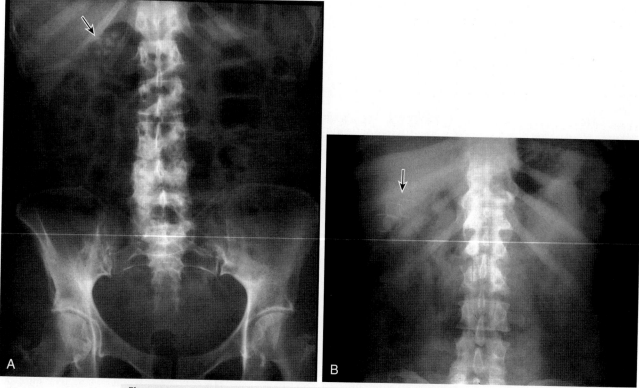

Figure 38-10 Radiographs of gallstones (*arrows;* **A** and **B**). (Courtesy Dr. Perry Pernicano.)

presence of stones by itself does not ensure the diagnosis of acute cholecystitis. Only 10% to 15% of gallstones are visible on plain radiographs (Figure 38-10). A CT scan of the upper abdomen is more sensitive than conventional radiography but may miss a significant amount of cholesterol gallstones and biliary sludge readily seen on ultrasonography (Figure 38-11). Biliary scintigraphy (HIDA scan) uses technetium 99m (^{99m}Tc)–labeled derivatives of excreted bile acids to determine CBD obstruction. Endoscopic retrograde cholangiopancreatography (ERCP) with stent placement or sphincterotomy (or both) is useful in identifying and treating CBD stones but is invasive; expensive; and often fraught with complications, including iatrogenic pancreatitis (Figure 38-12).

Endoscopic ultrasonography is a widely used, noninvasive method with excellent sensitivity and specificity for detecting and evaluating CBD stones. Magnetic resonance cholangiopancreatography (MRCP) is another noninvasive modality for identifying gallstones and CBD stones, but it often has lower sensitivity and specificity than ultrasonography and is more costly (Browning and Sreenarasimhaiah, 2006). The natural history of CBD stones suggests that 70% will pass safely into the duodenum and will not require ERCP for stone extraction.

Most surgeons advocate expectant management in patients with asymptomatic gallstones. Nonsurgical treatments include pain relief with narcotic analgesics, excluding morphine and its derivatives (which may precipitate sphincter of Oddi spasm and worsen symptoms), extracorporeal shock-wave lithotripsy, and gallstone dissolution using oral bile acid therapy and contact solvents such as methyl tert-butyl ether (MTBE). Numerous RCTs have

confirmed the adoption of laparoscopic cholecystectomy as the gold standard for the treatment of gallstone disease over the open procedure (Glasgow and Mulvihill, 2006).

Liver

HEPATITIS

Hepatitis is defined as acute inflammation of hepatic parenchyma. In the United States, the most common types of hepatitis are secondary to viral etiologies and are labeled as hepatitis A, B, and C. Table 38-10 outlines the various serologic markers for viral hepatitis. Viral hepatitis is less frequently attributed to Epstein-Barr virus, toxoplasmosis, and cytomegalovirus. Additional causes of hepatitis include bacterial and fungal sources, autoimmune and metabolic disorders, toxic poisoning, and various hepatotoxic medications (e.g., isoniazid, acetaminophen) and alternative supplements. Acetaminophen overdose should be considered in acute nonviral hepatitis and treated immediately with N-acetylcysteine to avoid permanent hepatic damage and death. Patients presenting with acute hepatitis often exhibit low-grade fever, fatigue, lethargy, anorexia, RUQ pain, nausea, vomiting, diarrhea, arthralgias and myalgias, and (in severe cases) dark urine and jaundice.

Serum bilirubin, transaminases, and ALP levels can be greatly elevated in all forms of acute hepatitis, but the specific values have poor prognostic value. Alarm symptoms of severe hepatic parenchymal destruction include mental status changes (hepatic encephalopathy), asterixis, ascites, and prolongation of prothrombin time (PT). These patients

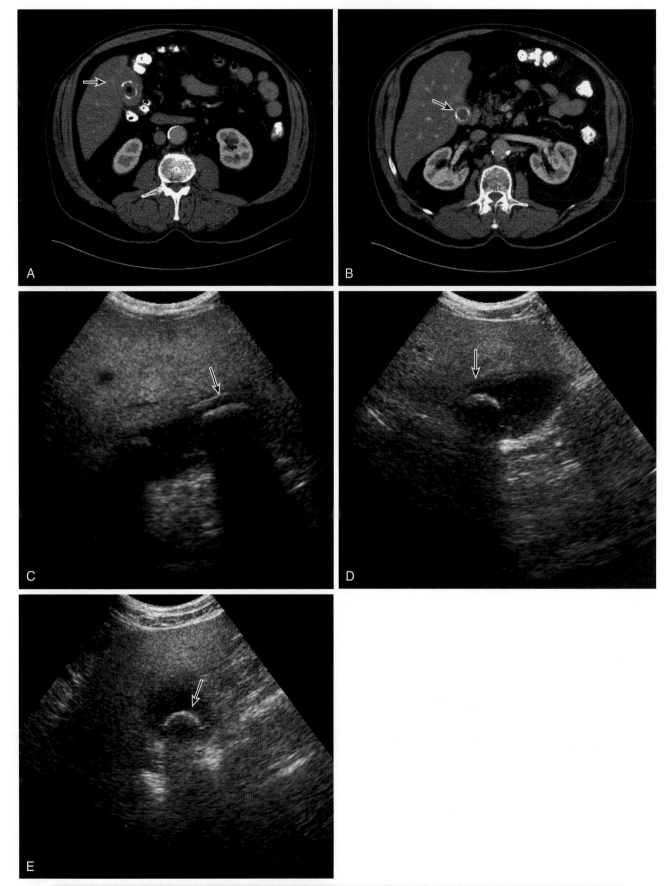

Figure 38-11 Computed tomography scans (**A, B**) and ultrasonography (**C-E**) of gallstones *(arrows)*. (Courtesy Dr. Perry Pernicano.)

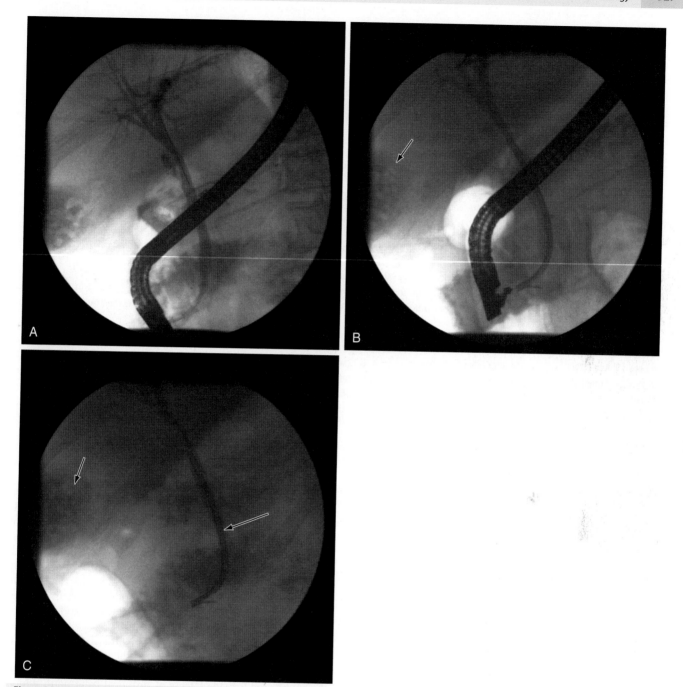

Figure 38-12 A to C, Endoscopic retrograde cholangiopancreatography (ERCP) with stent placement to identify and treat gallstones *(arrows)*. (Courtesy Dr. Perry Pernicano.)

may require hospitalization, with attention toward improving nutritional status and specialist referral for liver transplantation evaluation. Most cases of acute hepatitis resolve without complications, so most patients can be managed as an outpatient, although they must take proper contact isolation precautions and allow for a slow return to usual activity. A patient's symptomatic improvement usually precedes the resolution of liver function serologies.

Viral Hepatitis

Hepatitis A is endemic worldwide, with 10% of U.S. children seropositive and up to 100% of preschool children seropositive in areas where sanitation and socioeconomic status

are poor in less developed countries (Marsano, 2003). The virus has received sporadic national attention in the United States from outbreaks in restaurants from undercooked meat and vegetable sources. Spread through the fecal–oral route, severe hepatitis can be seen after an incubation period of 2 to 6 weeks, but the vast majority of patients recover completely within this time frame and without permanent hepatic damage. When a patient contracts hepatitis A, immunity follows with the appearance of anti–hepatitis A virus (HAV) IgG antibodies, and there is no chronic carrier state. If exposed to HAV during a known incubation period, the patient should be passively immunized with immune globulin. Vaccination is recommended in high-risk

Table 38-10   Viral Hepatitis Serologic Tests and Definitions

Test	Description
HEPATITIS A VIRUS (HAV)	
Anti-HAV IgM	Immunoglobulin M (IgM) antibody to hepatitis antigen. Antibody of IgM class signifies recent acute infection. This develops at onset of symptoms and resolves in <1 yr.
Anti-HAV IgG	Immunoglobulin G (IgG) antibody to hepatitis A antigen. With negative anti-HAV IgM result, this indicates past HAV infection and that the patient is immune. It appears 1 to 2 weeks after IgM antibody.
HEPATITIS B VIRUS (HBV)	
Hepatitis B surface antigen (HBsAg)	HBsAg is the earliest indicator of acute infection. It can be present for several months before symptoms and may remain detectable for up to 6 months. Persistence after 6 months may indicate a chronic carrier state.
Antibody to hepatitis B surface antigen (Anti-HBs)	Anti-HBs is an indicator of clinical recovery and subsequent immunity. It appears 1 to 2 months after HBsAg disappears, and it may be present for life.
HBcAg	No clinical significance; not readily available.
Anti-HBc IgG	Antibody to hepatitis B core antigen is an early indicator of acute infection. It is also a lifelong marker that represents past exposure. It may precede the detection of HBsAg. This persists for years but does not necessarily confer immunity.
IgM Anti-HBc	Early indicator of acute active infection; usually short lived (3-6 wk).
HBe g	Active infection is present, and patient is highly contagious.
Anti-HBe	Seroconversion from antigen to antibody is prognostic for resolution of infection and, in a carrier, means very low infectivity.
IgM anti-HBc	IgM fraction of antibody to hepatitis B core antigen is test of choice to rule out acute HBV infection. IgM fraction disappears in first few months.
Hepatitis C Anti-HCV	An antibody to HCV that appears 3 to 12 months after exposure.
Hepatitis D Anti-HDV	This antibody to HDV may appear late and may be short-lived.
Hepatitis E (non-A, non-B)	No markers detectable; epidemiology parallels that of hepatitis B.

Modified from Rodney WM. Gastrointestinal disorders. In Rakel RE, ed. *Textbook of family medicine.* 6th ed. Philadelphia: Saunders; 2002.

populations and before travel to endemic areas (Fiore et al., 2006).

Despite the availability of a highly effective vaccine against *hepatitis B,* approximately 2 billion people worldwide are infected, 350 million with chronic active infection accounting for 600,000 attributable deaths annually worldwide (World Health Organization, 2009). Hepatitis B is spread via blood and body fluid contact through heterosexual and homosexual relations, by sharing of needles by infected drug abusers, and by accidental needle sticks in the medical setting. In areas of high disease prevalence (e.g., Southeast Asia, China), transmission is primarily from mother to child during childbirth or in early childhood. The vaccination for hepatitis B uses recombinant DNA, requires three doses on a set schedule, and confers immunity in the majority of recipients (CDC, 1999). In a child born to a mother positive for hepatitis B surface antigen (HBsAg), in addition to the vaccine, hepatitis B hyperimmune globulin should be administered during the first 12 hours of life. Patients with chronic infection can develop cirrhosis and end-stage liver disease. Antiviral treatments for hepatitis B are indicated for patients with moderate to severe disease activity diagnosed on liver biopsy. Current therapies include interferon and, more recently, lamivudine and adefovir (Marsano, 2003).

Hepatitis C affects more than 300 million people worldwide and 4 million people in the United States. At least six genotypes and 100 subtypes have been identified (Bukh, 2000; Hepatitis C Statistics, 2009). The diagnosis is established with serum testing for HCV RNA antibodies; although an antibody is induced, it is not protective against disease contraction and progression. Transmission occurs via blood or body fluid contamination through IV and intranasal drug use, blood transfusions, and in health care workers (e.g., needle stick or skin disruption with contaminated instrument). Data on sexual transmission and through tattooing have been inconsistent. Co-infection with human immunodeficiency virus (HIV) increases the risk of transmission sexually, as well as vertically from mother to child. In patients with chronic hepatitis C, alcohol use rapidly accelerates liver damage and cirrhosis. Many experts believe lifelong abstinence from alcohol and IV and intranasal drugs should be immediate on diagnosis and enforced before initiating antiviral therapies.

Therapy with pegylated interferon and ribavirin has been shown to achieve sustained viral eradication in almost 50% of patients with hepatitis C (Shehab, 2004). Patients should be monitored for side effects of antiviral treatment, which may require dose adjustments or discontinuation of therapy. The duration and success of therapy depend on viral genotype and possible downward adjustments in therapeutic doses. Sustained virologic response ranges from 42% in genotype 1 to 80% in genotypes 2 and 3 (Marsano, 2003).

Hepatitis D virus (delta hepatitis) is usually only seen in IV drug users and in former carriers of hepatitis B as a co-infection. *Hepatitis E* is an enteric virus only rarely identified in the United States, characterized by an acute self-limited illness without a chronic carrier state.

CIRRHOSIS

Cirrhosis and chronic liver failure rank as the 12th leading causes of death in the United States, accounting for 27,555 deaths (9.2 per 100,000 population) in 2006, with a slight

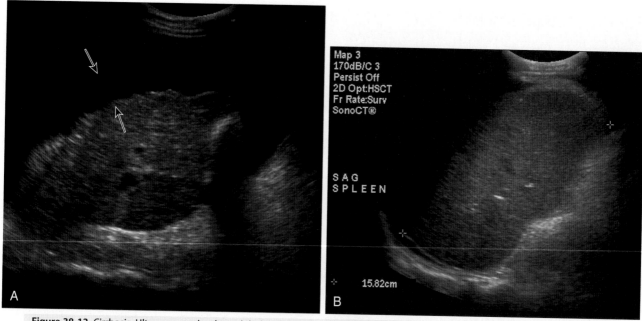

Figure 38-13 Cirrhosis. Ultrasonography shows lobulated shrunken liver with ascites and splenomegaly. (Courtesy Dr. Perry Pernicano.)

male predominance (National Center for Health Statistics, 2009). The vast majority of cirrhosis-related morbidity and mortality is secondary to excessive alcohol consumption, hepatitis B and C, and obesity (nonalcoholic fatty liver disease [NAFLD]) and is theoretically preventable. The term *cirrhosis* refers to a progressive diffuse, fibrosing, and nodular condition that disrupts the entire normal architecture of the liver. Portal hypertension ensues with multiple long-term complications. Approximately 40% of patients are asymptomatic, with cirrhosis often discovered during a routine examination, including laboratory and radiographic studies (Figures 38-13 and 38-14), or often at autopsy. Mortality rates in patients with alcoholic liver disease are considerably higher than in those with other forms of cirrhosis.

The incidence of NAFLD depends on definitions and populations. Risk factors include obesity, metabolic syndrome, dyslipidemia, and type 2 diabetes mellitus. Conditions with emerging association include polycystic ovary syndrome, hypothyroidism, sleep apnea, and hypogonadism. When patients with unsuspected hepatic steatosis detected on imaging have symptoms or signs attributable to liver disease or have abnormal liver biochemistries, they should be evaluated as though they have suspected NAFLD and worked up accordingly (SOR: A). Screening for NAFLD in adults attending primary care clinics or high-risk groups attending diabetes or obesity clinics is not advised at this time because of uncertainties surrounding diagnostic tests and treatment options along with lack of knowledge related to the long-term benefits and cost-effectiveness of screening (SOR: B; Chalasani et al., 2012). Treatment is aimed at weight loss (e.g., Mediterranean diet) and omega-3 fatty acid supplementation (e.g., >830 mg/day). There are no current recommendations for continued monitoring of patients with NAFLD, specifically with monitoring of serum transaminases or liver ultrasonography.

The major complications of cirrhosis that affect HRQOL and survival include ascites formation, spontaneous bacterial peritonitis, hepatorenal syndrome, encephalopathy, and GI bleeding secondary to portal hypertension and varices. Another serious complication of cirrhosis is the development of hepatocellular carcinoma, for which screening protocols with ultrasonography and serum α-fetoprotein testing are effective (Marrero, 2005). All patients with ascites should be evaluated for liver transplantation because of poor 5-year survival rates (30%-40%) (Gines et al., 2004) (Figure 38-15).

Pancreas

ACUTE PANCREATITIS

Acute pancreatitis continues to cause significant morbidity and mortality despite dramatic advances in the understanding of its pathophysiology and its critical care management. Some studies suggest a high rate of undiagnosed pancreatitis, with approximately 40% of acute cases recognized only at autopsy. Thus, it is imperative for primary and emergency care physicians to make the diagnosis of pancreatitis within the first 48 hours of admission (AGA, 2007). The diagnosis of acute pancreatitis is typically defined by at least two of the following criteria: (1) abdominal pain consistent with the disease, (2) serum amylase or lipase greater than three times the upper limit of normal, or (3) characteristic findings from abdominal imaging (Tenner et al., 2013). In severe acute pancreatitis, parenchymal and fat necrosis ensues, as well as profound multisystem organ failure, infection, and life-threatening hemodynamic instability.

The causes of acute pancreatitis are diverse and demonstrate changing trends over time and variation by geography. Gallstones, biliary sludge, and microlithiasis are

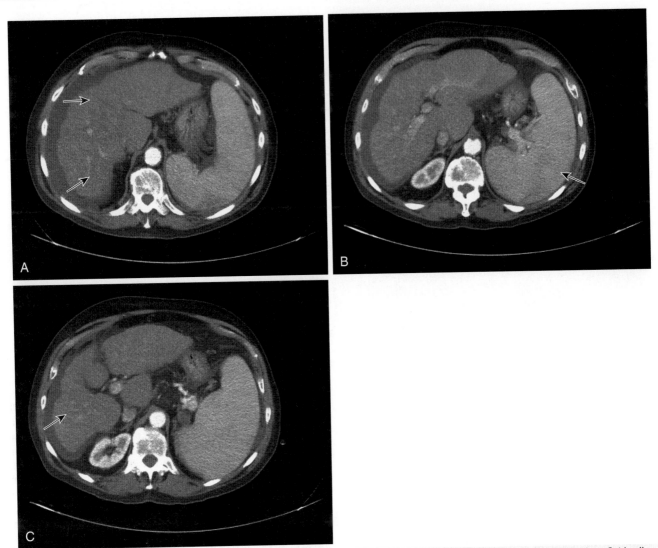

Figure 38-14 Cirrhosis. Computed tomography scans show lobulated contour of liver (**A**), splenomegaly (**B**), and ascites (**C**). *Arrows* show fluid collections (ascites). (Courtesy Dr. Perry Pernicano.)

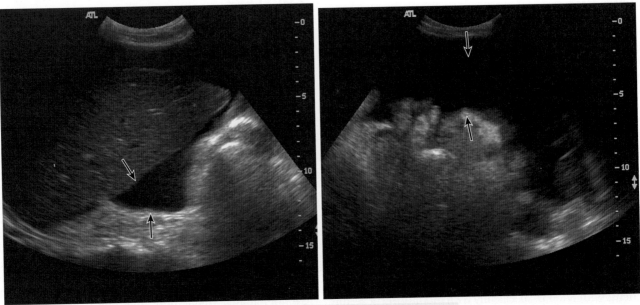

Figure 38-15 Ascites *(arrows)*. (Courtesy Dr. Perry Pernicano.)

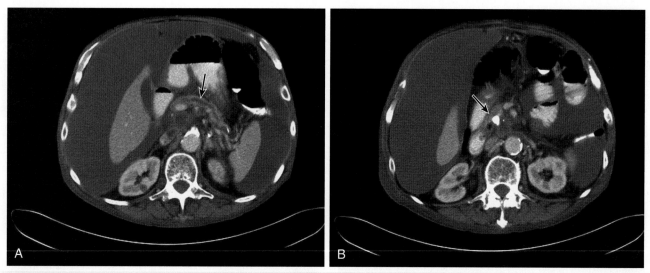

Figure 38-16 Computed tomography scans (**A** and **B**) of dilated pancreatic duct secondary to stone pancreatitis *(arrows)*. (Courtesy Dr. Perry Pernicano.)

recognized as the proximate cause in more than half of reported cases, and therefore, abdominal ultrasonography is recommended in all patients with acute pancreatitis (Tenner et al., 2013). Ethyl alcohol ingestion is the second most common reported cause of acute pancreatitis (≈30% of cases), although it is unclear whether alcohol is a toxin or an exacerbating factor in individuals who have compromised pancreatic function. The remaining causes of acute pancreatitis account for fewer than 15% of total cases, including hypertriglyceridemia, trauma, medications, ERCP, neoplasms, perforated PUD, viral infection, and idiopathic causes. Hypertriglyceridemia should be considered the etiology when serum triglycerides are greater than 1000 mg/dL and there is no evidence of cholelithiasis or significant alcohol use (Tenner et al., 2013). Pancreatic neoplasm should be considered on the differential especially in anyone older than the age of 40 years (Tenner et al., 2013).

Serum markers of acute pancreatitis have high sensitivity and specificity but no role in predicting the severity or course of disease. The most common enzymes assayed, amylase and lipase, are released at approximately the same time after the initial insult to the pancreas but are cleared from the bloodstream at different rates. Therefore, relying on total serum amylase alone to make an accurate diagnosis of acute pancreatitis is error prone because it is cleared almost totally from the blood within 48 to 72 hours. The sensitivity of pancreatic amylase for the diagnosis of acute pancreatitis decreases to less than 30% between the second and fourth day after onset of the acute episode. By contrast, an elevated serum lipase level can be detected up to 14 days after the acute event and has sensitivity greater than 90% for acute pancreatitis (Orbuch, 2004).

Hemodynamic status should be assessed immediately on patient presentation and resuscitative measures begun as needed. Risk assessment should be performed to stratify patients into higher and lower risk categories to assist triage, such as admission to an intensive care setting (Tenner et al., 2013). Early prognostic factors that can be measured and indicate severity of disease include the Acute Physiology and Chronic Health Evaluation II (APACHE II) score.

The overall success at prediction of mortality from acute pancreatitis at hospital admission remains at 40%, and even at 48 hours, it is no better than 80% when all diagnostic strategies of morbidity and mortality prediction are compared (Papachristou and Whitcomb, 2004). The most important factor in the management of patients with acute pancreatitis is maintaining appropriate intravascular volume status (AGA, 2007). Aggressive hydration, defined as 250 to 500 mL/hr of isotonic crystalloid solution, should be provided to all patients unless cardiovascular or renal comorbidities exist. Those with hypotension and tachycardia may require even higher infusion rates (Tenner et al., 2013). Many predictors of pancreatitis severity are directly related to "third spacing" of fluids and include hemoconcentration and rising creatinine level. The goal of aggressive hydration should be to decrease blood urea nitrogen (Tenner et al., 2013). The hematocrit may be high as a result of hypovolemia secondary to third spacing of fluids. Early aggressive hydration is most beneficial in the first 12 to 24 hours (Tenner et al., 2013) because this may minimize or even prevent pancreatic necrosis.

If the bilirubin, liver transaminases, and ALP increase, a CBD stone may exist (Figure 38-16). It is recommended that patients with acute pancreatitis and concurrent acute cholangitis undergo ERCP within 24 hours of admission. ERCP is not needed in most patients with gallstone pancreatitis who lack laboratory or clinical evidence of ongoing biliary obstruction. In the absence of cholangitis or jaundice, MRCP or endoscopic ultrasonography, rather than ERCP, should be used to screen for choledocholithiasis if highly suspected (Tenner et al., 2013). Similar laboratory abnormalities with a less acute presentation may occur in patients with chronic pancreatitis when bile duct stricture occurs.

Contrast-enhanced computed tomography (CECT) is the most extensively studied modality for the confirmation of acute pancreatitis (Figure 38-17) (Papachristou and Whitcomb, 2004). CECT or magnetic resonance imaging of the pancreas should be reserved for patients in whom the diagnosis is unclear or who fail to improve clinically within the first 48 to 72 hours after hospital admission (Tenner et al., 2013). Sensitivities using ultrasonography for the

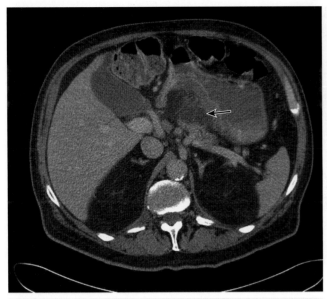

Figure 38-17 Pancreatitis (computed tomography scan) *(arrow).* (Courtesy Dr. Perry Pernicano.)

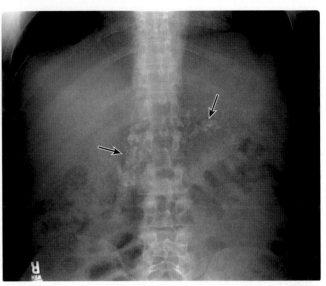

Figure 38-18 Chronic pancreatitis with calcifications *(arrows).* (Courtesy Dr. Perry Pernicano.)

diagnosis of acute pancreatitis range between 62% and 95% and probably reflect the failure to visualize the organ in as many as 30% of cases. When the pancreas is visualized in the setting of acute disease, tissue abnormalities are detected in 90% of those studied. The milder the disease presentation, the less likely it is that abnormalities will manifest that are detectable on CT examination.

Medical therapy of acute pancreatitis is primarily supportive, with the major objective being hemodynamic stabilization. Antibiotics should not be started routinely but should be given for extrapancreatic infection. In mild acute pancreatitis, oral feedings can be started immediately if there is no nausea and vomiting and abdominal pain has resolved. In mild pancreatitis, initiation of a low-fat solid diet appears as safe as a clear liquid diet (Tenner et al., 2013). Nutritional support should be provided for patients likely to remain "nothing by mouth" (NPO) for more than 7 days. Enteral feeding is preferred over parenteral nutrition to help prevent infectious complications. Nasogastric and nasojejunal delivery of enteral feeding appear comparable in safety and efficacy (Tenner et al., 2013). Pain management in the hospital setting is best achieved using morphine derivatives. Infrequently, patient-controlled anesthesia may be used for severe abdominal pain, and alternative diagnoses and complications should be considered.

CHRONIC PANCREATITIS

Permanent pathologic damage to the pancreas results in chronic pancreatitis. In addition to exocrine deficiency (with malabsorption, diabetes, or both), a chronic pain syndrome may evolve and become a management challenge. Many patients have substance abuse and other behavioral problems that require time, patience, compassion, and skill to resolve. Patients who continue to consume alcohol are more likely to have recurrent attacks. Carefully selected patients may benefit from therapeutic ERCP or pancreatic surgery, with some pain relief. Exocrine deficiency may be treated with pancreatic enzyme supplementation with each meal (Apte et al., 1999).

Chronic pancreatitis indicates some degree of progressive and permanent damage to the pancreas, usually visualized as calcifications on radiographs and CT (Figures 38-18 and 38-19). This damage often leads to diabetes and pancreatic insufficiency, resulting in malabsorption with chronic diarrhea. Patients with chronic pancreatitis present with repeated attacks of abdominal pain and are often admitted for acute or chronic exacerbations. Potential complications include pseudocyst (Figure 38-20) and abscess formation, fistula formation between pseudocysts and the gut, persistent pancreatic ascites caused by a disrupted pancreatic duct system, communication with the peritoneal cavity, mesenteric venous thrombosis, and arterial pseudoaneurysm (Apte et al., 1999).

PANCREATIC CANCER

More than 37,000 people in the United States were diagnosed with pancreatic cancer in 2008, and more than 34,000 died from their disease (Cancer Facts and Figures, 2008). The major risk factors are advancing age and a history of tobacco and alcohol use; the diagnosis is rarely made early in the disease course because of vague presenting symptoms of nonspecific abdominal pain, weight loss, cachexia, and painless obstructive jaundice. Approximately 85% of patients present with locally advanced or metastatic disease, with median survival period of 3 to 12 months. For these patients, conventional treatments include palliative surgery. Radiation and chemotherapy have not substantially impacted survival. Endoscopic ultrasonography and high-resolution CT allow for better preoperative selection for patients likely to benefit from exploration for resection (Figure 38-21).

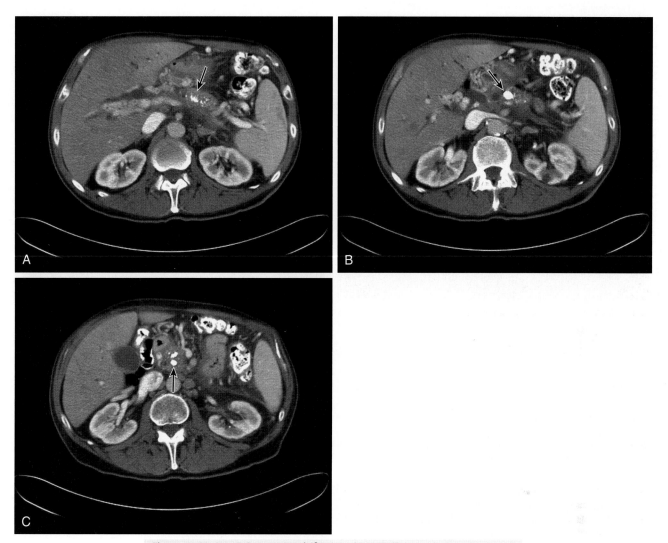

Figure 38-19 **A** to **C,** Pancreatic calcifications *(arrows).* (Courtesy Dr. Perry Pernicano.)

Lower Gastrointestinal Tract

INFLAMMATORY BOWEL DISEASE

Key Points

- Steroids are effective for inducing but not maintaining remission in IBD.
- The 5-aminosalicylic acid (5-ASA) medications are effective in ulcerative colitis (UC) for therapy induction and maintenance therapy but largely are ineffective for Crohn disease.

Inflammatory bowel disease is a chronic condition that often requires long-term maintenance therapy for the majority of the half-million Americans affected. The two major categories include UC and Crohn disease; a more recent and less common third category of *microscopic colitis* has also been identified. The incidence of UC and Crohn disease is 1.5 to 8 new cases per 100,000 U.S. population per year, more often in whites and with no specific gender predominance, although some suggest a male predominance in Crohn disease and a female predominance in UC. Most patients are diagnosed with IBD between ages 15 and 25 years, with a second peak between 55 and 65 years. The incidence of microscopic colitis is most likely underestimated because it is not well known; the estimated incidence ranges from 4.3 to 9.2 per 100,000 in Western European and Icelandic population studies (Loftus, 2003).

Genetic factors play an important role in the development of IBD. First-degree relatives of patients with either form of IBD have been shown to have an almost 10% lifetime risk of developing disease and often present with a similar disease type and course as the affected family member (Higgins and Zimmerman, 2004).

Ulcerative colitis involves the mucosal layer of the sigmoid colon and rectum in the vast majority of cases, causing proctitis and proctosigmoiditis (Figure 38-22). When there is proximal spread, it tends to be continuous and symmetric, causing intestinal mucosal inflammation with edema and friability that is visualized from the rectum proximally. Pancolitis is caused by inflammatory exudates producing a backwash ileitis by way of a patent ileocecal valve and can cause small bowel involvement.

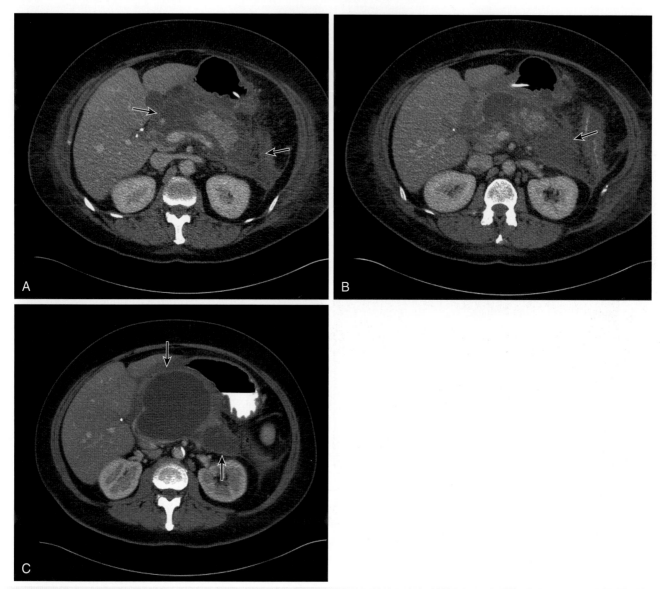

Figure 38-20 A to **C,** Computed tomography scans showing severe pancreatitis evolving into pseudocysts *(arrows)* over 2 months. (Courtesy Dr. Perry Pernicano.)

Crohn disease differs from UC in that it may involve any part of the GI tract from the mouth to the anus, including the gallbladder and biliary tree, and involves the entire thickness of the bowel wall. It is most often found in the immunologically rich terminal ileum, and Crohn disease involves the rectum in less than 50% of cases. In contrast to UC, the mucosal abnormalities are discontinuous ("skip lesions"), asymmetric, and patchy, which account for obstruction, abscesses, and perianal fistulas to other organs and skin. Recurrent disease flares and healing can result in significant muscular hypertrophy and fibrosis of the intestinal wall, leading to small bowel strictures, upstream dilation of intestine and increased fistula formation, and eventual bowel obstruction and the imminent need for surgical intervention (Higgins and Zimmerman, 2004).

Most patients with UC present with mild to moderate diarrhea without constitutional symptoms. Typically, the more severe the illness, the greater the number of bowel movements and the more likely that constitutional symptoms such as fever, fatigue, dehydration, and weight loss will also occur. UC can be intermittent with flare-ups, and remission can occur without therapy. A minority of patients with UC present with severe or fulminant panniculitis, ranging from an acute abdomen to toxic megacolon. Frequent urgent and bloody diarrhea usually suggests rectal disease and is most consistent with UC.

In patients with mild Crohn disease, abdominal pain may be vague, the diarrhea intermittent, and weight loss absent. Postprandial crampy pain can suggest transient small bowel obstruction from inflamed or fibrotic, narrowed small bowel segments. Colonic involvement with Crohn disease may present similar to UC, with predominantly bloody diarrhea. Rectal involvement produces more urgent and frequent small, bloody stools as a result of an inflamed, nondistensible rectum. Mucus in the stool is nonspecific and is found in both IBD and IBS (Higgins and Zimmerman, 2004).

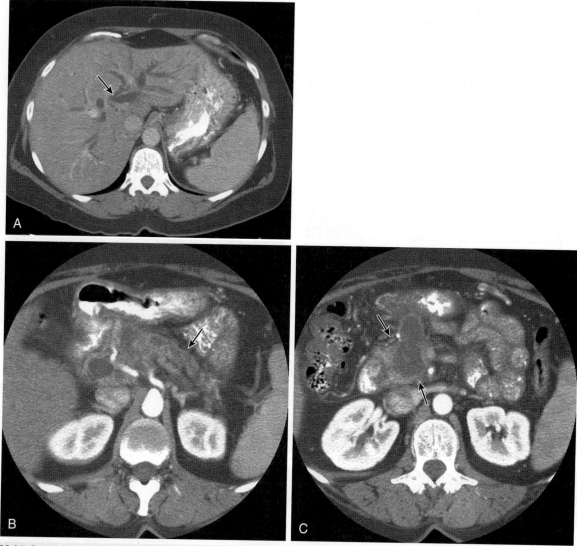

Figure 38-21 A to C, Pancreatic cancer, pancreatic head mass, with biliary and pancreatic ductal dilation. *Arrows* show fluid collections (ascites). (Courtesy Dr. Perry Pernicano.)

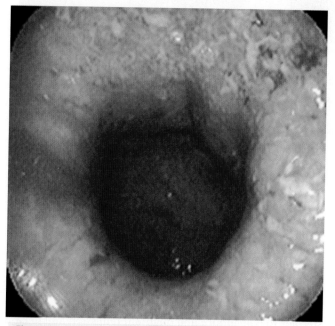

Figure 38-22 A to C, Severe colitis. (Courtesy Dr. Erik-Jan Wamsteker.)

Extraintestinal manifestations may be the presenting symptoms of UC or Crohn disease. Uveitis, iritis, or episcleritis often flares concomitantly with intestinal symptoms. Large-joint pain and sacroiliitis may be a form of enteropathic arthritis. Common skin manifestations include erythema nodosum, perianal fistulas, and pyoderma gangrenosum. IBS is much more prevalent than IBD, and thus a major pitfall in the diagnosis of IBD is the mislabeling of patients with IBS.

The finding of confluent erythematous rectal inflammation is most consistent with UC and infectious colitis. Whereas pseudopolyp formations indicate chronic inflammatory colitis (Figure 38-23), solitary aphthous ulcers, "rakelike" lesions, strictures, and rectal sparing are consistent with Crohn disease. Colonoscopic evaluation should include ileal intubation and biopsies of both normal and abnormal mucosa. Anal or perianal lesions, including sinus tracts, rectovaginal fistulas, and abscesses, is consistent with Crohn disease but not with UC. The mucosa in a patient with Crohn disease may appear cobblestoned or nodular. Loss of haustra, distortion of normal architecture, or both may be found (Figures 38-24 and 38-25).

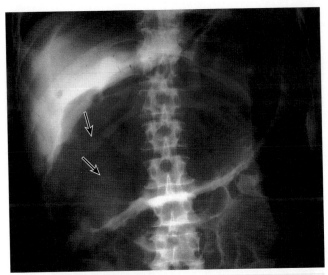

Figure 38-23 Ulcerative colitis, pseudopolyps *(arrows)*. (Courtesy Dr. Perry Pernicano.)

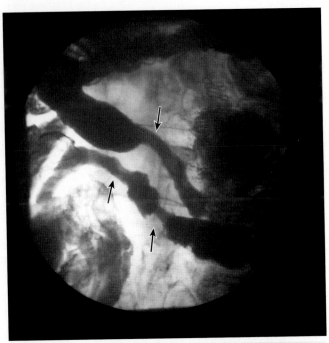

Figure 38-24 Crohn disease. *Arrows* point to colonic wall thickening, which is indicative of Crohn disease. (Courtesy Dr. Perry Pernicano.)

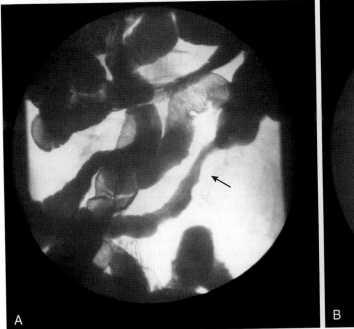
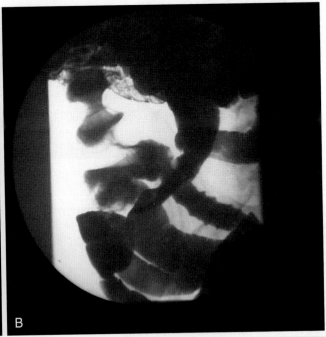

Figure 38-25 A and **B,** Crohn disease. The *arrow* points to colonic wall thickening, which is indicative of Crohn disease. (Courtesy Dr. Perry Pernicano.)

Pharmacologic treatment of IBD is aimed at inducing remission and maintaining a symptom-free life, often after consultation with a gastroenterologist. Treatment of active flares with systemic steroids has been the mainstay of remission induction therapy, producing remission rates up to 70% in Crohn disease versus 30% with placebo; similar results have been shown in the remission of UC. Budesonide, a nonsystemic steroid used in an enema formulation, has been effective for induction of remission in Crohn disease and distal UC flares. Mild flares of UC are usually treated with 5-ASA derivatives such as sulfasalazine, although RCTs have shown 5-ASA only marginally superior to placebo at controlling flare-ups of Crohn disease. 5-ASA products are thought to be inferior to budesonide and systemic steroids for remission induction in Crohn disease and generally are not used (Higgins and Zimmerman, 2004).

Azathioprine and its metabolite, 6-mercaptopurine, are slow-acting compounds proved effective for inducing remission in Crohn disease. They often are added to systemic steroids to help induce and maintain remission and to ease steroid tapering. Methotrexate is also effective for remission induction in Crohn disease. Close monitoring of CBC and serum transaminases is recommended, with monthly testing on initiation and with dosage changes. Pregnancy and exposure to live-virus vaccines should be avoided. Infliximab, an anti–tumor necrosis factor α antibody, is remarkably effective in treating approximately 60% of steroid-resistant patients with Crohn disease. Infliximab has significant side effect risks, including infusion reactions, and, rarely, worsening of heart failure, activation of latent tuberculosis, serum sickness, and invasive fungal infections (Feagan, 2003).

KEY TREATMENT

- Systemic steroid therapy is effective in the treatment of active flare-ups of Crohn disease and UC (Hanauer and Baert, 1994) (SOR: A).
- Budesonide is effective for remission induction in Crohn disease and distal UC flares (Kuhbacher and Fölsch, 2007) (SOR: A).

IRRITABLE BOWEL SYNDROME

Key Points

- IBS likely represents the clinical expression of multiple potential pathophysiologic factors, including a genetic predisposition to the disease, disturbed central nervous system (CNS) pain processing, visceral hypersensitivity, mucosal inflammation, abnormal colonic motility, and emotional stress.
- Anxiety disorders, somatoform disorders, and a history of physical or sexual abuse have been identified in 42% to 61% of patients with IBS referred to gastroenterologists.

Irritable bowel syndrome is one of the most common conditions encountered in family practices, with a prevalence ranging from 1% to 20% worldwide and approximately 7% in the United States. IBS is characterized by abdominal pain, bloating, and disturbed defecation in the absence of known structural or biochemical abnormality. It typically appears in the late 20s, although it may present in teenagers and in patients as old as age 45 years; patients older than 45 years with suspected IBS should be evaluated for organic disease. IBS is responsible for more than $20 billion in direct and indirect expenditures annually in the United States, and patients with IBS consume 50% more health care resources than matched control participants without IBS (ACG, 2009).

Irritable bowel syndrome likely represents the clinical expression of multiple potential pathophysiologic factors, including a genetic predisposition to the disease, disturbed CNS pain processing, visceral hypersensitivity, mucosal inflammation, abnormal colonic motility, and emotional stress. Given the degree of variation of IBS symptoms in affected patients, it is likely that the etiology of IBS is a heterogeneous combination of these factors, as well as other

Table 38-11 Diagnosis of Irritable Bowel Syndrome: Rome III Criteria

Symptoms of recurrent abdominal pain or discomfort and a marked change in bowel habit for at least 6 months, with symptoms experienced on at least 3 days of at least 3 months.

Two or more of the following must apply:
- Pain is relieved by a bowel movement.
- Onset of pain is related to a change in frequency of stool.
- Onset of pain is related to a change in the appearance of stool.

Modified from Longstreth GF, Thompson WG, Chey WD, et.al. Functional bowel disorders. *Gastroenterology* 2006;130:1480-1491.

undetermined mechanisms. Psychosocial stressors likely exacerbate symptoms in patients with functional GI disorders. Anxiety disorders, somatoform disorders, and a history of physical or sexual abuse have been identified in 42% to 61% of patients with IBS who have been referred to gastroenterologists (Miller et al., 2001).

The physical examination in patients with IBS is often nonspecific and may demonstrate a normal abdomen examination, a diffusely tender abdomen, or a focally tender abdomen. Multiple diagnostic screening tests have been recommended, including a CBC, erythrocyte sedimentation rate, serum chemistries, thyroid function tests, stool cultures (including ova and parasites), fecal occult blood test, colonoscopy, and hydrogen breath testing, specifically to rule out other causes of disease (ACG, 2009). Despite these recommendations, diagnostic testing should depend on the pretest probability of organic disease.

The differential diagnosis of IBS includes IBD, lactose intolerance, acute gastroenteritis, celiac disease, small intestinal bacterial overgrowth, colorectal cancer (CRC), and motility-altering metabolic disturbances (e.g., from hypo- or hyperthyroidism). Currently, the Rome III criteria are the most widely accepted symptomatic classification of IBS (Table 38-11) (Longstreth et al., 2006).

There is no single evidence-based, consistently successful therapeutic approach for patients with IBS. Because it is largely a chronic condition, the goals of therapy should focus on patient reassurance, education about the natural course of the syndrome, and global symptomatic improvement rather than on disease cure. This is best achieved through a well-developed physician–patient relationship with a clear delineation of realistic goals and expectations.

Newer treatments of IBS include tegaserod (Zelnorm), a 5-HT4 receptor agonist shown to be more effective than placebo in relieving global symptoms in women with constipation-predominant IBS. Alosetron (Lotronex), a 5-HT3 antagonist, is indicated for women with diarrhea-predominant IBS and is more effective than placebo in RCTs. Reports of ischemic colitis have limited the use of alosetron to physicians participating in the manufacturer's risk management program. Treatment of diarrhea-predominant IBS can be achieved with loperamide, although no effect over placebo for global IBS symptoms has been reported (Brandt et al., 2002). Interestingly, open-label studies in which the study subjects were told they were receiving a placebo for their IBS showed similar benefits as the best alosetron study.

To date, all other classes of medications used in the management of IBS have more limited impact on the global symptoms of IBS. The tricyclic antidepressants (TCAs) and selective serotonin reuptake inhibitors have been shown to reduce abdominal pain, although global symptom reduction and HRQOL did not significantly improve compared with placebo. Treatment of constipation-predominant IBS can be achieved with fiber-bulking agents but has not improved global IBS symptoms over placebo.

Cognitive-behavioral therapy (CBT), interpersonal psychotherapy, group therapy, biofeedback, and hypnosis have been shown to improve individual aspects of diarrhea-predominant IBS (see Key Treatment). Complementary and alternative medicine (CAM) techniques include acupuncture, enteric-coated peppermint oil, probiotic therapy, and Chinese herbal medicine. CAM therapies are becoming increasingly popular in the treatment of GI disorders and have shown some limited symptomatic improvement in select patients with IBS (ACG, 2009).

KEY TREATMENT

- CBT for IBS (efficacy defined as >50% reduction of symptoms) showed significant benefit with a mean number needed to treat (NTT) versus control participants of approximately two (two patients NTT for one to benefit) (meta-analysis of 17 studies; Lackner et al., 2004) (SOR: A).
- Gut-directed hypnotherapy can have long-lasting effects; of 204 patients with resistant IBS symptoms, 81% of initial responders had benefit 5 years after completion of treatment (Gonsalkorale et al., 2003) (SOR: B).
- Fiber bulking agents can help treat constipation-predominant IBS (Mertz, 2003) (SOR: B).
- Enteric-coated peppermint oil (0.2-0.4 mL [200-400 mg] three times daily in adults) reduced pain and spasm of IBS (Ford et al., 2008; Merat et al., 2009) (SOR: B).
- The TCAs should be considered in the treatment of pain-predominant IBS (Mertz, 2003) (SOR: B).
- Tegaserod is more effective than placebo at relieving global IBS symptoms in female patients with constipation-predominant IBS (ACG, 2009) (SOR: A).
- Alosetron is more effective than placebo at relieving global IBS symptoms in female patients with diarrhea-predominant IBS (ACG, 2009) (SOR: A).

LOWER GASTROINTESTINAL BLEEDING

Lower GI bleeding (LGIB) is defined as bleeding arising from a source distal to the ligament of Treitz, with the resultant potential for rapid hemodynamic instability. Physical signs of hemodynamic compromise include orthostatic hypotension, fatigue, pallor, palpitations, chest pain, dyspnea, tachypnea, and tachycardia. Hemodynamic stabilization through large-bore IV fluid resuscitation should be initiated immediately if acute LGIB is suspected, and blood transfusion may be necessary. Laboratory testing should include CBC, comprehensive panel, coagulation profile, iron studies (including transferrin saturation), reticulocyte count (before transfusion), and blood type and crossmatch. Clotting disorders and anticoagulant use, including daily

Table 38-12   Causes of Massive Acute Rectal Bleeding

Cause	Frequency (%)
UPPER GI TRACT	
Peptic ulcer disease	40-79
Gastritis, duodenitis	5-30
Esophageal varices	6-21
Mallory-Weiss tear	3-15
Esophagitis	2-8
Gastric cancer	2-3
Dieulafoy lesion	<1
Gastric AVMs	<1
Portal gastropathy	<1
LOWER GI TRACT	
Small Bowel	
Angiodysplasia	70-80
Jejunoileal diverticula	<1
Meckel diverticulum	<1
Neoplasms or lymphomas (benign and malignant)	<1
Enteritis, Crohn disease	<1
Aortoduodenal fistula in patient with synthetic vascular graft	<1
Large Bowel	
Diverticular disease	17-40
AVMs	2-30
Colitis	9-21
Colonic neoplasms, postpolypectomy bleeding	11-14
Anorectal causes (hemorrhoids, rectal varices, fissures)	4-10
Colonic tuberculosis	<1

AVM, arteriovenous malformation; *GI,* gastrointestinal.
Modified from Manning-Dimmitt LL, Dimmitt SG, Wilson GR. Diagnosis of gastrointestinal bleeding in adults. *Am Fam Physician* 2005;71:1339-1346.

aspirin or NSAIDs, should be identified during history taking. Figures 38-26 and 38-27 provide a detailed algorithm for the workup of LGIB.

The American Society for Gastrointestinal Endoscopy Standards of Practice Committee recommends colonoscopy as the preferred modality for the evaluation and treatment of LGIB, allowing for direct visualization of the source of bleeding in more than 70% of cases, as well as therapeutic intervention and tissue biopsy. Table 38-12 lists the frequency of the most common causes of LGIB. When no obvious colonic source of bleeding is discovered on lower endoscopy, upper endoscopy is done to evaluate potential causes of rapid, significant UGIB interpreted as LGIB. If there is still no identifiable source of bleeding, examination of the small intestine using enteroclysis or capsule endoscopy should be considered. Intubation of the terminal ileum at the time of colonoscopy may be useful, particularly when there is blood throughout the colon; fresh blood emanating from the ileum indicates small intestinal bleeding (Eisen et al., 2001).

The combination of an overall higher diagnostic yield and a lower rate of complications makes colonoscopy the preferred choice over angiography as the initial test in most patients with suspected GI bleeding. Colonoscopy may

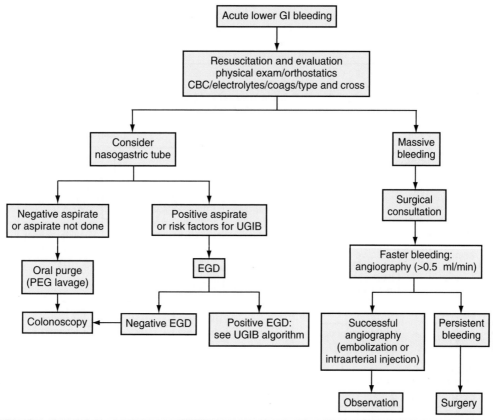

Figure 38-26 Algorithm for the management of acute lower gastrointestinal bleeding (part 1). *CBC,* Complete blood count; *EGD,* esophagogastroduodenoscopy; *PEG,* percutaneous endoscopic gastrostomy; *UGIB,* upper gastrointestinal bleeding. (Modified from Eisen GM, Dominitz JA, Faigel DO, et al; American Society for Gastrointestinal Endoscopy, Standards of Practice Committee. An annotated algorithmic approach to acute lower gastrointestinal bleeding. *Gastrointest Endosc.* 2001;53:859-863.)

be performed urgently or electively, depending on the patient's hemodynamic status and risk-stratification criteria. Comorbid risk factors for GI bleeding severity, including advanced age, presence or absence of shock, congestive heart failure, ischemic heart disease, and stigmata of recent hemorrhage, accurately predict the likelihood of death or rebleeding (Rockall et al., 1996). In patients with LGIB who are hemodynamically stable, a clean-out preparation (e.g., GoLytely) should be used before colonoscopy to increase visibility and diagnostic yield. In patients with hematochezia and hemodynamic compromise, consideration should be given to a rapidly bleeding upper GI source, the patient should be kept NPO, and a nasogastric tube should be placed. A bloody aspirate or one without blood or bile, a history of NSAID use or previous PUD, or a patient with massive bleeding may prompt performance of upper endoscopy before evaluation of the colon (Eisen et al., 2001).

The ^{99m}Tc pertechnetate–labeled red blood cell (RBC) scan is a safe and noninvasive alternative to angiography. Slower rates of bleeding may be detected with this technique, but it is not as accurate in identifying the exact location of a bleeding site. When arteriography is used in association with a ^{99m}Tc-tagged RBC blush, the sensitivity of the arteriogram is increased to 61% to 72% (Zuckerman et al., 2000). A retrospective study using these scans showed that an "immediate blush" (positive scan) had 60%

predictive value for an associated positive angiogram, and a "delayed blush" correlated with 93% predictive value for a negative angiogram.

Preoperative localization of the origin of LGIB is the standard practice, except in life-threatening cases of massive GI hemorrhage that necessitate emergency surgical exploration. Directed segmental resection is advised when the bleeding site is identified preoperatively, as seen in adenocarcinoma of the colon or diverticular disease limited to the left colon with persistent or recurrent bleeding. The removal of identified colonic lesions does not always result in effective treatment of the underlying source of bleeding. In these cases, arteriography can be used intraoperatively as an adjunct to localize a source of bleeding, facilitate segmental resection of the bowel, and prevent "blind hemicolectomy" (Manning-Dimmitt et al., 2005). A transfusion requirement of greater than 4 units of packed RBCs in 24 hours and recurrent diverticular bleeding (seen in up to 30% of patients) are common indications for surgical intervention. Other factors, such as comorbidities and individual surgical practices, play a significant role in this decision (Eisen et al., 2001).

In patients with chronic intermittent rectal bleeding, upper endoscopy is the preferred test for evaluation, with sensitivity and specificity of 92% and 100%, respectively. A barium-contrast upper GI series with small bowel follow-through (SBFT) may be considered if there is a relative

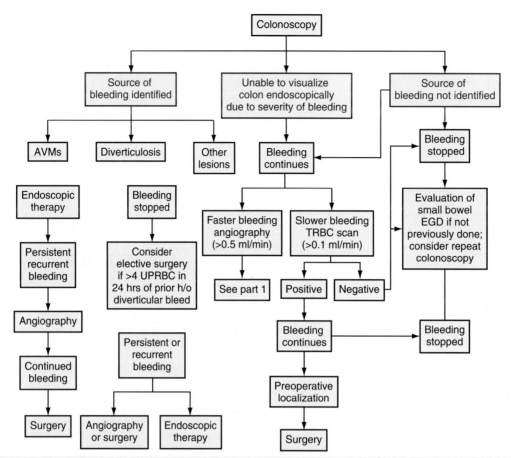

Figure 38-27 Algorithm for the management of acute lower gastrointestinal bleeding (part 2). *AVM,* Arteriovenous malformation; *TRBC,* tagged (radio-labeled) red blood cell; *UPRBC,* units of packed red blood cell. (Modified from Eisen GM, Dominitz JA, Faigel DO, et al; American Society for Gastrointestinal Endoscopy, Standards of Practice Committee. An annotated algorithmic approach to acute lower gastrointestinal bleeding. *Gastrointest Endosc.* 2001;53:859-863.)

contraindication to endoscopy (e.g., anticoagulation therapy, high risk for complications with conscious sedation, endoscopist unavailable). This test has sensitivity and specificity of 54% and 91%, respectively, in the detection of upper GI lesions located above the ligament of Treitz (Zuckerman et al., 2000). Transcatheter embolization is an alternative when vasopressin is unsuccessful or contraindicated but carries a risk of acute abdominal pain and intestinal infarction (Eisen et al., 2001).

Small intestinal sources of GI bleeding account for fewer than 10% of all cases. When upper and lower endoscopy have failed to determine the suspected cause of bleeding, the physician should consider *push enteroscopy* (extension of upper endoscopy that allows visualization of up to 160 cm of small bowel distal to ligament of Treitz), although this procedure is limited by its inability to visualize the entire small bowel and thus carries a low diagnostic yield. The barium-contrast upper GI series with SBFT carries a very low sensitivity of zero to 5.6%. *Enteroclysis* (endoscopic placement of radiopaque contrast directly into proximal small bowel) also has low sensitivity but has a shorter procedure time and can be used in the unconscious or uncooperative patient. Enteroclysis combined with push

enteroscopy has higher diagnostic sensitivity than either method alone. Arteriography can be used in challenging cases to evaluate bleeding not identified by endoscopy. It is particularly helpful in the evaluation of older patients in whom arteriovenous malformations or neoplasms are suspected because both of these lesions are associated with characteristic vascular patterns that can be identified on arteriography. Capsule endoscopy is being studied as another modality for identifying small bowel bleeding and neoplastic pathology but is limited in that biopsy samples cannot be obtained. Enhanced helical CT scanning is being explored as an alternative means of evaluating GI bleeding. Laparotomy with intraoperative enteroscopy should be considered a last resort in the diagnostic evaluation of nonemergent cases of GI bleeding because it is associated with higher rates of morbidity and mortality (Zuckerman et al., 2000).

KEY TREATMENT

• Colonoscopy is the preferred modality used in the treatment of lower GI bleeding (Zuccaro, 1998) (SOR: A).

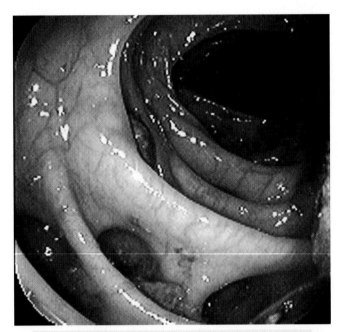

Figure 38-28 Diverticulosis. (Courtesy Dr. Erik-Jan Wamsteker.)

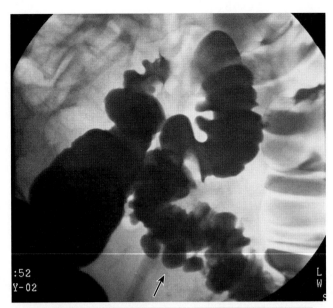

Figure 38-30 Sigmoid diverticula. (Courtesy Dr. Perry Pernicano.)

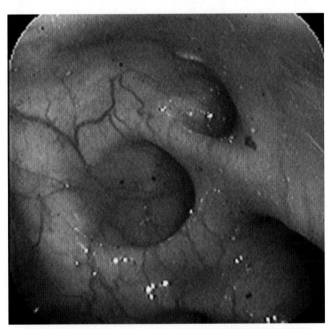

Figure 38-29 Diverticulosis. (Courtesy Dr. Erik-Jan Wamsteker.)

DIVERTICULAR DISEASE

Diverticulosis refers to the presence of diverticula, or herniations of the intestinal mucosa and submucosa, most often in the sigmoid colon (Figures 38-28 and 38-29). More than half of patients older than age 50 years have incidental colonic diverticula. *Diverticulitis* is the most common complication of diverticulosis, occurring in up to 20% of patients, and results from a microperforation of a diverticulum from inspissated fecal material that often becomes a phlegmon, or a pericolic or intraabdominal abscess.

The initial assessment of the patient with suspected diverticulitis should include a thorough history and physical examination, including abdominal, rectal, and pelvic examinations. The majority of patients have LLQ pain (93%-100%), fever (57%-100%), and leukocytosis (69%-83%). Other associated features include nausea, vomiting, constipation, diarrhea, dysuria, and urinary frequency. The differential diagnosis includes IBS, IBD, colon cancer, ischemic colitis, bowel obstruction, and gynecologic and urologic disorders (American Society of Colon and Rectal Surgeons [ASCRS], 2000). Initial evaluation of the patient with abdominal pain and suspected diverticulitis includes CBC, urinalysis, and flat and upright abdominal radiographs.

The ASCRS Standards Task Force for the treatment of diverticulitis state that if the patient's clinical picture clearly suggests acute diverticulitis, the diagnosis can be made on the basis of clinical criteria alone (ASCRS, 2000). The need for additional tests in the patient with suspected diverticulitis is determined by the severity of the presenting signs and symptoms and diagnostic confidence. When the diagnosis of diverticulitis is in question, other tests may include water-soluble contrast enema, abdominal CT, or ultrasonography.

Criteria for the diagnosis of diverticulitis on water-soluble contrast enema include the presence of diverticula (Figures 38-30 and 38-31), mass effect, intramural mass, sinus tract, and extravasation of contrast. Ultrasonography may reveal bowel wall thickening, abscess, and rigid hyperechogenicity of the colon caused by inflammation and may be helpful in female patients to exclude pelvic or gynecologic pathology. CT with oral and IV contrast is increasingly used as the initial imaging test for patients with suspected diverticulitis, particularly if disease of moderate severity or abscess is anticipated. Endoscopy is usually avoided in the setting of acute diverticulitis because of the risk of perforating the inflamed colon, either with the instrument itself or by insufflation of air. When the diagnosis of acute colonic diverticulitis is uncertain, limited flexible sigmoidoscopy with minimum insufflation of air may be performed to exclude other diagnoses.

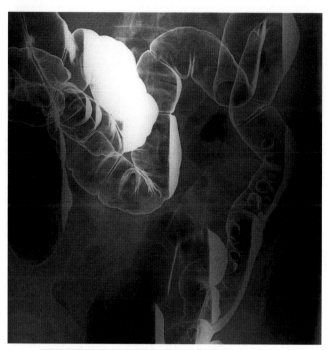

Figure 38-31 Diverticula. (Courtesy Dr. Perry Pernicano.)

Conservative medical management of uncomplicated diverticulitis without associated abscess, fistula, obstruction, or perforation includes bowel rest and IV fluoroquinolones or extended-spectrum penicillins. If the patient does not improve after several days, an abscess should be suspected and diagnostic imaging considered. Conservative treatment results in resolution in 70% to 100% of cases (ASCRS, 2000). After recovery from an initial episode of diverticulitis, when the inflammation has subsided, the patient should be reevaluated. Appropriate examinations include a combination of flexible sigmoidoscopy and single- or double-contrast barium enema or colonoscopy. Eventual resumption of a high-fiber diet is recommended after acute inflammation resolves; long-term fiber supplementation after the first episode of diverticulitis has been shown to prevent recurrence in more than 70% of patients followed up with for more than 5 years.

The decision of whether to proceed with inpatient or outpatient treatment of diverticulitis depends on the clinical judgment of the physician, the severity of the disease process, and the likelihood that the patient's condition will respond to outpatient therapy. Patients who are able to tolerate a diet, who do not have systemic symptoms, and who do not have significant peritoneal signs may be treated on an outpatient basis with TMP-SMX or a fluoroquinolone plus metronidazole (Gilbert et al., 2009).

Primary resection and anastomosis without a protective stoma has become the surgical treatment of choice for uncomplicated diverticulitis and may also be performed for patients with localized pericolic or pelvic abscess. A single-stage procedure is associated with decreased hospital stays and has lower mortality and morbidity rates than two- and three-stage procedures. The most common two-stage operation is the Hartmann procedure, which carries a mortality rate of 2.6% to 36.8% (ASCRS, 2000). Surgical treatment of diverticulitis, in both acute and chronic settings, has been successfully accomplished by laparoscopic and laparoscopic-assisted means.

Treatment of the patient with multiple attacks of diverticulitis or recurrent diverticulitis is individualized to minimize the morbidity and mortality of intervention. Factors considered when deciding whether to proceed with resection include the patient's age; number, severity, and interval of attacks; rapidity and degree of response to medical therapy; and persistence of symptoms after an acute attack. The risk of recurrent symptoms after an attack of diverticulitis ranges from 7% to 45%. With each episode, the patient is less likely to respond to medical therapy (70% respond to medical therapy after first attack vs. 6% after third). Thus, after two attacks of uncomplicated diverticulitis, resection is usually recommended (ASCRS, 2000).

KEY TREATMENT

- Patients who can tolerate a diet and do not have systemic symptoms or significant peritoneal signs may be treated as outpatients with TMP-SMX or a fluoroquinolone plus metronidazole (Gilbert et al., 2009) (SOR: B).
- Surgery may be necessary in some patients both in uncomplicated and complicated diverticulitis and should be individualized (Stollman and Raskin, 2004) (SOR: B).

CELIAC DISEASE

Key Points

- Tests to consider in testing for celiac disease include transglutaminase immunoglobulin (IgA), antiendomysial antibody, antigliadin antibody, and the genetic test human leukocyte antigen (HLA) DQ2/DQ8.
- A negative HLA DQ2/DQ8 test result is most helpful in ruling out celiac disease. A positive test result does not rule it in but is associated with an increased risk.
- Consider an elimination or challenge diet for 2 weeks. If symptoms improve, a rechallenge with gluten-containing foods will cause a recurrence of symptoms.
- The antibody test results (tissue transglutaminase antibody [TTG] IgA, antiendomysial, antigliadin) can become negative after elimination of gluten protein and may be false negative.

There has been a substantial increase in the prevalence of celiac disease over the past 50 years and an increase in the rate of diagnosis in the past 10 years. The adult presentation of celiac disease is characterized by weight loss, diarrhea, fatigue, and anemia. Children frequently present with failure to thrive, vomiting, diarrhea, muscle wasting, signs of hypoproteinemia (including possible ascites), and general irritability. Common comorbidities include type 1 diabetes mellitus, cerebral calcifications, Sjögren syndrome, and thyroid disease. Celiac disease should be considered in cases of unexplained folic acid, iron or vitamin B_{12} deficiency, reduced serum albumin concentration, osteoporosis, and osteomalacia. Other presentations may include infertility or recurrent miscarriage. Splenic atrophy commonly occurs in celiac sprue, and pneumococcal immunization should be administered in these patients.

Immunoglobulin A antiendomysial antibodies are currently the most accurate serologic test for diagnosing celiac sprue with a sensitivity of 97% to 100% and specificity of 98% to 99%. Antigliadin antibodies are also usually quantified. Enzyme tissue transglutaminase, the antigen for antiendomysial antibodies, has a sensitivity of 95% and specificity of 94% in diagnosing celiac disease (Rubio-Tapia, 2013). HLA testing can now be done to evaluate persons at risk for celiac. About 95% of patients with celiac disease are positive for HLA-DQ2 and 5% for HLA-DQ8. The majority of people who test positive for HLA-DQ2/DQ8 are at risk, but only 2% to 3% actually develop celiac disease. Celiac disease is rarely seen with a negative test result, and thus this test is most useful when the result is negative. A positive test result does not make the diagnosis. A CBC, comprehensive biochemical profile (including serum albumin concentration), transferrin saturation, serum or RBC folate, vitamin B_{12}, and liver function tests should also be obtained on diagnosis. Deficiencies of iron, folic acid, calcium, and vitamins B_{12} and D frequently often correct after initiating a gluten-free diet (GFD) without the need for vitamin supplementation.

The diagnostic standard for celiac disease is a small intestinal biopsy using endoscopy, although this is usually not necessary to establish an accurate diagnosis. Characteristic changes include damage to the normal villous morphology with decreased villous height or crypt depth, decreased epithelial surface cell height, and increased lymphocytic infiltration of the intestinal mucosa. The accepted AGA diagnostic criteria state that small intestinal mucosa should be abnormal while patients continue on a gluten diet. A repeat biopsy should be taken 4 to 6 months after induction of treatment, and if there has been no improvement in the small intestinal mucosal morphology, the original diagnosis should be questioned. Many gastroenterologists do not obtain a subsequent biopsy specimen, and the cost effectiveness of this approach has not been demonstrated. A gluten challenge is recommended if there is any doubt concerning the correct diagnosis (AGA, 2006).

The AGA guidelines state that the cornerstone of treatment of celiac disease and its resultant complications is GFD therapy under a nutritionist's guidance. Patients should completely omit wheat, rye, barley, beer, and breakfast cereals from their diets. It is important to explain the disease process and toxicity of gluten-containing foods to the patient, including the potential for the reversal of current celiac disease–related problems, including anemia, depression, and infertility. Gluten-free breads, pasta, and other products are commercially available and should be recommended as substitutes. Given the incomplete response of many patients to a GFD as well as the difficulty of adherence to the GFD over the long term, development of new effective therapies for symptom control and reversal of inflammation and organ damage are needed.

Patients with celiac disease usually experience rapid symptomatic improvement within weeks of the exclusion of dietary gluten, providing additional diagnostic confirmation. Monitoring of antiendomysial or TTG IgA titers, which usually normalize with the institution of a GFD, may prove useful to check dietary compliance but have neither become

standard practice nor been cost effective. Life-threatening hypokalemia or hypomagnesemia rarely occurs and should be appropriately corrected. Expert panels suggest that yearly weight, CBC, ferritin, folate, calcium, and ALP levels should be obtained for disease monitoring. Oral corticosteroids may be used in unresponsive patients but only when other causes of small intestinal villous atrophy have been excluded (AGA, 2006).

Dermatitis herpetiformis is a common extraintestinal manifestation of gluten-sensitive enteropathy characterized by a pruritic, blistering, and vesicular rash. The diagnosis is made with immunofluorescent staining of granular IgA after skin biopsy. Treatment involves oral dapsone and a GFD, and with sufficient symptom relapse after 6 months, dapsone can be withdrawn and the GFD continued indefinitely. Osteopenia and osteoporosis, as well as bone pain, pseudofractures, and orthopedic deformities, are common features of celiac disease. Osteoporosis carries a significant fracture risk, and thus dual-energy x-ray absorptiometry screening of patients with celiac disease is recommended yearly. If osteoporosis is discovered, measures include strict adherence to a GFD, calcium supplementation of up to 1500 mg/day, bisphosphonate or calcitonin therapy, or consideration of hormone replacement therapy in postmenopausal women. Smoking cessation should be encouraged and an exercise regimen advised in all patients.

Ulcerative jejunitis is a serious complication of celiac disease that carries a high mortality risk after intestinal hemorrhage, perforation, or obstruction in patients with a history of significant malnutrition. The diagnosis can be challenging, and small intestine radiography often is not helpful. If small intestinal ulceration or lymphoma is suspected, enteroscopy may be used to obtain biopsy specimens for histologic assessment. Surgical resection of the ulcer, especially if localized to one part of the intestine, can be curative. Again, a strict GFD should be initiated, and treatment with steroids has shown significant benefit. If a diagnosis of enteropathy-associated T-cell lymphoma is made, the patient should be referred to an oncologist for appropriate chemotherapy.

Overall mortality risks are higher in patients with celiac disease, attributed to malignant intestinal lymphoma and adenocarcinoma. One study found a fivefold increased risk of developing malignancy in patients with celiac disease, with a relative risk of 40 for developing non-Hodgkin lymphoma. These risks decreased to the level of the normal population after patients maintained a GFD for 5 years (AGA, 2006).

COLORECTAL CANCER

Key Point

- Average-risk individuals should begin CRC screening at age 50 years and at age 45 years in African Americans.

Colorectal cancer is the third leading cause of cancer death in the United States, accounting for an estimated 9% of all cancer deaths in 2009. Risk factors include increasing age,

Table 38-13   Current Colorectal Cancer (CRC) Screening Recommendations

Preferred screening tests	Cancer prevention tests should be offered first. The preferred CRC prevention test is colonoscopy every 10 yr, beginning at age 50 yr. Screening should begin at age 45 yr in African Americans.
	Cancer detection test should be offered to patients who decline colonoscopy or another cancer prevention test. The preferred cancer detection test is annual FIT for blood.
Alternative CRC prevention tests	Flexible sigmoidoscopy every 5 to 10 yr CT colonography every 5 yr
Alternative cancer detection tests	Annual Hemoccult Sensa Fecal DNA testing every 3 yr
Positive family history but HNPCC evaluation not indicated	Single first-degree relative with CRC or advanced adenoma diagnosed at age 60 yr or older: *Recommended screening:* Same as average risk Single first-degree relative with CRC or advanced adenoma diagnosed before age 60 yr or two first-degree relatives with CRC or advanced adenomas: *Recommended screening:* Colonoscopy every 5 yr beginning at age 40 yr or 10 yr younger than age at diagnosis of the youngest affected relative
Familial adenomatous polyposis (FAP)	Patients with classic FAP (>100 adenomas) should be advised to pursue genetic counseling and genetic testing if they have siblings or children who could potentially benefit from this testing. Patients with known FAP or who are at risk of FAP based on family history (and genetic testing has not been performed) should undergo annual flexible sigmoidoscopy or colonoscopy, as appropriate, until colectomy is deemed by physician and patient to be the best treatment. Patients with retained rectum after subtotal colectomy should undergo flexible sigmoidoscopy every 6 to 12 mo. Patients with classic FAP, in whom genetic test results are negative, should undergo genetic testing for biallelic MYH mutations. Patients with 10 to 100 adenomas can be considered for genetic testing for attenuated FAP and if the result is negative, MYH-associated polyposis.
Hereditary nonpolyposis CRC	Patients who meet the Bethesda criteria should undergo microsatellite instability testing of their tumor or a family member's tumor or tumor immunohistochemical staining for mismatch repair proteins. Patients with positive test results can be offered genetic testing. Those with positive genetic testing or those at risk when genetic testing is unsuccessful in an affected proband should undergo colonoscopy every 2 yr beginning at age 20 to 25 yr until age 40 yr and then annually thereafter.

CT, Computed tomography; *FAP,* familial adenomatous polyposis; *FIT,* fecal immunochemical test; *HNPCC,* hereditary nonpolyposis colorectal cancer.
Modified from Rex DK, Johnson DA, Anderson JC, et al. American College of Gastroenterology guidelines for colorectal cancer screening 2008. *Am J Gastroenterol* 2009;104:739-750.

a family history of CRC, obesity, a sedentary lifestyle, a diet high in red meat and low in vegetables, and excessive alcohol or tobacco use. Diets high in fiber, fruits, vegetables, and calcium may be protective, but data are inconclusive. African Americans have a 50% higher likelihood of dying from CRC than whites because they may have more proximal distribution of colonic adenomas and carcinomas than the general population, and these may be missed more often on suboptimal screening (ACS, 2009).

Approximately 75% of CRCs are diagnosed in individuals who have no risk factors other than advanced age; 90% of patients are older than 50 years. Other risk factors include prior or family history of CRC or adenomatous polyps, chronic IBD, and genetic syndromes. Several case-control and cohort studies found an inverse association between physical activity and risk in men and women of all ages and in various racial and ethnic groups in diverse geographic areas worldwide. The long-term use of aspirin may be associated with a decreased risk of CRC, yet the risk-to-benefit profile for chemoprevention cannot justify broad recommendations for its use in the general population (Nease et al., 2004).

Up to 30% of CRCs are believed to arise secondary to a genetic predisposition. Approximately 20% of cases occur among patients who have a history of CRC in a first-degree relative. About 6% are attributable to identifiable, inherited genetic mutations known as *hereditary CRC syndromes,* including familial adenomatous polyposis and hereditary nonpolyposis colorectal cancer. Although these syndromes are relatively uncommon, they confer a lifetime risk of CRC ranging from 80% to 100%.

Currently accepted methods for screening of CRC include the digital rectal examination (DRE), fecal immunochemical test (FIT), double-contrast barium enema (DCBE), flexible sigmoidoscopy, and colonoscopy. According to the AGA, "the relative virtues of each screening test can be debated, but the best test is the one that gets done" (Burt et al., 2004). Screening should begin by classifying a patient's level of risk based on personal, family, and medical history, which together determine the approach to screening in that person. Table 38-13 details current CRC screening recommendations.

The DRE is a simple, inexpensive, and minimally invasive test that can be routinely performed in the office during yearly health maintenance examinations. It allows for palpation of the internal anal canal and examination of the prostate. Along with DRE, FIT should be performed to assess for occult blood. The DRE itself has a very low diagnostic yield, identifying fewer than 10% of colorectal tumors. Sensitivity of DCBE varies widely, ranging from 50% to 80% for polyps smaller than 1 cm, 70% to 90% for polyps larger than 1 cm, and 55% to 85% for Dukes stage A and B colon cancers (Winawer et al., 1997). In a comparison study with colonoscopy, sensitivity of barium enema for neoplasia was significantly lower (32% for polyps ≤5 mm, 53% for polyps 0.6-10 mm, 48% for polyps >1 cm) (Winawer et al., 2000). Any suspected lesions identified by DCBE need to be confirmed, biopsied, and removed by colonoscopy. Rarely, the classic "apple core" hallmark sign of a colonic mass may be visualized on DCBE (Figure 38-32).

Flexible sigmoidoscopy is an efficient screening tool for individuals at an average risk for CRC, allowing for direct

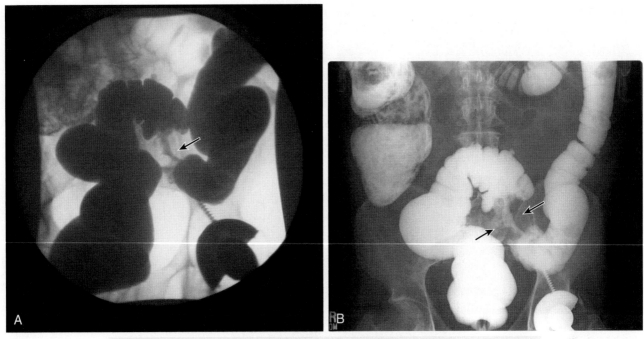

Figure 38-32 A and B, "Apple core" lesion *(arrows)* in colon cancer. (Courtesy Dr. Perry Pernicano.)

visualization and biopsy of the colonic mucosa in the rectosigmoid, descending, and distal transverse colon. To date, no RCTs or case-control studies have shown that screening with this method decreases CRC mortality for tumors within the reach of the standard 60-cm scope. The limitation of this method is that advanced lesions may be missed in the ascending and proximal transverse colon in individuals who do not have distal polyps. Although advocated as being more convenient than colonoscopy, because it is generally done in the office without the need for conscious sedation, only an estimated 30% of eligible patients undergo screening with flexible sigmoidoscopy (Nease et al., 2004). If polyps are identified during flexible sigmoidoscopy, a full colonoscopy is required to visualize the remaining colonic segments and to remove any remaining identified polyps.

Colonoscopy provides the most complete visualization of the entire colon and is the gold standard test for CRC screening. Because more than half of all individuals who have advanced proximal adenomas may not have distal polyps, many investigators advocate the use of colonoscopy as the primary modality for CRC screening. The removal of precancerous adenomas decreases CRC incidence by as much as 76% to 90% compared with no screening methodology (Figures 38-33 and 38-34). One study using colonoscopy as a screening tool in U.S. military veterans discovered advanced villous adenomas in 10.5% of subjects (Figure 38-35). Colonoscopy carries a higher risk of adverse events attributed to therapeutic interventions such as biopsy and polyp removal, compared with FIT, DCBE, and flexible sigmoidoscopy, specifically bowel perforation and postpolypectomy hemorrhage.

Newer modalities for CRC screening are being developed. Virtual colonoscopy, or CT colonography, uses thin-section helical CT scans to generate high-resolution two-dimensional images that are reconstructed into three-dimensional images of the colon to evaluate for the presence

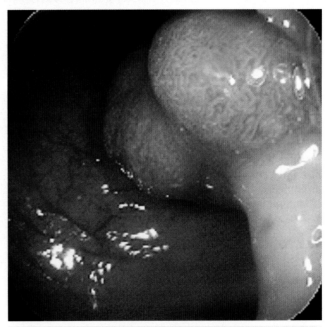

Figure 38-33 Precancerous adenomas. (Courtesy Dr. Erik-Jan Wamsteker.)

of polyps. Direct comparison of CT colonography with colonoscopy in asymptomatic adults has shown sensitivity and specificity for polyp detection comparable with that of colonoscopy for polyps larger than 6 mm. CT colonography may be viewed as a more acceptable approach for CRC screening because it is less invasive and requires less time without the potential adverse risks of sedation or bowel perforation. Most patients prefer conventional colonoscopy, reporting more pain, more discomfort, and less respect from staff with CT colonography. As with conventional

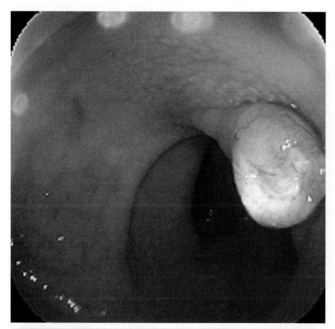

Figure 38-34 Precancerous adenomas. (Courtesy Dr. Erik-Jan Wamsteker.)

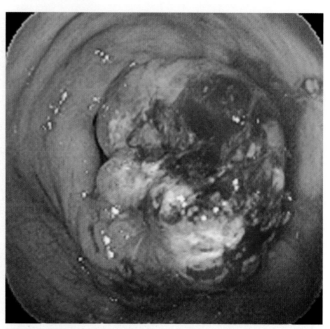

Figure 38-35 Advanced villous adenomas. (Courtesy Dr. Erik-Jan Wamsteker.)

colonoscopy, CT colonography is limited by quality of the bowel preparation, procedural cost, lack of insurance coverage, variable physician training, and procedural time.

Capsule endoscopy is another emerging technology in the detection of CRC. The patient fasts overnight, ingests a disposable capsule, and begins water intake 2 hours after the capsule is ingested; the capsule is usually expelled within 48 hours of ingestion. The recorded information from the capsule is then downloaded and reviewed for abnormal pathology. Capsule endoscopy has become an accepted method for screening the small intestine for obscure GI bleeding. For colonic imaging, however, its use has been limited because of the larger colonic diameter, residual stool, and limited battery life of the capsule.

KEY TREATMENT

- The removal of precancerous adenomas can significantly decrease CRC incidence by as much as 76% to 90% (SOR: A).

References

The complete reference list is available at www.expertconsult.com.

Web Resources

www.aafp.org American Association of Family Physicians. Topic-specific search of *American Family Physician* articles provides a concise overview of various diseases.

www.acg.gi.org The American College of Gastroenterology's site contains useful practice parameters and position statements.

www.gastro.org The American Gastroenterological Association's site contains useful practice parameters and position statements.

www.guideline.gov The National Guideline Clearinghouse provides evidence-based practice guidelines.

www.nlm.nih.gov The National Library of Medicine provides a thorough overview of disease processes.

39 *Hematology*

ETHAN A. NATELSON, ISABELLE CHUGHTAI-HARVEY, and SANA RABBI

Clinical hematology encompasses a broad domain that involves, in major part, the study of the cellular elements in the circulating blood and bone marrow, mechanisms of hemostasis and thrombosis, and features of transfusion medicine. The specific disorders that involve the hematopoietic system include both hereditary and acquired illnesses, neoplasms, autoimmune conditions, vitamin and other elemental deficiency states, and consequences of pharmacologic and environmentally encountered hematopoietic toxins. Aspects of both autologous and allogeneic bone marrow transplantation also represent an important subset of modern clinical hematology. The recognition, diagnosis, and treatment of common hematologic disorders may involve interactions among physicians practicing in all medical and surgical specialties. A detailed review of the entire field of hematology is beyond the scope of this brief chapter, and we reference useful major and abbreviated modern texts for such detailed information (Greer et al., 2013; Hillman et al., 2010; Hoffman et al., 2012; Rodgers and Young, 2013). Rather, this chapter focuses on the principles of a hematologic evaluation and potential mechanisms leading to hematologic aberrations and reviews some aspects of the more commonly seen hematologic disease states, illustrating their diagnostic features, potential complications, clinical courses, and the approach to modern therapy. Because of the importance of obstetrics in the field of family medicine, aspects of hematologic diagnosis in this area are also emphasized.

Normal hematopoiesis reflects a complex production system that, in an adult, is confined to the bone marrow, with mature cells entering the peripheral blood to carry out their specific functions during a varied finite survival. In the bone marrow, a small number of pluripotential and self-renewing stem cells give rise to modified stem cells committed to either myeloid or lymphoid development. The process is nurtured by a variety of cytokine stimuli emanating from the bone marrow stromal microenvironment. The myeloid stem cells produce the highly specialized cell lines, including the erythroid, megakaryocyte, and granulocyte precursors. The lymphoid stem cells produce a variety of B- and T-cell progenitors that confer tissue-based immunity and direct immunoglobulin synthesis. The net production of blood cells by the normal bone marrow is massive and amounts to more than 10^{11} cells/kg/day.

In considering disease states involving blood cell production, the hematopoietic system may be divided into disorders primarily affecting erythrocytes, granulocytes, platelets, and lymphoid cells. In some instances, expression of the illness may be highly specific, involving only one of these cell lines. Frequently, however, multiple cell types are involved either as a primary consequence of the disorder or as a secondary phenomenon, such as occurs with hypersplenism or postchemotherapy transient myelosuppression after treatment of a nonmyeloid malignancy.

In a general hematology practice, perhaps 60% to 70% of consultations involve nonmalignant conditions. Successful therapy for all of these circumstances begins with a differential diagnosis of causation, which should direct the selection of useful confirmatory diagnostic tests. In the modern era, an increasingly complex array of molecular-based laboratory studies and specialized imaging studies may be ordered at a keystroke of the computer but often at great expense. However, often a comprehensive history and physical examination associated with a routine blood count and a careful inspection of the peripheral blood film provides a logical direction to the next level of more sophisticated diagnostic study and, ultimately, to successful evidence-based therapy.

Terminology

In clinical medicine, each specialty acquires a unique descriptive language set that allows ease and accuracy of communication among physicians and in publications. Some of these commonly used terms involving hematology are defined as follows; primary care physicians should be generally conversant with their usage:

- **Agranulocytosis:** A sudden and selective absence of granulocytes from the circulating blood usually associated with a similar absence of granulocyte precursors in the bone marrow. In an adult, this condition is most often drug related.
- **Amegakaryocytic thrombocytopenia:** Thrombocytopenia consequent to a virtual absence of megakaryocytes and their platelet production. This is a rare entity, either congenital or more often acquired, and may be

associated with tumors of the thymus or a consequence of autoimmune illness.

- **Anemia:** A reduction in circulating erythrocyte mass below the normal range, adjusted for age and sex, and typically expressed in terms of hemoglobin concentration, red blood cell (RBC) count, or hematocrit value (the percentage of RBC volume in whole blood).

- **Anisocytosis:** Variation in the size of the erythrocytes, which should be uniform. Anisocytosis is characteristic of iron deficiency and many other forms of anemia. It is often accompanied by anisochromia, which refers to color variation in RBCs often striking in sideroblastic anemias in which there may be a dimorphic erythrocyte population consisting of both normochromic and hypochromic RBCs reflecting erythrocyte production by separate hematopoietic clones within the bone marrow.

- **Aplastic anemia:** A marked and persistent reduction in all bone marrow cellular precursors. The term *bone marrow hypoplasia* is applied to describe both transient episodes after chemotherapy and a persistent reduction in normal bone marrow cellularity but typically not to the profound degree present in aplastic anemia.

- **Cytopenia:** A reduction in circulating numbers of a specific blood cell line, for example, the terms *thrombocytopenia* to categorize a reduction in platelets, *neutropenia* to indicate a reduction in neutrophils, *lymphocytopenia* for a reduction in lymphocytes, and *pancytopenia* to signify a simultaneous reduction in erythrocytes, leukocytes, and platelets.

- **Cytosis:** An increase in numbers of a specific blood cell line. Thus, *erythrocytosis* for an increase in circulating erythrocytes, *leukocytosis* for an increase in total white blood cells (WBCs), *thrombocytosis* to signify an increase in the platelet count, but *thrombocythemia* when the cause for thrombocytosis is a myeloproliferative neoplasm (MPN). Similarly, the designation of *philia* to a cell line description also indicates an increase in numbers, such as *eosinophilia* to designate an increase in eosinophils, *basophilia* to indicate an increase in circulating basophils, and *thrombocytophilia* for an increase in platelet count.

- **Hematopoiesis:** Also referred to as *myelopoiesis*, it is the process by which stem cells may self-renew and differentiate into a variety of highly specialized blood cells, which then continuously populate the bone marrow and peripheral blood. On occasion, this process may occur outside the bone marrow and in the liver, lymph nodes, and spleen, for example, and is then referred to as *extramedullary* hematopoiesis.

- **Hypersplenism:** The consequence of an overactive and usually enlarged spleen that may remove, sequester, or destroy normal blood cells during their passage through the spleen. The process may be selective, as in idiopathic thrombocytopenic purpura (ITP) for platelets, or involve all cell lines, as is common in advanced hepatic cirrhosis with portal hypertension.

- **Ineffective hematopoiesis:** The normal bone marrow is highly efficient, and more than 90% of cells produced exit into the peripheral blood and circulate for their normal life span. The process is so effective that even with reduction in bone marrow cellularity to 20% of normal, the peripheral blood counts may remain in the normal range. With ineffective erythropoiesis, even with normal bone marrow cellularity, only 5% to 10% of hematopoietic cells produced may actually exit the bone marrow and support cell functions; the remainder undergo premature intramedullary cell death by various apoptotic mechanisms.

- **Karyorrhexis:** Abnormal condensation and fracture of nuclear chromatin characteristic of senescent blood cells and often evident among the atypical nuclei of granulocytes of some individuals with myelodysplastic syndromes (MDS) and acute myeloid leukemia (AML) syndromes.

- **Leukemia:** The presence of circulating malignant cells derived from hematopoietic tissues. These illnesses are generally divided into four broad categories, which include acute myeloid leukemia (AML), acute lymphoid leukemia (ALL), chronic myeloid leukemia (CML), and chronic lymphocytic leukemia (CLL). Many other neoplastic hematopoietic disorders may manifest a leukemic phase, and these consist primarily of B-cell neoplasms such as variants of non-Hodgkin lymphoma (NHL), hairy cell leukemia, and multiple myeloma (MM).

- **Lymphoma:** A large and diverse group of malignancies of both B and T lymphocytes and often involving the bone marrow and inhibiting normal bone marrow function. They are generally divided into Hodgkin lymphoma (HL) and the far more common NHL, which includes both B- and T-cell subtypes.

- **Myelodysplasia:** Frequently, terms such as *myelodysplasia, dysplasia, dyspoiesis,* and *dysmyelopoiesis* are used by hematopathologists and clinical hematologists to describe morphologic aberrations in precursor hematopoietic cells. Many confuse myelodysplasia as equivalent to the grouping of disorders classified as the MDS, which is incorrect. Even bone marrows from patients with simple iron-deficiency anemia may exhibit marked dyspoiesis among erythroid precursors.

- **Myelodysplastic syndromes:** The MDS are generally described as clonal myeloid disorders characterized by progressive peripheral blood cytopenias typically noted early as unexplained macrocytic anemia associated with ineffective myelopoiesis. These syndromes demonstrate variable degrees of morphologic cellular dysplasia in the bone marrow and peripheral blood cells that may affect a single or multiple cell lines. They are often considered neoplasms because of frequently associated genetic mutations and patient-limited survival with progression to AML or death related to the consequences of bone marrow failure, including infection, hemorrhage, and iron overload. However, not all of these disorders are neoplasms, and some MDS respond favorably to immunosuppressive therapy (Epling-Burnette et al., 2012; Natelson et al., 2013).

- **Myeloproliferative neoplasms:** Hematopoietic states characterized by overproduction of one or more of the three major cell lines. The classical forms are polycythemia vera, essential thrombocytosis, and primary myelofibrosis. These disorders are linked by a molecular mutation in the JAK-2 locus. Originally, CML was placed in this classification, but it is now a stand-alone illness characterized by the Philadelphia chromosome t(9:22) translocation. The World Health Organization (WHO) currently considers all of these disorders and a separate group of atypical myeloproliferative syndromes as neoplasms (Swerdlow et al., 2008).

- **Myelophthisic anemias:** The bone marrow may become infiltrated with reticulin fibrosis, metastatic tumor, or abnormal storage histocytes, reducing the capacity for normal blood production. In these circumstances, nucleated erythrocytes and early myeloid cells may circulate in the peripheral blood, producing a *leukoerythroblastic* reaction.
- **Panmyelosis:** A marked overproduction of all bone marrow cellular precursors.
- **Poikilocytosis:** Variation among RBC shapes on the peripheral blood film and particularly striking in severe iron-deficiency anemia and RBC fragmentation syndromes.
- **Polycythemia:** This term and *erythrocytosis* have become synonyms for excess RBCs, and polycythemia does not imply simultaneous increases in multiple cell lines that may occur during the course of the MPN polycythemia vera.
- **Pure RBC aplasia:** Absence of RBC precursors from an often otherwise normal bone marrow and typically occurring on an autoimmune basis consequent to an adverse drug reaction or the presence of a thymoma. This state may also appear during the course of CLL. Other potential causes include parvovirus infection, particularly in immune-compromised individuals and riboflavin deficiency.
- **Rouleaux:** The description of groups of RBCs assuming an association on a peripheral blood film resembling a roll of coins. This is typically related to elevated plasma globulin levels, monoclonal or polyclonal, and brings to mind disorders such as MM, chronic hepatitis, Waldenström macroglobulinemia (WM), sarcoidosis, or the presence of erythrocyte cold agglutinins.
- **Xenobiotics:** Chemical compounds and their metabolites not native to the body that may interfere with normal hematopoiesis, causing various forms of *myelotoxicity*. Such chemicals may be found as therapeutic drugs, foods, and occupational or environmental chemical exposures.

Specific Hematologic Disease States

The following section describes toxicity targeting the cellular elements in the circulating blood and bone marrow by affecting their numbers, their function, or both. Such hematotoxicity may be a direct chemical consequence of various xenobiotics in the form of either an idiosyncratic host response or with an effect related to dose and duration of the toxic exposure. In some instances, the toxicity may be mediated through stimulation of the immune system, inducing production of autoantibodies in a fashion that may cause a selective cellular breakdown or with a more broad toxicity affecting all cellular elements. Deficiency of limiting reagents to blood production such as certain vitamins and iron may also cause hematologic disease. Typically, hematotoxicity is manifest by a reduction in blood cell production, but under certain circumstances, the introduction of toxic agents may stimulate excessive production of blood cells and result in clinical illness. Neoplastic diseases of the blood-forming elements may result in a variety of cytopenias, as in MDS and AML, as well as increases in circulating blood cells, as in the MPN. Metastatic neoplasms such as breast and prostate cancer may also involve the bone marrow, crowding out or suppressing normal function and causing a myelophthisic form of anemia.

DISORDERS OF RED BLOOD CELLS

Key Points

- A diagnosis of iron-deficiency anemia mandates the search for a cause in addition to initiating therapy.
- Chronic ice hunger or other forms of pica suggest a diagnosis of iron deficiency.
- Oral preparations of iron salts such as sulfate, fumarate, and gluconate are generally equally effective, but timed-release iron formulations should not be prescribed.
- Patients with chronic iron deficiency consequent to bariatric surgery with roux-en-y anatomy and some individuals with celiac sprue may need periodic intravenous infusion of iron conjugates to avoid iron deficiency and anemia.
- Patients with sickle cell disease should receive the pneumococcal vaccination.
- Patients with sickle cell trait are typically not anemic from the illness but may experience episodic gross hematuria thought consequent to small renal infarcts.
- Chronic uncontrolled autoimmune hemolytic anemia is associated with an increased incidence of venous thrombosis.
- Corticosteroids are a primary therapy for autoimmune hemolytic anemia but may not alone effect a satisfactory remission of the illness.
- Anemia may be conveniently grouped as disorders involving reduced production, excessive hemolysis, or blood loss, recognizing that more than one mechanism may be present in any individual case.
- A very low serum ferritin level essentially confirms iron deficiency, but a markedly elevated serum ferritin level does not always indicate iron overload states.

The circulating blood cell present in greatest numbers is the erythrocyte, which, in humans, is a non-nucleated cell that contains the hemoglobin stores that are responsible for proper tissue oxygen delivery. A reduction in circulating erythrocyte mass below the normal range, adjusted for age and sex, and typically expressed in terms of hemoglobin concentration, RBC count, or hematocrit value is described as anemia. The most common acquired cause of anemia worldwide is iron deficiency, and this will be discussed in some detail, *vide infra*. Thalassemia syndromes are the most common hereditary causes of anemia. The normal mean peripheral blood values for men are a hemoglobin concentration of 15.5 g/dL, a hematocrit value of 47%, a RBC count of 5.2×10^{12}/L, and a platelet count of 250,000/mm^3. Particularly, the hemoglobin concentration is lower among women, and the comparable normal mean values for blood counts in healthy adult women are 14.0 g/dL, 41%, 4,600/mm^3, and 250,000/mm^3. With aging, there is a significant but variable decrease in the hemoglobin concentration, particularly among men. Normal finite RBC survival in the circulation is about 120 days or with a half-life of 60 days and a substantially shorter cell life span in hemolytic states.

A very useful metric in the analysis of anemia is the mean corpuscular volume (MCV), with a normal range of 86 to 90 fl. Other calculations often present on automated blood count laboratory slips, such as the mean corpuscular hemoglobin (MCH) and mean corpuscular hemoglobin concentration (MCHC), are not clinically useful. Dr. Maxwell Wintrobe, who conceptualized these measurements and wrote the first clinical textbook in hematology, was later quoted as being sorry he suggested the latter two calculations. The reticulocyte count is also a useful index of erythrocyte production and may be corrected by a simple formula to provide the reticulocyte index (% Reticulocytes × Hematocrit/45 = Absolute reticulocyte percentage); this may be an automatic calculation performed by some laboratory equipment. An elevated reticulocyte count is usually manifest by polychromasia or a bluish hue among some erythrocytes on the stained peripheral blood film. Reticulocytes may be extremely increased in certain forms of hemolytic anemia and virtually zero in the unusual circumstance of pure RBC aplasia. Modern automated cell counters also typically provide a graphic representation of cell count versus cell volume, which can visually demonstrate a skewed erythrocyte and platelet size, although this and considerable additional information is evident on inspection of a well-prepared and well-stained blood film.

An isolated anemia may result from reduced RBC production, a shortened RBC life span generally reflecting a hemolytic state, blood loss, or some combination of these mechanisms. Of the selective acquired toxicities affecting the erythroid cell line, iron-deficiency anemia primarily is a consequence of chronic blood loss and repeated pregnancies in women. It is occasionally seen in frequent blood donors. However, malabsorption of iron occurs in children with heavy milk intake; in adults with celiac sprue; and in recent years, as a consequence of now frequently performed bariatric surgery, which bypasses the predominant sites of iron absorption in the duodenum. Inadequate nutrition in developing countries also contributes to iron deficiency. Aside from blood loss, iron is well conserved, and the oral requirement is less than 4 mg/day. Individuals with chronic iron deficiency often develop pica, which may be manifest as ice hunger (*pagophagia*) and an urge to chew on something, including clay, starch, paper, or even rubber bands. Such cravings rapidly disappear shortly after treatment is begun and long before the hemoglobin concentration returns to normal. There may also be some cheilosis and glossitis, creating oral symptoms associated with severe iron deficiency.

In iron-deficiency anemia, we think of hypochromic and microcytic erythrocytes, which are typically evident when the hemoglobin concentration falls below 10 g/dL. However, the appearance of abnormal erythroid shapes such as elliptical erythrocytes and occasional teardrop forms are common. In very severe iron-deficiency anemia, the peripheral blood film may somewhat resemble a microangiopathic hemolytic process with fragmented appearing forms (Figure 39-1). The platelet count often becomes elevated with a mean value of 450,000/mm³ in iron-deficiency anemia, and the total leukocyte count typically remains normal.

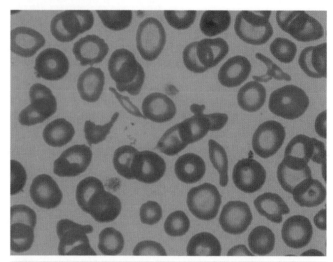

Figure 39-1 Peripheral blood film in severe iron-deficiency anemia (mean corpuscular volume, 57 fl; serum ferritin value, 3 ng/mL) showing misshapen and hypochromic erythrocytes.

It is good clinical practice to always obtain a serum ferritin value in the evaluation of patients with anemia. When the ferritin concentration is greatly reduced, iron deficiency is virtually always confirmed. Ferritin is an acute phase reacting protein. Although it is greatly elevated in hemochromatosis and transfusional iron overload, where it reflects a nonlinear increase in tissue iron stores, the highest ferritin values are seen in inflammatory illnesses such as juvenile rheumatoid arthritis and occasionally in NHL and the rare hemophagocytic syndromes. The ferritin molecule's structural configuration resembles a cylinder and may contain quite variable amounts of iron. The serum iron and iron-binding capacity are also helpful measurements in the evaluation of anemia and demonstrate a reduced serum iron and elevated iron-binding capacity with a reduced iron saturation of less than 16%.

It is well to always remember that iron deficiency should not simply be treated without consideration as to the cause. In addition to a careful history, this evaluation should involve a rectal examination, multiple stool tests for occult blood, and often a gastroenterology consultation seeking to demonstrate a potential site of intermittent blood loss. Occasionally, when upper and lower endoscopy is unproductive, the disposable so-called pill camera, which may take several hundred photos during its transit through the gut, may reveal a potential bleeding source. Although iron is a limiting reagent in blood production, individuals with an increased hemoglobin concentration may also be iron deficient. For example, patients with untreated polycythemia vera are virtually always iron deficient with low serum ferritin values and absent bone marrow iron stores. This is in contrast to a secondary polycythemia consequent to chronic hypoxemia, as in advanced lung disease, in which bone marrow iron stores and serum ferritin values are typically normal.

Treatment of iron-deficiency anemia is with oral iron salts, such as ferrous sulfate, fumarate, or gluconate. Timed-release preparations are to be avoided because the stool will turn dark, but the iron release will bypass the duodenum, and the anemia will not improve. Several intravenous iron preparations are available, and their use may be necessary in patients with celiac sprue and after bariatric surgery because oral iron absorption may be insufficient and ineffective. Their use may also be necessary in chronic bleeding states such as Osler-Weber-Rendu disease (hereditary hemorrhagic telangiectasia) and so-called watermelon stomach, in which oral iron is not sufficient to maintain a satisfactory hemoglobin concentration because of continuous blood loss from the friable gastric mucosa. If bleeding is the source of iron deficiency and this has ceased, the hemoglobin level will rise about 0.9 g/dL/week with oral iron preparations and may rise as rapidly as 1.5-1.9 g/dL/week after intravenous iron. Although the reticulocyte count will rise mildly with appropriate treatment, the bone marrow in iron deficiency is not hypercellular, and posttherapy reticulocyte counts would not be expected to rise to more than 4% or 5%, but they might reach 20% or more after appropriate treatment for megaloblastic anemia or in chronic hemolytic states in which the bone marrow is hypercellular.

Regulation of RBC synthesis is driven by erythropoietin production from the juxtaglomerular cells in the renal cortex, responding to variation in tissue oxygen delivery. In the case of chronic renal insufficiency, there is not a direct correlation between the rising serum levels of urea nitrogen and creatinine and the ability to produce erythropoietin. This disparity may be striking in patients with polycystic kidney disease and those who may have advanced renal failure without significant anemia. Thus, it is not unusual to encounter individuals with anemia responsive to parenteral erythropoietin who are not yet in need of chronic dialysis therapy. Erythropoietin levels in serum may be measured, but occasionally a therapeutic trial of parenteral erythropoietin is required to prove this mechanism for an isolated anemia in a patient with some degree of renal insufficiency. Erythropoietin is routinely given to patients receiving hemodialysis, often along with parenteral iron to maximize the response, but anemia in chronic renal disease may be multifactorial.

Another type of a selective deficit in erythroid cellular production is characterized by the disappearance of RBC precursors from the bone marrow and severe anemia referred to as pure RBC aplasia. This situation may occur as an idiosyncratic reaction to certain prescription medications, as an autoimmune illness, particularly associated with tumors of the thymus; as a consequence of infection with parvovirus; and as an association with certain neoplasms, such as CLL. It may also be induced by iatrogenic creation of a selective deficiency of the vitamin riboflavin. Selective riboflavin deficiency may be accomplished by administering an isocaloric diet very low in riboflavin and adding a competitive inhibitor of the residual dietary riboflavin, galactoflavin. Within a 3-week period, virtually all RBC precursors disappear from the bone marrow with no effect on WBC or platelet production. Even the aberrant and dyspoietic bone marrow RBC precursors present in forms of MDS and erythroleukemia will disappear with this therapy, revealing a background population of the accompanying myeloblasts, formerly hidden by the major overproduction of aberrant erythroid precursors. Aside from a sore tongue and cracking at the lip margins (cheilosis), there are surprisingly few short-term clinical symptoms from this unusual dietary treatment, which was used many years ago in early

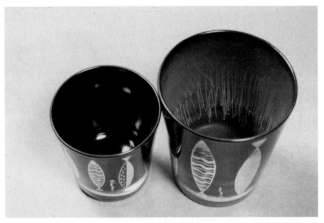

Figure 39-2 Cocktail glasses with the original interior shellac coating *(left)* removed by dishwasher heat *(right)*, exposing the dull lead-based paint lining (scratches made for sampling analysis).

approaches to cancer therapy in an attempt to "starve" rapidly growing tumor cells and possibly make them more sensitive to cytotoxic chemotherapy agents.

A classic example of chemical-induced selective hematotoxicity affecting the erythroid cell line is anemia consequent to lead poisoning. Excess lead may be assimilated through inhalation from refinery dusts, welding fumes and pesticides, or by ingestion of pigments used in lead-based paint or pottery or lead salts present as a contaminant in traditional medications, for example (Figure 39-2). The excess lead is incorporated into developing RBC precursors, where it interferes with several enzymes necessary for heme synthesis, including aminolevulinic acid (ALA) dehydrogenase, ferrochelatase, coproporphyrinogen oxidase, and porphobilinogen deaminase.

The mechanism of the resultant anemia is complex, as there is both a reduction in blood production by the bone marrow despite greatly increased erythroid precursors *(ineffective erythropoiesis)* and a reduction in the life span of circulating RBCs *(hemolytic anemia)*. The leukocytes and platelets are not affected. The illness may be suspected by the presence of basophilic stippling or multiple bluish cytoplasmic dots commonly evident in RBCs on stained peripheral blood films (Figure 39-3). It is proven and quantified by a whole blood lead level. Urinary coproporphyrins and urobilinogens are also greatly elevated in this illness. Lead poisoning may also be suspected by the presence of ringed sideroblasts (erythroid precursors containing three or more blue-staining iron granules associated with cytoplasmic mitochondria), as highlighted by iron stains of bone marrow (Figure 39-4). Treatment with chelating agents, such as calcium disodium EDTA (ethylenediaminetetraacetic acid), is highly effective after the source of lead exposure has been identified and eliminated (Natelson et al., 1976). Over time, without specific therapy, lead may be stored in the cortex of bone and does not produce toxicity because it is hidden from the hematopoietic elements. An incorrect diagnosis leading to treatment of occult lead poisoning with corticosteroids, effective in certain types of immune hemolytic anemias, may aggravate lead poisoning by causing the lead to be mobilized from the bone cortex and again become available to cause bone marrow toxicity. An interesting feature of the

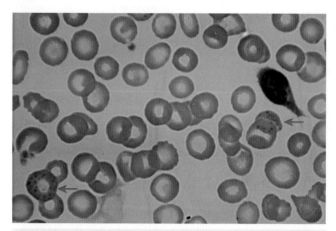

Figure 39-3 Peripheral blood film in lead poisoning showing erythrocyte basophilic stippling *(arrows)*.

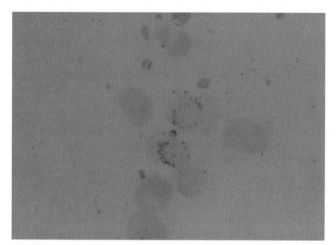

Figure 39-4 Iron stain of a bone marrow aspirate demonstrating multiple blue cytoplasmic granules ringing the nucleus in two erythroid precursor cells, confirming ringed sideroblasts.

sideroblastic anemia of lead poisoning in comparison with the sideroblastic anemia in MDS is that in lead poisoning, the MCV is usually normal, but it is typically increased in MDS.

A selective depletion primarily of circulating RBCs may also occur in most forms of hemolytic anemia, both congenital and acquired. Of the congenital types, hereditary spherocytosis is most common among white individuals and sickle cell syndromes among black individuals. In the acquired types of hemolytic states, such as autoimmune hemolytic anemia, the illness is mediated through antibody (*immunoglobulin*) production directed against antigenic sites on RBC membrane proteins, which are typically part of the Rh complex, causing breakdown of the erythrocytes, both directly in the bloodstream (*intravascular hemolysis*) or in the reticuloendothelial cells of the liver, spleen, or lymph nodes (*extravascular hemolysis*). Such events may occur as a consequence of an underlying immune-modifying illness such as lupus or CLL or by introduction of an antibody-provoking toxin in the form of prescription medications. A classic medication-induced example involves the antihypertensive drug, α-methyldopa, which may generate formation of typically IgG immunoglobulins directed against RBC

surface antigens. Such immunoglobulins, which become immobilized on the RBC surface membrane, create a positive antiglobulin (*direct Coombs*) test result and, occasionally, significant hemolysis of the targeted cells. Only the erythrocytes are involved, and the antibody titer eventually falls with discontinuation of the medication, allowing complete hematologic recovery. Many other drugs, particularly a variety of nonsteroidal antiinflammatory drugs (NSAIDs), may cause immune-related hemolysis in a similar fashion. Occasionally, the drug must remain in the circulation as a hapten for hemolysis to be sustained by the offending immunoglobulin.

In addition to inspection of the peripheral blood film, useful laboratory tests to suggest hemolysis and its cause are the direct and indirect antiglobulin tests (Coombs tests), serum lactate dehydrogenase (LDH), total and indirect bilirubin level, and haptoglobin concentration. The latter test is very sensitive and not quantitative in terms of how much hemolysis has occurred. Free hemoglobin and haptoglobin form a complex in the plasma after intravascular hemolysis, which is removed by the liver. It takes some weeks to recover a normal serum haptoglobin level after sudden hemolysis, as may occur with a transfusion-related episode of hemolysis. With intravascular hemolysis, the LDH level is markedly elevated. However, some elevation of the serum LDH will occur even with extravascular hemolysis occurring in the spleen or with intramedullary hemolysis in the bone marrow. The LDH is a useful test to follow the results of therapy in certain chronic hemolytic states and is a good indicator of the degree of hemolysis caused by a malfunctioning mechanical heart valve, for example.

In autoimmune hemolytic anemia, the classic peripheral blood findings involving the erythrocytes include large numbers of spherocytes. Spherocytes are small cells when examined on a peripheral blood film, sometimes referred to as microspherocytes, and it may be surprising to find the MCV normal on an automated blood cell counter in an immune-related hemolytic anemia after reviewing the blood film. This occurs because the detection physics of automated cell counters oversize spheres and provide a false reading in this circumstance. Also evident on the peripheral blood film may be erythrophagocytosis by monocytes of the immunoglobulin-coated erythrocytes (Figure 39-5). In some instances of autoimmune hemolytic anemia, a second cell line is involved, and frequently antibody is also directed against the platelets, as occurs in Evans syndrome and in systemic lupus, causing thrombocytopenia. Generally, a dual autoimmune cytopenia suggests a more aggressive illness, but typically both cytopenias are improved by therapy with immunosuppressive agents (Gómez-Almaguer et al., 2010). Most examples of autoimmune hemolytic anemia are caused by "warm" reacting antibodies, meaning they are active at 37° C. Some autoantibodies are referred to as "cold" acting because their ability to attach to the RBC membrane is better demonstrated at colder temperatures. Such cold antibody or cold agglutinin autoimmune hemolytic disease is more often associated with underlying lymphoproliferative disorders and is more difficult to treat successfully (Swiecicki et al., 2013).

Successful treatment of patients with autoimmune hemolytic anemia may require prolonged or recurrent therapy. Aside from attempts to eliminate any underlying

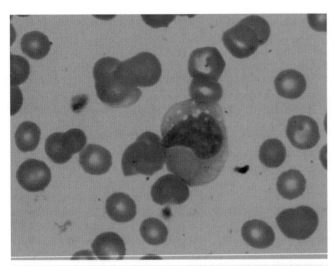

Figure 39-5 Erythrophagocytosis by a peripheral blood monocyte in autoimmune hemolytic anemia.

and causative disorder, drugs such as corticosteroids, immune-modifying and immunosuppressive agents such as Imuran, Rituxan, Campath, and mofetil mycophenolate may be helpful. Splenectomy has also been advocated in refractory autoimmune hemolysis. However, although highly effective in hereditary spherocytosis, in autoimmune hemolytic states, the hemolysis may not lessen and, as a consequence of an absent spleen and a continuing hemolytic state, the platelet count may greatly increase, further predisposing to thrombosis. Indeed, the most common cause of death in patients with autoimmune hemolytic anemia is not anemia but the development of thromboembolic complications causing pulmonary thromboemboli and pulmonary hypertension. In patients with uncontrolled chronic hemolysis, oral anticoagulants are often added to the therapy until the hemolysis subsides.

In sickle cell syndromes, such as classical SS sickle cell disease, some hemolysis is constant as a consequence of the variant hemoglobin. Over time, the spleen is destroyed by the hemolytic process and by small splenic infarcts. There are many adverse clinical manifestations in addition to anemia, including cholelithiasis, pain crises, bone marrow infarction, priapism, the so-called acute chest syndrome, and even stroke. Because of the loss of the spleen and the opsonizing antibodies it produces, there is an increased risk of infection related to infections with encapsulated organisms such as pneumococcus.

The presence of fetal hemoglobin in the erythrocyte, even in small amounts, is somewhat protective against sickling. Its concentration in the sickle-cell erythrocyte may be increased by continuous use of the oral drug hydroxyurea. In some sickle syndromes, such as S-C disease and S-thalassemia, the spleen actually enlarges, causing some degree of hypersplenism, usually manifest as mild to moderate thrombocytopenia. Because of the need for frequent blood transfusion in some patients with sickle cell disease, antibodies generated to minor blood group antigens such as Kell may cause a type of alloimmune hemolysis. There also may be hemolysis consequent to alloantibodies generated against components of the Rh system (Chou et al., 2013). If transfusions are infrequent, the titer of the offending antibody may fall below the level of detection during the routine cross match, but 10 to 14 days after transfusion, the antibody titer rises in response to the presence of the offending RBC antigen as an anamnestic response. Then what is referred to as a delayed hemolytic transfusion reaction may occur, causing severe hemolysis and destroying all of the transfused cells and even some of the native erythrocytes, worsening the anemia. Further transfusion becomes very difficult for several weeks.

Tissue iron overload is a common problem in patients with both sickle cell disease and thalassemia major syndromes consequent to increased absorption of iron, frequent blood transfusion, and the inability of the body to rid itself of excess iron. Early on, the storage sites of excess iron are primarily in the reticuloendothelial cells throughout the liver and differ from genetic hemochromatosis where iron deposition occurs first primarily in the hepatic parenchymal cells and in the pancreas. However, late in the course of all iron deposition syndromes, the liver biopsy in patients with transfusional iron overload may be difficult to distinguish from that of advanced hemochromatosis. Chelating agents may reduce iron overload by the removal of iron in the stool and urine, and the advantages of this are clear in patients with severe thalassemia, who cannot be phlebomized periodically to reduce excess iron, in contrast to those with hemochromatosis, in whom the hemoglobin concentration is normal. In the hemochromatosis group, many blood banks are now able to use this blood for transfusion as they would normal donor blood. Iron chelators may be given by prolonged, intermittent parenteral administration for maximal effect, and newer chelators, such as Exjade, may be given orally.

Individuals with sickle cell trait such as AS hemoglobin typically will have a distribution of hemoglobin concentrations on hemoglobin electrophoresis showing a moderate increase of A over S hemoglobin and will not experience sickle crises unless placed in extremely low oxygen circumstances, such as a nonpressurized high altitude. However, they do have a propensity for episodes of periodic hematuria consequent to microinfarcts in the kidney. Experienced urologists are well aware of this phenomenon and will order a hemoglobin electrophoresis in black individuals with unexplained gross hematuria regardless of the blood count. The life span of an individual with sickle trait is the same as that observed in the general population.

Many variant hemoglobins may be associated with anemia and an abnormal peripheral blood film result. With C hemoglobin trait, target cells are frequent, and virtually all of the erythrocytes are target cells with CC hemoglobin, although the anemia is generally mild. Certain ethnic groups have particular frequency of specific aberrant hemoglobins such as hemoglobin E in Thailand, which affects about 40% of the population, producing a mild anemia with target cells. In this population, there may be various combinations of hemoglobin E and thalassemia minor syndromes producing a varying severity of anemia.

Hereditary defects in RBC enzyme systems may cause a chronic hemolytic state. The two most frequent circumstances are with pyruvate kinase deficiency and with glucose-6-phosphate dehydrogenase (G-6PD) deficiency. G-6PD deficiency is sex linked, so most affected individuals are men. The enzyme defect allows increases in oxidative stress to affect the erythrocyte, causing hemolysis. Precipitated hemoglobin may be identified in the circulating erythrocytes with a Heinz body stain. The defect may cause continuous hemolysis among white individuals, but in black individuals, hemolysis may be more episodic and limited and seldom causes life-threatening anemia. Certain antimalarial drugs may precipitate hemolytic crises in those with G-6PD deficiency states.

Hemolysis and anemia is also a major component and consequence of a group of disorders associated with a variable degree of thrombotic microangiopathy. In this case, the hemolysis is intravascular and not immune related but rather caused by the shear stress applied to the erythrocytes as they traverse partially occluded small arterioles. Complement may play a role in the hemolytic process. The most frequent of these syndromes are thrombotic thrombocytopenia purpura (TTP); hemolytic uremic syndrome (HUS) linked to the verocytotoxin associated with acute bacterial diarrhea, sometimes occurring in an epidemic pattern; and atypical HUS. The pattern of the anemia is microangiopathic, with abundant fragmented-appearing erythrocytes evident on the peripheral blood film. A similar but less severe fragmentation pattern may also be seen in various forms of vasculitis, flares of chronic ulcerative colitis, and malignant hypertension.

Thrombotic thrombocytopenia purpura is usually associated with deficits of the plasma ADAMTS-13 enzyme, which regulates the size of circulating von Willebrand factor multimeric subunit proteins. The illness may be congenital or acquired in various clinical settings. On occasion, an autoantibody to ADAMTS-13 can be demonstrated along with a reduction in the concentration of the enzyme, suggesting an immune-related etiology. The congenital form may be controlled by periodic infusions of plasma to raise the ADAMTS-13 level. In the more common acquired form of the illness, which typically begins abruptly, the most effective initial therapy is repeated plasma exchange. If the ability to conduct an exchange is not immediately available, infusions of fresh-frozen plasma provide benefit until a formal exchange can be initiated. Corticosteroids are effective in about 25% of cases and are typically given along with the plasma exchanges. Some patients with TTP have modest favorable responses to antiplatelet aggregating agents, such as Aggrenox (aspirin + Persantine), which may be added to the treatment regimen. Platelet transfusions are to be avoided despite the often severe thrombocytopenia because they may precipitate intracerebral arterial thrombosis and seizures. Moreover, despite thrombocytopenia, life-threatening bleeding is only rarely present in TTP. Particularly in individuals with antibodies to ADAMTS-13, infusions of Rituxan, as an immune-modulating agent, have been added to the treatment program in recent years and may prevent relapses. The effects of therapy are monitored by following the hemoglobin concentration, platelet count, and the serum LDH. In the recovery phase, the platelet count begins to rise first, but hemolysis does not acutely abate, and the elevated LDH may take time to slowly recede as the partially occluded blood vessels recover. Some patients exhibit a relapsing course after months in unmaintained remission, and in many of these individuals, further recurrences may be aborted by splenectomy during a stable phase of the illness. The cause of TTP is uncertain but has clearly been associated with pregnancy, a familial link, and certain medications such as quinine (McMinn et al., 2001), Plavix, and ticlopidine. It also may appear during the course of HIV infection, where it seems very responsive to therapy.

Hemolytic anemia simulating TTP but with a greater predilection for often irreversible renal damage may occur after infections with organisms, including strains of *Escherichia coli*, which can produce a *Shiga* toxin referred to as verocytotoxin. This illness has occurred in epidemic form with food contamination. Plasma exchange is not as effective in this group but is usually initiated. The inhibitor of the C-5 complement protein eculizumab, effective in reducing hemolysis in patients with paroxysmal nocturnal hemoglobinuria (PNH), also has a beneficial effect in some atypical HUS. A microangiopathic process simulating TTP and HUS may occur abruptly during chemotherapy treatment with certain agents, but standard therapy is not highly effective in this group.

Less common causes of major hemolysis include the rare illness of paroxysmal nocturnal hemoglobinuria (PNH). In PNH, the cytoskeleton of the erythrocyte is abnormal and sensitive to complement-induced hemolysis. PNH may arise during the course of aplastic anemia or spontaneously appear. The diagnosis may be easily made by modern flow cytometry studies identifying certain cluster designation (CD) markers present on the erythrocytes. Iron deficiency is occasionally present consequent to chronic urinary iron loss from the hemoglobinuria. However, the hemolytic state may be set off by therapy with intravenous iron, which causes a sudden outpouring of reticulocytes from the bone marrow, with these younger RBCs more sensitive to hemolysis. The C-5 complement inhibitor eculizumab may greatly lessen the severity of hemolytic episodes but must be infused every 2 weeks at a massive cost. Successful therapy of PNH also has followed allogeneic bone marrow transfusion, which may eliminate the abnormal clone producing the complement-sensitive erythrocytes. Individuals with PNH are susceptible to thrombophlebitis because of the chronic intravascular hemolysis, which has a thromboplastin-like effect. Most individuals with PNH have a normal total leukocyte count and platelet count, but others may have periodic episodes of mild pancytopenia. Marked splenomegaly may occur in patients who have had the illness for many years.

In contrast to hemolytic states and anemia, a significant increase in the numbers of RBCs may occur among chronic smokers as a consequence of increased levels of carboxyhemoglobin, reducing oxygen-carrying capacity and interfering with tissue oxygen delivery. Oxygen sensors in the kidney respond to the lack of oxygen tension by augmenting production of erythropoietin from the juxtaglomerular cells, stimulating RBC production by the bone marrow. A similar effect may by produced by the administration of certain anabolic steroids, as used among bodybuilders and other athletes. In these situations, hemoglobin concentrations may exceed 20 g/dL, increasing circulating blood viscosity. Affected individuals may experience headache and sluggishness and appear flushed. Rarely, such secondary erythrocytosis, if marked, may result in venous or arterial thrombosis (or both).

Perhaps not widely appreciated is the effect of various types of anemia on the HgA_{1c} level often used to monitor mean blood glucose levels over the preceding several weeks in patients with diabetes mellitus. In part, this measurement depends on RBC turnover rates, which may vary widely among patients with chronic hemolytic anemias, iron-deficiency anemia, and MDS. For example, the HgbA$_{1c}$ level is falsely elevated in iron-deficiency anemia and in pure RBC aplasia and falsely lowered in hemolytic anemias and MDS, with ineffective erythropoiesis (Okawa et al., 2013). It may also be lowered in the anemia of renal disease under treatment with erythropoietin preparations. In some instances, the artifactual aberrations in HgA$_{1c}$ values are trivial, but in sickle cell disease, some rely on glycosylated albumin values rather than HgA$_{1c}$ levels for monitoring control of diabetes.

DISORDERS OF LEUKOCYTES AND PLATELETS

Key Points

- Splenectomy for treatment of ITP should be preceded by vaccinations for pneumococcal, hemophilus, and meningococcal infections at least 2 weeks before surgery.
- Although plasma exchange is the primary therapy for TTP, plasma infusions are of benefit and should be started immediately, along with corticosteroids, pending transfer to a facility equipped to perform apheresis (*plasmapheresis*).
- Patients with chronic thrombocythemia associated with an MPN may be treated with either hydroxyurea or anagrelide or combinations of both drugs to reduce the platelet count and reduce the risk of thrombosis and excessive postsurgical bleeding.
- Colony-stimulating factors such as Neupogen and Neulasta are helpful in chemotherapy-induced myelosuppression but generally should be avoided in those with autoimmune neutropenias.

The WBCs, or leukocytes, comprise several specialized forms. Granulocytes are the predominant circulating normal leukocyte type. These cells contain a variety of packaged cytoplasmic enzymes and are responsible for the phagocytosis and subsequent destruction of foreign organisms. In this regard, they work directly with opsonizing immunoglobulin antibodies produced by the lymphoid cells, particularly those present in the spleen, which help to immobilize encapsulated organisms such as the pneumococcus. Most of the granulocytes are mature neutrophils with lesser numbers circulating as monocytes, eosinophils, and basophils. The lymphoid cells are divided into B- and T-cell forms and have to do with support of a normal immune system. The platelets are non-nucleated cells derived from the parent bone marrow megakaryocytes by programmed fractionation and extrusion of their cytoplasm into the capillaries throughout the bone marrow. Some further division of the platelets occurs in the circulating blood. The platelet functions to ensure normal hemostasis, often acting in concert with the coagulation proteins or factors. Under normal conditions in adults, the production site for erythrocytes, granulocytes, and platelets is restricted to the bone marrow, although in certain disease states,

extramedullary hematopoiesis may occur in the liver, lymph nodes, and spleen, for example. Lymphoid cells may also be produced in the bone marrow but are primarily generated in the lymph nodes throughout the body.

A selective absence of granulocytes may occur abruptly and in this circumstance is typically consequent to various medications. Certain cardiac and antithyroid medications, for example, may cause agranulocytosis, presumably through an immune mechanism. In these cases, the period of agranulocytosis is generally short, typically around 2 weeks, after the offending medication is stopped. Similarly, a wide number of medications may cause isolated thrombocytopenia, which may be profound but is also typically a temporary phenomenon. In clinical practice, severe granulocytopenia is most commonly a predictable consequence of chemotherapy for both hematologic and solid tumor malignancies. Although recovery is expected within 10 to 14 days, depending on the type and dose of chemotherapeutic agents used, the period of severe neutropenia may be shortened by several days with the use of colony-stimulating factors such as Neupogen or Neulasta.

In thrombocytopenia consequent to a drug reaction, such as with quinine, a spontaneous recovery is predictable, and the drug should be avoided in the future. Selective thrombocytopenia is common with ITP. Here, IgG immunoglobulin coats the platelet, which usually does not interfere with its function, but the complex is removed by the spleen and other elements of the reticuloendothelial system. The process may be self-limited, particular after viral infections, in children, but in adults, remission may require therapeutic intervention. ITP may be the first sign of an underlying illness such as in systemic lupus, NHL, or HIV disease. Aside from the potential for bleeding problems, affected individuals are typically asymptomatic, a contrast with those with a sudden onset of TTP who often manifest a systemic illness as a consequence of the disease state. In the therapy of ITP, the first consideration is if any treatment is even indicated. This depends on the level of thrombocytopenia and the clinical circumstances. An individual with a chronically low but stable platelet count in the 60,000/mm^3 range may require no therapy unless a surgical procedure is required, and then some intervention may become necessary.

The initial approach to treatment in ITP is with corticosteroids, which will almost immediately lessen the bleeding tendency before any rise in the platelet count as a vascular effect. A significant rise in the platelet count seldom occurs for several days and may take 2 weeks for a major improvement. In part, this may be related to corticosteroid dose and type. However, only perhaps 25% of individuals who respond will actually attain unmaintained remission when the steroids are discontinued. Infusions of large amounts of intravenous immunoglobulin (IVIG) may improve the platelet count more rapidly but seldom give a sustained response. The oral drug Promacta, which stimulates platelet production, works promptly in most individuals, but in many, the thrombocytopenia will relapse abruptly when the drug is discontinued. Immunosuppressive drugs such as the monoclonal anti-CD-20 agent Rituxan do provide favorable responses, but relapse is common. Splenectomy remains a useful therapy for ITP, with remission rates in those younger than 40 years of around 80% to 85% and around 60% in those older than 40 years. Prophylactic immunizations against the encapsulated bacteria such as pneumococcus, *Haemophilus* spp., and meningococcus should be administered ideally at least 2 weeks before the surgery. These immunizations administered after the procedure yield a reduced serum immune titer response because splenic lymphocytes have been removed. With the advent of laparoscopic surgery, the risks of the procedure and the length of stay in the hospital are both less than with an open procedure.

Autoimmune neutropenia is occasionally seen as an isolated finding in otherwise healthy individuals and in those with underlying rheumatoid disorders and lupus. Occasionally, in those with rheumatoid disease, the neutropenia is profound and associated with some splenomegaly and referred to as Felty syndrome. Despite profound neutropenia in the peripheral blood, bacterial infections are rather uncommon in this group, but if they do present a problem, splenectomy is also effective, as in ITP. Generally, it is thought that granulocytopenia below 500 cells/mm^3 strongly predisposes to infection, but this is more applicable to the myelosuppression of chemotherapy than in idiopathic autoimmune neutropenia. This may reflect the observation that neutrophils may move from the bone marrow into the tissues in an adequate manner to combat infection but cannot easily continue to circulate for their normal life span in the peripheral blood because of the presence of the autoantibodies.

PANCYTOPENIA

Hematotoxicity may affect all three cell lines simultaneously. For example, the broad-spectrum antibiotic Chloromycetin (chloramphenicol) may damage the bone marrow permanently, causing aplastic anemia by an idiosyncratic form of toxicity that is poorly understood or by a dose-related reduction in bone marrow cellularity, which often slowly recovers after the drug is discontinued. In each instance, all three cell lines are affected, and pancytopenia occurs. The bone marrow histology in chloramphenicol poisoning is unique and illustrates the presence of multiple vacuoles in the nucleus and cytoplasms of both erythroid and myeloid precursors along with the presence of occasional ringed sideroblasts. Similar but less striking bone marrow toxicity is noted with the modern-day antibiotic linezolid, which also may cause pancytopenia. Aplastic anemia may occur from other prescription medications, including the formerly used NSAID Butazolidine and currently available products such as indomethacin. Alcohol is a prominent hematotoxin and may produce a typically reversible pancytopenia or selective thrombocytopenia. Its actions as a hematotoxin may occur through associated dietary deficiency of folic acid by induction of a sideroblastic process in the bone marrow erythroid precursors or a direct toxic effect on circulating platelets. Acute alcoholic thrombocytopenia is short lived after ingestion has ceased, but sideroblastic bone marrow toxicity is only slowly reversible upon discontinuing alcohol exposures.

The megaloblastic anemias are also often associated with pancytopenia and may be caused by deficiencies in folic acid or vitamin B$_{12}$. The peripheral blood film may show marked macrocytosis with the normal RBC volume (MCV) increasing from around 86 fl to as much as 125 to 130 fl. The bone marrow is hypercellular with marked ineffective erythropoiesis causing intramedullary cell breakdown associated with elevated serum LDH and indirect bilirubin values. Treatment with the appropriate depleted element is characterized by a rapid recovery of bone marrow function, with reticulocyte counts reaching 20% to 25% in about 5 to 7 days in contrast with iron-deficiency anemia, in which the bone marrow is mildly suppressed, and correction with iron supplements, even given intravenously, seldom generates a reticulocyte response above 4-5%.

In hereditary vitamin B$_{12}$ deficiency, pernicious anemia, the illness in black individuals may occur at an early age whereas in white individuals, it is unusual to detect its presence before age 60. Therapy is typically parenteral with vitamin B$_{12}$ injections but can be effectively given with various intranasal sprays, at much greater expense. The liver stores vitamin B$_{12}$ very well and, although monthly injections of vitamin B$_{12}$ are recommended, it actually takes several years for relapse to occur after treatment is stopped and the blood counts normalize. However, if neurologic disease is present, it is important to continue a frequent administration of vitamin B$_{12}$ because neuropathic recovery is very slow.

Because the causes of pancytopenia are multifactorial, the indication for a diagnostic bone marrow study is far more often necessary than with investigation of a single cytopenia. Particularly if malignancy is suspected, such as MDS or AML or a form of NHL, the addition of flow cytometric studies and chromosome analysis greatly increases the ability to confirm a specific diagnosis and direct appropriate therapy. It is also useful to obtain ultrasonography of the abdomen in the investigation of pancytopenia, which is the most cost-effective and accurate way of measuring spleen size. The length of the spleen is normally 9 to 10 cm and correlates well with its total volume.

LATENT HEMATOTOXICITY

Key Points

- The diagnosis of AML does not always rely on a particular number of myeloblasts in the peripheral blood or bone marrow but can be established by the presence of certain chromosomal aberrations.
- Secondary forms of AML after chemotherapy and radiation exposures are generally a more aggressive illness than de novo forms of AML.
- Advancing age, prior exposure to chemotherapy, cigarette smoking, and underlying autoimmune disorders are major risk factors for the development of MDS.
- The currently available therapy for acute promyelocytic leukemia (APL) makes this illness the most curable form of adult AML.

Certain compounds used therapeutically as anticancer agents and immunosuppressive drugs are mutagens and may cause various cytopenias by damage to the DNA through a variety of mechanisms. These include interference with the enzyme topoisomerase II, which allows the programmed DNA fracture necessary to sustain the rapid pace of hematopoietic cell duplication under normal circumstances. Other antineoplastic drugs such as alkylating agents, including cyclophosphamide and Alkeran, may intercalate DNA and cause stem cell genetic damage that may initially appear as a reversible pancytopenia but later predisposes the individual to AML despite apparent recovery of normal bone marrow function. Still other compounds may interfere with enzymes necessary for cell division by acting as fraudulent metabolites or interfering with the actions of vitamins such as folic acid that are necessary for normal cell division. In these circumstances, all three hematopoietic cell lines are variably affected, and although a period of pancytopenia is common, with removal of the offending agent, sustained bone marrow aplasia from chemotherapy administration is rare.

Benzene, an early and long-obsolete chemotherapeutic agent, is a mutagen that may also cause an initially reversible pancytopenia at very high dosage (Gailbraith et al., 2010; Natelson, 2007). The specific mechanism causing its hematotoxicity remains unknown. Prolonged exposure to benzene may result in a persistent pancytopenia characterized by bone marrow hypoplasia associated with atypical eosinophilia and erythrophagocytic histiocytes, suggesting an immune-related process. A true aplastic anemia from benzene would require exposures to the chemical now not likely possible in developed countries.

Acute pancytopenias consequent to mutagenic compounds may fully resolve, but years later, hematotoxicity may reappear and become progressive in the form of certain types of MDS and even AML. This event occurred after the administration of mitoxantrone, a topoisomerase II inhibitor, used as an immune-modulating agent for the treatment of multiple sclerosis. Here a significant incidence of AML involving balanced translocations, such as the t(15:17) translocation of APL, occurred within 5 years of initiating therapy.

Blood cell production requires replacement of the entire granulocyte population in the body multiple times per day, and genetic damage to precursor cells may escape the normally efficient reparative mechanisms. This may lead to continued production of small clones of hematopoietic cells with disordered sequences of maturation and natural cell death. If the abnormal clone expands, with time, it may develop additional molecular aberrations, which allow a favored growth, a reduced process of cell death, or both, creating a growth and proliferation advantage over the normal cell population. This may become evident first as a single cytopenia, often associated with subtle morphologic aberrations distinct from the normal cell line. Such a circumstance is referred to as MDS.

In MDS, ultimately, all myeloid bone marrow cell lines become affected, cell maturation may be trapped at an immature stage, and ineffective myelopoiesis becomes prominent. In MDS, aberrant cell morphology in both the peripheral blood and the bone marrow is common. Useful, although not specific, clues to the presence of MDS on the peripheral blood film are a progressive macrocytosis and the acquired Pelger-Huët bilobed neutrophil (Figure 39-6). This nuclear aberration is a robust marker for MDS, but it may be caused by medications and is reversible when they are discontinued, and it is important to be aware of this phenomenon (Wang et al., 2011). Ultimately, the presence of

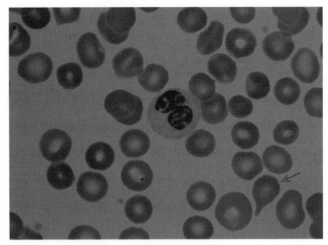

Figure 39-6 Peripheral blood film in myelodysplastic syndrome showing a teardrop erythrocyte *(arrow)* and acquired or pseudo Pelger-Huët neutrophil aberration with a bilobed nucleus and hypogranular cytoplasm.

large numbers of immature myeloid cells, referred to as blasts, becomes the hallmark for the progression to AML. Depending on the nature of the chromosomal aberrations in the abnormal cell line, the clinical manifestations, prognosis, and treatment of the AML syndrome may vary. MDS and AML arising without known causes are referred to as de novo, or primary, and account for the majority of adult AML/MDS. A chemical or radiation-induced form of AML is referred to as secondary, and amounts to about 10% to 15% of all AML syndromes. A secondary form of MDS/AML generally carries a more ominous prognosis than de novo disease. It is often characterized by complex (>3) separate clonal chromosomal aberrations and is associated with a poor response to therapy. Prolonged cigarette smoking may also predispose to MDS/AML, but the mechanism is uncertain and the cytogenetic manifestations differ from those seen in a chemical induced secondary MDS/AML, resembling those of de novo MDS/AML (Vardarajan et al., 2011). Many studies have shown that the prognosis for remission induction and ultimate survival in AML is worse for a smoker versus a nonsmoker (Vardarajan et al., 2011). Figure 39-7 illustrates the frequency of causation, age, and other associations as risk factors for MDS. Figure 39-8 provides similar information for AML.

Acute myeloid leukemia and MDS syndromes caused by drugs and chemicals do not appear as an idiosyncratic reaction to brief or low-level toxic exposures and typically require a cumulative threshold dose (CTD) necessary to exceed in order to predispose to disease (Natelson, 2007; Natelson et al., 2010). Such a potentially leukemic threshold dose varies considerably among known leukemogenic chemicals, and certain agents appear potentially far more leukemogenic, milligram for milligram, than others (Table 39-1). Thus, mutagenic chemicals such as methotrexate and hydroxyurea rarely, if ever, cause AML syndromes as monotherapy, but exposures to alkylating agents such as melphalan and nitrogen mustard may cause AML in as many as 10% or more of all recipients, depending on the cumulative dose of drug received. Environmental or occupational potential leukemogens, such as benzene,

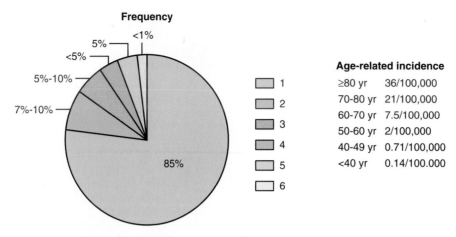

Frequency

	Age-related incidence	
1	≥80 yr	36/100,000
2	70-80 yr	21/100,000
3	60-70 yr	7.5/100,000
4	50-60 yr	2/100,000
5	40-49 yr	0.71/100,000
6	<40 yr	0.14/100.000

1. De novo MDS (primary): Estimates are 85% of all MDS. About 45% to 50% manifest cytogenetic abnormalities evident by standard analysis with recurring examples being del (5q), del (7q), del (20q), and trisomy 8.

2. Secondary MDS: Estimates are 7% to 10% of all MDS, with greater than 80% relating to prior therapy with mutagenic chemicals or radiation (therapy-related, t-MDS). Chromosome aberrations are present in greater than 90%, particularly involving chromosomes 5 and 7, and are often associated with complex cytogenetics and a poor prognosis.

3. Cigarette smoking is strongly associated with MDS/AML and directly relates to the total amount smoked and current smoking at diagnosis.

4. Subsets of MDS characterized by ringed sideroblasts may have different causation from other MDS syndromes, as virtually all are associated with the driver mutation SF3B1.

5. Perhaps 5% of individuals with MDS, as defined only by morphologic aberrations and cytopenias and with associated clinical features suggesting autoimmune disease, may respond favorably to immunosuppressive therapy.

6. Occupational or environmental chemical exposures are thought to cause less than 1% of all MDS with benzene-related disease some fraction of this amount.

Figure 39-7 Age-related incidence of myelodysplastic syndrome (MDS) and frequency estimates of MDS subsets. *AML,* Acute myeloid leukemia.

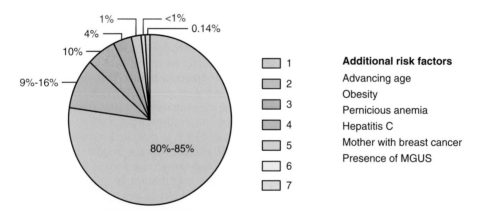

	Additional risk factors
1	Advancing age
2	Obesity
3	Pernicious anemia
4	Hepatitis C
5	Mother with breast cancer
6	Presence of MGUS
7	

1. De novo (primary, endogenous): Estimate are in the 80% to 85% range, particularly associated with normal cytogenetics or balanced translocations with absence of a prodrome of myelodysplasia (MDS).

2. Smoking-induced: Estimates are in the 9% to 16% range. Aberrations of chromosome 8 are specifically cited but almost half normal cytogenetics. Risk is directly related to amount smoked and with current smoking.

3. Therapy-induced AML/MDS: Estimates are 10%. Frequent cystogenetic aberrations involve chromosomes 5 and 7. Normal routine cytogenetics in greater than 10%. Two thirds with a history of MDS.

4. Evolution from de novo MDS: Perhaps 4%. Cytogenetics are normal in greater than 50%, and balanced translocations are uncommon.

5. Evolution from MPN: With effective therapy of CML, perhaps 1%.

6. Association with underlying genetic aberrations such as familial AML, Li Fromeni syndrome, Lynch syndrome, Down syndrome, Bloom syndrome, and so on: Frequency is less than 1%.

7. Environmental or occupational exposure: Rare, with estimates from benzene exposures only 0.14%

Figure 39-8 Frequency of etiology and risk factors for acute myeloid leukemia (AML). *CML,* Chronic myeloid leukemia; *MDS,* myelodysplastic syndrome; *MGUS,* monoclonal gammopathy of unknown causation; *MPH,* maternal past history.

Table 39-1   Estimated Cumulative Threshold Dose for Several Potentially Leukemogenic Agents

Compound	Activity	CTD (mg/m²)	Latency to MDS/AML (yr)
Temozolomide	Alkylating agent	18,000-20,000	0.75-3
Cyclophosphamide	Alkylating agent	8000-10,000	2-10
Alkeran	Alkylating agent	80	2-10
Mechlorethamine	Alkylating agent	60	2-10
Etoposide	Topoisomerase II inhibitor	2000	1-4
Mitoxantrone	Topoisomerase II inhibitor	60	0.5-5
Fludarabine	Nucleoside analog	750	0.75-7
Benzene	Unknown	46,000	2-10

AML, acute myeloid leukemia; *CTD,* cumulative threshold dose; *MDS,* myelodysplastic syndromes.

require a very large CTD to predispose to AML, and even then do so rarely. Aside from exposure to cigarette smoke, AML and MDS from potential environmental chemical exposures are thought to make up only a tiny fraction of all secondary MDS/AML syndromes (Natelson et al., 2013). There is also a latency window to MDS/AML after the CTD has been reached. Generally, most secondary forms of AML/MDS appear within 10 to 12 years of the last exposure (Natelson, 2007). Remote occurrence of AML/MDS in such exposed populations may simply reflect the greatly increasing risk of MDS/AML in the general population with advancing age.

What constitutes appropriate criteria to warrant a diagnosis of AML has undergone modifications over the years, and the initial requirement of 30% blasts in a cellular bone marrow was reduced to 20% blasts. Currently, the diagnosis of AML may be established simply by the presence of certain specific chromosome aberrations such as the t(15;17) translocation in APL and inversion 16 AML, which is often associated with an atypical eosinophilic population in the peripheral blood (Pulsoni et al., 2008). Simply the presence of the chromosome aberration without any particular increase in blast forms satisfies a diagnosis of AML in these circumstances. A full discussion of AML syndromes and their therapy is beyond the scope of this chapter but is covered in the referenced major texts.

The most important recent therapeutic breakthrough in the treatment of AML has occurred in the treatment of the t(15;17) APL variant with long-term survival rates of greater than 90% (Lo-Coco et al., 2013). Unfortunately, survival in other forms of AML, particularly cases that are secondary to chemotherapy, remains dismal. APL has a strong ethnic predisposition and is particularly common among Hispanic and Chinese populations, where it is the most common form of de novo AML. Therapy initially improved for this particular form of AML when it was demonstrated that all-trans retinoic acid (ATRA) served as a maturation agent, allowing the aberrant promyelocytes of APL to mature normally without first obliterating the bone marrow with intensive chemotherapy, as is the usual practice in AML, and that predictably caused acute disseminated intravascular coagulation (DIC) in APL. However, the major increase in survival resulted from the work with arsenic trioxide, which can be given either orally or by intravenous infusion in concert with or in sequence with ATRA and other drugs and produces sustained remissions and probable cures. The doses of arsenic trioxide given in the modern era are not those used decades ago as an early chemotherapeutic agent and that caused major neurologic and hematologic toxicity. In fact, arsenic is not measurable in the blood a few weeks after administration of the current doses of arsenic trioxide in the treatment of APL.

CYTOPENIAS VERSUS CYTOPATHIES

Certain compounds may directly impair the function of each of the three circulating cellular elements without necessarily directly interfering with bone marrow function or through reductions in the numbers of circulating cellular elements. For example, a primary benefit of the circulating erythrocyte mass involves oxygen transport to the tissues and return of carbon dioxide to the lung. In carbon monoxide, cyanide, and hydrogen sulfide poisoning, the toxic compounds can bind with the hemoglobin molecule and prevent its normal function with gas exchange, causing an acute illness associated with severe tissue hypoxia. Similarly, platelet function may be adversely affected by commonly used medications such as aspirin and NSAIDs as well as in disease states, leading to abnormal renal function in which the accumulation of nitrogenous waste products adversely affect platelet adhesion to bleeding sites and the ability of the platelets to aggregate to each other at the site of bleeding, forming a platelet plug. In terms of the leukocytes, corticosteroids may impair granulocyte phagocytosis, prevent egress of granulocytes into the tissues, and promote infection. Such impairments in phagocytosis and destruction of bacterial pathogens are also present in granulocytes from patients with MDS, which often lack normal amounts of cytoplasmic enzyme-containing granules.

Anticoagulant Therapy

Key Points

- Although warfarin may be antagonized by vitamin K in circumstances of excessive anticoagulation and bleeding, specific antagonists for the newer direct oral anticoagulants are not yet available.
- The lupus anticoagulant is not associated with excessive bleeding but may be associated with both venous and arterial thrombosis.

Table 39-2   Oral Anticoagulants

Feature	Warfarin	Dabigatran	Rivaroxaban	Apixaban
Target	Vitamin K	Factor IIa	Factor Xa	Factor Xa
Plasma half-life (h4)	40-60	12-16	7-13	8-15
Elimination	92% renal	80% renal 20% fecal	66% renal 33% fecal	27% renal 63% fecal
Monitoring	PT/INR	Not required	Not required	Not required
Antidote	Vitamin K	None	None	None
Hemodialysis reversal	No	Yes	No	No
Typical daily dose	7.5 mg in men 5 mg in women	150 mg twice daily	20 mg daily	5 mg twice daily
Use of PT/aPTT in therapy	Yes	Yes, not linear	Yes, not linear	Weakly affected

aPTT, Activated partial thromboplastin time; *INR,* international normalized ratio; *PT,* prothrombin time.

The application and monitoring of anticoagulant therapy in clinical medicine has undergone a major change in recent years with the introduction of newer drugs that are beginning to slowly replace the vitamin K antagonist warfarin, the standard for more than 50 years (Tripodi et al., 2013). Even certain indications for low-molecular-weight heparin (LMWH) and the necessity for hospital admission in cases of thrombophlebitis and pulmonary emboli have been affected by these newer agents, which are direct anticoagulants rather than a prodrug such as warfarin (Coumadin).

The primary need for oral anticoagulant therapy is in the prophylaxis against thrombosis in high-risk circumstances such as chronic atrial fibrillation, mechanical heart valve replacement, and the continuing treatment of thrombophlebitis and pulmonary thromboembolism. Postoperative use of anticoagulant therapy has become a common event after orthopedic surgery to lessen the risk of venous thrombosis. Warfarin is a cost-effective medication, but it is a prodrug and takes several days of administration to achieve an effective steady state of full anticoagulation. Moreover, there are many drug interactions with warfarin that can modify its metabolism and activity, either lessening or potentiating its anticoagulant effect. It has a prolonged half-life in the blood, but its effects on blood coagulation can be antagonized by administration of vitamin K, although this reversal will take several hours for full effect. Thus, in circumstances of major bleeding, plasma may need to be administered to replace reduced levels of clotting factors. Warfarin administration also must be monitored with the use of the prothrombin time (PT) test to ensure an effective degree of anticoagulation as reflected in the standardized INR measurement, or a calculation that accounts for laboratory variation based on types of equipment and reagents used in performing the study. A comparison of warfarin with the properties of several now-approved oral anticoagulant drugs is shown in Table 39-2.

Dabigatran (Pradaxa), rivaroxaban (Xarelto), and apixaban (Eliquis) are all approved for use in patients with atrial fibrillation and could replace warfarin in some instances because the bleeding risk and need for follow-up laboratory monitoring are reduced (Gonzalves et al., 2013). The significant renal excretion of dabigatran and rivaroxaban would make apixaban a safer option in patients with renal insufficiency. Rivaroxaban is the only one of the three newer anticoagulants yet approved for pulmonary embolism

treatment and prevention and may be the initial therapy in uncomplicated patients presenting to the emergency department with acute-onset thrombophlebitis. This is because of its favorable pharmacodynamics and the rapid development of full therapeutic anticoagulation a few hours after an oral dose. This would eliminate the necessity of LMWH as a bridge and eliminate the necessity for inpatient admission to begin warfarin along with LMWH. Here, the dose of rivaroxaban is 15 mg twice daily for 3 weeks, which is then modified to 20 mg once daily for long-term use. If one feels the necessity to monitor or prove the anticoagulant effect of rivaroxaban or apixaban is in effect, the activated factor X assay used to monitor heparin therapy can be modified to quantify their activity as well. The thrombin time may be used to document the anticoagulant effect of dabigatran, but because the thrombin time may be prolonged for many reasons, including a low serum albumin level, such assays would not be linear or useful for anticoagulant control.

Although the effects of most anticoagulants seen in clinical practice are consequent to their therapeutic use, spontaneously occurring circulating anticoagulants may occur in certain circumstances and may or may not cause excess bleeding and may or may not require specific therapy for their control. The two most common are the lupus anticoagulant and the circulating inhibitor of factor VIII. The lupus anticoagulant is often brought to light by performance of a routine screening test such as PT, activated partial thromboplastin time, or both, which are found to be prolonged. Well less than half of the patients seen with the lupus anticoagulant actually have lupus, and the anticoagulant may have no apparent underlying causation and disappear spontaneously. There is no bleeding diathesis associated with their presence, but in some instances, there is an increased risk of thrombosis, primarily venous but occasionally arterial. The inhibitor action is caused by antibodies to the complex of phospholipid and activated factors V and X, which convert factor II to thrombin. These are immediate-acting anticoagulants and are easily identified in the laboratory by mixing studies of patient plasma with normal plasma. Their return to normal values suggests a deficiency state, and a continued prolonged result indicates the presence of an anticoagulant. Certain other tests may be done to confirm this type of anticoagulant.

The spontaneous factor VIII anticoagulant is more of a delayed action anticoagulant in the test tube, and an incubation phase with normal plasma is necessary to document its presence and full activity. This circumstance may appear in patients with classical hemophilia consequent to antibodies generated to factor VIII after transfusions of plasma products. Rarely, such antibodies may also occur spontaneously in pregnancy and, after remission, recur again with a subsequent pregnancy. They also may appear in elderly individuals with no apparent underlying illness but occasionally are consequent to NHL or other malignancy or appear as a drug reaction. The use of combinations of corticosteroids, cyclophosphamide, and Rituxan is very effective in eliminating the circulating anticoagulant in elderly persons but is less effective if the problem is pregnancy related.

Hematologic Malignancies

The wide application of flow cytometry in the clinical laboratory has made the classification of disorders such as CLL and other B-cell and T-cell neoplasms more specific than by the simple morphologic examination of peripheral blood and bone marrow by providing a precise fingerprint of each individual disease. Lymphoid and myeloid cells bear a variety of specific antigenic surface proteins given the designation of CD markers. The application of several of these numbered markers to a peripheral blood or tissue biopsy sample identifies a typical pattern of both positive and negative reactions for each illness. As new markers are identified, the process becomes more specific. Flow cytometry is also useful in the diagnosis and treatment of myeloid malignancies along with major improvements in cytogenetic analysis, which now allow a more precise diagnosis of various forms of AML as well as among the lymphoproliferative disorders.

As the use of diagnostic cellular markers becomes more precise, the classification of hematologic malignancies will undergo constant change, seeking to identify the origin of disease and precise treatments most likely to be successful. For example, in the most recent (2008) edition of the *World Health Organization Classification of Tumours of Haematopoietic and Lymphoid Tissues*, more than 80 distinct types of neoplastic lymphoproliferative disorders are discussed making up the spectrum of HL and NHL (Swerdlow et al., 2008). Only a few of the more frequently encountered illnesses in this class are commented on here. Although we recognize general commonalities among the B-cell neoplasms, the clinical features of each specific illness may differ widely, and thus, most hematologists continue to think of each of these diseases as unique entities, particularly CLL, hairy cell leukemia, MM, WM, and so on, in the approach to diagnosis and therapy. The name may change with time, but the illness and its natural history remain constant.

In many examples of B-cell neoplasms, causation is unknown, although in certain categories, such as HL and CLL, there is a strong familial influence that is not modified by occupation (Altieri et al., 2005). This finding is much less evident among those with MM and hairy cell leukemia, for example. In selected B-cell neoplasms, infectious agents such as hepatitis C, Epstein-Barr virus, various bacteria, autoimmune illness, immunosuppression associated with posttransplantation disease, and the use of biologic disease modifiers are strong associations. In some types of NHL, specific causation is identified in the disease designation, such as EBV-positive diffuse large B-cell lymphoma of elderly adults.

CHRONIC LYMPHOCYTIC LEUKEMIA

Chronic lymphocytic leukemia is an easily recognized hematologic disorder characterized by the accumulation, over time, of mature-appearing B lymphocytes in various body tissues, including the circulating blood, bone marrow, spleen, and multiple lymph nodes. It is the most common form of leukemia seen in the United States, with perhaps as many as 18,000 to 19,000 new cases identified per year. The finding of a persistent lymphocytosis without a known underlying causation immediately suggests the diagnosis, but before the routine application of flow cytometry, inspection of the peripheral blood counts and blood film was accurate in confirming CLL perhaps only about 80% of the time. This is because other lymphoproliferative disorders such as mantle cell and marginal cell lymphoma and even WM and hairy cell leukemia could manifest a similar peripheral blood appearance and clinical presentation. Currently, the technique of rapidly quantifying various CD and other markers on millions of cells allows the diagnosis of CLL to be confirmed accurately and reproducibly even with only moderate elevations of the total lymphocyte count in the circulating blood. The pattern or signature of these immunochemically measured CD and other cell markers on lymphocyte clones in the circulating blood or solid tissues not only easily separates CLL from other B-cell neoplasms but also provides information pertinent to the probable course of the illness and may guide therapy.

About 10% of individuals with the typical CLL flow cytometry pattern only have this finding in lymphoid cells infiltrating lymph nodes or other tissues and do not manifest a leukemic picture in the peripheral blood. These individuals are considered to have small cell lymphocytic lymphoma rather than CLL. The prognosis and treatment of the two conditions are similar.

Chronic lymphocytic leukemia is often a very indolent illness, and as many as one third of affected individuals may never require specific therapy for the disorder during their lifetimes, and it is not a cause of their deaths. An example of this course in terms of the total leukocyte count is shown in one of the senior authors' patients in Figure 39-9. Indeed, for about half of patients, the diagnosis of CLL will not affect morbidity or mortality. However, depending on certain factors, including the cytogenetic pattern of the neoplastic cells and the uncommon transformation to a more aggressive cell type that occasionally is therapy related, the illness may progress rapidly in some individuals. CLL is often associated with immune-related clinically important manifestations, including thrombocytopenia and autoimmune hemolytic anemia. Herpes zoster is also common during the course of the illness. Hypogammaglobulinemia is typical among individuals with long-standing CLL. Because of the immune defects in CLL, it is inadvisable to administer live vaccines to such individuals because severe local reactions may occur, and there is the potential for complications of viremia.

The cause of CLL is entirely unknown, aside from a strong genetic familial risk. In some families, there are multiple

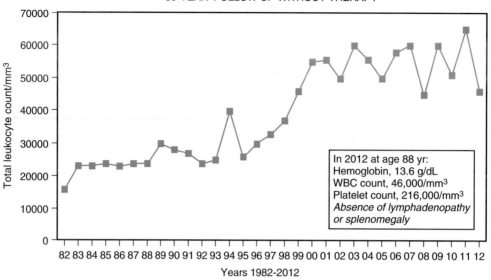

CHRONIC LYMPHOCYTIC LEUKEMIA
30-YEAR FOLLOW-UP WITHOUT THERAPY

In 2012 at age 88 yr:
Hemoglobin, 13.6 g/dL
WBC count, 46,000/mm³
Platelet count, 216,000/mm³
*Absence of lymphadenopathy
or splenomegaly*

Figure 39-9 Peripheral blood total leukocyte count in untreated chronic lymphocytic leukemia. *WBC,* White blood cell.

types of B-cell neoplasms in different individuals. There is no evidence that radiation or chemotherapy or occupational or environmental toxins may cause CLL, and it is not related to smoking. In recent years, it has been well documented that a surprising number of individuals in the general population, particularly individuals who are first-degree relatives of patients with CLL, may have a clone of circulating lymphocytes that type with flow cytometry analysis such as CLL. However, the very small clone may be stable and not necessarily proliferate during life or cause the total leukocyte count to increase to clinically evident levels. This state is referred to as monoclonal B-cell lymphocytosis (MBL) and requires no therapy, only observation (Te Raa et al., 2012). For this reason, currently, CLL is defined by the presence of 5000/mm³ or greater B lymphocytes with a characteristic CLL flow cytometry phenotype in the peripheral blood.

In patients with CLL who do require therapy, there are a wide variety of active drugs of different classes, including monoclonal antibodies, corticosteroids, alkylating agents, antimetabolites, and newer medications that interfere with particular molecular pathways controlling cell growth. In selected younger patients with high-risk chromosome aberrations, allogeneic bone marrow transplantation has been used.

WALDENSTRÖM MACROGLOBULINEMIA

Similar to CLL, about 20% of individuals with WM have a family history of the illness. The WHO has established a new NHL category of lymphoplasmacytic lymphoma, in which WM is the major tenant. The presentation is variable with predominant associated features, including weakness, fatigue, and unexplained anemia or lymphadenopathy. Some patients have unusual complications relating to the very high concentrations of the characteristic IgM paraprotein, such as venous retinal thrombosis or progressive deafness. The laboratory may first call attention to the marked rouleaux on the peripheral blood film and notify the

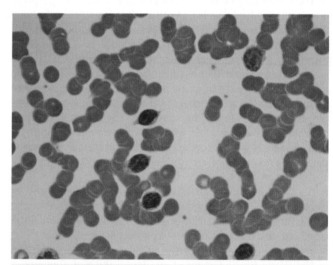

Figure 39-10 Peripheral blood in Waldenström macroglobulinemia demonstrating erythrocyte rouleaux formation and mature-appearing lymphoid cells.

ordering physician (Figure 39-10). As with CLL, the course is often indolent, and a decision to treat may be somewhat subjective and not based on a single factor. The neoplastic lymphoid cells are variable in appearance, ranging from a near normal morphology to plasmacytoid cells or even larger cells with cytoplasmic features very close to those found in hairy cell leukemia (Figure 39-11). Aside from causing an increasing viscosity and plasma volume, the IgM paraprotein may complex with plasma clotting factors, creating a bleeding diathesis. In contrast to CLL, the flow cytometry fingerprint of this illness is not uniform; however, the involved lymphoid cells are usually CD-5 and CD-10 negative. A low serum ferritin level and reduced iron stores are common findings but do not appear to represent chronic blood loss as causative, and the mechanism of iron deficiency is uncertain.

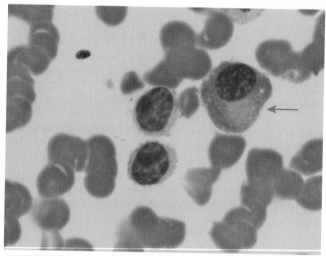

Figure 39-11 Bone marrow aspirate in Waldenström macroglobulin-emia demonstrating two atypical plasmacytoid lymphocytes with irregular cytoplasmic borders and a plasma cell *(arrow).*

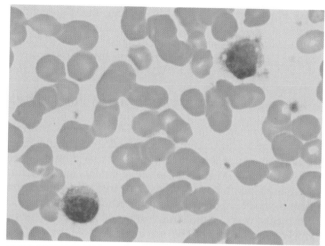

Figure 39-12 Peripheral blood film in hairy cell leukemia demonstrating the characteristic atypical B lymphocytes.

Many drugs are active in the treatment of WM, including corticosteroids, Leustatin, pentostatin, cyclophosphamide, chlorambucil, Velcade, and Rituxan. Unlike IgG parapro-teins, IgM paraproteins are confined in the circulating plasma volume and can be reduced dramatically by plasma exchange (apheresis, plasmapheresis) as dictated by the clinical circumstances. If the patient is not highly symp-tomatic, observation is not unreasonable to assess the pace of progression. On occasion, the neoplastic lymphocytes may transform, and the illness will then resemble a diffuse large cell form of NHL and require aggressive treatment.

HAIRY CELL LEUKEMIA

This is a usually indolent B-cell neoplasm with a striking male over female predominance, at least five to one, and classically presenting as a pancytopenia associated with unexplained splenomegaly and the absence of lymphade-nopathy. To an experienced observer, the diagnosis may often be made immediately by careful examination of the peripheral blood, although it is unusual for large numbers of hairy cells to circulate (Figure 39-12). By flow cytometry, the diagnosis can be confirmed by the typical pattern of positive markers, including CD-20, -22, -25, -103 and -123. Formerly, the tartrate resistant acid phosphatase stain, positive in virtually all cases, was used as a diagnostic aid, but the slides must be freshly prepared for best results, and there must be some dedication by the laboratory to carry this study out properly. It has largely been replaced by flow cytometry fingerprints to more conveniently vali-date the diagnosis. Reticulin fibrosis is often present in the bone marrow.

A family history of the illness has been rarely reported, but most cases are sporadic and diagnosed among individu-als older than 50 years. Splenectomy formerly was the treatment of choice but has largely been replaced by the use of drug combinations such as Leustatin or pentostatin and Rituxan, which will rapidly reduce the size of an enlarged spleen and typically produce a remission in the range of 10 years, at which time a second course of treatment may

become necessary. Patients with this illness are susceptible to granulomatous diseases, both fungal and tubercular, but are unable to form tissue granulomas, and the organisms must be identified by culture, special stains, and molecular studies. Secondary malignancies appear to be increased among patients with hairy cell leukemia.

MULTIPLE MYELOMA

Multiple myeloma is a specific B-cell neoplasm affecting about 20,000 new patients per year in the United States. Typical incidence figures reported are about 4.3 cases per 100,000 individuals. The median survival period after diag-nosis remains about 4 to 7 years, although some patients may follow an indolent course and survive longer than 10 years (Alexander et al., 2007; Kyle et al., 2007; Rajkumar, 2011). It is generally considered to be an incurable illness despite recent advances in chemotherapy and bone marrow transplantation techniques. MM has its peak incidence around age 66 to 70 years and is typically sporadic in appearance. It is very unusual in individuals younger than age 40 years. The incidence of MM is higher among black individuals, and the age of onset is slightly lower than in white populations; the frequency is still lower among Chinese individuals. A known familial incidence of MM is well described but quite uncommon. There is a strong asso-ciation of MM with Gaucher disease, but the mechanism is uncertain. In the case of MM, a B-lymphocyte neoplasm, the illness may be preceded by the presence of a small clone of monoclonal immunoglobulin (*monoclonal gammopathy of unknown causation* [MGUS]), which may suddenly prolifer-ate after many years of stability, causing a major plasmacy-tosis in the bone marrow, replacing normal hematopoiesis and creating bone destruction. It is now well accepted that a preceding period of MGUS has been in place in virtually all newly diagnosed patients with MM (Zingone et al., 2011). Moreover, as long as 16 years may elapse before MGUS progresses into an MM phase. MGUS may occur after hepatitis B and C and be sustained or disappear. It also is seen with some frequency in liver transplantation and does not appear to predispose to MM in this setting (Naina et al., 2012). The peer-reviewed scientific medical literature has consistently indicated that the etiology of MM remains unknown, or as stated in typical review articles from prominent medical journals, its epidemiologic pattern remains obscure (Alexander et al., 2007). No chemical exposures are known to predispose to MM, and its incidence is not increased among smokers.

Many organ systems may be affected by myeloma with anemia caused by infiltration of the bone marrow and reduced erythropoietin output by renal damage. Multiple bone fractures are frequently caused by loss of calcium from the bone matrix and isolated plasmacytomas. Renal failure may be multifactorial in causation in patients with MM but can relate to continuous excretion of free light chains and intact monoclonal proteins causing tubular damage.

In recent years, some stratification of risk is evident by cytogenetic analysis of the myeloma cells. Moreover, the availability of a number of new agents clearly has improved long-term survival. Active drugs include corticosteroids, protease inhibitors such as Velcade, alkylating agents including Alkeran, and cyclophosphamide and compounds such as lenalidomide and thalidomide. Bisphosphonates offer some bone protection and lessen the risk of hypercalcemia. The use of autologous bone marrow transplantation after high doses of intravenous chemotherapy with Alkeran may also offer a prolonged remission. Cure of the illness is rare.

CHRONIC MYELOID LEUKEMIA

The modern treatment of CML is a remarkable success story in an illness that formerly carried a uniformly fatal diagnosis. CML affects about 5000 individuals each year in the United States and is an acquired illness, present in only one of identical twin, not both. The etiology is unknown, but exposure to excess radiation is thought causative in rare circumstances. The characteristic t(9:22) chromosome aberration typically is evident in the laboratory analysis about 1 to 2 years before the disease becomes clinically evident as a rising total granulocyte count and often a rising platelet count. The illness is not familial and is not caused by chemotherapy, smoking, or any known potential environmental or occupational chemicals. CML and CLL were not increased in frequency among Aksoy's cohort of 29,000 shoe workers in Turkey who were chronically exposed to massive levels of pure benzene in the preparation of glues used in the shoe industry.

For many years, CML was placed in the category of classical MPNs because it is often associated with both marked thrombocytosis and bone marrow fibrosis, the latter two findings present in all types of MPN. The natural history of the illness is for the elevation of the total leukocyte count to plateau at around 300,000 to 350,000/mm^3 associated with progressive splenomegaly and anemia. The initial therapy to reduce the total leukocyte count was with benzene, taken orally with the liquid placed in capsules. Later, drugs such as hydroxyurea and Myleran were used to control the myeloproliferation and progressive splenomegaly, but conversion to an acute leukemic state, known as blast crisis, generally occurred within a 4-year period. Cures of CML were first obtained after allogeneic bone marrow transplantation, but the long-term survival rate was only in the 65% range. With the introduction of oral tyrosine kinase inhibitors, which antagonize the products of the BCR/ABL fusion gene produced by the translocation, long-term survival is now greater than 85%, with minimal drug-related side effects. Some patients may be cured after several years with such therapy and ultimately be able to stop all treatment. Several tyrosine kinase inhibitors are available, and some cause fluid retention and pleural effusions, which may be temporary. Today, when encountering a patient with persistent elevation in granulocytes or platelets, the BCR/ABL study on peripheral blood will easily establish the diagnosis of CML. However, classical cytogenetics and fluorescent in situ hybridization (FISH) studies on bone marrow cells are often applied to confirm the specific chromosome aberration and to quantify the percentage of affected bone marrow cells to monitor the effect of specific therapy.

The Myeloproliferative Neoplasms

The original designation of the MPN proposed by Dr. William Dameshek specifically included polycythemia vera, primary myelofibrosis, essential thrombocytosis, and CML because these disorders shared a number of clinical and laboratory features. Other known hematologic diseases involved a myeloproliferative state, but their appropriate classification was debated. As commented upon, the classification system for the MPN has been extensively revised by the WHO, with the exclusion of CML as a distinct entity separate from the other classical forms of MPN. Still other MPNs have been grouped in a diverse category referred to as MDS/MPN to emphasize that some MPN exhibit morphologic myelodysplasia of the type seen in MDS syndromes (Anderson et al., 2012; Orazi et al., 2008; Natelson, 2012; Schmidt and Oh, 2012). Nevertheless, they are MPNs and not MDS (Orazi and Germing, 2008). The most common entity among this nonclassical group of MPNs is chronic myelomonocytic leukemia. The etiology of the MPN is unknown, but all may eventuate in an illness resembling AML, often referred to as blast crisis. Although all of these illnesses are considered neoplasms, the risk for conversion to AML is very low in essential thrombocytosis, but the marked elevation in platelet counts often requires specific therapy and can cause major disability, particularly with surgery (Natelson, 2012).

Clonal or Myeloproliferative Eosinophilic Neoplasms

Key Points

- All patients with myelodysplasia do not necessarily have the MDS.
- All individuals with MPNs have an increased risk of an acute leukemia referred to as blast crisis.
- In patients with MPN, the most effective drugs for continuous use to suppress a massively elevated platelet count are anagrelide and hydroxyurea.
- Several oral tyrosine kinase inhibitor drugs are now approved for the treatment of CML.

Persistent eosinophilia of moderate degree is not an unusual finding among a general clinic population undergoing routine blood counts and only occasionally, when striking, should prompt a referral for hematologic consultation. The vast majority of such cases are reactive or polyclonal processes and generally driven by interleukin-5 (IL-5), a cytokine that promotes proliferation of eosinophilic precursor cells. Causative associations include drug reactions, asthma, a variety of dermatologic conditions (e.g., bullous pemphigoid), and allergic pulmonary conditions. Parasitic infections such as strongyloidiasis should always be considered as potential causes of eosinophilia because therapy with corticosteroids may worsen this condition. Eosinophilia is occasionally present in patients with advanced HL and solid tumors. It is also occasionally a predictable finding in certain types of AML in which it is considered a clonal event caused by specific genetic aberrations associated with the AML (Montgomery et al., 2013; Natelson et al., 2013; Pulsoni et al., 2008). Here the eosinophils are both increased in numbers and abnormal in morphology with large granules.

Some reactive hypereosinophilic syndromes are not neoplasms but may produce pulmonary, cutaneous, and other systemic symptoms that require intermittent therapy with corticosteroids or with currently available steroid-sparing molecularly targeted agents. For example, the monoclonal antibody mepolizumab is directed against IL-5 and has been effective in reducing the eosinophil count and lessening symptoms in such circumstances.

Reactive and idiopathic eosinophilia must be differentiated from the far less common myeloid neoplasms causing marked eosinophilia and sometimes referred to as myeloproliferative eosinophilia (Noel et al., 2013). Over time, these syndromes may cause irreversible tissue damage with infiltration by eosinophils and, if a consideration, require complex cytogenetic diagnostic studies, which may point the way to useful therapeutic interventions. In some affected individuals, a 4q12 chromosome deletion occurs and is involved by translocation and the creation of a fusion gene, *FIP1L1-PDGFRA*, generating a product driving the eosinophilic proliferation. In this instance, treatment with low doses of the tyrosine kinase inhibitor Gleevec may result in a complete remission of the hypereosinophilic state, as it does in CML by blocking of the fusion gene product. Not all of the currently approved tyrosine kinase inhibitor drugs are as effective as Gleevec in this particular circumstance.

Hematology and Pregnancy

Certain features of pregnancy affect the hematologic system on a physiological basis, but other hematologic circumstances, more specific to pregnancy, are important to recognize and require comment. Plasma volume greatly increases during pregnancy, causing a reduction in the hematocrit value and creating an apparent anemia or magnifying an existing anemia on the basis of dilution. The latter circumstance is frequently noticed in women with thalassemia minor who begin pregnancy with a lower hemoglobin concentration than normal. In addition, many women of childbearing age have borderline iron stores, and a pregnancy may transfer as much as 500 mg of iron, or an equivalent iron mass of 2 units of blood, to the fetus. Thus, it is important to provide iron supplements during pregnancy and well into the postpartum period. Various forms of thrombocytopenia are seen with some frequency in pregnancy and are dealt with as a separate entity.

Thrombocytopenia in Pregnancy

Key Points

- Bleeding from thrombocytopenia during pregnancy is unusual with platelet counts above 50,000/mm^3.
- In preeclampsia and the HELLP (hemolysis, elevated liver enzymes, and low platelets) syndrome, the most effective therapy is to facilitate delivery when safely allowed by fetal maturity.
- A bone marrow examination would be necessary to accurately separate pancytopenia of pregnancy from aplastic anemia or bone marrow infiltrative disorders.
- Gestational thrombocytopenia is the most common cause of reduced platelets during pregnancy.
- Vaginal delivery is preferred over cesarean section in acute fatty liver of pregnancy (AFLP) to reduce the risk of intraabdominal bleeding.
- A diagnosis of ITP is not a reason for cesarean section.

In addition to a marked increase in plasma volume, a modest reduction in the platelet count is a normal physiologic event during pregnancy (Gauer and Braun, 2010; Gernsheimer, 2012). Thrombocytopenia, as defined as a platelet count below 150,000/mm^3, occurs in almost 10% of all pregnant patients (Gernsheimer, 2012). In a study of 6670 pregnant patients, a platelet count greater than 115,000/mm^3, late in pregnancy, did not appear to cause adverse events and appeared to not require further evaluation (Boehlen et al., 2000). This should not be a surprising conclusion because a platelet count in the 75,000 to 100,000/mm^3 range is not considered a significant surgical risk in a normal individual unless the platelets are dysfunctional.

The most common form of thrombocytopenia specific to pregnancy is gestational thrombocytopenia. Other well-known pregnancy-induced thrombocytopenic disorders are preeclampsia and a subset, referred to as the HELLP syndrome. Because ITP frequently affects young women, it also is not unusual for this illness to complicate pregnancy (Gauer and Braun, 2010; Gernsheimer, 2012; Webert et al., 2003). Information on previous platelet counts, particularly those before the onset of pregnancy, and a detailed medical history and examination may provide useful diagnostic information in forming a clinical differential diagnosis. Examination of the peripheral blood film is essential and may immediately suggest a specific category of disease. It will also exclude spurious thrombocytopenia, a benign phenomenon often due to transient platelet cold agglutinins causing platelets to clump with each other or to granulocytes and causing an apparent reduction in the platelet count measured in automated equipment.

Depending on its degree and causation, specific therapy for thrombocytopenia may or may not be necessary during the course of the pregnancy, but the provider must be

Table 39-3 Considerations in the Differential Diagnosis of Thrombocytopenia in Pregnancy

Gestational thrombocytopenia	DIC
ITP	Nutritional deficiency
Preeclampsia	Alcohol abuse
AFLP	Drug-induced thrombocytopenia
HELLP syndrome	Certain viral infections
TTP	Pseudothrombocytopenia
HUS	Pancytopenia of pregnancy
SLE	Antiphospholipid antibody syndrome
A primary bone marrow disorder including AML and aplastic anemia	Lupus anticoagulant

AFLP, Acute fatty liver of pregnancy; *AML,* acute myeloid leukemia; *DIC,* disseminated intravascular coagulation; *HELLP,* hemolysis, elevated liver enzymes, and low platelets; *HUS,* hemolytic uremic syndrome; *ITP,* idiopathic thrombocytopenic purpura; *SLE,* systemic lupus erythematosus; *TTP,* thrombotic thrombocytopenic purpura.

familiar with the differential diagnosis of thrombocytopenia in order to make appropriate recommendations to optimize the health of both the mother and fetus (Table 39-3).

Gestational thrombocytopenia accounts for 75% of all pregnancy-related thrombocytopenia. There is no specific diagnostic test to establish this diagnosis, which is possibly related to some combination of increased platelet turnover, dilution, or decreased production. Immune-based platelet destruction that may be difficult to differentiate from that seen in ITP may also be present in gestational thrombocytopenia, and platelet-associated antibodies are found at similar levels in both circumstances (Bockenstedt, 2011). Gestational thrombocytopenia usually presents in the second or third trimester and is typically mild and not typically associated with any adverse fetal or maternal outcome. It usually resolves spontaneously within days to weeks after delivery (Gernsheimer, 2012). Because of the benign nature of the disorder, routine obstetric management is appropriate with the caveat that a neonatologist should evaluate the newborn. There is not an absolute platelet count that defines gestational thrombocytopenia, but according to the American Society of Hematology's guidelines, if the platelet count is below the 70,000 to 80,000/mm^3 range, gestational thrombocytopenia is less likely.

Severe ITP is unusual in pregnancy-associated thrombocytopenia occurring in one to two per 1000 live births (Gill and Kelton, 2000). Neither the incidence nor the severity of ITP increases in pregnancy, but it is a common condition in women of childbearing age (Sukenik-Halevy et al., 2008). Thus, it accounts for about 5% of cases of pregnancy-associated thrombocytopenia and usually presents early in pregnancy with a platelet count below 70,000/mm^3. Although rare in frequency compared with gestational thrombocytopenia, it is the most common pregnancy-associated thrombocytopenia occurring in the first trimester and can be typical ITP or secondary to medications, viral illness, and neoplastic and other immune-related processes (Stavrou and McCrae, 2009).

The pathophysiology and clinical presentation of ITP in pregnancy is similar to ITP in nonpregnant patients. It is a disorder of increased platelet destruction with an inadequate compensatory response by the bone marrow caused by the formation of IgG antiplatelet antibodies leading to the accelerated clearance of platelets by macrophages, typically most prominent in the spleen. Thrombocytopenia may be found incidentally by routine blood count or can present clinically as bruising, bleeding, or petechial lesions. The peripheral blood film will show increased numbers of enlarged platelets and typically an increased mean platelet volume. ITP remains a clinical diagnosis and, hence, it is a diagnosis of exclusion. Pregnant women with ITP may have a history of thrombocytopenia, menorrhagia, or epistaxis. Additionally, a history of excessive bleeding in the mother or fetus in previous pregnancies or a falling platelet count with onset in the first trimester makes ITP more likely.

Treatment of ITP is indicated for pregnant women with thrombocytopenia and bleeding, a platelet count less than 10,000/mm^3, and for platelet counts less than 30,000/mm^3 in the second and third trimesters. Generally, platelet counts above 50,000/mm^3 are thought safe. Corticosteroids are the first line of treatment and, although commonly used, may be associated with pregnancy-specific side effects that include hypertension, premature labor, placental abruption, and gestational diabetes (Gernsheimer, 2012; Gill and Kelton, 2000). IVIG is also a first-line agent. The benefits and risks of each agent should be considered before initiating treatment. A combination of corticosteroids and IVIG may be used if the patient is not responding to either agent alone (McCrae, 2010). In the setting of treatment failure and severe thrombocytopenia, laparoscopic splenectomy can be performed in the second trimester.

Idiopathic thrombocytopenic purpura, per se, is not an indication for cesarean section, and fetal outcome is not determined by maternal severity of disease (Gernsheimer 2012). Rather, the best predictor of neonatal thrombocytopenia is a history of thrombocytopenia in a previous infant sibling. Neonatal thrombocytopenia with a platelet count less than 100,000/mm^3 occurs in only 15% pregnancies with ITP, and the risk of neonatal intracranial hemorrhage is 1% to 2% (Bockenstedt, 2011; McCrae, 2010). The platelet count should be monitored in the neonate for about 1 week after delivery of mothers with ITP (Sukenik-Halevy et al., 2008).

As previously discussed, TTP and HUS are not unique to pregnancy, but the incidence of both increases during pregnancy. Microangiopathic hemolytic anemia (MAHA) and thrombocytopenia are seen in both disorders, as well as in preeclampsia, HELLP syndrome, and acute fatty liver, which can make distinguishing among these disorders difficult (Sibai, 2004). The pentad of MAHA, thrombocytopenia, neurologic abnormalities, fever, and renal dysfunction is classically seen in TTP, but renal dysfunction may be a later complication of the illness. HUS has a similar presentation except that renal dysfunction is more dominant and more commonly has its onset in the postpartum period (Stavrou and McCrae, 2009). The pathophysiology of TTP in nonpregnant patients has previously been discussed. HUS associated with pregnancy is generally not caused by *Shiga* toxins found in epidemic bacterial-related causes of HUS, and the etiology is unknown (McCrae, 2010).

If the diagnosis of TTP is strongly suspected, then plasma exchange should be initiated urgently. HUS, which often results in chronic kidney disease, usually responds poorly to plasma exchange. Nevertheless a trial of plasma exchange is a reasonable approach given the overlapping features of TTP and HUS and the difficulty distinguishing between the two entities. If the diagnosis of TTP-HUS is uncertain, then efforts should also be made to distinguish these disorders from preeclampsia, eclampsia, and HELLP syndrome, and urgent delivery should be considered. Spontaneous resolution of symptoms after delivery generally excludes HUS as a diagnosis. If the MAHA and thrombocytopenia continue postpartum, infusions of the anti-CD 20 antibody Rituxan may be helpful in resolving the illness, particularly if the plasma level of the ADAMTS-13 enzyme is reduced in concentration and accompanied by antibodies to ADAMTS-13.

Preeclampsia is a syndrome that affects multiple organ systems and is the second most common cause of thrombocytopenia in pregnancy, affecting 3% to 14% of pregnancies (Bockenstedt, 2011). Thrombocytopenia, which correlates with the severity of the disorder, occurs in about half of the cases of preeclampsia and occasionally may precede the characteristic findings of proteinuria and hypertension. The onset of preeclampsia is usually in the third trimester.

The American College of Obstetricians and Gynecologists' criteria for the diagnosis of preeclampsia includes a persistent blood pressure elevation of 140 mm Hg systolic or 90 mm Hg diastolic or higher that occurs after 20 weeks of gestation in a woman with previously normal blood pressure and urinary protein excretion of 0.3 g or greater in a 24-hour collection. This latter finding usually correlates with a 1+ or greater reading on a urinary dipstick.

The pathogenesis of preeclampsia is not fully understood, but it is initiated by an abnormal placental implantation process early in pregnancy leading to fetoplacental ischemia that is responsible for the abnormal release and metabolism of prostaglandins. This in turn leads to hypertension, vascular damage, platelet activation, and placental hypoperfusion. Risk factors for preeclampsia are age younger than 20 or older than 30 years, a previous personal or family history of preeclampsia, presence of the antiphospholipid syndrome, a high body mass index, hypertension, and nongestational diabetes. The goal of management is to stabilize maternal blood pressure and proceed with immediate fetal delivery. Usually preeclampsia presents after 34 weeks when the fetal lungs are already mature, but if preeclampsia presents before 34 weeks, delivery may be undertaken after administration of betamethasone to enhance fetal lung maturity, provided maternal and fetal status is reassuring (McCrae, 2010).

HELLP syndrome is a serious obstetric complication that is characterized by a microangiopathic peripheral blood picture and emphasizing hemolysis, elevated liver enzymes, and low platelets. It shares clinical characteristics of severe preeclampsia, and the two are often placed in a spectrum of similar disorders. Interestingly, not all patients with HELLP have hypertension or proteinuria. HELLP syndrome occurs in 0.5% to 0.9% of all pregnancies and complicates 10% to 20% of cases of severe preeclampsia or eclampsia (Bockenstedt, 2011; Schmidt et al., 2012). It presents at an older maternal age compared with preeclampsia, and most affected white women are multiparous.

The pathophysiology of HELLP syndrome is not clearly understood, but it is a multisystem disease similar to preeclampsia and eclampsia. It occurs before delivery in about 70% of cases and usually occurs between the 27th to 37th weeks of gestation. It can also present in the immediate postpartum period, usually within the first 48 hours. Some women manifest incomplete criteria for a HELLP syndrome, and historically, varying diagnostic criteria have been used for HELLP syndrome, making comparison of different studies on the disorder challenging. Common associated signs and symptoms of HELLP syndrome include malaise, right upper quadrant pain, nausea, vomiting, edema, headache, and nonspecific symptoms suggestive of a viral syndrome. The symptom intensity may wax and wane.

The evaluation of a patient with suspected HELLP syndrome includes determining gestational age and fetal status with ultrasonography, cervical bishop score, and maternal status including blood pressure. Laboratory studies should include complete blood count, evaluation of a peripheral blood film, LDH, haptoglobin, transaminase values, coagulation parameters, and urinalysis. Patients should be stabilized with fluids, blood pressure management, and magnesium sulphate, with close monitoring of vital signs and volume status. The goal of treatment is to facilitate delivery, which needs to be done promptly if the gestational age is more than 34 weeks or if maternal or fetal distress is present. If the gestational age is less than 34 weeks and there is no maternal or fetal distress, then corticosteroids should be administered to promote fetal lung maturity followed by delivery within 48 hours (Katz et al., 2008). If the gestational age is less than 27 weeks, expectant management for longer than 48 hours may be considered. The routine use of corticosteroids in HELLP syndrome has not consistently been shown to improve maternal or fetal outcome, although studies have shown improvement in maternal platelet counts. In HELLP syndrome, the rapidity in the resolution of markedly elevated transaminase and LDH values after delivery is striking.

Maternal complications of HELLP syndrome include placental abruption, DIC and hemorrhage, rupture of a subcapsular liver hematoma, acute renal failure, pulmonary edema, life-threatening neurologic complications, and maternal death. As in preeclampsia, there is an increased maternal risk of recurrent disease with subsequent pregnancies. HELLP syndrome is also associated with increased perinatal morbidity and mortality, with a perinatal death rate of 7.4% to 34% and neonatal thrombocytopenia in 15% to 50% of cases. Because of the high rate of preterm deliveries, most fetal complications are related to prematurity.

Acute fatty liver of pregnancy is a rare disorder that usually presents in primiparas in the third trimester. It has an incidence of one in 10,000 to 15,000 pregnancies, and the maternal and fetal mortality rates are 18% and 23%, respectively (Bockenstedt, 2011). Patients present with nausea, vomiting, malaise, right upper quadrant pain, and signs and symptoms of cholestasis. Most patients with AFLP develop DIC. The management of AFLP is immediate resolution of pregnancy, and vaginal delivery is preferred to reduce the incidence of maternal intraabdominal hemorrhage (McCrae, 2010).

Antiphospholipid syndrome (APS) may present as a venous or, rarely, arterial thrombosis. The frequency of thrombocytopenia in APS is usually less than that seen in ITP and occurs in 30% to 46% of patients with primary APS. Treatment includes management of thrombocytopenia as well as thrombotic risk. In a woman with a history of thrombocytopenia and previous miscarriage(s), consideration should be given to underlying disorders such as APS or systemic lupus erythematosus. The frequency of miscarriage in the APS and with the lupus anticoagulant may have been overestimated (Clark et al., 2013).

A very unusual complication of pregnancy is a progressive pancytopenia with cellular bone marrow that is easily initially mistaken for either aplastic anemia or MDS and tends to recur and become more severe with successive pregnancies (Natelson, 2006; Natelson et al., 2013). The entirely different syndrome of aplastic anemia also may occur or worsen during pregnancy, but this illness is easily documented by the character of the bone marrow, which shows severe hypoplasia or aplasia. Its treatment is similar to that of idiopathic aplastic anemia and may respond favorably to immunosuppressive therapy or require allogeneic bone marrow transplantation after the pregnancy has been concluded.

In the less common instance of pancytopenia of pregnancy, there is a progressive macrocytic anemia with frequent teardrop RBCs and often profound thrombocytopenia and significant neutropenia. The bone marrow is normo- to hypercellular, with striking erythroid dyspoiesis and ringed sideroblasts. Megakaryocytes are greatly reduced in numbers. Similar to idiopathic aplastic anemia, this illness also responds to immunosuppressive therapy, but only drugs such as prednisone and cyclosporine may be used during pregnancy, and a satisfactory remission will not occur until the pregnancy has been completed. After the pregnancy has been concluded, more potent immunosuppressive drugs such as antithymocyte globulin may be used, and typically there will be a full hematologic recovery over several months. However, relapse is predictable with subsequent pregnancies and may become more profound and not spontaneously remit. The infant is typically not affected and has a normal blood count.

References

The complete reference list is available at www.expertconsult.com.

Web Resources

www.cancer.gov/cancertopics/pdq/cancerdatabase The National Cancer Institute provides information on clinical trials, references for staging hematologic cancers, and patient handouts.

www.IDsociety.org and www.asco.org The Infectious Disease Society of America and American Society of Clinical Oncology have developed guidelines for the treatment of neutropenia in patients with acute febrile episodes and those receiving chemotherapy.

www.wadsworth.org/chemheme/heme/microscope/celllist.htm Pictures of normal and abnormal blood cells and specific hematologic disease states.

40 *Urinary Tract Disorders*

CHUCK CARTER

Urogenital health care concerns account for 4.1% of all ambulatory patient visits in the United States, more than half with primary care physicians (Schappert and Rechtsteiner, 2011). Disease in the urogenital system can be categorized into anatomic, functional, infectious, and neoplastic disorders. Although there is inevitable overlap among these categories, as in benign prostatic hyperplasia (BPH) (neoplastic) causing outflow obstruction and incontinence (functional), this framework is useful for characterizing urinary tract abnormalities.

Evaluation of the Urinary Tract

The urinary system includes the kidneys, ureters, bladder, and urethra; a system history most often focuses on *voiding*, its primary function. Other issues may include *sexual function* or areas of overlap with other systems (e.g., abdominal pain). Patients often present with or are found to have common concerns specific to the urinary tract (see later discussion). A thorough drug history is critical because many common medications have urologic side effects (Thomas et al., 2003) (see eTable 40-1 online).

PHYSICAL EXAMINATION

Physical examination is limited with urinary tract disorders, but special techniques are available. Many physical findings are helpful, if present, although their absence does not imply normalcy. For example, a renal bruit may indicate arterial stenosis, but its absence does not rule out the condition. Variations in examiner skill and patient factors also limit the accuracy and reliability of physical findings.

The kidneys are retroperitoneal organs and are difficult to palpate, except in very thin persons and children. The right kidney sits more inferior than the left because of the liver. The ureters are nonpalpable but, as with the kidneys, may radiate pain to the flank area. The bladder is typically nonpalpable unless distended with at least 150 mL of urine, and percussion is preferred over palpation for diagnosing distention (Gerber and Brendler, 2011). In women, an enlarged bladder may also be noted on bimanual examination.

Pelvic examination is useful for diagnosing *cystocele* in women. Two fingers can be placed in the introitus and opened to visualize the vaginal cavity. The patient then performs the Valsalva maneuver. The anterior wall dipping down into the vaginal cavity may signify a cystocele. Placing a lubricated cotton swab in the urethral meatus and having the patient perform the Valsalva maneuver can detect more subtle cystoceles. If the swab moves upward (anteriorly), it may indicate movement of the bladder neck with straining.

Examination of the external genitalia in men may reveal penile lesions, regional adenopathy, or disorders of the scrotum and testicles. Uncircumcised men should have the foreskin retracted to rule out phimosis and visualize the glans. Careful palpation of the testicular complex is needed to detect and differentiate masses and anatomic abnormalities. Digital rectal examination (DRE) can estimate prostate size and detect masses or inflammation. It is usually performed with the patient leaning forward on the examination table with his elbows bent. Prostate tenderness, warmth, or a boggy consistency suggests prostatitis. Prostate enlargement consistent with BPH is typical in older men. Masses or asymmetry may indicate a tumor.

LABORATORY TESTS

> **Key Points**
>
> - Routine screening urinalysis is not recommended for adult or child preventive care.
> - Evaluate for sexually transmitted infections (STIs) in patients with urinary tract infection (UTI) symptoms, positive leukocyte esterase results, and negative urine culture results.
> - Do not use urine from a catheter bag for culture.
> - Microalbuminuria screening is routine in diabetes care.

Urinalysis

Urinalysis is one of the most common office laboratory tests, with dipstick urinalysis most often used (Hsiao et al., 2010). Urinalysis is inexpensive, noninvasive, and easily carried out, and it can indicate a number of urinary and systemic conditions. Performing urinalysis in otherwise healthy people as a preventive health service is commonplace. However, screening is not recommended in asymptomatic adults for many of the conditions that urinalysis can identify (e.g., asymptomatic bacteriuria, bladder cancer; see later). Routine urinalysis lacks evidence of benefit, and guidelines recommend against routine urinalysis as part of adult or child preventive care, suggesting it only be done if clinically indicated (Hagan 2008; Stephens and Wilder, 2003; Wilkinson et al., 2013a, 2013b).

Although urinalysis can detect occult disease, most positive results will not yield this outcome; more patients would incur unnecessary or potentially dangerous medical evaluations than would benefit. Thus, the potential value is elusive, and there is the possibility of harm. It is important, however, not to confuse broad population screening recommendations with those specific to certain patients or problems. For example, microalbuminuria screening is routine in diabetes care (American Diabetes Association, 2014).

Physicians should be aware that there is a good chance of false-positive and false-negative results with dipstick tests. Thus, abnormal results are not necessarily indicative of disease and may need confirmatory testing (Gerber and Brendler, 2011; Simerville et al., 2005).

Specimen Preparation. A midstream clean-catch specimen is the recommended standard for urinalysis. Uncircumcised men should retract the foreskin before urinating. Urine should be examined immediately, if possible, and should be refrigerated if it will not be examined in 1 to 2 hours.

Inspection. Normal urine color varies from clear (dilute) to yellow to deep golden and cloudy. Many substances can cause urine color to appear abnormal (Table 40-1). Cloudy urine may be caused by infection (*pyuria*), but the most common cause is *phosphaturia*, in which phosphate crystals precipitate in alkaline urine. Microscopic analysis can differentiate between these two entities. A strong or foul-smelling sample does not necessarily indicate infection. Urine odor may change because of dietary intake (e.g., asparagus), medications, illness, or concentration. Fecal odor suggests gastrointestinal-vesical fistula.

Dipstick Urinalysis

SPECIFIC GRAVITY. Urine specific gravity ranges from 1.001 to 1.035. It reflects the urine concentration and is a marker of hydration status. However, conditions affecting renal functions, such as chronic kidney disease (CKD) and syndrome of inappropriate antidiuretic hormone secretion (SIADH), alter specific gravity and its relation to hydration. The glomerular filtrate has a specific gravity of 1.010, and urine with this fixed specific gravity may indicate renal dysfunction.

PH. Average urinary pH is usually acidic, ranging from 5.5 to 6.5. It reflects the serum pH except in patients with *renal tubular acidosis* (RTA) (Simerville et al., 2005). These patients have alkaline urine because the kidneys cannot acidify urine. Whereas type 1 RTA will always have alkaline urine, urine in type 2 RTA may become acidic as the acidosis worsens. Urine infected with urease-producing organisms such as *Proteus* spp. becomes alkaline.

BLOOD. Dipstick urinalysis has a sensitivity of 91% to 100% and a specificity of 65% to 99% for microscopic hematuria (Grossfeld et al., 2001a). Myoglobin and hemoglobin can cause a false-positive dipstick reaction. Thus, heme-positive urine specimens require microscopic examination (Davis et al., 2012).

GLUCOSE. Glucose in the urine (*glycosuria*) occurs when the glucose concentration of the glomerular filtrate exceeds the proximal tubule's ability to resorb it. The dipstick only reacts to glucose. A finding in uncontrolled diabetes mellitus, glycosuria occurs when the serum glucose level exceeds 180 mg/dL.

KETONES. Urinary ketone bodies are a main feature of diabetic ketoacidosis. They may also be found in starvation states and pregnancy. Dipsticks detect acetoacetic acid. False-positive results may occur with very concentrated or acidic urine.

LEUKOCYTE ESTERASE. Leukocyte esterase is a substance produced by neutrophils that signifies possible pyuria. The likelihood a positive test result for leukocyte esterase indicates UTI improves if urinary nitrite is also positive (Simati et al., 2013). Urine contamination by vaginal cells is the most common reason for false-positive results. Patients with typical UTI symptoms, positive leukocyte esterase, and negative urine cultures should be evaluated for STIs (Graham and Galloway, 2001).

NITRITE. The finding of nitrites in the urine is 92% to 100% specific for a UTI (Simerville et al., 2005). However, many patients with UTIs will not be nitrite positive (i.e., low sensitivity). Gram-negative coliform organisms convert urinary nitrates to nitrite but not *Staphylococcus saprophyticus* or enterococci. The test loses accuracy with lower bacterial colony counts. The reagent is air sensitive, so a dipstick may yield false-positive results if strips in the container are not tightly sealed (Gallagher et al., 1990).

PROTEIN. Urine dipsticks are very sensitive and specific for albuminuria. The reagent color change roughly corresponds to the protein concentration in the sample (Table 40-2). Very dilute, alkaline, or nonalbumin proteinuria

Table 40-1	Factors Affecting Urine Color
Color	**Causative Factor**
Colorless	Very dilute urine; overhydration
Cloudy, milky	Phosphaturia; pyuria; chyluria
Red	Hematuria; hemoglobinuria, myoglobinuria; anthocyanin in beets and blackberries; chronic lead and mercury poisoning; phenolphthalein (in bowel evacuants); phenothiazines (e.g., prochlorperazine [Compazine]); rifampin
Orange	Dehydration; phenazopyridine (Pyridium); sulfasalazine (Azulfidine)
Green-blue	Biliverdin; indicanuria (tryptophan indole metabolites); amitriptyline (Elavil); indigo carmine; methylene blue; phenols (e.g., IV cimetidine [Tagamet]; IV promethazine [Phenergan]); resorcinol; triamterene (Dyrenium)
Brown	Urobilinogen; porphyria; aloe, fava beans, rhubarb; chloroquine, primaquine; furazolidone (Furoxone); metronidazole (Flagyl); nitrofurantoin (Furadantin)
Brown-black	Alkaptonuria (homogentisic acid); hemorrhage; melanin; tyrosinosis (hydroxyphenylpyruvic acid); cascara, senna (laxatives); methocarbamol (Robaxin); methyldopa (Aldomet); sorbitol

IV, Intravenous.
From Hanno PM, Wein AJ. *A clinical manual of urology.* Norwalk, CT: Appleton-Century-Crofts; 1987:67.

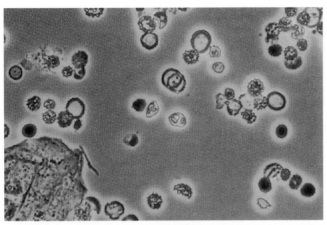

Figure 40-1 Urinalysis: dysmorphic red blood cells. (From Gerber GS, Brendler CB. Evaluation of the urologic patient. In Wein AJ, ed. *Campbell-Walsh urology.* 10th ed, vol 1. Philadelphia: Saunders; 2011:95.)

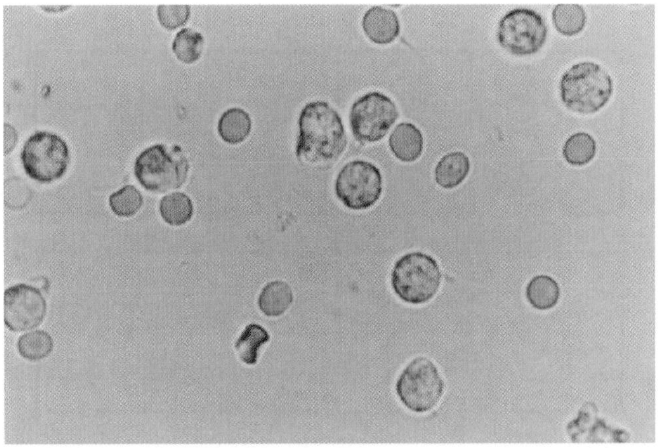

Figure 40-2 Urinalysis: white blood cells. (From Gerber GS, Brendler CB. Evaluation of the urologic patient. In Wein AJ, ed. *Campbell-Walsh urology.* 10th ed, vol 1. Philadelphia: Saunders; 2011:107.)

Table 40-2 Dipstick Protein Findings

Dipstick Color	Estimated Corresponding Protein Level (mg/dL)
Yellow	Negative (no protein)
Yellow-green	Trace (10-20)
Green	1+ (30)
Dark green	2+ (100)
Green-blue	3+ (300)
Blue	4+ (>1000)

From Simerville JA, Maxted WC, Pahira JJ. Urinalysis: a comprehensive review. *Am Fam Physician.* 2005;71:1153-1162.

may cause false-negative results. Microalbuminuria screening usually requires a separate dipstick designed specifically for this purpose. A urine protein electrophoresis is needed to evaluate nonalbumin proteinuria, such as globulinuria or Bence Jones protein.

UROBILINOGEN. Urobilinogen is a breakdown product of conjugated bilirubin. There is normally a small amount present, but elevations indicate possible hemolysis or liver disease. Conjugated bilirubinuria is abnormal and signifies hepatic disease or biliary obstruction. Unconjugated bilirubin is not filtered by the glomerulus.

Urine Microscopy. To prepare a urine sample for microscopic analysis, centrifuge 10 mL of urine for 5 minutes at 2000 rpm. After centrifugation, pour off the supernatant and resuspend the remaining sample (0.5-1.0 mL). Place a drop of this sample on the slide and focus up to high power. Samples showing probable skin or vaginal contamination should be retested or a catheterized specimen obtained (Grossfeld et al., 2001a). Sediment counts should be estimated as the average number of elements viewed per high-power field (hpf).

RED BLOOD CELLS. Urine specific gravity may affect findings because red cells may lyse at values lower than 1.007 (Vaughan and Wyker, 1971). Whereas normal-appearing red blood cells (RBCs) suggest a lesion in the urinary tract, dysmorphic RBCs are probably of glomerular origin (Figure 40-1). RBC casts are typically found at the edges of the

glass coverslip and are highly suspicious for renal parenchymal disease.

WHITE BLOOD CELLS. Normal urine samples may show some white blood cells (WBCs) on high-power examination (Figure 40-2). For women, fewer than 5 WBCs/hpf is normal; for men, fewer than 2 WBCs/hpf is normal (Simerville et al., 2005). Values in excess of these limits constitute microscopic pyuria. Purulent, cloudy urine with WBCs too numerous to count describes gross pyuria.

White blood cells are inflammatory markers, so infection cannot be confirmed by their presence or ruled out by their absence. Common causes of sterile pyuria include STIs, kidney stones, prostatitis, and urinary tract neoplasms. In children, pyuria may occur during a febrile illness even if a UTI is not present (Graham and Galloway, 2001).

CASTS. Red blood cell casts signify a nephritic or vasculitic process. WBC casts are often considered pathognomonic for pyelonephritis, but they may be found in other types of nephritis. Granular and waxy casts signify renal parenchymal disease. Hyaline casts may be normal in concentrated specimens or a marker of renal infection or disease.

CRYSTALS. Various crystal morphologies may be seen in urine samples (Figure 40-3).

URINARY EPITHELIAL (UROTHELIAL) CELLS. Transitional epithelial cells are normally found in microscopic specimens. They are uniform in shape and have large, central nuclei. In contrast, squamous cells have irregular borders and small nuclei. Squamous cells indicate skin contamination.

BACTERIA. Bacteria may signify bacteriuria, but in women, vaginal contamination is also likely. A urine Gram stain is also helpful for identifying bacterial characteristics in urine samples in which infection is suspected.

FUNGI. Yeast seen in urine specimens most likely indicates contamination from the skin or vagina. However, it may signify systemic *Candida* infection if found in a catheterized specimen (Graham and Galloway, 2001).

TRICHOMONADS. These motile organisms signify a common STI and may be seen in urine samples. Treatment with metronidazole (2 g as a single dose or 500 mg twice daily for 7 days) is effective. Patients should be evaluated for other STIs.

Crystals

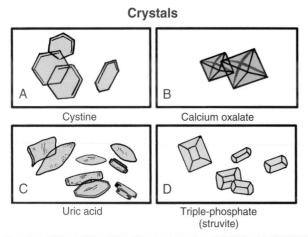

Figure 40-3 Crystal types found in urine samples. **A,** Cystine. **B,** Calcium oxalate. **C,** Uric acid stones found in acidic urine. **D,** Triple-phosphate crystals found in alkaline specimens. (From Gerber GS, Brendler CB. Evaluation of the urologic patient. In Wein AJ, ed. *Campbell-Walsh urology.* 10th ed, vol 1. Philadelphia: Saunders; 2011:96.)

Urine Culture

Urine culture is the "gold standard" test for diagnosing UTIs. Many sources have emphasized the midstream clean-catch technique as necessary for preventing contamination, although the value of this practice is uncertain in adults (Lifshitz and Kramer, 2000). However, genital cleansing may be more important in children (Vaillancourt et al., 2007). Bladder aspiration and catheterization are invasive sampling techniques. Urine from a catheter bag should not be used for culture because bacterial contamination is typical.

More than one bacterial isolate on culture suggests contamination. Controversy exists regarding the threshold colony counts that define bacteruria consistent with infection. Although more than 10^5 colony-forming units per milliliter (CFU/mL) is a well-known cutoff, lower values are meaningful in certain patients. In patients with typical UTI symptoms, counts as low as 10^2 CFU/mL signify infection if *Escherichia coli* or other Enterobacteriaceae are isolated. A cutoff of 10^3 CFU/mL is appropriate in men with symptoms (Graham and Galloway, 2001).

Other Diagnostic Tests

Postvoid Residual Measurement. Postvoid residual measurement assesses the volume of urine in the bladder after voiding and can be performed in the office. One method is to have the patient void and then measure any residual urine by catheterization. Less than 50 mL of residual urine is normal, and 200 mL or greater is abnormal (Kobashi, 2011). Portable ultrasound units can also estimate bladder urine volume as well as postvoid residual urine. *Urodynamics* refers to a battery of tests examining micturition, which may include postvoid residual measurement as well as various tests of bladder and sphincter pressures.

Endoscopy. Urinary endoscopy (cystoscopy) provides visual diagnosis and the opportunity for intervention. Rigid or flexible endoscopic procedures are available. Common interventional techniques include stone retrieval, stent placement, tumor biopsy and resection, and laser

treatment. Risks include infection, bleeding, urethral damage, and bladder perforation.

IMAGING STUDIES

> ### Key Points
>
> - Ultrasound studies are ideal for evaluating renal parenchymal disease and testicular disorders.
> - Computed tomography (CT) is a better choice for evaluating solid renal masses, renal infections, perirenal masses, and renal calculi.

Intravenous Urography

Once the standard method of upper urinary tract imaging, intravenous urography (IVU), also known as intravenous pyelography (IVP), has fallen out of favor for many indications in lieu of CT.

Ultrasonography

Ultrasonography has many applications for evaluating urinary tract disease. It is the method of choice for imaging renal cysts and the renal parenchyma as part of a renal disease workup. Ultrasonography is also the test of choice for evaluating scrotal and testicular disorders. It can usually differentiate masses such as hydrocele, inguinal hernia, and varicocele. Furthermore, regular and color Doppler ultrasonography are essential parts of evaluating acute scrotal pathology, such as epididymitis, orchitis, and testicular torsion.

Ultrasonography is almost 100% sensitive for testicular tumors (Dogra et al., 2003). However, it does not provide tissue diagnosis. Rather, ultrasonography helps define the nature of the suspected lesion, differentiating it from the many other conditions that might mimic an intratesticular tumor.

Computed Tomography

Computed tomography urography has replaced IVU as the test of choice for evaluating hematuria (Davis et al., 2012). It is a better choice for evaluating solid renal masses, perirenal masses, and renal infections (Grossfeld et al., 2001b). Noncontrast CT is the test of choice for adults in evaluating renal calculi (White, 2012). Other uses include CT angiography, trauma imaging, and cancer staging.

Other Techniques

Magnetic resonance imaging (MRI) is an option comparable with CT for detecting renal masses. MR urography is also available. MRI studies are more expensive than CT, however, and availability varies (Brehmer, 2002). Thus, this modality is often used when CT examination is equivocal or contraindicated. MRI is used for staging prostate cancers (Harisinghani et al., 2003).

Voiding cystourethrography (VCUG) uses contrast imaging of the bladder and urethra during urination. Contrast material is delivered via catheter, and the images are obtained while the patient voids. It is most often used to diagnose suspected vesicoureteral reflux (VUR). Nuclear medicine studies may also be used to examine possible VUR, as well as renal function or suspected testicular torsion.

COMMON URINARY TRACT CONCERNS

Key Points

- Dysuria most often indicates UTI, vaginitis, or STI.
- Gross hematuria requires aggressive evaluation.
- Urine microscopy is required to diagnose hematuria. In adults, risk factors for malignancy should be assessed; isolated hematuria is most common in children.
- Hematuria of renal origin often has dysmorphic red cells. Hematuria of bladder origin should show normal RBCs.
- Nocturia is common in both genders and increases the risk of falling in older adults.
- The urine protein-to-creatinine (UPr/UCr) ratio correlates well with a 24-hour urine and is much easier to obtain.
- Proteinuria in children is most often orthostatic.

Dysuria

Urinary burning or pain most often represents UTI or vaginitis. It is common in middle-aged and sexually active women. In men, it is more likely to occur as they grow older (Bremnor and Sadovsky, 2002). Both voiding history and sexual history are essential. Questions regarding vaginal symptoms are important in women. Also, use of medications and personal hygiene products should be reviewed.

Dysuria significantly increases the chance that a patient has a UTI. However, there are many potential causes of dysuria (Table 40-3), and empiric treatment based on this symptom alone leads to unnecessary antibiotic use. Incorporating other symptoms increases the likelihood that a UTI is the cause (see Urinary Tract Infection) (Bent et al., 2002; McIsaac et al., 2002).

Flank Pain

Flank pain may be a presenting complaint indicating urinary tract disorder. It is typically not relieved by position changes and is colicky in nature. Nausea and vomiting may

coincide. Obstruction (e.g., kidney stones) and inflammation (e.g., pyelonephritis) are the two most common causes. The location may help localize the underlying cause (Figure 40-4). Tumors are less likely because they are usually only symptomatic if they distend the renal capsule or obstruct the ureter.

Urinary Frequency

As a complaint, urinary frequency implies a deviation from a patient's normal urination pattern. Thus, it may either be truly abnormal or simply more than the patient's custom (but still normal). It may exist alone or in concert with other symptoms. For example, UTI often causes urinary frequency, urgency, and dysuria.

Adults typically urinate five to six times a day (Gerber and Brendler, 2011). Frequency usually represents an increased number of episodes with small volumes of urine as opposed to increased urine volumes, such as in polyuria. These factors help narrow the differential diagnosis (Table 40-4).

Hematuria

Hematuria is often an incidental finding on urinalysis, and evaluation depends on whether it is gross or microscopic and whether it occurs in adults, children, or adolescents. Most patients with hematuria do not have significant pathology, but this depends on the type of hematuria and underlying risk factors. One prospective study found that 61% of patients with hematuria had no finding after evaluation (Khadra et al., 2000). However, the malignancy rate in screening studies is 2.6%, suggesting the need for workup in patients demonstrating this finding (Davis et al., 2012).

Gross hematuria is blood in the urine visible to the patient or physician. Microscopic hematuria is the more common entity. Microscopic hematuria in adults is defined as 3 or more RBCs/hpf (Davis et al., 2012). In children, clear consensus is lacking, although more than 5 RBCs/hpf found in at least two weekly urine samples is considered abnormal (Dodge et al., 1976; Vehaskari et al., 1979). The reasons for the different definitions may reflect a lower evaluation

Table 40-3 Differential Diagnosis of Dysuria

Calculi
Meatal stenosis
Medications
Neoplasm—bladder, benign prostate hyperplasia, prostate, penile, vulvovaginal
Prostatitis
Sexually transmitted infection—*Chlamydia*, gonorrhea, herpes simplex virus, *Mycoplasma* spp., *Trichomonas* spp.
Somatization
Trauma—foreign body, mechanical, masturbation, postcoital
Urethral syndrome
Urethritis—infectious, irritant, chemical, spondyloarthropathy
Urinary tract infection—cystitis, pyelonephritis, prostatitis
Vaginitis—allergic, atrophic, bacterial vaginosis, candidiasis, chemical

Modified from Seller RH. Urethral discharge and dysuria. In *Differential diagnosis of common complaints*. 3rd ed. Philadelphia: Saunders; 1996 and Brenmor JD, Sadovsky R. Evaluation of dysuria in adults. *Am Fam Physician*. 2002;65:1589-1596.

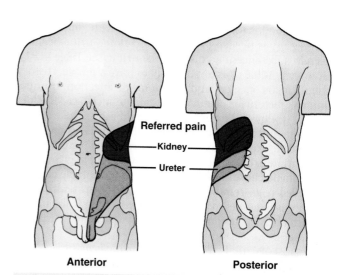

Figure 40-4 Localization of flank pain. (From Anderson JK, Kabalin JN, Cadeddu. Surgical anatomy of the retroperitoneum, adrenals, kidneys, and ureters. In Wein AJ, ed. *Campbell-Walsh urology*. 10th ed, vol 1. Philadelphia: Saunders; 2011:32.)

Table 40-4 Differential Diagnosis of Urinary Frequency

Anxiety
Bladder calculus
Bladder outlet obstruction
Chemical irritation
Cystitis
Diabetes insipidus
Diabetes mellitus
Detrusor instability
Diuretics
Excessive fluid intake
External genital lesion
Habit
Pelvic mass
Pregnancy
Somatization
Upper motor neuron lesion
Urethritis
Urinary tract infection
Vaginitis

From Hanno PM. Interstitial cystitis and related disorders. In Walsh PC, ed. *Campbell's urology*. 8th ed, vol 2. Philadelphia: Saunders; 2002:661.

threshold in adults because of the larger spectrum of potential causes.

Dipstick urinalysis alone is insufficient for diagnosing hematuria because certain substances (e.g., myoglobin) and test characteristics (e.g., specificity) can cause false-positive results. Thus, microscopic analysis is necessary and inherent in the definition.

Hematuria in Adults

GROSS HEMATURIA. Gross hematuria is a common presenting symptom for patients with bladder or renal cancer (Yun et al., 2004). The sensitivity of gross hematuria for bladder cancer is 83%, and the positive predictive value (PPV) is 22% (Buntinx and Wauters, 1997). However, the studies generating these values were of low quality and based on referral populations. No studies are available on the likelihood that family medicine patients with this finding will have serious pathology. Pending this research, the approach to gross hematuria should remain aggressive (Khadra et al., 2000).

Confirmation of blood in the urine with dipstick and microscopy is needed in cases of red-tinted urine because certain substances can discolor the urine (see Table 40-1). However, visible clots are unlikely to have a mimic. History should focus on signs and symptoms of infection, trauma, and risk factors for urinary tract malignancy (see "Bladder Cancer"). Physical examination should assess the external genitalia and include a pelvic examination in women and a prostate examination in men. Urology consultation is appropriate except when an obviously benign (e.g., menses) or treatable cause is found. Even when a treatable cause is identified (e.g., renal calculi), close follow-up with repeat urinalysis is needed because gross hematuria is frequently a harbinger of serious urinary tract pathology (Khadra et al., 2000).

MICROSCOPIC HEMATURIA. *Asymptomatic hematuria* potentially signals serious urinary tract disease, although there are many causes, often benign. Hematuria may occur in 9% to 18% of normal subjects (Grossfeld et al., 2001a). Most studies evaluating and defining this problem were not performed in typical family medicine populations, are of

lower quality, or both. No prospective studies demonstrate an improved outcome from routine screening; as noted earlier, routine urinalysis is not recommended for adults. For the general population, finding asymptomatic microscopic hematuria carries a predictive value of only 0.5% (Brehmer, 2002). Thus, benefit from routine microhematuria screening is unlikely (Kryszczuk et al., 2004).

Family physicians encountering microhematuria should consider patient risk characteristics and systematic laboratory testing and imaging (Figure 40-5). The first step in approaching asymptomatic microscopic hematuria is to assess whether a benign cause such as menses, sexual activity, vigorous exercise, viral illness, or trauma is the explanation, as this may preclude further workup. However, repeat urinalysis is often needed to verify the hematuria has resolved. A caveat is a patient at risk for bladder cancer because intermittent hematuria can precede this finding, and more extensive follow-up may be warranted (Davis et al., 2012; Grossfeld et al., 2001b). Family physicians should be cautious not to misattribute certain causes as benign. For example, warfarin (Coumadin) could cause hematuria if the patient is excessively anticoagulated, but it should not cause hematuria within its goal international normalized ratio (INR) range. Hematuria in this setting is often a sign of urologic disease (Culclasure et al., 1994). Thus, patients taking anticoagulants should be evaluated if they develop hematuria (Davis et al., 2012).

If hematuria is consistently found, the next step is to risk stratify the patient based on history, physical, and baseline laboratory findings. Initial laboratory testing should include urinalysis, urine culture (if indicated), and renal function assessment. If UTI is present, patients should be reassessed at a later date as they would for a benign cause. High-risk patients are those at increased risk for urologic malignancy—men, age older than 35 years, tobacco use history, analgesic abuse, pelvic irradiation, occupational exposures (see Bladder Cancer), prior urologic disease, irritative voiding symptoms, history of UTIs, history of urologic disease or gross hematuria, chronic indwelling device, and cyclophosphamide use (Davis et al., 2012). Hematuria of renal origin may be associated with microscopic RBC casts or dysmorphic RBCs. Other findings may include proteinuria, elevated serum creatinine, or a physical finding such as hypertension or edema. These patients need evaluation for renal disease, including urine protein quantification. Some patients will have risk factors and findings for both renal and urologic disease or may already have a history of CKD, so simultaneous evaluations for both causes may be necessary.

The evaluation for microhematuria includes upper urinary tract imaging (CT urography), and cystoscopy. Cystoscopy is necessary to rule out bladder cancer confidently because no imaging study is adequate for evaluation. However, cystoscopy is optional in low-risk patients because it is unlikely to yield a definitive finding (Davis et al., 2012). Urine cytology is no longer recommended as part of the routine workup but may be used for patients with negative evaluation findings who have ongoing hematuria and risk factors. Urine tumor markers are not routinely recommended either (Davis et al., 2012).

A cause of hematuria is often not found even after a complete evaluation. Isolated hematuria is *asymptomatic*

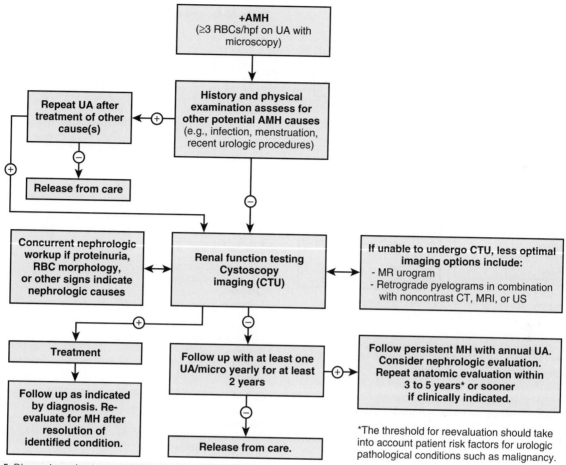

Figure 40-5 Diagnosis, evaluation, and follow-up of asymptomatic microscopic hematuria. *AMH,* Asymptomatic microscopic hematuria; *CT,* computed tomography; *hpf,* high-power field; *MH,* microscopic hematuria; *MRI,* magnetic resonance imaging; *RBC,* red blood cell; *UA,* urinalysis; *US,* ultrasonography. (Copyright ©2012 American Urological Association Education and Research, Inc.)

microscopic hematuria with a normal urologic evaluation and no signs of systemic disease or microscopic evidence of intrinsic renal disease (the definition slightly differs for children). The prognosis is good, although some studies indicate a high proportion of renal abnormalities (e.g., IgA nephropathy). Thus, surveillance for signs of renal disease is appropriate (Grossfeld et al., 2001b). Persons with negative evaluation findings can be followed with annual microscopic urinalysis. If results are normal for 2 years, they need no further testing because their risk approaches that of the general population. Those with ongoing hematuria need regular follow-up and may need a repeat urologic evaluation (Davis et al., 2012).

Evaluation and treatment of *symptomatic microscopic hematuria* is directed at the condition. However, family physicians should consider the underlying risk of urinary tract abnormalities when deciding on follow-up. For example, a patient with a symptomatic kidney stone may have microhematuria. Although this provides the most likely explanation for the bleeding, if the patient has a background risk for malignancy (e.g., smoking) or renal disease, repeat urinalysis is needed to ensure resolution.

Hematuria in Children and Adolescents. Hematuria is a relatively common finding in children, with an estimated prevalence of 0.5% to 2% of asymptomatic school-age children (Dodge et al., 1976). Those with hematuria and proteinuria, particularly when associated with hypertension, edema, or urinary casts, need aggressive evaluation for underlying glomerular disease or uropathy. The vast majority of children with hematuria, however, present with isolated hematuria. This is typically detected on a random urine sample obtained in the context of a routine physical examination but may also present as asymptomatic gross hematuria. In children, the term *isolated* refers to the complete absence of symptoms, significant past medical or family history, physical examination findings, or other abnormalities on urinalysis. This distinction often separates children with benign processes from those with underlying pathology.

After the diagnosis of hematuria has been confirmed, a complete history obtained, and a physical examination performed, a staged evaluation should ensue (Figure 40-6). Significant underlying renal or urologic disease is highly unlikely in children with isolated microscopic hematuria (Bergstein et al., 2005). A more thorough evaluation is indicated for asymptomatic macroscopic hematuria.

The most common glomerular diseases associated with isolated hematuria are subclinical postinfectious glomerulonephritis, IgA nephropathy, and Alport syndrome. In the

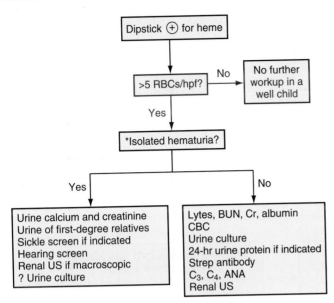

Figure 40-6 Approach to a child with hematuria. *ANA,* Antinuclear antibodies; *BUN,* blood urea nitrogen; *CBC,* complete blood cell count; *Cr,* creatinine; *hpf,* high-power field; *HTN,* hypertension; *RBC,* red blood cell; *US,* ultrasonography.

*Negative history; normal physical exam findings; and absence of symptoms, HTN, pyuria, proteinuria, and cellular casts

Table 40-5   Lower Urinary Tract Symptoms

Voiding	Hesitancy
	Poor urinary flow
	Straining
	Incomplete bladder emptying
	Terminal or postmicturition dribbling
	Prolonged urination
Storage	Urinary frequency
	Nocturia
	Urgency
	Urge incontinence

Modified from Thorpe A, Neal D. Benign prostatic hyperplasia. *Lancet.* 2003;361:1359-1367.

Table 40-6   Causes of Nocturia

Alcohol consumption
Anxiety
Benign prostatic hyperplasia
Bladder outlet obstruction
Caffeine
Calculi
Chronic heart failure
Cystitis
Detrusor instability
Diabetes insipidus
Diabetes mellitus
Diuretics
Dysfunctional voiding
Edema
Excessive nighttime fluid consumption
Myeloneuropathy
Nephrotic syndrome
Neurogenic bladder
Obstructive sleep apnea
Overactive bladder syndrome
Sleep disorders
Somatization
Stroke
Urologic cancer

From Weiss JP, Blaivas JG. Nocturia. *J Urol.* 2000;163:5-12.

absence of proteinuria or more advanced disease, there is no treatment given for these conditions. Yearly follow-up with blood pressure and urinalysis is indicated for all forms of persistent hematuria.

Hypercalciuria may or may not be associated with pain. The exact mechanism by which hypercalciuria causes hematuria is unproven but probably is secondary to crystalluria (Stapleton, 1994). Hypercalciuria is generally defined by a urinary calcium excretion higher than 4 mg/kg/day or a random UPr/UCr higher than 0.2. Higher excretion rates are expected in infants and toddlers. Patients with documented hypercalciuria should undergo renal ultrasonography to rule out nephrocalcinosis or significant stone disease. The treatment is to increase fluid intake and restrict dietary sodium (<3 g/day) while maintaining the recommended daily allowance of calcium (Escribano et al., 2014; Srivastava and Alon, 2005). This dietary intervention may lower the urine calcium concentration and ultimately result in resolution of the hematuria. A thiazide diuretic should be considered if there is evidence of nephrocalcinosis or nephrolithiasis.

Lower Urinary Tract Symptoms

Lower urinary tract symptoms (LUTS) are the symptoms traditionally associated with BPH. Many subcategories of LUTS exist, but the two most prominent are storage and voiding symptoms (Table 40-5). *Voiding* symptoms imply obstruction, but physical obstruction may not be responsible. In men with BPH, for example, detrusor overactivity, neurologic disorders, or age-related smooth muscle dysfunction may be the cause. Thus, LUTS should shift attention toward a larger symptom complex with many potential causes. This is particularly important when dealing with urinary tract disorders such as BPH, incontinence, and overactive bladder.

Nocturia

Nocturia describes waking at night to urinate. It is more common in older adults, but no population data define a normal range for any group; therefore, the complaint implies a deviation from a perceived norm. Furthermore, the primary complaint often centers on a sleep disturbance rather than on urination. It may represent frequent nocturnal urination or excessive nocturnal urine production (nocturnal polyuria). Although often thought of as a prostatic symptom, it is common in both men and women. The many secondary causes in addition to local causes include prostatic hyperplasia and bladder dysfunction (Table 40-6). In patients with prominent LUTS, the problem is compounded by urination difficulty. Furthermore, studies in older adults indicate that nocturia or LUTS increases the risk of falling (Parsons et al., 2009). Age-related variations in arginine vasopressin secretion may play a role in nocturnal polyuria (Weiss and Blaivas, 2000).

Treatment centers on the underlying cause, and a voiding diary may aid clinical decisions. Prostate hyperplasia or bladder dysfunction often receives first attention. Treating BPH may help, although BPH often does not result in true physical obstruction, and epidemiologic data have indicated

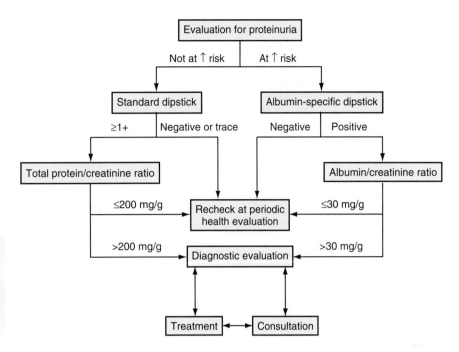

Figure 40-7 Approach to proteinuria in adults. (Modified from Levey AS, Coresh J, Balk E, et al. National Kidney Foundation practice guidelines for chronic kidney disease: evaluation, classification, and stratification. *Ann Intern Med.* 2003; 139:137-147, E148-E149. Redrawn from National Kidney Foundation/Kidney Disease Quality Initiative. See Web Resources.)

that nocturia is common in men without prostatic obstruction. Thus, family physicians should consider the contribution of nocturnal polyuria. For example, patients with chronic heart failure and leg edema may benefit from fluid restriction and napping with leg elevation during the day. Treating obstructive sleep apnea helps alleviate the increased urine production resulting from increased atrial natriuretic peptide production. Behavioral interventions include avoiding excess nighttime alcohol or fluid intake and afternoon napping. Adjusting diuretic doses so they are given earlier in the evening should negate medication effects during sleep (Weiss and Blaivas, 2000).

Proteinuria

The kidneys normally excrete a small amount of protein daily, usually glycoproteins. Only very small amounts of globulins, light-chain proteins, or albumin are released. Functional proteinuria may result from physiologic changes in glomerular filtration, as occurs with exercise (Venkat, 2004). However, consistent albuminuria implies glomerular or tubular dysfunction.

The urine dipstick is the most convenient measurement, but a more accurate test is the UPr/UCr ratio, obtained by dividing the random urine sample protein level by the urine creatinine level (both in milligrams per deciliter). This ratio has proven correlation with 24-hour excretion rates (Ginsberg et al., 1983). Thus, random urine samples are the best way to identify and follow proteinuria, and 24-hour collections are usually not needed (Levey et al., 2003) (Table 40-7). However, results from those with low or high levels of muscle mass may not correlate as well with 24-hour measurements (Venkat, 2004).

Proteinuria in Adults. Proteinuria is a marker of kidney disease in adults and may actually contribute to renal impairment. Patients with diabetes should be periodically tested for microalbuminuria. Others at risk for kidney disease, such as patients with hypertension, should also be tested.

Table 40-7 Proteinuria Values

Test	Protein Value
Dipstick	≥1+ if urine specific gravity ≤1.015 *or* ≥2+ if urine specific gravity >1.015
UPr/UCr ratio	**CHILDREN** >0.5 (age 6 mo to 2 yr) >0.25 (>2 yr)
	ADULTS: >0.2
24-hour urine assay	**CHILDREN** >4 mg/m²/hr >100 mg/m²/day
	ADULTS 30-300 mg/24 hr—microalbuminuria >300 mg/24 hr—albuminuria >3.5 g/24 hr—nephritic-range proteinuria

UPr/UCr, Urine protein/creatinine.

Adults with proteinuria need their UPr/UCr ratios determined. Those with values outside the normal range should undergo an evaluation for CKD (see later). Patients with dipstick proteinuria but normal-range UPr/UCr values should be rechecked at periodic follow-ups (Figure 40-7).

Proteinuria in Children and Adolescents. Most proteinuria in children is transient when followed up with weekly urine sample testing. Persistent proteinuria found in at least two of three weekly urine samples warrants further evaluation to identify children who may have chronic renal disease.

Proteinuria in children may be classified as functional, isolated, or symptomatic. *Functional* proteinuria may occur with fever or exercise. *Isolated* proteinuria is defined by the absence of abnormal history, physical examination findings, symptoms, or other urinary abnormalities. The most common cause of this form is *benign orthostatic proteinuria,*

Table 40-8   Causes of Pathologic Proteinuria in Children

Glomerular disease	Minimal-change disease
	Focal segmental glomerulosclerosis
	Membranous nephropathy
	Membranoproliferative glomerulonephritis
	IgA nephropathy
	Lupus nephritis
	Alport syndrome
	Diabetic nephropathy
	Hypertensive nephropathy
Tubulointerstitial disease	Obstructive uropathy
	Reflux nephropathy
	Polycystic kidney disease
	Interstitial nephritis
	Pyelonephritis
	Acute tubular necrosis
	Proximal tubulopathy

defined by normal protein excretion overnight or in the supine position. The initial evaluation for isolated proteinuria involves obtaining a first-morning urine sample for protein and creatinine as well as a formal urinalysis for microscopy review (Hogg et al., 2000). The absence of morning proteinuria, as evidenced by normal UPr/UCr ratio, supports the diagnosis of benign orthostatic proteinuria. A more accurate assessment is a split 24-hour urine collection for protein. Benign orthostatic proteinuria may be transient or fixed and in either case has an excellent prognosis (Springberg et al., 1982). In contrast, *nonorthostatic* isolated proteinuria with a duration of 1 year or longer may represent significant renal pathology (Trachtman et al., 1994). Thus, these patients need yearly or twice-yearly clinical follow-up with assessment of blood pressure, renal function, serum albumin, urine microscopy, and urine protein.

Pathologic proteinuria, whether isolated or symptomatic, occurs in the setting of a variety of glomerular and tubulointerstitial diseases (Table 40-8). Some children may present with the *nephrotic syndrome* (proteinuria, hypoalbuminemia, edema). Depending on the degree of proteinuria and the results of the initial laboratory evaluation, a renal biopsy may be indicated (Figure 40-8).

Anatomic Disorders

Key Points

- Underlying urinary tract obstruction may cause prenatally identified hydronephrosis. These infants need close follow-up with ultrasonography in the first week of life.
- Hydroceles in infants often resolve by age 2 years. Hydroceles in adults may have a secondary cause.
- Peyronie disease is usually self-limited but may require urology consultation when treatment is considered.
- Testicular torsion is a medical emergency. Torsion of the appendix testis is less severe and can be managed with supportive care.

Anatomic urinary tract disorders involve various congenital and acquired abnormalities, most notably of the

Table 40-9   Selected Differential Diagnosis of Scrotal Masses with Physical Findings

Abnormality	Physical Finding
Epididymitis, orchitis	Tender mass
Hydrocele	Transilluminates
Inguinal hernia	Does not transilluminate
Testicular torsion	Pain and loss of cremasteric reflex
Torsion of the appendix testis	Blue dot sign
Trauma	Tender scrotum, edema, trauma history
Tumor	Solid mass
Spermatocele	Nontender cystic mass
Varicocele	Bag of worms appearance

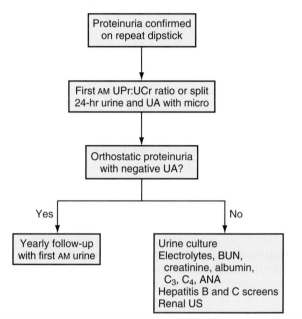

Figure 40-8 Approach to the child with proteinuria. *ANA,* Antinuclear antibody; *BUN,* blood urea nitrogen; *UA,* urinalysis; *UPr:UCr,* urine protein/urine creatinine.

external genitalia. Testicular disorders are seen more often than abnormalities of the penis, particularly undescended testes. Anatomic derangements of the bladder, ureter, and kidney are often only discovered incidentally or during an evaluation for UTIs, voiding problems, CKD, or pain possibly related to the urinary tract. For example, posterior urethral valves cause VUR and may contribute to recurrent UTIs (see "Urinary Tract Infections in Children").

Scrotal masses are frequently encountered in family medicine. Anatomic causes of scrotal masses are not limited to the urinary tract, and neoplastic and infectious causes are also in the differential diagnosis (Table 40-9). Scrotal or testicular pain, the so-called acute scrotum, implies a more urgent or emergent cause (e.g., testicular). Because the history and physical examination may not be adequate to differentiate certain conditions (e.g., epididymo-orchitis from testicular torsion), adjunctive imaging such as ultrasonography is often used.

FETAL HYDRONEPHROSIS

With the pervasive use of fetal ultrasonography, hydronephrosis is more often diagnosed prenatally. A dilated renal collecting system is often the only indication of a number of congenital uropathies (Ismaili et al., 2004). Although transient hydronephrosis is most common, two processes cause hydronephrosis: reverse urine flow (VUR) and impaired forward urine flow (obstruction) (Yamacake and Nguyen, 2013). VUR occurs as an isolated entity or can be associated with a more complicated uropathy, such as bladder outlet obstruction with VUR. Obstructive uropathy may occur at different sites along the urinary tract, most often the ureteropelvic junction.

Infants with fetal hydronephrosis need ultrasonography in the first week of life. If results are normal, repeat ultrasonography should be done in 4 weeks and 1 to 2 years (Yamacake and Nguyen, 2013). After the diagnosis is confirmed, evaluation includes a urinalysis, urine culture, basic metabolic panel (if bilateral), and a VCUG. If the VCUG results are normal, furosemide renography is needed to determine the presence and degree of obstruction.

HYDROCELE

Hydroceles are fluid accumulations in the tunica vaginalis and can result from a failure of the processus vaginalis to close during development, or secondary to epididymitis, orchitis, testicular torsion, trauma, or tumors (Barthold, 2011). Whereas hydroceles typically transilluminate, inguinal hernias do not. In young children, management is supportive, with the hydrocele often resolving by age 2 years. Hydroceles presenting beyond 2 years or those associated with inguinal hernias require surgical consultation. Also, some hydroceles are communicating; that is, fluid can pass from the peritoneal cavity into the hydrocele. These may change in size with activity or during the day and need surgical evaluation (Schneck and Bellinger, 2007). Hydroceles arising de novo in adults often have a secondary cause and require evaluation (Dogra et al., 2003).

HYPOSPADIAS

Hypospadias, in which the urethra opens on the underside of the penis, is infrequently seen (Figure 40-9). However, it is important that hypospadias is recognized early, preferably at the initial newborn examination. It can occur with or without chordee (curvature). Circumcision should be withheld and a urology consultation obtained. Hypospadias must be differentiated from ambiguous genitalia, which implies an intersex disorder. *Epispadias*, in which the meatus is located on the dorsal surface of the penis, is uncommon and is usually associated with extrophy of the bladder.

LABIAL ADHESIONS

Labial adhesions may be seen in young girls and may be partial or complete (fusion) and asymptomatic. However, labial adhesions can be associated with difficult or abnormal urination and may contribute to the development of UTIs. It is important to perform an external genital examination in a girl with her first UTI (Figure 40-10). Retrospective data and case series support topical estrogen cream to the affected areas, with gentle traction until the adhesions have separated (Bacon, 2002; Tebruegge et al., 2007). However, labial separation occurred more quickly

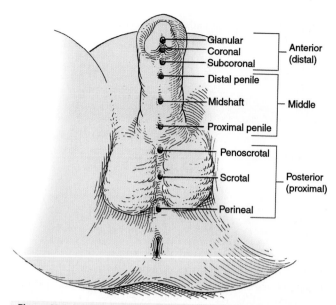

Figure 40-9 Hypospadias. (From Borer JG, Retik AB. Hypospadias. In Wein AJ, ed. *Campbell-Walsh urology.* 9th ed, vol IV. Philadelphia: Elsevier; 2007.)

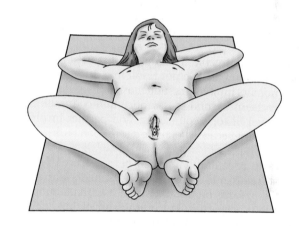

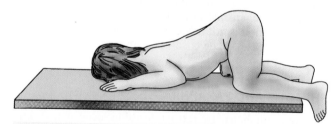

Figure 40-10 Techniques for pediatric female genital examination. (From Canning DA, Nguyen MT. Evaluation of the pediatric urologic patient. In Wein AJ, ed. *Campbell-Walsh urology.* 9th ed, vol 4. Philadelphia: Elsevier; 2007.)

and with less recurrence in patients treated with betamethasone than in those treated with estrogen cream (Mayoglou et al., 2009).

PEYRONIE DISEASE

Peyronie disease is characterized by formation of fibrosis in the tunica albuginea, with resulting penile deformity and pain. Symptoms include painful erection, physical penile deformity (often curvature), palpable penile plaque

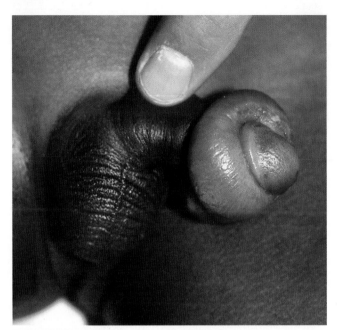

Figure 40-11 Paraphimosis. (From Kleigman R, Behrman RE, Jenson HB, et al. *Nelson textbook of pediatrics*. ed 18. Philadelphia: Saunders; 2007:2256.)

(fibrosis), and erectile dysfunction (ED). Pain is typically transient, most cases do not result in a deformity so severe that it impairs intercourse, and most patients do not require any treatment beyond reassurance and counseling. However, sexual history, counseling, and partner involvement are important because Peyronie disease can be disruptive to a relationship.

Urologic consultation should be considered before exploring treatment. Nonsurgical treatments are available and tend to focus on treatments with antiinflammatory or antioxidant properties, but overall supporting evidence is limited. Vitamin E and colchicine have uncertain efficacy. Pentoxifylline and phosphodiesterase-5 (PDE-5) inhibitors show promise. Intralesional verapamil is also an option. Steroid injection is not recommended. Surgery is an option in severe cases (Lewis and Munarriz, 2007; Shaw et al., 2013).

PHIMOSIS AND PARAPHIMOSIS

Phimosis (inability to retract foreskin over glans) and paraphimosis (inability to return retracted foreskin over glans) are possible complications seen in uncircumcised boys (Figure 40-11). About 50% of boys typically are able to retract their foreskins by 1 year of age and 80% by age 3 years (Anderson and Anderson, 1999). Low-potency topical corticosteroid therapy (0.05% betamethasone) combined with daily prepuce retraction appears effective for phimosis (Reddy et al., 2012; Zampieri et al., 2005).

Because vascular engorgement leads to necrosis of the glans, acute paraphimosis needs urgent medical attention. A dorsal slit procedure may be required if other reduction techniques are unsuccessful. Ice packs and plastic wrap may reduce the edema enough to allow manual reduction (Choe, 2000). Circumcision is generally indicated after the reduction and edema resolution. Methods of reduction

included manual, osmotic, puncture, and aspiration (Little and White, 2004).

SPERMATOCELES

Spermatoceles (epididymal cysts) are painless cysts filled with sperm and can be palpated distinct from the testis. They transilluminate, are generally of no consequence, and do not affect fertility.

TESTICULAR DISORDERS

Testicular Torsion

Although occasionally seen in newborn boys, testicular torsion is an acquired condition seen during puberty and is an emergency (Ringdahl and Teague, 2006). It usually presents with an abrupt onset of severe scrotal pain, at times waking the patient up in the early morning. Associated signs and symptoms include fever, nausea, vomiting, and abdominal pain. Intermittent testicular torsion has been described. On physical examination, the testis may lie in a more horizontal position, caused by a lack of normal attachment to the tunica vaginalis ("bell clapper" deformity), and demonstrate a loss of the cremasteric reflex. The diagnosis of testicular torsion can be made by physical examination or with the assistance of color Doppler ultrasonography; however, physical examination is unreliable for ruling torsion in or out (Schmitz and Safranek, 2009). Timeliness of the diagnosis is critical because testicular viability declines to 0% if detorsion occurs 24 hours after the onset of symptoms (Brenner and Ojo, 2004). Testicular torsion can occur in systemic illnesses, such as Henoch-Schönlein purpura, or can mimic the symptoms of other conditions, such as appendicitis or nephrolithiasis.

Torsion of the appendix testis presents similar to testicular torsion, although the symptoms are not as severe. The classic patient is a boy age 7 to 12 years. Palpation of the testis is normal except for a small, tender, palpable mass located on the superior or inferior pole. The cremasteric reflex is intact. The "blue dot" sign may be present and represents the compromised appendix testis as viewed through the scrotum. The diagnosis is generally made clinically, and treatment is supportive, including analgesia and scrotal elevation. It is not unusual for the pain to last 5 to 10 days, but chronic pain may occur and warrants urology consultation.

Undescended Testis

Undescended testis (testes) occurs in 2.7% to 5.9% of full-term male infants, decreasing to 1.2% to 1.8% by age 1 year (Pillai and Bassner, 1998); the incidence is higher in premature infants. An undescended testis must be differentiated from a *retractile* testis, which may occur as the cremasteric reflex is developed. As opposed to an undescended testis, a retractile testis can be manually coaxed into the scrotum. In general, the patient with truly undescended testes needs urology evaluation. Failure to respond to human chorionic gonadotropin (hCG) is an indication for orchiopexy, especially if the testes have not descended by the first birthday. This should be accomplished before the child is 6 years old (Job et al., 1982). Although it is uncertain that a contralateral normal testicle is at increased risk, testicular examination should be taught to orchiopexy patients because of the increased risk of testicular cancer (Altman, 1967; Wood and Elder, 2009).

Varicoceles

A varicocele is a collection of dilated and tortuous veins surrounding the spermatic cord. It is most often asymptomatic and left sided. Varicoceles arise in adolescence and are estimated to occur in 10% to 15% of the male population (Schneck and Bellinger, 2007). Evidence that varicoceles cause infertility is limited, but they are found in 12% of men presenting with infertility, and in mature adolescents with varicoceles, 26% had abnormal semen analyses (Biyani et al., 2009; Brenner and Ojo, 2004). The "bag of worms" appearance on scrotal examination is the hallmark of this diagnosis. Inferior vena cava obstruction should be considered if the varicocele is right sided, of acute onset, or occurs in a prepubertal boy.

Functional Disorders

Key Points

- Patients with proteinuria and elevated UPr/UCr ratios should be evaluated for CKD. The serum creatinine level may not correlate with glomerular filtration rate (GFR); GFR estimates are adequate to diagnose kidney disease, and 24-hour urine testing is usually not needed.
- Patients with CKD need systemic management.
- Enuresis typically resolves with age. A bedwetting alarm is effective if treatment is needed.
- ED has many causes and is associated with cardiovascular disease.
- Pelvic floor muscle exercises are the first-line treatment for urinary incontinence.
- Anticholinergic drugs and trospium are effective treatments for urge incontinence.
- Anticholinergic drugs for an overactive bladder can be beneficial but often cause dry mouth.
- Men with recurrent kidney stones and idiopathic hypercalciuria should be on low-sodium, low-protein diets. Low-calcium diets do not reduce stone formation.
- Non–contrast-enhanced CT is the test of choice for diagnosing kidney stones.

CHRONIC KIDNEY DISEASE

Renal disease is a significant public health burden, with almost 20 million persons in the United States having CKD (Coresh et al., 2003). The National Kidney Foundation's guidelines on the evaluation and management of CKD defines CKD as kidney damage or decreased kidney function for 3 months or longer (Levey et al., 2003).

Proteinuria is a clinical sign of kidney disease. Patients with proteinuria should be approached as described earlier. Patients with abnormal urinary protein values (e.g., UPr/UCr ratio) or other markers of kidney damage should be assessed for CKD (Johnson et al., 2004). The primary measure of kidney function is the GFR, and the stages of CKD are based on GFR (calculated by Cockcroft-Gault or

Table 40-10 Stages of Chronic Kidney Disease

Stage	Defining Features	GFR[†] (mL/min/1.73 m²)
1	Kidney damage,* normal GFR	≥90
2	Kidney damage, mild decrease in GFR	60-89
3	Moderate decrease in GFR	30-59
4	Severe decrease in GFR	15-29
5	Kidney failure	<15

*Pathologic renal abnormalities; markers of damage: abnormal blood, urine, or imaging study results.

[†]Glomerular filtration rate (GFR) equations:
Cockcroft-Gault equation:

$$CCr (mL/min) = ([140 - Age] \times Weight)/72 \times SCr$$
$$(\times 0.85, if female)$$

Abbreviated MDRD:

$$GFR \ (mL/min/1.73m^2) = 1.86 \times (SCr)^{1.154} \times (Age)$$
$$(0.742 \ [if \ female] \times 1.210 \ [if \ black])$$

CCr, Creatinine clearance; MDRD, modification of diet in renal disease study equation; SCr, serum creatinine level (mg/dL).
Calculators for office use are available from the National Kidney Disease Education Program (NKDEP). http://www.nkdep.nih.gov/professionals/gfr_calculators/index.htm.
From Johnson CA, Levey AS, Coresh J, et al. Clinical practice guidelines for chronic kidney disease in adults. Part II. Glomerular filtration rate, proteinuria, and other markers. Am Fam Physician. 2004;70:1091-1097.

Table 40-11 Serum Creatinine Levels and Chronic Kidney Disease*

	Serum Creatinine (mg/dL) MDRD Study Equation					
Age (yr)	European American		African American		Cockcroft-Gault Equation	
	Men	Women	Men	Women	Men	Women
30	1.47	1.13	1.73	1.34	1.83	1.56
40	1.39	1.08	1.65	1.27	1.67	1.42
50	1.34	1.03	1.58	1.22	1.50	1.28
60	1.30	1.00	1.53	1.18	1.33	1.13
70	1.26	0.97	1.49	1.15	1.17	0.99
80	1.23	0.95	1.46	1.12	1.00	0.85

*These values correspond to a glomerular filtration rate of 60 mL/min/1.73 m².
MDRD, Modification of diet in renal disease.
Modified from Levey AS, Coresh J, Balk E, et al. National Kidney Foundation practice guidelines for chronic kidney disease: evaluation, classification, and stratification. Ann Intern Med. 2003;139:137-147, E148-E149.

modification of diet in renal disease [MDRD] equation) (Table 40-10). The MDRD equation performs as well or better than measured creatinine clearance (Levey et al., 1999). However, physicians should be aware that the values obtained by the equations may differ slightly, and the Cockcroft-Gault equation is the primary measure used when validating recommended medication dosing adjustments for creatinine clearance. Slightly elevated (or even "normal range") serum creatinine levels may correlate with impaired GFR, depending on factors such as age or race (Table 40-11). Thus, the serum creatinine level alone is an inadequate clinical marker for a patient's risk for, or the presence of, renal impairment (Levey et al., 2003).

Workup of persons identified as having CKD (by GFR) includes a complete urinalysis, renal ultrasonography, and determination of the serum creatinine and serum electrolyte levels and albumin-to-creatinine ratio. Patients should also be assessed for background risk factors that may worsen their disease. Particular emphasis should be placed on the most common problems—diabetes, hypertension, and tobacco use. Patients with class 1 CKD have evidence of renal disease (e.g., diabetes, proteinuria) but a normal GFR. Patients with type 2 diabetes and nephropathy clearly benefit from treatment with an angiotensin-converting enzyme (ACE) inhibitor or an angiotensin receptor blocker (ARB). Furthermore, blood pressure control is critical for preventing nephropathy progression. ACE inhibitors have stronger evidence for treatment in patients with CKD without diabetes. ARBs are of uncertain benefit in this group. However, it is not clear if either drug is effective at reducing mortality rates (Clase, 2011; Sharma et al., 2011). The evidence is stronger for ARBs for preventing end-stage failure in patients with advanced nephropathy (Shlipak, 2009).

Management of patients with stage 1 or 2 CKD focuses on risk factors and preventing disease progression. Particular attention should be directed toward controlling diabetes and hypertension, if present. It is unclear if treating to certain albumin targets is helpful (Clase, 2011). CKD has numerous complications requiring regular assessment. In stage 3 CKD, family physicians should assess for anemia, neuropathy, nutrition, and disorders of bone metabolism. Patients with a GFR less than 30 should be referred to a nephrologist. Stage 4 patients should be proactively prepared for dialysis or transplantation. Patients in stage 5 should be monitored for uremia and dialysis initiated at that point (Levey et al., 2003).

CHRONIC NONBACTERIAL PROSTATITIS

The term *prostatitis* means prostate inflammation but often also implies infection (infectious causes are discussed later). However, prostatitis encompasses many different clinical entities (Table 40-12). Chronic nonbacterial prostatitis, also known as *chronic pelvic pain syndrome*, is poorly understood and better classified as a *functional* urinary tract disorder. Patients with chronic nonbacterial prostatitis can experience genital, ejaculatory, perineal, back, pelvic, or rectal pain; irritative voiding symptoms; and sexual dysfunction. Unlike those with category II prostatitis, however, patients with nonbacterial prostatitis do not experience recurrent UTIs (Stevermer and Easley, 2000). Physical examination results may be normal or reveal a tender prostate.

Chronic nonbacterial prostatitis negatively affects quality of life and is associated with depression, anxiety, and somatization (McNaughton-Collins, 2003). A potentially helpful clinical tool is the validated National Institutes of Health (NIH) Chronic Prostatitis Symptom Index, which can help define a patient's symptoms (McNaughton-Collins et al., 2007). Treatment is problematic because the underlying pathogenesis is uncertain and the evidence base poor. α-Adrenergic blockers are often initially considered because some data show reduced pain and improved quality of life. However, the evidence supporting this is inconsistent, so

Table 40-12   NIH and NIDDK Classification System for Prostatitis

Category	Name	Defining Characteristics
I	Acute bacterial prostatitis	Acute prostate infection
II	Chronic bacterial prostatitis	Recurrent prostate infection
IIIa	Chronic nonbacterial prostatitis—inflammatory chronic pelvic pain syndrome	No infection; WBCs evident in semen, prostatic secretions, or postprostate massage voided urine
IIIb	Chronic nonbacterial prostatitis—noninflammatory chronic pelvic pain syndrome	No infection; no WBCs in semen, prostatic secretions, or postprostate massage voided urine
IV	Asymptomatic inflammatory prostatitis	No subjective symptoms; WBCs in prostatic secretions or prostate tissue

WBC, White blood cell.
From McNaughton-Collins M, Joyce GF, et al. Prostatitis. In Litwin MS, Saigal CS, eds. *Urologic diseases in America.* US Department of Health and Human Services, Public Health Service, National Institutes of Health (NIH), National Institute of Diabetes and Digestive and Kidney Diseases (NIDDK). Washington, DC, US Government Printing Office, 2007; NIH Pub No 07-5512, p 13.

the benefit is uncertain (Le and Schaeffer, 2011). Routine antibiotic use is not beneficial (McNaughton-Collins et al., 2001). Patients with NIH category IIIa prostatitis can receive a trial of a fluoroquinolone antibiotic for 2 to 4 weeks or a prolonged course (4-6 weeks total) if they benefit. However, antibiotics in categories IIIb and IV prostatitis appear ineffective (Le and Schaeffer, 2011; Wagenlehner and Naber, 2003). Allopurinol, 5α-reductase inhibitors, antiinflammatory drugs, biofeedback, pentosan (Elmiron), pregabalin, prostate massage, quercetin, thermotherapy, and Sitz baths are alternatives of uncertain effectiveness (Aboumarzouk and Nelson, 2012; Le and Schaeffer, 2011; McNaughton-Collins and Wilt, 2002). As in other somatic syndromes, patients benefit from a supportive physician relationship focused on quality of life rather than cure.

ENURESIS

Nocturnal Enuresis

Enuresis is a common childhood complaint. Distinguishing *primary* enuresis (children who have never achieved a satisfactory period of nighttime dryness) from *secondary* enuresis (return of nighttime wetting after 6 months of nighttime dryness) is important; secondary enuresis indicates possible dysfunctional voiding or other pathologic condition. A child needs to be 5 years old to be considered enuretic, and children younger than 7 years may not exhibit the commitment necessary for treatment to be effective (Kiddoo, 2011). It is more common in boys and has a genetic tendency. The exact cause is unknown. Family background, life stressors, and psychological problems have not shown a causal relationship (Theidke, 2003). Enuresis typically resolves with age, although 1% of adults may have an average of 2 wet nights per week (Kiddoo, 2011).

History should focus on birth and development, family history, voiding and defecation history, signs of abnormal voiding, and parental response to the problem. A voiding diary may be helpful (Theidke, 2003). Evaluation with a urinalysis and an age-appropriate neurologic examination, including gait and anal reflex (wink), as well as close examination of the lumbosacral area, is mandatory to determine the need for further evaluation in a patient with primary nocturnal enuresis. If the history, physical examination, and urinalysis are normal, usually no further workup is indicated.

Interventions found to be beneficial for managing nocturnal enuresis include decreasing fluids at night, medications such as desmopressin and tricyclics, and conditioning therapy with nighttime bedwetting alarms with or without dry-bed training. Waking children age 4 to 5 years after 1.5 to 2 hours of sleep ("lifting") may help reduce the number of wet nights (Caldwell et al., 2013; vanDommelen et al., 2009). A bedwetting alarm is the most effective treatment for nocturnal enuresis (Glazener et al., 2005b). Desmopressin and tricyclic medications are effective, but the effects are temporary, with a high relapse rate once discontinued (Glazener and Evans, 2002; Glazener et al., 2003; Kiddoo, 2011). Tricyclic medication side effects, such as anorexia, drowsiness, and cardiac arrhythmias, limit their use. Other medication options lack adequate evidence of efficacy (Deshpande et al., 2012). Complementary therapies and dry bed training alone have uncertain efficacy (Glazener et al., 2004; Huang et al., 2011; Kiddoo 2011). Because most children will be dry by 7 years old, reassurance may be most appropriate until that point (Kiddoo, 2011).

DYSFUNCTIONAL VOIDING

Dysfunctional voiding, a term used to describe impairments of micturition, encompasses a wide array of symptoms and can lead to significant morbidity. The typical patient is a school-age girl who may be enuretic or have recurrent UTIs. Parents will often give a history that the child "holds her urine" or demonstrates urgency with infrequent voiding. *Vincent's curtsy* is a well-known posture assumed by these girls to help alleviate the pressure of a full bladder, which can result in a non-neurogenic neurogenic bladder. The dysfunctional voiding scoring system (DVSS) is a validated tool that can be used to diagnose and evaluate children with dysfunctional voiding (Farhat et al., 2000). Urodynamic studies, cystoscopy, and imaging studies are available in the workup of voiding dysfunction, if indicated by the history and physical examination. Treatment is designed to improve bladder tone by placing the patient on a timed voiding schedule.

ERECTILE DISORDERS

Erectile Dysfunction

Erectile dysfunction refers to "the inability to attain and/or maintain penile erection sufficient for satisfactory sexual performance" (NIH Consensus Development Panel on Impotence, 1993). Sexual function declines with age, and normal erectile function depends on a number of body systems, including cardiovascular, endocrine, muscular, nervous, and psychological (Lue, 2000). Disorders in any of these can lead to ED, although many factors often are involved.

Risk factors include diabetes, cardiovascular diseases (e.g., hypertension, coronary heart disease, hyperlipidemia), lifestyle (e.g., alcohol, obesity, smoking), depression, neurologic disease or damage, pelvic or vascular surgery, and medications, and other endocrine and urologic disorders (Fink et al., 2002). Medications such as antidepressants and antihypertensives are often implicated, and medications play a role in as many as 25% of cases (McVary, 2007) (see eTable 40-1). Men with cardiovascular disease often experience ED before the onset of cardiac symptoms (Billups, 2005). This association suggests that ED and cardiovascular disease may be part of the same continuum for many men and that men with ED should undergo cardiac risk assessment (Gandaglia et al., 2014).

The assessment should include a general health history, with a particular focus on risk factors and psychosocial issues, such as substance use, libido, and partner relationship. Clinical survey tools such as the Sexual Health Inventory for Men (SHIM) can aid in diagnosis and treatment (Cappelleri and Rosen, 2005). Surgical and medication history is essential. The examination should focus on genitourinary, endocrine, and vascular function. Laboratory work includes urinalysis; blood count; and assessment of renal function and glucose, lipid, and serum testosterone levels. Hyperprolactinemia may cause ED, although this occurs in fewer than 2% of cases (Mikhail, 2005). Thus, determination of prolactin levels, along with free testosterone and luteinizing hormone levels, should be reserved for patients with signs or findings consistent with hypogonadism (e.g., low serum testosterone level) (Lue, 2000).

Alprostadil (intracavernosal, intraurethral), apomorphine, and PDE-5 inhibitors are effective ED treatments (Table 40-13) (Montague and Jarow, 2007). Potentially beneficial alternative therapies include yohimbine and Korean red ginseng, with ginseng having the stronger evidence base (Khera and Goldstein, 2011). Attention to lifestyle issues is important. For example, weight loss may improve sexual function in obese patients (Esposito et al., 2004). Discontinuing potentially causative medicines is an option, although the risks and benefits of this choice and its effect on other conditions must be considered. The advent of oral treatment with PDE-5 inhibitors has made these medications the drugs of first choice (Table 40-14). Cardiovascular disease is a concern with PDE-5 inhibitors because these patients may be taking nitrates or may experience cardiac symptoms from sexual exertion. The medicine itself does not cause ischemia. Furthermore, no increase in cardiovascular events or death was found in randomized trials (Fink et al., 2002). Patients with antidepressant-induced ED, primarily from selective serotonin reuptake inhibitors (SSRIs), may benefit from the addition of a PDE-5 inhibitor, a switch to a different antidepressant (e.g., bupropion), or a drug holiday (Rudkin et al., 2004; Sturpe et al., 2002). PDE-5 inhibitors may also be beneficial in patients with ED from diabetes or spinal cord injury.

One unintended consequence of widely publicized ED treatments is the negative emotions when these treatments fail, which they often do (Fink et al., 2002; Tomlinson and

Wright, 2004). Psychosexual counseling may be beneficial, although evidence is limited (Khera and Goldstein, 2011).

Premature Ejaculation

Although various definitions exist, premature ejaculation is "a male sexual dysfunction characterized by ejaculation always or nearly always occurs prior to or within about 1 minute of vaginal penetration; inability to delay ejaculation on all or nearly all vaginal penetrations; and negative personal consequences, such as distress, bother, frustration and/or the avoidance of sexual intimacy" (McMahon et al.,

2008). Sexual history, psychological history, and differentiation from ED are essential. Treatment should be tailored to the individual patient. Psychological interventions are options for willing patients, although the evidence base supporting this approach is poor (Melnik et al., 2011). No medicines are U.S. Food and Drug Administration (FDA) approved for this problem; however, exploiting side effects of SSRIs and topical anesthetics is an option (American Urological Association [AUA], 2004).

INCONTINENCE

Urinary incontinence is defined by the involuntary loss of urine. Many systems for classifying incontinence exist, but the most widely accepted divides the problem into stress, urge, and mixed incontinence (Abrams et al., 2010). *Stress* incontinence is the loss of urine with effort, exertion, or the Valsalva maneuver (e.g., coughing). *Urge* incontinence is urine leakage preceded by an urge to void. *Mixed* incontinence describes patients with symptoms from both categories. *Functional* incontinence can be used to describe patients who have incontinence with clear functional causes and who do not fit the previous categories (e.g., spinal cord injury, bedridden patient).

Urinary incontinence negatively affects quality of life through social isolation, depression, sexual dysfunction, and impaired activities of daily living (Scottish Intercollegiate Guidelines Network [SIGN], 2004). Women are more likely to experience incontinence at a younger age than men. Risk increases with age, increased weight, depression, hysterectomy, smoking, and childbirth (Melville et al., 2005; Onwude, 2009). Causes for men are not well defined but include prostate procedures. Women are less likely than men to seek medical advice for this problem (SIGN, 2004). In community-dwelling elderly persons, the rates may approach 35%, up to 60% in those at long-term care facilities (Griebling, 2009).

The evaluation should address bowel and bladder history, symptom characteristics, surgical history, and medication review. A voiding diary may be helpful in characterizing the

---

Table 40-13 Erectile Dysfunction Treatment Options

ATLPROSTADIL*[*][†]

Intracavernosal (Caverject, Edex)*
Intraurethral (Muse)*
Topical

APOMORPHINE (SUBLINGUAL)*

COGNITIVE-BEHAVIORAL THERAPY

GINSENG

PHOSPHODIESTERASE (TYPE 5) INHIBITORS
Avanafil (Vivus)
Sildenafil (Viagra)*
Tadalafil (Cialis)*
Vardenafil (Levitra)*

YOHIMBINE (YOCON, YOHIMEX, GENERIC)

PAPAVERINE[‡] **(ALONE OR MIXED WITH PHENTOLAMINE OR PHENTOLAMINE AND ALPROSTADIL)**

PENILE PROSTHESIS SURGERY

PSYCHOSEXUAL COUNSELING

THERAPEUTIC LIFESTYLE CHANGES—SMOKING CESSATION, WEIGHT LOSS, LIMITED ALCOHOL CONSUMPTION

VACUUM DEVICE*

*These treatments have good evidence of benefit.
[†]Harms may limit use. Alprostadil may cause penile pain.
[‡]Harms may limit use. Papaverine injections may alter liver function and cause penile bruising or fibrosis.
Modified from Tharyan P, Gopalakrishanan G. Erectile dysfunction. *Clin Evid.* 2009;05:1803.

Table 40-14 Oral Phosphodiesterase Inhibitors for Erectile Dysfunction

Drug	Doses	Dosing	Side Effects, Precautions, Drug Contraindications
Avanafil (Vivus)	50, 100, 200 mg	100 mg/24 hr; 0.5 hr before intercourse; 50 mg if on α-blocker or CYP3A4	Common—headache, flushing, dyspepsia, nasal congestion, abnormal vision; serious—priapism, nonarteritic anterior ischemic optic neuropathy
Sildenafil (Viagra)	25, 50, 100 mg	50 mg (25 mg if >65 yr); 100 mg/24 hr; take 0.5-4 hr before intercourse	Caution if sexual activity or exertion risky because of existing cardiovascular disease; caution with potent CYP3A4 inhibitors; caution in renal, hepatic impairment; caution in anatomic penile deformity or risk for priapism; caution in older adults (>65 yr); caution with α-blockers*
Tadalafil (Cialis)	2.5, 5, 10, 20 mg	Daily use: 2.5 mg; may increase to 5 mg PRN use: 10 mg, 1 dose/24 hr; take before intercourse	
			Nitrates
Vardenafil (Levitra)	2.5, 5, 10, and 20 mg	10 mg (5 mg if >65 yr); 1 dose/24 hr; take 1 hour before intercourse	Avoid in patients with prolonged QT taking class IA or III antiarrhythmics

*Phosphodiesterase-5 (PDE-5) inhibitors should be used with caution in patients taking α-adrenergic blockers. This is no longer a contraindication based on labeling, but a number of precautions are based on potential for additive vasodilation in concomitant use:
  1. Patients should be on α-blocker therapy and stable before starting PDE-5 inhibitor.
  2. Patients who already have hemodynamic instability on α-blockers are at increased risk of additive vasodilatory effects.
  3. Use the lowest recommended dose to start.
  4. If starting α-blocker in a patient on a PDE-5 inhibitor, use the lowest dose of α-blocker.
  5. Other medications or volume status may also contribute to vasodilation and should be considered.
PRN, As needed.
From *Physicians' desk reference.* 64th ed. Montvale, NJ: Thompson, 2010. http://www.pdr.net.

type of incontinence and possible overlap with syndromes such as overactive bladder. Genitourinary and neurologic examinations as well as urinalysis should be performed. A postvoid residual urine measurement is useful for men with obstructive symptoms and patients with voiding difficulty (SIGN, 2004). Urodynamic studies are of uncertain benefit. Available data suggest that these test do alter clinical approach but may not improve outcomes (Clement et al., 2013; Lemack, 2004). Urodynamics may be helpful if the cause of incontinence is uncertain (Lopez et al., 2002). Children who are thought to be incontinent—that is, those who cannot be categorized as simply enuretic or dysfunctional voiders—need more extensive evaluation.

Incontinence treatment should focus on improving quality of life. Stress and urge incontinence may be treated differently, depending on the underlying cause. Physical therapies, medications, alternative treatments, and surgery are options. Pelvic floor exercises are effective and a reasonable first choice for stress, urge, and mixed symptoms (Dumoulin et al., 2014) Available evidence suggests that bladder training is effective for urge incontinence (Teunissen et al., 2004; Wallace et al., 2004). Other options include biofeedback and electrical stimulation (Onwude, 2009). Evidence does not currently support acupuncture treatment (SIGN, 2004).

Medications include α-agonists, anticholinergics, β-agonists, estrogen, serotonin and norepinephrine reuptake inhibitors, and tricyclic antidepressants (TCAs). Oral estrogen replacement therapy should not be used because of the underlying cardiac and cancer risk, as well as the finding that it worsens incontinence (Cody et al., 2012; Hendrix et al., 2005). Topical vaginal estrogen appears effective; however, data on long-term use and effects after treatment cessation are limited or lacking. Thus, short-term use is likely most prudent at present (Cody et al., 2012).

For stress incontinence, some evidence has shown that α-agonists are more effective than placebo, but the only available form in the United States is pseudoephedrine, and side effects limit its use. TCAs are an option, but no randomized controlled trials (RCTs) have evaluated this use (SIGN, 2004). Duloxetine (Cymbalta) improves stress incontinence compared with placebo, but long-term data are lacking (Guay, 2005; Onwude, 2009). Anticholinergic drugs such as oxybutynin, tolterodine, fesoterodine, solifenacin, and darifenacin are effective for urge incontinence (Table 40-15). Trospium, a quaternary ammonium compound, is also effective (Athanasopoulos and Perimenis, 2009). Mirabegron is a newer option that works on β3-adrenergic receptors in the detrusor (Hersh and Salzman, 2013). Preventing incontinence would be ideal. Methods such as pelvic muscle exercises are often recommended for women after childbirth, and evidence supports this approach, which may also be beneficial before childbirth (Boyle et al., 2012). Episiotomy does not appear to reduce urinary incontinency in women (Hartmann et al., 2005).

INTERSTITIAL CYSTITIS AND BLADDER PAIN SYNDROME

Interstitial cystitis is a chronic, noninfectious bladder disorder predominantly diagnosed in women. Symptoms mimic those of a UTI (urgency, frequency) with the addition of pelvic pain or pressure, dyspareunia, or both and varying with bladder filling. Although not associated with cellular change, epithelial inflammation and prolonged symptoms can lead to epithelial damage (Kahn et al., 2005). Two forms are identified: "classic" interstitial cystitis, demonstrating inflammatory bladder wall changes identifiable on cystoscopy, and *bladder pain syndrome*, defined by the symptoms of interstitial cystitis in the absence of any objective cystoscopic findings (Marinkovic et al., 2009).

The main impact of interstitial cystitis is on quality of life. Patients often express somatization and depression or anxiety; as with other somatic pain syndromes, its pathogenesis is unclear. The differential diagnosis includes other somatic syndromes such as fibromyalgia, irritable bowel, and chronic pelvic pain, as well as UTI, overactive bladder, uterine fibroids, and endometriosis. Interstitial cystitis should be considered in any patient presenting frequently with UTI symptoms. There may also be association with autoimmune disorders. Coexisting somatic syndromes are also common (Hanno et al., 2011).

Pentosan polysulfate sodium (Elmiron), 100 mg three times daily, is the only FDA-approved medication for interstitial cystitis. Adjunctive medications include antihistamines, TCAs, gabapentin, anticholinergics, and cyclosporine (Marinkovic et al., 2009). Urologic consultation should be considered. Physical therapy, counseling, and bladder training may help (Kahn et al., 2005). Pelvic floor muscle exercises are not recommended (Hanno et al., 2011). Many dietary avoidance recommendations have focused on acidic,

Table 40-15	Medications for Urinary Incontinence
Medication	**Dosage**
STRESS INCONTINENCE	
Duloxetine (Cymbalta)*	40 mg twice daily
Pseudoephedrine	30, 60 mg every 4-6 hr 120 mg SR daily
Estrogen*	Topical
URGE INCONTINENCE OR OVERACTIVE BLADDER	
Tolterodine (Detrol, Detrol LA)	1, 2 mg twice daily 2, 4 mg/day (LA)
Trospium (Sanctura, Sanctura XR)	20 mg twice daily 60 mg/day (XR)
Solifenacin (Vesicare)	5, 10 mg/day
Darifenacin (Enablex)	7.5, 15 mg/day
Mirabegron (Myrbetriq)	25, 50 mg/day
Oxybutynin (Ditropan, Ditropan XL)	5 mg twice daily 5, 10 mg/day (XL)
Oxybutynin transdermal (Oxytrol)	3.9 mg transdermal patch twice weekly available over the counter
Oxybutynin transdermal gel (Gelnique)	100 mg/g topical daily
Imipramine (Tofranil)*	10, 25, 50 mg at bedtime; max dose 150 mg

SR, Sustained release.
*Use not approved by the Food and Drug Administration.
Modified from Athanasopoulos A, Perimenis P. Pharmacotherapy of urinary incontinence. *Int Urogynecol J Pelvic Floor Dysfunct.* 2009;20:475-482; *Physicians' desk reference.* 64th ed. Montvale, NJ: Thompson, 2010. http://www.pdr.net; and Hersh L, Salzman B. Clinical management of urinary incontinence in women. *Am Fam Physician.* 2013;87(9):634-640.

high-potassium foods and drinks with acid, caffeine, or alcohol. However, prospective data on dietary interventions are lacking, so such restrictions should be individualized to each patient.

OVERACTIVE BLADDER

Overactive bladder describes a clinical syndrome characterized by lower urinary tract voiding dysfunction. The International Continence Society has defined overactive bladder as "urinary urgency, usually accompanied by frequency and nocturia, with or without urgency urinary incontinence, in the absence of UTI or other obvious pathology" (Haylen et al., 2010). The lack of specificity inherent in this definition creates potential for overlap with other urinary tract symptom complexes (e.g., LUTS) and diseases. The pathogenesis is uncertain, and urinary tract abnormalities that could cause symptoms should be ruled out. The primary dysfunction revolves around improper detrusor muscle activity and functional reductions in bladder volume. However, the definition does not exclude patients with the symptoms who do not have objective bladder hypercontractility. Furthermore, voluntary control of bladder contraction may be impaired so that the urge to void cannot be controlled (Herbison et al., 2003).

Neurologic conditions may contribute. For example, patients with multiple sclerosis, stroke, or diabetic neuropathy might manifest an overactive bladder. This might be better described as *neurogenic detrusor overactivity*, but patients without a cause or contributor might be described as having *idiopathic* detrusor overactivity (Herbison et al., 2003). Thus, overactive bladder is best viewed as a descriptive, symptom-driven complex rather than a disease.

Overactive bladder affects approximately 7% to 27% of men and 9% to 43% of women (Gormley et al., 2012). However, women are more likely to experience urge incontinence as a feature (Stewart et al., 2003). Patients may plan their days around issues such as restroom access or avoiding social settings because of incontinence. Patients may be reluctant to discuss these symptoms because of embarrassment, so family physicians may not detect the true impact of these symptoms without specific inquiry.

Physical and behavioral treatments, such as bladder training and pelvic floor exercises, are recommended as the initial approach because they are equal or superior to medications (Gormley et al., 2012). There have been no systematic reviews comparing these treatments, although incontinence data have suggested that physical therapies are a reasonable option. Many pharmacotherapy options are available for overactive bladder (see Table 40-15). Anticholinergic treatment can reduce leaking or likely voiding episodes, with dry mouth being a common side effect. A systematic review of anticholinergic medications versus placebo shows statistically significant effectiveness. However, the clinical significance is uncertain, with the exception of side effects, and long-term treatment effects are unknown (Herbison et al., 2003; Madhuvrata et al., 2012). There are small differences in effectiveness among medications, with extended-release products seeming to provide better efficacy with less dry mouth (Madhuvrata et al., 2012).

RENAL CALCULI

Adults

Approximately 9% of adults will have a kidney stone, and the chance of a recurrent stone is 50% (Parmar, 2004; Pearle et al., 2014; Teichman, 2004). Whites have the highest risk, particularly men. Family history increases the risk threefold and is present in 55% of recurrent stone formers (Teichman, 2004).

A classic history suggesting renal calculi is the abrupt onset of unilateral flank pain. It often radiates into the groin and may be accompanied by nausea and vomiting. Patients with kidney stones typically have great difficulty finding a comfortable position. On examination, there may be costovertebral angle or lower abdominal pain, and hematuria occurs in 90% of patients (Teichman, 2004). Patients may experience UTI symptoms such as dysuria, frequency, and urgency as the stone passes from the ureter into the bladder. However, patients with fever, microscopic signs of infection, or signs of systemic sepsis may have superimposed UTI. Complete obstruction and hydronephrosis can result in renal failure.

Helical non–contrast-enhanced CT is the test of choice for diagnosing renal calculi in adults (White, 2012). Renal ultrasonography may be helpful for children and pregnant women (Sheafor et al., 2000; White, 2012). Stones smaller than 5 mm are more likely to pass without intervention, and most do so within 6 weeks (Preminger et al., 2007; Teichman, 2004). Stones 5 mm to less than 10 mm also have a reasonable chance of passing spontaneously (47%) and observation with pain control is an option. Medical treatment with α-blockers should be considered to increase the chances of stone passage (Preminger et al., 2007; Tseng and Preminger, 2011). Stones 10 mm and greater likely require intervention (Preminger et al., 2007).

Treatment initially focuses on analgesia and relieving nausea and vomiting. Pain results from ureteral obstruction and renal capsular distention or hydronephrosis. Pain can be effectively managed with narcotic analgesics or nonsteroidal antiinflammatory drugs (diclofenac, indomethacin) (Tseng and Preminger, 2011). Ketorolac (Toradol) is more effective than meperidine (Demerol) and probably as effective as narcotics (Larkin et al., 1999; Teichman, 2004). α-Blockers such as terazosin or tamsulosin increase the likelihood of a stone passing (Tseng and Preminger, 2011).

Two thirds of stones pass spontaneously. Stones that have not passed within 4 weeks are unlikely to pass (Teichman, 2004). Urine straining is important because a captured stone can be analyzed for content (Pearle et al., 2014). Repeat imaging is needed when stone passage has not occurred or is uncertain.

It is debatable whether all patients should receive an evaluation for metabolic disorders after a first kidney stone. A reasonable workup includes an electrolyte panel, urinalysis, blood urea nitrogen, creatinine, calcium, parathyroid hormone (if calcium elevated), and stone analysis if possible. Calcium oxalate is found in 60% to 80% of stones (Parmar, 2004). Patients with recurrent stones need a more extensive evaluation, including urine culture and a 24-hour urine study to determine calcium, oxalate, uric acid, citrate, phosphate, sodium, and creatinine levels (Teichman, 2004).

Proper hydration may help prevent recurrent stones, although this has not been tested in randomized trials. Patients should aim for urine output of 2.5 L/day (Bao and Wei, 2012; Pearle et al., 2014). Cost-effectiveness data suggest that dietary intervention is appropriate for first episodes (Lotan et al., 2004). Patients with recurrent stones need dietary intervention, a metabolic evaluation, and potassium citrate measurement. Hypercalciuria is an indication for prophylaxis with thiazide diuretics, which effectively reduce the recurrence of calcium oxalate stones. Calcium oxalate stone formers with low urinary citrate benefit from potassium citrate treatment (Pearle et al., 2014). Men with recurrent stones and idiopathic hypercalciuria will have fewer stones on a low-sodium, low-protein diet than men on a low-calcium diet (number needed to treat, 5.5 for 5 years). Low-calcium diets do not reduce stone formation (Borghi et al., 2002).

Patients with uric acid stones respond to urinary alkalinization with potassium citrate (Pearle et al., 2014).

Children

Although usually considered an adult problem, children are not immune to urolithiasis. Older children present with typical symptoms, and younger children may have signs mimicking those of colic. About 15% of children presenting to the emergency department who were ultimately diagnosed with urolithiasis by CT did not have hematuria (Persaud et al., 2009). Metabolic disorders are often the cause of pediatric stones, most often hypercalciuria (Peitrow et al., 2002).

The mainstay of treatment is a high fluid intake. Urinary alkalinization inhibits cystine and uric acid stones. For calcium-based stones, a diet low in sodium and oxalate and high in potassium is recommended. Excess intake of vitamins D and C is discouraged. Thiazide diuretics are also a treatment option. Gated and ungated shockwave lithotripsy has been successful treatment in children, with minimal morbidity (Shouman et al., 2009).

KEY TREATMENT

- ACE inhibitors and ARBs should be used for nephropathy prevention in diabetes (Shlipak, 2009) (SOR: A).
- Antibiotics are ineffective for chronic nonbacterial prostatitis (category IIIb, IV) (Le and Schaeffer, 2011) (SOR: A).
- Enuresis alarm helps manage nocturnal enuresis (Kiddoo, 2011) (SOR: A).
- Pelvic floor muscle exercises are used for urinary incontinence (Dumoulin et al., 2014) (SOR: B).
- Duloxetine is effective for stress incontinence (Onwude, 2009) (SOR: A).
- Anticholinergics (oxybutynin, tolterodine, solifenacin, darifenacin) and trospium are effective for urge incontinence (Madhuvrata et al., 2012) (SOR: A).
- PDE-5 inhibitors are used for ED (Khera and Goldstein, 2011) (SOR: A).
- Men with ED should be evaluated for cardiovascular disease (Gandagila et al., 2014) (SOR: B).

Infectious Disorders

Key Points

- *Neisseria gonorrhoeae* and *Chlamydia trachomatis* cause most cases of urethritis and often coexist.
- Identifying and treating asymptomatic bacteriuria is only important in pregnant women.
- Evaluate for urethritis, prostatitis, or both in men with UTI symptoms.
- Women with dysuria and frequency without vaginal symptoms have a 90% chance of UTI.
- Cranberry juice does not prevent UTIs
- The ideal evaluation of children with UTIs is controversial.

BALANITIS

Balanitis refers to inflammation of the glans penis (Figure 40-12). It may occur as a local infectious process, as part of a urethritis syndrome (e.g., Reiter syndrome), or as a skin disease (e.g., lichen sclerosis). In uncircumcised men, yeast balanitis may result from poor hygiene. Consideration should be given to dermatologic conditions and immunodeficiency (including diabetes) in circumcised men.

EPIDIDYMITIS

Epididymitis (epididymo-orchitis) often presents with testicular pain or swelling. It is usually unilateral, with a palpable, tender epididymis and possibly hydrocele. Risk factors include STI, insertive anal intercourse, invasive urinary tract procedures, and anatomic urinary tract disorders. Anatomic abnormalities are the most likely explanation in children. The differential diagnosis includes trauma, infarction, testicular cancer, and testicular torsion. Testicular cancer can be misdiagnosed as epididymitis. Thus, family physicians should emphasize close follow-up.

Chlamydia trachomatis and *N. gonorrhoeae* cause most cases in men younger than 35 years of age and usually

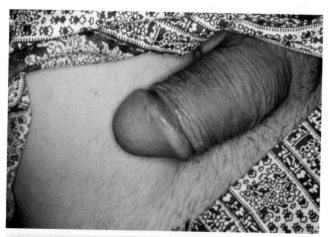

Figure 40-12 Circinate balanitis in a patient diagnosed with Reiter syndrome (arthritis, conjunctivitis, urethritis). (From the CDC Public Health Image Library image 5806. Courtesy Susan Lindsley and Dr. M. Rein.)

coexists with urethritis (Centers for Disease Control and Prevention [CDC], 2010). Other causative organisms include gram-negative enteric bacteria acquired during insertive anal intercourse. In men older than 35 years, causes include obstructive uropathy and invasive procedures (e.g., cystoscopy). Fungi and tuberculosis are other possible infectious causes and present as chronic epididymitis (CDC, 2010).

Treatment includes antibiotics, analgesia, and scrotal elevation. In patients in whom gonorrhea or chlamydia is the likely cause, ceftriaxone (single dose, 250 mg intramuscularly) and doxycycline (100 mg twice daily for 10 days) is the treatment of choice. In patients who are allergic to these or likely to have an enteric organism as the cause, 10 days of treatment with ofloxacin or levofloxacin is appropriate (CDC, 2010; del Rio, 2007).

PROSTATITIS

Prostatitis is a fairly common urinary tract disorder in men (Krieger et al., 2003) (see Table 40-12). Categories I (acute) and II (chronic) prostatitis are treated as infectious disorders. The four-glass method for diagnosing and localizing prostatitis is often recommended but has not been prospectively validated. A two-glass method, before and after prostate massage test, has good correlation with the four-glass method (Nickel, 2006; Sharp et al., 2010).

Acute Bacterial Prostatitis

Acute bacterial prostatitis should be suspected in men presenting with symptoms of UTI. Age and immunodeficiency contribute to men having UTIs, so prostatitis is more likely in otherwise healthy men with these symptoms (Lipsky, 1999). Patients may have UTI symptoms (e.g., dysuria, frequency, urgency) and typically systemic symptoms of acute illness, such as fever, chills, and myalgias. Local discomfort in the form of pelvic or back pain is also typical. Examination reveals a tender, boggy prostate. Most experts have recommended against prostate massage in acute prostatitis because it would be very uncomfortable and theoretically could disseminate the infection (Benway and Moon, 2008; Wagenlehner and Naber, 2003).

Abnormal urinalysis results showing nitrite and leukocyte esterase carry a 95% predictive value, but a negative test result does not rule out prostatitis. Urine and blood culture, blood count, and testing for STIs in at-risk patients are appropriate (Lipsky et al., 2010). Treatment is empiric pending the results. Depending on the degree of illness, patients may need an intravenous broad-spectrum penicillin or third-generation cephalosporin, possibly with an aminoglycoside, or a fluoroquinolone (Wagenlehner and Naber, 2003). Less severe cases can be managed with oral antibiotics. Fluoroquinolones are generally the choice, with options including trimethoprim–sulfamethoxazole (TMP-SMX) (Lipsky, 1999; Lipsky et al., 2010). An alternative when STI is likely is intramuscular (IM) ceftriaxone followed by oral doxycycline. Antibiotic therapy is typically 14 days, although some recommend 4 weeks because of concerns about antibiotics poorly penetrating prostatic tissue. Obstructive uropathy may result from prostatic enlargement; thus, assessment for this clinically or with postvoid residual assessment should be considered (Benway and Moon, 2008).

Chronic Bacterial Prostatitis

Chronic bacterial prostatitis may manifest with irritative voiding symptoms, prostatitic obstruction, or recurrent UTIs (Lipsky, 1999). Patients may have microscopic pyuria but negative culture results. Other symptoms include hemospermia, penile discharge, and systemic symptoms.

Longer courses of antibiotics are necessary for treatment, although the ideal duration is uncertain. Generally, treatment is for a minimum of 4 weeks, with fluoroquinolones being the treatment of choice. If an atypical infection such as chlamydia is a consideration, then a macrolide is likely more effective (Perletti, 2013). α-Adrenergic blockers may provide benefit when added to antimicrobials, but this has not been assessed in RCTs (Le and Schaeffer, 2011). Patients with recurrent symptoms may need longer antibiotic courses, urologic consultation, or reconsideration of their diagnosis.

SEXUALLY TRANSMITTED INFECTIONS

Chancroid

Chancroid is caused by infection with *Haemophilus ducreyi.* A clinical syndrome of painful genital ulcers and adenopathy (the patient does not have syphilis; ulcers are herpes negative) allows for presumptive diagnosis (Figure 40-13). Many treatment options exist (Table 40-16).

Gonorrhea and Nongonococcal Urethritis

Urethritis may present as a urethral discharge or simply dysuria. Family physicians should suspect urethritis in patients with symptoms of UTI, pyuria, presence of leukocyte esterase, and negative urine culture results. *N. gonorrhoeae* and *C. trachomatis* are the most important causative organisms. Gonococcal urethritis is typically symptomatic. Chlamydia causes most cases of nongonococcal urethritis (CDC, 2010). Patients need to be tested for both organisms because co-infection is common (CDC, 2010). Various treatment options exist (see Table 40-16). Patients with gonorrhea should be treated with IM ceftriaxone plus oral treatment with either azithromycin or doxycycline. Fluoroquinolones are no longer recommended because of

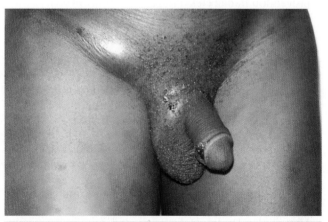

Figure 40-13 Chancroid: penile lesions and inguinal adenopathy. (From the CDC Public Health Image Library image 4419. Courtesy Pledger.)

Table 40-16   Treatment for Selected Sexually Transmitted Infections*

STI	Medication	Dose	Route*	Duration
Chancroid	Azithromycin	1000 mg	PO	Single dose
	Ceftriaxone[†]	250 mg	IM	Single dose
	Ciprofloxacin	500 mg	PO	Twice daily for 3 days
	Erythromycin base	500 mg	PO	Three times daily for 7 days
Chlamydia	Azithromycin	1000 mg	PO	Single dose
	Doxycycline	100 mg	PO	Twice daily for 7 days
Gonorrhea	Ceftriaxone[†] plus	250 mg	IM	Single dose
	Azithromycin or	1000 mg	PO	Single dose
	Doxycycline	100 mg	PO	Twice daily for 7 days
Syphilis, primary	Penicillin	2.4 million U	IM	Single dose

*For full recommendations including treatment alternatives, see Centers for Disease Control and Prevention (CDC). Sexually transmitted disease treatment guidelines, 2010. *MMWR Recomm Rep.* 2010;59(No. RR-12):1-109. Available at www.cdc.gov.
[†]Cefixime 400 mg is optional if ceftriaxone is not available. However, patients need a test of cure 1 week after treatment.
IM, Intramuscular; *PO,* oral.

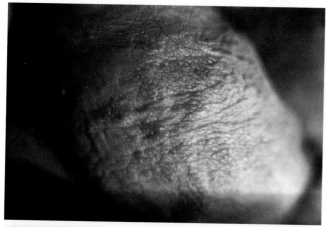

Figure 40-14 Crusted lesions of genital herpes on the penile shaft. (From CDC Public Health Image Library image 6480. Courtesy Susan Lindsley.)

Table 40-17   Treatment Options for Genital Warts

Treatment	Dose or Form	Notes
Imiquimod	1%, 5% cream	5% more effective but greater skin irritation Unknown effectiveness in patients with HIV
Interferon	Topical	Expensive
Podophyllotoxin	Topical	Skin burning, bleeding
Bichloracetic acid, trichloracetic acid	Topical	Office application
Cryotherapy		Office treatment
Surgical excision, electrosurgical excision		Office treatment

Buck HW. Warts (genital). *Clin Evid (Online).* 2010;2010:1602.

resistance rates (CDC, 2010; Del Rio et al., 2007). Furthermore, oral cephalosporins are no longer recommended as first-line treatment (Del Rio et al., 2012).

Herpes Genitalis

Herpes simplex virus type 2 (HSV-2) causes most genital herpes infections, although HSV-1 is increasingly a cause (CDC, 2010). An estimated 20% of those older than 12 years have it, and infection is often asymptomatic (U.S. Preventive Services Task Force [USPSTF], 2005). Symptoms, if present, may present as multiple, small, painful ulcers or vesicles (Figure 40-14). The causative virus is prognostically important, so confirmatory testing is recommended. Polymerase chain reaction testing is recommended, but a Tzanck preparation is not (CDC, 2010). Serologic tests for herpes IgG are available but do not differentiate acute from remote infection. Herpes IgM testing does not reliably differentiate HSV-1 from HSV-2 (CDC, 2010). The USPSTF recommends against routine screening for HSV in asymptomatic adults because there is no evidence that this decreases disease transmission or reduces morbidity (USPSTF, 2005). Antiviral medications can treat initial and recurrent acute outbreaks and can be used as prophylaxis to prevent recurrent outbreaks (Hollier and Straub, 2011).

Human Papillomavirus

Human papillomavirus (HPV) may cause symptomatic genital warts, although most patients do not manifest them. HPV types 6 and 11 cause most visible warts (CDC, 2010). Certain HPV types are associated with genital squamous neoplasia. Placing an acetic acid solution on the plaque and looking for an acetowhite change is not a sensitive test (CDC, 2010). Untreated warts will regress, remain stable, or spread; treatment is primarily symptomatic (Table 40-17).

Syphilis

Primary *Treponema pallidum* infection manifests as a painless genital ulcer known as a *chancre* (Figure 40-15). The diagnosis combines nontreponemal screening tests (rapid plasma reagin, Venereal Disease Research Laboratories) with confirmatory treponemal-specific tests (fluorescent treponemal antibody absorption, *Treponema pallidum* passive particle agglutination, and immunoassays). *T. pallidum* is difficult to culture, so darkfield microscopy or fluorescent antibody testing of a tissue specimen provides definitive diagnosis. Primary syphilis is treated with a single dose of

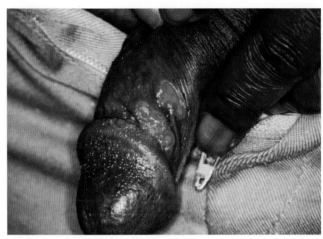

Figure 40-15 Chancre of primary syphilis. (From CDC Public Health Image Library image 6803. Courtesy Dr. M. Rein.)

Table 40-18   Treatment Options for Acute Uncomplicated Urinary Tract Infections*

Medication	Dose	Regimen	Duration
Trimethoprim–sulfamethoxazole (Bactrim DS, Cotrim DS, Septra DS)	160/800 mg	Twice daily	3 days
Nitrofurantoin monohydrate macrocrystals (Macrobid)	100 mg	Twice daily	7 days
Ciprofloxacin (Cipro)	250 mg	Twice daily	3 days
Levofloxacin (Levaquin)	250 mg	Once daily	3 days
Norfloxacin (Noroxin)	400 mg	Twice daily	3 days
Ofloxacin (Floxin)	200 mg	Twice daily	3 days
Fosfomycin (Monurol)	3 g	Single dose	Single dose

*β-Lactams agents may be used as an alternative to quinolones, but amoxicillin or ampicillin should be avoided.
DS, Double strength.
Adapted from Gupta K, Hooton TM, Naber KG, et al. International clinical practice guidelines for the treatment of acute uncomplicated cystitis and pyelonephritis in women: a 2010 update by the Infectious Diseases Society of America and the European Society for Microbiology and Infectious Diseases. *Clin Infect Dis.* 2011; 52(5): e103-e120 and Grabe M, Bjerklund-Johansen TE, Botto H, et al. *Guidelines on urological infections.* European Association of Urology; 2011.

penicillin (2.4 million units IM in adults and 50,000 to 2.4 million U/kg IM in children) (CDC, 2010). Penicillin remains the primary treatment option for all populations, although there is limited evidence supporting alternatives such as doxycycline and tetracycline for penicillin-allergic patients (CDC, 2010).

URINARY TRACT INFECTIONS

Urinary tract infections are the most common urologic issue encountered by family physicians and one of the most common diagnoses overall (Stange et al., 1998). Most are uncomplicated lower UTIs, such as cystitis.

Asymptomatic Bacteriuria

Approximately 5% of reproductive-age women have asymptomatic bacteriuria (Bent et al., 2002). It is also common in older adults. This is important for understanding the community risk of UTI when evaluating a patient with UTI symptoms. However, although asymptomatic bacteriuria may conceptually place a patient at risk for UTI, identification and treatment do not appear to affect morbidity or mortality (Lin and Fajardo, 2008). Thus, bacteriuria screening is not recommended (USPSTF, 2008).

In contrast, pregnant women do benefit from screening. Testing with urine culture should be done in all pregnant women at 12 to 16 weeks of gestation (USPSTF, 2008). Urine culture is the best method because dipstick testing and microscopy are not accurate enough tests to predict this condition.

Uncomplicated Cystitis

Most UTIs manifest as acute uncomplicated bacterial cystitis, and women experience most of these episodes. *E. coli* causes up to 90% of cases, with the rest probably caused by *Staphylococcus saprophyticus.* Other causative organisms include *Proteus mirabilis,* enterococci, and *Klebsiella* spp. (Fihn, 2003). To have "uncomplicated cystitis," women must have no underlying urinary tract abnormalities or immune compromise (Bent et al., 2002).

Dysuria, frequency, and urgency are the classic clinical triad. The condition most commonly mimicking UTI is vaginitis. Other conditions have been described (see "Dysuria").

Patients may also experience back or flank pain and suprapubic abdominal pain. Dipstick urinalysis may show leukocyte esterase or nitrite or may be heme positive. Microscopic analysis should assess for pyuria, hematuria, and bacteriuria. The gold standard for diagnosis is urine culture.

Women presenting with at least one UTI symptom have a 50% chance of having a UTI. The combination of dysuria and frequency without vaginal symptoms increases the chance to 90% (likelihood ratio, 24.6). Four symptoms significantly increase the chance of UTI—dysuria, frequency, hematuria, and back pain (Bent et al., 2002). Overall, no clinical symptom strongly indicates UTI. Nitrite-positive or leukocyte esterase–positive dipsticks are the most accurate tests but cannot rule out a UTI if negative (Medina-Bombardó and Jover-Palmer, 2011).

Antibiotics are the mainstay of treatment (Table 40-18). A shorter duration is as effective as longer therapy for most women, including older adult women (Lutters and Vogt, 2002; Milo et al., 2005). In the southeastern and southwestern United States, there is growing *E. coli* resistance to TMP-SMX, leading some to recommend that this should no longer be first-line treatment for UTIs. However, many women treated with TMP-SMX who have a resistant organism on culture achieve clinical cure (Fihn, 2003). Compared with quinolones' propensity for resistance, TMP-SMX is still a reasonable first choice for many patients, and family physicians should base treatment choices on documented local resistance patterns. If resistance to TMP-SMX exceeds 20%, an alternative treatment should be used (Gupta et al., 2011).

Complicated Infection

Complicated UTIs are characterized by signs and symptoms of upper tract (i.e., renal) involvement or by factors that predispose to upper tract involvement. UTIs with signs of renal or systemic involvement are also called *pyelonephritis.* Most cases of pyelonephritis are caused by ascending bacterial infection from the bladder (Ramakrishnan and Scheid, 2005).

Symptoms include fever, flank pain, nausea, vomiting, and costovertebral angle tenderness. Findings such as pyuria are typical, and urine culture results are usually positive. WBC casts may be present on urine microscopy. Hospitalized patients with UTIs are best managed based on culture results. *E. coli* is the typical pathogen for uncomplicated outpatient UTIs and pyelonephritis. *E. coli* is still the most common isolate in hospitalized patients, but now to a lesser extent as *Enterococcus, Pseudomonas,* and *Staphylococcus* spp. have become more likely (Graham and Galloway, 2001; Scholes et al., 2005). Blood cultures do not necessarily change management (Ramakrishnan and Scheid, 2005). Imaging, such as renal ultrasonography, is sometimes recommended, but it also does not necessarily change management and thus can be used at clinical discretion (Nicolle, 2008).

Outpatients can be managed with an oral fluoroquinolone. Hospitalized patients should receive a fluoroquinolone, an aminoglycoside with or without ampicillin, or an extended-spectrum cephalosporin with or without an aminoglycoside. Patients with cultures showing gram-positive cocci should receive an aminopenicillin along with a β-lactamase inhibitor (Grabe, 2011). Treatment for 7 to 14 days is usually adequate; however, an optimum treatment course is unknown because randomized trials of antibiotic treatment are lacking (Neumann and Moore, 2011). Resistant bacteria and renal calculi are the most common causes of treatment failure (Ramakrishnan and Scheid, 2005).

Recurrent Infections

In healthy, nonpregnant women, recurrent UTI can be defined as three episodes in 1 year or two episodes in 6 months (Sen, 2008). Patients with urinary tract pathology or other conditions impacting urinary function (e.g., neurogenic bladder) may require consultation. Self-diagnosis has an 84% PPV in women with recurrent UTIs (Bent et al., 2002). Cultures are helpful in guiding antibiotic choice (Table 40-19). Prophylactic antibiotics are effective for the subset of women with recurrent symptomatic UTI, although

Table 40-19 Selected Antibiotics for Uncomplicated Urinary Tract Infection Prophylaxis*

Drug	Pediatric Dose	Adult Dose*
Amoxicillin	10 mg/kg once daily	N/A
TMP-SMX	2 mg/kg once daily based on TMP	Single strength (80/400 mg), half-tablet at night or three times weekly
Trimethoprim	N/A	100 mg nightly
Nitrofurantoin	1-2 mg/kg once daily	50 or 100 mg nightly
Ciprofloxacin	N/A	125 mg/day
Norfloxacin	N/A	200 mg nightly

*Postcoital prophylaxis options: TMP-SMX, nitrofurantoin, fluoroquinolones.
N/A, Not applicable; *TMP-SMX,* trimethoprim–sulfamethoxazole.
Adult dosing adapted from Grabe et al., 2011.

choice of patient and duration is uncertain. Because sexual activity is associated with developing UTIs, many physicians recommend that women void immediately after intercourse. However, the poor-quality study examining this practice found no significant effect (Beisel et al., 2002). Thus, no evidence supports recommending this practice to patients. In contrast, postcoital antibiotic prophylaxis reduces the incidence of cystitis (Sen, 2008). Furthermore, it may be as effective as continuous prophylaxis at reducing recurrence because women in one RCT comparing these methods showed no difference in UTI rates (Albert et al., 2004). In postmenopausal women, topical estrogen is often proposed, but this also lacks good supporting evidence (Sen, 2008).

Cranberry juice is promoted as a potential preventive treatment for recurrent UTI because of chemical effects inhibiting bacterial adherence to uroepithelial cells (Raz et al., 2004). However, meta-analysis revealed a lack of efficacy in preventing recurrent UTIs (Jepson, 2012).

Urinary Tract Infections in Children

An estimated 3% to 8% of girls and 1% to 2% of boys will have a UTI (Foxman, 2002; Hellstrom et al., 1991). *Pyelonephritis* is a clinical diagnosis and is the most common documented serious bacterial infection in febrile infants. *Cystitis* is common in school-age children and adolescents and, as a general rule, is not a condition of infants or pre–toilet-trained toddlers. Risk factors for UTI range from constipation and dysfunctional voiding to congenital uropathies. Presenting symptoms vary with age and site of infection and may be nonspecific in younger children. Pyelonephritis in infants, for example, may present with fever, irritability, vomiting, diarrhea, poor feeding, or failure to thrive. School-age children and adolescents may present with fever, vomiting, and flank pain. Symptoms of cystitis are more common after age 2 years and may include dysuria, frequency, urgency, and low-grade fever (<38.3° C).

As with adults, the gold standard test in children is an appropriately obtained urine culture. In neonates and young infants, it is the ideal collection method. Either catheterization or a suprapubic aspiration is needed until the child is old enough to collect a midstream clean-catch specimen. Bag urine collections are unreliable and increase the number of ambiguous cultures (American Academy of Pediatrics [AAP], 2011; Schroeder et al., 2005). Many elements of the urinalysis have been viewed as tools for aiding diagnosis of UTI. Inadequate sensitivity and specificity continue to support use of urine culture (AAP, 2011). Furthermore, no RCTs have evaluated clinical empiric treatment versus awaiting culture results (Larcombe, 2010). However, pyuria (>5 WBCs/hpf) and a positive Gram stain result are helpful in making the decision to initiate early antibiotic therapy, pending culture results.

Treatment remains somewhat controversial, particularly the choice between parenteral and oral antibiotics in the setting of pyelonephritis. For children with pyelonephritis, therapeutic goals include treating or preventing systemic complications of bacteremia, preventing renal sequelae, and ameliorating acute symptoms. Historically, parenteral antibiotics have been the preferred option, particularly in younger children with pyelonephritis. This remains true for infants younger than 4 weeks, who should be hospitalized and receive parenteral therapy. This is also true for older infants and children assessed at high risk because of a septic appearance, vomiting or inability to take oral fluids and medications, dehydration, or concerns regarding compliance. However, most children can be treated with oral antibiotics (AAP, 2011). The choice of parenteral antibiotic includes ampicillin in combination with gentamicin or cefotaxime for neonates and third-generation cephalosporin alone for older children. In these cases, transition to oral therapy follows when culture results and sensitivities are known and signs of systemic infection have resolved. Follow-up urine cultures to test for cure are unnecessary in patients with good clinical response, although advice regarding reevaluation for febrile illnesses should be provided (AAP, 2011). Prolonged parenteral therapy is indicated for septic infants. For children 1 month and older not assessed as high risk, it now appears that oral antibiotics are equally effective not only regarding course of illness but also in preventing renal scarring (Montini et al., 2007). Options for initial oral therapy include amoxicillin–clavulanic acid, TMP-SMX (>2 months), and cephalosporins. Because of the increasing incidence of UTI with ampicillin-resistant *E. coli*, amoxicillin is no longer the preferred initial choice. The recommended length of therapy is typically 7 to 10 days for an uncomplicated UTI (i.e., cystitis) and 10 to 14 days for pyelonephritis (AAP, 2011; Larcombe, 2010).

The most appropriate evaluation after a child's first UTI is controversial (Layton, 2003). Traditionally, children have undergone a complete evaluation for underlying urologic abnormalities that would increase the risk of further infections and renal scarring, including renal ultrasonography and VCUG. In 309 children younger than 24 months with their first febrile UTI, ultrasonography was of limited value because it did not change management, and other tests may be obviated by routine cultures for children with a febrile illness after a prior UTI (Hoberman et al., 2003). However, 29% of 390 children younger than age 5 years with a first-time febrile UTI had abnormal renal ultrasound findings (Huang et al., 2008). Therefore, renal and bladder ultrasonography is recommended (AAP, 2011).

The most common uropathy associated with pediatric UTI is VUR, occurring in 30% to 40% of cases. Reflux is diagnosed by VCUG and graded on a scale of 1 to 5, with grade 5 being the most severe. The degree of VUR is directly proportional to the incidence of renal scarring. In addition to the standard fluoroscopic VCUG, radionuclide cystography may be performed. This test has the advantage of less radiation exposure but is lacking in anatomic detail and is most often used for follow-up studies. The traditional approach to a patient with VUR has been prophylactic antibiotics, with surgical intervention reserved for complicated patients with breakthrough UTIs and evidence of renal injury (see Table 40-19). Deflux is a newer, less invasive procedure performed using cystoscopy and is proving to be highly effective in the treatment of reflux. However, the management of VUR is a rapidly evolving field and remains controversial. Evidence supporting prolonged antibiotic prophylaxis is weak because of a lack of properly designed RCTs (Williams and Craig, 2011). Also, evidence is lacking showing that surgical repair is superior to medical management for reducing negative outcomes in children with moderate to severe VUR (Larcombe, 2010). The Randomized Intervention for Children with Vesicoureteral Reflux (RIVUR) study is a multicenter, randomized, double-blind prospective study currently in progress in the United States designed to assess the efficacy of prophylactic antibiotics in the treatment of grade 1 to 4 VUR in children age 2 months to 6 years. Initial findings show that children receiving prophylaxis have fewer UTIs but not reduced renal scarring (RIVUR Trial Investigators, 2014). Present guidelines do not recommend VCUG after the initial febrile UTI, but evaluation should be considered in recurrences, if there are findings on ultrasonography, or in special clinical situations (AAP, 2011). Renal scintigraphy (dimercaptosuccinic acid [DMSA] scan) has been recommended to help diagnose pyelonephritis. This is also controversial because false-negative results could lead to undertreating children with pyelonephritis. DMSA scanning has shown promise in predicting higher grades of reflux in older infants and children (Lee et al., 2009), but this has not been true in neonates (Siomou et al., 2009). DMSA scans are not recommended routinely in children with UTI (AAP, 2011).

The ultimate goal in the approach to patients with UTI is to prevent morbidity. Renal scarring may ultimately manifest as hypertension, proteinuria, or both. The incidence of renal scarring in patients with UTI is increased in children younger than 3 years, presence of VUR proportional to grade of reflux, recurrent UTI, and delayed or inadequate therapy.

KEY TREATMENT

- Continuous and postcoital antibiotics are equally effective for recurrent UTI (Sen, 2008) (SOR: A).
- IM ceftriaxone plus azithromycin or doxycycline is used for gonorrhea (CDC, 2010; Del Rio et al., 2012) (SOR: C).
- Fluoroquinolones should not be used to treat gonorrhea (CDC, 2010; Del Rio, 2007) (SOR: C).
- Screen for asymptomatic bacteriuria in pregnant women at 12 to 16 weeks (USPSTF, 2008) (SOR: A).

Neoplastic Disorders

Key Points

- BPH is a finding in many, but not all, men experiencing LUTS. LUTS vary and may not correlate with prostate size.
- α-Adrenergic antagonists and 5α-reductase inhibitors are effective for BPH and LUTS.
- Smoking is the top risk factor for bladder cancer, and hematuria is the most common presenting sign.
- Prostate cancer is the most common cancer in men and second most common cause of male cancer death.
- There is no prostate-specific antigen (PSA) value that is both sensitive and specific for prostate cancer.
- When ordering a PSA test, family physicians should discuss the risk, benefits, and uncertainties with patients so a shared decision can be made.
- The value of testicular self-examination is unknown.

BENIGN NEOPLASIA: BENIGN PROSTATIC HYPERPLASIA

Benign prostatic hyperplasia is a common problem for men. More than 50% of men older than 60 years have BPH, and this reaches 80% by 80 years of age (Dull et al., 2002; Thorpe and Neal, 2003). The exact pathogenesis of BPH is uncertain, but it is characterized by epithelial and stromal cell proliferation in the periurethral prostate tissue.

The LUTS syndrome (see earlier) overlaps with BPH because up to 30% of men have LUTS (Thorpe and Neal, 2003). The symptoms defining LUTS were once thought to be solely indicative of BPH. However, LUTS may arise from other disorders (e.g., detrusor dysfunction), and there is a lack of symptomatic correlation with prostate size. However, outflow obstruction from an enlarged prostate may contribute to the development of detrusor dysfunction and urinary retention, referred to as LUTS-BPH. More specifically, BPH refers to a histologic abnormality, and LUTS describes the symptom complex that may result (AUA, 2010).

The diagnosis focuses on patient history, rectal examination, and impact on quality of life. Symptoms can vary over time even without treatment; however, the course is typically progressive, and 1% to 2% of men with BPH experience acute urinary retention annually (McNicholas and Kirby, 2011). Various measures exist for measuring symptom severity. The most widely used and well validated is the International Prostate Symptom Score. This scoring system can discriminate the severity of symptoms and treatment response. However, it does not correlate with anatomic findings or objective measures of urinary flow (Barry and O'Leary, 1995). PSA values may increase with prostate hyperplasia, but the overlap with prostate cancer makes this of limited use in managing BPH (Barry, 2001).

Medical therapies have overtaken surgical as the most common treatments. α-Adrenergic blocking drugs improve urinary symptoms in BPH (McNicholas and Kirby, 2011; Wilt et al., 2008). α-Adrenergic antagonists block adrenoreceptors in the prostate and bladder neck (Table 40-20). They may also induce prostate epithelial apoptosis (Thorpe and Neal, 2003). Side effects, particularly blood pressure effects, are important because these drugs will most often be used in older adults (Schulman, 2003). Furthermore, α-blockers carry labeling cautioning use around the time of cataract surgery (AUA, 2010; Bell, 2009).

Prostate tissue is androgen responsive throughout life. 5α-Reductase inhibitors inhibit the conversion of testosterone to dihydrotestosterone, leading to glandular atrophy and reduced prostate volume (20%-30%) (Thorpe and Neal, 2003). It takes many months for these medicines to become effective. Sexual side effects are the most prominent. These drugs also reduce PSA by up to 50%. Based on the Prostate Cancer Prevention Trial, family physicians should discuss potential benefits and harms of 5α-reductase inhibitors (see "Prostate Cancer") when using these medications for BPH and LUTS (Kramer et al., 2009). Given that these drugs address prostate size, they are not recommended for treating LUTS absent prostate enlargement (AUA, 2010).

Prostate enlargement can progress enough to obstruct the bladder outlet completely, leading to acute urinary retention. If this occurs, catheterization is warranted. The addition of an α-blocker may aid in voiding after the

Table 40-20 Pharmacotherapy for Benign Prostatic Hyperplasia

Drug	Dosage	Adverse Effects
α-ADRENERGIC BLOCKERS		
Alfuzosin (Uroxatral)	10 mg/day	Cardiovascular: dizziness, postural hypotension, syncope
Doxazosin (Cardura, generic)	1-8 mg/day	
Terazosin (Hytrin, generic)	1-10 mg at bedtime	Ocular: warning for use around cataract surgery, intraoperative floppy iris syndrome
Tamsulosin (Flomax)*†	0.4 mg/day	
Silodosin (Rapaflo)	8 mg/day	Sexual: ejaculatory dysfunction
		Systemic: asthenia, drowsiness, fatigue, headache
5α-REDUCTASE INHIBITORS		
Dutasteride (Avodart)	0.5 mg/day	Sexual: impotence, decreased libido, ejaculatory dysfunction
Finasteride (Proscar)	5 mg/day	

*α-1 adrenoreceptor selective.
†Hypotension risk is greatest during the first 8 weeks of treatment.
From Schulman CC. Lower urinary tract symptoms/benign prostatic hyperplasia: minimizing morbidity caused by treatment. *Urology.* 2003;62:24-33; Schwinn DA, Price DT, Narayan P. α₁-Adrenoreceptor subtype selectivity and lower urinary tract symptoms. *Mayo Clin Proc.* 2004;79:1423-1434; Thorpe A, Neal D. Benign prostatic hyperplasia. *Lancet.* 2003;361:1359-1367; American Urological Association guideline: management of benign prostatic hyperplasia (BPH). American Urological Association Education and Research, Inc; 2010; and Bird ST, Delany JAC, Brophy JM, et al. Tamsulosin treatment for benign prostatic hyperplasia and risk of severe hypotension in men aged 40-85 years in the United States: risk window analyses using between and with patient methodology. *BMJ.* 2013;347:f6320.

catheter is removed (Thorpe and Neal, 2003). A randomized, double-blind trial of doxazosin and finasteride over 4 years showed that combining these two medications significantly slowed symptomatic progression and reduced the risk of urinary retention and invasive treatment. Treatment was safe, and the effect of combined treatment on symptom scores was greater than the effect of either agent alone (McConnell et al., 2003).

Given the commonality of BPH and LUTS, there is interest in alternative therapies. Saw palmetto extract *(Serenoa repens)* once held promise; however, high-quality evidence shows that it is not an effective treatment (Tacklind et al., 2012). β-Sitosterols may be effective, and pygeum (African plum, *Prunus africanus)* and rye grass pollen (cernilton) have uncertain efficacy (McNicholas and Kirby, 2011).

MALIGNANT NEOPLASIAS

With the exception of prostate cancer, urologic malignancy is relatively uncommon in the general population. After prostate cancer, which is the most common cancer diagnosed in men, the next most common cancers are bladder and kidney cancers (American Cancer Society [ACS], 2013). Testicular cancer is relatively common in young men compared with other cancers in that age group.

Bladder Cancer

Bladder cancer incidence increases with age and occurs four times more often in men than women. Its incidence in white men is twofold higher than in African American men (ACS, 2013; National Cancer Institute [NCI], 2013a).

Cigarette smoking is the most prominent risk factor, increasing the risk four- to sevenfold. Aminobiphenyl is a cigarette carcinogen linked to bladder cancer. Smoking cessation decreases the risk, although it still remains twofold higher 10 years after cessation. Other risk factors include exposure to the aromatic amines used in the dye and rubber industry, benzidine production, paint, metal, and petroleum manufacturing. Medical risks include cyclophosphamide, radiation, and prolonged exposure to foreign bodies (e.g., catheter). Finally, aristolochic acid, found in certain weight loss supplements and traditional Chinese herbal compounds containing *Aristolochia fangchi*, may increase the risk. Banned in many Western countries, it is still available in the United States (NCI, 2013a).

Hematuria is the most common sign of bladder cancer (NCI, 2013a), and the diagnosis is most often made by direct bladder visualization (cystoscopy) and biopsy. However, the prevalence of bladder cancer is low, and most patients with hematuria do not have bladder tumors. Positive urine cytology results are essentially diagnostic, although false-negative results limit the usefulness of this approach alone. No imaging test can reliably detect bladder cancers.

The USPSTF (2011a) does not recommend for or against screening asymptomatic persons for bladder cancer because of insufficient evidence.

Penile Cancers

Penile cancers are rare, with 1570 new U.S. cases in 2013 (ACS, 2013). Penile cancers are most often squamous cell, and there may be a connection to HPV infection. As expected from this cell type, lesions may appear as a superficial plaque or ulcer. Biopsy or consultation is appropriate in the evaluation of a suspicious penile lesion.

Prostate Cancer

Prostate cancer is the most common cancer diagnosed in men and is the second most common cause of cancer death in men after lung cancer. The gap between the annual numbers of diagnoses (238,590) and deaths (29,720) is wide (ACS, 2013). Major risk factors include age, African American race, and family history. Most cases occur in men older than 65 years of age. African Americans have a 70% higher incidence than whites and experience a disproportionate share of prostate cancer deaths (ACS, 2013).

Dietary factors may play a role, including an elevated risk with proandrogenic effects of dietary fat and carcinogenic compounds in grilled meats and a reduced risk with antioxidants in vegetables (Nelson et al., 2003). Dietary antioxidants such as lycopene show epidemiologic links supporting a preventive effect, with possible mechanisms including androgen inhibition (Wertz et al., 2004). However, an RCT using vitamin E and selenium, alone or in combination, showed that vitamin E increases the risk of prostate cancer (Klein et al., 2011; Lippman et al., 2009). Furthermore, there is a lack of evidence to know whether lycopene provides preventive benefit (Ilic et al., 2011). Given these results and prior disappointing results of other antioxidant trials, clinicians should not recommend supplements for prostate cancer prevention.

Prostate cancer is most often indolent, with symptoms typically arising later in the disease course (Johansson et al., 2004). Physical examination is most often unrevealing. A firm nodule on DRE may indicate a tumor. However, DRE accuracy depends on the performing physician and is imprecise. An abnormal DRE predicts prostate cancer in 18% to 28% of cases (Schwartz et al., 2005). Furthermore, up to 25% of biopsy-detected cancers after an abnormal DRE occur on the side opposite the palpated nodule (McNaughton-Collins et al., 1997). Thus, although DRE may be a potentially useful examination in a symptomatic patient, it does not play a prominent role in general population prostate cancer screening.

Prostate-specific antigen is a glycoprotein produced by prostatic epithelial cells. Its level increases with prostate adenocarcinoma, hyperplasia, inflammation, procedures, ejaculation, and massage. However, clinical DRE should not affect the PSA level (Barry, 2001). The most widely accepted upper limit of normal for total PSA is 4.0 ng/mL. The Prostate Cancer Prevention Trial, using a biopsy standard, indicated that as PSA levels increase, sensitivity declines and specificity increases, and at no point is there a good balance between the two (Thompson et al., 2005). Thus, cancer appears ubiquitous—men with normal-range PSA levels may have prostate cancer; 15% of men with a PSA less than 4.0 ng/mL have cancer, 15% of which are high-grade tumors (Thompson et al., 2004). Furthermore, although some studies have concluded that a lower abnormal PSA cutoff level would detect more cancer (Punglia et al., 2003), these findings indicate that more men would have unnecessary biopsies. Thus, PSA testing suffers from both a high false-positive and a false-negative rate (Harvey et al., 2009). Emerging data suggest that less frequent testing and adjusting the cutoff point for further testing upward could be helpful (Hayes and Barry, 2014).

Tumors are most often diagnosed after biopsy for an abnormal screening result. The Gleason score grades cellular differentiation of the two most common patterns seen in a biopsy specimen. Scores range from 2 to 10, with higher scores indicating a more poorly differentiated tumor (Schwartz et al., 2005). The risk of prostate cancer death is higher with poorly differentiated cancer. Whereas men with low Gleason scores (2-4) have a low risk of death, those with higher scores (8-10) had a high probability of dying from prostate cancer within 10 years (Albertson et al., 2005).

Treatment options for patients with prostate cancer include watchful waiting, brachytherapy, external-beam radiation, prostatectomy, androgen ablation, and combinations of these options. High-grade tumors receive aggressive treatment, but the ideal treatment for intermediate-grade tumors (Gleason score of 5 to 7) is controversial. Low-grade tumors are candidates for watchful waiting. Treatment for localized disease, regardless of method, carries the risk of persistent negative effects on quality of life, such as sexual, urinary, and bowel dysfunction (Smith et al., 2009). An RCT of prostatectomy versus watchful waiting for low-grade tumors in Scandinavian men found little difference in outcomes during early follow-up, but at 15 years, the prostatectomy group had a lower risk of prostate cancer death and lower overall mortality (Bill-Axelson et al., 2005, 2014; Holmberg et al.,

2002). The U.S Prostate Cancer Intervention Versus Observation Trial (PIVOT) found no improvements in all cause or prostate cancer–specific mortality at 12 years from prostatectomy versus observation in men with localized tumors (Wilt et al., 2012).

Men may be more comfortable with an aggressive approach to even localized prostate cancer and choose treatment accordingly (Xu et al., 2012). Because PSA testing will detect cancers early, patients may live longer with the disease but not actually live longer lives (lead-time bias). Also, some patients treated for PSA-detected cancer may not have aggressive tumors. Treating them may artificially elevate treatment success and survival rates (length-time bias). Thus, mortality rate reductions may reflect the success of screening, misattribution of cause of death, research bias, improved treatments, or changing disease patterns. The most significant challenge remains that there is no way to differentiate patients with aggressive disease from those with clinically unimportant disease using current screening tools. Until this is resolved, controversy surrounding prostate cancer screening will persist.

Two large, randomized screening trials, the Prostate, Lung, Colorectal, and Ovary (PLCO) trial and the European Randomized Study of Screening for Prostate Cancer (ERSPC), evaluated the impact of screening on mortality. ERSPC did not show an overall mortality benefit but did show a 20% relative reduction in prostate cancer death (absolute risk reduction, 0.07%); 1410 men would need to be screened and 48 prostate cancer cases treated to prevent one death in 10 years. Overdiagnosis of clinically insignificant prostate cancer was a problem (Chou et al., 2011; Schroder et al., 2009). In contrast, the PLCO trial found no differences in prostate cancer or all-cause mortality between the test and control groups (Andriole et al., 2009). A meta-analysis of prostate cancer screening failed to show a significant impact on prostate cancer mortality (Ilic et al., 2013).

Despite any clear evidence showing that screening saves lives, PSA testing remains common (Thompson et al., 2005). PSA testing is a well-known test, with men possibly believing that being screened is beneficial and responsible behavior (Chapple et al., 2002). Furthermore, the PSA test has accuracy problems, which makes reassuring patients with normal-range results difficult. As with any screening method, false-positive test results have potential for physical and psychological harm. Prostate biopsy carries procedural risks as well as the risk of discovering and treating a cancer that would not be significant in the patient's lifetime. Present data suggest that the number needed to screen to prevent possibly one prostate cancer death is 1000, and the potential for harm is significant. Furthermore, because of the inherent properties of the test, there will be significant overdiagnosis and overtreatment because of screening (Chou, 2011; USPSTF, 2012). However, some data suggest that men ages 55 to 69 years may be candidates for a risk-versus-benefit discussion, and this is reflected in certain guidelines (Hayes and Barry, 2014).

The controversies surrounding screening are reflected in the disparate prostate cancer screening guidelines (Table 40-21). The USPSTF recommends against PSA testing to detect prostate cancer for general population screening (USPSTF, 2012). Other bodies recommend

Table 40-21 Prostate Cancer Screening Recommendations

Organization	Recommendation
USPSTF (2012)	Recommends against screening with PSA (USPSTF D recommendation)
American Cancer Society (Wolf et al., 2010)	Recommends giving asymptomatic men with a 10-year life expectancy the opportunity to consider screening
	High-risk men before age 50 yr; average risk at 50 yr
	Recommends against testing without informed decision making and mass screening
	Screening uses PSA with or without DRE
American Academy of Family Physicians (2013)	Recommends against PSA screening
American Urological Association (Carter et al., 2013)	Recommends against screening men younger than age 40 yr
	No recommendation for screening average risk men 40-54 yr, men older than 70 yr, and men with less than a 10- to 15-yr life expectancy
	Recommends individualized screening decisions for high-risk men age 40-54 yr
	Recommends shared decision making for men age 55-69 yr; if PSA is performed, it should occur every 2 yr

DRE, Digital rectal examination; *PSA,* prostate-specific antigen.

different approaches. However, there is emerging consensus that mass PSA screening (by physicians, health fairs, and so on) should be avoided and that the decision to screen with PSA should not occur without an informed-consent discussion. The risks, benefits, and limitations should be discussed so that patients are fully informed and can incorporate their personal preferences into the screening decision.

Although older men have a higher prostate cancer risk, competing causes of death and the low chance of progression make screening men with less than 10 years in remaining life expectancy of little benefit (Fisher, 2002; Ilic et al., 2013).

Preventing prostate cancer with prophylactic measures has been suggested. The Prostate Cancer Prevention Trial showed that finasteride significantly reduced cancer compared with placebo in an RCT (absolute risk reduction, 6% at 7 years). However, patients taking finasteride had an increased risk of high-grade cancer (Thompson et al., 2003). The American Society for Clinical Oncology (ASCO) and AUA joint guideline previously recommended that clinicians consider discussing the risks and benefits of 5α-reductase inhibitors for men as chemoprevention. However, using these drugs for chemoprevention is not FDA approved, and the recommendation has been revised to reflect this (ASCO/AUA, 2012). Clinicians with patients taking 5α-reductase inhibitors should consider the impact on PSA values, and how PSA screening is interpreted must also be considered (Kramer et al., 2009).

Renal Cancers

Renal cancers are twice as common in men as in women; more than 40,000 cases are diagnosed annually in men (ACS, 2013). Risk factors are less well understood than for other urologic cancers. Heavy tobacco use (>20 packs/year) is a risk factor in men, and severe obesity is a risk in both genders. Risks from occupational or medication exposure are less certain (Dhote et al., 2004).

The diagnosis of renal cancer is often incidental to an imaging study (e.g., ultrasonography) obtained for another reason. Hematuria is also a clinical sign that may lead to the diagnosis. Localized renal cell cancers have a favorable outlook (91% at 5 years); however, overall survival rates (40% at 5 years) are not as encouraging as in other urologic cancers (ACS, 2013; Dhote et al., 2004; NCI, 2013b).

Testicular Cancer

Approximately 7900 men were diagnosed with testicular cancer in 2013 (ACS, 2013). It is unusual in that it occurs mostly in young men (15-35 years) and is the most common cancer in this group. Orchiopexy in children with cryptorchidism does not necessarily prevent cancer, so these patients should be followed closely (NCI, 2013c).

Most testicular tumors are initially discovered by patients. Typical presentations include painless testicular lumps or scrotal pain, edema, or hardness. Symptoms can mimic those of epididymitis, and tumor should be in the differential diagnosis of this condition (Kinkade, 1999). Ultrasonography is the initial study of choice for suspected testicular masses. Most tumors are germ cell neoplasms. Thus, serum tumor markers (β-hCG, lactate dehydrogenase, α-fetoprotein) are important in the diagnosis, prognosis, and monitoring aspects of care (NCI, 2013d). However, normal values do not rule out cancer in patients with a mass, and they are not appropriate as screening tools, so they should not be used to decide whether a confirmed mass is cancerous (Kinkade, 1999). Patients are typically followed for many years for treatment failure or recurrence, and family physicians play an important role in ensuring that patients participate adequately with follow-up.

Testicular self-examination or clinical examination might detect cancer at an earlier stage but is highly unlikely to have a significant impact on testicular cancer mortality because survival rates are already so high. Thus, the USPSTF does not recommend testicular cancer screening in the general population (USPSTF, 2011b).

Wilms Tumor

Wilms tumor presents in childhood as an abdominal mass. It is a rare cancer, with approximately 500 cases annually. Wilms tumor has good cure potential, with survival rates greater than 90% at 4 years (NCI, 2013e).

KEY TREATMENT

- Use of 5α-reductase inhibitors is effective for BPH (AUA, 2010; Kramer et al., 2009; Thorpe and Neal, 2003) (SOR: A).
- α-Adrenergic blockers are also used to treat BPH (AUA, 2010; Wilt et al., 2000) (SOR: A).
- 5α-Reductase medications are not FDA approved for prostate cancer prevention (SOR: C).
- Surgical treatments may be needed for BPH (SOR: A).

Summary of Additional Online Content

The following content is available at www.expertconsult.com:

eTable 40-1 Medications with Urologic Side Effects

References

The complete reference list is available at www.expertconsult.com.

Web Resources

nkdep.nih.gov/lab-evaluation/gfr-calculators.shtml National Kidney Disease Education Program's glomerular filtration rate calculators.

nkdep.nih.gov/professionals/index.htm National Kidney Disease Education Program site on chronic kidney disease with guidelines and glomerular filtration rate calculators for adults and children.

phil.cdc.gov/phil The Centers for Disease Control and Prevention's Public Health Image Library.

www.aafp.org/online/en/home/clinical/exam/p-t.html American Academy of Family Physicians. Recommendations for clinical preventive services.

www.auanet.org American Urological Association. Guidelines and patient education resources.

www.cancer.gov The National Cancer Institute's main site, with information on various cancers and treatment.

www.cancer.org/docroot/PED/content/PED American Cancer Society. Guidelines for early cancer detection.

www.cdc.gov/STD/treatment/default.htm Centers for Disease Control and Prevention. Guidelines for treating sexually transmitted diseases.

http://www.ncbi.nlm.nih.gov/pubmedhealth/PMH0033859/ International Prostate Symptom Score.

www.kidney.org/professionals/kdoqi/guidelines_ckd/p9_approach.htm. National Kidney Foundation/Kidney Disease Quality Initiative. Clinical practice guidelines for chronic kidney disease, including evaluation, classification, and stratification.

www.prostatitis.org/symptomindex.html The National Institutes of Health's Chronic Prostatitis Symptom Index.

http://www.prostatitis.org/symptomindex.html The National Institutes of Health's Chronic Prostatitis Symptom Index.

41 *Neurology*

DAVID R. MARQUES and WILLIAM E. CARROLL

Family physicians regularly encounter and manage a range of neurologic conditions. Many are fairly common in certain age groups, such as febrile seizures in children and Alzheimer dementia in older adults. Other conditions, such as dysautonomia, are less common but present first to primary care physicians. This chapter discusses the neurologic disorders that family physicians are most likely to encounter, with guidelines for assessment and management.

Neurologic Examination

The neurologic examination begins with information obtained from the neurologic history, which is similar to a general medical history. The chief complaint is determined by asking open-ended questions. Analysis of the chief complaint should include the following:

- Date of onset
- Character and severity
- Location and extension
- Time relationship (acute, subacute, or chronic)
- Associated complaints
- Aggravating and alleviating factors
- Previous treatment and effects

Knowing the sequence of the events and their progression is helpful in localizing the lesion and developing a differential diagnosis. A brief neurologic review of systems should include questions about headaches, visual changes, weakness, sensory changes, gait disturbances, and bowel and bladder function. The past medical history, social history, and family history are reviewed as well.

Much of the initial neurologic examination, including cranial nerve (CN) testing, carotid artery auscultation, and reflex and sensory assessment, can be conducted with the patient seated in a chair, on the bed, or on the examination table. Superficial reflexes, tests for meningeal irritability, and rectal examination are performed with the patient lying down. Gait, strength, and coordination can subsequently be evaluated with the patient standing. Traditionally, the neurologic examination is divided into five major areas: mental status, CNs, motor system, sensory system, and reflexes.

MENTAL STATUS EXAMINATION

The mental status examination assesses appearance and behavior (including level of consciousness), speech and language, mood, thoughts and perceptions, and cognition. Speech abnormalities can interfere with the initial history. Abnormalities of speech include hearing deficits, aphasia (problems with understanding, thought, and word finding), and dysarthria (problems with articulation). *Aphasia* results from damage to the dominant hemisphere. *Wernicke* aphasia refers to poor comprehension, with fluent but often meaningless speech. In *Broca* aphasia, comprehension is preserved, but speech is nonfluent. Repetition, naming, reading, and writing are impaired in Wernicke and Broca aphasia. With *conductive* aphasia, there is a loss of repetition but preserved comprehension. Reading comprehension is thus relatively preserved, but reading aloud and writing are impaired. *Dysarthria* refers to difficulties with the production of speech caused by injury to the vocal cords, larynx, palate, tongue, or facial muscles. It is also seen with extrapyramidal or cerebellar lesions. Cognitive function is often assessed by tools such as the Mini–Mental State Examination, a simple, quick screening test for cognitive function. Errors in copying several simple drawings can be indicative of organic brain damage, particularly in those with dementia or parietal lobe damage.

CRANIAL NERVE EXAMINATION

The CN examination usually evaluates all CNs, with the exception of CN I. CN I testing is generally reserved for patients with complaints of loss of smell or a closed-head injury. Smell can be decreased or lost in degenerative diseases, such as Parkinson or Alzheimer disease.

Cranial Nerve II (Optic Nerve)

The principal function of the optic nerve is vision. Testing of the optic nerve includes assessment of visual acuity and visual fields, funduscopic examination, and pupillary light reflex. Visual acuity is assessed in each eye individually. Visual fields are evaluated by confrontation. When performing the funduscopic examination, look for papilledema, hemorrhages, cholesterol emboli, and atrophy. Atrophy is characterized by a small, pale disc. Pupillary function assesses CNs II and III as well as sympathetic activity. The direct and consensual responses require CNs II and III to work correctly. If CN II is damaged, an afferent pupillary defect is often present. If the optic nerve is damaged, the light reflex is sluggish.

Cranial Nerves III (Oculomotor), IV (Trochlear), and VI (Abducens)

The principal functions of these nerves include ocular rotation, eyelid elevation (III), and pupillary constriction. CN III innervates the medial, inferior, and superior rectus muscles; the inferior oblique, which allows inward and upward gaze; and the levator palpebrae superioris muscle, which raises the upper eyelid. It also innervates the pupillary constrictor muscle. CN IV innervates the superior oblique muscle, which causes the eye to look inward and down. CN VI innervates the lateral rectus muscle.

To test ocular rotation, the patient should first be examined by looking straight ahead to note any imbalances between the eyes. Next, ocular rotation of each eye is tested separately. First, abduction is tested with the patient following the examiner's finger horizontally; this tests the lateral rectus muscle. The patient then looks laterally and upward to test the superior rectus and downward to test the inferior rectus. Adduction of the eye tests the medial rectus muscle. With the eye adducted, the patient looks up to test the inferior oblique and downward to test the superior oblique.

The pupils should be observed for symmetry. Most unequal pupils (anisocoria) are congenital and not clinically significant. The light reflex, direct and consensual, is checked by shining a bright light directly into the pupil. The response to light should be brisk.

Cranial Nerve V (Trigeminal)

The principal functions of the trigeminal nerve include control of the muscles of mastication and sensation in the face; anterior half of the scalp; and mucous membranes of the mouth, nose, and sinuses. The nerve also mediates the afferent arc of the corneal reflex. The three sensory divisions are ophthalmic, maxillary, and mandibular. Each division is tested by light touch, pinprick, and temperature. The motor division of CN V can be assessed by palpating the jaw as the patient bites down. CN V is the afferent limb of the corneal reflex, and CN VII is the efferent limb. This reflex is tested by lightly touching the cornea with a wisp of cotton; the reflex, integrated through the pons, results in brisk, bilateral eye closure.

Cranial Nerve VII (Facial)

The principal functions of the facial nerve are control of the muscles of facial expression and provision of taste for the anterior two thirds of the tongue. It also innervates the lacrimal, sublingual, and submaxillary glands. To test the facial nerve, the patient is asked to smile, close the eyes tightly, and wrinkle the forehead. Taste is tested on each side separately using bitter and sweet substances.

Cranial Nerve VIII (Vestibulocochlear Nerve)

The principal functions of the vestibulocochlear nerve are hearing and vestibular function. Hearing is tested one ear at a time. Testing of hearing can be done by comparing each side with a finger rub, watch tick, or vibration of a tuning fork. The Rinne test compares bone conduction with air conduction on both sides. A tuning fork is placed on the mastoid process to assess bone conduction and then in front of the ear to assess air conduction. Air conduction should be louder than bone conduction. The Weber test evaluates middle ear conduction. A vibrating tuning fork is placed on the forehead. With normal hearing, there should be equal sound in both ears. Sound lateralized to one side indicates a conductive loss on that side or a neural loss on the opposite side. Vestibular function is not routinely tested.

Cranial Nerve IX (Glossopharyngeal)

The principal function of CN IX is to supply sensation to the pharynx and tonsillar fossa and taste to the posterior third of the tongue. Clinical testing is done by eliciting a gag reflex. It should be done on both sides of the pharynx.

Cranial Nerve X (Vagus)

The principal functions of the vagus nerve are motor control to the pharynx, palate, and larynx and parasympathetic innervation of the thoracic and abdominal viscera. Motor control is tested by observing for symmetric elevation of the palate. The uvula should not deviate. Vocal cord paralysis can present with hoarseness or dysphonia and can occur with injury to the recurrent laryngeal branch.

Cranial Nerve XI (Spinal Accessory)

The principal functions of this nerve are to allow turning of the head and assist in shrugging of the shoulders. It innervates the sternocleidomastoid and upper trapezius. Strength is tested by shrugging the shoulders and turning the head to both sides against resistance.

Cranial Nerve XII (Hypoglossal)

The principal function of the hypoglossal nerve is innervation of intrinsic muscles of the tongue. To test this nerve, ask the patient to protrude the tongue. It should be midline. If not, it protrudes to the paretic side. Also, observe for atrophy or fasciculations of the tongue.

MOTOR EXAMINATION

The motor examination includes assessment of body position, strength, tone, involuntary movements, coordination, and gait. Strength is graded as follows:

5—Normal
4—Weak but can overcome gravity plus some additional resistance
3—Can overcome gravity but not additional resistance
2—Can move joint but cannot overcome the force of gravity
1—Muscle contracts but with little or no joint movement
0—No muscle contraction

Muscle tone is tested by passively flexing and extending the arm or wrist. Abnormal responses include spasticity, rigidity, and flaccidity. *Spasticity* refers to increased muscle resistance when the muscle is passively stretched. This is seen with lesions to the cortical spinal tract. *Rigidity* or *cogwheeling* is observed with extrapyramidal lesions and Parkinson disease. *Flaccid* refers to the absence of muscle tone.

Muscular weakness can result from upper motor neuron (UMN) lesions, lower motor neuron (LMN) lesions, muscle disease, neuromuscular junction disorders, or functional weakness. Whereas UMN disease is characterized by increased tone and reflexes, LMN disease presents with wasting, fasciculations, decreased tone, and absent reflexes. With neuromuscular junction disorders, the patient complains of fatigable weakness but has normal or decreased tone and normal reflexes. A patient with functional weakness has normal tone, normal reflexes without wasting, and erratic power. The motor examination also includes observation for any abnormal movements, including tremors, choreiform movements, myoclonus, and dystonia.

Gait should be examined even if assistance is needed. Assessment includes stride length, arm swing, posture, and turning, starting, and stopping. Watch for specific gait abnormalities, such as *hemiplegia*, which is seen with unilateral UMN damage; *spasticity*, in which both legs have UMN lesions; *steppage*, in which there is footdrop; *waddling*, caused by weakness of the trunk and pelvic girdle; and *parkinsonism*, characterized by a stooped posture, short steps, and flexed arms with decreased arm swing.

Balance is maintained by the cerebellum, proprioceptive system, basal ganglia, and vestibular system. The Romberg sign is tested with the patient standing with the feet together and then with eyes closed. If the patient falls with eyes closed, the test result is considered positive. A positive test result indicates proprioceptive loss, which can be from a peripheral cause or a posterior column lesion. The result of the Romberg test can be positive with cerebellar or vestibular disease. Postural stability can be checked by gently pushing the patient while the feet are together.

Coordination can be tested with simple tests. For the finger-to-nose test, ask the patient to extend the arm, touch the tip of the nose, and then touch the examiner's index finger. This is repeated after the examiner has moved the index finger several times. The heel–knee–shin test is performed by asking the supine patient to slide one heel smoothly down the opposite leg from the knee to the shin. Two other tests of coordination are finger tapping and rapidly alternating hand movements. Injury to the cerebellar hemisphere impairs smooth coordination of limb movements on the same side of the body. With cerebellar lesions, these tests will be inaccurate, will have increased amplitude, and will be initiated more slowly.

SENSORY EXAMINATION

The sensory examination requires an alert and cooperative patient. Sensory testing includes light touch, pinprick, proprioception, and vibration. Start by testing for light touch using a wisp of cotton or tissue on the major dermatomes of the extremities and trunk (Figure 41-1). Observe for dermatomal losses or a distal-to-proximal gradient. The same areas are then tested for superficial pain with a pin. Temperature is mediated by the same pathway as pain, so any deficits of pain sensation should have a corresponding deficit in temperature sensation. Vibration is tested by placing a 128-cycles/sec tuning fork on the bony prominences of the extremities and asking the patient to identify when it stops vibrating. Comparisons are made side to side. If there is a question of myelopathy, a vibration level may be noted as the tuning fork is moved up the spinous processes. Position is best tested using the great toe and distal phalanx of the thumb or another finger. The digit is grasped on the sides and moved up and down. Even a very slight movement of a finger should be detected. Proprioception, vibration, and light touch are functions of the dorsal column, and pain, temperature, crude touch, and pressure are functions of the spinothalamic tract.

Stereognosis, graphesthesia, and touch localization are integrated cortical sensations and are difficult to test if primary sensations are impaired. To test *stereognosis*, several small familiar objects are placed in the patient's hand, and the patient is asked to identify them. To test *graphesthesia*, the examiner writes numbers on the patient's palm and asks the patient to identify them.

Table 41-1 Nerve Root Innervations and Main Reflexes

Root	Movement	Reflex
C5	Shoulder abduction, elbow flexion	Biceps
C6	Elbow flexion	Supinator
C7	Finger extension, elbow extension	Triceps
C8	Finger flexors	Finger
T1	Small muscles of hand	None
L1, L2	Hip flexion	None
L3, L4	Knee extension	Knee
L5	Extension of great toe	None
S1	Hip extension, knee flexion, plantar flexion	Ankle

C, Cervical; T, thoracic; L, lumbar, S, sacral.

REFLEXES

The reflex examination includes the deep tendon reflexes (DTRs) and the pathologic reflexes. In testing the DTRs, it is important to look for symmetry. DTRs are graded using the following scale:

0—Absent
1—Present but diminished
2—Normal
3—Normal but brisker than average
4—Increased and pathologic, with one or more beats of clonus

The DTRs assist with localization of a lesion because these reflexes are integrated at different levels of the spinal cord. DTRs help in distinguishing whether a lesion is a UMN lesion with pathologic hyperreflexia or possibly an LMN lesion with hyporeflexia. Table 41-1 summarizes the most important reflexes and their nerve root innervations.

The Babinski sign, or extensor toe sign, is tested by stroking the sole of the foot with a sharp object. A normal response is toe flexion. A pathologic response is extension of the great toe and flaring of the other toes. A positive response is always abnormal in patients older than 3 years and is a sign of pyramidal tract disorder.

Neurologic Conditions

HEADACHES

Key Points

- More than 90% of men and women will have at least one headache each year.
- If there is a history typical of a particular primary headache with a normal examination, neuroimaging and electroencephalography (EEG) are not necessary.
- Prophylactic treatment of migraine headaches is recommended when they occur with increasing frequency and there appears to be a potential overuse of acute therapies.
- Giant cell or temporal arteritis is a serious headache to consider in older adults and can be associated with blindness.

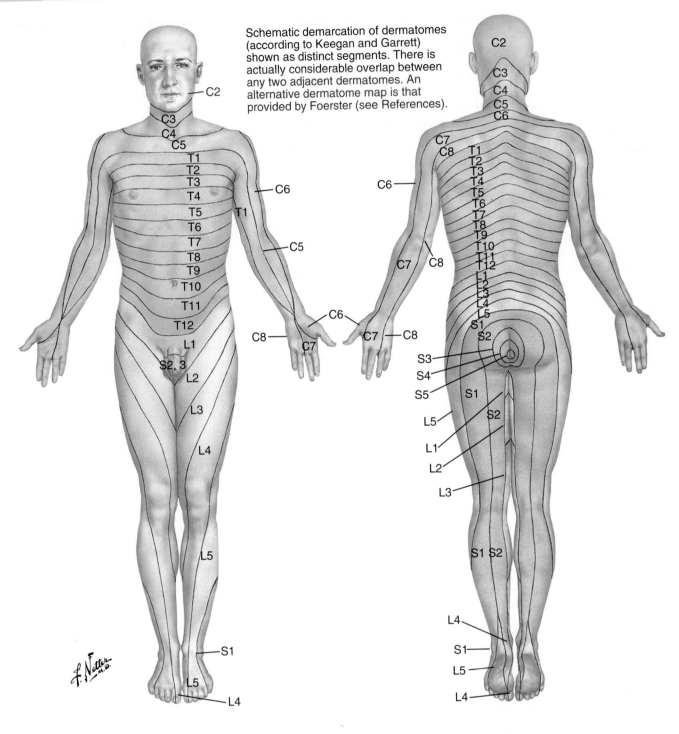

Schematic demarcation of dermatomes (according to Keegan and Garrett) shown as distinct segments. There is actually considerable overlap between any two adjacent dermatomes. An alternative dermatome map is that provided by Foerster (see References).

Levels of principal dermatomes

C5	Clavicles
C5, 6	Lateral sides of upper limbs
C8, T1	Medial sides of upper limbs
C6	Thumb
C6, 7, 8	Hand
C8	Ring and little fingers
T4	Level of nipples
T10	Level of umbilicus
L1	Inguinal or groin regions
L1, 2, 3, 4	Anterior and inner surfaces of lower limbs
L4, 5, S1	Foot
L4	Medial side of great toe
L5, S1, 2	Lateral and posterior surfaces of lower limbs
S1	Lateral margin of foot and little toe
S2, 3, 4	Perineum

Figure 41-1 Dermatomes. (Reused with permission from Netter FH. *Atlas of human anatomy.* 6th ed. Philadelphia: Saunders; 2014.)

Headaches are a common problem encountered by family physicians. More than 90% of men and women will have at least one headache each year, and as many as 4.5 million Americans will experience recurrent headaches. The International Headache Society established a system for the classification of headaches to assist in diagnosis and treatment with a standard of care for family physicians. Migraine with aura, migraine without aura, tension, and cluster headaches constitute most primary headaches. Secondary headaches are symptoms of organic disease (Sarchielli, 2004). The initial evaluation of a patient with headache requires a complete history and physical examination with the following information:

- Age at onset
- Location, frequency, and duration
- Intensity and character
- Associated symptoms
- Triggering and ameliorating factors
- Medications
- Associated physical and neurologic symptoms
- Impact on work and family
- Psychological symptoms
- History of head trauma
- Previous imaging results
- Family history

Features of the history that should warn of an ominous cause for headache include the following:

- Sudden onset of headache or headache that reaches maximal intensity within seconds or minutes of onset
- Worst (or first) headache ever
- Late onset of new headache (after age 50 years)
- Headache associated with fever, rash, or a stiff neck
- Progressively worsening headache
- Headache associated with neurologic signs and symptoms other than aura
- Headache associated with mental status changes
- Headache associated with papilledema
- Headache with exertion, sexual activity, coughing, or sneezing

The physical examination of a patient first presenting for evaluation of headache should include vital signs; cardiac examination; cervical spine examination, including nuchal rigidity; and ophthalmologic examination, including the optic fundi, pupils, and visual fields. The neurologic examination should include an assessment of cognitive function, motor function, reflexes, plantar response, CNs, coordination, and gait.

If there is a history typical of a particular primary headache with a normal examination, neuroimaging and EEG are not necessary. A lumbar puncture (LP) after neuroimaging is recommended only if there is suspicion of subarachnoid hemorrhage, infection, or idiopathic intracranial hypertension (pseudotumor cerebri). Routine EEG is not indicated but may be useful in evaluating patients with associated mental status or consciousness changes, a history of head injury, or a history of syncope.

Migraine

Migraine headaches include migraine without aura, migraine with aura, and other migrainous disorders. Women have migraines three times as often as men, and 90% of those with migraines have a positive family history. Migraines can begin in childhood, and as many as 4% to 10% of school-age children have migraines. The International Headache Society has developed diagnostic criteria for these types of headaches (Sarchielli, 2004). To establish a diagnosis of *migraine without aura*, there must have been at least five attacks fulfilling the following criteria:

1. Headache attacks lasting 4 to 72 hours
2. Headache with at least two of the following characteristics:
   a. Unilateral location
   b. Pulsating quality
   c. Moderate or severe intensity (inhibits or prohibits daily activities or causes avoidance of routine)
   d. Aggravated by physical activity such as walking or climbing
3. During the headache, at least one of the following occurs:
   a. Nausea and vomiting
   b. Photophobia and phonophobia

Migraine with aura has comparable diagnostic criteria but includes an aura. *Auras* can be visual, sensory, motor, or speech auras. Visual changes include parallel zigzag lines and are often associated with scotomatous defects. Sensory deficits can involve an ipsilateral arm or periorbital numbness or tingling. The tongue may be involved in some patients. The sensation has a marching characteristic. Motor deficits can be similar to sensory in that the deficits spread from one area to another. Speech problems may manifest as a mild dysphasia.

Other migraine types include basilar-type migraine, retinal migraine, status migrainosus, and migrainous infarction. *Basilar-type migraine* aura symptoms are referable to the brainstem or bilateral hemispheres, including dysarthria, vertigo, tinnitus, diplopia, and bilateral paresthesias. Reversible monocular, positive or negative visual disturbances associated with migraine are characteristic of *retinal migraine*. A diagnosis of *status migrainosus* requires an ongoing migraine of at least 72 hours in duration. Neuroimaging evidence of a cerebral infarct associated with a migraine is indicative of *migrainous infarction*.

Treatment. Migraine headache management includes acute analgesia, pharmacologic prophylaxis, and nonpharmacologic management. Factors to consider before starting prophylactic medications include frequency, severity, and lack of response or contraindications to analgesic medications. Nonpharmacologic management includes identification and avoidance of triggering factors, stress management, regular sleep and exercise, and physical therapy. Factors that can aggravate or trigger migraines include alcohol, oral contraceptives, hormonal replacement, caffeine or caffeine withdrawal, stress, changes in weather, strong scents, foods (nitrates, dairy products, chocolate, aged cheese), and fasting or missing meals.

The goal of pharmacologic treatment is to reduce the patient's disability and maintain an acceptable quality of life. The choice of abortive drug therapy depends on the severity of the patient's symptoms. A plan can be developed with the patient to use some medications for mild to

Table 41-2   Symptomatic Migraine Medications

Drug Name	Dose Range	Adverse Effects
Acetaminophen, 325 mg; isometheptene, 65 mg; and dichloralphenazone, 100 mg (Midrin)	2 capsules at onset, then qh PRN; max 5 caps/12 hr	Liver toxicity, dizziness
Lidocaine 4% aqueous solution for nasal spray (Xylocaine)	0.5 mL to nostrils; may repeat after 15 min	None known
Ergotamine, 1 mg with caffeine, 100-mg oral tablets (Cafergot)	2 tablets; then 1 every 30 min four times PRN; max 6 tabs/attack or 10 tabs/wk	Nausea, vasoconstriction, fetal harm
PARENTERAL AGENTS		
Dihydroergotamine, 1 mg/mL (DHE 45)	1 mg IV, IM, or SC qh, maximum, 2 mg IV, 3 mg IM or SC	Nausea, vasoconstriction
Dihydroergotamine, 0.5 mg/mL (Migranal)	0.5 mg spray in each nostril; may repeat in 15 min	
Ketorolac (Toradol)	15-30 mg IM or IV q6h	GI upset, renal toxicity
SELECTIVE SEROTONIN (5-HT) AGONISTS		
Sumatriptan (Imitrex)		
Autoinjector	6 mg qh PRN	Chest and neck discomfort
	Maximum, 12 mg/day	
Nasal spray	5 to 20 mg q2h PRN	
	Maximum, 40 mg/day	
Tablet	25-100 mg q2h PRN	
	Maximum, 200 mg/day	
Naratriptan (Amerge)	1 to 2.5 mg q4h PRN	
	Maximum, 5 mg/day	
Rizatriptan (Maxalt)	5 to 10 mg q2h PRN	
	Maximum, 30 mg/day	
Tabs	1.25 to 2.5 mg q2h PRN	
	Maximum, 10 mg/day	
Orally disintegrating tabs (ZMT)	2.5 mg q2h PRN	
	Maximum, 10 mg/day	
Nasal Spray	5 mg (1 spray) in one nostril q2h PRN	
	Maximum, 10 mg/day	
Zolmitriptan (Zomig)	2.5 to 5 mg q2h PRN	
	Maximum, 10 mg/day	
Eletriptan (Relpax)	20 to 40 mg q2h PRN	
	Maximum, 80 mg/day	
Frovatriptan (Frova)	2.5 mg q2h PRN	
	Maximum, 7.5 mg/day	
Almotriptan (Axert)	6.25 to 12.5 mg q2h PRN	
	Maximum, 25 mg/day	
Sumatriptan 85 mg and naproxen sodium 500 mg (Treximet)	1 tablet q2h PRN	
	Maximum, 2 tablets/day	

5-HT, 5-Hydroxytryptamine; *GI,* gastrointestinal; *IM,* intramuscular; *IV,* intravenous; *qh,* every hour; *q2h,* every 2 hours; *PRN,* as needed; *SC,* subcutaneous.

moderate attacks and other medications for more severe attacks. For mild attacks, combination medicines, such as aspirin, acetaminophen, and caffeine (Excedrin or generic equivalent), are effective. For more severe headaches, the triptans are the drugs of choice (the triptans are not indicated for basilar migraines or hemiplegic migraines) (Polizzotto, 2002).

Dihydroergotamine (DHE) and other ergotamine compounds are useful. Aqueous lidocaine applied intranasally is another option. Briefly, 0.5 mL of a 4% aqueous solution of lidocaine is slowly dripped into one nostril with the patient supine and the head hyperextended 45 degrees and rotated 30 degrees toward the side affected by the headache (Maizels et al., 1996). Antiemetics, such as metoclopramide or chlorpromazine, can be used in conjunction with most abortive medications (Table 41-2).

Prophylactic treatment of migraine is recommended when headaches occur with increasing frequency and the patient may be overusing acute therapies. The daily use of symptomatic medications, including acetaminophen and nonsteroidal antiinflammatory drugs (NSAIDs), can cause liver and kidney injury. Also, regular use of certain medications (e.g., propoxyphene, butalbital, ergotamines, triptans) can result in habituation or rebound headaches. Preventive treatment is also recommended for patients who have fre-

quent attacks, often four or more, throughout the month or when headaches are so severe that acute treatment is no longer completely effective. The overall goal of preventive treatment is to reduce the frequency and severity of migraine attacks. Prophylactic agents include β-adrenergic blockers, calcium channel blockers, selective serotonin reuptake inhibitors (SSRIs), tricyclic antidepressants (TCAs), and anticonvulsant medications (Table 41-3). β-Blockers such as propranolol have proven efficacy in this role (Polizzotto, 2002). For patients requesting alternative therapies, there is level B evidence for the effectiveness of petasites (purified extract from the butterbur plant), 75 mg twice a day for migraine prophylaxis (Lipton et al., 2004; Schapowal, 2002).

Tension-Type Headaches

Tension-type headaches can be episodic or chronic. There is a slight female preponderance, and the prevalence may be directly related to socioeconomic status. Chronic tension headaches can sometimes develop in migraine patients and are frequently associated with overuse of analgesics. The International Headache Society has further subdivided tension-type headaches into those with and without *pericranial tenderness* (Sarchielli, 2004). Headaches can be classified by cause, such as temporomandibular joint

Table 41-3 Preventive Antimigraine Therapy

Type of Drug	Dose Range	Adverse Effects
β-ADRENERGIC BLOCKERS		
Propranolol (Inderal)	40-240 mg/day	Bronchospasm, bradycardia, hypotension, fatigue, depression
Timolol (Blocadren)	10-60 mg/day	Bronchospasm, bradycardia, hypotension, fatigue, depression
CALCIUM CHANNEL BLOCKERS		
Verapamil (Calan)	240-480 mg/day	Hypotension, constipation, edema
TRICYCLIC ANTIDEPRESSANTS		
Amitriptyline (Elavil)	10-100 mg/day	Sedation, dry mouth, weight gain, tremor, cardiac arrhythmias, difficulty voiding
Nortriptyline (Pamelor)	10-150 mg/day	Sedation, dry mouth, weight gain, tremor, cardiac arrhythmias, difficulty voiding
ANTICONVULSANTS		
Divalproex sodium (Depakote)	250-1000 mg/day	Nausea, fatigue, weight gain, hair loss, tremor, liver toxicity, fetal harm
Gabapentin (Neurontin)	100-3600 mg/day	Fatigue
Topiramate (Topamax)	25-200 mg/day	Fatigue, paresthesias, weight loss, memory loss, nephrolithiasis
Cyproheptadine	4-16 mg/day	Drowsiness, dizziness, constipation, urinary retention
BOTANICALS		
Petasites extract (Butterbur)	75 mg BID	Potential allergic reaction to the plant

BID, Twice a day.

dysfunction, psychosocial stress, and analgesic overuse. Tension-type headaches require a comprehensive assessment to determine whether any comorbid conditions exacerbate the headache. The diagnostic criteria for episodic tension-type headaches include at least 10 previous headache episodes fulfilling the following criteria:

1. Headaches lasting for 30 minutes to 7 days, with at least two of the following pain characteristics:
   a. Pressing or tightening (nonpulsating) quality
   b. Mild or moderate intensity
   c. Bilateral location
   d. No aggravation by walking, climbing stairs, or similar routine physical activity
2. Both of the following:
   a. No nausea or vomiting
   b. Photophobia and phonophobia—both absent or only one present

Frequently, the initial symptoms of a tension headache are described as a bandlike, squeezing, or tight pressure sensation. It is generally diffuse, often concentrated in the occipital region or in the temples. This can also be associated with depression or anxiety and aggravated by stress. No neurologic abnormalities should be noted in the history or physical examination.

A chronic tension headache requires that the pain be present for 15 days a month for more than 3 months. The other criteria are the same as those for episodic tension-type headaches.

The treatment for tension-type headaches is generally difficult. There is always the concern of analgesic abuse. Amitriptyline is frequently a reasonable drug choice, 10 to 100 mg/day. Muscle relaxants can be helpful as a short-term intervention when the pain extends into the shoulder trapezius muscles. In addition to therapeutic options, it is beneficial to use relaxation therapy, physical therapy, and stress management programs. Improvement of posture, stretching exercises, and even traction can be beneficial. On occasion, relief can be obtained with injections or occipital nerve blocks.

Medications can be used for abortive treatment and can include NSAIDs and analgesics with caffeine. The choice of medication depends on the severity and frequency of the headaches. Care needs to be used when prescribing butalbital-containing compounds because their addiction potential is high. In addition, there is always the problem of analgesic overuse, which could lead to the development of chronic daily headaches.

Cluster Headaches

Cluster headaches are less common than migraines, and almost 80% of patients are male. Cluster headaches present with unilateral pain. Attacks may last 15 to 180 minutes and can occur every other day to up to eight times daily. The cycle may last for 4 to 12 weeks. These headaches frequently are triggered by alcohol, with some nausea. They tend to occur at a similar time during the day or night. The pain is frequently in the orbital or periorbital region. It is an extremely sharp, continuous, incapacitating pain. The criteria for diagnosis include at least five attacks with the following elements:

1. Severe unilateral orbital or supraorbital pain lasting 15 to 180 minutes
2. Headache associated with at least one of the following ipsilateral signs in addition to the headache:
   a. Conjunctival infection
   b. Lacrimation
   c. Nasal congestion
   d. Miosis or ptosis
   e. Eye edema
   f. Forehead and facial sweating
   g. Sense of restlessness or agitation
3. Frequency from every other day to eight times a day

Cluster headaches are unusual in that they may come at certain intervals throughout the year. Headaches may last for a few weeks and then disappear or can become chronic and persist throughout the year.

Medications for the treatment of cluster headaches include some of the same drugs used for abortive treatment for migraines, including DHE, ergotamines, intranasal 4% aqueous lidocaine solution, and triptans. The nasal and injectable forms have a more rapid onset of action than the oral preparations. Cluster headaches are also unusual in that they may respond to oxygen. Inhaled 100% oxygen can relieve an attack within 10 to 15 minutes.

For headaches that are intense, do not respond to abortive treatment, or require excessive use of abortive treatment, prophylaxis is recommended. Divalproex (Depakote) can be used for the treatment of the chronic cluster headache. Dosages range up to 1000 mg/day in divided doses. A pulse dose of steroids can also be effective, as can verapamil.

Medication Overuse Headaches

Individuals with headaches can begin to experience daily or almost daily headaches when medication doses are excessive or too frequent. Rebound can occur with opioids, acetaminophen, aspirin, analgesic–codeine or analgesic–barbiturate combinations, NSAIDs, ergotamines, and triptans. Characteristics of rebound headaches include a diffuse, bilateral, almost daily headache, often aggravated by mild physical or mental exertion. The headache is frequently present on waking and can be associated with restlessness, nausea, forgetfulness, and depression. Tolerance develops to abortive medications, and there is a decreased responsiveness to preventive medications.

Treatment of rebound headaches can be difficult. The causative medications must be identified, and there may be some psychological as well as physical dependence. The key to treatment is to discontinue the overused medication and thus break the cycle. Stopping the medication may result in withdrawal symptoms and an initial period of increased headaches, with subsequent improvement. Although there is no significant difference in outcomes at 1 year with inpatient versus outpatient treatment, hospitalization to stop the medication should be considered for barbiturates, opioids, and benzodiazepines. Specific limits need to be set for the use of analgesics, ergotamines, and triptans to reduce the likelihood of rebound headaches.

Miscellaneous Headaches

Episodic and chronic *paroxysmal hemicrania* is an unusual headache that tends to occur in women. The attacks are short, and the pain is similar to that of a cluster headache. These headaches respond to indomethacin, with a maximum of 150 mg/day in divided doses (off-label usage).

Posttraumatic headaches can follow a head injury, with presentation similar to that of migraine headache. No clear correlation appears to exist between intensity of the head trauma and development of headache. These headaches may be associated with dizziness and impaired concentration. Treatment is difficult, but many of the migraine compounds are effective.

Trigeminal neuralgia is described as a piercing, sudden, severe pain that can last for seconds to minutes in the area of the cheek or jaw and can be aggravated by chewing or talking. Treatment options include carbamazepine, oxcarbazepine, baclofen, and gabapentin. Surgical intervention is an option when medical treatment fails.

Headaches in Older Adults

A serious headache that presents in the older adult population is *giant cell arteritis*, or temporal arteritis. The pain can be bitemporal or unilateral; is moderate to severe in intensity; is diffuse, not always throbbing; and persists throughout the day and often worsens at night. This headache is often associated with systemic complaints (e.g., weight loss, joint tenderness) and can be aggravated with jaw movement. It is important to treat giant cell arteritis because it can be associated with blindness. The Westergren erythrocyte sedimentation rate (ESR) is frequently elevated. If temporal arteritis is suspected, a diagnostic temporal artery biopsy is performed. It is important not to delay treatment while waiting for the biopsy. Steroid treatment can be initiated up to 2 weeks before the biopsy without compromising the results. A patient with a headache of giant cell arteritis requires high doses of prednisone, usually for several months or longer.

Ophthalmic zoster is another type of head pain in older adults. The pain is described as a burning, constant, piercing, shocklike pain. It follows the distribution of the trigeminal nerve. This is a difficult headache to treat, but it responds well to anticonvulsants, particularly carbamazepine and gabapentin.

Glaucoma can cause a migrainelike headache, with severe pain around the affected eye.

STROKE

> ### Key Points
>
> - Strokes usually occur without warning, and fewer than 20% of cerebrovascular accidents (CVAs) are preceded by a warning transient ischemic attack (TIA).
> - Stroke risk factors include hypertension, smoking, atrial fibrillation, internal carotid artery stenosis, and diabetes.
> - The time-related cellular death in areas of hypoperfusion requires reperfusing the ischemic penumbra.
> - Both dipyridamole (plus aspirin) and clopidogrel are reasonable first-line antiplatelet agents for secondary stroke prevention.
> - During the first day after an ischemic stroke, most patients with elevated blood pressure (BP) should not be treated unless the systolic blood pressure (SBP) is consistently higher than 220 mm Hg or the diastolic blood pressure (DBP) is consistently higher than 120 mm Hg.

Stroke is the fourth leading cause of death in the United States and the leading cause of significant disability in adults. Until the past few years, stroke was the third leading cause of death, but efforts to increase adherence to risk factor modification as well as more extensive use of acute stroke treatments have reduced the number of deaths from stroke. The role of primary care in management of risk factors is paramount. Among women, stroke remains the third leading cause of death in the United States, however. Worldwide, stroke is the second leading cause of death, and in some countries, such as China, Japan, and Brazil, stroke is the leading cause of death.

About 750,000 new cases of stroke occur each year. Despite a decline in the stroke death rate, the absolute number of strokes in the United States continues to rise. This continued annual increase is the result of a rise in the mean age of the population. Current projections predict a 20% overall increase in stroke prevalence from 2012 to 2030. The mortality rate for CVA is about 15%, and only slightly less than one third of patients who have a stroke regain normal cerebral function. Furthermore, the recurrence rate for patients who survive a stroke is about 10% per year. Thus, stroke remains a major public health problem in the United States (Benavente and Hart, 1999; Hart and Benavente, 1999).

Stroke is defined as the sudden onset of neurologic dysfunction caused by focal central nervous system (CNS) infarction, which involves brain, spinal cord, or retinal cell death caused by ischemia. Evidence for the cell death can be determined by imaging, pathological data, or clinical presentation. A TIA is similarly characterized by the rapid onset of neurologic dysfunction but without permanent infarction. Previously, time-based definitions of stroke and TIA were used but are thought to be inadequate to reflect current understanding of the clinicopathological processes involved in cerebrovascular disease. Whereas strokes may be of ischemic or hemorrhagic origin, TIAs are generally ischemic events. Statistically, most patients have ischemic rather than hemorrhagic strokes. About two thirds of ischemic strokes are caused by thrombosis, and slightly less than one third are caused by embolus. *Ischemic* strokes result from many causes, including intracranial atherosclerosis; cervical carotid artery stenosis; and occlusive disease of the small, penetrating arteries, leading to lacunar infarcts. *Hemorrhagic* strokes are generally related to intracranial or subarachnoid hemorrhage, with intracranial hemorrhages being more common. No specific cause is identified in as many as 30% of patients with stroke; patients with cryptogenic stroke are often younger.

Strokes usually occur without warning, and fewer than 20% are preceded by a warning TIA. Patients with a previous TIA or CVA have a 4.5% to 6.6% annual risk for subsequent stroke. The risk for stroke after a retinal TIA (amaurosis fugax) is much lower than that after a hemispheric TIA.

Risk Factors

Hypertension. Patients with a SBP higher than 160 mm Hg or a diastolic DBP higher than 95 mm Hg have a fourfold increased risk of stroke compared with the general population. Decreasing DBP by as little as 5 mm Hg reduces the relative risk of strokes by 43%, and a decrease of 10 mm Hg results in a 50% relative risk reduction. Treatment of older adults with isolated SBP elevations higher than 160 mm Hg reduces their risk of stroke and is usually well tolerated if approached carefully.

Smoking. Cigarette smoking is an independent risk factor for stroke. The risk of stroke is almost twice as high for smokers, and the relative risk of subarachnoid hemorrhage is almost three times as high as for the general population. Patients who smoke should be encouraged to quit. It is also reasonable to avoid passive exposure to environmental tobacco smoke.

Atrial Fibrillation. Clinical trials continue to demonstrate the benefits of warfarin for primary and secondary stroke prevention among high-risk patients with nonvalvular atrial fibrillation. The stroke risk in patients with atrial fibrillation is reduced by about two thirds when they are treated with warfarin adjusted to achieve a target international normalized ratio (INR) of 2 or 3. Novel oral anticoagulants have become available and include dabigatran, rivaroxaban, and apixaban. These agents tend to have favorable safety profiles and do not require ongoing laboratory monitoring but with higher initial cost and inability to achieve emergent reversal. These newer oral anticoagulant agents tend to have less bleeding risk overall but a slightly higher risk of gastrointestinal bleeding than warfarin (Hankey, 2014).

These predictive tools can be found online and are useful in helping guide therapy:

- **ABCD2:** Estimates risk of stroke after a TIA (http://www.mdcalc.com/abcd2-score-for-tia/).
- **CHAD2DS2-VASc:** Estimates risk of stroke in those with atrial fibrillation and guides anti-platelet vs. anticoagulation therapy. A score greater than 2 suggests benefit from anticoagulation therapy (http://www.mdcalc.com/cha2ds2-vasc-score-for-atrial-fibrillation-stroke-risk/).
- **HAS-BLED:** Estimates risk of major bleeding with anticoagulation therapy. If the score is greater than 3, the risk of bleeding is significant with anticoagulation therapy (http://www.mdcalc.com/has-bled-score-for-major-bleeding-risk/).

Hypercholesterolemia. Modest stroke risk reduction has been demonstrated by the achievement of lower lipid levels. Statins are effective for the primary prevention of ischemic stroke for patients with a history of occlusive arterial disease, coronary artery disease (CAD), or diabetes without a history of cerebrovascular disease. Statins reduce the risk of ischemic stroke in hypertensive patients with multiple cardiovascular risk factors and nonfasting cholesterol levels lower than 250 mg/dL, reduce stroke risk for patients with CAD or equivalent (e.g., diabetes, peripheral artery disease), and prevent recurrent ischemic stroke in CAD patients (Busch et al., 2004). Statins have also been shown to reduce the incidence of stroke and TIA in patients without preexisting CAD (Amarenko et al., 2006).

Carotid Artery Stenosis. Patients with internal carotid artery stenosis of less than 75% have an annual risk of stroke of approximately 1.3%. In contrast, patients with internal carotid stenosis greater than 75% have annual TIA risk of 7.2% and annual stroke risk of 3.3%. Patients with asymptomatic carotid stenosis have a relatively low rate of ipsilateral stroke, probably about 2% per year (Norris et al., 1991). Select patients with asymptomatic carotid stenosis may benefit from carotid endarterectomy. The Asymptomatic Carotid Atherosclerosis Study (ACAS) showed a benefit from endarterectomy in patients with a stenosis more than 60%, although the overall benefit was relatively small (Young et al., 1996). A low perioperative complication rate is crucial if endarterectomy is to offer asymptomatic patients a beneficial option. Carotid angioplasty and stenting are viable alternatives to carotid endarterectomy but are limited to patients at high risk for endarterectomy. When used with an embolus protection device, the safety and efficacy of carotid stenting have been established, and the noninferiority of carotid stenting compared with endarterectomy has been demonstrated. When medical management is elected, it should include control of hypertension, smoking cessation, education regarding the symptoms of TIA, efforts to identify and treat existing CAD, antiplatelet therapy, statin therapy, and serial carotid ultrasound studies to monitor the progression of carotid stenosis.

The management of symptomatic carotid artery stenosis—that is, cervical carotid stenosis associated with ipsilateral focal ischemic events—is less controversial. Clinical trials consistently demonstrate the benefits of carotid endarterectomy for patients with high-grade (70%) cervical carotid stenosis who are symptomatic. Conversely, symptomatic patients with mild (<50%) carotid stenosis do not benefit from surgery. Patients with moderate stenosis obtain a moderate benefit from surgery. These patients may be appropriately treated with surgery or medical therapy, depending on the clinical judgment of the treating physicians. Physicians should remember that women have a lower incidence of subsequent stroke than men with similar degrees of carotid stenosis. Women also have higher rates of perioperative complications than men.

Diabetes. Patients with diabetes who have strokes tend to be younger and have a higher incidence of intracerebral bleeding. Diabetes is an established risk factor for initial strokes, but there is no evidence that intensive control of hyperglycemia decreases the incidence of recurrent stroke. Usual glycemic control remains a reasonable endeavor.

Acute Intervention

When oxygen deprivation occurs, neuronal cellular death occurs within minutes. Thus, in nonperfused areas of the brain, necrosis begins within minutes. These areas of necrosis are typically surrounded by areas of decreased blood flow. This diminished blood flow may be barely enough to keep the neurons in these areas alive. Such areas of hypoperfusion are electrically silent and are referred to as the *ischemic penumbra*. If timely reperfusion of the ischemic penumbra occurs, these neurons can recover. However, failure to reperfuse the ischemic penumbra promptly results in time-related neuronal cell death and transformation of an area of hypoperfusion into an area of frank infarction. Resuscitation of the ischemic penumbra is therefore a primary goal of acute stroke management. Because of the time-related cellular death that occurs in areas of hypoperfusion, interventions aimed at reperfusing the ischemic penumbra must be instituted expeditiously if maximal benefit is to be realized.

Many agents and interventions have been under investigation for the treatment of acute stroke. Although therapeutic options for acute stroke management are expanding, *tissue plasminogen activator* (t-PA) is currently the only specific medication validated for this purpose by clinical trials and labeled for this use by the U.S. Food and Drug Administration (FDA). The National Institute of Neurologic Disorders and Stroke recommends t-PA for acute intervention in select stroke patients (NINDS, 1995). The t-PA trials showed substantial improvement in long-term functional outcome for patients treated with t-PA within 3 hours of ischemic stroke onset compared with the placebo group (NINDS t-PA Stroke Study Group, 1997). For every 100 patients given t-PA, 12 more experienced complete neurologic recovery than those receiving placebo. However, there was an approximately 6% increase in intracerebral hemorrhage in t-PA recipients. This risk of intracerebral hemorrhage increased significantly if computed tomography (CT) demonstrated early infarction changes. More recently, the European Cooperative Acute Stroke Study III has

Table 41-4 Criteria for Tissue Plasminogen Activator Use in Patients with Thromboembolic Stroke

Considering t-PA as a treatment option	Age ≥18 years
	Noncontrast CT without evidence of hemorrhage
	Time since onset of symptoms clearly <3 hr (4.5 hr for select patients) before t-PA administration would begin
Excluding t-PA as a treatment option	**HISTORICAL AND CLINICAL FINDINGS**
	Clinical presentation suggests subarachnoid hemorrhage even if CT is normal:
	Sudden, severe headache, often with loss of consciousness at onset
	Vomiting common
	Active internal bleeding, increased risk of bleeding, or known bleeding diathesis, including:
	Recent use of warfarin with prolonged INR
	Use of heparin within 48 hr with prolonged aPTT
	Platelet count <100,000 cells/mm³
	History of intracranial hemorrhage
	Known arteriovenous malformation or aneurysm
	GI or GU bleeding in past 21 days
	Arterial puncture in past 7 days at noncompressible site
	Recent LP
	Stroke, intracranial surgery, or head trauma in previous 3 months
	Major surgery or serious trauma in preceding 14 days
	Persistent SBP >185 or DBP >110 mm Hg
	Seizure at stroke onset
	Rapidly improving neurologic signs
	Isolated, mild neurologic deficits
	Acute MI
	Post-MI pericarditis
	Blood glucose <50 mg/dL or >400 mg/dL
	Patient pregnant or lactating
	CT FINDINGS
	Evidence of intracranial hemorrhage
	Hypodensity or effacement of the sulci in one third of the region of the middle cerebral artery

aPTT, Activated partial thromboplastin time; *CT*, computed tomography; *DPB*, diastolic blood pressure; *GI*, gastrointestinal; *GU*, genitourinary; *INR*, international normalized ratio; *LP*, lumbar puncture; *MI*, myocardial infarction; *SBP*, systolic blood pressure; *t-PA*, tissue plasminogen activator (alteplase [Activase]).

demonstrated that the time window for administration of t-PA can be safely and effectively extended to 4.5 hours in select patients. Those older than 80 years, those with a history of stroke and diabetes, those taking oral anticoagulants, and those with NIH Stroke Scale score greater than 25 are excluded from this extended timeframe.

The administration of t-PA for the treatment of acute stroke requires strict adherence to established eligibility criteria, emergency CT capability with experienced interpretation, and 24-hour intensive care unit monitoring (Table 41-4). The limit from stroke onset to treatment with t-PA must be respected, whether the patient meets criteria for the 3-hour time window or the 4.5-hour time window. If a patient wakes from sleep with a neurologic deficit, the stroke must be assumed to have had its onset at the time sleep commenced. If the exact time of stroke onset is in question, t-PA should not be given. Patients and their families should understand that although treatment of acute ischemic stroke with t-PA is potentially beneficial, there is an approximately 1 in 15 chance of sustaining a serious cerebral hemorrhage even if t-PA is used in accordance with strict guidelines. They should also understand that although patients with severe ischemic strokes have the most to gain from t-PA, they also have a higher risk of t-PA–associated intracerebral hemorrhage. Finally, the CT must not demonstrate intracranial bleeding if t-PA is to be given, and some experts recommend withholding t-PA if the CT demonstrates evidence of early infarction.

In some referral centers, intraarterial t-PA is also a treatment option. Such intervention extends the treatment window to 6 hours, principally because of the lower dose of t-PA administered and the ability to deliver the agent directly into the clot. Additionally, mechanical removal of intraarterial thrombus is also a treatment option using a variety of devices such as a corkscrew-like mechanism (Merci device), a suction mechanism (Penumbra device), or a self-expanding stent retriever (Solitaire or Trevo device) to extract the clot and thereby reestablish blood flow to the ischemic penumbra. Whereas small series of patients and individual centers have shown favorable results using such revascularization techniques, no large randomized clinical trials have demonstrated improved outcomes. Additional studies to determine appropriate patient selection for intraarterial revascularization are ongoing.

Pharmacologic Therapy

Published studies to date overwhelmingly support the ability of *aspirin* to reduce stroke incidence and death in patients who present with TIA or CVA. Aspirin and other agents that affect platelet function are frequently used for long-term secondary stroke prevention. It therefore seems reasonable, after hemorrhage has been excluded by CT, to begin aspirin therapy in the setting of acute stroke, provided the patient does not have a contraindication to aspirin therapy. Aspirin doses between 50 and 1300 mg/day have been shown to be effective for stroke prevention. In the absence of convincing evidence favoring a specific dosage, most clinicians prescribe 81 or 325 mg/day. The FDA recommends that aspirin doses of 50 to 325 mg/day be used for stroke prevention.

Clopidogrel (Plavix) inhibits platelet function by irreversibly binding to adenosine diphosphate receptors. Compared with aspirin, clopidogrel significantly decreases the constellation of stroke, myocardial infarction (MI), and vascular death and has a toxicity comparable with that of aspirin. Thrombotic thrombocytopenic purpura has been reported after the initiation of clopidogrel, often within the first 2 weeks of therapy (Bennett et al., 2000).

Dipyridamole (Persantine) was widely used in combination with aspirin in the early 1980s for the prevention of stroke until critical analysis cast doubt on its efficacy. A European study found high-dose sustained-release dipyridamole plus aspirin to be superior to aspirin alone for the prevention of stroke (Diener et al., 1996). The side effects of this therapy included headache and required discontinuation in approximately 6% of patients.

Selection of the appropriate antiplatelet agent for stroke prevention can become complicated, especially for patients with comorbid cardiovascular disease. Both extended-release dipyridamole plus aspirin (Aggrenox) and clopidogrel (Plavix) are reasonable first-line antiplatelet agents for secondary stroke prevention, shown to be more effective than aspirin alone. Randomized controlled trials (RCTs)

Table 41-5   Cardiac Conditions Substantially Associated with Embolism

Atrial fibrillation
Mitral stenosis
Mechanical cardiac valves
Recent myocardial infarction
Left ventricular thrombus, especially if mobile and protruding
Atrial myxoma
Infective endocarditis
Dilated cardiomyopathy
Marantic (nonbacterial thrombotic) endocarditis

have shown no additional benefit of the combination of clopidogrel and aspirin, which only increase the risk of hemorrhage.

The use of *heparin* therapy for the prevention of recurrent TIA or stroke progression is limited. Progression of stroke is common, occurring in 15% to 20% of carotid-distribution strokes and 35% to 40% of vertebrobasilar strokes. Even in patients with angiographically minimal or absent cerebral artery occlusion, clinical worsening of neurologic findings frequently occurs. Furthermore, heparin has not been shown in adequate clinical trials to improve clinical outcome among patients with stroke. The International Stroke Trial Collaborative Group (1997) reported that patients receiving subcutaneous (SC) heparin had fewer recurrent ischemic strokes, but this improvement was offset by an increase in hemorrhagic strokes. There was no net benefit. Trials with heparinoids have also failed to demonstrate a clear benefit and have shown an increased risk of non-CNS bleeding. Studies have also failed to demonstrate a clear benefit for low-molecular-weight heparin (LMWH).

Currently, *warfarin* (Coumadin) cannot be recommended as initial therapy for most patients with stroke of primarily cerebrovascular origin. In two large-scale RCTs of warfarin compared with aspirin in the prevention of recurrent stroke (SPIRIT, WARSS), warfarin was not superior to aspirin for patients without cardioembolic disease or operable carotid stenosis (Sacco et al., 2006). Furthermore, the hemorrhagic risk with warfarin was higher than with aspirin. In contrast to ischemic stroke, there is good evidence that warfarin is beneficial for patients with several major cardiac disorders predisposing them to embolic stroke. Table 41-5 summarizes cardiac conditions that are substantially associated with cardioembolic stroke and often warrant prophylactic therapy with warfarin. Other cardiac conditions, such as mitral valve prolapse with or without myxomatous changes, severe mitral annular calcification, and calcific aortic stenosis, have a low or uncertain risk of embolism, and warfarin therapy is generally reserved for secondary prevention.

Management of Acute Stroke

Initial Management in Emergency Department. Patients suspected of having sustained an acute stroke should be stabilized in accordance with usual emergency management, which focuses initially on basic cardiopulmonary resuscitation and support. All patients should have a thorough but timely physical examination, looking especially for head and neck trauma and cardiovascular abnormalities, followed by neurologic evaluation, including assessment of mental status, CN function, cerebellar

Table 41-6   Initial Treatment Considerations for Stroke Patients

Provide initial care.	Stabilize the patient, secure the airway, and provide adequate oxygenation. Assess level of consciousness, language, visual fields, eye movements, and pupillary movements. Obtain history and perform physical examination. Perform CT of head without contrast. Obtain CBC with platelets and differential, electrolytes, creatinine, BUN, glucose, PT/PTT, and oxygen saturation.
Consider toxicology screen.	Consider special coagulation studies such as antiphospholipid antibodies, factor V Leiden assay, protein C and protein S, antithrombin III, ANA, fibrinogen, RPR, homocysteine, serum protein electrophoresis, prothrombin gene 20210.
Consider acute intervention with t-PA.	
Consider the following with admission orders.	TEE Carotid duplex ultrasonography Cardiac telemetry Supplemental oxygen and appropriate oxygen saturation monitoring Antiplatelet therapy Fluid restriction if infarct is large to reduce cerebral edema Close monitoring of intake and output Regular determinations of blood glucose levels to avoid hyperglycemia NPO until there is certainty about the gag reflex pending swallowing evaluation Elevate head of bed 20 to 30 degrees to reduce cerebral edema Bed rest for first 24 hr with fall precautions; then advance as appropriate Vital signs and neurologic checks every 2 hr × 4; then every 4 hr for 24 hr Prophylaxis for DVT while immobile Speech therapy consultation to evaluate swallowing Neurology, physical therapy, occupational therapy, nutrition, and social services consultations

ANA, Antinuclear antibodies; *BUN,* blood urea nitrogen; *CBC,* complete blood count; *CT,* computed tomography; *DVT,* deep vein thrombosis; *NPO,* nothing by mouth; *PT/PTT,* prothrombin time/partial thromboplastin time; *RPR,* rapid plasma reagin; *TEE,* transesophageal echocardiography; *t-PA,* tissue plasminogen activator.

function, and motor and sensory function using the NIH Stroke Scale. Initial laboratory studies should generally include determination of a complete blood count (CBC) with differential and platelet count; prothrombin time and partial thromboplastin time (PT/PTT); electrolyte, blood urea nitrogen (BUN), creatinine, and glucose levels; oxygen saturation by pulse oximetry; and a metabolic panel. Depending on the clinical history, some patients should have studies for possible altered coagulation or connective tissue diseases. A CT scan of the head should be obtained expeditiously to evaluate for hemorrhage. Most patients should have additional studies, including electrocardiography (ECG), chest radiography, echocardiography, and carotid duplex ultrasonography. Consultation with neurology, speech therapy, physical therapy, occupational therapy, and social services should be considered (Table 41-6).

Elevated Blood Pressure. During the first day after an ischemic stroke, elevated BP should not be treated unless the SBP is consistently higher than 220 mm Hg or the DBP is consistently higher than 120 mm Hg. There are exceptions to this recommendation. Patients who have received t-PA should have BP maintained below 185/110 mm Hg, and patients with MI, heart failure, aortic dissection, or renal failure should have more aggressive BP control. Areas of cerebral ischemia lose their normal autoregulatory capacity, and tissue perfusion becomes directly linked to mean arterial pressure. When cerebral ischemia occurs, BP elevations are often transient, and spontaneous declines common. Overzealous BP treatment can therefore convert an area of ischemia that retains the potential for recovery into an area of frank infarction with no potential for recovery.

When antihypertensive agents are used shortly after stroke, one with rapid action and predictable response, such

Table 41-7   Antihypertensive Agents for Patients with Acute Stroke

Labetalol (Normodyne)	10 mg IV over 1 to 2 min; may repeat or double dosage every 10 to 20 min until BP is controlled or a maximum dose of 300 mg has been reached 100 mg orally twice daily
Nicardipine (Cardene)	5 mg/hr IV, titrated upward as necessary, typically to a maximum of 15 mg/hr
Sodium nitroprusside (Nipride)	0.3 μg/kg/min IV, titrated upward as necessary, typically to a maximum of 10 μg/kg/min

BP, Blood pressure; *IV,* intravenous.

as nicardipine (Cardene), labetalol (Normodyne), or sodium nitroprusside, should be chosen (Table 41-7). Nicardipine is currently considered the first-line treatment in this setting. Labetalol is preferable to sodium nitroprusside because of nitroprusside's ability to cause cerebral vasodilation, which can worsen cerebral edema in some patients. Sublingual calcium channel antagonists should be avoided because of their ability to cause precipitous BP declines, which could significantly reduce cerebral blood flow and result in further ischemic damage.

Cerebral Edema. Cerebral edema usually peaks within 2 to 4 days after a stroke. It is seldom a problem during the first 24 hours, except in cases of large cerebellar strokes. Steroids are not used to treat cerebral edema related to thromboembolic strokes. Steroids are generally ineffective and may exacerbate hyperglycemia and raise BP. Cerebral edema related to thromboembolic stroke is first treated by raising the head of the bed 20 to 30 degrees. Hyperventilation can work rapidly to reduce *intracranial pressure* (ICP) but has only a transient effect. Mannitol can be given to lower ICP at 0.25 to 1 g/kg intravenously (IV) over 30 minutes, but its use is controversial because of possible pooling in the area of ischemia and potential worsening of edema. Mannitol can rapidly lower ICP and can be repeated every 6 hours. The maximum dose of mannitol is 2 g/kg IV. Hypertonic saline has also been used to reduce cerebral edema in this context. Hemicraniectomy with durotomy is performed for malignant middle cerebral artery-distribution infarct in select cases and has been shown to improve survival and functional outcome.

Other Management Issues. *Hypoxia* should be avoided. Any circumstance that is likely to impair oxygen delivery to the ischemic penumbra needs to be avoided. Patients with acute stroke should therefore have their oxygen saturation monitored and supplemental oxygen provided if desaturation occurs.

The use of SC heparin for the prevention of *deep vein thrombosis* (DVT) in nonhemorrhagic stroke patients has been well accepted. Heparin should be dosed based on weight. LMWH is a reasonable alternative in this setting. Intermittent pneumatic compression stockings are the best prophylactic alternative for patients unable to receive anticoagulants. Patients able to ambulate 50 feet daily are at low risk for venous thromboembolism.

Fever is seen quite often after an acute stroke. Regardless of cause, fever should be reduced because ischemic cerebral insults accompanied by even mild elevations in body temperature have been associated with less favorable outcomes in both experimental models and clinical studies.

Hyperglycemia can be harmful for the ischemic penumbra because it permits anaerobic metabolism, which results in local generation of lactic acidosis. Serum glucose levels should generally be maintained below 150 mg/dL. Nevertheless, it should be recognized that controlling blood glucose has not been shown to improve stroke outcome in humans.

Patients who have a *seizure* after a stroke have a higher mortality rate. Some believe that such patients should receive anticonvulsant therapy indefinitely, but others note that a trial off medication after several years without seizure activity seems reasonable.

DELERIUM

Key Points

- A confused older adult patient should generally be assumed to have delirium until proved otherwise.
- Delirium is a transient, global disorder of cognition and consciousness; changes in consciousness typically develop quickly and fluctuate during the day.
- Underlying dementia is a significant risk factor for delirium.
- The history, physical examination, and test results usually suggest a cause for delirium.
- Delirium is best managed by correction of the causative disturbances.
- Primary prevention of delirium is the most effective treatment strategy.

Table 41-8 Common Causes of Delirium

Dehydration
Electrolyte abnormalities
Infection
Myocardial infarction
Heart failure
Neurologic disorder (stroke, seizure)
Hypoxia
Medications (anticholinergics, antihistamines, antidepressants, benzodiazepines, narcotics)
Intoxication
Environmental changes (change in location or caregiver, overstimulation)
Pain
Sleep deprivation
Surgery
Urinary catheter
Urinary retention
Fecal impaction

Table 41-9 Factors for Development of Delirium

Age >65 years
Chronic kidney disease
Dehydration
Dependence with activities of daily living
Hearing impairment
Infection
Malnutrition
Multiple comorbid conditions
Polypharmacy
Underlying dementia
Vision impairment

Delirium is a common problem encountered in patients seen by family physicians, especially in hospitals and skilled nursing facilities. Delirium is characterized by a change in cognition and attention that develops rapidly, usually over hours to days, and fluctuates throughout the day. It may present as *hyperactive delirium*, with agitation, disorientation, and delusions; *hypoactive delirium*, demonstrated by a lethargic patient who is difficult to arouse and engage in conversation; or a mixed-type delirium with features of both. Hypoactive delirium is the most common encountered form of delirium, which may explain why it goes unrecognized in up to 70% of patients experiencing delirium (Gillis and MacDonald, 2006). Because of this, any confused older adult patient should generally be assumed to have delirium until proven otherwise. Delirium is a serious condition that has long-term ramifications, including increased hospital lengths of stay, increased mortality rates, failure to return to baseline cognitive and functional status, and increased need for prolonged, skilled nursing facility care. Table 41-8 summarizes risk factors for the development of delirium. Two thirds of delirium cases occur in patients with underlying dementia, placing these patients at significant risk when being treated for other health problems (Cole, 2004).

The mainstay of treatment for delirium is to identify and correct the underlying cause. This cause can usually be determined through a thorough history, physical examination, and evaluation of selected laboratory test results. Table 41-9 summarizes some of the common causes that should be considered. Special attention should focus on recently started medications. Although almost any medication can precipitate delirium, analgesics, antiarrhythmics, antidepressants, Parkinson medications, anticholinergic medications such as antihistamines, benzodiazepines, β-blockers, calcium channel blockers, steroids, diuretics, clonidine, and digoxin are common culprits. A targeted laboratory evaluation should be undertaken, including a CBC, determination of electrolytes, BUN, creatinine, glucose, calcium, magnesium, phosphate, and liver function tests (LFTs). Oxygenation should be assessed by oximetry or arterial blood gases (ABGs). ECG should be considered, especially for patients with angina, dyspnea, or a cardiac history. Chest radiography and urinalysis to evaluate for occult infection, especially in older adult patients, should also be considered.

If this evaluation does not elicit a likely cause for a patient's delirium, further testing may be necessary. Additional laboratory studies to consider include thyroid function tests, human immunodeficiency virus (HIV) testing, rapid plasma reagin (RPR) test, drug levels, toxicology screening, serum ammonia level, and serum vitamin B_{12} level. LP is usually reserved for patients with fever and signs suggesting meningitis. Neuroimaging may be indicated for patients with new neurologic signs or a history of head trauma. EEG may be helpful in the evaluation of patients with a suspected seizure disorder or to differentiate delirium from a functional psychiatric disorder.

Delirium can be treated with both nonpharmacologic and pharmacologic measures. Environmental modifications should be instituted early, before pharmacologic intervention or mechanical restraint is considered. A supportive and familiar environment should be created for the patient. Family members should be encouraged to remain nearby as much as possible. The staff should visit the patient frequently or move the patient to be near them. The room should be well illuminated, with a large, easily read clock and calendar. The family should bring familiar items from home to be placed in the patient's room. Whenever possible, normal sleep hygiene patterns should be maintained with minimal interruptions during the night hours.

Pharmacologic management of delirium should be considered when the previous treatments have failed to control agitation and should involve the use of antipsychotic medications. Among the antipsychotic agents, haloperidol (Haldol) at 1 to 2 mg orally every 4 hours as needed, or 0.25 to 0.5 mg orally every 4 hours for elderly patients, is recommended (American Psychiatric Association, 1999). Other antipsychotic medications, such as risperidone (Risperdal), 0.5 to 1 mg orally daily, and olanzapine (Zyprexa), 2.5 to 5 mg orally daily, may also be used; as yet, no RCTs have established the safety and effectiveness of one antipsychotic medication over another for the management of delirium symptoms (Seitz et al., 2007). Risperidone and olanzapine do not work as quickly as haloperidol, often require slow titration, and can be associated with significant orthostasis. Studies have also demonstrated a potentially elevated risk of death in older adults with dementia who were treated with atypical antipsychotics (Schneider et al., 2005). Therefore, these risks must be considered when initiating pharmacologic treatment for delirium. Further recommendations for initiating antipsychotics for the treatment of delirium include using the lowest possible doses, frequent reassessments to limit the duration of antipsychotic use, and a baseline ECG to rule out susceptibility to an arrhythmia from a prolonged QT interval (Seitz et al., 2007). Lorazepam (Ativan), a benzodiazepine, has also been used for the treatment of agitation associated with delirium, although a Cochrane review concluded that benzodiazepines cannot be recommended for the treatment of non–alcohol-related delirium (Lonergan et al., 2009). Physical restraints should be a last resort, reserved for the protection of patients who do not adequately respond to environmental and pharmacologic interventions.

Studies have shown that a multicomponent approach to reduce risk factors is the most effective for the prevention of delirium. Intervention strategies should be targeted toward orientation and therapeutic activities for cognitive impairment, early mobilization to avert immobilization, interventions to prevent sleep deprivation, eyeglasses and hearing aids if needed, early intervention for dehydration, minimization of the use of psychoactive drugs, pain management, nutrition, bowel and bladder function, oxygen delivery to the brain, and appropriate environmental stimuli (Inouye, 2006).

DEMENTIA

Key Points

- Dementia is a gradual, progressive impairment of memory and other cognitive functions that is severe enough to impact work, social activities, or relationships.
- Dementia can be divided into four categories: Alzheimer disease (60% of cases), dementia with Lewy bodies (15%), vascular dementia (15%), and all other causes (10%).
- Comprehensive, longitudinal, well-coordinated care delivered by the family physician for both the patient and the caregiver is the cornerstone of effective management of patients with dementia.
- The cholinesterase inhibitors are effective in slowing the progression of cognitive and functional decline and may be used in conjunction with memantine (an N-methyl-D-aspartate [NMDA] receptor antagonist) to treat moderate to severe dementia.

Dementia is characterized by the development of an acquired impairment in memory associated with impairment in one or more cognitive domains, including executive function, language (expressive or receptive), *praxis* (learned motor sequences), or *gnosis* (ability to recognize objects, faces, or other sensory information). The impairments are severe enough to interfere with work, social activities, or relationships (American Psychiatric Association, 1994). The course is usually one of gradual, progressive decline and causes impairment in the ability to perform activities of daily living (ADLs). The incidence of dementia increases with age. By 75 years, 10% to 15% of people have dementia, increasing to 35% to 50% for those older than 85 years.

Classification and Pathophysiology

Dementia is usually divided into four main categories. Dementia of the Alzheimer type accounts for approximately

60% of cases; dementia with Lewy bodies, 15%; and vascular dementia, 15%. The remaining category includes multiple other forms, including mixed dementias that exhibit components of both Alzheimer and vascular dementia and dementias resulting from CNS trauma, Parkinson disease, Pick disease, Creutzfeldt-Jakob disease, and Huntington disease.

Patients with *Alzheimer disease* have brains that demonstrate atrophy with ventricular and sulcal enlargement. They reveal evidence of neuronal loss as well as the presence of amyloid plaques and neurofibrillary tangles. Amyloid plaques are composed of misfolded β-amyloid that initiates a pathogenic cascade, resulting in neurotoxicity and nerve cell death.

Dementia with Lewy bodies is similar to Alzheimer disease, but visual hallucinations and motor symptoms similar to parkinsonism develop early in the course of the disease. Histologically, Lewy bodies are present; these are cytoplasmic inclusions found in the temporal, parietal, and paralimbic regions of the brain.

Vascular dementia is usually subdivided into multi-infarct dementia and subcortical vascular dementia. *Multi-infarct dementia* should be suspected when focal, asymmetric neurologic abnormalities accompany dementia. Neuroimaging may show multiple strokes. *Subcortical vascular dementia* should be suspected if the patient manifests significant problems with gait early in the course of the dementia. CT and magnetic resonance imaging (MRI) scans are usually normal in these patients, except for increased signal in the deep white matter, a nonspecific sign.

Evaluation

The diagnosis of dementia is still made clinically, so the evaluation of a patient with suspected dementia begins with a complete history and physical examination. The history should include questions regarding the time frame surrounding symptom progression. The relation to any recent vascular events such as stroke should be noted. Risk factors for vascular disease (hypertension, diabetes, hyperlipidemia, atrial fibrillation, smoking history) should be reviewed. Changes in the ability to perform ADLs should also be addressed. The patient's ability to perform dressing, eating, ambulating, toileting, and bathing tasks should be recorded as independent, requiring assistance, or dependent. The physical examination should include a thorough neurologic examination for signs of underlying vascular disease and stroke. Cognitive testing should be done, ideally with the Mini–Mental State Examination, which allows for quantification of cognitive impairment over time (Table 41-10). A score less than 24 is considered abnormal, but because of educational bias, highly educated patients may have inflated scores and those with limited education artificially low scores (Tombaugh, 1992).

When considering which tests to perform as part of the evaluation of a patient with dementia, physicians have traditionally been taught to search for reversible causes of dementia. It is now recognized that reversible dementia rarely occurs (Sloane, 1998). Current recommendations for laboratory testing generally recommend that all patients be evaluated with a CBC, thyroid-stimulating hormone (TSH), serum calcium, electrolytes, and fasting glucose, as well as a serum B_{12} level. Selective testing based on the presenting medical history, physical examination, and cognitive testing may include a red blood cell (RBC) folate level, RPR for syphilis screening, and HIV antibodies. Testing for homocysteine levels and genetic testing for apolipoprotein E gene is not recommended (Feldman et al., 2008). Although neuroimaging is not recommended for all patients in the workup of dementia, selective use of CT or MRI is recommended for patients with suspected tumor, subdural hematoma, or normal-pressure hydrocephalus (NPH) (Feldman et al., 2008). ^{18}F-florbetapir (Amyvid) was recently approved by the FDA for the detection of amyloid-β in the brain. Positive scans can be found in up to 30% of cognitively normal persons older than the age of 70 years. It is known that it can take up to 15 to 20 years for amyloid plaque density to increase to clinically apparent dementia. Thus, the majority of normal elderly persons with a positive scan are still normal in 5 to 10 years' time. The Society of Nuclear Medicine and Molecular Imaging and the Alzheimer's Association Joint Amyloid Imaging Task Force 2012 published appropriate use criteria to help guide cost-effective usage of this new modality (Rowe and Villemagne, 2013).

Management

Comprehensive, longitudinal, well-coordinated care delivered by the family physician for both the patient and the caregiver is the cornerstone of effective management of patients with dementia. Patients should be seen regularly in the office, and the physician should be readily available by telephone. The family should maintain frequent contact with the patient and physician. The family physician should update vaccinations, monitor visual acuity and hearing, and address other appropriate health issues. Families should be counseled regarding behavioral and environmental modifications that may be helpful, including reducing hazards in the home for falls and injuries. A discussion regarding the timing of cessation of driving should be undertaken early in the course of treatment. Decisions regarding advanced directives and planning for the later

Table 41-10 Mini–Mental Status Examination

Maximum Score*	Task
5	Orientation: year, season, date, day, and month
5	Orientation: state, county, town, building, and floor (as applicable)
3	Registration: Name three objects. Record the number of trials required to learn.
5	Attention and calculation: Serial 7 subtraction: Subtract from 100 by 7 (stop after 5 answers) *or* spell the word "world" backward (score number of correct letters in correct location).
3	Recall: Recall the three objects registered above.
2	Language: Name two objects (pencil and watch).
1	Repeat "No ifs, ands, or buts."
3	Follow a three-step command.
1	Read and obey: "Close your eyes" written in print large enough for patient to see clearly.
1	Write a sentence.
1	Copy a picture of intersecting pentagons.

*Total possible score: 30.
Modified from Folstein MF, Folstein SE, McHugh PR. Mini–Mental State: a practical method for grading the cognitive state of patients for the clinician. *J Psychiatr Res.* 1975;12:189.

stages of the disease should begin early in the process as well. The patient should legally designate a durable power of attorney for health care. The discussion of the placement of feeding tubes should begin before difficulties with feeding develop. Families should be aware that feeding tubes do not prolong life, are associated with discomfort and medical complications, and are generally not recommended for patients in the final stages of a dementing illness (Li, 2002). The role of palliative care and hospice care should also be discussed early in the course of the illness, when the patient has the opportunity to participate in the decision-making process.

Pharmacotherapy

The cholinesterase inhibitors donepezil (Aricept), galantamine (Razadyne), and rivastigmine (Exelon) have received FDA approval for the treatment of patients with Alzheimer disease. Tacrine (Cognex), which is associated with elevated liver transaminase levels in about 30% of patients, is rarely used. The cholinesterase inhibitors act by blocking acetylcholinesterase breakdown of acetylcholine, believed to increase acetylcholine in affected areas of the brain. All of these agents show comparable response rates, and choice is therefore individualized according to patient and caregiver needs as well as the drug's side effect profile. Pharmacologic effectiveness is measured by a slowing of the decline in cognitive and global functioning over 6 to 12 months. The cholinesterase inhibitors are generally well tolerated, although side effects include nausea, vomiting, diarrhea, dyspepsia, anorexia, weight loss, bradycardia, and agitation. When these medicines are discontinued, the patient may experience a rapid decline in global functioning.

Another medication, memantine (Namenda), an NMDA receptor antagonist, has been FDA approved for the treatment of moderate to severe dementia as monotherapy or in combination with a cholinesterase inhibitor (Reisberg et al., 2003). Memantine appears to have fewer side effects than the cholinesterase inhibitors, although dizziness, insomnia, and hallucination may be seen. Data for efficacy of alternative agents such as Ginkgo biloba, nicotine, vitamin C, and vitamin E for the treatment of Alzheimer disease has been mixed. A recent study found that long-term use of Ginkgo biloba failed to reduce the risk of progression to Alzheimer disease in elderly adults with memory complaints compared with placebo (Vellas et al., 2012). A Cochrane review in 2012 concluded that vitamin E should not be used for the treatment of mild cognitive impairment and Alzheimer disease. There is evidence that maintaining healthy vitamin C levels can have a protective function against age-related cognitive decline and Alzheimer disease, but maximal benefit is likely realized by avoiding vitamin C deficiency (Harrison, 2012). Because of the negative correlation between tobacco smoking and Alzheimer disease, there has been interest in nicotine as a potential therapeutic agent, but its use is limited because of toxicity and addictive properties. However, cotinine, the active metabolite of nicotine, has the benefits of nicotine and a much better safety profile, making it an ideal candidate for further study. At present, aside from avoiding vitamin C deficiency, no other prescribed medication, supplement, or herbal preparation can be recommended for the cognitive or functional manifestations of dementia.

SEIZURES

Key Points

- Febrile seizures usually occur between age 3 months and 5 years and represent the most common convulsive disorder of young children (2%-5%).
- Risk factors for a first febrile seizure include family history, developmental delays, high fever, and child care attendance.
- Initiation of treatment with anticonvulsant medication after a single seizure is not usually indicated if the initial workup is benign.
- Newer anticonvulsant medications tend to be better tolerated and have fewer adverse reactions than older, traditional medications and can be considered early in the course of treatment.

One in 11 Americans who lives to the age of 80 years experiences at least one seizure. About 1% of the U.S. population has epilepsy or recurrent unprovoked seizures. Treatment of patients with epilepsy reduces the risk of recurrent seizures while optimizing quality of life. This requires minimizing the adverse effects of antiepileptic medications and maximizing the patient's ability to engage in normal activities and responsibilities (Scheuer and Pedley, 1990).

Seizures are a manifestation of disturbed neurologic function and therefore are often associated with acute neurologic disorders such as meningitis. In some patients, the seizures are self-limited and resolve when an acute neurologic disturbance resolves. In others, the seizures persist and result in a diagnosis of epilepsy. Some patients who appear medically and neurologically normal after appropriate evaluation may experience a single seizure, and the cause is never determined. Such patients do not have epilepsy.

Seizures are typically classified as partial or generalized. Whereas *partial*, or *focal*, seizures arise in a portion of one cerebral hemisphere and are accompanied by focal EEG abnormalities, *generalized* seizures appear to involve simultaneously all or large parts of both cerebral hemispheres from their onset. Partial seizures are subclassified according to whether consciousness is preserved (simple partial seizures) or impaired (complex partial seizures). Generalized seizures are subclassified by their associated patterns of convulsive movements (Table 41-11).

It is not always possible to classify accurately a seizure based exclusively on clinical observations. A seizure with generalized convulsive activity may have a focal onset with rapid generalization. Such a seizure would best be classified as a partial seizure with secondary generalization rather than as a generalized tonic-clonic seizure. Accurate classification of such a seizure could not be accomplished, however, without EEG. Also, not every paroxysmal event that appears to be a seizure is actually a seizure. Movement disorders, psychological disorders, and sleep disorders can produce activity that is similar to seizure activity. Thus, accurate seizure diagnosis often requires both clinical observation and corroborative EEG. Because EEG is usually done in the absence of seizures, certain steps should be taken to increase its diagnostic yield. Both sleep and sleep deprivation increase the likelihood of recording

Table 41-11 Seizure Classification

Partial seizures	Simple (consciousness is preserved)
	Complex (consciousness is impaired)
	Secondarily generalized
	Simple partial seizures evolving to generalized tonic-clonic
	Complex partial seizures evolving to generalized tonic-clonic
	Simple partial seizures evolving to complex partial, then to generalized tonic-clonic
Generalized seizures	Tonic-clonic
	Absence
	Atypical absence
	Myoclonic
	Tonic
	Atonic

epileptiform abnormalities by EEG. Obtaining multiple recordings can also increase the diagnostic yield. In some cases, accurate diagnosis can be accomplished only with continuous video and EEG monitoring over several days during which the event of interest is recorded. Typically, this is accomplished in specialized epilepsy centers. A small number of patients with seizure disorders have normal interictal EEG recordings despite efforts made to record epileptiform abnormalities.

Febrile Seizures

Febrile seizures are seizures without a definite cause that are associated with fever. Febrile seizures, by definition, do not include seizures occurring in patients with an intracranial infection, such as meningitis or encephalitis, toxic encephalopathy, or any other neurologic illness. The definition also excludes seizures associated with fever that occur in patients who have a history of a previous nonfebrile seizure. Febrile seizures usually occur in children between the ages of 3 months and 5 years and represent the most common convulsive disorder of young children, affecting 2% to 5% of U.S. children. The most common age of onset is in the second year of life, and boys are affected slightly more often than girls (Freeman and Vining, 1995; Hirtz, 1997).

Risk factors for a first febrile seizure include a family history of febrile seizures, developmental delays, very high fever, and child care attendance. Approximately one third of children who experience a first febrile seizure will experience at least one more. The younger the child when the first febrile seizure occurs, the more likely the child is to have another febrile seizure. Most recurrences occur within 1 year. A family history of febrile seizures also increases the likelihood of recurrence. Fortunately, fewer than 5% of children who experience a febrile seizure develop epilepsy.

Febrile seizures can be of any type but are most often tonic-clonic. Febrile seizures are usually shorter than 6 minutes, and fewer than 8% last longer than 15 minutes. Most children therefore do not come to the attention of the family physician until after the seizure is over. Although it is commonly believed that the rate of fever increase is an important factor in the development of febrile seizures, no data support this as being more important than fever severity.

The evaluation of a child who has had a febrile seizure should begin with a careful history and physical examination. The history should include symptoms of infection, medication use, toxic ingestions, developmental and health problems, prenatal and birth history, family history, and detailed descriptions of the seizure by witnesses. The physical examination should pay particular attention to signs of severe illness, including petechiae, meningismus, tense or bulging fontanelle, Kernig and Brudzinski signs, and signs of neurologic abnormality (including decreased alertness or cognition and deficits of motor strength or tone). Even in children with a previous history of febrile seizures, a seizure associated with fever may be a sign of an intracranial infection. If intracranial infection is suspected, an LP should be performed. Otherwise, LP is not necessary. Children older than 18 months who have meningitis or encephalitis usually demonstrate typical clinical signs and symptoms. Many of these children lack histories, symptoms, or signs suggesting meningitis and thus do not require LP. However, children younger than 12 to 18 months may lack the typical clinical signs and symptoms of intracranial infection and are more likely to require LP. If a child is already taking antibiotics and experiences a seizure associated with fever, partially treated meningitis should be considered. The presence of a source of infection, such as otitis media, does not exclude the possibility of meningitis. Other features in the history that should also raise suspicion of meningitis in children with seizures and fever include evaluation for illness by a physician within the past 48 hours, a seizure that occurs in the office or emergency department (ED), or a focal seizure.

Most children with febrile seizures do not require routine laboratory testing. The only laboratory studies needed are those that will assist in evaluating the source of the child's fever. Radiography of the skull, neuroimaging studies such as CT and MRI, and EEG are not usually indicated. Children who are diagnosed with a febrile seizure should be observed in the ED or physician's office for several hours. These children may then be sent home, provided (1) they demonstrate satisfactory clinical improvement and are alert, (2) the fever has been appropriately evaluated and treated, and (3) close outpatient follow-up is possible. If there is any question about intracranial infection, if a child does not demonstrate expected clinical improvement during observation, or if follow-up cannot be ensured, hospital admission is recommended.

One of the most important components of outpatient management of children with febrile seizures is education of the parents. Seizures are frightening events for most parents. They should be reassured that febrile seizures do not result in brain damage and that the risk of epilepsy is very low. Slightly more than one in six children, however, experience another seizure within 24 hours, and about one in three experiences another febrile seizure at some point. If another seizure occurs, parents should be advised to place the child on his or her side or face down on the abdomen. Contrary to common belief, they should not attempt to place anything between the child's teeth during a seizure. The parents should carefully observe the child, and if the seizure does not spontaneously resolve after 10 minutes, they should call 9-1-1. Parents may have concerns about routine vaccinations for children with a history of febrile seizures. The diphtheria and tetanus toxoids and acellular pertussis (DTaP) and measles, mumps, and rubella (MMR) vaccinations are most likely to produce fever associated with seizure. If a febrile seizure is going to occur after vaccination, it is most likely to occur within 48 hours of the DTaP vaccination or within 10 days of the MMR vaccination.

Initial Diagnostic Evaluation of a First Seizure in Adults

A careful history and physical examination, along with routine blood work, can detect many medical problems that may be associated with seizures. Such problems include infection, electrolyte and glucose abnormalities, impaired hepatic or renal function, and cardiopulmonary disease. Most patients with new-onset seizures should have a CBC with platelet count and differential; toxicology screen; thyroid function testing; PT/PTT; determination of serum transaminase, electrolytes, calcium, magnesium, phosphorus, BUN, creatinine, and glucose; ABGs; or pulse oximetry. If cardiopulmonary disease is suspected, ECG and chest radiographs should be obtained. Meningitis or encephalitis suspected clinically indicates LP, which is otherwise not necessary. Patients usually recover rapidly after a first seizure, and their clinical progress can be gauged after several hours of observation. Hospitalization is not usually necessary after a first seizure unless an underlying illness is suspected and injury has been sustained or there are concerns about the patient's clinical progress, inadequate social support or observation, or a lack of the patient's ability or motivation to complete outpatient follow-up.

Patients with new-onset seizures should be scheduled for appropriate EEG and neuroimaging studies. MRI and CT are important complements to EEG because of their ability to identify structural abnormalities that may be related to the development of seizures. MRI is preferable to CT because of its superior ability to identify cortical architectural abnormalities, visualize the temporal lobes, detect gliomas, and identify cavernous malformations. CT, however, is appropriate in the emergency setting because it is readily available and can detect hemorrhages acutely. If the patient is seen in the office shortly after a first seizure, neuroimaging does not need to be performed immediately unless the history and physical examination suggest focal brain injury or marked cognitive impairment. In contrast to MRI and CT, positron emission tomography and single-photon emission CT can provide functional views of the brain. These studies can identify areas of relative hypoperfusion or hypometabolism that appear to be structurally normal but might play an important role in the development of partial seizures. Although such studies can be useful, especially for patients with conditions such as localization-related epilepsy, they are not routinely obtained or widely available.

Pharmacologic Therapy

Whether antiepileptic drug therapy should be initiated after a first seizure remains a topic of debate. The data regarding the likelihood of recurrent seizures after a first seizure are wanting or questionable, and estimates of the rate of recurrence after a single unprovoked seizure range widely. Certain findings and characteristics do seem to increase the likelihood of recurrence after a first seizure, including EEG abnormalities, previous neurologic injury, partial seizures, and a family history of seizures. Also, it is not known whether antiepileptic pharmacologic therapy after a single seizure alters the subsequent risk of epilepsy. Because of these uncertainties and because antiepileptic pharmacologic therapy is associated with a significant incidence of adverse effects, often exceeding the risk of recurrent seizures, many family physicians elect not to prescribe antiepileptic medications for most patients after a single seizure. Nonetheless, because of the unpredictable course of first-time seizures, patients should be cautioned against driving, according to local regulations, and engaging in other activities, which can present a danger should another seizure occur.

Although many agents are available for the treatment of seizures, carbamazepine (Tegretol), phenytoin (Dilantin), phenobarbital, and divalproex (Depakote) have been traditional first-line therapies for most patients with epilepsy. Increasing availability of newer agents to treat seizures has often resulted in more favorable side effect profiles. Phenobarbital is the oldest agent but has certain disadvantages. Its adverse effects include irritability, decreased cognition, and hyperactivity or lethargy. The degree of sedation and cognitive effects produced at therapeutic dosages are frequently significant enough that many family physicians do not prescribe phenobarbital as a first-line agent. The recommended dosage for common antiepileptics and adverse effects are summarized in Table 41-12. Most patients with epilepsy can achieve remission with the use of a single medication. Because the addition of another antiepileptic agent is usually associated with an increase in adverse drug effects, patients not controlled with one agent should be given a trial of a different agent rather than combining agents early in the course of treatment. Treatment with more than one agent is usually attempted only after a number of trials of monotherapy have failed.

Family physicians should exercise caution when measuring levels of antiepileptic drugs. Therapeutic ranges for most antiepileptics are only guidelines for treatment. Some patients achieve therapeutic remission without significant side effects with drug concentrations ordinarily toxic. Other patients develop intolerable side effects with subtherapeutic serum levels. Serum levels of most antiepileptic drugs should generally be determined when remission of seizures is achieved or the patient develops significant side effects. Drug concentrations can also provide evidence of compliance. More frequent serum testing is necessary for patients taking more than one agent, pregnant women, older adults, patients with hepatic or renal dysfunction, and patients taking medications for other medical problems. Table 41-13 lists drugs used to treat other medical conditions that can lower the seizure threshold. Nevertheless, serum levels should not be the primary basis for decisions regarding antiepileptic drug dosing. Seizure control and the development of adverse effects related to drug therapy are more important than serum levels alone.

Status Epilepticus

Status epilepticus is generally defined as more than 30 minutes of unconsciousness and continuous or

Table 41-12   Common Antiepileptic Agents

Agent	Usual Dosage	Adverse Effects
Carbamazepine (Tegretol)	Start: 200 mg twice daily (adults), 5 mg/kg/day (children) Maintenance: Increase by 200 mg/day weekly to max 1600 mg/day (adults), 20-35 mg/kg/day to max 1000 mg/day (children) Usually divided QID	Drowsiness or agitation, diplopia and blurred vision, disequilibrium, benign leukopenia, hepatic failure, rare SIADH, rare aplastic anemia
Phenytoin (Dilantin)	Oral loading dose: 400 mg, then 300 mg in 2 h and 4 h (adults) Maintenance: 300 mg/day (adults), 5 mg/kg/day to max 300 mg/day (children) Usually divided TID	Dose related: nausea and vomiting, nystagmus, ataxia Not dose related: gingival hyperplasia, hirsutism, acne, coarsening of features, hepatic failure, osteomalacia
Divalproex (Depakote)	Start: 10-15 mg/kg/day Maintenance: 15-60 mg/kg/day Usually divided BID-QID	Transient GI side effects Toxic effects: tremor, thrombocytopenia Side effects: weight increase, alopecia, hepatotoxicity (controversial whether LFTs detect in time to avoid), pancreatitis
Phenobarbital	Starting and maintenance: 100-300 mg/day (adults), 3-5 mg/kg/day (children) Usually given in single or divided doses	Lethargy, sedation, decreased cognition, decreased attention, hyperactivity, depression
Levetiracetam (Keppra)	Start: 1000 mg/day (adults), 20 mg/kg/day (children) Maintenance: maximum, 3000 mg/day (adults), 60 mg/kg/day (children) Usually divided BID	Depression, hostility, aggressive behavior, psychosis, somnolence, headache, URI symptoms, infection, fatigue, irritability
Oxcarbazepine (Trileptal)	Start: 600 mg/day (adults), 8-10 mg/kg/day (children) Maintenance: maximum, 2400 mg/day (adults), 45 mg/kg/day (children) Usually divided BID	Hyponatremia, hypersensitivity reaction, leukopenia, thrombocytopenia, angioedema, Stevens-Johnson syndrome, dizziness, somnolence, diplopia, headache, nausea, ataxia
Lamotrigine (Lamictal)	Start: dosing varies with concomitant antiepileptics Maintenance: maximum, 400 mg/day Usually divided BID	Rash, Stevens-Johnson syndrome, angioedema, neutropenia, pancreatitis, dizziness, headache, ataxia, nausea, somnolence
Tiagabine (Gabitril)	Start: 4 mg/day (adults and children >12 yr) Maintenance: maximum, 56 mg/day (adults), 32 mg/day (children) Usually divided BID-QID	CNS depression, seizures, weakness, rash, dizziness, asthenia, somnolence, nausea, diarrhea, tremor, confusion, impaired concentration
Gabapentin (Neurontin)	Start: 300 mg/day (adults), 10-15 mg/kg/day (children) Maintenance: up to 3600 mg/day (adults), 35 mg/kg/day (children) Usually divided TID	Leukopenia, depression, dizziness, somnolence, ataxia, fatigue, peripheral edema, weight gain, tremor, diarrhea
Topiramate (Topamax)	Start: 25 mg BID (adults, children >10 yr) Maintenance: up to 200 mg/day Usually divided BID	Nephrolithiasis, paresthesias, anorexia, ataxia, cognitive dysfunction
Zonisamide (Zonegran)	Start: 100 mg/day for 2 weeks (adults) Maintenance: up to 600 mg/day Usually divided BID	Nephrolithiasis, somnolence, anorexia, cognitive dysfunction
Pregabalin (Lyrica)	Start: 150 mg/day (adults) Maintenance: up to 600 mg/day Usually divided BID-TID	Thrombocytopenia, hypersensitivity reaction, angioedema, dizziness, somnolence, ataxia, peripheral edema, weight gain
Lacosamide (Vimpat)	Start: 100 mg/day (adults) Maintenance: up to 600 mg/day (300 mg/day in mild-mod hepatic failure or CrCl <30 mL/min) Divided BID	Syncope, atrial fibrillation (rare), dizziness, headache, diplopia, vomiting, fatigue, ataxia
Ezogabine (Potiga)	Start: 300 mg/day Maintenance: up to 1200 mg Divided TID	Psychosis, dependency, dizziness, somnolence, fatigue, cognitive dysfunction, weight gain
Rufinamide (Banzel)	Start: (Lennox-Gastaut) 400-800 mg/day (adults), 10 mg/kg/day (children) Maintenance: up to 3200 mg/day (adults and children) Usually divided BID	Suicidality, seizures, QT shortening, hypersensitivity reaction, leucopenia, somnolence, vomiting, headache, dizziness, nausea
Clobazam (Onfi)	Start: (Lennox-Gastaut) 10 mg/day (weight >30 kg) Maintenance: 40 mg/day Divided BID	Respiratory depression, dependency, suicidality, Stevens-Johnson syndrome, anemia, somnolence
Vigabatrin (Sabril)	Start: (infantile spasms) 40 mg/kg/day (children) Maintenance: up to 100-150 mg/kg/day Usually divided BID	(Restricted in United States) Permanent vision loss, anemia, neuropathy, headache, dizziness, fatigue, somnolence, weight gain

BID, Twice a day; *CNS,* central nervous system; *CrCl,* creatinine clearance; *LFT,* liver function test; *QID,* four times a day; *SIADH,* syndrome of inappropriate secretion of antidiuretic hormone; *TID,* three times a day; *URI,* upper respiratory infection.

Table 41-13   Drugs That Can Lower Seizure Threshold

Theophylline
Isoniazid
Tricyclic antidepressants
Penicillin
Phenothiazines
Diphenhydramine
Pseudoephedrine
Cocaine
Amphetamines
Alcohol (withdrawal)
Benzodiazepines
Barbiturates (including phenobarbital)

intermittent, generalized seizure activity. However, because most seizures last 2 minutes or less, any seizure longer than 5 minutes may progress to status epilepticus. Patients with recurrent seizures without recovery to wakefulness should also be considered to be in status epilepticus. Status epilepticus can be alarming to observe, even for experienced clinicians. A systematic approach to patients in status epilepticus can facilitate optimal patient care during such an episode. The first step in the management of patients with status epilepticus is to support vital functions. The airway should be protected. Although the patient should be intubated if necessary, this usually requires neuromuscular blockade, and bag and mask ventilation is often preferable. The patient's vital signs should be closely monitored, including continuous oximetry and ECG. Supplemental oxygen at a rate of about 4 L/min is recommended. IV access should be secured for the administration of parenteral medications and blood drawn for a CBC; toxicology screen; and determination of electrolyte, glucose, calcium, magnesium, and anticonvulsant drug levels. The patient should receive thiamine, 100 mg IV, followed by 50 mL of dextrose 50% with water.

If the patient continues to seize, parenteral agents may be given, including lorazepam, 0.1 mg/kg IV at 2 mg/min, or diazepam, 0.2 mg/kg (maximum, 10 mg) at a maximum rate of 5 mg/min. These agents have a relatively rapid onset and short duration of action. Simultaneous loading with phenytoin is therefore recommended. Phenytoin is loaded at 20 mg/kg IV at a rate of less than 50 mg/min through a line infusing glucose-free saline to avoid precipitation of phenytoin in the line. Fosphenytoin (Cerebyx) is the prodrug of phenytoin and has a more favorable safety profile than phenytoin, can be given at a faster rate (150 mg/min), and converts to phenytoin after first-pass metabolism, but it is more costly than phenytoin. BP and cardiac rhythm must be closely observed because of the ability of phenytoin to precipitate hypotension and heart block. If these side effects appear, they often resolve when the rate of administration is decreased. If seizures continue despite these measures, phenobarbital may be administered parenterally. As a last resort, barbiturate coma or general anesthesia can be instituted. Propofol (Diprivan) and midazolam (Versed) administered as continuous IV drips are often used in neurocritical care settings to induce coma for status epilepticus.

CENTRAL NERVOUS SYSTEM INFECTION AND INFLAMMATION

Key Points

- Bacterial meningitis is a neurologic emergency.
- Acute bacterial meningitis has high morbidity and mortality rates.
- Antibiotic therapy should be started as soon as possible after meningitis is considered likely, usually by cerebrospinal fluid (CSF) analysis.
- Knowing the most prevalent organisms that cause bacterial meningitis in different age groups is important in guiding therapy.
- Gram stain of CSF is recommended for all patients with suspected bacterial meningitis.
- Adjunctive dexamethasone therapy for infants, children, and adults who have already received antibiotics is not recommended.

Bacterial Meningitis

Acute bacterial meningitis has high morbidity and mortality rates even under the best circumstances. For this reason, prompt recognition of the clinical syndrome, performance of appropriate testing to confirm the diagnosis, and initiation of appropriate therapy are essential.

Most adult patients (85%) present with the classic triad of fever, headache, and neck stiffness (Roos et al., 1997). Other symptoms include nausea and vomiting (35%), seizures (30%), CN palsies, and other focal neurologic signs (10%-20%). Meningismus (50%) may be subtle or marked, as with Kernig sign (resistance to knee extension after flexion of hip and knees by examiner) or Brudzinski sign (involuntary flexion of knees in supine patient in response to rapid neck flexion by examiner) (Tunkel and Scheld, 1997). Other symptoms include nuchal rigidity, lethargy, photophobia, confusion, sweats, and rigors. Papilledema occurs in fewer than 1% of patients during the early phases of the disease. When papilledema is present early, an alternative diagnosis such as a brain abscess or mass lesion should be sought.

Not all patients present with the classic signs and symptoms. Neonates may present with poor feeding or weak sucking response, irritability, vomiting, temperature instability (hyperthermia or hypothermia), diarrhea, and apnea. Nuchal rigidity and meningismus are not reliable signs in children younger than 1 year (Prober, 1996). A bulging fontanelle may occur late in the disease, and seizures occur in 40% of neonates. A maculopapular rash that later becomes petechial and purpuric on the extremities should suggest meningococcal meningitis. Older adult patients may have a more insidious presentation, with variable meningeal signs, change in mental status, lethargy, obtundation, and no fever.

The host is an important determinant of susceptibility to meningitis. Obvious risk factors include a history of recent open trauma, surgery (especially neurosurgery), and burns. Closed-head trauma can cause CSF leaks, which have been associated with pneumococcal meningitis. Common predisposing factors include otitis media (most common);

Table 41-14 Common Pathogens of Bacterial Meningitis Based on Age

Age	Pathogens
0-1 mo	Group B streptococci, *Listeria monocytogenes*, *Streptococcus pneumoniae*, *Escherichia coli*
1-3 mo	Group B streptococci, *L. monocytogenes*, *S. pneumoniae*, *Neisseria meningitidis*, *Haemophilus influenzae*, *E. coli*
3 mo-18 yr	*S. pneumoniae*, *N. meningitidis*, *H. influenzae*
18-50 yr	*S. pneumoniae*, *N. meningitidis*, *H. influenzae*
>50 yr	*S. pneumoniae*, *L. monocytogenes*, gram-negative bacilli

Table 41-15 Criteria for Adult Patients with Suspected Bacterial Meningitis Recommended for Computed Tomography before Lumbar Puncture

Criterion	Comment
Immunocompromised state	HIV infection or AIDS, receiving immunosuppressive therapy, or after transplantation
History of CNS disease	Mass lesion, stroke, or focal infection
New-onset seizure	Within 1 week of presentation; some authorities would not perform LP on patients with prolonged seizures or would delay LP for 30 minutes in patients with short, convulsive seizures
Papilledema	Presence of venous pulsations suggests absence of increased ICP
Abnormal level of consciousness	—
Focal neurologic deficit	Includes dilated nonreactive pupil, abnormalities of ocular motility, abnormal visual fields, gaze palsy, arm or leg drift

AIDS, Acquired immunodeficiency syndrome; *CNS,* central nervous system; *CT,* computed tomography; *LP,* lumbar puncture; *HIV,* human immunodeficiency virus; *ICP,* intracranial pressure.
From Tunkel AR, Barry J, Hartman SL, et al. Practice guidelines for the management of bacterial meningitis. *Clin Infect Dis.* 2004;39:1267.

sinusitis; mastoiditis; alcoholism; perinatal exposure; and nonimmunized, immunocompromised, or asplenic status (Swartz, 1997).

Knowing the most prevalent organisms that cause bacterial meningitis in the various age groups is important in guiding empiric therapeutic choices (Table 41-14). The three most common pathogens for community-acquired bacterial meningitis are *Haemophilus influenzae*, *Neisseria meningitidis*, and *Streptococcus pneumoniae*, accounting for about 80% of cases in the United States. Until the development of the *H. influenzae* type b (Hib) vaccine in the early 1990s, this was the most common bacterial meningitis, occurring in almost 50% of cases. As a result, *S. pneumoniae* and *N. meningitidis* have become relatively more common, especially in the pediatric population. *Escherichia coli* has been superseded by group B streptococci as the most common cause in infants during the first months of life. Other common pathogens include *Listeria monocytogenes*, *Klebsiella pneumoniae*, *Staphylococcus aureus*, *Staphylococcus epidermidis*, other gram-negative bacilli, and other streptococci.

Initial Management. The Infectious Disease Society of America (IDSA) practice guidelines call for prompt blood cultures and LP for most patients with suspected acute bacterial meningitis (Tunkel et al., 2004). Nevertheless, emergency LP may not be successful or prudent because of overriding concerns about a CNS mass lesion or other cause of increased ICP, necessitating CT before LP. In these patients, blood samples should be drawn and appropriate antibiotic and adjunctive therapy provided before LP or CT (Table 41-15).

The LP is the foundation of the diagnosis of bacterial meningitis. In adults, opening pressure is typically 80 to 210 mm H_2O, although lower values may be observed in infants and children. Table 41-16 illustrates typical CSF findings. Gram stain is recommended for all patients because it permits rapid organism identification in 60% to 90% of patients with community-acquired bacterial meningitis, with a specificity of more than 97% (Tunkel et al., 2004). Other rapid diagnostic tests, such as latex agglutination, and limulus lysate assay have not shown clinical usefulness in diagnosis or management of bacterial meningitis. Polymerase chain reaction (PCR) assay to amplify DNA may be helpful, particularly for patients with negative Gram stains. The serum C-reactive protein (CRP) concentration may be particularly helpful for patients with findings consistent with meningitis but for whom the Gram stain is

Table 41-16 Typical Cerebrospinal Fluid Findings in Bacterial and Viral Meningitides

Parameter	Bacterial Meningitis	Viral Meningitis
Opening pressure (mm H_2O)	>180	Often normal or significantly elevated
Leukocyte count (cells/mm³)	1000-10,000 Median: 1195 Range: 100-20,000	<300 Median: 100 Range: 100-1000
Neutrophils (%)	>80	<20
Glucose (mg/dL)	<40	>40
Protein (mg/dL)	100-500	Often normal
Gram stain (% positive)	60-90	Negative
Culture (% positive)	70-85	50

negative and withholding antibiotics is being contemplated because a normal CRP result has a high negative predictive value (Tunkel et al., 2004).

Additional laboratory studies include CBC, platelet count, PT, PTT, and ABGs, as well as determination of electrolyte, protein, glucose, BUN, and creatinine levels. Further laboratory workup and imaging studies (chest radiography, sinus series, skull radiography) may be indicated, depending on the clinical setting.

Bacterial meningitis is a neurologic emergency. Accordingly, if the diagnosis is considered likely, antibiotic therapy should be started as soon as possible, usually immediately after the LP has been performed or as soon as blood cultures have been obtained if a CT of the head is warranted. Antibiotic therapy is generally targeted by the results of the Gram stain (Table 41-17) or may be chosen empirically based on age and predisposing conditions (Table 41-18). Table 41-19 outlines recommendations for specific

Table 41-17 Antimicrobial Therapy in Adult Patients with Presumptive Pathogen Identification by Positive Gram Stain Results

Microorganism	Recommended Therapy	Alternative Therapies
Streptococcus pneumoniae	Vancomycin plus third-generation cephalosporin*†	Meropenem (C), fluoroquinolone‡ (B)
Neisseria meningitidis	Third-generation cephalosporin*	Penicillin G, ampicillin, chloramphenicol, fluoroquinolone, aztreonam
Listeria monocytogenes	Ampicillin§ or penicillin G§	TMP-SMP, meropenem (B)
Streptococcus agalactiae	Ampicillin§ or penicillin G§	Third-generation cephalosporin* (B)
Haemophilus influenzae	Third-generation cephalosporin*	Chloramphenicol, cefepime, meropenem, fluoroquinolone
Escherichia coli	Third-generation cephalosporin*	Cefepime, meropenem, aztreonam, fluoroquinolone, TMP-SMP

*Ceftriaxone or cefotaxime.
†Some experts would add rifampin if dexamethasone is also given (B).
‡Gatifloxacin or moxifloxacin.
§Addition of an aminoglycoside should be considered.
Note: All recommendations are (A) unless otherwise indicated. In children, ampicillin is added to the standard therapeutic regimen of cefotaxime or ceftriaxone plus vancomycin when *L. monocytogenes* is considered and to an aminoglycoside if a gram-negative enteric pathogen is of concern.
TMP-SMP, trimethoprim–sulfamethoxazole.
Modified from Tunkel AR, Barry J, Hartman SL, et al. Practice guidelines for the management of bacterial meningitis. *Clin Infect* Dis. 39,1267, 2004.

Table 41-18 Empiric Antimicrobial Therapy for Purulent Meningitis Based on Patient Age and Specific Predisposing Condition (A)

Predisposing Factor	Common Bacterial Pathogens	Antimicrobial Therapy
AGE		
<1 mo	*Streptococcus agalactiae, Escherichia coli, Listeria monocytogenes, Klebsiella* spp.	Ampicillin *plus* cefotaxime or ampicillin *plus* an aminoglycoside
1-23 mo	*Streptococcus pneumoniae, Neisseria meningitidis, S. agalactiae, Haemophilus influenzae, E. coli*	Vancomycin *plus* third-generation cephalosporin*†
2-50 yr	*N. meningitidis, S. pneumoniae*	Vancomycin *plus* third-generation cephalosporin*†
>50 yr	*S. pneumoniae, N. meningitidis, L. monocytogenes,* aerobic gram-negative bacilli	Vancomycin *plus* ampicillin *plus* third-generation cephalosporin*†
HEAD TRAUMA		
Basilar skull fracture	*S. pneumoniae, H. influenzae,* group A ß-hemolytic streptococci	Vancomycin *plus* third-generation cephalosporin*
Penetrating trauma	*Staphylococcus aureus,* coagulase-negative staphylococci (especially *Staphylococcus epidermidis),* aerobic gram-negative bacilli (including *Pseudomonas aeruginosa)*	Vancomycin *plus* cefepime, vancomycin *plus* ceftazidime, *or* vancomycin *plus* meropenem
Postneurosurgery	Aerobic gram-negative bacilli (including *P. aeruginosa), S. aureus,* coagulase-negative staphylococci (especially *S. epidermidis)*	Vancomycin *plus* cefepime, vancomycin *plus* ceftazidime, *or* vancomycin *plus* meropenem
CSF shunt	Coagulase-negative staphylococci (especially *S. epidermidis), S. aureus,* aerobic gram-negative bacilli (including *P. aeruginosa), Propionibacterium acnes*	Vancomycin *plus* cefepime,‡ vancomycin *plus* ceftazidime,‡ *or* vancomycin *plus* meropenem‡

*Ceftriaxone or cefotaxime.
†Some experts would add rifampin if dexamethasone is also given.
‡In infants and children, vancomycin alone is reasonable unless Gram stain reveals gram-negative bacilli.
CSF, Cerebrospinal fluid.
Modified from Tunkel AR, Barry J, Hartman SL, et al. Practice guidelines for the management of bacterial meningitis. *Clin Infect Dis.* 2004;39,1267.

antimicrobial therapy based on isolates and susceptibility, and Table 41-20 recommends doses.

Role of Corticosteroids. The theoretic goal of using corticosteroids in bacterial meningitis is to minimize meningeal inflammation, thereby decreasing the severity and incidence of brain injury. However, the IDSA recommends adjunctive dexamethasone therapy in certain patients based on age.

NEONATES. There are currently insufficient data to make recommendations involving newborns (Tunkel et al., 2004).

INFANTS AND CHILDREN. Available evidence supports the use of adjunctive dexamethasone in infants and children with Hib meningitis initiated 10 to 20 minutes before (or at least concomitant with) the first doses of antibiotic at a dose

of 0.15 mg/kg every 6 hours for 2 to 4 days. However, adjunctive dexamethasone should not be given to infants and children who have already received antimicrobial therapy because it is unlikely to improve patient outcome (Tunkel et al., 2004). Adjunctive dexamethasone in infants and children with pneumococcal meningitis is controversial. On the use of steroids for pneumococcal meningitis, the Committee on Infectious Diseases of the American Academy of Pediatrics (AAP) stated, "For infants and children 6 weeks of age and older, adjunctive therapy with dexamethasone may be considered after weighing the potential benefits and possible risks. Experts vary in recommending the use of corticosteroids in pneumococcal meningitis; data are not sufficient to demonstrate clear benefit in children" (AAP, 2003). Also, data support adjunctive corticosteroids in children from high-income countries but

Table 41-19 Specific Antimicrobial Therapy in Bacterial Meningitis Based on Isolated Pathogen and Susceptibility Testing

Microorganism, Susceptibility	Standard Therapy	Alternative Therapies
STREPTOCOCCUS PNEUMONIAE		
Penicillin MIC		
<0.1 µg/mL	Penicillin G *or* ampicillin	Third-generation cephalosporin,* chloramphenicol
0.1-1.0 µg/mL[†]	Third-generation cephalosporin*	Cefepime (B), meropenem (B)
≥2.0 µg/mL	Vancomycin *plus* third-generation cephalosporin*‡	Moxifloxacin (B)
Cefotaxime or ceftriaxone MIC ≥1.0 µg/mL	Vancomycin *plus* third-generation cephalosporin*‡	Moxifloxacin (B)
NEISSERIA MENINGITIDIS		
Penicillin MIC		
<0.1 µg/mL	Penicillin G *or* ampicillin	Third-generation cephalosporin,* chloramphenicol
0.1-1.0 µg/mL	Third-generation cephalosporin*	Chloramphenicol, moxifloxacin, meropenem
Listeria monocytogenes	Ampicillin *or* penicillin G§	TMP-SMX, meropenem (B)
Streptococcus agalactiae	Ampicillin *or* penicillin G§	Third-generation cephalosporin* (B)
Escherichia coli and other Enterobacteriaceae‖	Third-generation cephalosporin	Aztreonam, moxifloxacin, meropenem, TMP-SMX, ampicillin
Pseudomonas aeruginosa‖	Cefepime§ *or* ceftazidime§	Aztreonam,§ ciprofloxacin,§ meropenem§
HAEMOPHILUS INFLUENZAE		
β-Lactamase negative	Ampicillin	Third-generation cephalosporin,* cefepime, chloramphenicol, moxifloxacin
β-Lactamase positive	Third-generation cephalosporin	Cefepime, chloramphenicol, moxifloxacin
STAPHYLOCOCCUS AUREUS		
Methicillin susceptible	Nafcillin *or* oxacillin	
Methicillin resistant	Vancomycin¶	Vancomycin, meropenem (B)
Staphylococcus epidermidis	Vancomycin¶	TMP-SMX, linezolid (B)
Enterococcus spp.		Linezolid (B)
Ampicillin susceptible	Ampicillin *plus* gentamicin	—
Ampicillin resistant	Vancomycin *plus* gentamicin	—
Ampicillin and vancomycin resistant	Linezolid (B)	

*Ceftriaxone or cefotaxime.
†Ceftriaxone- or cefotaxime-susceptible isolates.
‡Consider addition of rifampin if the MIC of ceftriaxone is >2 µg/mL.
§Addition of an aminoglycoside should be considered.
¶Consider addition of rifampin.
‖Choice of a specific antimicrobial agent must be guided by in vitro susceptibility test results.
Note: All recommendations are (A) unless otherwise indicated.
MIC, minimum inhibitory concentration; *TMP-SMX,* trimethoprim–sulfamethoxazole.
Modified from Tunkel AR, Barry J, Hartman SL, et al. Practice guidelines for the management of bacterial meningitis. *Clin Infect Dis.* 2004;39:1267.

show no beneficial effect for children in low-income countries (Cochrane review; van de Beek et al., 2007).

ADULTS. Adjunctive dexamethasone, 0.15 mg/kg every 6 hours for 2 to 4 days, with the first dose administered 10 to 20 minutes before (or at least concomitant with) the first dose of antibiotic, should be initiated in all adult patients with suspected or proven pneumococcal meningitis. Although data are insufficient to make this recommendation for other bacterial pathogens, many experts initiate dexamethasone in all adults because the cause of meningitis is not always ascertained at the initial evaluation. As in children, dexamethasone should not be given to adult patients who have already received antibiotics (Tunkel et al., 2004).

Dexamethasone should only be continued if the CSF stain reveals gram-positive diplococci or if the blood or CSF cultures are positive for *S. pneumoniae.*

ANTIMICROBIAL THERAPY. Prompt and accurate treatment of meningitis is essential to increase survival and reduce morbidity. Treatment recommendations for a known pathogen of community-acquired bacterial meningitis and for selected clinical settings are listed in Tables 41-21 and 41-22. Duration of therapy is based more on tradition than on clinical evidence and varies depending on the pathogen. Repeat LP for CSF analysis of response to therapy is not necessary for most patients who demonstrate clinical improvement within 24 to 48 hours. Patients who do not demonstrate significant clinical improvement and show high resistance on culture and sensitivity, as well as neonates with meningitis caused by gram-negative bacilli, should undergo repeat LP (Tunkel et al., 2004).

Prophylaxis and Prevention. Prophylaxis is indicated for any close contacts of persons with documented meningococcal meningitis or Hib meningitis. For meningococcal meningitis, adults should receive 600 mg of rifampin orally twice daily for 2 days; children older than 1 month should receive 10 mg/kg (up to 600 mg) every 12 hours orally for 2 days (5 mg/kg every 12 hours if younger than 1 month). Rifampin is not recommended for pregnant women, and the reliability of oral contraceptives may be affected by rifampin therapy. An alternative to rifampin is ceftriaxone intramuscularly as a single dose, 125 mg for those 15 years and younger and 250 mg for those older than 15 years.

Table 41-20   Recommended Dosages of Antimicrobial Therapy in Patients with Bacterial Meningitis (A)

| | Total Daily Dose (dosing interval in hr) | | | |
| | Neonates (age in days) | | | |
Antimicrobial Agent	0-7*	8-28*	Infants and Children	Adults
Amikacin	15-20 mg/kg (12)	30 mg/kg (8)	20-30 mg/kg (8)	15 mg/kg (8)
Ampicillin	150 mg/kg (8)	200 mg/kg (6-8)	300 mg/kg (6)	12 g (4)
Aztreonam	—	—	—	6-8 g (6-8)
Cefepime	—	—	150 mg/kg (8)	6 g (8)
Cefotaxime	100-150 mg/kg (8-12)	150-200 mg/kg (6-8)	225-300 mg/kg (6-8)	8-12g (4-6)
Ceftazidime	100-150 mg/kg (8-12)	150 mg/kg (8)	150 mg/kg (8)	6 g (8)
Ceftriaxone	—	—	80-100 mg/kg (12-24)	4 g (12-24)
Chloramphenicol	25 mg/kg (24)	50 mg/kg (12-24)	75-100 mg/kg (6)	4-6 g (6)[‡]
Ciprofloxacin	—	—	—	800-1200 mg (8-12)
Gatifloxacin	—	—	—	400 mg (24)[§]
Gentamicin[†]	5 mg/kg (12)	7.5 mg/kg (8)	7.5 mg/kg (8)	5 mg/kg (8)
Meropenem	—	—	120 mg/kg (8)	6 g (8)
Moxifloxacin	—	—	—	400 mg (24)[§]
Nafcillin	75 mg/kg (8-12)	100-150 mg/kg (6-8)	200 mg/kg (6)	9-12 g (4)
Oxacillin	75 mg/kg (8-12)	150-200 mg/kg (6-8)	200 mg/kg (6)	9-12 g (4)
Penicillin G	0.15 MU/kg (8-12)	0.2 MU/kg (6-8)	0.3 MU/kg (4-6)	24 MU (4)
Rifampin	—	10-20 mg/kg (12)	10-20 mg/kg (12-24)[‖]	600 mg (24)
Tobramycin[†]	5 mg/kg (12)	7.5 mg/kg (8)	7.5 mg/kg (8)	5 mg/kg (8)
TMP-SMX[§]	—	—	10-20 mg/kg (6-12)	10-20 mg/kg (6-12)
Vancomycin**	20-30 mg/kg (8-12)	30-45 mg/kg (6-8)	60 mg/kg (6)	30-45 mg/kg (8-12)

*Smaller doses and longer intervals of administration may be advisable for very-low-birth-weight neonates (<2000 g).
[†]Need to monitor peak and trough serum concentrations.
[‡]Higher dose recommended for patients with pneumococcal meningitis.
[§]No data on optimal dosage are needed in patients with bacterial meningitis.
[‖]Maximum daily dose of 600 mg.
**Maintain serum trough concentrations of 15 to 20 μg/mL.
MU, Million units; *TMP-SMX*, trimethoprim–sulfamethoxazole.
Dosage based on trimethoprim component.
Modified from Tunkel AR, Barry J, Hartman SL, et al. Practice guidelines for the management of bacterial meningitis. *Clin Infect Dis*. 2004;39:1267.

Table 41-21   Specific Antibiotic Treatments for Known Pathogens

Pathogen	Primary Therapy	Alternative*
Group B streptococci	Penicillin G *or* ampicillin	Vancomycin *or* third-generation cephalosporin[†]
Streptococcus pneumoniae (MIC <0.1)	Third-generation cephalosporin[†]	Meropenem penicillin
S. pneumoniae (MIC >0.1)	Vancomycin *plus* third-generation cephalosporin*	Substitute rifampin for vancomycin; *or* meropenem; *or* vancomycin as monotherapy if highly allergic to other alternatives
Haemophilus influenzae (ß-lactamase negative)	Ampicillin	Third-generation cephalosporin[†] *or* chloramphenicol *or* aztreonam
H. influenzae (ß-lactamase positive)	Third-generation cephalosporin[†]	Chloramphenicol *or* aztreonam *or* fluoroquinolones[‡]
Listeria monocytogenes	Ampicillin *plus* gentamicin	TMP-SMX
Neisseria meningitidis	Penicillin G *or* ampicillin	Third-generation cephalosporin[†]
Enterobacteriaceae	Third-generation cephalosporin[†] *plus* aminoglycoside	TMP-SMX *or* aztreonam *or* fluoroquinolones *or* antipseudomonal penicillin[§] (or ampicillin) *plus* aminoglycoside
Pseudomonas aeruginosa	Ceftazidime *plus* aminoglycoside	Aminoglycoside *plus* aztreonam *or* aminoglycoside *plus* antipseudomonal penicillin[§]
Staphylococcus aureus (methicillin sensitive)	Antistaphylococcal penicillin[‖] ± rifampin	Vancomycin *plus* rifampin *or* TMP-SMX *plus* rifampin
S. aureus (methicillin resistant)	Vancomycin *plus* rifampin	
Staphylococcus epidermidis	Vancomycin *plus* rifampin	

*If patient is highly allergic or intolerant of primary therapy.
[†]Ceftriaxone or cefotaxime.
[‡]Ciprofloxacin or levofloxacin.
[§]Piperacillin, mezlocillin, or ticarcillin.
[‖]Nafcillin, oxacillin, or methicillin.
MIC, Minimum inhibitory concentration; *TMP-SMX*, trimethoprim–sulfamethoxazole.

Table 41-22 Common Pathogens of Bacterial Meningitis and Empiric Treatment Based on Age

Age	Common Pathogens	Treatment*	Duration (days)
0-1 mo	Group B streptococci	Ampicillin *plus* third-generation cephalosporin[†]	14-21
	Listeria monocytogenes	*or* ampicillin *plus* aminoglycoside	14-21
	Escherichia coli		21
	Streptococcus pneumoniae		10-14
1-3 mo	Group B streptococci, *E. coli, L. monocytogenes*	Ampicillin *plus* third-generation cephalosporin[†]	14-21
	S. pneumoniae		10-14
	Neisseria meningitidis, Haemophilus influenzae		7-10
3 mo-18 yr	*H. influenzae, N. meningitidis*	Third-generation cephalosporin[†] *or* meropenem	7-10
	S. pneumoniae	*or* chloramphenicol	10-14
18-50 yr	*H. influenzae, N. meningitidis*	Third-generation cephalosporin[†] *or* meropenem	7-10
	S. pneumoniae	*or* ampicillin *plus* chloramphenicol	10-14
>50 yr	*S. pneumoniae*	Ampicillin *plus* third-generation cephalosporin[†]	10-14
	L. monocytogenes	*or* ampicillin *plus* fluoroquinolone[‡] *or*	14-21
	Gram-negative bacilli (other than *H. influenzae*)	meropenem	21

*Add vancomycin in areas where there is greater than 2% incidence of highly drug-resistant *S. pneumoniae*.
[†]Ceftriaxone or cefotaxime.
[‡]Ciprofloxacin or levofloxacin.

Ciprofloxacin, 500 mg orally as a single dose, is another alternative to rifampin in nonpregnant, nonlactating adults (Advisory Committee on Immunization Practices [ACIP], 2013; Centers for Disease Control and Prevention, 2000; Pickering, 2003).

Prevention of nasopharyngeal carriage in patients treated for meningitis is achieved by starting prophylaxis doses (same as earlier) before discharge. Prevention is also achieved by immunoprophylaxis. The Hib vaccine is now part of the primary vaccination series for children and has been immensely successful at almost eliminating *H. influenzae* meningitis. A vaccine for meningococcal disease is now a part of the standard immunization regimen for all children between the ages of 11 and 12 years, with a booster dose at age 16 years. It should also be administered to children between the ages of 13 and 18 years if not previously vaccinated (ACIP, 2013).

The 13-valent pneumococcal conjugate vaccine (PCV-13) is recommended for all children as part of the ACIP's immunization schedule. PCV-13 is also recommended for adults age 19 years or older with immunocompromising conditions, functional or anatomic asplenia, CSF leaks, or cochlear implant (ACIP, 2013).

KEY TREATMENT

- Evidence supports the use of adjunctive dexamethasone in infants and children with Hib meningitis (IDSA; Tunkel et al., 2004) (SOR: A).
- Adjunctive dexamethasone is recommended for adult patients with suspected or proven pneumococcal meningitis (IDSA; Tunkel et al., 2004) (SOR: A).

Recurrent Meningitis

Recurrent meningitis can have both infectious and noninfectious causes. A CSF leak accounts for approximately 75% of cases of recurrent meningitis. Clinically, it presents similar to aseptic meningitis. A careful history may detect a drug exposure, structural lesion, or associated systemic disorder. To be truly recurrent, the CSF must confirm pleocytosis. Between episodes, the CSF must also be documented to return to normal. The interval between recurrences can be months to years. Unless the source is bacterial, the course of recurrent meningitis is usually self-limited, and spontaneous recovery is generally the rule. Optimal treatment is aimed at the underlying cause.

Chronic Meningitis

There are no pathognomonic features of chronic meningitis. The classic symptoms, if present, may be extremely subtle and variable. There may be unusual symptoms such as psychoses, movement disorders, and parkinsonian syndrome. The average duration of symptoms is 17 to 43 months, during which symptoms may fluctuate or remain static. CSF that shows a mildly decreased glucose level in the setting of mononuclear pleocytosis should always raise the suspicion of chronic meningitis. The causes are numerous, and attention should be paid to a history of previous systemic diseases, specific infections that could involve the meninges, possible exposures, geographic risk factors, immunologic compromise, and concurrent extraneural involvement (Tables 41-23 and 41-24).

Viral Meningitis

Viral meningitis is actually a subset of aseptic meningitis. *Aseptic meningitis* antedates the modern science of virology and signifies an infection of the subarachnoid space and meninges with no obvious bacterial cause. *Encephalitis* occurs when there is inflammation of brain tissue. *Viral meningitis* presents with similar signs and symptoms as bacterial meningitis but with less severity. A history of a preceding viral respiratory infection is common. Obtaining LP for CSF evaluation is the only method for determining the difference. There are numerous causes of viral meningitis (Table 41-25). Outbreaks are often seasonal.

Treatment is mainly supportive, with the exception of herpes simplex virus (HSV) and HIV, for which specific antiviral therapy is available. Data regarding herpes meningitis treatment are limited, and both high-dose acyclovir (60 mg/kg/day) and lower-dose therapies have been advocated (Kohlhoff et al., 2004). For HIV and acquired

Table 41-23   Causes of Chronic Meningitis

Bacterial	Tuberculosis
	Brucellosis
	Nocardiosis
	Syphilis
	Lyme disease
	Actinomycosis
	Listeriosis
	Subacute bacterial endocarditis
	Tularemia
	Leptospirosis
	Meningococcal infection
Fungal	Cryptococcosis
	Coccidioidomycosis
	Histoplasmosis
	Blastomycosis
	Candida
	Aspergillus spp.
	Zygomycetes spp.
	Sporothrix spp.
Viral	Retroviruses
	Herpesvirus
	Enteroviruses
	Lymphocytic choriomeningitis
	Mumps
Parasitic	Cysticercosis
	Schistosomiasis
	Trichinosis
	Paragonimiasis
	Echinococcosis
	Toxoplasmosis
	Visceral larva migrans
Noninfectious	Neoplasm
	Vasculitis
	Chemical meningitis
	Collagen vascular disease
	Behçet disease
	Sarcoidosis
	Systemic lupus erythematosus
	Fabry disease
	Foreign body in central nervous system
	Vogt-Koyanagi-Harada syndrome
Other	Parameningeal focus
	Chronic lymphocytic meningitis

Table 41-24   Laboratory Evaluation for Chronic Meningitis

Blood	Complete blood count, differential
	Chemistries, ESR, ANA
	HIV serology
	RPR
	Consider ACE, antineutrophilic cytoplasmic antibodies, specific serologies, blood smears
Cerebrospinal fluid	Cell count with differential, protein, glucose
	Cytology
	VDRL
	Cultures (TB, fungal, bacterial, viral)
	Stain (Gram, acid fast, India ink)
	Cryptococcal antigen
	Oligoclonal bands, IgG index
	Consider ACE; PCR (viruses, mycobacteria, *Tropheryma whippelii*); *Histoplasma* antigen, immunocytochemistry (*T. whippelii* and other selected agents); paired antibodies for *Borrelia burgdorferi*, *Brucella* spp., *Histoplasma* spp., *Coccidioides* spp., other fungal agents; neoplastic markers
Neuroimaging	Brain MRI with contrast
	Consider CT, spinal MRI, angiography
Cultures	Blood (parasites, fungi, viruses, rare bacteria)
	Urine (mycobacteria, viruses, fungi)
	Sputum (mycobacteria, fungi)
	Consider gastric washings, stool, bone marrow, liver (mycobacteria, fungi)
Ancillary	Chest radiography
	Electrocardiography
	Select testing (e.g., mammography, chest or abdominal CT)
Biopsy	Extraneural sites (bone marrow, lymph node, peripheral nerve, liver, lung, skin, small bowel)
	Leptomeningeal or brain (with or without special stains)

ACE, Angiotensin-converting enzyme; *ANA,* antinuclear antibodies; *CT,* computed tomography; *ESR,* erythrocyte sedimentation rate; *HIV,* human immunodeficiency virus; *IgG,* immunoglobulin G; *MRI,* magnetic resonance imaging; *PRCR,* polymerase chain reaction; *RPR,* rapid plasma reagin; *TB,* tuberculosis; *VRDL,* Venereal Disease Research Laboratory.
Modified from Coyle PK. Overview of acute and chronic meningitis. *Neurol Clin.* 1999;17:691.

immunodeficiency syndrome (AIDS)–dementia complex (ADC), many antiviral combinations have been suggested. The factors to be considered when choosing a combination therapy for ADC include toxicity, the many potential drug interactions, CNS penetration, and resistance. Because the treatments for HIV and its complications are often changing, consultation with an infectious disease specialist should be considered.

With the exception of HSV encephalitis and ADC, the prognosis is generally very good for other viral meningitides. Children seem to recover within 1 to 2 weeks, but adults may take several months.

Brain Abscess

Brain abscess, a rare disease in the United States, can occur in single or multiple sites. It usually arises from a secondary focus outside the CNS. Examples may include upper or lower respiratory infection, intracardiac infection, penetrating skull trauma, local osteomyelitis, any source of bacteremia, or no source (20%). Risk factors include IV drug use, HIV infection, and any other immunocompromised

Table 41-25   Causes of Viral Meningitis

Enteroviruses
Echovirus
Poliovirus
Coxsackieviruses A and B
Herpesviruses
Herpes simplex virus types 1 and 2
Varicella-zoster virus
Lymphocytic choriomeningitis
Flaviviruses (St. Louis encephalitis)
Morbillivirus (measles)
Bunyaviruses (LaCrosse)
Epstein-Barr virus
Adenoviruses
Cytomegalovirus
Mumps
Hepatitis B virus
Human immunodeficiency virus

state. Common pathogens include streptococci, staphylococci, enteric gram-negative organisms, and anaerobes.

Clinically, brain abscess usually has a more aggressive onset of symptoms than bacterial meningitis. Symptoms usually present as typical meningeal irritation along with mental status changes that progress to stupor or coma, seizures, and focal neurologic findings. Laboratory studies are not impressive. Caution should be exercised before performing LP because brain edema is often present. Once past the initial cerebritis stage, CT or MRI of the brain often identifies the abscess. A search for a secondary cause is important. A radionuclide-labeled leukocyte scan may be needed to differentiate a brain tumor from infection. Aspiration or biopsy of the area in question usually confers a definitive diagnosis.

Treatment is directed toward the cause and lasts for 4 to 6 weeks. Drainage of the abscess is achieved by CT-guided needle aspiration or craniotomy. Recurrence can be expected in 5% to 10% of patients. Morbidity is significant and includes the risk of epilepsy (10%-70%), focal neurologic sequelae (25%), and cognitive impairment (15%). The overall mortality rate is 5% to 10%.

DIZZINESS

Key Points

- Dizziness is a risk factor for falls and functional decline in older adults.
- Characterizing the type of dizziness can narrow the differential diagnosis.
- Benign paroxysmal positional vertigo patients complain of episodic vertigo without aural symptoms.

Dizziness is a common problem encountered by family physicians. It is a typical complaint of elderly patients and has a broad differential diagnosis. Fortunately, dizziness is usually benign and self-limited. Nevertheless, it is a risk factor for falls and functional decline in the geriatric population and, in a small subset of patients, can signal a life-threatening condition.

Evaluation

The evaluation of dizziness is often frustrating for both patients and physicians. This frustration arises from the vast differential diagnosis, the potential for multiple etiologies, and the lack of a dependable method of diagnosing the more serious causes of dizziness. The initial step in the evaluation of a patient with dizziness is a thorough history. First, the physician should clarify the category of dizziness reported by the patient. Dizziness can be categorized as *vertigo*, which is the sensation of spinning or motion; *presyncopal lightheadedness*, which is a sensation of impending faint; *disequilibrium*, a sensation of unsteadiness and imbalance; or dizziness that cannot be adequately quantified, reported by patients as a feeling of lightheadedness or floating sensation. Categorizing the type of dizziness can limit the differential diagnosis (Table 41-26). Many patients, however, are unable to limit their dizziness symptoms to one specific category. Classically, the category of vertigo was further defined as peripheral or central vertigo based on

symptoms and signs, including nystagmus. This is not clinically useful, especially in the older adult population, because many of these findings are seen in normal patients as well.

After categorizing the type of dizziness experienced by the patient, the physician should next determine the temporal pattern of the symptoms. *Continuous* dizziness is typically produced by a stroke. *Episodic* dizziness lasting a few seconds to a minute and associated with head movement is usually a sign of benign positional vertigo. Meniere disease tends to cause dizziness lasting hours to days. Finally, the history should focus on the onset of the symptoms, alleviating or aggravating factors, and a review of the patient's medications (Table 41-27).

The physical examination should include orthostatic BP and pulse determinations; examination of the ears, nose, and throat for signs of infection; cardiovascular examination for murmurs and arrhythmias, with auscultation for carotid bruits; and neurologic examination, including evaluation of CNs, hearing and vision screening, observation of gait, cerebellar testing, and neuromuscular assessment of extremities. A Dix-Hallpike maneuver should be tested if the differential diagnosis includes benign positional vertigo because a positive test result confirms this diagnosis. Screening audiometry should be considered to rule out

Table 41-26 Types of Dizziness

Category	Differential Diagnosis
Vertigo (sensation of spinning)	Inner ear, vestibular, brainstem and cerebellar abnormalities, sinusitis, drug toxicity, panic disorder, cervical spine disease
Presyncopal lightheadedness	Cerebral hypoperfusion, venous pooling in extremities, low blood volume, cardiac abnormalities (arrhythmia, cardiac insufficiency), vasovagal phenomenon
Disequilibrium (unsteadiness more prominent when standing)	Broad differential—any disturbance of the neurosensory system
Other (vague descriptions of lightheadedness without presyncope, or a floating sensation)	Broad differential but often associated with psychological disorders

Table 41-27 Substances Associated with Dizziness

Alcohol
α-Blockers
Anticholinergics
Antihistamines
Tricyclic antidepressants
Meclizine
Anticonvulsants
β-Blockers
Caffeine
Calcium channel blockers
Cough and cold medications
Diuretics
Muscle relaxants
Nonsteroidal medications
Psychotropic medicines
Vasodilating agents

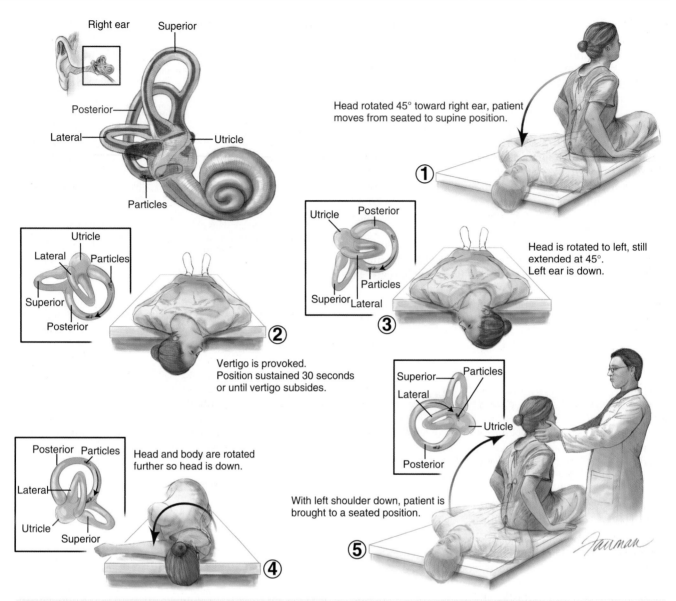

Figure 41-2 Epley maneuver. (Reused with permission from Jones HR, Allam G, Srinivasan J. *Netter's neurology.* 2nd ed. Philadelphia: Saunders; 2011:117.)

Meniere disease and acoustic neuroma if warranted by the type of dizziness described by the history.

Laboratory and imaging studies should be ordered based on history and physical examination findings. Laboratory tests frequently include CBC, electrolytes, BUN, creatinine, glucose, serum calcium, LFTs, and TSH. If neuroimaging is indicated, MRI is the preferred modality because of its superior ability to evaluate the posterior fossa and brainstem. In some patients, carotid Doppler evaluation, cardiac event monitoring, or echocardiography may be necessary. Subspecialty consultation should be considered before proceeding with further, extensive testing.

Conditions Associated with Dizziness

Benign Positional Vertigo. Benign positional vertigo is believed to be caused by a dislodged otolith from the semicircular canal. Symptoms include episodic vertigo without aural symptoms. Nausea and vomiting may also be present secondary to the vertigo. Common histories include vertigo precipitated by rolling over in bed or bending over to tie shoes. The diagnosis can usually be made by the history and eliciting a positive Dix-Hallpike maneuver. Patients can be expected to have gradual resolution of their symptoms over 4 to 6 weeks with supportive therapy. The canalith repositioning (Epley) maneuver (see Figure 41-2) provides short-term resolution of the vertiginous symptoms (Cochrane review; Pinder, 2004).

Postural Dizziness. Nonvertiginous postural dizziness suggests postural hypotension. *Orthostatic hypotension* is usually defined as a 20–mm Hg drop in systolic BP or 10–mm Hg drop in diastolic BP 2 minutes after moving from a recumbent to standing position. Older adult patients, however, can develop postural dizziness without apparent postural hypotension. In some cases, no BP decline occurs, although enough blood pools in the older adult's lower extremities to impair cerebral perfusion. When postural dizziness without postural hypotension is suspected, an evaluation of the cardiovascular system should be considered. If significant cardiovascular pathology, such as congestive heart failure, is not identified, a therapeutic trial of support stockings and optimized hydration can be contemplated.

Labyrinthitis, Vestibular Abnormalities, and Meniere Disease. A comprehensive review of these topics is beyond the scope of this chapter but should be considered when evaluating any patient with dizziness. Patients with the abrupt onset of a single episode of vertigo that gradually resolves over several days often have *labyrinthitis* or *vestibular neuronitis*, usually distinguished clinically by the presence or absence of hearing changes. Patients with labyrinthitis usually experience hearing changes, but those with vestibular neuronitis do not. Whereas a viral infection is the usual cause in younger patients, infarction becomes more likely in older adults. Older adult patients may recover more slowly and experience feelings of imbalance for several months. Treatment during the symptomatic period may include vestibular rehab exercises and pharmacologic agents such as meclizine, promethazine, or low-dose benzodiazepine (e.g., lorazepam). *Meniere disease* should be suspected when an older adult reports recurrent episodes of vertigo, tinnitus, gradual development of low-frequency hearing loss, and in some cases ear fullness before onset of vertigo.

Dizziness of Cervical Origin. Cervical spine problems, especially osteoarthritic changes, can cause dizziness that may be vertiginous in nature and of vascular or proprioceptive origin. In cases of vascular origin, flow through one or both of the vertebral arteries is temporarily disrupted by an osteoarthritic spur that compresses the vessel when the patient turns the head or looks up. In cases of proprioceptive origin, overstimulation of the proprioceptive receptors in the facet joints produces the sensation of dizziness. Either of these conditions can cause a "drop attack." These patients should avoid the position that precipitates the symptoms, and in some cases, cervical collars or cervical traction may be helpful.

Vertebrobasilar Transient Ischemic Attacks and Stroke. The TIAs that produce vertigo of abrupt onset lasting minutes to hours are a manifestation of ischemia in the distribution of the vertebrobasilar arteries, not the carotid arteries. Unfortunately, the TIA diagnosis can be difficult to make because vertigo may be the only symptom reported, and more definitive neurologic symptoms suggestive of a vertebrobasilar event may be absent, such as blurred vision, visual field deficits, diplopia, dysarthria, and unilateral motor or sensory changes. When a patient presents with symptoms of a vertebrobasilar TIA, the physician should consider causes such as cardioembolic disease, polycythemia, and subclavian steal syndrome. A significant BP difference in the arms and symptoms with arm abduction may signal subclavian steal syndrome, which may be corrected surgically. If the cause of these symptoms is related to vertebrobasilar vascular disease, treatment is usually medical with aspirin or other antiplatelet agents.

Vertigo is also a component of several well-recognized *vertebrobasilar stroke syndromes* (Table 41-28). *Lacunar strokes*, particularly those affecting the cerebellum, are also an important cause of dizziness. The dizziness associated with lacunar strokes is often reported as a sense of

Table 41-28 Vertebrobasilar Stroke Syndromes

Anatomy	Symptoms
Occlusion of vertebral artery	Lateral medullary syndrome: vertigo, nausea, ipsilateral facial numbness, Horner syndrome, contralateral body loss of pain and temperature sensation, tendency to fall to affected side
Occlusion of anterior inferior cerebellar artery: affects labyrinth, pontomedullary region, and inferolateral cerebellum	Lateral pontomedullary syndrome: severe vertigo, nausea, vomiting, unilateral hearing loss, tinnitus, facial paralysis, asymmetric cerebellar testing
Cerebellar infarction	Severe vomiting, vertigo, and ataxia; brainstem signs may be absent, making differentiation from labyrinthitis difficult or impossible

disequilibrium that is difficult to explain clinically. Such patients often report a sense of imbalance when standing that started when they were not feeling well and persists even after they return to their otherwise usual state of health. CT imaging is subject to excessive artifact in the posterior cranial fossa and is often inadequate to identify small cerebellar or brainstem infarcts. MRI is more useful for imaging this portion of the brain and should be considered as the initial imaging modality. Aggressive efforts to control BP are advised for patients believed to have experienced lacunar strokes.

PERIPHERAL NEUROPATHIES

Key Points

- In developed countries, diabetes and alcoholism are the most common causes of peripheral neuropathy in adults.
- Polyneuropathies are often inflammatory and caused by HIV infection, Lyme disease, and leprosy; no cause can be found in up to 20% of cases.
- There is no specific laboratory study or serum marker for the diagnosis of peripheral neuropathy.
- Electromyography (EMG) and nerve conduction studies (NCS) are most useful for evaluation of peripheral neuropathy and should be considered early.
- Mononeuropathies are usually caused by entrapment, compression, or other physical injury to a specific nerve.
- Carpal tunnel syndrome (CTS) is a common mononeuropathy caused by decreased tunnel size (Colles fracture, rheumatoid arthritis), enlargement of median nerve (diabetes, amyloidosis), or increased volume of other structures (tenosynovitis, gout).
- Common symptoms of CTS include numbness and paresthesias in the median nerve sensory distribution, pain at rest (especially at night), weakness in the thumb, and thenar atrophy.

The incidence of peripheral neuropathy is not known, but it is a common feature of many systemic diseases. In developed countries, diabetes and alcoholism are the most common causes of peripheral neuropathy in adults

(Poncelet, 1998). Worldwide, leprosy is the primary treatable cause of peripheral neuropathy, and HIV is one of the fastest growing causes (Sabin et al., 1993).

Peripheral neuropathies are frequently overlooked. The evaluation can be time consuming and costly without a systematic approach based on a careful history, clinical evaluation, and select studies. Despite a thoughtful approach, however, no cause can be found in up to 20% of cases (Dyck et al., 1981; McLeod et al., 1984). The goal in treating peripheral neuropathy should be to identify the treatable cause or underlying medical condition, such as diabetes, alcohol, drugs, or nutritional disorder. Hereditary neuropathies are uncommon but underdiagnosed; thus, a careful family history (e.g., long-standing distal neuropathy) should not be neglected.

Anatomy

The peripheral nervous system (PNS) consists of CNs III to XII, spinal roots (dorsal and ventral), spinal nerves, dorsal root ganglia, and most autonomic ganglia and roots. Because the motor neuron cell bodies are located in the spinal cord or CNS, diseases affecting these are considered separately. Peripheral nerves consist of different types of fiber bundles called *axons*. Large- and medium-sized axons are normally myelinated and carry information about proprioception, vibration, and light touch. Small axons, consisting of myelinated and unmyelinated types, are responsible for light touch, pain, and temperature, as well as autonomic information. These small, unmyelinated fibers of the autonomic PNS travel within most peripheral nerves and convey poorly defined visceral sensations and monitor autonomic functions. Most peripheral nerves carry incoming sensory information (afferent fibers) and outgoing motor and autonomic messages (efferent fibers).

Clinical Pathophysiology

Sensory Changes. Large- and small-fiber neuropathies can often be distinguished clinically by whether they affect proprioception and vibration or pain and temperature, respectively. Because processes that affect small fibers cause pain and sensory changes, symptoms may include reduced sensitivity to stimuli (hypoesthesia) or burning and tingling sensations (dysesthesias and paresthesias, respectively). There may also be impaired pain or temperature sensation and autonomic dysfunction. When large fibers are damaged, vibratory sense and proprioception are affected. This can lead to unsteady gait; complaints of coolness in the extremities; or *allodynia,* in which non-noxious stimuli such as light touch are perceived as pain. In polyneuropathies, pain and sensation are commonly affected in a stocking-glove distribution.

Motor Changes. Symptoms are usually most pronounced distally. This is especially true with polyneuropathies, in which symptoms of stumbling, clumsiness, and weakness are most common because of the effects on the intrinsic muscles. Motor symptoms can range from mild weakness to complete paralysis. Diminished DTRs may be one of the early signs of motor dysfunction. Denervation of muscles causes eventual atrophy. An example is the "sharp shin" sign, whereby atrophy of the tibialis anterior muscle gives a prominent appearance to the tibia. As the intrinsic muscles deteriorate, the wasting gives the hands and feet a skeletal appearance. In long-standing neuropathies, trophic changes such as high-arched feet (pes cavus), hammertoes, kyphoscoliosis, and hair loss with or without ulcerations can be seen. Cramps, fasciculations, and restless legs may also be present.

Autonomic Changes. Autonomic changes are especially common with diabetes. The skin may become smooth, cold, and shiny. It may be unusually dry and devoid of perspiration. Orthostatic hypotension is one of the most common autonomic symptoms associated with neuropathy from systemic disease. The genitourinary and gastrointestinal systems are also often affected.

Classification. Peripheral neuropathies are often categorized in terms of the anatomy affected, pathophysiologic process, temporal development, and functional outcome.

Anatomic Classification. The major anatomic patterns of peripheral nerve disease can be distinguished by the clinical presentation of mononeuropathy, multiple mononeuropathy, and polyneuropathy. *Mononeuropathies* occur when there is damage to a single peripheral nerve or root. This is seen with local entrapment from causes such as trauma (acute or chronic), tumor infiltration, or infarction. *Multiple mononeuropathies* (mononeuropathy multiplex) occur when several nerves are individually affected by a disease process. Involvement is usually asymmetric and noncontiguous. These mononeuropathies are much less common than other peripheral neuropathies and are more difficult to recognize and treat. Multiple mononeuropathies are usually seen with systemic diseases such as vasculitis, diabetes, and rheumatoid arthritis. *Polyneuropathies* occur in a symmetric, diffuse, bilateral pattern and produce a characteristic stocking-glove pattern of sensory changes. However, most polyneuropathies affect both sensory and motor nerves. Some can affect peripheral autonomic nerves. Many common peripheral neuropathies fall into this category.

Pathophysiologic Classification. Based on the primary site of involvement, peripheral neuropathies can be classified as neuronopathies, axonal neuropathies, and myelinopathies. Electrodiagnostic studies can help define this in a clinical setting. *Neuronopathies* result from damage to the sensory cell bodies in the dorsal root ganglia or motor neuron cell bodies in the spinal cord. Their location in the CNS usually results in a degenerative process that produces incomplete recovery. Diseases that specifically affect the motor neuron cell bodies in the CNS are usually not categorized as peripheral neuropathies. *Axonal neuropathies* occur when damage occurs at the level of the axon. When the axon is disrupted (e.g., by trauma), the axon and distal myelin sheath may degenerate distal to the site of injury (wallerian degeneration). In toxic or metabolic injuries, when the distal axon is injured and myelin degeneration spreads proximally, it is known as "dying back" neuropathy. With the dying back process, the longer nerves tend to be affected earlier and more severely. *Myelinopathies* (demyelinating neuropathies) result from a process affecting primarily the myelin sheath. They can result from

Table 41-29 Neuropathies Classified by Temporal Presentation

Acute onset (within days)	GBS Vasculitis Porphyria Diphtheria Thallium toxicity Ischemia Penetrating trauma Rheumatoid arthritis Diabetic plexopathy or cranial neuropathy Acute nerve compression Polyarteritis nodosa Burns Iatrogenic (e.g., improper injection techniques)
Subacute onset (weeks to months)	Most toxins Most drugs Nutritional deficiencies Abnormal metabolic state Diabetic plexopathy Neoplasms Uremia
Chronic course (months to years)	CIDP Alcohol Diabetes Hereditary neuropathies
Relapsing	GBS HIV Porphyria Refsum's disease CIDP

CIDP, Chronic inflammatory demyelinating polyradiculoneuropathy; *GBS*, Guillain-Barré syndrome; *HIV*, human immunodeficiency virus.

Table 41-30 Small-Fiber Neuropathies

Diabetes
Leprosy
Hereditary
HIV/AIDS
Amyloidosis
Alcoholism

HIV/AIDS, Human immunodeficiency virus/acquired immunodeficiency syndrome.
Modified from Poncelet AN. An algorithm for the evaluation of peripheral neuropathy. *Am Fam Physician*. 1998;57:755.

acute conditions such as Guillain-Barré syndrome (GBS), chronic inflammatory demyelinating polyradiculoneuropathies (CIDPs), and certain hereditary neuropathies.

Temporal Classification. Acute peripheral neuropathies develop over a few days. When motor signs are predominant, GBS should be suspected first. Vasculitic or toxic processes can also present acutely. A subacute presentation may be seen in toxic, inflammatory, infiltrative, or carcinomatous processes that develop over weeks. A chronic-onset neuropathy may develop gradually and progress over months to years, as is the case in metabolic or hereditary neuropathies. Peripheral neuropathies may also have a relapsing course (Table 41-29).

Laboratory Evaluation

There is no specific laboratory study or serum marker for the diagnosis of peripheral neuropathy. Information from the history and physical examination may direct specific laboratory tests (e.g., testing for specific toxins, infections, or inflammatory disorders). If the cause of neuropathy is not obvious, some screening laboratory studies should be considered, including ESR, CBC, LFTs, and determination of fasting blood glucose, glycosylated hemoglobin, BUN, creatinine, serum vitamin B_{12}, and TSH levels. Additional studies may be warranted, depending on the initial workup, such as chest radiography to rule out sarcoidosis, pulmonary function tests for GBS, or ECG for processes that affect cardiac conduction. An LP for CSF showing an elevated protein level with normal white blood cells (WBCs) may indicate an acquired inflammatory neuropathy (GBS or CIDP).

Electromyography and NCS are probably the most useful laboratory studies for the evaluation of peripheral neuropathy and should be considered early. They can confirm the presence of peripheral neuropathy and provide information about the type of fibers involved (sensory, motor, or both) and whether the problem is symmetric, asymmetric, or multifocal. EMG can define entrapment neuropathies and differentiate these from more proximal radicular compression. It can also help differentiate muscle wasting caused by neuropathic or myopathic disorders from simple disuse atrophy. NCS can help define pathophysiology (axonal loss vs. demyelination). EMG and NCS are useful but have limitations and should complement the history and examination. EMG is usually not as helpful in diseases that cause a diffuse small-fiber peripheral neuropathy, in which only pinprick and temperature sensation are affected (Table 41-30). In fact, the electromyography result may be normal. EMG needles also mildly inflame the muscles into which they are inserted. Thus, if a muscle biopsy is anticipated, that muscle should not be tested with EMG (Corse and Kuncl, 1999). NCS are most diagnostic with diseases affecting large, fast fibers and thus may be normal in patients with small-fiber neuropathies. Evaluation of small, proximal sensory nerves is not reliably done using EMG or NCS.

Nerve biopsy is helpful only in specific cases and is usually a last step in the workup. This includes patients with suspected amyloidosis, vasculitis, leprosy, leukodystrophies, sarcoidosis, or demyelinating disorders. Because the sural nerve, a sensory nerve, is generally used, disease affecting only motor nerves may be missed. Possible complications include permanent numbness or dysesthesia in the distribution of the excised nerve (typically lateral heel and ankle), infection, and poor wound healing.

In the evaluation of neuropathies, a carefully performed history that identifies key features of the presentation correlated with the findings of electrodiagnostic studies is the critical first step in developing a reasonable diagnosis. Questions include the following:

- Is the pattern of involvement focal or multifocal (Table 41-31)?
- Is the pattern symmetric (Tables 41-32 and 41-33)?
- Did symptoms evolve acutely, subacutely, or chronically? Was there a predilection for the upper extremities (Table 41-34)?
- Were the extremities affected in a distal versus a proximal distribution (see Tables 41-32 and 41-33)?

Table 41-31 Neuropathies by Pattern of Involvement

Focal	Multifocal
Common entrapment neuropathies: endocrine	Diabetes mellitus
Myxedema	Vasculitis
Acromegaly	Polyarteritis nodosa
Hypothyroidism	Churg-Strauss syndrome
Infection or inflammation	Giant cell arteritis
Septic arthritis	Wegener granulomatosis
Lyme disease	Rheumatoid arthritis
Tuberculosis	Sjögren syndrome
Histoplasmosis	Systemic lupus
Sarcoidosis	erythematosus
Rheumatoid arthritis	HIV (e.g., cytomegalovirus)
Amyloidosis	Leprosy
Tumors	Sarcoidosis
Ganglion	Cryoglobulinemia
Neurofibroma	Multifocal variant of CIDP
Lipoma	
Hemangioma	
Congenital: anatomic anomalies of muscles, bones, or vessels	
Trauma	
Fractures	
Hematoma	
Hemorrhage from anticoagulation	
Pregnancy	
Hemodialysis	
Idiopathic	
Occupational	
Repetitive stress	
Neoplastic infiltration or compression	
Leprosy	
Ischemic lesions	
Diabetes mellitus	
Vasculitis	

CIDP, Chronic inflammatory demyelinating polyneuroradiculopathy; *HIV,* human immunodeficiency virus.

- Are the symptoms sensory, motor, or both (Table 41-35; see also Tables 41-32 and 41-33)?
- Is there autonomic or CN involvement (Tables 41-36 and 41-37)?
- What did the EMG and NCS show? Were other significant laboratory studies done?

Taking this approach to peripheral neuropathies will prove to be more efficient and fruitful than less ordered approaches despite the often elusive nature of these diagnoses.

Mononeuropathies

Mononeuropathies are usually caused by entrapment, compression, or other physical injury to a specific nerve. Peripheral nerves most at risk are those that occupy spaces with confining borders. Electrodiagnostic studies are useful in confirming the diagnosis and quantifying the degree of injury. Treatment is generally conservative, involving protection of the affected nerve from further injury by the use of activity avoidance or modification, ergonomic workplace correction, and bracing. Local (by injection) or systemic antiinflammatory treatment is often helpful. Surgical intervention is usually reserved for patients who fail conservative therapy, have evidence of progressive weakness and atrophy, or have a significant focal conduction block on electrodiagnostic examination.

Table 41-32 Distal Symmetric Sensorimotor Polyneuropathies

Nutritional diseases
  B-complex deficiencies
  Vitamin E deficiency
  Folate deficiency
  Whipple's disease
  Postgastrectomy syndrome
  Alcoholism
  Gastric resection for obesity
  Endocrine diseases
  Diabetes mellitus
  Hypothyroidism
  Acromegaly
Neoplastic
  Multiple myeloma
  Lymphoma
  Carcinoma
Paraneoplastic
  Connective tissue disease
  Rheumatoid arthritis
  Cryoglobulinemia
  Polyarteritis nodosa
  Systemic lupus erythematosus
  Scleroderma
  Sarcoidosis
  Churg-Strauss vasculitis
  Medications and toxins (see Table 41-38)
Infectious
  Human immunodeficiency virus
  Lyme disease
  Hypophosphatemia
Metabolic
  Uremia
  Porphyria
  Gout
  Critical illness polyneuropathy
  Amyloidosis
  Metal neuropathy
  Thallium
  Gold
  Arsenic
  Mercury
  Inherited metabolic disease
  Refsum disease
  Adrenoleukodystrophy
  Hereditary neuropathies

Modified from Poncelet AN: An algorithm for the evaluation of peripheral neuropathy. *Am Fam Physician.* 1998;57:755.

Table 41-33 Distal Symmetric Motor Polyneuropathies

Lead neuropathy
Diphtheria
Guillain-Barré syndrome
Hereditary neuropathies
Diabetes mellitus
Lymphoma
Lyme disease
Vincristine toxicity
Hypothyroidism
Porphyria
Acute arsenic polyneuropathy
Osteoclastic myeloma
Human immunodeficiency virus
Waldenström macroglobulinemia
Chronic inflammatory demyelinating polyradiculoneuropathy
Monoclonal gammopathy of undetermined significance
Motor neuropathy with multifocal conduction block

Modified from Poncelet AN. An algorithm for the evaluation of peripheral neuropathy. *Am Fam Physician.* 1998;57:4755.

Table 41-34 Neuropathies with Predilection for the Upper Limbs

Diabetes
Porphyria
Hereditary neuropathies
Hereditary amyloid neuropathy type II (causes CTS from amyloid deposits)
Guillain-Barré syndrome
Myeloma
Lead neuropathy
Vitamin B$_{12}$ deficiency

CTS, Carpal tunnel syndrome.
Modified from Poncelet AN. An algorithm for the evaluation of peripheral neuropathy. *Am Fam Physician*. 1998;57:4755.

Table 41-35 Predominantly Sensory Neuropathies and Neuronopathies

Idiopathic sensory neuropathy
Paraneoplastic
  Pyridoxine toxicity
  Sjögren syndrome
  Primary biliary sclerosis
  Vitamin E deficiency
Medications
  Cisplatin
  Metronidazole
  Misonidazole
  Thalidomide
Carcinoma
  Lymphoma
Paraproteinemias
  Crohn's disease
Hereditary neuropathies
  Friedreich ataxia
  Chronic gluten enteropathy
  Nonsystemic vasculitic neuropathy
  Styrene-induced peripheral neuropathy

Modified from Poncelet AN. An algorithm for the evaluation of peripheral neuropathy. *Am Fam Physician*. 1998;57:755.

Table 41-36 Neuropathies with Autonomic Symptoms

Diabetic neuropathy
Amyloidosis
Thiamine deficiency
Alcoholic neuropathy
Guillain-Barré syndrome
Vincristine toxicity
Human immunodeficiency virus
Porphyria
Thallium, mercury, arsenic toxicity
Dysautonomia (Riley-Day)
Lymphoma
Paraneoplastic neuropathy

Modified from Poncelet AN. An algorithm for the evaluation of peripheral neuropathy. *Am Fam Physician*. 1998;57:755.

Table 41-37 Neuropathies with Cranial Nerve Involvement

Primary	Bell palsy
	Trigeminal neuralgia
Secondary	Diabetes mellitus
	Diphtheria
	Lyme disease
	Sarcoidosis with cranial invasion
	Guillain-Barré syndrome
	Human immunodeficiency virus

Brachial Plexus Neuropathy. Brachial plexus neuropathy (plexopathy) can result from blunt or penetrating trauma. The typical injury is directed into the axilla or violently increases the angle between the shoulder and head. In the latter case, *stingers* or *burners*, which frequently occur in football players, result in temporary paresthesias and diffuse weakness in the upper extremity. Recurrent stretch injuries to the brachial plexus can result in permanent weakness and atrophy. Also, apical lung tumors with direct extension or compression can cause pain in the upper extremity and hand numbness. Radiation therapy also can result in brachial plexopathies. *Idiopathic brachial plexopathy* (Parsonage-Turner syndrome) often occurs abruptly without any clear precipitating factor, although it can develop after an infection, injection, surgery, or childbirth. It typically begins with an aching sensation in the neck or shoulder and progresses over days to produce weakness, sensory loss, and diminished reflexes. Patients with brachial plexopathy often have considerable pain. Recovery is usually spontaneous but can take weeks to months. Some residual weakness may be present in a few patients.

Median Neuropathy (Carpal Tunnel Syndrome). Carpal tunnel syndrome is one of the most common mononeuropathies. It typically occurs within the confines of the carpal tunnel in the wrist. The median nerve can also be entrapped in the forearm as a pronator or interosseous syndrome. The entrapment can be caused by anything that causes a decrease in the size of the carpal tunnel (e.g., Colles fracture, rheumatoid arthritis, congenital carpal tunnel stenosis), enlargement of the median nerve (e.g., diabetes, amyloidosis, thyroid disease, neuroma), or an increase in the volume of other structures within the carpal tunnel (e.g., tenosynovitis, ganglion, gout, urate deposits, lipoma, hematoma, fluid retention in pregnancy).

Other risk factors include any tasks that require repeated or sustained stress over the base of the palm. Low-frequency vibration exposure is another well-recognized risk factor for CTS. Repetitive wrist and hand movements such as knitting, typing, painting, woodworking, and weightlifting are also implicated as high-risk factors.

Common symptoms include numbness and paresthesias in the sensory distribution of the median nerve (palmar surface of thumb, index finger, and middle finger; radial side of ring finger; radial two thirds of palm). The patient may also have pain at rest (especially at night), weakness in the thumb, and thenar atrophy. Signs include a positive Tinel sign at the wrist (tingling in median nerve distribution on percussion over ventral wrist), positive Phalen sign (similar findings within 45 seconds after placing patient's wrist in maximal flexion), pain or paresthesias in a median distribution with thumb pressure over the median nerve for up to 30 seconds, and thenar atrophy. CTS can present with many variations, including proximal pain in the arm and shoulder, and with normal EMG.

Ulnar Neuropathy. The most common place to have ulnar nerve injury is at the elbow, where the nerve is anatomically most exposed and vulnerable as it traverses superficially in the ulnar groove. Pressure at the elbow such as with prolonged elbow weight bearing, coma, intoxication, or anesthesia can account for this problem.

Cubital tunnel syndrome occurs when the nerve is compressed as it runs beneath the aponeurosis of the flexor carpi ulnaris just distal to the medial epicondyle (cubital tunnel). Activities that involve repetitive or sustained elbow flexion, such as baseball pitching, can injure and stretch the nerve. This results in hypermobility of the ulnar nerve and allows recurrent subluxation over the medial epicondyle. Common symptoms include paresthesias or pain in the ring and small fingers and dorsoulnar aspect of the hand and forearm. There may be generalized loss of grip or fine motor control in the hand because of impairment of the intrinsic muscles. Symptoms may improve with elbow extension. Recurrent subluxation of the ulnar nerve at the elbow, especially in young throwing athletes, often requires surgical intervention.

Ulnar neuropathy distal to the elbow usually presents as *ulnar tunnel syndrome* when the nerve is compressed within the Guyon canal in the wrist. Prolonged pressure over the hypothenar eminence, as occurs with cycling, is a common cause, as are similar causes listed for CTS. Dysesthesias may or may not be present in the ulnar regions. Depending on where the specific entrapment occurs, all the intrinsic hand muscles may be weak, or hypothenar function may be selectively preserved.

Radial Neuropathy. Radial nerve injuries are much less common than other upper extremity neuropathies. Proximally, the radial nerve is most vulnerable in the axilla, where it can be injured by hyperabduction of the arm, which puts traction on the nerve. This is the case with "Saturday night palsy," when an intoxicated person sleeps with an arm draped over a chair. A similar circumstance occurs when the nerve is compressed against the humerus at the spiral groove. It is also seen with improper fit or use of crutches. Other sources of compression that can injure the radial nerve along its course include lipoma, fibroma, and new or previous (from callus) humerus fracture.

The radial nerve is predominantly a motor nerve, so symptoms depend on the level of injury. If the compression is proximal enough, there will be sensory loss over the dorsum of the hand along with weakened triceps (elbow extension) and brachioradialis (elbow extension and supination) motor function. The most obvious finding in radial palsy is wristdrop and drop finger (digital extensor paralysis).

In *posterior interosseous syndrome* (radial tunnel syndrome) the compression is more distal; the purely motor branch of the radial nerve, the posterior interosseous nerve, is entrapped at the supinator muscle, causing only weakness in the finger extensors without affecting wrist extension.

Lumbosacral Neuropathy. Compared with the brachial plexus, the lumbosacral plexus is less susceptible to trauma. Injury caused by trauma or compression from surgery, pregnancy, childbirth, tumors, or aortic aneurysm can occur. Diabetes can also cause multiple mononeuropathy of the plexus (see later).

Meralgia Paresthetica. Compression of the lateral femoral cutaneous nerve as it passes over the anterior superior iliac spine at the lateral end of the inguinal canal is common. It is seen in those who have diabetes, are obese, or wear their pants too tight. Patients experience numbness, paresthesias, and pain over the anterolateral aspect of the thigh without weakness.

Femoral Neuropathy. Any blunt or penetrating trauma, surgery or angiography in the groin, prolonged lithotomy position, or hyperextension during dance or gymnastics can injure the femoral nerve. A tumor or inguinal hernia involving the plexus can also compress the nerve. The femoral nerve supplies the quadriceps muscles for knee extension and provides sensory information from the anterior medial thigh and medial leg. Dysfunction in this nerve can result in pain in the groin that radiates to the thigh, buckling of the knee caused by quadriceps weakness, and sensory loss over its area of distribution. Weakness in the hip flexors indicates a more proximal lesion in the lumbar plexus or roots. Diabetic lumbosacral plexopathy should also be distinguished from femoral neuropathies. With the former, patients are older than 50 years, have diabetes, and develop acute severe pain in the thigh that progresses over days to weakness in the femoral nerve distribution. Sensory symptoms are mild. EMG helps distinguish these different conditions.

Sciatic Neuropathy. The sciatic nerve arises from the sacral portion of the plexus. It leaves the pelvis through the sciatic notch and divides into the tibial and peroneal nerves at the popliteal fossa. The sciatic nerve provides sensation to the perineum, posterior thigh, lateral calf, and foot. It innervates the thigh extensors, hamstrings, and all the muscles of the lower leg and foot. Pain, weakness, and sensory changes caused by injury of the sciatic nerve or one of its two branches can be caused by trauma from gunshots, hip fracture or dislocation, compression from surgery or prolonged sitting on a hard edge, tumor, endometriosis, lipoma, aneurysm of the gluteal artery, or improper intramuscular injection into the gluteus. Symptoms of sciatic nerve compression can mimic L5 to S1 radiculopathy. Again, EMG is helpful in these clinical situations.

Peroneal Neuropathy. The common peroneal nerve is most often compressed as it passes close to the fibular head. Such compression occurs from prolonged leg crossing, squatting, or kneeling; an improperly fitted cast or stockings; or prolonged pressure in an intoxicated or comatose patient. Symptoms of peroneal palsy consist of sensory loss over the lateral calf and dorsum of the foot and a weakness of ankle dorsiflexion (footdrop) and foot eversion without pain. If a clear history of trauma or compression cannot be elicited, imaging of the posterior fossa is necessary to rule out a mass lesion. Patients with a more permanent injury to the peroneal nerve may need an ankle–foot orthotic device to provide ankle stability and prevent plantarflexion contractures.

Tibial Neuropathy (Tarsal Tunnel Syndrome). The tarsal tunnel is located at the inferoposterior margin of the medial malleolus. Its boundaries include the bones of the ankle and fibrous flexor retinaculum. The posterior tibial nerve and three flexor tendons of the foot and vessels lie within this tunnel. Compression can occur within the tunnel from tenosynovitis, enlarged veins, and fracture or dislocation of the ankle. Prolonged standing or walking may lead to vascular stasis and engorgement within the tunnel. A horse jockey is one of the few occupations associated with this syndrome. The primary symptom of tarsal tunnel syndrome is painful, burning paresthesias in the sole of the foot that are worse after a day of activity and may extend into the night. The symptoms can be reproduced or exacerbated by gentle percussion over the tarsal tunnel (Tinel sign). The patient may also have weakness in the intrinsic muscles of the foot, making it difficult to push off during walking. Definitive treatment is surgical decompression involving release of the retinaculum.

Interdigital Neuropathy. A common cause of foot pain, entrapment of an interdigital nerve is often caused by a Morton neuroma or benign swelling of the nerve. Tenderness is appreciated in the web space between the metatarsal heads. Any space can be affected, but the second and third web spaces are most often involved. Running, ballet dancing, and wearing tight shoes or high heels are all risk factors. Modifying risk factors, local corticosteroid injection, and surgical release are treatment options.

Polyneuropathies

Inflammatory Neuropathies. With inflammatory neuropathies, an inflammatory process is directed against the peripheral nerve; the most common causes follow. Treatment is usually directed toward the causative agent.

HUMAN IMMUNODEFICIENCY VIRUS. Several opportunistic infections of the PNS may result from HIV infection. HIV itself, cytomegalovirus, and herpes zoster are most common. Painful sensorimotor polyneuropathies or demyelinating polyradiculoneuropathies occur during the early and late stages of HIV disease. Symptomatic relief of neuropathic pain may be achieved with antidepressants (e.g., amitriptyline) or anticonvulsants (e.g., carbamazepine).

LYME DISEASE. The early stages of disseminated Lyme disease have resulted in Bell palsy or an inflammation of CN VII (facial nerve) in approximately 11% of patients with Lyme disease (Wilkinson, 1998). In the later stages of Lyme disease, a neuropathy mimicking CIDP can occur.

LEPROSY. Although uncommon in the United States, leprosy is the most common worldwide treatable cause of neuropathy. Symptoms of neuropathy can occur before the systemic manifestations of disease are present. As leprosy progresses, with its characteristic skin lesions, the risk for peripheral nerve injury increases. Sensory loss of some degree is expected. Treatment is directed toward the disease itself.

ACUTE INFLAMMATORY DEMYELINATING POLYRADICULONEU-ROPATHY. *Guillain-Barré syndrome*, or acute inflammatory demyelinating polyradiculoneuropathy, is a rapidly progressive paralytic syndrome affecting persons of all ages. GBS seems to occur through an immune-mediated process. Many cases follow a mild gastrointestinal or upper respiratory viral illness by 1 to 3 weeks. Other risk factors include pregnancy, influenza immunization, the postoperative period, and HIV infection. A particularly strong link between

Campylobacter jejuni infection and GBS has been suggested in up to 20% of cases (Dyck et al., 1993).

The traditional description of a rapid progression of ascending symmetric weakness starting in the lower extremities and moving to the upper extremities is often useful, *but variations are quite common*. Indeed, early development of proximal weakness is frequently seen, and involvement of upper extremities before lower extremities is not rare. In general, the presentation is one of rapid progression of an ascending symmetric weakness, usually starting in the lower extremities and moving to the upper extremities. Patients may initially complain of pain and paresthesias in the back and proximal limbs. The progressive weakness that involves the legs as well as the upper extremities, trunk, intercostals, head, and neck muscles may take several days to 4 weeks and often results in paralysis. There may be mild sensory impairment in the extremities, early loss of DTRs, and bilateral facial nerve palsy in up to 40% of patients. NCS demonstrate demyelination, and the CSF may show an increased protein level, with normal cell counts.

The differential diagnosis of a rapid-onset polyradiculoneuropathy includes botulism, diphtheria, hypophosphatemia, acute intermittent porphyria, poliomyelitis, Lyme disease, poisoning from contaminated shellfish (e.g., tetrodotoxin), and toxic neuropathies (e.g., arsenic, mercury, thallium).

Because of the rapidly progressive nature of GBS, patients should be monitored in the hospital for signs of respiratory failure and autonomic instability (arrhythmias, hypotension, hypertension, and hyperpyrexia in two thirds of patients). Treatment usually consists of plasmapheresis or intravenous human immune globulin (IVIG). There is no role for steroids in the acute treatment of GBS. In most patients, recovery is complete or nearly complete, although it may take a few weeks to 18 months. About 10% of cases result in severe permanent disability. Even under the best circumstances, 3% to 5% of patients do not survive.

CHRONIC INFLAMMATORY DEMYELINATING POLYRADICULO-NEUROPATHY. Chronic inflammatory demyelinating polyradiculoneuropathy is an acquired motor and sensory neuropathy of unknown cause. As with GBS, an immune-mediated pathogenesis is suspected. Unlike GBS, CIDP usually occurs in the absence of a preceding illness. Unusual exceptions include HIV infection, dysproteinemias, and lupus erythematosus. CIDP is predominantly a motor polyneuropathy affecting those of all ages, with a progressive or relapsing course. Weakness can be proximal or distal but usually develops in the legs over at least 2 months, distinguishing CIDP from GBS. Sensory changes include numbness or paresthesias but can be variable. DTRs are decreased or absent. Electrodiagnostic and CSF findings are similar to those found in GBS. Treatment includes prednisone, along with plasmapheresis or IVIG. CIDP should be distinguished from other acquired and hereditary neuropathies.

Metabolic Neuropathies

DIABETIC NEUROPATHY. Diabetes is the cause of the most common polyneuropathy seen by family physicians, occurring in up to 50% of all patients with diabetes. Its incidence usually rises with disease progression. Diabetic peripheral neuropathy has a widely variable presentation but usually is seen as a symmetric polyneuropathy, with predominant sensory signs and mild motor signs. Patients experience burning dysesthesias and pain in the soles of the feet. Impaired position sense leading to ataxia and arthropathy (Charcot joints) implies the involvement of large, myelinated sensory fibers. Patients with diabetic neuropathy experience bilateral symptoms that include burning pain in the back and thigh with proximal muscle weakness, decreased patellar DTRs, and normal sensory function. This is thought to be caused by microvascular ischemia of the proximal motor trunks. Diabetes is also associated with autonomic neuropathies. Symptoms may include postural hypotension; gastroparesis; intestinal dysmotility; atonic bladder; impotence; and loss of pain fibers in the cardiac sympathetic system, permitting silent MI.

URemic Neuropathy. Patients with chronic renal disease develop a symmetric sensorimotor neuropathy involving the upper and lower extremities. They complain mostly of burning paresthesias. Uremic neuropathy is thought to be secondary to a toxic effect on the peripheral nerves. Because many chronic renal patients also have diabetes, it is often difficult to isolate a single cause. However, patients with true uremic neuropathy who have undergone renal transplantation can have dramatic improvement of symptoms (Rees, 1995).

Nutritional Neuropathies. Most nutritional neuropathies involve one of the B-complex vitamins. Patients at risk for these neuropathies usually have chronic alcoholism, malabsorption syndrome, eating disorder, or unusual diet (food faddist). It presents as a symmetric polyneuropathy with burning in the feet. Weakness, atrophy, and hypoactive reflexes may also occur.

Alcoholic neuropathy is caused from inadequate intake and poor absorption. Treatment with multivitamin supplementation is usually adequate but may take time to be effective. Thiamine (vitamin B_1) deficiency, or beriberi, is seen most often with chronic alcoholism. It may present as a distal polyneuropathy or as a more serious Wernicke-Korsakoff encephalopathy, with mental status changes. In the latter case, intramuscular thiamine (100 mg/day) is preferred initially over oral administration. Pyridoxine (vitamin B_6) deficiency can be associated with the use of dapsone or isoniazid, which interfere with vitamin B_6 metabolism. Prevention requires supplementation with 50 mg of pyridoxine three times daily. Prolonged intake of pyridoxine of more than 2 g/day has also been associated with sensory neuropathy (Rostami, 1995). Vitamin B_{12} deficiency may present only with vague paresthesias. Determining the serum vitamin B_{12} level is the best way to assess a patient when this problem is suspected because abnormal RBC indices may not be apparent until irreversible neurologic symptoms have already occurred.

Hereditary Neuropathies. The hereditary neuropathies are often missed by family physicians and even by those close to the affected patient. These indolent, slowly progressive polyneuropathies may present with motor, autonomic, and less often, sensory symptoms. These include pes cavus, absent tendon reflexes, a high-stepping or slapping gait, footdrop, slowly progressive wasting and weakness of peroneal muscles, foot ulcers, joint arthropathy, and absence of sweating. Without a specific treatment for these

Table 41-38	Neuropathies Caused by Drugs and Toxins
Drugs	
Axonal	Amitriptyline
	Chloroquine
	Cimetidine
	Colchicine
	Dapsone
	Didanosine
	Disulfiram
	Ethambutol
	Hydralazine
	Interferon alfa
	Isoniazid
	Lithium
	Metronidazole
	Nitrous oxide
	Nitrofurantoin
	Paclitaxel
	Phenytoin
	Pyridoxine
	Procainamide
	Vincristine
Demyelinating	Amiodarone
	Colchicine
	Gold
Neuronopathy	Cisplatin
	Pyridoxine
	Thalidomide
Toxins	
Industrial	Organophosphates
	Lead, arsenic, mercury
	Thallium, methyl bromide
	Plastics, synthetic fabrics
	Carbon monoxide
	Ethylene oxide
Euphoriants	Glue
	Solvents

neuropathies, efforts are focused on management of physical disabilities, education, genetic counseling, and reassurance. Hereditary neuropathies and CIDP can both have a familial pattern, the important difference being that CIDP is treatable.

Toxic Neuropathies. Toxic neuropathies occur from repeated exposure to drugs, industrial toxins, or heavy metals (Table 41-38). The presentation depends on the exact exposure and what part of the nerve is affected. It may present as a progressive, symmetric, ascending polyneuropathy, as in many occupational exposures, or with vague sensory changes similar to those of nutritional neuropathies. Lead intoxication creates a motor neuropathy starting in the upper limbs, affecting the radial nerve and causing wristdrop. Many of these neuropathies slowly improve when the offending agent is removed; however, this is not always the case. A careful medical and occupation history is important. Treatment is directed accordingly.

Dysproteinemic Neuropathies. Dysproteinemias such as cryoglobulinemia, myeloma, amyloidosis, lymphoma, monoclonal gammopathies, and some leukemias are associated with peripheral neuropathy. In patients with idiopathic peripheral neuropathies, a *monoclonal gammopathy* can be identified in up to 10% (Kissel and Mendell, 1996).

Plasma exchange is useful as a treatment option for some of the dysproteinemic neuropathies.

CARCINOMATOUS NEUROPATHIES. Carcinomatous neuropathies may result from direct compression by a solid tumor or local infiltration of nerves. The most common association is lung carcinoma. Some chemotherapeutic agents, such as vincristine and cisplatin, have neurotoxic side effects. The most common presentation is that of a distal sensorimotor polyneuropathy. In up to 16% of patients with lung carcinoma and 4% of those with breast carcinomas, peripheral neuropathy preceded the actual signs of the disease.

CRANIAL NEUROPATHIES

Key Points

- Bell palsy is an acute unilateral paralysis of the facial nerve and involves the forehead muscles.
- Trigeminal neuralgia is usually a unilateral severe lancinating pain lasting a few seconds, triggered by innocuous stimuli (light touch to face, toothbrushing).
- Trigeminal neuralgia is rarely seen in patients younger than 40 years of age.

Many conditions or infections may affect the CNs and cause a peripheral neuropathy. Two common problems encountered by family physicians are idiopathic acute peripheral facial paralysis (Bell palsy) and trigeminal neuralgia (tic douloureux).

IDIOPATHIC ACUTE PERIPHERAL FACIAL PARALYSIS. *Bell palsy* is an acute, unilateral paralysis of the facial nerve of unknown etiology but possibly linked to an antecedent herpes infection (Adour, 1975). Bell palsy is likely the most common isolated cranial neuropathy (23 per 100,000) seen by family physicians (Hauser et al., 1971). Symptoms tend to develop over hours to days and may be associated with recent upper respiratory infection. Symptoms include partial or complete paralysis of the ipsilateral facial muscles, forehead involvement, otalgia, phonophobia, and cephalgia. If the forehead muscles are spared, one must consider a central etiology to the symptoms. Bilateral findings of Bell palsy should prompt consideration of GBS, sarcoidosis, disseminated Lyme disease, or diabetes.

Most patients with Bell palsy recover with only supportive therapy within a few days to a few months. This makes aggressive treatment controversial. A recent meta-analysis showed that whereas high-dose corticosteroids (>450 mg total dose) were associated with greater benefit and decreased risk of unsatisfactory recovery, antiviral agents showed no benefit alone but may have additional benefit when used with corticosteroids (de Almeida et al., 2009). A typical corticosteroid regimen may include oral prednisone, 60 mg/day (or 1 mg/kg/day) for 7 days, then tapering by 10 mg/day, with or without valacyclovir, 1 gram twice daily for 7 days.

KEY TREATMENT

- High-dose corticosteroids (>450 mg total dose) help reduce the risk of unsatisfactory recovery from Bell palsy (de Almeida et al., 2009) (SOR: A).

TRIGEMINAL NEURALGIA. Trigeminal neuralgia (tic douloureux) usually involves the second and third (maxillary and mandibular) divisions of the trigeminal nerve, causing pain of the innervated structures (lips, gums, teeth). It is almost always unilateral, with the pain sudden, sharp, and severe, lasting a few seconds at a time. This cycle of pain can occur hundreds of times a day. It may be described as lancinating, ice pick-like, or an electric shock and characteristically is precipitated by innocuous stimuli such as light touch to the face or toothbrushing. It is rarely seen in patients younger than 40 years. Pain that is longer in duration, bilateral, or described as more aching or pressure-like is usually not related to trigeminal neuralgia and should cause the physician to search for another cause. Other conditions that should be considered include multiple sclerosis (MS), acoustic neurinoma, aneurysm, meningioma, trigeminal neuroma, and early herpes zoster or postherpetic neuralgia. Herpes zoster should be suspected in patients younger than 40 years who present with pain following the upper division of the trigeminal nerve (forehead and eye). Neuroimaging with MRI scanning of the brain is recommended to exclude these causes from idiopathic disease.

A common initial pharmacologic treatment for idiopathic trigeminal neuralgia is carbamazepine (Tegretol), up to 1200 mg/day. Usually, it is started at relatively low doses (100-200 mg once or twice daily) and increased at 7- to 10-day intervals until adequate symptom control is achieved. Other medications that have been used but are not FDA approved include oxcarbazepine (Trileptal), up to 2400 mg/day, gabapentin (Neurontin), amitriptyline, and baclofen. Patients should be educated that these medicines will only work when taken on a consistent basis and not as an analgesic medication. Toxicities from these medications, including allergic reactions, bone marrow suppression, and liver toxicity, may develop and thus require close monitoring. Patients with refractory symptoms or who do not tolerate pharmacologic treatment should be considered for neurosurgical evaluation.

PARKINSON DISEASE

Key Points

- The hallmark clinical features of Parkinson disease include resting tremor, rigidity, and bradykinesia of asymmetric onset.
- Symptoms such as hallucinations, gait abnormalities, paralysis of upward gaze, early dementia, early postural instability, early autonomic dysfunction, involuntary movements other than tremor, and a failure to respond to levodopa suggest a parkinsonism-plus syndrome and require further evaluation.
- Drug therapy for Parkinson disease should be initiated when the symptoms are significant enough to cause functional impairment.

Parkinson disease is the second most common progressive neurodegenerative disorder in the United States after Alzheimer disease. Parkinson affects about 1% of the population older than age 60 years and 4% to 5% of those older than 85 years. The disease is uncommon before age 40 years, and the incidence is higher in men than women. A genetic predisposition to Parkinson disease may be present; up to 15% of patients have a first- or second-degree relative with Parkinson disease. At present, no clear environmental links to Parkinson disease have been identified. The disease is caused by a disruption of dopaminergic neurotransmission in the basal ganglia and the development of eosinophilic intracytoplasmic inclusions (Lewy bodies) in the residual dopaminergic neurons.

Symptoms and Signs

The hallmark clinical features of Parkinson disease include tremor, rigidity, and bradykinesia, usually of asymmetric onset. Tremor is the presenting symptom in up to 70% of patients, and in fact, an asymmetric rest tremor is virtually pathognomonic of Parkinson disease. Many patients present to family physicians complaining of a tremor and the concern they may have Parkinson disease. Most have *essential tremor,* which can be differentiated from the tremor of Parkinson disease in that whereas essential tremor is usually symmetric and exacerbated by action, the tremor of Parkinson disease is usually at rest and asymmetric.

Rigidity is often associated with *cogwheeling,* a ratchety quality during passive movement of the limb. *Bradykinesia* refers to the slowness of movements, which usually begins in an asymmetric fashion, described by the patient as "weakness" of an extremity, although no abnormalities are noted with strength testing. Other clinical features associated with Parkinson disease include micrographia, paucity of facial expression (masked facies), narrow shuffling gait, and postural instability (late finding). Behavioral and cognitive symptoms are frequently seen in patients with Parkinson disease as well.

Differential Diagnosis

Up to 20% of patients initially diagnosed with Parkinson disease ultimately have an alternative diagnosis. The term *parkinsonism-plus syndrome* is used for patients who have similar symptoms but also have additional abnormalities or do not respond to the usual medications. Symptoms that suggest a parkinsonism-plus syndrome include hallucinations, gait abnormalities, paralysis of upward gaze, early dementia, early postural instability, early autonomic dysfunction, involuntary movements other than tremor, and a failure to respond to levodopa (Italian Neurological Society, 2003). Conditions that frequently may be confused with Parkinson disease include progressive supranuclear palsy (PSP), dementia with Lewy bodies, multiple-system atrophy, vascular parkinsonism, and drug-induced parkinsonism.

Progressive supranuclear palsy may initially be mistaken for Parkinson disease. Patients have ophthalmoparesis of vertical gaze, primarily downward gaze. Early loss of postural reflexes, predominantly axial rigidity, pseudobulbar palsy, and frontal lobe signs are other characteristics of PSP. Response to dopaminergic medications is minimal.

Dementia with Lewy bodies has motor symptoms similar to those of Parkinson disease, and there may be a response to levodopa. Rigidity is usually more prominent than bradykinesia or tremor. Additionally, patients have early cognitive impairment and hallucinations early in the disease course.

Multisystem atrophy includes a number of diseases, and it is not clear if they represent distinct diseases or a single, pathologic continuum. This group includes olivopontocerebellar atrophy, striatonigral degeneration, and Shy-Drager syndrome. Symptoms are related to autonomic nervous system dysfunction and include orthostatic hypotension, cerebellar dysfunction, bladder dysfunction, and a poor levodopa response.

Vascular parkinsonism may be associated with multiple vascular lesions in the basal ganglia. There is usually a stepwise progression to the disease. Tremor at rest is not a common finding, and the bradykinesia and rigidity tend to be more significant in the legs. The gait is often broad-based. Associated symptoms include dementia, spasticity, and weakness. MRI studies show multi-infarct changes, and the response to levodopa is poor.

A final category of Parkinson-like conditions is *drug-induced parkinsonism.* It is important to identify this cause because it is usually reversible. Drug-induced parkinsonism accounted for 20% of cases of parkinsonism-plus conditions in a population-based study (Bower et al., 1999). Medications that can cause these symptoms include neuroleptics, atypical neuroleptics, antiemetic medications (e.g., metoclopramide, prochlorperazine), amiodarone, valproic acid, and lithium. Medicines that block the synthesis of dopamine, such as methyldopa (Aldomet), or deplete dopamine (e.g., reserpine) can also induce parkinsonism (Nutt and Wooten, 2005).

Diagnostic Evaluation

An extensive diagnostic evaluation is not necessary when the history and physical examination reveal classic findings of Parkinson disease. Imaging of the brain with CT or MRI may be performed if the diagnosis is in question and to rule out other conditions such as NPH or vascular parkinsonism. Consultation with a neurologist may be helpful, especially if the diagnosis is in question or a parkinsonism-plus diagnosis is likely.

Treatment

Currently, diagnosis of Parkinson disease does not relegate a patient to pharmacologic treatment. Drug therapy should be initiated when the symptoms are significant enough to cause functional impairment (Rao et al., 2006). Current therapies do not appear to slow the progression of the disease, and no studies have clearly demonstrated a best initial treatment for this condition (Schreck et al., 2003). Table 41-39 summarizes the pharmacologic agents available to treat Parkinson disease.

Pharmacotherapy. *Levodopa,* a precursor of dopamine, is the most frequently prescribed agent for the treatment of symptomatic Parkinson disease and is particularly effective at controlling bradykinesia and rigidity (Miyasaki et al., 2002). Alone, levodopa is absorbed but is peripherally metabolized to dopamine by dopa-decarboxylase enzymes. This peripheral conversion limits the overall effectiveness of levodopa and increases the side effects, including nausea, vomiting, and hypotension. To remedy this, levodopa is combined with carbidopa, which prevents this peripheral conversion. Dopa-decarboxylase is saturated with 70 to 100 mg of carbidopa. Thus the usual starting dose of

Table 41-39 Medications for Parkinson Disease

Generic Name	Recommended Dosage	Side Effects/Comments
ANTICHOLINERGICS		
Trihexyphenidyl (Artane)	1 mg TID; increase to 2 mg TID	Effective for tremor Side effects include impaired memory, blurred vision, urinary retention
Benztropine (Cogentin)	0.5 mg at bedtime; increase by 0.5 mg up to a maximum of 6 mg/day	Same as for trihexyphenidyl
CARBIDOPA–LEVODOPA COMBINATIONS		
Immediate release (Sinemet)	25 mg/100 mg initially ½ tablet TID; increase by ½ tablet every 4-7 days up to 1 tablet TID to QID	"Gold standard" of therapy Long-term therapy may result in motor fluctuations, dyskinesias, confusion, hallucinations
Controlled release (Sinemet-CR)	1 tablet BID	Same as for immediate release
Carbidopa–levodopa plus entacapone (Stalevo)	1 tablet TID (dosage based on titration of individual components)	Same as for other carbidopa–levodopa preparations, plus diarrhea
CATECHOL-O-METHYLTRANSFERASE INHIBITORS		
Tolcapone (Tasmar)	100 mg or 200 mg TID	Adjunct to levodopa to prevent motor fluctuations Monitor liver functions
Entacapone (Comtan)	200 mg with each dose of carbidopa–levodopa, up to 8 tabs (1600 mg) daily	Same as for tolcapone
DOPAMINE AGONISTS		
Bromocriptine (Parlodel)	1.25 mg with meals BID; increase by 2.5 mg every 2-4 wk to a maximum of 15 mg/day	Effective in monotherapy or as an adjunct to levodopa
Pramipexole (Mirapex)	0.125 mg TID; maximum, 1.5 mg TID	Side effects include excessive daytime somnolence, hypotension, confusion, hallucinations
Ropinirole (ReQuip)	0.25 mg TID; increase weekly by 0.25 mg TID to 3 mg TID Maximum dose, 8 mg TID	Same as for pramipexole
Rotigotine (Neupro)	Start 2 mg/24 hr patch daily; may increase by 2 mg weekly to a maximum of 6 mg/24 hr (start with 4 mg/24 hr to a maximum of 8 mg/24 hr for severe disease)	Contains sulfites; remove before MRI or cardioversion Side effects: sleep attacks, hypotension, psychosis, application site reactions
MONOAMINE OXIDASE TYPE B INHIBITORS		
Selegiline (Eldepryl)	5 mg at breakfast and lunch	Avoid use with SSRIs, TCAs, and meperidine Side effects: nausea, dizziness, hallucinations, abdominal pain, vivid dreams
Rasagiline (Azilect)	0.5 mg/day to 1 mg/day	Side effects: extrapyramidal symptoms, dyskinesia, hallucinations, hypotension, depression
N-METHYL-D-ASPARTATE ANTAGONIST (RECEPTOR INHIBITOR)		
Amantadine (Symmetrel)	100 mg twice daily	May be used as monotherapy Side effects: dizziness, confusion, livedo reticularis, hallucinations

BID, Twice a day; *MRI,* magnetic resonance imaging; *QID,* four times daily; *SSRI,* selective serotonin reuptake inhibitor; *TCA,* tricyclic antidepressant; *TID,* three times daily.

carbidopa–levodopa is 25 mg/100 mg three times daily (Rao et al., 2006).

Dopamine agonists directly stimulate dopamine receptors, thus bypassing the presynaptic synthesis of dopamine. These medications cause less dyskinesia and fewer fluctuations than levodopa. They can be used alone or in conjunction with levodopa. Currently, bromocriptine (Parlodel), pramipexole (Mirapex), and ropinirole (ReQuip) are oral medications in this class. Transdermal rotigotine (Neupro) is a once-daily patch available for the treatment of Parkinson disease. Apomorphine (Apokyn) is also available as a SC injection for the treatment of sudden, resistant "off" periods (Goetz et al., 2005). It has significant adverse effects and should only be used by individuals experienced with its use. Dopamine agonists should not be used in patients with dementia because of the high likelihood of producing hallucinations (Nutt and Wooten, 2005).

Monoamine oxidase type B (MAO-B) *inhibitors* were initially thought to provide a neuroprotective effect to patients with Parkinson disease. This has not been supported in the literature. Agents available in the United States in this class include selegiline (Eldepryl), orally disintegrating selegiline (Zelapar), and rasagiline (Azilect). A meta-analysis of 17 trials comparing MAO-B inhibitors with placebo or levodopa revealed that MAO inhibitors reduce disability, the incidence of motor fluctuations, and the need for levodopa (Ives et al., 2004).

Anticholinergic medications primarily work on the muscarinic acetylcholine receptors. These medications have low effectiveness and a high incidence of side effects, which limit their overall usefulness to patients younger than 70 years and with preserved cognitive function.

Degradation of levodopa in the periphery is known to be associated with motor fluctuations and dyskinesia in

Parkinson disease. The enzyme catechol-*O*-methyltransferase (COMT) is responsible for part of this degradation. *COMT inhibitors* prolong the dopamine response. Two medications in this category are tolcapone (Tasmar) and entacapone (Comtan). These medications reduced "off" time, reduced total levodopa dose, and improved motor symptoms in patients with advanced Parkinson disease and motor complications (Cochrane review; Deane et al., 2004). As such, COMT inhibitors are usually reserved for more advanced cases.

Among *NMDA antagonists* (NMDA receptor inhibitors), amantadine (Symmetrel), originally developed as an antiviral agent, is useful for tremor, rigidity, and bradykinesia associated with Parkinson disease, although few studies demonstrate its clear efficacy. Amantadine may also have a dopamine agonist effect as well as an anticholinergic effect. Side effects include dizziness, insomnia, nausea, and vomiting.

Surgical Treatment. Surgical treatments are options to be considered when tremor, motor fluctuations, and dyskinesia are not adequately controlled with medications alone. Early techniques such as unilateral pallidotomy or thalamotomy have fallen out of favor because of their irreversible nature. There is long-term, high-quality evidence for deep brain stimulation of the globus pallidus interna or subthalamic nucleus for improvement of motor features or stimulation of the thalamic ventralis intermedius for improvement of tremors (Fasano et al., 2012). Stimulation of other targeted centers needs further study. Patients with symptoms not controlled medically should be referred to specialized centers with surgeons experienced in performing these procedures.

Treatment of Nonmotor Symptoms. Patients with Parkinson disease frequently develop other comorbid conditions such as depression or dementia. In the case of depression, an SSRI can be used. Up to 40% of patients develop dementia (Aarsland et al., 2003). In these patients, the cholinesterase inhibitors can be effective. Parkinson disease is a progressive illness, so it is important for the family physician to discuss advanced directives, establishment of power of attorney for health care decisions, and the patient's wishes surrounding the use of artificial nutrition. Living wills and other legal documents should be prepared and appropriate discussions documented. Common symptoms such as constipation, sleep disturbance, and orthostatic hypotension should be aggressively treated.

KEY TREATMENT

- Levodopa, dopamine agonists, and MAO-B inhibitors, alone or in combination, are effective in treating the symptoms of Parkinson disease (Rao et al., 2006) (SOR: A).
- The usual starting dosage of carbidopa–levodopa is 25 mg/100 mg three times daily (Rao et al., 2006) (SOR: A).
- Surgical therapies (deep brain stimulation) are effective when medical therapy fails to control Parkinson symptoms (Fasano et al., 2012) (SOR: A).

MULTIPLE SCLEROSIS

Key Points

- The diagnosis of MS requires evidence of demyelinating disseminated disease.
- Optic neuritis, nystagmus from internuclear ophthalmoplegia, and Lhermitte sign are highly suggestive of MS.
- The currently most widely accepted diagnostic criteria for MS are the McDonald criteria, established by an international panel in 2001 and revised in 2005 and 2010.

Multiple sclerosis is a recurrent, chronic, demyelinating autoimmune disorder that affects the CNS. The mean age of onset for MS is 29 to 33 years, although the range is 15 to 50 years, which makes this the most common cause of neurologic disability in young adults.

Diagnosis

The diagnosis of MS is based on clinical signs and symptoms combined with diagnostic testing, which may include MRI, CSF analysis, and visual-evoked potentials (VEPs). Definitive diagnosis of MS requires evidence of demyelinating disease consisting of at least two attacks, disseminated over time and space (Polman et al., 2011). That is, clinical symptoms should last at least 24 hours in the absence of fever or infection and should be separated in time, and they should affect two different areas of the CNS: the brain, spinal cord, or optic nerves. The clinical symptoms vary, depending on which part of the CNS is involved. Three symptoms are highly suggestive of MS: optic neuritis, nystagmus resulting from internuclear ophthalmoplegia, and Lhermitte sign, which is an electrical sensation extending down the back and legs with flexion of the neck. The International Panel of the Diagnosis of Multiple Sclerosis developed criteria for the diagnosis of MS (McDonald et al., 2001), revised in 2005 and 2010 and summarized in Table 41-40 (Polman et al., 2011). It is important to remember that alternative diagnoses should be considered and excluded. These include CNS vasculitis, paraneoplastic syndromes, sarcoidosis, leukodystrophies, CNS tumors, infections, CNS lymphoma, and nutritional deficiencies (e.g., vitamin B_{12} deficiency). Neuromyelitis optica is considered a separate, although similar, entity in which there is demyelination predominantly in the spinal cord, often over multiple segments, in conjunction with unilateral or bilateral optic neuritis. Brain MRI is often normal and serum aquaporin-4 (AQP4) antibodies are detectable.

The precise relationship between clinical symptoms and MR findings is not well understood. Thus, MRI alone is not useful in predicting the clinical course of MS. T2-weighted MR images best define the size of white matter lesions, and gadolinium can reveal the disruption of the blood–brain barrier associated with an active MS lesion. In general, MR findings can be used to demonstrate evidence for dissemination in space and time when these features cannot be reliably determined clinically, such as when there is a clinically isolated syndrome. Dissemination in space is demonstrated by at least one lesion in two or more

Table 41-40 Criteria for Multiple Sclerosis

Clinical Presentation	Additional Data Needed
Two or more attacks (relapses); two or more objective clinical lesions	None; clinical evidence suffices (additional evidence desirable but must be consistent with MS)
Two or more attacks; one objective clinical lesion	Dissemination in space demonstrated by at least one T2 MRI lesion in at least two of four areas of the CNS
One attack; two or more objective clinical lesions	Dissemination in time demonstrated by a new T2- or gadolinium-enhancing lesion on follow-up MRI or simultaneous presence of asymptomatic gadolinium-enhancing and nonenhancing lesions at any time
One attack; one objective clinical lesion (monosymptomatic presentation)	Dissemination in space demonstrated by MRI findings described above *and* Dissemination in time demonstrated by MRI findings described above
Insidious neurologic progression suggestive of MS (primary progressive MS)	At least 1 year of progression of disease and two of the following three criteria: ■ Positive CSF ■ Dissemination in space demonstrated by MRI evidence of at least one T2 lesion in the periventricular, juxtacortical, or infratentorial region ■ At least two T2 cord lesions

CSF, Cerebrospinal fluid; *MRI,* magnetic resonance imaging; *MS,* multiple sclerosis.
Modified from McDonald WI, Compston A, Edan G, et al. Recommended diagnostic criteria for multiple sclerosis: guidelines from the International Panel on the Diagnosis of Multiple Sclerosis. *Ann Neurol.* 200;150:121.

regions of the CNS, which include the periventricular, juxtacortical, infratentorial, and spinal cord regions. Gadolinium enhancement is no longer a requirement. MRI criteria for dissemination in time are a new T2 or gadolinium-enhancing lesion on repeat MRI compared with a prior MRI (a 30-day interval is no longer necessary) or a single MRI study with simultaneous asymptomatic enhancing and nonenhancing lesions.

The CSF analysis of patients with MS generally demonstrates a normal opening pressure, cell count, glucose level, protein level, and culture. The most clinically useful CSF abnormality is the presence of oligoclonal immunoglobulin G (IgG) bands resulting from intrathecal IgG synthesis, which can be found in up to 90% of patients with MS (Freedman et al., 2005). IgG bands are not specific to MS and are also seen in sarcoidosis, AIDS, and subacute sclerosis panencephalitis. The value of CSF analysis is mainly limited to MS patients with only a few lesions on MRI or to make the diagnosis of primary progressive MS, as discussed later. Visual-evoked responses may also provide supporting evidence for MS, particularly in situations with few abnormalities on MRI. Other VEP analysis offers little in establishing a diagnosis of MS (Gronseth and Ashman, 2000).

Clinical Course

Four subtypes of MS are currently described: relapsing remitting, secondary progressive, primary progressive, and progressive relapsing. *Relapsing-remitting* MS accounts for about 85% of the initial diagnosis of MS patients and is characterized by acute attacks followed by full recovery. The interval between relapses can be variable and is characterized by a lack of disease progression. *Secondary-progressive* MS is characterized by a pattern that is initially relapsing remitting but then evolves into a pattern of progressive neurologic decline. MRI demonstrates more extensive lesions, and approximately 50% of patients initially diagnosed with relapsing-remitting MS will develop secondary-progressive disease. *Primary-progressive* MS, characterized by a gradual disease progression over at least 1 year from the initial onset, accounts for approximately 10% of MS diagnoses and has limited treatment options. Dissemination in space is demonstrated by at least one T2 lesion in the periventricular, juxtacortical, or infratentorial areas or at least two T2 lesions in the spinal cord, as well as the presence of oligoclonal bands in the CSF. *Progressive-relapsing* MS demonstrates a pattern of steady progression from the time of onset that may be punctuated by clearly defined relapses. The patients may or may not fully recover from these acute relapses.

Treatment

The treatment of MS can be divided into disease-modifying therapies, medications for acute relapses, and symptomatic management. Although there is no definitive cure, disease-modifying therapies may reduce the frequency of relapses, slow the rate of progression, and reduce the acute inflammatory response. Symptomatic therapy can improve the control of many of the functional disabilities and thus improve quality of life.

Disease-Modifying Therapies. It is generally held that disease-modifying therapy should be initiated immediately on the diagnosis of MS (Coyle and Hartung, 2002). Disease-modifying therapy has been shown to be more effective in preventing new lesion formation than repairing old lesions. These therapies include interferon β-1b (Betaseron, Extavia), interferon β-1a (Avonex, Rebif), and glatiramer acetate (Copaxone). The β interferons are immunomodulating medications that also have antiviral activities. They have been shown to reduce relapses in patients with the relapsing-remitting form of MS. Betaseron is given as an alternating-day SC injection, Rebif is a three-times-weekly SC injection, and Avonex is administered as a weekly intramuscular injection. All have similar side effects, including injection site reactions, influenza-like symptoms, and worsening of preexisting depression. Bone marrow suppression and transient elevation of liver enzymes may also occur.

Glatiramer (Copaxone) is a synthetic polypeptide consisting of four amino acids. It is thought to lead to the induction of antigen-specific suppressor T cells. It is administered as a daily SC injection and has been shown to reduce relapses by approximately 30% (Comi et al., 2001). Side effects include postinjection reactions and occasionally a reaction involving flushing, chest pain, anxiety, and dyspnea. The reaction is self-limited and does not require discontinuation of the medication.

Several orally administered disease-modifying treatments are now available. These include fingolimod (Gilenya), teriflunomide (Aubagio), and dimethyl fumarate (Tecfidera). Of these, fingolimod and teriflunomide require monitoring of baseline CBC and LFTs as well as other indices before the start of treatment because of associated toxicities.

Two other disease-modifying drugs for MS are mitoxantrone and natalizumab. Mitoxantrone is a synthetic anthracenedione given by IV infusion once every 3 months. It has been shown to reduce MS relapses by 67% (Hartung et al., 2002). Mitoxantrone is blue and can lead to transient bluish discoloration of the sclera and urine. It also can cause cardiotoxicity and as a chemotherapeutic agent should only be prescribed for worsening cases of MS not responding to first-line agents. Only health care professionals exprienced in the use of cytotoxic chemotherapy agents should administer mitoxantrone.

Natalizumab is a monoclonal antibody that blocks α_4-integrin. This molecule is involved in moving circulating leukocytes into the brain in response to inflammation. It is administered as a 1-hour infusion every 4 weeks. Natalizumab has been shown to reduce clinical relapses, slow the progression of disability, and reduce the development of new brain lesions (Polman et al., 2006). Complications that limit its use include a hypersensitivity reaction up to 1 hour after infusion. Natalizumab has also been associated with progressive multifocal leukoencephalopathy, a destructive brain infection caused by JC virus. Therefore, the distribution and use of natalizumab is closely monitored, and it can be administered only by registered physicians.

One treatment that has no prophylactic benefit but does potentially improve function is dalfampridine (Ampyra). Its effect is to facilitate nerve conduction by blocking potassium channels, which in the affected axon tend to function in an aberrant fashion. The result is improved motor function, typically assessed by a 25-foot timed walk. There is a risk of seizures, particularly with overdosing, so patients with coexisting epilepsy should not receive dalfampridine.

Medications for Acute Relapses. Glucocorticoids are still widely used for the treatment of acute exacerbations of MS. The principal effects of corticosteroids appear to be related to their antiinflammatory and antiedema effects. It is recommended as standard therapy for any patient with an acute attack of MS (Goodin et al., 2002). Treatment normally consists of 3 to 5 days of a 1-g/day IV infusion of methylprednisolone. Oral prednisone taper may or may not be used after infusion.

Symptomatic Management. Medications used for symptomatic management depend on the specific symptoms encountered by the patient. MS patients frequently develop spasticity, which can be treated with baclofen, tizanidine, or benzodiazepines. Physical therapy can also help with spasticity. Bladder dysfunction can also occur in patients with MS. New bladder symptoms should be evaluated with a urine culture to rule out infection. A postvoid residual should also be obtained, as well as urodynamic testing to determine whether the problem is overflow incontinence from urinary retention or urge incontinence from detrusor instability. In the presence of urge incontinence, the anticholinergics oxybutynin (Ditropan) and tolterodine (Detrol) may be useful. If the problem is urinary retention and overflow incontinence, patients will usually need to be treated with intermittent self-catheterization. Patients may also experience depression, constipation, and sexual dysfunction. The usual evaluation and treatment options should be considered for patients who experience these problems.

KEY TREATMENT

- Both β interferons as well as newly available oral medications have been shown to reduce the number of relapses in patients with the relapsing-remitting form of MS (Coyle and Hartung, 2002) (SOR: A).
- Glucocorticoids are recommended as standard therapy for any patient with an acute attack of MS (Goodin et al., 2002) (SOR: A).
- Disease-modifying therapy should begin at diagnosis of MS (Coyle and Hartung, 2002) (SOR: B).

References

The complete reference list is available at www.expertconsult.com.

Web Resources

www.cdc.gov/vaccines/schedules/index.html Centers for Disease Control and Prevention's recommended immunization schedule.

neuromuscular.wustl.edu/ Washington University Neuromuscular Disease Center. A comprehensive resource for disorders affecting the peripheral nerves, muscles, and neuromuscular junction.

www.aan.com American Academy of Neurology's practice parameters and neurologic news.

www.strokecenter.org/trials/ Internet Stroke Center. Updated resource for ongoing and completed trials related to stroke.

42 *Human Sexuality*

WENDY S. BIGGS and SULABHA CHAGANABOYANA

Overview

Sexuality is a fundamental aspect of human self-concept and a complex biopsychosocial process. Physiologic aspects of sexuality are interpreted within the patient's cultural and social context. Family physicians and primary care providers are well situated to offer patients basic information regarding human sexual health issues and to evaluate and treat most common sexual problems; however, they seldom ask patients about sexual functioning. This chapter describes the basic principles of evaluation of female and male sexual dysfunction and clinical management of common disorders.

SEXUAL SELF-CONCEPT

Humans possess a gender identity and a sexual orientation. *Gender* is the publicly and usually legally recognized perception of an individual as male or female and often is synonymous with chromosomal or genital phenotype (male or female sex). Gender when assigned at birth is an individual's "natal gender." *Gender identity* is a social identity, an internal self-perception of being male or female, masculine or feminine, or occasionally a category neither male nor female. Individuals may be androphilic (sexually attracted to men) or gynephilic (sexually attracted to women) toward sexual partners of their own or the other gender. If desired sexual partners are their own gender, individuals may self-identify as gay or lesbian or, if both genders, bisexual. Someone who falls outside the societal norms of gender or sexual attraction may self-identify as "queer," a more fluid or inclusive term for gender or sexual attraction (or both). Although many people remain either androphilic or gynephilic their entire lives, some individuals may have different predominant sexual attractions at different times in their lives. The terms "men who have sex with men" (MSM) and "women who have sex with women" (WSW) are used because the sexual activity defines the risks, not the gender identity.

MODELS OF HUMAN SEXUAL RESPONSE

Masters and Johnson first described the physiology of the "human sexual response cycle" in 1966. Based on the physical components of sexual functioning, they described four phases of the sexual response cycle: excitement, plateau, orgasm, and resolution (Figure 42-1). Helen Singer Kaplan subsequently described a more subjective, psychologically oriented sexual responsiveness model with three phases: desire, excitement, and orgasm. Nonlinear alternative models have been suggested, especially for women's sexual response (Basson and Schultz, 2007) (Figure 42-2). In certain settings, men may have similar nonlinear sexual responses.

INITIAL EVALUATION OF SEXUAL PROBLEMS

Many patients would benefit from detection and treatment of sexual problems; however, many clinicians do not ask, and patients may not volunteer the information. In the Global Study of Sexual Attitudes and Behaviors (GSSAB), which surveyed more than 27,000 adults age 40 to 80 years in 29 countries, 49% of women and 43% of men reported experiencing at least one sexual problem; fewer than 20% had sought medical assistance for sexual issues (Moreira et al., 2005). Health care providers should proactively and routinely address sexual health.

The sexual health interview may be approached with a screening or abbreviated method followed by in-depth questioning if necessary (Table 42-1). The answers on the detailed sexual history then direct the physical examination and appropriate laboratory testing. A physician may open the sexual history questioning with an *inclusion* technique. "Sexual health is important to overall health, so I ask all my patients about it. I'm going to ask you a few questions on sexual matters now." The clinician can use *normalization*, introducing emotionally laden or difficult subjects by implying these experiences are quite prevalent: "Many people have been sexually abused or molested as children. Did you have any experiences like that when you were young?" *Universalization* phrases questions as if everyone has done everything, making an affirmative answer easier for sensitive questions. For example, patients may be asked, "How often do you masturbate?" instead of "Do you masturbate?" The clinician should also reassure the patient about physician- or clinician-patient confidentiality. Physicians should avoid terms that make assumptions regarding patients' sexual behaviors. When inquiring about past or recent sexual encounters, the clinician may inquire "with men, women, or both?" Using the term "partner" instead of "husband," "boyfriend," "wife," or "girlfriend" may allow patients to discuss their sexual orientation openly. Slang words should be redefined in medical terminology so that the clinician and patient may communicate clearly.

In 1976, Jack Annon proposed the PLISSIT model to approach sexual concerns: permission, limited information, specific suggestions, and intensive treatment (Table 42-2). Many clinical cases can be managed with brief education or limited advice, such as discussing normal physiologic sexual changes with aging or recommending books or products (e.g., water-based lubricant for vaginal dryness). When a referral has been made, scheduled follow-up visits support the patient during the process. Counseling may be extremely important, and the physician should research

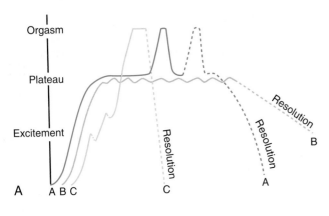

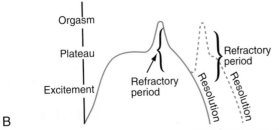

Figure 42-1 Female (**A**) and male (**B**) sexual response cycles. Desire precedes both cycles in this model. The phases illustrated are excitement, plateau, and orgasm. The length of the plateau phase is variable. Women may have a brief plateau followed by orgasm (cycle *C*) or a long plateau with no orgasm (cycle *B*). Women may have multiple orgasms before resolution, although many do not (cycle *A*). For men with premature ejaculation, the plateau phase is brief. After ejaculation, men enter a refractory period lasting minutes to hours during which they are unable to ejaculate.

Table 42-1 Questions for a Detailed Sexual History

Are you currently sexually active? Have you ever been sexually active?
Are your sexual partners men, women, or both?
How many sexual partners have you had in the past month? Past 6 months? Lifetime?
How satisfied are you with your (or your partner's) sexual functioning?
Has there been any change in your (or your partner's) sexual desire or the frequency of sexual activity?
Do you have, or have you ever had, any risk factors for HIV (blood transfusion, needle stick injuries, IV drug use, STIs, partners who placed you at risk)?
Have you ever had any sexually related diseases?
Have you ever been tested for HIV? Would you like to be?
What do you do to protect yourself from contracting HIV?
What method do you use for contraception?
Are you trying to become pregnant (or father a child)?
Do you participate in oral sex? Anal sex?
Do you or your partner(s) use any particular devices or substances to enhance your sexual pleasure?
Do you ever have pain with intercourse?
Women: Do you have any difficulty achieving orgasm?
Men: Do you have any difficulty obtaining and maintaining an erection? Difficulty with ejaculation?
Do you have any questions or concerns about your sexual functioning?
Is there anything about your (or your partner's) sexual activity (as individuals or as a couple) that you would like to change?

HIV, Human immunodeficiency virus; *IV,* intravenous; *STI,* sexually transmitted infection.
From Nusbaum MRH, Hamilton CD. The proactive sexual health history. *Am Fam Physician.* 2002;66:1705-1712.

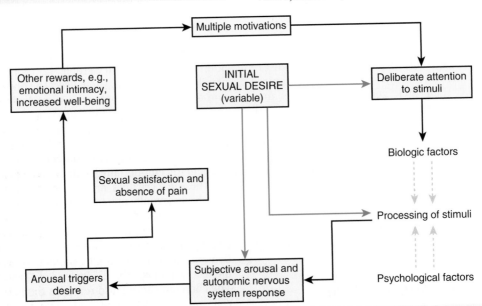

Figure 42-2 Circular model of female sexual response showing cycle of overlapping phases. (From Basson R, Schultz WW. Sexual sequelae of general medical disorders. *Lancet.* 2007;369:409-424.)

Table 42-2 PLISSIT Model for Approaching Sexual Problems

Permission	For physician to discuss sex with the patient For the patient to discuss concerns now or in the future To continue sexual behaviors not potentially harmful
Limited information	Clarify misinformation. Dispel myths. Provide factual information in a limited manner.
Specific suggestions	Provide specific suggestions directly related to the particular problem.
Intensive treatment	Provide highly individualized therapy for more complex issues.

Modified from Annon JS. *The behavioral treatment of sexual problems.* Honolulu: Enabling System; 1974-1975.

Table 42-3 Female Sexual Interest/Arousal Disorder

To be diagnosed with female sexual interest/ arousal disorder, a woman needs to lack or have significantly reduced sexual interest/arousal for at least a 6-month duration manifested by at least three of the following six criteria:	1. Absent or reduced interest in sexual activity 2. Absent or reduced sexual or erotic thoughts or fantasies 3. No or reduced initiation of sexual activity and typically unreceptive a partner's attempts to initiate 4. Absent or reduced sexual excitement and pleasure during sexual activity in almost all or all sexual encounters (in identified situational contexts or, if generalized, in all contexts) 5. Absent or reduced sexual interest or arousal in response to any internal or external sexual or erotic cues 6. Absent or reduced genital or nongenital sensations during sexual activity in almost all or all sexual encounters

local resources. The American Association of Sexuality Educators, Counselors and Therapists (AASECT) may be contacted for referral information (http://www.aasect.org).

the normal decrease in sexual response associated with aging and needs education, not a diagnosis of sexual dysfunction.

Sexual Dysfunction

Sexual functioning involves interactions among the physical, mental, and emotional aspects of an individual. The categorization outlined by the *Diagnostic and Statistical Manual of Mental Disorders,* fifth edition (DSM-5) is used to define sexual dysfunctions. To be a "disorder," the condition must cause the individual "clinically significant distress"; if an individual's sexual response or functioning is outside of the statistical norm but does not cause the person distress, it is not a disorder. The DSM-5 describes subtypes to designate the onset or situation of the sexual dysfunction. Sexual dysfunctions may be "lifelong," existing since the individual became sexually active, or "acquired," appearing after an interval of normal sexual functioning. The sexual dysfunction may be "generalized" or "situational," occurring in all instances or only with certain types of stimulation, situations, or partners, respectively. The DSM-5 also suggests defining the severity of the dysfunction as "mild," "moderate," or "severe" based on the distress of the individual regarding the dysfunction.

When evaluating a patient complaining of sexual dysfunction, a number of factors that may contribute solely or collectively to the individual's sexual dysfunction need to be considered: (1) partner factors, such as a partner's involvement or sexual response; (2) relationship factors, such as poor communication or emotional abuse; (3) individual vulnerability factors (e.g., body image), psychiatric comorbidity (e.g., depression, anxiety), and life stressors (e.g., unemployment); (4) cultural or religious factors; and (5) medical factors, such as physical disability or medications. Before a sexual dysfunction is diagnosed, the clinician must rule out that the patient's perceived sexual dysfunction is not better explained by a medical condition or treatment for a medical condition, such as a medication, or by a mental health disorder, such as depression. In addition, an individual's understanding of sexual functioning must be assessed. Occasionally, a patient complaining of a sexual dysfunction simply lacks the knowledge about effective modes of sexual stimulation or an understanding of

Female Sexual Dysfunction

Key Points

- Female sexual interest/arousal disorder in the DSM-5 recognizes the interaction between desire and arousal as the trigger for a woman's sexual response.
- Psychosocial interventions may be efficacious for the treatment of female sexual dysfunction.
- Selective serotonin reuptake inhibitor (SSRI) antidepressants delay or inhibit orgasm in women.
- The prevalence of genito-pelvic pain/penetration disorder ranges from 12% to 21% in the United States.

FEMALE SEXUAL INTEREST/AROUSAL DISORDER

For women, low sexual interest is the most frequently reported sexual problem. Four in 10 women state they have low sexual desire. The lack of or low sexual desire may not be distressing for all women; "distress" prevalence ranges in studies from 23% to 61% (Lindau et al., 2007; Shifren et al., 2008). Whereas in the DSM-IV-TR, women distressed by low or lacking sexual desire were diagnosed with "hypoactive sexual desire disorder," the DSM-5 recognizes the complex interaction between sexual interest and arousal in women and defines "female sexual interest/ arousal disorder." To be diagnosed with female sexual interest/arousal disorder, a woman needs to lack or have significantly reduced sexual interest or arousal for at least a 6-month duration manifested by at least three of six criteria (Table 42-3).

Female sexual desire is a complex interaction among biologic, psychological, social, interpersonal, and environmental components. Ovarian function, especially ovarian androgens, may play an important role. In women age 20 to 49 years, low or lacking sexual interest/arousal disorder is almost threefold more likely in surgical postmenopausal women than premenopausal women (Leiblum et al., 2006). Life stressors, health problems, and personality may play significant roles in the decrease in sexual interest or arousal of postmenopausal women, perhaps even more than the hormonal changes themselves (Ornat et al., 2013). Medical illnesses, such as thyroid disease, chronic pain conditions, urinary incontinence, and depression or anxiety, may negatively impact sexual interest or arousal. Medications can affect sexual interest or arousal, especially SSRI antidepressants, antihypertensives, antipsychotics, and narcotics. Fear of pregnancy or sexually transmitted infection (STI) and discord or communication difficulty in a couple's relationship may diminish sexual interest or arousal. The clinician must explore all aspects of the bio-psychosocial model when evaluating a woman distressed by her sexual interest or arousal functioning.

Evaluation

Evaluation for female sexual interest/arousal disorder includes a thorough history and physical examination to detect any gynecologic, neurologic, cardiovascular, or endocrine disorders. Laboratory testing should include thyroid function, fasting glucose, lipid profile, and liver function. If a hormonal problem is suspected, prolactin, total and free testosterone, sex hormone–binding globulin, dehydroepiandrosterone (DHEA), and estrogen levels may be drawn. Androgen levels in premenopausal women should be measured at the peak on days 8 to 10 of a 28-day menstrual cycle.

Treatment

The U.S. Food and Drug Administration (FDA) has not approved any medication specifically for treatment of female sexual interest/arousal disorder. Estrogen therapy improves vaginal dryness but may not affect sexual interest. For women within 5 years of amenorrhea (early menopause), treatment with estrogens alone or in combination with progestogens was associated with a small to moderate improvement in sexual function, particularly in pain (Nastri et al., 2013). Because the lack of ovarian androgens is implicated in sexual interest and arousal, testosterone replacement has been investigated for women. No FDA-approved testosterone formulation exists at the time of this writing. A randomized controlled trial (RCT) of sildenafil in postmenopausal women with SSRI-associated sexual dysfunction demonstrated a significant improvement in delayed orgasm and arousal (lubrication) but no improvement in desire (Nurnberg et al., 2008). In small studies, bupropion improves sexual interest and arousal in pre-menopausal women and women taking SSRIs (Segraves et al., 2004). The FDA-approved Eros Clitoral Therapy Device uses a silicon cup to apply a vacuum to increase blood flow to the clitoris and surrounding tissue. The device appears effective in women without detectable disease and after radiation treatment for cervical cancer (Munarriz et al., 2003; Schroder et al., 2005), although sample sizes have been small.

Given the lack of effective allopathic treatment for low or lacking sexual interest and arousal, many women turn to complementary and alternative therapies. Compared with placebo, daily local intravaginal application of prasterone (DHEA) for 12 weeks improved desire and interest, arousal, orgasm, and pain at sexual activity in 216 postmenopausal women with moderate to severe symptoms of vaginal atrophy (Labrie et al., 2009). Limited data exist for Ginkgo biloba, damiana leaf, ginseng, and other proprietary herbal blends that are marketed to improve female sexual interest and arousal (Simon, 2009). A review found psychosocial interventions in most published studies were reported efficacious for the treatment of female sexual dysfunction; however, the studies were heterogeneous and few in number, with multiple limitations (Gunzler and Berner, 2012).

FEMALE ORGASMIC DISORDER

Women demonstrate a wide range of orgasmic function, both subjectively and objectively. For a diagnosis of orgasmic disorder, women must have experienced a marked delay in orgasm, marked infrequency of or absence of orgasm, and markedly reduced intensity of orgasmic sensations over a 6-month time frame. Orgasmic dysfunction, the inability to reach orgasm when desired, may be lifelong or acquired. Some women may believe they have lifelong orgasmic disorder because, unlike many men, they do not reach orgasm solely with vaginal intercourse. A basic description of physical orgasm (i.e., pleasurable sensation in the genital area and contractions of the vagina followed by a feeling of physical and psychological relaxation) may facilitate discussion of orgasm. Many women prefer simultaneous vaginal and clitoral stimulation, oral-genital sex, or clitoral stimulation alone to have an orgasm and do not have an orgasmic disorder. In addition, the individual must express clinically significant distress regarding the diminished orgasmic sensations for an orgasmic disorder to be diagnosed.

In both lifelong and acquired orgasmic dysfunction, it is important to ask about past or current experiences of violence, victimization, and abuse. Social factors also affect a woman's experience of orgasm. Women taught negative messages regarding sexuality or with strict religious or cultural prohibitions on sexual attraction and thoughts may experience orgasmic difficulty even if the specified conditions for sexual behavior (e.g., marriage) have been fulfilled. Acquired orgasmic disorder can be caused by other medical illnesses and contributing contextual factors.

Evaluation

The clinical history in acquired orgasmic disorder should focus on the patient's perception of this dysfunction, including the time and circumstances of onset, possible causes, effect on relationship(s), and treatment goals. Physiologic functioning during sexual stimulation, including adequacy of lubrication and ability to sustain states of high arousal, should be explored. Contributing factors such as fatigue, depression, stress, substance abuse, and other medical illnesses should be considered. Contextual and relationship issues, including the possibility of abuse, should be discussed. Medications, especially SSRIs, may delay or inhibit orgasm in women. In most cases of orgasmic dysfunction, no specific physical examination or laboratory testing is necessary.

Treatment

Treatment of female orgasmic disorder usually involves increasing knowledge and sexual options for the patient and partner. Masturbation may provide information about sexual responsiveness and preferred stimulations. Partner education regarding clitoral stimulation and adequate pre-intercourse lovemaking (foreplay) can change the focus from intercourse to mutual pleasuring, spontaneity, and sexual satisfaction. Referral for more in-depth therapy is indicated if the evaluation reveals significant relationship dysfunction, past abuse, or other severe medical or psychosocial complications.

GENITO-PELVIC PAIN/PENETRATION DISORDER

Genito-pelvic pain/penetration disorder refers to four commonly comorbid symptoms: (1) difficulty having intercourse, (2) genito-pelvic pain, (3) fear of pain or vaginal pain, and (4) tension of the pelvic floor muscles. A diagnosis can be made with marked difficulty in only one of these areas. The prevalence of genito-pelvic pain in large North American studies ranges from 12% to 21% (Landry and Bergeron, 2009). Genito-pelvic pain is often idiopathic but may follow pelvic trauma, such as painful intercourse, childhood or adolescent sexual abuse, sexual assault, rough gynecologic examination, complicated episiotomy, vaginal infections, pelvic inflammatory disease, or pelvic surgery. Often an avoidance of sexual intercourse or even speculum medical examinations occurs in response to the genito-pelvic pain.

Evaluation

The diagnosis is usually made by history. Pain during tampon insertion or the inability to insert a tampon before a woman becomes sexually active may be an important risk factor for genito-pelvic pain/penetration disorder. Patients report pain and difficulty with, or inability to engage in, vaginal intercourse or digital vaginal stimulation, using tampons or vaginal contraceptives, or having a pelvic examination. Patients may demonstrate visible contraction of the pelvic floor musculature with anticipated speculum examination. Physical examination may detect pertinent anatomic abnormalities, such as vaginal septa.

Treatment

Few studies exist on treatment for genito-pelvic pain/penetration disorder. Uncontrolled reports suggest that sex therapy may be helpful (McGuire and Hawton, 2005). If vaginal muscle tightening or spasm is present, therapy must be directed at restoring conscious control of vaginal muscle relaxation under conditions that respect the patient's autonomy and maintain the patient's safety from further trauma. If the patient expresses fear or anxiety, pelvic examination may be deferred, and in severe cases, sedation may be necessary. Any physical abnormalities detected on pelvic examination, such as infections, should first be treated. After this, the patient may begin self-treatment with size-graded plastic or silicone vaginal dilators, gradually teaching her vagina to remain relaxed and receive nonpainful, self-controlled penetration. Specialized physical therapists teach patients to use biofeedback to relax the pelvic floor musculature; this can be more effective than treatment with dilators and is often preferred by patients. Treatment of posttraumatic stress disorder and other sequelae of past trauma may be crucial. Referral to a sex therapist is often helpful.

Male Sexual Dysfunction

Key Points

- The prevalence of erectile dysfunction (ED) increases with age.
- Vascular risk factors (e.g. diabetes, smoking, obesity, sedentary lifestyle) increase the risk of ED.
- Phosphodiesterase-5 (PDE-5) inhibitors (e.g., sildenafil) are the first-line therapy to treat ED.
- Premature (early) ejaculation (PE) is defined as a less than 1-minute intravaginal ejaculatory latency. SSRIs can delay ejaculation and can be used to treat PE.

ERECTILE DYSFUNCTION

The National Institutes of Health Consensus Development Conference (1992) defined ED as "the inability for a male to achieve an erect penis as part of the overall multifaceted process of male sexual function." The DSM-5 defines "erectile disorder" as ED accompanied by "clinically significant distress" that is not better accounted for by a nonsexual mental health disorder or the direct physiologic effects of a substance (e.g., drug of abuse, medication) or a general medical condition.

Both sympathetic and parasympathetic nerves regulate blood flow into the corpus cavernosum of the penis. Stimulation of the parasympathetic nerves causes release of nitric oxide (NO) from the noradrenergic, noncholinergic nerves and endothelial cells. NO increases the intracellular levels of cyclic guanosine monophosphate (cGMP) in the cavernosal smooth muscle, which relaxes the cavernosal tissues. With the resultant rapid blood flow into the corporal bodies of the penis, the small emissary veins that cross the tunica albuginea are occluded, and blood is trapped inside the corpus cavernosum, leading to an erection. The level of cGMP is also affected by prostaglandins. PDE-5 is the main cGMP-catalyzing enzyme in human smooth muscle. PDE-5 inhibitors increase cGMP levels and facilitate and maintain penile erection. The intact functioning of four body systems—vascular, neurologic, endocrine, and usually psychological—is necessary for a man to experience a penile erection.

Erectile dysfunction can occur at any age, but prevalence increases with age—2% for ages 40 to 49 years, 6% for 50 to 59 years, 17% for 60 to 69 years, and 39% for 70 years or older (Inman et al., 2009). Medical conditions associated with peripheral vascular disease, such as diabetes, coronary artery disease (CAD), stroke, and hypertension, increase the prevalence of ED. In men younger than 60 years, smoking, a sedentary lifestyle, and being overweight increased the risk for ED (Bacon et al., 2003).

Evaluation

Clinicians should carefully evaluate the patient's complaint of ED because some men consider PE as ED. Because penile erection depends on intact vasculature, the medical history is similar to one assessing cardiovascular risk factors: "What is bad for the heart is bad for the penis." Several common classes of medicines can cause sexual dysfunctions (Table 42-4). The social history should include the patient's smoking, alcohol, drug and marijuana use and important social and sexual relationships. The physician should also assess psychological factors such as depression and anxiety. Physical factors need to be considered. Some studies have shown that bicycle riding may cause ED

Table 42-4   Medications Affecting Sexual Function

Antihypertensives
β-Blockers (atenolol, metoprolol, bisoprolol, propranolol)
   Thiazide diuretics (hydrochlorothiazide, chlorthalidone)
   Sympatholytics (clonidine, methyldopa)
   Calcium channel blockers (nifedipine, amlodipine)
   ACE inhibitors (enalapril, lisinopril)
Antipsychotics
Antidepressants
   TCAs
   Selective and nonselective serotonin reuptake inhibitors
Anxiolytics and Tranquilizers
   Alprazolam
   Diazepam
Antiandrogens
   Ketoconazole
   Spironolactone
5α-Reductase Inhibitors
   Finasteride
   Dutasteride
Digoxin
Gonadotropin-Releasing Hormone Agonists
   Leuprolide acetate
   Buserelin
H₂blockers (cimetidine)
HIV retroviral medications
Fibrates (gemfibrozil, fenofibrate)
Opioid Narcotics
Statins
   Atorvastatin
   Pravastatin
   Rosuvastatin
   Simvastatin
Cytotoxic Agent
   Methotrexate

ACE, Angiotensin-converting enzyme; *HIV,* human immunodeficiency virus; SSRI, selective serotonin reuptake inhibitor; TCA, tricyclic antidepressant.

from perineal compression and hence decreased penile blood flow; however, more investigation is needed (Sommer et al., 2010).

Physical examination focuses on signs related to the vascular, neurologic, and endocrine systems. Peripheral pulses should be palpated and carotids auscultated for bruits. The thyroid should be examined for enlargement or nodular disease. A thorough genitourinary examination should be performed. The clinician can assess perineal enervation with anal sphincter tone, perianal sensation, and the bulbocavernosus reflex. The penile shaft may show Peyronie disease (fibrous plaques of corpus cavernosa affecting erectile function or causing pain with erection). The prostate should be evaluated. Testicular atrophy may indicate low testosterone levels. If secondary sexual characteristics are lacking or the patient has other signs of hypogonadism, further endocrine evaluation should be undertaken.

Vascular risk factors should be assessed with fasting glucose and lipid profile. Blood urea nitrogen (BUN) and creatinine, serum transaminases, thyroid-stimulating hormone, and prostate specific antigen (PSA) levels should be considered. If the patient is young, deficient in secondary sexual characteristics, or has other signs of hypogonadism, a testosterone level should be determined. A low testosterone level, however, cannot be considered a definitive cause of ED. Many men with very low levels of circulating testosterone have normal libido and erectile function. Testosterone is highly protein bound to sex hormone–binding globulin, with only about 2% circulating as free testosterone; therefore, total testosterone levels may not reflect the bioavailable testosterone. The prevalence of abnormally low serum testosterone levels, even among men with ED, is only about 7%. Testosterone supplementation can be considered in men with low testosterone (<300 ng/dl) and ED (Table 42-5).

Treatment

Phosphodiesterase-5 inhibitors are first-line therapy for ED and are effective in most cases. Sildenafil (Viagra),

Table 42-5   Testosterone Replacement Options

Route	Drug Dose	Estimated Monthly Cost	Advantages	Disadvantages
Oral	Testosterone undecanoate, 120-240 mg 2 to 3 times daily	Not approved in the United States	Oral	Serum testosterone levels vary
Intramuscular	Testosterone enanthate, 250 mg every 2-3 wk Testosterone cypionate, 50-200 mg every 2-4 wk	$100	Lower cost	Testosterone levels vary over the administration interval; higher risk of polycythemia; frequent injections
Subcutaneous	Testosterone pellets, two to six 75-mg implants every 3-6 mo	$150 plus physician fees	Continuous level	Expensive; needs a procedure to implant; can spontaneously extrude
Buccal	Testosterone, 30 mg every 12 hrs	$250	Self-administered	Twice-daily dosing oral irritation; bitter taste
Transdermal patch	5-10 mg/day	$250	Daily administration	Skin irritation; expensive
Transdermal gel—cutaneous	50-100 mg/day	$300	Daily administration; easy to adjust dose; no patch visible	Can take up to 10 minutes to dry; can transfer to contacts; expensive
Transdermal gel—axillary	2%: 30-120 mg/day 1.62%: 20.25-81 mg/day	$300	Smaller amount of gel to apply	Can transfer to contacts; expensive

Data from Seftel, 2007 and Corona, 2011.

Table 42-6   Phosphodiesterase-5 Inhibitors

Parameter	Sildenafil (Viagra)	Vardenafil (Levitra)	Tadalafil (Cialis)
Dosages	25, 50, 100 mg	2.5, 5, 10, 20 mg	2.5 mg (taken daily), 5 mg, 10 mg (as needed dosing)
Absorption	Decreased if taken with high-fat foods	Decreased if taken with high-fat foods	Unchanged with food; decreased if taken with antacids
Onset of action (min)	30-60	30-120	16-30
Length of effect (hr)	3-5	4-5	24-72
Side effects	Headache, flushing, nasal congestion, dyspepsia, abnormal color vision	Headache, flushing, dyspepsia, nasal congestion, abnormal color vision	Headache, flushing, nasal congestion, dyspepsia, back pain, myalgia 12-24 hr after dose, color vision changes very rare
Metabolism	Hepatic	Hepatic	Hepatic
Drug interactions	Strong CYP3A4 inhibitors (e.g., ritonavir, indinavir, ketoconazole, itraconazole), moderate CYP3A4 (e.g., erythromycin), nonspecific	Strong CYP3A4 inhibitors (e.g., ritonavir, indinavir, ketoconazole, itraconazole) increase plasma levels; potential hypotension with nitrates and α-adrenergic blockers	Strong CYP3A4 inhibitors (e.g., ritonavir, indinavir, ketoconazole, itraconazole) increase plasma levels; potential hypotension with nitrates and α-adrenergic blockers
Dose reduction	CYP450 inhibitor (cimetidine) causes significant increase in plasma levels; potential hypotension with nitrates and α-adrenergic blockers	Patients older than 65 yr; hepatic impairment; no adjustment for moderate to severe renal impairment (CrCl <30 mL/min)	No dosage adjustment for age; not recommended in patients with severe hepatic impairment Daily use: no adjustment for moderate to severe renal impairment (CrCl >30 mL/min); not recommended for CrCl <30 mL/min As-needed use; reduce dose for CrCl <50 mL/min
Additional information	Patients older than 65 yr; hepatic impairment; severe renal impairment (CrCl < 30 mL/min)	May prolong QT interval	Nitrates given no sooner than 48 hr after dose; substantial consumption of alcohol (e.g., 6 oz of 80-proof vodka) increases orthostatic hypotension; no blood pressure drop with tamsulosin (selective α-adrenergic blocker)

CrCl, Creatinine clearance
Data from Campbell, 2005.

vardenafil (Levitra), and tadalafil (Cialis) differ in their absorption, potential effective time interval, and some side effects (Table 42-6). All oral PDE-5 inhibitors are more effective than placebo, with tadalafil more effective followed by vardenafil (Yuan et al., 2013). All PDE-5 inhibitors can cause increased vasodilation with nitrates and should not be used concomitantly; fatalities have been reported. Use with α-adrenergic blocker medications should also be avoided because of the risk of significant hypotension. Human immunodeficiency virus (HIV) protease inhibitors significantly increase the half-life of PDE-5 inhibitors by interfering with hepatic metabolism. PDE-5 inhibitors may need titration to an effective dose or dose reduction for age and hepatic or renal impairment. PDE-5 inhibitors have also been found to reduce lower urinary tract symptoms associated with benign prostatic hypertrophy (BPH), and tadalafil was approved for treatment of BPH in 2012 (Miller, 2013). The FDA has issued a warning against consumption of dietary supplements that claim to increase sexual pleasure or claim to have sildenafil or tadalafil.

Prostaglandin E_1 (PGE$_1$; alprostadil) is second-line treatment for men who have a contraindication for or have failed PDE-5 inhibitors. In all patients with ED, regardless of its etiology, PGE$_1$ improves the dysfunction (Urciuoli et al., 2004). Intraurethral alprostadil (MUSE—medicated urethral system for erection) is a pellet of synthetic PGE$_1$ that is absorbed across the urethral mucosa and increases corpus cavernosum blood flow. Intracavernous self-injection of alprostadil (Caverject, Edex) is another alternative, especially for patients with mild to moderate vascular disease not responsive to PDE-5 inhibitors. Alprostadil along with

papaverine (parenteral vasodilator) and phentolamine (an α-adrenergic blocker) (Tri-mix) has been used for ED. Complications, although relatively uncommon, include ecchymosis, hematoma, and painful erection. Although priapism occurs in fewer than 1% of users, patients should be warned to seek prompt medical attention if an erection lasts longer than 4 hours. Injection can also cause minor bleeding, so condom use is advised if bloodborne infection risk is present. Long-term use can result in fibrosis of the corpus cavernosum, and administration more frequently than three times weekly is not recommended.

Vacuum erective devices (VEDs) can be used by men with ED from any cause. The penis is inserted into a tube in which a vacuum is applied, filling the corpus cavernosum with blood. A soft, constricting ring is placed at the base of the penis to prevent venous drainage from the corpus. Side effects include penile pain and numbness, bruising, and trapped ejaculation. Anticoagulant therapy is a relative contraindication. In men after a prostectomy or who cannot use a PDE-5 inhibitor, a VED should be first-line therapy (Brison et al., 2013).

Penile prostheses remains an option for men who find traditional treatment undesirable or men who have not responded to or have a contraindication to traditional treatment. The two types of prostheses are malleable rods and inflatable prostheses. Side effects are related to surgery and anesthesia along with mechanical failure, penile shortening, soft or hypoactive glans, or pencil-like penile syndrome (Vitarelli et al., 2013).

Men with ED may seek complementary and alternative medicine for treatment. A systematic review showed some evidence of effectiveness of red ginseng and yohimbine, although the studies were small and had limitations (Ernst et al., 2011). A study showed *melanocortin receptor agonists (PT-141)* along with a PDE-5 inhibitor to be safe and effective in men with minimal side effects in whom PDE-5 inhibitors were ineffective (Diamond et al., 2005).

Patients with ED primarily (or exclusively) of psychological origin may benefit from individual psychotherapy or pharmacologic therapy. Focused group therapy demonstrates greater efficacy than no therapy for ED. Group psychotherapy alone or with sildenafil significantly improves ED compared with sildenafil alone (Melnik et al., 2007). Men with sexual dysfunction often develop the "spectator effect," fear of recurrent failure or difficulty, and focus attention on self-performance rather than pleasuring and enjoyment, further decreasing arousal. Similarly, "performance anxiety" increases sympathetic tone, which physiologically impedes erectile function. Sensate focus exercises by both partners directed by a certified sexual therapy counselor can be helpful. Relationship conflicts, contraception or fertility concerns, and religious or moral conflicts regarding sexual activity can affect erectile function. Depression, anxiety, adjustment disorders, substance abuse, and other psychiatric symptoms should be evaluated and treated. Survivors of physical or sexual abuse may require long-term treatment and support with a therapist experienced in this area.

Testosterone Supplementation for Erectile Dysfunction

Testosterone supplementation may or may not improve erectile function in hypogonadal men. One study found that previously unresponsive hypogonadal men using testosterone supplementation responded to sildenafil or apomorphine (Foresta et al., 2004). A double-blind placebo-controlled trial comparing transdermal testosterone versus placebo in men with ED and low testosterone levels demonstrated a 30% increase in total testosterone versus placebo in the treated cohort but no significant difference in erectile function (Allan et al., 2008). Several options exist for testosterone supplementation (see Table 42-5).

PREMATURE (EARLY) EJACULATION

Premature (early) ejaculation is ejaculation that occurs before or shortly after vaginal penetration. Studies in heterosexual men suggest a 60-second or less intravaginal ejaculatory latency to define PE; the duration definition may apply to all men regardless of sexual activities and partners, but research is lacking (American Psychiatric Association, 2013). Using the new DSM-5 definition of ejaculation occurring within 1 minute of vaginal penetration, approximately 1% to 3% of men would be diagnosed with PE. When using the DSM-IV definition, which was ejaculation occurring more rapidly than desired, prevalence was 20% to 30%.

Evaluation

Evaluation of PE is by history. Onset, circumstances, and meaning (personal and relationship) of the dysfunction should be explored, as well as pertinent past sexual experiences. For example, young men whose first sexual experiences were rushed may later have difficulty establishing ejaculatory control in more relaxed contexts. Men having intercourse infrequently are more likely to ejaculate rapidly. The clinician should determine whether a patient can delay his ejaculation while masturbating. In addition, information regarding the patient's level of sexual knowledge and his partner's expectations may be significant. Evaluation for medical conditions such as hyperthyroidism or prostatitis that may shorten ejaculatory should occur.

Treatment

Selective serotonin reuptake inhibitor antidepressants can cause prolongation of the preorgasmic plateau and thus may delay ejaculation. Dapoxetine is a short-acting SSRI that can be taken as needed and is approved by the FDA for treatment of PE. RCTs show dapoxetine, 30 mg and 60 mg as needed, achieved statistically significant improvements in perceived control over ejaculation (Hellstrom, 2009). Using other SSRIs for PE is an off-label use. PDE-5 inhibitors added to SSRIs may further improve PE. Tramadol has been investigated as another oral agent; however, a large, international RCT of tramadol for the treatment of PE was stopped early (McMahon and Porst, 2011). Topical treatments that reduce the sensory stimuli to the penis (e.g., topical eutectic mixture of lidocaine-prilocaine spray) may increase ejaculatory latency time. Only weak or inconsistent evidence exists regarding the effectiveness of psychological interventions for the treatment of PE (Melnik et al., 2007).

DELAYED EJACULATION

Men who can sustain a full erection for a reasonable duration of sexual activity will usually be able to ejaculate. Only 75% of men report always ejaculating during sexual activity. Delayed ejaculation is diagnosed when the man has adequate sexual stimulation and the desire to ejaculate but subjectively has a delay or absence of ejaculation. Actual prevalence is unclear because the subjective definition and the time intervals to ejaculation vary. Alcohol use can cause difficulty with sustaining arousal or with orgasm. Contextual and partner issues may contribute to delaying ejaculation. Fewer than 1% of men will complain of delayed ejaculation lasting the 6 months needed for the diagnosis of delayed ejaculation disorder.

KEY TREATMENT

- PDE-5 inhibitors (sildenafil, tadalafil, vardenafil) are first-line therapy for ED (Yuan et al., 2013) (SOR: A).
- PGE_1, intraurethral or injected into the corpus cavernosum, is second-line treatment of ED (Urciuoli et al., 2004) (SOR: A).
- VEDs may help ED of any cause (Brison et al., 2013) (SOR: B).
- Men receiving group therapy plus sildenafil versus sildenafil alone showed significant improvement in erectile function (Melnik et al., 2007) (SOR: A).
- SSRI antidepressants improve PE by prolonging the preorgasmic plateau (Hellstrom, 2009) (SOR: A).

Substance- or Medication-Induced Sexual Dysfunction

The DSM-5 formalized the diagnosis of the sexual dysfunction that may be caused by medication or another substance. The sexual dysfunction must develop during or soon after the substance intoxication or withdrawal or after exposure to a medication. The substance or medication should be known to produce the symptoms for which the patient complains. Common substances are alcohol, opioid narcotics, amphetamines, and cocaine. Many common medications cause sexual dysfunction (see Table 42-4). Approximately 25% to 80% of individuals taking antidepressants, especially SSRIs or tricyclics, report sexual side effects, most commonly inhibited or delayed orgasm in both men and women and ED in men. Bupropion and mirtazapine do not appear to cause sexual side effects. For men with ED from SSRIs, administering sildenafil appears effective, but for women, adding bupropion at high doses may help (Taylor et al., 2013). Anticonvulsants, except for lamotrigine, have adverse effects on sexual desire. Gabapentin may affect orgasm. Chronic opioid use, even with appropriate use for pain management, lowers testosterone levels in men, which may cause decreased libido or ED. After discontinuing opioids, men may experience PE. Clinicians should inquire about sexual functioning in patients on medications or substances known to affect desire, arousal, or orgasm.

KEY TREATMENT

- For men with ED from SSRIs, administering sildenafil appears effective (Taylor et al., 2013) (SOR: B).
- For women with sexual dysfunction associated with SSRIs, adding bupropion at high doses appears most promising (Taylor et al., 2013) (SOR: C).
- Sildenafil may be a useful option in the treatment of antipsychotic-induced sexual dysfunction in men with schizophrenia (Schmidt et al., 2012) (SOR: B).

Gender and Sexual Orientation

Key Points

- Some individuals who have been sexually active with members of their own gender self-identify as heterosexual. Most clinicians overestimate the number of exclusively heterosexual patients in their practices.
- Women with same gender partners are less likely than heterosexual women to have had a mammogram or Pap smear recommended by a clinician in the past 3 years.
- Compared with heterosexual men and women, gay men, lesbian women, and bisexual women (LGB) are much more likely to have major depression and attempted suicide.
- The U.S. Preventive Services Task Force (USPSTF) suggests annual HIV screening in MSM.
- Preventive health care is important for transgendered individuals, and current guidelines should be consulted.

Sexual orientation is a social construct. Customs regarding which sexual acts are acceptable, with whom, and under what circumstances have varied in different cultures and eras. In *Sexual Behavior in the Human Male* in 1948, Kinsey and colleagues hypothesized that sexual orientation might be a continuous spectrum, from exclusive heterosexuality through exclusive homosexuality, and might vary across the life span in different people. Researchers have attempted to measure the prevalence of homosexuality and bisexuality in populations, with varying success and controversy. Some people who have been sexually active with members of their own gender self-identify as heterosexual. In one study, although only 2.8% of male respondents and 1.4% of female respondents self-identified as GLB, 10.9% of men and 4.3% of women ages 40 to 49 years reported having had at least one same-gender sexual experience since puberty (Laumann et al., 1994). Physicians likely overestimate the number of exclusively heterosexual patients in their clinical practices.

CARE OF LESBIAN, GAY, BISEXUAL, AND TRANSGENDERED PATIENTS

Lesbian, Gay, and Bisexual Patients

Lesbians are less likely to obtain health maintenance services, such as mammography and cervical cancer screening, than heterosexual women. Patients in same-gender couples are often not eligible for spousal health insurance benefits. Even when insurance status was the same, women with same-gender partners were less likely than heterosexual women to have had a mammogram or Pap smear recommended within the previous 3 years (Buchmueller and Carpenter, 2010). Many clinicians and lesbians mistakenly believe they do not need Pap smears. A woman self-identified as lesbian, however, may have been a victim of childhood sexual abuse, had a history of consensual male sexual contact, or may be bisexual. Nulliparous lesbians are at a high risk for cancers of the breast, endometrium, and ovary. Female-to-female transmission of STIs (including HIV/AIDS infection) is much less efficient than male-to-female transmission; however, genital–oral sex and fomites such as sex toys can transmit gonorrhea and *Trichomonas*, respectively. Mental health screening for depression and suicide should be considered, especially for "closeted" sexual minority women. Lesbians who had not disclosed their sexual orientation to a majority of friends, family, and coworkers were 90% more likely to have ever made a suicide attempt, and bisexual women were three times more likely to have made a suicide attempt than heterosexual women (Koh and Ross, 2006).

Gay men sometimes report difficulty in obtaining adequate health care caused by providers' bias and fear of discrimination. Any male patient who presents for treatment of urethritis should be asked about participation in oral-genital sex or receptive anal intercourse because some treatment regimens for urethral gonorrhea and chlamydia are not effective against pharyngeal and anal infections. A careful exposure history should be taken, even if the patient self-identifies as heterosexual, because some heterosexual-identified men have same-gender sexual experiences. Sixty percent of new HIV/AIDS infections in the United States are in MSM. In 2013, the USPSTF recommended universal screening for individuals between ages 15 and 65 years and suggested annual screening in high-risk groups, such as MSM. Men who self-identify as gay or bisexual are more likely than heterosexual men to have major depression, to admit to suicidal ideation, or to have attempted suicide. Mental health screening for depression may be prudent in this population.

Transgendered Patients

Transgendered individuals transiently or persistently identify with a gender different than their natal gender. A *transsexual* individual is one who seeks to take on the social role of the other gender, either full or part time, often with the assistance of hormone therapy, surgery, or both. *Cross-dressers* (previously referred to as "transvestites") are persons who at times may dress as the other gender to be publicly perceived as such or for sexual pleasure. *Intersex* is a different medical concept and refers to persons born with ambiguous genitalia or for whom phenotypic and chromosomal sex do not match (e.g., 5α-reductase deficiency). Some persons do not perceive themselves as being fully male or fully female and seek to create new gender identities, similar to those found in many indigenous cultures. The prevalence of transgendered individuals is difficult to assess because of cultural and reporting limitations. One study gives an estimate of one in 11,900 to one in 45,000 for male-to-female (MtF) individuals and one in 30,400 to one in 200,000 for female-to-male (FtM) individuals (De Cuypere et al., 2007). *Gender dysphoria* is clinically distressing incongruence between one's natal gender and one's expressed or experienced gender. People may seek medical assistance in changing their physical sex to be congruent with their internal self-perception. People who identify as transgendered or who cross-dress are likely to be more numerous than individuals seeking sexual reassignment surgery.

Family physicians and other clinicians may be involved in the treatment of transgendered individuals, both in their medical transformation to relieve their gender dysphoria and in their overall health. To relieve the distress associated with gender dysphoria, some individuals need hormone therapy and surgery, but others need only hormones or surgery. Transgendered people receiving hormones can present a blend of gender-associated physical characteristics. MtF sex reassignment surgery is currently technically advanced, with postoperative MtF individuals often not identified as such even on cursory gynecologic examination. FtM surgery is more complex and prone to complications with more variable results. Because of the fear of being stigmatized, some patients may seek medical services without revealing their hormone use or operative history. In one study, 26% of respondents reported being denied medical care because they were transgender (Kenagy, 2005).

The management of feminizing or masculinizing hormone treatment for transgendered individuals can be managed by primary care physicians with appropriate education, such as the primary care protocol from the University of California-San Francisco Center of Excellence for Transgender Health (see Web Resources) or the World Professional Association for Transgender Health Standard

of Care for Gender for Health of Transsexual, Transgender, and Gender-Nonconforming People, seventh edition (Coleman et al., 2012). Establishing routine visits for hormone management provides the opportunity to discuss routine health promotion and preventive services. Current guidelines should be consulted, such as one provided by the University of California-San Francisco's Center of Excellence for Transgender Health (http://transhealth.ucsf.edu). FtM reconstructive chest surgery does not remove all the glandular tissue as with a mastectomy; thus, FtM men who retain the axillary tail should at minimum continue self-examination. Clinicians should be alert for significant risks associated with feminizing or masculinizing hormones, such as increased risk of thromboembolic events with estrogen and increased cardiovascular events with testosterone.

The initiation of hormone therapy for modification of visible sex characteristics and sex reassignment surgery are life-changing medical interventions that should only be undertaken for patients who have completed an appropriate mental health evaluation and are in supportive mental health care. For clinical gender transition, a multidisciplinary team approach is ideal, such as in a comprehensive program or concurrent care from a mental health professional with experience in this area; a primary care physician knowledgeable about hormone supplementation and general transgender medical care; and urology, gynecology, and plastic surgery specialists. The World Professional Association for Transgender Health has resource links for patients (http://www.wpath.org).

Sexuality Issues at Specific Times of Life

ADOLESCENCE

Key Points

- Almost half (47%) of high school students report having experience sexual intercourse, with 15% reporting experience with four or more partners.
- Eight-four percent of high school students report being taught about HIV/AIDS in schools; however, only two thirds of sexually active male youth report condom use with their last sexual intercourse. The prevalence of condom use in adolescents has not changed significantly since 2003 (60%-63%).
- Twelve percent of female adolescents and 5% of male adolescents report being forced to have sexual intercourse they did not want. Almost 10% of adolescents report being hit, slapped, or physically hurt on purpose by a partner.
- Gender dysphoria can become apparent in young children or adolescents.
- Eight-four percent of LGBTQ (lesbian, gay, bisexual, transgender, and queer) youth report verbal harassment, 30% report physical abuse, and more than a quarter of them drop out of school because of harassment.

Although shyness, reticence, and embarrassment are common, most adolescents (77% in one survey) would like their health care providers to ask them directly about their sexual knowledge and experience (Rosenthal et al., 1999). Family physicians can use routine outpatient visits for school, camp, sports, or pre-employment physical examinations to offer medical information as it relates to the teenagers' current concerns.

Sexual Activity

The Centers for Disease Control and Prevention (CDC) conducts the Youth Risk Behavior Surveillance (YRBS) surveys every 2 years. In 2011, 15,503 questionnaires were completed in 43 states and 21 large urban school districts (158 high schools) nationally, with an overall response rate of 71%. Nationwide, almost half (47%) of all students reported having experienced sexual intercourse, with the prevalence by state ranging from 37% to 59%. Fifteen percent of teenagers reported experience with four or more sexual partners, ranging from 8% to 23% in the state surveys and 7% to 27% in the urban areas. Significantly more African American boys (32%) reported four or more sexual partners than Hispanic (20%) and white (13%) boys. Twice as many African American girls reported four or more sexual partners than Hispanic girls (18% vs. 9%) and one third more than white girls (13%). About one in five girls and boys report being sexually active (having sex with at least one person in the 3 months before the survey) in ninth grade, but by 12th grade, half of girls and 44% of boys reported being sexually active (Eaton et al., 2012).

Family physicians should remain mindful that teenagers may practice sexual acts other than intercourse. Some teens maintain sexual relationships involving mutual genital touching and masturbation for months or years before beginning intercourse. A significantly greater number of ninth grade students had engaged in oral sex than in vaginal sex (19.6% vs. 13.5%) and perceived fewer health, social, and emotional risks with oral sex than vaginal intercourse (Halpern-Felscher et al., 2005). Risks involved in oral–genital or anal sexual acts, such as oral transmission of gonorrhea or HIV infection with unprotected anal intercourse, should be discussed frankly with adolescents. Eight-four percent of high school students in the 2011 YRBS report being taught about HIV/AIDS in school, with 15% of girls and 11% of boys reported having had HIV testing. The prevalence of condom use has not changed significantly since 2003 (60%-63%), but use diminishes over time; 63% of sexually active 10th grade students reported condom use with sexual intercourse, decreasing to 61% and 56% of 11th graders and 12th graders, respectively (Eaton et al., 2012). Family physicians should remind sexually active adolescents to use a condom with each oral, genital, or anal intercourse to minimize HIV and other STI risk.

Family physicians should not assume that adolescent sexual experiences are consensual or desired. In the YRBS 2011, 8% of youth reported having been forced to have sexual intercourse they did not want (12% female, 5% male). Many teenagers who have had coercive sexual experiences do not identify these as rape or abuse. Asking a neutrally worded question (e.g., "Have you ever done anything sexual when you really didn't want to?") may open the door to further dialogue regarding exploitive or traumatic sex. Almost one in 10 of adolescents report being hit, slapped, or physically hurt on purpose by a partner (blacks, 12%; Hispanics, 11%; and whites, 8%; 9.4% overall). The prevalence of dating violence may be even higher, with the reported range from 8% to 24% in large urban school districts (Eaton et al., 2012).

For adolescent patients, drug and alcohol use is a significant risk factor for unprotected sexual activity. In the 2011 YRBS, 22% of teenagers reported alcohol or drug use immediately before they last had sexual intercourse. Almost one third of white girls (31%) report using oral contraceptives before their last sexual intercourse, but only one in 10 black and Hispanic girls report that use. Long-acting contraception is often the best option for young women who are at risk for pregnancy because of substance use. Referral for treatment of addiction should be considered for adolescents who combine drinking with driving or sex and who are unable to discontinue this risk behavior without assistance.

Lesbian, Gay, Bisexual, and Transgender and Questioning Youth

Sexual orientation has three dimensions: attraction, self-identification, and sexual behavior. During adolescence, these three dimensions may not be congruent or may be fluid. In pooled data from the 2001 to 2009 YRBS surveys, 53.5% of high school students reported having had sex with the opposite gender, 2.5% reported having had sex with the same gender, 3.3% reported having had sexual contact with both genders, and 40.5% reported having had no sexual contact (Kann et al., 2011). By maintaining an open questioning style, such as asking, "When you think of people to whom you are sexually or romantically attracted, are they male, female, or both, or are you not sure yet?," the health care provider gives the adolescent permission to express their sexual orientation freely. Some adolescents are uncertain of their sexual orientation and are considered "questioning." The inclusive acronym for sexual minority (nonheterosexual) individuals is LGBTQ.

Gender Dysphoria

Awareness of gender occurs very early in life. A toddler can be aware of the physical differences between the genders. By 3 or 4 years, a child self identifies as a boy or girl. Thus, some children may express gender dysphoria as early as preschool. Not all children who express distress over their natal gender continue to have gender dysphoria by adolescence. Gender dysphoric adolescents may have more anxiety and depression or oppositional defiant disorder than non–gender dysphoric adolescents (Coleman et al., 2012). In 2013, the American Academy of Pediatrics published a statement to help guide clinicians in the care of LGBTQ children and adolescents (Levine, 2013).

Health Risks for LGBTQ Youth

In an environment critical of their emerging sexual orientation, LGBTQ adolescents may experience harassment, profound isolation, and fear of discovery, which interfere with achieving the developmental tasks related to self-esteem, identity, and intimacy. Eight-four percent of adolescents who are open about their LGBTQ sexual orientation reported verbal harassment; 30% reported physical abuse. More than one quarter (28%) dropped out of school because of harassment (Levine, 2013). Censure, alienation, and abandonment by the family of origin represent a particularly devastating consequence for many LGBTQ teenagers. LGBTQ adolescents may become homeless after coming out to their families. Homeless LGBTQ adolescents may resort to the sexual trade to survive, risking STIs, HIV/AIDS, and pregnancy. LGBTQ adolescents are more likely to have had sexual intercourse, to have had three or more sexual partners, and to have experienced sexual intercourse against their will. Between 1997 and 2006, the rate of AIDS diagnoses reported among male adolescents 15 to 19 years nearly doubled, from 1.3 cases per 100,000 to 2.5 cases per 100,000 (CDC, 2009). LGBTQ teenagers are more likely than heterosexual peers to start using tobacco, alcohol, and illegal drugs at an earlier age.

Teenagers seeking family planning or obstetric services are not necessarily heterosexual; bisexual and lesbian respondents are two to seven times more likely to become pregnant than their heterosexual peers (Saewyc et al., 2008). Lesbian or bisexual young women have sexual intercourse with male partners at younger ages, more often engaging in sexual activity while under the influence of drugs or alcohol, and higher rates of forced or coerced sexual contact than heterosexual female adolescents (Tornello et al., 2013). Gay or lesbian youth were about half as likely to use a condom with their last intercourse than heterosexual youth (35.5% vs. 65.5%) (Kann et al., 2011). LGBTQ adolescents are twice as likely to have considered suicide in the past year as heterosexual youth (31% vs. 14%, 2007 YRBS). Primary care providers who care for adolescents, especially gay, lesbian, or bisexual youth, should be alert to the possibility of depression and suicide. For support, clinicians can suggest they contact the Gay, Lesbian, Bisexual, and Transgender National Hotline (888-843-4564 or http://www.glnh.org) or the Trevor Helpline (866-488-7386; 866-4UTREVOR), a 24-hour suicide prevention hotline that focuses on the needs of sexual minority youth.

OLDER ADULTHOOD

Key Points

- The likelihood of being sexually active correlates with good health status. Older women may be less likely to have a spouse or intimate partner because of their greater longevity.
- Testosterone levels are lower in men with chronic illnesses than in healthy men.
- Before testosterone replacement, men should have their prostates evaluated with a PSA and digital rectal examination. PSA should be drawn annually. Hematocrits should be monitored in men on testosterone.

Although the likelihood of being sexually active declines steadily with age, many older adults remain sexually active; 84% of men and 62% of women age 57 to 64 years and 67% of men and 40% of women age 65 to 74 years report being sexually active in the previous 12 months, with two thirds of both genders in each cohort sexually active more than two to three times a month. For those age 75 to 85 years, 39% of men and 17% of women reported sexual activity within 12 months (Lindau et al., 2007). Several factors impact the age related decline in sexual activity. As men and women age, physiologic changes in sexual functioning occur. During arousal, older men experience less scrotal vasoconstriction and testicular elevation, erection may be delayed or insufficient, and orgasm may be of shorter duration with less ejaculatory fluid. Women may have decreased labial engorgement and less vaginal lubrication during arousal and fewer and weaker uterine contractions during orgasm. Regardless of these physical changes, many older adults continue to have active sexual lives.

Approximately half of sexually active older adults reported at least one sexual problem, with almost two thirds having at least two bothersome sexual problems. Sexual problems most often reported by women were lack of interest (43%), difficulty with lubrication (39%), inability to climax (34%), finding sex not pleasurable (23%), and pain (17%). Among men, the most common sexual problems were difficulty in achieving or maintaining an erection (37%), lack of interest in sex (28%), climaxing too quickly (28%), anxiety about performance (27%), and inability to climax (20%) (Lindau et al., 2007). The likelihood of being sexually active is associated with good health. Men and women who reported good to excellent health were 80% and 70%, respectively, more likely to be sexually active than men and women with "poor" or "fair" health status (Lindau et al., 2007). Many common health conditions, such as arthritis or back pain, can inhibit sexual activity. Vascular disease and its risk factors, including CAD, stroke, diabetes, hypertension, hyperlipidemia, and smoking, correlate with ED (Laumann et al., 2005). Pudendal nerve disruption after hysterectomy and bladder, rectal, or prostate surgery may cause sexual dysfunction. Because they often take several medications, older adults may be particularly susceptible to medication-induced sexual dysfunction (see Table 42-4).

At all ages, women are less likely to be sexually active than men. However, 37% of women age 65 years or older reported some sexual activity, with 12% reporting at least weekly sexual activity (Huang et al., 2009). For women who reported no sexual activity in the previous 3 months, lack of interest (39%) was the most common reason followed by lack of a sexual partner (36%), physical problem of the partner (23%), and lack of interest by the partner (11%). Women may be more likely not to have a spouse or intimate partner because of their greater longevity. Between 75 and 85 years, men are almost twice as likely as women to have an intimate partner (78% vs. 40%) (Lindau et al., 2007). Lack of privacy may be problematic for elderly adults, who may live with family members or in long-term care settings.

A decline in sex steroid production is a factor in sexual dysfunction for both women and men. Postmenopausal estrogen deficiency is responsible for loss of vaginal lubrication and elasticity. The Women's Health Initiative raised concerns regarding deleterious effects of systemic estrogen replacement (Rossouw et al., 2002). Clinicians should counsel women, especially those older than 65 years, desiring long-term oral estrogen supplementation to diminish vaginal atrophy symptoms regarding the increased risk of CAD, thrombotic disease, and breast cancer. Vaginal estrogen supplementation by creams, tablets, or a vaginal ring may be helpful to decrease vaginal mucosal atrophy with much less systemic absorption. Women who remain sexually active may avoid significant vaginal atrophy through continued stimulation of the epithelium and vascular supply.

Testosterone levels do decline with age, eventually by 50% from midlife to old age. Free testosterone declines by 1.7% to 2.8% per year. Testosterone levels are lower in men with chronic illnesses than healthy men. Low testosterone levels associated with signs (increased abdominal fat, reduced muscle and bone mass, decreased body hair, gynecomastia, small testis) and symptoms (fatigue, weakness, decreased libido, decreased energy, erective dysfunction) comprise the clinical syndrome of late-onset hypogonadism, also called androgen deficiency in the aging male or colloquially "low T." Testosterone levels above 12 nmol/L (346 ng/dL) do not need supplementation, and testosterone replacement for levels below 8 nmol/L (231 ng/dL) is usually not controversial. Questions remain on treatment for testosterone levels between 8 and 12 nmol/L (231-346 ng/dL). In obese men, weight loss and increased physical activity can raise testosterone levels. Before testosterone replacement therapy (TRT), men should be screened with a PSA and a digital rectal examination and then have a PSA drawn annually. A PSA rise of 0.4 ng/mL over 2 years or an incremental rise of 1.4 ng/mL in 1 year should trigger further urologic examination (Mohr et al., 2005). Other risks of TRT are increased red blood cell mass. The hematocrit should be monitored regularly and TRT stopped if the hematocrit rises above 54%. Testosterone for replacement can be administered intramuscularly, subcutaneously, or transdermally (see Table 42-5). Replacement should only return testosterone levels to the physiologic level. Testosterone supplementation appears to have increased risk for men with cardiovascular disease. A study of testosterone supplementation in older men with CAD was halted early because of increased cardiovascular events in the treated cohort (Basaria et al., 2010). In a retrospective cohort study, men with known CAD by coronary artery catheterization using testosterone had a 5.8% increased absolute risk of death, myocardial infarction, or stroke than non-users of testosterone, with a 29% increased relative risk of adverse events (Vigeri et al., 2013). More research is needed on testosterone supplementation risks for older men.

Conclusion

Sexuality is a core aspect of personal identity. Knowledge regarding human sexual behavior in health and illness across the life span will enable family physicians to provide appropriate care to patients who are experiencing sexual difficulties. Many patients with sexual problems can be treated by family physicians and other primary health care providers without assistance. Referral to a certified sex therapist should be pursued for more complicated cases. Family physicians should maintain awareness of the health care needs of persons with same-gender sexual experiences or orientation. Transgendered persons may have the health care needs of their former and present gender. Sexual health issues are pertinent for adolescent and older adult well-health care. Family physicians should routinely include questions regarding gender identity, sexual behavior, and relationships during the clinical interview of all patients to help maintain their optimum health.

References

The complete reference list is available at www.expertconsult.com.

Web Resources

transhealth.ucsf.edu/trans?page=protocol-00-00 University of California, San Francisco Primary Care Protocol for Transgender Patient Care.

wpath.org World Professional Association for Transgender Health.

www.aasect.org American Association of Sexuality Educators, Counselors and Therapists. Can help locate local resources for sexual counseling.

www.cdc.gov/healthyouth/yrbs/data Centers for Disease Control and Prevention's Youth Risk Behavior Surveillance Survey. Data on adolescent high-risk behaviors.

www.endo-society.org/education-and-practice-management/clinical-practice-guidelines Endocrine Society Treatment Guideline (2010) for testosterone therapy in adult men with androgen deficiency syndromes.

www.uspreventiveservicestaskforce.org/uspstf13/hiv/hivfinalrs.htm#summary The U.S. Preventive Services Task Force's HIV screening recommendation.

43 Clinical Genomics

W. GREGORY FEERO, PHILIP ZAZOVE, and FREDERICK CHEN

Overview

Key Points

- Discoveries related to a wide variety of conditions are increasing the prominence of genomics in routine patient care.
- Primary care providers should be aware of what is known and not known about the benefits and harms of emerging genomic clinical technologies.
- Primary care providers should become familiar with supportive resources and, when appropriate, seek out expert consultation to help manage genetic conditions.

We stand at a remarkable time in history regarding our understanding of how variations in the human genome contribute to health and disease. At least some of this progress can be attributed to the technologies developed to complete the Human Genome Project. The tools of genomics and molecular biology are unlocking the fundamental underpinnings of previously enigmatic conditions, shedding light on the fundamental nature of the human species (Feero et al., 2010).

Some of the most exciting developments in genomics over the past decade relate to the genetics of common disease, cancer care, and microbial genomics. In the area of common conditions (e.g., diabetes, heart disease, asthma) in which multiple genes and environmental factors interact to cause disease, genetic scientists have been able to use a powerful technique known as a *genome-wide association study* to identify human genome variations associated with common disease risk. Thousands of risk markers known as *single nucleotide polymorphisms* (SNPs) have now been reliably associated with the presence of a long list of common conditions and traits. Although each individual marker confers only a small risk of disease (which greatly limits their use in the clinic to predict risk in individual patients), many have helped to better define disease pathogenesis (Kraft and Hunter, 2009; Manolio et al., 2013). This may lead to new interventions for multiple common diseases down the road.

Perhaps the biggest initial impacts of the expanding genomic knowledge are novel targeted therapies with improved efficacy and reduced toxicity compared with traditional chemotherapeutic agents. These are benefiting an increasing number of patients with cancer. This new generation of cancer treatments was made possible by insights into the pathological mutations responsible for tumorogenesis. Most of these insights could not have been achieved without the ability to sequence large numbers of samples of tumor and normal tissues from affected patients (McDermott et al., 2011). Application of rapid, accurate, and low-cost genotyping and sequencing technologies has also led to improved abilities to quickly identify and track emerging infectious disease threats in both the hospital setting and in international outbreaks (Relman, 2011).

We are at an early stage in the discovery process, and our embryonic knowledge of the human genome is not *easily* yielding rapid improvements in aspects of clinical care. This perspective is often lost in the media hype and attention given to the latest genetic discovery. The lack of a rapid translation from a new discovery to a proven clinical application (e.g., genetic test, targeted therapy) frustrates clinicians and patients alike and can lead to unrealistic and potentially harmful expectations. There is peril in the temptation to adopt promising, but as of yet unproven, clinical technologies. Primary care providers should recognize when the application of knowledge from genetic discovery is of proven benefit and when it is not. Perhaps most important, physicians should recognize that a substantial and rapidly expanding number of genomic applications fall into a gray area of unexplored benefit. The number of applications in this grey zone will continue to increase as fields such as epigenomics (the study of the consequences of chemical changes to DNA that don't affect the base pair sequence) mature. It is incumbent on providers to seek additional information from a reputable source when in doubt.

GENETICS VERSUS GENOMICS

The terms *genetics* and *genomics* are often used interchangeably in the literature, and this chapter is no exception. However, *genetics* is best viewed as the study of *single genes*, what they do, and how mutations in these genes cause disease. It is a snapshot of a specific situation, and environmental and behavioral factors often play a subordinate role. A prototypical genetic condition, cystic fibrosis (CF), is usually caused by a deletion mutation ΔF508 in the *CFTR*

Table 43-1 Select Evidence-Based Recommendations for Genetic/Genomic Applications

Condition	Clinical Scenario	Recommendation	Organization, Year of Recommendation
Breast cancer	Screening	Primary care providers screen women who have family members with breast, ovarian, tubal, or peritoneal cancer with one of several screening tools; women screening positive should receive genetic counseling and, if indicated after counseling, *BRCA* testing	USPSTF, 2013
	Screening	Recommend against using *BRCA1* and *BRCA2* testing as screening tool in average-risk populations	USPSTF, 2013
	Treatment	Insufficient evidence to recommend for or against routine use of expression profiles to guide care in specific populations of women with breast cancer	EGAPP, 2008
Colorectal cancer	Case finding	Recommend offering counseling and tumor sample testing for Lynch syndrome to all patients with newly diagnosed colorectal cancer, to reduce morbidity and mortality in relatives	EGAPP, 2009
	Pharmacogenetic testing	Insufficient evidence to recommend for or against *UGT1A1* testing for patients with metastatic colorectal cancer	EGAPP, 2009
	Pharmacogenetic testing	Recommend KRAS testing for patients with metastatic colorectal cancer who are being considered for treatment with cetuximab or panitumumab	EGAPP, 2013
Hemochromatosis	Screening	Recommend against screening for hemochromatosis in asymptomatic individuals	USPSTF, 2008
Hyperlipidemia	Screening	Recommend earlier screening for hyperlipidemia in patients with family history of premature cardiovascular disease	USPSTF, 2008
Diabetes	Screening	Insufficient evidence to recommend testing for variants TCF7L2 to assess risk for type 2 diabetes	EGAPP, 2013
Cardiovascular disease	Treatment	Recommend against routine use in adults with idiopathic VTE and family members to guide anticoagulation therapy	EGAPP, 2011
Prostate cancer	Testing	Recommend against routine use of the PCA3 genetic test for prognosis of progression	EGAPP, 2013

VTE, Venous thromboembolism.

From the U.S. Preventive Services Task Force (USPSTF) and CDC Evaluation of Genomic Applications in Practice and Prevention (EGAPP) Working Group relevant to primary care. http://www.uspreventiveservicestaskforce.org/uspstopics.htm#Btopics. EGAPP. http://www.egappreviews.org/workingrp/recommendations.htm.

gene. *Genomics* is the broader study of "the functions and interactions of all the genes in the genome," including how those genes interact with environmental and behavioral factors (Guttmacher and Collins, 2002). When considering genomics, it is important to recognize that environmental factors may be much more important in determining phenotype than genetic mutations. Common, so-called complex conditions, such as diabetes, cancer, and heart disease, are best considered from the perspective of genomics.

GENETICS AND EVIDENCE-BASED MEDICINE

As a discipline, *clinical genetics* originally developed in an environment that focused on the diagnosis and treatment of rare, or at least uncommon, disease. Often, large numbers of patients were not available for clinical trials, and in many cases, the severity of the conditions made randomized controlled trials (RCTs) untenable. This contrasts with *evidence-based medicine* (EBM), which primarily deals with common conditions and values large, prospective RCTs, as well as the public health consequences of individual medical choices. As genomic discoveries increasingly impact health care for common conditions, new

applications should be evaluated through a lens of *evidence of benefit*. Established groups that follow EBM precepts, such as the U.S. Preventive Services Task Force (USPSTF), for example, have issued recommendations on the potential of genomics for screening and testing for hereditary breast and ovarian cancer (HBOC) syndrome and hemochromatosis. The U.S. Centers for Disease Control and Prevention (CDC) has established newer groups such as the Evaluation of Genetic Applications in Practice and Prevention (EGAPP) specifically to review the evidence supporting genetic and genomic applications intended for health care use. Since 2005, the EGAPP has generated a number of evidence-based guidelines for the use of genomic technologies in patient care (Table 43-1). In 2013, the Office of Public Health Genomics (OPHG) at the CDC established a curated list of genomic technologies arranged into a three-tier system by available evidence of outcome benefits and the existence of guidelines regarding their use (OPHG, 2013). Considerable growing pains will occur as EBM and genomic medicine intersect, largely because the drive to adopt promising technologies outstrips the ability and resources to rapidly generate conclusive evidence of clinical benefit.

Family History: Best Guide to Genetic Components of Disease

Key Points

- Family history remains the best general tool for assessing a patient's risk for heritable conditions.
- Numerous guidelines relevant to primary care providers incorporate family history information.
- Evidence-based reviews have found that family history obtained from patients is generally accurate.
- Patient-completed web-based tools offer a convenient way to gather family history information.

Family history is arguably the single best tool for recognizing genetic components of disease in the primary care setting. Despite this, available evidence suggests it is very much underutilized in clinical care. In the context of single-gene disorders, family history has proved valuable for generations of clinicians and plays a major role in making a diagnosis and identifying at-risk individuals. Family physicians should be familiar with common patterns of inheritance of single-gene disorders, including X-linked recessive, X-linked dominant, autosomal dominant, autosomal recessive, and multifactorial or complex (Table 43-2). Classically, the three-generation genetic history known as a *pedigree* or *genogram* has been taught as the "gold standard" of family history collection. Certainly, after a potential genetic issue has been identified, a family physician should be comfortable in collecting and accurately representing a complete family history. However, taking a complete family history can be time consuming, and on a practical level, it is not always possible to collect in the context of a brief office visit. It is perfectly reasonable to gather, review, and update family history longitudinally.

Common diseases such as type 2 diabetes, coronary artery disease, and cancer also cluster in families. Family history captures both hereditary and environmental risks and is an important component of many validated risk algorithms for these and other conditions. Recent attention has focused on the systematic collection of family history as a screening tool in primary care settings, particularly via direct entry into electronic medical records. Family history information supplied by patients is generally fairly accurate for a wide range of conditions. However, few well-designed trials have examined health outcomes associated with use of family history as a screening tool (Berg et al., 2009; Wilson et al., 2009).

Given competing demands on family physicians' time and resources, what genetic family history is the most important to capture? A national collaboration of primary care and genetics professionals has developed mnemonics to help clinicians think genetically as they provide patient care (Burke et al., 2001). The mnemonic, "FamilyGENES" highlights "red flags" that signal a genetic concern, as follows (Whelan et al., 2004):

- **Family** history—multiple affected siblings or individuals in multiple generations
- **G**roups of congenital anomalies
- **E**xtreme (or **e**xceptional) presentation of common conditions
- **N**eurodevelopmental delay or degeneration
- **E**xtreme or exceptional pathology
- **S**urprising laboratory values

Another mnemonic is SCREEN (for familial disease), which uses the following set of family history questions to uncover genetic implications:

- **S**ome **c**oncerns: Do you have any (some) concerns about diseases or conditions that seem to run in the family?
- **R**eproduction: Have there been any problems with pregnancy, infertility, or birth defects in your family?
- **E**arly disease, death, or disability: Have any members of your family died or become sick at an early age?
- **E**thnicity: How would you describe your ethnicity? *or* Where were your grandparents born?
- **N**ongenetic: Are there any other risk factors or nonmedical conditions that run in your family?

Table 43-2 Patterns of Inheritance Often Encountered in Primary Care

Pattern of Inheritance	Characteristics of Family History	Example Conditions
X-linked recessive	Males affected more than females, maternal inheritance, 50% risk of female carrier sons affected	X-linked color blindness X-linked muscular dystrophy
X-linked dominant	Males and females may be affected, males more severe, daughters of affected males affected, male and female transmission	Fragile-X syndrome
Autosomal dominant	Affected individuals usually in every generation, 50% probability of affected individuals having affected offspring, M = F	Huntington disease Hyperkalemic periodic paralysis Lynch syndrome Marfan syndrome HBOC syndrome
Autosomal recessive	Often multiple affected individuals in same generation, skipped generations, 25% risk of affected child for carriers, M = F	α_1-Antitrypsin deficiency Cystic fibrosis Sickle cell disease Usher syndrome
Multifactorial	Clustering of cases in families, risk to first-degree relatives high, consequences of shared environment might be evident	Coronary artery disease Types 1 and 2 diabetes Many cancers

HBOC, Hereditary breast and ovarian cancer.

Electronic health record (EHR) systems seldom offer efficient and complete ways to collect and represent family history information. National efforts are underway to address this deficiency. Patient-completed paper and electronic tools provide another way to obtain a detailed genetic history. The U.S. Surgeon General's Family History Initiative (U.S. Surgeon General, 2013) includes a web-based tool that can be completed by patients, stored on their local computers, and shared with relatives and their health care providers in pedigree or table format (My Family Health Portrait; https://familyhistory.hhs.gov). This free, easy-to-use tool is an excellent way for patients with Internet access to record family history and is time saving for clinicians. The family history collected by the tool is now stored using emerging data standards that allow the data to be shared with EHR and personal health record systems. Alternatively, a number of organizations have created paper family history tools for patients and providers that are available on the Internet.

Genetic Testing

> ### Key Points
>
> - Knowledge of the indications for and limitations of genetic testing is relevant to common clinical situations in family medicine.
> - The context of testing and its limitations are important for proper interpretation.
> - Pretest and posttest counseling are currently recommended for genetic testing, although the need for such counseling in all testing situations is controversial.
> - Genetic testing results can have implications for the family, and providers generally have a duty to warn potentially affected members.
> - Family physicians should be involved in ordering, interpreting, and managing the consequences of genetic testing with health implications.

Identifying what constitutes a genetic or genomic test can be challenging. Traditionally, a genetic test measures changes in the sequence of DNA, but a "genetic test" can also be a measure of a protein or metabolite (Table 43-3). From this perspective, a fasting lipid panel could be

considered a genetic test. Also, a genetic test does not always need to be relevant to other family members, as when an individual's cancer cells are tested for mutations that affect prognosis and therapy. In some cases, a family physician's most important role is simply to reassure low-risk individuals that they do not need genetic testing.

The indications for genetic testing include confirming a diagnosis, identifying disease risk, and guiding therapeutic interventions. A genetic test can be done using many types of specimens, although testing for mutations in DNA is often done on DNA extracted from whole blood, saliva, or a cheek swab. Whereas some tests look for only specific mutations, others scan for all mutations in a specific DNA region. Testing costs can range from $100 to thousands of dollars, depending on the complexity and patent status of the test. Often, testing an affected family member first is the preferred strategy. Without knowing the mutation present in a family, an asymptomatic patient's negative test result may not be informative because the particular test done may not include the mutation affecting that family.

Family physicians should be aware that genetic testing may have implications for the extended family as well as the patient. For example, studies with patients with Huntington have shown that genetic test results, whether positive or negative, have significant implications for patients and their families. This includes depression, lifestyle behavior changes, and relationship changes among family members. Those testing negative may have survivor's guilt or may be treated as being outside the family. Patients can benefit from counseling about implications before undergoing genetic testing that is both highly predictive and associated with profound health consequences (Martin and Wilikofsky, 2004). For genetic tests that are less predictive or are associated with conditions with less profound health consequences, the benefits of formal genetic counseling are less clear-cut.

Obtaining and interpreting molecular tests for DNA mutations often has unique considerations. First, it is important to order the correct test for the patient's condition; this is not always obvious, particularly when multiple tests are available. Second, the presence of a mutation in an asymptomatic individual only rarely predicts disease onset, course, or severity. This is particularly true for the multitude of recently discovered SNP markers associated with risk for common complex conditions. Third, absence of a known causal mutation in a gene may not mean that an individual

Table 43-3 Types of Genetic and Genomic Testing

Test	Example Methods	Clinical Scenarios	Example Conditions
Chromosomal analysis	Fluorescent in situ hybridization, karyotype, array comparative genomic hybridization	Pediatrics, prenatal testing	Down syndrome, unexplained mental retardation
DNA analysis	Allele-specific oligonucleotide hybridization, sequencing, fluorescent PCR assays, DNA microarrays, high throughput exome or whole-genome sequencing	Adult, pediatric, prenatal testing, pharmacogenetic testing	HBOC syndrome, Huntington disease, CF, warfarin pharmacogenomics, unexplained developmental delay
Biochemical tests	Various	Adult, pediatric, prenatal	Hyperlipidemia, phenylketonuria, quadruple screen
Expression profiling	cDNA measurement on microarrays, quantitative PCR	Adult, pediatric	Breast cancer, melanoma, colorectal cancer

cDNA, Complementary (copy) deoxyribonucleic acid; *CF,* cystic fibrosis; *HBOC,* hereditary breast and ovarian cancer; *PCR,* polymerase chain reaction.

is at no or low risk of disease. For example, in families meeting the clinical criteria for HBOC syndrome, testing for mutations in the *BRCA1* or *BRCA2* occasionally fails to detect a mutation in affected members. The absence of detectable mutations in affected individuals means that the test is essentially uninformative, and the risk to asymptomatic family members needs to be estimated from the clinical scenario and is not that of the average population (GeneTests, 2013a).

Because of the complex factors involved, genetic tests are frequently ordered by physicians with particular expertise regarding the condition for which testing is being considered. Expert clinicians may be medical geneticists or other medical specialists (e.g., oncologists, neurologists, cardiologists) with specific interest and knowledge of genetic conditions affecting their specialty area; a few primary care physicians have also developed expertise with some genetic conditions. Genetic counselors are individuals with masters level training in genetics who are specifically trained to help manage individuals with genetic conditions. In many health care environments, these professionals provide the required pre and posttest counseling related to genetic testing under the supervision of an overseeing physician. Genetic counselors can be exceptionally valuable partners for primary care providers managing patients with suspected genetic conditions. Currently, there are insufficient genetics professionals in all U.S. regions; as a result, primary care physicians will most likely be providing more genetic counseling and testing in the future. The next section provides a more in-depth look at settings in which different types of genetic testing are relevant to primary care.

EXAMPLES OF GENETIC TESTING

Preconception and Prenatal Screening

Genetic screening or testing can occur either before conception or during the pregnancy. When possible, screening or testing before a pregnancy is ideal because this provides the broadest range of choices if increased risk of a genetic defect is detected. Preimplantation genetic testing is available for an increasing number of conditions but is costly and not accessible to many individuals. Most genetic evaluations occur after the pregnancy is established. The ability to detect genetic defects has grown rapidly over the past decade. Many ethical issues exist in both the preconception and the prenatal screening or testing environment, including the course of action if the fetus is found to have an incurable, life-altering condition. Common indications for prenatal testing are advanced maternal age, previous child with a chromosomal abnormality, family history of abnormality or single-gene disorder, family history of neural tube defect or other structural abnormality, abnormalities identified in pregnancy (e.g., on ultrasonography), parental consanguinity, recurrent miscarriages, previous unexplained stillbirth, parental ancestral origin, and use of certain medications. The American College of Obstetricians and Gynecologists (ACOG), March of Dimes, and American College of Medical Geneticists have developed or compiled guidelines for recommended tests. However, these guidelines are often based on consensus or expert opinion and do not always agree.

High-resolution ultrasonography, maternal serum marker testing, and maternal serum–based cell-free fetal DNA tests are screening tests for congenital anomalies associated with a variety of genetic conditions. More invasive testing, such as chorionic villus sampling and amniocentesis, can provide accurate diagnosis of genetic conditions but at the cost of a higher risk of complications. Available guidelines suggest that amniocentesis be offered to all pregnant women to aid in the detection of Down syndrome (ACOG, 2007). Rapid advances in cell-free fetal DNA testing of maternal serum may supplant more invasive testing. The family physician should evaluate the risks and benefits of all forms of prenatal genetic screening or testing, discuss them with the patient and her partner, and make referrals to health care providers with genetics expertise as appropriate.

Newborn Screening

The first genetic testing encountered by most individuals is the heel stick at 24 hours after birth. The advent of the Recommended Uniform Newborn Screening Panel and an improved evidence-based process for selecting conditions to add to newborn screening panels in the United States has led to a growing uniformity of newborn screening across the states (National Newborn Screening and Global Resource Center, 2013). The majority of conditions included on the panel are genetic, although testing for most conditions relies on measuring the presence of metabolites in newborn blood samples using gas chromatography mass spectrometry. DNA-based newborn screening protocols are being adopted nationally for conditions such as CF and severe combined immune deficiency.

Hearing screening in the newborn period has also been remarkably successful, and through such screening programs many heritable forms of congenital hearing loss are identified in time for early intervention and counseling of parents considering additional children. The Recommended Uniform Newborn Screening Panel has also been updated to include routine use of pulse oximetry screening to identify infants with serious congenital heart defects, which occur in up to 1% of newborns.

Pharmacogenetics

Pharmacogenetics is the study of genetically determined variations in response to medication. This can include variations in how a drug is metabolized as well as how drugs interact with intended as well as unintended targets in the body. Pharmacogenetic testing can be useful in ensuring accurate drug dosing, avoiding adverse side effects, and selecting drugs. The U.S. Food and Drug Administration (FDA) mandates that many drugs contain information referencing pharmacogenetic testing in their labeling. Although family physicians should be aware that such labeling exists, the evidence of benefit of testing for these variations is not uniform across drugs. For example, preliminary clinical data suggested that testing for variations in two genes related to warfarin treatment would improve care of patients requiring anticoagulation with this drug. This led to prominent inclusion of information regarding pharmacogenetic testing in the warfarin drug label by the FDA. Subsequently, a major study suggested that there was no appreciable benefit of adding pharmacogenetic testing

Table 43-4 Pharmacogenetic Testing

Drug	Gene	Notes
Abacavir	HLA-B*5701	HIV-1 patients
Aminoglycosides	A1555G	Not routinely
Antifolate chemotherapy	MTHFR	Not routinely
Azathioprine	TPMT	Not routinely
β-Blockers	CYP2D6	Not routinely
Irinotecan	UGT1A1	Not routinely
Opioids	CYP2D6	Not routinely
Oral contraceptives	FVL, prothrombin G20210A, others	Family and personal history of VT can be used
SSRIs	CYP450	EGAPP recommended against, 2007
Carbamazepine	HLA-B*1502	For Asian Americans
Warfarin	CYP2C9 and VKORC1	Algorithms may work as well or better

HIV-1, Human immunodeficiency virus type 1; *EGAPP*, Evaluation of Genomic Applications in Practice and Prevention; *SSRI*, selective serotonin reuptake inhibitor; *VT*, venous thrombosis.

to the initiation of warfarin anticoagulation. This being said, a variety of pharmacogenetic tests are routinely used to guide treatment of oncology and infectious disease patients based on evidence of clinical benefit. Current recommendations of pharmacogenomic tests for some conditions common in family medicine are in Table 43-4.

Recent promising applications of pharmacogenomics measure variations relevant to drug responsiveness in cancer. Often, cancer drugs are toxic and expensive, so more individually targeted therapy (personalized medicine) based on the mutations present in a patient's tumor prove valuable over time. Examples include testing breast cancer tumors for overexpression of HER2 receptor to guide use of targeted therapies and KRAS oncogene mutations testing to guide colorectal cancer (CRC) treatment (Allegra et al., 2009). Testing for mutations in patients' tumors is now a part of routine oncologic care for a growing variety of cancers, including breast, colon, lung, stomach, leukemia and lymphoma, and metastatic melanoma. The availability of low-cost sequencing of patient normal and tumor DNA is driving innovation in cancer care at a very rapid pace, and many more clinical applications of pharmacogenetic testing relevant to cancer care are in the pipeline for clinical release.

Direct-to-Consumer Testing

Since the completion of the Human Genome Project in 2003, more companies now offer direct-to-consumer (DTC) genetic testing. The public profile of DTC testing has increased dramatically over the past several years with the advent of inexpensive, genome-wide scans for SNPs. Tests that measure millions of genetic variations simultaneously can be obtained with a saliva sample and a few hundred dollars. The majority of these markers are probably of little significance to the tested individual's health, and patients may both overestimate and underestimate their personal risk of disease based on the results of such testing.

Other types of DTC genetic tests offered can be grouped into "medical" and "nonmedical" categories. Medical tests include highly validated DNA testing for specific mutations in classic single-gene mendelian disorders, pharmacogenetic testing, and paternity testing. Nonmedical testing ranges from determining one's ethnic and geographic origins or athletic prowess to ear wax type. DTC testing can offer advantages of anonymity for testing as well as easy access to genetic tests that might be difficult to obtain through routine health care channels. The consumer pays for most DTC genetic testing.

Clinicians should recognize that "buyer beware" applies to DTC genetic testing. National regulatory oversight ensuring the analytic and clinical validity of these tests is inadequate, although some states (California, New York) have enacted laws to increase scrutiny of consumer-oriented tests. Late in 2013, the FDA effectively stopped DTC SNP-based testing for common disease risk in the United States because of potential for harm from inaccurate or misleading results; it remains to be seen if consumer demand and advances in science will change this position. Even with accurate testing, there is no assurance that the result will be clinically useful to the individual. This is particularly problematic when a trained health professional is not available to help individuals appropriately select and interpret genetic testing. Companies now offer phone-based genetic counseling services independent of any testing services. Ideally, a trained health professional should be involved in ordering and interpreting any genetic or genomic testing with health implications.

Ethical, Legal, and Social Issues

Key Points

- Clinicians should consider potential ethical, legal, and social issues (ELSIs) when discussing genetic testing with patients.
- The Genetic Information Nondiscrimination Act (GINA) provides national protections against health insurance and employment discrimination based on genetic information. Health Insurance Portability and Accountability Act (HIPAA) provides insurance portability and privacy protections. Some states have more comprehensive statutes to prevent genetic discrimination.
- The Affordable Care Act (ACA) provides protection against discrimination in health insurance for individuals with preexisting genetic conditions.
- Case law suggests that family members have a right to know whether genetic information affects their personal health and that health care providers have a duty to warn family members of health risks.
- Minors incapable of providing informed consent should not be tested for conditions not immediately relevant to their health or not treatable in childhood.

Significant potential ELSIs are associated with the use of genomic technologies in health care, and funding for research regarding ELSIs was part of the Human Genome Project from the outset. ELSIs include concerns regarding potential for discrimination or stigmatization based on one's genome, the right to know or not know one's genetic status in family settings, potential adverse effects of genetic testing on reproductive decision making, and discomfort with genetic testing of conditions for which treatment in childhood is not recommended or is not available.

Many patients are concerned that genetic information could be used as a tool for discrimination by health insurers and employers. In 2008, the GINA became U.S. law and provides national protection against use of genetic and family history information as a basis for discrimination by health insurers or employers (Hudson et al., 2008). However, the law does not prevent use of genetic information by life, long-term care, or disability insurers. Some states have laws providing for more stringent protections than those afforded by GINA, and physicians should be aware of the protections their states provide. The passage of the ACA of 2010 has provided very important protections to individuals with genetic conditions that often require very costly care, by preventing insurers from denying coverage or setting rates based on preexisting conditions.

Family physicians must remember that a genetic diagnosis affecting a patient may have implications for the entire family. Before genetic testing, they should discuss the need to inform family members of abnormal results that might affect them. When a patient does not want family members to know that they have a genetic disease, the HIPAA has clarified and strengthened the patient's right to privacy of medical information. When knowledge of the patient's condition would not change health outcomes for the relative, the physician has no duty to warn. If the information can affect other family members' health, this presents a quandary. Some courts have ruled that physicians are liable for failure to inform other family members. Physician assistance in informing family members can also help the patient (Offit et al., 2004).

Several national groups of genetics professionals have developed consensus guidelines against genetic testing in *minors* unless there is a potential immediate benefit to the child's health. Experience in adult-onset conditions has revealed that many people choose not to know if they are at risk for a genetically determined condition. Knowing about the risk of developing an adult illness in childhood, when no treatment or intervention is available, may present unnecessary intrusion into normal child and family development. Consequently, rather than test minors, it is often advisable to wait until adulthood so that a fully informed decision can be made about testing.

Reproductive decision making can be complex. It is important to remember that the quadruple screen or high-resolution ultrasound during pregnancy is genetic testing. Before patients undergo preconception or prenatal screening or testing, family physicians need to discuss the patient's expectations about results and subsequent pregnancy planning. Counseling before fetal testing should include detailed information about risks; benefits to parents and infants; probability of abnormal results; and implications of possible results, including inconclusive results or those indicating alternate paternity. Reproductive counseling has followed a nondirective model in which the health professional avoids biasing the woman's or the couple's decision-making process.

Genetics in Primary Care Practice: Disease Illustrations

Key Points

- Health care providers should recognize when genetic factors contribute meaningfully to risk assessment, diagnosis, or disease management for rare conditions as well as common multifactorial conditions.
- Staying current with advances in diagnosis and treatment of genetic conditions challenges both genetic specialists and family physicians.
- Family physicians should identify and utilize credible and current information resources to support their care of patients with heritable conditions because proper diagnosis and management can be lifesaving.

Table 43-5 lists examples of multifactorial, single-gene, and chromosomal disorders seen in family medicine, including genetic information about each disease (Acheson and Wiesner, 2004; Christiansen et al., 2005; Gaston et al., 1986). In aggregate, single-gene and chromosomal disorders are relatively common. Physicians should remain alert for single-gene diseases when seeing patients, which can include causes of cancers, anemia, liver disease, developmental delay, and deep vein thrombosis. Making a correct genetic diagnosis can lead to lifesaving interventions for affected patients and their families.

Much research is needed regarding the genetics of multifactorial disorders, and predispositional genetic testing for such conditions using newer markers (e.g., disease-associated SNPs) is not currently recommended. A few examples illustrate what can currently be done with genetics and genomics in primary care.

HEREDITARY BREAST AND OVARIAN CANCER

A family history of premenopausal breast cancer in a first-degree relative doubles personal breast cancer risk. These women may benefit from earlier screening and should be counseled about the benefits of early detection. An autosomal dominant pattern of inheritance is seen in a much smaller number of families, perhaps 5% of women with breast cancer, known as HBOC syndrome. Current USPSTF guidelines suggest that physicians should recognize individuals from such families because they may benefit from counseling about HBOC and testing for mutations in the *BRCA1* and *BRCA2* genes. Risk factors include breast or ovarian cancer (or both) occurring at an early age in the family, in multiple individuals in the family, the presence of male breast cancer in a family, and Ashkenazi Jewish ancestry. The USPSTF recommends against using *BRCA1* and *BRCA2* mutation testing as a screening tool in the absence of a suggestive personal or family history.

Numerous *BRCA* mutations have been found, and their prevalence in the general population is about 1 in 800 but up to 1 in 40 in people of Ashkenazi Jewish descent. Pretest and posttest counseling is very important for HBOC testing. The ACA mandates that most insurers (with the notable exception of Medicare) cover genetic counseling for at-risk individuals and, when appropriate, *BRCA1* and *BRCA2*

Table 43-5   Multifactorial, Single-Gene, and Chromosomal Disorders Seen in Family Medicine

Condition	Inheritance Pattern	Genes Involved*
SINGLE-GENE DISEASES		
Early-onset Alzheimer disease	Autosomal dominant	*APP, PSEN1, PSEN2*
Breast cancer	Autosomal dominant with incomplete penetrance	*BRCA1, BRCA2*
Colon cancer (Lynch syndrome)	Autosomal dominant with incomplete penetrance	*MLH1, MSH2, MSH6,* and *PMS2*
Cystic fibrosis	Autosomal recessive	*CFTR*
Hemachromatosis, adult	Autosomal recessive	*HFE*
Marfan syndrome	Autosomal dominant	*FBN1, TGFBR2*
Sickle cell disease	Autosomal recessive	*HBB*
Tay-Sachs disease	Autosomal recessive	*HEXA*
β-Thalassemia	Autosomal recessive	*HBB*
Familial hypercholesterolemia	Various	*LDLR, ApoB, PCSK9, LDLRAP1*
CHROMOSOMAL DISEASES		
Down syndrome	Sporadic	Trisomy 21
Fragile X syndrome	X-linked dominant with incomplete penetrance	*FMR1,* with >200 CGG repeats
Turner syndrome	Sporadic	XO karyotype
XXY Males (Klinefelter syndrome)	Sporadic	XXY karyotype
MULTIFACTORIAL DISEASES		
Alzheimer disease	Multifactorial	*APOE4,* multiple SNPs
Asthma	Multifactorial	Multiple SNPs
Coronary artery disease	Multifactorial	Multiple SNPs
Depression	Multifactorial	Multiple SNPs
Type 1 diabetes	Multifactorial	HLA variants and multiple SNPs
Type 2 diabetes	Multifactorial	Multiple SNPs
Venous thromboembolism	Multifactorial/autosomal dominant	Factor V Leiden (FVL), proteins C and S, prothrombin G20210A, antithrombin III

*Most common mode of inheritance for each condition listed; for many common multifactorial conditions, there are rare instances of mutations in single genes causing a similar disease.
SNP, Single nucleotide polymorphism.
Data from Gene Tests (http://www.genetests.org); Online Mendelian Inheritance in Man (http://www.ncbi.nlm.nih.gov/omim); and National Human Genome Research Institute Genome Wide Association Study catalog (http://www.genome.gov/26525384).

mutation testing. The presence of many rare mutations and mutations of unknown clinical significance in the population can make interpretation of testing complicated, and involvement of a clinician with specialized knowledge is advisable.

Women with *BRCA* mutations may have up to an 80% lifetime risk of breast cancer and a 40% risk of ovarian cancer depending on the mutation. The risk of other cancers is also greater, although less so. It is important to recognize that men with *BRCA* mutations develop breast cancer at much higher rates than the general population. In fact, a diagnosis of male breast cancer should lead to a careful review of family history. Personal risk depends on the specific gene variant involved and other risk factors. Aggressive strategies aimed at early detection (e.g., breast magnetic resonance imaging [MRI]) are frequently recommended, but evidence of comparative effectiveness is not complete. Interventions such as bilateral mastectomy and oophorectomy have an enormous impact on women's lives, but evidence suggests these surgeries may confer up to a 90% reduction in cancer risk (National Comprehensive Cancer Network [NCCN], 2013).

Evidence regarding prophylaxis with tamoxifen or related agents is equivocal and may be related to the specific causal mutation. Although routinely offered to individuals with *BRCA* mutations, little evidence supports the use of annual CA-125 and transvaginal ultrasonography to screen for ovarian cancer. Options for prevention and treatment are increasing over time, and more targeted and less invasive options may become available.

KEY TREATMENT

- Women with a personal or family history suggestive of HBOC syndrome should be screened for breast cancer risk using a validated tool. Those screening positive should be offered genetic counseling and, when appropriate, testing for mutations associated with HBOC syndrome (USPSTF, 2013) (SOR: A).
- Enhanced breast cancer screening with annual mammograms and breast MRI starting at age 25 years or 10 years earlier than the age of earliest diagnosis in the family are recommended for individuals with *BRCA* mutations (NCCN, 2013; Saslow et al., 2007) (SOR: C).
- Prophylactic mastectomy and oophorectomy dramatically reduce the risk of breast and ovarian cancer in HBOC patients (NCCN, 2013) (SOR: B).

HEREDITARY COLORECTAL CANCER

About 10% of the general population has a first-degree relative with CRC; this history increases personal lifetime risk for CRC from 9% to 16%. Many guidelines recommend early screening for these individuals—by age 40 years or 10 years earlier than the age at diagnosis of a family member. Early detection and removal of adenomatous polyps have made determining family history more difficult. Patients should be asked about removal of polyps in relatives, and those who have adenomatous polyps should be encouraged to tell their families.

A family history that contains many relatives with CRC, adenomatous polyps, or endometrial cancer, especially in more than one generation or with early onset (age <50 years) suggests an autosomal dominant pattern of inheritance. Two relatively common, autosomal dominant, hereditary CRC syndromes account for about 3% to 5% of all CRC cases: Lynch syndrome and familial adenomatous polyposis (FAP).

Lynch syndrome, or *hereditary nonpolyposis colon cancer syndrome* (HNPCC), occurs in about 1 in 200 to 800 families and is underdiagnosed in primary care settings. Lynch syndrome is caused by mutations in mismatched repair genes and confers an approximately 80% lifetime risk of CRC. Often these cancers are right sided and occur at an earlier age than sporadic CRC. Women with HNPCC have an increased risk for endometrial cancer; the incidence of other gastrointestinal and central nervous system cancers is also increased but to a lesser degree. Evidence-based guidelines suggest that CRC screening with colonoscopy should begin in the 20s for affected individuals. Screening for endometrial cancer is also recommended, but there is less evidence of benefit. Evidence indicates that the disease burden could be reduced by screening tissue samples from all new CRC cases for molecular findings suggestive of Lynch syndrome. Family members of individuals testing positive then could be offered testing and enhanced surveillance if positive (EGAPP Working Group, 2009).

Familial adenomatous polyposis is seen in about 1 in 8000 families, and affected individuals have a 100% lifetime risk of CRC. Management usually involves early screening (age 10-12 years) with sigmoidoscopy and early colectomy. Chemoprophylaxis with nonsteroidal antiinflammatory drugs may also be of benefit.

Family physicians should recognize both FAP and HNPCC and ensure that genetic evaluation is offered to these families. If a specific mutation is identified, early screening of family members can be stopped for those testing negative. In the absence of a known mutation, all family members should be screened at an early age and the screening repeated at shorter intervals.

KEY TREATMENT

- Individuals with a single first-degree relative (parent, sibling, child) affected by colon cancer should be offered screening at 40 years of age or 10 years before the age at diagnosis of the affected relative (NCCN, 2013) (SOR: B).
- All colon cancer tumor samples should be tested for changes suggestive of Lynch syndrome (HNPCC) to reduce morbidity and mortality in family members (EGAPP Working Group, 2009) (SOR: A).
- Accelerated screening for colon cancer is recommended for individuals with Lynch syndrome (NCCN, 2013) (SOR: A).
- Colon cancer screening beginning in the second decade of life and early colectomy are recommended to reduce risk of CRC for individuals with FAP syndrome (NCCN, 2013) (SOR: A).

CYSTIC FIBROSIS

Cystic fibrosis is a relatively common autosomal recessive condition that causes progressive lung disease and exocrine pancreatic insufficiency. CF affects approximately 1 in 3200 U.S. whites but is less common in other population groups. CF results from inheriting two mutated copies of the *CTFR* gene, which is known to play a role in regulating chloride transport across epithelial membranes. More than 1000 *CFTR* mutations have been described, but the ΔF508 mutation accounts for the great majority of classic CF cases.

The diagnosis of CF in symptomatic individuals can be made by the chloride sweat test, transepithelial nasal potential difference measurement, or genetic testing for *CFTR* mutations. Once almost universally fatal in adolescence or early adulthood, improved management has resulted in more CF patients surviving well into adulthood. Patient management in specialized CF centers is common, although it is unclear to what extent management by a specialized center is associated with improved patient outcomes. Lung transplantation has been used as a "cure" for the pulmonary complications of CF.

All women should be offered CF carrier screening as part of prenatal or preconception care to determine risk, so that reproductive planning is an option (ACOG, 2011). It is important to recognize that the common panels offered for prenatal CF screening contain tests for a variety of CF mutations but perform less well in certain ethnic groups. This lowered sensitivity results in residual risk of having an infant with CF despite a negative screening test in certain population groups.

All U.S. states include CF in their newborn screening programs, and evidence suggests that screening is associated with improved outcomes (Grosse et al., 2006; Southern et al., 2009). Newborn screening for CF illustrates some important dilemmas. As a result of this screening, we now know that many patients with nonclassic *CFTR* mutations have only mild disease, such as congenital absence of the vas deferens or chronic sinus infections. Does diagnosis before the onset of symptoms improve outcomes for these individuals? What about the risks of informing parents of a serious disease in their apparently normal newborn—will it change parenting and child development? The answers to these questions are under investigation, but they are important factors to consider when assessing risks and benefits of early CF detection.

- Newborn screening for CF occurs in some U.S. states and is associated with improved outcomes (Grosse et al., 2006; Southern et al., 2009) (SOR: B).
- It is reasonable to offer CF carrier screening to women in the preconception or prenatal setting, regardless of race or ethnicity (ACOG, 2011) (SOR: C).
- Consensus guidelines suggest sweat chloride testing or genetic testing for *CFTR* mutations for CF diagnosis in symptomatic individuals (GeneTests/GeneReviews, 2013b) (SOR: C).

References

The complete reference list is available at www.expertconsult.com.

Web Resources

cancer.gov/bcrisktool/Default.aspx A tool from the National Cancer Institute to assess the risk of breast cancer.

familyhistory.hhs.gov My Family Health Portrait. This free, easy-to-use tool is an excellent way for patients to record family history and is time-saving for the clinician. The family history collected by the tool is now stored using emerging data standards that allow the data to be shared with electronic health record and personal health record systems.

genes-r-us.uthscsa.edu National Newborn Screening & Global Resource Center. Extensive information related to newborn screening, including links to the ACTion (ACT) sheets and general genetics resources.

genetests.org Detailed information on many genetic diseases, a genetics services searchable database, a list of laboratories performing specific genetic tests, and an illustrated glossary linked to text.

ghr.nlm.nih.gov Excellent and up-to-date basic resource for genetics and health, including a glossary.

www.cdc.gov/genomics Centers for Disease Control and Prevention (CDC) Office of Public Health Genomics. Extensive information on public health aspects of genetics and genomics, including family history and a listing of genetic applications by levels of available evidence of health benefit. Provides links to other CDC resources related to genomics.

www.egappreviews.org Evaluation of Genomic Applications in Practice and Prevention. Evidence-based guidelines for genomic applications.

www.genome.gov/Health National Human Genome Research Institute. Useful resources for patients and patient care, including links to family history tools and guidelines. the Genetics and Rare Disease website (genetics help desk), National Cancer Institute's cancer PDQ, and genetic professional locators.

www.ncbi.nlm.nih.gov/omim National Library of Medicine Online Mendelian Inheritance in Man. Compendium of information on most genetic diseases but may have more information than most nongeneticists need.

www.nchpeg.org National Coalition for Health Professional Education in Genetics, dedicated to educating health professionals about genetics and genomics.

44 *Crisis Intervention, Trauma, and Disasters*

ROBERT E. FEINSTEIN and EMILY COLLINS

Family medicine physicians are frequently asked to assist a patient who is in a crisis, whether a life-threatening illness; divorce; a sudden infant death; mental health crises such as depression or suicide attempt; or crises resulting from trauma such as rape, automobile accidents, natural disasters, or the trauma from terrorism. The *crisis intervention approach* provides both a theory and a treatment model that can be readily applied to patients in crisis, victims of disaster, and others who have been traumatized. This chapter reviews the development of crisis intervention theory, discusses current thinking about trauma and disasters, and presents a method for evaluation, formulation, and intervention in the biopsychosocial domains of a crisis.

Development of Crisis Intervention, Trauma, and Disaster Theory

HISTORICAL CONSIDERATIONS

Key Points

- A crisis is a brief psychological upheaval, precipitated by a stressor, resulting in an inability to cope, adapt, or function in daily life. A crisis may resolve with improved functioning, return to baseline functioning or stable functioning with a predisposition to a new crisis, or can be stabilized with the patient living at a lower level of functioning (Caplan, 1964).
- Crises can be effectively treated if patients are told that they can expect to recover, are treated immediately, and are returned to daily functioning as soon as possible (Salmon, 1917).
- A crisis typically lasts 6 weeks and can resolve spontaneously. Crisis resolution depends on the severity of precipitant, the personal reaction to the trauma, the support system helping the patient, and the effects of the trauma on the community (Lindemann, 1944).
- Some crises are precipitated by normal development, such as adolescence or marriage (Erikson, 1959).

Thomas Salmon (1917), a British military physician during World War I, was asked to evaluate patients with severe "shell shock" (traumatic neurosis), which was producing psychological paralysis in Allied soldiers. In this first medical description of the psychological effects of war, Salmon noted that French soldiers sustained fewer psychological casualties than British soldiers. Three factors seemed to account for the French advantage: (1) French soldiers were told that they could expect to recover from their psychological traumas; (2) soldiers received immediate psychological treatment close to the battlefront; and (3) soldiers were returned to battle as quickly as possible. These principles became the cornerstone of modern crisis theory and disaster management strategies. Patients entering crisis treatment can expect to be treated immediately in their natural environments with an expectation that they will recover from the crisis, trauma, or disaster. Efforts should be made to return patients to their normal lives and communities as soon as possible.

Eric Lindemann (1944) applied and expanded Salmon's theories. He studied the acute grief reactions of persons who lost family members in the Coconut Grove fire in Boston, which claimed 500 lives. Lindemann discovered that normal people surviving such trauma develop an emotional crisis of pain, confusion, anxiety, and temporary difficulty in daily functioning. Also, he discovered that the psychological trauma caused by the crisis had little relation to preexisting psychopathology and that only a small group of the victims declined after the event to a lower level of functioning. Generally, the outcome of a crisis was related to the severity of the stressor, personal reaction to the trauma, effect of the trauma on the person's family and friends, and degree of community disruption. Lindemann found that most crisis survivors recovered spontaneously within 6 weeks.

Erik Erikson (1959), a sociologist, introduced the idea of a life cycle composed of developmental stages and developmental crises. His eight stages were seen as normative processes during which age-specific psychological tasks, transitions, and crises were routinely encountered. A difficulty or inability to negotiate a stage successfully affects the ability to progress to the next stage. For example, an adolescent seeks an adult identity and redefines social roles that emphasize peer relationships and increasing autonomy from parents. Those who do not successfully traverse adolescence develop a childlike dependence on parental figures and often have difficulty developing a career, getting married, or developing autonomous social relations.

Other crisis practitioners have expanded Erikson's basic concept of eight developmental crises to include other crises, such as leaving home for the first time, the midlife crisis, and parents' experience of the "empty nest syndrome." For many patients, a transition from one life phase to the next, such as marriage, divorce, retirement, or an illness, may bring the potential for a new developmental crisis.

Gerald Caplan (1961, 1964) synthesized many of these earlier ideas into modern crisis theory and treatment. He defined the crisis state as a brief, personal, psychological upheaval precipitated by a stressor, or "hazard." A precipitant produces emotional turmoil so that the person is temporarily unable to cope, adapt, or function in daily activities. Caplan demonstrated that a crisis implies the potential for danger and an opportunity for growth. Although subscribing to Lindemann's theories of acute precipitants, Caplan believed that a person's preexisting psychiatric condition could influence the development, evolution, and resolution of a crisis. A crisis may be based on the failure of a person's individual coping style and ability to adapt. Caplan confirmed that most acute crises resolve in about 6 weeks, with four possible outcomes: improved functioning, functioning restored to precrisis levels, incompletely restored functioning with a susceptibility to the development of future crises, or a severely impaired but stable level of lower functioning. He corroborated Lindemann's findings that some people cope with a crisis by spontaneously and flexibly developing new coping or problem-solving styles. Caplan developed a crisis treatment focused on development of better coping mechanisms and adaptations to life's traumas.

CURRENT UNDERSTANDING OF CRISIS, TRAUMA, AND DISASTERS

Key Points

- Approximately 66% of patients will experience a traumatic event during their lifetimes.
- One-year prevalence rates for all forms of trauma are approximately 20%.
- Approximately 13% of the U.S. population has reported a lifetime exposure to natural or human-generated disaster.
- The U.S. National Comorbidity Survey has estimated that 18.9% of men and 15.2% of women reported a lifetime experience of a natural disaster.
- Posttraumatic stress disorder (PTSD) in the United States has an estimated lifetime prevalence of 8%, with women twice as likely as men to be affected at some time during their lives.
- The most common traumatic events include witnessing an injury, murder, fire, flood, or natural disaster; being in a life-threatening accident; or combat exposure.

The current understanding of "crisis" has been used as one of several core strategies in the management and treatment of trauma and disasters. The type of events which authors called "traumatic" defines the frequency of traumatic experiences. For example, whereas early studies limited traumatic events to wars, natural disasters, and plane crashes, more recent epidemiologic studies include intimate partner violence, car accidents, crime, and foreclosures. Estimates of lifetime trauma exposure vary with the definition of a "traumatic event," so community studies of exposure to lifetime trauma also vary (25%-90%). According to the American Psychiatric Association's (APA's) *Diagnostic and Statistical Manual of Mental Disorders,* 5th edition (DSM-5), the projected lifetime rate of PTSD is 8.7% at age 75 years. Additionally, the DSM-5 notes that the estimated 12-month prevalence rate among U.S. adults is 3.5%.

Natural disasters such as earthquakes, tsunamis, hurricanes, tornadoes, and volcanic eruptions can traumatize individuals, devastate whole communities, and disturb an entire population in a large geographic area. Human-made disasters, such as the September 11 attacks (2001), Oklahoma City bombing (1995), Newtown shooting (2012), suicide bombings, plane crashes, and environmental accidents, are all byproducts of the 21st century and, unfortunately, have become a part of modern life. The most common traumatic events that may cause PTSD include witnessing an injury, murder, fire, flood, or natural disaster; life-threatening accident; and combat exposure.

Evaluating the Crisis or Disaster

Key Points

A comprehensive evaluation of a crisis, trauma, or disaster includes assessment of the following:
- The normal equilibrium state
- The precipitant stressor or trauma
- The personal interpretation or meaning of the events
- The crisis state
- Preexisting personality or psychiatric conditions
- Selective past history
- System of social supports
- Effects on local society or community resources

Figure 44-1 presents an overview of a modern crisis intervention theory that is useful for the treatment of a crisis or trauma.

NORMAL EQUILIBRIUM STATE AND STRESSORS

Under normal circumstances, a person has a sense of internal psychological equilibrium and environmental support that generally permits activities of daily living, working, and experiencing pleasure. A delicate balance among the person's internal wishes and fears, skills and capacities, values, and ideals determines psychological equilibrium. *Environmental equilibrium* refers to a stable balance among basic needs for food, water, shelter, and physical comfort, as

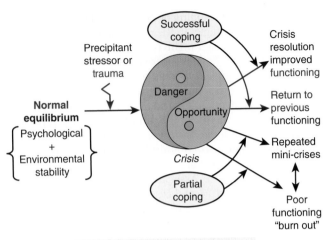

Figure 44-1 Crisis intervention theory.

well as the integrity of community and social supports for job, family, religion, and society.

A patient in crisis enters an emotional storm after a stressor disturbs the normal equilibrium. Environmental precipitants typically seen in a family physician's office include sickness and the stress of coping with death, divorce, marital separation, job loss, a financial crisis, traumas, intimate partner violence, and so forth. *Disasters* are acute environmental crises during which all concerned are focused on basic survival, acute medical care, and provisions of basic human needs. *Psychological stressors* may be related to events such as witnessing a trauma; surviving a disaster; loss of self-esteem; loss of love; a disturbing dream; sexual dysfunction; or sudden overwhelming fear, panic, or rage. *Developmental crises* such as latency, puberty, adolescence, marriage, birth of a child, midlife crisis, chronic medical illness, and retirement are common factors precipitating a crisis or may be comorbid factors.

Hobson and associates (1998) revised the Holmes and Rahe (1967) social readjustment scale. This newer scale lists 51 external life stressors that precipitate significant stress in most people. The top 20 items in this scale were in five separate domains: death and dying, health care issues, stress related to crime and the criminal justice system, financial and economic issues, and family stresses. This scale includes events that range in severity, from the most stressful being death of a spouse (rated as 1), divorce (7), experiencing domestic violence or sexual abuse (11), and surviving a disaster (16). It also includes events that many would consider positive yet stressful, such as getting married (32), experiencing a large monetary gain (42), and retirement (49). This list of stressors represents the most common external events that can cause a crisis. It is these types of stressors and the internally disturbing feelings attached to the events that produce emotional turmoil and a transient inability to adapt during the early stages of a crisis.

Most patients seeking treatment are surprised to discover that a major, unrecognized life stressor may have occurred on the same day or several days before the onset of the crisis. Less often, the stressor occurred sometime in the previous 6 weeks. Generally, events that occurred more than 6 weeks earlier are not acute stressors. Instead, these important past events may represent a previous crisis that was incompletely resolved and may be linked to the current crisis, as illustrated in Case Study 44-1.

Case Study 44-1

Lisa is a 28-year-old woman who presented to the office with increasing anxiety, irritability, and insomnia. Upon thorough questioning by her physician, Lisa revealed that her symptoms began about 4 weeks earlier when she saw the news and learned about a local shooting. Since seeing that news piece, Lisa has had an increase of anxiety in social settings, been more avoidant of family and friends, and had difficulty falling asleep and staying asleep. She has experienced great difficulty in concentrating at work and in her classes at school. She found that she had trouble focusing and her mind would often wander to an event from her past. She endorsed trying hard not to think about this event. When discussing her sleep, Lisa shared that she started to again have nightmares of this same experience from 10 years before in which a family she was living with was robbed and one of the family members killed by a firearm. Lisa had been out of the home during the robbery but returned to the police scene. She left that living situation shortly after this incident and subsequently developed symptoms of PTSD. She also realized that she had recently bumped into the mother of the family member who was killed in the incident 10 years earlier. She reported she had counseling at that time and was able to work through the trauma. Lisa had been living without symptoms for many years until recently.

Interpretation or Meaning of the Stressor

Whether a crisis is precipitated by an external life event or an internal psychological thought or feeling, each person interprets or adds meaning to the acute precipitant. For Lisa in Case Study 44-1, a news report of a shooting precipitated a major emotional crisis and a recurrence of her PTSD symptoms.

When listening for the precipitant of a crisis, it is important to understand the meaning of all stressors in the context of a patient's life. The report of a shooting in Lisa's local community had a personalized meaning to her that reawakened old wounds and PTSD symptoms, fueling a major emotional crisis. The following sequence of events, filtered through the lens of Lisa's select past personal experiences, created this current crisis. On learning of the shooting, Lisa perceived a personal threat. This current precipitant reawakened traumatic memories of the killing of a family member in the home in which she had lived 10 years earlier. She became avoidant of social situations, had traumatic dreams causing insomnia, and described difficulty with work and school. The report of the local shooting reawakened her internal reactions and her select past memories of the murder that happened 10 years earlier. This culminated in an acute crisis with a relapse of her PTSD symptoms associated with social and occupational dysfunctions.

Lisa presented to her physician with symptoms but was unable to articulate her problem. As they discussed her symptoms and situation, Lisa realized that her current reaction was rooted in PTSD symptoms returning from her past trauma. Her physician helped her recognize her reaction to the local report of a shooting in light of her past trauma. Lisa also realized with some surprise that meeting the mother of the family member who had been murdered also triggered the reemergence of her PTSD symptoms. With her physician's assistance, Lisa anchored her current fears in a reemergence of older PTSD symptoms. She felt more secure, her symptoms lessened, and she fully recovered.

CRISIS STATE

The crisis state can be defined as a brief psychological upheaval, precipitated by a stressor, that produces an intense state of inner turmoil or disorganization that overwhelms a person's ability to cope and adapt. As with Lisa, the crisis state can be experienced as symptoms of anxiety, nightmares, insomnia, and behavioral changes, resulting in social and occupational dysfunction. For some, the crisis state may be denied or experienced as psychological numbing.

Often, patients in a crisis or suffering from a trauma present to their family physicians with a confusing array of physical complaints (see Case Study 44-2). Patients typically experience four clusters of symptoms during a crisis or secondary to a trauma (Table 44-1).

Case Study 44-2

Mark, a 35-year-old real estate broker, presented to his family physician with anxiety and panic attacks, worrying about his performance at work, feeling depressed, and having 2 weeks of suicidal ideation. He noted that he was becoming so preoccupied with his decreasing performance that he was unable to get anything accomplished and feared he would be fired. Through careful questioning by his family physician, Mark admitted that these symptoms began 2 weeks earlier when his long-term girlfriend informed him that they would never get married. Mark became concerned that his girlfriend was going to leave him or be unfaithful. He described similar episodes in the past, noting that his first suicide attempt was in college after his first girlfriend left him for his roommate. He shared with his family physician that he wanted to get help because he did "not want to be like my father." Mark clarified that his mother left his father when Mark was a young boy. Mark's father began drinking and attempted suicide. Mark's father pursued other relationships and was often emotionally absent during those times. Inevitably, when these relationships ended, Mark's father would end up either attempting suicide or would be hospitalized for his recurrent depression.

Typically, a patient in crisis such as Mark cannot explain precisely what is upsetting him, although he was certainly aware that he was panicked and unable to concentrate. Mark's family physician asked, "Why now, at this point in time, are you anxious with suicidal thoughts and in crisis?" When asked, Mark initially felt distressed and confused. As he began to talk about his girlfriend, he recognized that he was panicked with the fear of losing her. He began to cry

Table 44-1 Common Symptoms Associated with a Crisis or Trauma

Physical	General	Insomnia
		Tremors
		Profuse sweating
		Chills
		Loss of or increased sexual drive
		Increased substance use or abuse
	Gastrointestinal	Nausea
		Vomiting
		Upset stomach
		Loss of or increased appetite
	Cardiac	Racing heart or palpitations
		Chest discomfort
	Neurologic	Headaches
		Dizziness
		Numbness, tingling
		Acute or chronic pain
Thoughts	Recurring traumatic dreams or nightmares	
	Difficulty with memory, attention, or concentration	
	Difficulty in making decisions	
	Obsessions or compulsions related to the trauma	
	Reconstructing the events of the crisis in an effort to master the trauma	
	Questioning spiritual or religious beliefs	
	Psychosis (extreme)	
	Suicidal ideation	
	Homicidal ideation	
Feelings	Numbness, irritability, restlessness	
	Anhedonia	
	Fear or anxiety when reminded of the traumatic event	
	Feeling sad, blue, or depressed	
	Emotional outbursts and angry feelings	
	Hopelessness or helplessness	
Behaviors	Overprotection of self and family	
	Easily startled	
	Isolation from others	
	Avoidance of activities associated with the event	
	Avoidance of places and people that trigger memories	
	Keeping busy to avoid thinking	
	Increase in conflict with family members	
	Agitation	
	Drug seeking	
	Suicidal behaviors	
	Acting out, violent behaviors	

with thoughts that he might be alone again. He became fearful he would follow in his father's footsteps of drinking, depression, repeated bouts of suicidal ideation, and never remarrying.

Frequently, people in crisis may not seek help by themselves and instead are brought in by concerned family members, lovers, friends, or perhaps the police or an ambulance. In these cases, it may take a while for the "Why now?" causes to be identified. Although symptoms often bring patients in to see their physicians, deeper unconscious levels of a crisis are often initially inaccessible to patients. Physician questioning and asking patients to retell the details of their experiences over the past 6 weeks and relevant past history is typically how the "Why now?" of the crisis emerges. This "Why now?" questioning is the first step in treating a crisis.

ACUTE CRISIS RESOLUTION AND ADAPTION TO THE CRISIS (WITHIN 6 WEEKS)

For many patients, the acute nature of the crisis is often resolved within 6 weeks as the patient learns to cope or adapt to the acute stress. The DSM-5 (APA, 2013) has classified the initial 1-month period of a crisis marked by impaired functioning as an "acute stress disorder." The DSM-5 specifies that the acute symptom picture must last more than 3 days and no more than 4 weeks and must cause clinically significant distress or impairment in social, occupational, or other important areas of functioning. The result of the acute stages of the crisis is one of four possible outcomes, as specified in Figure 44-1. Successful coping and adaptation to a crisis can lead to crisis resolution that ultimately promotes growth and can even lead to improved functioning. For most patients, however, crisis resolution means a return to a previous level of baseline functioning. Still other patients only partially resolve the crisis and instead "seal over" and deny the significance of their feelings or recent events, setting the stage for a future crisis. Those with the worst prognosis typically have poor adaptation skills and, at best, stabilize at a lower level of daily functioning. For example, an adolescent girl swallowed 30 pills after being left by her boyfriend. When questioned, she denied any suicidal intent and instead said, "I just had a headache." This patient has sealed over her crisis. Denial of her suicidal intent and anger with her boyfriend may lead to poor adaptation called a *missed* or *unresolved crisis*. This patient may continue to use unsuccessful coping strategies, such as drinking or cutting herself, as a way to deal with painful feelings. Unresolved crises predispose the patient to future episodes that may be caused by even less stressful precipitants. For example, this same patient may again become suicidal after a new date cancels their "hook-up." Fortunately, future crises often afford new opportunities to work past unresolved crisis, with better adaptation and coping.

SEQUELAE OF CRISIS, TRAUMA, OR DISASTER (6 WEEKS TO LIFETIME)

Although many patients completely recover from a crisis within 4 to 6 weeks, others may suffer with the sequelae of trauma or a crisis. The prognosis generally depends on three groups of factors: pretraumatic, traumatic, and posttraumatic risk factors (Ursano et al., 1995). *Pretraumatic* risk factors include prior psychiatric illness, genetics, typical coping styles, gender, and culture. *Traumatic* risk factors relate to the type of trauma, severity and duration of the trauma, and seriousness of a physical injury. *Posttraumatic* risk factors include dysfunctional coping styles, few resources available for repair, poor individual or community response, some incapacity for problem solving, and adaptation. In general, recovery is more likely if the crisis is not too severe and is short in duration. The crisis is often prolonged in victims of chronic abuse or torture or if a disaster is totally devastating to the fabric of a community (as with a hurricane or earthquake). After the crisis, the resources available for repair and the coping strategies used are the best predictors of outcome.

Table 44-2 Trauma and Crisis-Related Disorders

Adjustment disorder (309.XX; DSM-5, pp. 286-287)
Acute stress disorder (308.3; DSM-5, pp. 280-281)
Posttraumatic stress disorder (309.81; DSM-5, pp. 271-272)
Major depressive disorder (296.xx; DSM-5, pp. 160-161)
Substance-related and addictive disorders (DSM-5, pp. 481-585)
Dissociative disorders (301.14; DSM-5, p. 292)
Generalized anxiety disorder (300.02; DSM-5, p. 222)
Panic disorder (with or without agoraphobia) (300.01; DSM-5, pp. 208-209)
Specific phobia (300.xx; DSM-5, pp. 197-198)
Social anxiety disorder (social phobia) (300.23; DSM-5, pp. 202-203)
Brief psychotic disorder (298.8; DSM-5, p. 94)
Somatic symptom disorder (300.82; DSM-5, p. 311)
Conversion disorder (functional neurological symptom disorder) (300.11; DSM-5, p. 318)

DSM-5, Diagnostic and Statistical Manual of Mental Disorders, fifth edition. Diagnostic criteria available from American Psychiatric Association. *Diagnostic and statistical manual of mental disorders.* 5th ed. Arlington, VA: American Psychiatric Publishing; 2013.

When dealing with a patient who is in a crisis or has recently had a trauma, it is important for the family physician to assess for associated trauma-related conditions. This assessment begins with attention to physical illness or psychosomatic complaints and then focuses on basic health care needs (food, warmth, shelter, clean drinking water, good sanitation). From a psychiatric standpoint, the family physician must remember that it is normal to have symptoms of trauma after a crisis event. Most patients' symptoms will wane gradually or resolve spontaneously, and many patients may not require psychological treatment. At 1 year, however, 30% to 40% of those exposed to a disaster will show lingering evidence of psychiatric morbidity (Raphael, 1986). For example, 1 year after being involved in a car crash, about 25% of patients will show signs of a psychiatric disorder, and 11% will go on to develop PTSD (Mayou et al., 1993). Table 44-2 summarizes the spectrum of psychiatric disorders that can occur in the wake of a crisis or trauma.

PREVIOUS PSYCHIATRIC ILLNESS OR PERSONALITY DISORDER

For many people, there is little correlation between a previous psychiatric illness or personality disorder and their capacity to cope or adapt to an acute crisis or trauma. A person with schizophrenia may be just as capable of handling an acute crisis as others who do not have psychiatric disorders. How well a person handles an acute crisis or trauma depends primarily on the variables discussed earlier, including the precipitant, the meaning of the events, the crisis situation itself, the patient's coping skills and styles, and the effectiveness of the patient's support network.

However, there are many cases in which a preexisting psychiatric disorder or an unresolved trauma or crisis may influence the development of a new crisis. Consider the case of an intellectually disabled boy who becomes severely violent because his mother ran out of his favorite breakfast cereal. This change would be a minor stressor for most people, but for this boy, disruption of his daily breakfast food and routine are perceived as catastrophic. His low IQ and lack of verbal skills related to his intellectual disability predispose him to a crisis involving violence because he lacks the ability to consider other options. Patients with severe psychiatric illness or personality disorders, those with trauma-related disorders (see Table 44-2), and those who have rigid coping styles or poor adaptation skills all are at greater risk for future crises.

SELECTIVE PAST HISTORY

For an acute crisis, the patient's past history is relevant only in so far as it can help explain and resolve the current crisis. Many patients, wanting to avoid the pain of the current crisis, may unconsciously lead the family physician "down the garden path" with unexplained symptoms or other chronic problems, avoiding the pain of the current issues. To avoid the past history trap, the physician must try to understand the dynamics of the current crisis and then look for similar events in the patient's past that can be used to understand more about the current situation. For example, a selective past history of violence and the circumstances surrounding those events may provide valuable clues to understanding a current violent crisis. Taking a detailed selective history, discovering past events that are similar to the current crisis, will help the family physician assist in developing a deeper understanding of the "Why now?"

Additional events from the past history that might be helpful in understanding a violent event include a history of cruelty to animals; truancy; living in foster homes; childhood abuse or neglect; sexual abuse; a history of family violence; legal or severe financial problems; previous incarcerations; and a history of depression, substance abuse, or alcoholism. Selective past history that could be relevant for understanding an acute suicidal crisis might include a history of prior attempts, depression, bipolar disorder, substance abuse, chronic pain or disability, or severe neurologic or medical illness.

When dealing with trauma victims, it is important to ask about past trauma, previous successful coping styles or adaptations, and cultural and religious beliefs. This information can help promote recovery. The less severe the current traumatic event, the more critical are predisaster variables, such as prior social and occupational functioning or a history of a psychiatric illness.

Social Systems

Everyone lives within a network of social interaction, social support, and community and national resources. Most of our daily social interactions are with family, friends, and work colleagues. These daily social interactions are made possible by the community supports that enable a person to obtain clean water, adequate sanitation, housing, food, clothing, work, education, finances, and medical care. Community structures are generally made possible because of the support of the country or nation. National resources support the entire infrastructure of the civilization, from roads to a monetary system to constitutional protections. In general, stable social systems at different levels tend to provide the greatest buffers against crises or disasters of all types. An ecologic map (eco map) can be used to represent the patient's social network (review Figure 44-3 and Case Study 44-3).

Often, a patient goes into a crisis because the immediate social environment is threatened or disrupted by such issues as divorce, a dysfunctional family, drug abuse, unemployment, or an eviction notice. Relative damage to a local support network can have profoundly varied effects on a patient. For example, the death of a spouse produces a more severe crisis if the deceased person was also the sole financial provider. Even a minor disturbance in a small or dysfunctional support network can produce a major crisis. For example, an elderly woman who is housebound and without family, friends, or a telephone can experience a major crisis when her home health aide misses a scheduled visit.

When assessing the local support network of a patient, a family physician should consider whether the patient's network is interested, available, and competent to help. Some networks are helpful and should be included, but other networks may be harmful to the patient and need to be excluded from care. This determination may be especially complicated in intimate partner violence cases in which a marital separation is necessary but may also result in the woman needing to face financial stresses, loss of her home, and the loss of her social network. When a patient is in a crisis, the family physician can help the patient choose and mobilize the most helpful people in the patient's immediate support network and exclude others. Such helpful mobilizations may include calling in a specific family member, speaking to a supportive boss, helping the patient retain an attorney, establishing health care, or obtaining Medicaid.

In general, social disruptions at the local level of support (e.g., job loss) are less damaging than community-level disruptions (e.g., tsunami). National disruptions such as wars or earthquakes in poor countries cause a devastation from which many never recover. Disasters are long lasting when the needed resources remain greater than the available resources (Eranen and Liebkind, 1993). During a disaster, the social structure of a society can be damaged to such an extent that the existence and functioning of the entire community or nation can be threatened. This was experienced after Hurricane Sandy in 2012 and the earthquake in Haiti in 2010. Disasters of this magnitude require local, state, national, and even international support if there is to be a chance of restoring the social integrity of the community to predisaster levels of functioning.

Crisis Intervention Treatment in the Office Setting

BASIC CRISIS INTERVENTION APPROACH

Key Points

- Develop a timeline of events, starting with the "Why now?" and working from the initial presentation backward in time.
- Focus on acute risk assessment, including risk of suicide, violence, and acute medical conditions.
- Develop an eco map or support network map. This begins with a three-generational genogram and a list of other psychosocial supports, which may include friends, other medical professionals, medical insurance, religious

or community organization, and other people who could help the patient.

- Select a single problem or symptom to begin the treatment.
- Build a wheel-and-spoke treatment plan with the single problem or symptom in the center. List and prioritize all the spokes, which are the biopsychosociocultural factors that will need to be addressed to resolve the crisis.
- Treat the problem or symptoms by fostering the use of adaptive coping skills.
- Use a crisis resolution strategy.
- Use psychiatric medication for symptom-oriented crises.

The focus of a crisis assessment involves the evaluation and understanding of the precipitants of the crisis or trauma, personal meaning of the events, crisis state itself, selective past history, support network, and current psychiatric illness if relevant. These assessments are subsequently used to help formulate the causes of the crisis so that, if necessary, specific crisis intervention treatment and problem-solving approaches can be implemented.

A tailored crisis intervention treatment is typically one to five sessions offered on a voluntary basis, but this can be extended as needed. The treatment is specifically geared toward helping the patient survive and cope with the acute biopsychosocial or cultural effects of the crisis. The time required for each session depends on the complexity of the case and the practitioner's skill. A family physician can begin the crisis assessment and treatment by exploring the "Why now?" or the acute precipitants of the crisis. This inquiry can be followed by detective-style questioning designed to uncover the specific chronology and sequence of events, feelings, thoughts, and behaviors that led to the development of the acute crisis. Patients seeking help should be encouraged to tell the details of their acute crisis situation.

Helping the patient to describe the stressors and evolution of the acute problem may offer clues to developing problem-solving approaches for crisis resolution. Crises or disasters involving the lack of food, clothing, shelter, poor sanitation, or inadequate medical care should be given first priority. Crises involving violence, suicide, or a life-threatening medical illness have the next highest priority for focusing of the crisis treatment. Crises in everyday life can be treated according to the patient's preferences.

Crisis treatment focuses on the dynamic interplay of events from the most recent precipitants and days, the previous 6 weeks, and selective elements from the patient's past history that help frame the focus of immediate care. Important tools and approaches that can guide a crisis formulation and treatment are the timeline, eco map or support network tool, wheel-and-spoke formulation, symptom-oriented treatment, and assessment and development of more adaptive coping styles. All of these components can be used for the development of a general crisis resolution strategy.

TIMELINE

A timeline is a pictorial representation of the immediate, recent, and selective events from the past history

contributing to the current crisis. A family physician can build a timeline while interviewing the patient. The physician asks the patient to discuss the immediate events and precipitants of the crisis on the day of the office visit or events from the past week. Together, the physician and the patient reconstruct the history by working backward over the previous 6 weeks. Finally, the physician tries to elicit the selective past history that may relate to the current crisis. Use of the timeline is illustrated in Case Study 44-3. Developing a timeline with a patient helps both physician and patient focus on recent events and begins the process of formulating treatment, as illustrated in Figure 44-2 for Case Study 44-3.

Case Study 44-3

Joanne was an insurance adjuster who was assigned to work with families whose homes were destroyed after Hurricane Sandy in 2012. She began her job 6 weeks earlier, having had experience working with Hurricane Katrina families in the past. The fallen trees and damaged homes and cars after Sandy and the load of dealing with traumatized families left her distressed, feeling uncharacteristically anxious and overwhelmed, and with new-onset insomnia. Four weeks ago, she asked for help from work and was told several other adjusters would be available to help in a few weeks. Two weeks ago, her nanny threatened to resign for financial reasons. Her possible resignation raised the specter of a child care problem. This led Joanne to some binge overeating, drinking to help her insomnia, and migraines. She went to her family physician. During the office visit, her family physician helped her build her timeline (see Figure 44-2). Her family physician recognized the multiple levels of her distress and was able to help Joanne acknowledge that her migraines and insomnia were worsened by her drinking. The timeline also uncovered that 3 weeks earlier was the anniversary of her husband's death during Hurricane Irene. A tree fell on his car as he was returning home. The death of her husband left her alone as the sole provider, caring for her three children; her husband's mother, who had dementia; and her aging parents. Joanne and her physician did some problem solving, during which treatment of her migraines and insomnia was initiated. Exploring her eco map encouraged her to ask her siblings for help and discuss with her boss adding other adjusters to her current work site.

ECOLOGICAL MAP

An eco map is a pictorial representation of the patient's entire support network. Included in the eco map are a genogram and the immediate support network. This map can include the patient's current family, the family of origin for three generations, and all the people and community resources in the patient's immediate living environment (e.g., family, neighbors, nanny, physician, church, social services agencies). An eco map can be used by a family physician to help decide who can help the patient; who needs to be excluded; or what social, religious, legal, or

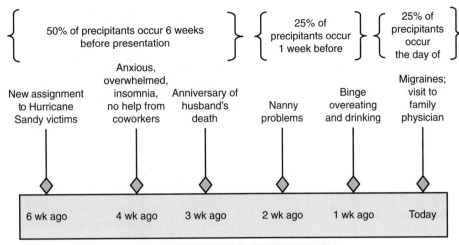

Figure 44-2 Crisis timeline: Case Study 44-3.

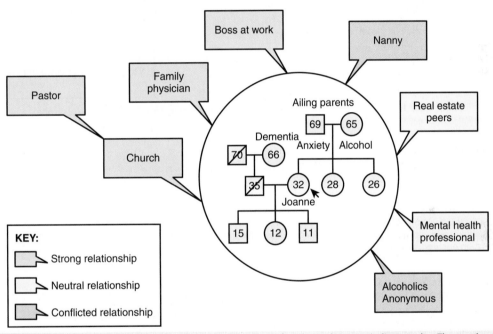

Figure 44-3 Ecologic or support network map: Case Study 44-3. *Circles* indicate females and *squares* indicate males. The *numbers* inside the circles and squares indicate the age. A *line across the square* indicates that the person is deceased, and the *arrow* represents the identified patient.

economic resources need to be mobilized to assist the patient in crisis.

Using Case Study 44-3, Joanne's eco map is illustrated in Figure 44-3. Her siblings, boss, and peers could be called on to assist her during this crisis. The decisions about which support members to use should be negotiated with the patient. Adding support in addition to the care offered by her family physician and the offer of additional mental health services was sufficient to help resolve this acute crisis.

Selecting the Problem or Symptom

Because most crises present with a number of problems and symptoms simultaneously, it is important to select the starting point of the treatment. Immediate survival and safety issues are almost always the first priorities. Providing food, shelter, safety, and medical care and preventing suicide risk or violence must supersede all other concerns. Less severe problems or symptoms can be handled according to the patient's preferences.

WHEEL-AND-SPOKE FORMULATION OF THE CRISIS

The wheel-and-spoke format is a useful tool to help develop a formulation that specifies the multiple causes of the crisis and can assist in the development of an effective, prioritized treatment plan. The acute crisis should be pictured as the center of a wheel. The spokes of the wheel are the problems or symptoms that are likely causing or contributing to the crisis. The physician can establish a numbered priority list for problem solving. For each problem listed, the family physician recommends a specific evaluation, test, or treatment approach designed to ameliorate the crisis. An application of the wheel-and-spoke diagram for Joanne's case is illustrated in Figure 44-4.

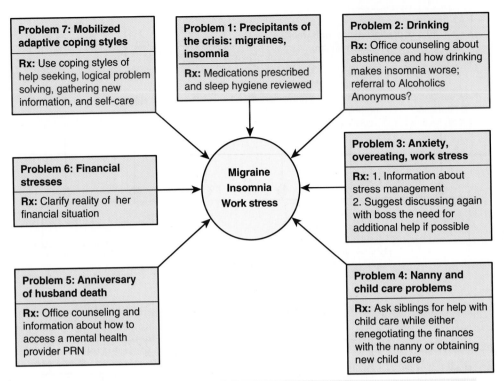

Figure 44-4 Wheel-and-spoke crisis formulation and treatment plan. *PRN,* As needed; *Rx,* prescribe.

Table 44-3   Coping Styles

Adaptive coping styles	Intuitive: using imagination, feelings, and perceptions to solve a problem Logical, rational: carefully reasoned, logical, deductive style Trial and error: trying a random solution; if it fails, modifying it and trying again Help seeking: gathering information and then proceeding Self-care: pursuing wellness through nutrition, exercise, stress management, or sleep hygiene Wait and see: allowing time or circumstance to determine the outcome Action oriented: taking action to rectify the problem immediately Contemplative: quietly thinking over the problem before acting Spiritual: asking for God's direction Emotional: using emotions such as tears, anger, or fear to help solve problem Controlling: controlling people or oneself to gain power to solve problem Manipulative: using various manipulative styles to resolve crisis
Pathologic coping styles	Use of alcohol and drugs Anxiety, panic, depression Deceptive, antisocial: use of dishonesty, lying, cheating, or stealing to resolve crisis Suicidal: using threat of suicide or suicide attempts to coerce someone or to solve problem Violent: using threat or actual violence to establish control and solve problem Avoidance or denial: failure to confront or acknowledge problems Somatization: displaying physical symptoms as a method of expressing emotions Impulsive: unpredictable or impulsive responses without anticipation of possible outcomes Random, chaotic: nonproductive and extreme form of trial and error and impulsive style; often seen in prolonged psychotic states

PROBLEM-FOCUSED OR SYMPTOM-ORIENTED TREATMENT

After the physician has formulated the case using the timeline and eco map and developed a wheel-and-spoke treatment plan, the problem-focused or symptom-oriented crisis treatment can begin. A family practitioner may use educational, psychotherapeutic, or supportive approaches with or without medications. The cornerstone approaches to crisis treatment are fostering coping skills and adaptive problem solving using a crisis resolution strategy. Medications may be necessary for symptom relief or as part of the treatment approach to related major psychiatric illness.

Coping Skills and Adaptive Problem Solving

Fortunately, most people find new ways to handle or cope with a crisis. Coping styles are the unique ways that patients deal with stress. For example, some cope with a stressful crisis by analyzing it, asking others for help, or gathering additional information. Some coping styles work better in certain situations than others. Table 44-3 lists some typical adaptive coping styles that can be suggested to patients, as well as pathologic coping styles that should be avoided whenever possible. Crisis resolution can be promoted by

Table 44-4 Crisis Resolution Strategy

Assess safety.	If a patient is in acute danger because of violence, suicide risk, or acute medical problems, more help may be required. Contact medical providers, law enforcement, or other resources as indicated.

1. Teach the patient to recognize the early warning signs of a crisis, which typically includes anxiety or depressive symptoms, occasional panic symptoms, feelings of being overwhelmed, a sense of urgency, vigilance, confusion, disorganization, intrusive thoughts, flashbacks, nightmares, self-defeating actions, and suicidal or homicidal feelings.
2. Set the patient's expectations for recovery.
3. Inform the patient that after an acute event, most acute life crises take approximately 6 weeks to subside, stabilize, or resolve.
4. Normalize the patient's symptoms. Patients need to know that, after an acute crisis or trauma, somatic and psychiatric symptoms and atypical daily routines (e.g., not going to work) are part of normal healthy coping.
5. It is important for patients to know that if problems and symptoms do not resolve after 6 weeks, they should obtain further evaluation and treatment as necessary.
6. If the patient desires, he or she can talk over the crisis with the family physician or a trusted friend. It is often best if these friends or family members are not directly involved in the crisis. For prevention or early intervention for the next crisis, the physician can assist the patient in developing a list of contacts of available friends, other physicians or specialists, and available community resources.
7. If a patient is overwhelmed with emotion, is coping poorly, or has a dysfunctional daily routine (beyond the typical norm of a posttraumatic reaction), she or he may benefit by sharing painful feelings or discussing recurrent or intrusive thoughts. This sharing may provide some immediate relief.
8. Identify the specific symptoms, problems, and areas of the patient's functioning that are most affected by the crisis (e.g., work, home, interpersonal, economic).
9. Identify the specific precipitants, other stressors, and symptoms (e.g., insomnia) that are currently contributing to the crisis. This can be done by helping the patient develop a timeline (see Figure 44-2).
10. Evaluate the support system by use of an eco map (see Figure 44-3). Using this support network tool, patients can be assisted in discovering who can help and who might exacerbate the situation.
11. Select the problem(s) or symptom(s) to treat first. This can be the most difficult part because it requires an accurate understanding or formulation of the causes of the crisis to prioritize what problem or symptom to treat first.
12. Use a wheel-and-spoke format (see Figure 44-4) to develop the treatment plan for a core crisis and prioritize the order of problems or symptoms that need to be treated.
13. Teach the patient to understand his or her current coping style and why and how it may not be working. Introduce other, more adaptive coping styles (see Table 44-3).
14. Obtain additional information from others who may be able to assist with crisis resolution. This should only be done after the crisis has been formulated and the focus of the treatment chosen.
15. Make a specific plan for crisis resolution based on additional information, newly discovered feelings, a crisis formulation, and treatment focus. This plan should involve the use of novel coping styles, a specific sequence of actions, and psychopharmacology as clinically appropriate (see Table 44-3).
16. The patient should implement the plan. Initially, it may be less overwhelming to resolve one cause of the crisis at a time instead of trying to handle many problems simultaneously.
17. Assess the results. Has the problem been resolved? If yes, go to step 1 and tackle a new symptom or problem. If not, go to step 18.
18. If the initial plan has not helped, try again, get additional help, or consult with a psychiatrist or other professionals.

evaluating a patient's coping style and, when necessary, suggesting an alternative or more adaptive coping style. These new skills facilitate a patient's adaptation to the stressful life circumstances. In general, those who can flexibly use many coping styles are the most successful at crisis resolution and problem solving. Often, patients in crisis rely too heavily on one coping style, which may not be the most adaptive for a particular situation. Those patients who lack the capacity to develop new, more adaptive coping styles may become dysfunctional when confronted with a crisis.

To illustrate coping styles and new coping skills, review Case Study 44-3. Joanne initially felt anxious and overwhelmed and began binge eating and drinking in her efforts to deal with her work stress, memories of the loss of her husband, and emerging problems with child care. As this progressed to symptoms of migraines and insomnia, she consulted her family physician. She realized she could ask for help from her physician, siblings, boss, and perhaps peers and she could get additional help as needed through a mental health professional or Alcoholics Anonymous. She mobilized her existing abilities to approach problems logically and work through alternative solutions as well as gather additional information about how to get

a new nanny. She also recognized her need to focus on self-care by using sleep hygiene and stress management techniques.

CRISIS RESOLUTION STRATEGY

In addition to teaching coping styles and coping skills, a family physician can provide a patient with general strategies for crisis resolution. A crisis resolution strategy, based on the crisis principles, consists of 18 steps (Table 44-4). The family physician may need to walk through some or all of these steps with the patient first before encouraging the patient to attempt some steps as a self-help strategy for the future.

Other Trauma Treatments

KEY TREATMENT

- Crisis intervention and psychotherapeutic techniques are a first-line approach for a crisis or mass trauma (Bradley et al., 2005; National Institute for Health and Care Excellence [NICE], 2005) (SOR: A). These include:

- Trauma-focused cognitive behavioral therapy (TFCBT) for adults and children is one of most beneficial forms of psychotherapy (Bisson et al., 2009; Foa et al., 2009; Forbes et al., 2010) (SOR: A).
- Eye movement desensitization and reprocessing is highly effective in some studies and less effective in others (Foa et al., 2009) (SOR: A or B).
- Exposure-based cognitive processing therapy is also one of the most beneficial form of psychotherapy (Bisson et al., 2009; Foa et al., 2009; Forbes et al., 2010) (SOR: A).
- Psychoeducation, breathing, relaxation training, and homework can be helpful for PTSD (Forbes et al., 2010) (SOR: B).
- Psychological first aid is helpful after mass trauma or disaster (Bisson et al., 2007) (SOR: B).
- Critical incident stress management (CISM), sometimes called debriefing, is not helpful (Benedek et al., 2009) (SOR: C).

Patients in an acute crisis or with disaster-related trauma may or may not require treatment. Crisis treatment is often necessary if the patient is suicidal or at risk for violence, has an acute medical emergency, or has a major psychiatric disorder (psychosis, PTSD, bipolar disorder, depression, overwhelming anxiety). All treatment is best when it is offered voluntarily or upon patient request.

Psychological treatment of patients with trauma can be offered immediately, with the patient allowed to pursue treatment voluntarily. Treatment should be vigorously pursued and possibly mandated if a major, life-threatening psychiatric illness appears acutely (APA, 2004; NICE, 2005).

No acute psychiatric treatment is often the best course of action if symptoms and non–life-threatening problems are resolving and if social and occupational functioning has remained intact over the first 6 weeks. Evidence indicates that mandatory crisis intervention in non–life-threatening circumstances, often called *critical incident stress management* (CISM) or "debriefing" (Mitchell et al., 1983), is not helpful (Rose et al., 2004). Patients who have experienced a mass trauma or disaster may benefit from "psychological first aid" (Bisson et al., 2007; Veterans Administration/ Department of Defense [VA/DoD] Management of Post-Traumatic Stress Working Group, 2012). This approach fosters safety, calmness, self and community efficacy, social connectedness, and optimism. In addition, psychoeducation, breathing, and relaxation training are often included as intervention that may be useful during the initial phases of exposure to traumas (APA, 2004; Benedek et al., 2009; NICE, 2005).

Seven major evidence-based guidelines are used to treat acute stress disorder and PTSD (Forbes et al., 2010). These practice guidelines do not always agree on the level of evidence for some treatments, which is why some forms of psychotherapy have two ratings in the key treatments crisis, trauma, disaster treatments. The current best recommendation for treatment of PTSD for adults (Foa et al., 2007) and children (AACAP Practice Parameters for PTSD, 2010) is TFCBT (Foa et al., 2009; Forbes et al., 2010) (SOR: A) as first-line preferential treatment rather than pharmacotherapy (Forbes et al., 2010). TFCBT includes exposure to past traumas through imagined, in vivo, and directed therapeutic, written, verbal, or taped narrative and use of cognitive-behavioral interventions. Exposure-based cognitive processing therapy is an evidence-based treatment with good efficacy (Foa et al., 2009; Forbes et al., 2010).

Eye movement desensitization and reprocessing is rated as either grade A (by Australian National Health, 2007; VA/DoD Management of Post-Traumatic Stress Working Group, 2012) or as grade B (by the Institute of Medicine, 2007). Because there are not enough experienced trauma therapists, pharmacotherapy is often used as the first-line treatment when trauma-based psychotherapy is not available.

Medications for Symptoms of Psychiatric Disorders

KEY TREATMENT

- First-line treatment for PTSD is with selective serotonin reuptake inhibitors (SSRIs), including sertraline and paroxetine, which are both approved by the U.S. Food and Drug Administration for PTSD (Friedman, 2013; Stein et al., 2003) (SOR: A). Venlafaxine (a serotonin–norepinephrine reuptake inhibitor [SNRI]) has also been shown to reduce symptoms similar to SSRIs (Friedman, 2013; Stein et al., 2003) (SOR: A), although the SSRIs and SNRIs may be less effective in combat veterans (Friedman, 2013; Hetrick et al., 2010).
- Mirtazapine and nefazodone are considered second-line agents. However, nefazodone is not often used because of concerns for liver toxicity (Friedman, 2013; Stein et al., 2003) (SOR: B).
- Benzodiazepines are not recommended for the treatment of PTSD unless being used for a comorbid disorder. Evidence has shown that this class of medication does not reduce symptoms and carries a high risk potential (Friedman, 2013; Stein et al., 2003) (SOR: B).
- Bupropion does not have any current consistent evidence as a treatment for PTSD (Friedman, 2013; Stein et al., 2003) (SOR: C).
- Topiramate is the only anticonvulsant that has consistently been shown to have efficacy as favorable as the SSRIs (Stein et al., 2003) (SOR: A).
- For PTSD nightmares, prazosin may be effective (Friedman, 2013; Stein et al., 2003) (SOR: B).
- Evidence is inconclusive regarding adjunctive treatment of PTSD with atypical antipsychotics in the absence of psychotic symptoms. Monotherapy is not recommended (Krystal et al., 2011; Stein et al., 2003) (SOR: B).
- There is currently insufficient evidence to determine if combined psychotherapy and pharmacotherapy is better than either modality alone (Hetrick et al., 2010) (SOR: A).

Although psychotherapeutic techniques are a first-line approach for a crisis or mass trauma (Forbes et al., 2010), use of medications for treatment of specific symptoms or psychiatric disorders can also be helpful. In general, pharmacology targeting symptom reduction parallels the pharmacology of the treatment for the major psychiatric disorders. For example, if a patient has an isolated sleep disturbance, use of the newer hypnotics is warranted. Similarly, for depressive or psychotic symptoms, antidepressants or antipsychotics can be used. This symptom-oriented approach has not been well studied.

During the acute crisis or immediate posttraumatic state, insomnia or other sleep disturbances may greatly affect coping. Use of a nonbenzodiazepine such as zolpidem, zaleplon, or eszopiclone can be considered as first-line pharmacologic treatment for acute sleep disturbances. The use of benzodiazepines for sleep or anxiety in the acute postcrisis state is questionable, with little support for efficacy and concerns that benzodiazepines may inhibit effective coping. Benzodiazepines also carry the risk of dependence and addiction, and data suggest that they do not reduce the progression to PTSD (Friedman, 2013). Although data are sparse regarding the effectiveness, trazodone is also often used clinically for chronic sleep difficulties because it carries no risk of dependence.

Thus far, no known interventions have prevented PTSD. For the primary treatment of PTSD, medications include SSRIs, prazosin, and topiramate. PTSD symptoms, including reexperiencing the trauma, avoidance, numbing, and hyperarousal, are effectively treated with SSRIs and SNRIs, including sertraline, paroxetine, venlafaxine, and fluoxetine (APA, 2004; Benedek et al., 2009; Forbes et al. 2010; Friedman, 2013; Stein et al., 2006). Prazosin has been shown to be effective in treating nightmares associated with PTSD, but its effects on other PTSD symptoms is not well studied (Friedman, 2013).

A distinction between non–combat-related and combat-related PSTD is warranted when considering pharmacologic therapy (Benedek et al., 2009). Non–combat-related PTSD includes civilian trauma, childhood or adult sexual assault, intimate partner violence, interpersonal trauma, or trauma caused by a motor vehicle crash. For non–combat-related PTSD, sertraline, paroxetine, fluoxetine, and venlafaxine are effective in short-term trials. These medications can either be a primary form of treatment if the patient does not want TFCBT or can be combined with TFCBT; no evidence yet shows that combined treatment is superior to SSRI or CBT alone (Hetrick et al., 2010). More recent studies suggest that topiramate is beneficial in the treatment of PTSD and is similar in efficacy to the SSRIs (Friedman, 2013). The efficacy of the antidepressant mirtazapine is equivocal but reportedly somewhat beneficial (Friedman, 2013). No efficacy for β-blockers or bupropion has been established.

The results for pharmacologic treatment of combat-related trauma are less convincing. It seems that younger veterans with PTSD from more recent wars are responsive to the same SSRIs and SNRIs as non–combat-related patients. However, older veterans from previous wars do not appear to respond to sertraline or fluoxetine. Thus, the common SSRIs may be only somewhat effective for this group (Benedek et al., 2009). For PTSD nightmares in both groups, prazosin (3-15 mg/night) has been used with some success.

Although the SSRIs are the first-line choice for the pharmacotherapy of PTSD, not all patients will have a full treatment response. Previously, it had been thought that adjunctive treatment with risperidone and olanzapine may be helpful. However, a recent large randomized clinical trial of veterans found that risperidone was no better than placebo (Friedman, 2013; Krystal et al., 2011). Augmentation with a mood stabilizer such as divalproex or lithium may be considered, but evidence for success is limited. Buspirone or benzodiazepines may also be used, but only sparingly and adjunctively, to decrease anxiety or panic attacks. These medications are not recommended as monotherapy.

Conclusion

Family physicians are routinely faced with a variety of acute crises, patient-reported traumas, and disaster situations that require a specialized knowledge to understand patient complaints and to successfully develop management and intervention strategies. The goals of crisis intervention and disaster management are to evaluate the precipitants of the crisis, understand the personal meaning of the events, deal with the crisis state itself, and use the selective past history to comprehend the current situation better. It is also important to mobilize the support network and, if relevant, diagnose and treat any comorbid psychiatric illnesses. A crisis evaluation strategy using a timeline, eco map, and wheel-and-spoke formulation can be used to help implement a specific problem-solving approach. Crisis treatment includes problem or symptom-oriented therapy, use of adaptive coping styles, 18-step crisis intervention approach, and medications when indicated. All of these interventions can be helpful when seeking a resolution of the crisis.

References

The complete reference list is available at www.expertconsult.com.

Web Resources

www.nice.org.uk/guidance/cg26 National Institute for Health and Care Excellence (NICE). Post-traumatic stress disorder (PTSD): the management of PTSD in adults and children in primary and secondary care, 2005. Clinical Guideline 26.

www.aacap.org/AACAP/AACAP/Families_and_Youth/Facts_for_Families/Facts_for_Families_Pages/Posttraumatic_Stress_Disorder_70.aspx American Academy of Child & Adolescent Psychiatry Practice Facts for Families page.

www.healthquality.va.gov/Post_Traumatic_Stress_Disorder_PTSD.asp U.S. Department of Veterans Affairs, Department of Defense. Clinical practice guideline for management of posttraumatic stress, version 2.0, 2010.

www.istss.org/TreatmentGuidelines/5168.htm International Society for Traumatic Stress Studies (ISTSS) Treatment Guidelines for PTSD.

www.nhmrc.gov.au/publications/synopses/mh13syn.htm Australian National Health and Medical Research Council Guidelines for the Treatment of Adults with Acute Stress Disorder and Posttraumatic Stress Disorder, 2007.

www.rehab.research.va.gov/jour/2012/495/pdf/VADODclinical guidlines495.pdf Review of Veterans Administration/Department of Defense Clinical Practice Guideline for the Management of Acute Stress and Intervention to Prevent Post-Traumatic Stress Disorder, 2012.

45 Difficult Encounters: Patients with Personality Disorders

ROBERT E. FEINSTEIN and JOSEPH CONNELLY

Patients with personality disorders are difficult to manage and can elicit intense reactions in the primary care physicians and medical staff who care for them. Patients with personality disorders have an unintentional ability to create problematic patient–physician–staff relationships. This covert pressure placed on the physicians and staff often affects how the medical team evaluates or diagnoses a patient and frequently affects physician orders, laboratory tests, suggested treatments, and recommendations. Up to 15% of primary care patients have a personality disorder (Moran et al., 2000; National Institute for Mental Health in England, 2003). However, patients with personality disorders often go unrecognized because they do not complain and often do not present with any overt symptoms. However, when interviewed, patients with personality disorders often reveal interpersonal failures and describe multiple social and occupation difficulties. Most patients with personality disorders are recognized after a problematic interpersonal interaction or are secondarily recognized by the complaints of others, especially complaints from spouses, family, or friends. Family physicians see these patients every day. Patients with personality disorders tend to consume a disproportionate amount of family physicians' time and emotional energy. Physicians with high numbers of difficult patients are more susceptible to low morale and burnout (An et al., 2013; Han, 1994, 1996, 2002).

Although family physicians do not treat the underlying personality disorder, recognition and effective management of these difficult patients is routinely possible and often necessary in medical settings. The goal in the management of patients with personality disorders is to provide or assist physicians or staff in the understanding and medical management of these patients so that optimal medical care can be delivered.

Personality Traits versus Personality Disorder

Personality traits are enduring. They describe a habitual way of coping that is manifested in how a patient feels, thinks, behaves, and interacts with others. Genetically determined personality traits are called *temperament*. Personality traits such as shyness or high stimulus barrier (the ability to stay focused and not be distracted by external stimuli) are often observable from birth and can be readily seen in a newborn nursery. Other personality traits that develop from the interaction with caregivers and the environment are called *character*. Character traits, such as the capacity to empathize or anxious or depressive tendencies, can be environmentally acquired through early parent–child experiences. The distinction between personality traits and a personality disorder is a matter of degree. Personality traits tend to be stable but can be more easily modified according to the needs of external reality. When personality traits combine and become rigid, extreme, and maladaptive and cause interpersonal, social, or occupational dysfunction, they are called *personality disorders* (Oldham et al., 2009; Skodal, 2009). These disorders are much harder to modify and typically require long-term psychotherapy, with or without pharmacotherapy, to facilitate change. Although everyone is unique, there seems to be a continuum of personality traits and disorders that are commonly encountered. Some personality disorders can be recognized in the movies. These include the narcissistic personality disorder as portrayed by Sharon Stone in *Basic Instinct*, the antisocial personality disorder played by Robert DeNiro in *Cape Fear*, and the schizotypal personality disorder portrayed by Karen Allen in *The Glass Menagerie*.

Classification and Diagnosis

Key Points

- A personality disorder is an enduring pattern of inner experience and behavior that deviates markedly from the expectations of the individual's culture.
- Problems are in at least two of these areas: cognition, affectivity, interpersonal functioning, and impulse control.
- An enduring pattern is inflexible and pervasive across a broad range of persona and social situations.
- The enduring pattern leads to clinically significant distress or impairment in social, occupational, or other areas of functioning.
- The pattern is stable and of long duration; onset can be traced back to adolescence or is diagnosed in adulthood.
- To diagnose, begin with dimensional measures: Cluster A, odd eccentric; Cluster B, dramatic emotional; and Cluster C, avoidant fearful (Table 45-1).

Table 45-1 Personality Clusters and Disorders

Cluster A (Odd, Eccentric)	Cluster B (Dramatic, Emotional)	Cluster C (Anxious, Fearful)
1. Paranoid (301.0; DSM-5, p. 649)	1. Antisocial (301.7; DSM-5, p. 659)	1. Avoidant (301.82; DSM-5, pp. 672-673)
2. Schizoid (301.20; DSM-5, pp. 652-653)	2. Borderline (301.83; DSM-5, p. 663)	2. Dependent (301.6; DSM-5, p. 675)
3. Schizotypal (301.22; DSM-5, pp. 655-656)	3. Histrionic (301.50; DSM-5, p. 667)	3. Obsessive-compulsive (301.4; DSM-5, pp. 678-679)
	4. Narcissistic (301.81; DSM-5, pp. 669-670)	

DSM-5, Diagnostic and Statistical Manual of Mental Disorders, fifth edition.
Personality disorder criteria are available from American Psychiatric Association. *Diagnostic and statistical manual of mental disorders.* 5th Ed. Washington, DC: American Psychiatric Association; 2013

> ■ Use the categorical classification systems to identify the specific personality disorder.
> ■ A particular patient may have traits from different clusters and may meet criteria for more than one personality disorder.

Patients with personality disorders are typically diagnosed using a categorical or a dimensional approach. The quasi-dimensional and *categorical* approach described in the *Diagnostic and Statistical Manual of Mental Disorders*, fourth edition, text revision (DSM IV-TR; American Psychiatric Association, 2005) and maintained in the *Diagnostic and Statistical Manual of Mental Disorders*, fifth edition (DSM-5; American Psychiatric Association, 2013), begins by identifying the appropriate dimensional cluster of a personality disorder. Each of these clusters broadly describes personality dimensions of the patient as either Cluster A, odd or eccentric; Cluster B, dramatic, emotional, or erratic; or Cluster C, anxious or fearful. After the dimensional cluster has been identified, the categorical approach describes 10 discrete "prototypes" or easily recognizable categories of personality disorders. This predominately categorical approach colorfully describes and differentiates 10 distinct personality disorders. This categorical approach has the advantage that it is easiest for clinicians to use. However, because personalities are complicated and often not discrete entities, it is not unusual for a patient to meet DSM-5 criteria for two cluster diagnoses and more than one specific personality disorder diagnosis. Because of these limitations in the current categorical system, the evolution within personality disorder research is to move toward a dimensional model for classification.

The DSM-5 has a dimensional "alternative DSM-5 model for personality disorders." This complex dimensional model describes Criteria A as the "level of personality functioning," which includes disturbances in the self (e.g., disturbances in experiences of self and others, problems with self-esteem, difficulty in regulating emotions, and difficulty being self-directed toward meaningful life goals) and disturbances in interpersonal functioning (e.g., problems with empathy and intimacy). Criteria B describes personality traits in five broad domains (e.g., negative affectivity, antagonism, detachment, disinhibition, and psychoticism). These domains consist of 25 specific personality traits that are described in detail. Although the DSM-5's *dimensional* approach has much to offer to psychiatrists and other mental health professionals who treat personality disorders, the approach is not yet validated for extensive or official use. Because the dimensional approach is still in development, this chapter uses the categorical approach

adopted by DSM-5, which is likely more useful for family physicians.

Management of Patients with Personality Disorders

Key Points

The following five-step process is useful as a management strategy for family physicians who wish to create therapeutic relationships with personality-disordered patients who might otherwise be experienced as difficult. (Tables 45-1 and 45-2 outline this process using the DSM-5 classification.)

1. Strive to understand the patient's core beliefs, irrational thoughts, and fears.
2. Identify the patient's defense mechanisms and coping style and use confrontation, clarification, and interpretation to modify these.
3. Recognize recurrent patient behaviors and how these will likely affect patient adherence and use of medical services.
4. Learn to use your own reactions to the patient to help identify the diagnosis and management strategy.
5. Recognize that specific interventions are helpful for different types of patients (Table 45-3).

PATIENT CORE BELIEFS, IRRATIONAL THOUGHTS, AND FEARS

Key Points

■ Patients have identifiable core beliefs (or worldviews) and fears.
■ These interact and can feed off each other in difficult patients.
■ Stress activates these core beliefs and precipitates intense and dysfunctional emotions, fears, thoughts, physical symptoms, or maladaptive behaviors that are characteristic for each specific personality disorder (see Table 45-2).
■ Adherence to medical recommendations and use of medical services are somewhat predictable based on the particular personality disorders.

The family physician can apply the principles of cognitive-behavioral therapy (CBT) to facilitate their management skills when working with patients with personality

Table 45-2   Schema for Managing Patients with a Personality Disorder

DSM-5 Disorder	Patient Core Beliefs	Patient Fears	Defenses	Coping Styles	Patient Health Behaviors
Paranoid	Others are adversaries and are to blame; I am being examined; They are out to get me; I can't trust anyone	Exploitation; slights; betrayal; humiliation; physical intrusions from medical procedures	Projection: ascribe one's impulses to others Projective identification: project one's impulse plus control of others as way to control one's own impulses Denial: refusal to admit painful realities Splitting: self and others seen as all good or all bad	Guarded and protective of their autonomy, often with an arrogant belief in their own superiority	Wariness, suspicion, mistrust, jealousy, self-sufficiency, counter-attacking, anger, violence
Schizoid	I need space; I need to be alone; people are replaceable or unimportant	Emotional contact; warmth; intimacy; caring; intrusions or violation of privacy	Isolation of affect: thoughts stored without emotion Intellectualization: replace feelings with fact Denial and splitting: see above Regression: revert to childlike thoughts, feelings, or behaviors	Inner world insulated from others	Withdrawal; seeking isolation and privacy
Schizotypal	Idiosyncratic, magical, or eccentric beliefs; I know what they're thinking or feeling; premonitions	Emotional contact; warmth; caring; violation of privacy	Schizoid fantasy: retreat to idiosyncratic fantasy when faced with painful experience Undoing: symbolic magical action designed to reverse or cancel unacceptable thoughts or actions Regression, denial, splitting: see above	Chaotic, disorganized	Withdrawal; odd, autistic, or magical behaviors and movements; seeks isolation and privacy
Antisocial	People are there to be used and exploited; I come before all others	Boredom; loss of prestige, power, or esteem	Acting out: expression in action or behavior rather than in words or emotions Splitting: see above	Seeks autonomy, freedom; seeks advantage or secondary gain	Lies, deceit, and manipulation; violence; seeks secondary gain
Borderline	I am very bad or very good; Who am I? I can't be alone	Separations, loss, emotional abandonment; not being loved and cared for; fluctuating self-esteem	Splitting, projection, projective identification, dissociation, regression, acting out (see above) Omnipotence: seeing self, others as all-powerful Idealization or devaluation: vacillates between seeing self or others as ideal and then deprecating self or others Mini-psychotic experiences	Hostile dependency; chaotic lifestyle; threatening or intimidating; seeking intimacy, dependency, or pseudo-autonomy	Impulsive behaviors; suicidal actions; cutting; anger or violence; panic; anxiety; poor reality; stormy relationships
Histrionic	I need to impress and to be admired or loved; I need to be taken care of or helped	Loss of love, admiration, attention, or dependent care	Sexualization: functions or objects changed into sexual symbols to avoid anxieties Regression, acting out, splitting: see above Dissociation: disrupted perceptions or sensations, consciousness, memory, or personal identity Somatization: physical symptoms caused by mental processes Repression: involuntary forgetting of painful memories, feelings, or experiences	Self-centered, emotion driven, flirtatious, flighty	Dramatics; exhibitionism; expressiveness; impressionistic
Narcissistic	I am special; I am important; I come first; The world should revolve around me	Loss of prestige, image, power, or esteem	Splitting, projection, projective identification, acting out, denial regression: see above	Superior and arrogant, self-aggrandizing, self-centered, self-protecting, demeaning, demanding, critical	Self aggrandizement; inflated or deflated self view; entitled; devalue or idealize; viciousness; envy; competitive
Avoidant	I must avoid harm or be cautious because I may get rejected or exposed or be humiliated	Rejection; embarrassment in social situations; humiliation; exposure of inadequacies	Inhibition: restriction of thoughts, feelings, behaviors to avoid shame, exposure of inadequacies, rejection or humiliation Phobias: fears of objects, people, situations; avoided to prevent anxiety Avoidance, withdrawal, regression, Somatization: see above	Withdraw or escape; avoid criticism	Avoidance; withdrawal; social timidity; caution; fear or anxiety

Table 45-2   Schema for Managing Patients with a Personality Disorder (Continued)

DSM-5 Disorder	Patient Core Beliefs	Patient Fears	Defenses	Coping Styles	Patient Health Behaviors
Dependent	I am helpless without others; I can't make a decision; I need constant reassurance and care	Separation, independence, making decisions, anger	Dependent: yearning for care, clinging, needing direction Passive-aggressive: superficial compliance and passivity disguising stubbornness and anger Reaction formation: unacceptable impulses expressed as the opposite Regression, splitting: see above	Passive, dependent, helpless	Unusually submissive; clinging; indecisive; childlike; needing to be taken care of
Obsessive-compulsive	People should do better or try harder; I must be perfect; I must make no errors or mistakes; details, not feelings, rule	Disorder, mistakes, imperfection, afraid of feelings, (especially rage or anger), anxiety, self-doubt, dependency	Isolation of affect, intellectualization, reaction formation, undoing: see above Controlling: efforts to regulate objects or others to avoid anxiety Displacement: transfer of one's feelings from one person on to another Dependent: see above Inhibition: restricting thoughts, feelings, or behaviors for fear that unacceptable impulses will erupt and create anxiety or damage Phobias, repression: see above	Inflexible; constricted; governed by rules, safety, or security concerns	Perfectionism; driven orderliness; logical; compulsions; controlling; critical; stubbornness or stinginess; workaholic; rational

DSM-5, Diagnostic and Statistical Manual of Mental Disorders, fifth edition.

Table 45-3   Personality-Disordered Patients: Adherence, Utilization, Physician Reactions, and Interventions

DSM-5 Disorder	Adherence	Utilization	Physician Reactions	Interventions
Paranoid	Difficult when requested by the physician because the patient is suspicious of the need for compliance Problematic but may be easier when the patient is seeking relief from symptoms	Limited utilization, or as a condition for medical service utilization, the patient may seek detailed explanations or reasons for the diagnostic testing or needs for other services	Fearful; sense of danger; mistrust; feeling accused, blamed, or threatened	1. Empathize with patient's fear of being hurt; acknowledge complaints without arguing or ignoring. 2. Openly and honestly explain medical illness. 3. Correct reality distortions and unreasonable patient expectations. 4. Gently question irrational thoughts and suggest more rational ones. 5. Do not confront delusions. 6. If the patient refuses care out of mistrust, rather than insist, ask if it is OK if you can disagree about the need for the test. 7. Interpret projection (blame) and other defenses.
Schizoid	May be difficult Will need reinforcement and monitoring; may need outreach services	Underutilization; outreach, if not too frequent, may help foster appropriate use of medical services	Detached or removed; wish to involve patient with others or to break through the isolation	1. Empathize with the patient's need for privacy and contact. 2. Accept the patient's unsociability. 3. Reduce the patient's isolation as tolerated. 4. Neutrally impart medical information. 5. Do not demand involvement nor permit total withdrawal. 6. Correct reality distortions and unreasonable patient expectations. 7. Gently question irrational thoughts and suggest more rational ones. 8. Interpret isolation and other defenses.
Schizotypal	May be difficult; may need outreach, visiting nurse, community resources, or case management	Underutilization; may need outreach to gain reasonable and appropriate utilization of medical services	Detached; removed; "weird and alone" feelings; wish to involve patient with others or to break through the isolation	1. Empathize with the patient's idiosyncratic style, magical thinking, and perceptions without directly confronting them. 2. Recognize the need for privacy and contact. 3. Accept the patient's unsociability; reduce the patient's isolation, as tolerated. 4. Neutrally impart information. 5. Do not demand involvement or permit total withdrawal. 6. Correct reality distortions and unreasonable patient expectations. 7. Gently question irrational thoughts and suggest more rational ones. 8. Interpret regression and other defenses.

Continued on following page

Table 45-3   Personality-Disordered Patients: Adherence, Utilization, Physician Reactions, and Interventions (Continued)

DSM-5 Disorder	Adherence	Utilization	Physician Reactions	Interventions
Antisocial	May be resistant, problematic, and intolerant of the need for ongoing compliance	May misuse medical resources for secondary gain	Used, exploited, or deceived; anger; a wish to uncover lies, punish, or imprison	1. Empathize with the patient's fear of exploitation and low self-esteem. 2. Determine if you are being used for secondary gain. If you suspect dishonesty, verify symptoms and illness progression with others. 3. Do not moralize. Explain that deception results in your giving the patient poor care. 4. Correct reality distortions and unreasonable patient expectations. 5. Gently question irrational thoughts and suggest more rational ones. 6. Interpret defenses. 7. Medications as adjunctive treatment.
Borderline	Inconsistent as adherence is easily Influenced by emotional storms, interpersonal conflicts, or chaotic lifestyles	Misuse or high use for maladaptive behaviors such as suicidal or disruptive behaviors	Feeling manipulated, angry, impotent, depleted, self-doubting; wish to rescue or get rid of the patient; guilty	1. Empathize with patient's fear of abandonment and separation and plan for absences by arranging coverage. 2. Express a wish to help and satisfy reasonable needs. 3. Ask the patient to monitor impulsive behaviors with a diary or log. 4. Set firm limits and do not punish. 5. Correct reality distortions and unreasonable patient expectations. 6. Gently question irrational thoughts and suggest more rational ones. 7. Interpret splitting and other defenses. 8. Negotiate emergency procedures in advance. If suicidal, the patient must go to the emergency room, if not safe. If the patient refuses emergency help when you offer, let the patient know in advance that this therapeutic breach may end the relationship. 9. Medications as adjunctive treatment.
Histrionic	Often dependent on others or inconsistent	May misuse or overuse medical resources to gain attention from the physician or staff	Flattered, captivated, seduced, or aroused; flooded by emotions; depleted; wish to rescue	1. Empathize with patient's fear of losing love or care. 2. Interact in a friendly way, not too reserved or too warm. 3. Discuss patient's fears; reassure when possible. 4. Use logic to counteract an emotional style of thinking. 5. Set limits if patient regresses. 6. Correct reality distortions and unreasonable patient expectations. 7. Gently question irrational thoughts and suggest more rational ones. 8. Interpret sexualization, regression, and other specific defenses.
Narcissistic	Can be problematic; intolerant of the need for ongoing compliance requirements	Entitled to use, or may abuse, medical services when needed	Devalued/ overvalued; inferior/superior; fearful of patient's criticism or anger; wish to retaliate, devalue, or get rid of the patient	1. Empathize with patient's vulnerability and low self-esteem. 2. Don't mistake patient's superior attitude for *real* confidence and don't confront entitlement. 3. When devalued or attacked, acknowledge the patient's hurt, your mistakes, and express your continued wish to help. 4. If devaluing continues, offer a referral as an option, not as punishment. 5. Correct reality distortions and unreasonable patient expectations. 6. Gently question irrational thoughts and suggest more rational ones. 7. Interpret splitting and other defenses.
Avoidant	Diverted or delayed by avoidant behavior; guided by a wish to avoid disapproval of medical staff	Seeks medical services to secure approval or avoid criticism, not necessarily seeking the health benefits	Frustrated because the patient often cannot articulate fears; annoyed at the patient's weakness	1. Empathize with patient's social fears, shame, shyness, and fears of revealing inadequacies, rejection, embarrassment, humiliation, and anger. 2. Help the patient describe in detail the feared situation(s). 3. Encourage and support the need for the patient to gradually face the fears and the tendency to avoid. If this seems overwhelming, choose smaller fears to confront or refer. 4. If frustrated or unclear about the nature of the fears, ask for detailed descriptions of the problem. 5. Gently elicit irrational thoughts and suggest more rational ones. 6. Correct reality distortions. 7. Interpret avoidance, phobias, and other defenses. 8. Medications as adjunctive treatment.

Table 45-3　Personality-Disordered Patients: Adherence, Utilization, Physician Reactions, and Interventions (Continued)

DSM-5 Disorder	Adherence	Utilization	Physician Reactions	Interventions
Dependent	Dependent on others for medical supervision and easily overwhelmed by the demands of self-monitoring compliance	Underuse when left to themselves, but may overuse service when physician or medical staff becomes the source of needed gratification	Depleted; annoyed at the patient's dependence; may deny the patient's reasonable needs	1. Empathize with the patient's need for care. 2. Frustrate total dependence. 3. Be careful to avoid telling the patient what to do. 4. Encourage independent thinking and action. 5. Realize that what the patient says that he or she wants (caretaking) is not necessarily what he or she needs. 6. Ask the patient what it is about independence that is so frightening. 7. Don't abandon or threaten termination because some very dependent patients need regular physician contact for life. 8. Correct reality distortions and unreasonable patient expectations. 9. Gently elicit irrational thoughts and suggest more rational ones. 10. Interpret regression and other specific defenses. 11. Prescribe medications as adjunctive treatment (see Table 45-4).
Obsessive-compulsive	Rigid and inflexibly follows the rules; disrupted or anxious if unexpected changes are required	Conflicted about utilization; fears of uncertainty may drive increased use, and fears of loss of control may decrease use	In a battle of control with negative reactions to patient stinginess, need for order, and stubbornness; distanced from feelings; bored with details	1. Empathize with the patient's logical, detailed, unemotional style of thinking. 2. If obsessive thoughts are interfering with medical care, ask about the patient's feelings. 3. Do not struggle with the patient over control or critical judgments. 4. Avoid abandoning the patient. 5. Correct reality distortions and unreasonable patient expectations. 6. Gently elicit irrational thoughts and suggest more rational ones. 7. Interpret specific defenses.

disorders. The theory of CBT (Beck and Freeman, 1990; Greenberger and Padesky, 1995) is that patients have a "worldview," or a set of "core beliefs," and personality-specific fears that can be identified and directly managed by the family physician who brings those worldviews to the patient's conscious awareness. When an environmental stress occurs against the background of the patient's core belief, a reinforcing feedback loop ensues. An external environmental stress or internal stress interacts with the core beliefs, and this triggers an irrational fear or thought. Irrational fears create negative emotions (e.g., depression or anxiety) that can lead to maladaptive behaviors or physical symptoms. Behaviors or symptoms can also feedback directly to confirm the patient's worldview and fears. Core beliefs and fears are readily activated in medical settings where patients are sick and vulnerable. For example, a patient with stomach distress may fear or believe that she has cancer. She may be anxious that she is dying as her mother recently did of a gastrointestinal cancer. By inquiring about the severity of the patient's fears and uncovering her irrational thoughts (that she too must have cancer), the physician can reassure her that this is unlikely and reduce her worry while also proceeding with the workup as indicated. Empathizing with the patient's core beliefs and fears will likely improve the doctor–patient relationship, which may allow the physician to help the patient recognize his or her irrational thoughts. The physician can then correct these distortions with facts, thereby relieving suffering and possibly improving the quality of medical care that takes place. The CBT sequences for each of the specific personality disorders are described in Table 45-2.

DEFENSES AND COPING STYLES

Key Points

- Defense mechanisms are automatic internal psychological processes that protect the patient from anxiety and stressors and help with adaptation to the environment.
- Patients with specific personality diagnoses use a known range of particular defense mechanisms (see Table 45-2).
- Patients with unexplained somatic symptoms tend to use denial, externalization, and somatization, converting psychosocial distress and problematic interpersonal relationships into unexplained physical complaints.
- Coping styles are typical behavioral ways of dealing with the external world.
- Patients with specific personality diagnoses tend to use a known range of coping styles (see Table 45-2).
- Patients with severe unexplained somatic symptoms tend to use high- or low-anxious coping styles or manipulative coping styles (see Table 45-2).

A family physician can attempt to relieve a core problem or a symptom presenting for medical care by fostering the patient's awareness of his or her problems. To do this, it is important to appreciate the unconscious psychological processes known as *defense mechanisms*. These unconscious psychological processes (e.g., denial, projection) are used to resolve internal conflicts, manage moods, mediate external dangers, and facilitate adaptations to reality. *Coping styles*, on the other hand, are typically behavioral patterns and methods of coping with the external environment.

Patients with personality disorders often present with unexplained symptoms. They tend to use defense mechanisms such as denial, externalization, and somatization, converting psychosocial distress and problematic interpersonal relationships into unexplained physical complaints. Patients with severe unexplained symptoms tend to use high- or low-anxious coping or manipulative coping styles (see Table 45-1). By understanding the constellation of defenses and coping styles used by personality-disordered patients, the physician may be able to modify the pathologic defenses or coping style that is interfering with the patient–physician alliance and the delivery of medical care. A physician can use clarification, confrontation, and interpretation (see Table 45-1). For example, a borderline patient may feel hurt and abandoned by the physician's vacation plans and accuse the physician of not caring. This patient may use a defense mechanism called *devaluation* (physician is deprecated as uncaring) and a coping style of manipulation (threatening suicide). With this understanding, the physician can begin to help the patient by not taking personally the patient's efforts to devalue or manipulate. The physician can respond to the patient by empathizing with the patient's fears of abandonment. The physician may clarify that the patient has a distorted belief and that the vacation is being incorrectly experienced as a personal abandonment of the patient. The physician may further clarify that the vacation does not communicate anything about the physician's future ability or wish to care for the patient. The patient can be reassured of the physician's return, future realistic medical availability, specific limits of availability, and medical coverage by another physician. In a preventive effort to allay a crisis and help a borderline patient manage separation fears, the physician (before the vacation) could also suggest that the patient use a new active coping style and schedule a meeting with a designated medical colleague who will provide coverage while the physician is away. Often, it is helpful to anticipate issues that may arise for the patient and suggest specific problem solving and coping.

PATIENT BEHAVIORS, ADHERENCE, AND USE OF MEDICAL SERVICES

Key Points

- Cluster A personality disorders (paranoid, schizoid, and schizotypal) tend not to adhere to medical recommendations and to underuse medical services.
- Cluster B patients (antisocial, histrionic, borderline, narcissistic) tend to have variable adherence to medical recommendations and may misuse, overuse, or underuse medical care.
- Cluster C patients (dependent, obsessive-compulsive, avoidant) tend to adhere to medical recommendations because of fear of the consequences of nonadherence.

Patients with personality disorders often display characteristic behaviors that affect their adherence to medical recommendations and use of medical services (Soeteman et al., 2008). Understanding these behaviors can also help physicians manage the expectations of these difficult patients and improve the chances for effective interventions that might improve medical adherence and health outcomes. In general, patients with Cluster A personality disorders (paranoid, schizoid, and schizotypal) tend not to adhere to medical recommendations and underuse medical services. They may require outreach to involve them in their own medical care. Cluster B patients (antisocial, histrionic, borderline, narcissistic, and self-defeating) tend to have variable adherence to medical recommendations and may misuse, overuse, or underuse medical care. Cluster C patients (dependent, obsessive-compulsive, avoidant) tend to adhere to medical recommendations because of fear of the consequences of nonadherence. They are ambivalent users of the medical system and tend to use medical services appropriately when others are involved in their care.

PHYSICIAN REACTIONS TO PATIENTS WITH PERSONALITY DISORDERS

Key Points

- Physician reactions are useful in recognizing, diagnosing, and managing difficult patients.
- Reactions stirred by the patient are referred to as *patient-generated countertransferences*.
- Physician reactions are often similar or shared in common by all physicians seeing the patient, with some elements peculiar to each individual physician.
- Difficult patients often generate intense physician feelings.
- There may be fantasies or thoughts about the patient that are uncharacteristic for the physician.
- The physician may engage in behaviors that would normally not be typical for him or her (see Table 45-3).

Although the DSM-5 is a useful aid for making a diagnosis, family physicians often recognize a patient with a personality trait or unexplained physical complaint by their own reactions to the patient. Physicians working with personality-disordered patients seem to have specific and characteristic reactions to these patients that need to be recognized, understood, and used for the patient's benefit. Patient-generated feelings provoked in the physician are created through the interpersonal interaction between patient and physician. These reactions to a patient should alert the physician to a possible diagnosis of a difficult patient. Typical physician reactions to patients that are provoked by the patient are also called *patient-generated countertransferences*. These include intense feelings, uncharacteristic fantasies, or atypical behaviors by the physician.

Intense Affects

Intense physician feelings elicited through patient interactions may include negative feelings such as active dislike, fury, or frustration toward a patient (Groves, 1978; Strous et al., 2006). Alternatively, the physician may have strong positive feelings of attraction, sexual arousal, wanting to rescue the patient, or wanting to provide exceptionally good medical care. These may alternate with other wishes to avoid the patient, terminate the relationship, or transfer the patient to a colleague. In extreme cases, intense feelings aroused in a physician can become a focal point for leading the physician into boundary violations with a patient. These are extremely damaging to both parties and violate the tenets of professional behavior.

Fantasies

Physicians may also recognize that they are interacting with a patient who has a personality disorder by recognizing their own fantasies. Fantasies described by family physicians that are commonly generated by patients with personality disorders may include excessive worrying about a patient after normal work hours; a wish to rescue a patient; a wish that a patient might die; dreaming about a patient; or experiencing unusually exaggerated, intrusive, angry, sexual, or curious fantasies about the patient when not at work and during personal private time.

Atypical Behaviors

A physician may also notice behaviors with certain patients that are atypical for his or her usual customary medical practice. These unusual physician behaviors should trigger self-examination by the physician and consideration that the patient may have a personality disorder. Frequently, difficult patients are capable of arousing unconscious reactions that lead to new and unusual physician behaviors.

Common atypical physician behaviors include ordering tests to placate a patient, asking for more than the usual number of consults on a patient whose care does not seem medically complicated, suggesting aggressive diagnostic testing or procedures when the yield of these tests is likely to be low, repeatedly extending the time spent with a particular patient or family, lowering the customary fee, offering free treatment, or developing a personal (not professional) relationship with a patient. Common physician reactions associated with difficult patients are reviewed in Table 45-2.

Physicians can use the scope of patient-generated countertransferences (their feelings, fantasies, and atypical medical behaviors) as a valuable diagnostic aid because difficult patients tend to provoke the same feelings in most physicians who deal with them. For example, a patient with a borderline personality disorder (BPD) often leaves many physicians exhausted and worried about the patient's suicidal threats. A patient with obsessive-compulsive personality disorder (OCPD) may argue over details of the treatment, fees, or scheduling. Physicians who learn to recognize feelings provoked by patients will find it easier to identify the subtype of personality disorder according to the feelings elicited. More important, physicians who can recognize their unusual reactions will be better able to tolerate them and avoid acting out their feelings with a patient. This will improve the physician–patient relationship, medical decision making, and ultimately patient care (Feinstein et al., 1999).

General Management Principles for Difficult Patients

ATTENDING TO A PROBLEMATIC ALLIANCE

To establish a good working alliance based on trust, acceptance, and confidence, the family physician should begin each patient encounter by listening, asking open-ended questions, and continually striving for empathy. The alliance is also fostered by the physician's own self-awareness, ability to acknowledge mistakes, and efforts to adapt to the patient's wishes or needs that will foster improved health outcomes. Problems often occur in developing an alliance with a patient who has a personality disorder. If tension develops in the alliance, the physician should ask what the patient thinks of the current problem. If the patient expresses the problem clearly, the physician should join with the patient in solving the problem to deliver effective medical care. If the problem is the physician–patient relationship, nondefensive reflective listening, clarifications, admitting mistakes, and initiating new efforts to improve the situation are often helpful. If the physician believes that there is a different problem affecting the alliance, the physician may say, "I believe that there is a different problem [identify the problem, e.g., psychosocial distress, problem drinking] that is affecting my ability to help you get well and offer you the best medical care available. We need to think about this problem and come up with some solutions."

CHOOSING A FOCUS FOR THE INTERVIEW

When delivering medical care with a patient with a personality disorder, it is important to be consistent, reliable, and predictable to avoid future problems. Patients with personality disorders often experience an inability to verbalize or prioritize their most important medical or psychosocial concerns. For these patients, it is particularly important to strive for a mutually agreed upon focus for short- and long-term medical treatment goals. It is often helpful to use a process called *informed shared decision making,* in which the physician takes time with the patient to discuss and negotiate the acute focus of medical care, short- and long-term medical goals, strategies to achieve these goals, and specific timelines for accomplishing the prioritized medical plan (Feinstein et al., 1999).

USING BASIC PSYCHOTHERAPY TECHNIQUES FOR INTERVIEWING A PATIENT

As is often the case, a general medical approach may not be sufficient to help a difficult-to-manage patient. After a brief period of immersion in the patient's complaints, the family physician can respond with empathic responses, initially acknowledging the patient's fears, core beliefs, and symptoms (see Table 45-1). If this is not helpful, the physician can use general psychotherapeutic techniques such as confrontations, clarifications, or interpretations directed toward the current problem interfering with medical care (Stoffers et al., 2012).

A *confrontation* is an observation by the physician offered to a patient for examination. It is usually a comment that draws attention to contradictions in the patient's beliefs, thoughts, feelings, or behaviors. For example, one might say to an anxious-somatic patient who denies that psychosocial factors might be contributing to her symptomatology that her physical complaints may be caused by medical, psychological, or social stresses and that her high levels of anxiety could be making her physical symptoms worse.

A *clarification* adds new information or perspective or elucidates misunderstandings, miscommunications, or other information that seems vague or confusing. The need for repeated clarifications occurs regularly with difficult patients. It is important to use clarifications before suggesting a new plan to correct the problem.

Interpretations are integrating comments that link confrontations and clarifications with the patient's current problem that is interfering with medical care. Interpretations can be made about the immediate medical situation and may address the patient's core beliefs, irrational thoughts, fears, maladaptive symptoms or behaviors, defense mechanisms, or coping style. Interpretations can also be directed at a difficulty in the physician–patient interaction, problems with the patient coping with the disease, problems in the patient's life circumstances, or patient refusal of a necessary medical workup or treatment. For example, an interpretation to a borderline patient with chronic pain might be:

I think you want relief from your pain. However, your refusal to adhere to my treatment recommendations makes relief from your pain unlikely (confrontation). You then get angry and suicidal with me because your pain is not relieved, so you do not keep your scheduled appointments (clarification). Instead of enlisting my help and using our services when the pain is overwhelming, you blame us for your pain and feel frustrated and suicidal. Your anger helps you avoid dealing with the chronic reality of your medical condition (interpretation), which is that we can make your pain manageable but not cure it.

Making interpretations takes practice but can powerfully restore a realistic and helpful physician–patient relationship.

ATTENDING TO THE PATIENT'S EMOTIONAL NEEDS

Patients with personality disorders are often exquisitely sensitive and distressed by internal emotional states, moods, desires, and physical complaints. At a basic level, attending to the patient's emotional needs means listening empathically, reflectively, and carefully before attempting an intervention. With many personality-disordered patients (e.g., avoidant, dependent, histrionic, or borderline), it may be initially more important to attend to the patient's emotional needs for contact, reassurance, or validation before addressing physical or somatic complaints. Alternatively, some other personality-disordered patients (paranoid or obsessive-compulsive personalities) may need the family physician to attend to pain or address physical complaints first before the patient can discuss anxious, depressed, or agitated moods.

MODIFYING THE PATIENT'S SURROUNDINGS

Patients with personality disorders often show fewer symptoms and a dramatic improvement in their acute emotional, physical, and behavioral functioning when the physician recruits additional support from the environment. This may mean bringing in a helpful spouse, friend, or other personal support into the patient's medical care. Other approaches to improving the patient's external environment may include allowing the nurse or office staff to spend more time with the patient, adding social services, offering self-help support groups, or recommending psychiatric care. In extreme situations, using psychiatric or medical emergency services can be helpful interventions. Some patients with personality disorders need to be managed with the help of the police.

IMPROVING THE PATIENT'S CAPACITY TO TEST REALITY

Patients with personality disorders typically have distorted views of realty. Stressed patients from the Cluster A and B groups may transiently hear voices, hallucinate, have brief episodes of delusional thinking, or have paranoia. Impairment in reality testing can occur with paranoid, schizoid, schizotypal, and borderline personality disorders. If psychotic disturbances in reality are present, assess and treat these first before providing the requested medical care. Mobilizing external supports, using medications, or placing the patient in a safe and calm environment is often sufficient.

A stressed patient can also present with a tenuous or disturbed relationship to reality. Cluster B patients may have a disturbance in the sense of reality, such as *derealization* (watching his or her own life as if it were a movie), *depersonalization* (not feeling a part of one's own life), dramatic distortions of what has been said, transient misperceptions of real events (interpreted according to core beliefs or irrational thoughts), or misunderstanding the physician or patient role. Such reality distortions are not usually dangerous but can lead to severe problems in the physician–patient relationship if they are not recognized and addressed. Helpful verbal techniques to improve reality testing include uncovering and clarifying the patient's irrational thoughts or core beliefs and using confrontation, clarification, and interpretation to improve the patient's reality distortions.

EMPATHIZING WITH THE PATIENT'S WORLDVIEW

Many patients need a focal physical examination first to believe that the physician is taking them seriously. Afterward, all psychological interventions used depend on the patient's feeling understood by the physician. Listening and reflecting back the problems identified by the patient while empathizing with the patient's worldview can be extremely helpful in management.

For example, an avoidant personality–disordered patient may refuse a prostate examination while having complaints of urinary hesitation and dribbling. The physician could say:

I am not trying to criticize you for your preference to avoid a physical exam. I understand your wish to avoid dealing with this problem. The testing (urinalysis and rectal examination) takes only a few minutes and is not terribly uncomfortable. This information will guide my treatment. I think it is in your interest to get these examinations. Could we do this today? Then we can plan a way to relieve your symptoms.

ACCEPTING THE PATIENT'S LIMITATIONS AND STRENGTHS

Patients with severe personality disorders are often rigid in their approach to the world and limited in their capacity for social and occupational functioning. They typically do not seek or make changes easily. In patients with the most severe personality disorders, it may be most effective to accept the patient's fixed and irrational beliefs and limited functioning. Focusing on the patient's strengths and how external circumstances (not the patient's beliefs) can be modified may be better strategies to help these most difficult patients.

MANAGING UNREASONABLE EXPECTATIONS AND SETTING REASONABLE LIMITS

Patients with personality disorders often have unreasonable expectations. They may expect an unrealistic cure, never-ending diagnostic testing, constant availability of the medical team, special treatment, an unwarranted disability diagnosis, excessive pain medication, or many consultations. The physician must set limits on a patient's unreasonable expectations. Effective limit setting involves exploring why the patient believes that his or her particular expectation can or should be met. This involves a reasonable physician response about what can or cannot be done. Ultimately, limit setting is about agreeing to a reasonable approximation of the patient's request and tactfully saying "no" to requests that are not appropriate.

QUESTIONING ILLOGICAL FEELINGS, THOUGHTS, AND BEHAVIORS

Patients often have irrational thoughts about their illnesses and the care that they will receive. They may also misunderstand the physician's efforts to communicate. For example, some patients may think that nothing can be done to ameliorate their physical complaints or that a prescribed medication may make them sick. Other patients may think that magnetic resonance imaging (MRI) will cure them or that the MRI may give them cancer. These types of irrational thoughts should be explored and the reality clarified. If done tactfully, this usually reduces anxiety in most patients. If a patient is frankly delusional, it is not useful to confront a patient's fixed belief. It is better to accept the patient's viewpoint while asking the patient's permission to have a different viewpoint.

DISCUSSING DEFENSE MECHANISMS AND COPING STYLES

Patients may benefit from discussing their maladaptive defenses and coping styles and exploring ways of effectively dealing with their situations. For example, an obsessive-compulsive patient has a high cholesterol level and is calling the physician's office for more details about other laboratory tests. The results of the lipid profile are given to the patient, who now wants to know whether a lifestyle change or a statin medication would work better. With the recommendation for an initial lifestyle plan of more exercise and nutritional counseling, the patient becomes concerned about how to pay for this. Repeated efforts to help the patient with additional information do not make the patient feel any better. In fact, more information just raises more requests for additional information. The patient is asked to come for another visit. At this visit, the physician might say, "I can continue to give you more information, but it seems that anxiety is driving your questions. What are you worried about?" In essence, this says, "Your coping style of seeking information and details is not helping you. If you can recognize your anxiety about this subject, you may feel calmer." Review Table 45-1 for specific defenses and coping styles. Interpreting defenses or modifying a coping style requires the ability to recognize these and then to implement the preparatory confrontations and clarifications before making an interpretation and subsequently suggesting new ways to cope with the situation.

KEY TREATMENT

- Attend to the doctor–patient relationship.
- Focus the interview on manageable goals within the time frame available.
- Use psychotherapeutic techniques of confrontation, clarification, and interpretation when interviewing the patient (Davanloo, 1990, 2001) (SOR: A).
- Attend to the patient's emotional needs (SOR: C).
- Modify the patient's surroundings (SOR: C).
- Improve the patient's capacity to test reality (Kernberg, 1975, 1984, 1992) (SOR: C).
- Empathize with the patient's worldview (Beck, 1990) (SOR: C).
- Accept the patient's limitations and strengths (SOR: C).
- Manage unreasonable patient expectations and set limits (SOR: C).
- Question illogical feelings, thoughts, and behaviors (Greenberg & Padesky, 1995) (SOR: C).
- Discuss defenses and coping style and interpret them (see Table 45-2) (SOR: C).
- Prescribe medications as needed (Markovitz, 2004; Soloff, 2000; Soloff, 2009) (SOR: A).
- Use specific interventions for each kind of difficult patient as detailed in Table 45-3 (SOR: C).

PSYCHOPHARMACOLOGY FOR PERSONALITY DISORDERS

Medication can be helpful at times in treating patients with personality disorders. Prescribing medication can be focused on (1) treating targeted traits or symptoms within the personality disorder, (2) the personality disorder itself, or (3) the comorbidity of any major psychiatric illnesses that coexists with the personality disorder.

Table 45-4   Pharmacotherapy for Symptomatic Treatment of Personality Traits and Disorders*

Anger and Impulsive Aggression	Suicidal Ideation	Psychotic Symptoms	Mood Instability and Interpersonal Problems	Anxiety	Depression
BORDERLINE PERSONALITY DISORDER (SOR: B)[†]					
Haloperidol	Flupenthixol	Aripiprazole	Aripiprazole	Aripiprazole	Aripiprazole
Aripiprazole	decanoate	Olanzapine	Olanzapine	Olanzapine	Divalproex sodium
Olanzapine	Olanzapine		Divalproex sodium	Topiramate	Amitriptyline
Lamotrigine	Fluphenazine		Topiramate		
Topiramate	decanoate				
	Paroxetine				
ANTISOCIAL PERSONALITY DISORDER (SOR: C)[‡]					
Lithium					
Phenytoin					
Citalopram					
Sertraline					
SCHIZOTYPAL PERSONALITY DISORDER (SOR: B)[‡]					
	Olanzapine	Olanzapine			
	Risperidone	Risperidone			
AVOIDANT PERSONALITY DISORDER (SOR: B), DEPENDENT TRAITS (SOR: C)[‡]					
			Brofaromine	Brofaromine	
			Citalopram	Citalopram	
			Sertraline	Sertraline	

*Doses of these medications are in the standard range that are used for the major psychiatric illnesses.
[†]Lieb et al., 2010; Soloff, 2000; Soloff, 2009; Nose et al., 2006; Ypriitham, 2004.
[‡]Markovitz, 2004; Soloff, 2000; Soloff, 2009.
SOR, Strength of recommendation.
Adapted from Triebwasser J, Siever LJ. Pharmacotherapy of personality disorders. *J Mental Health.* 2007;16(1):5-50 and Stoffers J, Völlm BA, Rüker G, et al. Pharmacological interventions for borderline personality disorder. *Cochrane Database Syst Rev.* 2010;6:CD005653.

Psychopharmacology targeting traits or symptoms of BPD has the most robust literature (Stoffers et al., 2010). The older approach of primarily using antidepressants and selective serotonin reuptake inhibitors for treating the multiple symptoms of BPD has not been replicated in the most recent literature. Medications shown to be somewhat effective in treating the multiple symptoms of anger and impulsive aggression, psychotic symptoms, and anxiety in BPD include aripiprazole and olanzapine. A medication somewhat effective at treating anger and impulsive aggression, disturbed interpersonal relationships, and anxiety of BPD is the mood stabilizer topiramate. Treatment of suicidal behaviors is best targeted with flupenthixol or fluphenazine decanoate, paroxetine, or olanzapine. Other medications that may be useful for treating a single targeted symptom of BPD are detailed in Table 45-4.

There is also some evidence for prescribing medication to treat antisocial personality disorders, avoidant personality disorder with dependent traits, and schizotypal personality disorder. These medications are also detailed in Table 45-4.

When using psychopharmacology to treat a patient with comorbid major psychiatric illness and personality disorder, it is most important to focus initial medication trials on the primary psychiatric illness, not the personality disorder. This is because many symptoms seen in major psychiatric disorders are the same as those seen in personality disorders. Some of the symptoms related to a personality disorder will completely remit when the primary psychiatric illness is treated first. If symptoms of the personality disorder remain after treatment of the primary psychiatric disorder, then the patient can be treated using the targeted symptom approach detailed in Table 45-4.

KEY TREATMENT

- Medications can target anger and impulsive aggression, suicidal ideation, psychotic symptoms, mood instability, interpersonal problems, anxiety, and depression (see Table 45-4) (Markovitz, 2004; Soloff, 2000; Soloff, 2009) (SOR: A).
- Doses for treating symptoms are the same as doses used for major psychiatric conditions (Markovitz, 2004; Soloff, 2000; Soloff, 2009) (SOR: B).
- Anger and impulsive aggression, psychotic symptoms, and anxiety in BPD can be treated with aripiprazole and olanzapine (Lieb et al., 2010) (SOR: A).
- Anger and impulsive aggression, disturbed interpersonal relationships, and anxiety of BPD can be treated with the mood stabilizer topiramate (Lieb et al., 2010; Nose et al., 2006; Ypriitham, 2004.) (SOR: A).
- Treatment of suicidal behaviors is best targeted with flupenthixol or fluphenazine decanoate, paroxetine, or olanzapine (Lieb et al., 2010; Soloff, 2009) (SOR: B).
- Irritability, anger, and mood symptoms in patients with personality disorders are *not* generally responsive to selective serotonin reuptake inhibitors (SSRIs) (Soloff, 2009) (SOR: A).
- Psychotic symptoms can be treated with low doses of typical or atypical antipsychotic medications (Soloff, 2009) (SOR: B).

Interventions for Specific Personality Disorders

Using specific interventions for each subtype of personality disorders is the art of medicine. A basic specific approach is outlined for each disorder in Tables 45-1 and 45-2. This schema includes choosing the correct DSM-5 cluster; identifying the specific personality diagnosis; understanding the patient's core beliefs, irrational thoughts, specific fears, main defense mechanisms, and coping style; and recognizing common physician reactions to each personality disorder. Using this knowledge, interventions are then tailored for each disorder (see Table 45-3). This conceptual framework allows the formulation of helpful interventions for the primary care management of specific personality disorders.

PARANOID PERSONALITY DISORDER

When interacting with a paranoid patient, the physician typically reacts with fear, mistrust, and a sense of danger. The physician may also feel blamed or accused. The patient may have a similar fear of being hurt, exploited, or invaded. Patients often react to suggestions for medical care with mistrust, excessive fault finding, sensitivity to criticism, or hypervigilance. They may collect small insults as proof of the world's injustices. When invasive medical procedures are performed, a paranoid patient may react with full-blown panic and anxiety; many paranoid patients unconsciously experience a body invasion as a homosexual assault. Patients with paranoid personality disorder rely most heavily on projection as their main defense. Using projection, they accuse the physician of hurts that reflect their own aggressive style of hurting others.

A physician working with the paranoid patient needs to empathize with the patient's mistrust and hypersensitivity. The physician should avoid arguing or attempting to reason the patient out of the paranoid worldview. It is extremely important to use confrontations and clarifications to help correct the patient's distorted perceptions about his or her medical care. Unfortunately, direct confrontation of a delusion or hallucinations (the most troubling deficits in reality testing) often has the paradoxical effect of making these patients more suspicious of the physician.

Acknowledging that the patient's suspicion has an emotional reality can be helpful. Rather than confronting mistrust or suspicions directly, the physician can acknowledge responsibility for any actions that the patient might have perceived as mistakes. For example, the physician could say, "I did not appreciate how it might hurt you when I ordered that lab test." It may also help to express understanding and concern for the patient's rights. If there is a medical need for special testing of which the patient is suspicious, acknowledge the patient's fears and describe openly and honestly the details of the procedures, potential for pain, and likely risks and benefits. If the patient still refuses to comply, do not use direct persuasion. Ask the patient, "Is it all right with you if we have different opinions?" With the patient's consent to hearing a different opinion, openly discuss the medical necessity of the testing without trying to resolve the problem. At future office visits,

attempt new and ongoing discussions of the patient's fears of complying with the request for specialized testing. It may take months for the paranoid patient to trust enough to consent to the appropriate treatment. Counterprojective statements by the physician can diffuse the projections and distortions directed at the physician. The physician can use counterprojective remarks to help the patient access his or her feelings while focusing angry or suspicious feelings away from the physician toward others who are not present. For example, a physician harassed by an angry, suspicious, or blaming patient could use a counterprojective statement such as, "You felt angry and hurt when the lab technician drew your blood. You must be fearful of the results of these tests."

SCHIZOID AND SCHIZOTYPAL PERSONALITY

Physicians typically feel uninvolved or detached or have a desire to break through the aloofness of schizoid and schizotypal patients. *Schizoid* patients may give the physician the impression that they are loners. A common physician reaction to *schizotypal* patients is a feeling that the patient is alone and "weird or strange." Superficially, patients with either diagnosis fear personal contact, emotional involvement, and invasion of their privacy. At the deepest level, they long for emotional contact that is not overwhelming. They may react to suggestions for medical care with avoidance, withdrawal, apparent emotional detachment, or denial of the medical problem. Schizotypal patients often function with impaired reality testing manifested by magical, odd, or psychotic modes of thinking. Schizotypal patients use regression to schizoid fantasy and, to a lesser extent, denial as their main defenses. They appear increasingly idiosyncratic and withdrawn when stressed. Schizotypal personality disorder appears to increase the risk for the future development of schizophrenia.

Schizoid patients do not appear psychotic or idiosyncratic in their behavior. They are disinterested in intimate contacts with others, appear detached and unemotional, and wish to be left alone. More infrequently than schizotypal personality disorder, the schizoid personality may also be associated with the future development of schizophrenia. When stressed by a medical problem, schizoid patients use isolation and intellectualization to hide their emotions. If necessary, they regress to childlike functioning or use psychotic denial of their illness as their main defenses.

Patients with schizotypal and schizoid personalities tend to experience their physicians as intruding into their privacy, which may drive them away from the physician. They are relieved when the physician is not present and prefer fewer medical appointments and contacts. It is generally helpful to accept their lack of sociability at a level that does not demand involvement or permit total withdrawal. Neutral or unemotional expressions of medical information are most likely to be heard and used.

ANTISOCIAL PERSONALITY DISORDER

Common physician reactions to a patient with antisocial personality disorder are feelings of being used, exploited, or deceived. This can lead to physician anger and wishes to be free of the patient, uncover lies, or punish or imprison the patient. These patients fear that they will become vulnerable, lose respect or admiration from others, and become easy prey to manipulation when they become ill. They expect to be exploited, demeaned, or humiliated. Similar to a narcissistic patient, they often have low self-esteem, excessive self-love, compensatory feelings of superiority, grandiosity, recklessness, and emotional shallowness, and they show a lack of concern for others. They often react to medical care with entitled demands for special treatment. When caught in dishonesty, they may angrily attack or devalue the physician. They may resort to other psychopathic manipulations of deception, lying, cheating, or stealing. In fact, their friendly, facile, slick, superficial charm and intelligent appearance is often beguiling for the physician. They can lose reality testing when stressed by the potential of getting caught in their deceptive practices. This is typically manifested by impulsive actions that reveal severely impaired or sometimes psychotic judgments. When receiving medical care for a legitimate illness, they typically function at the same level and often appear to have the same characteristic issues as the narcissistic personality disorder (Kernberg, 1992). They can often be managed similarly (see "Narcissistic Personality Disorder").

To intervene with an antisocial patient, the family physician needs to be alert and anticipate that the patient may be requesting unnecessary medical care or malingering or may present with a factitious disorder. Although setting strict limits and reasonable expectations is important when treating all patients with personality disorders, it is particularly important when dealing with a patient with antisocial personality disorder. This patient may be seeking the secondary gain of illegal disability benefits or money, excuses for work absenteeism, or avoidance of legal problems or may be just seeking caretaking. It is important not to inadvertently collude with the patient's plans for secondary gain. For example, if the physician thinks that a patient's request for disability is fraudulent or unwarranted, the patient should not be referred for additional disability evaluations. If deception is suspected, the physician can ask for verification of symptoms from other reliable sources. There is often dishonesty in a patient's communication in the form of withholding important information, partial truths, or outright lying, cheating, or stealing. If this occurs, avoid the common reaction of moralizing. Instead, grant the patient the reality that he has the ability to fool all the physicians if he or she wants. The patient can be told that the result of deception is that the physician may make poorly informed medical decisions. This will ultimately result in the patient's receiving inadequate or poor medical care. The physician can explore with the patient why he or she needs to act self-destructively. Patients may need to be reminded that the physician's role is to help with medical problems and not to pass judgment or help the patient obtain unfair medical benefits.

BORDERLINE PERSONALITY DISORDER

Patients with BPD have a high prevalence of somatic symptom and substance abuse disorders (Grant et al., 2004; Lubman et al., 2011). They frequently become dependent on their physicians in an extremely demanding, clinging, and helpless or self-destructive manner. Physicians may feel manipulated, angry, depleted, exhausted, or self-doubting. They may want to end the patient relationship or rescue patients from themselves, or they can be drawn into a cycle of extensive medical testing to try to explain many somatic complaints. Patients with BPD fear separation or abandonment and may react to potential losses with panic, emotional instability, anger, or impulsive (suicidal or self-destructive) actions. They may seek care and use defenses that appear as a somatic symptom disorder. These somatic symptoms and borderline personality structure often represent the sequelae of childhood abuse, sexual abuse, or other trauma (Kernberg, 1975; Sansone et al., 2001).

Use of parallel inquiry to uncover a history of trauma is often most helpful for a patient complaining of multiple somatic complaints. Borderline patients often react to medical care with an aggressive or dependent clinging to their physicians and other caretakers (Gross et al., 2002). They may angrily devalue a physician who does not adequately explain their symptoms and may make entitled demands for special treatment when they become worried or frustrated. They tend to relate to others as "all good or all bad," which significantly contributes to their poor life functioning.

Typically, reality testing is intact. However, under stress, patients with BPD may temporarily lose reality testing and have mini-psychotic breaks lasting minutes or hours. These patients may at times manifest severe distortions in perceptions or sense of reality. They may misunderstand the physician's intentions or instructions. They may also experience episodes of derealization or depersonalization. Patients with BPD have *identity diffusion*, extreme fluctuations in self-perception from the grandiose to an excessively harsh underestimation of their abilities. They also have stormy and chaotic relationships with others. They rely heavily on splitting, projective identification, projection, and devaluing.

Office management of patients with BPD involves an empathic understanding of their fears. These fears revolve around the threat to their security or fears of separation or abandonment and, secondarily, sensitivity to rejection or fears of humiliation. They require firm limit setting (e.g., what the physician can realistically offer). Attempts to satisfy these patients' intense needs often result in an exhausted or angry physician. This can be avoided by setting realistic limits while offering the patient different ideas or options for medical care and more adaptive behaviors. Initial interventions should attempt to establish reality testing or correct reality distortions. If reality testing is intact, the most helpful interventions can be aimed at attending to medical care while decreasing the pathologic splitting defenses by using confrontation, clarification, and interpretations of the problematic situation.

The primary treatment for BPD is psychotherapy complemented by symptom-targeted pharmacotherapy (APA, 2001). Four types of psychotherapy have been shown to be effective in treating this personality disorder (Stoffers et al., 2012). These are dialectical behavior training, transference-focused psychotherapy, mentalization-based psychotherapy, and supportive psychotherapy in conjunction with medications. Most patients with BPD need extended psychotherapy (twice per week for 1 to 2 years) with specially trained mental health professionals to attain and maintain lasting improvement in their personalities, interpersonal problems, and overall functioning. Pharmacotherapy often has an important adjunctive role, especially for diminution of symptoms such as affective instability, impulsivity, psychotic-like symptoms, and self-destructive behavior (see Table 45-4). Although caring for these patients can be exhausting for family physicians, it is important to know that the long-term remission rates for patients with BPD are quite good.

HISTRIONIC PERSONALITY DISORDER

Patients with histrionic personality disorder have an emotionally expressive style, seek excessive attention, are often dramatic, and may present with a conversion disorder. Physicians may feel flattered, captivated, seduced, or sexually aroused by these patients. Alternatively, the physician may feel overwhelmed by the patient's exaggerated or excessive emotions, embarrassed by the sexual overtures, depleted, or confounded by unexplained physical symptoms (e.g., pseudoseizures, paralysis, and mutism). These patients may unconsciously use their symptoms to elicit attention or support from the physician (Bornstein and Gold, 2008). They may also use their sexuality to recruit others to satisfy their needs to be taken care of or romantically pursued. They fear that they are not desired and will lose the care or admiration of others.

There are two different levels of functioning with the histrionic personality disorder. Kernberg (1984, 1992) describes a neurotically functioning "hysteric" who shows intact reality testing, defenses centered on repression, and stable and mature relations with others. The female hysteric has a flirtatious, clinging, childlike dependence in intimate relationships but can function at mature levels in social and work situations. Male hysterics have similar psychological conflicts but may appear as "macho" or "effeminate" (Kernberg, 1992). The hysteric of either sex often reacts to medical care with regression to a childlike, sexualized, dependent, and clinging position. They seek to gratify their wishes for dependent care by seducing or flattering others. Outside the office, they usually function well.

By contrast, a "histrionic patient" (Kernberg, 1984, 1992) can display transient losses of reality testing, defenses centered on splitting, chaotic sexualized relations with others, and a range of unexplained physical or somatic complaints. The histrionic patient is self-centered and self-indulgent, with a pervasive childlike dependence that extends from intimate relationships into all aspects of social and occupational functioning. Female histrionics typically act flirtatiously but may become indignant when a man shows sexual interest. Male histrionics also show the self-centered and dependent pattern but may also have hypochondriacal and antisocial features. Histrionics of both genders may seek medical care because of unexplained medical symptoms. They may react to medical care with regression but, unlike the hysteric, use defenses centered on "splitting"; they may see the physician as "all good or all bad" and can be extremely devaluing. They may appear severely self-centered, attention seeking, diffusely sexual, hypochondriacal, somatic, and exploitative. All of this may be coupled with an exhausting dependency on the physician.

In working with hysterics and histrionic patients, a physician needs to be friendly, neither overly warm nor reserved.

Hysterics and histrionics often are helped when the physician uses parallel diagnostic inquiry when they present with somatic complaints. Parallel diagnostic inquiry is a technique in which the clinician simultaneously explores potential physical and psychological factors involved in the patient's complaints. Hysterics also may benefit from some gratification of their dependent wishes and a free discussion of their fears and emotions. They can often be reassured by an educational and informational approach to their medical illnesses and are capable of expressing gratitude to the physician. In contrast, the intense dependency of histrionics is often made worse by gratifying the patient's needs. Offering excessive emotional care may make them greedy or demanding for satisfaction of their needs. Histrionics benefit from firm, kind limit setting (especially to their sexual overtures), with neutral acknowledgment and gratification of their reasonable needs. They may be further helped by focusing on their distortions in reality perception and through interpretation of their splitting mechanisms.

NARCISSISTIC PERSONALITY DISORDER

The family physician's reactions to the narcissistic patient are often difficult to manage. The superior, entitled, self-loving, arrogant attitude of these patients can be intimidating. They may elicit feelings in the physician of being devalued and inferior. The physician may have concerns about the patient's anger and criticism. Alternatively, the lack of empathy and interpersonal exploitation of these patients can readily provoke the physician to anger, a wish to retaliate with harsh criticism, or a desire to end the patient–physician relationship.

The core fears of narcissistic patients are the result of a fragile self-esteem and their need for constant approval and praise from others. They fear loss of admiration, potency, and power, and they fear being exploited when vulnerable. Any perceived insult to their "grandiose self" (Kernberg, 1984, 1992) makes them feel rejected, deflated, and criticized and frequently results in feelings of rage, shame, or humiliation.

A narcissistic patient generally has intact reality testing but can undergo severe reality distortions when he or she perceives slights, rejection, or competition from others with talent. Those narcissistic patients who have paranoid and antisocial features (Kernberg, 1992) have a worse prognosis. They often have a fragile identity that can swing from the grandiose to the worthless. They rely heavily on splitting mechanisms to regulate their self-esteem. They portray themselves as grandiose and superior. This helps defend against feelings of extreme inadequacy and vulnerability. They can devalue, viciously attack, or degrade those around them when they act in a self-important way. Alternatively, as splitting operates, they may idealize or be envious of others who are, for the moment, seen as more powerful or successful. In this position, their self-esteem plummets, as evidenced by their sense of worthlessness and their reports of deprecating and degrading self-attacks.

Office management of narcissistic patients, as well as many antisocial patients, requires that the physician not mistake the patient's superior and entitled manner for genuine confidence. When being verbally devaluing, it may help the physician to view the demeaning or verbally attacking patient as a wounded child having a "temper tantrum." This may prevent the physician from retaliating by demeaning the patient, which only escalates a maladaptive interaction. Intervening in the face of a devaluing attack involves acknowledging that the patient feels hurt and that the patient has a right to his or her opinions. If the patient can discuss his or her hurt feelings with a nonjudgmental and empathic physician, the problems generally resolve, and a good physician–patient alliance can be restored. If this is not possible, offer the patient the right to seek another expert for consultation. This offer needs to be made without malice, defensiveness, or apology. This may help the patient calm down and reconsider his or her position.

In a long-term relationship with a narcissistic patient, splitting can be interpreted. This can be done by reminding patients who are demeaning that they previously praised the skill and abilities of the physician. If hostile, patients can be asked why they are now so critical and angry. When this is effective, it will allow patients to discuss their perception of insults to their self-esteem.

AVOIDANT PERSONALITY DISORDER

Patients with avoidant personality disorder have feelings of inadequacy and fear of criticism. They have low self-esteem and believe that they are inept and inadequate. They believe that others are critical and disapproving until proved otherwise. Although avoidant patients crave human relationships and affection, their fear of being criticized, rejected, embarrassed, or hurt causes them to initially avoid social situations or meeting new people. Their shyness and avoidance protect them from their fears of being rejected or humiliated. In medical encounters, they often can seek psychosocial help through somatic complaints. This somatic approach of physical complaints can conceal psychological issues and makes them feel safer than revealing unconscious or unexpressed emotions. They prefer not to divulge personal aspects of themselves because this may leave them vulnerable. Their timidity, hypersensitivity, and cautiousness can generate feelings of frustration or annoyance in the physician. Patients with avoidant personality disorder typically use defense mechanisms based on denial; repression, including inhibition; phobia; and isolation.

Managing avoidant patients is more effective when the physician uses both parallel diagnostic inquiry and emotion-focused interviewing. It is most helpful when the physician can recognize and empathize with the patient's social fears, including the fear of the physician's criticism. Patients may minimize symptoms or delay seeking help because of fear of the physician or the feeling that they are unworthy or unimportant. Some avoidant patients do the reverse by asking for emotional help through their somatic symptoms. The physician should help the patient understand his or her symptoms and any specific fears revolving around the diagnostic or therapeutic plan. Irrational fears and thoughts can be gently corrected and alternative interpretations offered. Patients should be encouraged, with appropriate support, to face their somatic and other fears as the best way of mastering them. If the physician feels frustration or annoyance, it is often helpful to encourage the patient to describe what he or she is finding most difficult in the medical care or proposed medical plan.

DEPENDENT PERSONALITY DISORDER

Patients with dependent personality disorder may be characterized by an exaggerated need for care or a need for direction from another person (or both). Dependent patients may present initially with a physical illness. These initial medical complaints often elicit exaggerated caretaking response from physicians and may introduce into the medical relationship a tendency to return to the physician with increasing somatic complaints (Bornstein and Gold, 2008). Dependent patients often feel helpless and inadequate in making even minor decisions, such as what to do next medically, what to wear, or whom to befriend. They have a core belief that they cannot function alone, are completely incapable of taking care of themselves, and must have someone else provide care and make decisions. Their major fear is of independence.

Although both borderline patients and dependent patients are extremely dependent on others, they react very differently to the threat of losing a significant other. Whereas a borderline patient becomes angry or enraged, a dependent patient becomes submissive and obsequious. Patients with dependent personality disorder use defenses that include regression, passive aggression, and reaction formation.

Patients with dependent personality disorder are submissive and clinging with their caretakers because of fear of losing them. The dependence of these patients can make physicians feel annoyed, drained, or depleted. Physicians may tend to deny reasonable needs of an excessively dependent patient. The secondary gains that patients with dependent personality receive from an illness also create extra challenges for the physician. Use of parallel diagnostic inquiry and emotion-focused interviewing is helpful. The physician must understand and empathize with the patient's need for being taken care of while encouraging and fostering independent thinking and action by the patient. Because these patients often use medication, alcohol, food, and other means to satisfy their dependency needs, the physician must exercise caution in how these are used in the therapeutic plan. Unreasonable expectations for being taken care of should be gently discouraged by the physician.

OBSESSIVE-COMPULSIVE PERSONALITY DISORDER

Patients with OCPD are preoccupied with details, order, and control. Although their labels are similar, these patients differ in substantial ways from patients with obsessive-compulsive disorder (OCD). OCD patients have recurrent disturbing thoughts or obsessions that create marked subjective distress.

The core adaptive traits of patients with OCPD are orderliness, attention to detail, and an emphasis on rational thinking and logic. These traits are lifelong patterns that many patients use adaptively in their professional lives. Patients with OCPD often view these traits as a personal strength. However, often their attention to detail leads them to perfectionist beliefs, worry, or ruminations that they must not make mistakes or be imperfect. They can interpret rules, regulations, and values rigidly and stubbornly. Patients with OCPD often ruminate and are prone to interpret minor physical changes as worrisome somatic complaints (McGuire and Shore, 2001).

Because they are uncomfortable with feelings and emotions, patients with somatic presentations may be unconsciously motivated to seek reassurance from their physicians. They may fear disorderliness and dirt. The compulsive, critical, controlling, self-righteous side of their personalities often creates difficulty in relationships with physicians, coworkers, friends, and family. They can be stingy, orderly, and obstinate. Physicians, who often have obsessive-compulsive traits themselves, may feel irritated and competitive with these patients about who controls the diagnostic workup or treatment plan.

Patients with OCPD use defense mechanisms such as intellectualization, isolation, displacement, doing and undoing, and reaction formation. Using reaction formation, they may behave in a superficially deferential or obsequious manner to repress from themselves and hide from others their critical and self-righteous and indignant feelings. These defenses are used against their anger and dependency needs, which are often unconsciously denied. Illness may represent a dangerous threat to the sense of self-control in OCPD patients. A past illness can lead to a future somatic presentation. The physician should understand and empathize with this loss of self-control while helping patients regain some control in the management of their medical problems. Struggle or conflict with the patient over control of medical care should be avoided. Reality distortions, including excessive perfectionism, idealization of logic, and avoidance of feeling, can be gently elicited, explored, and worked through with the patient.

Conclusion

Patients with personality disorders often contribute significantly to physician dissatisfaction and burnout with medical practice. The negative effects of a personality disorder on the doctor–patient relationship are often so deleterious that many of these patients get less than optimal primary care. A unique approach to diagnostic, management, and intervention strategies is described in this chapter and summarized in Tables 45-2 and 45-3. This personality disorder schema combines DSM-5 diagnosis with cognitive-behavioral and psychodynamic viewpoints involving the patient's core beliefs and irrational thoughts, fears, defenses and coping style, behaviors, adherence to medical treatment, and use of medical services. Common physician reactions, general strategies, and specific physician interventions for 10 different personality disorders are addressed to help the family physician maintain a working physician–patient relationship that permits the delivery of needed medical care.

References

The complete reference list is available at www.expertconsult.com.

Web Resources

www.guideline.gov/search/search.aspx?term=personality+disorders National Guideline Clearinghouse. Practice guidelines for borderline and antisocial personality disorders.

www.ncbi.nlm.nih.gov/pubmedhealth/PMH0001935 National Center for Biotechnology Information. Reviews of the major personality disorders and treatments.

http://pathways.nice.org.uk/pathways/personality-disorders National Institute for Health and Clinical Excellence (NICE). Practice guidelines for personality disorders.

www.nimh.nih.gov/topics/topic-page-borderline-personality-disorder .shtml National Institute of Mental Health on Borderline Personality Disorders.

www.nmha.org/go/information/get-info/personality-disorders Mental Health America. Consumer information about personality disorders.

www.dsm5.org/Documents/Personality%20Disorders%20Fact%20Sheet .pdf American Psychiatric Association. Information on personality disorders.

46 Anxiety and Depression

BRIAN ROTHBERG and CHRISTOPHER D. SCHNECK

Overview

Key Points

- Depression and anxiety increase medical morbidity and mortality.
- Mood disorders comprise unipolar and bipolar disorders.
- Anxiety disorders comprise eight disorders, of which generalized anxiety disorder (GAD) and panic disorder are frequently encountered in primary care settings.
- Treatment of depression and anxiety improves overall health outcomes.
- The majority of patients with mood and anxiety disorders are treated in primary care settings.

Major depression and anxiety disorders are the two most common psychiatric illnesses in the United States and are particularly prevalent in primary care settings. Despite the relative availability of specialty psychiatric care in the United States, most patients with depression or anxiety disorder continue to receive their treatment from primary care physicians. Moreover, patients with both medical illness and comorbid mood or anxiety disorder frequently have poorer outcomes, experience more prolonged and difficult treatment, and have greater morbidity and mortality than patients without psychiatric illness (Katon, 2003). Conversely, treating underlying depressive and anxiety disorders not only improves the emotional well-being of patients but also improves overall health outcomes and lowers health care costs. Given their frequency, severity, prevalence, morbidity, and mortality, depression and anxiety disorders remain important illnesses for primary care physicians to identify and treat.

The broader categories of mood and anxiety disorders comprise a large number of specific illnesses. Describing the specific symptoms, epidemiology, assessment, and treatment of each illness is beyond the scope of this chapter; rather, we examine the illnesses that primary care physicians are most likely to encounter in clinical settings and provide the most common strategies used in assessment, diagnosis, and treatment. *Mood disorders* include major depression (also called unipolar depression), bipolar disorder (which includes bipolar I and bipolar II disorder),

cyclothymia, and dysthymia (also called pervasive depressive disorder). With the latest edition of the *Diagnostic and Statistical Manual of Mental Disorders*, fifth edition (DSM-5) (American Psychiatric Association [APA], 2013), several new mood disorder categories have been added, including disruptive mood dysregulation disorder (chronic, severe persistent irritability, along with severe temper outbursts, beginning at an early age), premenstrual dysphoric disorder, and two broad and nonspecific depressive diagnoses (other specified depressive disorder and unspecified depressive disorder). This chapter focuses on the major mood disorders of depression and bipolar disorder. The category of *anxiety disorders* in the new DSM-5 (APA, 2013) contains GAD, panic disorder, agoraphobia, specific phobia (e.g., fear of heights), and social anxiety disorder (social phobia). Obsessive-compulsive disorder (OCD) and posttraumatic stress disorder (PTSD) have been removed from the anxiety disorder category. This chapter focuses primarily on GAD and panic disorder.

EPIDEMIOLOGY

Key Points

- Major depression and anxiety disorders are the two most common psychiatric illnesses in the United States.
- The economic burden of anxiety and depressive disorders is substantial in terms of workdays lost, disability, health care expenditures, and mortality.
- Anxiety and depression are chronic illnesses that typically run a waxing and waning course.
- Prevalence rates for anxiety disorders appear to decline with advancing age, except for GAD, which may increase in geriatric populations.
- Depression is often a highly recurrent illness; each episode of depression increases the likelihood of future episodes.

Prevalence estimates of mental disorders in the United States continue to find that anxiety and mood disorders are the two most common mental disorders in the general population (Kessler et al., 2012). Lifetime prevalence for anxiety disorders is estimated at 16.6% to 28.8% (Conway et al., 2006; Kessler et al., 2005a) and for major depression is estimated at 14.9% to 16.2% (Kessler et al., 2003). Recent 12-month prevalence rates show a similar stratification, with anxiety disorders most common (18.1%) followed by mood disorders (9.5%). Lifetime prevalence rates of panic disorder and GAD are 4.7% and 5.7%, respectively (Kessler et al., 2005a). Anxiety disorders make up approximately 2% of all office visits to physicians in the United States, but almost 50% occur in primary care settings. In comparison, approximately 40% of patients presenting with anxiety disorders are seen by psychiatrists (Harman et al., 2002).

Major depression remains a common disorder and is associated with substantial symptom severity and role impairment (Kessler et al., 2003). One-year prevalence rates for major depression are approximately 6% in the general population followed by dysthymia (1.8%) and bipolar disorders (1%-2%). Rates in primary care settings remain substantially higher, with prevalence of 10% or greater (Spitzer et al., 1994), although many of these patients have depression that is unrecognized by their primary care physician (Schultheis et al., 1999).

COSTS

Both anxiety and depressive disorders account for substantial health care costs and thus constitute a major public health and economic concern. As of 2013, the cost of depression and anxiety disorders in the United States comes from data between 1990 and 2000 and was calculated to be $83.1 billion in 2000, of which $26.1 billion was for direct medical costs, $5.4 billion for suicide mortality costs, and $51.5 billion for work-related costs (Greenberg et al., 2003). Similarly, estimates from the 1990s placed the annual economic burden of anxiety disorders at $63.1 billion (in 1998 dollars), of which nonpsychiatric direct medical costs accounted for 54% of the total and direct psychiatric care accounted for 31% (Greenberg et al., 1999). Not surprisingly, patients with anxiety disorders are much more likely to see their primary care physicians or use emergency services. Patients with pure GAD (i.e., no comorbid medical illnesses), for example, were 1.6 times more likely to have seen a primary care physician four or more times in the past year than those without GAD or depression (Wittchen et al., 2002). Patients with panic disorder were almost twice as likely as controls to have visited an emergency department in the previous 6 months (Roy-Byrne et al., 1999).

DISEASE COURSE

Both anxiety and depressive disorders tend to run a chronic course, with waxing and waning symptomatology. Illness severity typically worsens the longer the illness remains untreated. The age of onset for anxiety disorders varies greatly, depending on the specific condition. Specific phobias and separation anxiety, for example, often begin in childhood (median age of onset, 7 years), but panic disorder (median age, 21 years) and GAD (median age, 31 years) are typically seen in early to mid-adulthood (Kessler et al., 2005b). In elderly persons (>65 years), the prevalence of all anxiety disorders appears to decline, except for GAD, which is maintained at 4% prevalence and may increase over time (Krasucki et al., 1998). GAD is often a recurring

illness in which patients may experience periods of residual symptoms and occasional interepisode remissions (Angst et al., 2009). More than one third of patients with panic disorder have full remission with treatment, but about 20% have an unremitting and chronic course despite treatment (Katschnig and Amering, 1998).

The onset of major depression can occur at any age, although the median age of onset is 30 years (Kessler et al., 2005b). Depression is a highly recurrent illness, and each episode increases the likelihood of future episodes. Whereas patients with a single episode have a 50% lifetime chance of recurrence, those with three or more episodes have an almost 100% chance of recurrence without treatment (Eaton et al., 2008). Untreated depressive episodes can last 6 months or longer (Kessler et al., 2003). The Sequenced Treatment Alternatives to Relieve Depression (STAR*D) study found that a substantial number of patients receiving first-line treatment may require 8 weeks or more of treatment to achieve response or remission (Trivedi et al., 2006b). Although most patients recover from their depressive episode and return to normal functioning with treatment, approximately 15% of patients continue to have an unremitting course, with worsening psychosocial functioning and a higher risk for suicide (Eaton et al., 2008).

NEUROBIOLOGY AND GENETICS

The neurobiology of both depressive and anxiety disorders is complex and incompletely understood. In contrast to illnesses such as Parkinson or Huntington disease, no single area of brain pathology or anatomic lesion has been implicated in the development of anxiety or depression; rather, these illnesses appear to be mediated by dysregulation of complex interactions between neural circuits (Nestler et al., 2002). In depression, most lines of investigation have involved dysregulation of the hypothalamic–pituitary axis (HPA) and hippocampus, along with investigations of neural circuitry mediating mood, reward, sleep, appetite, motivation, and cognition. In particular, hyperactivity of the HPA in some depressed patients has been found to lead to hippocampal volume reduction, likely by reduction of brain-derived neurotrophic factor (BDNF) and changes in the mechanisms that mediate BDNF expression. However, whether reduced hippocampal volume is a partial cause or merely a result of depression is currently unclear, and it is not seen in all patients diagnosed with depression. Although epidemiologic studies show that depression appears highly heritable, with some studies showing that 40% to 50% of the risk may be genetic, no one gene appears implicated, and depression likely is the phenotypic expression of multiple genetic vulnerabilities coupled with environmental stresses (physical or emotional trauma, viral illness), physical factors (e.g., preexisting or comorbid medical illnesses such as hypothyroidism or stroke), and random processes during brain development (Nestler et al., 2002).

Neurobiologic research in anxiety disorders has focused on elucidating the neural networks involved in the *fear response*, but despite advances in neuroimaging, the exact mechanism of each anxiety disorder has yet to be completely understood. Strategies to understand the neuroanatomic underpinnings of panic disorder have focused on translational research using conditioned fear in animals as a model for panic attacks in humans. Patients with panic disorder may have an especially sensitive fear mechanism involving the central nucleus of the amygdala, hippocampus, thalamus, hypothalamus, periaqueductal gray region, locus ceruleus, and other brainstem sites (Gorman et al., 2000). Other areas of focus in anxiety disorders have involved investigations into alterations of interoceptive processing of the anterior insula (Mathew et al., 2008). Both the insula and the anterior cingulate cortex are thought to be the regions of the brain that form a representation of the visceral state of the body. A heightened sensitivity of this region may underlie the misinterpretation of bodily signals in panic disorder.

Genetic epidemiologic studies have clearly documented that anxiety disorders aggregate in families and that this familial link primarily results from genetic factors (Smoller and Faraone, 2008). First-degree relatives of probands with the major anxiety disorders (panic disorder, social anxiety disorder, specific phobias, OCD) have a four- to sixfold increased risk of the index disorders compared with relatives of unaffected probands (Hettema et al., 2001). Genetic studies of GAD suggest that a common genetic susceptibility may apply to "clusters" of anxiety disorders and other comorbid disorders (Norrholm and Ressler, 2009). An overlap of genes may play a role in the development of multiple psychiatric conditions, including anxiety and depression.

Anxiety, Major Depression, and Medical Illnesses

Key Points

- Anxiety disorders and major depression often coexist.
- The more severe the anxiety disorder, the greater the likelihood of major depression.
- Medical illnesses are associated with higher prevalences of anxiety and depression and vice versa.
- Medically ill patients with comorbid anxiety or depressive disorders adapt more poorly to physical symptoms, complicating disease management.

INTERACTION OF DEPRESSION AND ANXIETY

Major depression and anxiety are often found together, and each illness complicates the course and outcome of the other. Studies have consistently shown that anxiety disorders are the most frequently occurring comorbid disorder with major depression, with 50% to 60% of major depressed patients with both illnesses (Zimmerman et al., 2002). Whereas anxiety can lead to depression in almost 60% of patients, depression leads to anxiety in only 15% of patients (Mineka et al., 1998). Not surprisingly, the more severe anxiety disorders, OCDs, and trauma related disorders are more likely to lead to subsequent depression; that is, panic disorder, agoraphobia, OCD, PTSD and GAD more frequently lead to depression than either social phobia or simple phobia. In addition, patients with both illnesses often have an increased severity of symptoms, increased frequency of

episodes (either mood or anxiety episodes), poorer response to treatment, higher suicide rates, more chronic course, and overall poorer prognosis.

Treatment is complicated by the fewer studies on coexisting depression and anxiety, providing clinicians with a smaller evidence base for treatment decisions. Based on DSM-IV criteria, patients with comorbid major depressive disorders are half as likely subsequently to recover from panic disorder with agoraphobia or GAD, and comorbid major depression almost doubles the likelihood of recurrence of panic disorder with agoraphobia (Bruce et al., 2005). In addition, children and adolescents with anxiety disorders are at eight times the risk of additional depression (Angold et al., 1999). Practitioners must therefore be aggressive in screening for anxiety disorders in patients reporting depressive symptoms, as well as screening for depression in patients reporting anxiety symptoms.

INTERACTION OF DEPRESSION, ANXIETY, AND MEDICAL ILLNESS

A complex and reciprocal relationship exists between medical illnesses and comorbid anxiety and depressive disorders. Medical illnesses are associated with higher prevalence rates of anxiety and depression, and anxiety and depression are associated with higher rates of comorbid medical illnesses. Studies of patients with diabetes, cancer, stroke, myocardial infarction, HIV-related illness, and Parkinson disease have higher rates of depression than patients without such illnesses (Katon, 2003). Common medical disorders seen in primary care settings have high comorbidity with anxiety disorders as well. Cardiovascular disease is associated with a 1.5 times greater risk of both GAD and panic disorder (Goodwin et al., 2008). Patients with back pain or arthritis are almost twice as likely to have panic attacks or GAD (McWilliams et al., 2004), and patients with asthma (pediatric or adult) may have a 30% increased likelihood of anxiety disorders (Katon et al., 2004). The prevalence of anxiety and depression in patients with diabetes is more than double that in the general population (Collins et al., 2009). Almost 100% of patients with irritable bowel syndrome have major depression, GAD, or panic disorder (Lydiard et al., 1993).

Medical illnesses are associated with a higher risk for mood and anxiety disorders, so the presence of these disorders places patients at higher risk for multiple medical conditions. Patients with GAD or panic disorder are almost six times more likely to have a cardiac disorder, three times more likely to have a gastrointestinal (GI) disorder, twice as likely to have respiratory difficulties, and twice as likely to have migraine headaches than patients without anxiety disorders (Harter et al., 2003). Depression may be a predictor for the subsequent development of medical illness. Several studies found an association between history of major depression and subsequent development of type II diabetes (Eaton et al., 1996; Kawakami et al., 1999) and coronary artery disease (Rugulies, 2002).

Management of patients with comorbid medical illness and anxiety or depression is complex. Such patients have higher rates of unexplained symptoms than patients without these disorders even after adjusting for the severity of medical illness (Katon and Walker, 1998). An increasing body of literature suggests that patients with medical illness and comorbid depression or anxiety adapt more poorly to chronic symptoms, such as fatigue or pain, and tend to focus on both symptoms of their physical illnesses and physical symptoms associated with other organ symptoms. Not surprisingly, patients with medical illness and comorbid depression have 50% higher medical costs than patients with medical illness alone (Katon, 2003). Comorbid patients are more functionally impaired and have more lost workdays, poorer quality of life, and higher rates of medical utilization (Simon, 2003). Disease management is also complicated by higher rates of nonadherence to treatment and self-care regimens, as well as higher rates of risk behaviors (e.g., smoking, overeating, sedentary lifestyle). Response to antidepressant treatment may be less robust, as evidenced by patients with cardiovascular disease, stroke, and diabetes (Katon, 2003).

Diagnosis and Screening of Mood and Anxiety Disorders

Key Points

- Distinguishing unipolar from bipolar depression is critical for the proper management of depressed patients. The Mood Disorder Questionnaire (MDQ) may aid practitioners in detecting bipolar disorder in primary care settings.
- The Patient Health Questionnaire 9 (PHQ-9) is a common and easy-to-use screening tool for depression.
- No standard screening instrument for anxiety disorders has currently been accepted in general practice.

DIAGNOSIS OF MOOD DISORDERS

Mood disorders are divided into depressive disorders, bipolar disorders, and disorders based on etiology (i.e., mood disorders caused by general medical conditions and substance-induced mood disorders). For primary care physicians, identification, treatment, and management of depressive disorders are essential. Bipolar disorders, which are typically more complex to identify and treat, are best referred to mental health professionals for ongoing treatment. Therefore, this chapter concentrates on identifying bipolar disorder and distinguishing between unipolar and bipolar depression, but it does not delve into the specifics of treating bipolar patients.

The essential feature of a *major depressive episode* is a period lasting at least 2 weeks during which the patient experiences depressed mood or loss of interest or pleasure in almost all activities, a distinct change in usual self, and clinically significant distress or changes in functioning. It is accompanied by a constellation of other symptoms, such as changes in sleep, eating, energy, motivation, and concentration; difficulty making decisions; and often feelings of hopelessness, worthlessness, and guilt (Table 46-1). Patients may ruminate about death, feel that life is not worth living, have thoughts about suicide, may make plans to kill themselves, or make suicide attempts. Many patients complain

of memory difficulties, become easily distracted, and describe an inability to think clearly. Patients often pace, wring their hands, or have an inability to sit still; conversely, they may become greatly slowed or immobilized. In some patients, irritable mood may predominate more than sadness, or they may have explosive, angry outbursts (Fava and Rosenbaum, 1999). Irritability is especially noted in depressed children and adolescents. In its most severe forms—major depression with psychotic features—patients may hear voices telling them to kill themselves or may develop delusional beliefs, such as having a serious illness despite numerous tests providing no evidence (APA, 2013).

The essential feature of *dysthymia,* also called persistent depressive disorder, is a chronically depressed mood that occurs most days for at least 2 years. Patients may have a variety of other symptoms, such as feelings of inadequacy; generalized loss of interest or pleasure; social withdrawal; feelings of guilt or brooding about the past; and decreased activity, productivity, or effectiveness (Table 46-2). Neurovegetative symptoms such as insomnia or hypersomnia, poor appetite or overeating, low energy, and poor concentration may be present but are less common than in major depressive episodes. These patients may state that they have been depressed for as long as they can remember and cannot recall episodes of recovery or remission of symptoms. In addition, dysthymic patients may periodically have superimposed major depressive episodes, often called "double depression" (APA, 2013).

Bipolar disorder is a chronic mood disorder characterized by the presence of mania (bipolar I disorder) or hypomania and depression (bipolar II disorder). Manic episodes are distinct periods of abnormally and persistent moods that can be euphoric, expansive, or irritable, co-occurring with persistently increased goal-directed activity or energy, lasting at least 1 week. Although manic patients are often thought to be always euphoric, only about 20% of patients experience pure euphoria; most describe a mix of severe irritability, severe emotional lability, and volatility (Goodwin and Jamison, 2007). Manic patients often have greatly inflated self-esteem, confidence, decreased need for sleep, pressured speech, racing or crowded thoughts, distractibility, increased involvement in goal-directed activities (e.g., starting many projects but being unable to finish any), hypersexuality, and excessive involvement in pleasurable activities with a high potential for painful consequences (APA, 2013). Patients can exert great levels of physical activity, appear tireless, and may become extremely physically agitated. Approximately 60% of bipolar I patients experience psychosis, which may involve delusions of grandeur (feeling omnipotent, having special powers or "gifts"), persecution, or hallucinations (more often auditory as opposed to visual) (Goodwin and Jamison, 2007). The DSM-5 recognizes that a patient can be diagnosed with bipolar disorder even when mania is thought to emerge during treatment with an antidepressant if the manic symptoms persist at a fully syndromal level beyond the physiological effects of the treatment. Despite mania being the defining characteristic of the disease, depressed moods tend to predominate, with bipolar I patients experiencing a 3 : 1 ratio of depression to mania over the course of the illness (Judd et al., 2003).

Primary care physicians are more likely to encounter patients with *bipolar II disorder* than bipolar I disorder.

Table 46-1 Diagnostic Criteria for Major Depressive Episode

A. Five (or more) of the following symptoms have been present during the same 2-week period and represent a change from previous functioning; at least one of the symptoms is either (1) depressed mood or (2) loss of interest or pleasure.

  Note: Do not include symptoms that are clearly attributable to a general medical condition or mood-incongruent delusions or hallucinations.

  1. Depressed mood most of the day, nearly every day, as indicated by either subjective report (e.g., feels sad, empty, hopeless) or observation made by others (e.g., appears tearful). (**Note:** In children and adolescents, can be irritable mood.)
  2. Markedly diminished interest or pleasure in all, or almost all, activities most of the day, nearly every day (as indicated by either subjective account or observation).
  3. Significant weight loss when not dieting or weight gain (e.g., a change of more than 5% of body weight in a month), or decrease or increase in appetite nearly every day. (**Note:** In children, consider failure to make expected weight gain.)
  4. Insomnia or hypersomnia nearly every day
  5. Psychomotor agitation or retardation nearly every day (observable by others, not merely subjective feelings of restlessness or being slowed down)
  6. Fatigue or loss of energy nearly every day
  7. Feelings of worthlessness or excessive or inappropriate guilt (which may be delusional) nearly every day (not merely self-reproach or guilt about being sick)
  8. Diminished ability to think or concentrate or indecisiveness nearly every day (either by subjective account or as observed by others)
  9. Recurrent thoughts of death (not just fear of dying), recurrent suicidal ideation without a specific plan, or a suicide attempt or a specific plan for committing suicide

B. The symptoms cause clinically significant distress or impairment in social, occupational, or other important areas of functioning.

C. The episode is not attributable to the physiological effects of a substance or to another medical condition.

  Note: Criteria A-C represent a major depressive episode.

  Note: Responses to a significant loss (e.g., bereavement, financial ruin, losses from a natural disaster, a serious medical illness or disability) may include the feelings of intense sadness, rumination about the loss, insomnia, poor appetite, and weight loss noted in Criterion A, which may resemble a depressive episode. Although such symptoms may be understandable or considered appropriate to the loss, the presence of a major depressive episode in addition to the normal response to a significant loss should also be carefully considered. This decision inevitably requires the exercise of clinical judgment based on the individual's history and the cultural norms for the expression of distress in the context of loss. In distinguishing grief from a major depressive episode (MDE), it is useful to consider that in grief the predominant affect is feelings of emptiness and loss, while in MDE it is persistent depressed mood and the inability to anticipate happiness or pleasure. The dysphoria in grief is likely to decrease in intensity over days to weeks and occurs in waves, the so-called pangs of grief. These waves tend to be associated with thoughts or reminders of the deceased. The depressed mood of MDE is more persistent and not tied to specific thoughts or preoccupations. The pain of grief may be accompanied by positive emotions and humor that are uncharacteristic of the pervasive unhappiness and misery characteristic of MDE. The thought content associated with grief generally features a preoccupation with thoughts and memories of the deceased, rather than the self-critical or pessimistic ruminations seen in MDE. In grief, self-esteem is generally preserved, whereas in MDE feelings of worthlessness and self-loathing are common. If self-derogatory ideation is present in grief, it typically involves perceived failings vis-à-vis the deceased (e.g., not visiting frequently enough, not telling the deceased how much he or she was loved). If a bereaved individual thinks about death and dying, such thoughts are generally focused on the deceased and possibly about "joining" the deceased, whereas in MDE such thoughts are focused on ending one's own life because of feeling worthless, undeserving of life, or unable to cope with the pain of depression.

From American Psychiatric Association. *Diagnostic and statistical manual of mental disorders.* 5th ed. Arlington, VA: American Psychiatric Association; 2013.

Bipolar II disorder is characterized by hypomanic and major depressive episodes, although over the course of the illness, it is primarily a disease of depression, with depressive episodes predominating over hypomanic episodes by a 37:1 ratio (Judd et al., 2003). Symptoms of hypomanic episodes are similar to full manic episodes, but the severity of manic behaviors is attenuated, and the extreme functional, occupational, and social impairments evident in manic episodes are absent in hypomania. Current DSM-5 criteria require that distinct elevations in mood must be present for at least 4 days, must be clearly different from the patient's usual nondepressed mood, and must be accompanied by a change in the patient's usual functioning. Because patients primarily seek help during their depressive episodes and typically do not report hypomanic episodes as abnormal, undiagnosed bipolar disorder remains a major difficulty in primary care settings (Manning et al., 1999). Moreover, bipolar disorder may be more common in primary care settings than in general populations. Of 649 patients being treated for depression in a primary care clinic, 21% screened positive for bipolar disorder (Hirschfeld et al., 2005), but 10% of patients screened positive for bipolar disorder in a general medical clinic, although 80% of these patients had been diagnosed with unipolar depression (Das et al., 2005).

The DSM-5 introduced several important conceptual changes in the subclassification of mood disorders and their accompanying symptoms. Because mood disorders are now thought to exist along a continuum, ranging from bipolar mania to unipolar depression, DSM-5 has recognized that patients with either diagnosis can have "mixed" symptoms of the opposite pole. That is, manic patients may also have accompanying depressive symptoms (e.g., depressed mood, suicidal thinking) and depressed patients may have some co-occurring symptoms of mania (e.g., racing thoughts, decreased need for sleep). Patients with either diagnosis (bipolar disorder or unipolar depression) may also have anxious distress, psychosis, or seasonal variation of mood. Clinicians should therefore recognize that patients with either unipolar depression or bipolar disorder may have a variety of accompanying symptoms associated with the opposite pole that ultimately may have an impact on prognosis or treatment. However, the clinical significance of these co-occurring symptoms and their implications for treatment are still being evaluated.

Unipolar Depression versus Bipolar Depression

Distinguishing unipolar from bipolar depression remains a critical distinction and poses one of the greatest clinical challenges for professionals who treat patients with mood disorders. Misdiagnosis of bipolar disorder can lead to mistreatment (typically with antidepressants alone), worsening of mood, switches into mania or mixed states

Table 46-2 Diagnostic Criteria for Dysthymic Disorder

Depressed mood for most of the day for more days than not as indicated either by subjective account or observation by others for at least 2 years.

Note: In children and adolescents, mood can be irritable and duration must last for at least 1 year.

A. Presence, while depressed, of two (or more) of the following:
1. Poor appetite or overeating
2. Insomnia or hypersomnia
3. Low energy or fatigue
4. Low self-esteem
5. Poor concentration or difficulty making decisions
6. Feelings of hopelessness
B. During the 2-year period (1 year for children or adolescents) of the disturbance, the person has never been without the symptoms in Criteria A and B for more than 2 months at a time.
C. No major depressive episode (see Table 46-1) has been present during the first 2 years of the disturbance (1 year for children and adolescents); that is, the disturbance is not better accounted for by chronic major depressive disorder or major depressive disorder in partial remission.
D. There has never been a manic episode, a mixed episode, or a hypomanic episode, and criteria have never been met for cyclothymic disorder.
E. The disturbance does not occur exclusively during the course of a chronic psychotic disorder, such as schizophrenia or delusional disorder.
F. The symptoms are not caused by the direct physiological effects of a substance (e.g., a drug of abuse, a medication) or a general medical condition (e.g., hypothyroidism).
G. The symptoms cause clinically significant distress or impairment in social, occupational, or other important areas of functioning.

From American Psychiatric Association. *Diagnostic and statistical manual of mental disorders.* 5th ed. Arlington, VA: American Psychiatric Association; 2013.

Table 46-3 Features Suggesting Bipolar Depression

Feature	Bipolar	Unipolar
Substance abuse	Very high	Moderate
Family history	Almost uniform	Sometimes
Seasonality	Common	Occasional
First episode before age 25 years	Very common	Sometimes
Postpartum illness	Very common	Sometimes
Psychotic features before age 35	Highly predictive	Uncommon
Atypical features	Common	Occasional
Rapid on/off pattern	Typical	Unusual
Recurrent major depressive episodes (>3)	Common	Unusual
Antidepressant-induced mania or hypomania	Predictive	Uncommon
Brief episodes (<3 mo)	Suggestive	Unusual (duration usually >3 mo)
Antidepressant tolerance	Suggestive	Uncommon
Mixed depression (presence of hypomanic features within depressive episode)	Predictive	Rare
Tension, edginess, fearfulness	More common	Less common
Somatic symptoms (muscular, respiratory, genitourinary)	Less common	More common

Modified from Kaye NS. Is your depressed patient bipolar? *J Am Board Fam Pract.* 2005;18:271-281; and Perlis RH, Brown E, Baker RW, Nierenberg AA. Clinical features of bipolar depression versus major depressive disorder in large multicenter trials. *Am J Psychiatry.* 2006;163:225-231.

(i.e., presence of both manic and depressive symptoms), rapid mood swings, worsening psychosocial impairment, more suicide attempts, and higher mortality (Goldberg and Ernst, 2002; Goldberg and Truman, 2003; Schneck et al., 2008). Treatment of patients with bipolar depression is rarely straightforward and often requires multiple medications and medication trials. Antidepressants do not appear to be especially helpful in the treatment of bipolar disorder, and antidepressants have not yet been shown to improve outcome compared with mood stabilizers alone (Sachs et al., 2007). Although no symptom is pathognomonic for bipolar depression, certain features of depression may suggest that a patient's depression is a manifestation of bipolar illness. Bipolar depression can present similar to unipolar depression, but some depression features may help distinguish the two (Ghaemi et al., 2004; Perlis et al., 2006) (Table 46-3). If a primary care physician makes a diagnosis of bipolar disorder, the patient is best served by referral to a mental health provider, preferably with expertise in treating mood disorders.

Screening Tools for Depression

Numerous screening measures have been specifically designed to detect depression, and many are sensitive to change over time when used repeatedly at follow-up visits. The integration of such tools into clinical practice, referred to as *measurement-based care,* may enhance care and improve clinical outcome. Measurement tools in the public domain and sensitive to change over time are most practical for

primary care physicians because they are a cost-effective way to manage depressed patients over time (Trivedi et al., 2006b). Self-report measures obviate the need for trained office personnel to administer tests. Depression screening measures do not diagnose depression but do provide critical information regarding symptom severity within a given period. Almost all measures have a statistically predetermined cutoff score at which depression symptoms are considered significant. When a depression screening result is positive, an interview is necessary because screening will not include many confounding diagnostic variables (e.g., substance abuse, hypothyroidism, bereavement), and physician judgment is required. Screening measures do not address important clinical features of psychiatric illnesses (e.g., total duration of symptoms, degree of impairment) from other comorbid psychiatric conditions.

Patient Health Questionnaire 9. The PHQ-9 is often used in primary care settings because of its ease of use, sensitivity to change over time, reliability, and validity (Kroenke et al., 2001). It uses only the nine depression items from the original self-report version of the Primary Care Evaluation of Mental Disorders Patient Health Questionnaire (PRIME-MD PHQ) (Spitzer et al., 1999). Major depression is diagnosed if five or more of the depressive symptoms have been present at least "more than half the days" in the past 2 weeks and if one of the symptoms is depressed mood or anhedonia. Other depressive syndromes (e.g., minor depression) are diagnosed if two, three, or four depressive symptoms have been present at least "more than half the days" in the past 2 weeks and if one symptom is depressed mood or anhedonia. One of the nine test items ("thoughts that you would be better off dead or by hurting yourself in some way") counts if present at all, regardless of duration. Using cutoff scores from 9 to 15, sensitivity ranges from 68% to 95%, with specificity from 84% to 95%. Using the cutoff score of 9, sensitivity is 95% and specificity 84%.

Quick Inventory of Depressive Symptomatology— Self Report. The 16-item Quick Inventory of Depressive Symptomatology Self Report (QIDS-SR$_{16}$) is an instrument designed to screen for depression and to follow the changes in severity of depression over time (Rush et al., 2006a). The QIDS-SR$_{16}$ is a shortened version of the original 30-item Inventory of Depressive Symptomatology (IDS). Whereas the IDS includes criterion symptoms and symptoms typically associated with depression, such as anxiety and irritability, the QIDS assesses only the nine symptom domains used to characterize depressive episodes (sad mood, concentration, self-criticism, suicidal ideation, interest, energy or fatigue, sleep disturbance, changes in appetite or weight, presence of psychomotor agitation or retardation). The total score on QIDS ranges from 0 to 27 (0-5, no severity; 6-10, mild; 11-15, moderate; 16-20, severe; 21-27, very severe). The QIDS was effective in assisting management of depression in the STAR*D study, the largest depression trial conducted thus far in the United States (Trivedi et al., 2006b).

Screening for Bipolar Disorder

Although no laboratory or imaging tests currently exist to distinguish unipolar depression from bipolar depression, screening questionnaires, as well as certain features of a patient's history and symptomatology, may prove helpful. The MDQ is a tool that combines DSM-IV criteria and clinical experience to screen for bipolar disorder in primary care settings (Hirschfeld et al., 2000). It is a brief, one-page self-report questionnaire with 13 yes-or-no items and two additional questions regarding functioning and timing of mood symptoms and typically can be completed in 5 minutes or less. Seven or more positive responses to questions about manic symptoms, plus positive responses to the severity of impairment (moderate or severe) and coincident timing of symptoms, yields a positive screen. The specificity and sensitivity of the MDQ vary widely by clinical setting, having the best combination of the two when given to patients with suspected mood symptoms (93% specificity; 58% sensitivity) but performs more poorly in general community samples (97% specificity; 28% sensitivity) (Hirschfeld et al., 2003, 2005). Other screening tools for bipolar disorder do not offer the ease of use and higher reliability and validity of the MDQ.

DIAGNOSIS OF ANXIETY DISORDERS

The essential feature of GAD is excessive anxiety and worry about a number of events or activities, occurring most days over 6 months. Patients have difficulty controlling the worry, report subjective distress, and may experience difficulties in social or occupational functioning. The intensity,

Table 46-4 Diagnostic Criteria for Generalized Anxiety Disorder

A. Excessive anxiety and worry (apprehensive expectation), occurring more days than not for at least 6 months, about a number of events or activities
B. The person finds it difficult to control the worry.
C. The anxiety and worry are associated with three (or more) of the following six symptoms:
   1. Restlessness and feeling keyed up or on edge
   2. Being easily fatigued
   3. Difficulty concentrating or mind going blank
   4. Irritability
   5. Muscle tension
   6. Sleep disturbance
D. The anxiety, worry, or physical symptoms cause clinically significant distress or impairment in social, occupational, or other important areas of functioning.
E. The disturbance is not caused by the direct physiological effects of a substance or a general medical condition.
F. The disturbance is not better explained by another mental disorder.

From American Psychiatric Association. *Diagnostic and statistical manual of mental disorders.* 5th ed. Arlington, VA: American Psychiatric Association; 2013.

Table 46-5 Diagnostic Criteria for Panic Attack

An abrupt surge of intense fear or intense discomfort that reaches a peak within minutes and during which time four (or more) of the following symptoms occur:

1. Palpitations, pounding heart, or accelerated heart rate
2. Sweating
3. Trembling or shaking
4. Sensations of shortness of breath or smothering
5. Feeling of choking
6. Chest pain or discomfort
7. Nausea or abdominal distress
8. Feeling dizzy, unsteady, lightheaded, or faint
9. Chills or heat sensations
10. Paresthesias (numbness or tingling sensations)
11. Derealization (feelings of unreality) or depersonalization (being detached from oneself)
12. Fear of losing control or "going crazy"
13. Fear of dying

From American Psychiatric Association. *Diagnostic and statistical manual of mental disorders.* 5th ed. Arlington, VA: American Psychiatric Association; 2013.

duration, or frequency of the worry is out of proportion to the actual likelihood or impact of the feared event. Patients must have at least three associated physical symptoms, including restlessness, irritability, muscle tension, disturbed sleep, fatigability, and difficulty concentrating. The list of associated symptoms can be thought of as symptoms of inner tension (restlessness or edginess, irritability, muscle tension) and symptoms associated with the fatiguing effects of chronic anxiety (fatigue, concentration difficulties, sleep disturbance) (Table 46-4).

Panic attacks, a collection of distressing physical, cognitive, and emotional symptoms, may occur in a variety of mental health disorders and are not limited to anxiety disorders. Panic attacks are discrete periods of intense fear in the absence of real danger accompanied by at least 4 of 13 cognitive and physical symptoms (Table 46-5). The attacks have a sudden onset; build to a peak quickly; and are often accompanied by feelings of doom, imminent danger, and a

Table 46-6 Diagnostic Criteria for Panic Disorder

A. Recurrent and unexpected panic attacks
B. At least one of the attacks has been followed by 1 month (or more) of one or both of the following:
   1. Persistent concern about having additional panic attacks or their consequences
   2. A significant maladaptive change in behavior related to the attacks
C. The disturbance is not attributable to the physiological effects of a substance or a general medical condition.
D. The disturbance is not better explained by another mental disorder.

From American Psychiatric Association. *Diagnostic and statistical manual of mental disorders.* 5th ed. Arlington, VA: American Psychiatric Association; 2013.

need to escape. Symptoms of panic attacks can include somatic complaints (e.g., sweating, chills), cardiovascular symptoms (pounding heart, accelerated heart rate, chest pain), neurologic symptoms (trembling, unsteadiness, lightheadedness, paresthesias), GI symptoms (choking sensations, nausea), and pulmonary symptoms (shortness of breath). In addition, patients with panic attacks may worry they are dying or "going crazy" or have the sensation of being detached from reality. Panic attacks can be listed as a specifier to all DSM-5 disorders and is not considered a stand-alone diagnosis.

Patients with *panic disorder* experience recurrent, unexpected panic attacks followed by at least 1 month of persistent worry that they will have another panic attack. Patients with panic disorder may begin to avoid places where a prior attack occurred or where help may not be available (Table 46-6). The DSM-5 has separated panic disorder and agoraphobia into two unique and distinct diagnoses.

Screening Tools for Anxiety Disorders

At present, screening tools for anxiety disorders have been developed to recognize anxiety as a broad syndrome, examining somatic symptoms (racing heart, lightheadedness) or cognitive symptoms (tendency to worry, intensity of worry). Other tools have been used to screen for single, distinct disorders, such as phobias or panic disorder. To date, no clear screening tool or symptom-severity measure has emerged for use in primary care settings, although newer instruments may be useful for primary care physicians. The Generalized Anxiety Disorder 7 (GAD-7) scale was developed and validated in primary care clinics and is a brief, seven-item self-report screening tool for GAD (Spitzer et al., 2006). The GAD-7 helps identify probable cases of GAD and measure symptom severity. A score of 10 or greater represents a reasonable cutoff point for identifying patients with GAD, and cutoffs of 5, 10, and 15 correlate to mild, moderate, and severe levels of anxiety, respectively. An extended version of the PHQ includes five questions for panic disorder (Spitzer et al., 1999), but its utility as a stand-alone tool is currently unclear. The Overall Anxiety Severity and Impairment Scale (OASIS) is a five-item continuous measure that can be used across anxiety disorders, with multiple anxiety disorders, and with subthreshold anxiety symptoms. OASIS can be used to measure the severity of anxiety symptoms, but it was not developed as a diagnostic tool for any specific disorder (Norman et al., 2006).

Assessment of the Depressed or Anxious Patient in Medical Settings

Key Points

- Patients with anxiety and depressive disorders often present with somatic complaints.
- Risk assessment includes identifying modifiable risk factors and developing a corresponding treatment plan.
- "Contracts for safety" have no empiric data to support their effectiveness in risk management.
- Worsening symptoms or suicidal ideation may require psychiatric hospitalization.

Diagnosing anxiety and depressive disorders may prove especially challenging in medical settings. The majority of patients with such illnesses more frequently present with somatic complaints; only a minority present with purely psychological symptoms and concerns (Bridges and Goldberg, 1985). Difficulties in diagnosis may be secondary to a patient's inability to articulate psychological problems, reticence to speak of emotional difficulties, the short time allowed for patient visits, or a primary care physician's relative lack of training in assessing and treating mental health disorders. Many presenting complaints may be consistent with symptoms of coexisting medical illnesses, further complicating assessment and likely requiring additional etiologic investigation. Of new patients presenting to an urban clinic, for example, only 17% presented with purely psychological symptoms. Of the remaining patients, 32% presented with pure somatization, 27% presented with symptoms for a coexisting medical illness, and 24% presented with an initial physical complaint that they were later able to relate to a psychological problem (Bridges and Goldberg, 1985). However, clinical clues in patients with physical complaints may identify a subgroup of patients who warrant further evaluation for an anxiety or depressive disorder. This includes patients who present with multiple physical symptoms (six or more), have higher ratings of symptom severity and lower ratings of overall health, and have an encounter that the physician perceives as "difficult" (Kroenke et al., 1997).

Assessment of anxious or depressed patients requires establishing specific psychiatric diagnosis (or diagnoses), providing a thorough risk assessment (i.e., suicidality, homicidality, ability or inability to care for self), assessing the severity of the illness, identifying specific target symptoms to track over time, assessing factors that are likely complicating or exacerbating the illness (e.g. medical disorders, substance abuse), and gathering collateral information whenever possible from family, friends, or other providers (Table 46-7). Distinguishing bipolar from unipolar depression, as discussed previously, is one of the most important distinctions when establishing a diagnosis. In addition, clinicians should look for the presence of comorbid anxiety disorders because patients with such disorders often require lower initial antidepressant dosing and may have their anxiety symptoms paradoxically worsen as treatment is initiated unless lower doses are used (Table 46-8). Education on the medical nature of depression and anxiety

Table 46-7 Initial Assessment of Anxious or Depressed Patients

1. Establish diagnosis.
2. Perform risk assessment:
   Suicide risk
   Risks to others
3. Establish severity of illness:
   Ability to care for self
   Functioning and functional impairment
4. Identify specific target symptoms:
   Neurovegetative symptoms (e.g., sleep, appetite, concentration)
   Use of measurement scales (e.g., Quick Inventory of Depressive Symptomatology [QIDS])
5. Assess factors complicating illness:
   Alcohol or drug use
   Comorbid or contributing medical conditions
6. Gather input from family and friends if possible.

Table 46-8 Dosing for Common Antidepressant and Antianxiety Agents

Medication	Usual Daily Starting Dose (mg)		Daily Dose Range
	Anxiety	Depression	
SELECTIVE SEROTONIN REUPTAKE INHIBITORS			
Citalopram	10	20	10-60
Escitalopram	5	10	5-30
Fluoxetine	10	20	20-80
Fluvoxamine	25	50	100-300
Paroxetine	10	20	20-60
Sertraline	25	50	50-200
SEROTONIN-NOREPINEPHRINE REUPTAKE INHIBITORS			
Desvenlafaxine	50	50	50-100
Duloxetine	30	30	30-120
Venlafaxine	37.5	75	150-300
TRICYCLIC ANTIDEPRESSANTS			
Amitriptyline	25	50	100-300
Imipramine	25	50	100-300
Nortriptyline	10	25	50-200
Desipramine	25	50	100-300
NOREPINEPHRINE-DOPAMINE REUPTAKE INHIBITORS			
Bupropion	—	150	300-450
NOREPINEPHRINE-SEROTONIN MODULATORS			
Mirtazapine	15	30	30-60

may prove extremely helpful because both patients and their families often believe that psychiatric illness is evidence of "weakness" or indicative of some other personal failing. Information on prognosis and the expected treatment course may lessen pressure and expectations for rapid improvement and let the patient know when to expect medication benefit.

Physicians should assess the severity of illness and develop a list of target symptoms to track and measure over time to better evaluate treatment response. Tracking specific symptoms particular to an individual patient's depression improves objective assessment of change. Often, patients' neurovegetative symptoms improve before the subjective experience of their mood improves. Assessing sleep, appetite, energy level, anxiety, and concentration allows the physician to select a more appropriate antidepressant or anxiolytic by targeting specific symptoms. This may include using a sedating antidepressant such as

mirtazapine for patients with insomnia or a more activating antidepressant such as bupropion for patients with lethargy or somnolence. Measurement tools that are symptom specific and sensitive to change over time (e.g., PHQ-9, QIDS-SR) may help the physician track such changes. In addition, assessing overall functionality (ability to shower, pay bills, shop, prepare meals) is equally important in establishing the degree of impairment caused by the patient's mood disorder.

DIFFERENTIAL DIAGNOSIS

Many medical conditions may cause or mimic depression. Physical disorders that have been associated with depression include Addison disease, acquired immunodeficiency syndrome (AIDS), coronary artery disease (especially in those with myocardial infarction), cancer, multiple sclerosis, Parkinson disease, anemia, diabetes, acute infection, temporal arteritis, hypothyroidism, and especially dementias. It is imperative that the physician complete a neurologic evaluation to rule out an underlying disorder as the cause of the patient's depression. In addition, many medications may worsen depression, especially cardiovascular drugs, hormones, typical antipsychotic agents, antiinflammatory agents, and anticonvulsants.

Anxiety disorders may be caused or exacerbated by medical conditions, medications taken for other psychiatric or medical disorders, and other substances with stimulant properties. For example, hyperthyroidism can mimic or exacerbate anxiety disorders, and therefore thyroid function should be carefully evaluated when patients present with anxiety symptoms. In addition, lifetime risk of thyroid dysfunction appears higher in patients with panic disorder or GAD (Simon et al., 2002). Physicians should also assess the patient's use of other medications, especially stimulants (whether prescribed or obtained from other sources), nicotine, illicit drugs, and caffeine.

SUICIDE SCREENING AND ASSESSMENT

Identifying patients at risk for suicide is a complex and difficult task, particularly in the setting of a busy medical practice. Suicide is currently the 10th leading cause of death for all ages and the third leading cause of death among the 15- to 24-year age group (Centers for Disease Control and Prevention, 2012). Older men (75 years and older) have the highest suicide rate, at 37.4 per 100,000. Men continue to take their lives at approximately four times the rate of women and account for almost 80% of all U.S. suicides. Women in their 40s and 50s have the highest rates of suicide among women (8 per 100,000), and women continue to make suicide attempts two to three times more often than men (Krug et al., 2002). Approximately 60% of all suicides are associated with patients with mood disorders (Isometsa et al., 1995a), and approximately 50% of patients who completed suicide had contact with professional help in the month before their death (Isometsa et al., 1995b).

Despite no definitive suicide assessment tool being available, risk factors have been defined that can help identify patients at risk for suicide. Suicide screening should include assessing current level of depression, severity of symptoms, feelings of hopelessness, current suicidal thoughts and behaviors (as well as past attempts), use of drugs or alcohol (which can increase levels of impulsivity and worsen dysphoria), current levels of anxiety and agitation, access to lethal means (especially firearms), presence of psychosis (command hallucinations, poor reality testing), recent acute stressors, and presence (or absence) of a psychosocial support system (APA, 2003). When possible, additional information from family or friends can be helpful in assessing statements or behaviors that may indicate a patient's intentions of committing suicide.

Physicians should be alert to suicide risk factors that can be modified. Although numerous historical and biologic risk factors cannot be modified (e.g., history of suicide attempts, family history of suicide, male gender, history of childhood trauma), other risk factors are amenable to intervention. Patients with mood, anxiety, and psychotic symptoms can be successfully treated with medications. Substance abuse referral may help a patient actively struggling with substance abuse or dependence or for relapse prevention. Encouraging the patient to mobilize psychosocial resources, such as contacting family members for support, can provide a measure of safety while the patient is recovering from depression. Removing access to firearms can be especially helpful in preventing rapid access to lethal means during episodes of acute distress and high levels of impulsivity. Physicians should be aware that "contracts for safety" have not been shown to be effective in preventing suicide and may provide a false sense of patient safety (Rudd et al., 2006). Continued assessment of mood, hopelessness, and suicidal ideation is required throughout the course of treatment. Worsening symptoms, along with plans or active preparations for suicide, may require increased observation or hospitalization.

Management and Treatment of Major Depression and Anxiety Disorders

The key objective in treating patients with depressive and anxiety disorders is remission of all symptoms. Studies in the treatment of major depression have consistently shown that a lack of remission is associated with higher relapse rates, more severe subsequent depressions, shorter durations between episodes, continued impairment in work settings and social relationships, increased all-cause mortality, and increased risk of suicide (Judd et al., 2000). Initiation of treatment should include education about the expected temporal course of improvement; importance of regular eating, activity, social interaction, and sleep; medication selection; follow-up schedule; and safety management if symptoms worsen or suicidal ideation is evident (Table 46-9).

DEPRESSION

Pharmacotherapy remains the mainstay treatment of depression. Treatment should be considered for the majority of depressed patients, especially those who are suicidal, functionally impaired from their depression, experiencing a recurrent episode, or who have comorbid medical or

Table 46-9 Initiation of Treatment for Major Depression and Anxiety Disorders

1. Educate the patient:
   Details of illness
   Treatment course, prognosis, goal of treatment (remission of symptoms)
   Importance of general health: exercise, sleep hygiene, nutrition
   Inclusion of family when possible
   Coordination with other providers
   Resource lists for support groups and therapy referrals
2. Select medication from reasonable choices:
   Patient history of antidepressant use and response
   Family history of antidepressant response
   Typical time course to antidepressant response
3. Administer starting dose and initiate dose titration:
   Common side effects of medications
4. Establish monitoring with measurement-based care (e.g., Quick Inventory of Depressive Symptomatology [QIDS]).
5. Schedule follow-up in 2 to 4 weeks.

psychiatric conditions likely to worsen unless their depression is treated (e.g., panic, GAD, chronic pain). Treatment of depression has clearly been shown to prevent relapse, shorten current episodes, decrease psychosocial impairment, decrease risk of suicide, and improve quality of life. Mild depression may be treated with symptomatic intervention alone (e.g., mild sedative for insomnia), although continuing depressive symptoms or inadequate response to purely symptomatic interventions warrants more aggressive treatment of the underlying depression. Patients with psychotic depression typically require treatment with both antidepressant and antipsychotic agents, or they may require electroconvulsive therapy (ECT). Often, psychotically depressed patients require hospitalization. Patients with psychotic depression should be referred to a psychiatrist, given the severity of illness and complexity of treatment.

Again, the aim of treatment is remission of all depressive symptoms and a return to the patient's previous baseline functioning. Pharmacotherapy combined with psychotherapy has been shown to be superior to either modality alone (de Maat et al., 2008; Thase, 1997); thus, referral to a psychotherapist may be helpful, especially for patients with moderate to severe depression. Some patients may choose psychotherapy alone to treat depression; psychodynamic therapy, cognitive-behavioral therapy (CBT), interpersonal therapy, and behavioral activation may prove as effective as medication alone.

Selection of Medication

The effectiveness of antidepressants is generally comparable across classes; therefore, selection of an antidepressant depends mainly on patient preference, side effect profile, drug interactions, previous response to a specific medication, treatment overlap with other psychiatric conditions, and cost (Tables 46-10 and 46-11). Minimal data support the increased efficacy or speed of onset for any particular agent, with response rates across clinical trials generally 50% to 75% for patients receiving active treatment. The onset of improvement typically takes 3 to 6 weeks, although the STAR*D study indicates that patients may require up to 12 to 14 weeks to achieve remission of symptoms. In fact, 40% of patients in the multiyear, multisite STAR*D study who eventually achieved remission in the first level of

Table 46-10 Food and Drug Administration Indications for Antidepressant Therapy

Medication	MDD	OCD	Panic	PTSD	GAD	Soc Anx	PMDD	Bulimia	Other or Off-Label Uses
Amitriptyline (Elavil)	X								Migraine prophylaxis, chronic pain
Bupropion (Wellbutrin)	X								Smoking cessation
Citalopram (Celexa)	X								
Desvenlafaxine (Pristiq)	X								
Desipramine (Norpramin)	X								
Duloxetine (Cymbalta)	X				X				Diabetic peripheral neuropathic pain, fibromyalgia
Escitalopram (Lexapro)	X				X				
Fluoxetine (Prozac)	X	X	X				X	X	Pediatric depression
Fluvoxamine (Luvox)		X							
Imipramine (Tofranil)	X								Enuresis
Levomilnacipran (Fetzima)	X								
Mirtazapine (Remeron)	X								
Nortriptyline (Pamelor)	X								
Paroxetine (Paxil)	X	X	X	X	X	X			
Sertraline (Zoloft)	X	X	X	X			X	X	Premature ejaculation
Venlafaxine (Effexor)	X		X		X	X			
Vilazodone (Viibryd)	X								
Vortioxetine (Brintellix)	X								

GAD, Generalized anxiety disorder; *MDD,* major depressive disorder; *OCD,* obsessive-compulsive disorder; *PMDD,* premenstrual dysphoric disorder; *PTSD,* posttraumatic stress disorder; *Soc Anx,* social anxiety disorder.

Table 46-11 Common Side Effects of Antidepressant Medications

Class or Drug	Side Effects	Comments
Selective serotonin reuptake inhibitor (SSRI)	GI side effects (nausea, diarrhea, heartburn); sexual dysfunction (decreased libido, delayed orgasm); headache; insomnia or somnolence	Likely little difference between SSRIs in rates of sexual side effects; SSRIs have been used to treat premature ejaculation
Serotonin-norepinephrine reuptake inhibitor (SNRI)	Hypertension, sweating, nausea, constipation, dizziness, sexual dysfunction	Risk of increased blood pressure escalates as dose is increased; abrupt withdrawal of venlafaxine may cause discontinuation syndrome
Tricyclic antidepressant (TCA)	Dry mouth, constipation, blurry vision, orthostatic hypotension, weight gain, somnolence, headache, sweating, sexual dysfunction	Use with caution in patients with cardiac conduction delays
Bupropion	Insomnia, dry mouth, tremor, headache, nausea, constipation, dizziness	Contraindicated in patients with seizure disorders or eating disorders; patients generally free of sexual side effects
Mirtazapine	Somnolence, increased appetite, weight gain, dry mouth	Sedation may be more pronounced at lower doses
Trazodone	Sedation, orthostatic hypotension, priapism	Usually used as a sedative–hypnotic
Benzodiazepines	Sedation, fatigue, ataxia, slurred speech, memory impairment, weakness	Risk of dependence or abuse, especially with shorter acting benzodiazepines

GI, Gastrointestinal.

treatment with citalopram did not show a response (i.e., 50% improvement in symptoms) until week 8 of treatment (Trivedi et al., 2006b).

For most patients, initial treatment with a selective serotonin reuptake inhibitor (SSRI), serotonin-norepinephrine reuptake inhibitor (SNRI), bupropion, or mirtazapine is reasonable. Tricyclic antidepressants (TCAs) are more often used as second-line agents in the treatment of depression because of their potential toxicity in overdose, greater side effect burden (largely from anticholinergic, antihistaminic, and antiadrenergic properties), and potential cardiac complications (conduction delays). Monoamine oxidase (MAO) inhibitors are complex drugs to use given their potentially fatal drug and dietary interactions and probably should not be prescribed in family practice settings. Most

antidepressant studies have been conducted in specialty settings, but a number of studies in primary care settings have also shown the superiority of antidepressants over placebo (Arroll et al., 2009). Thus, given the comparable speed and efficacy of antidepressants across classes and within classes, selection of an antidepressant agent may be primarily guided by side effect profile, possible secondary uses of antidepressants (e.g., treating pain or insomnia), and contraindications to particular agents (e.g., bupropion in seizure disorder patients). Table 46-8 gives the usual starting doses for treatment of major depression.

Serotonin reuptake inhibitors are safe, effective medications that can treat patients with a variety of psychiatric conditions. All SSRIs operate by the same mechanism of action and are considered equally effective in the treatment of depression. However, failure of one SSRI does not necessarily imply failure of all SSRIs; patients may respond preferentially to one SSRI over another (Rush et al., 2006b). The SSRIs differ substantially by their potential to inhibit particular hepatic cytochrome P-450 metabolic pathways and by half-life, potency, and presence or absence of active metabolites. Clinicians should check for drug interactions in patients receiving complex polypharmacy regimens because drug–drug interactions are constantly being updated and changing. For example, fluoxetine is a potent 2D6 inhibitor that can triple TCA and phenytoin levels or increase the anticoagulation associated with warfarin. Fluoxetine also has the longest half-life of any SSRI; its active metabolite norfluoxetine has a half-life of 10 days. The SSRIs have sexual side effects (decreased libido, delayed orgasm or anorgasmia) and GI side effects (nausea, diarrhea) (see Table 46-11). GI side effects likely will remit over time, but sexual effects typically do not attenuate and may require treatment with other agents, such as a phosphodiesterase inhibitor (e.g., sildenafil) or choosing an antidepressant less likely to cause sexual side effects.

The SNRIs (venlafaxine, duloxetine, desvenlafaxine, and levomilnacipran) are similar in efficacy to the SSRIs, although a few studies have suggested a mild advantage of SNRIs over SSRIs (Thase et al., 2001). Although the SNRIs by definition inhibit the reuptake of both serotonin and norepinephrine, dual-neurotransmitter reuptake inhibition does not occur with venlafaxine until doses reach approximately 150 mg/day; below this dose, it acts primarily as an SSRI. Venlafaxine is available in immediate-release and extended-release (XR) formulations, although most patients and clinicians favor use of the XR preparation, given its once-daily dosing and lower likelihood of provoking a withdrawal syndrome on discontinuation of the drug, more frequently observed with the immediate-release formulation. Desvenlafaxine, the active metabolite of venlafaxine, is more potent than its parent compound, but any advantages over venlafaxine are currently unclear. Unlike venlafaxine, duloxetine provides dual-neurotransmitter reuptake inhibition at any dose, although this does not appear to confer any advantage over other SNRIs in terms of efficacy or side effect profile. Duloxetine currently is indicated for treatment of chronic pain as well as depression, but this is likely a class effect of SNRIs and not unique to duloxetine. Levomilnacipran is an active enantiomer of the racemic drug milnacipran (approved by the U.S. Food and Drug Administration for the treatment of fibromyalgia). It is the most noradrenergically active of the SNRIs, but whether this will translate to unique clinical characteristics has yet to be determined. Side effects of SNRIs are similar to SSRIs (see Table 46-11), with the additional side effects with SNRIs likely caused by increased noradrenergic activity, including dose-related hypertension, excessive sweating, and dry mouth (Thase, 2008a; Thase et al., 2005).

Mirtazapine is a serotonin-norepinephrine modulator that also blocks postsynaptic hydroxytryptamine (HT) receptors, including those in the 5-HT-3 (serotonin) class. Mirtazapine is sedating and can increase appetite and therefore may be favored when patients have insomnia or decreased appetite and weight loss. Because of a dose-dependent ratio of neurotransmitter blockade involving histamine receptors, mirtazapine is generally more sedating at lower doses than higher. Although currently indicated only for depression, mirtazapine is reported to have general anxiolytic effects and may be beneficial for patients with mild to moderate anxiety. With its 5-HT-3 blockade, mirtazapine may be helpful when patients complain of nausea or other GI symptoms or side effects from SSRIs. Mirtazapine also has fewer sexual side effects than the SSRIs and SNRIs and has been tried as an antidote to SSRI-induced sexual side effects. Common side effects from mirtazapine include weight gain and daytime somnolence (see Table 46-11).

Bupropion is pharmacologically unique among antidepressants and is manufactured in immediate-release, slow-release (SR), and XR formulations. Although its primary mechanism of action is unclear, the drug has weak norepinephrine and dopamine reuptake inhibition. Bupropion is an activating drug, making it better suited for patients with poor energy or who believe they cannot tolerate a sedating medication. It is also virtually free from sexual side effects and has been used with limited success as an antidote for patients with SSRI-induced sexual side effects (Clayton et al., 2004). Bupropion rarely causes weight gain and is therefore a good choice for patients who are obese or who believe they cannot tolerate weight gain. Unlike the SSRIs, SNRIs, and TCAs, bupropion does not treat anxiety disorders and may even worsen anxiety in patients because of its activating properties. Bupropion carries a black box warning against its use in patients with a history of seizures or eating disorders; the latter group was shown to have a higher incidence of seizures in clinical trials. Given its greater propensity for seizures, bupropion dosing should not be pushed above the FDA-recommended dosing limits. Bupropion has also been approved for treatment of smoking cessation and therefore may have particular utility for depressed patients who also want to quit smoking.

Vortioxetine is the most recently FDA-approved drug for the treatment of major depression (FDA, 2013). Although it has unique pharmacologic characteristics, acting as an SSRI, a 5HT1A agonist, a partial agonist at 5-HT1B receptors, and an antagonist at 5-HT3, 5-HT1D, and 5-HT7 receptors, it is currently unclear to what extent these characteristics contribute to its antidepressant efficacy.

The TCAs are effective medications for treating depression and anxiety, with evidence of being more effective than the SSRIs for severe depression, but the TCAs confer a greater side effect burden than the newer antidepressants and can be fatal in overdose. TCAs are divided into tertiary and secondary amines. Tertiary amines, such as amitriptyline and imipramine, have greater anticholinergic, antihistaminic, and α-adrenergic blockade side effects than secondary amines, such as their respective metabolites nortriptyline and desipramine. The TCAs offer an advantage over other antidepressants in that blood levels can readily be checked and dosing individualized. Reasonable evidence suggests that the TCAs may be more effective in severely depressed patients (Gelenberg et al., 2010). In addition, nortriptyline has a therapeutic window, with superior antidepressant efficacy if levels are maintained at 50 to 150 ng/mL. Because of cardiac conduction side effects, however, the TCAs must be used with caution in patients with conduction delays or who are taking class I antiarrhythmic agents, and electrocardiograms should be checked and monitored in patients older than 50 years and in those with suspected cardiac disease. The TCAs also may cause tachycardia and orthostatic hypotension and thus should be used with caution in patients at risk for tachyarrhythmias or falls. The greatest single disadvantage to TCAs is their potential lethality in overdose; a typical 10-day supply can be lethal, and therefore TCAs should be prescribed cautiously in patients at high risk for suicide. The TCAs are also used in a variety of headache and pain syndromes and thus may be useful in patients with such comorbidities.

Trazodone is structurally distinct from the SSRIs, TCAs, tetracyclics, and MAO inhibitors, but it still inhibits neuronal uptake of serotonin. Although the FDA has approved it as an antidepressant, trazodone is most often used as a sedative–hypnotic. Whereas dosing as an antidepressant is usually 300 to 450 mg, sedative–hypnotic dosing is usually 50 to 150 mg. The risks and side effects of trazodone include sedation, priapism, and myocardial irritability; the latter effect includes the potential of inducing torsades de pointes.

KEY TREATMENT

- All antidepressants are generally equally effective; selection is most often based on side effect profile, previous response, comorbid conditions, drug interactions, and cost (Arroll et al., 2009; Trivedi et al., 2006b) (SOR: A).
- The SSRIs, the SNRIs, mirtazapine, and bupropion are first-line treatments for depression (Rush et al., 2006b) (SOR: A).
- Antidepressant doses should be increased every 2 to 4 weeks until remission of depressive symptoms is achieved or side effects become intolerable (Gelenberg et al., 2010) (SOR: A).
- Treatment of depressive episodes ranges from 6 to 9 months to years, depending on the number of prior episodes, severity of episodes, and risk of relapse (AHCPR, 1999; Geddes et al., 2003) (SOR:A).
- Psychotherapy has proved effective in treating depression, either as monotherapy or combined with pharmacotherapy (de Maat et al., 2008; Thase, 1997) (SOR: A).

Initiation of Treatment

After a patient has been initiated on an antidepressant, dosing should be optimized to treat depressive symptoms to remission while minimizing side effects (Table 46-12). Patients should be monitored for improvement in their mood and their specific array of depressive symptoms. Continued use of measurement-based care tools, such as

Table 46-12 Assessing Antidepressant Treatment

Monitor the effectiveness of treatment.
Continue assessment of specific symptoms.
Assess need for further titration of medication.
Continue to use measurement-based care.
Assess any worsening of mood, increased irritability, or worsening suicidal ideation.
Assess adherence to medication regimen.
Assess for medication side effects.
Continue to emphasize nutrition, physical activity, and caring for self.
Minimize complexity of medication dosing (e.g., once daily or nightly, when possible).

the PHQ-9 or QIDS, can aid in the objective assessment of improvement. Patients should be followed more frequently on initiation of treatment, increasing the time between appointments as the patient improves. Monitoring for side effects, particularly those that patients may be reluctant to bring up spontaneously, such as sexual side effects, can improve adherence and the therapeutic alliance. Patients should also be monitored for any worsening of mood, increased irritability, impulsivity, insomnia, sudden switches into euphoria, or suicidal ideation. Such symptoms may suggest *bipolar diathesis*, in which case discontinuing the antidepressant and changing to mood stabilizing agents may be indicated. Antidepressant doses should be increased every 2 to 4 weeks until the patient shows a response, maximum dose is reached, or side effects limit further dose changes. Antidepressant doses should continue to be pushed until remission is achieved or the patient has undergone an adequate antidepressant trial (i.e., continuation of a therapeutic dose for at least 4 to 8 weeks) (Nierenberg et al., 2000).

Continuation of Treatment

As noted, physicians are encouraged to push treatment until symptoms remit, maximum doses are achieved, or side effects become intolerable. After symptoms remit, medications should continue for 6 to 9 months because risk of relapse is greater if patients discontinue medications prematurely (AHCPR, 1999; Geddes et al., 2003). Patients who have had multiple episodes of depression should continue pharmacotherapy because lifetime relapse rates for such patients are 50% to 85% (Eaton et al., 2008), and the risk of recurrence increases by 16% with each successive episode (Solomon et al., 2000). Ongoing treatment should also be considered for patients who experienced severe functional impairment, severe suicidal ideation, or serious suicide attempts.

Discontinuation of Treatment

For patients who have achieved ongoing remission and want to discontinue their medications, withdrawal of treatment should be gradual and carefully monitored (Table 46-13). Timing of discontinuation often depends on a patient's current life stressors and the potential consequences of depressive relapse (e.g., loss of new job, stress on recently repaired relationship). Antidepressants should be gradually withdrawn to minimize potential withdrawal syndromes and allow for rapid upward titration if depressive symptoms recur. Physicians should discuss the early warning signs of relapse (insomnia, early-morning awakening, loss of interest in activities) and instruct patients to contact their physicians if such symptoms recur. The risk of relapse is greatest in the first few months of discontinuing antidepressants, and thus a scheduled appointment in this period is often needed to monitor for relapse. Patients who relapse after cessation of antidepressants should be

Table 46-13 Discontinuation of Antidepressant Treatment

Remission of symptoms for 6-12 mo
Tapering of medications rather than abrupt cessation
Discussion of relapse risks and early warning signs of recurrence

restarted on their previous medication and again titrated to remission of symptoms.

ANTIDEPRESSANT FAILURE

Patients who fail antidepressants should be carefully reevaluated, with reconsideration of medication adherence, adequacy of dosing and treatment duration, diagnosis, comorbid psychiatric illnesses, increased stressors, and unaddressed medical or substance comorbidities. Initial antidepressant failure may be relatively common; only one third of patients achieved remission after 12 to 14 weeks of treatment with citalopram in the STAR*D study (Trivedi et al., 2006b). If a patient fails an adequate antidepressant trial, the next strategy is (1) switching to a different antidepressant within the same class or across classes, (2) augmenting the existing antidepressant with a secondary agent, or (3) adding a second antidepressant to the first. The choice of strategy depends on patient preference, assessment of benefit from current antidepressant, current side effects, and psychiatric and medical comorbidities.

Switching antidepressants is generally considered when the patient has had little to no response to the first agent or is having intolerable side effects. Across-class switches are most often considered as an initial strategy (e.g., SSRI to SNRI), although within-class switches may also prove useful (e.g., fluoxetine to sertraline). Across-class or intra-class switching may yield response rates of 20% to 50% (Thase, 2008b). In the STAR*D study, switching from citalopram to either bupropion SR, venlafaxine, or sertraline yielded remission rates of 18% to 25% (Rush et al., 2006b). No clear guidelines exist as how best to cross-taper medications, although it is generally unwise to stop antidepressants abruptly because withdrawal syndromes may ensue. Medications with short half-lives, such as venlafaxine (immediate release) or paroxetine, have most often been associated with withdrawal syndromes. Typically, patients complain of flulike symptoms, electric-like shocks in the back of their heads, or dizziness (Taylor et al., 2006). Consideration of half-life and slow cross-tapers often yields the most tolerable switch.

Augmentation strategies involve adding a second agent with no intrinsic antidepressant properties to the existing antidepressant. These are often considered when a patient has had a partial response to an antidepressant but has not reached remission, and switching to an alternate antidepressant may risk loss of existing response. The two best studied augmentation strategies to date are adding lithium and triiodothyronine (T_3). Although many lithium augmentation studies are limited by methodologic considerations, response has been seen as quickly as 48 hours or as long as 2 to 4 weeks. Standard lithium levels of 0.5 to 1.0 mmol/L have most often been used. T_3 augmentation has yielded similar results, if often better tolerated than lithium, usually with doses of 25 to 50 µg/day. Overall remission rates in patients unable to achieve antidepressant-alone remission range from 15% to 50% (Nierenberg et al., 2006). Atypical antipsychotic drugs have also been used as augmenting agents in nonpsychotic major depression, with beneficial results. Aripiprazole currently has an indication as an augmenting agent, at 2 to 15 mg/day. To date, no other atypical antipsychotic has an FDA indication as an augmenting agent, although a meta-analysis of atypical antipsychotics as augmenting agents found their efficacy superior to placebo, with a number needed to treat (NNT) of nine for both response and remission (Nelson and Papakostas, 2009). Buspirone has also been used as an augmenting agent because its 5-HT-1A receptor agonism may enhance SSRI response. In the STAR*D study, 30% of patients who failed to achieve remission taking citalopram went on to remit with the addition of buspirone, up to 60 mg/day (Trivedi et al., 2006a).

Combining two antidepressants to treat refractory depression is based on the theory that targeting a greater number of neurotransmitters will lead to improved antidepressant response. Common strategies include combining mirtazapine and venlafaxine, bupropion and SSRIs, or bupropion and SNRIs. Combining drugs of similar class (e.g., SSRI + SSRI or SNRI + SNRI) currently has few data to support its use. Venlafaxine combined with mirtazapine and citalopram plus bupropion SR were effective in the STAR*D study when patients failed to achieve remission on their current regimen. Adding bupropion to citalopram achieved a remission rate of approximately 30% in patients whose symptoms failed to remit after 12 weeks of citalopram therapy. The combination of venlafaxine plus mirtazapine was used in a highly treatment-refractory group (failed three previous medication trials) and achieved remission of symptoms in approximately 14% of patients (McGrath et al., 2006).

KEY TREATMENT

- Patients who fail antidepressants should be carefully reevaluated for medication adherence, adequacy of dosing and therapy duration, diagnosis, comorbid psychiatric illnesses, increased stressors, and unaddressed comorbidities (Trivedi et al., 2006a) (SOR: A).
- Common strategies used when patients fail an initial antidepressant treatment are switching antidepressants (either within class or across classes) (Rush et al., 2006b; Thase, 2008b), augmenting with other agents (lithium, T_3, atypical antipsychotics) (Nierenberg et al., 2006; Trivedi et al., 2006a), or combining different antidepressants (McGrath et al., 2006) (SOR: A).

ANXIETY

There is significant pharmacologic overlap between the treatment of depression and anxiety disorders. Most antidepressants are also effective antianxiety agents, or anxiolytics (see Table 46-10), thus simplifying treatment strategies when patients have both disorders. In addition, significant overlap also exists between medications that effectively treat GAD and panic disorder. Treatment recommendations for both GAD and panic will be explored separately to highlight some of the treatment differences between the two disorders.

Generalized Anxiety Disorder

Antidepressants are generally considered first-line agents for treatment of GAD because of their efficacy and safety, effectiveness in treating comorbid major depression, and absence of addictive or abuse potential, as seen with benzodiazepines. As a general rule, starting antidepressant doses for patients with GAD should be approximately half the lowest starting dose for treatment of depression; many experience a paradoxical worsening of their symptoms on antidepressant initiation if doses are high (see Table 46-8). Patients with anxiety disorders are typically more sensitive to antidepressant side effects (see Table 46-11), and thus starting at lower doses and titrating slowly will likely yield better results.

The SSRIs and SNRIs are considered first-line treatments, with numerous studies demonstrating both efficacy and effectiveness (Hoffman and Mathew, 2008). A Cochrane review of antidepressant treatment of GAD that included paroxetine, sertraline, venlafaxine, and imipramine found a very large effect size, with an NNT of only five patients for one patient to receive benefit, with no clear evidence of one antidepressant superior to another (Kapczinski et al., 2003). At present, the SSRIs escitalopram and paroxetine and the SNRIs venlafaxine and duloxetine are the only antidepressants with an FDA indication for GAD (see Table 46-10). No randomized controlled trials (RCTs) have yet supported the efficacy of fluoxetine or citalopram in the treatment of GAD, although their clinical use is based on the assumption that SSRIs exert a class effect and are likely equally effective. The SNRI desvenlafaxine may be effective but currently is indicated only for major depression.

The TCAs, also effective agents for treating GAD, have been relegated to second-line treatment because of side effects (e.g., anticholinergic, sedative, orthostatic) and potential lethality in overdose. Imipramine has the strongest data to support its use in GAD (Kapczinski et al., 2003). Although used effectively in the treatment of anxiety disorders, MAO inhibitors have significant side effects (risk for hypertensive crisis, potential lethal interactions with other medications) and likely do not have a role in primary care and should be reserved for psychiatric practice. Mirtazapine has shown some efficacy in open-label trials (Gambi et al., 2005) but needs further study in RCTs to be considered a first-line agent in GAD. Bupropion has a less clear role in the treatment of anxiety disorders and may worsen rather than alleviate anxiety symptoms. However, a recent pilot study showed that bupropion XL had comparable anxiolytic efficacy with escitalopram in a 12-week, double-blind RCT and was well tolerated (Bystritsky et al., 2008). Bupropion may have a role in GAD treatment in the future but currently may be considered a second- or third-line agent.

Benzodiazepines are also extremely effective for treatment of GAD and offer the advantage of rapid effect. Their onset of action is typically within hours versus weeks with antidepressants. All benzodiazepines are theoretically equally effective in GAD, and thus selection of individual agents often involves comparing half-lives, metabolic pathways, the presence or absence of active metabolites (particularly in patients with liver disease), and the speed of onset of action. Benzodiazepines with shorter half-lives result in the inconvenience of multiple daily dosing, the risk of rebound anxiety, and the common need to use as-needed (PRN) doses as a "rescue" medication when symptoms are inadequately controlled. Medications such as clonazepam, with long half-lives, or alprazolam XR, with a slower and more prolonged onset of action, may be more effective than drugs with shorter half-lives, such as immediate-release alprazolam or lorazepam. Scheduled dosing of a benzodiazepine provides for a more consistent medication blood level and may also be a more effective approach than PRN dosing. The duration of therapeutic effect for benzodiazepines is determined by the rate and extent of drug distribution (lipophilicity) and not necessarily by the rate of elimination. Benzodiazepines such as diazepam have a longer half-life than lorazepam, but because diazepam is more lipophilic, it has a faster onset of action and shorter duration of effect after a single dose (Schatzberg and Nemeroff, 2009). Drug elimination occurs in the liver through microsomal oxidation or glucuronide conjugation. Oxidation is sensitive to liver disease and certain medical conditions and medications (e.g., cimetidine); therefore, benzodiazepines metabolized through hepatic oxidation are more likely to show unpredictability than those metabolized via conjugation. Benzodiazepines such as temazepam, lorazepam, and oxazepam are cleared through hepatic conjugation and are safer and better tolerated when oxidative elimination has been altered.

Even though the benzodiazepines offer the advantage of rapid onset and effectiveness, other disadvantages have relegated them to second-line agents. Benzodiazepines pose a significant risk of dependency and withdrawal, are potentially lethal in overdose if mixed with other sedating agents (especially alcohol), and are ineffective in treating comorbid depression. The benzodiazepines also can impair attention and vigilance and cause dose-dependent anterograde amnesia, with limited effect on psychic symptoms, including worry (Hoehn-Saric et al., 1988). Benzodiazepines should generally be considered second- to third-line agents as monotherapy in GAD, although they are often used as adjunctive agents when initiating antidepressant treatment to provide immediate relief of anxiety symptoms until antidepressant effects begin. Symptom severity and patient preference should be considered when deciding whether to use an antidepressant as monotherapy or to start a benzodiazepine with an antidepressant. A subset of patients may benefit from long-term treatment with both an antidepressant and a benzodiazepine.

Nonbenzodiazepine and nonantidepressant treatment may also be effective in the treatment of GAD, especially for patients with mild to moderate symptom severity. *Buspirone*, an azapirone that exerts 5-HT-1A receptor agonism, carries an FDA indication for GAD. Buspirone appears useful in the treatment of GAD, particularly for patients who have not yet received a benzodiazepine (Chessick et al., 2006). In clinical practice, buspirone can be used as monotherapy in patients with mild to moderate symptoms, and it is often considered an alternative to benzodiazepines as an augmenting agent to antidepressants. *Hydroxyzine*, an antihistaminic agent, also carries an FDA indication for GAD and has shown efficacy in RCTs (Llorca et al., 2002). Its sedative properties and lack of efficacy in comorbid disorders have relegated hydroxyzine to a second-line agent. Interestingly, a meta-analysis of effect sizes in pharmacotherapy of GAD recently showed that hydroxyzine had a larger effect size (0.45) than the SSRIs (0.36) (Hidalgo et al., 2007). At present, hydroxyzine may be considered an alternative to benzodiazepines when no comorbid illnesses are present as monotherapy. Recent studies of *pregabalin* have also shown efficacy in the treatment of GAD. In the meta-analysis cited, pregabalin was found to have the largest effect size (0.5) of all agents (SSRIs, SNRIs, benzodiazepines, azaspirones, antihistamines, complementary or alternative agents). The effect size of pregabalin was determined from two large RCTs. In addition, pregabalin was found to be effective in relapse prevention compared to placebo over a 6-month trial (Feltner et al., 2008). *β-Blockers* such as propranolol and pindolol have also been used in the treatment of GAD. Although these can block the physiologic effects of anxiety, such as sweating and increased heart rate, β-blockers appear ineffective in treating the underlying emotional component of anxiety, and little empiric evidence supports their use in GAD at present. In a recent Cochrane review, *quetiapine* is the only atypical antipsychotic to show effectiveness as a monotherapy in GAD (Depping et. al., 2010), but the FDA denied approval for this indication because of the side effect burden outweighing the benefit of the medication.

KEY TREATMENT

- The SSRIs and SNRIs are considered first-line treatments for GAD, with the starting dose typically half that used in patients with depression (Hoffman and Mathew, 2008) (SOR: A).
- The TCAs are effective in treatment of GAD (SOR: A), but their side effect profile and potential lethality have relegated them to second-line agents (Kapczinski, et al., 2003).
- The benzodiazepines offer the advantage of rapid effect and proven efficacy (Chessick et al., 2006; Schatzberg and Nemeroff, 2009) (SOR: A), but they carry risk of abuse and dependence.
- Other agents for the treatment of GAD include hydroxyzine (Llorca et al., 2002) (SOR: A), buspirone (Chessick et al., 2006) (SOR: B), and pregabalin (Feltner et al., 2008) (SOR: B).
- Maintenance treatment of GAD reduces the likelihood of relapse (Thuile et al., 2009) (SOR: B).

PANIC DISORDER

Similar to the treatment of GAD, SSRIs, SNRIs, TCAs, and benzodiazepines have all been found to be effective for the treatment of panic disorder. The effectiveness of these agents appears relatively equal, and thus selection of a particular agent is most often based on tolerability, cost, ability to treat comorbid disorders, potential for abuse and tolerance, and patient preference. First-line agents to treat panic are most often SSRIs and SNRIs. Fluoxetine, paroxetine, sertraline, and venlafaxine all have FDA indications for panic disorder (see Table 46-10), although all the SSRIs have data to support their use (Otto et al., 2001). The SNRIs duloxetine and desvenlafaxine do not currently have large RCT evidence to support their use in panic disorder but may have efficacy based on class effect. The TCAs are also as effective in treating panic as SSRIs but are less well tolerated because of their anticholinergic and antihistaminic side effects (Bakker et al., 2002). Both imipramine and clomipramine have the most data to support their use in panic disorder

(APA, 2009). Because of tolerability and toxicity in overdose, TCAs are second-line agents for panic.

The benzodiazepines offer several advantages over antidepressants in the treatment of panic, including rapid onset, PRN dosing schedules, and relief of insomnia and somatic symptoms (Bruce et al., 2003). Similar to use in GAD, selection of a particular benzodiazepine is based on half-life, speed of onset of action, presence or absence of active metabolites, and metabolic pathways (particularly in patients with liver disease). All benzodiazepines are likely equally effective in treating panic, although in clinical practice, higher potency benzodiazepines (e.g., alprazolam, clonazepam, lorazepam) are used more often than lower potency drugs (e.g., oxazepam). Clonazepam and alprazolam both are FDA approved for panic disorder, and some clinicians prefer clonazepam to alprazolam because of clonazepam's longer half-life, less frequent dosing, and slower onset of action. Lorazepam and diazepam do not have an FDA indication for panic but seem to be effective agents in RCTS and clinical practice (Mitte et al., 2005). The benzodiazepines may be considered as first-line monotherapy when no comorbid conditions exist with panic disorder. Agents with rapid onset (alprazolam, lorazepam) may be preferred if taken on a PRN basis or used as a rescue medication. However, shorter-acting agents can introduce problems with interdose rebound anxiety or more difficulty with adherence to multidose regimens. Agents with longer half-lives, such as clonazepam and alprazolam XR, may be scheduled once or twice daily to provide more even coverage throughout the day but do not provide immediate relief if taken on a PRN basis.

Although the benzodiazepines can bring quick relief from panic symptoms, their side effect profile and risk of dependency, abuse, and withdrawal must be considered when deciding on their use. Common side effects include sedation, fatigue, ataxia, slurred speech, memory impairment, and weakness. Geriatric patients taking benzodiazepines may be at higher risk for falls and fractures (Stone et al., 2008). Patients with a substance abuse history may need to be monitored closely for signs and symptoms of abuse; patients actively abusing substances should probably not be prescribed benzodiazepines. For many of these patients, discussing clear expectations that prescriptions will not be rewritten or refilled before a set date can limit later conflicts and improve treatment adherence.

Evidence for the use of β-blockers in panic disorder is sparse. β-Blockers have been used to reduce the somatic symptoms of panic attacks, such as palpitations, but do not seem to be effective in overall treatment of panic disorder.

KEY TREATMENT

- The SSRIs, SNRIs, TCAs, and benzodiazepines have all been found to be effective in the treatment of panic disorder (Otto et al., 2001) (SOR: A).
- The first-line agents for panic disorder are SSRIs and SNRIs, with starting doses typically half that for depression (APA, 2009) (SOR: A).
- Benzodiazepines can be used as first-line agents when no comorbid psychiatric issues are present, including issues of substance abuse and dependence (Mitte et al., 2005) (SOR: A).

- Maintenance treatment of panic disorder has been shown to reduce the likelihood of relapse (Thuile et al., 2009) (SOR: B).

CONTINUATION OF TREATMENT IN ANXIETY DISORDERS

Treatment for anxiety disorders should be continued for 6 months to 1 year; a more definitive time frame is not yet clear. Results from long-term RCTs of antidepressants in anxiety disorders indicate that maintenance treatment significantly reduces the risk of relapse, whatever the disorder (Thuile et al., 2009). Decisions on length of treatment are generally made on a case-by-case basis, taking into account the risk-to-benefit ratio of treatment versus no treatment. If the decision is to discontinue treatment, the medication should be tapered at a rate that takes into account its pharmacokinetics and whether the patient experiences withdrawal symptoms (see Table 46-13).

OTHER CONSIDERATIONS

Antidepressants and Suicidal Ideation

In 2004, the FDA added a black box warning to all antidepressants indicating that the use of antidepressants in children, adolescents, and adults younger than 25 years of age increased the risk of suicidal thinking and behavior. The warning on antidepressants was based on an analysis of 372 clinical trials involving 11 antidepressant medications noting an increase in the number of patients who experienced an increase in suicidal ideation and behavior, although no increase in actual suicides was observed. Further analysis of the FDA data revealed a strong age-dependent relationship, such that the greatest risk was in patients younger than 25 years old. In clinical terms, 4 additional patients in 1000, age 18 to 24 years, would be expected to experience suicidal ideation or behavior as a result of taking antidepressants, and an additional 14 patients in 1000 younger than age 18 years would be expected to experience worsening. Patients older than 30 years showed a reduction in suicidal ideation as a result of taking antidepressants, with a reduction of 6 patients of 1000 in adults older than 65 years. The net effect of antidepressant use in patients age 25 to 64 years seems moderately protective against suicidal ideation and more strongly protective for adults age 65 years and older (Levenson and Holland, 2006). Antidepressants should be used cautiously in patients younger than age 25 years, with close monitoring for worsening of mood or thoughts of suicide, particularly in the days and weeks after the drug is initiated. For the majority of depressed patients, the beneficial effects of antidepressants greatly outweigh the risks (Libby et al., 2007).

Nontraditional Therapy

Interest in complementary and alternative medicine (CAM) for health disorders has been growing steadily in the past several decades. As a result, a greater number of alternative or complementary agents are being tested in more methodologically rigorous ways, allowing greater scientific assessment of such treatments. Survey evidence suggests that as many as 40% to 60% of patients may be taking CAM therapies, although patients often do not disclose such use to their physicians (Elkins et al., 2005). In addition, because production of alternative agents is unregulated, variability in product strength, dosing, and purity is common, which in turn likely affects the predictability of their outcomes. Given the widespread use of CAM agents and patients' apparent reluctance to spontaneously disclose such use to their providers, it is incumbent on physicians to inquire about such use.

The majority of CAM treatments have been used to treat depression, including St John's wort (*Hypericum perforatum*), S-adenosyl-L-methionine (SAM-e), and omega-3 fatty acids. In a Cochrane review of St John's wort for treatment of major depression, great heterogeneity was found among the 29 analyzed trials (Linde et al., 2005). St John's wort was found to be superior to placebo and similarly effective as standard antidepressants, but findings were more favorable to St John's wort studies from German-speaking countries, where use of the extract has a long tradition. The more positive results may be caused by physician expertise with the medication, patient selection, or flawed methodologies in some research. The larger, placebo-controlled studies have yielded mixed results, although compared with antidepressants, St John's wort has generally been better tolerated (Shelton, 2009).

SAM-E, a dietary supplement, has been used to treat a variety of illnesses, ranging from major depression to osteoarthritis to liver disease. Clinical trials have shown SAM-e to be superior to placebo and equivalent to TCAs in treating patients with depression, although the most robust findings have been shown with parenteral administration of the drug. Studies using the oral form have yielded more variable results. In adjunctive use with antidepressants, only one open-label study has been published to date. SAM-e has been shown to be safe and well tolerated thus far (Papakostas, 2009).

Omega-3 fatty acids have a variety of health benefits and may be helpful as augmenting agents in the treatment of major depression. The best studied agents are eicosapentaenoic acid (EPA) and docosahexaenoic acid (DHA). Findings in depression are limited by variability in study design and small sample sizes, although the majority of evidence favors a positive effect in the treatment of mood disorders (Freeman, 2009).

At present, little robust evidence supports the efficacy of CAM agents in the treatment of anxiety disorders. Kava (*Piper methysticum*) has preliminary evidence of efficacy in GAD, but further testing is needed to determine its side effects and potential for hepatotoxicity (Sarris and Kavanagh, 2009). A meta-analysis found no statistically significant difference between kava and placebo (Hidalgo et al., 2007). Given the paucity of current evidence, caution should be used when considering kava as a therapeutic agent.

OTHER TREATMENTS

Electroconvulsive Therapy

Electroconvulsive therapy involves a brief electrical stimulation of the brain while the patient is anesthetized, inducing a seizure. ECT remains the most effective treatment for depression (UK ECT Group, 2003), although the stigma surrounding the treatment, misinformation about its practice, side effects, and cost have often made it a treatment of last resort. Although occasionally used as first-line therapy for severe depression, ECT is often used for multitreatment-refractory patients, those with psychotic depression, suicidal patients (imminent), and depressed patients with compromised oral intake. A typical course is 6 to 20 treatments, with patients receiving ECT three times a week during the acute phase, gradually increasing the time between treatments as improvement becomes apparent. After acute treatment, patients are often returned to antidepressant therapy, although medication efficacy after ECT does not appear to be enhanced (Kellner et al., 2006). Physicians should be aware that ECT is safe, well tolerated, humane, and effective.

Vagus Nerve Stimulation and Transcranial Magnetic Stimulation

Vagal nerve stimulation (VNS) involves the surgical implantation of a nerve stimulator for the left vagus nerve at the cervical level and has been approved for treatment of refractory depression. VNS is not an acute treatment but has shown some long-term benefit for depressed patients (George et al., 2005). Transcranial magnetic stimulation (TMS) involves the introduction of repetitive magnetic impulses to the right prefrontal cortex in a series of treatments over several weeks. TMS is approved for the treatment of unipolar depression for patients who have failed one trial of antidepressants or for those patients who have exhibited marked intolerance to antidepressants (O'Reardon et al., 2007).

Psychotherapy

In addition to pharmacologic interventions for depression, panic disorder, and GAD, psychotherapy continues to be an effective tool used by psychiatrists and psychotherapists for treating mood and anxiety disorders. Although primary care physicians will not administer such treatments, it is important to be aware of general psychotherapeutic concepts and strategies. Several types of therapy have strong evidence supporting their efficacy in treating both depression and anxiety disorders, including CBT, interpersonal therapy, psychodynamic psychotherapy, problem-solving therapy, and supportive therapy (Cuijpers et al., 2008). Some patients may prefer to begin treatment with medications alone, but others may prefer only psychotherapy or a combination. Combined pharmacologic and psychotherapeutic interventions have generally been shown to be superior to either approach alone in trials for both anxiety disorders and depression (Furukawa et al., 2007; Pampallona et al., 2004).

Referral to Mental Health Providers

Which patients should be referred to mental health providers? Referrals may be made because of patient preference or severity of illness or because of the complexity of comorbid illnesses. Patients who experience refractory depression or psychotic depression are best treated by specialty providers. Patients with bipolar disorder should be referred as well, especially those with bipolar depressions, because they are often especially difficult to treat, usually require complex polypharmacy, and worsen with inappropriate treatment. Patients requesting or needing psychotherapy or behavioral therapy may be referred to a mental health provider.

Summary

For the majority of depressed patients, the beneficial effects of antidepressants greatly outweigh the risks. CAM treatments for depression may be beneficial for some patients, but study methodology limits their generalizability. ECT is still considered the most effective treatment for severe depression. VNS and TMS are emerging therapies for the treatment of depression.

KEY TREATMENT

- Psychotherapy is an important and effective treatment strategy for both depression and anxiety. Psychotherapy combined with pharmacotherapy often yields results superior to either treatment alone (Furukawa et al., 2007; Pampallona et al., 2004) (SOR: A).

References

The complete reference list is available at www.expertconsult.com.

Web Resources

Patient Resources

freedomfromfear.org National nonprofit mental health advocacy organization focused on anxiety and depressive disorders.

www.nih.nimh.gov National Institute of Mental Health. Provides excellent up-to-date information on the symptoms, causes, course, and treatment of a number of illnesses. Provides numerous lists and links to resources.

www.ocdfoundation.org The Obsessive-Compulsive Foundation. Provides information and resources on obsessive-compulsive disorder and other mental health diagnoses.

Support for Patients, Family, and Friends

www.afsp.org American Foundation for Suicide Prevention. Leading national nonprofit dedicated to understanding and preventing suicide through education and research and to reaching out to people with mood disorders and those impacted by suicide.

www.coloradofederation.org The Federation for Families for Children's Mental Health. The mission of the federation is to promote mental health for all children, youth, and families. The website has numerous links to resources, articles, books, and support groups.

www.dbsalliance.org Depression and Bipolar Support Alliance. Provides education to patients and families about mood disorders. Advocates research funding, improving access to care, fostering self-help, and decreasing public stigma of these illnesses.

www.healthyminds.org Site created by the American Psychiatric Association to provide education and resources on mental health issues.

www.nami.org National Alliance on Mental Illness. Grass-roots, self-help, support, and advocacy group for people with severe mental illnesses, their family members, and friends.

www.webmd.com/depression Provides information on the diagnosis and treatment of mood disorders.

47 Delirium and Dementia

BIRJU B. PATEL, RINA EISENTEIN, and N. WILSON HOLLAND

Delirium

> ### Key Points
>
> - Delirium is often called altered mental status or acute confusional state.
> - There are two main subtypes of delirium: the hypervigilant and hypoactive types.
> - Hypoactive delirium is underdiagnosed because patients appear quiet, somnolent, or fatigued.
> - Delirium is never a normal occurrence.
> - Underlying cognitive impairment should be suspected in those with delirium.

Delirium is an abrupt change in brain function causing confusion that occurs from either physical or mental causes. Other terms used for delirium include *altered mental status, acute confusional state,* and *acute brain syndrome.* Making the diagnosis can often be difficult because most patients with delirium have comorbid physical and mental conditions. Delirium occurs in 31% to 66% of elderly adults either before or during a hospitalization (Flaherty, 2011). It is important to gain an understanding of this condition because it is often misdiagnosed. Mimickers may include dementia, depression, and acute psychosis. Delirium is often associated with poor outcomes. This includes prolonged hospitalizations, longer stays in skilled care facilities, and higher mortality rate (up to a 10-fold increase) (Inouye, 2006). It often leads to a functional decline that may not be reversible.

CLINICAL FEATURES

Delirium is often underrecognized and underdiagnosed. Even though it may be the most frequent type of acute-onset cognitive change, it is often misdiagnosed as depression, anxiety, psychosis, or other psychiatric disorders. Because it is frequently unrecognized, it has been called the "great imitator" (Caplan and Rabinowitz, 2010; Marcantonio, 2011). Delirium develops acutely and may be first recognized at night. The course of delirium typically shows diurnal fluctuations in symptoms. Many times there are rapid swings in mood and affect in the affected individual. Lucid intervals may occur intermittently in a 24-hour period. Alertness is the key clinical feature that should be carefully assessed. It may fluctuate between hypoactivity and hypervigilance. Individuals with hypoactive delirium may be mistaken as having depression, are harder to identify, and sometimes have worse outcomes than those with the hyperactive type (Table 47-1) (Caplan and Rabinowitz, 2010; Kiely et al., 2007). These individuals can be more sedated and do not bother the inpatient nursing staff, which results in difficulty in recognition. Another key clinical feature is change in attention. Attention span is always altered in delirium and fluctuates. Patients may show difficulty focusing, following commands, or carrying on conversations (Caplan and Rabinowitz, 2010; Inouye, 2006). Recent memory is usually impaired. An individual with delirium shows changes in thinking. Thinking is often disorganized and fragmented (Marcantonio, 2011). It may be slower, more hurried, or rambling in nature. Typically, there is alteration in levels of consciousness. Individuals show decreased awareness of their surroundings. Speech may be incoherent. Visual, auditory, or tactile hallucinations are often present in delirium (Flaherty, 2011). Delusional thinking is often present. For example, patients may have false interpretations such as thinking an intravenous line is a snake. They may be seen picking at the bed sheets looking for bugs or other objects that are not there (Alagiakrishnan, 2013). Emotional disturbances are often present and may manifest as depression, anxiety, anger, fear, or paranoia. Sleep–wake cycles are commonly disturbed and often reversed (Inouye, 2006).

Delirium is never a normal occurrence. Delirium usually implies an underlying cognitive impairment and may be the first sign of a deficit in the brain. Although in general, delirium develops acutely, there are reported prodromal phases lasting for days before it develops or becomes evident. During this prodromal phase, there may be sleep problems, vivid dreams, and heightened anxiety levels (Cole et al., 2003). Some patients with acute confusion may not meet the diagnostic criteria for delirium. This condition is termed *subsyndromal delirium.* It can have comparable outcomes to delirium and is treated similarly (Levkoff et al., 1992; Marcantonio, 2011; Quimet et al., 2007). Delirium in general lasts for days to weeks. However, it can be persistent, with symptoms lasting months to years (Levkoff et al., 1992; McCusker et al., 2003).

Table 47-1 Differentiating Delirium, Dementia, and Depression

Characteristic	Delirium	Dementia	Depression
Onset	Acute	Insidious	Acute or insidious depending on life situation
Duration	Generally hours to weeks; can be longer	Months to years	Weeks to years
Trajectory	Fluctuating and may be worse at night	Progressively worsening impairment later affecting function	Diurnal; worse in the morning; can have situational changes
Attention	Impaired and fluctuates	Normal; impaired in late stages	Minimal impairment; lack of motivation
Alertness	Hypoactive or hypervigilant; can fluctuate	Normal	Normal but may be impaired periodically
Consciousness	Fluctuates	Normal; can be impaired in late stages	Normal
Memory	Short-term memory usually impaired	Initially short-term memory impairment, which progresses to both short- and long-term memory impairment	Recent memory may be impaired; frequent "I don't know" answers; long-term memory intact
Hallucinations	Frequent visual, auditory, or tactile hallucinations	In later stages except in DLB, in which visual hallucinations occur early	Only in depression with psychosis

DLB, Dementia with Lewy bodies.

ETIOLOGY

> ### Key Points
>
> - Normal brains do not get delirium.
> - Functional impairment and sensory deficits can predispose to delirium in elderly adults.
> - Asymptomatic bacteriuria is commonly misdiagnosed as a cause of delirium.

Delirium often has multifactorial causations. A number of predisposing factors are seen with delirium, including age older than 65 years and more commonly occurring in men. Abnormal cognition, whether from dementia or depression, often underlies delirium. A good clinical pearl to remember is that normal brains do not get delirious. Alterations in functional status may predispose to delirium. These patients more commonly have history of falls and immobility.

Older individuals with diminished vision or hearing are more likely to develop delirium. A clinical pearl is always to remember to keep an older patient's glasses or hearing aids readily available and nearby while in the hospital. Older individuals physiologically have diminished thirst, and resulting dehydration can lead to the development of delirium.

Many coexisting medical conditions can predispose to acute confusion (Alagiakrishnan, 2013; Caplan and Rabinowitz, 2010; DesForges, 1989; Flaherty, 2011; Inouye et al., 2006; Marcantonio, 2011). These include but are not limited to hypoxia, hypothermia, hyperthermia, and alcohol withdrawal. Infection is another very common cause of delirium. Urinary tract and respiratory tract infections are the most common infections resulting in delirium. However, asymptomatic bacteriuria should not be attributed as a cause for delirium in elderly patients. Elderly adults many times present atypically and may have subtle findings such as silent cholecystitis, diverticulitis, or intraabdominal abscesses. Other infectious causes include encephalitis meningitis, human immunodeficiency virus (HIV), and bacteremia. Severe medical conditions such as myocardial infarctions, congestive heart failure, chronic hepatic disease, and chronic kidney failure can precipitate delirium. Asterixis may be a useful clinical sign in identifying chronic hepatic and chronic kidney disease as an etiology of delirium.

Metabolic abnormalities that should be considered include hyponatremia, hypernatremia, hypocalcemia, hypercalcemia, hypoglycemia, hypothyroidism, and hyperthyroidism. Selective serotonin reuptake inhibitors (SSRIs) used in the treatment of depression and anxiety should not be overlooked as a cause for hyponatremia. Malignancy, acute or chronic pain, and the postoperative period are also risk factors for development of delirium.

Falls resulting in fractures, especially hip fractures and subdural hematomas, cause delirium. Patients with subdural hematomas may initially have no focal neurologic signs. There should be a low threshold for doing a head computed tomography (CT) in elderly patients with delirium after a fall to evaluate for subdural hematomas.

Toxins and medications, including general anesthesia, illicit drugs, and withdrawal from alcohol, benzodiazepines, and opioids, should not be overlooked as potential causes for delirium. Anticholinergic medications predispose elderly patients to delirium. These may be prescribed drugs for urinary incontinence or may be found over the counter in many sleep aids. Tricyclic antidepressants should not be used in elderly adults for depression because of high anticholinergic side effects. Similarly, paroxetine, an SSRI, should not be used to treat depression in elderly adults because of anticholinergic side effects. Patients with a history of stroke and other neurologic diseases are also at risk. Individuals who are terminally ill are also more likely to develop delirium up to 83% of the time (Breibart and Strout, 2000; Casarett and Inouye, 2001). Iatrogenic factors that may predispose to delirium include use of physical restraints, indwelling urinary catheters, and polypharmacy. Often overlooked causes may be fecal impaction or urinary retention and should be ruled out in the setting of delirium (Blackburn and Dunn, 1990). There should be a high suspicion for underlying dementia in patients with delirium.

DIAGNOSTIC PROCESS

> ### Key Points
>
> - The Confusion Assessment Method (CAM) is a commonly used tool to evaluate for delirium.
> - Cognitive testing should also be used to evaluate for underlying deficits.
> - Neuroimaging, lumbar puncture, and electroencephalography (EEG) are not routinely required to evaluate for delirium unless focal findings are present.

Besides a thorough history and physical examination, diagnosis is made by short bedside evaluation exercises (Wong et al., 2010). The Mini-Mental Status Exam (MMSE) and Mini-Cog test cognitive function, including attention and visual spatial reasoning (Borson, 2000; Folstein et al., 1975). Other tests to measure attention include having the patient recite days of the week and serial numbers from 100 backward (Marcantonio, 2011). Neuroimaging, lumbar puncture, and EEG are not routinely needed unless focal neurologic findings are present. When EEG is done, findings supportive of a delirium diagnosis are generalized slowing in the theta-delta range and resolution with treatment (Caplan and Rabinowitz, 2010; Engel and Romano, 1959). The CAM developed by Inouye and colleagues is one of the most commonly used instruments in making a diagnosis of delirium (Inouye et al., 1990). It has a sensitivity of 94% to 100% and a specificity of 90% to 95% (Inouye et al., 1990; Marcantonio, 2011). The CAM can be administered in any setting within about 5 minutes (Table 47-2). Although it identifies the presence or absence of delirium, it is not reliable in assessing the severity. The CAM is a diagnostic tool and not one that should be used for following the patient for improvement or worsening of his or her delirium. There is also a CAM-ICU tool that uses nonverbal responses in the assessment of delirium (Ely et al., 2001). Clinical history and examination still remain of utmost importance in follow-up.

The *Diagnostic Statistical Manual of Mental Disorders*, fifth edition (DSM-5) diagnostic criteria for delirium include (A) disturbance in attention (i.e., reduced ability to direct, focus, sustain, and shift attention) and awareness (reduced orientation to the environment); (B) the disturbance develops over a short period (usually hours to a few days), represents a change from baseline attention and awareness,

and tends to fluctuate in severity during the course of a day; (C) an additional disturbance in cognition (e.g., memory deficit, disorientation, language, visuospatial ability, or perception); (D) the disturbances in criteria A and C are not better explained by another preexisting, established, or evolving neurocognitive disorder and do not occur in the context of a severely reduced level of arousal, such as coma; and (E) there is evidence from history, physical examination, or laboratory findings that the disturbance is a direct physiological consequence of another medical condition, substance intoxication, or withdrawal (i.e., caused by a drug of abuse or a medication) or exposure to a toxin or is from multiple causes. A substance intoxication delirium is further subclassified (American Psychiatric Association, 2013).

PREVENTION OF DELIRIUM

> ### Key Points
>
> - Multicomponent approaches targeting multiple etiologies and risk factors of delirium work best.
> - Proactive geriatric consultation may be helpful in preventing postoperative delirium.

Because delirium is generally multifactorial in etiology, a multicomponent management approach is most helpful in preventing it. One example of such an approach is the Yale Delirium Prevention Trial, which showed that targeting risk factors can be effective in helping prevent delirium. In their trial, intervention protocols were targeted toward six risk factors: (1) orientation and therapeutic activities for cognitive impairment, (2) early mobilization to help prevent immobility and falls, (3) nonpharmacologic approaches to lessen the use of psychoactive type medications and to reduce sleep deprivation, (4) communication strategies and adaptive equipment for hearing, (5) communication strategies and adaptive equipment for vision impairment, and (6) early intervention to prevent volume depletion.

In the Yale Delirium Prevention Trial, 852 patients 70 years and older were enrolled (Inouye et al., 1999). Half of these received usual hospital care for delirium, and half received the HELP (Hospital Elder Life Program) interventions as noted. These interventions resulted in a significant reduction in development of delirium (9% vs. 15%), total days of delirium, total number of episodes of delirium, and functional decline. HELP sites have subsequently been started in other hospitals across the United States showing similar results (Inouye, 2006).

Another approach that has been shown to be of benefit in preventing delirium includes using proactive geriatric consultation in older patients. One study using this approach showed a 36% reduction in the incidence of delirium for postoperative hip fracture patients. (Marcantonio, 2011; Marcantonio et al., 2011). Another study showed that using low-dose haloperidol, 0.5 mg three times per day for 3 days, started before the onset of delirium in elderly patients undergoing high-risk hip surgery reduced the severity and duration of postoperative delirium (Flaherty, 2011; Kalisvaar et al., 2005).

Table 47-2 Diagnosis of Delirium by the Confusion Assessment Method*

I. An acute and fluctuating course
II. Inattention
III. Disorganized thinking or
IV. Alteration in level of consciousness

*Diagnosis requires I and II and either III or IV.

TREATMENT OF DELIRIUM

> ### Key Points
>
> - Treatment of delirium starts with identifying and correcting the underlying cause.
> - Nonpharmacologic management should always precede management with medications, and different subtypes of delirium may require a different approach.
> - No medications have been approved by the Food and Drug Administration (FDA) to treat delirium, although several drugs (mainly antipsychotics and benzodiazepines) have been used with some success depending on the cause of delirium.
> - Medications should be used only when the risk of injury to self or others is significant and the behavior interferes with medical management.

Treatment of patients with delirium should always start with correcting potential causes: discontinuation of the offending medication, treatment of infection, correction of electrolyte imbalance, and treatment of pain. Correcting sensory deficits is very important (Khan et al., 2012). Family members or friends of patients with delirium should be encouraged to stay at the bedside and provide frequent orientation. Patients should be encouraged to maintain previous functional levels and independence in performing ADLs. Providing a room with adequately lighting, an accurate calendar, and a dry erase board for communication can be beneficial. Placing patients next to noisy areas and placing two delirious patients in the same room should be avoided. Lighting should be adequate during the day, and bright lights should be avoided at night to maintain circadian rhythm (Chong et al., 2013). External stimuli should be minimized at night (i.e., frequent awakenings should be avoided unless they are essential in guiding medical therapies). If possible, staff assignment should be consistent to maintain familiarity. Urinary catheters and restraints should be avoided if possible (Campbell et al., 2009). Using familiar objects brought from home, aroma therapy, and pleasant music might also be helpful. Environmental strategies are underused and should be used as first-line treatments because of a lack of adverse effects (Meagher, 2001).

It is important to note that there are no FDA-approved medications to treat delirium. However, with certain behavioral circumstances, such as hallucinations, delusions, and safety issues, or situations that hinder medical care, antipsychotics may need to be used. There are very limited data to support their use, but no good alternatives exist (Flaherty et al., 2011). Low doses of haloperidol (0.5-1 mg orally or intramuscularly) are usually used as a first-line treatment modality. Elderly patients can be very sensitive to these medications and may require lower doses. If intravenous haloperidol is used, there must be monitoring for development of QT prolongation and life-threatening arrhythmias (Huffman and Stern, 2003). Haloperidol should not be used in patients with parkinsonism, and consideration should be given to use of atypical antipsychotics (especially those with low extrapyramidal activity such as quetiapine). Hypo-

tension and sedation can occur as a result of use of antipsychotics, further complicating and prolonging the hospital stay. Use of antipsychotics can increase the risk of stroke and death; thus, short-term use is recommended only if absolutely needed. Metabolic abnormalities such as hyperglycemia and hyperlipidemia are also attributed to long-term antipsychotic use. It should be noted that patients with dementia with Lewy bodies (DLB) are extremely sensitive to antipsychotics and can have acute worsening of parkinsonism when these medications are used. Benzodiazepines are generally overused (but sometimes have to be used) in the management of delirium and have a shorter onset of action. Benzodiazepines with shorter half-lives (e.g., lorazepam) are preferred because these medications can cause significant sedation, confusion, and risk of falls in elderly adults. These medications are used primarily in alcohol and drug withdrawal-induced delirium as well as in situations when antipsychotics are contraindicated. Acetylcholinesterase inhibitors (AChEIs) generally do not have a role in treatment or prevention of delirium (van Eijk et al., 2010). In patients who present with nutritional deficiencies, thiamine should be supplemented because it is free of side effects, is cost effective, and is efficacious in terms of patients with delirium caused by alcoholism or thiamine deficiency.

> **KEY TREATMENT**
>
> - Low-dose antipsychotics (e.g., haloperidol) are used as first-line medical treatments (Huffman and Stern, 2003) (SOR: B).
> - Benzodiazepines should be avoided in most situations (SOR: B) except in alcohol withdrawal (Lonergan et al., 2009) (SOR: A).
> - Low-dose haloperidol used preemptively can be effective in reducing the severity and duration of delirium postoperatively (Kalisvaar et al., 2005) (SOR: B).

NATURAL HISTORY OF DELIRIUM

Delirium usually manifests as an acute (as opposed to gradual, as in dementia) change in mental status with a fluctuating course and variable duration. It can occur across all continuums of care: home, outpatient, long-term care, emergency department, intensive care unit, and hospice units. About one third of the hospitalized older patients in one study had symptoms of delirium at discharge, and longer initial episodes usually led to worse prognoses and worse clinical outcomes (McCusker et al., 2003). Patients with a protracted course of delirium can meet criteria for dementia (Fong et al., 2009). The frequency of delirium can be as high as 89% in hospitalized patients with dementia (Fick et al., 2013). Nursing home residents are three times as likely to develop delirium if they carry a diagnosis of dementia (Boorsma et al., 2011). Although delirium is a potentially reversible condition, it usually is a bad prognosticator for underlying or future dementia, worsening frailty, and increased short- and long-term mortality rates in elderly adults (Cole and Primeau, 1993).

Dementia

Key Points

- The prevalence of dementia is increasing as the elderly population increases.
- Cognitive evaluation involves the assessment of different domains (e.g., executive function, language).
- Age-associated memory impairment (AAMI), mild cognitive impairment (MCI), and depression can mimic dementia.

Dementia is a clinical syndrome with persistent intellectual decline that is severe enough to interfere with social or occupational functioning in an alert individual. The term *dementia* is taken from Latin, meaning "without mind." Subjective memory concerns typically bring patients to seek medical attention. A variety of different domains of cognition are important to recognize and are specified by the DSM-5 to include complex attention, executive function, learning and memory, language, perceptual-motor, and social cognition. When confronted with a patient with subjective memory concerns, clinicians must differentiate many conditions, including AAMI, MCI, depression, delirium, and dementia (Caplan and Rabinowitz, 2010). The workup helps to differentiate these and other conditions and ultimately identifies a specific etiology (e.g., Alzheimer disease [AD], vascular dementia [VD]).

CLINICAL FEATURES

The prevalence of dementia increases with age. About 5% to 10% of people older than the age of 65 years have dementia. This increases to about 30% to 50% of those older than the age of 85 years (Evans, 1996). A record number of people are getting older in the United States; some have termed this phenomenon "the silver tsunami" (Bartels and Naslund, 2013). Older people have more subjective cognitive concerns and a higher prevalence of dementia (Lliffe and Pealing, 2010). A survey by the MetLife Foundation (2011) found that AD is the second most feared disease among American adults, behind only cancer. Dementia has an increasing overall impact, including a societal, economic, health care–related, and emotional impact.

According to the DSM-5, the preferred term for dementia is *neurocognitive disorder*, which is defined as significant cognitive impairment and interference with independence not caused by delirium and not caused by other mental disorders. Cognitive impairment is quantified based on psychometric definitions in terms of standard deviations from the mean in testing. Whereas 1 to 2 standard deviations below the mean represent mild impairment, 2 to 3 standard deviations below the mean represent major impairment (Reisberg, 2006). In evaluating dementia, important consideration should also be given to function, behavior, and focal neurologic changes because these can be important clues as to the etiology as well as the prognosis. Both neuropsychiatric symptoms (wandering, agitation, changes in mood) and neurologic symptoms (gait imbalance, focal signs, seizures) may be present in individuals with dementia.

Frequently, elderly patients present with subjective cognitive concerns such as difficulty remembering names, slowing of processing speed, impaired recall, and forgetting and misplacing things such as keys. It is important to distinguish these subjective cognitive concerns related to normal aging (AAMI) from more serious conditions such as MCI that affect higher-level activities such as medication and financial management (impaired IADLs). Distinguishing MCI from AAMI can be very challenging (Table 47-3). Neuropsychological testing is used to distinguish these conditions after workup is done to rule out reversible medical conditions that can impact cognition (Pokorski, 2002). MCI has a significant risk to progress to dementia and is thus important to identify early.

Depression can also mimic dementia and must be ruled out. Known as "pseudo dementia," depression can affect cognition. Careful history taking as well as a thorough workup, including targeted evaluation of mood symptoms, can help differentiate these conditions. Those with untreated depression have an independent long-term increased risk of dementia.

Table 47-3   Distinguishing Mild Cognitive Impairment from Age-Associated Memory Impairment

Cognitive Concern	Age-Associated Memory Impairment	Mild Cognitive Impairment	Dementia
Complaints of memory concerns	Remembers details around memory concerns	May have delay but able to recall concerns	Problems remembering details; often lost
Short-term memory	Normal	Impaired in amnestic MCI subtypes	Impaired at first and later more profound
Cognitive evaluation	Normal	Mildly impaired	Impaired
Interpersonal and social skills	Normal	Usually normal	Impaired, especially in FTD
ADLs	Normal	Normal	Usually impaired
IADLs	Normal	Usually impaired	Impaired

ADLs, Activities of daily living; *FTD,* frontotemporal dementia; *IADLs,* instrumental activities of daily living.
Adapted from Patel BB, Holland NW. Mild cognitive impairment: hope for stability, plan for progression. *Cleve Clin J Med.* 2012;79:857-864.

DIAGNOSTIC PROCESS

> ### Key Points
>
> - Dementia evaluation should be prompted by a warning signs approach rather than screening.
> - Many different cognitive evaluation tools are helpful in evaluating cognitive deficits and support a diagnosis of dementia.
> - Functional assessment is an important aspect of evaluation of dementia.
> - Depression is the most common reversible etiology of dementia.

Detecting dementia in a busy clinical practice is a challenge. Often, patients with dementia do not present with memory loss complaints; instead, spouses or family members bring up concerns to the physician to be further evaluated. Importantly, cognitive concerns are incorrectly attributed to normal aging in some cases by patients and family members, as well as physicians. The U.S. Preventive Services Task Force has concluded that there is insufficient evidence to recommend for or against routine screening for dementia for any age group (Lin et al., 2013). Evaluation should be prompted by a warning signs approach. The Alzheimer's Association (2014) uses the "10 warning signs" that should prompt evaluation. Patient, caregiver, or clinician concerns regarding cognitive abilities should prompt further evaluation. Multiple different office cognitive evaluation tools are available that are beneficial in terms of quick assessment and identification of deficiencies affecting different domains of cognition. Among these are the Mini-Cog, MMSE, Montreal Cognitive Assessment (MOCA), St. Louis University Mental Status (SLUMS), and many others. Each of these tools has its pros and cons in terms of time needed to administer, cognitive domains evaluated, alternative versions available, and so on. The Mini-Cog is a good office screening tool for a busy practice. It involves a clock draw and three-item recall. The ease of scoring, briefness, and use in diverse ethnic populations make the Mini-Cog a useful tool (Borson et al., 2006). The SLUMS and the MOCA are more time-consuming tests and are more useful in evaluating MCI and early cognitive concerns. Both of these tests evaluate multiple cognitive domains. These brief office tests can be used to quantify deficiencies in cognition and to document change in cognition over time objectively (Patel and Holland 2012). They can be used to discuss the degree of cognitive impairment and thus reflect the stage of dementia when discussing this condition with care partners and family members. These tests should not be used in isolation to make the diagnosis of dementia and should be used in conjunction with functional assessment.

Functional assessment is also of vital importance when evaluating cognition. It is important to know if the patient is able to independently perform ADLs (bathing, dressing, feeding, toileting, transferring, grooming) and IADLs (shopping, cleaning, laundry, transportation, finances, medication management, using the telephone). With early cognitive impairment, there is trouble with IADLs, and patients who were previously independently able to do all of their higher-level activities now require assistance (especially with financial and medication management). Later, as

dementia progresses, ADLs become affected, which increases the care needs the individual has and increases the risk of placement. The short form of the Geriatric Depression Scale (GDS) can be used in the office setting to assess for depression (Sheikh and Yesavage, 1986). Evaluation focuses on trying to rule out reversible causes for dementia. A meta-analysis of 39 articles describing 5620 individuals with dementia-like symptoms reported that only 9% had potentially reversible dementia. These potentially reversible causes of dementia include delirium, depression, medications, thyroid problems, certain vitamin deficiencies, and excessive use of alcohol (Clarfield, 2003). A key clinical pearl is that the most common reversible cause of dementia is depression. Older patients are at a higher risk for depression and should be carefully evaluated for it.

HISTORY AND PHYSICAL EXAMINATION

Because chronicity of symptoms is of pivotal importance in terms of making the correct diagnosis, an accurate history of this must be obtained. Because dementia is of insidious onset, it is very difficult to clarify when deficits actually began. A cognitively impaired patient is often an unreliable source of information, and thus one must turn to caregivers, spouses, and friends to get further clarification and pinpoint the specific deficits.

The onset, clinical trajectory, and specific nature of symptoms are useful in making a determination of the etiology of the cognitive impairment. Further history of medications, both prescription and over the counter with emphasis on anticholinergic and psychoactive medications, should be an important aspect of assessment. Vascular disease such as diabetes, hypertension, stroke, coronary artery disease, and peripheral vascular disease should also be noted. A history of substance abuse, mental illness, head trauma, sleep concerns, seizure disorder, previous surgery, previous central nervous system infections, educational background with focus on deficiencies, occupational history, and family history of dementia are all important aspects of evaluation. Functional status as determined by ADLs and IADLs is a necessary component of the assessment. A general physical examination is a good starting point with further focused evaluations of the cardiovascular system looking for the presence of vascular disease as well as neurologic examination looking for focal deficits. Impairments in overall function raise safety and support concerns that often warrant additional evaluation (e.g., driving concerns, ability to live alone, medication management challenges, financial concerns) (McCarten, 2013).

LABORATORY AND IMAGING STUDIES

The usual laboratory workup for dementia includes a complete blood count, comprehensive metabolic profile, urinalysis, thyroid-stimulating hormone level, and vitamin B_{12} level. In appropriate high-risk populations, one may consider syphilis and HIV serology (Kelley and Minagar, 2009). All of these tests are done to determine the contribution of comorbidities to cognition and to look for reversible causes of dementia. Apolipoprotein E-e4 (ApoE-e4), located on chromosome 19, is linked to the greatest risk of development of AD. Those not expressing the ApoE-e4 allele have the least risk, followed by heterozygous patients with intermediate risk and then homozygous patients with greatest risk. Genetic testing for ApoE-e4 is controversial and should only be undertaken after considerable discussion of risks and benefits. After a decision is made to do this testing, a discussion with a genetic counselor may be beneficial (Ertekin-Taner, 2007). Cerebrospinal fluid (CSF) studies and structural imaging (structural magnetic resonance imaging [MRI] or CT and fluorodeoxyglucose positron emission tomography [FDG-PET]) have made great strides in terms of published research but have yet to become mainstream clinically (Mueller et al., 2012; Zetterberg and Blennow, 2013). These biomarkers hold promise for the future in terms of correctly diagnosing dementia of Alzheimer type. Imaging studies can be beneficial in the evaluation of focal neurologic deficits and should be used when suspicion is high for treatable cerebrovascular conditions such as brain tumors, normal-pressure hydrocephalus (NPH), traumatic brain injury, and so on. Thus, it is not necessary to do brain imaging in all patients being worked up for dementia. If an imaging study is warranted, it is recommended that CT or MRI be the imaging modalities of choice. Neuropsychological testing is very useful in the evaluation of cognitive deficits. It usually involves several hours of testing and completion of mentally challenging activities that the patient must be an appropriate candidate to complete, usually in one sitting. Severe visual or hearing deficits pose a challenge and make neuropsychological testing very difficult to complete. Furthermore, the patient must be willing to put forth his or her best effort in doing the testing to obtain results that can then be scored to determine deficits in different domains of cognition. Not all patients require neuropsychological testing, and only patients with challenging presentations who are not easy to diagnose should be referred. Generally, younger patients, those with very mild deficits, and those who rapidly develop dementia are good candidates for neuropsychological testing. This testing can also be useful as a baseline with which to compare for subsequent evaluations of cognitive abilities (Kulas and Naugle, 2003).

COMMON TYPES OF DEMENTIA

Alzheimer disease is the most common type of dementia, accounting for about 60% to 80% of cases with dementia, followed by DLB, which accounts for 10% to 22%. VD accounts for about 10% to 20% of all dementias, followed by more uncommon dementias. Autopsy studies done on patients with dementia usually show a mix in pathology between Alzheimer-type pathology and vascular changes (Nowrangi et al., 2011).

Alzheimer Disease

> ### Key Points
>
> - AD is the most common type of dementia.
> - Early memory impairment is the key clinical finding in AD.
> - AD is a slowly progressive dementia with an average life expectancy of 8 to 10 years from the time of diagnosis.

- Physical and mental activity is recommended to patients at risk for dementia.
- Caregiver stress and burnout should be evaluated and addressed to avoid long-term care placement.
- Feeding tubes are not indicated in late stage dementia.

Alzheimer disease is a degenerative disease diagnosed clinically, with definitive diagnosis made only through postmortem examination of the brain. Described first by Dr. Alois Alzheimer in 1906, AD has been extensively studied only in the past 30 years. The cause of AD is not well understood, but a great deal is known about the changes in the brain that occur in those with it. The classic neuropathological features in the brain include senile plaques and neurofibrillary tangles. The changes that occur in the brains of patients with AD start as many as 20 years before the first clinical manifestations of disease. The earliest clinically detectable point of deficits is known as MCI caused by AD. There is an accumulation of the β-amyloid protein outside neurons in the brain (β-amyloid plaques) and the accumulation of an abnormal form of the tau protein inside neurons (tau tangles). Gradually, information transfer at the level of synapses begins to fail, the number of synapses declines, and neurons ultimately die. β-Amyloid accumulation interferes with the interneuronal communication at synapses, leading to cell death. Tau tangles block the passage of nutrients and other necessary molecules in the neuron and contribute to cell death. These tangles are found in the hippocampus, medial temporal lobes, and amygdala. The rate of hippocampal atrophy correlates with change in clinical status. Notable brain shrinkage is evident on autopsies of brains of people with advanced AD from cell loss and debris from neuronal injury. The neuropathology of AD also involves neurotransmitters. With the loss of cholinergic neurons, there are decreased acetylcholine levels, and a decrease in the acetylcholine-synthesizing enzyme choline acetyltransferase levels in the brain. The loss of cholinergic neurons is most noted in the hippocampus and the nucleus basalis of Meynert. This alteration in levels of neurotransmitters contributes to the psychiatric symptoms in individuals with AD such as depression, anxiety, and agitation (Clark and Karlawaish, 2003; Jack et al., 2000).

The strongest risk factors for AD include advancing age and family history with a first-degree relative with early-onset type AD. The prevalence of AD doubles every 5 years, and it occurs more in women, likely because of their greater life expectancy. Additional risk factors include history of head trauma, vascular disease, presence of apoE-e4 gene, and low levels of education. Regular physical activity is the most protective factor. The course of AD is typically gradual in onset accompanied by continuing cognitive decline over many years. Behavioral concerns are also typical and include depression, anxiety, sleep disturbances, hallucinations, delusions, and agitation. The average duration of progression from onset to death is 8 to 10 years. AD is the sixth leading cause of death, which usually results from infection, cardiovascular disease, cachexia, or dehydration. Currently, about 5.2 million Americans have AD (Lindsay et al., 2002).

Memory impairment is the cornerstone of disease presentation from the start. It becomes more dramatic as the disease progresses, eventually leading to functional impairment (first IADLs and then ADLs become impaired). Early on in the disease, patients complain of difficulty remembering names and recent events (short-term memory). Depression and apathy can also complicate things and usually worsen prognosis. As the disease progresses, additional symptoms arise, including disorientation, confusion, impaired judgment, and behavior changes. Finally, during the late stages of AD, individuals have difficulty speaking, swallowing, recognizing loved ones, and worsening impairment in completing ADLs, and eventually the patient becomes bedridden, requiring total care. Individuals with AD progress from mild to moderate to severe stages at variable rates (Kelley and Petersen, 2007).

Pharmacotherapy. At the present time, there are no disease-modifying treatments for AD that slow or stop death or neuron damage in the brain. Managing AD is complex and must involve appropriate use of available treatment options; appropriate management of comorbid conditions; keeping the patient active mentally as much as possible; care coordination between caregivers and the health care team; and use of support groups, caregiver training, and supportive services to ease caregiver stress and burden. The goals of pharmacotherapy include improvement in memory and cognition, improving behavioral problems, easing caregiver stress and burden, and ultimately delaying long-term care placement. Many agents with the promise of being disease-modifying agents are being studied worldwide. Currently, the mainstay of treatment includes the AchEIs. Early detection is important so appropriate management strategies can be applied. Tacrine was the first AChEI developed, but it fell out of favor given that it has associated liver toxicity and frequent dosing and required monitoring. The other three AChEIs are donepezil, galantamine, and rivastigmine. Donepezil has been on the market since the mid-1990s and is a once-daily formulation. As a class, these medications have been well studied and show modest efficacy in managing the cognitive symptoms of AD. The most common side effects of the AChEIs include nausea, vomiting, and diarrhea. However, there are many other lesser known side effects of these medications, including rhinitis, nightmares, syncope, bradyarrhythmia, urinary incontinence, and weight loss (Patel and Holland, 2011). Side effects such as nightmares can respond to administration of the medication in the morning. Often, medication side effects lead to a prescription cascade whereby another medication is used to combat the side effect of one medication. The AChEIs are started at a lower dose and are then titrated slowly to avoid side effects. The length of response has been documented at 52 weeks, and benefit beyond that period is uncertain. It is worthwhile considering the risk versus benefits of these medications when used in patients with AD given that some of these patients may already have cachexia and poor appetite.

Another class of medications, the N-methyl-D-aspartate (NMDA) receptor agonists, are used in AD treatment as well. Memantine is currently the only NMDA agonist available and is indicated for moderate to severe AD. Some data show modest improvement in cognitive symptoms as well as quality of life. Generally, memantine has a better side effect profile than the AChEIs. Multiple different formulations of AChEIs exist, including transdermal patch, orally disintegrating pills, and liquid, thus improving compliance in patients with AD. All of these medications appear to be equally efficacious, and there is little evidence to recommend one over the other. They provide modest cognitive function enhancements but do not impact the underlying pathophysiological changes of AD. The decision to start therapy is very individual and should be made after full consideration of prognosis, comorbidities, side effects, and compliance, as well as caregiver education regarding risks and benefits in view of limited efficacy (Kelley and Petersen, 2007).

KEY TREATMENT

• AChEIs and NMDA agonists are only modestly effective and can be associated with significant side effects (Kelley and Petersen, 2007; Patel and Holland, 2011) (SOR: B).

Prevention. Many different studies have looked at the issue of prevention, and the data on AD prevention come primarily from observational studies. Prospective and randomized studies have shown no benefit from treatments such as vitamin E, nonsteroidal antiinflammatory drugs (NSAIDs), estrogen replacement, or AChEIs. The use of antioxidants in AD is an area of active research. A large clinical trial of patients with moderate AD found that vitamin E at a dosage of 1000 IU twice daily was effective at slowing the progression of moderate AD. This treatment modality fell out of favor after the well-known cardiovascular literature demonstrated an increased risk of death (from cardiovascular causes) with vitamin E dosages greater than 400 IU/day. Although observational studies also found NSAIDS to be modestly protective in dementia, their cardiovascular risk and long-term use risk preclude their use in AD. Ginkgo biloba, a popular neutraceutical, has also been studied in AD and has not shown to be of benefit. Additionally, it carries a risk of bleeding. Physical activity and exercise are well proven in terms of their health benefits, and evidence indicates that they benefit cognition as well. Cognitive leisure activities (e.g., playing cards, doing crossword puzzles) and social activities should also be recommended to those at risk of AD. Optimizing vascular risk factors (controlling blood pressure and diabetes) is also of great importance (Scarmeas et al., 2009).

Caregiver Education and Support. Health care teams must connect with and educate AD caregivers. Caregivers are of vital importance in keeping the patient with AD safe, compliant with treatment recommendations, and active. Caregiver education has been shown to reduce caregiver stress and burnout. It has been shown to reduce long-term care placement as well. Social work referral and referral to community programs and resources, such as the Alzheimer's Association, adult day health care, respite care, home health care, and hospice programs, are beneficial to caregivers and patients. Knowing about and inquiring about the health and personal challenges of AD caregivers is important. There are many tools and questionnaires available to assess caregiver burden and stress that can be used as well (Dang et al., 2008).

End-of-Life Care. Very commonly, family physicians lose focus in terms of viewing AD as a terminal illness. They wait until the later stages of the disease to discuss end-of-life issues and decision making, resulting in undue stress and expectations. Caregivers must be made aware of the prognosis of AD and the typical trajectory of it so that end-of-life decisions can be made earlier and can be planned for. Advanced care planning is much more than a living will and a power of attorney; it includes many decisions in terms of things such as hospitalization, comfort care, artificial nutrition, and placement. The insidious course of AD makes it more difficult for patients and families to accept that it is a terminal illness. Involvement of hospice services available through Medicare are reserved for very late AD patients. However, a palliative approach can be started much earlier. Loss of ADL function, loss of communication and understanding, loss of language, and being bedridden are some of the characteristics of a patient with AD who would qualify to receive the Medicare hospice benefit. Frequently, clinical dilemmas such as feeding an AD patient who cannot swallow, aspirates, and has weight loss are difficult to deal with without previous consideration. Feeding tubes should not be used in AD patients in the later stages of the disease. A palliative medicine team or specialist can be of benefit in consultation if these challenging situations arise.

Dementia with Lewy Bodies

> ### Key Points
>
> - Parkinsonian features and early visual hallucinations are common characteristics of DLB.
> - Patients with DLB have heightened neuroleptic sensitivity.

Dementia with Lewy bodies was first described in the 1960s as dementia with other important clinical features, including visual hallucinations, dysautonomia, parkinsonism, neuroleptic sensitivity, sleep disorders (e.g., parasomnias), and fluctuating cognition. Men are more commonly affected than women. Age is a risk factor for this disease as well. These patients are very sensitive to psychotropic medications, which can result in worsening parkinsonism and dysautonomia. The mainstays of treatment include cholinesterase inhibitors because the neurochemistry of DLB is similar to that of AD. Carbidopa–levodopa is used to treat the motor symptoms. It can be extremely challenging to manage patients with DLB, and caregiver education and training are very important to keep these patients functioning actively in the community as long as possible (Knopman et al., 2003).

Vascular Dementia

> ### Key Points
>
> - The course of VD is typically "stepwise" or associated with occurrence of strokes.
> - Optimizing vascular risk factors is the cornerstone of treatment.

There is a great deal of overlap between vascular and Alzheimer dementia in terms of comorbidities, risk factors, and pathogenesis. Cognitive deficits that occur in conjunction with a clinically obvious ischemic or hemorrhagic stroke or subclinical "silent" stroke represent the spectrum of VD. Usually memory impairment is mild early in the course of VD as opposed to AD, and executive dysfunction is present. The typical presentation of cognitive concerns occurs suddenly after a stroke or follows a "stepwise" course. Focal neurologic signs are frequently present such as hemianopsia, hemiparesis, and so on. The site and extent of the lesions determine the clinical presentation of disease. Chronic small vessel white matter ischemic disease is a common finding in elderly adults on brain imaging and may lead to mild cognitive deficits. Risk factors include hypertension, diabetes, hyperlipidemia, and atrial fibrillation. The mainstay of treatment includes control and optimization of vascular risk factors and AChEIs because patients with VD also have a deficiency in acetylcholine in the brain (De Leeuw and Gijn, 2003).

Less Common Causes of Dementia

Frontotemporal Dementia

> ### Key Points
>
> - Early mood and behavioral symptoms with disinhibition are characteristics of FTD.
> - There are no effective drug treatments for FTD.

Previously known as "Pick disease," FTD is an early-onset dementia with a mean age of onset of 58 years. About 20% to 40% of cases of FTD are familial. On neuroimaging, there is a gross degeneration of the frontal and temporal lobes, leading to clinical symptoms affecting personality and behavior. Cognitive impairment appears later and usually affects judgment and executive function. Social disinhibition and mood symptoms are prominent early on and help to distinguish this dementia from the others. Neuropsychological testing can be helpful in making the diagnosis. Currently, there are no effective treatments approved for FTD, but these patients are often treated with AChEIs because of the overlap of symptoms with other dementias (Snowden et al., 2002).

Normal-Pressure Hydrocephalus

> ### Key Point
>
> - The clinical triad of magnetic gait, dementia, and urinary incontinence is characteristics of NPH.

Normal-pressure hydrocephalus is an entity made of up of the clinical triad of dementia, urinary incontinence, and gait abnormalities (magnetic gait). Neuroimaging shows ventriculomegaly out of proportion to cerebral atrophy. These patients usually require neurology and neurosurgery referral to determine optimal treatment options. A large-volume CSF lumbar puncture in association with vestibular testing is done to determine if any of the symptoms are reversible. If so, the patient is referred to get a ventricular shunt procedure.

Creutzfeldt-Jakob Disease

> **Key Point**
>
> - Myoclonus and rapid progressive dementia over weeks are most characteristic of CJD.

Creutzfeldt-Jakob disease (CJD) is a rare neurodegenerative disorder resulting from prion infection of the brain. Cognitive decline in CJD occurs very rapidly (within weeks). Visual symptoms, ataxia, rigid posture, and myoclonus are associated symptoms. The diagnosis is usually made by the history characteristic of this disease, EEG, CSF analysis, and imaging. A brain biopsy provides a definitive diagnosis. Sporadic CJD accounts for 85% of the cases. Infectious CJD is rare and results from external sources of prions (medical procedures, transplanted organs, or infected animal products) (Knopman et al., 2003).

BEHAVIORAL AND PSYCHIATRIC SYMPTOMS OF DEMENTIA

> **Key Points**
>
> - Nonpharmacologic interventions should be attempted before the use of medications to control behavior.
> - Depression can coexist with dementia and should be treated to improve behavior.

In the dementia trajectory, most patients experience changes in mood, personality, thoughts, and perceptions, leading to behavioral changes, including wandering, repetitive questioning, paranoia, delusions, hallucinations, agitation, aggression, euphoria, apathy, disinhibition, irritability, resistance to care, and changes in circadian rhythm leading to sleepiness during the day and behavior disturbances at night (Fuh et al., 2005).

These symptoms usually manifest during moderate to severe stages of dementia and frequently cause significant distress to the patient, increase caregiver burden, and can result in long-term care placement. Early recognition and treatment of these symptoms is beneficial and can improve quality of life while decreasing caregiver burden. Caregivers should be educated on creating a structured environment and identifying and addressing the needs of the patient (including providing a comfortable room temperature, avoidance of noisy environment, minimizing background distraction, and being sure the patient gets adequate rest). Behavioral symptoms can result from new structural changes in the brain, environmental changes (moving to unfamiliar surroundings and having unfamiliar caregivers), and worsening comorbidities. These comorbidities may include fatigue; sleep disruption; physical discomfort such as fever, infection, pain, or constipation; adverse side effects of medications; and impaired vision or hearing. Evaluation and optimizing the comorbidities is important in improving the behavioral symptoms (Cerejeira et al., 2012). Depression can frequently coexist with dementia and when present leads to worsening of behavioral symptoms.

Many nonpharmacologic interventions have been evaluated and include cognitive-oriented interventions (e.g., reminiscence therapy), sensory stimulation interventions (e.g., acupuncture, aromatherapy, light therapy), behavior management techniques (e.g., cognitive-behavioral therapy, communication training, and individualized behavioral reinforcement strategies), and other psychosocial interventions (e.g., animal-assisted therapy, exercise). Overall, there is not sufficient strong evidence that shows positive effect of any of these nonpharmacologic modalities. However, some observational evidence suggests that light therapy, hand massage and touch, and exercise therapy could be helpful in reducing behavioral and psychiatric symptoms associated with dementia (O'Neil et al., 2011).

When nonpharmacologic therapies are ineffective and the patient's behavior is significantly problematic, drug therapies must be considered. Although many different classes of medications are used (antiepileptics, benzodiazepines, antidepressants, and antipsychotics), there is currently no FDA-approved drug treatment for the behavioral and psychiatric symptoms of dementia. Furthermore, there is significant evidence showing increased mortality risks with antipsychotics from cardiovascular and infectious causes. Antipsychotic medications are associated with short- and long-term risks and should be used sparingly. Certain behaviors, such as wandering, do not respond to antipsychotic treatment. When these medications are used, there should be a discussion with the caregiver about the risks and benefits, and the lowest effective dose should be used. When used for the long term, attempts to slowly wean these medications should be actively made.

CARE SETTINGS OF PATIENTS WITH DEMENTIA

> **Key Point**
>
> - Dementia is a terminal illness, and getting palliative care involved early on is important for advanced care planning.

Along the dementia trajectory, care settings can change as the dementia progresses. Patients with early stages of dementia are usually best managed in the outpatient setting. Ideally, a patient-centered, team-based approach to care should be used in the management of these patients. The role of the physician is to provide education, discuss the goals of care, discuss treatment options, explain the prognosis and the trajectory, and evaluate for optimal support in keeping the patient functioning in the community. Early completion of advanced directives, including a living will and especially the durable power of attorney for health care, will help identify the goals of care and guide future treatments. Palliative care should be introduced early to the patients and their caregivers, and discussion of resuscitation, tube feelings, laboratory testing, hospitalizations, intravenous therapies, and other aggressive interventions should start early to avoid unnecessary and inappropriate interventions over the course of disease progression.

Progression of the disease, especially functional and cognitive decline, often necessitates placement of the patient into long-term care facilities (assisted living facilities, personal care homes, and nursing homes). End-of-life care is ideally provided by hospice, which can take place in various settings from in-home services to long-term care facilities. Hospice provides valuable benefits for the patients with advanced dementia by educating and providing social support to families and caregivers as well as symptom management (e.g., pain, dehydration, constipation, depression, infection, and terminal delirium).

References

The complete reference list is available at www.expertconsult.com.

Web Resources

www.alz.org The Alzheimer's Association, an advocacy organization for patients and families dealing with Alzheimer's disease and other dementias. Includes useful patient and caregiver education materials. Also offers information for physicians and other professionals.

www.amda.com Professional organization for nursing home medical directors, attending physicians, and other members of the interdisciplinary team. Source of clinical and practice management information for care of patients in long-term care settings.

www.hospitalelderlifeprogram.org Description and supportive information for patients, families, and professionals about delirium and a program for its management in hospitals.

www.lbda.org Advocacy organization for patients and families dealing with Lewy body dementia. Useful patient and caregiver education materials. Also offers information for physicians and other professionals.

48 *Alcohol Use Disorders*

KEVIN SHERIN, STACY SEIKEL, and STEVEN HALE

Overview

Key Points

- Annual alcoholism-identified health costs are $223 billion.
- Alcoholic persons are heavy users of health care.
- Primary care screening is inadequate for patients with alcoholism.

Alcoholism is a chronic and pervasive medical disorder that adds enormous cost to the U.S. health care system. Alcohol use disorder (AUD) is among the top three preventable causes of death. The Centers for Disease Control and Prevention (CDC, 2004) estimates that for every alcohol-attributable death, 30 years of potential life is lost, accounting for 2.3 million years of potential life lost and 75,000 preventable deaths per year from identified cases. The total economic costs (2006 data) attributed to AUD are $223 billion, with 72% estimated from lost productivity, 11% from health care costs, 9.4% from criminal justice costs, and 7.5% from other effects. The economic cost of excessive alcohol consumption in this country is $746 per person, the majority from binge drinking (Bouchery et al., 2011).

Patients with alcoholism use health care resources disproportionately compared with other populations. The report from the 2006 data analysis above included 360,785 alcohol-attributable hospitalizations at community hospitals, 1.27 million emergency department (ED) visits, and 2.78 million physician office visits (Bouchery et al., 2011). Estimates of the extent of alcohol involvement in trauma include 39% of motor vehicle collision (MVC) fatalities (National Highway Traffic Safety Administration, 2006), 47% of homicides, 29% of suicides (Smith et al., 1999), 20% to 40% of fatal recreational injuries (Mayhew et al., 1986), and 10% to 25% of home injuries (CDC, 1983; Fell and Nash, 1989). Alcohol is involved in a substantial percentage of injuries caused by falls, drowning, and burns (Hingson and Howland, 1987, 1988). More than 5% of all hospital discharges other than childbirth include at least one alcohol-related diagnosis (Chen et al., 2005).

Cirrhosis of the liver continues to be largely attributable to alcohol use, with estimates of 60% to 90% of cirrhosis deaths being attributable to alcohol (Johannes et al., 1987).

Comorbidity with hepatitis C is frequently a factor in many of these alcoholic cirrhosis-related deaths. Hospitalizations for acute pancreatitis are frequently associated with AUD. Psychiatric comorbidity is common in the alcoholic population, especially depression and suicide. These sequelae have major implications for managed care organizations and federal and local payers alike. However, screening for alcoholism in primary care and emergency settings is not universal.

PREVALENCE

Key Points

- AUD is more common than diabetes mellitus (DM).
- Heavy alcohol use is more common in men.
- More screening and brief interventions (SBIs) are needed in primary care settings, which results in decreased drinking.
- Screening in hospitals, EDs, and trauma settings can be valuable, but brief interventions in these settings have produced inconclusive results.

In the United States, an estimated 140 million persons use alcohol, making it the most popular psychoactive substance (Baldwin et al., 1993). About 61% of the U.S. population drinks alcohol (CDC, 2003). A recent U.S. study using *Diagnostic Statistical Manual of Mental Disorders,* fifth edition (DSM-5) criteria and based on data from the National Epidemiologic Survey on Alcohol and Related Conditions (NESARC, Wave 2) placed the overall rate of past-year AUD at 10.8% (Agrawal et al., 2011). Ethnic variation is minimal in whites (6.4%), Hispanics (7.3%), and African Americans (4.8%) (Office of Applied Studies, 1995). The prevalence of binge drinking—that is, drinking five or more drinks at least once in the preceding month—is 14.2% (Winick, 1996). Heavy use is found more frequently in men (10.3%) than women (2.5%). Data also indicate that the greatest risk for AUDs occurs during young adulthood (Grant et al., 2008).

Compared with other chronic medical conditions in family medicine, AUDs appear to be of significant importance for early recognition and intervention. Hypertension is estimated to affect at least 50 million Americans, and DM type 2 affects more than 2% of the U.S. population, or 5.4 million adults. AUDs rank almost as high as hypertension and much higher than DM in terms of prevalence. The key for family physicians is to increase the screening, diagnosis, and treatment of AUD in the clinical setting to the level of importance attached to hypertension or DM. Screening in hospitals, EDs, and trauma care settings can add value (American College of Surgeons, 2008; Gentilello et al., 1999; Smothers et al., 2004). However, brief interventions for alcohol use in patients with acute injuries in the ED and in hospital admissions have been inconclusive (Dappen et al., 2007; Emmen et al., 2004). A meta-analysis of SBI was found effective in reducing alcohol consumption at 6 and 12 months among non–treatment-seeking primary care patients, regardless of gender (Fleming, 2002). Some evidence suggests that SBI for prevention is also effective in pregnancy care settings (Floyd, 2007).

CAUSATIVE FACTORS FOR ALCOHOL USE DISORDERS

See eAppendix 48-1 online.

DSM-5 CHANGES IN SUBSTANCE-RELATED AND ADDICTED DISORDERS

The DSM-5 was published by the American Psychiatric Association in 2013. The previous diagnoses of alcohol abuse and alcohol dependence were consolidated into a single disorder called *alcohol use disorder*. The "legal consequences" criteria previously used in DSM-IV was removed. An additional criterion, "craving or strong desire, or urge to use," was added to the DSM-5.

In DSM-5, there are 11 criteria, similar to DSM-IV (Table 48-1). Coding is based on *current* severity of symptoms:

- Mild: two or three symptoms
- Moderate: four or five symptoms
- Severe: six or more symptoms

For differences between DSM-IV and DSM-5, see http://pubs.niaaa.nih.gov/publications/dsmfactsheet/dsmfact.pdf.

Screening and Assessment

Key Points

- Apply CAGE screening to all patients older than 18 years of age.
- Be aware of a "negative" drinking history.
- Closely follow up positive responses.
- The AUDIT-C is a standard for quantifying AUDs in medical settings.

There is good evidence to support screening for AUD when using standard screening tools in practice. For a family physician, the diagnosis of alcoholism often depends on clues from the history and physical examination (Table 48-2). Possible clues may include a history of driving under the influence (DUI) or a MVC; history of repetitive trauma; new-onset hypertension, gastritis, or pancreatitis; otherwise unexplained liver disease (aspartate transaminase [AST] > alanine transaminase [ALT]); presence of depression; recent loss of employment or separation from family; unexplained tremor; upper gastrointestinal (GI) bleeding; recent falls or accidents; and a history of family or marital violence.

The four CAGE questions (cut down, annoyed, guilty, and eye opener) are adequate for screening purposes (Table 48-3), derived from the longer Michigan Alcoholism Screening Test (MAST) questions (see eTable 48-1 online) (Hays and Spickard, 1987; Powers and Spickard, 1984).

Table 48-1 DSM-5 Diagnostic Criteria for Alcohol Use Disorder*

A. A problematic pattern of alcohol use leading to clinically significant impairment or distress, as manifested by at least two of the following, occurring within a 12-month period:
1. Alcohol is often taken in larger amounts or over a longer period than was intended.
2. There is a persistent desire or unsuccessful efforts to cut down or control alcohol use.
3. A great deal of time is spent in activities necessary to obtain alcohol, use alcohol, or recover from its effects.
4. Craving or strong desire, or urge to use alcohol.
5. Recurrent alcohol use resulting in a failure to fulfill major role obligations at work, school, or home.
6. Continued alcohol use despite having persistent or recurrent social or interpersonal problems caused or exacerbated by the effects of alcohol.
7. Important social, occupational, or recreational activities are given up or reduced because of alcohol use.
8. Recurrent alcohol use in situations in which it is physically hazardous.
9. Alcohol use is continued despite knowledge of having a persistent or recurrent physical or psychological problem that is likely to have been caused or exacerbated by alcohol.
10. Tolerance, as defined by either of the following:
    a. A need for markedly increased amounts of alcohol to achieve intoxication or desired effect
    b. A markedly diminished effect with continued use of the same amount of alcohol
11. Withdrawal, as manifested by either of the following:
    a. The characteristic withdrawal syndrome for alcohol (refer to Criteria A and B of the criteria set for alcohol withdrawal).
    b. Alcohol (or a closely related substance, such as a benzodiazepine) is taken to relieve or avoid withdrawal symptoms.

*Review of data from the National Epidemiologic Survey on Alcohol and Related Conditions has shown that the similarities of the profiles from DSM-IV and DSM-V alcohol use disorder (AUD) far outweighed the differences and that the difference was mostly found at the lower end of the AUD severity spectrum (Dawson et al., 2013).
DSM, Diagnostic and Statistical Manual of Mental Disorders.
Reprinted with permission from American Psychiatric Association. *Diagnostic and statistical manual of mental disorders.* 5th ed. Arlington, VA: American Psychiatric Association; 2013.

Table 48-2 Screening Clues for Alcoholism

"Driving under the influence" arrest
Domestic violence
Unexplained trauma
Family stress
New hypertension
Gastritis
Pancreatitis
Tremor

Table 48-3   Brief Screening Questions for Alcohol Use

CAGE*
1. Have you ever felt you should cut down on your drinking?
2. Have people annoyed you by criticizing your drinking?
3. Have you ever felt bad or guilty about your drinking?
4. Have you ever had a drink first thing in the morning to steady your nerves or to get rid of a hangover (eye opener)?

Scoring: Item responses on the CAGE are scored 0 for "no" and 1 for "yes" answers, with a higher score an indication of alcohol problems. A total score of 2 or greater is considered clinically significant.

The normal cutoff for the CAGE is two positive answers; however, the Consensus Panel recommends that primary care clinicians lower the threshold to one positive answer to cast a wider net and identify more patients who may have substance use disorders. A number of other screening tools are available.

CAGE Questions Adapted to Include Drugs (CAGE-AID)†
1. Have you ever felt you ought to cut down on your drinking or drug use?
2. Have people annoyed you by criticizing your drinking or drug use?
3. Have you felt bad or guilty about your drinking or drug use?
4. Have you ever had a drink or used drugs first thing in the morning to steady your nerves or to get rid of a hangover (eye opener)?

*Ewing JA. Detecting alcoholism: the CAGE questionnaire. *JAMA.* 1984;252: 1905-1907.
†Brown RL, Rounds LA. Conjoint screening questionnaires for alcohol and drug abuse. *Wisc Med J.* 1995;94:135-140.

Table 48-4   TWEAK Screening for Alcohol Use

TWEAK is a five-item scale developed originally to screen for risk drinking during pregnancy.

Points
(1-2) *Tolerance:* How many drinks can you hold? or How many drinks do you need to feel high?
(1-2) *Worried:* Have close friends or relatives worried or complained about your drinking in the past year?
(1) *Eye openers:* Do you sometimes take a drink in the morning when you first get up?
(1) *Amnesia* (blackouts): Has a friend or family member ever told you about things you said or did while you were drinking that you could not remember?
(1) *Cut down:* Do you sometimes feel the need to cut down on your drinking?

Administering and scoring
Before administering TWEAK, drinkers are identified by a positive response to the question, "Do you consume or have you ever consumed beer, wine, wine coolers, or drinks containing liquor (i.e., whiskey, rum, or vodka)?"
To score the test, a 7-point scale is used.
The "tolerance-hold" question scores 2 points if the respondent is able to hold six or more drinks.
The "tolerance-high" question scores 2 points if three or more drinks are needed to feel high.
A total score of 2 or more indicates that obstetric patients are likely to be risk drinkers. However, preliminary studies suggest that cutoff points of 3 or 4 are better than 2 for identifying harmful drinking or alcoholism.

Two positive responses are considered a positive screen and indicate that further assessment is warranted. An important point is that family physicians should not assume that someone does not have an AUD when that person answers negatively to questions about drinking. If such patients do not use alcohol at all, it may indicate that they had to quit because they had problems with alcohol. Given the prevalence of AUDs, it is recommended that the CAGE questions be applied to all patients older than 18 years. Another brief set of screening questions is the TWEAK questionnaire: tolerance, worries, eye openers, amnesia, and cut down (Table 48-4).

Longer screening questionnaires include the MAST and the Alcohol Use Disorders Test (AUDIT; see eTable 48-2 online) (Saunders et al., 1993). Both are considered higher in predictive value but more difficult to administer. Age-specific and population-specific survey tools are also available, including the Geriatric Alcoholism Screen and an adolescent alcoholism inventory. The 10-item core questionnaire includes three questions on alcohol consumption (the AUDIT-C) and seven on the impact of alcohol use. The AUDIT has been shown to have good sensitivity and specificity in medical and general populations and has recently been useful for screening patients with major psychiatric disorders and as an assessment instrument for patients seeking treatment for AUDs (Cassidy et al., 2008; Donovan et al., 2006). The AUDIT-C provides an efficient standardized method for assessing the quantity and frequency of alcohol use and accounts for much of the test's discriminative power in medical populations (Rodriguez-Marros and Santamarina, 2007).

BIOLOGIC MARKERS

Key Points

- The mean corpuscular volume is higher than 100 fL.
- The AST level is higher than the ALT level.
- There is an elevated saturation (>1.7%) of *carbohydrate-deficient transferrin* (CDT) level.
- Five drinks daily for 2 weeks elevates γ-glutamyltransferase (GGT) in most people.
- Using GGT and CDT in combination increases sensitivity over either marker alone by 20% without compromising specificity.

Diagnostic clues from the laboratory include a complete blood count (CBC) with an elevated mean cell volume, elevated GGT, AST level higher than ALT, unexplained leukopenia or thrombocytopenia, and positive response to the CDT level (Borg et al., 1992). It is estimated that 5 drinks per day for 2 weeks will yield an elevated GGT in most people (U.S. Department of Health and Human Services, Substance Abuse and Mental Health Services Administration, 2006). Using CDT and GGT together increases sensitivity by 20% over either marker alone without compromising specificity (Hitela et al., 2006).

Dose-response relationships are not well established, making it difficult to use these tests as a direct quantifier for alcohol consumption (SAMSHA, 2014).

INTERVIEW QUESTIONS

Guidelines for interviewing adolescents about alcohol have been reviewed (Speraw and Rogers, 1998). An atmosphere of trust and privacy must be conveyed (parents should be excluded). The questioning should be gradually moved from nonthreatening areas about general lifestyle to more specific questions about medications to questions about alcohol use. Standard interview questions for alcohol use include quantity of consumption, frequency of consumption, preference of alcoholic beverages, age at onset of drinking, attempts to cut down or quit, time of most recent drink, adverse sequelae related to drinking (or stopping drinking), and pattern of drinking (continuous, daily drinking, binge pattern). Quantity questions can classify binge drinking as never, less than one, one to three, three to five, and more than five per month. Vague or evasive answers, as well as rationalizations, should be "red flags." Patients can also be asked how much alcohol they purchase and how often. It is important to elicit specific, concrete information and not become derailed by certain responses.

A family history of alcohol problems must be detailed because it is a major predictive variable. When a clinician receives the answer that the patient does not drink at all, the line of questioning should still be pursued to determine whether cessation was problem based. After it has been established that the person has a history of binge drinking or continuous daily drinking, follow-up questions are in order. These questions may include role impairment, family concerns, amnesia, self-concern, and hangovers to determine the patient's sentiments about alcohol consumption.

DETAILED ASSESSMENT

After it has been established that the patient has problems with alcohol, more detailed assessment is in order. The history should then be focused on the known harmful consequences of alcohol use as related to the patient's history. (For a list of complications, see Woodard, 2003.) Major disorders include Wernicke encephalopathy, withdrawal seizures, cerebellar disease, peripheral neuropathy, cardiomyopathy, cirrhosis, pancreatitis, gastritis, bone marrow suppression, and aseptic necrosis of the hip. A careful history should include an assessment of tolerance and withdrawal symptoms, including shakes, hallucinosis, seizures, and delirium tremens (DTs). The time of the last drink and quantification of daily drinking are prerequisites. Alcohol withdrawal often includes anxiety, nausea, vomiting, diarrhea, tremors, and elevated pulse and blood pressure (BP). A history of blackout or amnesic episodes while drinking must also be elicited. A history of family, social, legal, and occupational complications should be obtained as part of the diagnosis of alcoholism.

A psychiatric evaluation is key in the assessment for AUD. Screening tools such as the Beck Depression Inventory can help identify underlying depression. Assessment of suicidal ideation must be documented because people with alcoholism are at much greater risk for suicide-related deaths. The Mini–Mental Status Examination (MMSE) can be useful for assessing possible dementia or delirium and pointing to the need for more extensive neuropsychiatric testing (see Chapter 42). Cognitive damage may be a factor in denial, a trait that characterizes many patients with known AUD. A sexual history should be included, with attention to multiple partners and human immunodeficiency virus (HIV) risk assessment. A history of comorbid polysubstance abuse and intravenous drug use should also be sought. Cough, hemoptysis, night sweats, fever, and weight loss suggest the need to investigate for tuberculosis.

PHYSICAL ASSESSMENT

The physical examination should pay close attention to vital signs. Elevated BP, pulse, or respiration can be a clue to the severity of alcohol withdrawal. The smell of ethanol on the breath will point to acute intoxication; the comorbid "dry mouth" may then be a local effect and not related to dehydration. Skin changes can be seen in people with alcoholism and may include rhinophyma, red swollen facies, and porphyria cutanea tarda. A thorough neurologic examination is in order, including cranial nerves, extraocular movements, gait, and cerebellar signs, as well as a sensory assessment of the lower extremities. Ataxia and nystagmus can be clues to possible intoxication or Wernicke encephalopathy. Percussion and palpation of the liver are important in alcoholism. Examination of the extremities can include visualization of Dupuytren contractures and palmar erythema. An irregular heart rhythm suggests atrial fibrillation, or "holiday heart."

In women, a diagnosis of pregnancy should also be excluded (see AUD in Women). Alcoholism in pregnancy has severe perinatal effects. Cardiovascular, liver, GI, neurologic, and other sequelae of alcohol and other drugs of abuse have been reviewed (Gordis, 2003). AUD is frequently associated with hypertension.

KEY TREATMENT

- Evidence on the effectiveness of counseling to reduce alcohol consumption during pregnancy is limited; however, studies in the general adult population show that behavioral counseling interventions are effective among women of childbearing age. The benefits of behavioral counseling interventions to reduce alcohol misuse by adults outweigh any potential harm (United States Preventive Services Task Force [USPSTF], USDHHS, 2006) (SOR: B).

Management

ALCOHOL INTOXICATION

Key Points

- Naive alcohol users are impaired at lower levels.
- Always give thiamine to patients with alcoholism.
- Urine toxicology is frequently helpful for concomitant drug use.

Alcohol intoxication is frequently seen as a component of trauma, domestic violence, or suicide attempts (McGinnis and Foege, 1993). The degree of intoxication is determined by the amount of alcohol ingested, the duration of the ingestion, and the patient's tolerance, if any, for the alcohol. Subtle effects occur at levels of 20 mg/dL and include mild euphoria, mild impairment of coordination, and mood alterations. At 80 to 100 mg/dL, delayed reaction times and slurred speech may be noted. This 80-mg/dL level is generally accepted as an unsafe level for motor vehicle operation. Between 100 and 200 mg/dL, ataxia, grossly slurred speech, and incoordination occur. As the level climbs to 300 mg/dL, the ataxia becomes more marked, and drowsiness, lethargy, and vomiting may occur. In naive drinkers, levels above 400 mg/dL are associated with coma, respiratory depression, hypothermia, and death from central nervous system (CNS) depression, loss of airway integrity, or pulmonary aspiration. Patients with chronic alcoholism have different tolerance responses than those just listed and may be in severe withdrawal at substantial levels.

Alcohol-induced coma can be managed by protecting the airway and performing basic resuscitation, if necessary. The patient should be placed in a warm protective environment, with careful monitoring of vital signs. Gastric emptying is rarely helpful because of the rapid absorption of alcohol, but it may be considered if the ingestion has occurred within 60 minutes. Alcohol is eliminated mostly by hepatic metabolism, which follows zero-order kinetics. The rate does not change with changes in the alcohol blood level. Fructose can enhance elimination but is not typically used. In extreme cases, hemodialysis may be effective in reducing the level quickly. Activated charcoal does not efficiently absorb ethanol but may be given if other toxins have been ingested (Mayo-Smith, 2009).

Thiamine and glucose should always be administered because chronic alcoholism is associated with hypoglycemia and thiamine deficient states such as Wernicke encephalopathy (mental confusion, cranial nerve palsies, ataxia). Thiamine should be given immediately before or with glucose to prevent hypoglycemia because glucose is metabolized with the enzyme thiamine pyrophosphorylase. The physician should look for additional drug use in all patients because the effects of other drugs may be obscured by the obvious alcohol intoxication (Mayo-Smith, 2009). The result of a urine toxicology screen may be positive for concomitant intoxicants.

OVERVIEW OF ALCOHOLISM TREATMENT

Alcoholics who are actively drinking are among the highest cost users of medical services in the United States. Several studies have documented that alcohol treatment has beneficial effects on health care expenditures, primarily as a result of decreased health care use by people with alcoholism and their families. A Harvard Study compared 587 lifesaving interventions and ranked all substance abuse interventions, including treatment of alcoholism, in the top 10% (Tengs et al., 1995).

Physicians interface with the medical or behavioral effects of alcoholism when patients deteriorate to the point

of trauma, end-organ damage, or behavioral impairment. As with other chronic disorders, alcoholism is slow but progressive. As the disorder progresses, the ability to control drinking diminishes, which distinguishes an alcoholic from a nonalcoholic. Many physicians view detoxification as the treatment for this disorder, which is similar to giving patients with DM one injection of insulin to control their diabetes. It treats the immediate problem but does little to address the chronic disorder in 1 week or 1 month. Although the goal for a patient with alcoholism is complete abstinence from alcohol, the norm is alcohol consumption in increasing amounts. The family physician can view intermittent periods of abstinence or reductions in alcohol consumption as progress in treatment of the disorder and encourage further efforts. Relapse must be evaluated carefully, and keys to change can open the door to further reductions or ongoing abstinence.

The American Society of Addiction Medicine (ASAM) has developed patient placement criteria (PPC) to better guide treatment of alcoholism (Mee-Lee et al., 2001). The PPC can help to assign the appropriate level of care for detoxification and subsequent rehabilitation of those with AUDs. The ASAM criteria reflect a consensus of expert opinion for adolescents and adults in treatment. Levels of care are differentiated by three criteria: (1) degree of direct medical management provided; (2) degree of structure, safety, and security provided; and (3) degree of treatment intensity provided. Special populations that need consideration include pregnant and nursing women; adolescents; older adults; HIV-positive patients; patients with neurologic, cardiovascular, hepatic, or renal disorders; patients with psychiatric comorbidities; and persons in criminal justice settings (Wright et al., 2009).

DETOXIFICATION

The *alcohol withdrawal syndrome* is a somewhat predictable series of events that have a temporal relationship to the use, decrease in intake, or cessation of alcohol consumption. Alcohol withdrawal may occur in a patient who has a reduction in alcohol intake from a previously significant level or an absolute absence of alcohol. The pharmacology of alcohol and its subsequent metabolism is well known and follows zero-order kinetics, primarily through the liver and cytochrome pathways (Mayo-Smith, 2009).

Patients with mild to moderate alcohol withdrawal symptoms and no serious psychiatric or medical comorbidities can be safely treated in the outpatient setting (Asplund et al., 2004). The severity of these symptoms varies greatly among individuals, but in a majority, they are mild and transient, passing within 1 or 2 days (Driessen et al., 2005; Mayo-Smith, 2009).

The signs and symptoms of alcohol withdrawal vary individually but tend to be repetitive in the same person. Most people with alcoholism who withdraw from alcohol experience minimal symptoms, such as sleep disturbance or anxiety. A small number may have tremulousness, agitation, diaphoresis, and cognitive impairment. The tremors or shakes typically begin 12 to 14 hours after a period of heavy drinking and are usually noted in the early morning. Tremulousness may be accompanied by *alcoholic hallucinosis*, a misperception of objects in the

Table 48-5 Alcohol Withdrawal Seizures

Peak seizure risk is 24 to 48 hours after cessation; may occur up to 2 weeks later.
Seizures are brief or occur in a "flurry."
Dilantin is ineffective.
Use caution with medications that lower seizure threshold (e.g., tricyclics, phenothiazines).

patient's sensory arena. Other symptoms of withdrawal include nausea, vomiting, poor oral intake, sweats, and anxiety. Seizures during alcohol withdrawal tend to occur as one isolated seizure or a brief cluster of seizures. Seizures are frequently preceded by tremors and tend to recur in a similar pattern in the same patient. Seizures may be the initial manifestation of alcohol withdrawal. Seizure activity is most common 24 to 48 hours after alcohol cessation, although seizures can occur as early as 24 hours or as late as 2 weeks after cessation of alcohol (Victor, 1983) (Table 48-5). Seizures may occur even later with concomitant benzodiazepine use. Withdrawal seizures are typically generalized, grand mal, and self-limited. Rarely, seizures may progress to status epilepticus (<3%). Physical signs include an elevated pulse and BP along with signs of autonomic hyperactivity.

The Clinical Institute Withdrawal Assessment for Alcohol scale, revised (CIWA-Ar) is a validated 10-item assessment tool used to quantify the severity of alcohol withdrawal syndrome and to monitor and medicate patients going through withdrawal (Bayard et al., 2004) (Table 48-6). Patients with moderate withdrawal should receive pharmacotherapy to treat their symptoms and reduce the risk of seizures and DTs during outpatient detoxification. Benzodiazepines are the treatment of choice for alcohol withdrawal, according to U.S. and Scottish guidelines (Scottish Intercollegiate Guidelines Network [SIGN], 2003). In healthy people with mild to moderate alcohol withdrawal, carbamazepine has many advantages, making it a first-line treatment for properly selected patients (Asplund et al., 2004).

Major alcohol withdrawal, also known as *delirium tremens*, occurs in fewer than 5% of patients with alcoholism in withdrawal. Delirium tremens is usually preceded by minor withdrawal symptoms, although they may appear frankly in a patient with minimal symptomatology. The delirium often begins 3 to 4 days after the last drink and is characterized by a marked change in sensorium with agitation, frank hallucinations, and severe disorientation (Table 48-7). Severe and potentially life-threatening autonomic hyperactivity leads to tachycardia, hypertension, and diaphoresis, frequently with low-grade fever. The severe disorientation may lead to self-injury or harm. Typically, the patient's actions may be appropriate to the context of the state of disorientation and hallucinosis. The patient's sleep activity is usually disturbed, along with excessive motor activity. Risk factors for DTs are a high blood alcohol level at the initial evaluation, an alcohol withdrawal seizure early in the withdrawal syndrome, and a previous history

of delirium (Victor, 1983). Concomitant infections or additional medical disorders may also predispose to severe alcohol withdrawal. Fever over 101°F (38.3°C) should be evaluated further. Before the treatment of alcohol withdrawal, a complete physical examination should be performed to assess the patient, including analysis for GI blood loss.

KEY TREATMENT

- Physicians should always use thiamine supplementation (Mayo-Smith, 2009) (SOR: A).
- Giving benzodiazepines is the treatment of choice of alcohol withdrawal and is supported by the latest systematic reviews (Ntais et al., 2005) (SOR: A).
- Carbamazepine is a first-line treatment for properly selected patients (Asplund et al., 2004) (SOR: C).
- Phenytoin (Dilantin) is ineffective in withdrawal seizures (Rathlev et al., 1994).

WITHDRAWAL TREATMENT

Treatment of alcohol withdrawal consists of supportive and pharmacologic interventions. Supportive interventions include fostering the patient's desire for abstinence during the withdrawal process. A calm, quiet environment and reassuring and reorienting the patient if confused decreases the risk of injury or relapse.

The preferred CNS agents for detoxification are the benzodiazepines, according to U.S. and Scottish guidelines (Asplund et al., 2004; SIGN, 2003) and Cochrane review (Ntais et al., 2005). They provide the best side effect profile and have a better risk-to-benefit profile than other agents. Benzodiazepines are not likely to be fatal in overdose unless mixed with another central depressant (check the urine toxicology screen). Chlordiazepoxide and diazepam are both effective agents. If liver disease is present, or to treat withdrawal in an older patient, oxazepam or lorazepam may be a safer choice because of shorter half-life. Additionally, β-blockers such as atenolol, 50 to 100 mg/day, may decrease tremulousness and sympathomimetic symptoms if there are no contraindications (Table 48-8). A scheduled regimen of chlordiazepoxide, 100 to 300 mg on day 1 followed by daily 50% dose reductions for 3 to 5 days, rather than "as needed" or on a symptom schedule, provides for a smooth withdrawal. Doses must be held for oversedation or somnolence. Monitoring for oversedation is necessary before each dosing (Sullivan et al., 1989). Aggressive regimens support patient comfort, help maintain compliance, and reduce the risk of seizures and major withdrawal. Outpatient detoxification can be performed; without supervision, however, some risk is present (e.g., seizures, self-injury, overdose), and relapse is likely if further alcohol is available.

Anticonvulsants such as phenytoin have not been demonstrated to reduce withdrawal seizures better than benzodiazepines. Anticonvulsants used for detoxification with a history of seizures received a level B of evidence in the Scottish guidelines (SIGN, 2003). Carbamazepine is superior to other anticonvulsants and results in less

Table 48-6   Clinical Institute Withdrawal Assessment of Alcohol Scale, Revised (CIWA-Ar)*

Patient: _____ Date: _____ Time: _____ (24 hour clock, midnight = 00:00)

Pulse or heart rate, taken for 1 minute: _____ Blood pressure: _____

Nausea and Vomiting

Ask, "Do you feel sick to your stomach? Have you vomited?" Observation.
0 No nausea and no vomiting
1 Mild nausea with no vomiting
2
3
4 Intermittent nausea with dry heaves
5
6
7 Constant nausea, frequent dry heaves, and vomiting

Tremor

Arms extended and fingers spread apart. Observation.
0 No tremor
1 Not visible but can be felt fingertip to fingertip
2
3
4 Moderate, with patient's arms extended
5
6
7 Severe, even with arms not extended

Paroxysmal Sweats

Observation.
0 No sweat visible
1 Barely perceptible sweating, palms moist
2
3
4 Beads of sweat obvious on forehead
5
6
7 Drenching sweats

Anxiety

Ask, "Do you feel nervous?" Observation.
0 No anxiety, at ease
1 Mildly anxious
2
3
4 Moderately anxious, or guarded, so anxiety is inferred
5
6
7 Equivalent to acute panic states, as seen in severe delirium or acute schizophrenic reactions

Agitation

Observation.
0 Normal activity
1 Somewhat more than normal activity
2
3
4 Moderately fidgety and restless
5
6
7 Paces back and forth during most of the interview, or constantly thrashes about

Total CIWA-Ar Score _____

Rater's Initials _____

Tactile Disturbances

Ask, "Have you any itching, pins and needles sensations, any burning, any numbness, or do you feel bugs crawling on or under your skin?" Observation.
0 None
1 Very mild itching, pins and needles, burning, or numbness
2 Mild itching, pins and needles, burning, or numbness
3 Moderate itching, pins and needles, burning, or numbness
4 Moderately severe hallucinations
5 Severe hallucinations
6 Extremely severe hallucinations
7 Continuous hallucinations

Auditory Disturbances

Ask, "Are you more aware of sounds around you? Are they harsh? Do they frighten you? Are you hearing anything that is disturbing to you? Are you hearing things you know are not there?" Observation.
0 Not present
1 Very mild harshness or ability to frighten
2 Mild harshness or ability to frighten
3 Moderate harshness or ability to frighten
4 Moderately severe hallucinations
5 Severe hallucinations
6 Extremely severe hallucinations
7 Continuous hallucinations

Visual Disturbances

Ask, "Does the light appear to be too bright? Is its color different? Does it hurt your eyes? Are you seeing anything that is disturbing to you? Are you seeing things you know are not there?" Observation.
0 Not present
1 Very mild sensitivity
2 Mild sensitivity
3 Moderate sensitivity
4 Moderately severe hallucinations
5 Severe hallucinations
6 Extremely severe hallucinations
7 Continuous hallucinations

Headache, Fullness in Head

Ask, "Does your head feel different? Does it feel like there is a band around your head?" Do not rate for dizziness or lightheadedness. Otherwise, rate severity.
0 Not present
1 Very mild
2 Mild
3 Moderate
4 Moderately severe
5 Severe
6 Very severe
7 Extremely severe

Orientation and Clouding of Sensorium

Ask, "What day is this? Where are you? Who am I?"
0 Oriented and can do serial additions
1 Cannot do serial additions or is uncertain about date
2 Disoriented for date by no more than 2 calendar days
3 Disoriented for date by more than 2 calendar days
4 Disoriented for place or person

*The CIWA-Ar is not copyrighted and may be reproduced freely. This assessment for monitoring withdrawal symptoms requires approximately 5 minutes to administer. The maximum score is 67 (see instrument). Patients scoring less than 10 do not usually need additional medication for withdrawal.
From Sullivan JT, Sykora K, Schneiderman J, et al. Assessment of alcohol withdrawal: the revised Clinical Institute Withdrawal Assessment for Alcohol scale (CIWA-Ar). *Br J Addict.* 1989;84:1353-1357.

Table 48-7   Delirium Tremens

Usually preceded by tremor or seizures
Usually begin 3 to 4 days after alcohol cessation
Delirium with severe disorientation
Autonomic hyperactivity
Disturbed sleep
Worsened by concomitant disorders (e.g., pancreatitis, pneumonia, gastrointestinal bleed)

Table 48-9   Components of Effective Brief Intervention

Feedback of physician's assessment
Emphasis on patient responsibility
Clear, direct advice to change
Nonconfrontational physician approach
Menu of options provided

From Bien TH, Miller WR, Tonigan JS. Brief interventions for alcohol problems: a review. *Addiction*. 1993;8:315-335.

Table 48-8   Alcohol Withdrawal: Stages and Treatment Summary

Stage	Intervention	Pharmacology
I. Mild	Be supportive Contact Alcoholics Anonymous Provide close follow-up	Thiamine, 100 mg/day Chlordiazepoxide, 25 mg three times daily if necessary, 3 days only
II. Moderate	Allow brief inpatient visit Make observations Check laboratory test results (e.g., magnesium, phosphate, electrolyte, glucose levels)	As above, *plus* chlordiazepoxide, 100-300 mg/day, 3 days only Atenolol, 50-100 mg/day, 3 days only
III. Severe	Hospitalize in ICU Delirium tremens, intermediate care Laboratory tests as above Monitor fluid status May need restraint Monitor for infection Prevent self-harm	As above, *plus* chlordiazepoxide, 100 mg hourly until asleep or subdued; then taper Antipsychotics: haloperidol, 2-10 mg/day Lorazepam, 1-2 mg intravenously prn if unable to take orally

ICU, Intensive care unit.

psychiatric distress, a faster return to work, fewer rebound symptoms, and reduced posttreatment drinking (Malcolm et al., 2001). Anticonvulsants are not generally indicated unless a concomitant seizure disorder is present.

Antipsychotic medications such as risperidone, olanzapine, and haloperidol have benefits in patients with hallucinosis and DTs but may reduce the seizure threshold (SIGN, 2003). Ear acupuncture has not shown efficacy in alcohol withdrawal in clinical trials. However, massage therapy has reduced withdrawal scores (Kunz et al., 2007; Reader et al., 2005).

INTERVENTIONS IN ALCOHOL USE DISORDER

Interventions by family physicians have the goal of changing the natural course or outcome of the alcohol use disorder (AUD) process. A family physician typically performs many interventions on patients with chronic disorders over time. Interventions generally follow an assessment and consist of advice about how to manage the disorder, may include a pharmacologic agent, and usually require some type of follow-up or ongoing monitoring.

Brief Interventions

Brief interventions can be very successful in primary care (SIGN, 2003) (Table 48-9). The father of the concept of *stages of change*, Prochaska (2009), reviews motivation to change in alcohol addiction. Family physicians can apply motivational interviewing in helping patients to move to the next level in stages of change (see Chapter 8). Part of any substance abuse intervention is the physician's assessment of the patient's readiness to change. First described by Prochaska and DiClimente (1983) while studying smokers, assessing the state of change assists the family physician in targeting the interventional approach to the patient. Change consists of the following six states:

1. *Precontemplation.* The physician can plant the seed of how alcohol is harming the patient (think of creative ways to list reasons) physically or emotionally. Written information is helpful, and support to the family and others involved must be offered. Further biologic or historical data should be collected, with follow-up at reasonable intervals and availability to help the patient when ready. A nonjudgmental approach is best.
2. *Contemplation.* The patient is aware that harm is occurring but is not yet ready for action. The physician tries to motivate the patient to the action phase by listing more reasons for urgency, such as bleeding, ulcers, pancreatitis, and family violence. The physician offers referral advice if the patient is interested, collects more data, performs follow-up at a short interval, and is ready to help the patient when ready to start.
3. *Preparation.* The physician assists the patient in preparing for reduction or cessation of use.
4. *Action.* The patient is ready for referral, has "hit bottom," or is otherwise ready for change. The physician arranges inpatient or outpatient detoxification and involvement in a treatment program and completes a history and physical examination, with laboratory studies as appropriate.
5. *Maintenance.* The physician performs follow-up on the patient; reviews participation in the self-help program and use of the 12 steps as well as the frequency of Alcoholics Anonymous (AA) attendance; monitors target organ issues; performs mental status and depression screening; counsels regarding relapse prevention; monitors laboratory values (e.g., GGT, CDT); prescribes vitamins, naltrexone, acamprosate, antidepressants, or disulfiram (Antabuse) as needed; monitors urine ethylglucuronide (ETG) to determine alcohol use in the previous 72 hours; monitors and schedules and performs follow-up regularly, as with any chronic disease.

6. *Relapse.* The physician anticipates relapse with any addictive disorder, is ready to help the patient again with entry into a recovery program, and offers nonjudgmental support.

Brief interventions can be carried out in the context of a routine office visit (Edwards and Rollnick, 1997; Fleming et al., 1999). Interventions can follow assessment of the patient. When the physician sees sufficient evidence to conclude or strongly suspect that an AUD is present, the brief intervention can be targeted to the patient's stage of change. An encounter with a precontemplative patient would include presentation of the physician's analysis of the problem in a supportive and nonconfrontational manner, with the goal of moving the patient to another state of change. For example:

Mr. Smith, your recent accident, alcohol use pattern, liver enlargement on physical examination, and abnormal laboratory test results lead me to conclude that your use of alcohol is a problem. As your family physician, I am concerned about your ongoing health risks. What can we do to deal with this problem?

Alternatively, a patient who is in the contemplation phase of change would be asked a different set of questions, such as:

Mr. Smith, I am glad that you are able to realize the impact that your alcohol drinking is having on your health, but we need to move forward and discuss treatment options.

An effective brief intervention should include *feedback* summarizing the physician's assessment; patient responsibility should also be emphasized, followed by clear, direct advice to change given in a nonconfrontational manner. The patient is given a menu of options from which to choose (Bien et al., 1993). Authoritative approaches are generally less effective than an empathetic approach. This type of approach will take practice and refinement for busy family physicians but can be integrated into the office practice without substantial time or expense. These techniques are more generally known as *motivational interviewing.* Motivational interviewing is effective in helping family physicians to engage patients in a variety of behavioral changes, including alcohol or tobacco use. Motivational interviewing has been a successful technique when used with brief interventions (Vasilaki et al., 2006).

Classic Intervention

When a brief intervention is not effective or if the circumstances demand more expeditious change, a classic intervention can be planned. The interventional goal is to break through the alcoholic denial system by providing an overwhelming amount of evidence and feedback to the patient with alcoholism. Classic interventions need to be carefully orchestrated by professionals trained in addiction treatment. Unless actively involved in alcoholism treatment, most family physicians will consult one of their referral treatment programs for assistance in developing a classic intervention. The family physician may be an appropriate member of the intervention group.

Treatment of Alcoholism

> ### Key Points
>
> - Try the least restrictive treatment first for the patient with alcoholism.
> - Long-term treatment is favored for alcoholism. Regular attendance to AA meetings is helpful.
> - The presence of other disorders increases acuity needs in patients with alcoholism.

The treatment options for alcoholism are extensive (Fuller et al., 2003; Kranzler et al., 2009). The medications most widely studied for AUDs are disulfiram, naltrexone, and acamprosate. Results from the Combining Medications and Behavioral Intervention for Alcoholism (COMBINE) study and trials of injectable naltrexone formulations and oral topiramate have provided important information on the use of these medications in alcohol rehabilitation. Long-acting formulations of naltrexone have been shown to reduce the adverse event profile compared with oral treatment and significantly decrease heavy drinking in men with AUD (Bankole, 2007).

A family physician is faced with several decisions when evaluating a patient for treatment of alcoholism after successful detoxification or if medically supervised detoxification is not needed. Should the patient go through a hospital or a nonhospital (residential) inpatient program, a day treatment program, or any outpatient program? Should the patient receive counseling, attend AA, or be involved in a cognitive program? Inpatient programs offer isolation from the drinking environment, intensive treatment, family involvement, in-depth assessment, and convenience for further medical or psychiatric assessment. However, they carry significant expense, typically occur after detoxification, remove the patient from the real-world environment, and have not been consistently shown to improve long-term outcomes. Patients who are suicidal or who have serious concomitant mental disorders that may impair recovery, as well as those unable to maintain abstinence in a less restrictive environment, should be considered for these facilities. Advantages of day treatment and outpatient treatment include reduced expense, ability to maintain work in some cases, and usually a longer period of treatment in a less restrictive environment. In general, as long as it is safe to try outpatient treatment initially, it is the least restrictive and most cost-effective method.

Access to relapse prevention treatments of established efficacy should be facilitated for alcohol-dependent patients. These therapies include outpatient programs, residential and "halfway house" milieu therapies, and partial hospitalization programs (SIGN, 2003).

ALCOHOL USE DISORDER AND PSYCHIATRIC COMORBIDITIES: DUAL DIAGNOSIS

Dual diagnosis is defined as AUD with one or more other psychiatric comorbidities. Frequently, people with alcoholism abuse other substances, such as crack cocaine, nicotine, and even opiates (Tallia et al., 2005). Comorbidity estimates among people with alcoholism, gender preferences for addictive substances, and patterns of progression vary widely (Crum, 2009). Assessment of long-term outcomes highlights the impact of comorbidities on level of functioning, educational achievement, occupation, and social relationships (Crawford et al., 2008).

Patients with alcohol problems and anxiety or depression should have their alcohol problem treated first. If depressive symptoms persist for more than 2 weeks after treatment for alcohol dependence, the physician should consider use of a selective serotonin reuptake inhibitor (SSRI) or tricyclic antidepressant (TCA) or referral for supportive psychotherapy and cognitive-behavioral therapy (CBT) along with relapse prevention (SIGN, 2003). CBT has been shown to be efficacious (Longabaugh and Morgenstern, 1999; Project MATCH Research Group, 1997).

Patients with psychotic disorder and alcohol dependence should be encouraged to address their alcohol use and may benefit from motivational, CBT, family, and nonconfrontational approaches. Structured settings may offer some advantage for patients with psychotic comorbidities. Another challenge with treating people with alcoholism with comorbid conditions is *impulse control disorders* (ICDs). Also known as "behavioral addictions," ICDs include pathologic gambling (PG) and many other conditions (Yip and Potenza, 2009). Of interest in the treatment of those with alcoholism is evidence that patients with PG can benefit from treatment with naltrexone (Kim et al., 2001).

ALCOHOLICS ANONYMOUS

Most physicians have heard of AA, and many may have suggested that patients with alcohol-related problems attend meetings. However, few physicians know much about AA. To prepare patients for their first AA meetings, it is important to be familiar with this organization (Table 48-10).

DRUG TREATMENT SPECIFIC TO ALCOHOL USE DISORDER AND RECOVERY

Key Points

- Disulfiram can be regarded as an aversive agent.
- Naltrexone produces a surmountable opiate blockage and diminishes the reinforcing effect of alcohol.
- Injectable naltrexone has greater efficacy than oral naltrexone in AUDs.
- Acamprosate reduces the urge to drink in some patients.

Treatment of AUD with medications has long been a challenging and controversial topic. Drug treatment of AUD can be divided into drugs used for detoxification (see earlier discussion) and those used to reduce or eliminate alcohol consumption after detoxification and for relapse prevention. Pharmacologic interventions for alcoholism have been reviewed (Fuller et al., 2003). The U.S. Food and Drug Administration (FDA) now approves three drugs for

Table 48-10   Information on Alcoholics Anonymous (AA)

- AA pamphlets to give to patients may be ordered from the AA's website at www.aa.org. Look for the AA Literature menu.
- AA meetings in your area may also be found on the AA's website.
- There are several formats of AA meetings. Open meetings may be attended by anyone interested in AA. Physicians are encouraged to attend at least one open AA meeting. The local area meeting lists designate whether a specific meeting is open or closed.
- Closed meetings may only be attended by alcoholics or those who have a "desire not to drink alcohol."
- Other types of meetings include those for women only, men only, meetings for the gay and lesbian population, and meetings in Spanish. Other types of meeting include step study, open discussion, and speaker meetings, as well as online meetings.
- Most patients will object to attending AA meetings for a variety of reasons. Some common objections to AA:
  - "It's too religious." AA is not a religious program but a spiritual fellowship. It refers to a "Higher Power" and "God as we understand Him," but no belief in God is necessary.
  - "I don't want to stand up and bare my soul in front of a lot of other people." Only those who wish to do so speak at AA meetings.
  - "I don't want to meet with a lot of losers. It's too depressing." AA more accurately represents a cross-section of "winners" in the sense that they have survived the disease. Those who go to enough meetings are sure to find people with whom they can identify.
  - "I can't go there. All those people are sober, and I'm not. I'd be too ashamed." The only requirement for membership is a desire to stop drinking. Members who are still drinking are encouraged to "keep coming back."
  - "I don't want everyone to know about my drinking." Anonymity is and always has been the basis of the AA program. Traditionally, AA members never disclose their association with the movement.

Common objections reprinted from Alcoholics Anonymous. *AA as a resource for the health care professional.* Alcoholics Anonymous World Services, Inc. 5-8. http://www.aa.org/assets/en_US/information-for-professionals/p-23-aa-as-a-resource-for-the-health-care-professional.

alcohol treatment to reduce or eliminate consumption—disulfiram (Antabuse), acamprosate (Campral), and naltrexone (ReVia)—as well as long-acting naltrexone (Vivitrol).

Disulfiram

Disulfiram has been available for the treatment of AUD since the late 1940s. Given as a single daily dose, disulfiram inhibits aldehyde dehydrogenase, the second alcohol degradation enzyme. This inhibition causes acetaldehyde to increase five to 10 times the usual level found after alcohol consumption. Symptoms that occur in patients acquiring alcohol from any source include flushing, palpitations, respiratory difficulty, nausea, vomiting, weakness, and general uneasiness. If alcohol consumption continues or a large volume is ingested, hypotension, syncope, loss of consciousness, and death may follow. Minor reactions may occur with inadvertent exposure from nonbeverage alcohol sources such as colognes, over-the-counter (OTC) medications, or foods with uncooked alcohol. Also used in attempted and completed suicides, disulfiram can be thought of as an "incomplete poison" that will become a "complete poison" if alcohol is added.

Disulfiram works on the patient's understanding and expectation of an adverse experience if alcohol is consumed. It can be given in dosages of 125 to 500 mg/day and can be safely started 24 to 48 hours after alcohol cessation. Avoidance or extreme caution should be used in patients with known or suspected coronary artery disease, those at risk for suicide or with serious mental illness, and those unable or unlikely to comply with a complete treatment plan that includes additional forms of treatment. Disulfiram should not be used as the only treatment for AUD; it is better considered as an adjunct for carefully selected patients. An often-quoted blinded placebo-controlled study of Veterans Administration patients found that doses of 250 mg, 1 mg, and no disulfiram produced no significant differences in total abstinence (Fuller et al., 1986). Higher doses were associated with fewer drinking days than in other groups. Adverse reactions include peripheral neuropathy; optic neuritis; drowsiness; fatigue; metallic aftertaste; and infrequent hepatotoxicity, probably resulting from hypersensitivity. Evaluation of liver enzyme levels before therapy and periodically is recommended.

Supervised treatment or directly observed therapy with oral disulfiram may be used to prevent relapse. However, patients must be informed that this treatment requires complete abstinence, and they should clearly understand the risks of disulfiram therapy.

Naltrexone

The euphoric effect of alcohol is mediated through the endogenous opioid system, with activation of the prefrontal cortex (Tuhonen et al., 1994). Naltrexone, an opioid antagonist, has documented beneficial effect in reducing relapse and craving in patients with alcoholism (O'Malley et al., 1992; Swift et al., 1994; Volpicelli et al., 1992). Alcoholics taking naltrexone report a less pleasurable effect or high from alcohol consumption and do not escalate their drinking as rapidly as control groups (Volpicelli et al., 1995). A decreased craving for alcohol has not been universally reported. Naltrexone is given as a daily 50-mg tablet or a 380-mg IM injection monthly. This dosage provides a surmountable opioid blockage that will render other opioids ineffective unless given in greatly increased doses. Naltrexone is not an aversive agent. Many patients with alcoholism report a less-than-expected pleasurable experience with alcohol consumption, but others report some mild aversive symptoms.

Naltrexone undergoes first-pass hepatic metabolism and is hepatotoxic in excessive doses. It should not be given to patients currently addicted to opiates because it will precipitate acute opiate withdrawal (Croop et al., 1997). The most common side effects at the usual dosage include nausea, headache, dizziness, anxiety, and somnolence. Good candidates for naltrexone are those likely to be compliant with therapy, those concomitantly addicted to opiates who have been detoxified and have not received opiate replacement therapy, and those with heavy alcohol cravings at entry to therapy (Volpicelli et al., 1997). Naltrexone should *not* be used as a single treatment agent but rather in conjunction with other behavioral or motivational treatment modalities. Questions remain about the duration of treatment with naltrexone in AUDs. Generally, prolonged

abstinence rates improve after 12 months of continuous abstinence.

Poor compliance with oral naltrexone reduces its potential benefits (Volpicelli et al., 1997). In a pilot study, alcohol-dependent patients treated with a subcutaneous long-acting formulation of naltrexone had detectable plasma concentrations of the medication for more than 3 days after injection and had reduced frequency of heavy drinking compared with the placebo group (Kranzler et al., 1998). A randomized clinical trial with injectable naltrexone monthly did not demonstrate reduced incidence of heavy drinking, although it did demonstrate significantly delayed onset of drinking, increased number of abstinent days, and increased abstinence (Kranzler et al., 2004). The FDA-approved long-acting naltrexone (Vivitrol), 380 mg each month intramuscularly in the buttock, for AUD in 2006. Patients should be abstinent when they are started on naltrexone.

According to the Agency for Health Care Policy and Research (AHCPR), there is good (level B) evidence to support the use of naltrexone to reduce craving and relapse (AHCPR, 1999). An alternative opioid antagonist with some success in patients with AUD, but not as well studied, is nalmefene (Kranzler et al., 2009).

Acamprosate

Acamprosate is one of the newest drugs to be added to the formulary for the treatment of AUD. The FDA has approved acamprosate for maintenance of abstinence from alcohol in patients with AUD who are abstinent at treatment initiation. This provision includes that patients also participate in a comprehensive alcohol treatment program. Acamprosate is reasonably well tolerated and without serious adverse effects (AHCPR, 1999). European trials of acamprosate showed efficacy in alcohol dependence; acamprosate enhanced abstinence and reduced drinking days in alcohol-dependent subjects.

Acamprosate is recommended in newly detoxified dependent patients as an adjunct to psychosocial interventions. Acamprosate is approved for use in alcohol-dependent and alcohol-abusing patients. Its mechanism of action is not well known, although there is fair evidence of its benefit. Acamprosate is an analog of homotaurine, a GABA-ergic agonist. The GABA-ergic system appears to affect the action of alcohol-induced behavior. Acamprosate also appears to have effects on glutamate and N-methyl-D-aspartate (NMDA) receptors. Chronic alcohol exposure is thought to alter the normal balance between neuronal excitation and inhibition, and acamprosate may help restore some of this balance. Several controlled clinical trials have demonstrated the effectiveness of acamprosate as an adjunct to psychosocial therapy for people with alcoholism who have undergone inpatient detoxification. In these studies, acamprosate was demonstrated to be superior to placebo. Acamprosate does not appear to be effective in the treatment of polysubstance abuse (Bouza et al., 2004; Mann et al., 2004). Evaluation of renal function for those at risk, including elderly patients, is indicated before initiating treatment with acamprosate.

Two U.S. multicenter trials, including the COMBINE study, failed to show an advantage of acamprosate over placebo on an "intent-to-treat" basis (Anton et al., 2006;

Mason et al., 2006). Discrepancies may be caused by differences in European studies, which included heavier drinkers with longer periods of abstinence before induction in trials (Kranzler et al., 2009).

Pharmacotherapy for AUDs with strength of recommendation (SOR) is as follows:
- Naltrexone (SOR: A)
- Long-acting naltrexone (Vivitrol) (SOR: A)
- Acamprosate (SOR: A)
- Disulfiram (SOR: B)

OTHER MEDICATIONS USED IN ALCOHOL TREATMENT

Anticonvulsants (Topiramate)

Anticonvulsants likely exert beneficial effects on GABA receptors. Placebo-controlled studies included carbamazepine (Mueller et al., 1997), divalproex (Brady et al., 2002), and topiramate (Johnson et al., 2003), with a multicenter study confirming the efficacy of topiramate and anticonvulsants for treatment of AUDs (Johnson et al., 2007). Topiramate was shown to decrease (1) drinks per day, (2) drinks per drinking day, (3) drinking days, (4) heavy-drinking days, and (5) GGT levels (Johnson et al., 2007). Side effects of anticonvulsants include numbness and tingling; metabolic acidosis; fatigue; dizziness; loss of appetite; nausea; diarrhea; weight loss; and difficulty concentrating, with memory, and in word finding. Suicidal thoughts or actions are infrequently reported, as are renal calculi and acute secondary glaucoma (Kranzler et al., 2009).

Baclofen

A GABA-B receptor agonist, baclofen has long been used as an antispasmodic. Only more recently has baclofen been investigated as a treatment for AUD. In a modest controlled trial of 1 month, baclofen was efficacious in achievement of total abstinent days compared with placebo (Addolorato et al., 2002). A follow-up study demonstrated efficacy in 84 patients with cirrhosis of the liver in maintaining abstinence (71% baclofen vs. 29% placebo) (Addolorato et al., 2007). There is potential for abuse of baclofen and withdrawal reactions, including delirium, which underscores the need for further research (Kranzler et al., 2009).

Serotonergic Agents

Most episodes of postwithdrawal depression will remit without specific treatment if abstinence from alcohol is maintained for days or weeks (Brown and Schukit, 1988; Schuckit, 1983). Patients with comorbid depression often require pharmacotherapy, and although the SSRIs have a low side effect profile, they can exacerbate the tremor, anxiety, and insomnia in early-recovering people with alcoholism. Recovering people with alcoholism with comorbid depression may actually do better with TCAs (Nunes and Levin, 2004).

Table 48-11   Characteristics of Women with Alcoholism

Lower rates of use than men
More hidden drinking than men
TWEAK screening better than CAGE
Less alcohol consumption than men may cause a significant disease progression
Treatment in all-women program is preferred

CAGE, Cut down, annoyed, guilty, and eye opener; *TWEAK,* tolerance, worries, eye openers, amnesia, and cut down.

Special Populations

ALCOHOL USE DISORDER IN WOMEN

Women have lower rates of AUD than their male counterparts, 1.5% overall and 1.5% in older adult women (Mouton and Espino, 1999) (Table 48-11). Women generally enter treatment later than men and have more psychiatric symptoms. Women seem to develop many pathologic effects of alcohol more rapidly than men (Blume and Zilberman, 2005), including fatty liver, hypertension, anemia, malnutrition, GI hemorrhage, and peptic ulcer requiring surgery (Zweben, 2009). For women, five to seven drinks daily is sufficient to cause significant disease progression.

Nonmedical use of prescription drugs in general and opioids in particular has been identified as a significant problem since the late 1990s. Women also have higher associated rates with first use of illicit drugs after age 24 years, serious mental illness, and cigarette smoking (Tetrault et al., 2008). Comorbid conditions for women include drug addiction, sexual abuse, intimate partner violence, borderline personality disorder, eating disorders, mood and anxiety disorders, and HIV infection. Women who drink alcohol may be more sensitive to the behavioral effects of concomitant cocaine use (Zweben, 2009).

Family physicians generally detect AUDs in women later than in men with alcoholism. Screening tests (e.g., CAGE) have less sensitivity in women and need to be interpreted differently, usually with lower cutoff points. This difference may result from the lower volume of alcohol consumed and the social stigmatization of these women (Bradley et al., 1998). Screening tests such as the TWEAK have performed better than the CAGE in women. It is important for physicians to educate women, even highly educated patients, about their greater risk (Green et al., 2007). Incarcerated women often begin using drugs and alcohol at very young ages and frequently require significant educational and job-training support to make successful transitions to recovery (Zweben, 2009). Women may have better treatment outcomes if referred to all-women programs or programs specializing in women's addictions (Hodgkins et al., 1997).

Alcohol Use Disorder and Pregnancy

The Institute of Medicine recognizes alcohol-related birth defects (ARBDs) and alcohol-related neurodevelopmental disorder (ARND) in addition to fetal alcohol syndrome (FAS) as potential effects of alcohol use in pregnancy and the periconception period (Muchowski and Paladine, 2004; Warren and Foudin 2001). A diagnosis of FAS requires characteristic facial anomalies, growth retardation, and neurodevelopmental abnormalities. In *partial* FAS, affected children have some of these characteristics, with no other explanation. ARBD includes a confirmed history of maternal alcohol use plus one or more congenital defects, most often cardiac, renal, vision, hearing, or skeletal. ARNDs require a confirmed history of maternal alcohol use and the neurodevelopment abnormalities or cognitive-behavioral abnormalities found in partial FAS.

The prevalence of FAS in the U.S. population is estimated at 0.5 to 2 per 1000 births, with up to 10 in 1000 newborns having some effect from alcohol exposure. The rate of FAS is more than 20 times higher in the United States compared with other countries, including European countries, partially because of differences in diagnosis (Muchowski and Paladine, 2004). Whether a safe threshold of alcohol consumption exists before or during pregnancy is controversial. Many U.S. authorities recommend against any alcohol intake before or during pregnancy. The effects of alcohol on a fetus depend on the amount of alcohol consumed at one time, timing of alcohol consumption in gestation, and duration of alcohol use in pregnancy. This is complicated by studies using various definitions of "light" and "heavy" alcohol use, with categories that often overlap among different studies. *Binge drinking,* defined as more than five drinks in a single day, even when episodic, is more dangerous to fetal brain development than non–binge drinking (Muchowski and Paladine, 2004).

Less severe problems can occur, although a high level of alcohol use in pregnancy is associated with more severely affected offspring. A 1984 study of 31,000 pregnancies showed a higher risk of growth retardation if a mother had even one drink a day. A 2001 study of more than 600 urban African American children showed continued behavioral effects of alcohol at age 6 to 7 years with low levels (one drink daily) of maternal alcohol consumption (Muchowski and Paladine, 2004).

Some intervention attempts show promise. A review of trials in which physicians briefly counseled nonpregnant women who were problem drinkers found no consistent decrease in drinking. Trials of personalized advice to pregnant women have also been found to be no more effective than written information alone. A written self-help manual, however, did improve cessation rates in women at a prenatal clinic. The CDC sponsored a pilot project to encourage alcohol cessation and effective contraception in women at risk for alcohol-exposed pregnancy (Muchowski and Paladine, 2004). Although not a controlled trial, this more extensive intervention showed promise. Of the 143 women enrolled, 68.5% had stopped their alcohol consumption or were using effective contraception by the 6-month follow-up. Women should not be discouraged from breastfeeding if they are not using illicit drugs and do not have specific contraindications such as HIV infection (McCarthy and Posey, 2000).

Applying the Evidence. Written information about the risks of alcohol use in pregnancy should be provided to pregnant women who consume alcohol (Floyd et al., 1999; Muchowski and Paladine, 2004). Data are insufficient to recommend physician counseling for alcohol cessation before or during pregnancy. More comprehensive interventions may be more effective but have yet to be fully studied.

No studies have evaluated neonatal outcomes with women counseled on alcohol cessation in the periconception period.

Emergency Contraception. The importance of making information and resources available for emergency contraception deserves more attention for women with addictions. Emergency contraception techniques are widely available and as OTC medications in some states. However, these are underused by women at risk for unintended pregnancy. An emergency hotline is available nationally for emergency contraception access for women: 888-NOT-2-LATE (888-668-2528) (http://not-2-late.com).

ADOLESCENTS

Family physicians should develop expertise for recognizing alcohol use in adolescents. According to the American Academy of Family Physicians Graham Center, 38% of ambulatory adolescent health visits in the United States are made to family physicians (American Academy of Family Physicians [AAFP], 2001). Specific screening tools are available for adolescents (Comerci, 2002). AUD in the family system can create several levels of dysfunction, including the use of alcohol or other drugs by adolescents. Approximately 3% of adolescents are addicted to alcohol or other drugs (National Institute on Alcohol Abuse and Alcoholism [NIAAA], 1997). Drinking is frequently a family matter, with 82% of drinking families raising children who drink and 72% of families who abstain raising children to abstain (Johnson and Leff, 1999). Environmental, physiologic, and genetic factors combine to place certain adolescents at risk.

Detection of AUD requires reliable information from the adolescent. An atmosphere of trust must be established, and more than one visit is often necessary. Urine drug screening can be effective but is controversial. The American Academy of Pediatrics (AAP) recommends involuntary testing only in limited emergency circumstances, such as altered mental status, inability to give consent (seizures, coma), acute medical problems putting the adolescent at serious risk, a preadolescent or very young adolescent, and court-ordered monitoring (AAP, 1998; Comerci, 2002). Family physician interventions for adolescents abusing alcohol or other substance must be tailored to the adolescent's specific needs. Appropriate treatment programs should have strong family involvement, total abstinence goals, and professionals experienced in adolescent care.

College student drinking is a major concern on U.S. campuses. An estimated 1700 unintentional college student deaths per year involve alcohol (Hingson et al., 2005). The NIAAA Task Force on College Drinking categorized college student drinking consequences as damage to self, others, or the institution as well as the overlapping categories of drinking and driving, high-risk sexual behavior, and physical and sexual aggression (NIAAA, 2002). College prevention strategies include cognitive-behavioral skills–based interventions, brief motivation interventions, feedback-only interventions, and environmental interventions. Underage drinking statutes, including penalties for servers, and comprehensive campus-community approaches that involve students, all campus stakeholders, and community leaders have proved beneficial (Larimer et al., 2009).

TREATMENT OF OLDER ADULTS

Alcohol use disorders and prescription drug abuse are prevalent in older adults (Blow et al., 2002). Specific "geriatric AUD" screening tests can be used by family physicians, including the SMAST-G, MAST-G, AUDIT, and CAGE (Blow et al., 2009). Older adults are often categorized as "binge drinkers." The NIAAA and the Centers for Substance Abuse Treatment (CSAT) have published alcohol use guidelines for older adults (National Institute on Alcohol Abuse and Alcoholism [NIAAA], 2008). Often, comorbid affective disorders are present in older adults. Premorbid AUDs predict a more severe course of affective disorders (Cook et al., 1991). Concomitant AUDs and depression increase late-life suicide risk, as does at-risk and problem drinking among elderly persons (Blow et al., 2004). Older persons with AUDs may respond well to brief interventions and increased socialization. The Guiding Older Adult Lifestyles (GOAL) study and Health Profile Project found brief interventions in older adults to be efficacious (Blow and Barry, 2000, 2009; NIAAA, 2008).

PHYSICIANS WITH ALCOHOL USE DISORDERS

See eAppendix 48-2 online.

Prevention

Primary prevention is the education of at-risk populations to avoid problems. Family physicians have the power to identify families with alcoholism and provide education to the children and adolescents who are at risk. Primary prevention includes the community; a Chinese proverb says the physician who also cares for the community is the "best physician." Family physicians can offer universal screening for alcoholism and AUD; this is an example of the secondary level of prevention in their practice. The evidence for effectiveness of "designated driver" and school-based drinking and driving prevention programs has been insufficient (Ditter et al., 2005). School prevention programs noted as effective include the Michigan Model for Comprehensive School Health Education (Shope et al., 1996).

PUBLIC POLICY RECOMMENDATIONS

Family physicians can affect public policy advocacy on issues of AUD through professional organizations such as the AAFP and state academies. The CDC (2004) recommends that states and local jurisdictions consider adoption of effective strategies aimed at reducing excessive drinking. Family physicians can advocate policies that include (but are not limited to) increasing alcohol excise taxes, reducing DUI limits to the 0.04 blood alcohol level, toughening DUI penalties, restricting advertising along highways or in ethnic minority communities, zoning restrictions on placement of points of sale, and increasing opportunities for screening in various settings (e.g., courts, jails, EDs).

Public policy interventions can be categorized as (1) measures to reduce the availability of alcohol, such as control of hours and days of sales, outlet-density restrictions, monopoly regulatory systems, and minimum-age drinking laws or as (2) penalties, such as increased DUI enforcement, server-liability laws, and altering the server environment through training. "Ecologic research" on environmental changes and prevention of AUD includes the Communities Mobilizing for Change on Alcohol Project, Community Trials Project, and Sacramento Neighborhood Alcohol Prevention Project (Treno et al., 2009). This emerging body of evidence should help communities in the future as they strive to create environments that reduce the frequency of AUDs.

Summary of Additional Online Content

The following content is available at www.expertconsult.com:

eAppendix 48-1, Causative Factors for Alcohol Use Disorders

eTable 48-1, Michigan Alcoholism Screening Test (MAST)

eTable 48-2, Alcohol Use Disorders Identification Test (AUDIT): Interview Version

eAppendix 48-2, Physicians with Alcohol Use Disorders

References

The complete reference list is available at www.expertconsult.com

Web Resources

www.AA.org Alcoholics Anonymous.

www.samhsa.gov/about-us/who-we-are/offices-centers/csat The Centers for Substance Abuse Treatment is part of Substance Abuse and Mental Health Services and offers resources for treatment guidelines of practical use to clinicians and treatment improvement protocols.

www.niaaa.nih.gov The National Institute on Alcohol Abuse and Alcoholism is a clearinghouse for information on alcohol use disorders and treatment resources and is part of the National Institutes of Health.

www.nida.nih.gov The National Institute on Drug Abuse is a clearinghouse for substance use disorders and offers benefits for dually dependent and dual-use disorder populations and is part of NIH.

www.samhsa.gov The Substance Abuse and Mental Health Services Administration has resources for mental health and substance use disorders.

49 *Nicotine Addiction*

ROBERT E. RAKEL and THOMAS HOUSTON

Overview

Key Points

- Tobacco use is the leading cause of death in the United States.
- Toxins from cigarette smoke cause disease in most organs of the body.
- Smokers die an average of 13 or 14 years earlier than nonsmokers, and 50% of continuing smokers will die of a tobacco-related disease.
- Smoking is responsible for 40% of all deaths from cancer and 21% of deaths from cardiovascular disease.
- Almost 10% of deaths attributable to smoking occur in nonsmokers exposed to secondhand smoke.

The power of nicotine addiction became clear when I saw malnourished and hungry people trading food rations for cigarettes.

—**WILLIAM FOEGE (1989), COMMENTING ON REFUGEE CAMPS DURING THE NIGERIAN CIVIL WAR**

Tobacco smoking leads to a dependence on nicotine that is indistinguishable from other forms of drug dependence. The *Diagnostic and Statistical Manual of Mental Disorders, Fifth Edition,* (DSM-5) classifies "tobacco abuse disorder" in the Substance Abuse Disorder category (APA, 2013). In such a dependency, the drug is needed to maintain an optimal state of well-being. *Nicotine,* the addictive constituent of tobacco, meets these criteria because a typical withdrawal syndrome occurs after smoking cessation; tolerance to its use develops; and most important, use persists after developing symptoms attributable to the substance and in the face of its known harm. Some believe that nicotine is more addicting than cocaine or alcohol (Kandel et al., 1997; Krasnegor, 1979; Lee and D'Alonzo, 1993).

Nicotine acts on specific $\alpha 4\beta 2$ nicotinic acetylcholine receptors in the mesocorticolimbic system through neural pathways that are now seen as a common pathway for addictive drugs. Nicotine modulates the release of dopamine in the brain's reward centers in the ventral tegmental area and the nucleus accumbens, decreasing the normal rate of degradation of dopamine as well. High concentrations of nicotine are delivered to the central nervous system (CNS) within seconds of a puff. Complete saturation of nicotinic receptors occurs with as few as three cigarettes and lasts as long as 3 hours (Brody et al., 2006).

It may take only one cigarette to hook an adolescent. About one fourth of young people experience a *first-inhalation relaxation experience* (FIRE) with their first cigarette, a large percentage of whom become addicted (DiFranza et al., 2007).

For tobacco-dependent persons, craving and withdrawal symptoms result when nicotine occupancy on receptors declines over time (e.g., during sleep at night). Relief from these symptoms requires that the smoker replenish the nicotine within the receptor as completely as possible, which is why the first cigarette of the morning is often the most "satisfying" to addicted smokers. Because the cigarette is the most efficient rapid-delivery device for nicotine and the concurrent relief of craving and withdrawal symptoms, physicians and patients need to understand that medicinal nicotine replacement products are quite inefficient, by comparison, delivering lower concentrations of nicotine and incompletely resolving cravings and nicotine withdrawal.

The sheer number of nicotine doses is also highly reinforcing. A typical one-pack-daily smoker receives about 100,000 reinforcing hits a year, much more than with cocaine or heroin (Brunton, 1999).

Smoking affects nearly every organ of the body. Active smoking is now causally associated with age-related macular degeneration, diabetes, colorectal cancer, liver cancer, adverse health outcomes in cancer patients and survivors, tuberculosis, erectile dysfunction, orofacial clefts in infants, ectopic pregnancy, rheumatoid arthritis, inflammation, and impaired immune function. In addition, exposure to secondhand smoke has now been causally associated with an increased risk for stroke (U.S. Department of Health and Human Services [USDHHS], 2014). Tobacco contributes to about 488,000 deaths annually in the United States (USDHHS, 2014) and has rightly been dubbed the "leading cause of death in the United States" (McGinnis and Foege, 1993; Mokdad et al., 2004). One third of these smoking-related deaths are from cardiovascular disease and cerebrovascular accident (CVA, stroke), 29% from lung cancer, 20% from chronic respiratory disease, and at least 8% from cancers other than lung (Figure 49-1). There are now 13 different cancers associated with smoking. The new report

ABOUT 443,000 U.S. DEATHS ATTRIBUTABLE
EACH YEAR TO CIGARETTE SMOKING*

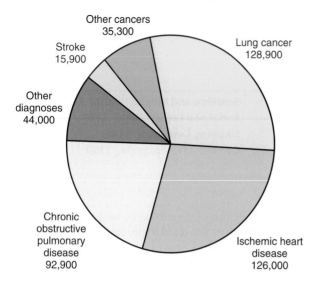

*Average annual number of deaths, 2000-2004.

Figure 49-1 Deaths attributable to smoking each year. (From Centers for Disease Control and Prevention Office on Smoking and Health. http://www.cdc.gov/tobacco/data_statistics/tables/index.htm.)

adds liver and colorectal cancer to that list. It also adds diabetes, rheumatoid arthritis, erectile dysfunction, impaired immune function, and cleft palate in infants (USDHHS, 2014). Just over 10% of deaths attributable to smoking occur in nonsmokers exposed to secondhand smoke, most from cardiovascular causes (Centers for Disease Control and Prevention [CDC], 2008). Each year, smoking is responsible for 18% of the total deaths in the United States—seven times more Americans than were killed in the Vietnam War. More than 10 times as many U.S. citizens have died prematurely from cigarette smoking than have died in all the wars fought by the United States during its history (USDHHS, 2014). Furthermore, cigarettes kill more Americans than alcohol, car accidents, suicide, AIDS, homicide, and illegal drugs combined (American Cancer Society [ACS], 2005).

As shown by the grim, disease-specific facts, most smokers do not understand the implications for longevity involved in continued tobacco use. On the average, male smokers in the United States die 13.2 years earlier and female smokers 14.5 years earlier than nonsmokers (Manson et al., 2000). Half of all continuing adult smokers will die of a cigarette-related illness (Doll et al., 2004). This relative lack of knowledge about tobacco harm may be in part because of the lack of publicity given to celebrities who die from smoking-related diseases (see eTable 49-1), although the death of news anchor Peter Jennings from lung cancer in 2005 received considerable attention and spurred increased interest in cessation.

The CDC (2012) estimated that in 2011, 19% of American adults smoked cigarettes (21.6% of men and 16.5% of women). Smoking prevalence is lowest among Asians (9.9%) and Hispanics (12.9%) and highest among American Indians and Alaska Natives (31.5%). Smoking prevalence is also higher among adults living below the poverty level (29%). Higher educational status confers additional protection against smoking, with persons holding a graduate degree smoking the least (5%). Thus, cigarette-related disease is increasingly becoming a set of afflictions suffered by the poor and undereducated, persons who understand the least about their risks and who have the poorest access to medical care resources (CDC, 2008).

Recent data show good news about teen smoking. The National Youth Tobacco Survey showed a drop in overall middle and high school youth tobacco use from 33.6% in 2000 to 20.4% in 2011; male use fell from 37.5% to 25.3%, and female use from 29.6% to 15.4%. Among non-Hispanic white youth, the drop went from 37.1% to 21.9%. Among black youth, tobacco use fell from 25.4% to 19.8%. About half of the current tobacco users consumed more than one form of tobacco (Arrazola et al., 2014). The tobacco industry spends more than $8 billion annually on marketing (>$24 million/day) (Campaign for Tobacco-Free Kids, 2013).

Although few people start smoking as adults, each day 4000 children and adolescents try smoking for the first time, and 3000 of them become regular users of tobacco. Half of high school seniors who smoke started by age 14 years. Most smokers start smoking before 18 years, and only 5% start after age 20 years. Each year, 70% of those who smoke say that they would like to stop, and about 50% attempt to quit, but fewer than 5% succeed (Fiore et al., 2008). The likelihood of success in smoking cessation increases with the number of attempts, and those with a college education are twice as likely to succeed as less educated smokers. Family physicians must view tobacco addiction as a chronic disease that requires frequent intervention.

Health Risks Associated with Smoking

Toxins from cigarette smoke go everywhere the blood goes and cause disease in almost every organ of the body.

CANCER

Key Points

- A dose-response relationship exists between the number of cigarettes smoked and the risk of cancer. For example, those smoking more than 1 pack a day have 20 times the lung cancer risk of nonsmokers.
- Smoking formerly labeled "low-tar" and "low-nicotine" cigarettes provides no benefit over smoking regular cigarettes.
- Fewer than half of all smoking deaths are from cancer; the rest are from heart disease, chronic lung disease, and stroke.
- Tobacco use increases the risk of cancer in most organs.

Table 49-1 Evidence-Based Relationship Between Smoking and Disease

The evidence is sufficient to infer a causal relationship between smoking and:	Cancer of the bladder, cervix, esophagus, kidney, larynx, lung, oral cavity, pharynx, pancreas, stomach Acute myeloid leukemia Abdominal aortic aneurysm Subclinical atherosclerosis Stroke (CVA) Coronary heart disease COPD Acute respiratory infections, including pneumonia Reduced lung function in infants Impaired lung growth during childhood and adolescence Respiratory symptoms in children and adolescents, including cough, phlegm, wheezing, and dyspnea Asthma-related symptoms (e.g., wheezing) in childhood and adolescence Premature onset of age-related decline in lung function All respiratory symptoms among adults, including coughing, phlegm, wheezing, and dyspnea Poor asthma control SIDS Reduced fertility in women Fetal growth restriction and low birth weight Premature rupture of membranes, placenta previa, and placental abruption Preterm delivery and shortened gestation Cataracts Increased absenteeism from work Adverse surgical outcomes related to wound healing and respiratory complications Hip fractures Low bone density in postmenopausal women Peptic ulcer disease
The evidence is suggestive of a causal relationship between smoking and:	Colorectal cancer Liver cancer Increased prostate cancer mortality Acute respiratory infections in persons with COPD Increased lower respiratory tract illnesses during infancy Impaired lung function in childhood and adulthood (with maternal smoking) Poorer prognosis for children and adolescents with asthma Increased nonspecific bronchial hyperresponsiveness Ectopic pregnancy Spontaneous abortion Cleft palate Low bone density in older men Dental caries Erectile dysfunction Macular degeneration Graves disease

COPD, Chronic obstructive pulmonary disease; *CVA,* cerebrovascular accident; *SIDS,* sudden infant death syndrome.
From U.S. Surgeon General. *The health consequences of smoking: a report of the Surgeon General, 2004.* Rockville, MD: U.S. Department of Health and Human Services, Public Health Service, Office of the Surgeon General; 2004.

About 30% of all cancer deaths are attributable to cigarette smoking. Table 49-1 lists diseases, including many cancers, for which the evidence is sufficient to *infer* a causal relationship, as well as those for which the evidence is sufficient only to *suggest* a causal relationship. Reviewing tobacco's role in carcinogenesis, Hecht (2008) discusses several mechanisms that contribute to cancer, including metabolic changes in DNA and formation of DNA-carcinogen adducts, leading to mutation, and inhibition of genes such as *p53,* a tumor suppressor; and mutations in the *K-RAS* oncogene (eFigure 49-1 online).

Lung

A clear dose-response relationship exists between lung cancer risk and daily cigarette consumption. From 1950 to 1990, the U.S. mortality rate for lung cancer increased four-fold for men and sevenfold for women. Although the mortality rates in men have been declining since 1990, lung cancer is still the principal cause of cancer death (28% of all cancer deaths) for both genders. In 1988, lung cancer passed breast cancer as the leading cause of death from cancer in women (Figures 49-2 and 49-3). For the first time ever, women are as likely as men to die from smoking-related diseases and they have about the same risk of death from lung cancer (USDHHS, 2014). Although the incidence rates have declined for most cancer sites, they are increasing for both men and women for melanoma and cancers of the liver and thyroid (see Figures 49-2 and 49-3). Although the incidence of squamous cell carcinoma of the lung declined as smoking rates dropped between 2000 and 2010, the incidence of adenocarcinoma of the lung increased dramatically. It is suggested that changes in the composition and design of the cigarette itself may have had some impact on the relative risk (RR) of lung cancer, as well as on the shift in the types of lung cancer occurring (Thun et al., 2013).

The 5-year survival rate for lung cancer is only 15% and has improved only slightly since the early 1960s (ACS, 2005). Almost 60% of lung cancer patients die from it within 1 year and 85% within 5 years. By the time the diagnosis is made, three of four patients already have metastases. However, the risk of death from lung cancer is substantially reduced when smoking is discontinued. Reducing smoking from an average of 20 cigarettes a day to less than 10 per day reduces the lung cancer risk by 25% (Godtfredsen et al., 2005). A diminished risk for lung cancer is experienced in former smokers after 5 years of cessation; however, the risk remains higher than that of nonsmokers for as long as 15 to 20 years (U.S. Surgeon General, 2004).

The U.S. Preventive Services Task Force (USPSTF) published draft recommendations (grade B) in August 2013 for early detection of lung cancer with annual low-dose computed tomography scans among high-risk smokers ages 55 to 79 years with a 30 pack-year history of smoking cigarettes, and less than 15 years since stopping smoking. The USPSTF's recommendations are based on evidence from clinical trials and modeling studies, finding that the benefit of early detection in this population of heavy smokers outweighs the risk of false positive findings and unnecessary further testing as well as radiation concerns. The USPSTF analysis shows a possible benefit as high as a 14% reduction in lung cancer mortality. Other groups, including the ACS, the American Thoracic Society, and the American College of Chest Physicians, have recently made similar recommendations (http://www.uspreventiveservicestaskforce.org/Page/Topic/recommendation-summary/lung-cancer-screening).

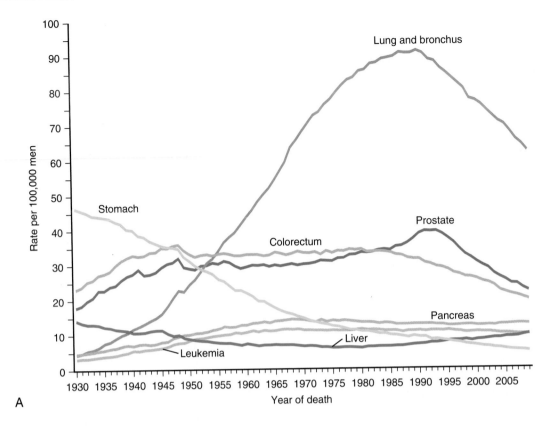

A

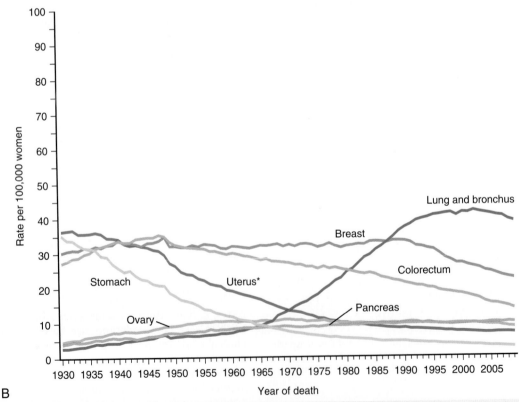

B

Figure 49-2 A, Trends in death rates among men for selected cancers, United States, 1930 to 2009. **B,** Trends in death rates among women for selected cancers, United States, 1930 to 2009. (Rates are age adjusted to the 2000 U.S. standard population.) *Asterisk* indicates that the uterus includes the uterine cervix and uterine corpus. Because of changes in International Classification of Diseases (ICD) coding, numerator information has changed over time. Rates for cancers of the uterus, ovary, lung and bronchus, and colon and rectum are affected by these changes. (From Siegel R, Naishadham MA, Jemal A. Cancer statistics, 2013. *CA Cancer J Clin.* 2013;63:11-30.)

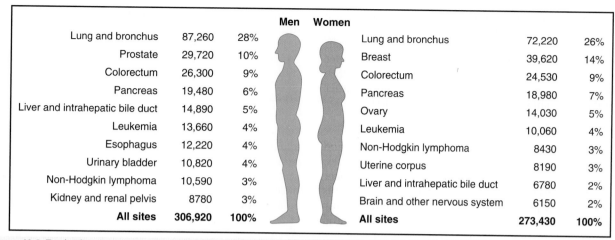

Men				Women		
Lung and bronchus	87,260	28%		Lung and bronchus	72,220	26%
Prostate	29,720	10%		Breast	39,620	14%
Colorectum	26,300	9%		Colorectum	24,530	9%
Pancreas	19,480	6%		Pancreas	18,980	7%
Liver and intrahepatic bile duct	14,890	5%		Ovary	14,030	5%
Leukemia	13,660	4%		Leukemia	10,060	4%
Esophagus	12,220	4%		Non-Hodgkin lymphoma	8430	3%
Urinary bladder	10,820	4%		Uterine corpus	8190	3%
Non-Hodgkin lymphoma	10,590	3%		Liver and intrahepatic bile duct	6780	2%
Kidney and renal pelvis	8780	3%		Brain and other nervous system	6150	2%
All sites	**306,920**	**100%**		**All sites**	**273,430**	**100%**

Figure 49-3 Ten leading cancer types for the estimated deaths by sex, United States, 2013. (Estimates are rounded to the nearest 10 and exclude basal cell and squamous cell skin cancers and in situ carcinoma except urinary bladder.) (From Siegel R, Naishadham MA, Jemal A. Cancer statistics, 2013. *CA Cancer J Clin.* 2013;63:11-30.)

Although the amount of tar in cigarettes has declined in recent years, the risk of lung cancer has not changed. Smoking formerly labeled "low-tar" and "low-nicotine" cigarettes provides no benefit over smoking regular cigarettes, and the uptake of carcinogens is no different in "regular," "light," and "ultralight" smokers (Hecht et al., 2005), as previously marketed. However, surveys show that most people believed "light" cigarettes to be less dangerous than regular cigarettes and regular cigarettes much more likely to cause illness. The recent federal legislation banning the use of words such as "light" from tobacco advertising is beginning to dispel this myth.

Increasing data regarding the genetic predisposition to lung cancer are emerging (see Smoking and Genetics, later in this chapter). Family aggregation related to lung cancer is likely multifactorial, including exposure to secondhand smoke, major genetic factors (e.g., chromosome 6p locus, *CYP1A1* gene), other genes that modify risk of lung cancer, and genes that may enhance nicotine addiction or modify nicotine metabolism (D'Amico, 2008; U.S. Surgeon General, 2004).

Larynx

The risk for laryngeal cancer is 20 to 30 times greater in smokers. About 70% of oral and 85% of laryngeal cancer deaths are directly attributable to smoking. The risks of cancer of the oral cavity, pharynx, and larynx drop sharply during the first 10 years after smoking cessation. There appears to be a synergistic, multiplicative effect between smoking and drinking, such that the risk for development of cancer of the larynx is as much as 75% higher in people who use tobacco and alcohol versus those exposed to either substance alone (U.S. Surgeon General, 1990, 2004).

Esophagus

Cigarette smoking is a casual factor in both squamous cell carcinoma and adenocarcinoma of the esophagus. Heavy smokers (>1 pack per day) have 10 times the mortality rate from esophageal cancer as do nonsmokers. Alcohol use is synergistic, with the combination of both heavy smoking and drinking greatly raising the risk of esophageal squamous cell carcinoma. This combination effect is stronger among men (Morita et al., 2010).

Head and Neck

Cancers of the head and neck account for about 5% of all cancers diagnosed and 3% of cancer deaths each year. Tobacco use, whether smoking or chewing, is a key causal factor, with excess risks ranging from five to 25 times that of persons not using tobacco. Smoking accounts for 45% to 75% of all head and neck cancers (Freedman et al., 2007). The risks are dose dependent, and concurrent alcohol use multiplies the risks of developing head and neck cancer.

Pancreas

An equally dismal picture occurs with cancer of the pancreas, for which the 5-year survival rate is only 2%. Because of the nonspecific nature of the initial symptoms and the difficulty in making a diagnosis, the mean survival time after diagnosis of pancreatic cancer is less than 6 months. Smokers have two to three times the risk of pancreatic cancer as nonsmokers, and the risk is proportional to the amount smoked. Increased risk persists at least 10 years after quitting. About one fourth of pancreatic cancer cases (20%-25%) are attributable to cigarette smoking (Maisonneuve and Lowenfels, 2010; U.S. Surgeon General, 2004).

Cervix, Uterus, and Ovary

Women who smoke cigarettes have four times the risk of cervical cancer as nonsmokers. Even women who smoke only 100 cigarettes during their lifetime more than double their risk of cervical cancer. The risk from smoking is greater in women younger than 30 years than in those older than 30 years (Slattery et al., 1989). Constituents from cigarette smoke, including mutagens and the carcinogen 4-(methylnitrosamino)-1-(3-pyridyl)-1-butanone (NNK), have been detected in the cervical mucus of smokers at levels 40 to 50 times those in serum. Smoking is a risk factor for cervical intraepithelial neoplasia (CIN) and cervical cancer among women who test positive as well as negative for human papillomavirus (HPV). The RRs for CIN and cervical cancer are two to four times greater for current and former smokers compared with never-smokers (U.S. Surgeon General, 2004). Although the risk of mucinous ovarian cancer has been shown to be as much as three times greater in women who smoke cigarettes (Qian et al., 1989; Tworoger et al., 2008), the evidence is inadequate to confer a causal relationship (U.S. Surgeon General, 2004).

Bladder and Kidney

Forty percent of bladder cancers are smoking related, and higher rates of kidney cancers are also noted in smokers. Smokers have two to four times the risk of bladder cancer as those who never smoked. The risk for kidney cancer is strongly dose dependent. Even one to nine cigarettes per day creates a 60% excess risk of renal cell cancer in men, and the risk doubles for men smoking more than one pack a day. Overall, the RR for women smokers is about 1.38 and 1.54 for men (Hunt et al., 2005). Smoking accounts for most cancers of the renal pelvis and ureter in the United States (McLaughlin et al., 1996; U.S. Surgeon General, 2004). The kidneys and bladder are the final common pathways for the concentration of toxic products of tobacco smoke and provide the longest direct exposure to carcinogens and radioactive substances, such as polonium 210, in tobacco smoke (Winters and DiFranza, 1982).

Colon and Rectum

A strong relationship has been noted between smoking and colorectal cancer, but the induction period is about 35 years. This lengthy induction would explain why it is just beginning to show up in women and indicates that efforts to prevent smoking among young people should be intensified (Giovannucci et al., 1994). The increased risk is about 20% higher for current smokers and appears to be stronger for rectal cancer. As with many other tobacco-related cancers, the risks are related to both intensity and duration of smoking, and decrease with early cessation. Although the evidence is suggestive but not conclusive, a causal relationship would mean that about 12% of the colorectal cancer burden would be attributable to smoking (Hannan et al., 2009; Tsoi et al., 2009; U.S. Surgeon General, 2004).

Liver

Although the 2004 Surgeon General's Report concludes that the relationship between smoking and liver cancer is suggestive but not causal, a meta-analysis from the World Health Organization International Agency for Research on Cancer found an RR of 1.55 among current smokers and 1.2 among former smokers for development of liver cancer (Lee et al., 2009). A recent European nested case-control study found that smoking had an increased risk for hepatocellular cancer (odds ratio [OR], 4.55 for current and 1.98 for former smokers) but a very high attributable risk (50%) as a contributing factor given the high smoking rates in the study population (Trichopoulos et al., 2011).

Leukemia

Overall, smoking cigarettes increases a person's risk for leukemia by 30%. The mortality rate from leukemia is increased 50% in cigarette smokers (RR, 1.53), the response is dose related, and the prognosis worsens for those with continued smoking after diagnosis and treatment. The risk is greatest for myeloid leukemia. The potent carcinogen *benzene*, a constituent of cigarette smoke, seems to be the major toxin responsible for leukemia among smokers. Approximately 14% of all cases of leukemia in the United States may be caused by cigarette smoking (Brownson et al., 1993).

Breast

Although smoking was not initially thought to be a risk factor for breast cancer, the evidence has grown over time and now suggests a causal relationship, particularly among women who start smoking early in life, are heavy smokers, and smoke for a long time. Both active and passive smoking have been implicated in breast cancer. This is still controversial, however, because some studies show the association to be quite small. The California Environmental Protection Agency and Canadian Task Force convened to study the problem both found significant relationships with both active and passive smoking, and the U.S. Surgeon General's report on passive smoking (USDHHS, 2006) found that mechanism to be suggestive (Reynolds, 2013).

Second Primary or Recurrent Cancers

Continued smoking interferes with both radiotherapy and chemotherapy used for cancer treatment. An increase in second primary tumors among continuing smokers is seen in lung (Lin et al., 2005) and head and neck cancer (Chuang et al., 2008). The emergence of contralateral breast cancer has also been linked to continued smoking among women (Li et al., 2009).

CHRONIC OBSTRUCTIVE PULMONARY DISEASE

> ### Key Points
>
> - Chronic obstructive pulmonary disease (COPD) is the leading cause of disability in the United States, and cigarette smoking is its main cause.
> - The risk of COPD is directly proportional to the number of cigarettes smoked, but lung function improves with cessation of smoking, even after age 60 years.

Cigarette smoking is the main cause of COPD, which includes emphysema and chronic bronchitis. COPD is the fourth leading cause of death and the leading cause of disability in the United States. Female smokers are 13 times more likely to die from COPD, and male smokers have about a 12-fold increased risk (U.S. Surgeon General, 2004). During their lifetimes, smokers have about a 40% chance of developing chronic bronchitis. There may also be important racial differences, with African Americans, particularly women, having a higher risk than white smokers (Dransfield et al., 2006; Pelkonen, 2008). COPD among women is rising more quickly than among men, and since 2000, more women than men have died each year from COPD (CDC, 2008). Patients who smoke and present with COPD are also at substantially higher risk for tobacco-related cancers.

Changes in bronchi and the lung parenchyma are proportional to the duration and intensity of smoking. Cigarette smoke inhibits ciliary activity of the bronchial epithelium and phagocytic activity of macrophages in the alveoli, resulting in decreased clearance of foreign material and bacteria from the lung, which leads to increased infection and tissue destruction. Smoking also releases inflammatory mediators, including oxidases and proteases, and inhibits pulmonary repair mechanisms. Even after age 60 years, smokers who quit have better pulmonary function than those who continue smoking. Lung function is inversely related to the number of cigarettes smoked over a lifetime. The rate of decline in pulmonary function is arrested by smoking cessation, the earlier the better.

CARDIOVASCULAR DISEASE

Key Points

- The risk of myocardial infarction (MI) is proportional to the number of cigarettes smoked.
- More than half of deaths from coronary artery disease are sudden, but the risk of sudden death is reduced immediately on cessation of smoking.
- Filter cigarettes and those with "low tar" or "low nicotine" do not reduce the risk of MI.

Coronary Heart Disease

Heart disease is the leading cause of death in the United States, and tobacco use is a major risk factor. Up to 30% of all deaths from heart disease are caused by smoking, with a strong dose-dependent relationship. In general, smokers have two to four times the risk of coronary heart disease as nonsmokers. For women smokers, the risk may be even higher. Women who smoke only one to five cigarettes a day have 2.5 times the risk of developing coronary heart disease as nonsmokers, rising to 75 times the risk in those who smoke 40 or more cigarettes a day. Three fourths of MIs in women younger than 50 years have been attributed to smoking (Dunn et al., 1999; Slone et al., 1978). Women who smoke and use oral contraceptives (OCs) have up to 10 times greater risk of heart attack than women who do neither, depending on which generation of OC is used.

Smoking acutely raises systolic blood pressure, heart rate, and cardiac output and causes vasoconstriction. It increases inflammation, promotes thrombosis and platelet aggregation, increases atherogenesis and plaque destabilization, and promotes oxidation of low-density lipoproteins (LDLs). Both active and secondhand smoke exposure cause endothelial dysfunction, a key element in early atherogenesis. Increased levels of C-reactive protein (CRP) are found in smokers, and the low-grade inflammatory response associated with smoking also results in increased leukocyte counts. Increased blood viscosity and lower oxygen-carrying capacity from carbon monoxide (CO) in cigarette smoke further decrease the coronary reserve. CO has an affinity for hemoglobin (forming carboxyhemoglobin) that is 245 times stronger than that of oxygen. Thus, CO reduces oxygen delivery to the myocardium and has a decidedly negative inotropic effect. Carboxyhemoglobin also lowers the threshold for ventricular fibrillation and could help explain the higher incidence of sudden death in those who smoke.

More than half of all deaths from coronary heart disease are sudden deaths caused by cardiac arrhythmia. Nicotine is arrhythmogenic because it increases serum catecholamine concentration. Those who quit smoking reduce their risk of sudden death immediately; the decline is not time dependent (Goldenberg et al., 2003). The risk of sudden cardiac death from smoking applies to both men and women.

The risk of MI is proportional to the number of cigarettes smoked, but as few as one to four cigarettes a day raises the risk of dying from ischemic heart disease by 2.7 times in men and 2.9 times in women (Bjartveit and Tverdal, 2005). The risk of MI increases progressively to as much as 20-fold in persons smoking 35 or more cigarettes per day. Persons who smoke cigarettes containing "low" amounts of nicotine have the same degree of MI risk as those who smoke cigarettes containing larger amounts. Smokers of these "low-dose" cigarettes still have three times the MI risk as nonsmokers (Kaufman et al., 1983).

It has been observed that smoking seems to confer a protective effect on mortality after the first nonfatal heart attack, the so-called "smoker's paradox." This phenomenon may be explained by differentials in age (first MI 12-14 years earlier among smokers) and fewer other comorbid factors such as diabetes and hypertension. On the other hand, continued smoking in this group is associated with more frequent recurrence of cardiac events and lower long-term survival.

Continued smoking after coronary stent placement is an independent risk factor for restenosis, as well as for repeat thrombosis after coronary artery bypass graft surgery.

Within a few years of stopping, the risk of MI in men decreases to a level similar to that in men who have never smoked, even in heavy smokers who have a positive family history of coronary heart disease (Rosenberg et al., 1985). The risk of coronary heart disease is reduced by about half after the first year of cessation, falling to that of never-smokers after 15 years of abstinence (U.S. Surgeon General, 1990). Those who have coronary heart disease and stop smoking have a reduction of about 36% in both all-cause mortality and nonfatal MI (Crichley and Capewell, 2004). Women who follow lifestyle guidelines involving diet, exercise, and not smoking have a very low risk of coronary heart disease (Stampfer et al., 2000).

"Silent" ischemia probably accounts for most cardiac ischemic events. Patients with coronary heart disease who smoke have three times as many episodes of silent ischemia as nonsmokers, and the duration of each is 12 times longer (Barry et al., 1989). Frequent episodes of myocardial ischemia, even though asymptomatic, must damage the heart. Because smoking also increases platelet adhesiveness, increases levels of triglycerides and LDL cholesterol, and lowers high-density lipoprotein cholesterol, a higher incidence of MI would be expected (Chelland et al., 2008).

Benefits from stopping smoking can be demonstrated at all ages. No decrease in benefit is seen with age, so it is still worthwhile for someone older than 65 years of age to break the addiction. Men who continue smoking in their 70s are 50% more likely to die from cancer, cardiovascular disease, and respiratory disease compared with those who never smoked. (Hermanson et al., 1988; LaCroix et al., 1991).

Stroke (Cerebrovascular Accident)

Key Points

- Risk of stroke is six times greater in smokers (>1 pack/day).
- Smokers who are also hypertensive have a 20 times greater stroke risk.
- The risk of CVA declines rapidly after smoking cessation and at 5 years is the same as for a nonsmoker.
- Exposure to secondhand smoke increases the risk for stroke by an estimated 20% to 30% (USDHHS, 2014).

Stroke (CVA) is the third most common cause of death in the United States. Although hypertension is the greatest risk factor for stroke, cigarette smoking is also significant. The incidence of stroke in smokers is two to four times higher than in nonsmokers. Among those screened in the Multiple Risk Factor Intervention Trial (MRFIT), smokers had twice the risk of a nonhemorrhagic stroke, and smoking was strongly associated with all forms of stroke (Neaton et al., 1993). A more recent systematic review and meta-analysis published in 2013 also concluded that smoking about doubles the lifetime risk of stroke and that the risk for ischemic stroke is similar among men and women. For hemorrhagic stroke however, the risk among women was 17% higher than men who smoked (Peters et al., 2013).

The risk of stroke increases in proportion to the amount of smoking. Those who smoke more than 40 cigarettes a day have twice the stroke risk of those who smoke fewer than 10 cigarettes a day. Compared with women who have never smoked, the risk of stroke increases 2.2-fold in women smoking 1 to 14 cigarettes a day and 3.7-fold in women smoking 25 or more cigarettes a day (Colditz et al., 1988). Noting a clear dose-response relationship, Bonita and associates (1986) found a threefold increase in the risk of stroke in smokers versus nonsmokers (see eFigure 49-2 online). The risk is 5.6 times higher in persons smoking more than one pack daily. Cigarette smokers who are also hypertensive have a 20-fold increased risk of stroke (U.S. Surgeon General, 2004).

Sclerosis of the carotid arteries is directly proportional to the amount of smoke exposure. Smoking increases the risk of ischemic heart disease and cerebrovascular disease regardless of the level of serum cholesterol. A low cholesterol level did not protect against smoking-related arteriosclerotic cardiovascular disease in patients in South Korea, where the prevalence of smoking is among the highest in the world (72% of men) (Jee et al., 1999). Smoking may increase the likelihood of thrombosis by increasing serum fibrinogen, enhancing platelet aggregation, and increasing blood viscosity.

The risk of stroke declines rapidly after cessation of smoking. Older adults who stop smoking have significantly higher cerebral perfusion levels than those who continue to smoke. Even those who have smoked for 30 to 40 years have improved cerebral circulation within a relatively short time after stopping smoking (Rogers et al., 1985).

After 5 years, risk of CVA is at the level of nonsmokers, which emphasizes that "it is never too late to quit," no matter how long the patient has been smoking.

Subarachnoid Hemorrhage

A recent systematic review of the risk factors for subarachnoid hemorrhage (SAH) shows that smoking doubles the risk for SAH (Feigin et al., 2005). About one third of all SAH was found to be attributable to smoking in a smaller case-control study, and although the risk dropped within a few years after quitting, it may remain increased for up to 15 years in the heaviest female smokers (Anderson et al., 2004). For SAH associated with cerebral aneurism, smoking increases the risk of bleeding three to six times.

Older studies involving high-dose estrogen OCs showed a significant interaction with smoking, increasing the risk for stroke and SAH among women who both smoked and used OCs. Studies of women who use second- and third-generation OCs find no increased risk of stroke, even among smokers (Yang et al., 2009). However, the American College of Obstetricians and Gynecologists (2006) states that "practitioners should prescribe combination hormonal contraceptives with caution, if at all, to women older than 35 years who smoke." The overall mortality RR among OC users who smoke 15 or more cigarettes a day was 2.25 in a large cohort study (Vessey et al., 2010).

PERIPHERAL VASCULAR DISEASE

Smoking is strongly associated with other forms of cardiovascular disease, including abdominal aortic aneurysm (AAA) and peripheral vascular disease, in both men and women. Smoking causes as much as half of all peripheral artery disease and significantly increases the failure rates after lower-limb bypass surgery. As with coronary artery disease, secondhand smoke exposure is also associated with intermittent claudication. The risk of AAA rises in proportion to the duration and intensity of smoking and is up to sevenfold greater at 20 pack-years (U.S. Surgeon General, 2004). The USPSTF has recommended one-time screening for AAA by ultrasonography in men age 65 to 75 years who have ever smoked, including men who only smoked pipes or cigars. Consideration should also be given for screening women older than age 65 years with a history of smoking (Derubertis et al., 2007) because about 40% of the annual deaths from AAA occur among women, in whom the disease is more deadly than men. Smoking is also an independent risk factor for erectile dysfunction, an additional fact that may help motivate men to stop smoking.

Other Diseases and Conditions

Alzheimer Disease

Studies show conflicting evidence linking smoking with Alzheimer dementia and other causes of cognitive decline. However, a meta-analysis found that compared with never-smokers, current smokers had RRs of 1.79 for Alzheimer disease (AD) and 1.78 for vascular dementia. Smokers in this study also had greater yearly declines in Mini–Mental State Examination (Anstey et al., 2007). Another systematic review and meta-analysis also found significant risk for AD among smokers (RR, 1.59), as well as elevated risk for developing vascular dementia (1.35) and cognitive decline (1.20) compared with never-smokers (Peters et al., 2008).

Indeed, the risk of cognitive decline may begin among smokers as early as age 35 years, joining diabetes and age as variables in the Framingham Risk Score that impact cognitive function as well as heart disease (Jooseten et al., 2013).

Graves Disease

Smoking appears to be one of the many factors causing Graves disease, particularly among women, and includes a higher risk of Graves ophthalmopathy as well (Vestergaard, 2002).

Diabetes Mellitus

Diabetes is a rapidly growing worldwide pandemic, and cigarette smoking is responsible for about 10% of the incidence of type 2 diabetes. The risk of developing type 2 diabetes is 30% to 40% higher for active smokers than nonsmokers, and the risk is proportional to the number of cigarettes smoked. Smoking promotes central obesity, which is a well-established risk factor for insulin resistance and diabetes (USDHHS, 2014). People who smoke more than one pack a day have about double the risk for type 2 diabetes as nonsmokers, and the risk is still 1.5 times greater for those who smoke only 1 to 14 cigarettes a day (Manson et al., 2000; Willi et al., 2007). A recent meta-analysis examined the risk of secondhand smoke exposure and development of type 2 diabetes, finding a 28% increased risk for exposed individuals (Wang et al., 2013).

Smoking increases the risk for development of the metabolic syndrome and its attendant cardiovascular consequences (Chiolero et al., 2008).

Patients with diabetes who smoke are at increased risk for both micro- and macrovascular complications. Cigarette smoking increases the risk for diabetic nephropathy, retinopathy, and neuropathy. This association is strongest in patients requiring insulin for control. Stopping smoking reduces the risk of developing diabetes and is essential for preventing diabetic complications.

Depression

Smokers are more likely to experience major depression than nonsmokers, and the incidence increases steadily with the number of cigarettes smoked. This increased risk may result from genes that predispose to both conditions (Kendler et al., 1993). Smoking may predispose to depression and, conversely, may be an antecedent to smoking in the adolescent population (Brook et al., 2004; Goodman and Capitman, 2000).

Wrinkles

We are not very effective in getting the message about tobacco's hazards across to adolescents. By talking about disease, we may not be speaking their language. The fact that smoking causes wrinkles, bad breath, and yellow teeth may be a more effective message than evidence that smoking kills. Premature wrinkling (crow's feet) increases with the number of cigarettes smoked; heavy smokers are five times more likely to have wrinkles than nonsmokers (Kadunce et al., 1991).

Macular Degeneration and Cataract

Macular degeneration is the leading cause of blindness after age 65 years, and nothing prevents or delays its progression. Smoking 20 or more cigarettes a day increases the risk of macular degeneration two- to threefold. As with other smoking-related disorders, macular degeneration also appears to be dose related, with the incidence increasing with the number of pack-years (Christen et al., 1996; Thornton et al., 2005). Smoking is also a cause of nuclear cataract, with smokers having two to three times the risk of never-smokers.

Other

Smoking is a cause of rheumatoid arthritis, and it interferes with the effectiveness of certain treatments. Smoking increases the risk for tuberculosis and for dying from tuberculosis (USDHHS, 2014).

THE MYTH OF FILTERED CIGARETTES

There is a mistaken popular belief that filtered brands of cigarettes, which now account for more than 97% of those sold in the United States, are safer than nonfiltered cigarettes and that formerly labeled "light" cigarettes convey a degree of health protection. "Low-tar" and "low-nicotine" filtered cigarettes are now the most commonly purchased products. Because the addiction is to nicotine, people who smoke low-nicotine cigarettes undergo "compensatory smoking," in which they inhale more frequently and more deeply to maintain their blood nicotine levels. As a result, tar intake increases, so the cigarette changes from the low-tar to the high-tar category. Smokers who take 14 puffs per cigarette inhale 58% more tar than those taking the standard 8.7 puffs per cigarette. Most manufacturers create tiny perforations in the filter to dilute the smoke with air, thus creating their "light" and "ultralight" cigarettes. Many smokers, however, block the holes with their lips or their fingers to obtain undiluted smoke with a higher concentration of nicotine (Kozlowski et al., 1980).

Cigarettes with reduced yields of nicotine and CO are not safer. The fourfold increased risk of MI does not vary according to the nicotine content. The degree of risk is proportional to the number of cigarettes smoked (Palmer et al., 1989). Similar myths about "natural" and "organic" cigarettes should be dispelled because there is absolutely no evidence that these tobacco products confer any health protection compared with other brands.

CIGARS

Key Points

- Cigars are not a safe alternative to cigarettes and cause both cancer and heart disease.
- Cigar-related health risks are related to number smoked and depth of inhalation.
- The risk of tobacco-related disease is increased when smoking is combined with alcohol consumption.

In 2012, the CDC estimated that about 9.1% of men and 2.0% of women, and 12.6% of students in grades 9-12 were current cigar smokers (CDC, 2013) The mortality patterns from cigar smoking relate in part to the degree of inhalation by the smoker. Primary cigar smokers, or those who have never or rarely smoked cigarettes, inhale much less than secondary cigar smokers—those who have switched from or are concurrent cigarette smokers. The main reason for the difference is the pH of the smoke, which in cigars is higher than in cigarettes, allowing nicotine to be absorbed across the oral mucosa. Secondary cigar smokers, however, have learned to inhale smoke, increasing their risk of cancer and heart disease.

Cigar smokers have a risk of oral and pharyngeal cancer that is similar to cigarette smokers; their risk of esophageal cancer is several times that of never-smokers. As with cigarette smoking, the use of alcohol multiplies the risk of these cancers, accounting for about 75% of cases in developed nations (Pelucci et al., 2008).

Lung cancer risk varies with depth of inhalation and number of cigars per day. Primary cigar smokers with no or slight inhalation have about a 1.8 mortality ratio of lung cancer; moderate-deep inhalers increase this to 4.9, with an overall mortality ratio of 2.11 compared with nonsmokers. Secondary cigar smokers have a mortality ratio of 5.4; moderate-deep inhalers in this group increase the risk to 9.77. Combined cigarette–cigar smokers have an overall lung cancer mortality ratio of 11.20 (National Cancer Institute (NCI), 1998).

Cigar smokers are also at higher risk for both COPD (RR, 1.45) and coronary artery disease (RR, 1.27) compared with nonsmokers (Iribarren et al., 1999). As with the cancer risk, the level of inhalation increases risk; for example, secondary cigar smokers with moderate-deep inhalation patterns have a fivefold increased risk for COPD (NCI, 1998).

ELECTRONIC CIGARETTES

Electronic cigarettes (e-cigarettes), first developed in China in 2003, consist of a metal tube resembling a normal cigarette; a battery; an atomizer; and a replaceable cartridge containing liquid nicotine, propylene glycol, and flavoring. Examples of flavorings are chocolate, cherry, and bubblegum, all of which can be enticing to children. When a user puffs on the e-cigarette (called vaping), an indicator light at the tip glows, and the heating element vaporizes the solution from the cartridge containing nicotine and other substances. A mist is produced that is similar to cigarette smoke and contains the propylene glycol, a known pulmonary irritant used in antifreeze. Although a few other compounds, including acetaldehyde, benzene, cadmium, formaldehyde, lead, and contaminants such as metallic particles, have been found in the vapor, they are at much lower concentrations than in conventional cigarettes. Toxicology studies, however, are not yet available, and the health effects of long-term use are unknown.

Sales of these devices have grown rapidly, both through the Internet and increasingly at convenience stores and gas stations in the United States, with projections of $1 billion or more in sales by 2014. All of the major traditional cigarette companies have now entered the e-cigarette market and see this as a growing slice of the nicotine business through which to market new products. Television is again seeing ads for these new nicotine delivery devices. Youth uptake of e-cigarettes, although less than for conventional cigarettes, is increasing. Data from the 2012 National Youth Tobacco Survey show that the percentage of high school students who reported ever using an e-cigarette rose from 4.7% in 2011 to 10.0% in 2012. In the same time period, high school students using e-cigarettes within the past 30 days rose from 1.5% to 2.8%. Use also doubled among middle school students. Altogether, in 2012 more than 1.78 million middle and high school students nationwide had tried e-cigarettes.

Many questions remain unanswered about e-cigarettes, including whether they will help current smokers quit or lead to "dual use" and perpetuate nicotine dependence. Early studies have not shown them to be very effective for cessation. Adolescents who use e-cigarettes have an increased likelihood of smoking conventional cigarettes and are also more likely to smoke heavily.

Many states do not restrict the sale of e-cigarettes to minors. There has been a surge in the number of calls to poison control centers. More than half of the calls involve children five years of age and younger, with the most common symptoms being nausea and vomiting. The nicotine-containing liquid can be purchased in bulk (up to a gallon) and can cause vomiting and seizures when ingested or absorbed through the skin. A single teaspoon of the highly concentrated form can kill a small child.

SMOKELESS TOBACCO

Key Points

- Snuff users have a 50-fold increased risk of cancer of the cheek and gum.
- The carcinogens in smokeless tobacco have a greater concentration than in cigarette tobacco; the level of nitrosamines is more than 14,000 times that allowed in bacon and beer.

Smokeless tobacco comes in two types: *snuff*, which is dry or moist, and *chewing* (spitting) tobacco, which comes as a loose leaf, plug, or twist. Smokeless tobacco contains many of the same carcinogens as cigarette tobacco, but some are present in much greater concentrations. *Nitrosamines*, which are powerful chemical carcinogens, are present at levels up to 14,000 times higher than the federal government allows in bacon and beer (Connolly et al., 1986).

A variation on smokeless tobacco is called *snus*, which contains powdered, flavored tobacco in small satchets placed under the lip, releasing nicotine through the buccal mucosa. Because of differences in manufacturing, snus has comparatively small levels of the carcinogenic compounds found in traditional smokeless products. No spitting is required. Snus marketing campaigns emphasize its use when smoking is not allowed, and most U.S. snus users also smoke cigarettes. In Sweden, snus use has eclipsed smoking, and many smokers have used snus to quit smoking but have continued using snus, and many appear to be dependent. Again, in the United States, this has sparked a fierce debate about the use of snus and similar products as agents for "harm reduction," and whether smokers should be advised to switch as a means of smoking cessation because exclusive smokeless tobacco use avoids many of the dangers of combustible tobacco.

Treatment of smokeless tobacco use is difficult because none of the standard medications used for smoking cessation have shown effectiveness for smokeless tobacco users, although behavioral counseling has a modest effect (Fiore et al., 2008). The nicotine patch and lozenge have been suggested, and clinical trials of combination therapy are ongoing. Behavioral interventions such as mailings, oral or dental screenings, group discussions, workplace interventions, and telephone support showed the best evidence for smokeless tobacco cessation (SOR: B). There was no benefit from the use of bupropion sustained release (SR) or nicotine patches or gum (Cayley, 2009; SOR: A).

Use of smokeless tobacco increases the frequency of oropharyngeal cancer and causes gum recession and tooth loss. Overall, the RR for oral cancer among snuff users is 2.6; for esophageal and pancreatic cancer, it is 1.6 (Boffetta et al., 2008). Leukoplakia is found in 18% to 64% of users (Connolly et al., 1986). Snus has been associated with a higher risk of oropharyngeal cancer in some studies (Roosar et al., 2008) but not others (Luo et al., 2007) and has a small risk of pancreatic cancer. A systematic review and meta-analysis of the risk for MI and stroke among current smokeless tobacco users found small increases in RR for these conditions (Boffetta and Straif, 2009).

Although educational programs have been launched by the National Cancer Institute and Major League Baseball, smokeless tobacco use has trended upward in adolescents. College athletes often believe that male peers, coaches, and professional athletes are indifferent to the use of spitting tobacco (Hilton et al., 1994). An estimated 8.6% of high school students use smokeless tobacco, and its use is more common among high school boys (14%) than girls (2.2%). As with college students, many high school spit tobacco users participate in organized sports. Enlisting the support of coaches to help with tobacco use prevention is an untapped resource that should be explored.

INVOLUNTARY (PASSIVE) SMOKING

Key Points

- Secondhand smoke contains 7000 different chemicals, of which more than 70 are carcinogenic.
- About one third of lung cancers occur in nonsmokers who live with a smoker or work in a smoky environment.
- Passive smoking is the third leading preventable cause of death, after alcohol and smoking itself.
- Passive smoking increases the risk of sudden infant death syndrome (SIDS) in infants and otitis media, cancer, and respiratory disease in older children, in direct proportion to smoke exposure.

Secondhand smoke, also called *environmental tobacco smoke* (ETS), is the combination of smoke emitted from the burning end of a cigarette, cigar, or pipe and the smoke exhaled by a smoker. Two thirds of the smoke from a burning cigarette never reaches a smoker's lungs but instead goes directly into the air. *Sidestream smoke* is emitted into the air from a smoldering cigarette or cigar between puffs, and *mainstream smoke* is what the smoker inhales directly; the exhaled smoke also contributes to ETS. Although diluted by air before being inhaled, sidestream smoke contains greater concentrations of toxic substances than mainstream smoke because of a lower combustion temperature and lack of filtration through the cigarette.

The 2006 Report of the Surgeon General, *The Health Consequences of Involuntary Exposure to Tobacco Smoke* (USDHHS, 2006), concludes the following:

1. Secondhand smoke causes premature death and disease in children and adults who do not smoke.
2. Children exposed to secondhand smoke are at increased risk for SIDS, acute respiratory infections, ear problems, and more severe asthma. Smoking by parents causes respiratory symptoms and slows lung growth in their children.
3. Exposure of adults to secondhand smoke has immediate adverse effects on the cardiovascular system and causes coronary heart disease and lung cancer.
4. The scientific evidence indicates that there is no risk-free level of exposure to secondhand smoke.
5. Eliminating smoking in indoor spaces fully protects nonsmokers from exposure to secondhand smoke. Separating smokers from nonsmokers, cleaning the air, and ventilating buildings cannot eliminate exposures of nonsmokers to secondhand smoke.

Tobacco smoke contains more than 7000 different chemicals, at least 70 of which are known carcinogens. Nonsmokers exposed to secondhand smoke at home or at work increase their risk of lung cancer by 20% to 30% (USDHHS, 2014). The U.S. Environmental Protection Agency, (EPA) National Toxicology Program, U.S. Surgeon General, and International Agency for Research on Cancer have determined that environmental tobacco smoke is a class A (known) human carcinogen, in the same class as asbestos, mustard gas, arsenic, and benzene. In addition to the 3000 lung cancer deaths a year in nonsmokers, almost 40,000 heart disease deaths each year are linked to secondhand smoke. Secondhand smoke exposure also causes chronic otitis media, cough, and lower respiratory illnesses in children (e.g., asthma, bronchitis, pneumonia). It is estimated that tobacco smoke in the home and workplace could be responsible for the deaths of about 50,000 nonsmokers annually in the United States, making passive smoking the third leading preventable cause of death, after those from direct smoking and alcohol (Air Resources Board, 2005).

In a classic study, Hirayama (1981) was among the first scientists to demonstrate an increased risk of lung cancer in nonsmoking housewives exposed to the secondhand cigarette smoke of their husbands (see eFigure 49-3 online). Since then, many studies have shown an association between being married to a smoker and having an increased risk of lung cancer. The overall risk of lung cancer increases 20% to 30% in nonsmokers exposed to ETS in the home; combined home and work exposure further increases the risk (USDHHS, 2006).

A report from the California EPA's Air Resources Board is another well-researched review of the health effects of passive smoking. Their meta-analyses of the breast cancer risk indicate that the RR for breast cancer, particularly among premenopausal women, is between 1.68 and 2.20 (Air Resources Board, 2005; Miller et al., 2006). A 2009 Canadian task force report found a causal link between passive smoke exposure and breast cancer, especially in younger, premenopausal women, and a causal relationship between active smoking and breast cancer at all ages (Johnson et al., 2011). A meta-analysis of case-control studies found a significant relationship between passive smoke exposure and cervical cancer, with a 73% increased risk among exposed nonsmoking women (Zeng et al., 2012). It is estimated that the risk of MI is up to 70% greater for a woman whose husband smokes (Wells, 1994). RR estimates from meta-analysis indicate a 25% to 30% increase in the risk for coronary heart disease in exposed nonsmokers; as with lung cancer, multiple sites of exposure increase the risk (USDHHS, 2006). The cardiovascular effects of even brief exposure to secondhand smoke are often nearly as great as those of direct smoking, with platelet aggregation and arterial endothelial damage occurring within 30 minutes of exposure; furthermore, secondhand smoke induces oxidative stress and promotes vascular inflammation (Barnoya and Glantz, 2005). Exposure to secondhand smoke is associated with increased levels of inflammatory markers related to the development of atherosclerosis. People exposed have higher white blood cell counts and elevated CRP levels, oxidized LDL cholesterol, homocysteine, and fibrinogen. Even occasional exposure results in elevated levels. These increases are similar to those seen in active smokers.

Reports show that the health benefits of banning smoking in public places and the workplace include a reduction in heart attacks. Examination of community MI rates after implementation of strong smoke-free legislation found a pooled random-effects estimate of the rate of acute MI hospitalization 12 months later to be 0.83 (95% confidence interval, 0.80-0.87), with growth of this benefit expected over time (Lightwood and Glantz, 2009). With similar findings, systematic review and meta-analysis of 10 locations with smoke-free legislation concluded that the acute MI risk decreased by 17% overall, with the greatest effect in younger individuals and nonsmokers (Meyers et al., 2009).

Secondhand Smoke: Effects on Children

More than 50% of children younger than 5 years of age live in homes with at least one adult smoker. Children of smoking parents have more bronchitis and pneumonia during their first year of life and more otitis media when older. They have increased incidence of cough, bronchitis, and pneumonia proportional to the number of cigarettes smoked by the parents, particularly the mother. In fact, children of parents who smoke at least a half-pack a day have almost twice the risk of hospitalization for a respiratory illness. Secondhand smoke causes new-onset asthma in exposed children, and young persons with asthma have more asthma episodes (Charlton, 1994; Rantakallio, 1978; USHHS, 2006).

Passive smoking also increases the risk of sudden infant death syndrome. Infants exposed to secondhand smoke have twice the risk of SIDS, and infants whose mothers smoke before and after birth are three to four times more likely to die from SIDS (USDHHS, 2014).

Small children are victimized more by passive smoking than adults. Because of their more rapid breathing, children inhale larger amounts of harmful substances. Children exposed to their parents' cigarette smoke have six times the average number of respiratory infections. They also have deficits in growth and in intellectual and emotional development, as well as more behavior disorders, such as hyperactivity.

Physicians and health care providers who care for children should advise parents to quit smoking to limit their children's exposure to secondhand smoke and should advocate for smoke-free indoor air both at home and in cars when children are passengers because these two locations account for the majority of childhood exposure to secondhand smoke.

Thirdhand Smoke

Thirdhand smoke occurs when cigarette smoke reacts with nitrous acid on surfaces to form *tobacco-specific nitrosamines* (TSNAs). Nitrous acid is a common indoor pollutant and, when combined with cigarette smoke, forms a carcinogen that becomes more potent over time. Thus, nicotine is converted to a dangerous carcinogen after it is absorbed on indoor surfaces in automobiles and furniture. This can be especially hazardous to infants and children who live close to the floor because the TSNAs are especially concentrated in dust and carpeting. Smokers may believe that smoking only when others are not present (e.g., in car or home) creates no risk to nonsmokers who arrive later. In fact, the smoke clings to upholstery, cotton, and carpeting and actually builds up over time, exposing nonsmokers to potent carcinogens. This thirdhand smoke can be especially dangerous because TSNAs cannot be simply inactivated by dry cleaning or washing with soap and water. Most soaps are alkaline, and cleansers that dissolve nicotine must be acidic. Thus, it is almost impossible to remove TSNAs from carpeting, which will continuously uptake nicotine. Even washing smooth stone and metal with an alkaline soap will not remove nicotine residue (Dreyfuss, 2010; Sleiman et al., 2010).

PREGNANCY

See eAppendix 49-1 online.

Key Points

- The more a pregnant woman smokes, the greater the risk of premature delivery and low-birth-weight infants unless she stops smoking by the fourth month of gestation.
- Smoking during pregnancy increases the risk of congenital abnormalities, mental retardation, learning problems, and attention-deficit hyperactivity disorder (ADHD).
- The risk is increased for spontaneous abortion, placenta previa, and premature rupture of membranes.
- Reduced fertility is proportional to the number of cigarettes smoked.

KEY TREATMENT

- Because of the serious risks of smoking to the pregnant smoker and the fetus, whenever possible, pregnant smokers should be offered person-to-person psychosocial interventions that exceed minimal advice to quit (Fiore et al., 2008) (SOR: A).

- Although abstinence early in pregnancy will produce the greatest benefits to the fetus and expectant mother, quitting at any point in pregnancy can yield benefits. Therefore, physicians should offer effective tobacco-dependence interventions to pregnant smokers at the first prenatal visit and throughout pregnancy (Fiore et al., 2008) (SOR: B).

Smoking and Mental Health

Mental illness with substance abuse puts patients at particular risk for dying of tobacco-related illness because they are more likely to smoke and to smoke more heavily than others in the population. Patients with psychiatric illness consume up to 70% of the cigarettes smoked in the United States, with two to four times the general prevalence of smoking (Grant et al., 2004; Kalman et al., 2005). Among mentally ill and substance-abusing patients, as many as 200,000 die each year from tobacco-related causes—almost half the total U.S. tobacco-related mortality (Williams et al., 2004). Individuals in this special population of smokers do express strong interest in quitting smoking, however. Counseling and pharmacology that is useful with other smokers is effective in mentally ill and substance-abusing patients who smoke (Ranney et al., 2006), and just as with other smokers, this part of their health care must not be neglected.

Social and Legal Action

See eAppendix 49-2 online.

Smoking Cessation

Key Points

- Patients who smoke should receive advice and encouragement to stop at every visit.
- Take advantage of the teachable moment, when a patient who smokes is being treated for any medical condition.
- Multiple strategies and persistence are usually needed for successful cessation because tobacco dependence is a chronic disease.
- Brief counseling, usually lasting less than 3 minutes, is an effective way to begin intervention.
- In the United States, there are now more former smokers than current smokers. More than half of previous smokers have quit smoking (USDHHS, 2014).

Family physicians are in a unique position to assist their patients in smoking cessation. Because 7 of every 10 smokers visit their physicians at least once a year, this is a golden opportunity that should not be missed. Among smokers, 70% want to quit, and about 40% make an attempt each year, but fewer than 5% succeed. Even brief physician advice can double the quit rate (Fiore et al., 2008). Of those who try to quit on their own and do not use recommended cessation methods, most relapse within 8 days (CDC, 2008).

A survey by the Association of American Medical Colleges (2007) about physician behavior related to smoking cessation is summarized as follows:

Most physicians consistently ask patients who smoke about their smoking status and advise them to stop (86%), but only 13% say they usually refer smokers to others for appropriate treatment and only 17% say they usually arrange for follow-up visits to address smoking. Only 31% "usually" advised use of nicotine replacement therapy, and 25% "usually" prescribed other medication for cessation. Only 7% regularly referred patients to a quit line.

Patients should be asked about tobacco use at every visit because repeated screening increases rates of clinical intervention. Tobacco users should be advised to quit at every visit (SOR: A) because there is a dose-response relationship between the number of contacts and abstinence. Tobacco use screening coupled with brief advice is one of the top three clinical prevention measures and is cost-effective as well (Maciosek et al., 2006). Tobacco cessation treatment may include a variety of components: counseling for behavior change in both individual and group settings, such as motivational interviewing and problem solving or skills training, use of evidence-based pharmacotherapy, and proactive telephone quit line counseling (Fiore et al., 2008; USPSTF, 2009). Patients should receive at least minimal advice and encouragement at every visit based on the five A's approach (Table 49-2). The American Academy of Family Physicians (AAFP, 2005) has a campaign to encourage its members to engage themselves in smoking cessation interventions. Using two A's, ask and act, the AAFP program emphasizes brief counseling and effective follow-up. The AAFP emphasizes a team approach to tobacco use cessation in the office setting. It has many resources that can assist in developing effective approaches for the practice team. These materials can be accessed on the AAFP website.

As part of taking the history from a patient who smokes, clinicians should ask the following three questions to assess the patient's degree of nicotine addiction:

1. How much do you smoke? (How many cigarettes or cans of "dip" per day, for how many years?)
2. When do you smoke the first cigarette of the day?
3. How long is the period between cigarettes before craving another smoke?

Patients who smoke more than 20 cigarettes a day, who light their first cigarette within 30 minutes of waking, and who have cravings within 1 hour of the most recent cigarette are likely to have significant physiologic addiction to nicotine. Smoking fewer than 10 cigarettes a day suggests less addictive behavior, and a few patients report that they

Table 49-2 Five A's for Tobacco Users Willing to Quit

Ask about tobacco use at every visit.
Advise to quit through clear, personalized messages.
Assess about willingness to quit.
Assist efforts to quit.
Arrange follow-up and support.

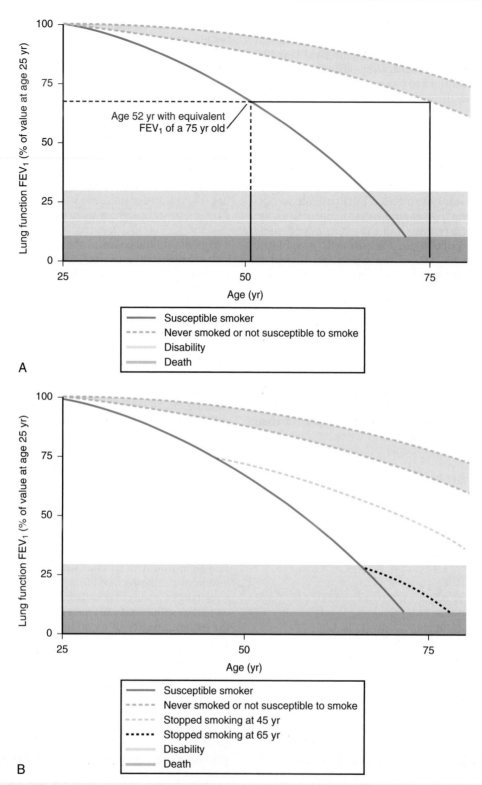

Figure 49-4 A, Explaining lung age to participants. **B,** Graph of lung function against age showing how smoking accelerates age-related decline in lung function. *FEV1,* Forced expiratory volume in 1 second. (From Parkes G, Greenhaigh T, Griffin M, Dent R. Effect on smoking quit rate of telling patients their lung age: the Step2quit randomized controlled trial. *BMJ.* 2008;336:598-600.)

smoke only during social situations and only 5 to 10 cigarettes a week. Determining the patient's pattern of smoking will provide clues into the level of addiction.

Office spirometry to obtain a forced expiratory volume in 1 second (FEV$_1$) can also be useful in motivating smokers to quit. Comparing the smoker's "lung age" with the age of a healthy individual who has the same FEV$_1$ and then showing the smoker a graphic display (Figure 49-4, *A*) more than doubled the rate of quitting smoking after 12 months (13.6% vs. 6.4%) in one study (Parkes et al., 2008). For example, a 52-year-old smoker with a 20-pack-year history (1 pack/day for 20 years) may have the lung age of a 75-year-old. Probable age at disability and death if the person continues smoking or stops smoking can be shown (Figure 49-4, *B*). Such a visual presentation is often effective in achieving cessation even if smokers have a normal lung age because he or she may think it is not too late to quit.

STAGES OF CHANGE

Patients who begin any major behavioral or lifestyle change go through successive stages in the process, as follows:

- **Precontemplation:** The patient is not interested in quitting smoking in the near future (within 6 months).
- **Contemplation:** The patient is thinking about quitting within the next few months but has taken no action.
- **Preparation:** The patient is planning to quit in the next 30 days.
- **Action:** The patient is in the process of quitting or has quit during the past 6 months.
- **Maintenance:** The patient has abstained for more than 3 months.

Family physicians should emphasize progression through the process of change to facilitate the patient's efforts to stop smoking. When a patient reaches the preparation stage, the physician can play a major role in motivating the patient, including counseling and routine use of pharmacotherapy. However, recent research indicates that many smokers do not go through sequential stages and are often successful in quitting during spontaneous, unplanned attempts, perhaps sparked by an illness or by policy changes such as price increases or clean indoor air laws. Physicians' continued support and encouragement may help increase the frequency and success of these efforts (Ferguson et al., 2009).

HELPING TO CHANGE BEHAVIOR

In addition to the support for smoking cessation activity described by the U.S. Public Health Service (PHS) (Fiore et al., 2008), *motivational interviewing* is a patient-focused approach to discussing patients' ambivalence about changing their tobacco use behavior. Motivational interviewing uses empathy and a nonjudgmental style to open a dialogue that can show the importance of change and build a patient's self-motivation. Patients can build on prior success (even brief) and become more active partners in the path to abstinence (Mallin, 2002; Miller and Rollnick, 2002). A clear relationship exists between the intensity of counseling and its effectiveness. Although even brief counseling (≤3 minutes) doubles the spontaneous quit rate, intensive therapy can be more effective and should be used whenever possible (Fiore et al., 2008).

Both physicians and their patients who smoke should think of nicotine dependence as a chronic disease, usually characterized by many episodes of remission and relapse. A number of strategies are often needed, and expectations must be realistic because smokers usually do not succeed on their first or even second attempt. Clearly, however, the chances of success increase with each attempt, and relapse should not be considered a sign of failure.

Intensive counseling is associated with a 22% smoking cessation success rate, and even minimal counseling (<3 minutes) has a 13% quit rate (Schroeder, 2005). Physicians should take advantage of the teachable moment, such as when a smoker is being seen for a respiratory or cardiovascular problem, an asthma attack in a smoke-exposed child, or the smoking-related death of a loved one (Miller and Wood, 2003). One of the most productive times for cessation advice to be received and effective is during prenatal care or after a nonfatal cardiac event. When intensive counseling and follow-up are provided to patients recovering from coronary bypass graft surgery or a heart attack, more than 60% stop smoking and stay off cigarettes, almost twice the rate of those who receive less definitive advice (Smith and Burgess, 2009; SOR A). A Cochrane review of cessation interventions among hospitalized patients shows that intensive interventions that begin in the hospital and have at least one supportive contact after discharge increase the odds of successful tobacco abstinence (Rigotti et al., 2007).

PHARMACOTHERAPY

The updated clinical practice guideline, Treating Tobacco Use and Dependence (Fiore et al., 2008), discusses the use of the different forms of nicotine replacement therapy and the other two FDA-approved prescription medications used for tobacco cessation, bupropion and varenicline (Table 49-3). Effective second-line agents include clonidine, delivered transdermally or orally, and nortriptyline (Fiore et al., 2008), but neither is FDA approved for this indication. All of these medications in randomized clinical trials have two to four times the odds ratio for success compared with placebo for smoking cessation. Medication and treatments to avoid include antidepressants such as selective serotonin reuptake inhibitors, benzodiazepines, mecamylamine, hypnosis, acupuncture, laser therapy, and β-adrenergic blocking agents, none of which has been found to have a beneficial effect (Fiore et al., 2008).

KEY TREATMENT

- Tobacco users attempting to quit should be prescribed one or more effective first-line pharmacotherapies for tobacco use cessation, including five nicotine replacement therapies (NRTs) (transdermal patch, gum, nasal spray, lozenges, or vapor inhaler) and non-nicotine replacement (bupropion SR or varenicline) (Eisenberg et al., 2008; Fiore et al., 2008) (SOR: A).
- Brief counseling (≤3 minutes) doubles the spontaneous quit rate; intensive therapy can be even more effective and should be used whenever possible (Fiore et al., 2008) (SOR: A).

Nicotine Patch

The nicotine patch is a mainstay of treatment, often combined with other short-acting forms of nicotine replacement therapy and counseling. The main advantages of the

Table 49-3   Clinical Guidelines for Nicotine Withdrawal

		Dosage
Nicotine patch	Patches should be applied as soon as patients waken on their quit day. At the start of each day, the patient should place a new patch on a relatively hairless location between the neck and waist. There should be no activity restrictions while using the patch. Treatment for 8 wk or less is as effective as longer treatment periods. New research indicates that starting the patch 2 wk before quit day increases success.	*Nicoderm, Habitrol:* 21 mg/24 hr for 4 wk; then 14 mg/24 hr for 2 wk; then 7 mg/24 hr for 2 wk. *Nicotrol:* 15 mg/16 hr for 4 wk; then 10 mg/16 hr for 2 wk; then 5 mg/16 hr for 2 wk. *ProStep:* 22 mg/24 hr for 4 wk; then 11 mg/24 hr for 4 wk.
Nicotine gum	Gum should be chewed slowly until a peppery taste emerges and then parked between the check and gum to facilitate nicotine absorption through the oral mucosa. The gum should be slowly and intermittently chewed and parked for about 30 minutes. Acidic beverages (e.g., coffee, juices, soft drinks) interfere with the buccal absorption of nicotine, so eating and drinking anything except water should be avoided for 5 minutes before and during chewing. Instructing patients to chew the gum on a fixed schedule may be more beneficial than ad lib use. Patients often do not use enough gum to obtain the maximum benefit.	*Nicorette:* Available as 2 mg and 4 mg per piece. Smokers of more than 1 pack a day, those who smoke within 30 minutes of awakening, and those with a history of severe withdrawal symptoms should use 4 mg; light smokers should use 2 mg. Chew one piece every 1-2 hr (at least 9/day) for 6 wk; then one piece every 2-4 hr for 3 wk; then one piece every 4-8 hr for 3 wk; then discontinue. For the 2-mg dose, do not exceed 30 pieces/day; for the 4-mg dose, 20 pieces/day.
Nicotine lozenge	Each lozenge is one 2- or 4-mg dose and should be dissolved in the mouth when the urge to smoke starts; lasts 20-30 minutes. Start with 4 mg if first cigarette is within 30 minutes of waking; others start with 2 mg. Use 9-20/day for up to 12 wk. No eating or drinking during use or 15 minutes before use. Side effects include sore teeth or gums, indigestion, throat irritation, and other symptoms similar to those with nicotine gum.	*Commit lozenge:* 2 mg and 4 mg per piece. Smokers of more than 1 pack a day who smoke within 30 minutes of waking and those with prior history of severe withdrawal should use the 4-mg form. Light smokers should start with the 2-mg strength. Do not swallow, bite, or chew the lozenge.
Nicotine inhaler	Local irritation in the mouth and throat occurs in 40% of patients. Coughing and rhinitis are also common. The severity and frequency of these symptoms decline with continued use. In cold weather, the inhaler and cartridges should be kept in an inside pocket or warm area because nicotine delivery declines significantly at temperatures below 40°F (4.4°C).	*Nicotrol inhaler:* 10 mg/cartridge (4 mg delivered and 2 mg absorbed). Each cartridge lasts about 20 minutes with frequent puffing and is equivalent to about two cigarettes. Use 6-16 cartridges/day for the first 12 wk; then reduce gradually over 12 wk.
Nicotine nasal spray	Moderate nasal irritation for first 3 wk or longer. Nasal congestion and transient changes in sense of smell and taste may also occur. Should not be used in patients with severe reactive airway disease. Do not sniff, swallow, or inhale through nose while administering doses. Deliver with head tilted slightly back.	*Nicotrol NS:* One spray (0.5 mg) to each nostril (1.0 mg total). Use 1-2 doses/hr and 8-40 doses/day (maximum, 5 doses/hr). Each bottle contains 100 doses. Usual maximum, 12 wk.
Bupropion SR	Contraindicated in patients with a history of significant head trauma, seizure disorder, or eating disorder and in those who have used a MAO inhibitor in the past 14 days. Side effects are insomnia and dry mouth. If insomnia is present, take the evening dose in the afternoon but at least 8 hours after the first dose.	150-mg tablets; one every morning for 3 days and then twice daily. Start 2 wk before the target quit date and continue for 12 wk.
Varenicline	Start 1 wk before quit date. Side effects are nausea (30% of patients), abnormal dreams, insomnia, headache, taste aversion, and flatulence. FDA warning addresses behavior changes and suicidal ideation.	*Chantix:* 0.5 mg (white tablet) once daily for 3 days; then twice daily for 4 days; then 1.0 mg (blue tablet) twice daily for a total of 12 wk.

FDA, Food and Drug Administration; *MAO,* monoamine oxidase.
*Some patients may prefer the nasal spray or inhaler because the more rapid delivery of nicotine better simulates smoking. Others may prefer bupropion because it is non-nicotine therapy. Bupropion should be considered especially in those with a history of depression.
Modified from U.S. Department of Health and Human Services. *Treating tobacco use and dependence: clinical practice update.* Rockville, MD: Agency for Health Care Policy and Research, Public Health Service; 2008.

patch are consistent delivery, easy use, and concealment. The major disadvantage is insomnia, which can be avoided by not wearing the patch at night.

In a study by Cornish and Gariti (2002), by the second day of patch use, nicotine levels are about half or greater than those achieved by smoking. Quit rates at 4 to 8 weeks (depending on the study) are about double the rate of success for placebo—that is, up to 70% for the nicotine patch versus up to 40% for placebo. After 1 year, the abstinence rates are about 25% for the gum and patch compared with 12% for placebo. The combination of a short-acting form of NRT (gum, lozenge, nasal spray) added to the patch increases the odds of success because it helps control cravings and gives the smoker the ability to titrate the dose. Combination therapy is becoming the standard approach for most patients using NRT. Recent evidence also indicates that smokers who begin the patch 2 weeks before the quit date may double the rate of abstinence (Rose et al., 2009). When dosing the patch, it is common to use 1-mg replacement per cigarette smoked in a day. For heavy smokers, that might mean "double patching" for 2 packs a day. High-dose patch therapy is not universally accepted, however, and there is less robust evidence for its routine use (Dale et al., 2000; Fiore et al., 2008).

Nicotine Gum

To obtain maximal results, the gum must be chewed slowly and then parked between cheek and gum to allow for buccal absorption. Although 2-mg and 4-mg strengths are available, the 4-mg strength is recommended for patients who smoke more than one pack a day. Absorption is decreased if the mouth is acidic, so the patient should avoid beverages such as coffee, tea, soda, and fruit juice. Abstinence rates at 4 to 6 weeks are 73% for nicotine gum compared with 49% for placebo gum. The duration of treatment, as with other NRT, should be at least 6 weeks, although a Cochrane review did not find evidence of enhanced success for the patch beyond 8 weeks (Stead et al., 2007). The gum is most useful when used in combination with the patch.

Nicotine Inhaler and Nasal Spray

The nicotine inhaler resembles a cigarette and mimics the act of smoking, thus permitting perpetuation of a behavioral ritual, but the nicotine is absorbed through the buccal mucosa rather than the lungs. Its efficacy is similar to that of the patch. The nicotine nasal spray is more rapidly absorbed than the other forms of NRT and should be a first-line treatment for heavier smokers. As monotherapy, the nasal spray has a higher odds ratio for success than the other NRTs used alone (Fiore et al., 2008).

Nicotine Lozenges

Nicotine lozenges deliver slightly more available nicotine than nicotine gum, are easier to use, and have fewer gastric side effects. The lozenge comes in several flavors and should be sucked like candy, slowly, until the flavor becomes intense. It is then held between the cheek and gums, similar to nicotine gum, and sucked again after the flavor has diminished. It should not be chewed or swallowed. The 4-mg strength lozenge should be used for those whose first cigarette is within 30 minutes of waking, with the 2-mg strength used for lighter smokers. Smokers should use seven or eight lozenges or more per day, up to 20. Although slightly more effective than gum as monotherapy, lozenges are most effective in combination with the patch.

Bupropion

Bupropion is a monocyclic antidepressant, thought to inhibit the reuptake of both dopamine and norepinephrine. It may exert multiple mechanisms, producing craving relief from dopaminergic activity, and antagonism of nicotinic acetylcholine receptors. The U.S. PHS guidelines and other analyses show that bupropion doubles long-term abstinence compared with placebo (Eisenberg et al., 2008; Fiore et al., 2008). Dosing begins 1 week before the quit date: 150 mg for 3 days and then 150 mg twice daily for the remainder of the week until quit day, with long-term maintenance at that dose. Bupropion may also be effective in relapse prevention, although a Cochrane review questions that conclusion (Hajek et al., 2008). Bupropion carries a small risk of seizures, as with other antidepressants, and is contraindicated in patients with a significant history of head trauma, eating disorders, or seizure disorders. Bupropion is effective in delaying weight gain

Table 49-4 Recommended Dosages for Nicotine Replacement Therapy

Cigarettes (per day)	Nicotine Patch Dose (mg/day)
<10	7-14
10-20	14-22
21-40	22-44
>40	44+

associated with smoking cessation. The FDA has issued a black box warning for both bupropion and varenicline, highlighting the risk of serious mental health events, including changes in behavior, depressed mood, hostility, agitation, suicidal thoughts, and attempted suicide.

Combination Therapy. Just as long-acting and short-acting NRT can be combined to augment cessation success, bupropion can be used with the patch or other forms of NRT. Combination therapy appears to be a promising approach. A 9-week study combining bupropion SR with transdermal nicotine found much greater efficacy than with either medication alone (Jorenby et al., 1999), and subsequent review in the PHS guidelines confirms the utility of combination therapy (Fiore et al., 2008). One might think of bupropion or the patch as the "controller" medication and the short-acting NRT as the "rescue" drug, much as dual therapy is used in asthma control. A trial of "triple therapy" using the patch, bupropion, and the nicotine vapor inhaler for up to 6 months showed a 2.57 odds ratio for abstinence compared with the patch alone (Steinberg et al., 2009).

Clinicians at the Mayo Clinic Nicotine Dependence Center have routinely used combination therapy and base initial NRT patch dosing on venous cotinine levels. If that is not available, the intensity of smoking or spit tobacco use can be a useful guide (Table 49-4) (Dale et al., 2000).

Varenicline

Varenicline is a partial agonist and antagonist that is selectively bound to the $\alpha 4 \beta 2$ nicotinic receptors, thus blocking nicotine from these brain cells, as well as stimulating them to release dopamine at lower levels than does nicotine itself. This leads to reduced cravings and fewer symptoms of nicotine withdrawal. A Cochrane review of its effectiveness concludes that it increases the odds of successful cessation two to three times more than attempts not using pharmacotherapy, with a pooled RR at 1 year compared with bupropion of 1.52 (Cahill et al., 2008). Varenicline is titrated over 1 week, mainly to help overcome its major side effect of nausea, ameliorated by taking varenicline with meals. Begin with 0.5 mg daily for 3 days, then 0.5 mg twice daily, and then 1 mg twice daily on day 8, which is quit day for the patient. Treatment should continue for at least 12 weeks; an additional 12 weeks may be useful in patients who are insecure in their attempts and are at high risk for relapse. The longer dosing schedule was shown to increase success in clinical trials.

Concern has been raised about varenicline and its potential to cause behavior changes and suicidal thoughts. In July 2009, the FDA issued a black box warning for both varenicline and bupropion, saying that patients taking either of these drugs should be observed for symptoms of behavior change, including hostility, aggression, depressed mood, and suicidal ideation or attempts. Patients should stop taking varenicline and contact their physicians if these or other unusual neuropsychiatric symptoms occur. In addition, patients should take precautions when driving or operating machinery until they know whether varenicline might adversely affect them. Pilots, air traffic controllers, and persons with commercial motor vehicle licenses cannot use varenicline, according to federal rules issued in 2008. A cohort study of more than 80,000 persons using different medications for smoking cessation, however, found no clear evidence that varenicline caused suicide or depression (Gunnell et al., 2009). The most recent study of varenicline and depression was a multicenter, double-blind, randomized trial of 525 persons with stable, treated depression or a history of depression. Varenicline had a significant cessation effect vs placebo (35.9% vs 15.6% continuous abstinence; OR, 3.35) with no differences between groups of suicidal symptoms or exacerbation of depression (Anthenelli et al., 2013).

Early evidence shows that using varenicline in combination with the nicotine patch and with bupropion appears to be safe and well tolerated; however, more investigation is needed before these combinations become a mainstay of smoking-cessation therapy (Ebbert et al., 2009a, 2009b).

Second-Line Medications

Clonidine and nortriptyline are listed in the PHS guidelines as second-line drugs, and both have been shown to have significant effects on cessation compared with placebo (Fiore et al., 2008). Nortriptyline is generally titrated up to 75 to 100 mg/day and used for 8 to 12 weeks. It has the advantage of being quite inexpensive, but drug levels may be needed to avoid toxicity. Clonidine patches, 0.2 mg/day, are recommended for up to 10 weeks and should be started 1 week before the quit date. Clonidine's side effects of drowsiness may limit its usefulness in many patients. Neither is FDA approved for smoking cessation.

Quit Lines

One of the least used methods, yet one of the most effective, is telephone quit lines. Surveys have shown that 70% to 85% of smokers prefer to use a quit line to seeing a clinician, perhaps because of the convenience, anonymity, and ability to obtain counseling in their native language. The toll-free number, 800-QUIT-NOW (800-784-8669), is a single access point to the National Network of Tobacco Cessation Quit Lines. Callers are automatically routed to a state-run quit line, if one exists in their area. If there is no state-run line, callers are routed to the NCI's quit line, where they may receive cessation services and other information. Quit lines are available in almost every state (Schroeder, 2005). There is also a California Smoker's Helpline at 800-662-8887, which links people nationwide to counselors who will give one-to-one support. Quit lines are even more effective when combined with NRT (Bush et al., 2008).

Relapse Prevention

Perhaps the most poorly understood element in smoking cessation is preventing relapse. Follow-up and ongoing contact with patients is essential, especially in the first few weeks of a cessation attempt. The first 2 weeks are the most crucial period, when smoking even one cigarette is a strong predictor of a return to regular smoking within 1 year. A return visit, proactive telephone call, or regular sessions with a quit line counselor in the early stages of cessation should be integrated into the patient's treatment. To be truly successful, family physicians should integrate tobacco dependence treatment into their practice (Solberg, 2000). The AAFP has created a toolkit that can be downloaded for this aim, called "Office Champions" (see Web Resources). A Cochrane review on relapse prevention found that although no definitive evidence yet exists for specific interventions to sustain abstinence, efforts to help smokers identify and deal with "tempting situations" show promise (Hajek et al., 2008). However, an excellent series of materials for patients is available from the NCI's website and may be very useful in helping patients with discussions of relapse issues ("Forever Free" at http://www.smokefree.gov/resources.aspx).

Current Developments

SMOKING AND GENETICS

Genetics plays a key role in a variety of issues related to tobacco dependence. Recent research has included the molecular basis for nicotine dependence, genetic influences on the family of nicotine receptors, genetic influences on tobacco-related cancer and heart disease, and treatment issues.

Genetic testing may be able to indicate persons most susceptible to becoming addicted to nicotine. Addictive individuals who have a particular gene and are trying to quit may be more responsive to nicotine patches than nonnicotine measures such as bupropion (Zyban). Multiple genes are involved, however, and considerable research will be needed to create practical applications for these discoveries.

Much work is currently underway regarding genes and gene mutations that predispose cigarette smokers to lung cancer. *Gene methylation* is a chemical modification that may be a marker for the early detection of lung cancer. The gene GPC5 has an important tumor suppressor–like function that, if insufficient, can promote lung cancer development. A variant of this gene has been found in one third of nonsmokers who develop lung cancer (Yafei, 2010).

Summary of Additional Online Content

The following content is available at www.expertconsult.com:

eFigure 49-1

eFigure 49-2

eFigure 49-3

eTable 49-1 Celebrities Who Died of Cancer or Other Smoking-Related Diseases

eAppendix 49-1 Health Risks with Smoking: Pregnancy

eAppendix 49-2 Social and Legal Action

References

The complete reference list is available at www.expertconsult.com.

Web Resources

www.aafp.org/patient-care/public-health/tobacco-nicotine/office-champions/training-resources.html Office Champions project training and resources.

www.aafp.org/patient-care/public-health/tobacco-nicotine/ask-act.html American Academy of Family Physicians' website for tobacco prevention and cessation.

www.cancer.gov National Cancer Institute site, with prevention and cessation information.

www.cdc.gov/tobacco Centers for Disease Control and Prevention Office on Smoking & Tobacco Use site. Contains fact sheets, U.S. Surgeon General reports, *MMWR* articles on tobacco, and much more.

www.cochrane.org/cochrane-reviews Evidence-based systematic reviews of the medical literature, with dozens of topics related to smoking and tobacco.

www.epa.gov/smokefree Advice on how to protect children from secondhand smoke. Also contains other tobacco-related materials.

www.lung.org The American Lung Association offers printed quit materials, some in Spanish. Provides a Lung Helpline to speak to someone directly or online. Also offers the tobacco cessation program "Freedom from Smoking Online" at www.ffsonline.org and support for smokers who want to quit at www.quitterinyou.org.

www.nicotine-anonymous.org Offers help to those who wish to stop using nicotine products and provides schedules of Nicotine Anonymous meetings in your area.

www.no-smoke.org The Americans for Nonsmokers' Rights site. A primary spot for information on secondhand smoke.

www.quitnet.com Offers free cutting-edge tobacco-cessation services to people worldwide, including the amount of money saved by quitting.

www.scenesmoking.org Annual monitoring of the amount of smoking in each movie category by the Breathe California of Sacramento–Emigrant Trails, Sacramento. Good video showing that 80% of PG-13 movies show smoking and that leading actors smoke in 82% of them.

www.smokefree.gov Evidence-based information and professional assistance to help support the immediate and long-term needs of people trying to quit smoking.

smokingcessationleadership.ucsf.edu University of California at San Francisco site, promoting health professionals to help patients with cessation.

www.thecommunityguide.org The Guide to Community Preventive Services, especially directed toward reducing tobacco use and secondhand smoke.

www.tobacco.org A daily news service with medical articles on tobacco issues from print and broadcast media.

www.tobaccofreekids.org Campaign for Tobacco-Free Kids. Useful reports and data on state and national issues.

50 Substance Use Disorders

ALICIA KOWALCHUK and BRIAN C. REED

Scope of the Problem

Key Points

- Approximately 9.2% of the U.S. population age 12 years or older, or an estimated 23.9 million Americans, reported being current users of illicit drugs in 2012.
- The prevalence of current illicit drug use is greatest in those 18 to 20 years of age, with a rate of 23.9%.
- Marijuana is the most frequently used illicit drug in the United States, and its use is increasing.
- Medical emergencies related to nonmedical use of pharmaceuticals have increased 132% between 2004 and 2011.
- In 2013, the diagnoses of substance use disorder (SUD), mild, moderate, or severe in the *Diagnostic and Statistical Manual of Mental Disorders*, fifth edition (DSM-5) replaced the diagnoses of substance abuse and dependence from the DSM IV.

According to the 2012 Substance Abuse and Mental Health Services Administration (SAMHSA) National Survey on Drug Use and Health (SAMHSA, 2012), an estimated 23.9 million Americans age 12 years or older, or 9.2% of the population, were current users of illicit drugs or reported having used an illicit substance 1 month before the survey. This rate is slightly higher than reported rates of illicit substance use of 7.9% to 8.3% between the survey years of 2002 and 2008. With an estimated 18.9 million current users, or 7.2% of the population age 12 years and older, marijuana was the most frequently used illicit drug and increased from 5.8% in 2007. Among people who used illicit drugs, marijuana was used by an estimated 79.0%, with many reporting daily or almost daily use. Following marijuana was nonmedical use of prescription psychotherapeutic drugs such as narcotic pain relievers or sedatives (6.8 million), cocaine (1.6 million), hallucinogens (1.1 million), methamphetamine (440,000), and heroin (335,000).

Individuals age 18 to 20 years, or 23.9%, have the highest rate of illicit drug use. The next highest rate, of 19.7%, was seen in individuals between 21 and 25 years of age. Rates of illicit drug use among youths age 12 to 17 years was approximately 9.5% in 2012.

The rate of substance use for boys and men age 12 years and older was almost twice as high as that for girls and women (11.6% vs. 6.9%). In general, men are much more likely to be current users of marijuana (9.6% vs. 5.0%), cocaine (1.0% vs. 0.3%), and hallucinogens (0.6% vs. 0.3%) compared with women. However, men and women have similar rates of nonmedical use of psychotherapeutic drugs, pain relievers, stimulants, and sedatives (2.8% vs. 2.4%).

The prevalence of illicit drug use varies by race and ethnicity. The rate of illicit substance use has been found to be highest among people reporting two or more races, at 14.8%. An estimated 12.7% of American Indians or Alaska Natives, 11.3% of blacks, 9.2% of whites, 8.3% of Hispanics, 7.8% of Native Hawaiians or other Pacific Islanders, and 3.7% of Asians were current illicit drug users in 2012. Illicit drug use also varies by education level. Among adults age 18 years or older, the prevalence of current illicit drug use was greatest among adults who did not complete high school, at a rate of 11.1%. The rate dropped to 6.6% in college graduates.

In 2012, an estimated 7900 people used an illicit substance for the first time each day. Most initiates were female and younger than 18. Of the estimated 2.9 million people age 12 years or older who used illicit drugs for the first time in 2012, approximately 65.6% of these individuals first used marijuana. Another 26% initiate illicit drug use by taking prescription drugs such as pain relievers in a nonmedical manner. The most recent Drug Abuse Warning Network (DAWN) 2011 national estimates of drug-related emergency department (ED) visits reveal that there were more than 2.5 million ED visits related to drug misuse or abuse, or an approximate rate of 790 ED visits per 100,000 people (DAWN, 2011). The most frequent reasons for ED visits related to drug misuse or abuse involved cocaine intoxication, marijuana intoxication, and nonmedical use of pharmaceuticals such as narcotic pain relievers.

Approximately 18.1% of unemployed individuals age 18 years and older were current illicit drug users. This was significantly higher than the prevalence of current drug use among individuals employed full time (8.9%) and part time (12.5%).

The prevalence of substance abuse was also significantly higher among individuals with serious mental illness. The most recent available analysis comparing prevalence of illicit substance use among individuals with comorbid

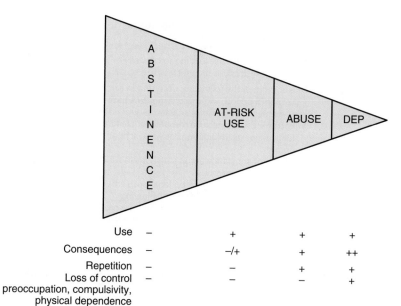

Figure 50-1 Continuum of drug use in patients with substance use disorders. *DEP,* **Dependence.** (Modified from Brown, RL Module III: Screening and Assessment, Project MAINSTREAM Syllabus Interdisciplinary Faculty Development Program in Substance Abuse Education, October 2005, last accessed from http://www.amersa.org/mainstream.asp 11/19/2014.)

serious mental illness comes from the 2011 National Survey on Drug Use and Health, which showed the rate of illicit drug use in the past year among adults age 18 years or older with serious mental illness was 25.2%, compared with a rate of 11.8% among same-age adults without serious mental illness.

TERMINOLOGY

The term *substance use disorder* implies a continuum of use, from abstinence to at-risk use to abuse and dependence (Figure 50-1). The majority of the general population, as well as family medicine patients, are "abstainers." The majority of users of illicit substances do not meet criteria for the diagnosis of an SUD. This model of substance use is important for family medicine physicians to keep in mind as they talk with their patients about substance use issues. It highlights the key role played by screening for substance use and early intervention at the at-risk use level before specialized treatment services are more likely needed.

The updated terminology of SUD diagnoses and criteria in the DSM-5 reflects this continuum as well. Table 50-1 lists the DSM-5 diagnostic criteria for SUDs, mild, moderate, and severe. Table 50-2 lists the older DSM-IV diagnostic criteria for substance abuse and dependence for reference because these terms are still frequently used in patient care settings and the medical literature. Other key changes with the DSM-5 are the inclusion of cravings in the diagnostic criteria, elimination of legal problems as a criterion, and the addition of a cannabis withdrawal diagnosis. DSM-IV abuse and dependence and DSM-5 SUD moderate and severe diagnoses for several substances have shown good correlation (Compton et al., 2013). The clinical significance in terms of appropriateness of current treatments developed for DSM IV abuse and dependence diagnoses for DSM-5 mild SUDs remains as yet unclear.

Table 50-3 shows some common drug street names. Comprehensive lists can be found on the Office of National Drug Control Policy's website (http://www.whitehousedrugpolicy.gov). Street names vary by region

Table 50-1 DSM-5 Diagnostic Criteria for Substance Use Disorders

Substances	Cannabis, hallucinogens (PCP or similarly acting arylcyclohexylamines), other hallucinogens such as LSD, inhalants, opioids, sedatives, hypnotics, anxiolytics, stimulants (including amphetamine-type substances, cocaine, and other stimulants), and other or unknown substances
Criteria	Mild if two or three of the following for at least 1 year, moderate if four or five, and severe if six or more 1. Taking the substance in larger amounts or for longer than you meant to 2. Wanting to cut down or stop using the substance but not managing to 3. Spending a lot of time getting, using, or recovering from use of the substance 4. Cravings and urges to use the substance 5. Not managing to do what you should at work, home, or school because of substance use 6. Continuing to use even when it causes problems in relationships 7. Giving up important social, occupational, or recreational activities because of substance use 8. Using substances again and again even when it puts you in danger 9. Continuing to use even when you know you have a physical or psychological problem that could have been caused or made worse by the substance 10. Needing more of the substance to get the effect you want (tolerance) 11. Development of withdrawal symptoms, which can be relieved by taking more of the substance
Modifiers	1. "In early remission": no criteria except craving for 3 to 12 months 2. "In sustained remission": no criteria except craving for at least 12 months 3. "On maintenance therapy": e.g., with methadone or buprenorphine containing medications 4. "in a controlled environment": e.g., incarcerated, in residential-based treatment

DSM-5, Diagnostic and Statistical Manual of Mental Disorders, 5th edition; *LSD,* lysergic acid diethylamide; *PCP,* phencyclidine.
Adapted from American Psychiatric Association. *Diagnostic and statistical manual of mental disorders.* 5th ed. Arlington, VA: American Psychiatric Association; 2013.

Table 50-2 Diagnostic Criteria for Substance Abuse and Dependence (DSM-IV)

A maladaptive pattern of substance use leading to clinically significant impairment or distress, as manifested by:

Abuse	One or more of the following, occurring in a 12-month period, and these symptoms have never met the criteria for substance dependence:
	1. Recurrent substance use resulting in a failure to fulfill major role obligations at work, school, or home
	2. Recurrent substance use in situations in which it is physically hazardous
	3. Recurrent substance-related legal problems
	4. Continued substance use despite having persistent or recurrent social or interpersonal problems caused or exacerbated by the effects of the substance
Dependence	Three or more of the following, occurring in the same 12-month period:
	1. *Tolerance,* as defined by either of the following: a need for markedly increased amounts of the substance to achieve intoxication or desired effect *or* markedly diminished effect with continued use of the same amount of substance.
	2. *Withdrawal,* as manifested by either of the following: the characteristic withdrawal syndrome for the substance *or* the same (or a closely related) substance is taken to relieve or avoid withdrawal symptoms.
	3. The substance is often taken in larger amounts or longer than intended.
	4. There is a persistent desire or unsuccessful efforts to cut down or control substance use.
	5. A great deal of time is spent in activities to obtain the substance, use the substance, or recover from its effects.
	6. Important social, occupational, or recreational activities are given up or reduced because of substance use.
	7. The substance use is continued despite knowledge of having a persistent or recurrent physical or psychological problem that is likely to have been caused or exacerbated by the substance.

Adapted from American Psychiatric Association. *Diagnostic and Statistical Manual of Mental Disorders.* 4th ed, text rev. Washington, DC: American Psychiatric Association; 2000.

and user group. The most useful information is obtained on the local level simply by asking patients what they call the drug they are using.

Screening

Key Point

- A single-question screen for drug use, comparable in sensitivity and specificity to the four-question CAGE-Adjusted to Include Drugs (CAGE-AID), has been validated for primary care: "How many times in the past year have you used an illegal drug or used a prescription medication for nonmedical reasons?" An answer of one or more is a positive screen.

Table 50-3 Common Drug Street Names

Substance	Street Names (NIDA website)	
Benzodiazepines	Candy, downers, sleeping pills, sticks, handlebars	
Cocaine	Blow, bump, C, candy, coke, crack, flake, rock, snow	
Codeine	Captain Cody, school boy, pancakes and syrup	
Dextromethorphan	Robotripping, Robo, Triple C	
Flunitrazepam (Rohypnol)	Roofies, rope, rophies, forget-me pill, Mexican Valium	
GHB	Liquid ecstasy, Georgia home boy, grievous bodily harm	
Heroin	Brown sugar, dope, H, horse, junk, skag, skunk, smack	
Ketamine	K, special K, vitamin K, cat Valiums	
LSD	Acid, blotter, boomers, cubes, microdot	
Marijuana	Blunt, dope, ganja, grass, herb, joints, pot, reefer, weed	
MDMA	Adam, clarity, ecstasy, Eve, lover's speed, Molly, peace, X	
Methamphetamine	Chalk, rank, crystal, fire, glass, go fast, ice, meth, speed	
Methylphenidate	Skippy, vitamin R, the smart drug, R-ball	
Oxycodone (OxyContin), hydrocodone (Vicodin)	Oxy, OC, killer, vike	
PCP	Angel dust, boat, hog, love boat, peace pill	

GHB, γ-Hydroxybutyrate; *LSD,* lysergic acid diethylamide; *MDMA,* methylenedioxymethamphetamine; *NIDA,* National Institute on Drug Abuse; *PCP,* phencyclidine.

Screening, brief intervention, and *referral to treatment* (SBIRT) for alcohol use disorders in primary care has been well studied and is recommended for incorporation into routine primary care by the U.S. Preventive Services Task Force (USPSTF, 2008; SOR B). However, SBIRT in primary care for drug use has been less studied to date, and the USPSTF states that there is currently insufficient evidence to recommend for or against routine screening for drug use in primary care.

With the recent increase in prescription drug misuse, interest in drug use SBIRT incorporation into primary care has broadened and is being studied for efficacy (Insight Project, 2009). Limitations on drug use SBIRT in primary care include lower prevalence of drug use in primary care patients compared with alcohol use as well as concerns about the practicality of use and positive predictive value (PPV) of available screening instruments in the primary care setting. The American Academy of Pediatrics, Bright Future Initiative, and American Medical Association Guidelines for Adolescent Preventative Services all recommend at least annual screening of adolescents for drug use. The American College of Obstetricians and Gynecologists advocates regular, periodic screening for all patients, regardless of pregnancy status, although no specific screening instrument is recommended and, to date, no screening instrument has been validated for pregnant women (Lanier and Ko, 2008). Common validated screening instruments for drug use are briefly discussed later.

The CRAFFT is the only screening instrument validated for adolescents and has shown an 83% PPV (Table 50-4). It screens for alcohol as well as drug use (Knight et al., 2002).

The ASSIST, CAGE-AID, and Drug Abuse Screening Test (DAST) have been validated in nonpregnant adults. PPVs for the Alcohol, Smoking and Substance Involvement Screening Test (ASSIST) are not currently available (Newcombe et al., 2005). It screens for tobacco and alcohol in addition to drugs. The ASSIST is available at no cost from the World Health Organization.

The CAGE-AID has shown 12% to 78% PPV, with PPV increasing with increasing prevalence of drug use in the study population (Brown and Rounds, 1995). It screens for both alcohol and drug use (see eTable 50-1 online).

The DAST has similarly shown a wide PPV range of 23% to 75% and is also in the public domain. It screens for drug use only (Staley and El-Guebaly, 1990).

The ASSIST and DAST are more lengthy screens than the CAGE-AID and CRAFFT and consequently have not been reproduced here. The SAMHSA SBIRT initiative recommends both the ASSIST and the DAST for drug screening (Lanier and Ko, 2008). SBIRT models vary but typically involve a brief screen of several questions regarding tobacco, alcohol, or drug use conducted by frontline staff. A single-question screen for drug use has been validated for primary care: "How many times in the past year have you used an illegal drug or used a prescription medication for nonmedical reasons?" An answer of one or more is a positive screening response (Smith et al., 2010). With sensitivity of 100% and specificity of 73.5%, this single-question screen is comparable to the four-question CAGE-AID.

Patients screening positive receive more in-depth screening with a self-administered or provider-administered screening instrument, such as the DAST or ASSIST, which both allow for stratification of each patient along the SUD continuum. The physician then scores the formal screen and reviews the results with the patient. Patients screening negative are given brief feedback about the results of their screen, and their healthy choices regarding substance use are reinforced by the physician. Patients screening positive for at-risk use but who do not meet criteria for an SUD receive a brief intervention, often using the FRAMES model (Table 50-5) or the "five A's" model (Table 50-6). Both are useful for patients receptive to change. Motivational interviewing techniques may be more useful than the FRAMES or five A's for patients who are more ambivalent about change (Searight, 2009).

Patients screening positive and meeting criteria for an SUD are offered referral to onsite or, more typically, community drug treatment programs. Referral to treatment can be time consuming and therefore is often done by ancillary staff with knowledge of local treatment resources or by referring the patient to a community-based agency that provides treatment-matching services.

Table 50-4 CRAFFT Screening Tool for Adolescents

CRAFFT	Question
Car	Have you ever ridden in a *car* driven by someone (including yourself) who was "high" or had been using alcohol or drugs?
Relax	Do you ever use alcohol or drugs to *relax,* feel better about yourself, or fit in?
Alone	Do you ever use alcohol or drugs while you are by yourself, or *alone?*
Forget	Do you ever *forget* things you did while using alcohol or drugs?
Friends	Do family members or *friends* ever tell you that you should cut down on your drinking or drug use?
Trouble	Have you ever gotten into *trouble* while you were using alcohol or drugs?

Scoring:
A "no" response = 0 points; a "yes" response = 1 point.
0-1 point = negative screen.
2-6 points = positive screen; consider a safety contract for "yes" response to "car" question regardless of total score.

Table 50-5 FRAMES Intervention Technique

Feedback about personal risk
Responsibility of the patient for change
Advice to change
Menu of strategies
Empathy: express empathy
Self-efficacy: elicit and support patient's self-efficacy for change

Table 50-6 Five "A's" Intervention Technique

Assess the risk of the behavior for the patient.
Advise the patient on his or her risk and how to modify it.
Agree: come to an agreement with the patient on treatment.
Assist the patient with the treatment plan.
Arrange follow-up or referral to treatment.

Laboratory Testing

Key Points

Any drug testing method involves several important considerations:

- Samples can be adulterated to mask true results; creatinine, pH, specific gravity, and temperature are often used to detect urine sample adulteration.
- A single test result is a marker of use at one point in time and does not itself make a diagnosis of an SUD; laboratory detection of drug use is one tool that may be used during screening, diagnosis, treatment, and relapse prevention of SUDs.
- Rates of false positives and false negatives depend on the drug ingested, quantity ingested, duration of use, and specific laboratory cutoffs used; it is important to know the cutoff values of the laboratory used and to obtain a comprehensive history of drug ingestion quantity and frequency over time.

Laboratory testing is frequently used in SUD screening, treatment, and monitoring for relapse. The most common testing method is the *urine drug test*. Other options include blood, sweat, hair, and oral fluid testing. Table 50-7 lists the advantages and disadvantages of each method (Ries et al., 2009).

Table 50-8 details typical detection times and causes of false-positive results for drugs that can be detected by readily available urine drug testing. Most urine drug tests use immunoassays because these are inexpensive, fast, and easily automated. Gas chromatography with mass spectroscopy is typically reserved for confirmation of a positive result. Methadone is not a part of most urine drug screen panels and does not show as a positive opiate test result. Separate testing for methadone is available. Separate testing is also needed for most "club drugs," including 3,4-methylenedioxymethamphetamine (MDMA), ketamine, and γ-hydroxybutyrate (GHB). Benzodiazepines have a wide range of potencies, half-lives, and metabolites, which makes urine drug screen results less reliable (Ries et al., 2009).

Pharmacology

COCAINE

Cocaine is a powerful and highly addictive stimulant derived from the leaf extract of the *Erythroxylon coca* bush. In 2012, there were an estimated 1.6 million current users of cocaine, or 0.6% of the U.S. population. Cocaine use is highest among individuals 18 to 25 years of age.

Table 50-7   Drug-Testing Methods: Advantages and Disadvantages

Test	Advantages	Disadvantages
Blood	Difficult to adulterate; detects very recent ingestion	Invasive; drugs clear blood more quickly after ingestion than urine
Hair	Noninvasive; difficult to adulterate; detects patterns of use over time; frequently used in forensics and research	Not useful for recent ingestion; more difficult to process than other methods
Oral fluids	Noninvasive; direct observation easy and makes adulteration more difficult; detects recent ingestion; rapid results	Unintentional contamination from recently ingested substances; drugs clear quickly after ingestion (see "Urine")
Sweat	Noninvasive; uses patch for collection; monitors for use over extended period	Quantification of drug levels difficult
Urine	Noninvasive; rapid results; relatively inexpensive vs. other methods	Easy to adulterate sample, even when observed collection method used

Table 50-8   Urine Drug Testing: Detection Times and Drugs Causing False Positives

Drug	Detection Time	False-Positive Result
Amphetamines, methamphetamine	1-3 days	Bupropion, chloroquine, chlorpromazine, ephedrine, labetalol, phenylpropanolamine, propranolol, pseudoephedrine, ranitidine, selegiline, trazodone, tyramine, Vick's inhaler
Barbiturates	Short acting: 1-4 days Long acting: several weeks	Phenytoin
Benzodiazepines	Highly variable	Oxaprozin, sertraline
Cocaine	3 days	None
LSD	2-5 days	Amitriptyline, chlorpromazine, doxepin, fluoxetine, haloperidol, metoclopramide, risperidone, sertraline, thioridazine, verapamil
Marijuana (THC)	Single joint: 2 days Heavy use: 27 days	Efavirenz, pantoprazole
Methadone	2-3 days	Quetiapine
Opiates	1-2 days	Gatifloxacin, levofloxacin, ofloxacin, papaverine, rifampicin, poppy seeds
PCP	7 days	Dextromethorphan, diphenylhydramine, thioridazine, venlafaxine
Propoxyphene	6 hours to 2 days	Cyclobenzaprine, diphenylhydramine, doxylamine, imipramine, methadone

LSD, Lysergic acid diethylamide; *PCP*, phencyclidine; *THC*, delta-9-tetrahydrocannabinol.

Cocaine causes a brief, intense feeling of euphoria by blocking the reuptake of dopamine, a neurotransmitter that is associated with pleasure and movement. This blockage accordingly increases the level of dopamine in the central nervous system (CNS). The more rapidly cocaine is absorbed into the bloodstream and delivered to the CNS, the more intense the "high" experienced by the user. Cocaine can be inhaled, injected, or smoked. Injecting or smoking cocaine produces an intense, 5- or 10-minute high that is much stronger than the sensation produced by snorting powder cocaine. The euphoria induced by snorting powder cocaine typically lasts 15 to 30 minutes but is slower in onset than injecting or smoking cocaine. Small amounts of cocaine give users feelings of euphoria, increased mental alertness, and energy.

Symptoms of cocaine intoxication include euphoria, agitation, impaired judgment, bizarre behavior, paranoia, tachycardia, elevated blood pressure, dilated pupils, and diaphoresis. Increased doses of cocaine cause some cocaine users to experience auditory hallucinations, tactile hallucinations, delusions, and aggressive behavior. Sudden cardiac arrest, seizures, and respiratory arrest are examples of fatal complications from cocaine overdose. Tolerance to cocaine causes addicts to binge on cocaine or take more cocaine at increasingly frequent intervals. Withdrawal from cocaine begins with a "crash," or excessive sleep. After 1 to 2 days, the user may feel anxious, irritated, fatigued, and depressed from the absence of cocaine and decreased dopamine levels, which can also cause intense cravings, depression, and suicidal ideation.

Although cocaine has legitimate medical uses, such as local anesthesia in eye, ear, and throat surgery, nonmedical use and importation were banned by the Harrison Act in December 1914.

MARIJUANA

Derived from a mix of flowers, stems, seeds, and leaves of the plant *Cannabis sativa*, marijuana is the most commonly abused illicit drug in the United States. Marijuana is classified as an illicit drug under federal law, and thus in national drug surveys; however, 20 states and the District of Columbia have passed legislation legalizing at least some form of marijuana use for medicinal purposes. In 2013, two states, Colorado and Washington, legalized recreational use of marijuana as well.

Nerve cells in the brain have receptors for THC (delta-9-tetrahydrocannabinol), the main active chemical in marijuana. After the drug enters the brain, THC causes the release of dopamine and produces feelings of euphoria. Smoking marijuana can produce a high that lasts 1 to 3 hours. Ingesting marijuana that has been mixed with food or brewed with tea can cause a longer high that lasts up to 4 hours. While high on marijuana, users may experience pleasant feelings, a feeling that time passes more slowly, and perceptions of heightened sensation with color and sound stimuli. Marijuana users may also have sudden hunger, thirst, and feelings of paranoia and anxiety. As the euphoria passes, marijuana users may feel depressed or sleepy. Long-term marijuana use can cause damage to short-term memory by altering the manner in which information is processed in the hippocampus.

Marijuana use can also cause respiratory problems such as chronic cough, recurrent lung infections, and lung cancer. The DSM-5 has added a diagnosis of cannabis withdrawal, defined as marijuana cessation in heavy, long-term users resulting in clinically significant distress or social, occupational, or other important functional impairment due to at least three withdrawal symptoms. There is currently no medication approved by the U.S. Food and Drug Administration (FDA) for the treatment of cannabis withdrawal, although studies are ongoing for several promising candidates, including gabapentin (Mason, et al., 2012).

METHAMPHETAMINE

Methamphetamine is a highly addictive stimulant that can cause increased alertness and increased physical activity with small doses by causing the release of high levels of the neurotransmitter dopamine in the brain. Abusers of methamphetamine experience a brief "rush" by smoking or injecting methamphetamine. Oral ingestion or snorting methamphetamine can produce a high that can last approximately half a day. Because of tolerance, chronic users of methamphetamine may take higher doses of the drug or binge for several days. Long-term use of methamphetamine can cause functional and molecular changes to the brain. Chronic methamphetamine users may exhibit anxiety, violent behavior, and symptoms of psychosis (e.g., hallucinations, paranoia, delusions). Fortunately, the use of methamphetamine in the United States has been decreasing. In 2012, there were approximately 440,000 users of methamphetamine.

HALLUCINOGENS

Hallucinogens alter mood and perception. Commonly abused hallucinogens include lysergic acid diethylamide (LSD), phencyclidine (PCP), MDMA, and hallucinogenic mushrooms. In 2012, there were 1.1 million current users of hallucinogens in the United States; use increased among youths age 12 to 17 years. LSD is sold as tablets, capsules, or liquids. It is often added to absorbent paper and dosed in small, decorated squares. Users of LSD experience unpredictable sensations of sound, color, hallucinations, and delusions. Long-term consequences of LSD usage include flashbacks, depression, and long-lasting psychosis. Users of PCP may smoke, ingest, inject, or snort it to experience hallucinations. PCP use may cause violent behavior, anxiety, and paranoia.

"CLUB DRUGS"

Ketamine, MDMA, GHB, and flunitrazepam (Rohypnol) are substances used in nightclubs, "raves," and dance parties to enhance feelings of intimacy and sensory stimulation. "Ecstasy," or MDMA, produces distorted perceptions of time, enhanced enjoyment of tactile sensations, and feelings of increased energy by increasing the release of serotonin, dopamine, and norepinephrine. MDMA is usually taken as a tablet or a capsule. The pure crystalline powder form of MDMA is often referred to as "Molly." The sympathetic overload caused by MDMA can produce hypertension, tachycardia, tremor, diaphoresis, and arrhythmias. MDMA intoxication is also associated with a potentially fatal serotonin syndrome that causes hyperthermia, autonomic instability, and myoclonus. Users of MDMA will typically experience severe depression 2 days after its ingestion.

Ketamine is a dissociative anesthetic derived from PCP. Usually stolen from veterinarian and physician offices, illicit supplies of ketamine are dried in powder form and smoked in nightclubs with tobacco and marijuana or inhaled. "Special K" can produce sensations of floating outside one's body, visual hallucinations, and dreamlike states that last for 30 to 45 minutes after ingestion.

Gamma-hydroxybutyrate can cause euphoria at lower doses and drowsiness, dizziness, visual disturbances, hypotonia, and amnesia at higher doses. Overdoses of GHB can cause seizures, severe respiratory depression, coma, and death. Because of its sedative and amnesic effect, GHB has been used as a "date rape" drug.

Flunitrazepam (Rohypnol) is a powerful benzodiazepine with 10 times the strength of diazepam that is capable of reducing anxiety, muscle tension, and inhibition. Higher doses of flunitrazepam can produce lack of muscle control, loss of consciousness, and anterograde amnesia. As with GHB, flunitrazepam has been used as a "date rape" drug (Gahlinger, 2004).

Bath salts are synthetic cathinone derivatives. These derivatives have psychoactive properties similar to cocaine and MDMA. These white or brown powder drugs are usually sold at convenience stores, smoke shops, and online. Bath salts can be taken orally, inhaled via smoking or vaporization, or injected intravenously. Users can experience euphoric feelings, increased sex drive, along with paranoia, agitation, hallucinations, and violent behavior. In 2011, intoxication with bath salts either alone or in combination with other drugs accounted for 22,904 ED visits.

BENZODIAZEPINES

Benzodiazepines are a family of depressants used therapeutically to produce sedation, relieve anxiety, induce sleep, control seizures, and alleviate muscle spasms. Abusers of benzodiazepines experience reduced inhibition and impaired judgment. Users of cocaine and amphetamines may take benzodiazepines to counter the stimulant effects. Concurrent use of benzodiazepines with alcohol and other depressants can be life threatening. Abrupt cessation of benzodiazepine use can cause seizures and a withdrawal syndrome similar to delirium tremens.

OPIATES (NONMEDICAL USE OF PRESCRIPTION DRUGS)

Hydrocodone (Vicodin) is the most frequently prescribed opioid in the United States. Oxycodone (OxyContin) and hydrocodone are prescribed in the treatment of acute and chronic pain. Abusers of hydrocodone and oxycodone experience euphoria, relaxation, and sedation. Long-term use can result in tolerance. Abusers may overdose as they take increasing doses of the medication while pursuing euphoric sensations that they previously experienced. Overdoses may result in severe respiratory depression, hypotension, coma,

and death. Recently, methadone, primarily diverted from prescriptions for chronic pain and not methadone maintenance treatment, has been linked to increased opiate overdoses as well. Its relatively long onset of action and long half-life make methadone-naive individuals more prone to overdose as they seek a stronger high with escalating doses, which accumulate, causing overdose. In 2011, there were 488,004 ED visits related to nonmedical use of prescription opioids.

HEROIN

Heroin, or diacetylmorphine, is a synthetic opiate, first created by Bayer in the late 1800s and marketed for pain relief and treatment of morphine addicts. It has a high abuse potential because of its rapid onset of action and short half-life. Heroin is therefore a Schedule I substance (i.e., not available for therapeutic use in the United States). The number of people that have used heroin in the past year has been increasing. In the 2012 SAMHSA National Survey on Drug Use and Health, an estimated 669,000 people used heroin within the last year. This increased use may be a consequence of the prescription drug epidemic as prescription drug users switch to heroin when tolerance to prescription opiates develops or when they are unable to gain access to prescription opiates. Heroin can be injected intravenously or subcutaneously ("skin popping"), snorted intranasally, as well as smoked in freebase form. Use of the intranasal route has greatly increased, along with the purity of street heroin and awareness of human immunodeficiency virus (HIV) infection risk associated with injecting. Heroin itself is an inactive prodrug with two active metabolites, one of which is morphine, and both of which are active at the μ-opioid receptor. After intravenous (IV) injection, users describe an intense rush within 1 to 2 minutes followed by a period of euphoric sedation lasting about 1 hour. In dependent users, withdrawal symptoms can begin within 4 to 6 hours (Ries et al., 2009).

Intoxication and Withdrawal

Signs and symptoms of intoxication and withdrawal and treatments are based on drug class. Generally, withdrawal symptoms are characterized by the opposite of intoxication, with their intensity inversely proportional to the duration of action of the drug and proportional to chronicity of use. Symptom onset is proportional to the half-life of the drug.

Treatment of intoxication for most substances is supportive and symptomatic and typically occurs in inpatient settings. Receptor antagonists are available for both opiate and benzodiazepine intoxication, with use reserved primarily for the overdose state. Treatment of withdrawal usually follows one of two principles: (1) substituting a longer-acting, less reinforcing equivalent and then tapering or (2) symptom control. Withdrawal treatment may occur in the inpatient or outpatient setting depending on the severity of the withdrawal anticipated, the underlying mental and physical health issues of the patient, and the level of support available to the patient in the outpatient setting.

OPIATES

Intoxication with opiates causes miotic pupils, euphoria, altered level of consciousness, constipation, and respiratory depression. Treatment of opiate overdose involves providing respiratory support and administering naloxone, a pure opiate antagonist. Naloxone is typically administered IV but may also be administered subcutaneously, intramuscularly, via endotracheal tube, or intranasally until IV access is established (Barton et al., 2005). The initial dose is typically 0.4 to 0.8 mg, with a 2-minute onset of action when given IV. Doses are repeated and escalated as needed to reverse the overdose. After reversal, patients need to be monitored for 1 to 3 hours for repeated dosing and sometimes longer if longer-acting opiates such as methadone have been used in the overdose. Naloxone treatment can initiate a rapid and intense withdrawal syndrome (Ries et al., 2009).

Opiate withdrawal is rarely fatal but is extremely uncomfortable and typically is accompanied by strong cravings. Withdrawal signs and symptoms include vomiting, diarrhea, body aches, rhinorrhea, thermoderegulation, insomnia, anxiety, dysphoria, gooseflesh, yawning, and pupil dilation. Treatment can be symptomatic, as with the α_2-adrenergic agonist clonidine, or can involve receptor agonist or antagonist activity. Methadone can be used with short- or long-taper protocols. Buprenorphine, a partial opiate agonist, can similarly be used. The antagonist naltrexone in combination with clonidine has been used effectively in both inpatient and outpatient settings (Ries et al., 2009).

SEDATIVE–HYPNOTICS (INCLUDING BENZODIAZEPINES)

Intoxication with the sedative–hypnotic drug class causes slurred speech, ataxia, respiratory depression, stupor, coma, and death (mostly with mixed overdose). Treatment of overdose involves providing respiratory support and gastrointestinal (GI) tract evacuation. Activated charcoal is particularly helpful for barbiturate overdose, as is urine alkalization for phenobarbital overdose. Flumazenil, a benzodiazepine receptor antagonist, can be used in benzodiazepine overdose but with caution because it can dramatically increase the risk of seizures and cardiac arrhythmias, especially in mixed overdoses and in patients physiologically dependent on benzodiazepines (Ries et al., 2009).

Withdrawal signs and symptoms from sedative–hypnotics include tachycardia, hypertension, fever, agitation, anxiety, hallucinations, insomnia, irritability, nightmares, sensory disturbances, tremor, tinnitus, anorexia, diarrhea, nausea, seizures, delirium, and death. Most sedative–hypnotic withdrawal is managed by either simple, slow, fixed-dose taper or substitution and taper. A *simple taper* involves decreasing the dose by no more than 10% every 1 to 2 weeks until the starting dose has been 75% decreased and then by 5% every 2 to 4 weeks for the last 25% until the taper is completed. *Substitution and taper* involves substituting a long-acting benzodiazepine (e.g., clonazepam) or phenobarbital for a shorter-acting drug and tapering as above. Conversion tables are available to calculate an approximate equivalent dose, and the dose is titrated over several days to a week to achieve good relief of withdrawal symptoms before tapering is begun of the substitute, as with the simple taper

method. Other adjunctive medications that have shown positive effects include carbamazepine, sodium valproate, propranolol, and trazodone. Because many patients dependent on benzodiazepines in particular have underlying anxiety and other psychiatric comorbidities and because withdrawal protocols are typically prolonged, anticipation and treatment of reemergence of these symptoms must be anticipated, or relapse is more likely (Ries et al., 2009).

OTHER DRUGS

eTable 50-2 online lists the signs and symptoms of intoxication and withdrawal of other drugs. There are no specific antidotes or reversal agents for the remaining drug classes. Care of overdose patients is largely supportive and aimed at treating the medical effects of the particular overdose, such as treatment of myocardial ischemia resulting from cocaine overdose. Currently, no FDA-approved medications are available for stimulant (including cocaine and methamphetamine), marijuana, hallucinogen (e.g., LSD, PCP), or club drug (e.g., MDMA) withdrawal. Behavioral therapies are the mainstay of treatment.

KEY TREATMENT

- Naloxone at 0.4 to 0.8 mg initial dose and repeated as needed is effective for opiate-intoxicated patients with inadequate spontaneous ventilation (Ries et al., 2009) (SOR: A).
- Sedative–hypnotic withdrawal is managed by simple taper or substitution to phenobarbital or longer-acting benzodiazepine and taper (SOR: C).

MEDICAL MANAGEMENT (BEYOND WITHDRAWAL)

Medical management of SUD after the acute withdrawal period for opiate dependence has a relatively long history, with various opioids being tried as maintenance therapies from the late 1800s until passage of the Harrison Act of 1914, which effectively outlawed prescribing opiates for treating addiction for nearly half a century. Currently, three pharmacologic interventions predominate: methadone, buprenorphine, and naltrexone. Of these three therapies, methadone is the most studied and the standard of care for patients with chronic relapsing opiate dependence. However, methadone is also the most stigmatized and has many regulatory barriers to access.

Naltrexone works as a competitive opiate receptor antagonist to block the effects of opiate agonists. It has been shown to be most useful in patients with a strong external motivator for treatment adherence, such as professionals with ongoing licensing board monitoring. In more generalized patient populations, retention in treatment with naltrexone is only 20% to 30% at 6 months. The usual dose of naltrexone is 50 mg/day or 350 mg weekly divided into three doses (100, 100, and 150 mg). A reduced starting dose of 25 mg on day 1 is used to minimize GI side effects such as nausea and vomiting, which occur in 10% of patients. Liver enzymes are monitored because liver toxicity is a rare but more serious side effect, shown to resolve after stopping naltrexone (Reis et al., 2009). A monthly depot injectable form of naltrexone was approved by the FDA for treating opiate-dependent patients in 2010. Studies of longer-acting naltrexone implants are ongoing for FDA approval.

Methadone is a long-acting opiate receptor agonist with strong affinity for its receptor and can be dosed once daily for most opiate-dependent patients. Currently, methadone may be used for treating opiate dependence in hospitalized patients (i.e., for withdrawal) or in licensed methadone treatment facilities. Take-home doses are regulated and depend on length of time in treatment and treatment response, including good attendance, adherence to program rules, lack of diverting behaviors, and abstinence, as verified by drug test results. Generally one take-home dose a week is allowed from the outset (many programs are closed on Sundays). Progression to increased take-home doses is determined by state and federal regulations, with the more restrictive statute taking precedent. For family physicians with patients in methadone maintenance, knowing a patient's take-home schedule can provide insight into how well they are doing in treatment. Recent increases in overdose deaths involving methadone have been explored and are more likely caused by an increase in misuse or diversion of methadone prescribed to treat chronic pain and less likely from an increase in opiate agonist treatment facility diversion (Center for Substance Abuse Treatment, 2004).

Buprenorphine is a partial opiate agonist that causes a 50% activation of the opiate receptors. This is typically enough to alleviate withdrawal symptoms and prolonged abstinence symptoms but not enough to induce euphoria for patients with opiate dependence. It binds more tightly than any of the opiate agonists and has a long half-life, making it a good candidate for blockade therapy. Buprenorphine is given as a sublingual tablet or film, most often compounded with naloxone *(Suboxone)*, to discourage IV use because the naloxone, a potent opiate antagonist, has little effect unless injected. Buprenorphine comes in 2-mg, 4-mg, 8-mg, and 12-mg strengths. Unlike methadone, the Drug Abuse Treatment Act of 2000 allows physicians to prescribe buprenorphine outside a methadone treatment facility, with the goal of bringing the treatment of opiate dependence into primary care, greatly expanding treatment availability. To prescribe buprenorphine for opiate dependence, a physician needs to take an 8-hour course, now available online, and submit his or her application for an additional "X" number from the U.S. Drug Enforcement Administration (DEA). Physicians also need to have a way to refer or provide behavioral health-based addiction treatment for their patients. The number of patients is proscribed by statute to 30 the first year and up to 100 patients at any given time past the first year if an additional waiver is submitted. Typical doses of buprenorphine range from 8 to 16 mg/day.

Many pharmacologic interventions have been studied for stimulant dependence, but to date, none have been FDA approved. Several anticonvulsants, baclofen, disulfiram, and antidepressants have shown promise in select patient populations, have shown little effect, or are still in clinical trials. Topiramate has recently been shown to decrease cocaine use compared with placebo, but FDA approval for this indication is still pending (Bankole et al., 2013). Research in treating stimulant dependence also includes

maintenance therapy, with sustained-released preparations of slow-onset stimulants such as modafinil (Ries et al., 2009). Vaccine therapy is also currently being studied and involves stimulating the patient's immune system to produce antibodies; for example, when bound to cocaine, antibodies prevent the drug from crossing the blood–brain barrier (Martell et al., 2009).

There is even less evidence for use of medications in the long-term management of other substances of abuse, such as hallucinogens, marijuana, and club drugs. Currently, behavioral therapies are the mainstay of treatment (Ries et al., 2009).

KEY TREATMENT

- Methadone maintenance is the most studied and effective medical treatment for opiate dependence (National Consensus, 1998) (SOR: A).
- Buprenorphine maintenance therapy, an alternative to methadone for treating opiate dependence, can be prescribed by appropriately trained and certified primary care physicians but is somewhat less effective than methadone prescribed at adequate doses (Mattick et al., 2008) (SOR: A).
- Oral naltrexone is typically reserved for use in patients with strong external motivators for treatment adherence, such as licensed professionals, because treatment retention is otherwise poor, and relapse is common (Minozzi et al., 2006) (SOR: B).

Behavioral Therapies for Substance Use Disorders

Behavioral therapies are a mainstay of SUD treatment. Common modalities include cognitive-behavioral therapy, contingency management, motivational enhancement therapy (MET), "therapeutic communities," and 12-step facilitation. Except for MET, these have not been adapted for use by family medicine physicians in routine office practice but are usually available as community-based referrals.

COGNITIVE-BEHAVIORAL THERAPY

Cognitive-behavioral therapy (CBT) is based on the assumption that the learning processes used by patients to initiate and continue their drug use behaviors can also be used to reduce or stop their drug use. CBT has been extensively studied, especially with cocaine users, and has shown good results. CBT is primarily used in the outpatient setting, usually with weekly individual sessions over several months. Sessions focus on patients learning to recognize the situations in which they are most likely to use drugs, learning to avoid those situations, and learning to cope with their problems without resorting to drug use. These lessons are accomplished through functional analysis and skills training. In functional analysis, each episode of drug use is analyzed in terms of what the patient was feeling, thinking, or doing before and after the use. This helps identify high-risk situations and coping issues. Skills training involves working on ways to avoid these situations and learn new (or reconnect with past) coping mechanisms for handling high-risk situations and other life stressors without using drugs (Carroll, 1998).

CONTIGENCY MANAGEMENT

Contingency management (CM) is based on operant conditioning and involves a structured and consistently administered system of consequences that are used to reinforce behaviors consistent with treatment goals. Basic principles include close temporal proximity of consequence to targeted behavior, performance of targeted behavior easy to verify and verified often, positive consequence given and escalated for continuous positive behavior change, and positive consequence removed when targeted behavior is not performed. CM has been shown to be more effective when a single targeted behavior is addressed at a time and when resumption of continuous positive change is reinforced after a brief slip. Barriers include funding sources to cover the cost of rewards and determining appropriate length of treatment for this method. Advantages of CM include the breadth of behavioral changes that can be targeted and its demonstrated success in patients with severe and complex SUDs (Petry et al., 2001).

MOTIVATIONAL ENHANCEMENT THERAPY

Motivational enhancement therapy engages patients in increasing their internal motivations for making healthy changes in their drug use and building on a patient's strengths and resources in making prior behavioral changes. Goals are set by the patient, although the counselor may advise specific goals when appropriate. This approach is nonconfrontational. The counselor elicits change talk—that is, positive statements about making a change—from the patient in a way that highlights discrepancies between the patient's life goals or beliefs and current drug use behaviors (Miller and Rollnick, 2013). Awareness of these discrepancies increases the patient's internal desire for change or discomfort with the status quo. A patient's stage of readiness to change, whether precontemplative, contemplative, preparation, action, maintenance, or relapse, may also be used to guide the session. In addition, assessment of a patient's self-efficacy for change can facilitate the patient discussing prior successful behavioral changes, and any optimism for change is reflected and highlighted (Prochaska et al., 1992). MET has been used in both inpatient and outpatient settings, from one session (brief intervention) to several months of weekly sessions.

THERAPEUTIC COMMUNITIES

Therapeutic communities (TCs) are traditionally residential facilities in which the community structure and function are agents of change, and 12-step–based self-help programs guide individual recovery. Average lengths of stay are about 12 months (6-24 months). Community members progress through varying roles and responsibilities in their recovery and collectively ensure day-to-day functioning of the community. Days are highly structured and involve group and individual sessions, as well as time for community and personal chores and self-development, such as exercise, vocational time, and educational time. TCs have been successfully adapted to serve special needs populations, such as adolescents, patients with concomitant mental health disorders, patients with HIV infection, and women with children. Successful completion of a TC program has been shown to lead to a significant decrease in SUD behaviors. Day treatment or nonresidential TCs are also available and may be more cost effective for patients with less severe social problems to address (National Institute on Drug Abuse, 2002).

TWELVE-STEP FACILITATION

Twelve-step facilitation (TSF) is a modality that seeks to increase the SUD patient's attendance and active involvement in 12-step self-help groups such as Cocaine Anonymous (CA) and Narcotics Anonymous (NA). TSF is used in residential treatment programs as well as outpatient settings. Sessions are highly structured, often workbook guided, and cast the counselor in the role of facilitator of change, with patient involvement the true agent of change. The underlying 12-step principles are the same: the patient's lack of control must be accepted, willpower is insufficient to stop use, and abstinence is desired. Research has shown that the more 12-step self-help group involvement, both in terms of number of meetings attended and, more robustly, the degree of active participation, the greater the success of achieving abstinence and recovery (McIntosh, 2009a).

Formal TSF counseling is outside the scope of most family medicine practices. However, physicians making a 12-step self-help group referral can increase the likelihood the patient will engage by (1) contracting with the patient to attend a certain number of meetings weekly, (2) having the patient call the local CA or NA hotline during the visit to set up his or her first meeting, and (3) encouraging attendance at several different meetings to ensure a "good fit." Checking in with patients previously referred or in long-term recovery on meeting attendance and 12-step involvement, such as sponsorship and step work, is supportive of recovery and easily integrated into the primary care visit.

KEY TREATMENT

- CBT and CM decrease cocaine use and increase treatment retention (Knapp et al., 2007) (SOR: B).
- Twelve-step involvement positively correlates with achieving abstinence and recovery (McIntosh, 2009b) (SOR: C).

PRIMARY CARE OF PATIENTS WITH SUBSTANCE USE DISORDERS

The primary care of SUD patients must take into account the systemic effects of the drug(s) ingested, route of administration, methods of drug procurement, illicit drug–prescription drug interactions, and typically higher rates of nonadherence to follow-up and prescribed regimens (Ries et al., 2009). Infectious diseases (e.g., HIV, hepatitis B and C, tuberculosis) and sexually transmitted infections (e.g., gonorrhea, Chlamydia, herpes, syphilis, human papillomavirus) are more common in SUD patients than in the general population, and patients should be screened routinely. Other infections common in IV drug users include skin abscesses, cellulitis, infectious endocarditis, and pneumonia.

Cocaine and other stimulants can cause myocardial infarction and stroke, raise blood pressure, and make essential hypertension resistant to treatment. Crack cocaine use, inhaled methamphetamines, and marijuana can lead to lung injury, chronic obstructive pulmonary disease, fibrosis, and pulmonary hypertension. Seizures can stem from stimulant use, benzodiazepine withdrawal, and "ecstasy" and other "club drug" intoxication (Ries et al., 2009).

Treatment for asthma, hypertension, chronic pain, and diabetes is complicated by the concomitant SUD. Patient adherence to treatment regimens is often compromised by the SUD, with "getting high" and minimizing withdrawal symptoms becoming the focus of their activities. Regular and nutritious meals may be difficult to access or may not be a priority for SUD patients, along with hygienic activities. Sleep disorders are common and can exacerbate health problems and their management. SUD patients' ability to store their medications safely and securely can be compromised by homelessness, diversion, and an unsafe living environment.

Ongoing SUDs can mask symptoms, leading to late presentation of diseases such as cancer. This masking often is compounded by lack of access or use of primary care and preventive services by SUD patients.

Special Populations

ADOLESCENTS

In 2012, approximately 9.5% of youths age 12 to 17 years were current users of illicit drugs. This continued a trend of decreased illicit substance use among adolescents. Compared with 2002 data, the prevalence of illicit drug use had decreased for several drugs, including marijuana (8.2%-7.2%) and nonmedical use of prescription drugs (4.0%-2.8%). Concern about performance-enhancing agents and steroid use among high school and junior high school students has led to surveillance of steroid use among teenagers since 1989. Compared with previous years, the overall use of anabolic steroids has decreased. Although predominantly found among young men, the proportion of anabolic steroid use attributable to young women has increased.

Most youths reported that drugs are readily available. For example, approximately 47.8% of teenagers 12 to 17 years old reported that it would be "fairly easy" to obtain marijuana, 16.0% reported they could obtain cocaine, and 11.5% reported that they could obtain LSD. In 2012, 13.2% of adolescents reported that they had been approached by someone selling drugs within the past month.

Because peer pressure is a significant factor for adolescents, their perceptions of risk associated with substance abuse and peer disapproval have also been surveyed. A majority of teenagers have strongly disapproved or somewhat disapproved of illicit drug use by their peers. However, the perceived risk of using marijuana, cocaine, hallucinogens, and other drugs has been lower in recent years. Teenagers may possess less knowledge about adverse drug effects than their predecessors and may display some "generational forgetting" (Johnston et al., 2008).

RACIAL AND ETHNIC MINORITIES

In 2012, the rate of current illicit drug use varied significantly among people of seven different major racial categories. Current drug use was highest among people who reported having two or more races (14.8%). An estimated 12.7% of American Indians or Alaska Natives, 11.3% of blacks, 9.2% of whites, 8.3% of Hispanics, 7.8% of Native Hawaiians or other Pacific Islanders, and 3.7% of Asians were current illicit drug users in 2012.

PREGNANT WOMEN

Approximately 5.9% of pregnant women age 15 to 44 years were current users of illicit substances in 2012. Compared with nonpregnant women, the rate of drug use is significantly lower for all age groups. Use of cocaine, heroin, methamphetamines, marijuana, MDMA, inhalants, and nicotine during pregnancy has been associated with adverse outcomes such as intrauterine growth retardation, delayed cognitive development, and difficulty with attention and learning. Effects vary by substance ingested, quantity and frequency of ingested drug or drugs, and stage of fetal development when ingestion occurs. Currently, methadone maintenance is the treatment of choice for opiate dependence during pregnancy, although buprenorphine has been used when methadone is not available. Newborns are monitored for signs of withdrawal and treated if symptoms are noted.

MENTAL HEALTH AND SUBSTANCE ABUSE

The prevalence of illicit substance abuse or dependence among patients with serious mental illness was 31.3% in 2011. Similarly, adults age 18 years and older with an episode of major depression within the past year had higher rates of illicit drug use than adults without a major depressive episode (28.5% vs. 13.4%). Having a major depressive episode within the past year was also associated with higher prevalence of dependence on illicit drugs.

Summary of Additional Online Content

The following content is available at www.expertconsult.com:

eTable 50-1 CAGE-AID Screening Tool for Adults

eTable 50-2 Signs and Symptoms of Intoxication and Withdrawal for Other Drugs

References

The complete reference list is available at www.expertconsult.com.

Web Resources

www.findtreatment.samhsa.gov Substance Abuse and Mental Health Services Administration. Treatment locator resource.

www.nar-anon.org 12-step–based resource for families.

nsduhweb.rti.org The National Survey on Drug Use and Health's website has a current and extensive database.

www.asam.org The American Society of Addiction Medicine's website with links to online buprenorphine training.

www.bu.edu/aodhealth/index.html Boston University's website offering periodic summaries of the latest SUD research findings.

www.cdaweb.org 12-step–based self-help organization.

www.drugfree.org/join-together Addiction medicine news and advocacy and research.

www.nida.nih.gov The National Institute on Drug Abuse's website has valuable resources for physicians and families.

Index

Page numbers followed by "f" indicate figures, "t" indicate tables, and "b" indicate boxes.